Ulrike Steinert

Women's Healthcare in Ancient Mesopotamia in the First Millennium BCE

Die babylonisch-assyrische Medizin in Texten und Untersuchungen

Begründet von Franz Köcher

Herausgegeben von
Nils P. Heeßel und Marten Stol

Band 12

Ulrike Steinert

Women's Healthcare in Ancient Mesopotamia in the First Millennium BCE

An Edition of the Textual Sources

DE GRUYTER

The work on this volume as part of the project BabMed – Babylonian Medicine has been funded by the European Research Council (ERC) under the European Union's Seventh Framework Programme (FP7/2007–2013; Project No. 323596).

European Research Council
Established by the European Commission

ISBN 978-1-5015-1525-5
e-ISBN (PDF) 978-1-5015-0647-5
e-ISBN (EPUB) 978-1-5015-0659-8
DOI https://doi.org/10.1515/9781501506475

Library of Congress Control Number: 2025946537

Bibliographic information published by the Deutsche Nationalbibliothek
The Deutsche Nationalbibliothek lists this publication in the Deutsche Nationalbibliografie; detailed bibliographic data are available on the internet at http://dnb.dnb.de.

Cover image: Symbols of the mother goddess Ninḫursaĝa (uterus and knife) on a socle; detail from the Kudurru of Meli-Šipak II;
Drawing by U. Steinert, after: E. D. van Buren 1933-1934, AfO 9, 169 Fig. 7
Typesetting: Integra Software Services Pvt. Ltd.
Printing and binding: CPI books GmbH, Leck

www.degruyterbrill.com
Questions about General Product Safety Regulation:
productsafety@degruyterbrill.com

Acknowledgements

This book would not have possible without the ground-breaking work and support of two eminent Assyriologists and specialists of the Mesopotamian cuneiform medical corpus: Irving Finkel and Mark Geller. It is to both these scholars that the present work is most deeply indebted. Irving Finkel must be regarded as a major pioneer in the study of women's healthcare texts who over the years had identified and joined numerous fragments in the British Museum's Babylonian Collection belonging to the corpus (as well as related fragments from other museums), and who had published sections of this material in the *Festschrift* for W. G. Lambert in 2000. In 2011, Mark Geller proposed the idea to me to undertake a study and edition of the first millennium BCE Mesopotamian women's healthcare texts and introduced me to Irving Finkel, who then kindly took me under his wing, made me acquainted with unpublished Babylonian women's healthcare texts in the British Museum collection known to him and who generously shared his transliterations of this material.

Work on the present publication began in 2011–2013 during a Medical History and Humanities Fellowship funded by the Wellcome Trust (Grant No. WT 094297) entitled "Gynaecology in the Medical Texts of Ancient Mesopotamia from the 1st Millennium BC". It was Mark Geller who emphatically supported the Wellcome application and made it possible for me to base that project at the University College London's Department of Hebrew and Jewish Studies. During my time in London, I had the chance to study and copy numerous cuneiform texts related to women's health in the Babylonian collection of the British Museum, and to identify other relevant fragments. I cannot thank Irving Finkel enough for his enormous and unending support in these two years, who sat down with me for hours on end in the Middle East Study Room to decipher and discuss difficult text passages. Mark Geller likewise shared several of his transliterations of Babylonian medical fragments on women in the BM collections with me and made numerous crucial suggestions on texts edited in this volume.

The completion of the text editions leading to the present volume continued during the years of the BabMed Project at Freie Universität Berlin (2013–2018), which was initiated and led by Markham J. Geller, and which was funded by the European Research Council as an Advanced Grant (Project No. 323596, "BabMed – Babylonian Medicine: Fragments of cuneiform medicine in the Babylonian Talmud: Knowledge Transfer in Late Antiquity"). I would like to thank all the colleagues involved in the BabMed project, for numerous discussions and suggestions relating to texts published here, which I had the chance to present during the regular meetings of the Keilschriftmedizin Seminar: especially Mark Geller, J. Cale Johnson, Eric Schmidtchen and Krisztián Simkó, as well as visiting scholars such as András Bácskay, Henry Stadhouders and Frans Wiggermann.

During 2016, I had the chance to carry out a visiting fellowship at the Institute of Social and Cultural Anthropology (School of Anthropology) of the University of Oxford and at Wolfson College, Oxford, which was funded by a Medical Humanities Small Grant of the Wellcome Trust (Grant-No. 200707/Z/16/Z). The research on female blood and menstruation in Mesopotamian medicine undertaken during that grant has contributed much to the presentation of these topics in the present volume. I am indebted to Elisabeth Hsu and Jacob Dahl for inviting me to Oxford and for giving me the opportunity to present my research at departmental seminars. Elisabeth Hsu also invited me to attend several of her courses and lectures on the body, gender, senses and medicine at the Institute of Social and Cultural Anthropology, which inspired me to embrace both historical and medical-anthropological perspectives more fully in my research on Mesopotamian (women's) medicine, and for which I will always be grateful.

I would also like to acknowledge the funding of the German Research Foundation (Deutsche Forschungsgemeinschaft, DFG) during my employment in the Research Training Group (GRK 1876) "Early Concepts of Humans and Nature" (Project No. 215342465/GRK 1876/2) at Johannes Gutenberg-Universität Mainz, in 2018–2022. During these years, especially Doris Prechel (JGU Mainz) and Tanja Pommerening (Marburg) supervised and supported the present work, which finally was completed and submitted in April 2025 as Habilitation dissertation at the Department of History and Cultural Studies of JGU Mainz. But the work on various issues relating to the women's healthcare texts and Mesopotamian medicine presented in this book also benefited from fruitful discussions and exchanges with many colleagues in the GRK 1876.

Several other scholars have supported the present work, for which I am extremely thankful. Jon Taylor, Christopher Walker, Marten Stol, Henry Stadhouders, Zsombor Földi, Enrique Jiménez, Klaus Wagensonner, Anmar Fadhil and Daniel Schwemer shared their discoveries of unpublished texts related to the women's health corpus, provided photos or information on joins. I would also like to thank Annie Attia, Gilles Buisson, Andrew George, Marie-Christine Ludwig, Diana Stein, Ronit Yoeli-Tlalim, Nathan Wasserman, Florentina Badalanova Geller, Rebecca Flemming and Lennart Lehmhaus for personal exchanges and helpful suggestions.

https://doi.org/10.1515/9781501506475-202

In the years between 2011 and 2024, I had the opportunity to collate and study cuneiform texts on women's health in the British Museum London, the Vorderasiatisches Museum, Berlin, the Musée du Louvre, the Oriental Institute of the University Chicago (now Institute for the Study of Ancient Cultures), the Yale Babylonian Collection, the Free Library Philadelphia, the Babylonian section of the Penn Museum (Philadelphia), the Anadolu Medeniyetleri Müzesi Ankara and the Arkeoloji Müzeleri Istanbul. I would like to thank J. Taylor, I. L. Finkel (London), J. Marzahn, H. Gries, J. Eule (Berlin), B. André-Salvini (Louvre), E. Frahm, A. W. Lassen, K. Wagensonner (New Haven), W. Farber, S. Paulus, R. Winters (Chicago), M. Arslan and M. Çifçi (Ankara), Z. Kızıltan and A. Dönmez (Istanbul) for granting access to the collections or permission to publish texts in their collections, and for their kind assistance during my stays at the museums or with providing detailed information on specific tablets.

I would like to express my sincere and deep gratitude to Marten Stol who over a process of several months sent extensive corrections and comments on the chapters of this book before being sent to press, to Nils Heeßel for critical feedback and to Mark Geller for proof-reading the manuscript prior to submission. Thanks also go to Albrecht Doehnert, Katrin Mittmann and Antonia Pohl from Walter de Gruyter who have seen this volume through to publication, and to Nils Heeßel and Marten Stol, the editors of *Babylonisch-assyrische Medizin in Texten und Untersuchungen*, for accepting the present work's publication within this series.

I also thank my husband Yves, for his support, love and companionship through all the years in which the present work has grown and taken shape.

Mainz, July 2025

Contents

Abbreviations

Bibliographical Abbreviations

See also R. Borger, *Handbuch der Keilschriftliteratur*, Vol. 2, Berlin/New York 1975, XI–XXXIII and http://www.rla.badw.de/reallexikon/abkuerzungslisten.html

AbB 9	M. Stol, *Letters from Yale*, Altbabylonische Briefe in Umschrift und Übersetzung 9, Leiden 1981.
ABIM	A. al-Zeebari, *Altbabylonische Briefe des Iraq-Museums (Baghdad)*. PhD Dissertation Münster. Köln 1964.
ABRT	J. A. Craig, *Assyrian and Babylonian Religious Texts Being Prayers, Oracles, Hymns Etc.* 2 Vol., Assyriologische Bibliothek 13/1–2, Leipzig 1895–1897.
AHw	W. von Soden, *Akkadisches Handwörterbuch*. 3 Vol., Wiesbaden 1965–1981.
AMT	R. C. Thompson, *Assyrian Medical Texts from the Originals in the British Museum*, London 1923.
ARM	Archives royales de Mari
ASKT	P. Haupt, *Akkadische und sumerische Keilschrifttexte nach den Originalen im British Museum*, Leipzig 1882.
BabMed	*BabMed Corpora Online* (https://www.geschkult.fu-berlin.de/e/babmed/index.html)
BAM	Babylonisch-assyrische Medizin in Texten und Untersuchungen
BE	The Babylonian Expedition of the University of Pennsylvania, Series A: Cuneiform Texts
BiOr	Bibliotheca Orientalis
BSA	Bulletin on Sumerian Agriculture
CAD	Gelb, I. J. et al. (eds.), *The Assyrian Dictionary of the Oriental Institute of the University of Chicago*. Chicago 1956–2010.
CAL	Comprehensive Aramaic Dictionary. https://cal.huc.edu.
CBT VI	E. Leichty, *Catalogue of the Babylonian Tablets in the British Museum. Volume VI. Tablets from Sippar 1* (with an Introduction by J. E. Reade), London 1986.
CBT VIII	E. Leichty, J. J. Finkelstein and C. B. F. Walker, *Catalogue of the Babylonian Tablets in the British Museum, Volume VIII. Tablets from Sippar 3*, London 1988.
CCP	*Cuneiform Commentaries Project* (https://ccp.yale.edu)
CDA[2]	J. Black, A. R. George and N. Postgate (eds.), *A Concise Dictionary of Akkadian*, 2nd (corrected) printing, Wiesbaden 2000.
CDLI	*Cuneiform Digital Library Initiative* (https://cdli.mpiwg-berlin.mpg.de)
CM	Cuneiform Monographs
CMAwR 1	see Abusch and Schwemer 2011
CMAwR 2	see Abusch and Schwemer 2016
CMAwR 3	see Abusch et al. 2020
CMAwR 4	see Luukko and van Buylaere 2020
CTMMA 2	I. Spar and W. G. Lambert (eds.), *Literary and Scholarly Texts of the First Millennium B.C.*, Cuneiform Texts in the Metropolitan Museum of Art, Vol. 2, New York 2005.
CT	Cuneiform Texts from Babylonian Tablets in the British Museum
CTN 4	D. J. Wiseman and J. A. Black, *Literary Texts from the Temple of Nabû*, Cuneiform Texts from Nimrud 4, Oxford 1996.
CUSAS	Cornell University Studies in Assyriology and Sumerology
eBL	*electronic Babylonian Library* (https://www.ebl.lmu.de)
ePSD2	Electronic Pennsylvania Sumerian Dictionary 2 (http://oracc.iaas.upenn.edu/epsd2/suxs)
eSAD	The Electronic Supplement to the Akkadian Dictionaries (https://www.gkr.uni-leipzig.de/altorientalisches-institut/forschung/supplement-to-the-akkadian-dictionaries)
ETCSL	The Electronic Text Corpus of Sumerian Literature (https://etcsl.orinst.ox.ac.uk)
GAG	see von Soden 1995
GKAB	CAMS Geography of Knowledge Corpus (https://oracc.museum.upenn.edu/cams/gkab/; https://oracc.org)
JANER	Journal of Ancient Near Eastern Religions
JMC	Le Journal des Médecines Cunéiformes
K.	Signature of cuneiform texts from Nineveh (Kuyunjik) in the British Museum
KADP	F. Köcher, *Keilschrifttexte zur assyrisch-babylonischen Drogen- und Pflanzenkunde*, Berlin 1955.
KAL	S. M. Maul (ed.), Keilschrifttexte aus Assur literarischen Inhalts, Wiesbaden 2007–.
KBo	Keilschrifttexte aus Boghazköi
KAR	E. Ebeling, *Keilschrifttexte aus Assur religiösen Inhalts*, 2 Vol., Leipzig 1915–1923.
LKA	E. Ebeling and F. Köcher, *Literarische Keilschrifttexte aus Assur*, Berlin 1953.
LKU	A. Falkenstein, *Literarische Keilschrifttexte aus Uruk*, Berlin 1931.
MCS	Manchester Cuneiform Studies
MDP 4	V. Scheil, *Textes élamities-sémitiques, deuxième série*. Mémoires de la Délégation en Perse 4, Paris 1902.

https://doi.org/10.1515/9781501506475-204

MDP 22	V. Scheil, *Actes juridiques*, Mémoires de la Mission Archéologique de Perse 22, Paris 1930.
MDP 57	see Labat 1974
MSL 3	R. T. Hallock and B. Landsberger, *Das Syllabar A, das Vokabular S^a und das Vokabular S^b*, Materialien zum sumerischen Lexikon 3, Roma 1955.
MSL 4	B. Landsberger, R. T. Hallock, T. Jacobsen and A. Falkenstein, *Vokabulare und Formularbücher*, Materialien zum sumerischen Lexikon 4, Roma 1956.
MSL 8/1	B. Landsberger (in cooperation with Anne Draffkorn Kilmer and Edmund I. Gordon), *The Fauna of Ancient Mesopotamia, First Part. Tablet XIII*, Materialien zum sumerischen Lexikon 8/1, Roma 1960.
MSL 8/2	B. Landsberger, *The Fauna of Ancient Mesopotamia, Second Part. ḪAR-ra = ḫubullu XIV and XVIII*, Materialien zum sumerischen Lexikon 8/2, Roma 1962.
MSL 9	Landsberger, Benno, *The Series ḪAR-ra = ḫubullu, Tablet XV and Related Texts, with Additions and Corrections*, Materialien zum sumerischen Lexikon 9, Roma 1967.
MSL 10	B. Landsberger, E. Reiner and M. Civil, *The Series ḪAR-ra = ḫubullu, Tablets XVI, XVII, XIX and Related Texts*, Materialien zum sumerischen Lexikon 10, Roma 1970.
MSL 11	E. Reiner and M. Civil, *The Series ḪAR-ra = ḫubullu, Tablets XX-XXIV*, Materialien zum sumerischen Lexikon 11, Roma 1974.
MSL 12	M. Civil, R. D. Biggs, H. G. Güterbock, H. J. Nissen and E. Reiner, *The Series lú = ša and Related Texts*, Materialien zum sumerischen Lexikon 12, Roma 1969.
MSL 13	B. Landsberger, M. Civil, H. G. Güterbock, W. W. Hallo, H. A. Hoffner and E. Reiner, *Izi = išātu, Ká-gal = abullu and Níg-ga = makkūru*, Materialien zum sumerischen Lexikon 13, Roma 1971.
MSL 14	M. Civil, M. W. Green and W. G. Lambert, *Ea A = nâqu, Aa A = nâqu, with Their Forerunners and Related Texts*, Materialien zum sumerischen Lexikon 14, Roma 1979.
MSL 15	M. Civil, G. Farber and D. A. Kennedy, *The Series DIRI = (w)atru*, Materialien zum sumerischen Lexikon 15, Roma 2004.
MSL 16	I. L. Finkel and M. Civil, *The Series SIG₇.ALAN = Nabnītu*, Materialien zum sumerischen Lexikon 16, Roma 1982.
MSL 17	A. Cavigneaux, H. G. Güterbock, M. T. Roth and G. Farber, *The Series Erim-ḫuš = anantu and An-ta-gál = šaqû*, Materialien zum sumerischen Lexikon 17, Roma 1985.
OECT 11	O. R. Gurney, *Literary and Miscellaneous Texts in the Ashmolean Museum*, Oxford Editions of Cuneiform Texts 11, Oxford 1989.
PBS 1/1	D. W. Myhrman, *Babylonian Hymns and Prayers*, Publications of the Babylonian Section 1/1, University of Pennsylvania Museum, Babylonian Section, Philadelphia 1911.
PBS 1/2	H. F. Lutz, *Selected Sumerian and Babylonian Texts*. Publications of the Babylonian Section 1/2, University of Pennsylvania Museum, Babylonian Section, Philadelphia 1919.
PBS 2/1	A. T. Clay, *Business Documents of Murashû Sons of Nippur Dated in the Reign of Darius II*, Publications of the Babylonian Section 2/1, University of Pennsylvania Museum, Babylonian Section, Philadelphia 1912.
PIHANS	Uitgaven van het Nederlands Instituut voor het Nabije Oosten te Leiden
PNA	K. Radner and H. Baker (eds.), *The Prosopography of the Neo-Assyrian Empire*. 6 Vol., Helsinki 1998–2011.
PSD	Å. Sjöberg (ed.), The Sumerian Dictionary of the University Museum of the University of Pennsylvania, Philadelphia 1984–.
RA	Revue d'assyriologie et d'archéologie orientale
RAcc.	F. Thureau-Dangin, *Rituels accadiens*, Paris 1921.
RIME 4	D. R. Frayne, *Old Babylonian Period (2003–1595 B.C.)*, The Royal Inscriptions of Mesopotamia, Early Periods 4, Toronto 1990.
SAA 1	S. Parpola, *The Correspondence of Sargon II, Part 1. Letters from Assyria and the West*, State Archives of Assyria 1, Helsinki 1987.
SAA 3	see Livingstone 1989
SAA 7	F. M. Fales and J. N. Postgate, *Imperial Administrative Records, Part 1*, State Archives of Assyria 7, Helsinki 1992.
SAA 8	H. Hunger, *Astrological Reports to Assyrian Kings*, State Archives of Assyria 8, Helsinki 1992.
SAA 10	S. Parpola, *Letters from Assyrian and Babylonian Scholars*, State Archives of Assyria 10, Helsinki 1993.
SAA 13	S. W. Cole and P. Machinist, *Letters from Priests to the Kings Esarhaddon and Assurbanipal*, State Archives of Assyria 13, Helsinki 1998.
SAA 16	M. Luukko and G. van Buylaere, *The Political Correspondence of Esarhaddon*, State Archives of Assyria 16, Helsinki 2002.
SAA 21	S. Parpola, *The Correspondence of Assurbanipal, Part 1. Letters from Assyria, Babylonia and Vassal States*. State Archives of Assyria 21. Helsinki 2018.
SAAB	State Archives of Assyria Bulletin
SAD	M. P. Streck et al. (ed.), *Supplement to the Akkadian Dictionaries*, Wiesbaden 2018–.
SEAL	M. P. Streck and N. Wasserman, *Sources of Early Akkadian Literature*. http://seal.huji.ac.il.
SpTU 1	see Hunger 1976
SpTU 2	see von Weiher 1983
SpTU 3	see von Weiher 1988
SpTU 4	see von Weiher 1993
SpTU 5	see von Weiher 1998
STT I	O. R. Gurney, J. J. Finkelstein and P. Hulin, *The Sultantepe Tablets* I, London 1957.
STT II	O. R. Gurney and P. Hulin, *The Sultantepe Tablets* II, London 1964.
TCL	Musée du Louvre, Département des Antiquités Orientales, Textes Cunéiformes

TLHdig	Thesaurus Linguarum Hethaeorum digitalis, hethiter.net/: TLHdig – *Beta Version* (2023-07-26)
UET	Ur Excavations, Texts
VS 17	J. J. A. van Dijk, *Nicht-kanonische Beschwörungen und sonstige literarische Texte,* Vorderasiatische Schriftdenkmäler der Königlichen Museen zu Berlin 17, Berlin 1971.
YOS 3	A. T. Clay, *Neo-Babylonian Letters from Erech,* Yale Oriental Series, Babylonian Texts 3, New Haven 1919.
YOS 6	R. P. Dougherty. 1920. *Records from Erech, Time of Nabonidus (555–538 B.C.),* Yale Oriental Series, Babylonian Texts 6, New Haven 1920.
YOS 11	J. J. van Dijk, *Early Mesopotamian Incantations and Rituals,* Yale Oriental Series, Babylonian Texts 11, New Haven 1985.
ZA	Zeitschrift für Assyriologie und Vorderasiatische Archäologie

Symbols and Other Abbreviations

x	undecipherable damaged sign
:	division marker (disjunction sign)
|	vertical division marker
[ ]	break
[x]	indicates space available in the break
⸢ ⸣	partially broken sign(s)
< >	signs to be added to the text
<< >>	sign(s) to be deleted from the text
{ }	indicates now lost signs that are still visible on older photographs or hand copies
(( ))	indicates a variant reading in the transcription
…	untranscribed, untranslated sign(s), word(s) or text passage(s)
---	indicates a missing word or passage in a given manuscript in relation to a duplicate edited in the same score
* *	signs written over an erasure
šu$^{!}$	emended sign with certain reading
šu$^{!?}$	emended sign with uncertain reading
šu$^{!}$(ma)	emended sign (against an identifiable sign on tablet)
/	indicates the end of the line in a given manuscript (if two or more lines are transliterated in sequence)
//	duplicate of
\	indentation
+	joined to
(+)	indirectly joined to
adv.	adverb
caus.	causative
col.	column
coll.	collated
conj.	conjunction
cont.	indicates that transliterated text is not found at the beginning of a new line but continues in a given line
fem.	feminine
iter.	iterative
LB	Late Babylonian
l. e.	left edge
lit.	literally
lo. e.	lower edge
MA	Middle Assyrian
masc.	masculine
MB	Middle Babylonian
ms(s).	manuscript(s)
NA	Neo-Assyrian
NB	Neo-Babylonian
OA	Old Assyrian
OB	Old Babylonian
obv.	obverse
pass.	passive
pl.	plural

prep.	preposition
r. e.	right edge
rev.	reverse
s.v.	sub voce
sg.	singular
u. e.	upper edge
var.	variant
vent.	ventive

Introduction

The corpus of medical cuneiform texts on women's health from ancient Mesopotamia forms the largest ancient medical text corpus devoted to women, beside comparable material preserved in the Egyptian medical papyri and the gynaecological treatises in the Hippocratic Corpus. The present book presents an edition and discussion of all texts from the first millennium BCE Mesopotamia identified to date that deal with female health matters, a corpus of more than 100 texts and fragments. Cuneiform healing texts devoted to women, like the Mesopotamian medical corpus in general, can be divided into several distinct "genres" or text groups: a) diagnostic texts, giving a symptom description, diagnosis and prognosis, but usually excluding a therapeutic recommendation, b) therapeutic texts, which comprise medical prescriptions, incantations and ritual procedures. In addition, Mesopotamian healing specialists collected compendia on *materia medica*, which can take the form of drug descriptions or pharmaceutical handbooks that list plant names together with their uses and forms of applications, including their usages for women's conditions.[1] Finally, in the first millennium BCE, scholarly commentaries on medical texts were written, among which are also a few commentaries on medical compendia and treatises concerned with women.

1 Previous Studies

Among the first publications of medical cuneiform texts containing material relating to women's conditions are Thompson's *Assyrian Medical Texts* (1923), Ebeling's *Keilschrifttexte aus Assur religiösen Inhalts* (1919–1923) and Falkenstein's *Literarische Keilschrifttexte aus Uruk* (1931). Among the pioneering works, R. Labat presented an edition of the *Diagnostic Handbook* SA.GIG in 1951, which included text witnesses for Tablet 36 and 37, which deal with pregnant women, birth prognoses and medical diagnoses for female patients. New texts from the second and first millennium BCE were steadily added in the following years and decades, for instance in *The Sultantepe Tablets I* and *II* by Gurney, Finkelstein and Hulin (1957–1964) and in Lambert's (1965, 1969) contributions to the subject. In 1964 and 1971 F. Köcher published copies of a group of 20 tablets and fragments of therapeutic women's healthcare texts mostly from Assur including material previously found in KAR and LKU in his *Assyrische and babylonische Medizin*, Volumes 3 and 4 (BAM 235–251, BAM 347, BAM 363 and BAM 408). Further key publications that contributed new material to the corpus of women's healthcare texts are found in the editions of tablets from Late Babylonian Uruk by Hunger (1976) and von Weiher (1993, 1998), in Finkel's (2000) publication of a medical archive from Sippar, as well as in Reiner (1982), Schwemer (2007, No. 41), Steinert (2012b), Scurlock (2014a, 245–257, 571–619), Farber (2014, "RA" and "SpTU"), Meinhold (2017, no. 16), Bácskay (2018a, 108–112), Abusch et al. (2020, CMAwR 3, texts 5.1–5.6, 5.8–5.10), to name but a few.

Incantations devoted to women's health matters have also been the subject of numerous Assyriological publications and studies through the years. Important contributions are found in van Dijk (1972; 1973; 1975); Finkel (1980), Krebernik (1984), van Dijk, Goetze and Hussey (1985), Röllig (1985), Veldhuis (1991), Cunningham (1997), Collins (1999), Michel (2004), Rudik (2011), Barjamovic (2015), George (2016), Wasserman and Zomer (2022) as well as via the website of *Sources of Early Akkadian Literature* (SEAL). Another fundamental study on women, reproduction and medicine in Mesopotamian cultures to this day is Stol's *Birth in Babylonia and the Bible* (2000), complemented by his much broader monograph on *Women in the Ancient Near East* (2016).

The available textual material on women's health has steadily grown over the years, and several studies discuss selected texts or offer overviews (e.g. Veldhuis 1989; Stol 2000; 2016, 436–458; Scurlock and Andersen 2005, 259–283; Böck 2010; Scurlock 2014b; Minen 2018; Steinert 2021a), or discussions of specific topics, such as the scope of Mesopotamian medicine for women and underlying gender constructions (Heeßel 2006; Couto-Ferreira 2018d), concepts of the female body (Böck 2013; 2014–2016; Steinert and Paoletti 2014–2016; Steinert 2017a; 2017b; Couto-Ferreira 2017, 2018a; 2018c), fertility and con(tra)ception (Böck 2013; Couto-Ferreira 2013), embryology (Stol 2008; Couto-Ferreira 2015–2016), pregnancy (Couto-Ferreira 2013), birth (Stol 2000; 2012; Volk 2004; Couto-Ferreira 2014), female blood and body fluids (Steinert 2012b,

1 For discussion of pertinent passages, see e.g. Stol 2000, 52–55; Couto-Ferreira 2014, 309. On Mesopotamian pharmaceutics, drug compendia and on practical issues connected to the preparation and administration of medical substances, see e.g. Attia and Buisson 2012; Böck 2010b; 2011; 2015; Fincke 2021; Goltz 1974; Herréro 1984; Rumor 2017a, 2024; Scurlock 2014a: 273–293; 2017: 277–280; Stadhouders 2011; 2012; Stol 2002–2005a; 2002–2005b.

https://doi.org/10.1515/9781501506475-001

2013, 2023), therapeutic strategies (Steinert 2017a; 2020; 2021a). However, no attempt at an edition and systematic study of the *complete* corpus of women's healthcare texts so far identified has ever been undertaken before, and many issues, details and topics linked to the texts are still little understood. The present book hopes to fill some of these gaps and present a somewhat more comprehensive picture of Mesopotamian women's healthcare in the first millennium BCE.

2 Historical Overview of the Ancient Mesopotamian Women's Healthcare Texts

2.1 The Earliest Texts (3rd Millennium to First Half of the 2nd Millennium BCE)

From a diachronic angle, spells countering diseases and drug lists with short therapeutic instructions are the texts genres related to healing/medicine with the longest history in Mesopotamia. The former started to be written down already in the mid-third millennium (during the Early Dynastic period), while the earliest examples of pharmaceutic-therapeutic texts come from Ebla (ca. 24th cent. BCE, written in Semitic Eblaite). A few medical prescriptions in Sumerian are attested from the end of the third millennium (Ur III period), but from the Old Babylonian period onward (ca. 1900–1600 BCE), prescriptions from Mesopotamia are exclusively written in the Akkadian language.[2]

The earliest texts related to women's health issues are a few Sumerian and Semitic incantations on tablets from the cities of Fara and Ebla dating to the Early Dynastic period (ca. mid-third millennium BCE), which were recited in the context of childbirth or address the topic of gynaecological bleeding.[3] These compositions were included within collections of various incantations and do not yet feature prescriptions. Among the incantations related to women's health from the end of the third millennium and the first half of the second millennium BCE (Ur III period, Old Assyrian and Old Babylonian periods), we encounter examples in the Sumerian, Akkadian or Elamite language, inscribed on small tablets as single text as well as spells found on tablets with multiple compositions.[4] In some cases, short therapeutic instructions in Akkadian are now appended to the spells, usually consisting of only a few words or a single sentence. Often, however, the therapeutic procedure to be applied together with the spell is integrated and described in the incantation itself. The most common poetic form within spells used for embedding the therapy is the so-called 'Marduk-Ea-dialogue' or 'communication formula'.[5] In this formula, a junior divinity (such as Marduk/Asalluḫi) reports the encountered medical problem to a senior deity (such as Ea/Enki) and asks for advice as to what shall be done to treat the patient. The senior deity then communicates the remedy to be applied. This passage from a Sumerian birth incantation known from manuscripts dating to the Ur III and the Old Babylonian period can be taken as an example:

> "Enki answered his son Asalluḫi:
> 'My son, what do you not know, what shall I add for you?
> Asalluḫi, what do you not know, what shall I add for you?
> Whatever I know you know too.
> After you have received fat from a pure cow, cream from a mother-cow,
> after you have taken what is in the (sleeping) chamber of the agrun[6],

2 For early examples of medical texts, see e.g. Fronzaroli 1998; Bonechi 2003; Civil 1960; 1961; van Dijk and Geller 2003, 75–76; Haussperger 1997; Geller 2006, 7–12; Attinger 2008, 9–18; Neumann 2010, 3–7; Schwemer 2010b; George 2016, CUSAS 32, No. 72–73; Geller and Panayotov 2020, 1–8. For incantations from the third millennium, see e.g. Cunningham 1997, 5–97; George 2016, No. 1–4; Krebernik 1984; Neumann 2008, 1–15; Rudik 2011.

3 See Cunningham 1997, 34; Krebernik 1984, No. 6A+B, No. 23c, No. 37; Rudik 2011, 318–326, FSB 56–57. The spells against haemorrhage may have been used in the context of pregnancy, as in later texts.

4 For Ur III incantations in Sumerian (birth/bleeding), see e.g. Rudik 2011, 327–336 FSB 58–59; van Dijk 1975, 53–57; Cunningham 1997, 69–75, 96–97. For Old Babylonian incantations in Sumerian, see Finkel 1980 (bleeding); for birth incantations: van Dijk 1975, 62–63 (VAT 8381 (= VS 17, 33)); van Dijk 1975, 66–67 (MLC 1207 (= YOS 11, 85); G. Farber 1984 (E 47.190); Wilcke 1973, 13–14 (John Rylands Library Box 24 E6 (24)); Cohen 1976 (bilingual); Cunningham 1997, 107–108, 131, 134, 137–138, 148–149. For Old Assyrian birth incantations, see Michel 2004; Kouwenberg and Fincke 2012–2013; Barjamovic 2015. For Old Babylonian birth incantations in Akkadian, see van Dijk 1972, 343–344 (VAT 8539 (= VS 17, 34)); van Dijk 1973, 503–507; George 2016, No. 26a, 28a, 29b; Wasserman 2018, *BiOr* 75, 15-20; Wasserman and Zomer 2022, No. 1–14 (OB/OA Akkadian birth incantations); Cunningham 1997, 153, 155–156. For Elamite birth incantations on Old Babylonian tablets, see George 2016, No. 21b; Krebernik 2018, No. 13–14, 45; Cunningham 1997, 99–100, 157, 158; Scurlock 1991, 136–137; Stol 2000, 60–64; Bergmann 2008, 18–19, 22–23.

5 For the 'Marduk-Ea-formula' see e.g. Falkenstein 1931; George 2016; Rudik 2011.

6 The Sumerian word agrun stands for Enki's domain, the subterranean water (abzu), but also denotes the deity's sleeping chamber in temples. In Sumerian birth incantations, the term can metaphorically refer to the womb as a 'chamber' in the body, where the foetus dwells, see Steinert 2017a, 297.

> after you have cast the incantation of Eridu over the vulva of the troubled woman from which a cord hangs (variant: after having recited the incantation of Eridu over the back, thighs and flanks of this woman),
> may it (the baby) be released like rain from heaven,
> may it run down like drainpipe water from a high roof,
> . . .
> may it [*gush forth*] like a river pouring into a swamp,
> . . .
> may it be smashed like a pot! . . .'
> Recitation for a 'hastened woman' (viz. a woman in labour) (*šipat aruḫtim*)."[7]

The appended short Akkadian prescription following the spell gives a slightly varying, straightforward instruction compared with the poetic wording of the incantation:

> *ki-ki-ta-ša* Ì.GIŠ *ù* Ì.NUN / *tu-ba-al-la-al-ma i-na* ⌈KUŠ/SU⌉ *bu-di-im ba-am-ti-ša* / *ki-la-ti-in ta-pa-aš-ša-aš-ma it-ta-aṣ-ṣa-a*
> "The procedure for it: you mix oil and ghee, apply (it) to the skin/flesh of the shoulder(s) (and) both her flanks and it (the baby) will come out."[8]

Although it is very short compared with later prescriptions, the instruction contains most of the salient elements of Mesopotamian medical formulae: an introductory rubric marking the beginning of the prescription, the ingredients, instructions for their preparation and administration, and the expected effect of the treatment (prognosis).[9] The only missing element in comparison with later therapeutic texts is a description of the symptoms or a purpose statement, but these elements are expressed in the incantation itself, which begins with a description of the woman's conception, pregnancy and delivery, including an allusion to a complication ('a cord', i.e. the umbilical cord, is hanging down from the woman's vagina). Enki's instructions to Asalluḫi in the spell above provide more detailed information on the treatment that is not conveyed in the recipe, for instance that the spell should be recited over the woman's body, presumably whilst massaging the woman with the ointment.

As examples of the early traditions of therapies for women, the present volume presents two Old Babylonian texts, both of which are related to the context of delivery. The first (text II.1.1, BM 97093) contains a Sumerian incantation for a woman having difficulty in delivery (*šipat mušapšiqtim*) with an appended therapeutic instruction, and an Akkadian birth incantation. The Sumerian incantation features the "classic" dialogue between Enki and Asalluḫi and presents parallels to other birth incantations from Old Babylonian and later times. The prescription is remarkable not only because it is reminiscent of the intervention recommended by the god Enki within the spell (in the dialogue with his son), but also because the prescription recurs in its essence in the Neo-Assyrian Birth Compendium (see Wasserman and Zomer 2022, No. 10; Steinert 2017a, 336–339; *infra* text D.1.1 and below for discussion). The second Old Babylonian text edited in this volume (text II.1.2, BM 115745; Wasserman and Zomer 2022, No. 4) is presumably a re-used(?) school tablet inscribed with an arithmetical exercise and an Akkadian birth incantation that is known in varying versions that are found on three other Old Babylonian tablets, all beginning with the well-known sentence: "From the fluids of intercourse, the bone was created" (*ina mê nâkim ibbani eṣemtum*).[10]

Notably, among the preserved Old Babylonian medical texts containing prescriptions known to date, remedies for conditions specific to women seem so far to be absent. One exception may be found in CUSAS 32, No. 73 obv. 14 (George 2016, 167, pl. CXLIII–CXLIV; Bácskay 2018, 33 No. 0), a damaged, one-line prescription possibly treating fever (*išātum*) in a postpartum(?) woman (restore MUNUS *mus*[*ukkatim*] "impure woman"?).

---

7 See UM 29-15-367 ii 14–iii 9; var. VS 17, 33: 15–28 (van Dijk 1975; Cunningham 1997, 69–75).

8 VS 17, 33: 28–30; see van Dijk 1975, 63–64; George 2016, 142.

9 In Old Babylonian texts, the instruction may consist merely of the rubric KÌD.KÌD.BI "the procedure for it" and the ingredient oil (Ì.GIŠ), as in George 2016, No. 29b: 30. Other examples of short remedies appended to Old Babylonian spells for women in labour are found in George 2016, 142–143 No. 21b, lines 28'–29', following an Elamite incantation: "You cast (the spell) on oil and massage her[!] belly (with it) seven times straight down, and massage her[!] shoulders seven times straight down" (*ana* Ì.GIŠ *ta-na-ad-di-ma* 7-*šu mi-š*[*a-r*]*a-am pa-ap-pa-al-li-ib-bi-šu ta-pa-aš-ša-aš* / 7-*šu mi-š*[*a-r*]*a-am bu-di-šu ta-pa-aš-ša-aš*). Cf. further E 47.190 rev. 7', bottom edge and left edge (G. Farber 1984, 313–316), which lists merely ingredients and a short instruction: "The procedure: reed and ghee, carnelian and lapis lazuli, [. . .] he/she will pour out for you[?] (fem.)" (*ki-ik-ki-ṭi-um* ^{giš}GI *ù* Ì.NUN / *sa-am-tum ù uq-ni-um* / [. . . m]u[?] mu *i-na-ad-di-*⌈*ki*[?]*-im*⌉).

10 For the other texts, see Wasserman and Zomer 2022, No. 6, 7, 14.

2.2 The Second Half of the 2nd Millennium BCE

Women's healthcare texts from the second half of the second millennium BCE are fewer compared with what is preserved from the preceding and following centuries. However, during the Middle Babylonian and Middle Assyrian period important developments took place in the realm of cuneiform medical texts (including materials relating to female conditions), such as the expansion of corpora and the formation of larger compendia or handbooks that include treatises concerned with women.[11]

The following texts from the latter half of the second millennium known to me are concerned with therapies for women. They come from Assur, Nippur as well as from Hattuša and Ugarit, the latter being a witness to the transmission of Babylonian medical texts, including material linked to women's healthcare, to the Western periphery during the Late Bronze Age.[12]

- **BAM 241 (+) VAT 9543** and **BAM 242** (edited as text II.1.3 and II.1.3.1):
  The three fragments in Middle Babylonian script were found at Assur and presumably belonged to the same two-column tablet. The tablet which must have been imported following Tukulti-Ninurta's I conquest of Babylon (late 13th century BCE) and integrated into the so-called library of Tiglath-pileser I (M2), forms the oldest fragmentary compendium that may have exclusively contained therapies for women (incantations and prescriptions).[13]
- **CBS 10911** (photo CDLI P266104):
  This fragment from Nippur (courtesy of H. Stadhouders) perhaps dates to the Kassite period.[14] The obverse preserves eight fragmentary lines with prescriptions; the reverse appears to contain remnants of an Akkadian incantation (rev. 11': TU_6 ÉN) invoking the healing goddess Gula (rev. 9', 11').[15] The text is difficult to read; the scribe inserted small explanatory glosses above or below specific words (rev. 5', 7'). The prescriptions on the obverse seem to deal with pregnancy-related issues, i.e. protecting from miscarriage and expelling a foetus:

Beginning of the obv. lost

Obv. 1'	[DIŠ MUNS *lu* (*ša*) ITI *lu* 2 ITI *lu*] 3 ⸢ITI⸣ *ša* ⸢ŠÀ⸣-*šá* Š[UB? . . .]
Obv. 2'	[. . . . . .]x *la pa-tan* NAG-*ši-ma* [*ša* ŠÀ-*šá* NU ŠUB?]
Obv. 3'	[. . . GI]G? ÉLLAG? GU_4 ḪÁD.DU SUḪUŠ GÚR.GÚR šimLI.DUR? G[AZ? . . .]
Obv. 4'	[(. . .) *ina* . . .] x KAŠ.SAG NAG-*ši-ma ša* [Š]À?-*ša ár-ḫiš* IGI-⸢*mar*⸣ [. . .]
Obv. 5'	[. . . . . .] ⸢ú⸣ḪAR.ḪAR ⸢ú⸣KUR.KUR ú⸢KUR⸣.R[A? . . . .]x x[. . . . . .]
Obv. 6'	[. . . . . .] x-*su tur-<ár> tu*-x[. . . . . .]
Obv. 7'	[. . . . . .-*ḫ*]*u*? *ana* ŠÀ?.[TÙR-*ša*? . . . .]
Obv. 8'	[. . . . . .] x [. . . . . .]

Obv. breaks

1' "[If a woman who is one month, two months or(?)] three months (pregnant), misc[arries] her foetus [. . .], 2' [. . . . . .]. . . you have her drink (it) on an empty stomach. Then [she will not miscarry her foetus(?)].

11 For these developments and medical texts from that period, see e.g. Attinger 2008, 18–24; Abusch and Schwemer 2011; 2016; Abusch et al. 2020; Heeßel 2000, 97–109; 2009; 2010b, 10–15; Schmidtchen 2021, 2–3; Geller and Panayotov 2020, 6–8; Finkel 2018. For incantations, see Zomer 2018.

12 For healing texts of the Mesopotamian tradition in the Western periphery, see e.g. Tsukimoto 1999; Marquéz Rowe 2014; Schwemer 1998; 2010c; 2013.

13 Library M2 incorporated texts that can be dated between the 13th and the 11th centuries BCE (Weidner 1952–1953, *AfO* 16, 197–215; Pedersén 1985, 31–42 Library M2; Zomer 2018, 39).

14 A transliteration is available via the website of the *Electronic Babylonian Library* (https://www.ebl.lmu.de/library/CBS.10911). CDLI and eBL give an early Old Babylonian (2000–1900 BCE) date to the fragment; however, sign forms and the frequency of logographic writings suggest a later (i.e. Middle Babylonian) date. The thickness of the fragment suggests that like BAM 241 (+), CBS 10911 must have belonged to a large tablet.

15 In rev. 9', one finds the phrase d*gu-la bulliṭī*(DIN)-*ma qīšta*(NÍG.BA) *le-q*[*í-i*] "Gula, heal and take (your) gift!" known from other incantations addressing Gula, see e.g. Böck 2014a, 114; Sibbing-Plantholt 2022, 80 n. 189. In rev. 11', one may restore [*a-zu-gal-l*]*a-tu* d*gu-la* "chief female physician Gula" (for this epithet, see e.g. Böck 2014a, 110 (K. 6057+ ii 32); Zomer 2018, 328–329 (Rm. 376 iv 22); Sibbing-Plantholt 2022, 80.

3' [. . . . . .]. . . you dry the kidney of an ox, you po[und] (*tahaššal*) root of *kukru*-plant (and) *abukkatu*-aromatic [. . .], 4' [. . . . . .] . . . you have her drink it [in . . .] (and) beer. Then she will quickly see (*immar*) her [foe]tus(?) [. . .].

5' [. . . . . .] *hašû*-plant (thyme), *atā'išu*-plant, *nīnû*-plant(?), . . . [. . .]. . .[. . .] 6' [. . .] . . . you parch(?), you [. . . . . .] 7' [. . . . . .] . . ., [you . . .] into [her] wo[mb(?) . . .].

8' *traces*

Notes

The prescription in lines 1'–2' is restored after BM 42313+ rev. 9–11 // (text A.2.2 lines 50–52). The expression "she will quickly see her [foe]tus(?)") is reminiscent of similar expressions in first millennium BCE women's healthcare texts. The phrase *arhiš ullad* "she will deliver quickly" is attested in texts to ease a difficult delivery; on the other hand, one finds the verb *amāru* "to see, experience" with terms referring to the menses, in prescriptions to induce menstrual bleeding, when it is delayed (*sagûša/maruštāša/damāša immar* "she will see her menses / 'trouble' / blood" (see e.g. BM 61975 line 7' (text C.2.4); BM 38624+ line 54''', 63''' (text A.2.1), BM 47578 line 1 (text C.2.2); SpTU 1, 59: 12' (text C.2.1) and *passim* Chapter C.2.

- ***Iraq* 31, pl. V–VI** (Lambert 1969):
  This Middle Assyrian text (re-edited as text II.1.4) may likewise have been part of the so-called library of Tiglath-pileser I at Assur (as suggested by Fales 1989, 195). The text, which may be described as an excerpt compiled from at least two different sources, begins with prescriptions for women after delivery suffering from symptoms of intestinal blockage and retention of the lochia (postpartum blood/fluids). The remedies are followed by two Akkadian birth incantations used to speed up difficult labour. The second of these incantations is a version of the incantation "A Cow of Sîn" known from the so-called Neo-Assyrian Birth Compendium (BAM 248 and parallels (text D.1.1) as well as from two other Middle Babylonian fragments that were found at Ugarit and Hattuša (see below, RS 25.436 and KUB 4, 13).
- **Rm. 376 (*AS* 16, 287–288):**
  This fragment of a Middle Assyrian two-column tablet (ca. 1100 BCE) was excavated in the area of the Kidmuru temple at Nimrud (Kalhu) dedicated to Ištar of Kidmuru. The preserved text is a collection of incantations for different purposes, e.g. against Lamaštu and *maškadu*-disease (Zomer 2018, 270–272, 326–330, 341–342). The last section on the obverse (obv. ii 19–36) contains a close variant of the birth incantation "Cow of Sîn" (see *infra* text D.1.1).[16]
- **KUB 4, 13 (CTH 810):**
  This is the first of two medical fragments found at the Hittite capital Hattuša containing Akkadian material from the Mesopotamian tradition concerned with women's healthcare. Written in a 'non-Hittite' script, KUB 4, 13 preserves remnants of two Akkadian birth incantations, the first of which parallels a couple of lines of the famous incantation "Cow of Sîn". The second composition is closely related to another spell in the Neo-Assyrian Birth Compendium (BAM 248 obv. i 36–50 //) focusing on the cow in travail beloved by the moon god, which also has precursors in Old Babylonian birth incantations (see text D.1.1; Veldhuis 1991, 12–13; Schwemer 2013, 156; Zomer 2013; 2018, 382–383).
- **KUB 37, 189 (CTH 537.I.14):**
  The second fragment from Hattuša connected to the corpus of women's healthcare preserves twenty lines of diagnostic omens that form a close parallel to a section of the standard recension of *Diagnostic Handbook* Tablet 36, attesting to a Middle Babylonian precursor of these omens. Although KUB 37, 189 reflects an earlier and shorter version, the omens on the fragment closely match several consecutive diagnostic entries in the first millennium BCE sources of Tablet 36. The fragment presents the oldest known example of a diagnostic text concerned with women (see Wilhelm 1994, 69–72 and *infra* text I.1.1).[17]
- **RS 25.436** (Arnaud 2007, AuOr Suppl. 23, pl. 11 (no. 20)):
  The tiny fragment from Ugarit, found in the so-called "House of the Lamaštu tablets", preserves part of a Middle Babylonian precursor of the birth incantation "A Cow of Sîn" (see Marquéz Rowe 2014, *SANER* 4, 77–78; Zomer 2018, 342–343; *infra* text D.1.1).

16 For discussion, see also Arbøll 2018, 270–272; 2023, 273.

17 Several other diagnostic texts bearing close parallels to entries from the later *Diagnostic Handbook* were discovered at Hattuša (Wilhelm 1994, 104–106).

- **RS 17.081:**
  This poorly preserved fragment from Ugarit contains several lines of prescriptions for a female patient. The text, which may have been a student's copy, was found in a residential building designated as the "House of the Scholar".[18] The fragment preserves fourteen damaged lines of text that display elements resembling passages in first millennium BCE prescriptions and ritual procedures to protect women from haemorrhage during pregnancy and miscarriage. Lines 1'–6' contain instructions for making amulet necklaces with stones and knots that are attached to different parts of the woman's body, similar to instructions found in texts such as STT 241: 1–8 (text C.1.1), AO 6473: 1–7 (C.3.9), BAM 237(+) (text C.1.4) and *passim* in Chapters C.1, C.3 and F). Lines 7'–13' contain instructions for a ritual procedure (including a short recitation by the patient) that mention a holy water vessel (*agubbû*) and a door. These lines are reminiscent of a ritual procedure to stop bleeding during pregnancy in BAM 237 obv. i 9'–16', in which a door in the patient's house forms the locus of the ritual actions (see text C.1.4). The last preserved line 14' contained a recipe for a potion.

Apart from the Middle Babylonian and Middle Assyrian fragments with precursors of first millennium BCE incantations and treatments for women, another hint to the Late Bronze Age as the crucial formative period of the first millennium BCE texts on women's health is encountered in an incantation within the Neo-Assyrian Birth Compendium BAM 248 rev. iii 3–5 // (text D.1.1, on which see also section 2.3). Thus, the legitimizing formula at the end of a lengthy Akkadian incantation (D.1.1 lines 128–130) appears to mention the famous scholar and exorcist Bullussa-rabi, who may have lived in the Kassite period and is known as the author of a hymn to the healing goddess Gula (Lambert 1967, 129; the end of the composition mentions his name) and of three other (unidentified) compositions.[19] The passage in question reads:[20]

> ^{128} [ÉN] *šá* ^{d}*asal-lú-ḫi ni-ṣir-tu šá eri-*[*du*$_{10}$^{ki}] ^{129} [*an-nu k*]*i-nu šá* ^{d}*é-a i-di-tu*$_{4}$ ÉN *šá* ^{d}*ma-mi i-ri-šú ana* $^{(m)}$*bu-luṭ-sa*$^{?}$-GA[L]$^{?}$ ^{130} [^{d}40-LU]GAL *id-di-nu ana šu-te-šur* ŠÀ.TÙR
> ^{128} (It is) the incantation of the god Asalluḫi, a secret of Eridu,
> ^{129} the reliable approval of the god Ea, the renowned incantation which (the birth goddess) Mami requested, (and which)
> ^{130} (the god) Ea-šarru gave ^{129} to (the exorcist) Bullussa-ra[bi(?)], ^{130} to let the womb give birth easily."

The appearance of a famous scholar and exorcist from Babylon (given the name is read correctly) in a highly poetic birth incantation of the Neo-Assyrian Birth Compendium is remarkable. The legitimizing formulas at the end of incantations usually attribute spells exclusively to deities. The formula in BAM 248 rev. iii 3–5 // (= lines 128–130) may be seen as presenting the ideological model of scribal succession as discussed by Lenzi (2008a, 67–128; 2008b; 2015, 172, 178–180), in which knowledge of the arts of healing, magic and divination are said to have been transmitted in an unbroken chain from the gods (especially from Enki-Ea) to the *apkallu*-sages from before the flood and finally to the *ummânu*-scholars. In our case, the text appears to say that Bullussa-rabi received the spell from the gods Ea, Asalluḫi and Mami for use in healing. If the reading Bullussa-rabi is correct, the occurrence of his name could be regarded as a hint to a Middle Babylonian origin of the present incantation or possibly even as a hidden hint to the authorship of the composition. However, the suggestion remains tentative for the time being.

---

18 Nougayrol 1968, *Ugaritica* V, 29 No. 15, 375, 629–630 fig. 18; Clemens 2001, 695–705; Marquéz Rowe 2014, *SANER* 4, 78–80; Del Olmo Lete 2014, *SANER* 4, pl. XI (photo).

19 This information is found in a Neo-Assyrian catalogue of texts and authors, where he is designated as an exorcist (^{lú}MAŠ.MAŠ) and a scholar (*ummânu*) of Babylon (Lambert 1962, *JCS* 16, 62, 66–67; Lambert 1967, 107–109). Z. Földi (in Jiménez et al. 2019, *KASKAL* 16, 81–83) presents several attestations of the personal name Bullussa-rabi in documents from the Middle Babylonian (Kassite) period, which lend further support to the suggestion that the exorcist/*ummânu* Bullussa-rabi may have lived in the same period. Because in the administrative documents (e.g. ration lists), the name bearers are always female, Földi proposes that the author of the Gula hymn may in fact have been a woman – an interesting question which is left open in the present discussion.

20 The reading $^{(m)}$*bu-luṭ-sa*$^{?}$-GA[L]$^{?}$ in line 129 was first suggested to me by I.L. Finkel (personal communication).

2.3 The First Millennium BCE

Texts dating to the first millennium BCE form the lion's share of the preserved sources on women's health and the focus of the present volume. Mesopotamian medical texts from this era reflect a number complex and significant developments that are visible in other areas of scholarly texts but that can also be grasped to some degree in the sources on women's healthcare. One such development is the formation of larger serialized compendia (or text series) on diagnosis and therapy, including several compendia of incantations and medical-therapeutic material, which can be grasped through the colophons of text manuscripts as well as through catalogues that list the contents of the serialized compendia in question (see Steinert 2018 for an overview). Several concerted edition projects with the aim to assemble medical materials into handbooks or longer compendia were undertaken during this era at different places. The most important work happened under the aegis of the Neo-Assyrian king Ashurbanipal (668–631 BCE) for his royal library at Nineveh, but we also have attestations for similar serialized compendia from Late Babylonian times (Panayotov 2018).

As is known from a series catalogue and other sources, diagnostic texts were redacted into a handbook known under the title SA.GIG (*Sakikkû*), here referred to as the *Diagnostic Handbook*. The compiling and editing of SA.GIG and other canonical texts were attributed by the ancients to the scholar Esagil-kīn-apli who (according to the scholarly tradition) lived and worked under the reign of the Babylonian king Adad-apla-iddina in the 11th century BCE.[21] The *Diagnostic Handbook* SA.GIG known from first millennium BCE sources consisted of forty tablets (or chapters) that were grouped in six treatises or sections with distinct topics and an organised structure. The sixth treatise contained four tablets (chapters 36–39) concerned with women, of which only two are partially preserved in actual manuscripts. From these sources and the series catalogue we know that these tablets dealt with predictions and birth prognoses for pregnant women, with health problems during pregnancy, delivery and in the postpartum period, as well as with diseases and health problems manifesting in female patients that are not "gynaecological" *per se*.

The medical-therapeutic sources from Nineveh and from other sites in Assyria and Babylonia (most of which are from the first millennium BCE) were collected and reconstructed over several decades by F. Köcher (published as the first six volumes of BAM between 1963 and 1980). Parts of this material have been edited and studied recently (e.g. Abusch and Schwemer 2011; 2016; Abusch et al. 2020; Geller 2005a; Geller and Panayotov 2020; Johnson and Simkó 2024; Maul 2019). The present volume presents all women's healthcare texts known from previous publications as well as numerous hitherto unpublished texts, many of which come from first millennium BCE Babylonia. The material is divided into diagnostic texts and therapeutic texts, including commentaries on the former materials.

A glimpse on the therapeutic women's healthcare texts in the Neo-Assyrian period (9th–7th cent. BCE) can be grasped from two scholarly catalogues, the so-called Exorcist's Manual and the Assur Medical Catalogue.[22] The Exorcist's Manual lists the titles of series or text genres pertaining to the discipline of *āšipūtu* "the art of the conjurer, ritual healer" – titles that are also used as rubrics to classify certain groups of incantations and rituals pertaining to them. The first part of the catalogue lists components of *āšipūtu* in a narrower sense, such as temple and healing rituals, diagnostic and physiognomic omens (Frahm 2018, 42–43). It includes as relevant genre titles ^{munus}PEŠ$_4$.KÉŠ.DA "(spells/rituals) to bind a pregnant woman", ^{munus}LA.RA.AḪ "(spells/rituals for) a woman in difficult labour", flanked by related genres of ŠÀ.ZI.GA "(spells/rituals for) arousing (sexual) desire", ^{d}KAMAD.ME "(spells/rituals against) Lamaštu" (a demoness predominantly attacking pregnant women and infants) and LÚ.TUR.ḪUN.GÁ "(spells/ritual) to calm a (crying) infant" (Geller 2018a, 298 KAR 44: 14–15 and dupl.; Heeßel 2023, 294). Spells bearing the rubric ^{munus}LA.RA.AḪ.(A.KAM) are found in first millennium BCE texts dealing with (difficult) delivery. The genre title ^{munus}PEŠ$_4$.KÉŠ.DA, referring to spells to protect pregnant women from haemorrhage and miscarriage, is attested only in older texts from the second millennium BCE,[23] although it also occurs in the Assur Medical Catalogue (see below). However, several texts edited in this volume presumably contain incantations that have a relation to the genre designated by the ancient healers with that title (see Chapters C.1 and C.3). The second part of the Exorcist's Manual comprises additional fields of knowledge to be mastered by the *āšipu*, especially medical-therapeutic treatises, among which the catalogue lists *šipir sinništi* (KIN MUNUS) "treatment(s) for women", which may be a

21 Finkel 1988; Heeßel 2010e, 139–143, 154–171; Rutz 2011, 294–296, 299; Schmidtchen 2018a; 2018b; 2021.

22 For the Assur Medical Catalogue, see Steinert et al. 2018. For the Exorcist's Manual, see Bácskay and Simkó 2012; Frahm 2011, 325–332; 2018; Geller 2000a; 2018; Jean 2006, 62–82; Heeßel 2023.

23 For OB Sumerian spells with the rubric MUNUS.KÉŠ.DA.KAM "to bind a woman" and similar rubrics, see Finkel 1980, 38–39, 42–43 text C (CBS 1509 i 20, iii 25); Steinert 2018, 183; Steinert et al. 2018, 272.

reference to medical remedies for female conditions that were incorporated in the treatises PREGNANCY and BIRTH of the Assur Medical Catalogue (Geller 2018a, 301: 35; Heeßel 2023, 295; Steinert 2018, 185, 187).

The Assur Medical Catalogue (AMC) is a key document and piece of evidence for the organisation of medical-therapeutic materials concerned with women's health matters in Neo-Assyrian times. The texts listed in the AMC belong to a large medical compendium that is closely associated with the large-scale edition project in Nineveh in Ashurbanipal's reign (668–631 BCE), witnessed in numerous tablets excavated there that bear colophons with catchlines and titles following those outlined in the AMC and that are now referred to by Assyriologists as the *Nineveh Medical Compendium* (also *Nineveh Medical Encyclopedia*). The therapeutic compendium outlined in AMC consists of two parts organised in thematic sections or treatises. The catalogue lists two treatises toward the end of Part II of AMC comprising eleven tablets that are concerned with female health matters. These two treatises have been given the titles PREGNANCY / OFFSPRING and BIRTH for easy reference (Steinert et al. 2018, 217–218 lines 109–120). The lines in question are worth repeating here:

XXI PREGNANCY/OFFSPRING

109) [(. . .) DIŠ NA *a-na* ^{d}*ni*]*n-kar-ra-ak* ⸢*pa*⸣*-qid* : DIŠ NA *mi-iḫ-ra im-ḫur-ma* DUMU.MEŠ-*šú ana* ŠU-*šú* È.MEŠ
[(. . .) If a man] is entrusted to the goddess [Ni]nkarrak. If a man is confronted with (a *carrier of*) misfortune with the consequence that his sons are lost for him (i.e. have died).

110) [*ana* ^{munus}PEŠ$_4$ UŠ$_{11}$.ZU NU T]E$^!$-*ši-ma ana šà* ŠÀ-*šà* NU$^!$ (DIŠ) ⸢ŠUB⸣-*e*
[For witchcraft not to] approach [a pregnant woman] and to prevent her from having a miscarriage.

---

111) ⸢NÍGIN⸣ [3 DUB.MEŠ DIŠ N]A *a-na* ^{d}*nin-kar-*⸢*ra-ak*⸣ ⸢*pa-qid*⸣
Total of [three tablets (of the section) "If a] man is entrusted to the goddess Ninkarrak."

112) *ša*$^?$ x x x[. . . EN DIŠ ^{munus}PEŠ$_4$] ⸢A⸣.MEŠ-*šá* DU-*ku* : DIŠ ^{munus}PEŠ$_4$ MÚD.MEŠ-*šá* DU-*ku*
. . . [. . ., including (prescriptions) for the case that a pregnant woman's] (amniotic) fluid flows, for the case that a pregnant woman's blood flows,

113) DIŠ ^{munus}PEŠ$_4$ *i-*⸢*sa-ap*⸣*-*[*pid*$^?$. . .]x : DIŠ ^{munus}PEŠ$_4$ *kun-nu-*⸢*kàt*⸣ ⸢:⸣ DIŠ ^{munus}PEŠ$_4$ *kul-lu-mat*
for the case that a pregnant woman [mour]ns [. . .], for the case that a pregnant woman is sealed up (i.e. cannot deliver), for the case that a pregnant woman is *bewitched* (lit. was shown something),

114) DIŠ MUNUS Ù.TU-*ma kul*$^?$*-l*[*u-mat*$^?$ . . . (:) . . . (*ana*) *ḫ*]*a-riš-te* ⸢*ša*$^!$⸣ ⸢*kul-lu-ma-tú*⸣ ⸢BÚR⸣ : *ù* ^{munus}PEŠ$_4$.K[ÉŠ.DA.KÁM (x x)]
for the case that a woman gives birth and is *bewitched*, [. . . (treatments)] for releasing a woman in confinement who has been *bewitched* and (spells) to bind a pregnant woman (. . .).

XXII BIRTH

115) DIŠ ^{munus}PEŠ$_4$ *ina a-la-d*[*i-šá šu-up-šu-qat a-n*]*a šu-up-šu-ḫ*[*i*]
If a pregnant woman [is suffering severely during her] delivery, [in] order to calm (her) down.

116) ÉN *ina* A *na-*⸢*a*⸣*-*[*ki-im ib-b*]*a-ni* GÌR$^!$.PAD.D[U]
Incantation: "From the fluids of intercourse the bone was created."

117) DIŠ MUNUS *ina* Ù.TU *uš-*[*tap-šiq* : DIŠ MUNUS Ù.T]U-⸢*ma*⸣ *ni-ip-šá ina kir-ri-š*[*á* x x (x)]
If a woman suffers [severely during delivery. If a woman delivers] and then a smell [. . .] in her throat.

118) DIŠ ^{munus}Ù.TU Ù.T[U-*ma* . . . : DIŠ MUN]US$^?$ *šá-gu-šá*$^?$ *p*[*e-lu-ú*$^?$]
If a fertile woman delivers [and . . . . If a] woman's *menstrual discharges* [*are* bright r]ed$^?$.

119) DIŠ MUNUS GIN$_7$ *ri-ḫu-ut* GÌŠ T[A$^?$ GAL$_4$.LA-*šú* DU-*ku*$^?$: . . . Š]À MUN[US$^?$ . . .]
If a semen-like discharge [flows] from a woman's [vagina]. [. . . the] belly of a wo[man. . .].

---

120) NÍGIN 8 DUB.MEŠ *ša* ^{munu}[^{s}PEŠ$_4$ *ù* ^{munus}Ù.TU$^?$]
Total of eight tablets (of the section) concerning [pregnant$^?$] women [and women in childbirth$^?$].

The incipits and additional keywords listed in these lines of the AMC reveal several focal topics and texts groups that are represented by women's healthcare texts published in this volume (for detailed discussion, see Steinert et al. 2018, 269–276 and *infra*). The treatise PREGNANCY / OFFSPRING with the title "If a man is entrusted to the goddess Ninkarrak" focuses on rituals and treatments for families affected by the death of children, either born or unborn (due to the woman's repeated miscarriages). The tablet incipits in AMC 109–110 and 113–114 allude to some of the possible causes of the infant death and miscarriage mentioned in the texts pertaining to this treatise: the wrath of the goddess Ninkarrak, who is a healing and oath deity associated with the goddess Gula, and witchcraft.[24] Notably, the title of the treatise, the titles of the listed chapters as well as several of the topics enumerated in AMC 109–114 are attested in the textual sources on women's health from the first millennium BCE (although not necessarily as tablet incipits). The majority of these sources stem from Late Babylonian manuscripts as well as from several Neo-Assyrian manuscripts from Assur, Sultantepe and Nineveh.

Most of the text sources pertaining or related to PREGNANCY / OFFSPRING are assembled in Chapters C.1 and C.3 focusing on bleeding and protection from miscarriage, but some related materials (e.g. treatments against loss of amniotic fluid) are also found in texts edited in Chapter A. Closely related to the theme of protection from bleeding (during pregnancy) and miscarriage are the texts on amulet necklaces edited in Chapter F, which the ancient scholars collected in a separate compendium on amulets entitled *kunuk ḫalti* (see previously Schuster-Brandis 2008).

The treatise BIRTH outlined in AMC 115–120, which comprised eight tablets (chapters), seems to have contained materials dealing with delivery, including birth incantations and treatments to ease a difficult delivery (chapters 1–3 in AMC 115–117), texts concerned with postpartum problems (chapters 4–5, AMC 117–118) and topics that could be described as gynaecological and included treatments dealing with the menstrual flow (*sagû*) and with other morbid genital discharges (chapters 6–8, AMC 118–119). In this light, the summary rubric in AMC 120 may have referred to women in childbirth, but perhaps also to women's diseases.

The sources linked to BIRTH chapters 1–3 referenced in AMC 115–117 are assembled in Chapter D.1 focussing on treatments for delivery. Several sources in Neo-Assyrian and Neo-Babylonian script from Nineveh, Assur and Babylonia focusing specifically on delivery are preserved including a well-known collection of materials called here the Neo-Assyrian Birth Compendium (text D.1.1), a text that was also the subject of scholarly commentaries (edited in Chapter G). None of the preserved sources can definitely be identified as being witnesses for the recension of texts described in AMC, although it is clear from identical phrases matching two of the incipits that the preserved texts have an intimate connection to the materials referenced in AMC 115–117. That the preserved texts and fragments represent only a fraction of the complete transmitted textual lore, is seen in the title of BIRTH chapter 2, which is the title of an Akkadian birth incantation that is only known so far from Old Babylonian tablets (see text II.1.2) but must still have been known and transmitted in the first millennium BCE.

The incipit of BIRTH chapter 4 in AMC 117 is currently attested only in one Late Babylonian tablet fragment (text A.2.7), but not as an incipit. However, treatments for postpartum conditions are preserved in several first millennium BCE text sources edited in this volume (e.g. texts D.2.1, A.1.2, A.1.4, A.2.1, A.2.2). The treatments deal with different serious symptoms and problems such as fever, infection, retention of the afterbirth, retention of the lochia, and pain. The textual material referenced in the incipit of BIRTH chapter 6 (AMC 118) may have been related to texts edited in chapter C.2 that deal with regulating the menses (see further below), while treatments against abnormal genital discharges similar to the ones referred to in the incipit of BIRTH chapter 7 (AMC 119) are encountered in several texts edited here (e.g. texts C.1.1–C.1.2, C.1.4).

Multiple other topics and female health problems than those referenced in AMC 109–120 are encountered in the texts from the first millennium BCE (for which see further below). At this point it is useful to give a brief overview of the geographical and temporal distribution of the sources, on the formats of the texts, on their proveniences and archival contexts as well as some information on scribes and scholars gleaned from colophons or occasional rubrics.

Table 1 presents an overview of the number and distribution of the first millennium BCE sources on women's healthcare. The count excludes texts that integrate prescriptions for women but whose focus is not on gender-specific conditions, e.g. the texts on hair loss included in the Appendix (Chapter H) that belong to a different compendial context altogether. Included however are texts on amulet necklaces for women (edited in Chapter F). Although these procedures were inte-

24 The appearance of Ninkarrak in this context also alludes to the attribution of infant death to the "Ban" (NAM.ÉRIM; *māmītu*) encountered in some of the texts in question.

grated into the compendium *kunuk ḫalti*, they also circulated in manuscripts that only contain a group of amulets specifically designed for pregnant women and that have close connections to women's healthcare texts on matters of pregnancy and bleeding edited in Chapters C.1 and C.3 of the book.

Table 1: Number of first millennium BCE women's healthcare texts according to text groups and provenience (52 of them have been previously edited).

Text group	Assyria	Babylonia	Total
Diagnostic Texts (SA.GIG 36–39)	2	7	**9**
Therapeutic Texts (including amulet texts)	55	44	**99**
Commentaries	1	4	**5**

The distribution reveals that for the diagnostic texts and commentaries, few manuscripts are preserved from the Neo-Assyrian period, and that the majority of the sources comes from Babylonia (and from the Late Babylonian period). The number of therapeutic texts is higher for Assyrian findspots. However, of the 55 therapeutic texts from Assyria, 17 found in Ashurbanipal's library at Nineveh are written in a Babylonian ductus and were either copied by Babylonian scribes or were brought from Babylonia to Nineveh in connection with Ashurbanipal's collecting efforts.

Table 2 gives an overview of the number of sources according to proveniences within Assyria and Babylonia (note that among the tablets counted for Babylon are a couple of texts of uncertain provenience, which may stem from different locations in Babylonia).

Table 2: The proveniences of the first millennium BCE women's healthcare texts.

Assyria		
	Assur	24
	Nimrud	2
	Nineveh	33
	Sultantepe	4
Babylonia		
	Babylon	18(?)
	Borsippa	2
	Dilbat	1
	Nippur	2
	Sippar	12
	Ur	2
	Uruk	14

As with cuneiform medical texts in general, the women's healthcare texts edited here display different formats that can be linked with specific contexts in which such texts were used, and with different purposes for which they were written down or copied.[25] The various manuscripts can be loosely classified as a) *handbooks* or *collections* (sometimes part of larger compendia) inscribed on large single- or multi-column tablets which served as reference works for healing specialists and other scholars, drawn on for teaching and professional practice; b) shorter *extracts* (of selected prescriptions, incantations or ritual procedures) linked to concrete events of healing and practical application on a specific patient; c) small *students' or apprentices' tablets* (linked to contexts of knowledge transfer, i.e. teaching and learning of the healing

25 On tablet formats, see in general Schnitzlein 2023.

crafts and related scholarly knowledge), usually containing only a few prescriptions.[26] The medical commentaries can also be placed in a teaching context, as their colophons indicate (see e.g. Frahm 2011; Clancier 2014; Gabbay 2016; Wee 2019a; 2019b). An example is encountered in text G.1, a Late Babylonian commentary from Nippur on a compendium of texts for a woman in (difficult) labour (referred to here as the Neo-Assyrian Birth Compendium), which is described in its colophon as "oral explanations, and (materials for) a 'questioning', following the sayings of a (master)-scholar" (*šūt pî u maš'altu ša pī ummâni*).

We have only few examples of women's healthcare texts with colophons identifying the text as part of a larger compendium. SpTU 1, No. 59 (text C.2.1), the fragment of a tablet copied by the exorcist Anu-ikṣur (belonging to the Šangû-Ninurta family) with remedies to regulate the menses, is designated in the colophon as the 41st tablet of the therapeutic series *šumma amēlu muḫḫašu umma ukâl* "if a man's skull contains heat", i.e. a Late Babylonian recension of the therapeutic series (or compendium) with the same title known from the AMC and the Nineveh texts (see e.g., Heeßel 2010c, *TUAT NF* 5, 31–35; Panayotov 2018; Steinert 2018; Steinert et al. 2018). BM 42327+ and SpTU 3, No. 84 (texts C.3.3 and C.3.4) present textual evidence for the section PREGNANCY/OFFSPRING listed in the AMC 109–114 (see above), with BM 42327+ featuring the matching incipit of Tablet 3 (*ana erīti kišpī lā ṭeḫê-ma ša libbīša lā nadê* "so that witchcraft not come near a pregnant woman and for her not to have a miscarriage") as well as a corresponding catchline and series title in the colophon. Other examples of tablets or fragments with women's healthcare texts that may have belonged to a serialized compendium are BM 61975 (text C.2.4) and BM 47801 (text E.2.3). Several single- or two-column tablets from Nineveh, Assur and Babylonian sites (e.g. Uruk) that either do not preserve a colophon or do not give a catchline matching the recension of therapeutic materials listed in AMC but deal with a specific topic (e.g. bleeding, delivery) may also represent compilations on women's health that belonged to a longer compendium (e.g. BAM 237(+), BAM 244, BAM 248 // K. 2413(+), K. 11647 (AMT 66/3), BM 51246+, SpTU 4, No. 153, SpTU 5, 253).

It is noteworthy that when one looks at the preserved first millennium BCE sources, it is only in exceptional cases that we find two duplicating manuscripts of the same text. One example is the Neo-Assyrian Birth Compendium (text D.1.1), for which we have two duplicating manuscripts, one from Assur (BAM 248) and one from Nineveh (K. 2413+); another example is found in two duplicating copies of a Šamaš prayer from Nineveh recited in the context of childbirth (K. 897 and K. 3025, text D.1.8). It is more common for a given manuscript that it shares one or several procedures or a text section with one or more parallel sources. Thus, we see relatively fluid and flexible textual traditions that are characterised by diffuse long-term processes of transmission, local differences and influences from diverse groups, "schools" or members of healing professionals (see further below). Within the materials on women's healthcare written down and copied in the first millennium BCE one finds older components that stem from the second millennium as well as newer materials added to these older components over time. Among the Late Babylonian texts, there are also sources with prescriptions that contain many Aramaic loanwords or other linguistic features pointing to links with oral traditions and the contemporary healing practices of the day. The impact of astro-medicine or astro-magic can be discerned rarely, among Late Babylonian women's healthcare texts (as in BM 47491, text A.2.6).

In the corpus edited here, texts are only rarely designed as excerpts (*nisḫu*) belonging to a longer series. BM 51246+ (text A.2.7), a fragment of a single-column tablet with a selection of treatments for women, ends with a damaged one-line colophon designating the tablet as a "34th excerpt (*nisḫu*) of remedies (*bulṭū*)" (line 41').[27] Another Late Babylonian text (BM 47578, text C.2.2), a small, almost oval tablet with prescriptions to induce the flow of the menses showing signs of re-use, is designated as a "40th extract" (*nisḫu*) that was "quickly excerpted" (*zamar nasḫi*), suggesting that the copied text stemmed from a larger compilation, although the tablet may have been an exercise of some kind. Another manuscript in the corpus that was "excerpted" (*nasāḫu*) is UET 7, No. 123 (text B.2.2), a text with tests and treatments for fertility. In some cases, texts designated as "excerpted" may have served for treating a specific patient. A few tablets containing only one ritual procedure or incantation for a female patient may likewise be seen as excerpts copied by a practitioner to prepare a remedy or a ritual performance on a specific occasion, e.g. AO 4425A+B (text B.2.6), STT 241 (text C.3.1), or K. 11956 + 14200 (text D.1.2). One Late Babylonian tablet containing a birth incantation/ritual mentions the treated patient by name (BM 54846, text D.1.10).

26 For studies of medical texts as documents written by students or apprentice healers as well as questions of curricula, see e.g. Finkel 2000; Maul 2010; Clancier 2014; Arbøll 2021.

27 For similar designations in colophons of Late Babylonian medical texts or commentaries referring to "remedies (*bulṭū*) from the house of Dābibī", see Panayotov 2018, 115; SpTU 1, No. 59: 15' (text C.2.1).

Students' or school tablets with remedies for women are relatively frequent among the first millennium BCE sources. As previously discussed by Finkel (2000, 171–173), among the Late Babylonian texts from Sippar (booked in the 81-7-1 collection of Babylonian texts in the British Museum) that can be linked with the family archive of Bēl-rēmanni (a wealthy scribe associated with the Ebabbar temple) are examples of students' tablets with prescriptions for women. One of these tablets duplicates passages from a longer collection of "gynaecological" prescriptions likewise attributed to the same collection, which presumably served as the teaching source, attesting to activities of medical training (see text A.2.2, BM 42313+ and BM 42333+). Other such school tablets from the Bēl-rēmanni archive with prescriptions for women are BM 42450+ (text B.2.3), BM 42507, F 238 (+) BM 43268, BM 43229 (text E.2.1) and BM 43110+ (text E.2.2). A similar Late Babylonian tablet containing only one or a few recipes is BM 59710 (text B.2.5), but examples can also be encountered among the Neo-Assyrian medical texts for women (e.g. BAM 250 from Assur, text B.1.4). If the features of the tablet or script do not reveal a beginner's work, it cannot always be decided whether such manuscripts are school exercises or extracts selected by a practitioner for preparing a remedy on a specific occasion. In one instance, an apprentice scribe copied a text that he dedicated to the temple of Nabû, as a pious act to promote his career (BM 92694, a Late Babylonian copy of Tablet 36 of the *Diagnostic Handbook*).

2.4 Archives and Libraries, Scribes and Colophons

Several of the texts on women's health edited in this volume can be assigned to specific archaeological contexts and archives. The texts from Nineveh are attributed to "Ashurbanipal's library" located on mound Kuyunjik and thus date to the 7th century BCE.[28] The majority of the Nineveh sources is fragmentary, but some of the texts (belonging to large two-column tablets) very likely have close connections to the treatises on women outlined in AMC. The preserved material (which includes several tablets and fragments written in a Neo-Babylonian ductus, which were either brought to Nineveh from Babylonia or copied in Nineveh by Babylonian scribes) shows that the royal tablet collection included a range of therapeutic texts as well as a copy of the sixth section of the *Diagnostic Handbook* dealing with women and infants (Minen 2020).[29] The surviving fragments cover topics such as bleeding, miscarriage, difficult delivery, postpartum conditions, amulets for women and often have parallels in texts from Assur, Sultantepe and Babylonia. Notably, the Neo-Assyrian Birth Compendium, a collection of incantations and remedies to ease difficult delivery, is attested in at least two duplicating copies from Nineveh and Assur (K. 2413+ and BAM 248; text D.1.1). Only two of the Nineveh texts on women's health preserve a colophon marking the tablets as property of Ashurbanipal's palace: K. 11956 + 14200 (text D.1.3) and Sm. 157 + 1134 (text D.1.6), both of which deal with difficult delivery. One text (Rm. 376, a Middle Assyrian tablet with incantations) that was originally catalogued among tablets from Nineveh has been identified as actually stemming from the Kidmuru temple at Nimrud (Kalḫu); a second text from Nimrud (CTN 4, No. 105; text C.3.6) was found at the temple of Nabû.[30]

The second most important collection of Neo-Assyrian women's healthcare texts comes from Assur. Almost all of the women's healthcare texts found at Assur are known to originate from library N4 of the so-called "House of the incantation priest" belonging to the family of Kiṣir-Aššur, whose male members served as exorcists (*mašmaššu*) of the Aššur temple over four generations during the 8th–7th century BCE (BAM 235–240, BAM 243–246, BAM 248–251; BAM 346, BAM 363; KAR 223, KAR 247; KAL 2, No. 41, KAL 7, No. 16; LKA 9).[31] The texts deal with a broad range of topics (e.g. fertility, haemorrhage, pregnancy, delivery, abortion, postpartum issues, amulets) and several of them are related to the treatises outlined in the

28 Many of the scholarly tablets were excavated in the South-West Palace, but it is known that some were stored in other archives/libraries on mound Kuyunjik (e.g. in the North Palace, the Nabû temple or the Ištar temple). For discussion of the different archives and Ashurbanipal's tablet collection, see e.g. Reade 1986; 1998–2001, 421–424; Lieberman 1990; Pedeŕsen 1998, 161–165; Frame and George 2005; Schnitzlein 2023, 257–358. For texts in Babylonian script from Kuyunjik, see Fincke 2003–2004; 2017a; 2017b.

29 Two small fragments of *Diagnostic Handbook* Tablet 36 (K. 7071 and K. 17663) and a fragment of a *mukallimtu*-commentary on Tablet 37 (K. 11939) have been identified among the diagnostic materials concerned with women (see *infra* text I.1.1 and I.1.5).

30 Reade 1986, 218.

31 For this library and the family members' activities associated with it, see Pedersén 1986, 41–76; 1998, 135–136; Maul 2010; Arbøll 2021. Kiṣir-Aššur's active years were during the reign of Ashurbanipal.

AMC.[32] Only one of these texts preserves a colophon that includes the name of the scribe: KAR 223 (text D.3.1) was copied by Kiṣir-Nabû, son of Šamaš-ibni and nephew of Kiṣir-Aššur.

Four Neo-Assyrian tablet fragments on women's health were discovered at Sultantepe (ancient Ḫuzirina near Ḫarran), in a hoard of several hundred tablet fragments of medical-magical and other scholarly contents that belonged to an archive associated with a private house (the so-called House of Qurdi-Nergal): STT 241, STT 98 (+) 284, STT 278.[33] Only STT 241 (text C.1.1), a tablet with an incantation and amulet prescription to protect a pregnant woman from miscarriage, preserves a colophon mentioning the scribe (a certain Sîn-iddina). STT 278 is a fragment on amulet necklaces for women connected to the series *kunuk ḫalti* (text G.1), while STT 98 (+) 284 (text A.1.1) belonged to a tablet with a collection of medical prescriptions for women (on topics such as fertility and difficult delivery).

Turning to the women's healthcare texts from first millennium BCE Babylonia, the best documented evidence for a library context comes from Uruk and Sippar during the Achaemenid and Hellenistic period. The tablet collections in the houses of the *āšipus* in Uruk (which contained texts from all branches of scholarship including magic, medicine, divination, astrology) have yielded both therapeutic texts and fragments of commentaries on tablets of the *Diagnostic Handbook* concerned with women.[34] Among the tablets in the library of the descendants of Šangû-Ninurta (active in the 5th–4th cent. BCE) is SpTU 3, No. 84 (text C.3.4) written by Šamaš-iddina, son of Nādinu. Anu-ikṣur, son of Šamaš-iddina, was the scribe of SpTU 1, No. 59 (text C.2.1) and SpTU 5, No. 248 (text C.3.10). Further, SpTU 1, No. 39 and 40, two fragments of commentaries on *Diagnostic Handbook* Tablet 36 and 39, were found together with other texts and commentaries preserving colophons mentioning Anu-ikṣur as their scribe and can thus be identified as coming from the same archive. The second Uruk library associated with a family of exorcists can be dated to the 4th–3rd cent. BCE and belonged to the descendants of Ekur-zakir. SpTU 4, No. 153 (texts C.1.10 and D.1.11) and SpTU 5, No. 253 (text E.2.6), possibly fragments of one and the same tablet, can be attributed to this archive. The latter two fragments are collections of prescriptions for topics such as haemorrhage, difficult delivery and conditions of the uterus, which are written in a particular discursive style that makes repeated references to orally transmitted lore. From three women's healthcare texts in the Šangû-Ninurta collection, especially SpTU 3, No. 84 and SpTU 5, No. 248, two tablets with ritual ceremonies to counter repeated miscarriages and infant death, have intimate links to other Neo-Assyrian as well as Babylonian sources that can be associated with the treatise PREGNANCY/OFFSPRING in the AMC (see above).[35]

An interesting Late Babylonian archive associated with scribal and medical training has been already mentioned above: the archive of Bēl-rēmanni from Sippar (Jursa 1999; Finkel 2000) dating to the Achaemenid period (ca. 500 BCE). This collection included ca. 90 medical texts, among them seven tablets with prescriptions for women (BM 42313+, BM 42333+ (text A.2.2), BM 42450+ (text B.2.3), BM 42507, F 238 (+) BM 43268, BM 43229 (text E.2.1), BM 43110+ (text E.2.2)). The teaching handbook BM 42313+ is an important collection of prescriptions for various conditions and medical issues concerning women's health and body care. Some of the prescriptions on smaller tablets have unique purposes not attested elsewhere, e.g. text E.2.1 (preserved in three copies) dealing with pain in the breasts.

Other Babylonian texts in the corpus from the British Museum's Sippar collection do not have a certain provenience. At least one fragment with prescriptions (BM 57853, text E.2.5) can be attributed to the Ebabbar temple.

A substantial number of Late Babylonian tablets and fragments on women's health are found in the Babylon collection of the British Museum; some of these texts stemming from the excavations of Hormuzd Rassam may come from other places in Babylonia (e.g. Sippar). A few of these texts preserve colophons mentioning the scribe or owner. The owner/scribe of BM 42327+ (text C.3.3), a certain Itti-Marduk-balāṭu, may be identical with Itti-Marduk-balāṭu, son of Nabû-aḫḫē-iddin and a member of the prominent Babylonian Egibi family, who was active in the latter half of the 6th century BCE; this Itti-Marduk-balāṭu is known as the owner of other medical texts (Bácskay and Simkó 2021). Two texts in the Babylon group, BM 47459 (text D.3.1) and BM 47491 (text A.2.6), were written by the scholar Iprā'ya, son of Zababa-pir'u-uṣur and member

32 May (2018a, 69–74) proposes the AMC, which was copied by an apprentice physician and son of a *šangû* priest of Baba/Bau, may have belonged to the N4 library as well.

33 See e.g. Pedersén 1998, 178–181.

34 For these tablet collections, see e.g. Clancier 2009a; 2014.

35 The fragment A. 3438 containing the beginning of *Diagnostic Handbook* Tablet 37 likewise stems from Uruk. According to its colophon, it was owned by the Eanna temple and written by an apprentice exorcist, Itti-Marduk-balāṭu, son of Mušallim-Marduk of the Šangû-parakki family.

of the Ēṭiru family, which had ties to Borsippa and Babylon.[36] The latter of the two texts is quite special in its combination of recipes for love magic (*ša šudbubu*) with astrological allusions and treatments for women's conditions, specifically types of fever (*ummu* "heat"). The former text is a tablet with procedures to avoid a delivery in the month Nisannu that is known in five other manuscripts (from Neo-Assyrian and later times). One tablet, BM 40152 (text C.1.8), designates a section of remedies as having been copied from a wooden writing board (*lēʾu*) owned by a scholar (*ummânu*) from Babylon named Nūr-Marduk. Although not preserved, such writing boards (wax tablets) are occasionally mentioned as *Vorlage* in colophons of women's healthcare texts as well as in tablet inventories.[37]

Furthermore, there are examples women's healthcare texts from Nippur and Ur with colophons. A remarkable tablet is N. 4001 (text B.2.1) from Nippur, which contains a procedure against infertility and pregnancy prognoses (tests). Its unusual colophon mentions a *Vorlage* owned by Sîn-multēšir, son of Gaḫul-Tutu, grandson/descendant of Gula-balāssu-iqbi). Interestingly, this tablet was written by a physician "for his learning" (*ana lamādīšu*). Sîn-multēšir is mentioned as the copyist of an older *Vorlage* in the colophon of another remarkable tablet of medical content, BM 78158 (Stadhouders 2018a, 169–170). It may be that the damaged colophon of UET 7, No. 123 (text B.2.2), a fragment from Ur likewise with treatments for infertility and test procedures, refers to the same Sîn-multēšir son of Gaḫul-Tutu, although this remains a guess. Moreover, we possess two medical commentaries on the so-called Neo-Assyrian Birth Compendium, one from Ur (UET 6/3, 897) and one from Nippur (11N-T3, see Chapter G).

3 The Scope of Mesopotamian Women's Healthcare in the First Millennium BCE

This section aims to give a brief overview of the contents of the therapeutic texts edited in this volume and comments on the scope of Mesopotamian women's healthcare reflected in them. In this study, I prefer to use the term women's healthcare (texts), although one may speak of "gynaecological" texts in a broader sense of the word.[38] This follows a critical trend that regards the application of the term "gynaecology" as a branch of specialized medicine to sources from the ancient world as problematic and too limited (Gourevitch 1996; Couto-Ferreira 2018c, 110–112). Linked to the question of a medical sub-domain concerned with female patients is the question of Mesopotamian healers' understanding of the relationship between male and female bodies, anatomies and physiologies, i.e. whether they regarded them as similar or radically different.[39] Thus, the texts presented here clearly show that Mesopotamian women's healthcare was a branch of healing connected to a delimited text corpus, the focus of which was clearly on specific issues related to the female physiology, on topics linked to women's reproductive processes and problems encountered in this connection: (in)fertility, menstruation, abnormal bleeding, pregnancy, birth.

If we compare incantations and prescriptions from a diachronic angle, four cardinal topics or groups are represented in both genres: fertility, pregnancy, delivery and bleeding. The purposes of the incantations are often apparent from rubrics appended to the compositions. While spells identified by rubrics as belonging to the context of childbirth and bleeding (during pregnancy or after delivery) are attested in texts from the second and first millennium,[40] spells to enhance fertility

36 On the reading of the name, see Schwemer 2009, 58. This scholar who lived in the fifth or fourth century BCE is known from colophons of several other scholarly texts, especially commentaries and texts of magico-medical, astrological and divinatory content (Frahm 2011, 307; Jiménez 2014, 218; Ossendrijver 2019, 66–68). One text written by Iprāʾya, a commentary on *Marduk's Address to the Demons*, was housed in the Ezida temple in Borsippa.

37 E.g. SpTU 3, No. 84 (text C.3.4). BM 57373 (= CT 55, 411: 3–5) from Sippar, a short inventory listing wax tablets of different content, refers to a polyptych of 13 writing boards of (prescriptions for) a woman who does not bring (her pregnancies) to term (13 ^{giš}IG ^{giš}DA *šá* MUNUS NU SI.SÁ), together with one polyptych of 11 boards of medical remedies (11 ^{giš}IG ^{giš}DA *šá bul-ṭu*), writing boards containing other magical procedures or rituals (anti-witchcraft ceremonies, washing of the mouth (cultic rituals), house-building rituals and further materials.

38 See also Lehmhaus 2023, 75. A similar expression to the ancient Greek term *gynaikeia* which was used for texts dealing with this area of medicine, was perhaps found in the Assur Medical Catalogue (see above line 120).

39 Ancient views on the issue of sexual difference give a range of diverging answers. Some views distinguish two sexes and emphasize the need to evaluate women's ailments in line with their physiology, as different from that of male bodies (e.g. the Hippocratic texts). Other views embrace a one-sex model that regarded female sexual anatomy as an introverted version of the male body and differentiated both sexes merely in their level of internal heat, although recognizing a limited set of bodily functions peculiar to women (such as conception, giving birth, and lactation). For discussion, see Lehmhaus 2023, 6–7, 31–33 with further references.

40 Rubrics of birth incantations encountered already in second millennium BCE texts are KA.INIM.MA MUNUS.Ù.TU.(UD.DA.KAM) "recitation for a woman in childbirth", *šipat aruhtim* "spell for a hastened woman" (viz. a woman in labour) and KA.IMIM.MA/*šipat mul/š(t)apšiqtim* "recitation/

or enable conception and spells to protect a woman from miscarriage can so far only be identified through their respective rubrics in texts from the first millennium.[41] In comparison, the topics of the medical prescriptions from the second and first millennium cover a much wider range of specific conditions and medical problems affecting women (see Table 3):

Table 3: Conditions and problems treated in Mesopotamian therapeutic texts for women.

– To promote fertility/conception (also after menopause)	– To expel a dead foetus(?)
– Lack of desire for intercourse	– To relief pain after childbirth
– Fertility tests/pregnancy prognoses	– Prolapse of the uterus
– Contraception and abortion	– Prolapse of the rectum (postpartum)
– To provoke the menstrual flow	– Puerperal sepsis/infection
– To regulate the menses	– Vaginal/uterine discharges
– To stop (abnormal) haemorrhage	– Fevers
– To prevent miscarriage	– Urological complaints
– Bleeding during pregnancy (*naḫšātu*)	– Uterine tumours(?) ("crab disease")
– Preterm/premature rupture of the membranes (flow of amniotic fluids)	– Uterine ulcers(?) (*tikpū*)
	– Breast pain
– Dystocia (to ease/speed up difficult delivery)	– Skin diseases
– Acute bleeding during/after delivery	– Gastrointestinal complaints (diarrhoea, 'wind', constipation, colic, during pregnancy or postpartum)
– To expel the afterbirth/placenta	– Epilepsy / seizures
– Retention of the lochia (postpartum blood)	– To improve body odour

Most of the conditions listed in the table have a connection to the realm of women's reproductive life or occur as symptoms that are discussed in the context of pregnancy and childbirth (e.g. gastrointestinal problems, fever, infection). The focus of the texts was clearly on women of childbearing age or young women (*sinništu, ālittu, ardatu*). No texts appear to concern pubescent girls or menarche, and problems of menopausal women are not explicitly treated except the decline of fertility and perhaps the ceasing of the menses.[42] A few texts deal with specific diseases of the uterus (ulcers, tumours?) and with urological conditions (common problems affecting women until today), while ailments linked to the breasts, lactation or breastfeeding are almost completely absent: only one Late Babylonian text (BM 42507 and duplicates, text E.2.1) has so far been identified that contains a prescription for breast pain.[43] This finding is surprising, since one expects problems affecting women's breasts to have been common and represented to a greater extent in the Mesopotamian medical literature on women's healthcare (the scarcity in comparison with Greco-Roman and Egyptian medical texts is noteworthy, see e.g. Westendorf 1999, 427–428). Different interpretations for this lacuna may be offered. The lack of textual sources may merely be coincidental (the sources have just not yet come to light). However, other factors may be at play, e.g. having to do with different specialisations of healthcare professionals. Treatments for the breasts and for lactation may have been one domain of expertise of midwives and wet-nurses, and women who encountered such problems may have commonly

spell for a woman in difficult labour". For the latter genre, first millennium BCE texts also use the logographic rubric KA.INIMA.MA ^{munus}LA.(-)RA.AḪ.A.KAM. Rubrics for Sumerian spells to stop bleeding from the second millennium are KA.INIM.MA IDIM.(KA).KÉŠ.DA.KAM 'recitation for sealing (lit. binding) the source (at the mouth)' or KA.INIM.MA MUNUS.KÉŠ.DA.KAM "recitation to seal (lit. bind) a woman", while the first millennium BCE therapeutic texts use the labels KA.INIM.MA MÚD MUNUS KUD-*si* "recitation for stopping a woman's blood" and KA.INIM.MA MUNUS *ša nahšāte* GIG "recitation for a woman who is sick with *nahšātu*".

41 The first millennium BCE texts offer the rubric KA.[INIM].MA ^{munus}NU.Ù.TU *ana urrî* "recitation to enable a barren woman to get pregnant" (N. 4001: 13 (and duplicate); text B.2.1) in the context of treatments for fertility, and the rubric KA.INIM.MA MUNUS NU S[I].SÁ.[KAM] "recitation for a woman who does not bring (pregnancies) to term" (*sinništu lā muš(t)ēšertu*, STT 241: 29; text C.3.1) in the context of therapies protecting women from repeated miscarriage.

42 For a discussion of menarche (only rarely mentioned in cuneiform textual sources), the question of puberty rituals and conditions interpreted as befalling adolescent girls and boys, see e.g. Scurlock and Andersen 2005, 272–274; Scurlock 2014b; Steinert 2023, 244–248 with further references.

43 According to Asher-Greve (1997, 438), the female body/sex was "essentially defined by the vulva and womb", while breasts were "not conceived of as primary distinction between the sexes". The physical appearance of women's breasts was observed in Mesopotamian diagnostic and physiognomic texts for making predictions about a woman's reproductive capacities, about the sex of a pregnant woman's foetus, or about the wellbeing of the expecting mother and her child (see Böck 2000; Scurlock and Andersen 2005, 669–670; Minen 2020, 11–15 and *infra* on *Diagnostic Handbook* Tablet 36).

turned to such women for help and advice.[44] Among the "non-gynaecological" conditions surprisingly attested, albeit rarely, in therapeutic texts dealing with a female patient is epilepsy. Thus, a fragment from Assur contains treatments for epilepsy in a female patient (BAM 245; text A.1.3), but the context of the fragment, whether it belonged to a text focusing exclusively on women's health or on treatments for epilepsy, is not completely certain.

The texts edited for the first time in this volume fill considerable gaps in the documentation of the spectrum of Mesopotamian women's healthcare. For example, a few prescriptions for contraceptives have been identified for the first time in a Late Babylonian text (BM 51246+, text A.2.7). New are also prescriptions to improve a woman's body odour and to treat a woman's lack of desire for sexual intercourse, called "doing the work/duty of women" (*šipir sinnišāti epēšu*, see BM 42313+, text A.2.2).[45] Vice versa, there are also a few conditions affecting women that are still exclusively attested in sources outside the text corpus edited here, e.g. in drug compendia or related texts highlighting the uses of specific *materia medica*.[46]

In connection with evaluating the scope of ancient Mesopotamian women's healthcare as a sub-field of medical practice, it is further remarkable that women's healthcare texts were occasionally assembled with other materials. There are a few examples of therapeutic tablets with "mixed" content, i.e. procedures or prescriptions for women's health matters combined with procedures for problems that are not peculiar to women or are not strictly medical in nature.[47] Thus, one text combines recipes for love magic and prescriptions for treating *ummu* "heat" (fever) in women (BM 47491), but also texts combining treatments for rectal diseases, the hips and women's health (K. 8678+), skin conditions and women's health (BM 50700; BM 61975), dream rituals(?) and women's health (BAM 249, text D.1.3). A fragment from Assur contains prescriptions for a female patient suffering from "non-gynaecological" conditions (e.g. epilepsy, in BAM 245 (text A.1.3)), which could suggest that Mesopotamian women's healthcare was a branch of medicine that had a much broader scope than treating merely female reproductive health (gynaecology) and thus develops towards a form of gender-specific medicine. This finding may hint at underlying developments within Mesopotamian medicine towards more differentiated views of male and female bodies and their physiologies, linked to increasingly differentiated knowledge about conditions that women are more prone to develop than men (and vice versa), having specific causes, as well as towards differentiated, gender-specific treatments for the same pathologies and diseases.[48]

Judging from the evidence of medical texts and other written discourses beyond this corpus, it seems that in Mesopotamian medicine, the female body was seen as standing in a kind of parallelism to the male body, although women's anatomical differences, their gender-specific roles in reproduction, the existence of gender-specific complaints as well as the necessity of context-specific treatments are also clearly recognised (Steinert 2023).[49] For example, the most important body metaphors encountered in women's healthcare texts to describe irregular processes in the female body (vessels and agricultural landscapes, canals, crafts and technologies) also served to conceptualize other types of conditions such as intestinal/digestive ailments, which are not restricted to women.[50] Haemorrhage and genital discharges form examples for conditions, in which male and female bodies were seen as behaving in a similar manner and as comparable with each

44 For textual hints to ailments affecting women connected to breastfeeding/wet-nursing, cf. Stol 2000, 184; 2016, 378, 616.

45 There are no references to "(sexual) arousal" (ŠÀ.ZI.GA, *nīš libbi*) in women's healthcare texts so far, cf. Zisa 2021 for discussion.

46 For example, the term *šalputtu* "ruined" and the expression "to be touched by a touch" (TAG TAG.TAG-*at*), both referring to a complication during delivery, perhaps meaning a woman having a protracted delivery whose foetus has died in utero and needs to be removed (BAM 380 rev. 38–41 // BAM 381 iii 33–36; BAM 422 rev. iii 4' // BAM 421 i 27; KADP 22 ii 2; Stol 2000, 53–54; Mirelman 2015, 177–178, 181 K. 4206+ rev. 28). Likewise attested only in drug compendia is prolapse of the uterus, perhaps referred to in KADP 22 ii 4 (commentary): DIŠ MUNUS ḪÁŠ[⸢*šap-ru*⸣] GIG : ḪÁŠ ŠUB ŠÀ.TÙ[R] "if a woman suffers in her *thigh* (Akk. gloss: *šapru*) : *šapru* (means) dropping (*nadû*) of the uterus". Cf. below on a similar expression for expelling the afterbirth (ÙŠ, *silītu*).

47 A unique assemblage of materials is LKA 9 from Assur, which combines extracts of different texts associated with stones and amulet necklaces (e.g. an extract from Tablet 2 of the mythological composition Lugale), including amulets and other prescriptions to protect pregnant women (text C.3.5).

48 For sick women in letters and other texts outside the medical corpus, see Stol 2016, 441–446. Some of them are treated by physicians and suffer from conditions such as abscesses, fevers, colic.

49 In that study, I argue based on the creation account in the *Atramḫasīs* myth that Mesopotamian traditions may have embraced a view of simultaneous similarity and difference between male and female bodies: they were created from the same (human) prototype and material substances, but men and women were equipped with anatomical differences marking their diverging roles in sexual reproduction. For the male body as the normative (or "default") body in Mesopotamian medicine, and the subordinate position of the female body in the medical compendia, see Heeßel 2006. See further Couto-Ferreira 2018c for discussion.

50 See e.g. Johnson and Simkó 2024; Steinert 2013; 2020; Steinert and Vacín 2018.

other (Steinert 2023). For example, a few texts compare female genital haemorrhage with nosebleed in men and recommend the same treatment for either condition (see e.g. texts C.1.4 and C.1.8). Haemorrhage from the penis and anus in male patients is often compared with blood flows from the vulva (be it menstrual or irregular), and abnormal genital discharges or urological problems are recognized as affecting both male and female patients.[51] The Late Babylonian disease taxonomy SpTU 1, No. 43 (Geller 2014, 4: 25–30; Steinert 2016, 231, 238; Wee 2021, 325, 329–333) also points to a similar reasoning that male and female reproductive processes and irregularities in these bodily processes have a parallel or common physiological basis, since it views both infertility (in women) and lack of sexual desire (in men) as being caused by the kidneys.

However, therapeutic texts from the first millennium BCE deal with topics such as genital haemorrhage and urological problems in gender-specific ways, and remedies for these conditions in men and women were collected in different treatises. Treatments for urological problems affecting women are included in "gynaecological" recipe collections (e.g. BM 42313+ (text A.2.2); BAM 237(+) iv 9–12 (text C.1.4)) rather than in the therapeutic treatise dealing with renal diseases (Geller 2005a). One of these passages is worth quoting as an example:

BM 42313+ rev. 1–6 (text A.2.2); var. BAM 237 iv 9–10 (text C.1.4); BAM 241(+) ii 9'-10' (text II.1.3):
"If a woman suffers from NI.NE (a burning sensation?) and *binding* of the urine (DIŠ MUNUS NI.NE *ki-is*[!] KÀŠ GIG-*at*), (and) her blood [. . .] into [. . .] (and) there is [. . .], this woman suffers from NI.NE. You tie ashes of *urbatu*-rush (and) ashes of poplar (var. one litre ashes of *amḫara*-plant) (into) fourteen knots of cloth, [you insert (them) one by one into her womb (i.e. vagina)].
If ditto, **she shall drink 'white drug' in grape juice, [. . .].**
If ditto, **you crush *murru*-plant with oil (and) pour (it) into her urethra (var. womb) with a bronze tube**.
. . .
If a woman suffers from (uncontrollable) discharging (and) 'seizing' of urine (DIŠ MUNUS ŠUB DAB KÀŠ[!] GIG-*at*), you wrap *imbû tâmti*-mineral in a wad of wool and put it into her womb."

The condition NI.NE mentioned in this passage is only known from women's healthcare texts and thus appears to be a specifically female ailment associated with symptoms affecting urination (see further below).[52] Retention of urine and incontinence are also dealt with in the treatise KIDNEY on renal diseases (cf. Steinert et al. 2018), where one can at times find similar prescriptions with identical drugs or forms of treatment, but also differences (in the terminology and applied treatments). The prescriptions for women quoted above are gender-specific, in that they treat the condition with vaginal suppositories. The other two modes of treatment, potions and injection of *materia medica* into the urethra with a bronze tube, are also prominent in renal disease texts:

AMT 31/1+ 59/1+ 61/1 i 16–21, 23 (Geller 2005a, No. 2):
"If a man suffers from 'stricture of the bladder' (*ḫiniqti elabuḫḫi*), crush shell of ostrich egg and *imbû tâmti*-mineral, he shall drink it in oil (and) beer.
If a man has *difficulty* with urine . . ., he suffers from stricture of the bladder. He shall drink seed of wild melon (*irrû*) in beer.
You crush *murru*-plant, mix it in oil, blow it through a bronze tube in his urethra, ...
. . .
You crush juice of *kasû*-plant, date juice, pressed oil, fish sauce, river locust **and 'white' drug, and he drinks it in milk.**
. . .
You **crush 'white' drug and mix it in oil** and blow it through a copper tube into his urethra."

Other glimpses of a differentiated understanding of male and female bodies and their pathologies (at least in some contexts) are found in diagnostic and therapeutic texts. A few diagnostic entries in the *Diagnostic Handbook* add a comment that certain diagnoses (for specific symptoms/conditions) are "the same for a man and a woman" (*ana zikari u sinništi ištēnma*, e.g. *muruṣ râmi* "love sickness"), which may express an exception (i.e. that the sections in the *Diagnostic Handbook* for-

51 For example, BAM 205: 40–41 refers to abnormal genital secretions (*suḫsu, su'su*) as a flow of semen (*riḫûtu*) affecting both male and female patients: "(If) either a man's or a woman's seminal fluids (*su'su riḫûssunu*) flow *copiously*(?), (and) they spill them while urinating" (Biggs 1967, 68; Scurlock and Andersen 2005, 89 sub 4.3). See also Steinert 2017a, 310–311; Zisa 2021, 413 for discussion. Note also the parallel reference to *mūṣu*-discharge "from the vagina" (*šá* ŠÀ GAL$_4$.LA) and "from the penis (urethra)" (*šá* ŠÀ GÌŠ) in Uruanna III 161–162 (quoted in MSL 10, 70: 19ff.; cf. CAD S, 293a sub b; CAD M/2, 246b sub 2). Related to symptoms of genital discharges may be sexually transmitted diseases, which were known to affect both sexes and referred to with terms such as *muruṣ nâki* "disease(s) of illicit intercourse", linked to the "Hand of the goddess Ištar" (cf. Stol 2016, 444; Scurlock and Andersen 2005, 88–97).

52 Another disease name only encountered in women's healthcare texts is NI.RA (see text D.2.1), which is a condition linked to the postpartum period.

mulated for a male patient were usually thought to apply only to men) or confirm a general rule (that omens formulated for a male patient are also valid for women).[53] More common are examples of diagnostic entries that give differentiated diagnoses or aetiologies, i.e. gender-specific causes or disease agents responsible for the same sickness in male and female patients:[54]

Diagnostic Handbook Tablet 26: 82'–83' (see also lines 45'–47', 48'–49'; Stol 1993, 46; Heeßel 2000, 285, 291; Scurlock 2014a, 199, 204):
DIŠ *pa-rid-ma it-te-né-et-bi ma-gal* DUG_4.DUG_4-*ub u i[g-d]a-na-al-lu-u[t] ana* MUNUS LÍL.L[Á].EN.NA *ana* NITA MUNUS.LÍL.LÁ.EN.NA
"If he shudders (with fear) and gets up time and again, he talks a lot and jerks continually: for a woman (it is) a *lilû*-demon; for a man, a *lilītu*-demon."

Diagnostic entries for women outside *Diagnostic Handbook* Tablets 36–39 that complement identical or similar symptoms for male patients are rare.[55] However, several diagnostic entries pertaining to "sick women" in Tablet 37 are variants of diagnostic omens in sections dealing with the same conditions or symptoms affecting male patients (see text I.1.3–I.1.4 for detailed discussion). The following examples may illustrate the point:

Diagnostic Handbook Tablet 11: 22, 24 (Scurlock 2014a, 83; Scurlock and Andersen 2005, 19.41–19.42; Schmidtchen 2021a, 459):
DIŠ ŠU.MIN-*šú ina* UGU-*šú* NU DU_8.MEŠ MÁŠKIM SÌG-*s[u*? . . .]
"If his hands never leave his skull, a lurker-demon (*rābiṣu*) has struck hi[m . . .]."
DIŠ ŠU.MIN-*šú ina* SAG.DU-*šú* GAR-*na-ma la ur-ra-da-ni* ŠU ^{d}*lugal-ir*$_9$*-ra u* ^{d}*mes-la[m-ta-è-a]*
"If his hands are placed on his head and they don't come down: Hand of Lugalirra and Meslamtaea [. . .]".

Diagnostic Handbook Tablet 37: 10 (see *infra*):
DIŠ MUNUS GIG-*ma* ŠU.MIN-*šá ina* SAG.DU-*šá* GAR-*na-ma la ur-ra-da-ni* ŠU EN ÙR KI.MIN MAŠKIM ÙR SÌG-*aṣ* UG_7
"If a woman is sick and her hands are placed on her head, and they don't come down: hand of the "Lord of the roof" (*bēl ūri*). Alternatively, the 'Lurker of the roof' has struck (her); she will die."

Within therapeutic texts, it can occasionally be observed that variant, but differentiated treatments were prescribed for the same or similar medical problem in a male and female patient. Examples can be found, for example, in the context of digestive ailments, haemorrhage, urological conditions, or in remedies for hair loss. For instance, BAM 240 obv. 26' and 28' (text D.2.1) contains a slight variant of a remedy for intestinal bloating due to 'wind' in the body found in BAM 575 ii 54–55 (= STOMACH Tablet 2; Johnson and Simkó 2024, 127–128 lines 124–125). In BAM 240, the remedy is recommended for a pregnant woman, in BAM 575, it is prescribed for a male (or generalized) patient. As a second example, specific remedies for hair loss in women were included in therapeutic texts or treatises focusing on diseases of the head (rather than in the women's healthcare texts), and these remedies are differentiated from the treatments for male patients with hair loss (see the *Appendix*, Chapter H for discussion).[56] Rarer statements to be found in the therapeutic texts are warnings to administer a certain remedy only to a male, but not to a female patient.[57]

---

53 See Heeßel 2000, 43. Note *Diagnostic Handbook* Tablet 14: 212' (Schmidtchen 2021, 577, 588); Tablet 18: 8–9, 30 (Heeßel 2000, 218–220; Scurlock 2014a, 173–175, Tablet 22: 6–9 (Heeßel 2000, 251–252, 258; Scurlock 2014a, 185–186, 189). For "love sickness", see also Couto-Ferreira 2010; 2018c. Some diagnoses add instead "it is the same for an adult and a child".

54 See also *Diagnostic Handbook* Tablet 3: 40 (Scurlock and Andersen 2005, 432 19.5; Scurlock 2014a, 14, 20 (lines 41–42); Schmidtchen 2021, 250, 259, 271–273; Wee 2018, 156), a diagnostic entry that links a set of symptoms with persecution by the goddess Ištar but stipulates differentiated causes (broken taboos?) in the case the patient is a man, a woman or an adolescent girl (*batultu*).

55 E.g. Tablet 3: 29 concerning sparse hair (cf. lines 24–28 for men); Tablet 13: 124' (concerning the belly (*libbu*), cf. lines 115'–125'); Tablet 14: 28 concerning paralysis of the hips (cf. lines 25–27); see Schmidtchen 2021, 249, 258, 525, 535, 565, 581.

56 The first entry in *Diagnostic Handbook* Tablet 30 (lines 1–4) contains a short prescription, which stipulates that the patient should be rubbed with gazelle horn, *ankinūtu*-plant, nine times if it is a man, and seven times if it is a woman (Scurlock 2014a, 223–224, restored from CTN 4, 72 vi 1'–8'; Stadhouders 2011, 39–51).

57 For example, a Nineveh text on respiratory ailments (BAM 554–556) features a recipe for a special potion (*sahunu*) for "all constrictions of the lungs", specifying that it should only be administered to a man, but not to a woman (BAM 555 ii 15: *ana zikari teppuš ana sinništi lā teppuš*).

4 Women's Healthcare in Ancient Mesopotamia: Concepts and Practices

4.1 Concepts of the Female Body

Medical knowledge about women's bodies, the anatomy of women's genital organs and the conceptualization of physiological processes in the female body reflected in Mesopotamian medical texts has been the subject of previous studies (e.g. Steinert 2013; 2017a; 2020; 2023; Couto-Ferreira 2013; 2017; 2018a; 2018c) and is discussed in detail within the different chapters of this volume. Here, I will only briefly summarise the most important and new findings of the present study.

As mentioned above, due to the lack of theoretical discourse in Mesopotamian medical literature, concepts of the female body and its processes have to be gleaned from the vocabulary and descriptions of bodily processes found in the diagnostic and therapeutic texts themselves. The language of these texts is often ambiguous, euphemistic or metaphorical, but paradoxically the metaphors (e.g. in the medical incantations) give important clues for unravelling some of the underlying concepts. Furthermore, knowledge about normal processes linked to the female body such as menstruation often has to be inferred from the descriptions of abnormal and irregular processes (e.g. lacking or excessive menses). The preceding section showed that Mesopotamian women's healthcare texts focus primarily on conditions linked to reproduction, with the womb (*rēmu, šassūru*) featuring as the central organ of femininity associated with these processes.[58] However, the treatments for women suggest that Mesopotamian healers often understood and treated women's bodies and their ailments in a holistic manner, as is suggested by the concepts underlying therapeutic interventions for these female conditions (see further below).

Menstruation and Notions of Blood and Female Genital Bleeding

Many ancient medical traditions closely associate menstruation with female "nature" and women's reproductive capacities. Mesopotamian women's healthcare texts from the first millennium BCE attest to developments in the terminology and concepts of female genital bleeding: the appearance of specific terms and expressions to mark women's menstrual discharges from irregular and abnormal occurrences of genital bleeding and a discernible growing interest in regulating women's menstrual discharges (Steinert 2023). The most common expression in women's healthcare texts, *dām sinništi* "a woman's blood", is vague and ambiguous, although it is usually found in delimited contexts of prescriptions that either seek "to stop a woman's blood" (*dām sinništi parāsu*) or "to make a woman's blood appear" (*dām sinništi kullumu*). The causes behind cases of abnormal haemorrhage and amenorrhoea referred to with these expressions can be manifold and are rarely specified in the texts. Amenorrhoea may be due to pregnancy, poor diets, menopause or other bodily disturbances. The expression "to stop a woman's blood" may relate to cases of acute haemorrhage during or after delivery (as texts occasionally specify) or describe a symptom of some other gynaecological affliction, but less likely unusually heavy menstrual periods (menorrhagia), since these would stop by themselves (while the prescriptions often mention the contrary). Texts from the first millennium BCE show some terminological and conceptual differentiation, as they also use more specific expressions such as *dām ḫarišti* "the blood of a woman in childbed" to refer to the lochia (the postpartum discharges). A group of texts are concerned with the condition *naḫšātu* which refers to bleeding during pregnancy (for texts dealing with these problems, see Chapter C.1; text D.2.1 *passim*).[59] From the contexts in which the latter terms are used it is clear that Mesopotamian healers understood that it is normal for a pregnant woman not to menstruate,[60] and that women should emit postpartum discharges (see further below). Another expression for a genital haemorrhage that is used in reference to female as well as male patients is "to be struck/hit by the weapon" (*kakka maḫāṣu*), which should most likely be understood as a euphemistic expression for an abnormal haemorrhage and symptom of sickness, although the ancient healers appear to see it as a typical condition of women.[61]

58 For knowledge of female anatomy and the terminology for the genitals and reproductive organs, see e.g. Böck 2014–2016; Steinert and Paoletti 2014–2016; Steinert 2017a. Neither the hymen nor the ovaries seem to have been known or designated by specific terms. A term for the clitoris not yet recognised as such in the dictionaries may be *pingu/pinku* "knob" (Stol 2020a, *BiOr* 77, 109).

59 The term is understood here as a derivation from the verb *naḫāšu* "to prosper, thrive" used in a euphemistic fashion (i.e. meaning that the foetus of a woman who suffers from *naḫšātu* does not prosper, but is in danger of being aborted before term); cf. Butz 1982, 221–222; Finkel 1980, 41–42; Scurlock and Andersen 2005, 260 ("menorrhagia"); Steinert 2023, 241. The condition was understood as a "sickness" (*murṣu*).

60 For a passage attesting to exceptions from this rule, see the discussion of *Diagnostic Handbook* Tablet 36 in this volume.

61 Men with a haemorrhage from the penis or anus are said to be "struck by the weapon like a woman" (Steinert 2023, 253–254).

In addition to these terms denoting genital bleeding, a few more words and expressions appear to refer to the menses more specifically, although the Akkadian terms in question do not refer to a typical monthly occurrence (as is the case in the ancient Greek counterpart terms *epimenia* and *katamenia*, for example). The word *maruštu* (NÍG.GIG) "trouble" is encountered both in Late Babylonian therapeutic texts and in the *Diagnostic Handbook* and refers to the menses in a euphemistic fashion that may express a view of this blood flow as unpleasant (although not polluting or impure), as does the word *sagû* (also *šagû* in Assyrian texts) "(menstrual) flow", which may be connected with the verb *sagû* "to cause distress, trouble". Both terms are only attested in first millennium BCE texts. The term *sagû* denotes a woman's menstrual flow in several Late Babylonian women's healthcare texts that aim at provoking (*kullumu* "to make appear") *sagû*, when a woman "does not see" (*amāru*) her menstruation.[62] Some scholars connect this word with a term for menstrual bandage, and it is possible that the meaning "menses" developed from a more concrete meaning "(menstrual) bandage".[63] However, in the attestations of *sagû* in the late women's healthcare texts this word clearly refers to a flow of blood that is normal and expected to occur. It is explained as *dām ardati* "a young woman's blood" in SpTU 1, No. 39: 6', a Late Babylonian commentary on *Diagnostic Handbook* Tablet 36 (see *infra* text I.1.1). In BAM 235 obv. 1, 7 (text C.1.1), a Neo-Assyrian text to stop female bleeding from Assur (ca. 8th/7th cent. BCE), the variant (dialectal) forms *šagû/šugû* are used instead of the usual term *dām sinništi* "a woman's blood", and a "bright red" (*pelû*) discharge is described.[64] Here, *šagû* seems to refer to a haemorrhage or discharge that is perceived as abnormal.[65] The meaning of the term *sagû* may therefore have developed towards a more specific meaning "menses" in the Late Babylonian period (in the 6th/5th cent. BCE).

A third and very rare term attested only in three Late Babylonian texts so far, however, may express a notion of the menses as something typical for women and allude to a notion of regularity, which is an exciting new insight. Thus, the word *kibsu* means "step, track, route" and can metaphorically denote the typical behaviour of a person. Like *dām sinništi* and *sagû*, the term *kibsu* is attested in formulations with the verb *parāsu* "to stop", referring to the case that a woman's menses, i.e. her normal "*course*", has stopped. More significantly, one text (BM 47491, text A.2.6 lines 25–26) also links the stopping of *kibsu* with the decline of a woman's fertility, thus clearly referring to a menopausal woman: *sinništu ša alāda u kibsa taprusu* "a woman who has ceased to bear and (to experience) the (normal) *course* (of women's menses)".[66] Thus, *kibsu* offers the semantic equivalent to the Hebrew expression *derekh ha-nashim* "the way of women" in Biblical texts.[67] Like its Hebrew counterpart, *kibsu* may mark the menses as something typical for women of childbearing age (as does the ancient Greek medical term *gynaikeia* "women's things"), but not in terms of an ideal regular monthly occurrence (which is something never stated as such in Mesopotamian women's healthcare texts).

A second significant idea or ideational complex that emerges from the present study of Mesopotamian women's healthcare texts is the notion of (menstrual) blood or bleeding as a "hot" state (simultaneously linked to an excess of moisture in contexts concerned with stopping an excessive or abnormal flow of blood) and hence a notion of menopausal women as being "cooler" than women in their reproductive age or during childbirth in particular. This idea can be grasped in a Late Babylonian text from Uruk (SpTU 4, No. 153 obv. 7–9, text C.1.10), in a passage that describes the effect of a treatment applied to stop a woman's blood as "cooling" (*kaṣû, takṣâtu*), a process that results in the blood being held back (*kalû*). This idea of blood as hot and moist (which finds a fascinating parallel in Graeco-Roman medical theories based on the system of the humours) can be traced in some of the *materia medica* applied to stop gynaecological haemorrhage, which can be

62 See text C.2.1 for discussion of the different attested spellings and the texts BM 45736 obv. i 4' and 5' (text A.2.5); BM 38624+ ii 20', 28', 30' (text A.2.1); BM 54587+73802 obv. 6', 8', 9', rev. 3, 9 (text C.2.3); BM 61975 obv. 5', 7' (C.2.4).

63 Cf. CAD S 27 sub *sagû* B, translating "flow of blood(?)", while AHw 1003 sub *sagû* II and CDA^2 310, among others, regard *sagû* as a menstrual rag. Wasserman (2019, 1135) includes *sagû* in a survey of Akkadian words for underwear but notes possible confusion or overlap with the lemma *sāgu*, referring to a garment and sackcloth used as a piece of clothing worn around the hips ("kilt"), e.g. by soldiers and workers. For discussion, see AHw 1003 sub *sāgu* I CAD S, 27–28; Postgate 2001, 384–385; Gaspa 2018, 99, 184–185, 260–261; Steinert et al. 2018, 218, 275 on line 118 (for the occurrence of *sagû* instead of *dāmu* "(menstrual) blood" in an entry of the Assur Medical Catalogue); Steinert 2023.

64 For written *š* pronounced as /s/ in Neo-Assyrian texts (and vice versa), cf. Hämeen-Anttila 2000, 9–10; Luukko 2004, 74–75, with spellings such as *pa-ri-iš-tú* for *paristu*, and ^{túg}*ši-ši-ik-ti-šú* for *sissiktu*.

65 For the concept of menses (*sagû*) that are not regular/normal (*lā išaru*), see BM 40152 (text C.1.8) line 15'.

66 The expression relates to another term for a (post-)menopausal woman, *pariš/stu* "(woman) who has stopped" (CAD P, 187a). More commonly a menopausal woman is designated as a woman "who has stopped to bear" (*ša alāda parsat*).

67 E.g. Gen. 31:35 and 18:11; see Philip 2006, 19–25; Lehmaus 2023, 34. The noun *derekh* has a similar meaning spectrum ("way, road, journey" as well as "(typical) manner, customary experience, condition or habit") and is derived from a verb *darakh* meaning "to tread, to march" (Gesenius 1930 [1906], 202–203), as in the case of Akkadian *kibsu*, which is derived from *kabāsu* "to tread, step".

regarded as signature ingredients evoking notions of dryness and heat or coolness (see Steinert 2020 and *infra*). The same logics of "like cures like" or treating a state of excess with a substance of opposite properties can also be traced in treatments for other conditions classified as hot, most prominently fevers. Thus, BM 47491 (text A.2.6), a Late Babylonian text already referred to above, applies substances with "cooling" properties to treat fever in a female patient, such as algae (an ingredient of aquatic origin) and "dust from underneath a woman who has ceased to bear and (to experience) the (normal) *course* (of women's menses)". The same ingredients as well as numerous other ingredients that underline the application of a hot-cold-reasoning are encountered in prescriptions against fever (see Bácskay 2018 and *infra* for examples). Moreover, additional evidence for the application of a reasoning in terms of hot-cold can be found in prescriptions treating a reverse gynaecological condition, namely the retention of postpartum blood. In several texts, heat or hot substances are applied to induce the lochia, especially fumigations (see e.g. texts 0.4 and A.1.4 for discussion).

A debated aspect linked to (women's) blood, menses or other genital discharges is to which extent these flows were regarded as polluting or impure in ancient Mesopotamia. These questions have been discussed recently (Steinert 2023); therefore, only a brief summary is given here. From medical and other textual sources, which reflect a dominance of scholarly and male views on the subject omitting the experiences of women, it can be gleaned that genital discharges in general (including flows of blood and emissions of semen) were regarded and evaluated in ambivalent terms, and that such discharges (especially abnormal ones) were associated with disease, dirt and decay and led to cultic or ritual impurity. There are several hints that ritual impurity/pollution was believed to affect women with flows of blood, especially women in childbed in the period after delivery when they discharged the lochia (and referred to with terms such as *musukkatu* "impure woman") and women who suffered from *naḫšātu* (bleeding during pregnancy). But the conception of ritual or cultic impurity may have included menstruants. Since ritual pollution could be transmitted to other persons through physical contact and was seen as defiling, it would need to be avoided for any direct contact with the divine and cultic sphere. The extent to which menstruants or postpartum women were required to go into seclusion or separated themselves in ancient Mesopotamia is uncertain and debated, and one expects that such practices were not uniform through time and dependent on social contexts. Reviewing the textual sources that come from the realm of healing professionals and scholars, including the women's healthcare texts themselves, one has the impression that male healers did not generally avoid direct contact with patients (whether male or female) suffering from conditions of a defiling character, including women with discharges, although we know very little in detail about healers' bedside manners and hands-on contact while examining and treating female patients. It is also remarkable that female body fluids associated with reproduction and childbirth are also seen as positive in some contexts and used as curative agents and as powerful substances to repel evil. This is especially apparent in the case of breast milk, in particular the milk of a *musukkatu* (i.e. a woman who has recently given birth), which was used in a range of medical contexts, e.g. in treatments against inflammation, fevers, epilepsy/seizures, in eye remedies (e.g. Steinert 2023, 276–280). This ingredient also occurs occasionally in women's healthcare texts, including milk of an "impure (*musukkatu*) cow".[68]

Beside blood, Mesopotamian women's healthcare texts also mention other genital secretions and fluids, mostly referred to vaguely as *mû* "water, fluid", a term that can stand for amniotic fluid, at times for other (normal or abnormal) discharges[69], e.g. after childbirth (see *infra* and the next paragraph for further discussion).

4.2 Health Problems and Diseases Specific to the Female Body

Whereas some earlier scholarship on ancient Mesopotamian medical texts tried to identify the conditions described in women's healthcare texts in terms of modern biomedical diseases and modern biological knowledge (Scurlock and Andersen 2005), this study follows trends critical toward an approach of retrospective diagnosis and rather seeks to investigate the emic concepts and interlinked health practices as culturally embedded. This section outlines the most prominent issues and problems dealt with in the women's healthcare texts and highlights important insights as well as difficulties of interpretation.

68 See text A.2.6 and *passim.* Other ingredients related to female body parts or fluids (human or animal) attested in Mesopotamian medical texts are placenta (of animals), urine of a postpartum woman, and an ingredient referred to as "soiled (menstrual) rag" (*ulāpu lupputu*), of which at least the latter may be an alias name (*Deckname*) for a plant (see Steinert 2023, 280–290).

69 An example of an abnormal vaginal discharge are "fluids" (*mû*) caused by sorcery (affecting a woman who has been given "drugs of hatred" (*šammī zērūte*) to eat (BAM 237 iv 29; text C.1.4).

Infertility and Conception

In Mesopotamian medicine, infertility (here understood merely as the inability to conceive and not in terms of more detailed modern definitions) is usually attributed to the woman and her womb and appears to be a gendered condition.[70] Mesopotamian women's healthcare texts allow us to trace multifaceted and quite complex concepts of female (in)fertility that revolve around dominant views of the womb and the physiology of the female body (e.g. Steinert 2017a; 2020). The metaphors and imagery encountered in this context view the womb as a receptacle or vessel for the male semen and assume that conception takes place when the womb is in a condition that it can receive (*maḫāru*) and retain (*kalû*) the semen.[71] Consequently, notions of openness and closure are part of the treatment strategies for treating infertility or the inability to conceive. Some remedies are explicitly said to bring about an "opening" (*petû*) of the womb, while infertility may be addressed as being caused by a blockage (*sekēru*) (see Chapter B). The inability to receive or retain the semen in Mesopotamian women's healthcare texts (see BAM 240: 71'ff.; text D.2.1) may also be compared to similar notions encountered in the Hippocratic treatise *Diseases of Women* I (Chapters 10–13; see Potter 2018, 42–55), where a woman's inability to conceive is connected to the observation that the patient discharges the semen within the first seven days after intercourse, which the Hippocratic doctors linked to closure of the cervix (mouth of the uterus) or to excess moisture in the womb.

Comparable causes of infertility envisioned in Mesopotamian texts are deformations or dislocations of the womb which hinder the semen from reaching the interior of the womb. The womb may be "twisted" (*zīr*; SpTU 1, No. 43 rev. 31) or "knotted" (*kuṣṣuru*; Lambert and Millard 1969, 108ff. K. 3399+ iv 51, 61) or "turned over; lying flat down" (*saḫāpu*) rather than being in a normal state of straightness/uprightness (see UET 7, No. 123; text B.2.2 for discussion). Such conceptions of subtle movements or dislocations of the womb leading to infertility and to other problems such as pain and suffocation are also encountered in ancient Egyptian texts and in Graeco-Roman (e.g. Hippocratic) texts.[72] Moreover, infertility may be caused by impurities or some kind of physical "matter" in the woman's womb or body. Mesopotamian healers often attributed such impurities to adverse influences such as witchcraft or demonic attacks (see e.g. BAM 244 (text B.1.1) and UET 7, No. 123 for discussion); sometimes infertility is attributed to the anger of the personal god (BAM 240, text D.2.1; Steinert 2012a, 238, 398–399). The elimination of such "matter" and bodily impurities can be grasped from the therapeutic interventions applied to treat infertility, which consist of many purifying substances and treatments (such as baths, bandages, ointments as well as tampons).[73] Mesopotamian healers also sought to extend or restore a woman's fertility beyond menopause (see e.g. BAM 243; text B.1.2).

Closely linked to treatments to promote conception and remove infertility are tests with pregnancy prognoses, which are usually found in conjunction with such therapies (see N. 4001 and UET 7, No. 123; STT 98 (A.1.1)). It is difficult to decide in most cases whether these tests evaluated a woman's ability to conceive or detected signs of pregnancy (from the neighbouring ancient cultures both fertility tests and signs to establish whether a woman was pregnant are known). The Mesopotamian tests usually consist in tampons or suppositories filled with different (mostly unidentified) drugs, which were inserted into the vagina, removed after some time and examined, mostly for colour changes. These procedures differ from test procedures found in Egyptian papyri (and Graeco-Roman sources), which observed whether the woman suffered from an internal obstruction (detected by inserting a strongly smelling substances into the vagina and checking whether the woman later emitted the smell from her mouth) or whether the woman's urine caused seed of cereals to sprout. Both Mesopotamian texts and Egyptian papyri also employed tests where the woman's reaction to some ingested substance was observed (e.g. Westendorf 1999; Pommerening 2015; 2023).

---

70 E.g. Stol 2000; Böck 2013; Steinert 2017a, 303–314. Female infertility was associated with serious distress: in prayers, the weeping infertile woman (*lā ālittu/ālidat*, lit. "woman who does not conceive/bear") serves as a point of comparison with the suffering petitioner (e.g. Oshima 2011, 164–165: 132). The corresponding (largely gendered) ailment in men was lack of sexual desire (ŠÀ.ZI.GA) linked to impotence (inability of male sexual performance), see Zisa 2021. The male counterpart to an infertile woman is the eunuch (see Steinert 2027a, 312 with n. 74).

71 While the dominant view regards the role of the man (male semen) to "engender" (*reḫû*) and the role of the woman to "give birth" ((*w*)*alādu*) to the offspring, a few texts suggest an alternative view that assumes a female contribution to the foetus, either in the form of seminal fluids (mingling with male semen) or in the form of other body substances (flesh, muscles, (menstrual) blood), see Stol 2000, 1–12; 2008. The processes of gestation were regularly described as an active, "productive" contribution of the womb that is compared with processes in agriculture (e.g. plant growth) and in craft production (e.g. pottery, textile industries); see e.g. Couto-Ferreira 2015–2016; Steinert 2017a.

72 See e.g. Pommerening 2023; Potter 2018, *Diseases of Women* I, Chapters 10, 14–15; *Diseases of Women* II, Chapters 14–32, 95; *infra* text B.2.2.

73 See also Böck 2013; Steinert 2020; 2021a for discussion. Since offspring was also a gift bestowed by deities, women and men (household heads) also turned to such deities with prayers and ritual offerings to receive help, see e.g. text B.2.6 with further discussion. Such practices are also mentioned in letters (e.g. SAA 10, No. 294 rev. 23–25; Parpola 1993, 234).

Pregnancy and Miscarriage

Pregnancy and miscarriage form a second thematic focus of Mesopotamian women's healthcare texts. Other texts beyond these sources make it clear that the ancients saw pregnancy and childbirth as a prolonged period of risk and dangers to women and their babies. Infant mortality is believed to have been high in ancient Near Eastern societies, and the death of the mother in childbirth was presumably also not uncommon, as these subjects are also addressed in literary works (e.g. George 2010), in the so-called oracle queries (*tāmītu*) to the sun god and in letters.[74] While news of a woman's pregnancy were a reason for joy, the months of pregnancy also seem to have been accompanied by worries and uncertainties, and a host of different measures were undertaken to deal with these uncertainties. The diagnostic texts (*Diagnostic Handbook* Tablet 36–37) suggest that pregnant women's physical and psychological state, habits and behaviour (including sexual intercourse) were closely monitored for signs of risk (such as miscarriage, death of the mother or child; Minen 2020). A host of rituals, apotropaic measures and treatments was designed to protect pregnant women from evil influences causing miscarriage (especially witchcraft and demons such as the child-snatcher Lamaštu).

Furthermore, there are complex rituals and other therapies for women who had experienced repeated miscarriages in the past, referred to as (*sinništu*) *lā muš(t)ēšertu* and *lā mušallimtu* (also written logographically, MUNUS NU SI.SÁ)[75] "(a woman) who does not bring (her pregnancy) to term", a condition that is usually attributed to external agents including divine punishment for misdeeds that happened in the women's family (see Chapters C.1, C.3 and G in this volume). Several therapeutic texts contain prescriptions to prevent miscarriage, some of which mention miscarriage in the first, second or third month of pregnancy (e.g. BM 42313+, text A.2.2).[76] Other symptoms treated to avoid a miscarriage are bleeding during pregnancy and loss of amniotic fluid. A few medical texts contain treatments for other medical problems during pregnancy (e.g. BAM 240, text D.2.1), such as intestinal bloating or "wind".

Recipes for contraception (MUNUS NU PEŠ$_4$ "to cause a woman to not get pregnant") and abortion (*ša libbīša nadû/šuddû*(ŠUB)) "to cause a woman to expel her foetus") are rare in the preserved women's healthcare texts, which is in accordance with the Mesopotamian cultures' predominant pro-natalist attitudes, but nonetheless highly remarkable (see also below). The recipes for abortive remedies consist in potions or tampons inserted into the vagina, while the only text containing contraceptives (BM 51246+) appears to administer these as potions.[77] We have no information in which situations it would have been permitted for a woman to procure an abortion, and no written discourses are preserved about such ethical questions as to the exact moment when a foetus was regarded as a living human being and abortion prohibited by law.[78] From all the Mesopotamian legal texts, only the *Middle Assyrian Laws* (§53) contain a paragraph prohibiting women from procuring an abortion at their own initiative, under the threat of capital punishment by impaling and being denied proper burial; the same punishment was performed even if the woman died as a result of the abortion (e.g. Stol 2000, 41; Peled 2020, 196). The law thereby sought to protect male rights to offspring, regarding abortion initiated by the woman as an offence against the family. A few literary texts blame female professionals involved in midwifery, nursing, and women's healthcare of performing abortion or infanticide (see below).[79]

Abortion was presumably delimited from inducing delivery (of a full-term foetus) by its premature date (i.e. before the tenth month which was normally regarded as the proper month of delivery).[80] One situation in which assisted abortion

74 E.g. Lambert 2007, No. 12a i 11–16, No. 12b ii 4–14, No. 13 rev. 12–17; Stol 2000, 36; SAA 10, No. 187, 293 (Parpola 1993, 154, 229–230).

75 These terms are derived from the verbs *ešēru* "to be/go well, to be straight" and *šalāmu* "to be healthy, intact" in the meaning "to bring to term". Another term encountered in this context is *šuklulu* "to complete, to create perfectly; to carry a child to full term". The verb *ešēru* in the Š- and Št-stems can also mean "to give birth easily, promptly."

76 Miscarriage is referred to as "dropping" (ŠUB, *nadû*) the foetus (*ša libbīša* "that of her womb"); the aborted foetus is called *nīd libbi* "dropped from the womb", *kūbu* (a foetus of human shape) or *kirṣu* "nipped off"; a Sumerian expression is saĝ-iti-nu-til-la "one who doesn't complete the months" (Stol 2000, 28–29).

77 For contraceptive drugs, see further below. It is likely that other contraceptive methods were known and used in ancient Mesopotamia, e.g. wiping the vulva after intercourse, sterile forms of sexual intercourse or perhaps even condoms made from animal gut, see e.g. Stol 2000, 37–38; 2016, 571–572; cf. CAD Š/3, s.v. *šuḫḫu* A, a term for a part of the gut (of animals), which can also refer to the buttocks, and is equated in lexical texts with the penis and vulva.

78 For texts that express concepts of foetal development and embryology, see e.g. Stol 2000, 1–12; 2008; Couto-Ferreira 2015–2016; Steinert 2017a and Chapter C4 in this book.

79 For these professionals who are connected to specific deities and cults, see e.g. Westenholz 1989, 250–260; Böck 2014a, 30–32; Civil 2011, 281–284; Stol 2016, 605–616; Steinkeller 2022, 21–32 and below.

80 Mesopotamian texts mention nine or more often ten months as the normal length of pregnancy (Stol 2000, 22–25 for discussion). Examples of Late Babylonian birth horoscopes and other astrological texts state that pregnancy lasted 273 or 277 days from the moment of conception, which

may have been legitimate could have been the premature death of the foetus in utero.[81] However, remedies to speed up delivery and recipes for abortion employed several identical drugs, which means that Mesopotamian healers knew about *materia medica* that caused uterine contractions. One of the texts with prescriptions for abortion (BAM 246 (text B.1.6) from the library N4 at Assur) also contained prescriptions to expel the placenta, which suggests the scribe who copied these remedies saw both contexts as related, and some of the drugs used to induce an abortion or to speed up a difficult delivery may also have been useful for expelling the afterbirth (see also below).

Concepts and knowledge about foetal development or embryology gleaned from cuneiform textual sources have been discussed elsewhere (Stol 2000, 9–26; Stol 2008; Couto-Ferreira 2015–2016; Steinert 2017a, 303–318, 320–322), so I will be brief here. Ancient Mesopotamian scholars haven not written down theoretical treatises on embryology, but in birth incantations one encounters images for the foetus (*ša libbīša*) *in utero*. The embryo is built up from procreative fluids and body substances of both parents (semen, blood, muscles, sinews) and shaped into a baby (*šerru*) of human form by the woman's womb (see BM 115745, text II.1.2), although deities are regularly seen as participating in this creation process. The foetus is depicted as "fish roe of the sea" (*niššulāt tâmātim*), a "creature of the flood" (*binīt edêm*), as an aquatic animal living in a shell (*dādum*) or as a prisoner (sitting in the dark, *āšib ekleti*); occasionally, a foetus is said to be "sleeping" (*ṣalālu*, see *infra*, *Diagnostic Handbook* Tablet 36, lines 5, 94; Stol 2000, 25–26).[82] In birth incantations, the baby is often described as an animal; there, especially snakes and wild animals (gazelles) embody models of easy birth (Steinert 2017b; Wasserman and Zomer 2022, No. 7, 9, 11–12; *infra* Chapter D).

The most important models of foetal development stem from crafts production and from agriculture, by analogy with the growth of plants from seed; the uterus may be likened to a fertile field, which makes the seed "sprout" (*šūṣû*, see texts A.2.7 and B.2.1). The latter model is also applied in a Late Babylonian mathematical text that envisages a scheme of foetal growth, from conception to the moment of birth (for discussion and a new text manuscript, see BM 37014 (Chapter C.4) in this volume). This scheme calculates the gradual growth by stipulating the size of the foetus at different points of the gestation period, with units of measurement (length): on the day of conception, the foetus is "half a barley corn" long, and it grows steadily half a barley corn per day, reaching "five barley corns" on the tenth day of gestation. After one month the foetus reaches a length of three "fingers" (ca. 5 cm), and after ten months, when it has reached full term and birth is expected to take place, it reaches a size of one "cubit" (ca. 50 cm).

Delivery and Problems in the Postpartum Period

As discussed in section 2 of this introduction, remedies to assure a smooth delivery (*alādu*, *ešēru* Š(t)-stem) and to ease difficult labour (dystocia) are attested from very early on and form the topic of specific thematic treatises on women's health in first millennium BCE sources. Treatments for problems during the postpartum period are regularly included in remedy collections for women, in texts from the Middle Babylonian and Middle Assyrian period (late second millennium BCE) onward (e.g. text II.1.4).[83] Beside terms for a woman having difficulty in delivery (^{munus}LA.RA.AḪ, *muš(t)apšiqtu* and related expressions with the verb *pašāqu* "to be narrow, to have difficulties"), the texts refer to birth pangs (*ḫīlū*) and being in labour (*ḫâlu*, *ḫiālu*), pain, screaming in labour, and the breaking amniotic fluids (*mû*).[84] A few texts speak of the woman "entering" (*erēbu*) the (stipulated) month of her delivery. One Late Babylonian tablet (SpTU 4, No. 153) seems to suggest the application of remedies to initiate delivery, in the case that a woman had not delivered in the expected month (text

comes close to the normal term of pregnancy considered in modern medicine (i.e. 280 days or 40 weeks (= nine months and one week), counting from the last menses), see Rochberg 1998, 49–50, 74; Reiner 1995, 115; Stol 2000, 22.

81 Such a life-threatening situation is mentioned in an Old Babylonian letter (see ABIM 15: 8–9 and the discussion on text D.1.6).

82 Various features and (partially imagined) shapes of malformed foetuses or preterm miscarriages are described in the teratological omen series *Šumma izbu* on malformed births among humans and animals (especially in Tablet 1, see de Zorzi 2014).

83 The woman in childbed (confinement) is designated with the word *ḫarištu*, which is derived from the verb *ḫarāšu* "to lie in childbed" (AHw 326; CAD Ḫ, 103-104; cf. Stol 2000, 123 n. 82). The word *ḫarištu* occurs beside the terms *ālittu* "woman in labour" and *mušēniqtu* "nursing (mother)" and is associated with "lying in her blood" (i.e. the discharges of delivery and the postpartum period), and with a bandage (*kannu*) absorbing this blood, but also being confined to bed (i.e. sickness), see also Steinert 2023, 281–282; Stol 2000, 125 n. 103. Note an oracle query for a woman in childbed (whether she will survive) in Lambert 2007, 90–91 No. 12c: rev. iii 17.

84 See chapter D for discussion. Old Babylonian birth incantations use another word for the woman in labour, *aruḫtum*, which has been connected with the words *arāḫu* "to hurry, hasten" (i.e. hastened), (*w*)*arḫu* "month" (i.e. one who has gone through the months) or *arḫu* "cow" by different scholars, see e.g. Stol 2000, 20, 123; Wasserman and Zomer 2022, 70; *infra* text II.1.2 (BM 115745).

D.1.11). Vice versa, the textual record also preserves a group of rituals for the case that the calculated month of a woman's delivery fell in Nisannu, the first month of the Babylonian calendar (text D.3.1). According to the hemerological tradition, the birth of a child in Nisannu foreshadowed grave disaster for the parents, and therefore the rituals in question sought to postpone the delivery with divine help (of the sun god and moon god).

Delivery is an arena in which both male and female professionals were engaged, sometimes collaborating with each other (see e.g. SpTU 4, No. 153, text D.1.11; Stol 2000; Sibbing-Plantholt 2022, 291–302 and below). These sources suggest that the midwife (*šabsūtu*) functioned as the true "obstetrician" who monitored the progress of labour and could manually and by other means intervene in the delivery process in case of complications.[85] This is suggested by a fragment from Ashurbanipal's library in Nineveh, a text which appears to focus on the midwife (*lamittu* "wise woman"), giving instructions for interventions in the case of obstructed labour, e.g. when the baby was stuck in the womb or birth pangs had ceased (Sm. 157 + 1134, text D.1.6). This text appears to advocate actions such as reaching for the child in the womb, perhaps to turn a foetus with a malpresentation or pull it out from the womb.[86] The midwife was also responsible for cutting the umbilical cord (an action associated with the determination of the newborn's destiny), for depositing the afterbirth and taking care of the newborn infant, e.g. washing it, rubbing it with oil and removing stuff from its mouth to let it breathe freely (see e.g. texts D.1.5, D.1.9).[87] Occasionally, therapeutic texts for women or easy delivery include apotropaic or prophylactic treatments for the newborn infant, usually to protect it from divine or demonic agents responsible for causing disease (e.g. epileptic seizures) in babies (texts D.1.1, D.1.3).

Remedies to speed up difficult labour in Mesopotamian therapeutic texts (transmitted by male healing specialists) often combine incantations with the administration of drugs, which were administered as potions or other ingested remedies, rarely tampons, as well as ointments and massages applied to the woman's belly and trunk. The ingredients often carry a symbolic or metaphorical meaning alluding to the imagery of birth found in the incantations[88] that were recited over the remedy before application:

> BAM 248 i 52–52; var. BM 36339 obv. 2'–3' (text D.1.1):
> "The procedure for it: You stir oil-from-the-jar with an arrow that has [gon]e out from the *mouth* of a bow, you recite the incantation three times (over the oil), you massage (her) from the top (of her belly) downwards, and the child will come straight out."

> BAM 248 i 68–69 (text D.1.1):
> "The procedure for it: (You take) dust from a crossroads, dust from the front (door) threshold, dust from the upper and lower drainpipe, dust from the door socket; you cut off a very thick reed (at) top and bottom, you throw (all the mentioned types of) dust into oil, you recite this incantation over it seven times, you fill the thick reed (with the oil) and rub it over her bulging belly from top to bottom."

> BAM 248 iv 13–15 and dupl. (text D.1.1):
> "If a woman has difficulty in delivery, you pound fox grape-plant, 'dog's tongue'-plant, *tuḫlu*-plant, you fill a bottle with beer from an innkeeper, you whisk these plants into it. She shall drink (it) on an empty stomach, and she will give birth quickly."

Some of the drugs used as *materia medica* to speed up labour are also recommended for inducing an abortion, which suggests these were substances that caused contractions of the uterus (see below). A Late Babylonian text from Uruk (SpTU 4, No. 153: 25, text D.1.11) prescribes vaginal suppositories to "dilate" (*petû* "to open") the woman's birth canal. Other actions to promote labour recommended in this text consist in having the woman walk around or ride in a wagon (text D.1.11). The Neo-Assyrian Birth Compendium (BAM 248 and dupl., text D.1.1) also contains a section recommending specific types of meat (turtle, pig, fox) to be consumed by the woman for easy delivery.

---

85 For a possible instrument (*palû*) used by the midwife to "open the womb" (membranes), see Stol 2000, 83, 115, 171. For birthing postures and the brick of birth, see Stol 2000, 118–124. The birth brick (well-known also from ancient Egypt, where it is a physical support for the woman during delivery) is only mentioned in myths (*Atramḫasīs*) and hymns to mother goddesses but never occurs in Mesopotamian medical texts or birth rituals. Thus, we are little informed about its actual use in daily practice.

86 Birth incantations speak of the foetus being stuck (*kânu*) or lying crosswise (*parāku*) in the womb, or the opening of the womb as being blocked (*kalû, sanāqu*), see Chapter D and text II.1.4. For a discussion of questions of agency (of mother or child) in the delivery process, see e.g. Steinert 2017a, 323–326. It is not uncommon for birth incantations to address the baby in the womb to come out.

87 The performance of surgical techniques such as embryotomy (cutting up a (dead) foetus in utero to remove it) or caesarean sections could not be verified in cuneiform sources (see also Stol 2000, 127–128 on the expression *šilip rēmi* "pulled out from the womb").

88 For imagery and tropes of birth (e.g. the woman in labour as a boat loaded with a cargo going downstream, the woman in labour as a cow in dire straits, images relating to locked doors and passageways etc.), see Couto-Ferreira 2014; Steinert 2017a and *infra* for discussion.

A few sources outside the women's healthcare texts mention additional terms that appear to refer to complications related to difficult labour and are phrased in euphemistic and ambiguous terms. The word *šalputtu* "ruined (woman)" and the expression "to be touched by a touch" (TAG TAG.TAG-*at*), may perhaps designate a woman in a protracted delivery whose birth pangs have stopped or whose foetus has died in utero and needs to be removed (Stol 2000, 53–55; Mirelman 2015, 177–178, 181 K. 4206+ rev. 28 and below).

Remedies to expel the afterbirth (*silītu*) (which is delayed) are likewise found in a few texts (including specific drugs for this purpose listed in drug compendia)[89], as are treatments that concern the retention of the lochia or postpartum discharges. In this context, one encounters several formulations that seem to be used interchangeably and refer to blood or fluids. The Neo-Assyrian text BAM 240: 40' explains symptoms such as fever and vomiting in childbed to be due to "the blood of the woman in confinement (i.e. the lochia), which is locked in her belly" (*dām ḫarištīša ša ina libbīša itteskiru*). Several texts use the verb *târu* "to turn around/back" in the D-stem together with *mû* "fluids", presumably in a similar meaning "to block" (e.g. *Iraq* 31, 31: 2–3 (text 0.4): A.MEŠ-*ša u* MÚD.M[EŠ-*ša ina* ŠÀ-*bi-ša*?] GUR.MEŠ-*ru* "(if a woman gives birth and then) . . . her fluids and [her] blood are *blocked* [in her belly(?)]"). In other texts (e.g. BM 38624+ obv. i 24'–25', 30'–31', ii 19'ff.; K.8678+ rev. 3', texts A.2.1 and A.1.4), we find the phrase "she is *blocked* regarding (her) fluids" (*mê turrat*); BAM 240: 67' (text D.2.1) speaks of "*blocked* fluids" (*mê turrēti/turrūti*). NBC 4211, an unpublished Late Babylonian extract or excerpt from Uruk with medical passages, appears to differentiate these fluids further:

rev. 17 DIŠ MUNUS *šá ina* Ù.TU A.MEŠ-*šú* ⌜*tu*?⌝-*ru-ú-ma ana* ŠÀ-*bi-šú* [x]
"In the case of a woman whose fluids are *blocked* (*turrū*) during delivery and [. . .] into her belly (. . .)"

rev. 18 [DIŠ] MUNUS Ù.TU-*ma* A.MEŠ-*šú ú-ta-ri ana* ŠÀ-*šú* x[x]
[If] a woman delivers, and subsequently *she is blocked regarding* (or: *turns back*) her fluids, (so that they?) [. . .] into her belly (. . .)"

rev. 19 [DIŠ] ⌜MUNUS⌝ A.MEŠ-*šú tu-<<tu>>-ú-ru ana* ŠÀ-*bi-šú* [x]
[If] a woman's fluids are *blocked/turned back*(?) (and) [. . .] into her belly (. . .)"

The exact nuance of these expressions with *turru* (blockage or reverse movement?) remains difficult to grasp.[90] Treatments for this condition include tampons, washes, bandages, as well as fumigations from below and other forms of "heat treatment" seeking to release the fluids (see e.g. text II.1.4 and A.1.4). Other symptoms that are mentioned together with retention of the postpartum fluids are pain in the abdomen and pubic region[91], fever, and "blocked intestines". The recurring mention of fever in childbed suggests that infections caused during delivery were a common problem; more serious cases also mention pus inside the womb, which additionally points to injuries during delivery (BAM 240: 65'). Further treated postpartum ailments are prolapse/dislocation of the anus/rectum, diarrhoea, sweating and a "loose" navel (BAM 240: 29', 30', 33'–35'; BM 38624+ i 34').

Other Ailments

Apart from conditions associated directly with reproduction, several other ailments and health problems are encountered in the women's healthcare texts (see also above). A brief comment on these conditions needs to suffice here (for detailed discussion, see the editions of the texts in question).

Of a gynaecological nature is a serious condition referred to as *tikpū* "spots" on the womb, found in a Late Babylonian text from Uruk (SpTU 5, No. 253, text E.2.6). An exact interpretation is difficult, but the symptoms and treatments may perhaps be compared to the treatments for ulceration of the uterus in Hippocratic gynaecological texts (e.g. *Diseases of Women* I). This text has been taken as an indication that Mesopotamian healers undertook examinations of female patients' vagina and cervix with the help of an instrument to spread open the vagina (Scurlock and Andersen 2005, 259).

89 See e.g. BAM 246 rev. (text B.1.6); BM 38624+ i' 14'–15'; ii 23'–24' (text A.2.1).

90 The verb *târu* "to return; to make turn back" in the D-stem can have the sense of "to be locked, closed (from the inside)" in connection with doors or gates, see CAD T, 273b sub 11d; CAD S, 143 sub 11; Steinert 2013, *JMC* 22, 7–8. However, another nuance of *târu* in the D-stem with reference to body parts is further "to turn around".

91 The text BAM 240: 17'–18' (text D.2.1) associate the peculiar disease term NI.RA with these symptoms: "If a woman gives birth and subsequently feels a piercing pain (in) her pubic region (and) her lower abdomen continually hurts her, that woman is afflicted by NI.RA-disease" (NI.RA DAB-*si*). Cf. Scurlock 1991, 173 n. 133; Scurlock and Andersen 2005, sub 12.120.

Such instruments are attested from Roman medical practice (the so-called *speculum*), but no comparable instruments have been identified in the archaeological record from ancient Mesopotamia.

Puzzling is also an ailment befalling women called "crab-(disease)" (*alluttu*), which is treated in a text from Assur that deals mainly with remedies against bleeding during pregnancy (*naḫšātu*) and other morbid discharges from the vagina (BAM 237(+), text D.1.4). Different interpretations of this disease have been suggested (including body parasites such as lice). However, the disease term *alluttu* is the same word that is used for the zodiac sign Cancer, as is the case with ancient Greek *karkinos* "cancer", which in Graeco-Roman medical texts is the term for malignant tumours (often of the female breasts). Therefore, the disease *alluttu* may be the Babylonian counterpart of Greek *karkinos*, and the disease concept may therefore have a Mesopotamian precursor (Steinert 2021a, 64–65; Stol 2016, 448).

As mentioned above, urological (or renal) conditions also receive some attention in therapeutic texts for women. A few texts include treatments against uncontrollable releasing of urine and difficulty urinating. Some form of incontinence may also be implied in the expression *tattīkāt ūri* "dribbling from the vulva". Another condition encountered in this context and already highlighted above in section 3 is NI.NE. The exact reading and etymology of the disease term NI.NE is uncertain, and several diverging interpretations have been proposed.[92] Labat (1953–1971a, 109b) interpreted the term NI.NE as an inflammation of the uterus. A reading of the signs as Ì.KÚM has been proposed by Scurlock and Andersen (2005, 281 with n. 96), interpreting Ì.KÚM as childbed or puerperal fever (connected to Akkadian *emēmu* (KÚM) "to be hot; feverish").[93] However, the condition NI.NE is never mentioned with symptoms of fever, but beside the symptom *kīs šīnāti* "binding of the urine" (i.e. difficulty of emptying the bladder).[94] This symptom may thus have been a typical complaint associated with NI.NE-disease. It is therefore suggested here that NI.NE (or Ì.KÚM) may refer to a burning sensation during urination.

The prescriptions often mention febrile conditions in female patients, which can be treated on their own or as one among other symptoms that are part of context-specific female ailments (e.g. postpartum infection, childbed fever). More specific terms attested in the corpus are *li'bu*-disease/fever (BAM 240: 59'; cf. Stol 2007a, 11–15; Scurlock and Andersen 2005, 29–32; Bácskay 2018a, 5–6) and tertian fever (*ummu šalšu*), the latter of which is unique to a single Late Babylonian text (BM 47491, text A.2.6).[95]

Furthermore, women's healthcare texts feature prescriptions to treat skin conditions or lesions in a female patient, some of which are among the symptoms occurring after delivery, e.g. *sikkatu* "pock, pimple", *ruṭibtu* "dampness", *rišûtu* "itching" (BM 50700: 6', 12' (text A.2.3)), or *birdu*-pustules (BAM 240: 29' (text D.2.1); BM 79061: 15 (text A.2.8).

4.3 Treatment Strategies, Medical Practices and *Materia Medica*

4.3.1 Therapeutic Strategies and Types of Treatment

The women's healthcare texts have proven to be a highly fruitful and significant sub-corpus of Mesopotamian medicine for investigating medical practices, treatment strategies as well as therapeutic agents (*materia medica*) and their interrelations with body and disease concepts (see e.g. Böck 2013; Steinert 2012b; 2020; 2021a). Here I will summarize the most important findings and new insights stemming from research in previous works and in the present study.

Table 4 gives an overview of the therapeutic techniques and other measures encountered in women's healthcare texts with a selection of conditions treated with them. The chart illustrates the relative importance of some medical techniques employed to treat female conditions (e.g. a high frequency of tampons / suppositories (Akkadian *itqu*, *allānu*, *ubānu*, *maššītu*) and potions (*mašqītu*) as well as a range of alternative therapeutic options that are representative of Mesopotamian therapeutics in general and not exclusive to treating women. Therapies for women's specific health conditions were selected and applied in context-dependent ways, as can be seen from the table (see also Steinert 2020):

---

92 Kirsch (1996) suggested to read the disease term NI.NE as *ni-ṭè* (CAD N/II, s.v. *nīṭu* "bloody excrement"); followed by Rumor 2016, *Studies L. Milano*, 596 n. 55. For example, in BAM 159 ii 49 and iii 10, the latter word occurs in connection with a disease of the anus. Cf. Finkel 1980, *AfO* 27, 45 note 13.

93 See also Scurlock 1991, 173 n. 133; Scurlock 2014a, 576.

94 See BM 42313+ rev. 1–6 (text A.2.2) quoted in section 3. Variants of the prescription are found in BAM 237 iv 9–10 (text C.1.4); BAM 241(+) ii 9'–10' (text II.1.3).

95 See also SpTU 5, No. 253 (text E.2.6), *ummi irrī* "intestinal fever" (BAM 240: 39'; text D.2.1).

Table 4: Types of treatments and their application in women's healthcare texts.

Treatment Type	Purpose of Application
Tampons/Suppositories (inserted into vagina)	Fertility / conception; stopping bleeding; stopping loss of amniotic fluid; avoiding miscarriage; genital discharges; intestinal trouble; "wind"; postpartum fever and retention of the lochia; inducing the menstrual flow; inducing abortion; speeding up delivery (rare); tests (pregnancy prognoses)
Potions	fertility / conception; stopping bleeding; stopping loss of amniotic fluid; avoiding miscarriage; vaginal discharges; "wind"; diarrhoea; postpartum fever and retention of the lochia; inducing the menstrual flow; induing abortion; easing difficult labour; tests (pregnancy prognoses)
Ingesting (rarely fasting)	fertility / conception; swelling / inflammation; diarrhoea; easing difficult labour
Ointments	fertility / conception; bleeding during pregnancy; avoiding miscarriage; fever; "wind", postpartum infection and retention of the lochia; easing delivery
Bandages/Poultices	fertility / conception; bleeding during pregnancy - avoiding miscarriage; pain in pubic region after delivery; postpartum fever; "wind"; diarrhoea; postpartum infection with skin spots
Fumigations	bleeding during pregnancy; intestinal trouble after delivery; retention of the lochia
Lotions/Bathing	fertility / conception; avoiding miscarriage; "wind"; postpartum infection (pus) and retention of the lochia; easing delivery
Enemas (into urethra, vagina or anus)	fertility / conception; pain in pubic region after delivery; "wind"; postpartum fever and retention of the lochia; pain in breasts/genitals (anus); NI.NE (problems with urination)
Sniffing substances (to induce sneezing)	being bloated with "wind"
Massage	easing delivery
Amulet necklaces and medicine bags	fertility / conception; stopping bleeding (also during pregnancy); avoiding miscarriage; vaginal discharge; easing delivery (rare)
Rituals / symbolic actions / spells	fertility / conception; stopping bleeding (also during pregnancy); avoiding miscarriage; vaginal discharge; easing delivery

The present study contributes to refining the understanding of medical terminology in Mesopotamian women's healthcare texts in the first millennium BCE. For example, systematic inquiry of the prescriptions for preparations inserted into the vagina revealed that Mesopotamian women's healthcare texts differentiate between tampons (Akkadian *itqu*) and suppositories which are called *maššītu* lit. "that which is worn/applied", or more specifically *allānu* "acorn" or *ubānu* "finger". Tampons and suppositories both ensure medical ingredients are absorbed by mucous tissues inside the body. The term tampon refers to ingredients wrapped into a tuft of wool or into a piece of cloth that are inserted into the vagina (or anus); suppository (or pessary) refers to a solid preparation of medical ingredients mixed with fat, wax or resin and brought into a conical or cylindrical shape. An additional function of tampons is to absorb body substances. Tampons are removed after a certain time, while suppositories are designed to dissolve after insertion into the vagina (or anus). The present study revealed the significance of the term *maššītu* (lit. "that which is worn", derived from the verb *našû* "to carry; to wear; to apply", also "to insert a medication into a body opening") as a general term for "suppository", used beside the more specific synonyms *allānu* "acorn", *ubānu* "finger").[96] This meaning has not yet been recognized in the Akkadian dictionaries, which translate the term as "mixture" or "ingredients".[97] It is important to highlight the meaning of *maššītu*, since this term is often translated as "tampon", which is in many cases a misleading and technically inexact rendering.[98] The designation "tampon" should be reserved for preparations that mention wrapping into wads of wool (*itqu*) or a similar

96 For *našû* (ÍL) in instructions specifying that the patient applies or inserts a tampon or suppository into the vagina, see e.g. BAM 240: 22', 57' (text D.2.1); SpTU 4, No. 153 obv. 4, 6 (text C.1.10).

97 See AHw 629-630, s.v. *maššītu* I sub 3 "Ingredienziengemisch"; cf. CAD M/1 389–390, suggesting the translations "ingredients; mixture". For the equation of the spelling ḪI-*tú* with *maššītu*, see Köcher 1963, BAM III, p. xxii. Goltz (1972, 75–78) does not discuss *maššītu* among the terms for suppositories and tampons.

98 For example, the term *maššītu* is translated as "tampon" in Geller's discussion of UET 7, No. 123 (Geller 2023, *JMC* 41, 1–14). Similarly, Stol 2000, 130; Geller 1995–1996, 246.

textile, while *maššītu* should be translated as "suppository", since it usually consists of a mixture of pulverized drugs that is blended with a fatty or sticky substance introduced into the vagina (less often into the anus).[99]

The application of vaginal treatments in Mesopotamian women's healthcare texts is based on an understanding of the womb as the central organ connected to female health and affected in gynaecological conditions, while their interchangeability with potions points to an understanding of internal ailments affecting the inner organs as treatable by administering medicine via the main orifices leading to the inside of the body (belly), especially via the mouth/anus in men and the mouth/vagina in women (i.e. from above and from below). The focus of the texts on the reproductive organs and on conditions associated with them explains the importance of treatments introduced into the vagina. The preference for potions and ointments/massage to ease delivery indicates that the prescriptions focused on directing the downward movement of the baby by applying treatments that supported this movement, while vaginal suppositories are only prescribed rarely in this context, explicitly to effect dilation of the birth canal (SpTU 4, No. 153, text D.1.11).

Apart from potions, gynaecological texts sometimes prescribe other oral medicaments to be eaten or consumed (*akālu*) by the patient, consisting of different types of food. Fumigations from below form another type of treatment administered to the vagina, in other cases also to the mouth or nostrils. The application of the fumigants to the mouth, nostrils and vagina again suggests the idea of a central passageway connecting these body openings and the womb. This therapy was used, for instance, to dislodge fluids retained in the womb, such as postpartum blood, but also to stop bleeding (Steinert 2014a; 2014b; see text II.1.4, text C.1.4 (lines 26'–27'), text A.1.4). As elucidated in the present study, the uses of fumigation from below in these cases may be based on a reasoning in terms of the properties hot/cold and moist/dry. Since fumigants are both heating and can also have a drying effect, they seem adequate both to stop a flow of blood (excess moisture) and to release retained blood (since blood is regarded as hot in Mesopotamian texts, heating up promotes the flow of blood).

In some gynaecological texts, medicaments in liquid form are also administered via enemas, i.e. they are "poured" (*tabāku*) into the vagina or anus. In addition, medicaments could be "blown" (*napāḫu*) into the vagina or urethra with a bronze tube (*uppu*). Rarely, a substance would have to be sniffed (*eṣēnu*) by the patient through the nostrils to induce sneezing, to release a pathogenic substance (wind):

> BAM 240: 26' (text D.2.1):
> "If a woman gives birth and subsequently is distended and bloated with wind (*ṣemrat u šāra uddupat*), you have her sniff (lit. smell) the dust from a copper bell(?) and she will get well."

External treatments in women's healthcare texts often consist of ointments/salves (*napšaltu*), with which the patient is rubbed (*pašāšu*) or massaged (*muššu'u*), e.g. in the context of delivery, to ease labour. Also popular are recipes for baths or lotions (*narmaktu*, *marḫaṣu*) and recipes for poultices or bandages (*naṣmattu*, *lubku*), in which semi-solid, paste-like ingredients are smeared on a piece of cloth or leather and applied as a bandage (*ṣamādu*). Examples of washes, bandages and poultices applied in the context of postpartum conditions are associated with symptoms of infection and demonstrate that these treatments were intended to cool down fever, to treat associated skin conditions and probably also to cleanse the body from the outside. Enemas applied to the vagina as an alternative treatment for the same problem were presumably likewise intended to cleanse and cool the uterus and reproductive organs. Of interest in this context are also examples for treatments to enable conception and enhance female fertility, making use of external remedies such as washes, ointments and bandages (in addition to vaginal suppositories).

Gynaecological prescriptions for purposes such as enhancing fertility (promoting conception), protecting from miscarriage, stopping bleeding or other discharges also recommend amulets (mostly consisting of various stone beads, metals or plants strung on strings of wool or animal tendons) and medicine bags (drug ingredients wrapped up in leather, called *mêlu*) worn around the neck or other body parts. While such practices appear to a modern eye as purely "magical", such amulets were prescribed by Mesopotamian healers for various medical purposes from headache, hair loss to epilepsy

99 An exceptional Late Babylonian text with prescriptions for women (BM 42450+ lines 14"–15", text B.2.3) speaks of a "suppository with wool" (*maš[šītu] ša šīpāti*), which suggests *maššītu* could serve as an overarching inclusive term that could be specified to refer to a tampon. The Greek term in Hippocratic gynaecological treatises corresponding to *maššītu* is *prostheton* "suppository", which, like *maššītu*, is derived from a verb meaning "to bring; to apply; to insert" (*prostithenai*; Goltz 1974, 226–228). See e.g. a group of suppositories in *Diseases of Women* I, 74 (Potter 2018, 161–167). Another direct correspondence between Akkadian and Greek terminology is found in Akkadian *allānu* and Greek *balanon*, both meaning "acorn-(shaped suppository)".

or nightmares.[100] On the one hand, the amulet necklaces had protective and apotropaic functions, especially against evil forces such as sorcery, believed to cause a range of serious health problems as well as miscarriage and other female conditions such as abnormal genital discharge (Schwemer 2007; CMAwR 1–3). The belief in the healing powers of stones and other minerals links the Mesopotamian medical texts with other ancient and later traditions, but it is also tied to knowledge about medicinal and other (e.g. external) properties of the minerals and other ingredients (see e.g. Steinert 2020).

Last, but not least, for a truly representative picture of healing in Mesopotamian medicine, we should emphasise the important role of ritual procedures, specifically in dealing with women's health problems.[101] Such ritual procedures consist of recitations (prayers, incantations) addressed at (often superhuman) agents of disease and healing, and various symbolic and magical actions (sometimes including offerings). Moreover, incantations were often recited over remedies before application, to boost their powers and efficacy. In addition, healers sometimes observed specific ritual actions when procuring healing plants, the latter of which they also sometimes invoked before using them (e.g. Böck 2014a).

Ritual procedures usually deal with external agents responsible for health and disease: they seek to expel agents of disease and to remove their damaging influences from the patient, reaching out to deities and positive forces to get their help and support (e.g. Schwemer 2011). Symbolic actions often involve rites of transfer or substitution (e.g. Scurlock 2002; Couto-Ferreira 2013; Maul 2019; Abusch et al. 2020), in which the evil affecting the patient was transferred to an object and removed in exchange for some positive property, or in which a substitute (e.g. a figurine) replaces the patient. Specific objects and settings (places, locations) often play central roles in these rituals (see e.g. texts, C.1.4, C.3.10; D.3.1). It is also important to stress the psychological importance of such performances for the patient and her family, e.g. in such burdensome, distressful and frightening circumstances as infertility or loss of one's offspring (e.g. due to miscarriage), or in coping with risks and anxieties of pregnancy and childbirth and with problems that may have involved social stigma. Thus, it is a common element in the ritual performances that the patient was either allowed or required to express her feelings verbally, e.g. by repeating preformulated prayers or recitations (Couto-Ferreira 2015, 193–196).

Moreover, incantations recited by the healer can be ascribed ritual efficacy through several interlinked mechanisms. Healing spells are loaded with divine power and presence because they are said to have been communicated to the healer by the deities of his craft; they are composed in an unusual, poetic language or use mumbo-jumbo words to emphasize their power over demonic agents of disease (Veldhuis 1999). Mesopotamian incantations used in medical contexts also feature *historiolae* explaining the origin of the treated condition (often linked to the actions of deities) or present a prototypical patient that was healed. Thus, a famous and popular *historiola* transmitted in birth incantations from the second and first millennium BCE is that of the cow of the moon god who had difficulties in delivery and gave birth successfully through divine help (Veldhuis 1991; *infra* text D.1.1 and *passim*). Furthermore, Mesopotamian healing spells use (conceptual) metaphors as important epistemic devices to express conceptions about the body, disease and healing processes. By drawing on processes in other domains of experience these metaphors help to describe and explain processes in the healthy and sick body, while at the same time providing models or guides for choosing therapeutic interventions (e.g. Collins 1999; Böck 2014a; Steinert 2013; 2017a; Johnson and Simkó 2024).[102]

On the other hand, Mesopotamian healing spells were performative instruments of healing. Spells were believed to establish control over the disease entity and to have an immediate (activating) effect on the applied therapeutic agents, both of which served together as mediators that could bring about a change in the patient's condition. To this end, not only the agency of healing deities addressed in the spells was instrumental. Metaphors in healing spells function as clever devices that were intended to trigger anticipated changes in the patient's state by equating the patient's state with processes in other domains of experience (e.g. in the natural environment) that were seen as parallel.

---

100 See Schuster-Brandis 2008.

101 Although several textual sources contain only medical prescriptions (and no incantations/rituals, or vice versa), it is important to emphasize the equal status of "magical/symbolic/ritual" and "medical" practices in Mesopotamian healing practices from a general point of view. Thus, any type of treatment applied in healing texts could be referred to as "remedy" (*bulṭu*) or "procedure" (DÙ.DÙ.BI/KÌD.KÌD.BI) in the texts.

102 For metaphors in medical cultures, see e.g. van Rijn-van Tongeren 1997; Martin 1987; Nerlich 2011; Pritzker 2003; Yu 2008; Horstmanshoff et al. 2012; Wee 2017b; Lehmhaus 2023. These studies show that metaphors highlight certain aspects, while hiding others, and that metaphors of the female body in the past and present often served certain ideologies by corroborating views of women (and their bodies) as inferior to or different from men.

4.3.2 Technical Medical Terminology in First Millennium BCE Women's Healthcare Texts: Some New Terms and Meanings

In addition to the terms for types of medical preparations and treatments discussed in the previous section, several new or rare technical terms occur especially in Late Babylonian women's healthcare texts, which deserve to be briefly highlighted here.[103]

***ribīku* "paste"**

This term is found in BM 50700 (text A.2.3, perhaps from Dilbat), a Late Babylonian medical text with prescriptions for women that features several rare technical terms that are possibly loanwords from Aramaic. The term *ribīku*, occurring in this text as a designation for a type of treatment, is likely a variant form of the words *rabīku* or *ribku*, which dictionaries render as "decoction" or "mash".[104] The related Akkadian verb *rabāku* "to stir" often found in medical prescriptions has cognates in Hebrew and Aramaic that mean "to mix". It has been argued that the mixture produced by the action of *rabāku* is rather a thicker, semi-liquid, soft paste than a liquid, since in many recipes the produced drug mixture is applied in the form of a poultice or salve.[105] The context of some attestations of *rabīku* imply a mash that is eaten, although in other instances, the action of *rabāku* produces a potion (cf. CAD R, 8 sub b, 20). In BM 50700, the term *ribīku* most likely refers to a paste that was eaten by the patient after delivery and that was applied to the skin to treat skin conditions in women.

paṣû

The term *paṣû* occurs in two Late Babylonian tablets as a type of potion administered to a female patient. In BM 45736 line 4' (text A.2.5), a preparation designated as *paṣû* is good or prescribed "as a potion for [provoking?] the menstrual flow" (*pa-ṣu-ú šá ana maš-qut šá sa-ge-⌈e⌉ [kul-lu-mu* SIG_5/SUM[?]]). In BM 45559 + 45574 (text A.2.4), a *paṣû zukkû* "cleansing/purifying(?) *paṣû*" is prescribed as a potion for a woman after delivery, which consists of a mixture of (date) syrup and oil. The notion of purification or cleansing in the latter text may be linked with promoting the flow of the lochia after a woman's delivery, a period during which women were regarded as impure (*musukkatu*).

The word *paṣû* itself is a variant of *peṣû* "white, pale, light-coloured", which is usually an adjective, but here occurs in the function of a noun. A type of beer called (*šikaru*) *paṣû* is often encountered in Neo-/Late Babylonian texts (see CAD P, 330–331 sub 1d). It was made from dates and is mentioned beside "date beer" (KAŠ ZÚ.LUM.MA; see Landsberger 1967, 56; Stol 1994, 166–167). However, in the two texts under discussion *paṣû* has a more restricted meaning. The commentary HAR-gud B VI 82 gives the equation of kaš-babbar = *pe-ṣu-ú* "white/light-coloured (beer)", which is further explained as *ribku* "decoction".[106] In BM 45559+ and BM 45736, *paṣû* could be close in meaning to the word *ribku* explaining *peṣû* in HAR-gud.[107]

muttapiḫtu

This word is a newly attested term (hapax) not yet picked up in the dictionaries. It is found in the gynaecological compendium BM 38624+ (text A.2.1, line 87''''') and appears to refer to a type of treatment or form of application. The term itself is derived from *napāḫu* "to blow; to ignite; to rise"; the form *muttappiḫtu* suggests a feminine noun formed from the Gtn- or

103 Note also the following attestations of new terms for drugs: *kal-damiq* "good-for-everything-plant" (BM 79061 (text A.2.8) line 2), *riqqi ḫīlī* "aromatic plant for the birth pangs" (BM 79061 (text A.2.8) lines 3, 5, 34'), *ḫamedīrānu*-plant (BM 79061 (text A.2.8) line 6).

104 CAD R, 20 and 321; AHw 935a "ein Absud" and AHw 980b "ein (Drogen-) Absud". The cognate Aramaic term *rbyk*, *rbykh*, which means "flour paste" (*Comprehensive Aramaic Dictionary* (CAL)), designates "a pulp of flour mixed with hot water or oil" (Jastrow 1903, *A Dictionary of the Targumim*, 1442b).

105 See e.g. Goltz 1974, 47–48, 70 (glossing *rabāku* with German "verrühren"); Attia 2021, *JMC* 38, 77–78. Böck (2009, 116) suggests a meaning "to mix; to moisten". For *ribku* in eye recipes, cf. Geller and Panayotov (2020, 259 comment on line 78' and *passim*), translating "infusion", with IGI 1 line 33', IGI 2 lines 7, 99, IGI 3 lines 43', 98', 103' (*ribku ša īnī* "infusion for the eyes"); see also BAM 3 ii 46, Worthington 2006, *JMC* 7, 22. Scurlock (2006, No. 126) translates "balm" in this context.

106 MSL 11, 89, there read as *labku*; cf. also HAR-gud B VI 71; AHw 857b sub 4.

107 For *peṣû*/*paṣû* in medical prescriptions, see further BM 78963: 35, 50 (Stadhouders and Johnson 2018, in: *FS Geller*, 574, 578).

Dtn-stem participle of *napāḫu* (cf. GAG 81 § 56g, sub *muttapris(t)* < **muntapris(t)*). The literal meaning of *muttappiḫtu* may be "that which constantly flares up/produces heat"; it might be a by-form of *munappiḫtu* "bellows" (AHw 672b). Since the term seems to designate a specific type of treatment or application form for listed *materia medica* in BM 38624+, *muttapiḫtu* refers perhaps to an intended effect (a "heating treatment" aimed at producing sweat?).

taḫsistu "memorandum"

The Late Babylonian text BM 45559 + 45574 line 16' (text A.2.4) features the word *taḫsistu* "memorandum, aide-memoire" in an unusual context introducing minute instructions about the use and processing of salt (*ṭābtu*), presumably for application in a medical context. Unfortunately, the passage is very fragmentary. Significantly, however, the term *taḫsistu* is not common at all as a rubric in medical texts – the word is predominantly known from first millennium BCE text colophons referring to the purpose of a copied text.[108] The usage of *taḫsistu* in BM 45559 + 45574 therefore signals a subtle change in the application of technical terminology, marking a piece of important information to be remembered or kept in mind by the practitioner.

kuṣāru

This term designating amulet necklaces worn by pregnant women, literally meaning "knotting" (and derived from the verb *kaṣāru* "to knot; to tie"), is attested only once in a Neo-Assyrian memorandum from Assur (BAM 363, text G.2).[109] It has not yet been included in the Akkadian dictionaries. The word is a synonym to the cognate noun *takṣīru* lit. "knotting; attachment" used interchangeably for "amulet necklace".

Verbs for Processing Medical Ingredients with Uncertain Meaning

A few Late Babylonian women's healthcare texts edited here also attest to hitherto unknown verbs describing steps in the processing of medical ingredients, or they offer new or rare meanings for known Akkadian verbs. Two new terms that may be Aramaic loanwords are *seḫû* (or *saḫû*)[110] and *ḫapû*[111]. They are found in a text from Uruk dating to the fourth or third century BCE (text E.2.6), in a context that suggests meanings such as "to mix" and "to pour over", respectively. A second text (A.2.3) known from three manuscripts features the verbs *sapānu* and *naṭāpu*[112] as two subsequent steps in a preparation procedure, perhaps referring both to a drying process. The first verb *sapānu* usually means "to lay flat; to flatten" or "to pluck", but for some occurrences in medical texts, a special meaning "to dip(?) (in a liquid)" has been proposed.[113] The medical context may specifically refer to laying something out flat to dry or perhaps to draining a washed ingredient. The Akkadian verb *naṭāpu* usually means "to tear out; to pluck", but in the passage in question the word (a D-stem form) may rather be related to the Aramaic verb *nṭp* means "to drip".[114]

Other Textual Features and Scribal Peculiarities

Apart from new technical terminology, some of the texts edited in this volume also display other unusual linguistic features or scribal peculiarities worth noting, e.g. references to oral lore.

108 See e.g. Hunger 1968, No. 336: 1: *ana taḫsisti zamar nasḫa* "quickly excerpted as an aide-mémoire"; No. 323: 4 *ana taḫsisti tāmartīšu išṭur* "as a memorandum and for his reading he has written (it)", no. 324: 2; [*a*]*na taḫsisti* [*š*]*itassīšu išṭur* "as a memorandum and for his reading out loud he has written (it)"; all examples are from texts from Ashurbanipal's library. For earlier (second millennium BCE) attestations of the word, see SAD Vol. 2, 52.

109 For nouns with the form *purās*, see GAG § 55k sub 15.

110 SpTU 5, No. 253: 24', 26', 35' (text E.2.6), spelled *ta-se-ḫi* and *te-se-eḫ-hi*. Cf. the Aramaic verb *sḥy* "to wash; to bathe" (Jastrow 1903, 971; Sokoloff 2002, 797; Geller 2024, 206).

111 SpTU 5, No. 253: 31', spelled *ta-ḫap-pu*. Cf. the Aramaic verb *ḥph* / *ḥpy* "to cover; to strew/spread over" (Jastrow 1903, 491; Sokoloff 2002, 477).

112 BM 50700: 7', 10' (text A.2.3).

113 CAD S, 158–161 sub 3.

114 *nṭp* means "to drip", in the D-stem "to drip copiously" or "to make drip" (see the *Comprehensive Aramaic Dictionary* (CAL); Jastrow 1903, 901; Sokoloff 2002, 745). For another conspicuous verbal form *tu-še-ep-su* referring to administering a remedy, see BM 42507 and dupl. (text E.2.1: 14').

Several first millennium BCE women's healthcare texts mark specific information contained in them, e.g. particular remedies, as oral tradition (*šūt/ša pî; šum'uttu*).[115] The origin of such knowledge marked as "oral lore" was presumably diverse and included information stemming from folk medicine or lay healing practitioners (see below section 5). However, labels such as *šūt pî* can also refer to a stream of knowledge that was not (yet) included in the "canonical" scholarly compendia and series of the first millennium BCE.[116]

A few manuscripts refer to oral information that is omitted in medical prescriptions but assumed to be common knowledge of the healer. Such information is marked by the phrases *ša/mala iqbâkka* "(of) which/as much as one has told you".[117] These expressions resemble similar statements in commentaries (cf. Gabbay 2016, 201–260, esp. 212–213, 238–240), but the form *iqbâkka* with the pronominal suffix in the second person masc. singular is not common in commentaries. The usual phrase found in commentaries is *mala/ša iqbû* "as much as/of which it (= the base text) said", which serves to introduce textual citations from the base text or explanations commenting on the base text.[118] In one instance in the text SpTU 4, No. 153, a comparable usage of *ša iqbû* is found, in which the phrase refers back to written information encountered earlier in the text:

SpTU 4, No. 154 obv. 13 (text C.1.10):
KU ^{giš}ÙR ***šá* E-*ú*** *ul šá* ^{giš}GIŠIMMAR {(KU) *šá* ^{giš}ÁS[AL]}
"The powder of the beam **that is prescribed (lit. 'that it (= the text) said (above)')**, shall not be of the date palm, (but) [(powder)] of poplar wood."

Here, *ša iqbû* resumes the substance "powder of a beam" referred to a line before in the text and introduces an additional piece of information on the kind of wood that the log should be of. This information added in the comment may stem from oral tradition. In contrast, the phrase *mala iqbâkka* usually refers to information on drug dosages not written down in the text, but communicated orally ("these drugs, as much as one has told you (to use)"), while *ša iqbâkka* refers to lore associated with the uses of specific *materia medica*:

SpTU 4, No. 153 obv. 4 (text C.1.10):
Ú.MEŠ *an-nu-tu* ***ma-la iq-bak-ka*** 1.TA.ÀM *ina-aš-ši*
"(Of) these drugs, **as much as one has told you** (to be appropriate), she applies one unit (i.e. the same amount) of each."

BM 45736 obv. 9'–10' (text A.2.5):
K[U$^{?}$.K]U$^{?}$ *ṣar-bat* ŠIKA NUNUZ ⌈*lu*⌉-*ur-mu*$^{?}$ KA *tam-tim* / **[m]*a*-⌈*la*$^{?}$⌉ *iq-bak-ka*** 1.⌈TA⌉.ÀM SUM-*in gab-bi* [1]-*en-šú la* SUM-*in*
"⌈Powder(?)⌉ of poplar (wood), ostrich eggshell, *imbu' tâmti*-mineral, 10' (apply of them) **as much as one has told you** (to be appropriate). You administer (these ingredients) one by one/separately, you should not administer (them) all at once."

BM 45736 obv. 7'–8' (text A.2.5):
ŠIKA G[A.N]U$_{11}$⌈$^{mušen?}$⌉ [*l*]*u*$^{?}$ A.⌈MEŠ$^{?}$⌉ ***šá iq-bak-k*[*a*]** / *šá i-ṣi giš-ma-ru u te-e*[*l-la*]-*tú*$^{?}$
"(Or you apply) os[tri]ch (egg)shell or the sap(?), **as one has told you to,** 8' from the wood of date palm or grapevine (. . .)."

A third nuance with an explanatory or cross-referential function is encountered in the expression *ša ana . . . iqbû* "which is prescribed (lit. said) for . . .", which can be illustrated by the following instances:

SpTU 4, No. 153 obv. 5 (text C.1.10):
^{ú}KUR.KUR ^{ú}MAŠ.TAB.BA ^{ú}*sim-bir-ri* ^{šim}GAM.MA 4 Ú.MEŠ ***šá ana maš-ši-ti*** **E-*ú*** *šá* ÚŠ-*e*
"*Atā'išu*-plant, *māštu*-plant, *simbirru*-plant (and) *ṣumlalû*-plant: (these) four drugs **which are prescribed for a suppository** (are good) for blocking."[119]

SpTU 4, No. 153 obv. 17 (text C.1.10):
⌈^{na4}KUR⌉-*nu* DAB ***šá ana*** *maš-qit* *erasure* *šá* MÚD MUNUS KUD-*si* **E-*ú*** . . .
"The magnetic haematite, **which is prescribed for** a potion *erasure* for stopping a woman's blood, . . ."

---

115 See e.g. BM 38624+ iv 3' (text A.2.1); BM 50700 obv. 11' (text A.2.3); SpTU 5, No. 253: 3' (text E.2.6); BM 45736 iv 12 (text A.2.5); BAM 240: 16' (text D.2.1).

116 The expression *šūt pî* occurs otherwise in the subscripts of scholarly commentaries, where it indicates explanations that go back to oral teachings by master scholars in a teaching context (Frahm 2011, 44–45, 51–52 *passim*; Gabbay 2016, 51–52).

117 SpTU 4, No. 153 obv. 4 (text C.1.10); BM 45736 obv. 7', 10' (text A.2.5).

118 Gabbay proposes that *mala* could refer to a lemma that occurs several times in the base text ("as many times as it (is) said (in the text)".

119 See also SpTU 4, No. 153 obv. 7 (text C.1.10): "*Maštakal* (and) *simbirru*-plant(?) are prescribed (*iqbû*) for cooling a pregnant woman."

In the first passage quoted above, the expression *ša ana . . . iqbû* serves to explain and specify the application method and therapeutic effect for a group of plants with haemostatic properties. In the second passage, with the comment concerning the use of magnetic haematite, the text lacks a prescription fitting the reference. However, since recipes with magnetite to stop bleeding are known from several other gynaecological manuscripts, the comment seems to draw on a pool of textual information that was probably established and known among the healers of the time.

Beside references to oral knowledge not written down, a few text passages also contain discursive statements referring to information not copied from the *Vorlage* and omitted from the manuscript (e.g. BM 45736 line 14'; text A.2.5). Sometimes, an incantation recited with a remedy was omitted in a manuscript (compared with the duplicating text copies) without special notice by the copyist (see e.g. texts A.2.7 and C.3.3).

The Late Babylonian medical prescriptions reflect a less strict and more variable format than texts from the Neo-Assyrian period. Among the scribal peculiarities of some Late Babylonian medical manuscripts edited in this volume are rare instances in which the text of a prescription does not conclude at the end of a line (as is usually the case in cuneiform medical texts, which often even rule off prescriptions from each other with horizontal rulings). In these exceptional cases, the following prescription starts in the middle of a line without interruption (e.g. BM 45559+ line 12', 16'; text A.2.4); in one instance, the scribe impressed a small vertical stroke with the stylus as a disjunction sign to mark the end of the preceding remedy and the beginning of the next prescription (BM 79061 line 36'; text A.2.8).

4.3.3 Ingredients as Healing Agents in Women's Healthcare Texts

Mesopotamian texts such as pharmaceutical compendia and medical prescriptions show that healing professionals had detailed and complex knowledge about the properties and characteristics of a broad range of *materia medica*. However, the reconstruction and evaluation of this knowledge is often considerably hampered by the difficulties involved in identifying many of the ancient Akkadian and Sumerian terms for plants, minerals etc. and in trying to link them with modern taxa or species (see Böck, Ghazanfar and Nesbitt 2023; Rumor 2024 for recent overviews). Until now, only few of the hundreds of drugs mentioned in prescriptions and compendia on *materia medica* have been identified with certainty. Due to these uncertainties, it is also difficult to evaluate the pharmaceutical efficacy of the remedies and drugs employed in Mesopotamian medical texts (including women's healthcare) from a modern biomedical perspective. The same difficulties are discussed by scholars working on other ancient medical text corpora.[120]

However, all these difficulties and our distance from the Mesopotamians and their practices should not make us exclude the possibility that the ancients had some empirically valid knowledge and insights into the efficacy of healing substances in the treatment of specific health problems, even if some of the treatments recommended in ancient texts look overtly bizarre, or may have been of limited pharmaceutical effect, or were based to some extent on belief.[121] Seeing efficacy as a process arising from a bio-cultural nexus of interactions between humans and their environment, I regard these interactions involving patients, practitioners, drugs and environments as part of a "skilled practice" (Hsu 2010, 16), which integrates knowledge about the therapeutic, phytochemical effects of plants and other healings substances, but also culturally mediated concepts concerning the body, diseases and the healing processes effected by the properties of drugs.

Mesopotamian therapeutic texts often appear to be based on such a holistic or integrated understanding of therapeutic processes, drugs and their efficacy, which sees *materia medica* as *agents and mediators* of these processes rather than mere objects with certain properties.[122] The agency of *materia medica* as well as other objects and entities used for rites of transfer is underlined in the procedures themselves by direct invocations addressing these healing agents, referring to

120 See e.g. Totelin 2009 and Flemming 2021 on gynaecological recipes in Graeco-Roman medicine. For recent discussions of issues of efficacy in ancient Mesopotamian medicine, see e.g. Rumor 2021; Zisa 2021. Studies on plants and healing practices in medical anthropology remind us that the efficacy of drugs is "a cultural construction with biological and social dimensions" (van der Geest et al. 1996, 167), which includes social expectations and cultural beliefs in the effectiveness of drugs beyond their pharmaceutical properties.

121 For the (limited) efficacy of some medical practices in ancient and folk-medical traditions, see e.g. Root-Bernstein and Root-Bernstein 1997. For example, Pommerening (2006) investigated remedies from Egyptian medical papyri focusing on examples with identified ingredients and exact quantities, comparing them with modern pharmaceutical uses and recommended dosages. The selected remedies, drug uses and dosages corresponded quite well with today's pharmaceutical standards, thus implying that they could have been potentially effective for the indicated complaints. See also Pommerening and Steinert 2019.

122 For concepts of agency and personhood attributed to healing plants in Mesopotamia, see e.g. Perdibon 2019.

their positive properties, powers or to their links with deities.[123] Another recurring action in medical procedures that was intended to boost the efficacy of healing substances was to let them stand under the stars (or certain stars) overnight – a procedure that may have been applied not only for technical reasons, but that may have served, according to E. Reiner (1995, 48–60), to "load" the remedy with divine powers.

As recent studies into Mesopotamian medical remedies including the present work show, the uses of curative agents in treatments were informed by empirical knowledge of pharmaceutical properties, but these often overlap with "symbolic", "sympathetic" or "magical" uses based on other (material) properties of the *materia medica*, involving analogical reasoning or thinking in correspondences.[124] Thus, Mesopotamian remedies draw on multiple relations or "resonances" between significant properties of *materia medica*, the distinctive logics of their perceived effects unfolding through specific treatment regimes, and the perceived nature and properties of the treated conditions (e.g. Steinert 2020).

One promising approach to tracing emic conceptions of ancient medical prescriptions and *materia medica* that has great potential for the study of Mesopotamian therapeutic texts including women's healthcare texts is the concept of "medical (re)-enactment", described by Pommerening (2017) for ancient Egyptian medical remedies. "Medical (re)-enactment" refers to the phenomenon that certain properties of healing substances and applied procedures physically enact or mimic characteristics of the treated ailment or anticipate the outcome of the therapy, similar to a "signature" ingredient. Elucidating the concepts underlying these "re-enactments" allows glimpses of an emic understanding of medical treatments and disease conditions. This approach can enrich our view of Mesopotamian prescriptions for women, offering an alternative perspective on ancient recipes as encoding knowledge about the various (e.g. material, pharmaceutical) properties of healing agents, their associated cultural meanings and how they are linked to concepts of the female body and its conditions.[125]

On a general level, Mesopotamian medical texts apply substances stemming from plants, minerals, animals and more rarely, the human body.[126] One recurring difficulty for a modern interpreter of Mesopotamian *materia medica* is that one plant may be known by many names and that some drug names are metaphorical or refer to animals or to body parts and substances. However, a section in the drug compendium Uruanna Tablet III explains that terms such as "dog's tongue", "human bone" or "sailor's excrement" (also designated as *Dreckapotheke*) can refer to plants and should not be understood literally.[127] As a consequence, however, the exact nature of some drug designations in medical texts can be ambiguous and not completely transparent, since Mesopotamian medicine actually also employed a range of substances of animal origin such as hair, horn, blood, urine, milk, fats or meat.[128]

---

123 On such invocations of healing agents (often simultaneously used in ritual or cultic contexts), which are traditionally referred to in Assyriology as "Kultmittelbeschwörungen", see e.g. Cunningham 1997; Perdibon 2019, 162–169; Maul 2019. In the present corpus, see e.g. SpTU 5, No. 248 (text C.3.10); BAM 248 iv 34–38 (text D.1.1). For example, in a procedure in BM 51246+ (text A.2.7), the "dog's tongue-plant" (*lišān kalbi*) used in a treatment is referred to as "your plant" within an address to the sun god. See further on this below.

124 Systematic correspondences in the uses of *materia medica* are attested in Late Babylonian Mesopotamian astro-medicine and astro-magic, in which plants, minerals and parts or substances of specific animals are chosen because of their association with zodiac signs or astral constellations (see e.g. Reiner 1995; Heeßel 2005; 2008; Geller 2014; Schreiber 2018a; 2018b). For such astrological allusions, see e.g. BM 47491 (text A.2.6) in the present volume.

125 Examples of medical re-enactment in Mesopotamian women's remedies have been discussed in Steinert 2020. This study is drawn on in the following discussion.

126 For overviews on Mesopotamian medical technology, pharmaceutical knowledge and literature, see e.g. Böck 2009; 2010b; 2011; 2013; 2021; Rumor 2018; 2021; 2024; Stol 2002–2005a; 2003–2005b. For healing substances in women's healthcare texts, see Böck 2013; Steinert 2020; 2021a; for animal substances see Herréro 1984, 50–53; Chalendar 2016; 2017; for the use of human body substances (e.g. urine, breast milk), see Biggs 2006; Steinert 2023.

127 This phenomenon of alternative/alias names (or *Decknamen*) has been clarified through equations in drug compendia which list alternative names for the same plant. The explanation for the use of alias names is debated in Assyriological research. Franz Köcher (1995) sketched an interpretation of such names as *Decknamen* (secret names or coded names) used by medical specialists to hide specific knowledge from non-insiders. Others (e.g. Kinnier Wilson 2005; Rumor 2020; 2024) have argued that the matter is more complex and that such descriptive names for plants may often have had a popular character (i.e. that some such names may have been commonly known alternative designations for one and the same drug rather than secret names known only to medical practitioners).

128 Suspicions of an ingredient being an alias name are often raised in cases pointing to repulsive body substances (so-called *Dreckapotheke*) such as animal excrement, urine or blood. However, whether such an ingredient is a "coded" name or whether it should be understood literally needs to be assessed on a case-to-case basis, considering criteria such as access to the substance/animal in question, feasibility of the drug in the light of the instructions given in a prescription, and the possible motivations for the use of a substance (Chalendar 2016; 2017). On the other

As elucidated by studies of ancient prescriptions for gender-related conditions, the uses of curative agents such as plants and animals often display symbolic connotations or analogical reasoning. Treatments often aim at transferring a specific property associated with the animal to the patient, as seen, for example, in Mesopotamian treatments to stimulate sexual desire and potency, which often employ ingredients derived from male animals known for their sexual vigour (Zisa 2021). Similarly, Totelin's (2007; 2009, 197–224) investigations of Hippocratic gynaecological prescriptions elucidate ingredients with sexual or fertility connotations. Mesopotamian women's healthcare texts likewise offer ample evidence for such connotations and culturally based connections between medical ingredients and concepts of the female body, its physiology and dysfunctions in connections with reproductive processes (e.g. Steinert 2020; 2021a).

That Mesopotamian healers were aware of such hidden meanings and associations underlying the selection of *materia medica* employed in their therapeutic procedures can be seen in two commentaries on a therapeutic treatise for childbirth (referred to here as the Neo-Assyrian Birth Compendium) from the first millennium BCE (see text D.1.1 for the base text and Chapter G for the commentaries). Thus, the commentaries go into great length to explain links between the *materia medica* employed to ease difficult labour on the one hand and the patient, her foetus and the birth situation on the other, underlining and bolstering their ritual/symbolic efficacy in the context. For example, one passage (11N-T3: 8–10; text G.1) explains the use of a reed and dust from a crossroads, by pointing out associations that are offered by the cuneiform script and the bilingualism of the texts, namely by analysing the components of Sumerian words in the base text in terms of equations in the Akkadian language that provide a direct relation to the woman, the baby and a prompt delivery ("to go straight"):

> "(In the Sumerian phrase) gi èn-bar bàn-da šu u-me-ti ('Take a small reed from the marsh'), gi ('reed') means 'woman'; bar (the second element of the word èn-bar 'marsh') means 'to go out', bàn-da ('small') means 'baby' (or) 'small (child)'. (In) 'dust (saḫar) from the street (sila)', saḫar means 'dust'. 'Dust' (saḫar) and 'baby' (*ṣahar*) are one and the same (phonetically). (In) 'crossroads' (Sumerian sila-lam$_4$-ma), si means 'to go straight'', said of 'going'; *la* means 'child' (*la'û*, which means) 'little one'; and 'people' (*ammu*, written *amma*) means 'seed'."

The range of plant-based ingredients in Mesopotamian gynaecological texts includes grasses, rushes, reeds, thorny plants, soapworts, trees and their fruit, as well as vines, cereals, vegetables, and plant resins/gums. The *materia medica* thus includes many spices and foods, as well as liquids such as different kinds of beer, beer mash, grape juice/wine, vinegar and plant oils (perfumed oils produced by adding aromatic plants), which play an important role as carrier substances in medical preparations. Less numerous, but of considerable importance in the women's healthcare texts are also minerals and animal-based ingredients.[129] Concerning the latter group of ingredients, most frequently attested in these texts is the use of wool (especially for making tampons), shells, animal fats, horn, and eggshell. Shells (and cowry snails), which tended to be classified as "stones/minerals" (using the classifier for minerals) rather than animals, are used in Mesopotamian women's healthcare texts especially for amulets (together with other stones). However, shells, eggshells (of birds) and animal horn are likewise attested recurringly in treatments to stop bleeding, as are animal bones. Animal fats are encountered as carrier or lubricating substance for suppositories and tampons, while ghee or cream occur predominantly as component of oral remedies or ointments.

In the following, a few significant examples of *materia medica* for specific female health issues are discussed. Drug handbooks listing the most important simple drugs according to their indications or medical uses often also contain a section on women's ailments. These sections together with the prescriptions for the same purposes reflect a differentiated knowledge of the salient pharmaceutical properties of specific plants, while the prescriptions themselves also reveal complex cultural associations and logics (of analogical reasoning or thinking in terms of properties) underlying *materia medica* and their uses.

---

hand, animal ingredients (including repulsive ones) are widely attested in traditional medical systems throughout the ages; and such uses may sometimes be based on "perfectly valid medical reasons" (Scurlock 2006, 63).

129 The women's healthcare texts alone mention ca. 48 different animals (including mammals, birds, fish, insects, reptiles, crustacea and mollusks (shells) as a source of an ingredient and ca. 20 different animal products, body parts or substances.

Contraceptives and Fertility Enhancers

Beside fertility enhancers, which play a considerable role in Mesopotamian prescriptions for women as seen in the texts edited in Chapter B of this volume, the present study has identified the first examples for contraceptive remedies.[130] Both types of *materia medica* are also included in the "gynaecological section" of drug handbooks. One such gynaecological section in a list of simple drugs gives a sequence of herbal drugs for conception ("drug for acquiring seed/offspring", Ú NUMUN TUKU, *šammi zēra rašî*), to treat infertility ("drug for a barren woman", Ú munusNU.Ù.TU, *šammi lā ālitti*), followed by plants used for contraception ("drug for preventing a woman from getting pregnant", Ú MUNUS NU $PEŠ_4$, *šammi sinništi lā šūrî*).[131] The expression Ú MUNUS NU $PEŠ_4$ has been interpreted differently as "plant for a woman who does not (or cannot) get pregnant," i.e. as a synonym for a (fertile) woman who has difficulties conceiving a(nother) child. Yet, given the section of contraceptives in BM 51246+ and the similarity between the formulations it seems more likely that Ú MUNUS NU $PEŠ_4$ should be understood as a "drug for (the purpose that) a woman does not get pregnant/for not letting a woman get pregnant" (*šammi sinništi lā erî/šūrî*).

One of the plants with the indication Ú MUNUS NU $PEŠ_4$ in the lists of simple drugs is the *ankinūtu*-plant. Interestingly, this unidentified plant is an ingredient in a prescription for abortion (BAM 246: 3; text B.1.6) and is prescribed as a simple drug in a recipe for contraception in BM 51246+ (rev. 11'; text A.2.7).[132] Its use both as a contraceptive and abortifacient may indicate that the healers saw these purposes as related (e.g., for ejecting the male semen after intercourse, or the foetus, when conception had already occurred). A second drug for MUNUS NU $PEŠ_4$ is (seed of) *ḫaluppu*-tree, perhaps to be identified with the willow, which would be significant, since the bark of the willow (white willow or weeping willow (*Salix babylonica*)) was used in other ancient cultures as a contraceptive drug.[133] Interestingly, some plants are recommended for different or even contradictory uses in women's healthcare texts and drug compendia. One example is *pillû*-plant, the suggested identification of which with mandrake is uncertain (Stol 2000, 57–58). Thus, the root of male *pillû*-plant is recommended in a potion for contraception in BM 51246+ but also occurs as the main ingredient in a salve to speed up difficult labour (BAM 248 rev. iv 19–20 //; text D.1.1), and as a fertility-enhancing ingredient (BAM 244 obv. 4; text B.1.1). While this evidence is perplexing, the fact that male *pillû*-plant does not bear fruit makes it a suitable drug for ending a pregnancy, but also even more so for contraception (if we assume this choice applies analogical reasoning).[134]

Among the numerous herbal drugs recommended for promoting fertility, one may highlight that lists of simple drugs prescribe plant seeds (of the *atkam* and *kamantu*-plant) "to acquire seed" (i.e. offspring); thus, the part of the plant standing for fertility and reproduction was chosen to bring about female fecundity.[135] A couple of plants employed as fertility enhancers have widespread associations with fecundity in Mesopotamian cultures, such as the fruit-bearing date palm and pomegranate tree (Steinert 2021a, 64–69).[136] Furthermore, the prescriptions for fertility and conception show a pre-

130 These contraceptive remedies are, interestingly, oral applications. Beside oral contraceptive preparations, other methods used by women in the past include vaginal suppositories as barriers that block the cervix (e.g. wool, absorbent cotton) or douches after intercourse (e.g. Riddle 1992; Root-Bernstein and Root-Bernstein 1997, 149–165; Westendorf 1999, 426; Stol 2000, 37–39; Totelin 2009, 214–219; Flemming 2021).

131 BAM 380 rev. 25–41 (esp. 25–29) // BAM 381 iii 17–36 (esp. iii 17–22). The passage continues with drugs in the context of pregnancy, delivery and postpartum conditions; Stol 2000, 53–54; Couto-Ferreira 2014, 309. For discussion, see also Böck 2013, 29–36; Steinert 2021a, 57–60.

132 The following prescription in BM 51246+ rev. 12', actually preserving the prognosis NU $PEŠ_4$ "she will not get pregnant", recommends the *ašqulālu*-plant, which like the *ankinūtu*-plant grows in swamps, see Stol 2000, 54 with n. 35. The *ašqulālu*-plant is classified as a "drug for (inducing?) labour pains" (*šammi ḫâli*) in Uruanna II 39, see CAD Ḫ 55.

133 See Thompson 1949, 291; Stol 2000, 42, with Riddle 1992, 31–33 (citing e.g. Dioscorides); Duke 2008, 404–411.

134 Contrary to Riddle (2010, 15–18), there is no direct evidence so far for pomegranate (Akkadian *lurmû*) as a contraceptive in ancient Mesopotamian medical texts. Riddle's identification of the *ḫaluppu*-tree with pomegranate should be refuted (see Steinert 2021b, 58 n. 87, 64–66).

135 For the text passage, see BAM 380 rev. 25–26, duplicated in BAM 381 iii 17–19; cf. also the drug list BAM 1 i 18–20, prescribing the same two plants for getting seed, to be drunk in beer or inserted into the vagina (Attia and Buisson 2012, 26). Other plants recommended for fertility and conception in plant lists are *imhur-līm*-plant (lit. "it heals thousand (diseases)", a very common medicinal plant), *išin eqli* (lit. "(grain) stalk of the field-plant") and *lišān kalbi* "dog's tongue-plant" Böck (2014a, 141, 154, 157–158) suggested an identification of *lišān kalbi* with *Cynoglossum officinale*, but Böck, Ghazanfar and Nesbitt (2023, 118–123) now propose it could be *Plantago major*. See further Stadhouders 2011, 38 lines 46–48 and 40–42 with parallel KADP 4 lines 36–37; Stadhouders 2012, 17; Stol 2000, 52–53.

136 E.g. BM 79061 obv. 5–8 (text A.2.8); BAM 408 i' 2'–3' (text A.2.9). Pomegranate and date were also used as aphrodisiacs in Mesopotamia, see Biggs 1967; Zisa 2021. Pomegranate seeds contain oestrogens; and modern trials confirmed the plant's potential to reduce fertility (in mice). Pomegranate has also been employed as an abortifacient (the bark has toxic properties and its consumption is contraindicated in pregnancy), as an emmenagogue, to ease delivery, stop bleeding, to treat cancer (e.g. of the breasts, genitals, uterus), venereal diseases, infections, inflammation, infertility, and to manage menopause and irregular gynaecological bleeding (Biggs 2000, 9; Duke 2008, 364–367; Riddle 1992, 25–26, 32–33, 40–44, 51–53, 94–97 and *passim*; King 1998, 147–148; Totelin 2009, 209–211, 222). Dates and their oestrogen-containing seeds and pollen were used in

ponderance for aromatic plants and for medicinal plants that are associated with cleansing and purifying properties and are used to neutralise evil and defiling forces, especially witchcraft. Among these plants are cedar (*erēnu*) and *kurkānû*-plant (for which an identification with turmeric has been suggested)[137], tamarisk (*bīnu*), juniper (*daprānu, burāšu*), *šambaliltu* (fenugreek) and various other aromatics.[138]

Several of the animal ingredients found in this context may have been used because of their associations with fertility or potency, such as (the edible) *ušummu*-dormouse and types of locust (*erib turbu'ti* "dust-locust", *erib-tâmti* "sea locust") employed in tampons.[139] The use of *pizallurtu* "gecko" in a tampon for fertility mirrors the use of this animal in prescriptions to promote potency / male sexual desire (especially "copulating geckos of the steppe").[140] Other conspicuous ingredients for female fertility are "mongoose excrement" (*zê šikkî*, perhaps an alias name for a plant ingredient), "gazelle dung" (as a component of an amulet, perhaps a leather bag worn around the neck)[141] as well as prescriptions using animal bones (BAM 240: 71'–74' (text D.2.1); BM 42313+: 67–68 (texts A.2.2). Bone may have been regarded as a substance resembling semen, since according to a birth incantation the bone of the foetus was believed to be built up from semen (see text II.1.2; Steinert 2020, 63–64). Moreover, some details in the methods of administration of fertility-enhancing remedies point to concepts of the female body and to metaphors of the womb linked to vessels (e.g. the notion of "opening" the womb for conception), to analogies from the domain of agriculture (e.g. notions of "irrigation" or "moistening") as well as to notions of purification (Steinert 2017a, 303–318; 2020, 60–64).

Menstrual Regulators, Drugs for Abortion and Delivery

Studies on birth control in historical perspective have noted a close connection in medical and folk-medical practices between abortive remedies and so-called menstrual regulators, i.e. drugs that induce the menses when they are delayed (emmenagogues), which may have involved uses as abortifacients interrupting an early term pregnancy (e.g. Riddle 1992; Böck 2013, 39–40). Both types of prescriptions "to cause a woman to abort her foetus" and for "making the menses appear" are attested in the Mesopotamian women's healthcare texts (see Chapters B and C.2), but the ingredients elucidated from these texts show only few commonalities so far (e.g. *nuḫurtu*-plant is attested in both contexts).[142] Interesting is the attestation of *ašqulālu*-plant to induce the menses, which fits its other attested uses as a contraceptive and as a drug to induce labour (see above).[143]

It has been noted however that several of the drugs encountered in Mesopotamian recipes for abortion are also recommended in prescriptions to promote (difficult) delivery, which suggests that these drugs caused uterine contractions. For example, the *nabruqqu*-plant (also *namruqqu*) occurs as a simple drug for abortion in BAM 246 (text B.1.6) but is known as

folk-medical traditions as an aphrodisiac and for enhancing fertility, but also as a contraceptive, to treat genital sores, cancer (e.g. of the uterus or vagina) and venereal diseases, see e.g. Duke 2008, 327–328; Riddle 1992, 33, 51–53, 85.

137 For *kurkānû*-plant as a drug promoting fertility, see BM 79061 obv. 11 (text A.2.8); N. 4001 obv. 15 // BM 51246+ obv. 11; N. 4001 rev. 2 (text A.2.7, B.2.1); BM 42313+ obv. 7 (text A.2.2), BAM 244: 31, 33, 37 (text B.1.1); BAM 247: 8 (text B.1.3), attested in two varieties, domesticated and wild. Scurlock (2020, 57–58) connects this use of *kurkānû* with the anti-androgenic properties of turmeric identified in modern studies. For critique concerning Scurlock's identification of *kurkānû* with turmeric (curcuma), see Jursa 2009, 162 n. 74. See further BM 79061 obv. 11 (text A.2.8) for discussion.

138 There are several identical ingredients and similarities in the use of herbal drugs for female infertility and for stimulating (male) sexual desire (ŠÀ.ZI.GA). For example, the "dog's tongue-plant" is attested as a drug for both these purposes and for a woman in difficult labour, see Böck 2014a, 141; Zisa 2021, 160–164; BAM 380 rev. 31–31 // BAM 381 iii 25–26 (Stol 2000, 52–53); BAM 248 iv 13, 21–22 (text D.1.1) and below.

139 For locusts in fertility treatments, see e.g. N. 4001: 16 (text B.2.1); BM 42450+: 17'–20' (text B.2.3); BM 45559+: 12'–16' (text A.2.4).

140 See e.g. STT 98: 21' (text A.1.1); Zisa 2021, 167, 408–409 Text K Prescription 31: 135–140 = Text N Prescription 8 (ii 3–8). For mice and fertility, see also Böck 2013, 32–33. It may not be a coincidence that mice, geckos and lizards are associated with the female sexual organs in Mesopotamia, see Rumor 2017b, 200 n. 71; Zisa 2021, 98 n. 208.

141 See BM 38624+: 7' (text A.2.1); AMT 66/9: 6'-8' (text B.1.5). Dung pellets (of a gazelle, sheep or an unspecified animal) occur several times in Mesopotamian prescriptions (e.g. Geller 2005a, in treatments for rectal diseases, in bandages, fumigations, suppositories). In the context of women's prescriptions, dung may have been regarded as a fertilizing substance, by analogy with its uses in agriculture, see Steinert 2020, 61–62.

142 See BM 47578 obv. 4 (text C.2.2); K. 8678+ rev. 13' (text A.1.4).

143 See BM 47578 obv. 3 (text C.2.2). Another example for a drug used as contraceptive and to induce the menses is *imḫur-līm*-plant ("it heals thousand (diseases)" (BM 47578 rev. 1; BM 51246+ rev. 6'). However, the *imḫur-līm*-plant is also recommended as a plant for an infertile woman (^{munus}NU.Ù.TU) in BM 380 rev. 27 // BAM 381 iii 20. That the same plant seems to be used for opposite purposes in two different texts is surprising and needs to be investigated further. For a suggested identification with red bryony (*Bryonia multiflora*), see Böck, Ghazanfar and Nesbitt 2023, 155–159.

a plant for a woman who is *šalputtu*[144], and used to induce the flow of postpartum blood (lochia) (BM 38624+ rev. iv 5'; text A.2.1). Similarly, the *ēdu*-plant (lit. solitary plant) is found among the drugs for abortion in BAM 246, while it is designated as a drug for a woman who is *šalputtu* (BAM 380 rev. 39 // BAM 381 iii 34). A conspicuous ingredient found in remedies to induce abortion and ease difficult labour is "(excrement of multicoloured) wall-lizard" ((*zê*) *ṣurār igāri* (*barmi*), which may be an alias name for an herbal drug.[145] The occurrence of "(wall) lizard" as an abortifacient may be compared with use of *anduḫallatu*-lizard to induce menstrual bleeding (BM 42313+ obv. 16; text A.2.2), which recalls similar associations of geckos and lizards with fertility and potency.[146]

In a few cases, herbal drugs with expellant properties in Mesopotamian texts may be linked to abortifacients known in other traditions, although the suggested identifications of these drugs are not certain and need to be viewed with caution. For example, the *šunû*-plant (suggested identification: chaste tree (*Vitex agnus-castus*)) occurs as a drug to induce abortion in a manuscript from Nineveh.[147] This plant is also employed for different postpartum complaints, including gastrointestinal problems, fever and retained lochia (BAM 240: 23', 41, 58'; text D.2.1). Another plant associated with abortion in the text BAM 246 is *azupīrānu*.[148] As a related example, the use of *kamūnu*-plant (usually identified with cumin) in prescriptions to speed up delivery (e.g. SpTU 4, No. 153 obv. 22, 25) fits in with the use of cumin as abortifacient and utero-contractant in other Near Eastern cultures.[149]

Looking closer at drugs for a woman in hard labour ([munus]LA.RA.AḪ), two plants which are attested both in the prescriptions and in drug handbooks are "fox grape" (*karān šēlebi*) and "dog's tongue"-plant (*lišān kalbi*).[150] Conspicuous are two further ingredients referring to an animal: *rikibti arkabi* "*spur* of a bat" and "excrement of *ḫurru*-bird" (*zê iṣṣūr ḫurri*).[151] The first ingredient is attested as a simple drug for difficult labour in BAM 248 iv 23 // (text D.1.1) and BM 38624+ obv. ii 26' (text A.2.1: 59'"). In a medical text from Nineveh, *rikibti arkabi* appears as a gloss above the plant name *urânu* (probably a type of fennel or anise), which could indicate that the former might be used as an alias name for the latter.[152] The drug "excrement of *ḫurru*-bird" (*zê iṣṣūr ḫurri*) is encountered as an ingredient for a tampon to dilate the birth canal in a Late Babylonian text from Uruk (SpTU 4, No. 153 obv. 21, 24–25, text D.1.11). It is possible that this drug is likewise an alias name, since we know other plant designations with this naming principle.[153]

---

144 Stol 2000a, 53–55 for discussion, with BAM 380 rev. 40 // BAM 381 iii 35.

145 See BAM 246 obv. 2, 8; BAM 248 iv 16 //. Böck (2013, 37–39) discusses the possibility that "wall lizard" or similar terms encountered here may indeed be alternative designations for an herbal drug, used to keep the actual identity of the most efficacious ingredient to cause an abortion secret and inaccessible to non-specialists. This interpretation raises the question how to explain the occurrence of "uncoded" plant names such as *nabruqqu* side-by-side with bizarre or "coded" drug names such as "wall lizard" in the same context.

146 See above; Zisa 2021, 98, 408–409 Text K Prescription 31: 135–140 = Text N Prescription 8 (ii 3–8)).

147 K. 8678+ rev. 13'–20' (text A.1.4). The proposed identification is based on the similarity of the word *šunû* to Syriac *šūnājā* (CAD Š/3, 309–310). Chaste tree was used as a contraceptive and abortifacient plant in the Graeco-Roman world, see Riddle 1992, 61, 78–79 and *passim*.

148 The name *azupīrānu* means "resembling *azupīru*-plant", and the latter plant is traditionally identified with saffron or safflower on etymological grounds (CAD A/2, 530–531; AHw 93; Thompson 1949, 159). Saffron was known as an abortifacient elsewhere in ancient times (Pangas 1990, 216 with n. 29; Riddle 1992, 244, Index).

149 For identification (based on connections to the Greek and Arabic terms for cumin), see Böck, Ghazanfar and Nesbitt 2023, 90–93. For cumin as abortifacient, see Duke 2008, 159–160.

150 BAM 380 rev. 31–35 // BAM 381 iii 25–40 (Stol 2000, 52–53); BAM 248 iv 13, 21–22, 24 // (text D.1.1); STT 98 rev. 2', 4' (text A.1.1); SpTU 4, No. 153 obv. 23, 26 (text D.1.11); BAM 248 rev. iv 13, 21, 22, 24 (text D.1.1) and *passim*. For "dog's tongue"-plant and "fox grape", cf. Böck 2014a, 140–158; Böck, Ghazanfar and Nesbitt 2023, 67–71, 118–122. The drug *karān šēlebi* "fox grape" is linked to black nightshade (*Solanum nigrum*) by the latter authors, due to the parallel Arabic term *'inab al-ṯal'ab* which has exactly the same meaning as the Akkadian.

151 I retain the conventional reading *rikibtu* for U_5, although as Chalendar (2018, *JMC* 32, 24–45) has argued that U_5 should be read *rikbu* rather than *rikibtu*, since direct lexical equations are so far only known for U_5 = *rikbu* (cf. CAD R, 343–344 and 344–345). Both terms are derived from the same verb *rakābu* "to ride; mount (sexually)"; but *rikbu* seems to have a completely different range of meanings (including "pollen of the date palm"), while *rikibtu* lit. "copulation, pollination" occurs as a term for a body part/substance specifically of either the stag (*ayyalu*) or the bat (*arkabu*). The exact meaning of the word *rikibtu* is disputed and different suggestions have been pronounced about its interpretation; it is at least clear that *rikibtu* refers to a body part or substance. Some think *rikibtu* refers to guano, semen or musk (secreted by musk deer), others suggest an identification with the dewclaw (of deer) and bat thumb, respectively. It has been noted that *rikibti arkabi/ayyali* occur both as aphrodisiac substances in Mesopotamian medical texts (see Zisa 2021, 165–173; Biggs 2002, 75–76).

152 AMT 47/1+ ii 12 (Geller 2005a, text No. 24); for *urânu*, see CAD U/W, 206–208; Civil 2008, ARET 4, 105 No. 223; see also Maul 2019, 300 note on Text 78 line 76 (BAM 168); Heeßel 2016, 32–33). The *urânu*-plant occurs as a simple remedy to induce the menses in BM 47578 obv. 7 (text C.2.2) Interestingly, *rikibti arkabi* may occur for the same purpose in SpTU 1, No. 59 4'–6' (text C.2.1).

153 For instance, "dove excrement" (*zê summati*) is an alias name for the seed of *ašāgu*-thorn; "dog excrement" (*zê kalbi*) is an alternative name for the *nikiptu*-plant (a strongly smelling plant).

Ingredients to Stop Gynaecological Haemorrhage and to Protect from Miscarriage

One of the central topics of Mesopotamian gynaecological remedies is abnormal bleeding, in particular haemorrhage during pregnancy and delivery.[154] The most prominent type of treatment for gynaecological bleeding in these texts are tampons or suppositories inserted into the vagina and potions. The recipes apply a variety of different (plant, mineral, or animal) substances, some of which have astringent or haemostatic properties (e.g. alum). Numerous parallels to identified ingredients encountered in these prescriptions can be found in other ancient medical traditions as well as in folk-medical practices, and many of the drugs prescribed for stopping haemorrhage or similar discharges in female patients also occur in therapeutic texts concerned with similar conditions in men (Steinert 2012b). Beside haemostatic properties, several ingredients encountered in the context of gynaecological haemorrhage provide signature elements alluding to the haemorrhage (as hot and moist). Thus, ingredients having a red colour obviously highlight this connection, such as the reddish pigment *kalgukku*, used beside yellow ochre (*kalû*) and haematite (*šadânu*, also known as haemostatic "blood stone" in the Egyptian, Graeco-Roman, Arabic and Western traditions), the root of *ḫûratu*-plant (madder) which contains a red colourant, *illūru*-plant (which has a red flower/fruit), or red-coloured wool used for tampons into which ingredients were wrapped and then inserted into the vagina. Sometimes, also the name of the drug (e.g. a substance referred to as Akkadian as "cedar blood" (*dām erēni*))[155], provides a link between the drug and the treated condition.

The insertion of tampons/suppositories into the vagina as a prominent therapeutic strategy in the context of gynaecological bleeding can be seen as corresponding to the metaphors comparing the female body to a leaking vessel or to a field or meadow flooded by the river, with its bank / dike having collapsed through the excessive flooding (e.g. BAM 237(+), text C.1.4). Suppositories (*maššītu*) and particular *materia medica* administered with them were explicitly prescribed for the purpose of "damming up/blocking" (*peḫû*) the blood flow, thus enacting the goals of sealing a leaking body opening, as well as of containing and stopping the body fluids.[156] In this context, another term *lubbuku* occurs together with *peḫû*. For example, the remarkable Late Babylonian text SpTU 4, No. 153 obv. 2, 6, 9, 11, 14 (text C.1.10) also speaks of suppositories and medical substances with the effect of "*absorbing*" (*lubbuku*). This verb occurs in the meanings "to lubricate; to soften; to make supple" in other medical texts, when it refers to therapeutic effects of remedies on the body.[157] As in SpTU 4, No. 153, *lubbuku* is encountered together elsewhere with the term *maššītu* "suppository". For example, BAM 303 (a Neo-Assyrian extract tablet copied by the healer Kiṣir-Aššur), contains four different *maššāti ša lubbuki* "suppositories for *softening*", including a *maššītu* for making stiff (muscles) supple (*šaggi ana lubbuki*, line 22') and a *maššītu* for releasing 'wind' (line 21'; cf. Arbøll 2021, 285–286). While the meanings "to soften" or "to lubricate" fit well for *lubbuku* in the context of stiff muscles, it is suggested that in connection with stopping bleeding, this verb may have the specific meaning "to absorb" (body fluids).[158]

Interestingly, prescriptions against bleeding in the text SpTU 4, No. 153 (text C.1.10) speak not only of damming up (*peḫû*) and absorbing (*lubbuku*) but also recommend drugs that "dry up" the wetness (*abālu*, obv. 4 and 14) and "cool down" (*kaṣû*, obv. 9, 14; *ana takṣâti* "for cooling", obv. 7) the patient, so that "the blood will be held back" (*dāmū ikkallû*, obv. 9). The latter notion of a "cooling" effect associated with halting a haemorrhage is remarkable, given the occasional characterization of menstrual blood as hot in ancient Greek medicine.[159] In SpTU 4, No. 153 obv. 7–8, *maštakal*-soapwort (an astringent substance) and *simbirru*-plant are recommended "for cooling a pregnant woman" (with a haemorrhage during the first trimester) or for acute bleeding after delivery, and the former plant is also among the drugs for treating *naḫšātu* (bleeding during pregnancy) in the gynaecological sections of drug lists.[160]

Moreover, several elements in the remedies for gynaecological haemorrhage can be read as "medical re-enactments" using signature ingredients and forms of preparation that present a link to the intention of "drying" an excessive wetness implied by the haemorrhage. Thus, the use of dry ingredients (such as powder of *šupuḫru*-cedar or powder from an old

154 See for previous discussion, Steinert 2012b; 2020, 57–60.

155 For *dām erēni*, usually interpreted as cedar resin, but perhaps to be identified as cedar tar, a liquid substance of brown or black colour produced through heating of cedar wood (a process called pyrolysis), see Böck 2023, 121–125; Böck, Ghazanfar and Nesbitt 2023, 78.

156 SpTU 4, No. 153 (text C.1.10) obv. 2, 5, 10. The verb *peḫû*(ÚŠ) "to block; to bar; to lute" occurs elsewhere in connection with stopping gynaecological haemorrhage, see e.g. K. 263 + 10934 rev. 42–44 (text C.1.5); Steinert 2012b.

157 In instructions for the preparation of medical substances, *lubbuku* also means "to soak; to macerate ingredients in a liquid" (Goltz 1974, 43; Herrero 1984, 43, 68).

158 For this expression in women's healthcare texts, see also BM 38624+ obv. i 10' (text A.2.1); BM 50700 obv. 11' (text A.2.3).

159 See King 1998, 32–33, 90; Totelin 2009, 197.

160 BAM 380 rev. 30 // BAM 381 iii 23–24 (Stol 2000, 52–53).

wooden beam) and the use of roasted materials devoid of moisture, signal the aim of the treatments (absorbing and drying out, or balancing excessive moisture). Another ingredient "enacting" the aims of treatment (absorbing, drying and cooling) is found in the potsherd from the opening of an oven, since the oven and potsherd both stand for an object (container/vessel) that gets hot and cold again, in a way signalling the intended cooling of the patient's "hot" body state. Roasting of the drugs could likewise be understood as an action enacting the patient's hot state:

> SpTU 4, No. 153 obv. 10–12, 14–15:
> "Powder of *kanaktu*-aromatic and *šupuhru*-cedar, . . . you will always find (to be good) for damming up. . . .
> *Kanaktu*-aromatic will *absorb*, *šupuhru*-cedar will dry (out). You (can also) roast resin of(?) *maštakal*-plant (and) sheep bone over the fire. You (can also) administer to her (lit. 'give her') the shell of an ostrich egg, *imbû tâmti*-mineral (and) powder of an old log, one (unit, i.e. the same amount of) each (ingredient) . . .
> A new(?) pot (*diqāru eššu*) or a porous potsherd (*haṣbu šaharru*) from the opening of an oven (*utūnu*) is very good (as well): it *absorbs*, cools and dri[es out(?) . . .].
> A sheep's eye (and) sheep's horn, which have been roasted on embers, are very good (as well). Their ashes . . . [. . .]."

The use of a porous potsherd is based on complex analogies. On the one hand, potsherds are associated with obstruction and thus play a role in therapies to stop irregular bleeding.[161] On the other hand, porous vessels have a cooling effect on their contents, which again points towards the idea of cooling of a haemorrhaging pregnant woman (i.e. a hot state) encountered in SpTU 4, No. 153.[162]

Ingredients of animal origin in Mesopotamian prescriptions to stop gynaecological bleeding are also interesting in connection with the notion of "signatures" and analogical reasoning. Among the popular ingredients occur shells (often pulverized), eggshells (of ostrich, dove, turtledove), horn (of gazelle, cow, goat, stag), excrement (of a *ṣurāru*-lizard), and blood (of *ḫurru*-bird, goat).[163] Some of the ingredients may indeed have been effective: shells, eggshells and animal horns contain as main component calcium carbonate, which in modern trials has been shown to have haemostatic properties that improve wound healing (He et al. 2021).[164]

Eggshells (like shells) are reported to have an astringent effect.[165] For example, in ancient Egyptian sources, ostrich eggshells are applied in the Papyrus Smith as an astringent to dry a skull wound on the forehead (Westendorf 1999, 720). Dioscorides ascribes an astringent effect to *chalkitis* (mineral calcium carbonate) and recommends it for discharges of blood from the womb (*De Materia Medica*, Book 5–115). Furthermore, he writes about fossilized oyster shells (*ostrakites lithos*) (Book 5–165):

> "A teaspoonful (taken in a drink with wine) stops the menstrual flow. If anyone drinks two teaspoonfuls after the menstrual flow, it prevents conception."

The use of deer horn to treat abnormal fluxes in women is also attested in ancient Greek sources. For example, in the Hippocratic text *Diseases of Women* 2 (83 (1), 90 (4)), a potion of incinerated deer horn mixed with barley flour and wine/water is recommended (Potter 2018, 411, 423). Similarly, Dioscorides in *De Materia Medica* 2–63 writes: "It is . . . good for women troubled with excessive [menstrual] discharge, given in some liquid suitable for that suffering."

---

161 For potsherds found standing upright on a street used in amulets and other treatments, see e.g. BAM 237 i 9'–16', ii 41'–44', iii 6–7, iv 23, iv 35 (text C.1.4); BM 40152 iii 1–5 (text C.1.8).

162 For a parallel use of a sherd from an oven to decrease fever/heat of the head/skull, see e.g. BAM 3 i 12–14, with variant in BAM 480 i 8–9 // BAM 4: 5'–6' (CRANIUM Tablet 1, see Worthington 2005, 7, 16; Worthington 2006, 19, 27; Scurlock 2014a, 307, 319; Bácskay 2018, no. 12). In other examples the sherd as an ingredient stemming from a "hot container" (oven) is applied topically to cool another "container" (body part), see further BAM 3 iv 11 (Worthington 2006, 24, 31; Stol 2009, 39; Bacskáy 2018, 105–106 No. 38).

163 The use of animal blood in potions against female haemorrhage (e.g. K. 263+ obv. 8–10, rev. 2; BAM 235: 4–6; texts C.1.1 and C.1.5) could be seen as replacement for the blood loss, i.e. as a restorative treatment (based on the principle "like cures like"). In a similar fashion, bull's blood is given to drink in a prescription against bleeding from the rectum for a male patient (BAM 99: 30–32 // BAM 152 iii 11–12; Geller 2005a, No. 35).

164 It is noteworthy that several of the ingredients to stop gynaecological bleeding are also recommended in texts dealing with renal and rectal diseases, such as ostrich eggshells, "donkey-vulva shell" (*biṣṣūr atāni*), *ayyartu* (shell or coral), *yānibu*, for conditions such as calculus, stricture of the bladder and blood in the urine (Geller 2005a).

165 Cf. Steinert 2012b, 83 n. 82. In addition to empirical knowledge, the use of eggshells to stop bleeding in pregnancy in Mesopotamian sources may have been bolstered by analogy and associations: eggshell surrounds and protects the bird foetus and, in the case of ostrich eggs, they are also quite thick and hard (vessels were made from them).

Moreover, shells may have been particularly popular in Mesopotamian remedies against female bleeding (including haemorrhage during pregnancy), since they were associated with the female genitals; the foetus is compared with the animal inside the shell in a first millennium BCE birth incantation.[166] The aquatic origin of shells (and therefore their assumed cooling properties?) may have been likewise significant for their use against a "hot" body state.

A remarkable ritual involving a treatment to stop loss of amniotic fluid (and to prevent miscarriage) found in a Late Babylonian text (BM 51246+; text A.2.7 lines 37'–40') involves the "dog's tongue-plant" (*lišān kalbi*). Its use for stopping the loss of amniotic fluid and preventing miscarriage in the present text is noteworthy. In other women's healthcare texts, "dog's tongue-plant" is known as a drug to speed up or ease difficult labour (Ú ^{munus}LA.RA.AḪ), suggesting that "dog's tongue-plant" had abortifacient properties (see above). These properties seem contrary to its use to preserve pregnancy in BM 51246+. The application form required by the remedy in BM 51246+ may have involved external application of the plant's root (unfortunately this information is lost), in contrast to texts recommending "dog's tongue-plant" (and sometimes its root) to speed up delivery (where it is given in a potion). The association of the "dog's tongue-plant" with Šamaš in BM 51246+ is well-suited, since the sun god played a crucial role as a protector of pregnant women and their foetuses and appears in several pregnancy- and birth-related incantations and prayers (see section 5). One may ask whether the root of the "dog's tongue-plant" symbolized the foetus in the womb. Both the root and the foetus exist in the darkness (of the earth / womb); and another analogy between them is that both should only "see the sunlight" when the proper time has come (i.e. for being born and harvested, respectively; see text A.2.7 for discussion).

5 Practitioners Involved in Women's Healthcare

The cuneiform textual sources concerned with healing have been linked with two professions that were either performed exclusively by men (i.e. the function of the *āšipu/mašmaššu* "conjurer; exorcist") or were largely male occupations (i.e. the *asû* "physician"), although the prominence of female healing deities and birth goddesses in Mesopotamian cultures reflects a deep-rooted and long-standing connection of women with the realm of healing and midwifery.[167] This connection can be further supported by scattered textual evidence documenting the performance of these roles by women. Since there is a growing amount of historical evidence (e.g. from Graeco-Roman, Christian, Jewish backgrounds) for women as medical experts in and beyond the field of women's healthcare (and occasionally as medical authors) whose knowledge left traces in the male-dominated medical literatures (Lehmhaus 2023, 61–75), this section rounds up the introduction by briefly reviewing the evidence for male and female expertise in the Mesopotamian women's healthcare texts edited in this volume. Additional information on female professionals in the fields of healing and midwifery beyond these texts is summarised cursorily.[168]

The conjurer/exorcist (*āšipu/mašmaššu*) is undoubtably the most prominent healing professional when it comes to attestations of conjurers as owners and copyists of women's healthcare texts from the first millennium BCE, as the sources from the so-called "House of the incantation priest" at Assur (library N4) and from the libraries of the conjurers' families at Late Babylonian Uruk show (see above). The texts owned by these scholarly healers included both tablets containing medical prescriptions as well as incantations and healing rituals (beside other genres such as literary and divinatory texts, astrology/astronomy), which underlines their broad qualifications as men of learning as well as practitioners.

166 See Bergmann 2008, 52–54; Couto-Ferreira 2014, 310; Steinert 2017a, 323–326, 332–335. The connection is revealed in two commentaries (11N-T3 and UET 6/3, 897, see Chapter G). I quote the latter of these passages (rev. 2'–4'): "(The phrase) 'let him (the sun god Šamaš) show the one inside the shell the light' – it (the base text) said it in reference to the pregnant woman. ^{na4}PEŠ$_4$(IŠKILA) (means) 'shell'; secondly, (it means) 'mother', thirdly (it means) 'pregnant woman'."

167 Both conjurers and physicians acted as specialists in the diagnosis and treatment of diseases affecting humans and animals, including male and female adults as well as children. Each of the two disciplines had traditional areas of expertise and was linked to different patron deities representing the respective craft. The *asû* was primarily an expert on drugs and their medical uses in remedies (*bulṭu*) whose knowledge included some surgical interventions (as is clear from the Laws of Hammurapi), while the conjurer or ritual specialist (*āšipu*) served basically as a mediator between the human and divine sphere who was able to identify and interpret any sign in the environment indicative of divine anger, as well any kind of illness, misfortune and evil, and to counter them with the help of incantations, rituals and medical healing procedures. For debates concerning the relationship between the disciplines of *āšipūtu* and *asûtu* and for discussion of their historical developments, see e.g. Attinger 2008, 71–77; Fales 2018; Geller 2010, 43–88; 2018; Jean 2006; Ritter 1965; Scurlock 1999; Sibbing-Plantholt 2022; Steinert 2018.

168 For discussion, see e.g. Stol 2000, 171–192; 2016, 371–372, 375–381, 605–615; Sibbing-Plantholt 2022, 188–192, 217–218.

In contrast, male physicians (*asû*) are only rarely attested directly in the women's healthcare texts. Only a single colophon (N. 4001; text B.2.1) mentions a physician as the copyist/scribe of a text dealing with infertility and tests for pregnancy prognoses, saying that he copied the text "for his learning" (*ana lamādīšu*). This expression suggests that the scribe may have still been an apprentice in his craft but also shows that physicians acquired knowledge in the treatment of women's ailments. The colophon includes secrecy statements that strictly interdict to share this precious knowledge with outsiders to the craft or scholarly circles. Letters from physicians at the Neo-Assyrian royal court rarely refer to their treatment of female members of the court or royal family.[169] In SAA 16, No. 26, the prince Šamaš-mētu-uballiṭ writes to his father Esarhaddon about a sick court woman and requests a physician (*asû*) to come and examine (*amāru*) her.[170] In SAA 10, No. 316 (rev. 22–23), the chief physician Urad-Nanāya informs Esarhaddon that he sends him two plants which are good for a woman in childbirth (*ana sinništi ša tāl[itte] danqū*). Remarkable is a letter (unfortunately very fragmentary) by the medical expert Urad-Gula (SAA 10, No. 293), in which he reports about rituals being performed for a pregnant member of the court (whose name is not preserved).[171] Interestingly, this letter mentions that Urad-Gula brought the patient to the temple of Gula where she was attended to by women(?) who worship different divine avatars of Gula (lines 23'–26'; their exact function cannot be determined). The fragmentary passage also discusses a basket (*masabbu*) that was taken to the temple (presumably with offerings).

Attestations of female physicians (^{munus}a-zu$_{(5)}$; *asâtu*/*asûtu*) are limited to the third and second millennium BCE, with the latest evidence found in Hittite sources. Some of these professional healers are known to have worked for the royal courts (e.g. at Ebla, Mari) and received goods from the queen. Although it has been concluded that the female *asûs* were specialized in healthcare for women and have even been referred to as "gynaecologists", it is likely that they performed very much the same functions as male *asûs*, although their patients may often have been women (Sibbing-Plantholt 2022, 217–218). In one Old Babylonian attestation a female physician was listed together with a midwife (*šabsūtu*) (Stol 2016, 371). Female physicians are not found in first millennium BCE sources and never show up anywhere in the medical texts.

The midwife (^{munus}šà-zu lit. "the one who knows the inside", from which the Akkadian counterpart *šabsūtu* is derived) is the best-attested female professional associated with women's health in the Mesopotamian sources throughout the millennia, whose roles are also highlighted in numerous literary and mythological texts (often via their divine counterparts, the mother or birth goddesses).[172] Other terms and epithets associated with the midwife mark her as a wise (*erištu*) or experienced (*lamittu*) woman. In lexical texts, the profession of the midwife is listed with professions meaning "barber; shaver" (Akkadian *gallābu*), an association that may stem from the shared use of knives and cutting techniques in both professions, as well as from a perception of both professions as health-related occupations (cf. Stol 2000, 172; Sibbing-Plantholt 2022, 184–188, 189).

There are other terms for female occupations associated with midwifery, wet-nursing or childcare in cuneiform textual sources. These include the *qadištu* "holy woman" (Sumerian nu-gig), *kulmašītu* (Sum. nu-bar), *nadītu* lit. "uncultivated (childless) woman" (Sum. lukur), *ištarītu* "the woman of Ištar", *mušēniqtu* "wet-nurse" (Sum. um-me, um-me-ga-lá), and the *tārītu* "nursemaid" (Sum. um-me-da).[173] Of prominent interest here are the Sumerian terms nu-gig (lit. "one who is taboo, sacrosanct", corresponding to Akkadian *qadištu* "holy one") and nu-bar (lit. "one who is set aside"). Literary texts connect these female professions to specific goddesses, especially Inanna and Ninisina, who are said to perform the func-

169 For the Middle Babylonian letters written by medical specialists mentioning treatments for sick female singers, see Waschow 1936; Sibbing-Plantholt 2014.

170 Letters by the exorcists Adad-šumu-uṣur and Marduk-šākin-šumi report about healing rituals that were performed for the queen mother Naqi'a (e.g. SAA 10, No. 200) and about her recovery from illness (SAA 10, No. 244).

171 Urad-Gula who bears the title *āšipu* but is once designated as deputy of the chief physician and as *asû*, may in fact be two different individuals with the same name (Parpola 1983a, Vol. II, 470 Appendix O; PNA 3/2, 1402 no. 5-6). The letter SAA 10, No. 293 may imply that Urad-Gula had connections to the Gula temple, which could point to his profession as an *asû*.

172 On mother and birth goddesses, see e.g. Jacobsen 1973; Krebernik 1993–1997; Stol 2000, 74–82, 109–118; Asher-Greve and Westenholz 2013; Rodin 2014; Steinert 2017b. On the healing goddesses (Gula, Ninisina, Ba'u) as midwives, see Böck 2014a, 30–34; Sibbing-Plantholt 2022, 48–50, 103–104, 130, 141–142. On midwifery in Mesopotamia, see e.g. Civil 2011, 281–284; Karahashi 2017; Stol 2000, 171–181; 2016, 375–381; Sibbing-Plantholt 2022, 188–192; 291–302; Steinkeller 2022. For midwives in the Hittite world, see Beckman 1993, 38–39.

173 For these professions, see Bird 2019, 209–336; Civil 2011, 251, 281–284; Karahashi 2017; Stol 2000, 172–192; 2016, 375–381, 605–616; Steinert 2023, 245, 246–247; Steinkeller 2022, 21–32; Westenholz 1989, 250–260.

tion of the nu-gig among the gods (and therefore serve as patron deities of the human craft).[174] At the same time, these titles may mark the functions performed by these women euphemistically as connected to the liminal and potentially defiling realm of childbirth (associated with impure substances such as the parturient's blood).

Sumerian sources such as the Laws of Ur-Namma portray the nu-gig as a professional performing midwifery and wet-nursing (for a defined wage).[175] In the Sumerian myth *Enlil and Sud* (line 154), the function of the nu-gig is assigned to the mother goddess and is subsumed as "the function(s) of the nu-gig (nam-nu-gig), everything pertaining to women (níĝ-nam munus-e-ne) (which) is something that no one must see (lú igi nu-bar-re-dam)" (Civil 1983, 157; 2011, 282). The passage suggests that these women possessed specific knowledge linked to their craft that was guarded from men.[176] Reviewing the sources from the third and early second millennium BCE, Steinkeller (2022, 25–26) even defined the nu-gig as a professional "concerned with women's health in general, . . . comparable with the modern gynecologist, who provides care during pre-conception, pregnancy, childbirth and immediately after delivery but also deals with all of women's reproductive health issues, including menstruation and breast-related problems."[177] Steinkeller suggests that in the early periods the services of the nu-gig were broader than those of the šà-zu "midwife" (with the latter operating specifically in the context of delivery) and that the activities of the nu-gig had an additional ritual/religious dimension.[178] However, the women's healthcare texts from later centuries suggest that the activities of the midwife were neither limited to the delivery, but that her advice was also sought in the context of treatments for fertility, during pregnancy and in the postpartum period (see below).[179]

Our image of the occupations of the *qadištu, kulmašītu* and *ištarītu* and their activities are unfortunately blurred and patchy, although they are mentioned in texts from the second to the first millennia BCE. It is clear, however, that these professionals were involved in both religious/cultic and secular activities and that the *qadištu, kulmašītu* and *ištarītu* were usually devoted or dedicated to a deity. The *qadištu* appears in texts from the second and first millennium BCE, where she is connected to midwifery and wet-nursing (against a fee), as well as to purifications, participation in exorcistic rites, cultic and musical performances (e.g. Westenholz 1989, 250–260; Macgregor 2012, 12–15; May 2022, 141–144). The reference in the *Atramḫasīs* myth to the "house of the *qadištu*" where the midwife assisted women giving birth may not correspond to reality, however. Thus, the *qadištu* is never mentioned in birth rituals, and no other textual source informs us that women in Mesopotamia gave birth at a place outside their home.[180]

---

174 For the latest discussion, see Steinkeller 2022, 26–29. For Ninisina performing the office of the nu-gig, see the hymn *Ninisina* A, lines 64–81 (Römer 2001, 113; Civil 2011, 282; Böck 2014a, 30–31; ETCSL text 4.22.1; Steinkeller 2022, 26–27). This passage describes the nu-gig's competences linked to fertility, preserving pregnancy and midwifery: manipulations to assist delivery (directing the foetus downward, opening the mouth of the uterus), severing the umbilical cord and caring for the neonate (e.g. cleaning the breathing passage). In the myth *Enki and the World Order* 394–400, paraphernalia including the brick of birth and an umbilical cord-cutter used by the midwife (šà-zu) are assigned to the mother goddess Aruru/Nintur (ETCSL c.1.1.3; Stol 2000a, 111–112).

175 Civil 2011, 245, 251 section E, §E2.

176 Cf. Westenholz 1989, 250–260. Steinkeller (2022, 23–24, 26) surmises that the interdiction expressed here refers to the professional exclusivity of performing the nu-gig's functions and their guild-like organization. The nu-gig also operated in the context of sanctuaries called NÌGIN.GAR (nigar$_x$), localities linked exclusively with the cult of Inanna and Ninisina and metaphorically associated with the womb and foetus (Sjöberg 1969, 92–93; Stol 2000, 29; Steinkeller 2022, 29–31 for the etymology "(place where) the foetus/newborn are placed"). For the nu-gig/*qadištu* as wet-nurses, see Stol 2000, 186–187.

177 Similarly, Civil (2011, 282): "The conclusion is that the *nugig* was a midwife, with duties not limited to the parturition but extending all through pregnancy, administering the physical preparations and care given to pregnant women in traditional societies: massages and manipulations presumed to place the fetus in a favorable position for birth, dilation of the cervix by insertion of certain plants or stones, etc."

178 The midwife and the nu-gig/*qadištu* are mentioned side by side in a few sources from the second millennium (Stol 2000, 173), e.g. in *Atramḫasīs* (Lambert and Millard 1969, 62: 290), which hints at overlapping professional profiles and occasional collaboration of both professionals. Steinkeller (2022, 24) assumes the profession of the midwife was less prestigious and her position subordinate to the nu-gig. In contrast, Stol (2000, 187) assumes that the *qadištu* in Old Babylonian times did not have a high social status; she often worked as a paid wet-nurse for income.

179 Note in this connection the negative depiction of the female demon Lamaštu as the "anti-midwife", from which the essential activities of a real midwife can be gleaned: "counting the months", "opening" the 'door' (of the womb) during delivery, and "wiping clean" (*kuppuru*) the baby (Farber 2014, 260, 282–283 OB$_3$ lines 3–6): "Although not a physician (*asâtu*), she puts on bandages, although not a midwife (*tabsât*), she wipes the baby clean. She keeps counting the months of the pregnant women, constantly blocking the 'door' of the women about to give birth (*wālidātum*)".

180 Lambert and Millard 1969, 62–63 I 290, with Macgregor 2012, 13.

Interestingly, the nu-gig/*qadištu* and nu-bar/*kulmašītu* are also associated with infanticide or abortion in a few literary texts, e.g. in the *Curse over Agade* 241.[181] It is not entirely clear whether this passage refers to infanticide or to abortion of premature foetuses, but the line is formulated as a curse negating the usual pronatalist role of the nu-gig and the nu-bar. The connection between these and other female occupations and abortion also seems to be alluded to in a first millennium BCE incantation to Šamaš (SpTU 3, No. 67 iii 9–12). Here, *qadištu* and *kulmašītu* appear together with other female titles: "It is in your power, o Šamaš, to call the names of the foetuses (*kūbu*) of the *nadītu*, the *qadištu*, the *kulmašītu*, the *ištarītu* of Anu, the little ones who never knew their own names, who (never) saw the sunlight!"[182]

It is difficult to draw definite conclusions from such literary passages about these female occupations in the first millennium BCE. Passages such as the Šamaš incantation quoted above may allude to sexual taboos that women like the *nadītu* had to observe, while also pointing to a "devaluation" of old titles and changes in the roles of such female professions in the later periods of Mesopotamian history (Stol 2016, 426). In Old Babylonian times, the *nadītu*, *qadištu* and *kulmašītu* were groups of women dedicated by their parents to a god or temple; their rights of inheritance, possibilities of marrying and providing offspring for their husbands (through a secondary wife or female slave) are detailed in legal texts.[183] The *nadītus* were dedicated to a deity (e.g. Šamaš at Sippar; Marduk at Babylon) and were generally not allowed to bear children. Some *nadītus* were allowed to marry, while others led a celibate, pious life in a "convent" or "cloister" (*gagû*) linked to temples; both cloistered and married *nadītus* could adopt children (Stol 2016, 584–604).

The *qadištu*, although devoted to a deity (usually Adad), could marry and have children and is mentioned in connection with wet-nursing (for a fee), especially in Old Babylonian sources. The participation of the *qadištu* in cultic and other ritual activities is documented in Middle and Neo-Assyrian texts, e.g. in a ritual in the Adad temple at Assur.[184] A Neo-Assyrian letter to Esarhaddon by his chief exorcist Marduk-šākin-šumi specifies that a *qadištu* should perform exorcistic rituals for the male royal offspring (SAA 10, No. 246).[185] In another late text (a hymn praising the inhabitants of Babylon), the *qadištu* is linked with purifications. Here she appears beside the *nadītu* and the *entu*-priestess as classes of pious, respectful women who are characterised in more favourable terms as beneficial and knowledgeable. Unusually, the *nadītu* is linked to midwifery or the care for pregnant women in this text:

> "Women who have learned insight at their work (*sinnišātu ša ina šiprīšina tašīmta aḫzū*): the *entu*-votaries (NIN.DINGIR.RA) who are faithful(?) to their husbands, the *nadītu*-women who keep the womb healthy through (their) wisdom (*nadâte ša ina nēmeqi uballaṭā rēmu*), the *qadištu*-women who [per]form purifications with water. They respect the taboo, they observe the interdict, they pray . . . They are reverent, observant, minding the good. Daughters of the gods . . ." (KAR 321: 6–9; Lambert 1960, pl. 36; Foster 1996, 756; Stol 2000, 172)

While this passage contrasts with the Šamaš incantation quoted above, the negative image of these female functions associated with knowledge about matters of ritual and women's reproductive health is also communicated in other first millennium BCE learned or literary texts. Thus, the *ištarītu*, *qadištu*, *nadītu* and *kulmašītu* are depicted as witches performing sorcery (*Maqlû* III 40–55) and are mentioned together with the prostitute (*ḫarimtu*) in negative terms as dubious marriage partners.[186] As Sibbing-Plantholt (2022, 191–192, 297–302) underlines, these negative images may point to competition between male, learned healers (especially *āšipus*) and female lay healers who often were experts in women's

181 Cooper 1983, 240–241 (lines 244–245); ETCSL text 2.1.5; Attinger 2007, 13 with n. 122–123; Stol 2016, 421: "May the prostitute hang herself in the door of her drinking house, may your mother the nu-gig and your mother the nu-bar kill their children."

182 The foetuses (*kūbu*) of the *nadītus* and *qadištus* are also invoked in incantations (Farber 2014, 266, 294–295 "Ug" III 8', "ND" 11'-12'; 328); one passage (SpTU 1, No. 44: 67) claims that the child of a *nadītu* does not thrive, followed by a reference to an aborted foetus (*nīd libbi*) that will never suckle its mother's breast. Little is known about the function of the nu-bar/*kulmašītu*. The nu-bar is mentioned side by side with the nu-gig, see e.g. in an Ur III-period incantation against the demon Samana (Nougayrol 1949, pl. III–IV lines 14–15; Finkel 1998, 72–76 No. 1; Stol 2016, 438; Beck 2015, 35).

183 Stol 2016, 422; see e.g. Laws of Hammurapi §§144–146, 181-182; Laws of Lipit-Ištar §22 (Roth 1997, 30, 198, 118). In Old Babylonian times, the *kulmašītu* is found among other groups of dedicated women, and in a few sources, she is associated with breastfeeding (Stol 2016, 605–607, 615–616). The exact occupation of the *ištarītu* in the cult remains obscure but her designation implies a link to the goddess Ištar; she may have served as wet-nurse (cf. Stol 2016, 425, 612). Women with the title *ištarītu* are occasionally mentioned beside the midwife or the *qadištu* in second millennium BCE texts, which may indicate that they could have a similar role.

184 Menzel 1989, II T2–T4 (KAR 154); Westenholz 1989, 254; Macgregor 2012, 13. See also May 2022, 142 for another Neo-Assyrian text describing role of the *qadištu* in the context of purifications during the New Years Festival.

185 See May 2022, 143 for discussion.

186 For texts that give the *ištarītu*, *nadītu* and *kulmašītu* a bad reputation of being promiscuous and witches performing sorcery, see Stol 2016, 604, 611–612, 615–616; Schwemer 2007a, 76–77; MacGregor 2012, 10–12.

health matters and presumably provided services for the lower strata of society to which they themselves often belonged. One may see here a desire to marginalize such female professionals and their knowledge, apparently perceived as a threat by male experts.[187]

The reviewed sources leave us with a contradictory and patchy image of female occupations in the realm of midwifery and lay healing, in terms of their specific activities, social esteem and evaluations. Thus, over the course of three millennia we need to reckon with changes and differences in the meanings of such terms (as *nadītu*, *qadištu*) and with changes in social roles, status and settings associated with these women. Furthermore, several of the key sources quoted for these professionals are literary texts whose historical accuracy may be questioned, and which may reflect specific (often male-biased) perspectives. Nonetheless, the overview of sources has shown that women in ancient Mesopotamia could potentially turn to several different female lay practitioners in matters of reproduction and female health for their services, beside the male healing experts *āšipu* and *asû*.

Female healers involved in women's healthcare did not write down their knowledge and may often have been illiterate, as far as we know (cf. May 2018b; 2022, 141, 143). There are occasional remarks in women's healthcare texts that mark certain prescriptions or procedures as oral lore (*šūt/ša pî*; *šum'uttu*).[188] Unfortunately, the origin of this oral lore is never specified, although passages may at times record household remedies stemming from the sphere of folk healing practices, which would prominently have been the realm of female lay healers and midwives (e.g. Stol 2007b, 1). Intriguing, however, are first millennium BCE women's healthcare texts that mention the midwife's presence and collaboration with the male healer in treating female patients.[189] These references draw attention to the midwife's intimate knowledge of the female body and her practical expertise and knowledge of remedies. For example, in the fragment UET 7, No. 123 (text B.2.2), which contains tests for pregnancy prognoses and treatments to promote female fertility, the midwife had to examine (*ḫâṭu*) the patient, presumably to check the effect of an ongoing treatment procedure:

> *ša qerbīssa(!) innassaḫu u šabsūtu iḫâṭāšu maltaktāšu* [22'] *kī irrû kī lā irrû . . .*
> "(When) that which is (in) her womb is removed, then the midwife should examine her. (This is) the test for her(?) (or: her test?) (to see) [22'] whether she will conceive or whether she will not conceive . . ."

Unfortunately, the details of this examination or the reason why the midwife was required to do it (and not the male healer), remain shadowy. Was a manual examination of the patient's womb required, and this close-up inspection was not appropriate or allowed to be carried out by a male healer? Or does it imply specific insider knowledge that only the midwife possessed? The following sentence is likewise ambiguous: Does "*her* test" (*maltaktāšu*) refer to the patient (i.e. the test for her?), or could it refer to a test used and communicated (to the male healer) by the midwife, which is then reported in the following lines of the text?

This text passage also throws up the unresolved question as to whether male healers had unrestricted direct access to female patients' bodies, performed physical examinations of women's private parts or indeed applied remedies (such as tampons) in these body zones with the same freedom as they would when treating male patients (cf. Heeßel 2006: 12–13). Unfortunately, we are left in the dark about such potential restrictions (e.g. the presence of other persons during male healers' treatment of female patients (such as female household members or the woman's husband) may perhaps have been silently assumed). It is also unknown whether the male healer would regularly collaborate with a midwife. While male healers doubtlessly had anatomical knowledge of women's bodies, the fact that some instructions in women's healthcare texts for applying remedies (such as tampons) are formulated in the third person rather than the second person singular, may suggest that patients may have possessed some (limited) agency to apply these remedies by themselves. In contrast to the Hippocratic or Rabbinic texts, Mesopotamian women's healthcare texts never explicitly mention or require the (manual) self-examination by the patient, and they refer to the patients' own experience or knowledge of bodily processes only indirectly or laconically.

---

187 For similar strategies of othering in Graeco-Roman medical authors who attribute negative practices (such as abortion) or repulsive superstitious remedies to prostitutes, see e.g. Flemming 2000, 40–42; 2007, 273–275; Lehmhaus 2023, 68; Steinert 2023, 277, 290.

188 See e.g. BM 38624+ iv 3' (text A.2.1); BM 50700 obv. 11 (text A.2.3); SpTU 5, No. 253: 3' (text E.2.6); BM 45736 iv 12 (text A.2.5); BAM 240: 16' (text D.2.1) and the discussion above.

189 The midwife is also mentioned in birth incantations both from the second and first millennium BCE (e.g. BAM 248 iii 35 // (text D.1.1 lines 160): "May the midwife not be kept (waiting), may the pregnant woman be all right!" (*šabsūtu ay ikkali erītu līšer*).

A second text mentioning the midwife is SpTU 4, No. 153 obv. 23–26 (text D.1.11) from the exorcists' library of the descendants of Ekur-zakir, this time in a birth context. Here, the midwife's examination of the patient is required to confirm the progress of labour and the appropriate moment for administering a specific remedy to speed up the delivery:

> "You let her walk around. Her baby will start to approach (come out) and [when(?)] the midwife examines (the woman), she will tell you, thus: "Birth is near!" (*šabsūtu tammaru-ma iqabbâkka umma alādu qerub*) Afterwards you administer to her (another?) suppository of *ḫur*[-*ru*-bird] excrement (and) cumin. The *ḫurru*-bird excrement and cumin should dilate (lit. "open") (her) considerably. You (also) administer (it) to her when [she has] a lot of pain(?) (lit. "is in difficulty"). Should she let her (amniotic) fluid flow out completely, her baby will die."

Further evidence for the activities of the midwife in the context of delivery is found in two Neo-Assyrian texts from Nineveh. K. 11530 (text D.1.5) refers to actions of neonate care performed by the midwife: she "wipes off" (*kuppuru*) the newborn and rubs (*muššu'u*) "his chest" with oil, puts her fingers into "his mouth", so that *mucus* (*nīṣu*) is discharged (for unhindered breathing). The fragment Sm. 157 + 1134 (text D.1.6) appears to give instructions for the midwife's practice during delivery and in the postpartum period. In this unfortunately very fragmentary text, the midwife seems to be the key expert able to deal with dangerous complications in childbirth and to perform obstetric interventions. The texts mentioning the midwife within women's healthcare texts do not evoke the impression that the midwife acted merely in an assistant role to the male healer (cf. Sibbing-Plantholt 2022, 300–301). The discussed examples rather suggest a division of labour between male healer and midwife and may underline the indispensable roles and expertise of the midwife in the context of delivery, in particular.[190] It is possible that male healers absorbed or adopted some practices and techniques of midwives, as mentioned above. This may also apply to the practice of massage (*muššu'u*) attested in women's healthcare texts in the context of delivery (beside anointing the woman in labour), since this technique is also associated with midwives in other cultures.[191]

The multitude of male and female professionals involved in women's healthcare in Mesopotamia is also reflected in the appearance of the different patron deities associated with healing professions, in addition to other deities connected to women and to reproduction, in the women's healthcare texts themselves.

The gods Marduk/Asalluḫi and Enki/Ea as the divine patrons of the conjurer (*āšipu*) naturally play a prominent role in the women's healthcare texts. Both deities feature in incantations for women that use the classic format of the Marduk-Ea dialogue, for example in BM 97093 (text II.1.1), BAM 244: 41ff. (text B.1.1); BM 34208 (text D.1.)) and in BAM 248 (and dupl.), the Neo-Assyrian Birth Compendium (text D.1.1). The god of magic *par excellence* Marduk/Asalluḫi is clearly the most important deity in the spells of the Neo-Assyrian Birth Compendium, while the mother goddess and other birth goddesses (more prominent in earlier texts) even appear in a subordinate role. Marduk/Asalluḫi clearly seems to have absorbed traditional roles of the mother/birth goddesses, since he is called or calls himself "(male) midwife" (ŠÀ.ZU, *šabsû*) in at least two incantations (D.1.1 lines 194–195, 197–198). Ea and Asalluḫi occur together in this role (e.g. "opening the path" for the baby) already in Ur III-period and Old Babylonian birth incantations (see e.g. UM 29-15-367 // VS 17, 33 (van Dijk 1975; Cunningham 1997, 69–75); BM 97093 (text II.1.1); BM 115745, text II.1.2).

Two other significant male deities in the women's healthcare texts are the sun god (Utu/Šamaš) and the moon god Nanna(r)/Sîn. The moon god's links to fertility, pregnancy and birth can be traced back at least to Old Babylonian times and are underlined in birth incantations (see e.g. text D.1.1) and in rituals for female fertility and offspring (N. 4001 (text B.2.1) // BM 51246+ (A.2.7); AO 4425A+B (text B.2.6), where Sîn is invoked via prayers and offerings, sometimes together with the sun god.[192] Sîn and Šamaš also play the leading role in a group of rituals to postpone an ill-omened birth in the month Nisannu (KAR 223 //, text D.3.1). The moon god as luminary is associated with the month (and therefore a regulator of female bodies during pregnancy), but also with cows and boats, two important motifs representing the woman in labour/pregnancy. The sun god as divine judge appears in many different contexts and rituals within women's healthcare texts, in which his intervention and help are requested. Notably, Utu/Šamaš as a god who oversees the realms of heaven, earth and netherworld, is intimately linked to taking care of human foetuses during pregnancy and delivery and to determining human destiny. Several birth incantations from the second and first millennium BCE invoke the sun god to set the baby free from the womb and to show it the daylight (Polonsky 2006; Wasserman and Zomer 2022, No. 8, 12; BAM 248 obv. ii 23

190 Rare images depicting scenes of delivery from Mesopotamia show both male and female birth attendants, but these date almost exclusively to the third and early second millennium BCE (Battini 2006, 6 fig. 6; 14 fig. 19; Otto 2016, 135–142).

191 For massage as an important cross-cultural element in traditional birth practises, see Kuntner 1994.

192 See also Stol 2000, 61–62, 63–64, 66–68, 71; Hätinen 2021.

(text D.1.1)). A bilingual prayer (K. 3025 // K. 879; text D.1.8) seeks Šamaš's help during a delivery that is hindered by the machinations of sorcery. In two rituals, Šamaš is approached as the guardian of healing plants ("dog's tongue-plant" and "shepherd's staff-plant") that are used to stop bleeding during pregnancy (BM 40152 (text C.1.8); BM 51246+ (text A.2.7). Together with Ea and Asalluḫi, the sun god receives offerings and is also addressed in a ritual for a woman affected by an ominous eclipse which resembles Namburbi rituals (BM 47801; text E.2.3).

Unsurprisingly, female deities are well represented in women's healthcare texts in their functions as mother and birth goddesses as well as goddesses of healing, all of whom could perform the function of a divine midwife (Stol 2000, 74–83).[193]

The most important healing goddesses performing midwifery are Gula, Ninisina and Nintinuga. Another goddess syncretised with Gula and taking on her roles as female healer is Ninkarrak, originally an oath deity.[194] Ninkarrak appears (interchangeable with Gula) in texts concerned with rituals dealing with repeated infant death and miscarriages, in which Ninkarrak and Gula are identified as divine agents responsible for the problem (SpTU 3, No. 84 (text C.3.4); BM 42327+ (text C.3.3); SpTU 5, No. 248 (text C.3.10 lines 62–67)). Gula is mentioned again in a similar context in KAR 247 (text C.3.6, line 41'''). One spell to stop gynaecological bleeding is specifically attributed to Gula in BM 40152 ii 14' (text C.1.8), and she is mentioned together with Bēlet-ilī, Ištar and Šamaš in another incantation for this purpose (BAM 237; text C.1.4 line 53''); she thus is linked with powers to interrupt as well as to preserve pregnancy and bring it to full term. More common in the texts is the instruction to leave medicine outside overnight before Gula or the Goat Star (Lyra) equated with her (e.g. STT 98 obv. 8' (text A.1.1)). While Gula is encountered as divine midwife cutting the umbilical cord and determining the child's destiny in birth incantations as early as the Ur III-period (UM 29-15-367 iii 13–14 // VS 17, 33: 25–26; van Dijk 1975; Cunningham 1997, 69–75), other avatars of Gula occur in this role in later texts, especially Ninisina. Thus, Ninisina's assigned role as divine nu-gig (midwife) and her competences are specified in the Sumerian hymn *Ninisina* A (from the Old Babylonian period; Civil 2011, 282; Steinkeller 2022, 26–27; Sibbing-Plantholt 2022, 130), and she still appears in this role together with Nintinuga in a bilingual birth incantation from the first millennium BCE (BM 34208, text D.1.9).

The function of the midwife in a broader context of creating human beings is also performed by mother and birth goddesses such as Nintur, Aruru, Bēlet-ilī, Mami, Ninḫursaĝa and Nimaḫ (Stol 2000, 74–83; Asher-Greve and Westenholz 2013; Steinert 2017b); several of these goddesses feature in birth incantations and in other spells within the women's healthcare texts. In birth incantations, delivery is sometimes imagined as taking place in the temple of the mother goddess (e.g. BM 34208 (text D.1.9); K. 11530 (text D.1.8)). Bēlet-ilī is invoked in her capacity as "mistress of the womb" (*bēlet rēmi*) in the Neo-Assyrian Birth Compendium BAM 248 (text D.1.1 lines 48–52), but she is also referred to as the one who created human beings' blood (alluding to myths in which the mother goddess creates the first human beings together with Enki/Ea) in an incantation to stop bleeding during pregnancy (BAM 237; text C.1.4 line 49''). The titles "creatrix of humankind" (*bāniat awīlūtim*) as well as *asûtum* "female physician" are given to Bēlet-ilī and Ninḫursaĝa in Old Babylonian birth incantations, where they act as midwife (CUSAS 32, 26a: 8'–9'; CUSAS 32, 28a: 13–14; YOS 11, No. 86: 18; Wasserman and Zomer 2022, No. 6, 7, 14). A special link to human offspring is drawn with Ninmaḫ in rituals like SpTU 3, No. 84 (text C.3.4) and KAR 247 // (text C.3.6), performed against cases of repeated miscarriage, in which her powers over foetal growth and pregnancy are invoked (which is reminiscent of the goddess' creating several abnormal foetuses in the Sumerian myth *Enki and Ninmaḫ*).

Although the Venus goddess Inanna/Ištar was not a birth or mother goddess, she was intimately linked with sexuality, fecundity, human reproduction and womanhood, which explains her repeated appearance in the corpus of texts edited in this volume. In a couple of texts, she takes on the roles of a midwife, wet-nurse or protectress (especially of rulers) and her help and protection was sought by women in matters of reproduction and pregnancy.[195] For example, among the rituals and incantations against bleeding during pregnancy in BAM 237(+) (text C.1.4), Ištar is invoked through incantations and *šigû*-prayers uttered by the patient. Relatedly, the constellation "Wagon" (Ursa Major) associated with Venus/

193 The goddess Ningirim(a), a deity of purification and incantations, is further attested occasionally in expressions attributing spells recited for women (e.g. in labour) to her, often together with Ea, Asalluḫi, Gula and Damu (e.g. Rudik 2011, 318 FSB 56 (D); STT 241 (text C.3.1: 27); LKA 9 // CUNES 52-15-029 (text C.3.5: 29'); SpTU 5, No. 248 (text C.3.10: 18).

194 For detailed discussion of these goddesses and their relationship, see Sibbing-Plantholt 2022.

195 For Inanna as nu-gig, which is linked to midwifery and nursing, see Zgoll 1997 and above. For more on Inanna and Ištar, see e.g. Groneberg 1997; Lapinkivi 2004; Leick 1994, 80–169; Matsushima 2014; Parpola 1997, xxi–xlviii; Stol 2000, 269 *passim*; 2016, 405–409, 419-435, 638-661. For women's prayers to Ištar requesting offspring, see Zgoll 2003, "Ištar 4" and "Ištar 23". For links of Inanna/Ištar to menstruation, menarche and female sexual organs, see also Steinert 2017b, 212–214; 2023, 247 n. 50.

Ištar is addressed or receives offerings in protective rituals against miscarriage (SpTU 3, No. 84 (text C.3.4); BM 48030 (text C.3.8)). A manifestation of Ištar venerated in Assyria (Nimrud), Šarrat-kidmuri (Queen of the Kidmuru temple), is invoked in a similar context in an incantation in STT 241 (text C.3.1, line 20), together with the god Lillu (a son of the mother goddess).[196] A birth incantation on a fragment from Nineveh (K. 11530, text D.1.5) mentions the goddess Bēlet-ēkalli ("Lady of the Palace"), who belongs to the circle of Inanna/Ištar, in association with a cow pen and birthing among cows. Interestingly, a few older Sumerian birth incantations equate or identify the women in labour with the goddesses Aruru, Nintur, Inanna and Ninḫursaĝa, underlining their motherly nature or their connection with creating offspring.[197]

Last but not least, a special feature of incantations for women (especially of birth incantations) is the invocation of Elamite deities (Kiririša, Napiriša, Naḫḫunte, Narunde) acting as intermediaries or messengers (of Sîn or Marduk) in two incantations of the Neo-Assyrian Birth Compendium (text D.1.1 lines 40–47, 163–172; see also A.3461 (text A.1.2)), which seems to be a reflex of an old tradition of birth incantations in the Elamite language (attested on Old Babylonian tablets) which feature the same deities (Krebernik 2018, 31).

6 Directions for Future Research

In conclusion to this overview of Mesopotamian women's healthcare, it is hoped that the present volume of text editions will contribute to the study of cuneiform healings texts as well as to the history of ancient medicine concerned with women more generally. Due to constraints of feasibility, this work necessarily had to focus on the reconstruction and decipherment of textual sources and on philological analyses and interpretations of the immediate contents of the texts under study. Due to the fragmentary state of the source texts, numerous textual difficulties could not be resolved satisfactorily, leaving us with ambiguities and several possible interpretations or readings. These difficulties are addressed extensively in the philological notes of the text editions, and alternative views proposed in previous studies or suggested to me through personal communications with colleagues are pointed out. Hopefully, some of the gaps and uncertainties in our knowledge can be filled in the future, through the discovery of new text sources.

Many issues and broader questions could only be touched on briefly and could not be explored in detail. It is hoped nonetheless that the sources presented here will be useful for future research into women's healthcare in ancient Mesopotamia and beyond. Much work still needs to be done in several directions. For example, the interrelations or specificities of Mesopotamian women's healthcare texts vis-à-vis other areas of cuneiform medical texts as well as the question of gender-specific medicine(s) deserve more attention in the future. A second promising area of research would be a more systematic exploration of *materia medica* in women's healthcare texts and its uses in comparison to applications beyond conditions specific to the female body.

Undoubtably, a third important avenue for further exploration is offered by comparisons, both synchronic and diachronic, between Mesopotamian women's healthcare texts and other medical traditions in the ancient Near East and Mediterranean world. Thus, cross-cultural similarities (at times substantial ones) as well as differences in concepts of the female body and in the ways of treating its conditions and their development in the *longue durée* promise to be a vast and fruitful area for research and cross-disciplinary collaboration (see e.g. Stol 2000; Couto-Ferreira and Verderame 2018; Lehmhaus 2023). This should include further explorations of cross-cultural transfers of medical lore on women's health in the ancient world, of which previous scholarly work in this direction has offered glimpses (e.g. Geller 2004, 34–36; Geller 2021).

The present study of Mesopotamian women's healthcare has highlighted several close similarities with Hippocratic views of the female body and treatments for specific conditions such as infertility and its causes (see Chapter B; Steinert 2020; 2021a for discussion). Especially Late Babylonian texts which are roughly contemporary with Hippocratic medicine raise the question of cross-cultural transfers of knowledge. For example, through the texts edited here it has become clear that notions suggesting thinking in correspondences with the qualities hot, cold, wet and dry, which is one of the most characteristic elements of Greco-Roman medicine (including Hippocratic gynaecological works), also appear to play a considerable role in first millennium BCE Mesopotamian women's healthcare. This can be seen most clearly in the notion of blood and bleeding as hot (and wet) encountered in several cuneiform medical texts edited in this volume. Relatedly,

196 Meinhold 2009, 110.

197 See e.g. BM 97093: 1–4 (text II.1.1); E 47.190: 1–3 (G. Farber 1984, *JNES* 43, 313ff.); AUAM 73.1425 v 4–5 (Rudik 2011, 327–331 FSB 58).

notions of heating, cooling, drying and moistening can be seen to play a key role in Mesopotamian treatments for women and their use of signature ingredients, for example in remedies for stopping or inducing the flow of blood, but also in prescriptions against fevers. Should such similarities be seen as independent or as interconnected phenomena and developments? Other, more specific elements encountered in Late Babylonian texts edited here raise questions about possible borrowings or adaptations of medical terms and concepts during this period, such as the occurrence of the term *ummu šalšu* "tertian fever" not previously known from Babylonian texts but perhaps a calque translation of the corresponding Greek term *tritaios pyretos* (see text A.2.6). Another aspect of Late Babylonian medical texts highlighted by examples edited in this volume and in need of further study is the increasing use of new and rare technical terms (as well as names of ingredients) that may stem from Aramaic or Greek.

A final note on the presentation of the text editions in this work, which adopts the basic format and structure applied in the volumes of CMAwR 1–3 (Abusch and Schwemer 2011; 2016; Abusch et al. 2020). Thus, each text is introduced in a brief overview of the manuscript(s) and their contents in a "synopsis", followed by a (score) transliteration, a bound transcription with translation, and philological notes. The Akkadian transcriptions attempt to capture variant (e.g. dialectal) forms or aberrant spellings gleaned from syllabic renderings, without strictly seeking to harmonize morphological or other grammatical variations. For example, the singular accusative case ending *-a* is added in the case of nouns written logographically to assist understanding of syntax, although most syllabic spellings in first millennium BCE texts do not differentiate nominative and accusative anymore or mark case endings in a haphazard manner. No attempt was made to render Sumerian texts in normalized, bound transcriptions.

Addendum:

One recently identified text belonging to the corpus of first millennium BCE women's healthcare texts that could not be included in this volume is Ashm. 1971-405 (courtesy of H. Stadhouders), a Neo-Babylonian fragment with simple prescriptions resembling remedies and ingredients to stop bleeding and related conditions in BAM 237 (text C.1.4). A transliteration is available via the website of the electronic Babylonian Library project (https://www.ebl.badw.de/library/Ashm-1971.405).

Text Editions

Part I: **Diagnostic Texts Concerned with Women**

I.1 *Diagnostic Handbook* (SA.GIG) Tablets 36–39 and Related Material

This chapter offers a survey of first millennium BCE Mesopotamian diagnostic texts concerned with women. In this period, women's health issues were collected in the final subsection of the diagnostic series with the ancient title *Sakikkû* (SA.GIG) "Symptoms", also referred to as the *Diagnostic Handbook* by modern scholars. The last subsection of the *Diagnostic Handbook* consisted of five chapters (Tablets 36–40), of which Tablets 36–39 dealt with women, while Tablet 40 was concerned with conditions of infants. The *Diagnostic Handbook* has repeatedly been in the focus of intense study by Assyriologists since Labat (1951), but due to the patchy preservation of the sources our knowledge of Tablets 36–39 is still incomplete.[198] This chapter presents a treatment of all currently known sources related to first millennium BCE Mesopotamian diagnostic texts concerned with women: an edition of *Diagnostic Handbook* Tablets 36 and 37 (unequally well preserved) as well as two fragments of related content.[199] These materials are complemented by three fragments of commentaries (one Neo-Assyrian and two Late Babylonian fragments) on *Diagnostic Handbook* Tablets 36, 37 and 39. These scholarly commentaries offer additional insight into parts of the *Diagnostic Handbook*'s "gynaecological" chapters still unknown to us, as well as glimpses of the textual hermeneutics that Babylonian and Assyrian scholars and medical specialists applied to the "classical" or canonical texts of their tradition.[200]

The tablets on women in the *Diagnostic Handbook* SA.GIG reflect a roughly logical organisation of the topics included in the last section of the handbook. Tablet 36, the first chapter of the sixth section of the series, had the title (incipit) *Šumma ālittu erâtma* "If a fertile woman is pregnant". Its main concern are predictions based on the observation of conspicuous external features of a pregnant woman's body. *Diagnostic Handbook* Tablet 37, of which only a fraction of the text is preserved, had the title "If a pregnant woman is sick" (*Šumma erītu marṣatma*). It begins with predictions related to engaging in intercourse with a sick pregnant woman. The tablet then continues with symptom descriptions that are introduced with "If a woman is sick" and therefore deal with female patients in general (instead of pregnant women in particular). No manuscripts of Tablets 38–39 identified with certainty are known to date, but their titles are preserved in an ancient series catalogue (Schmidtchen 2018b, 316). These two incipits, "If a woman's (amniotic) fluid flows for three days" (*Šumma sinništu mûša šalāšti ūmī illakū* = Tablet 38) and "If a woman in confinement is bloated and belches" (*Šumma sinništu iddip u igeššū* = Tablet 39), suggest that their respective topics were concerned with specific pregnancy-related symptoms and problems surrounding delivery on the one hand, as well as with postpartum complications on the other.[201] The final Tablet 40 dealing with health problems of babies forms a logical conclusion of the sixth section of the *Diagnostic Handbook*.

I.1.1 *Diagnostic Handbook* Tablet 36: Prognoses for Pregnant Women and Their Unborn Children

Diagnostic Handbook Tablet 36 with the title (incipit) *Šumma ālittu erâtma* "If a fertile woman is pregnant" has come down to us in an almost completely preserved manuscript. As mentioned above, the tablet focuses on predictions based on the observation of conspicuous external features of a pregnant woman's body, but it also includes entries describing symptoms indicating a health issue, conspicuous or abnormal behaviour, as well as attitudes and emotional states of a pregnant woman. One section towards the end of the tablet deals with the positive or negative consequences of sexual intercourse for a pregnant woman.

While the contents of the sixth section as a whole embrace women and babies, Tablet 36 shows a particularly strong interest in predicting the sex, well-being, chances of survival, future fate and social position of the unborn child, while only a minority of entries consists in predictions concerning the health, well-being or survival of the pregnant woman.

198 See e.g. Heeßel 2000; 2010b, 28; Stol 2000a, 193–203; Scurlock 2014a, 13–271; Schmidtchen 2018a, 2018b, 2021; Fales 2016, 2018; Minen 2018, 2020; Steinert 2021b, 143, 147, 150, 154–171.

199 Including LKU 126, a fragment with birth omens that may belong to *Diagnostic Handbook* Tablet 38.

200 For general surveys of cuneiform commentaries and hermeutic techniques, see Frahm 2011; Gabbay 2016; for commentaries on the *Diagnostic Handbook*, see Wee 2019a, 2019b.

201 Schmidtchen 2021a, 45, 48–50; see also LKU 126, edited in section 5 of this chapter.

https://doi.org/10.1515/9781501506475-002

More than fifty of the 115 entries of the tablet make predictions about the sex of the foetus (Minen 2020, 15 n. 36). Since the focus was on pregnant but healthy women, only few of the omens in Tablet 36 report actual symptoms of disease or make medical diagnoses, while the selection of observed body parts and physical features as well as certain hermeneutic patterns show similarities with the observations and predictions about female reproductive capacities in physiognomic omens for women (Couto-Ferreira 2008; Minen 2020).

Tablet 36 is the only one of the four tablets of the *Diagnostic Handbook* (Tablets 36–39) concerned with women that is almost completely preserved. The main witness is a skilfully written tablet from the Achaemenid period (ms. a, BM 92694). According to its colophon, ms. a was copied by Nabû-kuṣuršu, a brewer-apprentice of the god Nabû (i.e. of the Ezida temple in Borsippa) and was intended for his study (Hunger 1968, 51 No. 127; the colophon refers to an original from Borsippa). The tablet is dated to the 11th year of an Achaemenid king Artaxerxes (either Artaxerxes I (453 BCE) or II (393 BCE)). Other tablets written by Nabû-kuṣuršu are known, among them several lexical texts (Hunger 1968, Nos. 124–126, 128–130, 132) such as A = *nâqu* and Ur$_5$-ra = *ḫubullu*). He also copied Tablet 2 of the *Diagnostic Handbook* (BM 76022; TDP, 6–16; pl. 3: 22–25; Hunger 1968, No. 131).

To date, four more fragments, two from the Late Babylonian period (mss. b and c) and two Neo-Assyrian exemplars from Ashurbanipal's library at Nineveh (mss. D and E), have been identified as witnesses for Tablet 36. Ms. b (whose exact provenience is uncertain) presents a large fragment of a portrait-shaped tablet almost identical in layout and spacing of the cuneiform signs to ms. a. The upper portion of the obverse and lower portion of the reverse of ms. b are missing; no colophon is preserved. Both mss. a and b have horizontal guiding lines drawn out between empty spaces over the tablet, and their text presents only minimal variants. However, the switch between obverse and reverse occurs at different points in mss. a and b. On the reverse, ms. b omits two lines encountered in ms. a; in a few lines ms. b shows a differing text layout (where two entries are combined in one line).

Ms. c (from Uruk) is a small fragment preserving about ten lines of text. Compared with the main manuscript, ms. c seems to present an abbreviated version of Tablet 36, omitting several lines encountered in ms. a, as well as a few omens with diverging text unknown from ms. a.

On the other hand, mss. D and E attest to the presence of Tablet 36 in Ashurbanipal's library in the seventh century BCE. These two fragments feature a few variant spellings and slight textual divergences in comparison with the Late Babylonian witnesses, but the preserved fragmentary lines run parallel to a section on the reverse of ms. a.

Ms. F from Hattuša preserves twenty lines of diagnostic entries which form a close parallel to a section of Tablet 36, attesting to a Middle Babylonian precursor of these omens. Although ms. F reflects an earlier version, the omens on the fragment closely match diagnostic entries in lines 26–55 of ms. a. Sometimes several consecutive lines run parallel in mss. a and F, but the standard version presented by mss. a and b adds additional omens not found in ms. F. Because of the close similarities to the standard version of Tablet 36 and because the fragment presents the oldest known example of a diagnostic text concerned with women, the omens of ms. F have been included here, although strictly speaking the manuscript does not belong to the first millennium BCE diagnostic series. Several other diagnostic texts bearing close parallels to entries from the later *Diagnostic Handbook* were discovered at Hattuša (see Wilhelm 1994, 104–106).

The omens of Tablet 36 focus on prognoses concerning the well-being, future fate and sex of the woman's foetus, or they give prognoses concerning the woman's well-being or health. The tablet contains four ruled-off section of differing length. The first long section (lines 1–71) is roughly organised "from head to foot": lines 1–8 are concerned with the top of the forehead, lines 9–14 with the muscles or blood vessels of the forehead or temple; lines 15–23 concern the nose; lines 24–25 deal the lips and face. Lines 26–48 treat the nipples; lines 49–51 the veins(?) of the breasts; lines 52–55 the top of the breast; line 56 the epigastrium; lines 57–71 the abdomen. The following section (lines 72–105), which has no apparent structure, was designated by Stol (2000a, 194) as "an interesting collection of folk wisdom known among midwives". Yet, the lore found in these lines may just as much have been at home among male healing specialists. The third section (lines 106–113) contains predictions about the consequences of intercourse during pregnancy on different days of the month, which may have been influenced by hemerological traditions or by behavioural omens found in tablets of the omen series *Šumma ālu*. The last two lines of Tablet 36 (114–115) are drawn and adapted from entries in the teratological omen series *Šumma izbu*.

Some textual features presented by ms. a may point to a long textual tradition. For example, some syllabic spellings (e.g., *eb-ṭù* in line 66, *qá-du* (lines 80, 83), *e-ra-at u mu-šal-li-mat* and *ma-lu-ú* (lines 99 and 100)) are reminiscent of a syllabary and dominantly syllabic spellings typical for texts from the Old Babylonian period. The regular occurrence of textual variants and variant formulations (integrated into the manuscript by the scribe) points to the compilation of textual material from multiple traditions or sources. As another significant feature, several entries in ms. a contain unusual logograms and fanciful spellings, as a witness to the learned character of this kind of literature in the first millennium BCE. For example, *ša libbīša* "her foetus" is spelled *šà* ŠÀ-*šà* (in mss. a and b). Other rare logograms are presented by PEŠ for $PEŠ_4$ "to be pregnant" (lines 57–76), as well as by MU.TIN (Emesal) and MU.PA for *zikaru* "male" (lines 58–60).

List of Manuscripts

Siglum	Museum Number	Copy	Collation	Format; Ductus	Provenience
a	BM 92694 (83-1-18, 1341)	TDP II, pl. LII–LVI	Coll.	Single-column tablet; Late Babylonian script; 5th/4th cent. BCE	Borsippa
b	BM 65450 (82-9-18, 5437) + BM 76497 (AH 83-1-18, 1867)	Pl. 1–2	Coll.	Fragment of a single-column tablet; Late Babylonian script; 6th-3rd cent. BCE[202]	Sippar
c	W. 17360f	TDP II, pl. LXVI	–	Fragment; Late Babylonian script; 6th-3rd cent. BCE	Uruk
D	K. 7071	Geers, Folio N034 Pl. 3	Coll.	Fragment; Neo-Assyrian; 7th cent. BCE[203]	Nineveh
E	K. 17663	–	Coll.	Fragment; Neo-Assyrian; 7th cent. BCE[204]	Nineveh
F	372/f	KUB 37, 189	Photo coll.	Fragment of a single column tablet; ca. 13th cent. BCE	Boghazköy (Hattuša)

Overview

Lines 1–8	Predictions based on observations of a pregnant woman's forehead a obv. 1–8
Lines 9–14	Predictions based on observations of a pregnant woman's temples (blood vessels) a obv. 9–14 // b obv. 1'
Lines 15–23	Predictions based on observations of a pregnant woman's nose a obv. 15–23 // b obv. 2'–10'
Lines 24–25	Predictions based on observations of a pregnant woman's lips and face a obv. 24–25 // b obv. 11'–12'
Lines 26–48	Predictions based on observations of a pregnant woman's nipples a obv. 26–48 // b obv. 13'–32' // F obv.? 4'–17'
Lines 49–51	Predictions based on observations of a pregnant woman's breasts (blood vessels/muscles) a obv. 49–51 // b obv. 33'–35'
Lines 52–55	Predictions based on observations of a pregnant woman's breasts a obv. 52–55 // b obv. 36'–39' // F obv.? 18'-20'
Line 56	Predictions based on observations of a pregnant woman's epigastrium a obv. 52 // b obv. 40'
Lines 57–71	Predictions based on observations of a pregnant woman's abdomen ("insides") a obv. 53–rev. 10 // b obv. 41'–rev. 13
Lines 72–76	Predictions based on observations of a pregnant woman's abdomen ("muscles"; "insides") a rev. 11–15 // b rev. 14–16
Lines 77–80	Predictions based on observations of a pregnant woman's face a rev. 16–19 // c rev.? 4'–7' // E rev.? 1'–4'

202 Measurements ca. 7.5 x 13 x 2.5 cm.

203 Measurements ca. 4.4 x 6.0 x 1.5 cm; fragment from the middle of a tablet.

204 Measurements ca. 4.9 x 5 x 0.9 cm.

Lines 81–83	Predictions based on observations of body fluids discharged from the "mouth" a rev. 20–22 // E rev.$^{?}$ 5'–6'
Lines 84	Prediction based on the paralysis of hands and feet a rev. 23
Lines 85–86	Predictions based on observations of a pregnant woman's navel a rev. 24–25 // b rev. 24–25 // E rev.$^{?}$ 7'
Lines 87–89	Predictions based on observations of blood flowing from a pregnant woman's nostrils a rev. 26–28 // b rev. 26–28 // c rev.$^{?}$ 8'–9'
Lines 90–93	Predictions based on observations of a pregnant woman's ankles (blood vessels) a rev. 29–32 // b rev. 29–32
Lines 94–99	Predictions based on observations of a pregnant woman's gait and feet a rev. 33–38 // b rev. 33–38
Lines 100–102	Predictions based on observations of a pregnant woman's genital discharges(?) a rev. 39–41 // b rev. 39–40
Lines 103–105	Predictions based on observations of a pregnant woman's emotional state a rev. 42–44 // b rev. 40$^{cont.}$–41 // D rev.$^{?}$ 1'–2'
Lines 106–113	Predictions derived from sexual intercourse with a pregnant woman on different days of a month a rev. 45–52 // b rev. 42–45 // D rev.$^{?}$ 3'–10'
Lines 114–115	Predictions based on the birth of twins a rev. 53–54 // D rev.$^{?}$ 11'–12'
Lines 116–118	Colophon a rev. 55–57

Previous Edition and Discussion

Labat 1951, *TDP* I, 200–212 ("Tablette 35"; mss. a, c)
Wilhelm 1994, 69–72 Fragment M; pl. IX (ms. F, edition photo)[205]
Stol 2000a, *Birth*, 193–202 (translation; discussion)
Scurlock 2014a, *Sourcebook*, 245–255 (transliteration; translation)
Heeßel 2000, 137–138, 145–146 (list of sources)
Heeßel 2010b, 28 (translation of lines 1–12)
Heeßel 2017 (CRRAI 60), 61 (lines 52, 83, 98)
Scurlock and Andersen 2005, xiii (reference to mss. b and D), 259–283 (discussion of various lines from Tablet 36)
Schmidtchen 2018a, 142 (discussion of the incipits of Tablets 36–39 of *Sakikkû* and *Alamdimmû*)
Schmidtchen 2018b, 316, 324–325 (discussion of the incipits of Tablets 36–39 of *Sakikkû*)
Wee 2019a, 43, 47, 50 (discussion of lines 4–5, 65)
Minen 2018, in: F.M. Fales, *La medicina assiro-babilonese*, 188–192
Minen 2020, *JMC* 36, 10–22 (discussion)
Schmidtchen 2021a, 46–47, 244 (list of sources)
Electronic Babylonian Library (eBL) (https://www.ebl.lmu.de/library/BM.92694; ms. a) (https://www.ebl.lmu.de/library/BM.65450; ms. b) (https://www.ebl.lmu.de/library/K.7071; ms. D, photo, transliteration) (https://www.ebl.lmu.de/library/K.17663; mss. E, photo, transliteration)
CDLI P273373 (ms. a), P397007 (photo ms. D), P402974 (photo ms. E)

205 For photos of the tablet see Hethitologie Portal Mainz (http://www.hethport.adwmainz.de/fotarch/bildausw.php?n=372/f&b=+N07275+N07276+N07277+N07278+N07279+BoFN06018a). Photos of mss. a (rev.), D and E are available via the British Museum online database.

Transliteration

1	a obv. 1	*šum*$_4$*-ma* TU PEŠ$_4$*-ma* UGU SAG.KI*-šá* SIG$_7$ *šà* ŠÀ*-šà* NITA : *i-kar-ri-iṣ*
2	a obv. 2	DIŠ TU *mu-úḫ* SAG.KI*-šá* BABBAR *na-mir šà* ŠÀ*-šà* MUNUS : *i-šár-rù*
3	a obv. 3	DIŠ GI$_6$ *šà* ŠÀ*-šà* MUNUS : SILIM*-im*
4	a obv. 4	DIŠ SA$_5$ *šà* ŠÀ*-šà* NITA : UG$_7$
5	a obv. 5	DIŠ GÙN.A : *ba-ru-um šà* ŠÀ*-šà* NÁ
6	a obv. 6	DIŠ *uṭ-ṭe-ti* DIRI *šà* ŠÀ*-šà* NITA : NÍG.TUK
7	a obv. 7	DIŠ *uṭ-ṭe-ti* SA$_5$.MEŠ DIRI *šà* ŠÀ*-šà i*$_{11}$*-šár-rù*
8	a obv. 8	DIŠ *bar-mat šà* ŠÀ*-šà* NITA
9	a obv. 9	DIŠ TU SA SAG.KI*-ša* SA$_5$ *šà* ŠÀ*-šà* NITA
10	a obv. 10	DIŠ BABBAR *šà* ŠÀ*-šà* MUNUS
11	a obv. 11	DIŠ KI.TA*-nu* ZAG *te-bi šà* ŠÀ*-šà* MUNUS
12	a obv. 12	DIŠ KI.TA*-nu* GÙB *te-bi šà* ŠÀ*-šà* NITA
13	a obv. 13	DIŠ TU ⸢SA$^{?}$⸣.DIDLI SAG.KI*-ša* SA$_5$.DIDLI *šà* ŠÀ*-šà* NITA
14	a obv. 14	DIŠ SAG.KI*-šá* BABBAR.DIDLI ⸢*šà*⸣ ⸢ŠÀ*-šà*⸣ ⸢MUNUS⸣
	b obv. 1'	[DIŠ S]AG.⸢KI*-šá*⸣ BA[BBAR ....]
15	a obv. 15	DIŠ TU K[IR$_4$]*-šá ṣa-pir* : *za-qir* AŠ *šà* ŠÀ*-šà* NITA [TI/UG$_7$]
	b obv. 2'	[DIŠ ....*-p*]*ir* : *za-qir* AŠ [....................]
16	a obv. 16	DIŠ TU S[AG K]IR$_4$*-šá* ZAG ZI*-ma u* GI$_6$ *šà* ŠÀ*-šà* U[G$_7$$^{?}$]
	b obv. 3'	[........................]*-šá* ZAG ZI*-ma u* GI$_6$ [...................]
17	a obv. 17	DIŠ -*šá* GÙB ZI*-ma u* GI$_6$ *šà* ŠÀ*-šà* UG$_7$: TI
	b obv. 4'	[DIŠ]*-šá* GÙB ZI*-ma u* GI$_6$ [................]
18	a obv. 18	[DIŠ] ⸢TU⸣ [x] K]IR$_4$*-šá* KI.TA*-nu* 15 SA$_5$ *šà* ŠÀ*-šà* UG$_7$
	b obv. 5'	[DIŠ ....]*-šá* KI.TA*-nu* 15 SA$_5$ [...............]
19	a obv. 19	[DIŠ] KI.TA*-nu* 150 SA$_5$ *šà* ŠÀ*-šà* NITA
	b obv. 6'	[DIŠ] KI.TA*-nu* 150 SA$_5$ [................]
20	a obv. 20	[DIŠ] KI.TA*-nu* 15 GÙN.A *šà* ŠÀ*-šà* TIN
	b obv. 7'	[DIŠ] KI.TA*-nu* 15 GÙN.A *š*[*à* ŠÀ*-šà* ...]
21	a obv. 21	[DIŠ] KI.TA*-nu* 150 GÙN.A *šà* ŠÀ*-šà* UG$_7$
	b obv. 8'	[DIŠ] KI.TA*-nu* 150 GÙN.A *šà* Š[À*-šà* ...]
22	a obv. 22	DIŠ KI.TA*-nu* 15 *te-bi šà* ŠÀ*-šà* NITA
	b obv. 9'	[DIŠ] KI.TA*-nu* 15 ZI*-bi šà* ŠÀ*-š*[*à* ...]
23	a obv. 23	DIŠ KI.TA*-nu* 150 *te-bi šà* ŠÀ*-šà* MUNUS
	b obv. 10'	[DIŠ] KI.TA*-nu* 150 ZI*-bi šà* ŠÀ*-šà* [...]
24	a obv. 24	DIŠ TU ⸢NUMDUM⸣.MEŠ*-šú uq-tal-la-pa u* IGI.MEŠ*-šú* SIG$_7$ *šà* ŠÀ*-šà* NITA
	b obv. 11'	[x x N]UMDUM.MEŠ*-šá uq-tal-la-pa u* IGI.MEŠ*-šú* SIG$_7$ *šà* ŠÀ*-šà* [x]

25	a obv. 25	DIŠ *u* IGI.MEŠ-*šú* SA$_5$ *šà* ŠÀ-*šà* MUNUS
	b obv. 12'	[DIŠ] *u* IGI.MEŠ-*šú* ⸢SA$_5$⸣ *šà* ŠÀ-*šà* [x]
26	a obv. 26	DIŠ TU *ap-pi* UBUR-*šá zi-i-ir*$_9$ *šà* ŠÀ-*šà* NU SI.SÁ
	b obv. 13'	[x x *a*]*p-pi* UBUR-*šá zi-i-ir*$_9$ *šà* ŠÀ-*šà* NU S[I.SÁ]
	F obv.$^?$ 3'	[DIŠ TU] ⸢*e*⸣-*ra-at* KIR$_{14}$ UBU[R-*ša* ....][206]
27	a obv. 27	DIŠ *pa-ṭi-ir*$_9$ *šà* ŠÀ-*šà* SI.SÁ
	b obv. 14'	⸢DIŠ⸣ ⸢*pa*⸣-*ṭi-ir*$_9$ *šà* ŠÀ-*šà* SI.[SÁ]
	F	(*omits*)
28	a obv. 28	DIŠ GI$_6$ NITA PEŠ$_4$-*at*
	b obv. 15'	DIŠ GI$_6$ NITA PEŠ$_4$-[...]
	F obv.$^?$ 5'	[DIŠ MIN] GI$_6$ [......]
29	a obv. 29	DIŠ SA$_5$ MUNUS PEŠ$_4$-*at*
	b obv. 16'	DIŠ SA$_5$ MUNUS PEŠ$_4$-[...]
	F obv.$^?$ 6'	[DIŠ MIN] SA$_5$ [.........]
30	a obv. 30	DIŠ BABBAR ⸢NU⸣ ⸢SI⸣.SÁ PEŠ$_4$-*at*
	b obv. 17'	DIŠ BABBAR NU SI.SÁ PEŠ$_4$-[...]
	F obv.$^?$ 4'	[DIŠ] ⸢MIN⸣ BABBAR [.......]
31	a obv. 31	DIŠ ⸢MÚD$^!$⸣ SA$_5$ NITA ⸢PEŠ$_4$⸣-*at*
	b obv. 18'	DIŠ MÚD SA$_5$ NITA PEŠ$_4$-[...]
	F	(*omits*)
32	a obv. 32	DIŠ SIG$_7$ *šà* ŠÀ-*šà* ŠUB
	b obv. 19'	DIŠ SIG$_7$ *šà* ŠÀ-*šà* [x]
	F obv.$^?$ 7'	[DIŠ MIN] SIG$_7$ [.......][207]
33	a obv. 33	DIŠ SAMAG.MEŠ BABBAR.MEŠ DIRI SI.SÁ PEŠ$_4$-*át*
	b obv. 20'	DIŠ SAMAG.MEŠ ⸢BABBAR⸣.MEŠ DIRI SI.SÁ PEŠ$_4$-[x]
	F	(*omits*)
34	a obv. 34	DIŠ SAMAG.MEŠ SA$_5$.MEŠ DIRI NU SI.SÁ PEŠ$_4$-*át*
	b obv. 21'	DIŠ SAMAG.MEŠ SA$_5$.MEŠ DIRI NU SI.SÁ PEŠ$_4$-[...]
	F	(*omits*)
35	a obv. 35	DIŠ SAMAG.MEŠ GI$_6$.MEŠ DIRI NITA PEŠ$_4$-*át*
	b obv. 22'	DIŠ SAMAG.MEŠ GI$_6$.MEŠ DIRI NITA PEŠ$_4$-[x]
	F	(*omits*)
36	a obv. 36	DIŠ 3 BÙRU-*šu šà* ŠÀ-*šà* ÚKU
	b obv. 23'	DIŠ 3 BÙRU-*šu šà* ŠÀ-*šà* [...]
	F obv.$^?$ 8'	[DIŠ TU *e-r*]*a-at* <<UGU>> KIR$_{14}$ UBUR 3 *pa-liš ša* [ŠÀ-*ša* ...]
37	a obv. 37	DIŠ 4 BÙRU-*šu šà* ŠÀ-*šà* ÚKU
	b obv. 24'	DIŠ 4 BÙRU-*šu šà* ŠÀ-*šà* [...]
	F obv.$^?$ 9'	[DIŠ MIN] 4 *pa-liš ša* ŠÀ-[*ša* ...]

206 In ms. F, this line forms the beginning of a new topic, marked by a ruling preceding it. Of the first two lines (obv.$^?$ 1'–2'), only identical beginnings of the protases are preserved (reading ⸢DIŠ⸣ ⸢MIN⸣ ⸢*iš*⸣-*t*[*u* ...], which does not seem to match any entries in mss. a and b.
207 Ms. F inserts a ruling after line 7', signalling the beginning of a new topic.

38	a obv. 38	DIŠ 5 BÙRU-*šu šà* ŠÀ-*šà* UG$_7$
	b obv. 25'	DIŠ 5 BÙRU-*šu šà* ŠÀ-*šà* [...]
	F obv.$^?$ 10'	[DIŠ MIN] 5 MIN MIN [...]
39	a obv. 39	DIŠ 6 BÙRU-*šu šà* ŠÀ-*šà* NU SI.SÁ
	b obv. 26'	[DIŠ] 6 BÙRU-*šu šà* ŠÀ-*šà* NU SI.[SÁ]
	F obv.$^?$ 11'	[DIŠ MIN] 6 MIN MIN [...]
40	a obv. 40	DIŠ 7 BÙRU-*šu šà* ŠÀ-*šà* TI-*uṭ*
	b obv. 27'	[DIŠ] 7 BÙRU-*šu šà* ŠÀ-*šà* T[I-*uṭ*]
	F obv.$^?$ 12'	[DIŠ MIN] 7 MIN MIN [...]
41	a obv. 41	DIŠ 8 BÙRU-*šu šà* ŠÀ-*šà* TI-*uṭ*
	b obv. 28'	[DIŠ] 8 BÙRU-*šu šà* ŠÀ-*šà* T[I-*uṭ*]
	F obv.$^?$ 13'	[DIŠ MIN] 8 MIN MIN [...]
42	a obv. 42	DIŠ 9 BÙRU-*šu* DUMU.MEŠ-*šá ina* IGI-*šá ú-na-ka-ru* : DU.ME
	b obv. 29'	DIŠ 9 BÙRU-*šu* ⸢DUMU.MEŠ-*šá*⸣ [*ina*] ⸢IGI-*šá*⸣ [*ú-n*]*a*-⸢*ka-ru*⸣ : D[U.x]
	F obv.$^?$ 14'	[DIŠ MIN] 9 MIN MIN [...]
43	a obv. 43	DIŠ 10 BÙRU-*šu* DUMU.MEŠ-*šá ú-šal-lam*
	b obv. 30'	DIŠ 10 BÙRU-[*š*]*u* [.............................]
	F obv.$^?$ 15'	[DIŠ MIN] 10 MIN DUMU.MEŠ-[*ša* ....]
44	a obv. 44	DIŠ 14 BÙRU-*šu* DUMU.MEŠ-*šá* NU *ú-šal-lam*
	b obv. 31'	DIŠ 14 [BÙRU-*š*]*u* [.................................]
	F	(*omits*)
45	a obv. 45	DIŠ 15 BÙRU-*šu ù* URUxKEŠDA-*šú-nu* SA$_5$ NITA PEŠ$_4$-*at*
	b obv. 32'	DIŠ 15 [BÙRU-*š*]*u* [.................]
	F obv.$^?$ 16'	[DIŠ MIN] 15 MIN DUMU.MEŠ-[*ša* (*ul*) *ú-šal-lam*(?)]
46	a obv. 46	DIŠ 15 BÙRU-*šu ù* MIN GI$_6$ *šà* ŠÀ-*šà* MUNUS
	b obv. 33'	[...............-*š*]*u* [...................................]
	F obv.$^?$ 17'	[DIŠ MIN] 16 MIN *ḫe-pí* [............................][208]
47	a obv. 47	DIŠ 5 BÙRU-*šu ù* MIN SA$_5$ *šà* ŠÀ-*šà* NITA
	b obv. 34'	[...............-*š*]*u* [..............................]
	F	(*omits*)
48	a obv. 48	DIŠ 5 BÙRU-*šu ù* MIN GI$_6$ *šà* ŠÀ-*šà* MUNUS
	b obv. 35'	[...............-*š*]*u* [.................................]
	F	(*omits*)
49	a obv. 49	DIŠ TU SA UBUR-*šá šú-šú-ru* MUNUS PEŠ$_4$-*at*
	b obv. 36'	⸢DIŠ⸣ TU SA UBU[R-*š*]*á šú-šú-ru* [..........]
	F	(*omits*)
50	a obv. 50	DIŠ GU.MEŠ DAB.DAB NITA PEŠ$_4$-*at*
	b obv. 37'	DIŠ GU.MEŠ D[A]B.DAB NITA PEŠ$_4$-*at* :
	F	(*omits*)
51	a obv. 51	DIŠ SA$_5$ NÍTA PEŠ$_4$-*at*
	b obv. 37'$^{cont.}$	[.............................]
	F	(*omits*)

208 Ms. F inserts a ruling after line 17'.

52	a obv. 52	DIŠ TU *mu-úḫ* UBUR-*šá* SA.MEŠ SA$_5$.MEŠ *pur-ru-ku* MUNUS PEŠ$_4$-*at*
	b obv. 38'	⸢DIŠ⸣ TU *mu-úḫ* U[B]UR-*šá* SA.MEŠ S[A$_5$].M[EŠ ....]
	F obv.$^?$ 18'	[DIŠ TU *e-ra-a*]*t* UGU <<KIR$_{14}$>> UBUR DARA$_4$$^!$-⸢*im*⸣ DUMU.MEŠ [(...) Ù.TU$^?$]
53	a obv. 53	DIŠ GI$_6$.MEŠ *pur-ru-ku* NITA PEŠ$_4$-*at*
	b obv. 39'	DIŠ GI$_6$.MEŠ ⸢*pur*⸣-*ru-ku* [...............]
	F obv.$^?$ 19'	[DIŠ MIN ...]x MIN SA$_5$ [(x)] ⸢*ša*⸣ [ŠÀ-*ša*$^?$ (*ul*) *ú-šal-lam*$^?$]
54	a obv. 54	DIŠ BABBAR.MEŠ *pur-ru-ku* NU SI.SÁ PEŠ$_4$-*at*
	b obv. 40'	DIŠ BABBAR.MEŠ ⸢*pur*⸣-*ru-ku* [....................]
	F	(*omits*)
55	a obv. 55	DIŠ SIG$_7$.MEŠ *pur-ru-ku šà* ŠÀ-*šà* NU SI.SÁ
	b obv. 41'	DIŠ SIG$_7$.MEŠ ⸢*pur*⸣-*ru-ku* [......................]
	F obv.$^?$ 20'	[DIŠ MIN ...]x MIN *ur-q*[*a* ....][209]
56	a obv. 56	DIŠ TU *ina* SAG ŠÀ-*ša* SA.MEŠ SIG$_7$.MEŠ ŠUB-*ú šà* ŠÀ-*šà* SI.SÁ
	b obv. 42'	DIŠ TU *ina* ⸢SAG⸣ ⸢ŠÀ-*ša*⸣ [SA.M]EŠ ⸢SIG$_7$⸣.ME[Š ....]
57	a obv. 57	DIŠ TU ŠÀ.MEŠ-*ša paṭ-ri* NITA PEŠ-*at*
	b obv. 43'	DIŠ TU ⸢ŠÀ.MEŠ⸣-*ša* [...................]
58	a obv. 58	DIŠ *zaq-ru* : *na-šal-lu-lu-nim* MU.PA PEŠ-*at*
	b obv. 44'	DIŠ *zaq-ru̥* : ⸢*na*⸣-*šal-l*[*u-* ....]
59	a obv. 59	DIŠ TU ŠÀ.MEŠ-*ša ana em-ši-ša na-šal-lu-lu-nim* MU.TIN PEŠ-*at*
	b rev. 1	DIŠ TU ⸢ŠÀ.MEŠ⸣-*š*[*a* ....]
60	a obv. 60	DIŠ *ana em-ši-ša zaq-ru* : *ana* ḪAŠ$_4$-*šà* MU.TIN PEŠ-*at*
	b rev. 2	DIŠ *ana em-ši*-⸢*ša*⸣ [...]
61	a obv. 61	DIŠ *ana em-ši-ša* GAR-*nu šuk-ku-ku* Ù.TU
	b rev. 3	DIŠ *ana* ⸢*em-ši-ša*⸣ [..........................]
62	a rev. 1	DIŠ *ana em-ši-ša* ŠUB-*ú* ŠU.BI.AŠ.ÀM
	b rev. 4	DIŠ *ana* [*em*]-⸢*ši*⸣-[..........................]
63	a rev. 2	DIŠ *ana em-ši-ša* ZAG ŠUB-*ú* NITA PEŠ-*at*
	b rev. 5	DIŠ ⸢*ana*⸣ [......................................]
64	a rev. 3	DIŠ *ana em-ši-ša* AN.TA *zaq-ru* MUNUS PEŠ-*at*
	b rev. 6	DIŠ [..]
65	a rev. 4	DIŠ *ana em-ši-ša* KI.TA *zaq-ru* : *saḫ-ru* NITA PEŠ-*at*
	b rev. 7	DIŠ [...]
66	a rev. 5	DIŠ *eb-ṭù* NITA PEŠ-*at*
	b rev. 8	DIŠ [.....................]
67	a rev. 6	DIŠ *nap-ḫu* MUNUS PEŠ-*at*
	b rev. 9	[.................................]
68	a rev. 7	DIŠ *ma-a'-du* MUNUS PEŠ-*at*
	b rev. 10	[..................................]
69	a rev. 8	DIŠ SIG$_7$ ŠUB-*ú šà* ŠÀ-*šà ú-šak-lal*
	b rev. 11	[..]

209 Ms. F adds three more lines on the breasts before a ruling (obv.$^?$ 21'–23'), which are very fragmentarily preserved and do not correspond to mss. a and b. After a ruling and traces of one more line, the fragment breaks off.

70	a rev. 9	DIŠ GIN$_7$ *ap-pi-šá za-qip* MUNUS PEŠ-*at*
	b rev. 12	[...]
71	a rev. 10	DIŠ *ma-a'-du* GÌR.DIDLI-*ša u* ZI.IN.GI.DIDLI-*šá nu-up-pu-ḫa* ZAG *u* GÙB ZUKUM-*as* MAŠ.TAB.BA PEŠ-*at*
	b rev. 13	DIŠ [...]
a		____
72	a rev. 11	DIŠ TU ŠU.MIN-*šá* ŠÀ.ME-*šá ú-kal-la* NITA PEŠ-*at*
	b rev. 14	DIŠ [T]U [...]
73	a rev. 12	DIŠ TU SA.MEŠ-*šá ana* SAG ŠÀ-*šá zaq-ru* MUNUS PEŠ-*at*
	b rev. 15	⸢DIŠ⸣ ⸢TU⸣ [..]
74	a rev. 13	DIŠ *ana em-ši-šá zaq-ru* NITA PEŠ-*at*
	b	(*omits*)
75	a rev. 14	DIŠ *ma-a'-du* MUNUS PEŠ-*at*
	b	(*omits*)
76	a rev. 15	DIŠ TU ŠÀ.MEŠ-*ša nap-ḫu* NITA PEŠ-*at*
	b rev. 16	⸢DIŠ⸣ ⸢TU$^{?}$⸣ [....................................]
77	a rev. 16	DIŠ TU IGI.MEŠ-*šá ik-ki-ru ina šà* ŠÀ-*šà* UG$_7$
	b rev.	(*breaks*)
	c rev.$^{?}$ 4'	[................] ⸢x x⸣-*ru* : *ik-ki-r*[*u* ....]
	E rev.$^{?}$ 1'	[.......................... *ik-k*]*i-ru* x[..........................]
78	a rev. 17	DIŠ TU IGI.MEŠ-*šá ne-e-ḫu ina šà* ŠÀ-*šà ú-šal-lam*
	c rev.$^{?}$ 5'	[...........................-*š*]*á ne-ḫu* : *re-*[.........................]
	E rev.$^{?}$ 2'	[........................ *n*]*e-e-ḫu i*[*na* ....]
79	a rev. 18	DIŠ TU KUŠ.TAB IGI.<MEŠ>-*šá ma-lu-ú šà* ŠÀ-*šà* GAM
	c rev.$^{?}$ 6'	[.............]-*šá* KUŠ.TAB *ma-lu-ú* [......................]
	E rev.$^{?}$ 3'	[...................... IGI.M]EŠ-*šá ma-lu-ú ina š*[*à* ŠÀ-*šà* GAM$^{?}$]
80	a rev. 19	DIŠ TU KUŠ.TAB IGI.<MEŠ>-*šá* DIRI-*ú* IGI.DIDLI-*šá tur-ru-pa qá-du šà* ŠÀ-*šà* GAM
	c rev.$^{?}$ 7'	[.............]-*šá* KUŠ.TAB *ma-lu-ú ù* [...]
	E rev.$^{?}$ 4'	[.......................................] DIRI-*ú* IGI.DIDLI-*šá tur-ru-pa qá-*[*du* ....]
81	a rev. 20	DIŠ TU *ip-ta-na-ar-ru ul ú-šal-lam*
	E rev.$^{?}$ 5'	[....... *ip-ta-nar*$^{?}$]-*ra-ar ul ú-*[*šal-lam*]
82	a rev. 21	DIŠ TU MUD *ina* KA-*šú* DU-*ku ina* PEŠ$_4$-*šú* NU TIN
	E	(*omits*$^{?}$)
83	a rev. 22	DIŠ TU LUGUD *ina* KA-*šú* ŠUB.ŠUB-*a qá-du šà* ŠÀ-*šà* GAM
	E rev.$^{?}$ 6'	[...] x x [x x] x x x *šà* ŠÀ-*š*[*à* ...]
84	a rev. 23	DIŠ TU GÌR.MIN-*šá u* ŠU.MIN-*šú it-te-nen-ṣi-la* U U DIŠ (= 21$^{?}$) PA.AN
	E	(*omits*$^{?}$)
85	a rev. 24	DIŠ TU SAG *a-bu-un-na-ti-šá pa-ši-ir šà* ŠÀ-*šà ú-šal-lam*
	b rev. 24	[DIŠ TU SAG *a-bu-u*]*n-na-t*[*i-šá* ....]
	E rev.$^{?}$ 7'	[... *š*]*à* ŠÀ-*š*[*à* ....]
86	a rev. 25	DIŠ *zi-ir*$_9$: *pa-ši-ir šà* ŠÀ-*šà* NU TIN
	b rev. 25	[..........] : *pa-*⸢*ši-ir*⸣ [.....................]

87	a rev. 26	DIŠ TU *ina* KIR$_4$-*šá ša* ZAG MUD DU *šà* ŠÀ-*šà* GAM
	b rev. 26	[..................]-*šá ša* ZAG MUD DU [..................]
	c rev.$^?$ 8'	[.....................]-*šá* 15 MÚD DU-*ku* [.........................]
88	a rev. 27	DIŠ ⸢TU⸣ *ina* KIR$_4$-*šá ša* GÙB MUD DU *šà* ŠÀ-*šà* GAM
	b rev. 27	[.......................]-*šá ša* GÙB MUD DU [.................]
	c rev.$^?$ 9'	[..........................]-*šá* 150 MÚD DU-*ku* [....................]
89	a rev. 28	DIŠ TU ⸢IGI.MIN⸣-*šá* [B]AL.BAL.MEŠ *ar-na* AB.BA ÍL *šà* ŠÀ-*šà* GAM
	b rev. 28	[...........................] BAL.BAL.MEŠ *ar-na* AB.[BA ....]
	c rev.$^?$	(*breaks*)
90	a rev. 29	DIŠ TU SA *k*[*i-ṣil*]-⸢*li-šá*⸣ ⸢ZAG⸣ ⸢ZI-*bi*⸣ MUNUS PEŠ$_4$-*at*
	b rev. 29	[............ *ki*]-*ṣil-li-šá* ZAG ZI-*b*[*i* ....]
91	a rev. 30	DIŠ [................ N]ITA PEŠ$_4$-*at*
	b rev. 30	[DIŠ] GÙB ZI-*b*[*i* ....]
92	a rev. 31	DIŠ TU SA *ki*-[*ṣil-li-šá* ZAG *u* GÙ]B ⸢ZI-*bi*⸣ MAŠ.TAB.BA NU SI.SÁ PEŠ$_4$-*at*
	b rev. 31	[DIŠ TU SA *ki-ṣil*]-⸢*li*⸣-<*šá*> ZAG *u* GÙB ZI-[*bi* ....]
93	a rev. 32	DIŠ TU SA *ki-ṣil-li-šá* MÚD DIRI.MEŠ NITA PEŠ$_4$-*at*
	b rev. 32	[........................-*š*]*á* MÚD DIRI.MEŠ [.............]
94	a rev. 33	DIŠ TU *ina* ŠÀ *ma-ru-uš-ti-šá* ZAG ZUKUM-*as* NÁ PEŠ$_4$-*at*
	b rev. 33	[................. *ma-ru-u*]*š-ti-šá* ZAG ZUK[UM ....]
95	a rev. 34	DIŠ GÙB ZUKUM-*as* MUNUS PEŠ$_4$-*at*
	b rev. 34	[DIŠ] GÙB ZUKUM-*a*[*s* ....]
96	a rev. 35	DIŠ TU ZAG ZUKUM-*as u* GÌR-*šá* DUGUD-*at* NITA *u* MUNUS PEŠ$_4$-*at*
	b rev. 35	[.................................... GÌ]R-*šá* DUGUD-*at* [...............]
97	a rev. 36	DIŠ GÙB ZUKUM-*as u* KI.MIN MUNUS PEŠ$_4$-*at*
	b rev. 36	[.........................] *u* KI.MIN [.........................]
98	a rev. 37	DIŠ ZAG *u* GÙB ZUKUM-*as* MAŠ.TAB.BA PEŠ$_4$-*at*
	b rev. 37	[....................] ZUKUM-⸢*as*⸣ M[AŠ.TAB.BA PEŠ$_4$-*at*]
99	a rev. 38	DIŠ TU GÌR.MIN-*šá* TUR.MEŠ *e-ra-at u mu-šal-li-mat*
	b rev. 38	[.......................]-*šá* TUR.MEŠ ⸢*e*⸣-[......................]
100	a rev. 39	DIŠ TU ŠÀ.KU.SA *sa-a-mu* NITA *ir-ḫi*
	b rev. 39	[...........................-*m*]*u* NITA *ir-ḫi* :
101	a rev. 40	DIŠ TU ŠÀ.KU.SA *pe-lu-ú* NITA *ir-ḫi*
	b rev. 39$^{cont.}$	DIŠ T[U ....]
102	a rev. 41	DIŠ TU ŠÀ.KU.SA *nam-ru* NU SI.SÁ *ir-ḫi*
	b rev. 40	[........................-*r*]*u* NU SI.SÁ *ir-ḫi* :
103	a rev. 42	DIŠ ⸢TU⸣ ⸢*mé*⸣-*ra-a pal-ḫat ina šà* ŠÀ-*šà i-šal-lim*
	b rev. 40$^{cont.}$	DIŠ T[U ....]
104	a rev. 43	DIŠ [TU *mé*]-*ra-a še-la-at ina šà* ŠÀ-*šà* UG$_7$
	b rev. 41	[.........................]-*at ina šà* ŠÀ-*šà* UG$_7$:
	D rev.$^?$ 1'	[..........................]x-⸢*at*⸣ *ina š*[*à* ŠÀ-*šà* ...]

105 a rev. 44 DIŠ T[U ŠÀ.MEŠ$^?$]-*šá i-ta-na-aš-šá-šu šà* ŠÀ-*šà* UG$_7$
b rev. 41$^{cont.}$ DIŠ T[U ....]
D rev.$^?$ 2' [......................-*š*]*á i-ta-na-aš-šá ina šà* Š[À-*šà* ...]

a, b, D ____

106 a rev. 45 DIŠ T[U PEŠ$_4$-*ma š*]*a* <<5>>$^?$ ITI 3 *u$_4$-mi iq-ri-bu-niš-šú* NAM.TI.[LA]
b rev. 42 [...................................] *u$_4$-mi iq-ri-bu-niš-*[*šú* ....]
D rev.$^?$ 3' [.............................. *š*]*a* ⸢ITI⸣ U$_4$.3.KÁM *iq-ri-*⸢*bu-niš-ši*⸣ [..........]

107 a rev. 46 DIŠ TU ⸢PEŠ$_4$-*ma*⸣ ⸢*ša*⸣ ITI 4 *u$_4$-mi* KI.MIN NAM.TI.[LA]
b rev. 43 [.............................] ⸢*u$_4$*⸣-*mi* KI.MIN [.................]
D rev.$^?$ 4' [..................... *š*]*a* ⸢ITI⸣ U$_4$.4.KÁM *iq-ri-bu-niš-ši* [...]

108 a rev. 47 DIŠ TU PEŠ$_4$-*ma ša* ITI 5 *u$_4$-mi* KI.MIN *ša na-aḫ-šá-ti* [GIG]
b rev. 44 [..............................-*m*]*i* KI.MIN *ša na-aḫ-šá-*[*ti* GIG]
D rev.$^?$ 5' [.....................] ⸢ITI⸣ ⸢U$_4$⸣.5.KÁM *iq-ri-bu-niš-ši* [...........]

109 a rev. 48 DIŠ TU PEŠ$_4$-*ma ša* ITI 6 *u$_4$-mi* KI.MIN KI.MIN
b rev. 45 [...................................] KI.MIN [........]
D rev.$^?$ 6' [.....................] ⸢ITI⸣ ⸢U$_4$⸣.6.KÁM *iq-ri-bu-niš-ši* [...]

110 a rev. 49 DIŠ TU PEŠ$_4$-*ma ša* ITI 7 *u$_4$-mi* KI.MIN NAM.TI.[LA]
b rev. (*breaks*)
D rev.$^?$ 7' [..................... I]TI U$_4$.7.KÁM *iq-ri-bu-niš-ši* [......]

111 a rev. 50 DIŠ TU PEŠ$_4$-*ma ša* ITI 8 *u$_4$-mi* KI.MIN ḪUL *a-bi* NAM.ÉRIM DAB-*su*
D rev.$^?$ 8' [......................... IT]I U$_4$.8.KÁM *iq-ri-bu-niš-š*[*i* ....]

112 a rev. 51 DIŠ TU PEŠ$_4$-*ma ša* ITI 9 *u$_4$-mi* KI.MIN BA.UG$_7$
D rev.$^?$ 9' [..................... ITI U$_4$].⸢9⸣.KÁM *iq-ri-bu-niš-š*[*i* ...]

113 a rev. 52 DIŠ TU PEŠ$_4$-*ma ša* ITI 10 *u$_4$-mi* KI.MIN TI.LA
D rev.$^?$ 10' [..................... ITI U$_4$.10].KÁM *iq-ri-bu-niš-š*[*i* ...]

a, D ____

114 a rev. 53 DIŠ MUNUS 2 NITA.ME Ù.TU KUR *su-un-qam* IGI-*mar*
D rev.$^?$ 11' [.....................................] KUR *su-*[..................]

115 a rev. 54 DIŠ MUNUS 2 MUNUS.ME Ù.TU É BI *ana* IGI-*šú* DU-*ak*
D rev.$^?$ 12' [.....................................] ⸢É⸣ BI [...................]

a, D ____

Colophon:

116 a rev. 54 DIŠ ^{munus}PEŠ$_4$ GIG-*m*[*a*] 1 UŠ 54 MU.ŠID.BI *tup-pi* IGI-*ú šum$_4$-ma* TU PEŠ$_4$-⸢*ma*⸣

117 a rev. 55 DUB 36.KÁM.MA *e-nu-*⸢*ma*⸣ *ana* É LÚ.GIG KA.PIRIG DU-*ku* SA.GIG NU AL.TIL GABA.RI BÁR.SIPA^{ki} GIN$_7$ SUMUN-*šú*

118 a rev. 56 ^{md}AG-*ku-ṣur-šú* A-*šú šá* ^{md}EN-SU A ^{m}*ḫu-ṣa-bi* ^{lú}LUNGA ^{d}AG TUR *a-na* GÙ.DÉ-*šú* DU-*ma bir*(*i*) *pa-liḫ* ^{d}AG *ina sar-tú* NU GUR$_{17}$ MU 11.KÁM ^{m}*ar* LUGAL AŠ.AŠ

210 After the ruling in ms. D, there are traces of two more ruled lines, which should belong to a catchline and colophon.

Bound Transcription and Translation

1 *šumma ālittu erât-ma muḫ pūtīša aruq ša libbīša zikar : ik(k)arriṣ*	1 If a childbearing woman is pregnant and the top of her forehead is yellow-green (livid): her foetus (lit. that of her womb) is male, var. he will *be pinched off*.
2 *šumma muḫ pūtīša peṣi namir ša libbīša sinnišat : išarru*	2 If the top of a childbearing woman's forehead is white (and) shiny: her foetus is female, var. he/she will be rich.
3 *šumma ṣalim ša libbīša sinnišat : išallim*	3 If it is black (dark): her foetus is female, var. he/she will be healthy.
4 *šumma sām ša libbīša zikar : imât*	4 If it is red: her foetus is male, var. he/she will die.
5 *šumma* GÙN.A : *barum ša libbīša ṣalil(?)*	5 If it is GÙN.A, (which means) spotted/multi-coloured: her foetus sleeps(?).
6 *šumma uṭṭēti mali ša libbīša zikar : mašrû*	6 If it is full of 'grains': her foetus is male; var. wealth.
7 *šumma uṭṭēti sāmāti mali ša libbīša išarru*	7 If it is full of red 'grains': her foetus will be rich.
8 *šumma barmat ša libbīša zikar*	8 If it (the forehead) is multi-coloured: her foetus is male.
9 *šumma ālittu šer'ān nakkaptīša(?) sām ša libbīša zikar*	9 If the *blood vessel* of a childbearing woman's temple(?) is red: her foetus is male.
10 *šumma peṣi ša libbīša sinnišat*	10 If it is white: her foetus is female.
11 *šumma šaplānu imna tebi ša libbīša sinnišat*	11 If the area below (the blood vessel of the temple) on the right side pulsates: her foetus is female.
12 *šumma šaplānu šumēla tebi ša libbīša zikar*	12 If the area below (the blood vessel of the temple) on the left side pulsates: her foetus is male.
13 *šumma ālittu šer'ānū nakkaptīša sāmū ša libbīša zikar*	13 If the *blood vessels* of a childbearing woman's temple(?) are red: her foetus is male.
14 *šumma (šer'ānū) nakkaptīša peṣû ša libbīša sinnišat*	14 If (the *blood vessels*) of her temple are white: her foetus is female.
15 *šumma ālittu ap[pa]ša ṣapir : zaqir* AŠ *ša libbīša zikar [iballuṭ/imât]*	15 If a childbearing woman's n[ose] is pinched (flat), var. pointed: ... her foetus is male, [he/she will live/die].
16 *šumma ālittu r[ēš ap]pīša imna tebī-ma u ṣalim ša libbīša i[mât(?)]*	16 If the t[ip] of a childbearing woman's no[se] is elevated to the right and is black (dark): her foetus w[ill die(?)].
17 *šumma (rēš appī)ša šumēla tebī-ma u ṣalim ša libbīša imât : iballuṭ*	17 If (the tip of) her (nose) is elevated to the left side and is black: her foetus will die, var. he will live.
18 *šumma ālittu* [...] *appīša šaplānu imitta sām ša libbīša imât*	18 [If the ... of] a childbearing woman's n]ose is red on the lower side, on the right: her foetus will die.
19 *šumma šaplānu šumēla sām ša libbīša zikar*	19 If it is red on the lower side, on the left: her foetus is male.
20 *šumma šaplānu imitta barum ša libbīša iballuṭ*	20 [If] it is multi-coloured on the lower side, on the right: her foetus will live.
21 *šumma šaplānu šumēla barum ša libbīša imât*	21 [If] it is multi-coloured on the lower side, on the left: her foetus will die.
22 *šumma šaplānu imitta tebi ša libbīša zikar*	22 If it is elevated on the lower side towards the right: her foetus is male.
23 *šumma šaplānu šumēla tebi ša libbīša sinnišat*	23 If it is elevated on the lower side towards the left: her foetus is female.
24 *šumma šapātūša uqtallapā u pānūša arqū ša libbīša zikar*	24 If a childbearing woman's lips of are peeled off and her face is yellow-green (livid): her foetus is male.
25 *šumma u pānūša sāmū ša libbīša sinnišat*	25 If (ditto, i.e. a childbearing woman's lips of are peeled off) and her face is red, her foetus is female.

[26] *šumma appi tulîša zīr ša libbīša ul uštešser*

[26] If the nipple of a childbearing woman's breast is twisted (shut?): she will not bring her foetus to term.[211]

[27] *šumma paṭir ša libbīša uštešser*

[27] If it is loose (open?): she will bring her foetus to term.

[28] *šumma ṣalim zikara erât*

[28] If it is black: she is pregnant with a male (child).

[29] *šumma sām sinništa erât*

[29] If it is red: she is pregnant with a female (child).

[30] *šumma peṣi lā išara(?) erât*

[30] If it is white: she is pregnant with a (foetus who is) *not in a good condition* (lit. straight, normal).

[31] *šumma dāma sām zikara erât*

[31] If it is blood-red: she is pregnant with a male.

[32] *šumma aruq ša libbīša inaddi*

[32] If it is yellow-green: she will abort her foetus.

[33] *šumma umṣāti peṣâti mali išara(?) erât*

[33] If it is full of white moles: she is pregnant with a (foetus who is *in*) *a good condition* (lit. straight, normal).

[34] *šumma umṣāti sāmāti mali lā išara(?) erât*

[34] If it is full of red moles: she is pregnant with a (foetus who is) *not in a good condition.*

[35] *šumma umṣāti ṣalmāti mali zikara erât*

[35] If it is full of black moles: she is pregnant with a male.

[36] *šumma* 3 *pilšū* (var. [*šumma ālittu er*]*ât appi tulî šalāš*(*īšu*) *pališ*) *ša libbīša ilappin*

[36] If it has three 'holes' (var. ms. F: [If a childbearing woman is pre]gnant and the nipple has three holes): her foetus will be poor.

[37] *šumma* 4 *pilšū* (var. *pališ*) *ša libbīša ilappin*

[37] If it has four holes: her foetus will be poor.

[38] *šumma* 5 *pilšū* (var. *pališ*) *ša libbīša imât*

[38] If it has five holes: her foetus will die.

[39] *šumma* 6 *pilšū* (var. *pališ*) *ša libbīša ul uštešser*

[39] If it has six holes: she will not bring her foetus to term.

[40] *šumma* 7 *pilšū* (var. *pališ*) *ša libbīša iballuṭ*

[40] If it has seven holes: her foetus will live.

[41] *šumma* 8 *pilšū* (var. *pališ*) *ša libbīša iballuṭ*

[41] If it has eight holes: her foetus will live.

[42] *šumma* 9 *pilšū* (var. *pališ*) *mārūša ina pānīša unakkarū* : *ittallakū*

[42] If it has nine holes: her sons/children will be estranged to her; var. they will go away.

[43] *šumma* 10 *pilšū* (var. *pališ*) *mārīša ušallam*

[43] If it has ten holes: she will bring her children to term.

[44] *šumma* 14 *pilšū mārīša ul ušallam*

[44] If it has fourteen holes: she will not bring her children to term.

[45] *šumma* 15 *pilšū u ...-šunu sām zikara erât* (var. *mārī*[*ša* (*ul*) *ušallam*?)])

[45] If it has fifteen holes and their ... is red: she is pregnant with a male (var. ms. F: [she will (not) bring her] children [to term(?)]).

[46] *šumma* 15 *pilšū u* MIN *ṣalim ša libbīša sinnišat*

[46] If it has fifteen holes and ditto (their ...) is black: her foetus is female.[212]

[47] *šumma* 5 *pilšū u* MIN *sām ša libbīša zikar*

[47] If it has five holes and ditto (their ...) is red: her foetus is male.

[48] *šumma* 5 *pilšū u* MIN *ṣalim ša libbīša sinnišat*

[48] If it has five holes and ditto (their ...) is black: her foetus is female.

[49] *šumma ālittu šer'ān tulêša šūšurū sinništa erât*

[49] If the *muscles/blood vessels* of a childbearing woman's breast run in a straight line: she is pregnant with a female.

[50] *šumma qê ṣubbutū zikara erât*

[50] If they are surrounded (lit. held) by 'threads': she is pregnant with a male.

[51] *šumma sāmū zikara erât*

[51] If they are red: she is pregnant with a male.

[52] *šumma ālittu muḫ tulîša šer'ānū sāmūtu purrukū sinništa erât*

[52] If on top of a childbearing woman's breast red veins lie crosswise: she is pregnant with a female.[213]

[53] *šumma ṣalmūtu purrukū zikara erât*

[53] If black ones lie crosswise: she is pregnant with a male.[214]

[54] *šumma peṣûtu purrukū lā išara erât*

[54] If white ones lie crosswise: she is pregnant with a (foetus who is) *not in a good condition.*

---

211 The variant line in ms. F reads: "[If a childbearing woman] is pregnant (and) the nipple [of her] breast [...]".

212 The variant line in ms. F reads: "[If ditto (i.e. the nipple has)] sixteen ditto, *broken* (original) [...]".

213 The variant line in ms. F reads: [*šumma ālittu erâ*]*t muḫ*(*ḫi*) *tulî da'im mārī*[*ša* (*ul*) *ušallam*(?)] "If a childbearing woman is pregnant (and) the upper side of the breast is dark (brown): [she will (not) bring her] children [to term?]".

214 The variant line in ms. F reads: [If ditto ...] ... ditto is red (*sām*): [her] fo[etus (*ša libbīša*) ...]".

55 *šumma arqūtu purrukū ša libbīša ul ušteššer*	55 If yellow-green ones lie crosswise: she will not bring her foetus to term.[215]
56 *šumma ālittu ina rēš libbīša šer'ānū urqī nadû ša libbīša ušteššer*	56 If the *muscles/blood vessels* on a childbearing woman's epigastrium of are tinged with yellow (spots): she will bring her foetus to term.
57 *šumma ālittu qerbūša paṭrū(?) zikara erât*	57 If a childbearing woman's insides are loose: she is pregnant with a male.
58 *šumma zaqrū : našallulūni zikara(?) erât*	58 If they protrude, variant: *undulate*: she is pregnant with a male(?).
59 *šumma ālittu qerbūša ana emšīša našallulūni zikara erât*	59 If a childbearing woman's insides *undulate*(?) towards her lower abdomen: she is pregnant with a male.
60 *šumma ana emšīša zaqrū : ana ḫallīša(?) zikara erât*	60 If they are protruding towards her lower abdomen, variant: towards her crotch(?): she is pregnant with a male.
61 *šumma ana emšīša šaknū sukkuka ullad*	61 If they are packed into her lower abdomen: she will give birth to a deaf/retarded (child).
62 *šumma ana emšīša nadû* ŠU.BI.AŠ.ÀM	62 If they *hang down* (lit. drop) towards her lower abdomen: ditto.
63 *šumma ana emšīša imna nadû zikara erât*	63 If they *hang down* (lit. drop) towards her lower abdomen, on the right side: she is pregnant with a male.
64 *šumma ana emšīša eliš zaqrū sinništa erât*	64 If they protrude towards her lower abdomen, (pointing) upwards: she is pregnant with a female.
65 *šumma ana emšīša šapliš zaqrū : saḫrū zikara erât*	65 If they protrude, var.: are turned/curved towards her lower abdomen (pointing) downwards: she is pregnant with a male.
66 *šumma ebṭū zikara erât*	66 If they are cramped: she is pregnant with a male.
67 *šumma napḫū sinnšta erât*	67 If they are swollen/bloated: she is pregnant with a female.
68 *šumma ma'dū sinništa erât*	68 If they are enlarged: she is pregnant with a female.
69 *šumma urqa nadû ša libbīša ušaklal*	69 If they are coloured unevenly with yellow (spots): she will bring her foetus to perfection.
70 *šumma kīma appīša zaqip sinništa erât*	70 If it (the belly?) is as pointed as her nose: she is pregnant with a female.
71 *šumma ma'dū šēpāša kiṣallāša nuppuḫā imitta u šumēla ikkabbas māšī erât*	71 If they (her insides) are enlarged, her feet and ankles are swollen, she *tends to* tread with the right, (and another time) with the left (foot): she is pregnant with twins.

---

72 *šumma ālittu qātāša qerbīša ukallā zikara erât*	72 If a childbearing woman holds her insides (belly) with her hands: she is pregnant with a male.
73 *šumma ālittu šer'ānūša ana rēš libbīša zaqrū sinništa erât*	73 If the *muscles/blood vessels* of a childbearing woman protrude towards her epigastrium: she is pregnant with a female.
74 *šumma ālittu ana emšīša zaqrū zikara erât*	74 If they (the muscles/vessels) protrude toward her lower abdomen: she is pregnant with a male.
75 *šumma ma'dū sinništa erât*	75 If they are numerous: she is pregnant with a female.
76 *šumma qerbūša napḫū zikara erât*	76 If a childbearing woman's insides are bloated: she is pregnant with a male.
77 *šumma ālittu pānūša ikkirū ina ša libbīša imât*	77 If a childbearing woman's face has an unhealthy appearance: she will die as a result of her being with child.
78 *šumma ālittu pānūša nēḫū ina ša libbīša ušallam*	78 If a childbearing woman's face is peaceful/calm: she will stay healthy as a result of her being with child.

---

215 The variant line in ms. F reads: "[If ditto ...] ... ditto [...] a yellow-green (spot) (*urqu*) [...]".

79 *šumma ālittu* KUŠ.TAB *pānūša malû* (var. adds *ina*) *ša libbīša imât*	79 If a childbearing woman's face is full of (patches resembling tanned) ox-hide: her foetus will die (var. [she will die(?)] as a result of [her being with child]).
80 *šumma ālittu* KUŠ.TAB *pānūša malû u īnāša turrupā qadu ša libbīša imât*	80 If a childbearing woman's face is full of (patches resembling tanned) ox-hide (and) her eyes are mottled (with spots): she will die together with her foetus.
81 *šumma ālittu iptanarru* (var. [*iptana*]*rrar*(?)) *ul ušallam*	81 If a childbearing woman vomits continually (var. is [always] weak(?)): she will not bring (her foetus) to term.
82 *šumma ālittu da'mu ina pîša illaku ina mērêša ul iballuṭ*	82 If dark (blood) flows from a childbearing woman's mouth(?): she will not stay alive in her pregnancy.
83 *šumma ālittu šarku ina pîša ittanaddâ qadu ša libbīša imât*	83 If a childbearing woman repeatedly discharges pus from her mouth(?): she will die together with her foetus.
84 *šumma ālittu šēpāša u qātāša ittenenṣilā* ...	84 If a childbearing woman's hands and feet become repeatedly paralysed: ... .
85 *šumma ālittu rēš abunnatīša pašir ša libbīša ušallam*	85 If the top of a childbearing woman's navel is 'unravelled': she will bring her foetus to term.
86 *šumma zīr* : *pašir ša libbīša ul iballuṭ*	86 If it is twisted, var. 'unravelled': her foetus will not live.
87 *šumma ālittu ina appīša ša imitti da'mu illak* (var. *dāmū illakū*) *ša libbīša imât*	87 If dark blood (var. ms. c: blood) flows from a childbearing woman's right nostril: her foetus will die.
88 *šumma ālittu ina appīša ša šumēli da'mu illak* (var. *dāmū illakū*) *ša libbīša imât*	88 If dark blood (var. blood) flows from a childbearing woman's left nostril: her foetus will die.
89 *šumma ālittu īnāša ittanablakkatā arna abi inašši ša libbīša imât*	89 If a childbearing woman's eyes keep rolling back: she bears the guilt of (her) father; her foetus will die.
90 *šumma ālittu šer'ān k*[*iṣil*]*līša imitti tebi sinništa erât*	90 If the blood vessel of a childbearing woman's right ankle pulsates: she is pregnant with a female.
91 *šumma šumēlu tebi zikara erât*	91 If the left one pulsates: she is pregnant with a male.
92 *šumma ālittu šer'ān ki*[*ṣil*]*līša imitti u šumēli tebi māšī lā išarūti*(?) *erât*	92 If the blood vessel of a childbearing woman's right and left ankle pulsates: she is pregnant with abnormal(?) twins.
93 *šumma ālittu šer'ān kiṣillīša dāma malû zikara erât*	93 If the blood vessel(s) of a childbearing woman's ankle are full of blood: she is pregnant with a male.
94 *šumma ālittu ina maruštīša imitta ikkabbas ṣālila*(?) *erât*	94 If during her "trouble" a childbearing woman *tends to tread* with the right (foot): she is pregnant with a sleeping (foetus?).
95 *šumma imitta ikkabbas sinništa erât*	95 If she *tends to tread* with the left (foot): she is pregnant with a female.
96 *šumma ālittu imitta ikkabbas u šēpša kabtat zikara u sinništa erât*	96 If a childbearing woman *tends to tread* with the right (foot) and her foot feels heavy: she is pregnant with a male and a female.
97 *šumma šumēla ikkabbas u* KI.MIN *sinništa erât*	97 If she *tends to tread* with the left (foot) and ditto (her foot feels heavy): she is pregnant with a female.
98 *šumma imitta u šumēla ikkabbas māšī erât*	98 If she *tends to tread* with the right and (sometimes with the) left (foot): she is pregnant with twins.
99 *šumma ālittu šēpāša ṣeḫrā erât u mušallimat*	99 If a childbearing woman's feet are small: she is pregnant and she is one who brings (her foetus) to term.
100 *šumma ālittu sagûša*(?) *sāmū zikara irḫi*	100 If a childbearing woman's (menstrual) *discharges*(?) are red: she was impregnated with a male.
101 *šumma ālittu sagûša*(?) *pelû zikara irḫi*	101 If a childbearing woman's (menstrual) *discharges*(?) are light-red: she was impregnated with a male.
102 *šumma ālittu sagûša*(?) *namrū lā išara irḫi*	102 If a childbearing woman's (menstrual) *discharges*(?) are bright/light-coloured: she was impregnated with (a foetus who is) *not in a good condition*.

103 *šumma ālittu mērâ palḫat ina ša libbīša išallim*	103 If a childbearing woman is fearful of pregnancy: she will be well with(?) her foetus.
104 *šumma [ālittu mē]râ šelât ina ša libbīša imât*	104 If a [childbearing woman] is careless of [preg]nancy: she will die through her foetus.
105 *šumma ālit[tu qerbū]ša(?) ītanaššašū (ina) ša libbīša imât*	105 If childbearing woman's [insides(?)] are continually upset: her foetus will die (var. ms. D: [she will die] through [her] foetus).

---

106 *šumma ālit[tu erât-ma š]a* <<5>> *arḫi šalši(?) ūmi iqribūniššī balāṭu*	106 If a childbearing [woman is pregnant and] one approaches her (sexually) (on) the third day of the <<fifth>> month(?): life/wellbeing.
107 *šumma ālittu erât-ma ša arḫi rebî(?) ūmi* KI.MIN (var. *iqribūniššī*) *balāṭu*	107 If a childbearing woman [is pregnant and] and ditto (var. one approaches her (sexually)) on the fourth day of the month(?): life/wellbeing.
108 *šumma ālittu erât-ma ša arḫi ḫamši(?) ūmi* KI.MIN (var. *iqribūniššī*) *ša naḫšāti imarraṣ*(?)	108 If a childbearing woman is pregnant and ditto (var. one approaches her (sexually)) (on) the fifth day of the month(?): she will get sick with *naḫšātu*-disease (haemorrhage).
109 *šumma ālittu erât-ma ša arḫi šešši(?) ūmi* KI.MIN (var. *iqribūniššī*) KI.MIN	109 If a childbearing woman is pregnant and ditto (var. one approaches her (sexually)) (on) the sixth day of the month(?): ditto (she will get sick with *naḫšātu*-disease).
110 *šumma ālittu erât-ma ša arḫi sebî(?) ūmi* KI.MIN (var. *iqribūniššī*) *balāṭu*	110 If a childbearing woman is pregnant and ditto (var. one approaches her (sexually)) (on) the seventh day of the month(?): life/wellbeing.
111 *šumma ālittu erât-ma ša arḫi samānî(?) ūmi* KI.MIN (var. *iqribūniššī*) *lumun abi māmītu iṣabbassu*	111 If a childbearing woman is pregnant and ditto (var. one approaches her (sexually)) (on) the eighth day of the month(?): the evil of (her) father (in the form of) the Ban will seize her.
112 *šumma ālittu erât-ma ša arḫi tišî(?) ūmi* KI.MIN (var. *iqribūniššī*) *imât*	112 If a childbearing woman is pregnant and ditto (var. one approaches her (sexually)) (on) the ninth day of the month(?): she will die.
113 *šumma ālittu erât-ma ša arḫi ešrî(?) ūmi* KI.MIN (var. *iqribūniššī*) *iballuṭ*	113 If a childbearing woman is pregnant and ditto (var. one approaches her (sexually)) (on) the tenth day of the month(?): she will live/be well.

---

114 *šumma sinništu šina zikarī ūlid mātu sunqa immar*	114 If a woman gives birth to two males: the country will experience famine.
115 *šumma sinništu šīna sinnišāti ūlid bītu šū ana pānīšu illak*	115 If a woman gives birth to two females: that house will prosper.

Colophon (ms. a):

116 *šumma erītu marṣat-m[a]* 114 MU.ŠID.BI *tuppu maḫrû šumma ālittu erât-ma*	116 (Catchline:) "If a pregnant woman is sick." 114 (sic!) lines. First tablet of "If a childbearing woman is pregnant".
117 *tuppu* 36.KÁM.MA *enūma ana bīt marṣi āšipu illaku Sakikkû ul qati gabari Barsipa kīma labirīšu*	117 36th tablet of "When the exorcist goes to a sick man's house", (of the series) *Sakikkû*. Not finished. A copy of an original from Borsippa. (Written) according to its original.
118 *Nabû-kuṣuršu māršu ša Bēl-erība mār Ḫuṣābi sīrašû Nabû ṣeḫru ana šitassîsu išṭur-ma biri pāliḫ Nabû ina sarti lā inašši šattu ištēnšerû Ar(takšatsu) šar mātāti*	118 Nabû-kuṣuršu, son of Bēl-erība, descendent of Ḫuṣābi, the young brewer of Nabû, wrote and checked (the tablet) for his reading. Anyone who revers Nabû must not take away (this tablet) by stealth. Eleventh year of Artaxerxes, king of the lands.

Notes

Line 1: The verb *karāṣu* in the variant of the apodosis means "to break off; to pinch off (clay)". The cognate noun *kirṣu* means "abortion, aborted foetus" (synonym to *nīd libbi*); it occurs beside the terms *izbu* and *kūbu* referring to stillborn foetuses in lexical sources (MSL 9, 29: 1–4). Stol (2000a, 194) wonders whether this verb may refer to embryotomy, an abortion by cutting up the foetus (Hebr. *ḥātak*), thus translating "he will be cut up" (N-stem, not attested according to the dictionaries). Scurlock (2014a, 248) instead translates "it will be fully formed". Both translations suggest an underlying N-stem of *karāṣu* (not attested elsewhere so far). Interestingly, the verb *karāṣu* is also found in the context of anthropogony, for example in the *Gilgamesh Epic* (Tablet I 102), where the mother goddess Aruru "pinches off" (*iktariṣ*) clay and throws it down in the desert to create Enkidu (see George 2003, 544–545; for the phrase *ṭiṭṭa karāṣu* see also Mayer 1987, *OrNS* 56, 62 (line 14')). This line is quoted in a commentary on Tablet 1 of the *Diagnostic Handbook* (George 1991, *RA* 85, 146, 2b 4'–5'; Wee 2019b, 30, 32 SA-GIG 1B obv. 4'–5'). For further attestations of the divine creative act of pinching off clay in anthropogonic myths, see Wee 2019b, 20.

The verb *karāṣu* also features in a second passage in a parallel commentary on *Diagnostic Handbook* Tablet 1, where the term is associated with a kiln-fired brick and pregnancy. There, the omen "if he sees a kiln-fired brick (*agurru*): the patient will die" is explained as follows: "Thirdly, (the brick means) a pregnant woman: (this is because the sign) A (means) 'son', and gur$_4$ (when read KÌR means) 'to pinch off' (*karāṣu*)" (see George 1991, *RA* 85, 146 4b rev. 22; Frahm 2011, 38; Wee 2019b, 6, 10, 19–20 SA-GIG 1A: 11–12). The underlying logic of this association is therefore that a pregnant woman is "one who will pinch off a son (from her body?)" (Wee 2019b, 10). According to Wee (2019b, 20), the association of *karāṣu* with birth and creation makes it unlikely that *ikarriṣ* in our omen entry refers to abortion or stillbirth; however, the meaning of the verb in this passage remains ambiguous (see also Schmidtchen 2021a, 46 n. 341).

In the Late Babylonian manuscript BM 92694 (ms. a), the expression *ša libbīša* "her foetus" (i.e. that of her womb/belly) is written *šà* ŠÀ-*šà* instead of *šá* ŠÀ-*šá*, a spelling that is attested in other women's healthcare texts (reminiscent of similar artificial spellings such as *šá* ŠÀ-ŠÀ-ŠÀ-*šú*, see *infra* text A.2.2).

Line 2: The colour white is often associated with females, and the colour red with males (see e.g. line 4). The sign BABBAR (*na-mir*) in line 2 could alternatively be read as *pūṣu* "white spot" (thus Stol 2000a, 194 *pūṣa namir* "is bright with a white spot"). However, references to spots of different colour are usually expressed with the verb *nadû*. Thus, the interpretation of BABBAR as a stative form of *peṣû* "white" is preferred here.

Line 3: The entry plays with similar keywords in the protasis and apodosis: *ṣalim* "it is black" and *išallim* "it will be healthy/ will prosper".

Line 4: The association of the variant apodosis in line 4 may have been triggered by the homophony of the phonetic values of the cuneiform signs NITA (= UŠ) and UG$_7$ (= ÚŠ) used in the protasis and apodosis. Lines 3 and 4 clearly form contrasting pairs of prognoses.

Lines 1–4 present the following correlations between colours and sex of the foetus:
black and white = female
red and yellow-green = male
Such correlations also occur in other entries in Tablet 36 (see below).

Line 5: In the protasis, logographic GÙN.A is followed by the variant *barum*, which may be understood as a gloss or syllabic realisation of GÙN.A (cf. CAD B, 103 s.v. *barāmu* sub a, reading the signs GÙN.A together as SU$_9$ = SU$_4$.A). But it is also possible that GÙN.A stood for the D-stem *burrumu*. The colour term *barmu* "multihued, versicoloured" can indicate multiple hues, but also changeability of colour (shimmering appearance, mostly of the eyes), see Thavapalan 2020, 79–89. The terms *barmu/burrumu* can describe the mottled or speckled appearance of animals, minerals or plants. For example, the speckled coat of the panther (*nimru*) is described as GÙN.A = *barāmu* (SpTU 1, No. 27: 27). "Multi-coloured" also belongs to the standard sequence of colour terms in some omen texts; however, *barmu/burrumu* does not usually feature among the diagnostic colours listed in diagnostic and physiognomic texts (Heeßel 2000, 43–44).

The characterization of the unborn child as "lying down" or "sleeping" in the apodosis is unusual; it is found a second time in line 94 (see below). The logogram NÁ can correspond to Akkadian *ṣalālu* "to sleep" or *nâlu* "to lie down (to sleep)". The exact meaning of the logogram in this passage is uncertain. If NÁ stands for *inâl* "it will lie down", the verb could be used euphemistically, in the sense of "to be bed-stricken" or "to lie down in the grave" (die). However, the meaning could also be more technical. In favour of a possible interpretation of NÁ as *ṣalil* "he sleeps", Stol (2000a, 25–26, 194) notes that in Arabic folklore, a woman can be pregnant with a "sleeping" foetus for several years without being aware of it. See also line

94 below. Scurlock and Andersen (2005, 12.114) and Scurlock (2014a, 248) translate "the child in her womb will lie down" and understand this as a reference to a neurological disease interfering with normal movement and standing.

Lines 6–7: The word *uṭṭētu* "grains", which refers to grain or kernels of plants, may be understood as a mole, wart or pimple (CAD U/W, 357 sub 4). A seemingly corresponding omen to line 7 is found in the physiognomic omen series (*Alamdimmû* Tablet 8; Böck 2000, 110–111: 22): *šumma uṭṭēti* [*sāmāti* MIN (= *malû*(?) *i*]-*šarru*(LUGAL) "If (his face) [is full of red(?)] 'grains', he will get rich". The analogy between grain and wealth is obvious.

The cryptographic spelling of *i*$_{11}$-*šár-rù* and similar renderings are also encountered in physiognomic omens (and related Late Babylonian commentaries), see CAD Š/2, 132 sub 1b.

Line 8: The feminine stative form *barmat* should refer to *pūtu* "forehead" (fem.) instead of the "top of the forehead" in the preceding lines (see also Stol 2000a, 195). Cf. also *Diagnostic Handbook* Tablet 4: 129 (Scurlock 2014a, 33, 40; Schmidtchen 2021a, 300, 307): *šumma pūssu barmat* "if his forehead is multi-coloured".

Lines 9–10: The exact denotation of SA and SAG.KI is ambiguous here, since *šer'ānu* (SA) can refer to blood vessels and muscles, and SAG.KI can be *pūtu* "forehead" or *nakkaptu* "temple". Stol (2000a, 195) translates "vein of the forehead" and regards the whole section from lines 1–14 as concerned with the forehead. Scurlock (2014a, 248) understands SA SAG.KI in lines 9–10 as "muscles of the forehead" but regards lines 11–14 as concerned with the temple(s), differentiating between "muscles" in lines 13–14 concerned with colours and "veins" in lines 11–12 referring to pulsation (*tebû*), cf. below.

The opposition between the colours white and red is common in the omen and ritual literature (Scurlock and Andersen 2005, 276ff.). In SA.GIG Tablet 36 red/black often stands for a male baby, white for a female one (see also lines 13–14, 28, 31), but there are also examples where red predicts a female baby, cf. line 29 below.

Lines 11–12: The term *tebû* "to rise, stand up" refers to pulsating bloods vessels (*šer'ānu*) or throbbing temples (e.g., in descriptions of headaches). For this reason, the reading *nakkaptu* "temple" for SAG.KI seems more likely here than a reading *pūtu* "forehead", since especially the right and left side are differentiated here (cf. CAD Š/2, 311–312 sub 1f; CAD P, 547–548 sub 1; note for example *Diagnostic Handbook* Tablet 12: 6 (Schmidtchen 2021a, 483, 494; Scurlock 2014a, 79: 7) for a case where the blood vessels on the right and left side of the throat's upper part (*rēš napišti*) throb but those of the forehead (*pūtu*) are calm).

Observations of pulsating vessels play quite an important role in diagnostics. Scurlock and Andersen (2005, 274–275) point out a parallel from Chinese medicine, where the sex of the foetus was similarly predicted through pulse diagnosis, e.g. by a stronger pulse in the right or left finger. Interestingly, in the present lines pulsating of the right temple signals a girl and a pulsating left temple a boy, which is contrary to the usual association of the right side with the male and the left with the female. See further lines 90–91 below for the pulse of the right and left ankle.

Scurlock and Andersen (ibid.) further suggest this divergence caused by the application of a relative reference frame in the diagnostic context, meaning that "right" and "left" in the present entries refer to the observer's right and left side (or perspective looking at the patient), and not to the patient's intrinsic right and left body sides. Thus, the terms *imittu* and *šumēlu* in the present omens would in fact refer to their direct opposite and the predictions would conform with the usual gender associations. For critical comments on this interpretation, see Heeßel 2010a.

The exact meaning of *šaplānu* "below, underneath" (written KI.TA-*nu*) in lines 11–12 is not entirely clear (cf. CAD T, 318 sub 9; CAD Š/1, 461 sub 1a-2'). Perhaps the area below the *blood vessel* of the temple is meant.

Lines 13–14: In line 13, Scurlock and Andersen (2005) read ⌜SA.MEŠ⌝ "the muscles (of her temple)", but a reading ⌜SA?⌝. DIDLI parallel to SA$_5$.DIDLI "they are red" is suggested (see also line 14). DIDLI can indicate plurality or duality (thus Stol 2000a, 195 translating "both …s of her forehead"). Again, SAG.KI could be read *nakkaptu* "temple" or *pūtu* "forehead" in both entries. Cf. also Scurlock and Andersen 2005, 12.87 and 12.88.

Lines 15–17: The reading KIR$_4$ "nose" follows Stol 2000a, 195 and CAD T, 317 sub 8a), which is in line with the order "from head to feet" applied in this section of Tablet 36.

In line 15, the sign AŠ following *za-qir* in both mss. is difficult to interpret, since *za-qir-rù* does not seem likely. As a logogram, AŠ can mean *ištēn* "one", *aplu* "son" or *magir* "propitious". Note perhaps the lexical equation AŠ = *edēdu* // MIN // *ṣapāru* (cited CAD Ṣ, 97 sub *ṣapāru*; cf. AHw 185, 1082). Both verbs describe features of body parts and horns, but while *edēdu* means "to be pointed", *ṣapāru* means "to be flat; to press down" (AHw 1082a "eindrücken", see G sub 1a). Since the verb *ṣapāru* is also found line 15, followed by a verb describing a contrasting feature (*zaqāru* "to be pointed; to stick up, project"), AŠ may have been used as a logogram for all these verbs.

In lines 16–17, ZI-*ma* most likely stands for the stative *tebī-ma*, parallel to *te-bi* in ms. a lines 22–23.

Lines 22–23: Since this section of Tablet 36 seems to follow roughly the order from "head to toes" (as often in sections of the *Diagnostic Handbook*), a feature of the head should be described here, since the tablet starts with the forehead/temples, and the lips/face follow in lines 24–25. Thus, I understand the entries up to line 23 literally, as dealing with the nose. My interpretation diverges from Scurlock and Andersen (2005, 275 sub 12.81) and Scurlock 2014a, 249 (cf. above comments on lines 15–17).

Line 24: Labat (*TDP* I, 202: 24) reads the third sign in this line as tentatively SAMAG (= DUB), which can stand for *umṣatu*, a mole or wart, a term often found in physiognomic omens and medical texts (cf. Scurlock and Andersen 2005; CAD U/W, 135–136). This reading is followed by Stol 2000a, 195 and Scurlock 2014a, 245. However, the sign in question looks different from the SAMAG-sign found in ms. a obv. 33ff. // ms. b obv. 20'ff.; and we expect a body part term here rather than a conspicuous feature. Thus, I suggest reading NUMDUM (= KAxNUN), "lip(s)" here, which also fits in with the order of body parts, i.e. ⸢NUMDUM⸣.MEŠ-*šú* "her lips" (see also ms. b).

The following verb *qalāpu* "to peel (off), to skin" is attested in connection with *bubu'tu* "boils; blisters" and other body parts (cf. BAM 35 ii 8, 10; CAD Q, 59a sub 3a; AHw 894a). Stol (2000a, 195) wonders whether a pock-pitted appearance could be meant here. The form *uq-tal-la-pa* can be interpreted as a Dt-stem durative (3rd person pl. fem.).

Lines 26–32: These lines deal with the different colours of the woman's nipples. The section shows several divergences in ms. F obv.? 3'–7'. The entries are arranged in a different order than in mss. a and b, and ms. F omits a few lines in comparison with the first millennium BCE version. Moreover, the protasis in ms. F obv.? 3' differs in its formulation and is longer: *šumma ālittu erât appi tulêša* ... "If a childbearing woman is pregnant (and) the nipples of her breast ...". Instead of KIR_4 for Akkadian *appu*, ms. F (obv.? 3', 8') uses the more unusual logogram KIR_{14}(= KAxGAG), cf. Rüster 1989, *Hethitisches Zeichenlexikon*, Nr. 140; Wilhelm 1994, 71 comment on lines 3', 8', 18'.

Lines 26–27: For *zi-i-ir*$_9$ (*zīr*) from *zâru* "to be twisted", see AHw 1516a, sub 2b ("umdrehen; verdrehen"); cf. CAD Z, 72–73 *zâru* A and B. The verb contrasts with *paṭir* "it is loose" (open?) in this pair of lines. For another attestation of *zīr* "it is twisted" (variant: *pašir*) is found in line 86 (see below), with reference to the woman's navel. Similar predictions on a woman's ability to bear and bring pregnancies to term based on the appearance of her nipples are found in physiognomic omens for women. Thus, lines 163–175 of the treatise *Šumma sinništu qaqqada rabât* deal with the nipples (KIR_4 UBUR), and the majority gives apodoses about the woman's procreative abilities: nipples that are white, yellow, black, dark-red/brown (*da'mu*) or pinched (*ṣapir*) signal that the woman is *lā mušallimat* "she is one who does not bring to term" or *lā ālidat* "infertile" (Böck 2000, 161ff. lines 163–166, 169). If they are small, the woman "will not bring to term" (*ul ušallam*). For *šalāmu* in D-stem, see also lines 43–44 below; for *mušallimtu* see line 99.

The two contrasting apodoses in lines 26–27, however, use the logogram SI.SÁ, the Akkadian reading of which is ambiguous. Most likely it should be interpreted as a Št-stem form of *ešēru* "to be straight", which occurs in connection with delivery and with the ability of bringing a pregnancy to term (see e.g., BAM 248 and dupl. iii 9, iv 12; SpTU 3, No. 84 line 11, and the corresponding noun (MUNUS) NU SI.SÁ, (*sinništu*) *lā muš(t)ēšertu*), see e.g. SpTU 5, No. 248: 1). Syllabic renderings of the verb (*uštešser*) "she will bring to term" are found in other apodoses (e.g. DA 96, 25 // CT 30, 30a: 5 (liver omen); quoted in Stol 2000a, 103–104 with fn. 72). Similarly, Stol 2000a, 195–196. For further examples, see CAD E, 359 sub 10. For this apodosis, see also lines 39 and 55–56 below.

Lines 30, 33–34: The formulations (NU) SI.SÁ *erât* in the apodoses of these lines have been interpreted in different ways. Stol (2000a, 196) tentatively reads (*lā*) *išaru* "(she is pregnant) with a normal/abnormal one", referring to the foetus. Labat (1951, *TDP* I, 203) suggests rendering the apodoses as (*lā*) *išariš erât* "she is pregnant in a normal manner" ("elle est enceinte de façon normale"). Similarly, Scurlock (2014a, 249) translates line 30 as "she is pregnant with a foetus which will not do well" and lines 33–34 as "the delivery will (not) be easy" (literally "she is pregnant with (a delivery that) will (not) be easy"), see also Scurlock and Andersen 2005, 10.120, 10.121. See also Schmidtchen 2021a, 46 n. 341 for discussion. Note that the expression *lā išarūtu* "abnormal ones" occurs among other terms for disabled or crippled people in the omen series *Šumma ālu* (see CAD I/J, 226 sub 1a for references; the phrase *lā išaru* "not straight/normal/in a good condition" is also used in references to grain of bad quality to which the field/furrow "gives birth").

Line 31: This line is omitted in the earlier version from Hattuša and thus may be a later addition to the text. The reading MÚD SA_5 is confirmed by ms. B. The signs could be understood as *dāma mali*(DIRI) "(If) it is full of blood" (cf. Stol 2000a, 196). However, the fact that this line occurs in a row of omens describing the colour of the nipples, MÚD SA_5 may refer to a shade of red (*sāmu*) the colour of blood (*dāmu*), although one would rather expect a formulation "is red like blood" (*kīma dāmi sām*). See also Scurlock 2014a, 245. Thus, a somewhat unusual construction "red (as) with blood" may lie behind the logographic spelling. Note for a similar connection the occurrence of "blood-(red) carnelian" (*sāmtu ša dāmi*) in BAM 237(+) iv 40 (see *infra* text C.1.4).

Lines 33–35: For *umṣatu*, a mole or wart, see Böck 2000, 28–29; CAD U/W, 135–136; George 2016, CUSAS 32, 73: 19 (OB): *umṣatu* "growing/coming out on (a man's) body" (*ina zumrīšu ittaṣiam*); Fincke 2018, *FS Geller*, 216, 219–220, 225 ii 9; SpTU 5, No. 260: 9 (commentary; reading NA *ša um-ṣa-a-tú* ...).

Lines 36–48: These entries are concerned with "holes" (*pilšu*) of the nipples. According to Labat (1951, *TDP* I, 203 n. 363), these could refer to openings of the milk vessels which, coming from the mammary gland, open separately on the surface of the nipple. He adds that usually the number of these openings can vary between 15 and 18. Wilhelm (1994) similarly speaks of "Öffnungen der Milchkanäle". Mss. a and b deal with cases, in which there are between 3 and 10 as well as 14 or 15 of these "holes"; ms. F closes with an entry concerned with 16 holes as maximum number.

Although the sign BÙRU can be read *šīlu* "hole" or *pilšu* "breach, opening, hole, perforation", the former term is only attested in extispicy (and exceptionally in *Šumma izbu*); the latter is often found in genitive expressions with body part terms (e.g. in Ugu-mu for the nostrils, the opening of the ears, the urethra, see CAD P, 378–379; CAD Š/2, 352–352). The older ms. F (obv.$^?$ 8'-9') uses the verb *palāšu* "to pierce" (the stative form *pališ*) with numerals instead of a nominal sentence with *pilšu*. Since ms. F obv.$^?$ 3' introduces KIR_{14} UBU[R] as the topic and the parallel mss. a and b have *appi tulî* "tip of the nipple(s)" and *muḫ tulî* "upper side of the breast" in the parallel lines 26 and 52, the sign sequence UGU KIR_{14} UBUR in lines 8' and 18' is presumably a scribal mistake and needs to be emended (see also Wilhelm 1994, 71–72). In line 8', the text should read KIR_{14} UBUR, and in line 18' UGU UBUR.

Line 42: The apodosis in ms. F obv.$^?$ 14' differs, starting with *ša libbīša* [...] "her foetus [...]" (resumed by the sign MIN "ditto") instead of *mārūša* "her children" in mss. a and b.

Lines 43–44: For *šalāmu* in the D-stem in the meaning "to bring to term", see also CAD Š/1, 226 sub 11f.; SpTU 5, No. 248: 10, 30; BM 51246+ rev. 14' and *passim* in this volume. Note also the derived noun *mušallimtu* "a woman who brings to term" in line 99 below. Cf. further line 103 below, with *šalāmu* in the G-stem, in the meaning "she will do well" (*išallim*). M. Stol (personal communication) suggests that the association of ten "holes" with the prediction that the woman will bring her pregnancy to term is due to the tenth month of pregnancy being regarded in Mesopotamian sources as the month of delivery (when the foetus has been brought to full term).

Line 45: Note that in ms. b the second half of the protasis seems to be omitted. The reading of the compound sign in ms. a as URUxKEŠDA$^?$ follows Scurlock 2014a, 246. The meaning of this logogram and its Akkadian correspondence remain unknown. But as noted by Schmidtchen (2021a, 46 n. 342), the sign in question could be a variant form of UKKIN, which stands for *puḫru* "assembly; group; totality" (for *puḫru* referring to a group of body features or body parts such as muscles (*šer'ānu*), cf. CAD P, 492 sub 2; AHw 877a sub C, 2. Alternatively, URUxKEŠDA may be a mistake for KA.KEŠDA = *kiṣru* "knot; concentration; group".

Lines 49–51: These three lines concern features designated as "veins" or "muscles" (*šer'ānū*) visible on the breast. The omens describing "veins" or "muscles" (*šer'ānu*) located on the breast in lines 49–51 and on the belly (lines 56, 69 below) could all refer to stretch marks (stria), which occur on the belly and the breasts (also on arms and thighs) of pregnant women.

For line 49, see CAD Š/3, 388a; for line 50, see CAD Ṣ, 37a; CAD Q, 288b. For lines 49–51, see also Scurlock and Andersen 2005, 274 12.77 and 12.78. The word "threads" (*qû*) found here perhaps refers to smaller capillary vessels surrounding larger veins visible on the surface of the skin.

Lines 52–55: Apparently, these entries continue with the appearance of "veins" on the woman's breast; however, line 52 uses a variant protasis beginning with *šumma ālittu muḫ tulîša* "if on top of a childbearing woman's breast ...". Ms. F obv.$^?$ 18'ff. from Hattuša presents a variant version of these lines.

Line 56: For the meaning of *nadû* in this context, cf. CAD N/1, s.v. *nadû* sub 3b-3' "to have a feature"; CAD U/W, 239–240 s.v. *urqu* sub 1 and 2. According to Scurlock and Andersen (2005, 217), *nadû* with colour terms refers to uneven colouration of the skin (e.g., *Diagnostic Handbook* Tablet 9: 29 Scurlock 2014a, 70, 250 *passim*). Scurlock and Andersen (2005, 277 12.93) see in the protasis a description of abdominal stretch marks (see also line 69 below) and translate: "If on the upper abdomen of a woman of childbearing age, the muscles are unevenly coloured with yellow/tan" (see also 12.94). I.e., the word *šer'ānu* "muscles/blood vessels" would refer here to stretch marks looking similar to veins.

Line 57: From this line onward, ms. a uses the logogram PEŠ for *erû* "to be pregnant" instead of $PEŠ_4$. The reading of the verb in the protasis, *paṭ-ri*, is problematic, since one would expect be stative masc. pl. *paṭrū* here (as in the following lines), see Stol 2000a, 197. Scurlock and Andersen 2005, 12.97 and Scurlock 2014a, 246, 250, read *pat-tal* "(if the insides) feel balled up(?)". The verb *patālu* "to be entwined, twisted" occurs in omen texts, where it describes the appearance of the gut or intestines (e.g. of a malformed foetus, see CAD P, 271 sub 1b), but in our example, the correct stative form should likewise be plural (*pat-lu*). The noun *qerbū* (ŠÀ.MEŠ) usually refers to the intestines or insides, but the word here and in the following lines must refer *pars pro toto* to the area of the belly where the intestines are situated. The entries concerning the "insides" may describe visual or tactile information that the healers gained from visual inspection or palpation of the woman's belly.

Line 58: The Akkadian reading of the logogram MU.PA is uncertain. Stol (2000a, 193, 197) tentatively suggests MU.PA is a rare logogram for *zikaru* "male". MU.PA seems to be used as a variant to the Emesal term mu-tin, which is found as a logogram for *zikaru* in an analogous position in the apodosis of the next two lines (59–60). Moreover, the protases in lines 59–60 feature the same verbs found in line 58 as textual variants (*zaqāru* and *našallulu*), which suggests that line 58 and lines 59–60 are variants from different manuscripts that were combined in a sequence here. In the Emesal dialect, mu-PA corresponds to Sumerian ^{giš}gidru(PA) and Akkadian *ḫaṭṭu* "staff, stick", which may be a euphemistic term for "male" (cf. Emesal Voc. II 150; MSL 4, 21).

The exact meaning of *našallulu* "to slither" in medical or physiognomic omens, where it characterises different body parts, is likewise unclear. Stol (2000a, 197) proposes translating "are hanging down(?)" from the context. In *Diagnostic Handbook* Tablet 5: 55' *našallulu* characterises a part of the lips. Schmidtchen (2021a, 333, 339, 347) translates that occurrence with "*schlüpfrig/gewellt*", i.e. to be slippery or wavy. In an Old Babylonian omen text (Köcher, Oppenheim and Güterbock 1957–1958, *AfO* 18, 64 i 24), this verb describes the testicles. This verb primarily describes the gliding movement of snakes, worms (and demons) and is grouped with *pašālu* "to crawl; to wriggle" and *ḫalāpu* "to slip (into/through)" in lexical lists (CAD N/2, 55–56); cf. also the Gt-stem stative of *ḫalāpu*, which means "tangled" (said of intestines). In the protases of lines 59 and 60, the verbs *zaqāru* "to protrude" and *našallulu* are used again, possibly as a pair of contrasting features, but in this case paired with *ana emšīša* "towards her lower abdomen". Whatever their exact meaning, both lines 58–60 describe variations in the external shape of the pregnant woman's enlarged belly.

Line 59: mu-tin in the Emesal dialect can stand for *zikaru* "male" (Schretter 1990, 236; MSL 13, 202). It is apparently used here as a logogram. See also Stol 2000a, 197.

Line 60: For $ḫaš_4$ (also ḫáš) as a Sumerian equivalent for *ḫallu* "crotch; thigh", cf. Alster 1972, *Dumuzi's Dream*, 102, 121. Another Akkadian equivalent for $ḫaš_4$ attested in lexical sources is *biṣṣūru* "vulva" and *šassūru* "womb" (SpTU 2, 209 No. 54: 31; see further CAD Š/2, s.v. *šassūru* A lex. sect.). Both Stol (2000a, 197) and Scurlock (2014a, 246) read $ḪAŠ_4$(ZUM) ŠÀ, translating this as "crotch of the belly" and "her womb", respectively. Although "crotch of the belly" may be a synonym for *emšu* "lower abdomen", it is not excluded that ŠÀ is used here, maybe by mistake, to indicate the pronominal suffix *-ša*, analogous to the phrase *šà* ŠÀ-*šà*, and that the signs should be rendered as $ḪAŠ_4$-*šà* "her crotch".

Lines 61–71: With the exception of line 69, the entries in lines 61–71 are concerned with different external shapes of the pregnant woman's enlarged belly (*qerbū* "insides"), using terms and expressions denoting subtle differences in curving, elevation, size etc. The verbs (stative forms) encountered in the protases are *šakānu* "to be placed", *nadû* "to pour out; to drop, hang down (said of parts of the body, CAD N/1, 90–91 sub 4b), *zaqāru* "to stick up, protrude", *saḫāru* "to be turned", *ebēṭu* "to be swollen", *napāḫu* "to rise; to be swollen, bloated", *mâdu* "to be very large; to increase" and (*kīma appi*) *zaqāpu* "to be upright, erect; to protrude (like a nose)". Line 69 inserts an unrelated entry about skin colour (uneven colour), which appears here because of the verb *nadû* (which here means "to be covered with spots, discolorations").

Line 61: My translation follows Scurlock and Andersen 2005, 280 12.111 and Scurlock 2014a, 250.

Lines 62–65: Scurlock and Andersen (2005, 280 12.112) and Scurlock (2014a, 250) translate *nadû* as "they are poured (into her lower abdomen)". In lines 64 and 65, the directions "above" and "below" are added to the protasis. Scurlock (2014a, 251) translates here: "they protrude/are turned from above/below towards her hypogastric region".

Line 66: The spelling *eb-ṭù*(DU) encountered here preserves an Old Babylonian (southern) orthography (Stol 2000a, 197).

Line 67: The same omen occurs once more in line 76 (ms. a), with an extended protasis (DIŠ TU ŠÀ.MEŠ-*ša nap-ḫu*), and with a contrasting prognosis (she is pregnant with a male).

Line 69: The verb *šuklulu* "to bring to perfection" may refer to the foetus having a perfect bodily form or being brought to term (CAD Š/3, 225a sub g). The stative sg. form *zaqip* instead of plural *zaqpū* is unexpected here and probably a mistake.

Line 71: In ms. b, no traces of a section ruling are visible after this line, so possibly, none was inserted here. For the reading ZUKUM = *kabāsu* "to step" in lines 71 and 94–98, see Reiner 1971, *RA* 65, 180–181. For *kabāsu* with named directions in another Late Babylonian omen fragment, see also SpTU 5, No. 249: 4'–7' (unclear context). The topic of line 71 is further developed in lines 94–98. The verb is interpreted here as an N-stem with an ingressive meaning. Apparently, healers observed whether a pregnant woman habitually started walking with her right or left foot, to make predictions about the sex of the foetus. If she started walking with her right foot, the foetus was believed to be male; if she did so with her left foot, the foetus was female. These predictions may have been linked with the idea (found also in the Graeco-Roman world) that a male foetus is located in the right, and a female foetus in the left side of the womb; thus, because the weight of the foetus was unevenly distributed in her belly, the woman would tend make a first step with the foot where the main weight of the foetus was felt. In the present case, since the woman started walking equally with her right and left foot, and her feet and ankles were also swollen, it was concluded that she carried the additional weight of a second foetus, thus predicting twins. For discussion, see also Steinert 2017b, *FS* Wiggermann, 231–232; cf. Scurlock and Andersen 2005, 279 12. 110 with n. 92 and comments on lines 94–98 below.

Line 72: Scurlock and Andersen (2005, 278 sub 12.96 with n. 86) connect this omen with the folklore belief that male babies are more active in the womb. Alternatively, the prediction is based on the belief that a male foetus is larger than a female one, and that the bigger weight causes the woman to hold (support) her belly with her hands.

Line 74: Since ms. b seems to begin with ⸢DIŠ TU$^{?}$⸣ [...], it probably belongs together with line 76, and lines 74–75 were omitted in this manuscript. In ms. b, probably only 4 or 5 lines are missing between the corresponding lines 76 and 85 in ms. a, which means that ms. b must have been a few lines shorter than ms. a in this section of Tablet 36.

Line 77: As in line 78, ms. c in rev.$^{?}$ 4' appears to have incorporated a textual variant for part of the protasis, which is not found in ms. a. Moreover, I have not been able to place the first three lines of ms. c, which do not appear to fit any entries in ms. a. The traces read:

c rev.$^{?}$ 1' [..........]x x[.................]
c rev.$^{?}$ 2' [.....] ⸢x x⸣-⸢*na*$^{?}$⸣-*šá* G[I$_6$$^{?}$ ...]
c rev.$^{?}$ 3' [.....]-⸢*a*$^{?}$⸣ *mi-iḫ-ra* x[..........]

For *miḫru* "mishap, adversity, unfortunate incident" in ms. c rev.$^{?}$ 3', see e.g. *Diagnostic Handbook* Tablet 40 lines 7, 9 (Scurlock 2014a, 258, 263, apodosis): *miḫru* DAB-*su* "a *miḫru* afflicts him (the baby)", which appears to be the only passage in SA.GIG with this diagnosis known so far. The phrase *miḫra maḫāru* "to be confronted with (an object inflicting) *misfortune*" is attested in therapeutic texts dealing with the "Ban", see Maul 2019, Text 3 obv. 1 and *passim* for discussion; SpTU 3, No. 84 (text C.3.4). The textual differences between mss. a and c and the peculiar features of ms. c let one wonder whether ms. c may not even be the fragment of a commentary on Tablet 36. Moreover, ms. c also omits several lines of the text (ms. c rev.$^{?}$ 4'–7' = lines 77–70; c rev.$^{?}$ 8'–9' = lines 87–88).

Both lines 77–78 and 103 feature the phrase *ina ša libbīša* in the apodosis. Ms. E rev.$^{?}$ 2'–3' confirm this reading in ms. a lines 77–78. Line 77 has *ina ša libbīša imât* "she will die through her foetus" and line 103 *ina ša libbīša išallim* "she will be well with(?) her foetus"; for line 78, see the next note below. Stol (2000a, 197) translates *ina ša libbīša* as "(she will die) with her foetus"; Scurlock (2014a, 251–252) renders it as "from/as a result of her being with child". Perhaps, these expressions are analogous to *ina mērêša ul iballuṭ* "she will not stay alive/be healthy in her pregnancy" in line 82. Note further a similar apodosis in an Old Babylonian omen text (Nougayrol 1963, *OrNS* 32, 384: 34–35): *erītu ina ša libbīša ul iballuṭ* "a pregnant woman will not stay alive/be healthy through her foetus" (Nougayrol translates "en sa grossesse", i.e. "in her pregnancy").

For *ikkirū* (with *pānū* "face") from *nakāru* in the meaning "to have an unhealthy appearance", see CAD N/1, 163a sub 2d (the contrasting term is *nēḫū* "(the face) is calm/peaceful" in line 78; see also CAD N/1, 145a sub 1b).

Line 78: As in the preceding line, the traces in ms. c suggest that this manuscript incorporated a textual variant for the predicate of the protasis, which is not included in ms. a.

Since *ša libbīša ušallam* is a common phrase found in other apodoses in Tablet 36 meaning "she will will bring her foetus to term", the *ina* preceding it seems superfluous, see also Stol 2000a, 197; CAD Š/1, 226a sub 11f. The repetition of *ina* may have been inspired by the use of *ina* in the apodosis in line 77. Note, however, that ms. E also preserves the *ina*, which leads me to refrain from emending ms. a.

Lines 79–80: KUŠ.TAB in these two lines seems to be an abbreviation of KUŠ.TAB.BA, which in first millennium BCE texts is found as a logogram referring to "plucked wool" (*qerdu*) or to "ox-hide" in the context of tanning (see CAD Q, 228a; Stol 1980–1983, "Leder(industrie)", *RlA* 6, 528a, §3; Stol 2000a, 198). The Akkadian reading of the latter may have been *gildu* (which is an Aramaic loanword). For translation and discussion, cf. also Scurlock and Andersen (2005, 271 12.65 and 12. 66) and Scurlock (2014a, 251), translating "If the face of a woman of childbearing age is full of (patches of what look like) ox-hide treated with depilatories". Ms. a presents an unusual word order in the protasis with the subject (IGI.<MEŠ>-*šá* "her face") preceding the verb, while ms. c places the direct object KUŠ.TAB before *malû* in the regular manner. The spelling *qá-du* in line 80 reflects an Old Babylonian orthography (see Stol 2000a, 193).

The terms *tarāpu* and *turrupu* "to be discoloured" often refer to an abnormal form of pigmentation and can be rendered "to be mottled (with spots)" or "to have streaks (of some colour)" (see Thavapalan 2020, 63–65; Scurlock and Andersen 2005, 218).

Line 81: This entry (ms. a) presents an interesting analogy between vomiting and miscarriage, where opposite body openings (mouth and the female reproductive organs/vagina) are seen in correspondence (i.e. ejecting food via the mouth signals the loss of the foetus). A similar logic may be found in lines 82–83 (see next note).

Ms. E presents a varying verb in the protasis, which is not completely preserved, but may perhaps be restored as [*iptanar*]*rar*, in contrast to *iptanarru* "she keeps on vomiting" (Gtn-stem of *parû*) in ms. a. If read correctly, *iptanarrar* would be a Gtn-stem of *parāru* "to be dissolved, broken up". This verb is attested a few times in the G-stem in medical texts (CAD P, 162 s.v. *parāru* I sub 1). Heeßel (2000, 302, 305) renders an occurrence of the G-stem in *Diagnostic Handbook* Tablet 27: 26 as "kraftlos werden" ("to become weak, powerless"), see also SAD Vol. 1, 67; Stol 2008, 351; AHw 829b.

Lines 82–83: Stol (2000a, 198) notes that the signs MÚD.BABBAR, literally "white/light blood", usually stand for LUGUD = *šarku* "pus", but suggests the meaning "light-coloured blood" here, in contrast to dark blood in line 82 (see also CAD N/1 89b; CAD Š/2 64a, however, read "pus"). Both interpretations are equally possible. Because the sign KA is ambiguous and can stand either for "mouth" or "nose", Stol (ibid.) further draws attention to a difference in phraseology in medical texts: blood (*dāmu*) usually flows (*alāku*) from the nose (KIR_4), but is "ejected, discharged" (*nadû*) from the mouth (KA). However, Scurlock and Andersen (2005, 268 12.47, 12.48) and Scurlock (2014a, 251) read KA "mouth" in both lines and suggest this stands for the mouth of the uterus (cervix). They identify the described symptoms as endometritis (intrauterine infection). In this connection, it is worthy to note that Mesopotamian healers drew connections between nosebleed and bleeding during pregnancy, since incantations to stop gynaecological bleeding could also be used against nosebleed (see BAM 237(+) and dupl. (text C.1.7); Steinert 2017a, 318–320). Interestingly in this regard, lines 82–83 use the 3rd sg. masc. pronominal suffix -*šú* in reference to the patient instead of feminine -*šá*, which is used in most other entries of Tablet 36, which suggests that these lines may have been borrowed or adapted from other sections of *Diagnostic Handbook* in which the subject is a male patient and in which body emissions occur from mouth or nose. It is thus possible that Mesopotamian healers associated discharge of blood or other body fluids from mouth and nose by analogy with uterine bleeding during pregnancy, which was known to be linked to miscarriage. However, the symptoms invoked here are even more fatal. In line 82, the woman's death, in line 83, both the death of woman and child are predicted. Although an extended meaning of "mouth" for the mouth of the womb might be suggested by the context, a literal interpretation following Stol (2000a, 198) remains equally possible here.

Line 84: The cryptic spelling U U DIŠ PA.AN in the apodosis is difficult to understand, see Stol 2000a, 198–199. Scurlock (2014a, 247, 251) reads 21 PA.AN and translates "twenty-one (possible) prognoses", which would be a rather unusual apodosis. Labat (*TDP* I, 208) similarly interpreted the passage as 21 *têrēti*(?) "21 pronostics(?)". However, the word *têrtu* rarely refers to portents not obtained through extispicy, while in medical and other omen texts, "prognosis" or "prediction" is Akkadian *qību* (written ME-*a* or DUG_4.(GA)). The sign sequence U U DIŠ could stand for the number 21, but PA.AN usually corresponds to Akkadian *napāšu* "to breathe freely; to relax, ease" (said of diseases, afflictions), which would make good sense as an apodosis, if it wasn't preceded by a number. Another possibility would be to read *pa-an* as Akkadian *pānu*. However, none of the attested meanings ("front; surface; plan; consideration; opinion") offer a convincing meaning. Stol (2000a, 198–199) further wondered whether *pa-an* might be a gloss or phonetic complement to the sign DIŠ. This may indicate either a verbal form ending in *–pan* or a noun ending in *–ānu*. Perhaps, read *il*$_4$*-pa-an*, for *ilappan* "he/she will become poor", but this again leaves the signs U.U unexplained.

Lines 85–86: In line 86, Scurlock and Andersen (2005, 265 12.29–12.30) emend to <NU> *pa-ši-ir* as a contrast to *zīr* "twisted" (i.e. shut), understanding *pašir* as "unravelled", meaning a protruding navel as a normal sign of an enlarged uterus (also Minen 2018, 189). However, the duplicate ms. b neither has a negated form in line 86. Scurlock (2014a, 252) translates *pašir* in lines 85–86 as "unravelled" and "loose". Thus, it seems that the bodily feature of a "loose" navel is associated with contradictory outcomes, receiving a positive prognosis in line 85 and negative one in line 86. The verb *pašāru* "to loosen, undo, relax, unravel (a thread)" seems mark a contrasting state to *zīru* "twisted" (cf. CAD P, 236ff.; AHw 1516 *zâru* I; CAD Z, 72–73 *zâru* A and B). Incidentally, *zīru* "twisted" (a synonym of *kapālu, kitpulu* "to coil; to entwine") is also used with reference to the womb as an expression for infertility in the Late Babylonian disease taxonomy SpTU 1, No. 43: 30 (Geller 2014, 4: ARḪUŠ *šá zi-i-ri* "a womb which is twisted").

Line 89: For the verb *nabalkutu* "to cross over, turn over" in the sense of "to roll one's eyes", see CAD N/1, s.v. *nabalkutu* sub 3d; e.g. *Diagnostic Handbook* Tablet 5: 115'–120' (Schmidtchen 2021a, 341, 353); Tablet 10: 1 (with diagnosis AN.TA.ŠUB.BA; Schmidtchen 2021a, 440); Tablet 26: 30' (Heeßel 2000, 280, 288).

The interpretation of the apodosis follows Stol 2000a, 199 and CAD A/2, 296a sub 1a-6' (reading *ar-na* AB.BA ÍL "she bears the guilt (for the wrongdoing) of her father"). For *arna našû* "to bear guilt", see also AHw 70 sub 4b; CAD A/2, 299 sub 2d; CAD N/2, 103. Compare, for example, *Šumma ālu* Tablet 104 (CT 39, 46: 64): NAM.TAG.GA DINGIR-*šú na-ši* "(If (a man)'s wife curses his god), he bears the punishment of his god". The differing interpretation in Labat (*TDP* I, 208–209), Scurlock and Andersen (2005, 280 12.115) and Scurlock (2014a, 252), reading *ar-na-ab-ba* ÍL "she carries a hare" (*arnabu*) and interpreting this as a reference to a foetus with a hare's lip, is not followed here.

For the "evil" (*lumnu*) or "ban" (*māmītu*) of the father as a consequence of sexual intercourse during pregnancy, see also line 111 below and *Diagnostic Handbook* Tablet 37: 6: *māmīt abīša* "the ban of her father (will afflict her)". The "Ban" (NAM.ÉRIM, i.e. punishment caused by swearing a false oath)) and *arnu* (NAM.TAG.GA) "guilt" are equated in *Diagnostic Handbook* Tablet 22: 28, 30 (apodosis; Heeßel 2000, 254), and "the guilt of the father" (and other family members) is often referred to in rituals against the "Ban" (cf. Maul 2019). The "evil" or "guilt" of the father may allude to a belief that the consequence would be the birth of a child with abnormalities (cf. Scurlock and Andersen 2005, 266).

Line 93: Scurlock and Andersen (2005, 278 12.102) understand the protasis as a description of varicose veins, a frequent occurrence in pregnancy, although they are more likely to occur on the calves.

Line 94: I follow Stol's (2000, 25–26, 199) interpretation of this line and understand *maruštu* "trouble, distress" as a term for "menstrual period". See further SpTU 1, No. 59 rev. 12' (*infra* text C.2.3), where the logogram (NÍG).GIG is used instead in connection with a missed period. If this interpretation is correct, it would mean that Mesopotamian healers believed that a woman could be pregnant and continue to menstruate. This unusual phenomenon may have been explained in the apodosis of line 94 with the presence of a "sleeping" foetus. Stol (2000a, 25–26, 199) proposed the translation of NÁ (Akkadian *ṣalālu*) as a "sleeping (foetus)" and linked this with a belief found in the Arab world (especially in Northern Africa) about foetuses who dwell for a long time in their mothers' womb without being noticed (a similar apodosis occurs in line 5 above: *šà* ŠÀ-*šà* NÁ "her foetus sleeps/lies down").

The folk theory of a "sleeping" foetus may have been applied to women who were unsuccessful in getting pregnant for a long time, especially in a society where female infertility was associated with social stigma. This belief can be compared with the culturally-bound illness called "arrested pregnancy syndrome", "a culturally recognized state in which a woman is thought to be carrying a child, but the normal progression of pregnancy is arrested. The condition ... may persist for months or even years, during which time the physical symptoms of pregnancy are absent, yet the woman is considered to be 'with child'" (Coreil et al. 1996, 425). Arrested pregnancy syndrome seems to be linked with infertility or subfecundity and is interpreted as a face-saving strategy for women in cultural settings that place high social pressures on women to bear children.

The line commenting on this entry in the commentary SpTU 1, No. 39: 3' is unfortunately fragmentary (see below).

Lines 94–98: In the *Diagnostic Handbook*, the left side of the body is often associated with the female and the right with the male reflected, e.g. in the gender of the deity identified as the sender of certain afflictions/symptoms (for right and left in omen texts, see also Schmidtchen 2021a, 197–200, 205; Guinan 1996, *SAAB* 10, 5–10). In Tablet 36, features observed on the right side of a pregnant woman's body are in most cases associated with the presence of a male foetus, and features on the left side with a female one. Scurlock and Andersen (2005, 732 n. 79) interpret the omen protases in lines 94–98 as describing a pregnant woman's "listing" gait ("stepping to the right/left") and compare them with similar Persian and Arabic folklore practices related to predicting the sex of the foetus. In fact, these examples associate the woman's preference to start walking with the right foot with a male foetus, and the preference for the left foot with a female foetus, as appears to be case also in the present lines of Tablet 36. For discussion of the passage, see also Steinert 2017b, *FS Wiggermann*, 231–232 and the note on lines 96–98 below. For a differing interpretation of the passage, see Scurlock and Andersen (2005, 275–276, 280 with 12.84, 12.85, 12.86, 12.113).

Lines 96–98: The commentary SpTU 1, 39: 3'–4' (see below) gives a syllabic spelling for the sign ZUKUM, the keyword of the protases in lines 94–98, rendering it as *ik-ka-ba*[!]*-sa*[!]. This should be understood as an N-stem form of *kabāsu*, used with an ingressive meaning (i.e. to start treading or walking). Although rarely attested with *kabāsu* (CAD K, 11 sub 8), an ingressive function of the N-stem is found in similar verbs such as *saḫāru* "to turn around/back" (Kouwenberg 2010, 297; CAD S, 52–53 sub 16). The protases of lines 94–98 imply that healers observed whether a (pregnant) woman, when called upon, habitually started walking with her left or right foot, to make predictions about her foetus. The commentary further adds an explanation for the phrase GÌR.MIN-*šú* DUGUD "her feet are heavy" found in line 96: [*šá ana da-k*]*e-e dan-na-áš-šú* "[(this) refers to the case when] they are (too) difficult for her [to lift] up."

The apodosis of line 96 probably refers to twins (a male and a female foetus), although the translation "or" for *u* is likewise possible. The former possibility is suggested by the elements of the protasis: the woman tends to start walking with the right foot (i.e. a male foetus) and additionally her feet feel heavy (i.e. she carries the heavy weight of a second foetus). The equal tendency to start walking with the right and left foot in line 98 similarly triggers the prediction that the woman bears twins (there is an equal weight on both sides of the woman's body, thus she does not favour one side over the other).

In line 97, the woman's habit of starting to walk with her left foot leads to the prognosis of a female child. The additional element, that the woman's feet feel heavy may imply the idea that women suffer more difficulties when they are pregnant with a female foetus (than when they bear a male one). Similar views are attested in ancient Greek medical authors (see e.g. Temkin 1991, 44–45 *Soranus, Gynaecology* Book I, 45; Flemming 2002, 108–109 on Galen and *Hippocrates' Aphorisms* V 42). Moreover, similar to ideas encountered in ancient Graeco-Roman texts, the group of omens in lines 94–98 may also be based on the belief that a male foetus develops in the right side of the womb, and a female foetus in the left, which would lead to a preference for one foot over the other in the mother's gait (cf. *Hippocrates, Aphorisms* V 48 (Jones 1931); Flemming 2000, 308–309).

Line 99: The same apodosis is also encountered in a physiognomic omen in the series *Šumma sinništu qaqqada rabât* concerned with female bodies (Böck 2000, 166 line 222); the protasis of that omen is not preserved, but the omen belongs to a fragmentary section preceding entries about a woman's toes. It is thus possible that this omen in Tablet 36 was borrowed from the diagnostic series. The commentary SpTU 1, 39: 5' comments on the protasis of line 99 (see below text I.1.2).

Lines 100–102: The reading of the sign sequence ŠÀ KU SA in the protases of these three lines is either cryptographic or corrupt. Scurlock and Andersen (2005, 259 12.2 and 12.3) and Scurlock (2014a, 247–248) read ŠÀ.SUR$_{11}$-*sa*, interpreting the term as an unusual logogram for *šassūru* "womb". However, this reading leaves unexplained why the pronominal suffix attached to the subject is *–sa* instead of *–šá* (which would indicate that the preceding noun ends in a sibilant or a dental (see also Frahm 2011, 228 n. 1062). It is possible that the scribe did not have the word *šassūru* in mind here, but a synonym, e.g. *qerbītu*. For other possibilities of analysing the sign sequence, see Stol (2000a, 200–201) for discussion.

The commentary SpTU 1, No. 39: 6' comments on the passage in question, but does not quote the signs ŠÀ KU SA. Instead, it renders the corresponding keyword syllabically as *sa-gu-u* and explains this word as *da-mu a*[*r-da*]*-tu*$_4$ "the blood of a [you]ng woman" (see below). Thus, the signs ŠÀ.KU.SA in ms. a lines 100–102 may be a corrupt rendering of an expected phrase *sagûša* "her *sagû* (i.e. menses)" (in other Late Babylonian attestations of the term in gynaecological texts, we usually find the spelling *sa-gu-šá*. But variant attested spellings are *šá/ša-gu-šá* and *sa/šá-gu*$_5$(KU)-*šá*, of which the sign sequence ŠÀ.KU.SA is reminiscent (cf. SpTU 1, No. 59: lines 6'; BM 40152 ii 15'; BAM 235: 7 for discussion). The commentator's explanation of the word *sagû*, however, corresponds well with the reference to different colours in line 100–102 (especially *sāmu* "red" and *pelû* "light-red" are known as colours of blood, see e.g. BAM 235–236), but also with other attestations of the word *sagû* in a few Late Babylonian gynaecological prescriptions, where it is apparently used as a term for the menses, in a context where the regular menses are absent and need to be induced (see e.g. BM 38624+ ii 28', 30' (text A.2.1), texts C.1.1–C.1.2, chapter C.2 and *passim*). For further discussion, see the commentary SpTU 1, No. 39 (edited below). The synonym list *Malku* = *šarru* VIII 150–152 (Hrůša 2010, 247) equates *sagû* with *qablu* "waist" and *ḫanṣātu* "hips", which has led to the suggestion that *sagû* was a term for a menstrual bandage or piece of underwear worn around the hips/genitals (see Wasserman 2019, *FS Charpin*, 1135, 1138–1139). It is possible that the meaning of the term *sagû* became extended or changed in the course of the first millennium BCE, from a piece of clothing that may have served as a menstrual bandage to a word for the menstrual discharge itself. Moreover, *sagû* may be related to the term *sāgu*, which is a piece of clothing tied around the waist (a workers' apron?), cf. CAD S, 27–28 s.v. *sagû* B and *sāgu*; AHw 1003a s.v. *sāgu* and *sagû* II.

If the present understanding of *sagû* as "(menstrual) discharge" in the context of lines 100–102 is correct, these entries may refer to a haemorrhage during pregnancy (usually designated as *naḫšātu*, see line 108 below). This would underline that the Mesopotamian healers only vaguely differentiated between (normal) menstruation and abnormal bleeding (e.g. during pregnancy). In the cases encountered here, a red flux in pregnancy signalled a male foetus; a "bright/light-coloured" (*namru*) discharge signalled an "abnormal" foetus (for similar apodoses, see also lines 30, 34, 54, 92). The verb *reḫû* "to inseminate; to impregnate" normally refers to the man's activity; thus, we understand the G-stem form *irḫi* here exceptionally in a passive sense ("she was impregnated").

Lines 103–104: These two entries associates contrasting attitudes or moods of the pregnant woman with contrasting outcomes. The verbal form *palḫat* can be rendered as "she is fearful" or "she is respectful"; the contrasting word *šelât* (from *šelû*) means "she is negligent, careless". Instead of the latter, Stol (2000a, 201) reads *ḫe*[!]-*la-at* "(if a fertile woman) enjoys pregnancy" instead (from *ḫelû* "to be bright, merry", with AHw 339 s.v. *ḫelû* II). Note that *šelû* is usually not construed with a direct object in the accusative, but with a prepositional phrase with *ina muḫḫi* (cf. CAD Š/2, 274–275).

Line 105: In ms. a, the verbal form *i-ta-na-aš-šá-šu* (Gtn or Ntn-stem of *ašāšu*, meaning "to become constantly distressed, upset", cf. AHw 79; CAD A/2, 424a sub 2a-2') indicates a masculine plural subject (thus ŠÀ.MEŠ most likely stands for Akkadian *qerbū* or *irrū* "insides, entrails"). Ms. D, however, presents a variant *i-ta-na-aš-šá*, which should presumably be interpreted as a Gtn-stem of *našû*, i.e. "it constantly rises up", which may have to be restored according to similar formulations referring to an urge to vomit: *libbašu* (*ana arê/parê i-ta-na-*(*áš*)*-šá-a* "his belly continually heaves (rises up to vomit)" (see e.g. *Diagnostic Handbook* Tablet 22: 26 (Scurlock 2014a, 186); SpTU 1, No. 33: 2).

Furthermore, the verb *ašāšu* "to be upset, tormented" in ms. a can refer to somatic (e.g. intestinal) as well as emotional disturbances. In attestations from medical texts, these two levels of meaning are often difficult to differentiate (see Attia 2018, *JMC* 31, 83–88 for discussion). Emotional distress as the cause of a fatal outcome of pregnancy would in fact fit well with the contrasting affective dispositions of the woman described in lines 103–104. In line 105, *ašāšu* describes a problematic behaviour, while *palḫat* "fearful, respectful" in line 103 denotes a positive behaviour corresponding with social conventions and expectations.

For this line, cf. Attia 2018, 83–84. Heeßel (2000, 223 notes 8–9) compares the form *i-ta-na-aš-šá-aš* in *Diagnostic* Handbook Tablet 17: 9 with the present line 105. However, the present passage differs (plural subject).

Lines 106–113: The fact that this section is set apart from the preceding and following lines in all three manuscripts may signal that these lines originally stemmed from a different source or collection of material than the preceding sections. The lines resemble the beginning of Tablet 37 (lines 1–7), which make predictions about the positive or ill consequences of sexual intercourse with a sick pregnant woman in different months of pregnancy (using the verb *ratāpu* "to continue" instead of *qerēbu* "to approach" line Tablet 36, cf. below). The concern with certain days in the present lines suggests a connection with hemerological or menological thinking.

The wording of the protases in lines 106–113 has been interpreted in differing ways. The Neo-Assyrian ms. D differs slightly from its Late Babylonian duplicates. I follow Stol's (2000, 201) suggestion to delete the number 5 before ITI in ms. a in line 106, on the basis that it is not present in ms. D. Stol translates the protasis as "one approaches her (sexually) on three days per <<5>> month" (following Kraus 1986, 131–132), while Scurlock and Andersen (2005, 267 12.39–12.43) and

Scurlock (2014a, 253) translate "at five months (and) three days". However, since in ms. D, KÁM is added to the number of the day, "on the third day of the month" may be meant here. The elision of the number 5 seems likely, since it is difficult to explain why the fifth month would have been picked out as particularly critical or relevant. Perhaps the date formula in ms. a should be understood as "during the days of month 3 (of pregnancy)". In this case, we would have a parallel set of predictions compared with Tablet 37: 1ff., but Tablet 36: 106–113 were meant to cover the cases of intercourse with a healthy pregnant woman. Thus, lines 106–113 use the same number scheme as Tablet 37: 1–7, from the third to tenth month of pregnancy. It is difficult to explain why the passage in Tablet 36 does not treat all days of the month, but only days three to ten.

It is interesting that the general (positive/negative) value of the apodoses attached to the numbers 3–10 in both passages are identical in almost all cases: months (day) 3 and 4 are positive, 5 and 6 are negative, 7 is positive. The only divergence is presented by the final months (days): in Tablet 36, the numbers 8 and 9 are negative and 10 is positive, while in Tablet 37: 6–7, one variant is positive for month 8, while months 9 and 10 are both negative. Scurlock and Andersen (2005, 265) propose that intercourse during the first and second month of pregnancy was not contemplated due to the danger of miscarriage, and for this reason omens for intercourse in months 1 and 2 were not included in the list of cases. They also point out that lines 106–113 in Tablet 36 are modelled after the month-scheme in Tablet 37. However, Scurlock and Andersen (ibid., 266ff.) regard the section in Tablet 36 as a day-to-day scheme for the fifth month of pregnancy because it was regarded as a particularly "problematic" month. They explain that the number scheme for the first ten days would have been repeated for the rest of the days of the month.

Line 108: The commentary SpTU 1, No. 39: 7'–8' comments on the apodosis of line 108 "she will get sick with *naḫšātu*-disease", by reference to the phrase *šá na-*[*aḫ-š*]*á-a-tú* GIG-*át* "she is sick with *naḫšātu*-disease" known from therapeutic texts (see e.g. BAM 237(+) (text C.1.7) in this volume). The commentary explains this with *sinništu ša ina mērêšu dāmu ītanammaru* "a woman who keeps discovering blood during her pregnancy" (see below). Therefore, I regard *naḫšātu* as a form of abnormal haemorrhage (during pregnancy) rather than "excessive bleeding" (contra Biggs 2006, 43 note 29).

Line 111: The prognosis given in this line, "the evil of the father (in the form of) the 'Ban' will afflict her" (ḪUL *a-bi* NAM.ÉRIM DAB-*su*) is similar to the corresponding prognosis for intercourse in the eighth month of pregnancy in Tablet 37: 6: "the ban of her father will afflict her" (NAM.ÉRIM AD-*šú* DAB-*si*), see below. The 'Ban' affliction (caused by a broken or falsely sworn oath) is often described as affecting not only the person guilty of the offense, but also his/her family and descendants (see Maul 2019).

Lines 114–115: These two entries are quotations or adaptations from *Šumma izbu* Tablet 1. Line 114 resembles *Šumma izbu* 1: 83, while line 115 duplicates *Šumma izbu* 1: 100 (de Zorzi 2014, II 360, 365), with the well-known exception that the sign DIŠ is used for *šumma* in the diagnostic text (instead of BE in *Šumma izbu*). *Šumma izbu* Tablet 1: 83 has a varying apodosis: *dannatu ina māti ibaššī-ma mātu lumun libbi immar lumnu ana bīt abīšu iššakkan* "there will be hardship in the land, and the country will experience distress; evil will beset the house of their (the children's) father."

Lines 116–118: For the colophon see Hunger 1968, 51 No. 127. The catchline of Tablet 37 is also quoted in the colophon of the commentary on Tablet 36, SpTU 1, No. 39: 13' (see below). For the correct reading DUB 36.KÁM.MA "36th Tablet" in line 117, see already Hunger 1975, *ZA* 65, 68 n. 11, which corresponds with the tablet number assigned by the catalogue of *Sakikkû* and *Alamdimmû* (Schmidtchen 2018b, 316). However, the catalogue witnesses give a much higher number of 147 [149] entries (omens) for Tablet 36 instead of the 114 (sic!) lines counted in the colophon of ms. a. In fact, ms. a contains 115 omens, not 114 (cf. Schmidtchen 2018a, 142 n. 42; 2018b, 324). A similar divergence in the number of lines is found between the catalogue and the main witness of Tablet 37 (see below).

In line 118, *bir(i)* could be a sign play for *bari* or *ibri* "collated", since it is found in the usual position following *išṭur*. AŠ.AŠ is an abbreviation for KUR.KUR = *mātāti*.

I.1.2 SpTU 1, No. 39: A Commentary Fragment on *Diagnostic Handbook* Tablet 36

This fragmentary commentary on *Diagnostic Handbook* Tablet 36 was found at Uruk (Area U18, Level V), together with a group of other commentaries and texts with colophons by Anu-ikṣur, which suggests that the tablet belonged to the library of the descendants of Šangû-Ninurta dating to the latter half of the Achaemenid period (Clancier 2009, 64, 388). The colophon designates it as an oblong (IM.GÍD.DA) tablet of Šamaš-aḫa-iddina. The fragment preserves the lower part of the tablet's reverse, with twelve lines of commentary on selected lines from Tablet 36 (lines 94–99, 100, 108), concerned with birth prognoses and omens for pregnant women.

List of Manuscripts

Siglum	Museum Number	Copy	Collation	Format; Ductus	Provenience
a	W. 22307/23+74	SpTU 1, No. 39	Photo coll.	Fragment of a single-column tablet; Late Babylonian script; 5th/4th cent. BCE	Uruk; library of the descendants of Šangû-Ninurta

Previous Edition and Discussion

Hunger 1976, SpTU 1, 48, 138 No. 39 (edition; copy)
Clancier 2009c, *GKAB* P348460 (edition)
Wee 2019b, 323–329 (edition), 433 pl. 29 (photo of the reverse)
CDLI P348460 (copy)
Frahm, Frazer and Jiménez 2013a, *CCP* 4.1.36 (copy)
Clancier 2009a, 388
Frahm 2011, 228, 291, 315 n. 1500
Genty 2010, *JMC* 16, 14, 16, 26–27
Heeßel 2000, 95–96 n. 103, 137, 146
Maul 1994, 162
Scurlock and Andersen 2005, 260 n. 4
Schmidtchen 2018b, 327 n. 40
Steinert et al. 2018, 275
Wee 2017, *ZA* 107, 240

Transliteration

Ms. a obv. not preserved
Beginning of the reverse lost

1' a rev. 1' [........-*u*]*s*(?) : *šá* S[AG$^?$ ......]

2' a rev. 2' [.........]-*šu* : *i-li* x[........]

3' a rev. 3' ***ina* ŠÀ *ma-ru-uṣ-ti-šú*** : x[...... **ZUKU]M**(?)[216]

4' a rev. 4' *ik-ka-ba*$^!$(zu)-*as*$^!$(ta) : **GÌR.MIN-*šú* DU[GUD** : *šá ana da-k*]*e-e*

5' a rev. 5' *dan-na-áš-šú* : **MUNUS GÌR-*šú* TUR** [: *ṣe-eḫ-ra* :] *qal-la-la*

6' a rev. 6' *sa-gu-u* : *da-mu a*[*r-da*]-*tu*$_4$: sa [: *d*]*a-mu* : gi

7' a rev. 7' *ar-da-tu*$_4$: ***šá na-*[*aḫ-š*]*á-a-tú* GIG-*át***

8' a rev. 8' MUNUS *šá ina me-re-e-šú da-mu i-ta-nam-ma-ru*

9' a rev. 9' SA.GIG : *ri-*[*kis m*]*ur-ṣu* : *nap-ḫar mu*[*r-ṣ*]*u*

10' a rev. 10' gul-la : gú [: gú]-sa-a : ki-šá-ra :

216 Bold characters indicate quotes from the base text.

11' a rev. 11' *kul-lat* : *na-[ga]b* : *nap-ḫar* : *kiš-šat* : gú-sa-a

12' a rev. 12' gú : *nap-ḫar* : sa : *[n]ap-ḫa-rù*

Colophon:

13' a rev. 13' DIŠ ^{munus}PEŠ$_4$ GIG-*ma šum-ma šá* ITI 3.KAM *ir-ṭú-pu-niš-ši*

14' a rev. 14' IM.GÍD.DA ^{md}20-PAP-MU DUMU.A.NI ^{md}KÁR.ŠUL-*id*-[....]

15' a rev. 15' *pa-liḫ* ^{d}60 *u* $^{d+}$INANNA NU TÙM *ina* ITI-*šú ana* UMUN-*šú* GUR-[*šú*]

Bound Transcription and Translation
Ms. a obv. not preserved
Beginning of the reverse lost

1' *too fragmentary for transcription*	1' [...] ... [...]
2' *too fragmentary for transcription*	2' [...] ... [...]
3' *ina libbi maruštīšu* : ...[... ZUKU]M(?)	3' during her trouble (means) [...; ZUKU]M (means)
4' *ikkabbas* : *šēpāšu ka[btā* : *ša ana dak]ê*	4' *she tends to tread.* "Her feet are heavy" [refers to the case when] they are (too) 5' difficult for her 4' [to lift] up.
5' *dannāšu* : *sinništu šēpšu* TUR [: *ṣeḫrā* :] *qallalā*	5' "(If) a woman's feet (lit. foot) are TUR" [means they are small, which means] they are little.
6' *sagû* : *dām a[rda]ti* : sa [: *d*]*āmu* : gi	6' *sagû* refers to the blood of a young woman; sa means "blood"; gi means
7' *ardatu* : *ša n[aḫš]āti marṣat*	7' "young woman" (in the Emesal dialect). One who is sick with *naḫšā-tu* (refers to)
8' *sinništu ša ina mērêšu dāmu ītanammaru*	8' a woman who keeps seeing blood during her pregnancy.
9' SA.GIG : *ri[kis m]urṣī* : *napḫar mu[rṣ]ī*	9' SA.GIG (*Sakikkû*) refers to the *collection* concerning (all) sickness(es); which refers to all sickness.
10' gul-la : gú [: gú]-sa-a : ki-šá-ra :	10' gul-la, gú, [gú]-sa-a (and) ki-šá-ra
11' *kullat* : *na[ga]b* : *napḫar* : *kiššat* : gú-sa-a	11' mean "all" (*kullatu*), "the whole" (*nagbu*), "total" (*napḫaru*), totality (*kiššatu*). In gú-sa-a,
12' gú : *napḫar* : sa : *[n]apḫaru*	12' gú means "total"; sa (also) means "total".

Colophon:

13' *šumma erītu marṣat-ma šumma ša* ITI 3.KAM *irṭupūnišši*	13' (Catchline:) "If a pregnant woman is sick and if (one) continues (to have sexual relations) with her in the third month (of pregnancy)."
14' *imgiddû Šamaš-aḫa-iddina mār Ištar-id*-[....]	14' Oblong tablet of Šamaš-aḫa-iddina, son of Ištar-...[...].
15' *pāliḫ Anu u Ištar lā itabbal ina arḫīšu ana bēlī-šu utâr[šu]*	15' Who revers Anu and Ištar must not carry off (this tablet). He shall return [it] to its owner within the same month.

Notes

Lines 3'–4': These lines comment on line 94 of Tablet 36, which in the main manuscript (ms. a) reads: DIŠ TU *ina* ŠÀ *ma-ru-uš-ti-šá* ZAG ZUKUM-*as* NÚ PEŠ$_4$-*at* "If a fertile woman during her trouble treads to the right, she is pregnant with a 'sleeping one'." The restoration of [ZUKU]M at the end of line 3' and the emendation at the beginning of line 4' follow Wee (2019b, 323, 326–327), who understands *ikkabbasa* as an N-stem durative form of *kabāsu* "to tread" (with a meaning "she tends to tread"), which explains the logogram ZUKUM (corresponding to ZUKUM-*as* in the protasis of Tablet 36: 94). Note that 3rd person feminine pronominal suffixes referring to the patient in the base text are replaced by masculine suffixes in the Uruk commentary, a phenomenon that can be observed also in SpTU 1, No. 40, the commentary on Tablet 39 (see below). Wee (2019b, 326) proposes that the commentator's usage may have been intended to signal that the medical terminology commented on could be potentially applied to both male and female patients. It should be noted, however, that many of the observed phenomena in medical texts concerned with women deal with issues that are specific to the female body (e.g. pregnancy, birth, menstruation).

Lines 4'–5': The restorations in the breaks follow Wee 2019b, 323. The restoration in line 4' [*šá ana da-k*]*e-e dan-na-áš-šú* follows the similar phrase *ša ana dakê u šakānu dannāniššu* in the Uruk commentary on Tablet 39 (SpTU 1, No. 40), found there with reference to the thighs (see below). The form *dannāšu* is thus analysed as a 3rd person feminine plural stative with a resumptive suffix *-šu* (see also Finkel 2000, *FS Lambert*, 181–182 obv. 9 with note). For explanations in commentaries introduced by the relative pronoun (*ša ...-šu/-ša*), see Gabbay 2016, 109–110. The resumptive *-šu* refers back to the antecedent of *ša*.

The quotation MUNUS GÌR-*šú* TUR stems from line 96 of Tablet 36 (ms. a): DIŠ TU ZAG ZUKUM-*as u* GÌR-*šá* DUGUD-*at* "If a fertile woman has a tendency to tread with the right side (foot) and her foot feels heavy". For other instances of "heaviness" of the limbs, linked with difficulties of movement and expressed with the verbs *kabātu* "to be heavy" and *danānu* "to be difficult", see also Wee 2019b, 327. The phrase "the woman's feet (lit. foot) are small (TUR)" is quoted from line 99 of the base text (ms. a): DIŠ TU GÌR.MIN-*šá* TUR.MEŠ "If fertile woman's feet are small". For the adjective *qallalu* "little, small", see CAD Q, 60.

Lines 6'-7': This commentary entry on the key term *sagû*, "flow of blood" (referring to menstrual blood) relates to lines 100–102 of Tablet 36, where this word is however written pseudo-logographically or erroneously as ŠÀ.KU.SA (ms. a). In lines 100–102, the colours of the discharge are described as red-brown (*sāmu*), bright red (*pelû*) or bright/shiny (*namru*). Since the commentator analyses the signs SA and GI as components of the word *sagû*, he probably had a varying manuscript at his disposal that did not have the spelling ŠÀ.KU. In all other medical texts known to me, in which this word occurs, *sagû* (or *šagû* in Neo-Assyrian texts) is written syllabically (cf. above, with notes on SA.GIG Tablet 36: 100–102). The commentary passage is crucial for its explanation of *sagû* as *dām ardati* "blood of a young woman", suggesting that this term refers to women's regular menstrual discharges.

Sumerian sa is also equated with *dāmu* "blood" in the lexical list Nigga 298 (MSL 13, 104) and in the Standard Babylonian *List of Diseases* (MSL 9, 95 line 156 (216)). The meaning "blood vessel" connected with the Sumerian word sa (beside the meanings "muscle" and "tendon") may have influenced this equation (Wee 2019b, 327–328). The correspondence of Sumerian gi (or gi_4) with *ardatu* "young woman" is found in bilingual and lexical texts (CAD A/2, 242; Emesal Vocabulary II 71 (MSL 4, 17)). Compare also the Nippur Commentary on the birth compendium, 11N-T3: 8 (see *infra* text G.1), which equates gi with *sinništu* "woman; female".

Lines 7'–8': SAD Vol. 4, 109 s.v. *naḫšātu* differently interprets the verbal form *i-ta-nam-ma-ru* in line 8' as an Ntn-stem, with *dāmu* as subject. In contrast to Wee (2019b, 325, 328), I do not understand lines 6'–8' as continuous explanations, but regard lines 7b'–8' beginning with *ša naḫšātu marṣat* "she suffers from *naḫšātu*-haemorrhage" as a new commentary entry beginning with an expression related to the apodosis of SA.GIG Tablet 36 line 108 (ms. a), which reads: DIŠ TU $PE\check{S}_4$-*ma ša* ITI 5 u_4-*mi* KI.MIN *ša na-aḫ-šá-ti* [GIG] "If a childbearing woman is pregnant and ditto (i.e. they approach her (sexually) at (five) months and five days), she will get sick with *naḫšātu*-disease". In my view, the commentator did not regard *naḫšātu* as a synonym for *sagû* or as just another term for "menstrual flow". That *naḫšātu* denoted a pathological condition, is clarified by the commentator's explanation that it is an irregular haemorrhage during pregnancy, which differs from that given for *sagû* in line 6'. For *naḫšātu* see further the discussion on BAM 237(+) (text C.1.4). The condition is also mentioned in the drug list BAM 381 iii 24 (see Stol 2000a, 53–54).

Line 9': The last lines of commentary in SpTU 1, No. 39 rev. 9'–12' focus on the title of the *Diagnostic Handbook* SA.GIG, which was probably motivated by the occurrence of the title SA.GIG in the colophon of the base text (see ms. a line 117). The interpretation of the title SA.GIG (*sakikkû*, the literal meaning of which is "sick string(s); symptom(s)") as *rikis murṣī* "the compilation/collection/bundling of (all forms of) sickness(es)" is also found in other commentaries on the *Diagnostic Handbook* and stems from editorial note (also called "Esagil-kīn-apli's Manifesto" by Wee) in the catalogue of the diagnostic series, the oldest text offering this equation (Finkel 1988, 148–150; Heeßel 2000, 95–96; Schmidtchen 2018b, 318, 327 line 65; Wee 2019a, 13–26; 2019b, 7, 16, 27, 171, 176, 183 Commentary Sa-gig 1A line 47; Sa-gig 5 lines 33–34). The understanding of the *Diagnostic Handbook* of a text collecting information on all kinds of diseases is further underlined by the following equation *napḫar murṣi* "the totality/sum of (all) sickness" in line 9' of SpTU 1, No. 39.

Lines 10'–12': These lines form the continuation of the commentator's analysis of the sign SA, aiming to show that it has the meaning "all, totality" (Wee 2019b, 325, 328–329). As Wee points out, the commentator draws on four lexical equations found in Erimhuš V 43–46 (MSL 17, 68): there, gul-la = *kullatu*, gugú = *nagbu*, gú- di-ir dir = *napḫaru*, ki-šár-ra = *kiššatu*. Gul-la is attested in Erimḫuš V 43 as sumerogram for *kullatu* and synonyms (MSL 17, 68). The commentator's variant [gú]-sa-a used instead of gú-dir(SI.A) in Erimḫuš V 44 may be based on a misreading (Wee 2019b, 328–329; cf. further gú-si-(a) = *napḫaru*/*nagbu* "total", attested in Izi Bogh. A 91 (MSL 13, 135) and Antagal G 31 (MSL 17, 222)). The spelling ki-šá-ra in the commentary likewise seems to be a mistake for ki-šár-ra. The following analysis of the signs gú and sa found in gú-sa-a in lines 11'-12' are probably inspired by the analysis of *sagû* in the preceding lines (see Frahm 2011, 228). For the logic applied by the commentator, showing that gú and sa both mean "all", see Wee 201b, 325, 329.

Line 14': For dKÁR.ŠUL as a cryptographic logogram for the goddess Ištar, see Erimhuš V 4 (MSL 17, 67) and the god list An = *Anu ša amēli* 87 (Litke 1998, 234; Lambert and Winters 2023, 248); Lambert 1976–1980, "Karašul," *RlA* 5, 408; Frahm 2011, 228 n. 1061.

I.1.3 *Diagnostic Handbook* Tablet 37: Women's Afflictions and Pregnancy

Tablet 37 of the *Diagnostic Handbook* is still poorly known. The two identified fragments a and b preserve only the first 28 entries in a more or less fragmentary state. Schmidtchen (2021a, 245) proposes that the small fragment W. 17630i (TDP II, pl. LXVII) may likewise belong to Tablet 37 (and should be placed after line 28). This fragment is edited as an appendix below.

List of Manuscripts

Siglum	Museum Number	Copy	Collation	Format; Ductus	Provenience
a	A. 3438	TDP II, pl. LVII	Photo coll.	Fragment of a single-column tablet; Neo-Babylonian script; ca. 7th/6th cent. BCE	Uruk
b	W. 17360q	TDP II, pl. LXVIII	–	Fragment; Late Babylonian script; ca. 6th-3rd cent. BCE	Uruk

Overview

Lines 1–7	Omens concerning sexual intercourse during pregnancy (months 3–10) a obv. 1–7
Line 8	Fever a obv. 8–9
Line 9	Symptom of the hair a obv. 10
Line 10	Sickness due to the "Lord of the roof" a obv. 11
Lines 11–13	Affliction in the night/evening due to the *lilû*-demon a obv. 12–14
Lines 14–15	Strange behaviours (jerking, biting the hands) a obv. 15–16
Line 16	Affliction due to the Hand of Ištar a obv. 17

Line 17	Affliction in the night a obv. 18
Line 18	Affliction by wind a obv. 19
Lines 19–20	Staying awake all night a obv. 20–21
Lines 21–23	Strange behaviours a obv. 22–24 // b obv.$^?$ 1'
Lines 24–28	Fragmentary omens a obv. 25–29 // b obv.$^?$ 2'–4'
Lines 29'-30'	Fragmentary omens a rev. 1'–2'
Lines 31'–37'	Colophon a rev. 3'–9'

Previous Edition and Discussion

Labat 1951, *TDP* I, 212–216 (edition)
Stol 2000a, 202–203 (translation)
Heeßel 2000, 137, 146
Scurlock and Andersen 2005, 264–281 (12.31, 12.32, 12.34–12.38, 12.42, 12.68–12.70, 16.28–16.29, 16.58, 19.16, 19.18)
Scurlock 2014a, 255–257 (edition)
Minen 2018, 188–192
Minen 2020, *JMC* 36, 13–14
Schmidtchen 2021a, 245 (discussion)
Wee 2019b, CM 49/2, 44–45 (discussion of lines 18, 20)
CDLI P273373 (photo)

Transliteration

1 a obv. 1 DIŠ ^{munus}PEŠ$_4$ GIG-*ma šum-ma šá* ITI 3.KAM *ir-ṭú-pu-niš-ši* : *iq-ru-bu-niš-ši* MUNUS BI AL.TI

2 a obv. 2 *šum-ma ša* ITI 4.KAM *ir-ṭú-pu-niš-ši* MUNUS BI AL.TI

3 a obv. 3 *šum-ma ša* ITI 5.KAM *ir-ṭú-pu-niš-ši* MUNUS BI *na-a'-da-át*

4 a obv. 4 *šum-ma ša* ITI 6.KAM *ir-ṭú-pu-niš-ši* MUNUS BI *na-a'-da-át*

5 a obv. 5 *šum-ma ša* ITI 7.KAM *ir-ṭú-pu-niš-ši* MUNUS BI AL.TI

6 a obv. 6 *šum-ma ša* ITI 8.KAM *ir-ṭú-pu-niš-ši* MUNUS BI TI-*uṭ* : *ma-mit* AD-*šú* DAB-*si*

7 a obv. 7 *šum-ma ša* ITI 9.KAM *ù* ITI 10.KAM *ir-ṭú-pu-niš-ši* MUNUS BI *ul* <<NIN>> TI-*uṭ* : *ul* Ù.TU

8 a obv. 8 DIŠ MUNUS GIG-*ma* ADDA-*šú* KÚM ÚḪ TUKU MURUB$_4$ ŠU-*šá šá* 150 *ku-uṣ-ṣu* UL$_4$.GAL *ba-li-*[*i*]*l*

9 a obv. 10 DIŠ MUNUS GIG-*ma ú-ru-úḫ-šá bé-e-er ana* U$_4$.2.KAM *ana* U$_4$.3.KAM-*ma* UG$_7$

10 a obv. 11 DIŠ MUNUS GIG-*ma* ŠU.MIN-*šá ina* SAG.DU-*šá* GAR-*na-ma la ur-ra-da-ni* ŠU EN ÙR KI.MIN MAŠKIM ÙR SÌG-*aṣ* UG$_7$

11 a obv. 12 DIŠ MUNUS GIG-*ma* DAB-*sa ina* GI$_6$ DAB.DAB-*si* DAB-*it* LÍL.LÁ.EN.NA

12 a obv. 13 DIŠ MUNUS GIG-*ma* DAB-*sa ina* AN.USAN DAB.DAB-*si u* TÚG-*sa* ŠUB.ŠUB-*di* DAB-*it* LÍL.LÁ.EN.NA

13 a obv. 14 DIŠ MUNUS GIG-*sa ina* GI$_6$ DAB.DAB-*si* DAB-*it* LÍL.LÁ.EN.NA

14 a obv. 15 DIŠ MUNUS *ina* GIG-*šá* ḪULUḪ.ḪULUḪ-*ut* ÚŠ *ina* SU UN.MEŠ-*šá* BAD-*ši*

15 a obv. 16 DIŠ MUNUS *ina* GIG-*šá* ŠU.MIN-*šá ú-na-aš-šak* ŠU.MEŠ *lu-'-a-ti* TAG-*ši*

16 a obv. 17 DIŠ MUNUS *ina* GIG-*šá lìb-bi ku-ri i-qab-bi* ŠU ^{d}15 AL.TI

17 a obv. 18 DIŠ MUNUS *ina* GI$_6$ GIG-*ma ina šèr-ti it-te-bi* GIG-*sà i-sa-dir-ši-ma* UG$_7$

18 a obv. 19 DIŠ MUNUS [*ina* MURU]B$_4^?$-*šá* SÌG-*át* SAG ŠÀ-*šá* TU$_{15}$ *le-qí* : ŠÀ-*šá* TU$_{15}$ *ṣa-bit* BA.UG$_7$

19 a obv. 20 DIŠ [MUNUS *ina bal-ṭ*]*ú-ti-šá ú-šam-šá u ina* GIG-*šá ú-šam-šá* DUMU DINGIR-*šú* TE-*ši*

20 a obv. 21 DIŠ MU[NUS x x x]x-⸢*ma*$^?$⸣ *lu* ŠU.MIN-*šá lu* GÌR.MIN-*šá ú-ṣa-*⸢*bi-ta*⸣-*ši* DUMU DINGIR-*šú* TE-*ši* : DIŠ KI.NÁ-*šá* ŠUB.ŠUB-*ši* É-*sà* ⸢BIR⸣

21 a obv. 22 DIŠ MU[NUS SÍG SAG.DU-*šá*$^?$] *ú-baq-qam* [x x x DAB$^?$-*s*]*i* ZÁḪ É AD-*šú*

22 a obv. 23 DIŠ MU[NUS x x x-*šá* IGI$^?$].BAR.MEŠ : x[x x x x x DAB-*s*]*i*$^?$ BIR-*aḫ* É AD-*šú*

23 a obv. 24 [DIŠ] MU[NUS x x GEŠTU.MI]N$^?$-*šá iš-ta-*[*na-as-sa-a*$^?$ x x]x *u* ZI.IR.MEŠ GIG-*sà* GÍD-*ma* UG$_7$
b obv.$^?$ 1' [............................... *i-nam*$^?$]-⸢*ga*$_5^?$-*ag*$^?$⸣ ⸢ZI.IR.ME⸣ GI[G-*sa* ....]

24 a obv. 25 [DIŠ MUNUS x x x x]-*šá* GI$_6$ x[x x x x] A ŠÀ GIG-*šá* DU-*ku*
b obv.$^?$ 2' [..] A ŠÀ GI[G-.........]

25 a obv. 26 [DIŠ MUNUS x x] ⸢x⸣-*šá* [*s*]*im-mi* ⸢DIRI$^?$⸣-*m*[*a*$^?$ ....] NÍG.GIG-*šá* Ì.GU$_7$
b obv.$^?$ 3' [...] NÍG.GIG-*š*[*á* ....]

26 a obv. 27 [DIŠ MUNUS x]x ⸢GÚ$^?$⸣-*šá* DU$_8$.M[E x].⸢MIN$^?$⸣-*šá za-*x[x x] x-⸢*šá*⸣ ⸢ÚŠ.MEŠ⸣-*ra* SÌG-*iṣ* ÚŠ-*šá* SÌ[G-*at*$^?$ x]
b obv.$^?$ 4' [..]x x x x[.................]

27 a obv. 28 [DIŠ MUNUS$^?$ (x)] ⸢*ana*⸣ IGI-*šá* ⸢DU$^?$⸣-[*ma* x x x x x] SÌG-*iṣ* ÚŠ-*šá* S[ÌG-*at*$^?$ x]

28 a obv. 29 [DIŠ MUNUS x G]Ù.⸢GÙ$^?$⸣-*s*[*i*$^?$ x x x x x x]x-*šá it-ti-x-x* ⸢*šà*$^?$⸣ ⸢ŠÀ-*šá*⸣ x x[x x x x]

Ms. a obv. breaks; gap of unknown length
Beginning of ms. a rev. lost

29' a rev. 1' [...............................] x [.......................]

30' a rev. 2' [DIŠ MUNUS$^?$ x x]x-⸢*su*$^?$⸣ ⸢NU⸣ [x x x (x)] MUNUS BI ⸢*ni-iḫ*$^?$-*lu*$^?$⸣ ⸢GIG-*át*⸣

Colophon:

31' a rev. 3' [DIŠ MUNUS A-*šá* U$_4$].⸢3⸣.KAM DU-*ku* GI$_6$ IGI GAR-*ši*

32' a rev. 4' DUB 2.KAM DIŠ *šum*$_4$-*ma* TU [PEŠ$_4$-*ma*] UGU SAG.KI-*šá* SIG$_7$

33' a rev. 5' DUB 37$^!$(36).KAM DIŠ *e-nu-*⸢*ma*⸣ ⸢*ana*⸣ É LÚ.GIG KA.PIRIG DU-*ku*

34' a rev. 6' 1 UŠ 4 MU.ŠID.BI NU AL.TIL

35' a rev. 7' GABA.RI UNUG^{ki} ^{m}KI-AMAR.UTU-TIN A-*šú šá* ⸢GI⸣-⸢^{d}AMAR⸣.[UTU]

36' a rev. 8' DUMU ^{lú}SANGA-BARAG-*ki* ^{lú}ŠÁMAN.LÁ MAŠ.MAŠ *ana* TIN Z[I-*šú* SAR]

37' a rev. 9' NÍG.GA *é-an-na*

Bound Transcription and Translation

1 *šumma erītu marṣat-ma šumma ša* ITI 3.KAM *irṭupūniššī : iqribūniššī šinništu šī iballuṭ*

1 If a pregnant woman is sick, and if when she is (in) the third month one (lit. they) continues (sexual intercourse) with her, var. one approaches her (sexually): that woman will get well.

2 *šumma ša* ITI 4.KAM *irṭupūniššī šinništu šī iballuṭ*

2 If one (lit. they) continues (sexual intercourse) with her when she is (in) the fourth month: that woman will get well.

3 *šumma ša* ITI 5.KAM *irṭupūniššī šinništu šī na'dat*

3 If one (lit. they) continues (sexual intercourse) with her when she is (in) the fifth month: that woman is in a worrisome condition.

4 *šumma ša* ITI 6.KAM *irṭupūniššī šinništu šī na'dat*

4 If one (lit. they) continues (sexual intercourse) with her when she is (in) the sixth month: that woman is in a worrisome condition.

5 *šumma ša* ITI 7.KAM *irṭupūniššī šinništu šī iballuṭ*

5 If one (lit. they) continues (sexual intercourse) with her when she is (in) the seventh month: this woman will get well.

6 *šumma ša* ITI 8.KAM *irṭupūniššī šinništu šī iballuṭ : māmīt abīšu iṣabbassi*

6 If one (lit. they) continues (sexual intercourse) with her when she is (in) the eighth month: that woman will get better/live, var. the 'ban' of her father will seize her.

7 *šumma ša* ITI 9.KAM *u* ITI 10.KAM *irṭupūniššī šinništu šī ul iballuṭ : ul ullad*

7 If one (lit. they) continues (sexual relations) with her when she is (in) the ninth or tenth month: that woman will not get well, var. she will not give birth.

8 *šumma sinništu marṣat-ma pagaršu umma ṣarḫa iraššī qabal qātīša ša šumēli kuṣṣu magal balil : imaqqut(?)-ma ēm magal lā iballal-ma imât*

8 If a woman is sick and her body has a burning fever, var. collapses(?) and is hot, (and) the middle of her left hand is very mixed with cold, var. not very mixed (with cold): she will die.

9 *šumma sinništu marṣat-ma uruḫša bēr ana šina ūmī ana šalāšat ūmī-ma imât*

9 If a woman is sick and her hair is *sparse*, (she will be sick?) for two (or) three days, and then she will die.

10 *šumma sinništu marṣat-ma qātāša ina qaqqadīša šaknā-ma lā urradāni qāt bēl ūri* KI.MIN *rābiṣ ūri imḫaṣ imât*

10 If a woman is sick and her hands are placed on her head, and they don't come down: hand of the "Lord of the roof". Alternatively, the 'Lurker of the roof' has struck (her); she will die.

11 *šumma sinništu marṣat-ma ṣibissa ina mūši iṣṣanabbassi ṣibit lilî*

11 If a woman is sick and her affliction always afflicts her in the night: seizure of a *lilû*-demon.

12 *šumma sinništu marṣat-ma ṣibissa ina šimētān iṣṣanabbassi u ṣubāssu ittanaddi ṣibit lilî*

12 If a woman is sick and her affliction always afflicts her in the evening und she keeps taking off her garment: (it is an) affliction of a *lilû*-demon.

13 *šumma šinništu murussa ina mūši iṣṣanabbassi ṣibit lilî*

13 If a woman's illness always afflicts her in the night: (it is an) affliction of a *lilû*-demon.

14 *šumma sinništu ina murṣīša igdanallut mūtu(?) ina zumur nišēša inessīši/unessīši*

14 If a woman in her illness jerks all the time, death(?) will take her away from her family (lit. "from the body of her people").

15 *šumma sinništu ina murṣīša qātīša unaššak qātā lu'âti ilputāši*

15 If a woman during her illness bites her hands, dirty hands have touched her.

16 *šumma šinništu ina murṣīša libbī kuri iqabbi qāt Ištar iballuṭ*

16 If a woman during her illness says, "My heart/inside is short!": Hand of Ištar; she will get better.

17 *šumma sinništu ina muši marṣat-ma ina šērti ittebi murussa isaddir-ma imât*

17 If a woman is sick at night, but gets up in the morning, (if) her illness becomes regular for her, she will die.

18 *šumma sinništu [ina qab]līša maḫṣat rēš libbīša šāra leqi : libbaša šāra ṣabit imât*

18 If a woman is affected (lit. "hit") [in] her h[ip region] (and) her upper abdomen holds (lit. is taken with) wind, var. her belly is afflicted with wind: she will die.

19 *šumma [sinništu ina balṭ]ūtīša ušamša u ina murṣīša ušamša mār ilīšu iṭḫēši*

19 If [a woman] stays awake all night [whether] she is w[ell] or sick: the 'son of her god' has approached her (sexually).

[20] *šumma sinn[ištu ......-m]a(?) lū qātāša lū šēpāša uṣab-bitāši mār ilīšu iṭḫēši : šumma mayyālša ittanassukši bīssa issappaḫ*

[20] If a wom[an ..., a]nd(?) either her hands or her feet afflict her: the 'son of her god' has approached her (sexually). If her bed keeps throwing her off: her household (family) will be scattered.

[21] *šumma sinn[ištu šārat qaqqadīša(?)] ubaqqam [... iṣbas-s]i(?) ḫalāq bīt abīšu*

[21] If a wom[an] tears out [the hair of her head(?)]: [... has seized(?) h]er, ruin of her father's household.

[22] *šumma sinn[ištu ...-šá itta]naplas(?) ...[... iṣbass]i(?) sapāḫ bīt abīšu*

[22] If a wo[man ...] constantly lo[oks at her ...(?)], var. ...[... has seized h]er(?); dispersal of her father's household.

[23] *[šumma] sinn[ištu ... uznā]ša išta[nassâ(?) inam]gag(?) u ītanaššaš murussa irrik-ma imât*

[23] [If] ... a wom[an]'s [ears(?)] ri[ng constantly, she] brays (like a donkey?) and is continually upset (agitated?): her illness will be prolonged and then she will die.

[24] *[šumma sinništu ...]-ša ṣalim/ṣalmū(?) ...[...] mê libbi maruštuša(?) illakū*

[24] [If a woman]'s [...] is/are black, ...[...]: the fluids of the *womb*(?), her 'trouble' (i.e. menses?), will flow(?).

[25] *[šumma sinništu ...]... simmī malû-m[a(?) ...] ikkibša īkul*

[25] [If a woman']s [...] are full of(?) lesions and [...]: she has done (lit. eaten) something forbidden to her.

[26] *[šumma sinništu ...]... kišādīša paṭrū(?) [...]-ša ...[...]-ša itteneskerā(?) miḫiṣ mūtīša(?) maḫ[ṣat ...]*

[26] [If the ... of a woman]'s neck(?) are continually loose(?), both her [...]s are ..., her [....] are blocked up continually(?): she has been [struck] by a 'blow' of her (personal) Death(?) [...].

[27] *[šumma sinništu ...] ana pānīša illak-[ma(?)...] miḫiṣ mūtīša(?) maḫ[ṣat ...]*

[27] [If the woman(?) (i.e. her condition) ...] improves, [but then ...]: she has been [struck] by a 'blow' of her (personal) Death(?) [...].

[28] *[šumma sinništu ... iš]tanassi(?) [...]-ša ... ša libbīša(?) ... [... ...]*

[28] [If a woman ... kee]ps crying out(?), [...] her [...] ..., her foe-tus(?) [... ...].

Ms. a obv. breaks; gap of unknown length

Beginning of ms. a rev. lost

[29'] *traces*

[29'] *Too fragmentary for translation*

[30'] *[šumma sinništu(?) ...]...-su lā(?) [... ...] sinništu šī niḫ-la(?) marṣat*

[30'] [If a woman(?) ...] ... not(?) [......]: that woman is sick with *niḫlu*-disease(?).

Colophon:

[31'] *šumma sinništu šalāšat ūmī mûša illakū ṣalām pānī iššakkanši* [32'] *tuppu šanû šumma ālittu [erât-ma] muḫ pūtīša aruq* [33'] *tuppu* 37[!].KAM DIŠ *enūma ana bīt marṣi āšipu illaku* [34'] 64 MU.ŠID.BI *ul qati* [35'] *gabari Uruk Itti-Mar-duk-balāṭu māršu ša Mušallim-Marduk* [36'] *mār Šangû-par-akki šamallû mašmaššu ana balāṭ nap[ištīšu išṭur]* [37'] *mak-kūr Eanna*

[31'] (Catchline:) "If a woman's (amniotic) fluids flow for three days, gloom(?) (lit. "darkening of the face") is set for her. [32'] Second tablet of "If a childbearing woman [is pregnant and] the top of her forehead is yellow-green". [33'] 37th! (text: 36th) tablet of "When the conjurer goes to the patient's house". [34'] Sixty-four are its lines. (Series) not completed. [35'] A copy (of an original) from Uruk. Itti-Marduk-balāṭu, the son of Mušal-lim-Marduk, [36'] a descendent of the Šangû-parakki family, the apprentice exorcist, has [written (this tablet)] for his well[be-ing]. [37'] Property of the Eanna temple.

Notes

Lines 1–7: Rabbinic sources contain similar predictions concerning the consequences of sexual intercourse during pregnancy (see Feldman 1975, 180ff.). In this tradition, intercourse is regarded as harmful for both woman and child in the first trimester; in the fourth month it is harmful for the woman, but good for the child; after that it is good for both woman and child. Apparently, there are a few differences in comparison with the significance attributed to the months in *Diagnostic Handbook* Tablet 37: here, months 3–4 and 7 are auspicious, and months 5–6 and 8–10 inauspicious. The first and second month of pregnancy are not considered at all in Tablet 37. For a similar concern with the first one hundred days of pregnancy, see AO 6473 (text C.3.9).

Presumably for semantic reasons, CAD R, 217b regards the form *ir-ṭú-pu-niš-ši* in lines 1–7 as a separate lemma *ratāpu* (with uncertain meaning), translating "(if (people) have sexual relations(?) with her", in view of the integrated variant *iqribūnišši* "they approach her (sexually)". However, von Soden (AHw 963b sub 3) includes our passage under a verb *raṭāpu* (or *ratāpu*), for which he assumes the general meaning "to continue" ("fortfahren"), and suggests a derived meaning "Geschlechtsverkehr fortführen mit (Dat.)" (i.e to continue intercourse with) for our attestation. In contrast to this, CAD R, 217 proposes to keep the lemma *ratābu* (*raṭābu*) "to proceed to do something" separate from the suggested verb *ratāpu* in Tablet 37. For further discussion of the verb *rat/ṭāb/pu*, see Kraus 1986; George and Krebernik 2022, *RA* 116, 145; Streck 2021, HdO 152/2, 1017.

Stol (2000a, 202) translates *šá* ITI 3.KAM as "three times a month", following Kraus (1986, 131–132). My interpretation of the numerals here and in the next lines follows Scurlock (2014a, 256) and Scurlock and Andersen (2005, 265–267 with 12.31–12.38; with Labat 1951, *TPD* I, 213; CAD Q, 233b), regarding ITI 3.KAM (and the parallel entries in lines 2–7) as a reference to the months of pregnancy, from the third to the tenth month (the latter of which is the usual maximum duration of pregnancy in Mesopotamian texts; cf. Stol 2000a, 21). See further the discussion on Tablet 36 lines 106–113 above.

The incipit of Tablet 37 is also quoted in the colophon of the commentary on Tablet 36 (see SpTU 1, No. 39: 13', edited above).

Lines 3–4: For *na'ādu* "to be attentive, concerned" in the apodosis, which in the stative can have the meaning "to be a cause for worry" (i.e. to be in a dangerous condition), see CAD N/1, 4 sub 3.

Line 7: The sign NIN before TI-*uṭ* seems to be superfluous and is therefore emended.

Line 8: From ms. a obv. 8 onward until the obverse breaks, all entries begin with DIŠ MUNUS (GIG-*ma*) instead of DIŠ ^{munus}PEŠ$_4$ GIG-*ma*, which suggests that Tablet 37 here left the realm of pregnancy and dealt with symptom descriptions and diagnoses for women in general. The symptoms and cases of sickness described in the following lines are not gynaecological in the strict sense, however. It rather seems that this section of Tablet 37 collected a variety of ailments or symptoms that could in theory also be observed in male patients, but for which healers gave a specific diagnosis, when they observed them in female patients.

For KÚM ÚḪ as a logographic writing for *ummu ṣarḫu* "burning fever" or *umma ṣariḫ* "he is burning with fever," see Heeßel 2000, 162–163, e.g. *Diagnostic Handbook* Tablet 15: 15' (Scurlock 2014a, 27); also Tablet 3: 61–62, 65–68; Tablet 13: 53, 56 (Schmidtchen 2021a, 252–253, 260, 520, 531–532) and the Middle Assyrian precursor KAR 211: 4 which has syllabic *ṣariḫ* instead of ÚḪ. For *ṣarāḫu* and cognate terms in the context of fever, see also Stol 2007, 7–8 (who defines this as a "flaring-up fever" that is remittent). For the expression "to have burning fever", see also BAM 401 obv. 23 (Bácskay 2018, No. 40): DIŠ NA KÚM *ṣar-ḫa* TUKU-*ma*; similarly BAM 66 obv. 21 (Bácskay 2018, No. 41).

Ms. a obv. 9 gives two variants for different parts of the protasis; each of the two variant phrases is positioned exactly below the passages in obv. 8 for which they are the alternative. I understand ADDA-*šú* "her body" as the subject of ŠUB-*ma* KÚM in ms. a obv. 9 (meaning "it collapses and is hot"), as a variant to "it has burning fever". The expression "to be very mixed (stative of *balālu*) with cold", referring here to the patient's left hand, is unusual. CAD B, 42 sub mng. 1h proposes the translation "to be numb(?) with(?) cold" in this context. For a similar passage, see however, *Diagnostic Handbook* Tablet 6: 29 (Scurlock 2014a, 57; Schmidtchen 2021a, 359, 367): "(if the tip of his nose) *ku-uṣ-ṣa ba-lil* "is mixed (i.e. *coated*?) with cold").

Line 9: For the phrase *uruḫša bēr* "her hair is *sparse*" (lit. "select"), cf. CAD U/W 270; CAD B 208a, s.v. *bēru* C adj.; Labat (1951, *TDP* I, 215) translated "blanchit (brusquement)"; Scurlock (2014a, 19, 236) renders it as "fine" (lit. select). A very similar protasis is encountered in *Diagnostic Handbook* Tablet 3: 27–30, from the male perspective: DIŠ *ú-ru-uḫ* SAG.DU-*šú bé-e-er* (...) "if the *uruḫḫu*-hair of his head becomes *sparse*". See also SA.GIG Tablet 4: 117 (Schmidtchen 2021a, 299, 307, 328). The commentary STT 403: 23 (on *Diagnostic Handbook* Tablets 1–3) explains this phrase as *perettu/berittu ša qaqqadīšu marṣat*, which is usually understood as "the hair (*pertu*) of his head is sick". Wee (2019b, 73, 77, 88–89) re-analyses *perettu* as *berittu/birītu* "in-between area", translating "the partition of his head is sick". Cf. further *Alamdimmû* II 33–39 (Böck 2000, 74). For the meaning of the verb *bêru* "to select", Wee (2019b) draws on SA.GIG Tablet 5: 94' where it is found with reference to the eyes, and on the commentary on SA.GIG Tablet 5: 30–31, which equates it with *bêšu* "to move apart" and *petû* "to open" (Wee 2019b, 171, 177, 182–183). Wee suggests the translation "(the hair) is parted" for *bēr*, possibly indicating a bald spot.

The second half of the protasis seems to be abbreviated; one expects GIG "she has been sick" after U$_4$.3.KAM.

The Neo-Assyrian fragment K. 11939: 8' with a commentary on Tablet 37 (Heeßel 2019, *JMC* 34; see below) cites the omen of line 9, but the following explanations on the entry are unfortunately too fragmentary.

Lines 10–15: These lines form a group of entries concerned with neurological and psychiatric conditions attributed to different deities and demons, including the "wind demon" (*lilû*).

Line 10: This entry presents an interesting correspondence with a slightly varying diagnosis (sender of the illness) in *Diagnostic Handbook* Tablet 11: 24 (Scurlock 2014a, 83; Scurlock and Andersen 2005, 19.41–19.42; Schmidtchen 2021a, 459):

> DIŠ ŠU.MIN-*šú ina* SAG.DU-*šú* GAR-*na-ma la ur-ra-da-ni* ŠU ^{d}*lugal-ir$_9$-ra u* ^{d}*mes-la*[*m-ta-è-a*]
> "If his hands are placed on his head and he does not bring them down: Hand of Lugalirra and Meslamtaea [...]".

Note also Tablet 11: 22 (within the similar cases in lines 21–25), where the patient's inability to remove his hands from his head are attributed to the *rābiṣu* ("lurker")-demon, similar to the "*rābiṣu* of the roof" encountered in the variant of Tablet 37: 10. The gods and demons in these omens are well-known senders of neurological disorders related to epilepsy, see Stol 1993, 16–19, 116–117, 119 for discussion.

Lines 11–13: For the group of wind demons (*lilû, lilītu, ardat lilî*), spirits of men and women or boys and girls who died before marriage, who typically afflict victims of the opposite sex and cause types of fevers and mainly psychiatric symptoms, including seizures, confusional dissociative states and strange or sexualized behaviours that are sometimes suggestive of possession phenomena, see e.g. Scurlock and Andersen 2005, 272–274, 434–436, with 12.69–12.70 and 19.18; Stol 1993, 46–49, 69–70; Steinert 2022. Women are attacked by the male *lilû*, men (predominantly) by the female *lilītu* and *ardat lilî*:

> *Diagnostic Handbook* Tablet 26: 82'–83' (see also lines 45'–47', 48'-49'; Stol 1993, 46; Heeßel 2000, 285, 291; Scurlock 2014a, 199, 204):
> DIŠ *pa-rid-ma it-te-né-et-bi ma-gal* DUG$_4$.DUG$_4$-*ub u i*[*g-d*]*a-na-al-lu-u*[*t*] *ana* MUNUS LÍL.L[Á].EN.NA *ana* NITA MUNUS.LÍL.LÁ.EN.NA
> "If he shudders (with fear) and gets up time and again, he talks a lot and jerks continually: for a woman (it is) a *lilû*-demon; for a man, a *lilītu*-demon."

For the night and evening as typical times of afflicting by the wind demons (connected to the demons' desire for human victims as sexual and marriage partners), see also *Diagnostic Handbook* Tablet 26: 39' (Stol 1993, 64; Heeßel 2000, 281, 288; Scurlock 2014a, 197, 202): DIŠ KI.MIN U$_4$ DAB-*šú an-nu-ú šu-ú i-qab-bi* ŠU KI.SIKIL.LÍL.L[Á.EN.NA] "If ditto (his affliction always afflicts him in the evening and) when it afflicts him, he says 'This is it/him': Hand of *ardat lilî* (wind maiden)." Note also Tablet 17: 78 (Heeßel 2000, 202, 210; Scurlock 2014a, 165, 170): DIŠ *ina* GI$_6$ GIG-(*ma*) *ina šèr-ti ba-liṭ u ú-šam-šá* ŠU LÍL.LÁ.[EN.NA] "If he is sick in the night and well in the morning and it keeps (him) awake all night: Hand of *lilû*."

For the symptom of taking or throwing off one's garment, which also occurs in other sections of the *Diagnostic Handbook*, see also Scurlock and Andersen 2005, 378, 16.56–16.59.

Line 14: The apodosis ÚŠ *ina* SU UN.MEŠ-*šá* BAD-*ši* is ambiguous. Labat (TDP I, 215) suggested "un mort, parmi ses ..., veut la faire mourir", interpreting the verb as *mâtu* (UG$_7$) "to die" (Š-stem). I have opted to understand the apodosis as one clause and suggest ÚŠ stands for *mūtu* "death", understood here as the personified Death known as the reaper of humankind from other cuneiform sources (see Sibbing-Plantholt 2021, 335–356). The phrase *ina* SU UN.MEŠ-*šá* as *zumur nišēša* "(from) the body of (i.e. from among) her people" as a phrase referring to one's family is not attested elsewhere (cf. CAD Z, 160 sub d for a "prepositional use" of *zumru*). Compare however the similar expression *zumur māti* "body of the land" referring to the collective of a country's inhabitants, and the expression *ina zumur* NN *nesû* "to depart/move away from someone" is not uncommon (CAD N/2, 187 sub 1b). Therefore, I interpret the logogram BAD-*ši* at the end of the line as the verb *nesû* "to be distant", which is also used in the transitive sense "to remove" in the G-stem (CAD N/2, 188 sub 2). The D- and Š-stem of *nesû* likewise have the senses of "to remove; to drive (far) away" and occur, for example, in passages referring to disease and evil driven away *ina zumri* NN "from the body (of NN)" (cf. CAD N/2, 188–189 sub 3–4; AHw 782). However, logographic writings with BAD appear to be restricted to the G-stem. Thus, we would have a somewhat poetic expression for "she will die (before her time)". Personified Death ($^{(d)}$*Mūtu*(ÚŠ)) as a reaper is often encountered in literary texts, but also occurs Late Babylonian commentaries on the *Diagnostic Handbook* and in ritual texts, where he is represented through protective figurines (see Wee 2019b, 31, 38 SpTU 1, 27 rev. 7–8 (SA-GIG 1B U1: 24); 185, 188 SpTU 1, 32 rev. 11–13 (SA-GIG 7A); Sibbing-Plantholt 2021, esp. 342–343, 350–356, also discussing the representation of *Mūtu* in the *Göttertypentext* (MIO 1)). In the *Elegy on the Death of a Woman in Childbirth* (Livingstone 1989, SAA 3, 15 rev. 20–23; George 2010, *FS Foster*, 212–213;

Sibbing-Plantholt 2021, 347–348), the deceased woman describes how Death (*Mūtu*) crept into her bedroom, "he drove me out of my home, he separated me from my husband, he set my feet in a land of no return" (*issu* (TA) *bēti*(É-*ti*)-*ia us-se-ṣa-an-ni a-a-ši* / *issu*(TA) *pa-an ḫa-bi-re-ia ip-tar-sa-an-ni* / *šēpē*(GÌR.MIN)-*ia is-sa-ka-na ina qaq-qar la* ⌜*ta-ia-re*⌝-*ia*).

Incidentally, the protasis of *Diagnostic Handbook* Tablet 17: 24 (Scurlock 2014a, 163, 167; Heeßel 2000, 197) begins with the same words (DIŠ *ina* GIG-*šú* ḪULUḪ.ḪULUḪ-*ut*) as in Tablet 37: 14, but the rest of the former entry differs.

For the symptom of "shivering" or "jerking" (ḪULUḪ, *galātu*), which is often found in the context of seizures, epileptic fits and attack by demons and said to occur at night in bed, see also Stol 1993, 6, 38, 72; Scurlock and Andersen 2005, 294–295; Steinert et al. 2018, 265 (line 95); Arbøll 2019, *JMC* 33, 16–17 rev. 5'; Steinert 2024, 125–127.

Line 15: This entry is quoted and commented on in K. 11939: 6'–7', a Neo-Assyrian fragment of a commentary on *Diagnostic Handbook* Tablet 37 (see Heeßel 2019 and below). The commentary appears to explain the apodosis as "someone with dirty hands [*has touched her*]" (see below for discussion).

Line 16: The patient's exclamation "my inside is short" (*libbī kuri*) may be an expression of an emotion or feeling rather than a purely physical sensation. In comparable contexts, *karû* "to be short" occurs with *ikku* "breath", which may refer to irritability, anxiety or moping; the verb *karû* "to become short" is also encountered with *napištu* "life, breath" (cf. CAD I/J, 59–60; Mayer 2010, *OrNS* 79, 320, 338; Steinert 2012a, 275–276; Attia 2018, *JMC* 31, 74–78). Stol (2017, *BiOr* 74, 376) interprets the expression "becoming short of life / breath" (with *napištu*, *ikku*) as being "very sad" or having "a disturbed spirit", drawing on Syriac / Aramaic cognate expressions (cf. also Mayer 2010, *OrNS* 79, 338). The expression *libbī kuri* could similarly refer to feelings of anxiety / panic or sadness. In an anti-witchcraft incantation (Abusch and Schwemer 2016 (CMAwR 2), text 8.20, 2 lines 33'''–34'''), the wish "let her heart/inside be 'short', let her heart/inside become 'short'" (*lū kuri libbaša likru libbaša*) is expressed against the witch, however, in fragmentary context; cf. Abusch and Schwemer 2016 (CMAwR 2), text 8.30 line 19 *takturu napištī* "my (breath of) life has become short".

Line 17: For a diagnostic entry with a similar protasis, see *Diagnostic Handbook* Tablet 17: 78 (Heeßel 2000, 202, 210; Scurlock 2014a, 154, 160): DIŠ *ina* GI_6 GIG-*ma ina šèr-ti ba-liṭ u ú-šam-šá* ŠU LÍL.LÁ.[EN.NA] "If he is sick in the night and well in the morning and it keeps (him) awake all night: Hand of *lilû*."

The verb *sadāru* means "to occur regularly, continually" (cf. CAD S, 11–15, sub 4b), and seems to be used in a similar sense as the term "chronic" (meaning regular re-occurrence of symptoms).

Line 18: For "wind" in the abdomen as part of symptom descriptions in women's healthcare texts, see also BAM 240: 20'–28' (text D.2.1); BM 50700: 28''' (text A.2.3).

Line 19: See also Scurlock and Andersen 2005, 16.28. For *šumšû* "to spend the night awake", CAD Š/3, 283 s.v. *šumšû* sub 1c. The apodosis explains the woman's illness as caused by the breaking of a taboo, namely having sexual relations with the "son of her god" (*mār ili*), who has "approached" her (*iṭḫēši*). This expression as well as the female counterpart *mārat ili* "daughter of one's god" have been discussed by Renger (1973, *AfO* 24, 103–107), arguing convincingly that both expressions refer to any member of one's patrilineal clan or lineage (connected by patrilineal descent from a common ancestor and by the shared veneration of the same clan deity), with whom marriage was prohibited, pointing to the practice to exogamy in some periods and places, going back at least to Old Babylonian times. A related passage is found in *Šurpu* IV 7 (Reiner 1958, 25), where sexual relations with a *mārat ili* are found in a group of other interdictions. A commentary (K. 4320: 19; Reiner 1958, 50) explains *mārat ilīšu* in this passage as *aḫassu* "his sister", but the underlying general idea of an incest taboo is the same (cf. Renger 1973, 107 arguing *aḫatu* can be understood in a classificatory sense, embracing a larger group of female relatives). See further Oppenheim 1956, *Dreams*, 291; Petschow, "Inzest", *RlA* 5, 149–150 §6.

Line 20: See also Scurlock and Andersen 2005, 16.29; Scurlock 2014a, 257 (line 21). A different interpretation of the omen variant is proposed in Wee 2019b, 45, which is not followed here. For the bed "throwing off" (*nasāku*; here in the Gtn-stem written logographically (ŠUB.ŠUB)) the patient (i.e. falling out of one's bed in one's sleep), see also Köcher, Oppenheim and Güterbock 1957–1958, *AfO* 18, 64 i 33–34 (Old Babylonian omen text): DIŠ LÚ *ma-ia-al-šu it-*[*ta-na-a*]*s-su-uk-šu* LÚ *šu-ú i-*[*x-x i-i*]*m-ma-ar* "If a man's bed keeps throwing him off: he will experience [...]". See also ibid., 74 K. 8821: 12–14 (fragmentary): DIŠ NA *ina* ^gišNÁ-*šú* KI.NÁ-*šú* ŠUB "If a man while lying in his bed, (his bed) throws (him) off". See further CAD N/2, 18 sub 2d; CAD M/1, 118 sub 1c; KAR 69 rev. 17 (Biggs 1967, 77): *mayyālu ana qaqqari lissukki* "may (your) bed throw you down to the ground".

Line 21: For the reconstruction of the apodosis, compare a similar entry in *Diagnostic Handbook* Tablet 13: 117' (Scurlock 2014a, 108 (line 134); Schmidtchen 2021a, 525, 535): *šumma*(DIŠ) *libbī*(ŠÀ) *libbī*(ŠÀ) *ištanassi*(GÙ.GÙ-*si*) *u šārassu*(SÍG-*su*) *ubaqqan* "If he cries 'my belly, my belly!' and tears out his hair" (with a different apodosis).

Line 22: The missing passage before BAR.MEŠ in the protasis could be restored according to the following parallels with the verb IGI.BAR.MEŠ (*naplusu*, Ntn-stem): *Diagnostic Handbook* Tablet 4: 117 (Scurlock 2014a, 32; Schmidtchen 2021a, 298: 109): AD_6-*šú* IGI.BAR.MEŠ "he continually gazes (*ittanaplas*) at his body"; or Tablet 11: 37, 38 (Scurlock 2014a, 84; Schmidtchen 2021a, 460): [DIŠ ŠU.MIN-*šú* IG]I.BAR.MEŠ "[If he] constantly gazes [at his hands]"; or Tablet 10 B rev. 5 (Scurlock 2014a, 76; Schmidtchen 2021a, 439: 72'): DIŠ Á.MIN-*šú* IGI.BAR.MEŠ "if he constantly gazes at his arms".

Line 23: Perhaps, restore [*ina* GIG-*šá* GEŠTU.MI]N-*šá iš-ta-*[*na-as-sa-a*?] "(If), [during her illness her ears] rin[g all the time]". Cf. *Diagnostic Handbook* Tablet 8: 12: DIŠ GEŠTU.MIN-*šú* GÙ.GÙ.MEŠ GIG-*su* DUGUD "If his ears ring continually, his illness will be difficult"; also Tablet 8: 15: DIŠ GEŠTU.MIN-*šú* GÙ.GÙ.MEŠ *i-nan-ziq* "If his ears ring continually, he will suffer distress" (Schmidtchen 2021a, 402–403).

The verb *nagāgu* "to bray (like a donkey)", restored tentatively in ms. b, is found as a symptom in psychiatric and epilepsy-related conditions, see e.g. *Diagnostic Handbook* Tablet 22: 61 (Scurlock 2014a, 188): DIŠ *i-nam-gag*; STT 89: 144 (Stol 1993, 94). The restoration of the present line remains tentative.

For *ašāšu* "to be upset, distressed, tormented" in medical texts, see Attia 2018, *JMC* 31, 83–89.

Line 24: The apodosis is difficult to interpret. The verb *alāku* "to go" probably should be understood in the sense of "to flow", which is usually found in the context of discharges of body fluids such as blood or other "fluids" designated as *mû*. The sign sequence A ŠÀ GIG-*šá* is not known from other women's healthcare texts and is ambiguous. Since a reading A.ŠÀ as Akkadian *eqlu* "field" seems unlikely, so I interpret the signs as A ŠÀ, for *mê libbi* "waters of the inside/belly" (i.e. womb). Akkadian *mû* (A.(MEŠ)) usually refers to the amniotic fluid. But in a few passages, it may refer to other fluids discharged from a woman's vagina resembling a watery discharge (e.g. BM 42313+ // rev. 36 (text A.2.1). The sign GIG (as a variant of NÍG.GIG) probably should be read *maruštu* "trouble" and is occasionally used as a euphemistic term for the menses in Late Babylonian texts. Thus, in SpTU 1, No. 59: 12' (text C.2.1), the purpose of a recipe is [DIŠ MUNUS?] *ša* GIG-*šá* NU *im-mar* <<*šá*>> GIG-*šá i*[*m*]-*mar* "[so that a woman] who does not see her 'trouble', will see her 'trouble'", which may be understood as a remedy to induce menstrual bleeding. In similar prescriptions, the word *sagû* occurs in the same position and with the same meaning (see e.g., BM 38624+ (texts A.2.1, C.1.1–C.1.2, chapter C.2 and *passim* in this volume). For a syllabic occurrence of *maruštu* see also *Diagnostic Handbook* Tablet 36: 94–96 (above).

Line 25: The usual expression encountered in similar apodoses is *ikkib*(NÍG.GIG) *ili*(DINGIR)-*šú īkul*(GU_7) "he has done (something) forbidden (lit. eaten the taboo of) his god", see e.g. *Diagnostic Handbook* Tablet 10: 26 (Schmidtchen 2021a, 436); Tablet 15: 7' (Heeßel 2000, 150); cf. Tablet 13: 116', 123' (Schmidtchen 2021a, 525); *Šurpu* IV 4 (Borger 2000, *FS Lambert*, 57): *ikkib ilīšu* <*ina*> *lā idê akālu* "to unwittingly eat (what is) taboo of one's god" (within a list of taboos). However, both mss. a and b in our text have NÍG.GIG-*šá* instead of NÍG.GIG DINGIR-*šá*. Perhaps the dropping of DINGIR is an abbreviation or a textual error that was transmitted through copying, and thus the text should be emended (see also Schmidtchen 2021a, 164 n. 745). For *ikkibu* "taboo, sacrilege, forbidden thing/action", see further Hallo 1985, *JQR* 76, 21–40; Geller 1990, *JCS* 42, 105–117; Feder 2010, *JANER* 10, 119–157; Böck 2016.

Lines 26–27: The apodosis *miḫiṣ*(SÌG-*iṣ*) NN *maḫiṣ*(SÌG-*iṣ*) "he was hit by a blow of NN" is well attested in diagnostic texts, combined with demons such as *rābiṣu* (MAŠKIM; "lurker") or *Namtaru* (NAM.TAR; "fate") or with deities (e.g. Sîn; Baba) as senders of disease. In many of these cases of disease caused by a "blow", the outcome is negative (death). See for instance, *Diagnostic Handbook* Tablet 4: 100, 105, 106, 117; Tablet 11: 13–14, 77' (*rābiṣu*); Tablet 14: 197' (Baba); Tablet 15: 4' (Namtar), 10' (Sîn), 91' (Lamaštu); see Heeßel 2000, 150–151, 155; Schmidtchen 2021a, 297–299, 459, 462, 576. The spelling SÌG-*iṣ* in lines 26–27 likewise suggests a genitive construction. The following signs BAD-*šá* could be read as ÚŠ-*šá*, with ÚŠ standing for *mūtu* (i.e. "her (personified) death"). The personified reaper Death (*Mūtu*) is equated with *Namtaru*, the personification of the ultimate, preordained fate of humankind (see Sibbing-Plantholt 2021, 335–356). Alternatively, BAD-*šá* could refer to a body part of the patient. Thus, reading SÌG-*iṣ sun-šá* S[ÌG] for *miḫiṣ sūnīša maḫṣat* "she was hit by a blow to her crotch" is not excluded.

In line 26, the protasis is unfortunately very fragmentary. If read correctly, the verbal form behind BAD.MEŠ-*ra* indicates a feminine plural or dual subject. The form BAD.MEŠ-*ra* could be an Ntn- or a D-stem of *sekēru*, both of which are attested with body parts in the sense "to be(come) blocked" in medical texts (cf. CAD S, 212–213 sub 3b, 5b). Note, for example, *Diagnostic Handbook* Tablet 14: 111 (Schmidtchen 2021a, 570): *šumma šīnātūšu itteneskerā imât* "if his urine (urinary tract) is blocked up, he will die". In this light, perhaps a restoration [KÀ]Š-*šá* "her urine" is thinkable before BAD.(-) MEŠ-*ra* in line 26. Consequently, one expects a lethal prognosis at the end of the line.

For *ana pāni*+pronominal suffix *alāku* in the sense "to prosper, to improve (physically)", in the protasis of line 27, cf. CAD A/1, 318 sub 4c-d; CAD P, 92b; Reiner 1982b, *FS Kraus*, 286 CT 51, 147 rev. 12 (behavioural omens); SAA 10, No. 329 rev. 3; ARM 33, No. 276: 13; Stol 2016, 159 n. 53 (for the Sumerian calque igi-šè du modelled on the Akkadian phrase, in the *Elegy on the Death of Nawirtum*; https://etcsl.orinst.ox.ac.uk text 5.5.3 line 61). See also *Diagnostic Handbook* Tablet 36: 115 (above).

Line 28': The reading [G]Ù.GÙ-*s*[*i*] "she cries out/screams continually" follows a suggestion by Schmidtchen (2021a, 245 n. 24), noting that this form can also be reconstructed in the fragment W. 17630i: 2'. Schmidtchen sees this as a hint that the latter fragment may likewise belong to Tablet 37 and represent hitherto unknown entries. For W. 17630i, see below.

Line 30': The disease name preceding *marṣat* may be *niḫlu* or *neḫlu*, a term for a morbid condition of the skin (cf. AHw 715a; 775a reading *né-eḫ-lu*). The word *niḫlu* is attested in *Šurpu* VII 88, also *Šurpu* I rev. ii 3 (catchline and incantation incipit), in a sequence of disease terms: ÉN *ni-'i-iš/ši ni-iḫ-lu/li gu-uḫ-ḫu ḫa-aḫ-ḫu ru-*[*u'-tu*] "Incantation: Sneeze, *niḫlu*, *guḫḫu*-cough, *ḫaḫḫu*-cough, sp[ittle/phlegm]" (Reiner 1958, 39).

Line 31': Interpretations of the expression *ṣalām/ṣulum pānī* "blackness/darkening of the face" (GI_6 IGI) in the omen apodoses are not entirely certain. For the reading, see Borger 2004, MZL, 398 (translating it as "Verfinsterung der Miene"). Attestations of the expression in Old Assyrian letters suggest the meaning "anger" (CAD Ṣ, 241 sub 1c-2'). AHw 1110b, s.v. *ṣulmu* sub 4 books logographic spellings (GI_6 IGI) in omen apodoses likewise under the meaning "anger, wrath". The expression also occurs in *Šumma ālu* Tablet 33: 51' (Freedman 2006, 208–209), but without the verb *šakānu*: "(If a lizard) is seen [...] a man [...]: GI_6 IGI". Borger (1954, *BiOr* 11, 89: 36) renders the phrase as Akkadian *ṣalām pāni* "distress, misery" ("Kummer"), assuming an infinitive *ṣalāmu* in a genitive construction instead of the noun *ṣulmu*. Freedman (2006, 209) instead interprets IGI in this apodosis as the verb *amāru* and translates "he will experience darkness". Two more occurrences are found in the *Assyrian Dream Book* (Oppenheim 1956, 316a: x+13; 317 y+11). In both passages, the expression is abbreviated as well and apparently has a negative connotation. Thus, the latter passage preserves the entry: DIŠ SAḪAR. ḪI.A GU_7 LÍL-*a'* DU_{11}.DU_{11} *i-ma-(ak)-ki qí-be* DINGIR-*šú* GAR-*šú* GI_6 IGI "If he eats dust (in his dream): he will become critically ill; what he says(?) will be negligent(?); an oracular decision(?) from his god will be in store for him; gloom(?)." Cf. Borger 1957–1958, *AfO* 18, 417–418. See further, for a syllabic spelling, BAM 513 iii 34 // BAM 514 iii 33' (Geller and Panayotov 2020, 91–92 IGI 1: 130'): *i-kil pa-ni ṣu-lu-u*[*m p*]*a-n*[*i*] "darkness of the face (gloom?), blackening of the face (anger?)" (within an incantation for sick eyes).

Lines 31'–37': For the colophon, see also Hunger 1968, No. 108; Schmidtchen 2021a, 515 n. 1200. The scribe Itti-Marduk-balāṭu, referred to in A. 3438 as apprentice exorcist, is also attested in the colophons of a copy of *Diagnostic Handbook* Tablet 12 (LKU 85 + 83), 22 (AO 6678, *TDP* II, Pl. XVII) and 30 (LKU 72), see Heeßel 2000, 257–258 262 (colophon A), 339–340 (colophon A); Schmidtchen 2021a, 493, 499, 514–515 (colophon G). Since LKU 85 + 83 was found in the Eanna temple (and can archaeologically be dated to the 7th/6th cent. BCE), also AO 6678 and A. 3438 can be attributed to this context, see Oelsner 1996, 431, 432, 436. For the Babylonian family name Šangû-parakki, see Wunsch 2014a, 310.

I.1.4 W. 17360i: Another Fragment of *Diagnostic Handbook* Tablet 37?

Following a suggestion by Schmidtchen (2021a, 245) this Late Babylonian fragment from Uruk may preserve a passage of Tablet 37 of the *Diagnostic Handbook*. In line with this proposition, the fragment is edited here for convenience of the reader. The partially preserved entries of W. 17360i present several parallels with omens from other sections of the *Diagnostic Handbook*, which are formulated from the perspective of a male patient, especially Tablet 11 (see the notes below for discussion).

List of Manuscripts

Siglum	Museum Number	Copy	Collation	Format; Ductus	Provenience
a	W. 17360i	TDP II, Pl. LXVII	–	Fragment of a tablet; Late Babylonian script; ca. 5th-3rd cent. BCE	Uruk

Overview

i' Fragmentary diagnostic entries 1'–11'
a obv.? 1'–11'

Previous Edition and Discussion

Labat 1951, *TDP* II, Pl. LXXVII (copy)
Schmidtchen 2021a, 245 n. 24 (discussion)

Transliteration

Beginning of ms. a obv. lost

1'	a obv. 1'	[............] x [.........................]
2'	a obv. 2'	[DIŠ MUNUS? ......] GÙ.G[Ù-*si* ....]
3'	a obv. 3'	[DIŠ MUNUS? ...... *u*]*š-ta-nab-l*[*ak-kát* ....]
4'	a obv. 4'	[DIŠ MUNUS? ....].MEŠ-*šá it-te-ne*[*n-ṣi-la* ....]
5'	a obv. 5'	[DIŠ MUNUS? ....]x-*na* GÁL? GAR-*an* x[............]
6'	a obv. 6'	[DIŠ MUNUS? ....]x GIG GÌR.MIN?-*šá nu-up-*[*pu-ḫa* .....]
7'	a obv. 7'	[DIŠ MUNUS? ....]x *ma-mit ṣar-ti* D[AB-*si*? ....]
8'	a obv. 8'	[DIŠ MUNUS? ....]-*šá*? *nu-up-pu-ḫa* ŠÀ-[*šá*? ....]
9'	a obv. 9'	[DIŠ MUNUS? ....-*šá i*]*t-ta-nak-n*[*a-na* ....]
10'	a obv. 10'	[DIŠ MUNUS? .... *i*]-*ta-nàr-ra-*[*ar*? ....]
11'	a obv. 11'	[..............] x x [.........................]

Ms. a obv. breaks; remainder lost

Bound Transcription and Translation

Beginning of ms. a obv. lost

1' [... ...] ... [... ...]	1' [... ...] ... [... ...]
2' [*šumma sinništu*(?) ... *iš*]*tanas*[*si* ... ...]	2' [If a woman(?) ... scre]ams all the time, [... ...].
3' [*šumma sinništu*(?) ...] *uštanabl*[*akkat* ... ...]	3' [If a woman(?) ...] keeps tossing [back and forth(?) ...].
4' [*šumma sinništu*(?) ...]-*ša ittene*[*nṣilā* ... ...]	4' [If a woman(?) ...] her [...] constantly [become] paralysed [... ...].
5' [*šumma sinništu*(?) ...]... *ibašši*(?) *šakān*(?) ...[... ...]	5' [If a woman(?) ...] ... there is [...], placing of(?) [... ...].
6' [*šumma sinništu*(?) ...] ... *marṣat*(?) *šēpāša nup*[*puḫā* ... ...]	6' [If a woman(?) ...] is sick(?), her feet(?) are inflam[ed/swollen ... ...].
7' [*šumma sinništu*(?) ...]... *māmīt sarti iṣb*[*assi*(?) ...]	7' [If a woman(?) ...] ... a ban due to treacherousness has sei[zed her(?) ...].

8' [*šumma sinništu*(?) ...]-*ša nuppuḫā libba*[*ša*(?) ... ...]
9' [*šumma sinništu*(?) ...-*ša i*]*ttanakn*[*anā* ... ...]
10' [*šumma sinništu*(?) ... *ī*]*tanarr*[*ar* ... ...]
11' [... ...] ... [... ...]

8' [If a woman(?) ...] her [...] are inflamed, [her] belly [... ...].
9' [If a woman(?) ... her ...] constantly become contracted, [... ...].
10' [If a woman(?) ...] trembles constantly, [... ...].
11' [... ...] ... [... ...]

Ms. a obv. breaks; remainder lost

Notes

Line 2': For screaming as a symptom, see e.g. *Diagnostic Handbook* Tablet 17: 15: DIŠ *ina* GIG-*šú* GÙ.GÙ-*si* "If he keeps screaming during his illness" (Scurlock 2014a, 163; Heeßel 2000, 196); Tablet 22: 59: DIŠ *ma-gal* GÙ.GÙ-*si* "If he screams a lot" (Scurlock 2014a, 188; Heeßel 2000, 256). See also Schmidtchen 2021a, Tablet 3: 8–12, Tablet 8: 10–15; Tablet 13: 115'–124', Tablet 14: 227'–229'. For the patient crying out in bed, see also Tablet 15: 90' (Scurlock 2014a, 143); BAM 30: 54 (Scurlock 2014a, 673). The verbal form GÙ.GÙ-*si* is possibly mentioned as well in Tablet 37: 28 (see above).

Line 3': Similar entries with the verb *nabalkutu* in the Štn-stem are found in *Diagnostic Handbook* Tablet 11: 37–39 (Schmidtchen 2021a, 460, 465): [DIŠ ŠU.MIN-*šú* (*u* G]ÌR.MIN-*šú*) IGI.BAR.MEŠ *uš-ta-nab-lak-kát* (var. BAL.BAL) "[If he keeps loo]king [at his hands (and his feet)], constantly tosses back and forth ...". CAD N/1, 20 sub 5e proposes to translate the Štn-stem of *nabalkutu* with "to stagger(?)"; Schmidtchen (2021a, 465) translates "(wenn) er sich immer wieder hin- und herwirft", close to the meaning of the N-stem "to turn over" (cf. CAD N/1, 17 sub 3b); Scurlock (2014a, 88) renders *uštanablakkat* as "he has changes of mood".

Line 4': The verb *eṣēlu* "to paralyse" in the Ntn-stem is also encountered in *Diagnostic Handbook* Tablet 36: 84 (see also above): DIŠ TU GÌR.MIN-*šá u* ŠU.MIN-*šú it-te-nen-ṣi-la* "if a childbearing woman's hands and feet become paralysed repeatedly". The feminine pronominal suffix -*šá* preceding the verb indicates a female patient. For similar occurrences mentioning the hands (and feet), see also *Diagnostic Handbook* Tablet 11: 18, 55 (Schmidtchen 2021a, 459, 461): DIŠ ŠU.MIN-*šú* (*u* GÌR.MIN-*šú*) *it-te-nen-ṣi-la-šú.*

Line 6': Diagnostic entries with a D-stem stative form of *napāḫu* "to become inflamed", referring to the hands, feet and fingers/toes, are also found in *Diagnostic Handbook* Tablet 11: 34, 53–54, 100' (Schmidtchen 2021a, 460, 461, 463); See also Tablet 6: 23 (Schmidtchen 2021a, 358).

Line 7': For *māmīt sarti* (also spelled *ṣartu*) "oath of falseness", see also *Šurpu* III 12 (Reiner 1958, 19); cf. Reiner 1956, *JNES* 15, 136: 94. Specific symptoms are attributed to *māmītu* (the Ban caused by a false oath) in healing texts including the *Diagnostic Handbook*; however, different formulations are used, cf. Heeßel 2000; Maul 2019; Schmidtchen 2021a for examples and discussion. For mentions of *māmītu* in *Diagnostic Handbook* Tablets 36–37, see above Tablet 36: 111, Tablet 37: 6.

Line 8': See also above line 6'.

Line 9': For *kanānu* (*qanānu*) "to roll up, to contract" in the Ntn-stem, in reference to the hands/feet, see also *Diagnostic Handbook* Tablet 11: 18, Tablet 14: 205' (Schmidtchen 2021a, 459, 576), both times encountered together with the verb *eṣēlu* "to become paralyzed".

Line 10': For another attestation of *arāru* "to tremble" (Gtn-stem), see *Diagnostic Handbook* Tablet 26: 81' (Heeßel 2000, 285; Scurlock 2014a, 199).

I.1.5 K. 11939: A Commentary Fragment on *Diagnostic Handbook* Tablet 37

This Neo-Assyrian fragment is currently the only identified commentary on the *Diagnostic Handbook* (SA.GIG) from Nineveh, and the first known commentary specimen on Tablet 37. Most other commentaries on the *Diagnostic Handbook* stem from Babylonia, with the exception of STT 403 from Sultantepe (Wee 2019b, 72–100; Frahm 2011, 220–229; Koch 2015, 281; Heeßel 2019). The discovery of a commentary on the gynaecological sections of the *Diagnostic Handbook* is the more remarkable, since so far, only two small fragments of the *Diagnostic Handbook* from Nineveh belonging to the tablets concerned with women have been identified (K. 7071 and K. 17663, belonging to Tablet 36; see above). Currently only a portion from the beginning of Tablet 37 is preserved on two Babylonian fragments; however, a few passages in K. 11939 can be identified as quotations from preserved lines (lines 1–7, 9, 15).

As Heeßel (2019, 1) points out, K. 11939 corresponds in layout to Nineveh commentaries in Neo-Assyrian script with the label *mukallimtu*, which mark comments on individual entries through indentation (see e.g. Frahm 2011, 42, 193, 199 on Rm. 122; CDLI P424630). Thus, the commentator first quoted an entry from the base text in one line, followed by comments on individual words or phrases in the following lines, which are indented.

List of Manuscripts

Siglum	Museum Number	Copy	Collation	Format; Ductus	Provenience
A	K. 11939	Heeßel 2019, 1	Coll.	Fragment of a single-column tablet; Neo-Assyrian script; 7th cent. BCE	Nineveh; Ashurbanipal's library

Previous Edition and Discussion

Heeßel 2019, *JMC* 34, 1–3 (copy; edition)
CDLI P3995329 (photo)
Electronic Babylonian Library (eBL) (https://www.ebl.lmu.de/library/K.11939; photo, edition)[217]

Transliteration

Beginning of ms. A obv.(?) lost

1' A obv.$^{?}$ 1' [........] ⸢***ir***⸣***-ṭ[ú-pu-niš-ši*** ....][218]

2' A obv.$^{?}$ 2' [........] *ir-ri-ma i-*⸢*na*⸣(-)x[.......]

3' A obv.$^{?}$ 3' [........] ^{ú}ḪAR.ḪAR ^{ú}[.......]

4' A obv.$^{?}$ 4' [........] **MUNUS BI *na-a'-da-at*** x[...]

5' A obv.$^{?}$ 5' [........] *mu-tu*$_4$ *ina* ZU-*šá* [.......]

6' A obv.$^{?}$ 6' **[DIŠ MUNUS *ina* G]IG-*šá qa-ti-šá ú-na-[aš-šak* ŠU.MEŠ *lu-'-a-ti* TAG-*ši*]**

6a' A obv.$^{?}$ 6'a *blank space (of half a line)*

7' A obv.$^{?}$ 7' [........] *mam-ma šá qa-ta-šú lu-'a-[a*$^{?}$*-ni*$^{?}$ ....]

8' A obv.$^{?}$ 8' **[DIŠ MUNUS GIG-*ma*] *ú-ru-uḫ-šá bé-e-[er ana* U$_4$.2.KAM *ana* U$_4$.3.KAM-*ma* UG$_7$]**

9' A obv.$^{?}$ 9' [....... *s*]*a-ra-as-sa* [...]

10' A obv.$^{?}$ 10' [......] ⸢*šá*⸣*-ra-as-sa* : MUNUS BI dub/u[m ...]

11' A obv.$^{?}$ 11' [........] ⸢x⸣*-ba-šá i-šiṭ/mèš i-la*(-)[...]

12' A obv.$^{?}$ 12' [........] x x ⸢ka⸣ šá x x x[...]

Ms. A obv.(?) breaks; remainder lost

---

217 A photo is also available via the digital database of the British Museum (https://www.britishmuseum.org/collection/object/W_K-11939).
218 Bold characters indicate quotes from the base text

Bound Transcription and Translation

Beginning of Ms. a obv.(?) lost

1' [...] *irṭ[upūniššī ... ...]* 2' [...] *irrī-ma ina*(?) ...[...] 3' [...] *ḫašû* ...[...]

1' [...] "(if) one con[tinues (to have sexual relations) with her" ...] 2' [...] she gets pregnant and *during*(?) [...], 3' [...] *ḫašû*-plant, [...]-plant, [...],

4' [...] *sinništu šī na'dat* ...[...] 5' [...] *mutu ina idîša*(?) [... ...]

6' [*šumma sinništu ina mur*]*ṣī-ša qātīša una*[*ššak qātātu lu"âti ilputāši*] 6a' [...] ... [...] 7' [...] *mamma ša qātāšu lu"â*[*ni*(?) ... ...]

8' [... *šumma sinništu marṣat-ma uruḫša bēr*(?) [*ana šina ūmē ana šalāšat ūmē-ma imât*] 9' [... *s*]*ārassa* [...] 10' [...] *šārassa sinništu šī* ...[... ...] 11' [...] ...-*ša išēṭ/imēs* ...[...]

4' [...] "that woman is in a critical condition" (means) [...], 5' [...] the husband, with her knowledge(?), [...].

6' ["If a woman during] her [illness], bi[tes] her hands, [dirty hands have touched her]." 6a' [...] ... [...] 7' [(...)] anyone whose hands are dir[ty ...].

8' [If a woman is sick, and] her hair is *spa*[*rse*, (and she has been sick?) for two or three days, she will die]. 9' [...] her hair(?) [...], 10' [...] her hair. (Concerning the phrase) "that woman [...]" 11' [...] (this means?) *she has despised/has disregarded* her ..., she [...].

12' *too fragmentary for transcription*

12' *too fragmentary for translation*

Ms. A obv.(?) breaks; remainder lost

Notes

Line 1': It cannot be established whether this line is quoting a complete entry from the beginning of Tablet 37 or whether this line belongs to the commentary and takes up a word from a diagnostic entry (*irṭipūniššī* "they continue (to have sexual relations) with her"), followed by a (lost) comment. However, the key phrase *irṭipūniššī* occurs in the first seven entries (lines 1–7) of Tablet 37. It is possible that line 1' is part of a commentary on the first entry (line 1).

Line 2': The phrase *irrī-ma ina* x[...] "she gets pregnant and in [...]" is probably part of a comment on the beginning of Tablet 37, e.g. on line 1, beginning with the phrase DIŠ ^{munus}PEŠ$_4$ GIG-*ma* "if a pregnant woman is sick". Perhaps the commentary may be restored as "she gets pregnant and during her pregnancy (*ina mērêša*) [...]".

Line 3': The reference to medical plants here must be part of the commentary. It looks a bit like a passage from a therapeutic text.

Line 4': This line preserves part of the apodosis of SA.GIG 37: 3 and 4 (see above). It is thus possible as well that K. 11939: 1'–5' as a whole comment on either of these two entries.

Line 5': Heeßel (2019, 3) notes that *mu-tu*$_4$ could be read either as *mūtu* "death" or *mutu* "husband". However, given the context, this line may present a comment on the negative evaluation of sexual intercourse in the fifth or sixth month of pregnancy, suggesting a reference to the woman's husband. The phrase *ina* ZU-*šá* can mean "with her knowledge", cf. *ina idê* "intentionally, knowingly" (an adverbial expression with the infinitive), CAD I/J, 29 sub 3a.

Lines 6'–7': The passage cited and commented on here is SA.GIG Tablet 37: 15:

Line 8': This line quotes SA.GIG Tablet 37: 9. For the phrase *uruḫša bēr* "her hair is *sparse*" (lit. "select"), cf. CAD U/W, 270. This diagnostic entry was presumably included in SA.GIG Tablet 3: 29 (cf. Schmidtchen 2021a, 249, 258, 269). The protasis is also encountered in SA.GIG Tablet 3: 24–27, formulated for a male-patient (see Schmidtchen 2021a, 248–249, 258 line 24). For further discussion, see above.

Line 9'–10': This passage appears to be part of the commentary on Tablet 37: 9 quoted in line 8'. If read correctly, the word *šārassa* "her hair" occurs twice in lines 9' and 10', as a synonym for *uruḫḫu* "hair", in the varying spellings *sa/šá-ra-as-sa*. Alternatively, the commentator may have commented on the near homonym *sartu* "misdeed; criminal act" (Heeßel 2019, 3). The sentence following the disjunction sign (*Trennungszeichen*; cf. Wee 2019b, 356–363) in line 10' looks like a citation from an apodosis beginning MUNUS BI "that woman ...". The only apodoses containing this phrase preserved in the fragmentary manuscript A. 3438 are found in lines 1–7, however (cf. *infra* text I.1.3).

Line 11': The reading of this line is provisional. It most likely forms part of the commentary since the text does not match a passage in the preserved entries of Tablet 37. Possibly, *i-šiṭ/mèš*(RID) can be read as *išēṭ* or *imēš* "she has been negligent/ has disregarded" (from *šêṭu* "to disdain, to be negligent" or *mêšu* "to despise, disregard").

I.1.6 LKU 126: A Fragment of *Diagnostic Handbook* Tablet 38?

No sources for Tablet 38 and 39 of the *Diagnostic Handbook* have been identified to date. However, judging from the topic of the protases, the fragment LKU 126 from Uruk[219] may represent a manuscript of either Tablet 38 or 39 of the series (Schmidtchen 2018a, 143 n. 51; 2021, 640), which justifies its inclusion in the present review of sources for diagnostic texts concerned with women.[220]

LKU 126 contains omens concerned with the circumstances of a woman's delivery. Unfortunately, none of the entries are completely preserved, but many of them feature the phrase *šumma sinništu … ūlid(ma)* "If a woman gives birth …". Several entries resemble omens in the teratomantic series *Šumma izbu*.[221] However, in contrast to *Šumma izbu* omens, the entries of LKU 126 begin with DIŠ rather than BE, which is an indicator that the text does not belong to the latter omen series (see de Zorzi 2014). According to the series catalogue listing the incipits of SA.GIG, the incipit of Tablet 38 is "If a woman's (amniotic) fluid flows for three days" (DIŠ MUNUS A-*šá ina* U_4.3.KÁM DU-*ku*). Thus, the beginning of this tablet still dealt with events prior to delivery. Tablet 39, however, bears the title "If a woman in childbed is bloated and belches" (DIŠ ^{munus}*ḫa-riš-ti i-di-ip i-geš-šú*), and thus seems to focus on postpartum conditions.[222]

Since a few lines of the fragment share close similarities or verbatim parallels to entries in *Šumma izbu* Tablets 1–4 (concerned with human birth), without running parallel to the canonical series (cf. the notes on lines 19'–22', 25'–26', 34', 36'), it is not excluded that the present tablet belonged to a collection of *aḫû*-omens related to *Šumma izbu* (Schmidtchen 2021a, 640 n. 1709). In particular, new fragments of *Šumma izbu* Tablet 4 recently published by Schmidtchen (2023) reveal further interconnections with LKU 126. These latter fragments include omens on labour pains, loss of amniotic fluid and blood, unusual places of a delivery in the street or a river (lines 66–81), in which one entry is identical with the incipit of *Diagnostic Handbook* Tablet 38. Three more lines on the appearance of the body of the newborn (lines 93–95) can now be shown to duplicate lines 19'–21' of LKU 126 (see the notes for discussion). It is not excluded that other entries of *Šumma izbu* Tablet 4 (lines 82–92) are parallel to LKU 126 (lines 8'–18'), but their fragmentary state does not allow a definite identification for the time being.

The partially preserved entries of LKU 126 deal with different times of birth (lines 12'–15', night, morning, daytime), with the colour of the baby's flesh at birth (lines 19'–21'), abnormal births (a stillbirth(?), line 22'), a child of six months (line 23'), birth feet first (*šēpānuššu*, lines 2'–26'), the birth of boys, girls and twins.

List of Manuscripts

Siglum	Museum Number	Copy	Collation	Format; Ductus	Provenience
a	VAT 14587	LKU 126	Coll.	Fragment of a single column-tablet; late Neo-Babylonian or early Achaemenid period; ca. 6th–5th cent. BCE	Uruk

Previous Edition and Discussion

Falkenstein 1931, LKU, 26, pl. 38 (copy)
Schmidtchen 2021a, 640–644 (edition)

219 The fragment was found in the north-eastern corner of the enclosure wall of the Eanna complex (Falkenstein 1931, *LKU*, 1 for comments), where it had been discarded together with other economic documents and scholarly texts.

220 It cannot be judged with certainty from the appearance of the fragment, whether the preserved text belongs to the obverse or reverse of the tablet. However, since the side in question looks quite flat, it is tentatively assigned to the obverse here.

221 Von Soden (1952, 185) assumed that LKU 126 belonged to the reverse of *Šumma izbu* Tablet 4.

222 Schmidtchen 2018b, 316: 46–47.

Stol 2000a, 202–203 (discussion)
Meissner 1932–1933 (review of Falkenstein, *LKU*), *AfO* 8, 62 (discussion)
von Soden 1952, *ZA* 50, 185 (discussion)
CDLI P414257 (photo)
Schmidtchen 2023, *NABU* 2023, 33–39 No. 18 (discussion)

Transliteration

Beginning of ms. a obv.(?) lost

1'	a obv.$^{?}$ 1'	⸢DIŠ⸣ [MUNUS ....]
2'	a obv.$^{?}$ 2'	DIŠ ⸢MUNUS⸣ [...]
3'	a obv.$^{?}$ 3'	DIŠ ⸢MUNUS⸣ x[...]
4'	a obv.$^{?}$ 4'	DIŠ ⸢MUNUS⸣ [x x x]-*qàt-ma* [...............................]
5'	a obv.$^{?}$ 5'	DIŠ [MUNUS *ú*]-⸢*šam*$^{?}$-*qàt*$^{?}$-*ma*⸣ x[..........................]
6'	a obv.$^{?}$ 6'	[DIŠ] ⸢MUNUS⸣ ⸢*ú-šam-qàt-ma*⸣ x[............................]
7'	a obv.$^{?}$ 7'	DIŠ MUNUS *ú*-⸢*šam-qàt-ma*⸣ *šá* Š[À-*šá*$^{?}$ ....]
8'	a obv.$^{?}$ 8'	DIŠ MUNUS MÚD [x x] ⸢ru$^{?}$⸣ [..............................]
9'	a obv.$^{?}$ 9'	DIŠ MUNUS MÚD ⸢*i*$^{?}$⸣-*pár*-⸢*rù*$^{!?}$⸣ ⸢Ù⸣.[TU$^{?}$ ....]
10'	a obv.$^{?}$ 10'	DIŠ MUNUS [(x)] x ⸢*ú*$^{?}$-*šam*$^{?}$⸣-<*šá*>-*ma*$^{?}$ ⸢Ù⸣.[TU$^{?}$.......]
11'	a obv.$^{?}$ 11'	DIŠ MU[NUS [(x)] za$^{?}$ x x-*ṣa-ma* Ù.T[U ....]
12'	a obv.$^{?}$ 12'	DIŠ MUNUS ⸢x x x⸣ Ù.T[U ....]
13'	a obv.$^{?}$ 13'	DIŠ MUNUS G[I$_6$ U$_4$.ZA]L$^{?}$ Ù.[TU ....]
14'	a obv.$^{?}$ 14'	DIŠ MUNUS GI$_6$ U$_4$.ZAL Ù.[TU ....]
15'	a obv.$^{?}$ 15'	DIŠ MUNUS *ina li-la-a-ti* ⸢Ù⸣.[TU ....]
16'	a obv.$^{?}$ 16'	[DIŠ MUNU]S *ina* AN.BIR$_9$ Ù.[TU ....]
17'	a obv.$^{?}$ 17'	[DIŠ MUNU]S *ina* 1/2 *u*$_4$-*mi* Ù.[TU ....]
18'	a obv.$^{?}$ 18'	DIŠ MUNUS Ù.TU-*ma* GIG *i-še*$^{!?}$-[*er-ši*$^{?}$ ....]
19'	a obv.$^{?}$ 19'	DIŠ MUNUS Ù.TU-*ma* UZU.MEŠ-*šú* *tar*-[*ku uq-ta-at-tar*]
20'	a obv.$^{?}$ 20'	DIŠ MUNUS Ù.TU-*ma* UZU.MEŠ-*šú* SIG$_7$.M[EŠ TIL *u*$_4$-*mi*]
21'	a obv.$^{?}$ 21'	DIŠ MUNUS Ù.TU-*ma* UZU.MEŠ-*šú* SA$_5$.M[EŠ NÍ-*šá* GU$_7$]
22'	a obv.$^{?}$ 22'	DIŠ MUNUS Ù.TU-*ma* BA.UG$_7$ [.................................]
23'	a obv.$^{?}$ 23'	DIŠ MUNUS *šá* 6 ITI Ù.TU x[....................................]
24'	a obv.$^{?}$ 24'	DIŠ MUNUS *še-pa-nu-uš-šu* Ù.TU x[............................]
25'	a obv.$^{?}$ 25'	DIŠ MUNUS *še-pa-nu-uš-šu* NITA Ù.TU x[.....................]
26'	a obv.$^{?}$ 26'	DIŠ MUNUS *še-pa-nu-uš-šu* MUNUS Ù.TU [..................]
27'	a obv.$^{?}$ 27'	DIŠ MUNUS NITA.MAŠ.TAB.BA Ù.TU [.....................]

28' a obv.? 28' DIŠ MUNUS MUNUS.MAŠ.TAB.BA Ù.TU [..................]

29' a obv.?29' [DIŠ MU]NUS 2 NITA.MEŠ Ù.TU [............................]

30' a obv.? 30' ⸢DIŠ⸣ [MUNUS] 2 MUNUS.MEŠ Ù.T[U ....]

____?

31' a obv.? 31' DIŠ MUNUS Ù.TU-*ma mi-it* x[.....................................]

32' a obv.? 32' DIŠ MUNUS Ù.TU-*ma* U_4.5.KAM! TI.[LA-*ma* UG_7 ....]

33' a obv.? 33' DIŠ MUNUS Ù.TU-*ma i-*⸢*qá*?⸣-*a*[*l*? ....]

34' a obv.? 34' DIŠ MUNUS Ù.TU-*ma* GÙ.G[Ù-*si*? ....]

35' a obv.? 35' DIŠ MUNUS *ina* IGI Ù.T[U-*ma* ....]

36' a obv.? 36' DIŠ MUNUS *lu*!? 11 ITI x[...]

37' a obv.? 37' DIŠ MUNUS Ù.TU-*m*[*a* ....]

38' a obv.? 38' DIŠ MUNUS Ù.[TU-*ma* ....]

39' a obv.? 39' [DIŠ MUN]US [..]

Ms. a obv.(?) breaks; gap of unknown length
Rev.(?) almost completely worn off and illegible

Bound Transcription and Translation
Beginning of ms. a obv.(?) lost

1' *šumma* [*sinništu* … …]	1' If [a woman … …].
2' *šumma sin*[*ništu* … …]	2' If a wo[man … …].
3' *šumma sinništu* …[… …]	3' If a woman …[… …].
4' *šumma sinništu* …[… …]	4' If a woman …[… …].
5' *šumma* [*sinništu*] *ušamqat-ma* …[… …]	5' If [a woman] *is struck down* and [… …].
6' *šumma sinništu ušamqat-ma* …[… …]	6' If a woman *is struck down* and [… …].
7' *šumma sinništu ušamqat-ma ša* [*libbīša*(?) … …]	7' If a woman *is struck down* so that [her foetus(?) … …].
8' *šumma sinništu dāma*(?) … [… …]	8' If a woman […] blood [… …].
9' *šumma sinništu dāma iparru*(?) *ull*[*ad*(?) … …]	9' If a woman voids blood(?) (while?) giving [birth(?) … …].
10' *šumma sinništu* […] *ušamšâ-ma*(?) *ull*[*ad*(?) …]	10' If a woman […] spends the night awake and then gives [birth(?) … …].
11' *šumma sinništu* […]…*-ma ull*[*ad*(?) …]	11' If a woman […] and then gives [birth … …].
12' *šumma sinništu* … *ūlid*(?) [… …]	12' If a woman … gives [birth … …].
13' *šumma šinništu mūša ur*[*ra*(?)] *ūl*[*id* … …]	13' If a woman gives [birth(?)] at night (or) early [morning(?)] [… …].
14' *šumma šinništu mūša urra*(?) *ūl*[*id* … …]	14' If a woman gives birth(?) at night (or) early morning(?) [… …].
15' [*šumma sinništu*] *ina līlâti ūl*[*id* … …]	15' [If a woman] gives [birth] in the evening [… …].
16' [*šumma sinni*]*štu ina muṣlāli ūl*[*id* … …]	16' [If a wom]an gives [birth] at noon [… …].
17' *šumma sinništu ina mišil ūmi ūl*[*id* … …]	17' If a woman [gives] birth at midday [… …].
18' *šumma sinništu ūlid-ma murṣu iššer*[*ši*(?) … …]	18' If sickness befalls(?) a woman as soon as she has given birth [… …].
19' *šumma sinništu ūlid-ma šīrūšu tar*[*kū uqtattar*]	19' If a woman gives birth and his(?) (i.e. the baby's) body is bruise-[coloured: he/she will become dejected].

20' *šumma sinništu ūlid-ma šīrūšu arq[ū gamār ūmī]*

20' If a woman gives birth and his(?) (i.e. the baby's) body is yellow-green: [end of days].

21' *šumma sinništu ūlid-ma šīrūšu sām[ū ramānša ikkal]*

21' If a woman gives birth and his(?) (i.e. the baby's) body is red: [she will *ruin* herself].

22' *šumma sinništu ūlid-ma imât* [... ...]

22' If a woman gives birth and then dies, [... ...].

23' *šumma sinništu ša šeššet arḫī ūlid* [... ...]

23' If a woman who is six months (pregnant) gives birth, [... ...].

24' *šumma sinništu šēpānuššu ūlid* ...[... ...]

24' If a woman gives birth (to a baby) with its feet first, [... ...].

25' *šumma sinništu šēpānuššu zikara ūlid* ...[... ...]

25' If a woman gives birth to a male with its feet first, [... ...].

26' *šumma sinništu šēpānuššu sinništa ūlid* [... ...]

26' If a woman gives birth to a female with its feet first, [... ...].

27' *šumma sinništu māšalrtū'ama ūlid* [... ...]

27' If a woman gives birth to male twins, [... ...].

28' *šumma sinništu māšta/tū'amta ūlid* [... ...]

28' If a woman gives birth to female twins, [... ...].

29' *šumma sinništu šina zikarī ūlid* [... ...]

29' If a woman gives birth to two males, [... ...].

30' *šumma sinništu šitta sinnišāti ūlid* [... ...]

30' If a woman gives birth to two females, [... ...].

?

31' *šumma sinništu ūlid-ma mīt* ...[... ...]

31' If a woman gives birth and (the new-born) is (already) dead(?) ...[...].

32' *šumma sinništu ūlid-ma ḫamšat ūmī iball[uṭ-ma imât* ...]

32' If a woman gives birth and (the new-born?) stays [alive] for five days and [then dies, ...].

33' *šumma sinništu ūlid-ma iq[âl* ...]

33' If a woman gives birth and (the new-born?) re[mains silent ... ...].

34' *šumma sinništu ūlid-ma ištana[ssi* ...]

34' If a woman gives birth and (the new-born?) constantly cries [out ... ...].

35' *šumma sinništu ina pān*(?) *alā[di* ...]

35' If a woman prior to(?) (her) giving birth [... ...].

36' *šumma sinništu lū* 11 *arḫū* [*lū* ... *ūlid* ...]

36' If a woman [gives birth] either (after) eleven [or after ...] month(s) [... ...].

37' *šumma sinništu ūlid-m[a* ...]

37' If a woman gives birth and [... ...].

38' *šumma sinništu ūlid-[ma* ...]

38' If a woman gives bi[rth and ......].

39' [*šumma sinn*]*ištu* [... ...]

39' [If a wo]man [... ...].

Ms. a obv.(?) breaks; gap of unknown length
Reverse(?) almost completely worn off and illegible

Notes

Lines 4'–6': The most probable restoration following line 7' is DIŠ MUNUS *ú-šam-qàt-ma*. However, a second possibility in line 4' could be [*šup-šu*]-*qàt-ma* "(If a woman) has difficulties during her delivery and ...". The form *ušamqat* is a Š-stem (present tense form) of *maqātu* "to fall", which is not otherwise attested in a comparable context. The common meanings of the Š-stem are "to overpower; to defeat; to strike down, destroy" and the subject usually assumes an active role (in a transitive construction), which does not fit the present context (cf. CAD M/1, 249–250 sub 7–8). So perhaps the (implicit) subject of *ušamqat* (lost in the gap?) is not the woman, but a sickness or a person who strikes down the woman. The translation "is struck down" is therefore tentative. Cf. Schmidtchen (2021a, 643) suggesting that the present lines may deal with a premature delivery due to injury inflicted on the woman (she has been "knocked down"). For the form, see also Stol 1985b, in: *Mélanges Birot*, 273: 7', with p. 275: ri-ri-ga = *ú-ša-<am>-qá-at* (referring to deaths among sheep).

Lines 8'–10': The proposed reading of these fragmentary lines is very tentative and partially follows Schmidtchen 2021a, 640. Cf. CAD P, 208–209 s.v. *parû* sub 1a; CAD Š/3, 283 s.v. *šumšû* sub 1c. For vomiting blood, see e.g. BAM 389: 5'. For *ú-šam-šá*, "to spend the night awake", see also *Diagnostic Handbook* Tablet 37: 19 (edited above). In line 8', perhaps restore MÚD [*i-par*]-*ru* "(If a woman) [vom]its blood", according to line 9' (which presents a different spelling).

The Akkadian reading of the verb form behind logographic Ù.TU "to give birth" (i.e. as a durative or a preterite tense form of *alādu*) in the omen protases of LKU 126 is ambiguous. I have opted for a preterite form *ūlid* (following conventional usage in second millennium BCE texts; GAG § 161). The syllabic spelling *ú-lid-ma* is still attested in a comparable context in a Late Babylonian therapeutic text, see BM 79061 obv. 15, rev. 1', 9' (text A.2.8).

Lines 13'–14': The signs GI_6 U_4.ZAL should refer to times of the day. The expressions $\hat{g}i_6$-zal and u_4-zal are known to correspond to early morning and dawn. Note $\hat{g}i_6$-zal-šè = *adi kaṣâti* "until the early morning", u_4-zal-šè = *adi urram* "until the early morning" and u_4-zal-(le) = *namāru* or *namārītu* "(to) dawn" (CAD K, 263b lex section; CAD N/1, 211a lex. section; CAD U/W, 240b, 243a lex. section; Attinger 2021, *Glossaire*, 1153 u_4-zal-(le) *"au point du jour, à l'aurore"*; Wilcke 1969, 149; Sjöberg and Bergmann 1969, TCS 3, 113b). Otherwise, $\hat{g}i_6$ u_4-zal corresponds to *mūša u urri* "night and day", cf. CAD M/2, 292a sub lex. section. Cf. Schmidtchen 2021a, 641, 643 for a different reading of the passage.

Lines 15'–17': The significance or interpretation of birth during different times of the day may have resembled hemerological or astrological considerations (stipulating auspicious or inauspicious dates and consequences for the fate of the newborn and his/her family), cf. Stol 2000a, 91–98.

Line 18': The protasis of this entry, appears to be cited in the principal commentary on *Šumma izbu*, albeit in a slightly varying spelling, in a section relating to Tablet 4 (de Zorzi 2014, 440 lines 27–29 with notes; CAD E, 353b): BE MUNUS Ù.[-TU]-*ma* GIG *i-ši-ir-ši* / SI.SÁ = *i-še-rù* / *šá a-la-ki* "If a woman gives birth and then sickness befalls her (lit. comes straight to her): SI.SÁ means "to direct oneself (toward something)" (*ešēru*), in the sense of "to come". The quoted line is not preserved in the manuscripts of *Šumma izbu* Tablet 4; presumably the entry is to be found in a section of Tablet 4 that has not been recovered yet. I suggest emending the verbal form in ms. a to *i-še*!(ḪI)-[*er-ši*] in line with the commentary's *i-ši-ir-ši*. The form could be interpreted as a preterite or present tense form. Instead of the emendation, it would be possible to read *i-šár*-[*ši*] (for the stative), although this reading is less likely (cf. AHw 254–255).

Lines 19'–21': These three lines can now be restored from three identical entries in a new fragment of *Šumma izbu* Tablet 4 published by Schmidtchen 2023, 36 (lines 93–95). The masculine pronominal suffix in UZU.MEŠ-*šú* "his body" (lit. fleshes) in the present lines leaves it open whether this observation refers to the appearance of the body of the new-born rather than to the woman's body. *Šumma izbu* Tablet 4 lines 2–15 includes similar entries on marks visible on the skin of the newborn having different colour (cf. de Zorzi 2014, 441–443).

The meaning of the apodosis *ramānša ikkal*, lit. "she will eat/consume herself" restored in line 21' (from *Šumma izbu* Tablet 4: 95) is interpreted here in the sense of "to destroy, ruin (oneself)" (see CAD A/1, 253–255 sub 5). The same apodosis is attested in another omen text (KAR 392 obv.(!) 15): DIŠ ^{d}DÌM.ME DAB-*su ra-man-šú* GU_7 "If Lamaštu seizes him, he will *ruin*(?) himself" (quoted in CAD R, 119 sub a-7'; CAD A/1, 253b sub sub 4 assumes the meaning "to bite oneself"). Note, however, a contextually similar omen apodosis in *Inbu bēl arḫi* (K. 2809 iv 9; Livingstone 2013, 226 rev. col. ii 8'; Labat 1965, *Calendrier*, pl. 45): [...] ^{d}DÌM.ME DAB-*su ra-man-šú* GAZ-*ak* "[If...], Lamaštu will seize him (and) he will kill himself". M. Geller (personal communication) suggests the expression "to eat oneself" may be idiomatic and refer to a psychotic state of mind (self-deprecating).

For *uqtattar* (Dt-stem of *qatāru* "to become dejected, despondent" (literally "to become blackened by smoke") in the restored apodosis of line 19', see CAD Q, 168a sub mng. 6; see also Labat 1965, *Calendrier*, 132–133 § 64: 5; Schmidtchen 2023, 38 (*Šumma izbu* Tablet 4) line 111: GENNA BI *uqtattar* "(If a child is born is month Abu), that child will become despondent".

Line 22': This entry is also found with minor variation in *Šumma izbu* Tablet 4: 40 (de Zorzi 2014, 446), where the apodosis is likewise lost: BE MUNUS Ù.TU-*ma* UG_7 *i*-[...] "If a woman gives birth and then dies ...[...]." Cf. Leichty 1970, 70. It is equally possible that the protasis refers to the death of the newborn during or immediately after birth (cf. Stol 2000a, 203 n. 21; Schmidtchen 2021a, 642). Cf. also line 31' below.

Line 23': The premature birth of a baby after six months of pregnancy is very likely described here (thus Stol 2000a, 203 with n. 21). In Greek and Jewish tradition, gods, heroes and other important and legendary persons are often born after six or in the seventh month, and both traditions regard a baby born after six months/in the seventh month viable (Stol 2000a, 21–22 for discussion).

Lines 24'–26': Two similar protases concerning multiple births are found in *Šumma izbu* Tablet 1: 85 and 103 (de Zorzi 2014, 360, 366). However, the cases of a single baby born with the feet arriving first, which are found in ms. a lines 24'–25', are not included in *Šumma izbu* Tablet 1. The entries in question read:

BE MUNUS 2 NITA.MEŠ *še-pa-nu-us-šú-nu* Ù.TU É BI BIR-(*aḫ*)
"If a woman gives birth to two males with their feet first: that household will be dispersed." (line 85)

BE MUNUS 2 (var. 3) MUNUS.MEŠ *še-pa-nu-ši-na* Ù.TU EN É BI (BA).UG$_7$
"If a woman gives birth to two (var. three) females with their feet first: the head of that household will die." (line 103)

Line 26' uses the masculine suffix *-šú* instead of correct *še-pa-nu-uš-šá* (cf. the correct feminine form in *Šumma izbu* Tablet 1: 103).

Line 27'–28': For omens on the birth of twins (MAŠ.TAB.BA), compare also *Šumma izbu* Tablet 1: 90–99. However, the present cases differentiating the birth of male and female twins are not included there.

Lines 29'–30': Compare the similar entries in *Diagnostic Handbook* Tablet 36: 114–115 and in *Šumma izbu* 1: 83 and 100 concerning the birth of two male or two female babies (cf. de Zorzi 2014, 360, 365, and *infra* for discussion). In the *Šumma izbu*-omens, the birth of two male babies signals hardship and distress (for the family/country), while the birth of two female babies means prosperity for their family. It is unclear why the omen series differentiates between male/female twins and the birth of two boys/girls (cf. Meissner 1932–1933, *AfO* 8, 62).

Line 31': This entry may be compared with a similar one in *Šumma izbu* Tablet 1: 100a (de Zorzi 2014, 265): BE MUNUS 2 MUNUS.MEŠ Ù.TU-*ma* UG$_7$.MEŠ [... ...] "If a woman gives birth to two females, but they are dead (*mītā*) [... ...]."

Line 32': Compare *Šumma izbu* Tablet 4: 41 (de Zorzi 2014, 446): BE MUNUS Ù.TU-*ma* 3 U$_4$-*me* TI.LA-*ma* UG$_7$ *i*-[...] "If a woman gives birth and (the newborn?) lives for three days but then dies [...]." As in line 22' above, the protasis is ambiguous and could refer to either maternal death or to the death of the newborn.

Line 33': This line could be a quote or adaptation from *Šumma izbu* Tablet 4: 43 (de Zorzi 2014, 446): BE MUNUS Ù.TU-*ma* ⌜*i*⌝-*qá-al bu-še-*[*e* ...] "If a woman gives birth and (the newborn) remains silent: the property [...]".

Line 34': The entry could be similar to *Šumma izbu* Tablet 4: 44: [BE] MUNUS Ù.TU-*ma* GÙ.GÙ-*si ṣal-tum* [*pu-uḫ-pu-ḫu-u* GAR-*nu-šú*] "If a woman gives birth and (the newborn?) constantly cries out – there will be squabbling and quarrelling for him (the child)". For restoration and commentary see de Zorzi 2014, 447, 459. The interpretation given by the omen is analogical.

Line 35': Schmidtchen (2021a, 442) translates: "vor dem Gebären", suggesting a reading *ina pān alādi* "(if a woman) prior to (her) giving birth ...". But the phrase *ina pāni*(IGI) could also be interpreted as an adverbial expression with a temporal meaning ("earlier; in the past", cf. CAD P, 90–92 sub 5a and c).

Line 36': The reading of this line follows *Šumma izbu* Tablet 4: 46 (de Zorzi 2014, 447): [BE MUNUS] *lu* ITI.11.KAM *lu* 12.KAM *ú-bi-il-ma* Ù.TU-[*ma* ...] "If a woman carries (a child) either eleven or twelve months and then gives birth [...]. Schmidtchen (2021a, 441) reads DIŠ MUNUS *ša* ITI x[...]; however, Falkenstein's copy looks more like DA than ŠA. On the photo, the sign in question is very broadly spaced and could alternatively be read as *lu* 11 or *lu* U$_4$.

I.1.7 SpTU 1, No. 40: A Commentary on *Diagnostic Handbook* Tablet 39

This Late Babylonian commentary on the still unpreserved Tablet 39 of the *Diagnostic Handbook* SA.GIG was found at Uruk (Area U18, Level V), close to the findspot of a few other commentaries on the *Diagnostic Handbook* (registered under the field number W. 22307) with colophons of the conjurer Anu-ikṣur, descendant of Šangû-Ninurta, which suggests that it also belonged to the same family library (Clancier 2009a, 388; Frahm 2011, 290–291; Wee 2019b, 330). In this case, the tablet could be dated approximately to the second half of the Achaemenid period (late 5th/early 4th cent. BCE).

The obverse of this tablet in landscape format is completely preserved, but the reverse is largely worn off. The commentary begins with the incipit of *Diagnostic Handbook* Tablet 39 known from the incipit catalogues of the compendium (Schmidtchen 2018b, 316: 47). SpTU 1, No. 40 can thus be assumed to comment on this chapter, although the pronominal suffixes referring to the patient in the base text quotations are masculine (*-šú*) rather than feminine (*-šá*). Wee (2019b, 334) draws attention to the possibility that masculine suffixes in this tablet could also refer to the newborn, given that Tablet 39 dealt with a postnatal situation (a woman in childbed). The Late Babylonian commentary on Tablet 36 (SpTU 1,

No. 39) likewise uses masculine suffixes, while the Neo-/Late Babylonian manuscripts of SA.GIG Tablet 36 and 37 are not consistent in their use (often feminine, sometimes masculine suffixes). Wee (2019b, 326, 334) further proposes that the commentator's use of masculine suffixes may have been intentional, signalling that the medical terminology commented on could potentially be applied both to male and female patients.

List of Manuscripts

Siglum	Museum Number	Copy	Collation	Format; Ductus	Provenience
a	IM 74452 W. 22311	SpTU 1, No. 40	Photo coll.	Fragment of a single-column tablet; Late Babylonian script; ca. 5th/4th cent. BCE	Uruk

Previous Edition and Discussion

Hunger 1976, 48–49 (edition), 138 (copy)
Clancier 2009b, *GKAB* P348461 (edition)
Wee 2019b, *CM* 49/2, 330–339 (edition), 434 pl. 30 (photo of the obverse)
Fincke 2000, *Augenleiden*, 155, 159, 163, 165, 183, 232
Frahm 2011, 66, 228–229, 291
Gabbay 2016, *The Exegetical Terminology*, 68, 74, 77, 107, 109, 229
Geller 2010, *Ancient Babylonian Medicine*, 141–160
Genty 2010, *JMC* 16, 14
Heeßel 2000, 137, 146
Panayotov 2017, in: *The Comparable Body*, 238 n. 10
Scurlock 2014a, 185 n. 8, 257 n. 1
Scurlock and Andersen 2005, no. 9.76
Bácskay 2019, *RA* 113, 180 (lines 1–6)
CDLI P348461 (copy)
Frahm, Frazer and Jiménez 2013b, *CCP* 4.1.39 (copy)

Transliteration

1 a obv. 1 **DIŠ** **^{munus}*ḫa-riš-ti i-di-ip u i-geš-sú*** **BA.UG$_7$**[223]

2 a obv. 2 ***ši-bit*** **SAG.DU-*šú* *nu-uḫ$_5$-ḫu-rat*** : saĝ ĝiš ra

3 a obv. 3 *nu-ú-ú-ru* : saĝ : *kak-ku* : ĝiš : *kak-ku*

4 a obv. 4 ra : *ma-ḫa-ṣu šá-niš* ra : *na-a-ra* : ra : *ma-ḫa-ṣu*

5 a obv. 5 *šal-šiš* gaz : *na-a-ra* : gaz : *ḫé-pu-u*

6 a obv. 6 *né-'i-ir* SAG.DU *ma-ḫi-iṣ muḫ-ḫi* : *ki ši-gu-ú*

7 a obv. 7 *al-si-ka*: *pe-ret* **SAG.DU-*šú* *sa-mat*(KUR)**: *sa-ma-ta*

8 a obv. 8 *sa-ap-ḫa-at* : ***ka-ra-an*** **IGI.MIN-*šú* *šad-du***

9 a obv. 9 *šá kak-kul-tu$_4$ i-ni-šú ú-ṣa-a* : **ÚR-*šú* *ta-a-ka***

10 a obv. 10 *šá ana da-ke-e u šá-ka-ni dan-na-niš-šú*

223 Bold characters indicate quotes from the base text.

11	a obv. 11	*šá ši-kin-šú*!(ni) NU *iš-nu-ú*: **KA-*šú ṣa-pir* UG$_7$**
12	a obv. 12	*ṣa-pa-ru* : *kub-bu-lu$_4$*: *ṣa-pa-ru* : *ṣu-un-du-ru*
13	a obv. 13	*ṣa-pa-ru* : *la ta-ra-ṣu*: sa : *šér-a-ni*
14'	a rev. 1'	x[........]
15'	a rev. 2'	x[........]
16'	a rev. 3'	i x[......]
17'	a rev. 4'	*šá* x[......]

18'	a rev. 5'	x[........]

Ms. a rev. breaks; remainder lost

Bound Transcription and Translation

1 *šumma ḫarištu iddip u igeššu imât*	1 "If a woman in childbed is bloated and belches, she will die".
2 *šibīt qaqqadīšu nuḫḫurat* : saĝ ĝiš ra	2 (With regard to) "her(?) fontanelle (lit. "seam of her head") has been struck", saĝ ĝiš ra means
3 *nu''uru*: saĝ : *kakku* : ĝiš : *kakku*	3 "to hit"; saĝ means "weapon"; ĝiš means "weapon";
4 ra : *maḫāṣu šanîš* ra : *nâra* : ra : *maḫāṣu*	4 ra means "to strike". Alternatively, ra means "to hit", (or) ra means "to strike".
5 *šalšiš* gaz : *nâra* : gaz : *ḫepû*	5 Thirdly, gaz (likewise) means "to hit", (or) gaz means "to break, to smash".
6 *nē'ir qaqqadi māḫiṣ muḫḫi* : *itti šigû*	6 (As in) "He who hits the head, who strikes the skull". (This is recited) together with "With a *šigû*-prayer
7 *alsīka*: *peret qaqqadīšu sa-mat*(KUR) : *samât(a)*	7 I have invoked you". (In) "the hair of her head is *sa-mat*(KUR)", (the latter is to be read as) *samât* ("faltering"),
8 *sapḫat* : *karān īnīšu šaddū*	8 (which means) "it is spread out (thinly)". (The expression) "the irises of her eyes are *stretched out*"
9 *ša kakkultu īnīšu uṣṣâ* : *pēnētūšu ta-a-ka*	9 (means) "(someone) whose irises are oriented outwards". (The phrase) "her thighs are *ta-a-ka*"
10 *ša ana dakê u šakāni dannānišşu*	10 (is said in the case that) that they (the thighs) are difficult for her to move or to set in position,
11 *ša šikinšu*(!) *lā išnû* : *pûšu*(?) *ṣapir imât*	11 (which means) that their(!) *position* does not change (anymore). (In) "(if) her mouth(?) is *pressed down*, she will die",
12 *ṣapāru* : *kubbulu* : *ṣapāru* : *ṣun-duru*	12 "to press down" (*ṣapāru*) means "to be paralysed" (*kubbulu*); *ṣapāru* (also) means "to twitch" (*ṣudduru*);
13 *ṣapāru* : *lā tarāṣu* : SA : *šer'āni*	13 "to press down" (also) means "not being able to stretch out". SA means "tendons".

Traces of five lines in ms. a rev.; remainder lost

Notes

Line 1: For the incipit of *Diagnostic Handbook* Tablet 39, see the SA.GIG catalogue discussed in Schmidtchen 2018b, 316 line 47. The verb *edēpu* "to inflate" is usually used in the stative (G- or D-stem), see CAD E, 28 sub mng. 1a-b; in the present line *i-di-ip* is interpreted as a present tense form, parallel to *igeššu* "she belches" (from *gešû*). For a similar problem affecting women in childbed treated in a therapeutic text, see BAM 240: 25', 26', 28' (text D.2.1): "(if a woman gives birth and subsequently) she is bloated with wind" (*šāra uddupat*).

Line 2: The commentator understood the stative form *nuḫḫurat* as *nu''urat*, i.e. as the D-stem of *nêru* "to smite, hit", rather than related to *naḫāru* D-stem (a verb with obscure meaning), see Wee 2019b, 331, 334; CAD N/2, 179b s.v. *nêru* lex. section; cf. CAD N/1, 127 s.v. *naḫāru* A; AHw 713 s.v. *naḫāru* I. This understanding is made apparent by the following explanation, in which the Sumerian phrase saĝ ĝiš ra is equated with Akkadian *nu''uru*. For *šibīt qaqqadi* "seam of the head" (fontanelle), see CAD Š/2, 381a sub mng. b, e.g. in *Diagnostic Handbook* Tablet 3: 21–23 (Schmidtchen 2021a, 248, 258, 268), Tablet 40: 44–45 (Scurlock 2014a, 14, 260), where the fontanelle is said to be "open, split" (*paṭāru*).

Lines 2–5: The commentator analyses the components of the phrase saĝ ĝiš ra "to smite (the head with a weapon)". In line 3, instead of the equation of the element saĝ with *kakku*, one would expect Akkadian *qaqqadu* "head." Wee (2019b, 331–332, 335) argues that the commentator may have had the following association in mind: since SAG.DU means "head" (Akkadian *qaqqa-du*), SAG could have been thought to stand for /*qaqqa*/, which sounds like *kakka* "weapon". Gabbay (2016, 68) and Hunger (1976, 49) assume a mistake for *qaq-qa-du*. GIŠ instead of ^{giš}TUKUL occurs occasionally as a logogram for *kakku* in lexical texts (e.g. Idu II 181 (CAD K, 51); Hh. VII A 7 (MSL 6, 84)).

In lines 4–5, the commentator supports his understanding of the term *nuḫḫurat* "it has been struck" by presenting semantically related Akkadian readings of the Sumerian verb ra, further extended by parallel equations for gaz, having the semantic range of "to hit, strike", "to break, smash" (see Wee 2019b, 332, 335).

Lines 6–7: In line 6, the commentator juxtaposes two equivalent Akkadian phrases, *nē'ir qaqqadi* "he who smites the head" and *māḫiṣ muḫḫi* "he who strikes the top (of the head)", lending further support to his interpretation of the phrase cited from the base text in line 2. Gabbay (2016, 68) proposes that these two phrases together present a quotation from a literary text. An exact correspondence is not known to me, but the phrase *māḫiṣ muḫḫi* is an address to malevolent demons or disease agents found in several apotropaic incantations. Within the women's healthcare texts, one spell to protect from miscarriage begins with this phrase, see AO 6473 obv. 26 (quoting the incipit), STT 241: 8–26 (incantation); for both texts, see C.3.1 and C.3.9 in this volume). For similar spells featuring *māḫiṣ muḫḫi*, see further STT 215 obv. iii 24 (in Ḫulbazizi, see Finkel 1976, 108, 184–186 No. 31: 172–174 and pl. 11); KUB 29, 58+59 (+) KUB 37, 84 iv 9–10 (Meier 1939, *ZA* 45, 206; Bácskay 2018, 168 No. 55); Wee 2019b, 336.

Concerning the phrase *šīgû alsīka* in lines 6–7, Wee (2019b, 332, 336) notes that *šigû*-prayers often begin with the statement *alsīka* "I have invoked you (with a *šigû*-prayer)" (cf. CAD Š/2, 413 s.v. *šigû* sub a). Following Gabbay (2016, 68), I understand the sign KI before *šīgû alsīka* as *itti* "with", used here to indicate a textual citation or contextualisation (instead of the complete phrase *ša itti … iqbû* "which is said with …", used in references to names of compositions or to a corpus to which a previous citation belongs, see Gabbay 2016, 228–230). Thus, *šigû alsīka* could be understood here as title/incipit of such a *šigû*-prayer, or an indication that the preceding *nē'ir qaqqadi māḫiṣ muḫḫi* forms an incantation incipit and that this recitation was performed with the prayer *šigû alsīka* or stemmed from a *šigû*-prayer. A prayer to Marduk with this incipit is known (Oshima 2011, 125 K. 2832+ i 5 (incipit), preserved in K. 2425 // K. 9252 (Oshima ibid., n. 119; van der Toorn 1985, 137–138 with pl. 2–3; Jaques 2015, 227–231). For *šigû*-prayers, see Mayer 1976, 111–113; van der Toorn 1985, 117–121, 125–139; Oshima 2011, 296–304; and discussion of BAM 237(+) obv. i 12' (text C.1.7).

Lines 7–8: The commentator picks out the verbal form *sa-mat* in the phrase *peret qaqqadīšu sa-mat* "the hair of his/her head is *sa-mat*", extracted from the base text. As Frahm (2011, 66) and Wee (2019b, 336–337) argue, the explanation *sa-ma-ta* is meant to clarify the reading of the syllable *mat* (written with the ambiguous sign KUR, which can also be read *lat*). As clarified by Wee, *sa-mat* is to be understood as *samât* derived from the verb *samû* "to be faltering", rather than *sāmat* from *sâmu* "to be red". Thus, *samû* is linked with *makû* "to become lacking", with reference to someone's hair, in a commentary on Tablet 21/22 of the *Diagnostic Handbook* (see Wee 2019b, 283, 285–286, 291–292 obv. 1–2). In line 8, the commentator equates *samât* with *sapḫat* "it is spread out (thinly)", to further clarify the meaning of the former.

Lines 8–9: The phrase *karān īnīšu šaddū* "the grape(s) of his/her eye(s) (irises) are stretched out" from the base text is explained as *kakkulti īnīšu uṣṣâ* "the iris goes out(ward)". A similar explanation for the phrase *karān īnīšu šaddū* (but this time with inward movement) is given in a commentary on SA.GIG Tablet 21/22, commenting on SA.GIG Tablet 21 line 3, see Leichty, 1973, *AfO* 24, 83: 3–4; Heeßel 2000, 247ff.; Frahm 2011, 226–227; Wee 2019b, 284, 293 lines 3–4). Fincke (2000, 19 with Abb. 2) and Wee (2019b, 293 note on obv. 3–4) identify the expression *kakkulti īni* (lit. "the fermenting vessel of the eye") with the iris rather than the whole eyeball (as CAD K, 59–60). The described symptom has been interpreted as a dilation or constriction of the pupil (i.e. perceived in terms of the iris moving inward or outward from the centre of the eyes), see thus Fincke 2000, 163–164 (*Seclusio pupillae*), accepted by Wee 2019b, 293, 333, 337–338; differently Frahm 2011, 227–229 (proposing a cross-eyed condition).

Lines 9–11: The verbal form in the phrase "his/her thigh(s) (ÚR-*šú*) are *ta-a-ka*" is difficult to identify with certainty. Wee (2019b, 338) considers *takkā* as the 3rd person fem. pl. G-stem stative of *takāku* (with *pēnētu* "thighs" as the subject), which refers to a physical feature or defect (CAD T, 61; Fincke 2000, 163 n. 1238; George 2013, CUSAS 18, 89 note on obv. 6'). Clancier (2009b) suggests reading *dá-a-ka*, from *dâku* "to kill, slay, beat," but the stative form of this verb should be *dīkā* rather than *dākā*. A completely different interpretation of the commentary passage as referring to the nose is proposed by Geller (2010, 145 with notes 195), emending to <*na*>-*ta-a-ka* "dripping".

The interpretation of the commentary's explanations of lines 10–11 largely follows Wee (2019b, 333, 338), understanding *dannāniššu* (line 10) as a fem. stative plural form of *danānu* "to be difficult" with ventiv (-*ni*(*m*)) and resumptive pronominal suffix -*šu*. For explanations in commentaries introduced by the relative pronoun (*ša* ...-*šu*/-*ša*), see Gabbay 2016, 109–110. The resumptive -*šu* refers back to the antecedent of *ša*. For different interpretations of the passage cf. Clancier 2009b; Geller 2010, 145 with note 196 (assuming *niš-šú* on its own stands for *ni'šu* "sneeze").

As proposed by Wee (2019b, 338), the noun *šikinnu* in line 11 suggests a meaning related to *šakānu* "to set in position" in line 10, rather than the specific meanings given for the terms in CAD Š/2, 429 s.v. *šikinnu* A and B). Clancier (2009b) translates the phrase *ša šikinni lā išnû* "whose nature does not change", suggesting *šikinnu* stands for *šiknu* "outward appearance, shape"; similarly, Geller 2010, 145 with n. 197, proposing emendation to *ši-kin-šú*!. My translation "position" is very close to Wee's "disposition".

Lines 11–13: For analysis, see Wee 2019b, 338–339. The exact reading of KA-*šú* in line 11 (his/her mouth/nose) is not certain. The verbs equated with *ṣapāru*, *kubbulu* "to be paralysed" and *ṣudduru* "to twitch", occur with the mouth and nose as subject, respectively.

Part II: **Therapeutic Texts**

II.1 Selected Texts from the Second Millennium BCE

The four texts presented in this chapter have been selected as examples representing therapies for women's health matters from the second millennium BCE and as precursors to the healing traditions that are much more amply attested in the corpus of the first millennium BCE medical cuneiform texts edited in this book. Two of the texts (II.1.1–II.1.2) date to the Old Babylonian period, the other two to the second half of the second millennium BCE. Of the former sources, text II.1.1 (BM 97093) has not been edited before. The two Old Babylonian tablets are witness to the flourishing tradition of Sumerian and Akkadian birth incantations known from that period and from earlier centuries (see e.g. Cunningham 1997, 40–43, 69–75, 96–97, 131–159; Rudik 2011, 318–331 FM 56–58; Wasserman and Zomer 2022, No. 1–14).[224] Texts II.1.3 and II.1.4 – the former written in a Middle Babylonian, the latter in a Middle Assyrian script – may both stem from Assur. Middle Babylonian scholarly texts including magico-medical tablets were imported to Assur following Tukulti-Ninurta's I conquest of Babylon (late 13th century BCE) and have been attributed to the so-called library of Tiglath-pileser I (Library M2), which incorporated texts that can be dated between the 13th and the 11th centuries BCE.[225]

Texts II.1.3 and II.1.4 display some general features that resemble first millennium BCE women's healthcare texts. Thus, they contain a mixture of incantations and medical prescriptions; they also contain several passages that duplicate or form close parallels to sources from the first millennium BCE. The medical prescriptions preserved in these two texts deal with a range of female conditions typical for texts from later periods (from fertility to delivery and other specific complaints). Moreover, while text II.1.4 can be described as an excerpt, text II.1.3 may present a compendium concerned exclusively with women's health inscribed on a two-column collective tablet (which is also the format of tablets of the later, serialized *Nineveh Medical Compendium* (also known as *Nineveh Medical Encyclopedia*) from the 7th century BCE (Panayotov 2018; Steinert et al. 2018). Thus, text II.1.3 is the oldest example of such a specialised gynaecological compendium attested from Mesopotamia known at present, reflecting processes of development and formation in ancient Mesopotamian medical literature that took place in the centuries of the Late Bronze Age.

II.1.1 BM 97093: An Old Babylonian Tablet with Birth Incantations

This Old Babylonian tablet contains two hitherto unknown birth incantations. The first of them is a Sumerian composition that shares similar passages with several other Old Babylonian birth incantations that begin with the phrase munus ù-tu-da-a-ni "the woman giving birth" and focus on the metaphor of the woman in delivery as a fully laden boat floating on water on its way to the quay (of successful birth). The incantation has the well-known format that includes the dialogue between the gods Enki and Asalluḫi (Falkenstein 1931b, 44–67; Rudik 2011, 46–63; George 2016, 2–4). A version of the spell with the incipit munus ù-tu-da-a-ni (with an interlinear Akkadian translation) was transmitted to the first millennium BCE and included in the so-called Neo-Assyrian Birth Compendium (see text D.1.1). The Sumerian incantation in BM 97093 is classified with the rubric *šipat mušapšiqtim* "spell for a woman who has difficulty in delivery", followed by an Akkadian prescription that is reminiscent of the intervention recommended by Enki within the spell (in the dialogue with his son). The prescription also recurs in its essence in the Neo-Assyrian Birth Compendium (see Wasserman and Zomer 2022, No. 10; Steinert 2017a, 336–339; *infra* text D.1.1 for discussion). The remedy is rather symbolic: a hollow reed is filled with oil over which the spell was recited and then broken above the woman's belly or umbilical area, thus releasing the oil. This performative action supposedly symbolised an easy and successful delivery of the baby released through the woman's narrow birth canal.

The Sumerian incantation in BM 97093 displays many unorthographic phonetic spellings that at times are difficult to understand. The use of such non-standard (syllabic) writings has been described as a feature of Old Babylonian Sumerian texts from the Northern Babylonian tradition.[226] Parallels from other contemporary tablets containing variations of the spell munus ù-tu-da-a-ni are at times helpful to elucidate the phonetic spellings in BM 97093 (see the notes below).

224 A second incantation genre already attested in the third and second millennium BCE are spells to stop bleeding (during pregnancy or delivery), see Krebernik 1984, No. 37; Finkel 1980; Scurlock 1991; Rudik 2011, 332–336 FM 59.

225 Weidner 1952–1953, *AfO* 16, 197–215; Pedersén 1985, 31–42 Library M2; Zomer 2018, 39.

226 As seen, for example, in the incantations from Tell Haddad published by Cavigneaux and al-Rawi 1993, 2002; Cavigneaux 1995a, 1995b; see also George 2016 for Old Babylonian incantations in the Schøyen Collection and Viano 2016.

https://doi.org/10.1515/9781501506475-003

From the Akkadian incantation on the reverse of BM 97093 unfortunately only the first lines are preserved. At the beginning of this composition the baby in the womb is addressed as "fish roe of the sea" and as a "creature of the flood". This conceptualisation of the foetus *in utero* as a marine creature is also encountered in other Old Babylonian birth incantations (Wasserman and Zomer 2022, 51, 92 No. 14: 26, on the term *dādu*, an aquatic animal with a shell). The appended colophon provides a date formula giving the year when the tablet was written as year 35 of the Babylonian king Ammiditana (ca. 1649 BCE).

List of Manuscripts

Siglum	Museum Number	Copy	Collation	Format; Ductus	Provenience
a	BM 97093 (1902-10-11, 147)	Pl. 4–5	Coll.	Single-column tablet in portrait format; 18th cent. BCE[227]	Unknown

Overview

i	Sumerian birth incantation a obv. 1–rev. 2	1–27
	Akkadian prescription a rev. 3–5	28–30
ii	Akkadian birth incantation a rev. 6–19	31–39'
iii	Colophon a rev. 20–u.e. 3	40'–44'

Previous Edition and Discussion

CDLI P527479 (without photo or transliteration)
British Museum Collection (https://www.britishmuseum.org/collection/object/W_1902-1011-147)

Transliteration

1	a obv. 1	[munus du-da]-an-ni[228] mi-ki a mi-ni$^{!}$(IR)-ri
2	a obv. 2	[kù ^{d}inann]a-ke$_{4}$ du-da-an-ni mi-ki a mi-ni-ri
3	a obv. 3	[munus d]u-da-an-ni mi-ki a mi-ni-ri
4	a obv. 4	[^{d}nin-hur]-saĝ-ĝá-ke$_{4}$ du-da-an-ni mi-ki a mi-ni-ri
5	a obv. 5	[m]á-gur$_{8}$ <gu>-ki gu-ki a-mi-íb-si
6	a obv. 6	[m]á še-em-ma-ak-ke$_{4}$ še-em-ma a-am-mi-íb-si
7	a obv. 7	[m]á ^{ĝiš}eren-na-ke$_{4}$ ^{ĝiš}eren-na a-am-mi-íb-si
8	a obv. 8	[má] ^{na4}za-gìn-na za-gìn-na a-am-mi-íb-si
9	a obv. 9	[x ^{n}]$^{a4?}$ku$^{?}$-ug nu-uz-zu za-gi-in nu-uz-zu
10	a obv. 10	[x x x x]x-dab-ba ag-ga-ab ú-ra gi-ba-a im-me-gi-bi

227 Measurements: ca. 4.5 x 7.5 x 1.5 cm.
228 The scribe uses several forms of the sign NI, writing it either without a vertical wedge, or with one/two verticals (see e.g. lines 1–4).

11 a obv. 11 [^{d}asal-lú-ḫi] igi-ni im-ma-an-zi a-a-ni ^{d}en-ki-ra

12 a obv. 12 [x x x x x] é ba-ši-in-ku$_{4}$ gù mu-un-na-de-e

13 a obv. 13 [^{d}en-ki . . . ^{d}]asal-lú-ḫi mu-un-na-ni-íb-gi$_{4}$-gi$_{4}$

14 a obv. 14 [dumu-ĝu$_{10}$ a-na-àm] nu-me-e-zu a-na-àm a-ra-ab-daḫ-ḫe-e

15 a obv. 15 [^{d}asal-lú-hi a]-na-àm nu-me-e-zu a-na-àm a-ra-ab-daḫ-ḫe-e

16 a obv. 16 [níĝ ì-zu-a]-ĝu$_{10}$ ù ze-e in-ga-ra-e-zu

17 a obv. 17 [x x ĝen-n]a$^{?}$ ^{d}asal-lú-ḫi

18 a obv. 18 [x x x x]x-bí-zu in-nu-zu

19 a obv. 19 x x [x x g]i sú-gu ba-an-du ap-pa-ar gi du-g[a]

20 a obv. 20 ì ⸢nu-ub-da-a⸣ ì-nun nu-ub-da-a [x x]

21 a obv. 21 gal$_{4}$-la si-pa-ad-da ri-a si$^{?}$-⸢in$^{?}$-da⸣-x[x x]

22 a obv. 22 tu-ku-u[b]-[b]i ni-in-ta tu-ku-⸢ub⸣-b[i . . . .]

23 a obv. 23 tu-k[u]-[ub]-[b]i mu-nu-ús x[. . . . .]

24 a lo. e. 1 tu-ku-ub-bi saĝ-lú-ti-la igi l[ú$^{?}$ x x x x]

25 a lo. e. 2 [mu-u]š$^{?}$-gin$_{7}$ ḫu-us-ḫu-us-ta ù-me-e-⸢ta$^{?}$⸣-⸢dirig$^{?}$⸣

26 a rev. 1 [x]-eš-ta lú pa-na-gin$_{7}$ si-sá-⸢e⸣-[dè]

27 a rev. 2 [t]u$_{6}^{!}$([K]A) én-[é-nu-ru]

28 a rev. 3 *ši-pa-at mu-ša-ap-ši-iq-tim* Ì.GIŠ *la*-x[x x x x]

29 a rev. 4 *a-na ki-iṣ-ri ša* GI *ta-ša-ap-pa-ak-m*[*a e-li a-bu-un-na-ti-ša*]

30 a rev. 5 *ta-ḫa-aṣ-ṣa-aṣ-ma mu-ša-ap-ši-iq-tum* ⸢*i*⸣-[*ša-al-la-am*$^{?}$]

---

31 a rev. 6 *ni-iš-šu-la-at* *t*[*a-ma-a-tim* (. . .)]

32 a rev. 7 *bi-ni-it e-de-e-em bi-ni-it e-s*[*u-ur-ra-ak-ki-im*]

33 a rev. 8 *li-i*[*š-ša-l*]*i-la-am ki-ma* MUŠ *ka-r*[*a-ni-im*$^{?}$]

34 a rev. 9 *li-l*[*i-id*$^{?}$ x x x x] x *a-na* MUNUS *ša* x[x x x x]

35 a rev. 10 ka [. . . . .] x *mu-*⸢*ša*⸣*-a*[*p-ši-iq-tum*$^{?}$ . . .]

36 a rev. 11 x [. . . . .] *ù* x [. . . . .]

37 a rev. 12 [. . . . .] x [. . . . .]x

Five lines lost

38' a rev. 18 [. . . . .] x

39' a rev. 19 [. . . . .]x x-*im*

Colophon:

40'	a rev. 20	[iti . . . . . .] ⸢u$_4$⸣ 15.kam
41'	a u. e. 1	⸢mu⸣ a[m-mi]-di-ta-na <<DI>>
42'	a u. e. 2	bàd-am-mi-di-ta-na^{ki}
43'	a u. e. 3	gú ⸢íd⸣-me-en-líl-lá-ke$_4$ bí-in-dù-a

Bound Transcription and Translation

1 [munus du-da]-an-ni mi-ki a mi-ni$^{!}$(IR)-ri	1 “[The woman giv]ing [birth] steers the boat (through) the water,
2 [kù ^{d}inann]a-ke$_4$ du-da-an-ni mi-ki a mi-ni-ri	2 [holy Inan]na giving birth steers the boat (through) the water.
3 [munus d]u-da-an-ni mi-ki a mi-ni-ri	3 [The woman] giving birth steers the boat (through) the water,
4 [^{d}nin-hur]-saĝ-ĝá-ke$_4$ du-da-an-ni mi-ki a mi-ni-ri	4 [Ninḫur]saĝa giving birth steers the boat (through) the water.
5 [m]á-gur$_8$ <gu>-ki gu-ki a-mi-íb-si	5 On a barge (carrying) carnelian(?) she has loaded carnelian.
6 [m]á še-em-ma-ak-ke$_4$ še-em-ma a-am-mi-íb-si	6 On a boat (carrying) aromatics she has loaded aromatics.
7 [m]á ^{ĝiš}eren-na-ke$_4$ ^{ĝiš}eren-na a-am-mi-íb-si	7 On a boat (carrying) cedar (wood) she has loaded cedar.
8 [má] ^{na4}za-gìn-na za-gìn-na a-am-mi-íb-si	8 On a boat (carrying) lapis lazuli she has loaded lapis lazuli.
9 [(x) ^{n}]$^{a4?}$ku$^{?}$-ug nu-uz-zu za-gi-in nu-uz-zu	9 (Yet) she does not know (whether it is) carnelian, (yet) does not know (whether it is) lapis lazuli.
10 [x x x x]x-dab-ba ag-ga-ab ú-ra gi-ba-a im-me-gi-bi	10 [. . .] . . . its (i.e. the baby's) skull(?) being stuck, lying crosswise in the *loins, it causes her to have difficulty* (delivering the baby).
11 [^{d}asal-lú-ḫi] igi-ni im-ma-an-zi a-a-ni ^{d}en-ki-ra	11 [Asalluḫi] saw her (there). To Enki, his father,
12 [x x x x x] é ba-ši-in-ku$_4$ gù mu-un-na-de-e	12 [. . .] he entered the house, telling him (the matter).
13 [^{d}en-ki$^{?}$ (. . .) ^{d}]asal-lú-ḫi mu-un-na-ni-íb-gi$_4$-gi$_4$	13 [Enki (. . .)] answered his son Asalluḫi:
14 [dumu-ĝu$_{10}$ a-na-àm] nu-me-e-zu a-na-àm a-ra-ab-daḫ-ḫe-e	14 ‘[My son, what is there that] you do not know? What further can I add for you?
15 [^{d}asal-lú-hi a]-na-àm nu-me-e-zu a-na-àm a-ra-ab-daḫ-ḫe-e	15 [Asalluḫi, what is there] that you do not know? What further can I add for you?
16 [níĝ ì-zu-a]-ĝu$_{10}$ ù ze-e in-ga-ra-e-zu	16 [What] I [know], you also know,
17 [x x ĝen-n]a$^{?}$ ^{d}asal-lú-ḫi	17 [. . . co]me, (my son) Asalluḫi,
18 [x x x x]x-bí-zu in-nu-zu	18 [. . . .] . . .,
19 x x [x x g]i sú-gu ba-an-du ap-pa-ar gi du-g[a]	19 [. . . *take*] a little reed from the marsh, the marsh of the sweet reed,
20 ì ⸢nu-ub-da-a⸣ ì-nun nu-ub-da-a [x x]	20 . . . oil, . . . ghee [. . .],
21 gal$_4$-la si-pa-ad-da ri-a si-in$^{!?}$-da-x [x x]	21 *poured* on the vulva of the hoopoe-bird(?), . . .[. . .]!
22 tu-ku-u[b]-[b]i ni-in-ta tu-ku-⸢ub⸣-b[i . . . . . .]	22 If (the baby) is male, if [. . . . . .].
23 tu-ku-[ub]-[b]i mu-nu-ús x[. . . . . .]	23 If (the baby) is female, [. . . . . .].
24 tu-ku-ub-bi saĝ-lú-ti-la igi l[ú$^{?}$-. . . . . .]	24 If it is a *stillborn child*(?), [. . .] the face of a human being(?) –
25 [mu-u]š$^{?}$-gin$_7$ ḫu-us-ḫu-us-ta ù-me-e-⸢ta$^{?}$⸣-⸢dirig$^{?}$⸣	25 when (the baby) has slid from (between) the *thighs* like a [sn]ake(?),
26 [x]-eš-ta lú pa-na-gin$_7$ si-sá-⸢e⸣-[dè]	26 [. . .] . . . the human being *shall* be straight(?) like a bow (string?)!”
27 [t]u$_6^{!}$([K]A) én-[é-nu-ru]	27 *Formula* of an [Enuru]-incantation.

28 *šipat mušapšiqtim šamnam*. . .[. . . . . .]
29 *ana kiṣri ša qanîm tašappak-m[a eli abunnatīša]*
30 *taḫaṣṣaṣ-ma mušapšiqtum i[šallam]*

28 Incantation for a woman who has difficulty during delivery. 29 You pour 28 . . . oil [. . . . . .] 29 into a reed node. Then 30 you break it 29 [above her navel] 30 and the woman who has difficulty in delivery will [be alright].

---

31 *niššulāt t[âmātim* (. . .)]
32 *binīt edêm binīt es[urrakkim]*
33 *li[ššal]ilam kīma ṣerri kar[ānim]*
34 *līl[id(?)* . . . . . .] *ana sinništim ša* . . .[. . .]

35 . . . [. . . . . .] *muš[apšiqtum*(?) . . .]
36–37 *only traces preserved*
Five lines lost
38'–39' *only traces preserved*

31 "Fish roe of the [(. . .)] s[ea],
32 creature of the flood, creature of sub[terranean waters]!
33 May it glide out like a vi[ne] snake!
34 May she give [birth(?), *may it* . . .] for the woman who . . .[. . .],

35 . . .[. . . . . .], the [woman] having [difficulty in delivery(?) . . .]
36–37 *too fragmentary for translation*
Five lines lost
38'–39' *only traces preserved*

Colophon:

40' [iti . . .] ⸢u$_4$⸣ 15.kam 41' ⸢mu⸣ a[m]-m[i]-di-ta-na <<KI>> 42' bàd-am-mi-di-ta-na^{ki} 43' gú ⸢íd⸣-me-en-líl-lá-ke$_4$ bí-in-dù-a

40' (Written on) the fifteenth day of [month . . .] 41' (in) the year (in which) Ammiditana 43' built 42' Dūr-Ammiditana 43' on the banks of the Me-Enlil-canal.

Notes

Lines 1–4: The phrase du-da-an-ni stands for (ù)-tu-da-ni, as parallels from similar Old Babylonian birth incantations confirm:

AUAM 73.3094: 2–10 (Cohen 1976, *RA* 70, 135–139; Wasserman and Zomer 2022, No. 10):
[munus du-d]a-a-ni ma-gi$_4$ a mi-ni-ri: [. . .] *ina a-ta-al-lu-ki-ša ki-ma e-le-pí i-te-i-il*
"The woman giving birth steers the boat through the water (Sum.); [the woman], in walking about, was *wobbling like a boat* (Akk.)."

E 47.190: 1–3 (G. Farber 1984, *JNES* 43, 313ff.):
munus du-da-an-ni má-ak-ki am-ni-ir-r[i] / kù ^{d}inanna-ki má-ak-ki am-ni-ir-r[i] / ^{d}nin-ḫur-saĝ-a-ak-ki má-ak-ki am-i-ni-ir-ri
"The woman giving birth steers the boat through the water. Pure Inanna giving birth steers the boat through the water. Ninḫursaĝa giving birth steers the boat through the water."

YOS 11, No. 85 obv. 4'–5' (van Dijk 1975, 66; reconstructed from obv. 13'–15'):
4' [x x **munus ù-tud]-⸢a⸣-[ni** ^{giš}má-gi a bí-ir-ri] 5' an-[úr-ra? munus ù-tu]d-a-ni ^{giš}⸢má-gi⸣ ⸢a⸣ [bí-ir-ri]
4' "[. . . The woman giving] birth [*steers* the boat through the water]. 5' [(From) the hor]izon [the woman giving] birth [*steers*] the boat through the water."

Notably, the Akkadian translation of AUAM 73.3094 interpreted the verb form du-da-a-ni as *atalluku* (Gtn-stem of *alāku*) "to walk about".

The phrase mi-ki a mi-ni-ri can be compared with similar spellings, showing that má "boat" has become mi in BM 97093. The element -ki in mi-ki interchanges with (-ak)-ki (má-ak-ki) and -gi/gi$_4$ in the parallel texts. Van Dijk (1975, *OrNS* 44, 67 n. 41) understands ^{giš}má-gi$_{(4)}$ as "bateau destiné à transporter du roseau"; G. Farber (1984, *JNES* 43, 314) translates the corresponding má-ak-ki in E 47.190 as "Gi-boat". The Akkadian translation in AUAM 73.3094, however, apparently understood the element -gi$_{(4)}$ as equative, rendered as *kīma* in the Akkadian interlinear translation (Cohen 1976, *RA* 70, 140 note on lines 2–9).

The incantation E 47.190: 1–3 is parallel to BM 97093: 1–4, equating the woman in labour with the goddesses Inanna and Ninḫursaĝa. BM 97093: 2 and 4 confirms that in the spellings ^{d}inanna-ki and ^{d}nin-ḫur-sag-a-ak-ki in E.47190: 2–3 –ki stands for –ke$_4$.

As BM 97093 and AUAM 73.3094 show, am-ni-ir-ri and am-i-ni-ir-ri stand for a mi-ni-ri (see also G. Farber 1984, 315 note on lines 1–3; Cohen 1976, 140). The phrase má—ri means "to direct, steer a boat" (Attinger 2021, *Glossaire*, 851). In text II.1.1 and the similar incantations reviewed here (see also text D.1.1 lines 1ff.), the boat is the pregnant woman's body; her "steering" of the boat signifies her agency in the process of labour (see Steinert 2017, 323–324).

Line 5: The sequence má-gur$_8$-ki could theoretically be interpreted as a deficient spelling of má-gur$_8$-gin$_7$ "like a barge".[229] However, the following word gu-ki is assumed to stand for gug "carnelian" (with directive case marker -e), because of the parallel $^{[n]a4?}$ku$^?$-ug "carnelian" in line 9. Since the following lines 6–8 are formulated in a parallel manner, má-gur$_8$-ki in line 5 should probably be emended to má-gur$_8$ <gu>-ki "on a barge of carnelian". The verbal form is parallel to lines 6–8 (a-<am>-mi-íb-si). For si "to fill, to become full" with directive case, see Attinger 2021, *Glossaire*, 897.

Lines 5–8: These lines equate the baby in the uterus with the precious cargo loaded onto a ship: in this incantation, these items are carnelian, lapis lazuli, aromatics and cedar. Variations of this passage are found in the following Old Babylonian incantations: YOS 11, No. 85 obv. 6'–7', l. e. (van Dijk 1975, 66); E 47.190: 4–6 (G. Farber 1984, 313ff.); AUAM 73.3094 obv. 18–19 (Cohen 1976, *RA* 70, 136; Wasserman and Zomer 2022, No. 10); UM 29-15-367: 14 (van Dijk 1975, 53ff.); VS 17, No. 33: 13 (van Dijk 1975, 62–63).

Carnelian and lapis lazuli (red stone and blue stone) function as objects signaling the gender of the baby, see Bergmann 2008, 43–44 for discussion. The phrases in line 9 expressing the mother's lack of knowledge whether she is expecting a girl or a boy also occur in the parallel birth incantations (e.g. YOS 11, No. 85: 9; van Dijk 1975, 66; AUAM 73.3094 obv. 20–21 (Cohen 1976, *RA* 70, 136; Wasserman and Zomer 2022, No. 10).

Line 10: The interpretation of this line is tentative. One expects here a brief description of the difficulties experienced by the woman in labour, e.g. about the baby being stuck in the birth canal. In this line of thought, the sequence ag-ga-ab may have to be read as aga-bi "its rear, back", or perhaps better as ugu-bi "its head/skull", referring to the baby (for /agu/ or /aga/ as variants of ugu "skull", cf. Attinger 2021, *Glossaire*, 1102 s.v. ugu$_6$; ePSD2 s.v. ugu). The following ú-ra gi-ba-a may be a phonetic spelling for úr-a gib-a "being blocked (lying crosswise) in the lap/loins (i.e. the birth canal)". The verb gib "to lie across; to block" is presumably also indicated in the form im-me-gi-bi in line 10. Sumerian gib corresponds to Akkadian *parāku* "to lie crosswise" (Attinger 2021, *Glossaire*, 407–408), the latter of which is also found in Akkadian birth incantations. In these passages, *parāku* usually has the foetus as its subject, not the woman in labour, e.g. BAM 248 obv. i 57 // (text D.1.1 line 43): [LÚ.TUR] *a-a ip-par-rik li-ṣa-a* "[the ch]ild shall not lie athwart, may it come out!"; Sm. 157 + 1134 obv. 7 (text D.1.6): ⌈GENNA⌉ *šá* ŠÀ-*šá la i-pár-ri-ku i*[*na*$^?$ ŠÀ.TÙR-*šá*$^?$] "(so that) the child of her womb will not get stuck (lit. lie crosswise) *i*[*n her womb*(?)]".

Lines 13–16: For the classical format of the dialogue between Enki and Asalluḫi in Sumerian incantations, its many variations and (often corrupt) orthographies in Old Babylonian incantations, see Falkenstein 1931b, 44–67; Rudik 2011, 46–63; George 2016, *CUSAS* 32, 2–4. The Enki-Asalluḫi-dialogue is found, for example, the following birth incantations: UM 29-15-367: 16–36 // (van Dijk 1975, *OrNS* 44, 55; Cunningham 1997, 70–71); VS 17, 33: 14–15 (van Dijk 1975, *OrNS* 44, 63); YOS 11, No. 85: 11–20 (van Dijk 1975, *OrNS* 44, 66); E 47.190 obv. 8–10 (G. Farber 1984, 314); AUAM 73.3094: 24–41 (Cohen 1976, *RA* 70, 136–138; Wasserman and Zomer 2022, No. 10); JRL Box 24 E6+24: 5'–9' (Wilcke 1973, *AfO* 24, 13–14).

Lines 19–21: In line 19, ap-pa-ar stands for ambar "marsh" (Akk. *appāru*). The "small reed from the marsh" is also encountered with a similar ritual procedure to promote labour in other birth incantations. In better understandable parallels of contemporary spells, a fatty substance is filled into the reed, which is then broken above the woman's navel or umbilical area. In BM 97093, the marsh is called the "marsh of the sweet reed" (gi du-ga for gi du$_{10}$-ga) (see also BAM 248 quoted below); in other instances, it is called the "marsh of Eridu" (alluding to the god Enki):

> AUAM 73.3094 rev. 42–53 (Cohen 1976, *RA* 70, 135–139; Wasserman and Zomer 2022, No. 10):
> gi sú-ug bàn-da eri$_4$-du$_{10}$-ga šu [ù-me-ti] / *qá-na-a ša sú-ug-bàn-da ša eri$_4$-du$_{10}$-ga i-na* [*le-qí-i*]
> ia-ab kù-ga ga-ra ab-ši-il-la-ma šà-ba [ù-me-ni-dub] / *ša-ma-an li-it-tim el-le-tim li-iš-da-am* [*ina libbi*$^?$] *šu-pu-uk*
> saḫar sila-⌈lam$_4$⌉-bi   *e-pé-er su-qí er-bé-e*[*t*]
> ...

229 Notably, the element -ki-im in the parallel sentence in E 47.190 obv. 4–5 (i.e. in má ši-im-má-ki-im and má i-ri-na-ki-im is interpreted as the equative case marker -gin$_7$ (G. Farber 1984, 314–315 "*as* on a boat carrying perfume/cedar wood"). The Akkadian translation in the parallel passage in AUAM 73.3094: 12–19 likewise rendered the corresponding phrases ma-še-ma-ta and ma-e-re-na-ta as *kīma eleppi* "like a boat" (Cohen 1976, *RA* 70, 136, 140; Wasserman and Zomer 2022, No. 10).

[. . .] x ḫé-en-[x]-ge$_4$ / [*e-li a-bu-un-na-ti*]-*ša ḫe-pé-e-ma*
"When [taking] a (Sum.) little reed from the marsh (Akk. a reed from the little marsh) of Eridu,
pour into it the milk fat of a pure cow and the cream of a mother cow,
(mix with) dust from a crossroads,
. . .
break it [above her navel]!"[230]

A similar procedure is described in the Neo-Assyrian Birth Compendium BAM 248 obv. i 52–53 // (text D.1.1 lines 38–39). For a Neo-Babylonian fragment from Nippur (N. 1568) with a bilingual incantation passage that corresponds to the procedure in BAM 248 obv. i 52–53 // and may represent part of the poorly preserved incantation in BAM 248 obv. i 1–35 //, see Jiménez 2019, *NABU* 2019/3, 140–141 No. 77; *infra* text D.1.1 (ms. e). The commentary 11N-T3: 9–12 (text G.1) quotes a corresponding passage in the Neo-Assyrian Birth Compendium (not preserved in BAM 248 //) that refers to breaking a reed filled with oil above the woman's belly. The ritual actions alluded to in lines 19–21 of BM 97093 and in the quoted textual parallels can also be gleaned from the Akkadian ritual instruction in lines 29–30 (see below).

Other birth incantations from Ur III and Old Babylonian times present variations of the procedure, making use of fat, cream (or similar fatty substances)[231] as *materia medica* which are applied to the woman's body to promote labour (see UM 29-15-367: 37–41 // (van Dijk 1975, *OrNS* 44, 56–57, 60–61; Cunningham 1997, 70)[232]; JRL Box 24 E6+24: 10'–13' (Wilcke 1973, *AfO* 24, 13–14).

The form nu-ub-da-a in line 20 is difficult (the prefix nu- suggests a negated form), but from the context da-a may stand for dé-a "to pour out" (Attinger 2021, *Glossaire*, 240–241).

Line 21: Interpretation of this line is again difficult. The interpretation of si-pa-ad-da as "hoopoe-bird" (sipad) is not entirely certain (one would expect the classifier mušen to follow). The whole expression gal$_4$-la si-pa-ad-da ri-a "poured over the vulva of a sipad-(bird)" is somewhat unexpected. Alternatively, si-pa-ad-da may stand for zi-pà-da "(of) the truly chosen one(?)".

Lines 22–24: Similar passages referring to the sex of the newborn are found in other birth incantations. Usually, these passages refer to symbolic actions relating to gender-specific objects or attributes that express the determination of the baby's gender (especially a spindle/dress pin for girls and weapons for boys, see SF 54 vii 1–4 // TSŠ 170 v 7–vi 4 (Krebernik 1984, no. 6A–B; Rudik 2011, 321–326 (FSB 57)); AUAM 73.1425 iv 6–12 (Sigrist 1980, 157–158; Rudik 2011, 327–332 (FB 58)); UM 29-15-367: 46–47 // (van Dijk 1975, 57, 61; Cunningham 1997, 70–71); YOS 11, No. 85: 27'-28' (van Dijk 1975, 67); AUAM 73.3094 rev. 54–57 (Cohen 1976, *RA* 70, 138; Wasserman and Zomer 2022, No. 10 For discussion, see also *infra* text D.1.1 (note on line 12) and text G.1 (line 14).

Line 24: A comparable passage referring to the possibility of a stillborn child (following a healthy boy or girl) is encountered in the Old Assyrian birth incantation Kt 90/k 178 (Michel 2004; Wasserman and Zomer 2022, No. 9: 17–18): *šu-ma* : *sà-ak-pu-um* : *sà-ki-ip* / *i-li-šu* : *li-šé-lá-ma* "if it is a stillbirth (*sakpum*, from *sakāpu* "to lie down/still"(?)) – rejected by his god – may they (the Daughters of the Womb) let it come up". The sequence saĝ-lú-ti-la in BM 97093 may be an aberrant or erroneous spelling for the Sumerian term saĝ-iti-nu-til-la, which corresponds to Akkadian *kūbu* "premature birth, stillborn child", see CAD K, 487 lex. section. The following igi l[ú . . .] is perhaps to be read as "[who has] the face of a human being(?)". The sign traces do not support the restoration igi ^{d}[utu . . .] "[who has never seen] the [sun]light" (cf. SpTU 3, No. 67 rev. iii 1–2, 9–12).

Line 25: The form ḫu-us-ḫu-us is interpreted as reduplicated ḫáš/ḫaš$_4$ "thigh", signaling a plural, i.e. "(from) the (two) thighs", cf. Attinger 2021, *Glossaire*, 522 (a non-standard spelling ḫu(s) is attested in an Old Babylonian Sumerian proverb, SP 28.27). For the verb diri(g) "to drift (said of clouds), to float, glide along/down", see ePSD2; Attinger 2021, 258–259. It is

230 See also YOS 11, No. 85: 22'–24' (van Dijk 1975, 67–68 with n. 39).

231 For these products, see further Stol 1993–1997b, "Milch(produkte). A. In Mesopotamien," *RlA* 8, esp. §§ 2, 7–8.

232 The parallel VS 17, 33: 16–18 (van Dijk 1975, 63–64) reads: [ì] áb-kù-ga ^{ra}gára-áb-⸢šilam⸣-ma ù-me-ni-dib / [dag-ag]run-na-ka im-mi-gub-ba šu um-me-te^{ti} / [nam-šu]b-eridu^{ki}-ga murgu$^{mu-ur-gu}$ sa-sa-al ti-ti munus$^{mu-nu-ús}$-bi ù-me-ni-dib . . . "When you have taken the fat of a pure cow (and) the cream of a mother-cow, when you have taken what has been placed in(?) the (sleeping) chamber of the agrun, when you have *applied* (it with) the incantation of Eridu to the back, the thighs and flanks of that woman . . .".

equated with Akkadian *alāku* "to go" and *neqelpû* "to go downstream"; the verb is presumably used here in reminiscence of the boat theme in the first lines of the incantation.

Line 26: Interpretation of this line is difficult. For $^{(\text{ĝiš})}$pana (PAN) "bow", spelled pa-na, see Attinger 2021, *Glossaire*, 835 n. 2538. The simile in this line is perhaps to be understood as "to be straight (si-sá) like a bow (string)". The verb si-sá "to be/make straight" corresponds to Akkadian *ešēru*, which has the meaning "to deliver easily" or "to come out quickly, be born easily" in Akkadian birth incantations. Could the line possibly refer to a preferred vertical (head-down) posture of the foetus in the birth canal that allows an easy birth?

Line 27: One expects the rubric tu_6 én-é-nu-ru "formula of an Enuru-incantation" here, but the traces of the first sign look more like [K]A than KAxLI. Perhaps this is a simple mistake for tu_6.

Lines 28–30: The Akkadian rubric *šipat mušapšiqtim* "incantation for a woman who has difficulty in (her) delivery" is attested in another Old Babylonian tablet with a version of the spell munus ù-tu-da-a-ni, in E 47.190 rev. 6' (G. Farber 1984, 314): MU-Ú (presumably standing for mu_7 = *šiptum* "incantation") *mu-ša-ap-ši-iq-tum*. The more usual rubric following birth incantations in Old Babylonian texts is ka-inim-ma munus ù-tu-(da-kam) "incantation for a woman in labour" (see Wasserman and Zomer 2022, Nos. 6, 8, 10, 12–14, corresponding to ka-inim-ma *[ālit]tum* in No. 7). In later texts, the rubric *šipat mušapšiqtim* is replaced by logographic KA.INIM.MA ^{munus}LA.RA.AḪ.KAM/KÁM (see text D.1.1 line 37 for discussion). For attestations and discussion, see the Middle Assyrian birth incantation *Iraq* 31, 31: 33–50 having the rubric *šiptu ša multapšiqte*, as well as KUB 4, 13: 13': KA.INIM.MA ÉN *mušapš[iqti]* (see text D.1.1 line 161 ms. b).

The reconstruction of the prescription follows the parallel incantation passage in AUAM 73.3094: 42–53 (Cohen 1976, *RA* 70, 138; Wasserman and Zomer 2022, No. 10) and in BAM 248 obv. i 52–53 (text D.1.1 lines 38–39). See also Steinert 2017a, 336–339 for discussion.

Another Old Babylonian text (VS 17, 33: 28–30; van Dijk 1975, 63–64) appends an Akkadian instruction to the text of a related Sumerian birth incantation. That prescription focuses on anointing the woman's body with oil and ghee (Scurlock 1991, 144–145; Stol 2000a, 63, 124): *ki-ki-ta-ša* Ì.GIŠ *ù* Ì.NUN / *tu-ba-al-la-al-ma i-na* ⸢KUŠ/SU⸣ *bu-di-im ba-am-ti-ša* / *ki-la-ti-in ta-pa-aš-ša-aš-ma it-ta-aṣ-ṣa-a* "The procedure for it: you mix oil and ghee and apply it to the skin/flesh of the shoulder(s) (and) both her flanks, and it (the baby) will come out." In BM 97093 as well as VS 17, 33, the appended prescription draws directly on the instruction within the incantation given by Enki to his son Asalluḫi in their dialogue. An even more concise variation of the prescription follows another version of the spell munus ù-tu-da-a-ni in E 47.190 (G. Farber 1984, 314 rev. 7', lower edge and left edge): *ki-ik-ki-ṭi-um* ^{giš}GI *ù* Ì.NUN / *sa-am-tum ù uq-ni-um* / [. . . m]u$^?$ mu *i-na-ad-di-*⸢*ki*$^?$*-im*⸣ "The procedure: reed and ghee, carnelian and lapis lazuli. [. . .] . . . he/she will pour out/cast for you(?) (fem.)."[233]

For the verb *ḫaṣāṣu* "to cut; to break (reeds)" in BM 97093 line 30, see also George 1992, 276; CAD Ḫ, 130–131; CAD G, 153a (additions to CAD Ḫ). For the ritual procedure of breaking a reed filled with an oily substance above the belly of the woman giving birth, see note on lines 19–21 above.

Line 31: For *nimšulu* (*niššulu*), pl. *niššulātu* "(fish) roe/spawn(?)", see CAD N/2, 235; AHw 790, 796. The word was previously only attested in lexical lists, where it is equated with *binītu* or *binâti* referring to fish eggs/spawn (cf. Landsberger 1962, MSL 8/2, 105).

Line 32: For *edû* "high water, flood" (from Sumerian a-dé-a "flooding"), see CAD E, 35–36; AHw 187b. The form *esurrakku* is a variant of *asurrakku* "depths; subterranean waters", see CAD A/2, 349–350; AHw 77a (a loan from Sumerian a-su(r)-ra "water from the depths"). For the use of the synonymous term *anzanunzû* in another Old Babylonian birth incantations, see text II.1.2 below (BM 115745 rev. 7).

Line 33: The prompt to the baby to glide out of the womb like a snake is a common passus in birth incantations (see also BAM 248 and dupl. (D.1.1 lines 35, 46, 171, 194)). The "wine/grapevine snake" (*ṣerri karānim*) is also mentioned, in a compa-

233 Note also the brief note KÍD.KÍD.BI Ì.GIŠ "the procedure for it: oil" in CUSAS 32, No. 29b: 30, following an Akkadian birth incantation (George 2016, pl. LXXVIII–LXXIX; Wasserman and Zomer 2022, 77) and the prescription following an Elamite incantation for a woman in labour (CUSAS 32, No. 21b: 28'–29'; George 2016, 142–143): "You cast (the spell) on oil and massage her(!) belly (with it) seven times straight down, and massage her(!) shoulders seven times straight down" (*ana* Ì.GIŠ *ta-na-ad-di-ma 7-šu mi-š[a-r]a-am pa-ap-pa-al-li-ib-bi-šu ta-pa-aš-ša-aš* / *7-šu mi-š[a-r]a-am bu-di-šu ta-pa-aš-ša-aš*).

rable context, in the Old Assyrian birth incantations Kt 90/k 178: 18–20 (Michel 2004; Wasserman and Zomer 2022, No. 9): *k[i]-i* / *ṣa-ru-ú* : *ki-ra-nim* : *li-i[m-q]ú-tám* / *qá-qá-ar-šu* "may (the baby) fall down to the ground like a vine snake". See also Kt 94/k 429: 21–22, Barjamovic 2015, 58, 75–77; Wasserman and Zomer 2022, No. 11.

Lines 40'–43': For the year formula, see https://cdli-gh.github.io/year-names/HTML/T12K9.htm (after MCS 2, 51).

II.1.2 BM 115745: An Old Babylonian Tablet with an Incantation for Easy Delivery

BM 115745 was purchased by the British Museum from the Paris dealer Élias Géjou in 1923. It was kindly brought to my attention by J. Taylor and I. L. Finkel. The large signs as well as the numerous mistakes and erasures point to a scribal exercise. The middle section of the reverse shows signs of re-use: one can observe sign multiple traces suggesting that the scribed had erased several lines of text and written over them.[234] Indicative of a school context is also the table with numbers arranged in four fields on the tablet's obverse, most likely presenting an arithmetical exercise. Remarkably, the obverse of the tablet is oriented at a 90° angle to the reverse. According to Christine Proust (personal communication), the layout of the table evokes an intermediate-level mathematical exercise of the Old Babylonian period, resembling exercises found at Nippur and Ur. Similar arithmetical exercises arranged in a table layout containing multiplications or squaring exercises with numbers have been published, e.g. by Friberg 2007, 13–15, 18–19, 466 (MS 2729, MS 2728, MS 3944, MS 2831).

There are other examples of Old and Middle Babylonian school tablets containing two different text types on the obverse and reverse, e.g. an incantation combined with a different kind of text (e.g. an extract from a lexical list).[235] Veldhuis (2000, *JCS* 52, 67) and Bartelmus (2018, 66–77) further report about a comparable format in Kassite period exercise tablets that are pillow-shaped and whose obverse and reverse are inscribed in different directions (i.e. one side is inscribed in a landscape orientation parallel to the longer side of the tablet (usually with a literary passage); the other side is inscribed in portrait orientation, usually with a lexical text). These features partially resemble BM 115745. Bartelmus (2018, 70 nn. 23–24) mentions that a few late Old Babylonian pillow-shaped school tablets with the same layout features have recently come to light which stem from sites in northern Babylonia (Sippar, Babylon). BM 115745 may thus come from the same background in terms of provenience and date.

The reverse of BM 115745 is inscribed with a version of the birth incantation *ina mê nâkim ibbani eṣemtum* "In the fluid of intercourse the bone was created", known in slightly different versions from three other Old Babylonian sources (YOS 11, No. 86, CUSAS 32, No. 26a and CUSAS 32, No. 28a; see Wasserman and Zomer 2022, Nos. 6, 7, 14; Veldhuis 1999, 39–41).

The parallel sources YOS 11, No. 86 and CUSAS 32, No. 26a identify the spell with the rubric ka-inim-ma munus ù-tu-da-kam "incantation for a woman in labour", while in BM 115745, the incantation is followed by the rubric *šipat aruḫtim* "incantation for a 'hastened' woman" (i.e. a woman in labour). The word *aruḫtum* is also known from the rubric ka-inim-ma *a-ru-úḫ-tum* in VS 17, 33: 28 (van Dijk 1975, *OrNS* 44, 63, 65), where the latter is appended to a Sumerian birth incantation. Therefore, the fragmentary rubric in CUSAS 32, No. 28a may be restored either as ka-inim-ma *[a-lit]-tum* "incantation for a woman giving birth" or ka-inim-ma *[a-ru-uḫ]-tum* "incantation for a 'hastened' woman".

The birth incantation must have been transmitted to the first millennium BCE, although no sources for this composition have been preserved or identified from that period. However, the so-called Assur Medical Catalogue quotes the incipit of the incantation as title of a chapter tablet of a medical treatise concerned with childbirth and women's diseases (Steinert et al. 2018, 218, 273–274, line 116 BIRTH).

234 As already observed by the Online Database of the British Museum (https://www.britishmuseum.org/collection/object/W_1923-0113-26).

235 E.g. OECT 5, 55, an OB lenticular tablet with four lines of an Lamaštu incantation on one side and traces of numerals on the other (CDLI P345836; Michalowski 1978, *JNES* 37, 345). *Emar* 737 contains a section of the lexical list ur$_5$-ra = *ḫubullu* and an incantation against gastrointestinal disease, separated by a colophon (Arnaud 1985, *Emar* 6/1, 105–109; Arnaud 1987, *Emar* 6/4, No. 737; Rutz 2013, 179–180; Zomer 2018, 12).

236 Measurements: ca. 5.0 x 7.6 x 2.0 cm.

List of Manuscripts

Siglum	Museum Number	Copy	Collation	Format; Ductus	Provenience
a	BM 115745 (= 1923-1-13, 26)	Pl. 6	Coll.	Single-column tablet; Old Babylonian period (ca. 18th/17th cent. BCE)[236]	Unknown

Previous Edition and Discussion

SEAL No. 7054 (transliteration; translation of the reverse)
Wasserman and Zomer 2022, 68–70 No. 4 (edition of the reverse)

Transliteration

Obv.

Numbers arranged in a table:

[x$^{?}$] ⸢2⸣5$^{?}$ 30 ⸢25$^{?}$⸣	⸢8$^{?}$⸣
⸢25⸣ ⸢1⸣ 23 20	⸢x⸣

Remainder of the obv. uninscribed

1 a rev. 1 [*ina m*]*e-e na-ki*$^{!}$(DI)-*im*

2 a rev. 2 ⸢*ib*⸣-*ba-ni e-ṣe-em-tum*

3 a rev. 3 *ši-ru-ú še*$_{20}$-*er-ḫa*-⸢*nu*⸣-*ú*

4 a rev. 4 *ib-nu li-li-da-am*

5 a rev. 5 *i-na me-e a-a-ba ša-am*-⸢*ru*⸣-*tim*

6 a rev. 6 *ša-ru-uḫ-tim*

7 a rev. 7 *i-na me-e* **an**-*za*-⸢*nu*⸣-*zi ru-qú-tim*

8 a rev. 8 *a-ša-ar še*$_{20}$-⸢*er-ru*⸣-*um*

9 a rev. 9 *ku-us-sà i-da-šu*

10 a rev. 10 *ka-at-ma i-na-šu la i-da-ga-la* ⸢*ḫa*$^{!}$-*ra*⸣-*na-am*

11 a rev. 11 *i-mu-ur-šu*-**ma** *é-a* ^{d}*a-sa-lu-ḫa*

12 a rev. 12 *ip-te-šu pa-da-na*-<*am*> *uš-ta-sí-iq-šu ṭù-dam*

13 a rev. 13 *a-na mi-ša-ri-im* ^{d}UTU *li-iš-ku*-<*un*>-*ka*

14 a rev. 14 tu en-ni-in-nu-ra

15 a l. e. 1 *ši-pa-at a-ru-uḫ-tim*

Bound Transcription and Translation (of the Reverse)

1 *[ina mê] nâkim* 2 *ibbani eṣemtum*	1[From the flu]ids of intercourse 2 the bone was created.
3 *šīrū šer'ānū* 4 *ibnû lillidam*	3 Flesh (and) *muscles* 4 have created the child.
5 *ina mê ayabba šamrūtim* 6 *šaruḫtim*	5–6 In the fierce, magnificent waters of the ocean,
7 *ina mê anzanuzî rūqūtim*	7 in the distant waters of the subterranean ocean,
8 *ašar šerrum* 9 *kussā idāšu*	8–9 where the baby's arms are bound,
10 *katmā īnāšu lā idaggalā ḫarrānam*	10 his eyes are covered, not seeing the road –
11 *īmuršu-ma Ea Asalluḫi*	11 Ea saw him (there). Then Asalluḫi
12 *iptēšu padānam uštassiqšu ṭūdam*	12 opened the path for him, prepared the way for him (saying):
13 *ana mīšarim Šamaš liškunka*	13 'May Šamaš set you to freedom!'"
14 tu-en-ni-in-nu-ra	14 Formula of an Enuru-incantation.
15 *šipat aruḫtim*	15 An incantation for a woman *in labour* (lit. the hastened one).

Notes

Obverse

I owe valuable suggestions for reading the numerals to Christine Proust (personal communication), who observes: "If it is a school exercise, we can expect to find regular numbers, and to observe that the different numbers are produced by multiplying or dividing some of the others." However, the connection between the numbers in the present table based on multiplication or division is not entirely transparent, except that 8 x 25 x 25 = 1.23.20 (5,000) (information courtesy of C. Proust).

Reverse

Line 1: The spelling *na*-DI-*im* is apparently a mistake for *nâkim* "intercourse". Other errors made by the scribe are found in lines 11 and 15 (see the notes below).

Lines 3–4: In contrast to BM 115745, the processes of foetus formation are described in a passive fashion in a similar passage in YOS 11, No. 86: 3–4: *i-na ši-i-ir* [*še*$_{20}$]*-er-ḫa-nim* / *ib-ba-ni* [*l*]*i-il-li-du-um* "from the *substance* of the *blood vessels/ muscles* the baby *was* created". In BM 115745, *šīru* "flesh" and *šer'ānu* "muscle, sinew, blood vessel" (here used in the plural) are the active agents in creating the baby. The meaning of *šer'ānu* is ambiguous here. Usually the term is translated with "sinews" or "muscles", but "blood vessels" may be a better rendering, given the idea found in other ancient traditions that the foetus is nourished by its mother's menstrual blood.

Line 6: The form *šaruḫtim* is a mistake for the correct masculine plural form *šarḫūtim* "splendid, magnificent" (CAD Š/2, 61ff.). However, the form may be used consciously as a word play on *ša aruḫtim* "of the woman in delivery" (cf. the incantation rubric *šipat aruḫtim* in line 15).

Line 7: The word *anzanu(n)zû* "subterranean water; deep water" is rather rare and poetic and has not been attested in Old Babylonian texts before, only in texts from later periods, see CAD A/2, 152–153. The parallel sources use more common terms (YOS 11, No. 86: 7 (Wasserman and Zomer 2022, No. 14): *ina mê tiāmtim rūqūtim*; CUSAS 32, 28a: 2 (Wasserman and Zomer 2022, No. 7): *ina* ⸢*mê apsîm*⸣ *rūqūt*[*im*]).

Line 8: Wasserman and Zomer (2022, 69) note the pun between *šīrum* "flesh" and *šerrum* "baby" in BM 115745, whereas YOS 11, No. 86: 8 uses *ṣehrum* "little one" instead.

Line 10: Wasserman and Zomer (2022, 68) propose emending the text to *lā idaggalā* ⸢*nu*$^{?!}$-*ra*⸣-<<am>>-*am* "they (the baby's eyes) are unable to see the light" instead of ⸢*ḫa*$^{!}$-*ra*⸣-*na-am* "the road", because the *nūram dagālum* "to see the light" seems to them the more pertinent image and expression in the this context. However, the two last signs NA and AM are quite clearly visible, although written so closely together that they overlap slightly. A similar image of the baby not finding the way out of the womb is also used in the parallel incantation CUSAS 32, 28a: 7: *mu-ṣa-a-am i-še*$_{20}$-⸢*e*⸣-[*am*] "he is looking for a way out". Looking for or not seeing the way fits the resolution of the situation in line 12, where Asalluḫi "opens the path (*padānum*), makes the road (*ṭūdum*) ready" for the baby.

Line 11: In all parallel texts, Asalluḫi is the sole helping agent, e.g. CUSAS 32, 28a: 8–9: *i-mu-ur-šu-ú-ma* ^{d}*asal-lú-*[*ḫi*] / *ip-te-šum- ṭù-da-am*. In YOS 11, No. 86: 11 we find *i-mu-ur-šu-ú-ma* ^{d}*asal-lú-*[*ḫi*] *ma-ri* ^{d}*en-ki* "Asalluḫi, son of Enki, saw him (there)". In BM 115745, however, Ea and Asalluḫi (the latter name is spelled syllabically as ^{d}*a-sa-lu-ḫa*) act together in facilitating the birth process. The syntax in line 11 is somewhat unusual (using a chiastic construction); one would expect *Ea īmuršu-ma Asalluḫi iptēšum*.

Line 12: Wasserman and Zomer (2022, 68) read *pa-da-na-*⸢*am*⸣; but there does not seem enough space for *-am* before the following *uš-*. I therefore restore *pa-da-na-*<*am*>. The scribe also omitted one sign in line 13.

For the Št-stem of *nasāqu* "to select", having the meaning "to make ready, to prepare; to bring/keep in order" (*šutassuqu*), cf. CAD N/2, 22–23; AHw 753. The verb occurs in a similar passage in the OB Gilg. Yale Tablet vi 259–261 (George 2003, 204–206): *li-ip-te-kum pa-da-nam pe-ḫi-tam* / *ḫarrānam*(KASKAL) *li-iš-ta-sí-iq a-na ki-ib-sí-ka* / *ša-di-a li-iš-ta-sí-iq a-na šēpī*(GÌR)*-ka* "May he (Šamaš) open for you the paths that are shut, may he make ready the road for your footsteps! May he make ready the mountain for your feet!" The Štn-stem forms (*lu*)*-uš-ta-*(*as*)*-sí-iq* are attested in other Old Babylonian texts, see e.g. Kutscher and Wilcke 1978, *ZA* 68, 115: 49; Kienast 1978, *Kisurra*, Vol. 2, 159–160 No. 178: 30: *eq-lam lu-uš-ta-*⸢*sí*⸣*-iq* "(one shall give me the workers and then) I shall put the field in order".

Line 13: The expression *ana mīšarim Šamaš lišku*<*n*>*ka* is not found in the parallel sources of the spell. The use of the phrase *ana mīšarim šakānu* "to render/establish justice (for someone)", usually referring to the sun god's role as a divine judge, is unexpected in this context and probably motivated by the link of *mīšaru* to the verb *ešēru* ("to be straight") and its use in connection with easy delivery (especially in the Š-stem). However, the role of Šamaš as a helper during birth (releasing the baby from the dark prison of the womb and showing him the light) is well known from other birth incantations and prayers, in Old Babylonian and later texts; see, for example, CUSAS 32, 29b: 26 (Wasserman and Zomer 2022, No. 8), Polonsky 2006; *infra* text D.1.1 BAM 248 obv. ii 23; texts G.1 (11N-T3 lines 37ff.) and G.2 (UET 6/3, 897 rev. 3'–4')).

Line 15: Wasserman and Zomer (2022, 70) regard the word *aruḫtum* (the feminine form of *arḫum* "quick") as a word play on, or a conflation of, several almost homonymous terms: *arītum* "pregnant (woman)", *arḫum* "quick" and *arḫum* "cow", (*w*)*arḫum* "month" and the *Araḫtum*-canal. For discussion see also Steinert 2017b, 224–225, with Kt 90/k 178 (Michel 2004, 397, 399; Barjamovic 2015, 74; Wasserman and Zomer 2022, No. 9).

II.1.3 BAM 241 (+) VAT 9543 and BAM 242: Fragments of a Middle Babylonian Tablet from Assur on Women's Health

These two fragments must have belonged to a tablet that contained a larger collection of medical remedies for women, which are otherwise rarely attested from the Middle Babylonian period. The fragment BAM 241 from Assur with prescriptions for women was published as copy by F. Köcher in BAM III (xviii and pl. 44–45). He noted that it belonged to a two-column tablet in Middle Babylonian script, and that based on its external features, it probably belonged to tablets imported from Babylonia that were integrated into the so-called library of Tiglath-pileser I.[237]

At the Vorderasiatisches Museum, VAT 10575 (BAM 241, ms. a_1) is now kept in a box together with VAT 9543 (ms. a_2). Both fragments probably belong to one tablet, although they do not join directly. VAT 9543 appears to be written by the same hand as ms. a_1, and both fragments have firing holes. It offers a fragment of the middle portion from the right side of a large two-column tablet, preserving part of a Sumerian incantation in column ii of the obverse, and fragmentary prescriptions in column iii on the reverse. Small pieces have fallen off from the middle of the tablet's reverse (which seem to have been glued to the tablet at some point). The original position of two of these flakes on the tablet could be tentatively determined (No. 2 contains the signs SUḪUŠ / [. . .]x ḪAR).

VAT 10575 (ms. a_1) is a fragment from the bottom of the tablet, preserving some lines of col. ii and the beginning of col. iii. These contain medical prescriptions, which are continued on the reverse of ms. a_2. The remedies concern promoting

237 For this library, see Weidner 1952–1953, *AfO* 16, 197–215; Pedersén 1985, 31–42 Library M2; Zomer 2018, 39.

female fertility, the condition NI.NE and *tattīkāt ūrīša* "dribblings from her vulva", perhaps referring to uncontrolled discharge of urine (or some other discharge from the vagina). Two of the prescriptions for NI.NE-disease are duplicated in texts from the first millennium BCE: BAM 237(+) (text C.1.4), a Neo-Assyrian tablet from Assur with therapies for *naḫšātu* (bleeding during pregnancy) and other female conditions, and BM 42313+ (text A.2.2). This continuity underlines once more that first millennium BCE healing traditions concerned with women's health, like other cuneiform medical texts, go back to the second millennium BCE.

The fragmentary Sumerian spell in col. ii of ms. a_2 reflects the features of (post)-Old Babylonian Sumerian incantations using difficult-to-understand, unorthographic or phonetic spellings, showing numerous alterations from standard orthography in the use of syllabic spellings.[238] Interestingly, the composition shares a number of similarities with the beginning of the first incantation of the first millennium BCE series SAG.GIG.(GA.MEŠ) "Headache" (I/a), which was incorporated in the therapeutic series *Muššu'u* "Massage; Rubbing" and has the title saĝ-gig é-kur-ta nam-ta-è "Headache has come out from the Ekur" (Linton 1970, 45–60; Böck 2007, 24, 93–111). A little fragment of a Middle Babylonian forerunner to SAG. GIG I/a is known from Emar (*Emar* 732; Zomer 2018, 208–209, 264–265). The preserved lines of the spell in VAT 10575 (BAM 241) (+) VAT 9543 evoke images of sickness as a demonic attack, including a longer litany of disease agents. It is possible that the incantation accompanied one of the treatments for fertility on the tablet.

Another Middle Babylonian medical fragment that F. Köcher (1964, xxviii) proposed could belong to the same tablet as BAM 241 is BAM 242. The script of this small Middle Babylonian fragment looks very similar to that of BAM 241. The fragment is added as an appendix below.

List of Manuscripts

Siglum	Museum Number	Copy	Collation	Format; Ductus	Provenience
a_1 (+)	VAT 10575	BAM 241	Coll.	Fragment of a two-column tablet; Middle Babylonian script; ca. 12th/11th cent. BCE	Assur
a_2	VAT 9543	Pl. 7–8	Coll.	Fragment of a two-column tablet; Middle Babylonian script; ca. 12th/11th cent. BCE	Assur
B	VAT 8577 + 13655 + 13671 + 13706 + 13707 + 13708 + 13828 + 14177 + 14185	BAM 237	Coll.	Two-column tablet; Neo-Assyrian script; 8th/7th cent. BCE	Assur, N4 library
c	BM 42313 + 42427 + 42585 + o.N.(81-7-1,353) + 43174 + 43215 + 43274 + 43279 + 43281 + 43439 + 43483+ 43595 + 43766 + 43803	Pl. 14–15	Coll.	Single-column tablet in portrait format; Late Babylonian script; ca. 6th/5th cent. BCE	Sippar

Overview

i'	Fragmentary prescription a_1 obv. i 1'	. . .]1'–[. . .]
ii'	Fragmentary prescription a_2 obv. ii 1'–2'	. . .]2''–3''
iii'	Sumerian incantation a_2 obv. ii 3'–26'	4''–26''[. . .
iv'	Fragmentary prescription to promote female fertility a_1 obv. ii 1'–4'	. . .]27'''–30'''
v'	Fragmentary prescription against NI.NE-disease a_1 obv. ii 5'–8' // B rev. iv 9–10	31'''–34'''
vi'	Prescription against NI.NE-disease a_1 obv. ii 9'–10' // c rev. 4	35'''–36'''

238 See e.g. Cavigneaux and al-Rawi 1993, 2002; Cavigneaux 1995a, 1995b; George 2016; Viano 2014, 2016.

vii'	Prescription against NI.NE-disease a_1 obv. ii 11'	37'''
viii'	Prescription against “dribblings from the vagina” a_1 obv. ii 12'–14'	38'''–40'''
ix'	Fragmentary prescription a_1 rev. iii 1–2	41'''–42'''
x'	Prescription to promote fertility after menopause a_1 rev. iii 3–6	43'''–46'''
xi'	Prescription to promote female fertility a_1 rev. iii 7–13	47'''–53'''[. . .
xii'	Fragmentary prescription a_2 rev. iii 1'–11'	. . .]54''''–64''''
xiii'	Fragmentary prescription a_2 rev. iii 12'–16'	65''''–69''''[. . .

Previous Edition and Discussion

Kirsch 1996, *Die Behandlung von Frauenkrankheiten*, 108ff. (edition of BAM 241)
Böck 2010a, *TUAT NF* 5, 114 (translation of BAM 241 iii 3–13)
Böck 2013, 31 n. 13, 35 with n. 31 (BAM 241 iii 3'–6' and 7'–11')
Minen 2018, 180 (translation of BAM 241 iii 7'–11')
CDLI P285327 (photo of VAT 9543 and VAT 10575)
Infra text C.1.4 (edition of BAM 237), text A.2.2 (edition of BM 42313+)

Transliteration

Beginning of ms. a_1 obv. i lost

1'	a_1 obv. i 1'	[. . . . .]x KI.MIN KI.MIN

Bottom of ms. a_1 obv. i
Beginning of ms. a_2 obv. i lost

2''	a_2 obv. ii 1'	[x x x x]x x[. . . . .]
3''	a_2 obv. ii 2'	[x x x x]x-*ma* [. . . . .]
4''	a_2 obv. ii 3'	[ÉN x x kur-ta$^{?}$] nam-ta-è ⸢min$^{?}$⸣ [x] x[. . . . .]
5''	a_2 obv. ii 4'	[x x x g]ig-ga-ta min a-ri-a-[ta$^{?}$ min x x x]
6''	a_2 obv. ii 5'	[x x x x] min kur-ra gu-ĝar-ra$^{!?}$ min k[i$^{?}$ x x]
7''	a_2 obv. ii 6'	[x x x x] ḫul-gig min é bar-gin$_7$$^{?}$ ⸢min$^{?}$⸣
8''	a_2 obv. ii 7'	[x x x x]x min nam-tar gig-ga-a-ta min
9''	a_2 obv. ii 8'	[na-á]ĝ$^{?}$-tag šu-re-dè min lugal-maš-pa-è-a min
10''	a_2 obv. ii 9'	[x saĝ ĝiš ra-r]a$^{?}$-e-dè min udug ḫul-ĝál
11''	a_2 obv. ii 10'	[x x udug ḫar$^{?}$]-ra-an-na min gidim saĝ ĝiš ra-ra <šu> nu-gu
12''	a_2 obv. ii 11'	[x x x lú]-lil-lá zu-zu min guruš-lil-lá ki-sikil-
13''	a_2 obv. ii 12'	[lil-lá$^{?}$ x]x min an-ta-šub-ba min *erasure?*

14''	a_2 obv. ii 13'	[ka-muš]-⸢ì⸣-gu$_7$ uš-šú-uš-ru min
15''	a_2 obv. ii 14'	[a-lá ḫul$^?$] šu nu-tuku nu gi du-du ki-⸢a$^?$⸣-ga
16''	a_2 obv. ii 15'	[tu-ra$^?$] ĝi$_6$-ù-na tu-ra nu-du$_{10}$-ga an-⸢ki⸣-⸢kam$^?$⸣-m[a$^?$]
17''	a_2 obv. ii 16'	[x-]x du$_{10}^?$ ^{d}kamad-me ^{d}kamad-duru$_5$ ^{d}⸢kamad⸣-[LAGAB$^?$]
18''	a_2 obv. ii 17'	[x]-bi-šè kur-ra-a ù nu-ga ù nu-d[u$_{10}$-du$_{10}$-da]
19''	a_2 obv. ii 18'	[sa]ĝ-bi ú-la-a alan(GÀR.GÀR)-bi ú-la-a [x x x]
20''	a_2 obv. ii 19'	[sa]ĝ gig-bi uš-šú-uš-ru-a igi-bi [x x x (x)]
21''	a_2 obv. ii 20'	ù ku-uk-ku ra-a á-šu-<<bi>> ĝìri-bi [x x (x)]
22''	a_2 obv. ii 21'	sa-ad-nim kur-ra a-zu-<<bi-šè>>-ĝìri-b[i ^{d}lugal-$^?$]
23''	a_2 obv. ii 22'	nam-me-en-na e-ne saĝ-gig dad[ag-ge-ta]
24''	a_2 obv. ii 23'	saĝ-gig dadag-ge-ta sa ki ⸢gurum$^?$⸣ x[x x x]
25''	a_2 obv. ii 24'	⸢sa$^?$⸣-umbin-⸢a-ni$^?$⸣ ⸢nam$^?$⸣-x[. . . . .]
26''	a_2 obv. ii 25'	[x x]x sùr$^?$-ri-r[i$^?$ . . . .]

Ms. a_2 obv. ii breaks; gap of unknown length

27'''	a_1 obv. ii 1'	[x x x x x x UR.BA]R.RA$^?$ [x x]
28'''	a_1 obv. ii 2'	[x x x x x x *ina* ^{sí}]^{g}ḪÉ.ME.<DA> *ta-*[*lam-mi*$^?$]
29'''	a_1 obv. ii 3'	[x x x x x x *ana*$^?$] ⸢U$_4$⸣.11.KAM 7-*šú* ÍL-*m*[*a* x x]
30'''	a_1 obv. ii 4'	[x x x x x] *ir-ri* [(x x)]
31'''	a_1 obv. ii 5'	[(DIŠ) MUNUS NI.NE GI]G 1 SÌLA *dì-iq-mé-*[*en*]
	B rev. iv 9	DIŠ MUNUS NI.NE GIG 1 SÌLA DÈ
32'''	a_1 obv. ii 6'	[^{giš}*ṣar-ba*]-*ti* 1 SÌLA *dì-iq-m*[*é-en*]
	B rev. iv 9$^{cont.}$	^{giš}ÁSAL 1 SÌLA DÈ
33'''	a_1 obv. ii 7'	[^{ú}*am-ḫa-r*]*a*$^?$ 14 KA.KÉŠ *šá* TÚG [*takaṣṣar*]
	B rev. iv 9$^{cont.}$–10	^{ú}*am-ḫa-ra* ḪI.⸢ḪI⸣ / 14 KEŠDA.MEŠ *šá* TÚG KÉŠ
34'''	a_1 obv. ii 8'	[1.TA.À]M$^?$ *ina šà-su-ri-šá* GAR-*an-m*[*a* TI-*uṭ*$^?$]
	B rev. iv 10	1.TA.ÀM *ana* ŠÀ.TÙR-*šá* GAR-*an*
35'''	a_1 obv. ii 9'	KI.MIN *mur-ra ta-ḫaš-šal ina* Ì *t*[*a-bal-lal*$^?$]
	b rev. 4	DIŠ KI.MIN ^{šim}ŠEŠ *ina* Ì SÚD
36'''	a_1 obv. ii 10'	*ina up-pí ina šà-su-ri-šá i-ta-b*[*a-ak* (x x)]
	b rev. 4$^{cont.}$	*ina* MUD ZABAR *ana múš-tin-ni-šú* DUB-[*ak*$^?$]
37'''	a_1 obv. ii 11'	KI.MIN ^{ú}ḪAB *ina* KAŠ GEŠTIN *ta-ma-ḫa-*[*aṣ* NAG$^?$]

38'''	a$_1$ obv. ii 12'	MUNUS *ta-ti-ka-at ú-ri-ša* GIG [x x x]
39'''	a$_1$ obv. ii 13'	ŠIM.MEŠ DÙ.A.BI *ina* T[ÚG *takaṣṣar* (x x)]
40'''	a$_1$ obv. ii 14'	*ina šà-su-ri-*[*šá* GAR-*an-ma* x x x x]

(Bottom of Ms. a$_1$ obv. ii)

41'''	a$_1$ rev. iii 1	MUNUS ⸢Ù⸣.[TU$^{?}$. . . . .]
42'''	a$_1$ rev. iii 2	NAG x[. . . . .]

43'''	a$_1$ rev. iii 3	MUNUS *a-la-da* KUD-*sà-*[*at* x x x x x x]
44'''	a$_1$ rev. iii 4	*ta-sà-ak ina* KA[Š x x x x x x]
45'''	a$_1$ rev. iii 5	*ana* IGI ^{mul}MAR.GÍD.DA *t*[*uš-bat*$^{?}$ x x x x x]
46'''	a$_1$ rev. iii 6	⸢*ana*⸣ TÚG.MEŠ-*šá* DU-*ku* NAG-*ma* [x x x x x]

47'''	a$_1$ rev. iii 7	[MUNUS N]U *a-li-da-at ana ur-re-*⸢*e*⸣ [x x x x x]
48'''	a$_1$ rev. iii 8	[^{ú}*k*]*a-am-kà-ta* ^{ú}*im-ḫur-aš-ra* [x x x x]
49'''	a$_1$ rev. iii 9	[*ta-sà-ak*$^{?}$] *ina* A *ta-la-áš ta-ta-*x-[x x x]
50'''	a$_1$ rev. iii 10	[x x *t*]*a-ḫaš-šal lu-ub-ki te-pu-u*[*š* x x]
51'''	a$_1$ rev. iii 11	[x x x x x] x ŠUB *ina še-e-ri* [x x x]
52'''	a$_1$ rev. iii 12	[x x x x x x] ⸢*ana*$^{?}$⸣ U$_4$.16.KAM MUNUS NU [x x]
53'''	a$_1$ rev. iii 13	[x x x x x x *ir*]-*ri* [x x x]

Ms. a$_1$ rev. iii breaks; gap of unknown length

54''''	a$_2$ rev. iii 1'	[. . . . .] x [. . . . .]
55''''	a$_2$ rev. iii 2'	[. . . . .]x x.ḪI.A *ana* x[x x x]
56''''	a$_2$ rev. iii 3'	[. . . . . *ina*] Ì ⸢GAZ$^{?}$⸣ x x [x x (x)]
57''''	a$_2$ rev. iii 4'	[. . . . .]x x [x x] NITA [x]
58''''	a$_2$ rev. iii 5'	[x x x x x x] še$^{?}$ x[x x x x] ⸢AL$^{?}$⸣.[Ú]S.SA$^{?}$ [x]
59''''	a$_2$ rev. iii 6'	[x x x]x x [GA]R$^{?}$-*an* KÉŠ-*r*[*a*$^{?}$] x x [*in*]*a* A KÚM [x x]
60''''	a$_2$ rev. iii 7'	[x]x KU$^{?}$ x x BU[RU$_5$.Ḫ]ABRUD$^{?mu}$[$^{šen?}$] *it-t*[*a*$^{?}$*-x*]*-aṣ-ma* [x]
61''''	a$_2$ rev. iii 8'	⸢x ga x x⸣ du [x] ⸢^{giš}GADA$^{sar?}$⸣ ^{ú}ḪU[R].SAG ^{ú}KUR.KUR.R[A]
62''''	a$_2$ rev. iii 9'	^{ú}*im-*⸢*ḫur*⸣*-lim* ⸢^{ú}⸣[x x x] ^{ú}IN.NU.UŠ [(x)]
63''''	a$_2$ rev. iii 10'	^{ú}KUR.⸢RA$^{?}$⸣ ^{ú}x[x x] ⸢^{ú}⸣NU.LUḪ.ḪA MUN$^{!}$ *ta-s*[*ak*$_6$$^{?}$]
64''''	a$_2$ rev. iii 11'	[(x) TÉ]Š.BI *te-ṭe*$_4$*-en* [x x x]-*šú*$^{?}$ *ta-ká*$^{?}$*-pár-ma* TI-*uṭ*

65''''	a$_2$ rev. iii 12'	[x]x x ŠID$^{?}$-*ti* x[x x x]x-*ma-tu*$_4$ NUMUN ŠE.LÚ
66''''	a$_2$ rev. iii 13'	[x]x ^{ú}SUR.SUR SAR [x x x]⸢^{ú}⸣KUR.KUR.RA
67''''	a$_2$ rev. iii 14'	[x]x ^{giš}ŠU.Ú[R.MÌN x x ^{giš}]MA.NU Ú.ḪI.A *an-*[*nu-ti*]

68'''' a$_2$ rev. iii 15' [.......................................]x i ḫu-x-[x x x]

69'''' a$_2$ rev. iii 16' [.......................................]x ⸢ḫu$^{?}$⸣ si$^{?}$[x x x x]

Ms. a$_2$ rev. iii breaks; remainder lost

Bound Transcription and Translation

Beginning of ms. a$_1$ obv. i lost

1' [.....] KI.MIN KI.MIN

1' [.....] ditto, ditto.

Bottom of ms. a$_1$ obv. i

Beginning of ms. a$_2$ obv. i lost

2''–3'' *traces*

2''–3'' *too fragmentary for translation*

4'' [ÉN$^{?}$ x x kur-ta$^{?}$] nam-ta-è ⸢min$^{?}$⸣ [x] x[.....]

4'' [Incantation(?). "[...] has come out [from the mountain(?)], ditto(?) (i.e., it has come out), ...[.....],

5'' [x x x g]ig-ga-ta min a-ri-a-[ta$^{?}$ min$^{?}$ x x]

5'' *from the troublesome* [...] ditto (i.e. it has come out), [from(?)] the wasteland(?) [ditto(?)...],

6'' [x x x x] min kur-ra gu-ĝar-ra$^{?!}$ min k[i$^{?}$ x x]

6'' [.....] ditto (i.e. it has come out), (from) a breach(?) in the mountains ditto (i.e., it has come out), ...[...]

7'' [x x x x] ḫul-gig min é bar-gin$_7$$^{?}$ ⸢min$^{?}$⸣

7'' [...] the hated one ditto (i.e., has come out), like a foster child ditto(?),

8'' [x x x x]x min nam-tar gig-ga-a-ta min

8'' [......] ditto. Together with the troublesome Namtar (Fate)-demon ditto (i.e., it has come out),

9'' [na-á]ĝ$^{?}$-tag šu-re-dè min lugal-maš-pa-è-a min

9'' [s]in(?) (and) crime ditto (i.e., have come out), Lugal-amaš-pa'e ditto (i.e., has come out),

10'' [x saĝ ĝiš ra-r]a-e-dè min udug ḫul-ĝál

10'' [the ... who commit]s murder ditto, the evil Udug-demon,

11'' [x x udug ḫar$^{?}$]-ra-an-na min gidim saĝ ĝiš ra-ra <šu> nu-gu

11'' [..., the Udug-demon(?)] of the [ro]ad(?) ditto, the murderous, *irresistible* ghost,

12'' [x x x lú]-líl-lá zu-zu min ĝuruš-líl-lá ki-sikil-

12'' [...], the well-known(?) wind-demon (*lilû*) ditto, the young man wind-demon (*eṭel lilî*), the maiden [wind]-demon (*lilītu*),

13'' [líl-lá$^{?}$ x]x min an-ta-šub-ba min

13'' [...] ditto, Antašubba-epilepsy ditto,

14'' [ka-muš]-⸢ì⸣-gu$_7$ uš-šú-uš-ru min

14'' 'Eaten [by the worm']-demon (and) debility ditto (i.e., have come out).

15'' [a-lá ḫul$^{?}$] šu nu-tuku nu gi du-du ki-⸢a$^{?}$⸣-ga

15'' [The evil Alû-demon(?)] who has no hands, *who loves to walk around at night*(?),

16'' [tu-ra$^{?}$] ĝi$_6$-ù-na tu-ra nu-du$_{10}$-ga an-⸢ki⸣-⸢kam$^{?}$⸣-m[a$^{?}$]

16'' [the sickness] of the early morning, it is the unpleasant sickness of heaven and earth(?).

17'' [x-]x ⸢du$_{10}$$^{?}$⸣ ^{d}kamad-me ^{d}kamad-duru$_5$ ^{d}⸢kamad⸣-[LAGAB$^{?}$]

17'' [...]..., Kamadme (Lamaštu), Kamadduru-demon (*labāṣu*), Kamad-[LAGAB]-demon (*aḫḫāzu*),

18'' [x-(x)]-bi-šè kur-ra-a ù nu-ga ù nu-d[u$_{10}$-du$_{10}$-da]

18'' who *enters through the* [...], who does not allow one to sleep, who does not let the sleep be good –

19'' [sa]ĝ-bi ú-la-a alan-bi ú-la-a [x x x]

19'' its [head] is the Alû-demon(?), its body (shape) is the Alû-demon(?) [. . .].

20'' [sa]ĝ gig-bi uš-šú-uš-ru-a igi-bi [x x x (x)]
21'' ù ku-uk-ku ra-a á-šu-<<bi>>-ĝìri-bi [x x (x)]
22'' sa-ad-nim kur-ra a-zu-<<bi-šè>>- ĝìri-b[i ^{d}lugal-]

20'' Its terrible head is debility, its face [is . . .],
21'' who pours out sleep (on the victim). Its limbs are [. . .]
22''–23'' sadnim-disease of the mountains. Its limbs(!) are those of [Lugal]namenna(?).

23'' nam-me-en-na e-ne saĝ-gig dad[ag-ge-ta]
24'' saĝ-gig dadag-ge-ta sa ki ⸢gurum?⸣ x[x x x]

23'' To purify (the patient suffering from) the head disease,
24'' to purify (from) the head-disease, [*to* . . .] the *sick*, twisted(?) muscles,

25'' <uzu>- ⸢sa?⸣-umbin-⸢a-ni?⸣ ⸢nam?⸣-x[. . . . . .]
26'' [x x]x sùr? ri-r[i? . . . . . .]

25'' his/her (the patient's) sinews . . . [. . . . . .],
26'' [. . .] . . . *release* [. . . . . .]

Ms. a₂ obv. ii breaks; gap of unknown length

27''' [. . . . . . *bar]bari* . . .[. . .] 28''' [. . . . . . *ina*] *tabarri ta*[*lammi*] 29''' [. . . . . . *ana*] *ištešser ūmī sebîšu inaššī-m*[*a* . . .] 30''' [. . . . . .] *irri*

27''' [. . . . . .] wolf's [. . .], 28''' [. . . .] you [wrap?] into red wool, [. . .], 29''' [. . . over(?)] eleven days(?) she shall apply (it) seven times, [. . .]. 30''' [. . .] (Then) she will get pregnant.

31''' [*šumma sinništu* NI.NE *marṣ*]*at išten qa diqmēn* 32''' [*ṣarba*]*ti ištēn qa diqm*[*ēn*] 33''' [*amḫar*]*a*(?) 14 *kiṣrī ša lubāri* [*takaṣṣar*] 34''' [*ištē*]*nâ ina šassūrīša tašakkan-m*[*a iballuṭ*(?)]

31''' [(If) a woman suff]ers [from NI.NE-disease]: (ms. B adds: you mix) one litre ashes of 32''' [*ṣarbat*]*u*-poplar (and) one litre ashes of 33''' [*amḫar*]*a*-[plant(?)]. [You tie (this into)] fourteen knots of cloth. 34''' You insert [one (piece of cloth) at a] time into her womb (i.e. her vagina), and [she will get well(?)].

35''' KI.MIN *murra taḫaššal ina šamni t*[*aballal*] (var. *murra ina šamni tasâk*) 36''' *ina uppi ina šassūrīša itabb*[*ak* (. . .)] (var. *ina uppi siparri ana muštinnīšu tatabbak*)

35''' Alternatively (lit. another (prescription)): you crush *murru*-plant, m[ix(?)] (it) with oil (var.: you pound *murru*-plant in oil). 36''') She shall po[ur] (it) into her womb with a tube, [(. . .)] (var. you pour it into her urethra with a bronze tube).

37''' KI.MIN *būšāna ina šikari karāni tamaḫḫa*[*ṣ išatti*(?)]

37''' Alternatively, you st[ir] *būšānu*-plant into beer (and) wine, [she drinks it(?)].

38''' *sinništu tattīkāt ūrīša marṣat* [. . .] 39''' *riqqē kalāma ina lub*[*āri takaṣṣar* (. . .)] 40''' *ina šassūrī*[*ša tašakkan-ma* . . . . . .]

38''' (If) a woman is sick with dribbling from her vulva [. . . . . .] 39''' [you tie] all (kinds of) aromatic plants into a (piece of) clo[th (. . .)], 40''' [you insert (it)] into [her] womb (viz. vagina). [Then . . . . . .].

41''' *sinništu ū*[*lid*(?) . . . . . .] 42''' *išatti* [. . . . . .]

41''' (If) a woman *giv*[*es birth*(?) . . . . . .] 42''' she drinks (it), . . .[. . . . . .].

43''' *sinništu alāda parsa*[*t* . . . . . .] 44''' *tasâk ina šika*[*ri* . . . . . .] 45''' *ana pān Ereqqi t*[*ušbât* . . . . . .] 46''' *ana lubārēša illakū išattī-ma* [. . . . . .]

43''' (If) a woman has stopped to bear: [. . . . . .] 44''' you pound, [you . . . (it)] with be[er . . . . . .]. 45''' You let [(it) stand outside overnight] before the Wagon star (Ursa Major). [. . . (*when*) . . .] 46''' *flow onto her cloth* (i.e. her menstrual bandage?), she shall drink (it). Then [. . . . . .].

47''' *[sinništu] lā ālidat ana urrê* [. . . . . .] 48''' *[k]amkadu imḫur-ešrā* [. . .] 49''' *[tasâk(?)] ina mê talâš* . . .[. . .] 50''' [. . .] *taḫaššal lubki teppuš* [. . .] 51''' [. . . . . .] . . . *tanaddi(?) ina šēri* [. . .] 52''' [. . . . . .] *ana sešŝer ūmī sinništu lā* [. . .] 53''' [. . . . . . *ir*]*ri* [. . .]

47''' [(If) a woman] is infertile, to make (her) get pregnant: [. . . . . .] 49''' [you pound(?)] 48''' *[k]amkadu*-[plant], 'heals twenty'-plant, [. . . . . .]. 49''' You knead (it) with water, you [. . . . . .], 50''' you pound [. . .]. You prepare a lubricant [. . . . . .], 51''' [. . . . . .] you add (to it?). In the morning [. . . . . .] 52''' [. . . . . .]. For sixteen days the woman *shall not*(?) [*remove it*(?)]. 53''' [. . . . . . she will get] pregnant [. . .].

Ms. a_1 rev. iii breaks; gap of unknown length

54''''–55'''' *traces* 56'''' [. . . . . . *ina*] *šamni taḫaššal(?)* . . . [. . . . . .] 57'''' *traces* 58'''' [. . . . . .] *šiqqu(?)* 59'''' [. . . . . . *taša*]*kkan(?) kiṣra(?)* [. . .] *ina mê baḫrūti* [. . .] 60'''' [. . . . . .] . . . *iṣṣūr ḫurri(?)* . . .[. . .] 61'''' [. . . . . .] . . . *kitû azupīru atā'išu* 62'''' *imḫur-līm* [. . .] *maštakal* 63'''' *nīnû* . . .[. . .] *nuḫurtu ṭābtu tas[âk]* 64'''' [. . . *išt*]*ēniš teṭên* [. . .]-*šu takappar-ma iballuṭ*

54''''–55'''' *too fragmentary for translation* 56'''' [. . . . . .] you crush(?) [in] oil, . . . [. . .] 57'''' *traces* 58'''' [. . . . . .] fish sauce(?), 59'''' [. . . . . . you] put(?). A knot/node(?) [. . .] with hot water [. . .]. 60'''' [. . . . . .] (with) [. . .] of a *ḫurru*-bird(?) *she/it shall* [. . .] and [. . .]. 63'''' You cr[ush] 61'''' [. . . . . .] flax, *azupīru*-plant, *atā'išu*-plant, 62'''' [. . . . . .], 'heals thousand'-plant, [. . .]-plant, *maštakal*-soapwort, 63'''' [. . . . . .] *atā'išu*-plant, [. . .]-plant, *nuḫurtu*-plant (and) salt. 64'''' [. . .] you grind together, you wipe her [. . .] (with it). Then she will get well.

65'''' [. . . . . .] . . . [. . .] *zēr kisibirri* 66'''' [. . . . . .] . . . *pizzer arqu(?)* [. . .] *atā'išu* 67'''' [. . .] *šur[mēnu* . . .] *e'ru šammī an[nûti]* 68''''–69'''' *traces*

65'''' [. . . . . .] . . . [. . .] . . . coriander seed, 66'''' [. . . . . .] . . . cobweb, garden green(s)(?), [. . .], *atā'išu*-plant, 67'''' [. . .] *šur*[*mēnu*-cypress, . . .], *e'ru*-wood – these plants 68''''–69'''' *only traces preserved*

Ms. a_2 rev. iii breaks; remainder lost

Notes

Lines 2''–3'': The double ruling following lines 2''–3'' indicates the end of a (thematic) section and the beginning of a new topic.

Lines 4''–26'': The first lines of this spell contain several phrases that seem to be reminiscent of the incantation saĝ-gig é-kur-ta nam-ta-è "Head disease has come out from the Ekur", which forms the beginning of the canonical series SAG.GIG.(GA.MEŠ) "Head disease" and *Muššu'u* (see Böck 2007: 24, 93ff. *Muššu'u* I; Linton 1970, 45). Note that the forerunner to SAG.GIG I/a from Emar (*Emar* 732; Arnaud 1987, 341 no. 732; Viano 2016, 321; Zomer 2018, 264) begins in a slightly different way: saĝ-gig kur-ta [. . .] "Headache [has come out] from the mountains (i.e. Netherworld)". Perhaps the latter variant also formed the begin of the present spell. See for the same motif of diseases coming out from the Netherworld or mountain (also referred to as Ekur, the house/temple of Enlil), the following lines from the incantation saĝ-gig gú-sa-àm "Head disease is (like) neck muscle-disease" in SAG.GIG.(GA.MEŠ) Tablet III and *Muššu'u* III (Böck 2007, 133ff. *Muššu'u* III/a 3–7; Linton 1970, 64): "Head disease has come out from the Ekur (saĝ-gig é-kur-ta nam-ta-e$_{11}$: *di-ḫu iš-tu é-kur it-ta-ṣa-a*), it has come out from the house of Enlil (é ^{d}en-líl-lá-ta nam-ta-è/e$_{11}$-[dè]: *iš-tu* É ^{d}*en-líl it-ta-ṣa-a*). It has come down from the midst of the mountains to the land (kur-ra kur šà-ta nam-ta-e$_{11}$-dè : *iš-tu qé-reb* KUR-*i ana* KUR *ur-da*). It has come down from the horizon of the mountains to the land (gilim ḫur-saĝ-ĝá-ta kur-ta nam-ta-e$_{11}$-dè : *iš-tu kip-pat* KUR-*i ana* KUR *ur-da*). It came down from the pasture lands, not to return (anymore)" (a-gàr nu-gi$_4$-gi$_4$-a-ta kur-ta nam-ta-e$_{11}$-dè : *iš-tu ú-ga-ri ana la ta-a-ri ur-da*).

Line 5'': For a-ri-a "desert, wasteland" as a place inhabited by demons or diseases to which they are banned in exorcistic rituals, see e.g. Udug-hul Tablet 8: 29, 48, 50 (Geller 2016, 296, 300–301). This reading is probably to be preferred over a-ri-a "offspring of . . ." (describing the origin of the demon).

Line 6'': The spelling gu-ĝar-ra$^{!}$ is interpreted as gú-ĝìri "breach" (suggestion courtesy of M. Geller). Alternatively, gu-ĝar may stand for gú-ĝar "entirety".

Line 7'': The sequence é bar is understood as a bar-ra "adopted child" (Akk. *liqûtu*).

Line 8'': In nam-tar gig-ga-a-ta, the suffix -ta is interpreted as an alternative spelling for -da (comitative).

Line 9'': If the restoration [na-á]ĝ$^{?}$-tag šu-re-dè at the beginning of the line is correct, it could be interpreted as a cryptographic spelling for nam-tag šu-re-da (= šer$_{7}$-da), corresponding to Akkadian *arnu šertu* "sin (and) crime".
The spelling lugal-maš-pa-è-a appears to be abbreviated for ^{d}Lugal-amaš-pa-è, a sickness and netherworld deity/demon, often mentioned beside Namtar and Lugalurra and associated with epilepsy (see Stol 1993, 20, 110 n. 119 for similar spellings also dropping the divine epithet). It has been proposed that the name may have to be read Lugal-ùtul-pa-è "the king shepherd shining forth", but in the light of the present spelling, the pronunciation must in fact have been amaš, i.e. "sheepfold" (see Krebernik 1987–1990b, "Lugal-AMAŠ-pa'e", *RlA* 7, 111).

Line 10'': The restoration is tentative, for similar passages, see e.g. Udug-ḫul Tablet 16: 4, 21 (Geller 2016, 502, 505).

Line 11'': For the udug-demon of the highway (udug ḫar-ra-an-(na)), see also Udug-ḫul Tablet 5: 146 (Geller 2016, 206). The proposed emendation <šu> nu-gu is tentative; the text seems to be corrupt. Possibly, <šu> nu-gu is an error for šu nu-kur$_{9}$ (šu ku$_{4}$-ku$_{4}$) "whom one cannot withstand; whom no one can approach". Other possible interpretations may be šu nu-gur "who does not wipe the hand (clean)" or šu nu-ĝar-(ra) "one who does not spare; merciless" (Akk. *lā gāmilu*).

Line 12'': The spelling zu-zu is understood as "well-known; recognised"; alternatively, it may perhaps be interpreted as šú-šú "to overwhelm" (šuš).

Line 14'': The entity ka-muš-ì-gu$_{7}$ corresponds to Akkadian *pāšittu* lit. "the extinguisher", a female demon associated with Lamaštu, in medical texts also known as a disease linked to bile. The Sumerian name ka-muš-ì-gu$_{7}$ is translated as "Wurmfraß" (Köcher 1978, 36 note 59) or as "the one who feeds (the victim) to the worms", see Wiggermann 2003–2005, *RlA* 10, 363–364; *Muššu'u* Tablet 1: 3 (Böck 2007, 94).

The spelling uš-šú-uš-ru stands for u$_{4}$-šú-uš-ru = Akk. *lu'tu* "debility, decay", often associated with *mungu/mangu* "paralysis, stiffness", see e.g. Jaques 2015, *Mon dieu*, 95 *ad* 67: 11; cf. AHw 565 (associating *lu'tu* with "dirt" and skin disease, because of its derivation from *lu''û* "to defile"); CAD L, 255–256 translates "softness, debility, decay".

Line 15'': The phonetic spelling nu gi du-du should presumably be interpreted as lú gi$_{6}$-a du-du "who walks around at night", usually equated with *ḫā'iṭu* "night watchman", also an epithet of gods and demons (CAD Ḫ, 32a). Perhaps ki-a-ga at the end of the line should be understood as ki-áĝ-ĝá "who loves". The epithet befits the description of the evil *Alû*-demon in Udug-ḫul, see e.g. Geller 2016, 288–289 Udug-ḫul Tablet 3: 5–9, 12: "whether you are the evil *Alû*-demon who has no mouth (ka nu-tuku-a), whether you are the evil *Alû*-demon who has no limbs (me-dím nu-tuku-a), whether you are the evil *Alû*-demon who cannot hear (ĝiš nu-tuku-a), whether you are the evil *Alû*-demon who has no face igi-kir$_{4}$ nu-tuku-a), whether you are the evil *Alû*-demon who is not visible (even) by daylight, . . ., whether you are the evil *Alû*-demon who is a god stalking at night" (diĝir gi$_{6}$-a du-du). For the *Alû*-demon as a demon attacking victims at night, see also Stol 1993, 41–42.

Line 16'': See also Böck 2007, 94 *Muššu'u* Beschwörung I line 5: [tu-r]a gi$_{6}$-u$_{4}$-na e-ne-bi-da-ke$_{4}$ "it is the illness of the early morning". The entity tu-ra gi$_{6}$-ù-na is equated with *muruṣ kaṣâti* in ASKT 11, p. 84–85 line 56 (zi-pà-incantations, see Borger 1969, *FS von Soden*, 5). See also the forerunner to SAG.GIG I/a *Emar* 732: 3 (Zomer 2018, 264; Viano 2016, 321): tu-ra nu-du$_{10}$-ga "an illness-not-improving".

Line 17'': For the reading of the Sumerian name of Lamaštu, ^{d}DÌM.ME, as Kamad-me, see George 2018. Lamaštu (^{d}DÌM.ME) forms a group of demonic, sickness-bringing entities together with ^{d}DÌM.(ME).A, now read Kamad-duru$_{5}$ (*Labāṣu*) and ^{d}DÌM.ME.LAGAB/ḪAB (= *Aḫḫāzu*).

Line 18'': The restoration at the beginning of the line is uncertain, but I suppose that kur-ra-a belongs together, perhaps representing a phonetic spelling for ku$_{4}$-r / kur$_{9}$ "to enter" (i.e. "one who enters . . ."). Compare, for example the phrase ab ku$_{4}$ "to slip in through the window (said of demons)" (usually construed with the locative, not the terminative).

The phrase ù nu-ga could be interpreted as an abbreviated spelling of ù-nu-ĝar-ra "impropriety". However, in terms of the context, a better interpretation is to assume an unusual spelling of ù nu-ku/ku$_{4}$ "it doesn't allow one to sleep". See for a parallel bilingual line, Böck 2007, 94 *Muššu'u* I Beschwörung I line 4: [ù] nu-ku-ku ù nu-du$_{10}$-du$_{10}$-da : [*u*]*l ú-šá-aṣ-lal šit-ta ul uš-ta-a-bi* "the one who does not allow (one) to sleep, who doesn't let the sleep be good (Akk.: it does not let one sleep, it did not let the sleep be good)".

Line 19'': Compare the similar sentence in Böck 2007, 94 *Muššu'u* I Beschwörung I line 6: [saĝ]-bi u$_{18}$-lu alan-bi ùru-àm : *qaqqassu alû lānšu abūbumma* "his head is (like that of) the *Alû*-demon, his body is the deluge". Thus, the spelling ú-la-a in line 19'' would stand for a- lá-àm "it is the *Alû*-demon" (for a similar alteration of *a* > *u* in Sumerian texts from the western periphery (Emar, Ugarit, Hattuša) in the latter half of the second millennium BCE, see Viano 2016, 211). It is not impossible, although unlikely, that ú-la-a here stands instead for the Ulāya river (Greek Eulaios). In Mesopotamian sources this river is mentioned as a holy river and a deity associated with purification and creating healing plants; it was also seen as a crossing point for demons and an entrance to the Netherworld; as a deified river Ulāya had an apotropaic function and was also a guardian of gates, see Frame 2014–2016, "Ulai, Ulaja," *RlA* 14, 302–303; Krebernik, 2014–2016, "Ulai, Ulaja" *RlA* 14, 303; Perdibon 2019, 130–131; Meinhold 2009, 105–106.

Line 20'': The spelling uš-šú-uš-ru is a phonetic variant of u$_4$-šú-uš-ru, which corresponds to Akkadian *lu'tu* "decay". The term often occurs in Udug-hul incantations (see e.g. Geller 2016, Udug-ḫul Tablet 3: 142).

Line 21'': The spelling ù ku-uk-ku is understood as ù ku-ku "sleep". The form ra-a is interpreted as ri-a, from ri "to cast, throw down; to pour out".

Line 22'': Sumerian sa-ad-nim is equated with several different Akkadian disease terms. Note sa-ad-nim = *bennu* "epilepsy" and *šaššaṭu* (MSL 9, 94: 83–84). A passage from a bilingual anti-witchcraft incantation offers a parallel (Abusch and Schwemer 2016, CMAwR 2, 115: 11): lú-ùlu-bi á-šu-ĝìri-ni sa-ad-nim im-šub : *i-⌜na⌝ ma-na-ni-⌜šu⌝* [*š*]*a-⌜áš⌝-š*[*a-tam id-di*] "she (the witch) cast sadnim-disease (Akk. *šaššaṭu*-disease) on that man's limbs (Akk. on his *muscles*)".[239] On *šaššaṭu*-disease (associated with jerking, spasms and rigidity), see e.g. Scurlock and Andersen 2005, 66–68 (interpreted as tetanus).

In the present text, sa-ad-nim is said to come from the mountain(s). Only few specific diseases are credited with this place of origin, especially the 'mountain fever' (*li'b*(*i*) *šadî*), also known as "seizure of the mountain" (*ṣibit šadî*), see e.g. Stadhouders 2018a, *RA* 112, 159–160 with further references. The association of this febrile condition with the "mountain(s)" may stem from its potential lethal outcome and from its occasional epidemic outbreaks. See further the "migraine of the mountain" (saĝ-ki-dab-ba ḫur-saĝ-ĝá) in SAG.GIG.GA.MEŠ Tablet VI Incantation 1 (CT 17, 23: 1 Linton 1970, 110).

The phrase a-zu-<<bi-šè>> is tentatively interpreted as a corrupt writing for á-šu-ĝìri-bi "limbs", already found in the previous line, where the scribe likewise wrote a superfluous sign (á-šu-<<bi>>-ĝìri-bi).

Line 23'': I owe the identification of nam-me-en-na at the beginning of the line with the name ^{d}Lugal-nam-en-na to a suggestion by Marten Stol, although the present text presents an unusual spelling ((Lugal)-nam-me-en-na). Lugal-nam-en-na (also Nam-en-na, Lugal-me(a)) is one of the lesser deities linked to epilepsy (*bennu*), beside Lugal-amašpa'ea, Šulpa'ea and the 'Lord of the roof' (Lugal-urra), see Stol 1993, 20–21; Lambert 1987–1990, *RlA* 7, 149; Geller 2016, 100 Udug-ḫul 3: 52 (with n. 52); CT 17, 4: 2 // (Linton 1970, 132) ^{d}lugal-nam-en-na (= *bennu*) beside dugud-da (= *miqtu*) and other demonic entities. It is uncertain, whether the name was indeed written out in full by the scribe of BAM 241(+), carrying over from line 22'' to 23'', or whether it was abbreviated (Nam-me-en-na). However, the same phenomenon can be observed in line 12''–13'' where the name ki-sikil-líl-lá is similarly split up between the end of line 12'' and the beginning of line 13'' (see above).

The spelling dadag-ge-ta in lines 23''–24'' should presumably be understood as dadag + -èd + -a "to purify".

Line 24'': For gurum (GAM) "to bend" (Akk. *kanānu* "to twist, contort") in connection with sa "muscle, sinew", see e.g. [sa ši-in]-gurum-ma : *še*[*r'ānī uka*]*nnan* "it (head disease) twists the sinews" (CT 17, 25: 23 //; Böck 2007, 96 *Muššu'u* I Beschwörung 1 line 14; MSL 9, 23–24). The element KI in sa ki gurum is interpreted here as a phonetic spelling of gig (ge$_{17}$-ga) "sick" (see e.g. Cavigneaux 1999, 258: 17 (Tell Haddad)).

239 Furthermore, sa-ad-nim (in first millennium BCE texts also saĝ-nim-(nim) and sa-niĝin) corresponds to Akkadian *rapādu*, a disease term associated with mental derangement (*šinīt ṭēmi*) (CAD R, 147; AHw 954). Especially when referring to a disease of sheep, *rapādu* has been interpreted as "staggers" (listeriosis), cf. CAD R, 147 sub 1. There appears to be a partial overlap with the condition of *ṣīdānu* "vertigo", which also corresponds to sa-ad-nim or saĝ-niĝin / sa-(ad)-niĝin (see AHw 1100a; Sjöberg 1973, *JCS* 25, 141 ad line 166, variant saĝ-nim-nim). The homonymous plant *rapādu* induces this state (i.e. a psychoactive plant); in a Late Babylonian anti-witchcraft incantation it is said to grow in the steppe and be of a purple colour, see Abusch and Schwemer 2016, CMAwR 2, 100, 103–104 text 7.24; Stol 2017, *BiOr* 74, 371–372; 2022, *BiOr* 79, 326–327.

Line 25'': Sumerian uzu-sa-umbin corresponds to Akkadian *manānu* "sinews, nerves", in Böck 2007, 96 *Muššu'u* I Beschwörung I line 16: [uzu-sa-um]bin an-lum-[mu]: [*man*]*āni ukannan* "it twists (all) the sinews". Cf. AHw 602a; CAD M/1, 208.

Lines 27'''–30''': In women's healthcare texts, the verb *našû* (ÍL) "to wear, to apply" regularly denotes the insertion of a tampon into the vagina, which is filled with medicinal ingredients and kept in place for a certain amount of time (CAD N/2, 100a; Reiner 1982, *ZA* 72, 131 with UET 7, No. 123 obv. 1–7 and dupl. (text B.2.2)). See e.g., a similar prescription to promote fertility in BAM 408 obv.? i' 1': MUNUS BI ÍL-*ma* ... *irri* "the woman applies it, ... (Then) she will get pregnant" (see *infra* text A.2.9, section B and *passim* for further discussion).

For the reconstruction [*ana*] U_4.11.KAM "for/over a period of eleven days", see also line 52''' below (ms. a_2 rev. iii 12): *ana* U_4.16.KAM "for sixteen days (the woman shall not [*remove* (the tampon)])".

Lines 31'''–34''': These lines have been restored according to the parallel prescription in BAM 237 rev. iv 9–10 (ms. B). Ms. a_1 seems to be slightly abbreviated, dropping the verb *tuballal*(ḪI.ḪI) "you mix", which is found in ms. B rev. iv 9. The rest of the recipe appears to be identical.

Because of the conspicuously high amount of two litres of ashes that are filled into the pieces ("knots") of cloth, only one piece of cloth can have been inserted into the woman's vagina at a time (which must be indicated by the expression 1.TA.ÀM "one by one; separately") in line 34'''. Therefore, the treatment was presumably spread out over a period of fourteen days. For the use of ashes in Mesopotamian medical texts, see further CAD Ṭ, 111b s.v. *ṭikmennu*. For discussion of the condition NI.NE treated with this remedy, see the edition of the parallel in BAM 237(+) and the text BM 42313+ (texts C.1.4 and A.2.2).

Lines 35'''–36''': The parallel in the Late Babylonian ms. b varies slightly from ms. a_1. Instead of the phrase DIŠ KI.MIN "alternatively" (perhaps to be read *ana šanî*) in ms. b, ms. a_1 only has KI.MIN, which presumably should be read *šanû* "another (prescription)". Secondly, in ms. b the medicine is introduced into the woman's urethra rather than her vagina, as the Middle Babylonian precursor recommends. The younger text explicitly prescribes the use of a bronze tube. It is interesting that the verbal form at the end of line 36''' in ms. a_1 is in the third rather than the second person, meaning that the patient applied the medicine herself, not the healer. Compare also BAM 237 rev. iv 12 (text C.1.4) using a similar procedure for the same condition (NI.NE), but here "white drug" is the simple and not *murru*-plant: Ú BABBAR *ta-sàk ina* Ì.GIŠ ḪI.ḪI *ina* MUD ZABAR *ina muš-tin-ni-ša* DUB-*ak* "You pound 'white drug', mix it with oil (and) pour (it) into her urethra with a bronze tube." For the use of a tube to apply a remedy, see also BAM 240: 46 (text D.2.1): *ina* MUD A.BÁR *ana pag-ri-šá i-nap-paḫ-ma* "she blows (the medication) into her body with a lead tube" (prescription against (intestinal) fever after delivery).

For the *murru*-plant (an aromatic), which is unlikely to be identified with myrrh, see Farber 1993–1997, "Myrrhe B. Philologisch", *RlA* 8, 536–537; Jursa 2009, *FS Sima*, 163; Kinnier Wilson 2011, *JMC* 17, 4–5 (proposing *murru* is a type of juniper); BAM 1 iii 12 ^{šim}ŠEŠ *šá* KUR "*murru*-plant of the mountain(s)" (i.e. a wild-growing variety?), Attia and Buisson 2012, *JMC* 19, 28. Stol (1980–1983, "Leder(industrie)", *RlA* 6, 533 § 16) suggests *murru* ("bitter plant)" may be aloe. This plant is often prescribed in women's healthcare texts, see e.g. BM 47578: 11 (text C.2.2, to induce bleeding), *Iraq* 31, 31: 5 (text II.1.4, to induce the lochia); K. 8893: 5' (text C.1.6, to stop haemorrhage), BM 54587 + 73802: 4' (text C.2.3, to stop bleeding); BM 38624+ : 86'''' (text A.2.1); BM 42313+: 24, 26, 30, 78 (bleeding, fertility; text A.2.2); BM 47491: 21 (text A.2.6); BM 48557: 8' (text A.2.10).

Line 37''': For *maḫāṣu* in the meaning "to stir (usually a powdered substance) into a liquid", see CAD M/1, 78–70 sub 3e. See also BAM 237 obv. ii 34' (text C.1.4 line 92'); K. 263+10934 rev. 12 (text C.1.5 line 35) and BM 40152 rev. iii 11 (text C.1.8 line 26').

Lines 38'''–40''': The form *tattīkātu* is a fem. pl. of *tattīk(t)u*, derived from the verb *natāku* "to drip" (CAD T, 299b). The expression *tattīkāt ūrīša marṣat* "she is sick with dribbling from her vulva" may not refer to a discharge from the vagina, but perhaps to urination (i.e. incontinence). Similar phrases found in texts dealing with male renal diseases explicitly speak of urine, however: see, e.g., BAM 396 i 10: *šumma amēlu tattīkam ša šīnāti maruṣ* "if a man suffers from dribbling of urine"; KAR 73: 2–3: [*šumma amēlu*] ... *lu mūṣu lu ḫiniqtu lu šuburra marṣa lu tattīkāte ša šīnāte irtanašši* "[If a man] (suffers) from *mūṣu*-discharge, from stricture (or) from rectal disease, or (if) he regularly has dribbling of urine" (see Geller 2005a, texts No. 1 and No. 10; CAD M/2, s.v. *mūṣu* mng. 1a).

Lines 41'''–42''': Instead of (*šumma*) *sinništu ūl*[*id*] "(If) a woman giv[es birth]", it is likewise possible to read ^{munus}Ù.[TU] = *ālittu* "(If) a fertile woman". In this case, the fragmentary prescription may have had a similar purpose as the following sections (promoting fertility). A similar introductory formula as in line 43''' is also not excluded (e.g., MUNUS Ù.TU KUD-*sà-at* "(If) a woman has stopped to bear").

Lines 43'''–46''': A different prescription for the same purpose (fertility after menopause), literally expressed with the phrase "(if) a woman stopped (lit. is cut off) to bear", is preserved in another fragment found at Assur, dating to the Neo-Assyrian period (BAM 243: 5': DIŠ MUNUS *a-la-da* ⌈KUD⌉-*at*; see text B.1.2). For discussion and further references, see CAD P, 167 sub 1b; Reiner 1982, *ZA* 72, 129, 131 n. 24; Volk 2004, 74 n. 17). Note the slightly varying formulation MUNUS *šà* Ù.TU *pa-ar-sà-at* in MDP 57, 11 vi 21 (Labat 1974, *Textes littéraires de Suse*, 246) and the logographic spelling *šá* MUD AL.KUD in AMT 20/1 obv. i(!) 30. These expressions may designate a woman who did not get pregnant for a long time or a menopausal woman. The verb *parāsu* "to be cut off" is also used in expressions referring to the stopping of the menses ("a woman whose blood is cut off"). Note also the cognate term (*sinništu*) *parištu* (logographic spelling MUNUS KUD-tu_4), which refers to a post-menopausal woman (see CAD P, 187; see also BAM 237 obv. i 22 (text C.1.4). See also BM 47491: 25–26 (text A.2.6) for discussion.

Line 45''': The constellation Ursa Major (*Ereqqu* "Wagon star") is addressed or receives an offering in other treatments or rituals for women, see SpTU 3, No. 84 line 89 (text C.3.4); BM 48030 (text C.3.8). The constellation is designated as "mother of all the gods" in KAL 4, No. 53 rev. 10 (Maul and Strauß 2011, 105–106). The "Wagon Star" is otherwise associated with Ninlil in MUL.APIN (Tablet I i 15), but mostly with Venus (i.e. the goddess Ištar) and with Antu (Reiner 1995, 57–58, 139).

Line 46''': The passage is difficult. The verb *alāku* (DU-*ku*) is often encountered in expressions referring to the haemorrhage or menstrual bleeding, usually in combination with the phrase "her blood" (MÚD.(MEŠ)-*šá*) or her "menses" (*sagûša*). However, the logographic spelling KU.MEŠ-*šá* in the present text does not yield a term for blood, unless the text is corrupt. I have opted for reading TÚG.MEŠ-*šá* "her cloth" (*lubāru*). If understood correctly, TÚG.MEŠ-*šá* could refer to a menstrual bandage (usually in this context, we find the spelling TÚG.ḪI.A instead of TÚG.MEŠ); a reference to the woman's blood is expected in the gap in the preceding line 45'''. This would mean that the patient took the medicament for fertility when she had her period.

Lines 47'''–53''': See also Reiner 1982, *ZA* 72, 128; Volk 2004, 74 n. 17. I interpret [ᵘ*k*]*a-am-kà-ta* in line 48''' as a variant spelling for the *kamkadu*-plant (cf. CAD K, 123–124).

For *lubku* "wet poultice, lubricant" in line 50''', which is also encountered with *napšaltu* "salve", see CAD L, 232. In line 52''', Böck (2013, 31 n. 13) restores ᵐᵘⁿᵘˢNU.[Ù.TU] "the in[fertile] woman . . ." (*lā ālittu*). The alternative reading suggested here leaves open the possibility that the lubricant (perhaps not a poultice, but a tampon?) was applied for sixteen days and then removed.

Lines 54''''–64'''': Several readings in these lines are highly provisional due to the poor state of preservation of Ms. a_2. ᵘKUR.(-)KUR.RA in lines 61'''' and 66'''' is a variant spelling for ᵘKUR.KUR (for the plant *atā'išu*), see CAD A/2, 481 sub f. This spelling is also attested in a Middle Babylonian collection of anti-witchcraft rituals from Hattuša (Abusch and Schwemer 2011, CMAwR 1, 29 text 1.1, 1: 22' (the duplicate writes *a-ta-i-ši*).

The reading *ta-ká*?-*pár-ma* "you rub" in line 64'''' is tentative, since the use of KÁ as a syllabic sign is otherwise rare (cf. Borger 2004, MZL 298). If the proposed reading is correct, one expects a body part as an object of *takappar* in the gap preceding the verb.

Lines 65''''–69'''': The logogram ᵘSUR.SUR (also written ZÚ.SUR) found in line 66'''' corresponds to *pizzir* (*pi/enzir*) "cobweb", see CAD P, 452 lex. section.

II.1.3.1 BAM 242: A Middle Babylonian Fragment from Assur

The script of this small Middle Babylonian fragment looks very similar to BAM 241 (see above), and Franz Köcher (BAM III, p. xviii) proposed that both fragments belonged to the same tablet, although this remains uncertain, since the fragments do not join. The preserved traces of the ten lines of text on BAM 242 give no definite clue that the prescriptions were concerned with treating women, although the ingredients and treatment (bandaging) may be compared with prescriptions against infertility in BAM 244 (see text B.1.1 and notes below).

List of Manuscripts

Siglum	Museum Number	Copy	Collation	Format; Ductus	Provenience
a	VAT 14389	BAM 242	Coll.	Fragment; Middle Babylonian period; ca. 12th/11th cent. BCE	Assur

Overview

i'	Fragmentary prescription (bandage) a obv.$^?$ 1'–3'	. . .]1'–3'
ii'	Fragmentary prescription a obv.$^?$ 4'–10'	4'–10'[. . .

Previous Edition and Discussion

Köcher 1964, xxviii, pl. 45
CDLI P285328 (transliteration; photo)
BabMed Corpora (https://www.geschkult.fu-berlin.de/e/babmed/Corpora/BAM-3/BAM-3_-242)

Transliteration

Beginning of ms. a lost

1' a obv.$^?$ 1' [. . . . .] x [. . . . .]

2' a obv.$^?$ 2' [. . . . .]-*su te-ṭe*$_4$*-e*[*n* . . . .]

3' a obv.$^?$ 3' [. . . . . *t*]*a-ṣa-*⸢*na*⸣*-mi-id-m*[*a* . . . .]

4' a obv.$^?$ 4' [. . . . .] 1 SÌLA ZÌ.DA [. . . . .]

5' a obv.$^?$ 5' [. . . . . 1 SÌLA] ZÌ.DA ^{ú}ḪAR.[ḪAR . . . .]

6' a obv.$^?$ 6' [. . . . . 1 SÌ]LA ZÌ.DA ^{ú}GADA x[. . . . .]

7' a obv.$^?$ 7' [. . . . . 1 SÌL]A ZÌ.DA *ka-*[*mu-nu*$^?$ . . . .]

8' a obv.$^?$ 8' [. . . . . 1 SÌL]A ZÌ.DA ^{ú}[. . . . .]

9' a obv.$^?$ 9' [. . . . . 1 SÌLA$^?$] KU PA x[. . . . .]

10' a obv.$^?$ 10' [. . . . . 1 SÌLA$^?$] ⸢KU⸣ GAM.M[A . . . .]

Ms. a breaks; remainder lost

Bound Transcription and Translation

Beginning lost

1' *traces* 2' [. . . . . .] . . . *ṭeṭên* [. . . . . .] 3' [. . . . . . *t*]*aṣṣanam-mid-m*[*a* . . .]

1' *traces* 2' [. . . . .] you grind, [. . .], 3' [. . .] you bandage (her) repeatedly, and [. . . .].

4' [......] *ištēn qa qēm* [......] 5' [... *ištēn qa*] *qēm ḫašî* [......] 6' [...... *ištēn*] *qa qēm kitê* [......] 7' [... *ištēn*] *qa qēm k*[*amūni*(?)......] 8' [...... *ištēn q*]*a qēm* [......] 9' [...... *ištēn qa*] *sīkti*... [......] 10' [... *ištēn qa*] *sīkti sumla*[*lê*......]
Ms. a breaks; remainder lost

4' [......], one litre flour of [...], 5' [... one litre] powder of *ḫašû*-plant, [...], 6' [... one lit]re powder of flax, [...], 7' [... one litr]e powder of c[umin(?), ...], 8' [... one litr]e powder of [...]-plant, [...], 9' [... one litre] powder of ... [...], 10' [... one litre] powder of *ṣumlalû*-plant, [......].

Notes

Line 3': The fragmentary verb is interpreted as a Gtn-stem durative form of *ṣamādu* (*taṣṣanammidma*). Cf. also the Middle Babylonian medical text BAM 398 rev. 46' from Nippur (Scurlock 2014a, 564): *ta-aṣ-ṣa-na-mid-su* "you bandage him repeatedly (with it)".

Lines 4'–10': The use of flours or powdered plant materials points to the preparation of a bandage. Cf. BAM 244: 21–30 (text B.1.1) for a similar prescription of a bandage using more than 20 different powders or flours (ZÌ.(DA) or KU). For discussion of the Akkadian readings of these logograms, see *infra* notes to text B.1.1.

II.1.4 A Middle Assyrian Tablet with Birth Incantations and Prescriptions for Problems after Delivery

Like the preceding text II.1.3, this Middle Assyrian tablet from the Giancarlo Ligabue Collection (Venice) may have originated from Assur, perhaps from the so-called library of Tiglath-pileser I (as suggested by Fales (1989, 195)).[240] The text, which can be described as an excerpt compiled from at least two different sources, begins with four sections with prescriptions for women after delivery suffering from symptoms of intestinal blockage and retention of the lochia (postpartum blood/ fluids). The treatments applied to counter these symptoms, especially fumigations, baths, bandages, share similarities with other medical cuneiform texts within and beyond the women's healthcare texts (see the notes below for discussion), but also with therapies for women in the Hippocratic gynaecological treatises (Steinert 2014a; 2014b). The present text describes a sequence of treatments (fumigations, tampon, ointment) that continued for two days, after which recovery was expected. For the case that the patient's state had not improved by then, the text provides a second sequence of treatments (bath, ointment, bandage) that had to be applied. The specific therapies used to induce the lochia attest to an underlying idea of applying heat to provoke the flow of blood/fluids locked in the body, making this remarkable text one of the earliest examples within the Mesopotamian women's healthcare texts in which pathological body states are conceptualized and manipulated in terms of the properties hot/cold (see the *Introduction* and the notes below for further discussion).

The remedies are followed by a scribal note and by two Akkadian birth incantations used to speed up difficult labour. The second of these incantations is a version of the incantation "A Cow of Sîn" (see BAM 248 (text D.1.1), the Neo-Assyrian Birth Compendium, with all parallels). Moreover, the first of both incantations, which describes the suffering of the woman in difficult childbirth with highly poetic imagery, also finds almost verbatim parallels in several lines of another birth incantation in BAM 248, suggesting processes of transmission and re-working of older forerunners in first millennium BCE texts. The text of ms. A contains several scribal mistakes and textual corruptions, perhaps being witness to an unexperienced scribe.

240 For this library, see Weidner 1952–1953, *AfO* 16, 197–215; Pedersén 1985, 31–42 Library M2; Zomer 2018, 39. Another Middle Assyrian medical-therapeutic text attributed to this library is BAM 208 (CDLI P281819) = Abusch and Schwemer 2011, CMAwR 1, text 2.4 (against witchcraft-induced ailments).

241 Photos of the tablet were published by Fales 1989, 195.

List of Manuscripts

Siglum	Museum Number	Copy	Collation	Format; Ductus	Provenience
A	Ligabue –	*Iraq* 31, Pl. V–VI	Photo coll.[241]	Single-column tablet in portrait format; Middle Assyrian script; ca. 12th/11th cent. BCE	Assur(?)

Overview

i	Prescription for a postpartum woman suffering from retention of the lochia (fumigation, tampon) A obv. 1–13	1–13
ii	Prescription for a postpartum woman suffering from retention of the lochia (fumigation, ointment) A obv. 14–18	14–18
iii	Prescription for a postpartum woman suffering from retention of the lochia (bath, ointment) A obv. 19–26	19–26
iv	Prescription for a postpartum woman suffering from retention of the lochia (bandage) A rev. 1–5	27–31
v	Scribal note A rev. 6	32
vi	Akkadian incantation for a woman in difficult labour: *multapšiqtu šapšuqat alāda* A rev. 6–24	33–50
vii	Akkadian incantation for a woman in difficult labour: *Gī-Sîn amtu ša Sîn alāda šapšuqat* A rev. 25–l.e. 4	51–62

Previous Edition and Discussion

Lambert 1969, *Iraq* 31, 28–39 (edition)
Albertz 1978, 52 with 230 (notes)
Finkel 1980, *AfO* 27, 45
Röllig 1985, *OrNS* 54, 260–273 (lines 51–62)
Fales 1989, 195–196 No. 62 (photo, translation)
Scurlock 1991, 146–148, 150–151, 173–174, 177–178 with notes 95–96, 107, 109, 114, 116–118, 141, 144–149, 153–155 (discussion)
Stol 2000a, 130 (with notes)
Foster 2005, 1006 (translation of lines 33–50)
Scurlock 2005, 311 (lines 1–3)
Scurlock and Andersen 2005, 282 12.122 (lines 1–3)
Attinger 2008, 21–22 (lines 1–3, 33–49)
Scurlock 2014a, 605–608 (edition)
Scurlock 2014b, 113–114 (translation of lines 1–31)
Marquéz Rowe 2015, *AuOr* 33, 51–62
Zomer 2018, 254–256 (lines 33–50), 363
SEAL Texts No. 7231 and 7232 (lines 33–50, 51–62)
CDLI P282478

Transliteration

1	A obv. 1	MUNUS Ù.TU-*ma em-rat šit-t*[*u*]-*š*[*a*$^{?}$ x (x)]
2	A obv. 2	ŠÀ.MEŠ-*ša es-lu* A.MEŠ-*ša u* MÚD.M[EŠ-*ša ina* ŠÀ-*bi-ša*$^{?}$]
3	A obv. 3	GUR.MEŠ-*ru ana šup-šu-ri-ša* ^{šim}GÚR.GÚR ⸢^{šim}LI⸣
4	A obv. 4	^{ú}KUR.KUR ^{šim}GAM.ME GI DU$_{10}$.GA ^{šim}BAL
5	A obv. 5	^{šim}ŠEŠ ^{šim}ḪAB ILLU *a-bu-ka-ta*
6	A obv. 6	ILLU ^{šim}BULUḪ SUḪUŠ ^{ú}KUR.KUR 11 Ú.ḪI.A
7	A obv. 7	*an-nu-ti* TÉŠ.BI *tu-sa-maḫ* DÈ ^{giš}KIŠI$_{16}$
8	A obv. 8	*ana* ^{dug}KÍR$^{!}$ *te-si-ip* Ú.<ḪI.A> *šá-šu-nu ana* ŠÀ ŠUB-*di*
9	A obv. 9	MUNUS *šá-ši ina* UGU *tu-še-šab ina* TÚG.ḪI.A *tu*-ŠIR-*ši*
10	A obv. 10	^{giš}*si-ḫa* ^{giš}*ar-ga-na* ^{ú}*ba-ri-ra-ta*
11	A obv. 11	ZÀ.ḪI.LI^{sar} DIDA *ina* Ì ÁB$^{!}$(AMAR) KÙ.GA
12	A obv. 12	ḪI.ḪI *ina* ^{síg}ÀKA$^{!}$(ÍL) NIGIN-*ma ana* ŠÀ GAL$_{4}$.LA-*ša* GAR.GAR-*ma*
13	A obv. 13	*ur-ra u* GI$_{6}$ *an-na-a* DÙ.MEŠ-*uš-ma* DU$_{10}$-*ba* IGI-*mar*
14	A obv. 14	*ina* 2 *u*$_{4}$-*me* ⸢x x x⸣ *tu-šab-šal* E$_{11}$-*la-ma*
15	A obv. 15	MUNUS *ina* UGU [*t*]*u-še-ša-ab ina* TÚG.ḪI.A *tu*-ŠIR-*ši*
16	A obv. 16	KAŠ *ana* UGU ⸢*qut*-PA$^{?}$⸣ ^{ri} *tu-sa-làḫ* ⸢*qú-ut*$^{?}$⸣-*ru*
17	A obv. 17	*ana* KA.MEŠ-*šá u na-ḫi-ri-ša e-ru-ub*
18	A obv. 18	Ì DU$_{10}$.GA ŠÉŠ.MEŠ *še-ḫa* NU IGI-*mar-ma* TI
19	A obv. 19	*šum*$_{4}$-*ma* DU$_{10}$-*ba* NU IGI-*mur* ^{urudu}ŠEN.TUR A.MEŠ *u* KAŠ DIRI
20	A obv. 20	^{šim}EREN.NA ^{šim}ŠUR.MÌN.NA ^{šim}*dáp-ra-na*
21	A obv. 21	^{šim}GÚR.GÚR ^{šim}LI ^{šim}GAM.ME ^{ú}KUR.KUR
22	A obv. 22	^{ú}*si-ḫa* ^{ú}*ar-ga-na* ^{ú}*ba-ri-ra-ta*
23	A obv. 23	GAZI^{sar} NUMUN *šu-ši* 11 Ú.ḪI.A *an-nu-ti*
24	A obv. 24	TÉŠ.BI *ana* ŠÀ ŠUB-*di tu-šab-šal ta-šá-ḫal*
25	A obv. 25	*ina* ŠÀ RA-*si* E$_{11}$-*ma* Ì.GIŠ ŠÉŠ *ana* É
26	A obv. 26	*pag-ri tu-še-rab-ši še-ḫa* NU IGI DU$_{8}$-*ma*
27	A rev. 1	⸢ŠEŠ⸣.MEŠ ŠIM.MEŠ DÙ.A.BI-*šu-nu* ^{giš}*ba*$^{!}$(SU)-*ri-ra*-[*t*]*a*
28	A rev. 2	KI DIDA BIL ḪI.ḪI *ana* ^{dug}BÁN *te-si-ip*
29	A rev. 3	*ina* ^{im}<ŠU>.RIN.NA *te*$^{!}$-*se-kér* E$_{11}$-*ma ina* TÚG.ḪI.A

30 A rev. 4 *te-ṭe*$_4$*-ri* ^{uzu}*em-ši-e-ša* ^{uzu}*šu-ḫe-e-ša*

31 A rev. 5 *u* ^{uzu}*ra-pal-te-ša* LÁL-*id-ma* TI

---

32 A rev. 6 *tup-pu ši-it up*$^{!}$(ŠA)*-pu-ša-ta la ga-am-rat*

---

33 A rev. 7 ^{munus}LA.<RA>.AḪ-*tu šap-šu-qa-at* Ù.TU.MEŠ-*da*

34 A rev. 8 Ù.TU.MEŠ *šap-šu-qa-at še-er-ra ku-na-at*

35 A rev. 9 *še-er-ra ku-na-at ana qa-tu-ú* ZI-*te* ŠU.RA ^{giš}SAG.KUL

36 A rev. 10 *sa-ni-iq* KÁ *ana ti-nu-qí ka*$^{!}$(la)*-lu-ú pi-it* ARḪUŠ-*mu*

37 A rev. 11 *ba-ni-tu u-bu-ḫa-at* SAḪAR$^{!}$(BA).MEŠ *mu-ú-te*

38 A rev. 12 *ki-i* ^{giš}GIGIR *u-bu-ḫa-at* SAḪAR$^{!}$(BA).MEŠ *ta-ḫa-zi*

39 A rev. 13 *ki-i* ^{giš}APIN *u-bu-ḫa-at* SAḪAR$^{!}$(BA).MEŠ GIŠ.ÙR$^{!}$(TIR).MEŠ

40 A rev. 14 *ki-i* UR.SAG *mu-ut-taḫ-iṣ ina* MÚD.MEŠ-*šá ṣa-la-at*

41 A rev. 15 *ú-ṭa-a* IGI.MEŠ-*šá ul ta-da-gal ka-at-ma šap-ta-šá*

42 A rev. 16 *ul ta-pa-te ši-mat mu-te u ši-ma-ta ša-pa-a* IGI.MEŠ-*šá*

43 A rev. 17 *ú-ia* KA-*ša ik-ta-na-at-tam ul* ŠE.GA-*a*

44 A rev. 18 GEŠTU.MEŠ-*šá ul sa-qa-at* ^{uzu}GABA-*sa sà-pu-ḫu ku-lu-lu-ša*

45 A rev. 19 *pu-ṣu-ni ul pa-ṣu-na-at bul-ta ul ti-šu*

46 A rev. 20 GUB-*za*-<<*ma*>>*-am-ma* DUG$_4$.GA.MEŠ-*si re-ma-nu-ú* ^{d}AMAR.UTU

47 A rev. 21 *an-nu-ú te-šu-ú la-a-ma-ku-ma ku-ul-da-a-ni*

48 A rev. 22 *še-li kak-ka ša-ti bu-nu-ut* DINGIR.MEŠ

49 A rev. 23 *bu-nu-ut* LÚ.U$_{18}$.LU *lu-ú-ṣa-ma li-mur* IZI.GAR

50 A rev. 24 ÉN$^{!}$(IGI) É.NU.RU *ši-ip-tu ša mu-ul-tap-ši-iq-te*

---

51 A rev. 25 *gi-se-en* <<^{d}30>> GÉME *šá* ^{d}30 *a-la-da šap-šu-qa-at še-er-ra*

52 A rev. 26 *ku-na-at še-er-ra ku-na-at ana qa-tu-ú* ZI-*te* ŠU.RA *si-ku-rum*

53 A rev. 27 *sa-ni-iq* KÁ-*bu ana ti*$^{!}$(nu)*-nu*$^{!}$(ti)*-qí la-ku*$^{!}$(lu)*-ú* IGI.DU$_8$-*ši-ma* ^{d}30

54 A rev. 28 *i-ra-'-ši ana nu-ru-ub* Ú.MEŠ *ir-ta-na-'i ina sa-ḫi m*[*aš-q*]*í*$^{?}$

55 A u. e. 1 NAG.MEŠ-[*ši* A].MEŠ *ana* UGU GU$_4$.ÁB *il-ti-ki-iṭ bu-ru*

56 A u. e. 2 *ek-du* U$_4$.MEŠ-*ša ana mu-le-e* ITI.MEŠ-*ša ana* [*ga-ma-ri*]

57 A u. e. 3 *ta-aḫ-ti-me-iš ta-ḫa-al bu-ur-tu ina i*[*k-ki-li-ša*$^{?}$]

58 A u. e. 4 *ina* GÙ.MEŠ *ḫi-li-ša* ^{d}30 *na-an-na-ar* AN-*e* [x x x x (x)]

59 A l. e. 1 2 *ši-na* DUMU.MUNUS ^{d}*a-nim* TA AN-*e ú-ri-da-a-ni* 1-*te na-ša-at* A.MEŠ [*ḫ*]*i-i-li ša-ni-tu*

60 A l. e. 2 *na-ša-at* Ì *pu-ú-ri* A.MEŠ *ḫi-li* <<*li*>> *il-pu-ut* SAG.KI.MEŠ-*sa* Ì *pu-ú-ri* <<x>> *ú*-<*šap*>-*pi*-<*ḫa*>

61 A l. e. 3 DÙ.A.BI SU.MEŠ-*ša* GIN$_7$-*ma gi-i-*^{d}30 GÉME *ša* ^{d}30 *e-eš-ri-ši* Ù.TU-*du lu*-Ù.TU-*id*

62 A l. e. 4 *ar-da-a-tu* ^{munus}LA.RA.AḪ.MEŠ ÉN!(IGI) É.NU.RU

Bound Transcription and Translation

[1] *sinništu ūlid-ma emrat šittūš[a . . .]* [2] *qerbūša eslū mûša u dām[ūša ina libbī-ša]* [3] *turrū ana šupšurīša kukru burāšu* [4] *atā'išu ṣumlalû qanû ṭābu ballukku* [5] *murru ṭūru ḫīl abukkati* [6] *ḫīl baluḫḫi šuruš atā'iši ištešššeret šammī* [7] *annûti išteniš tusammaḫ pēmti ašāgi* [8] *ana kirri tessip šammī šâšunu ana libbi tanaddi* [9] *sinništa šâši ina muḫḫi tušeššab ina lubāri tussarši(?)* [10] *sīḫa argāna barīrāta* [11] *saḫlê billata ina šaman litti(!) elleti* [12] *tuballal ina itqi talammī-ma ana libbi ūrīša taštanakkan-ma* [13] *urra u mūša annâ tētenepuš-ma ṭūba immar*

[1] (If) a woman gives birth and subsequently she is distended, her excrement(?) [. . .], [2] her intestines are constipated, her fluids and [her] blood are blocked [in her belly(?)], [3] to make her release (it): *kukru*-aromatic, juniper, [4] *atā'išu*-plant, *ṣumlalû*-aromatic, "sweet reed", *ballukku*-aromatic, [5] *murru*-aromatic, *ṭūru*-aromatic, *abukkatu*-resin, [6] resin of *baluḫḫu*-aromatic, root of *atā'išu*-plant – these eleven drugs [7] you mix together. You gather charcoals of *ašāgu*-thorn [8] into a *kirru*-vessel, you throw these drugs into it, [9] you have that woman sit down above it, you *wrap* her with cloth. [10] You mix *sīhu*-wood, *argānu*-conifer, *barīrātu*-plant, [11] *saḫlû*-cress, (and) *billatu*-substance with fat from a pure cow(!). [12] You wrap (this mixture) in a wad of wool and insert it repeatedly into her vagina. [13] You continue doing this for (one) day and (one) night, then she will experience improvement.

---

[14] *ina šanî ūme . . . tušabšal tušellâ-ma* [15] *sinništa ina muḫḫi tušeššab ina lubāri tussarši(?)* [16] *šikara ina muḫḫi qutārī(?) tusallaḫ qutru* [17] *ana pîša u naḫīrīša errub* [18] *šamna ṭāba taptanaššaš šēḫa lā immar-ma iballuṭ*

[14] On the second day, you boil . . . . (When) you have taken it out (of the fire), [15] you let the woman sit down over it, you *wrap* her with cloth. [16] You sprinkle beer on the fumigants(?); the smoke [17] should enter her mouth and nostrils. [18] You rub (her) repeatedly with fragrant oil. She should not catch a draft(?), then she will recover.

[19] *šumma ṭūba lā īmur tangussa mê u šīkara tumalla* [20] *erēna šurmēna daprāna* [21] *kukra burāša ṣumlalâ atā'iša* [22] *sīḫa argāna barīrāta* [23] *kasâ zēr šūši ištešššeret šammī annûti* [24] *išteniš ana libbi tanaddi tušabšal tašaḫḫal* [25] *ina libbi taraḫḫassi illī-ma šamna tapaššaš ana bīt* [26] *pagri tušerrabši šēḫa lā immar ippaššar-ma*

[19] If she does not experience improvement, you fill a *tangussu*-vessel with water and beer. [20] Cedar, cypress, *daprānu*-juniper, [21] *kukru*-aromatic, *burāšu*-juniper, *ṣumlalû*-aromatic, *atā'išu*-plant, [22] *sīḫu*-plant, *argānu*-conifer, *barīrātu*-plant, [23] *kasû*-plant, seed of *šūšu*-liquorice – these eleven drugs [24] you pour together into (the vessel). You boil (and) strain (it), [25] you wash her with it. (When) she comes out (from the bath), you rub (her) with oil. You take her into [26] (her) *own room*(?). She should not catch a draft(?), then she will find relief.

---

[27] *annûti riqqī kalīšunu barīrāta* [28] *itti billati qalīti tuballal ana sūti tessip* [29] *ina tinūri tesekker tušellâ-ma ina lubāri* [30] *teṭerri emšēša šuḫḫēša* [31] *u rapaltēša taṣammid-ma iballuṭ*

[27] Then you mix all the afore mentioned aromatics (and) *barīrātu*-wood [28] with roasted *billatu*-substance (instant beer mixture), you collect (it) into a *sūtu*-vessel. [29] You heat (lit. enclose it) in an oven. (Then) you take it out and *spread* (the mixture) on pieces of cloth. [30] You bandage her lower abdomen, her buttocks, [31] and her thighs (with it). Then she will recover.

---

[32] *tuppu šīt uppušat(!) lā gamrat*

[32] This tablet is executed (properly/ready for use?), but not finished.

33 *multapšiqtu šapšuqat alāda*	33 "The woman in hard labour has great difficulty giving birth,
34 *alāda šapšuqat šerra kunnat*	34 She has great difficulty giving birth, she is stuck with the baby.
35 *šerra kunnat ana qatû napište maḫiṣ sikkūru*	35 She is stuck with the baby to the point of ending (her) life. The door bolt is locked,
36 *saniq bābu ana tēnūqi kalû*(!) *pīt rēmi*	36 the door is *closed* (lit. fastened) against the suckling infant. The opening of the womb is blocked(!).
37 *bānītu ubbuḫat eprī mūte*	37 The (delivering) mother is covered with the dust of death.
38 *kī narkabti ubbuḫat eprī tāḫāzi*	38 Like a chariot, she is covered with the dust of battle,
39 *kī epinni ubbuḫat eprī šukkuki*(?)	39 like a plough, she is covered with the dust of harrowing(?),
40 *kī qarrādi muttaḫḫiṣi ina dāmēša ṣal'at*	40 like a fighting warrior, she lies in her blood.
41 *uṭṭâ īnāša ul tadaggal katmā šaptāša*	41 Her eyes are darkened, she cannot see; her lips are closed (lit. covered),
42 *ul tapatte šimat mūte u šimmata šāpâ īnāša*	42 she cannot open (them). Her eyes are *clouded* with the signs of death and with paralysis.
43 *ūya pīša iktanattam ul šemâ*	43 The woe of her mouth keeps covering (her),
44 *uznāša ul sāqat irassa sappuḫū kulūlūša*	44 her ears cannot hear. Her breast is not restrained, her headbands are loosened.
45 *puṣunnī ul paṣṣunat būlta ul tīšu*	45 She is not covered with a veil, (but) she feels no shame.
46 *izizam-ma ištanassi*(?) *rēmānû Marduk*	46 Stand by, oh merciful Marduk, *while she keeps calling out*:
47 *annû tēšû lamâku kuldanni*	47 'Here is confusion, I am surrounded, reach for me!'
48 *šēli kakka šâti bunût ilāni*	48 Bring forth that sealed one, a creation of the gods,
49 *bunût a'īli lūṣâ-ma līmur nūra*	49 a creation of humankind! Let it come out and see the light!"
50 ÉN É.NU.RU *šiptu ša multapšiqte*	50 Enuru-incantation. A spell for a woman having difficulty in delivery.

---

51 *Gī-Sîn amtu ša Sîn alāda šapšuqat šerra*	51 Gī-Sîn, the maidservant of Sîn, has difficulty in (her) delivery. The child
52 *kunnat šerra kunnat ana qatû napište maḫiṣ sikkūru*	52 is stuck, the child is stuck, to bring (her) life to an end. The bolt is lowered,
53 *saniq bābu ana tēnūqi lakê īmuršī-ma Sîn*	53 the door is *closed* (lit. fastened) for the suckling infant. Sîn saw her and
54 *irā'ši ina nurub šammē irtana''i ina saḫḫi m[ašq]î*	54 fell in love with her. Among the lushest grasses he always pastured her, at a meadow with a water[place]
55 *iltanaqqī[ši] mê ana muḫḫi litti iltikiṭ būru*	55 he always gave her water to drink. The wild bull mounted the cow.
56 *ekdu ūmēša ana mullê arḫēša ana [gamāri]*	56 When her days came to an end, her months were finished,
57 *taḫtimiš taḫâl būrtu ina i[kkillīša]*	57 the cow bent down (and) was taken with labour pains. At [her crying],
58 *ina rigmī ḫīlīša Sîn nannār šamê* [. . .]	58 at her screaming in labour, Sîn, the luminary of heaven, [*heard her screaming*].
59 *šittā šina mārāt Anim ultu šamê ūridāni ištēte našât mê ḫīlī šanītu*	59 Two are daughters of Anu. They descended from heaven. One carried water of labour, the second
60 *našât šaman pūri mê ḫīlī ilput pūssa šaman pūri ušappiḫa*(!)	60 carried oil-from-the-jar. One smeared her forehead with water of labour, with oil-from-the-jar (the other) sprinkled(!)
61 *kala zumrīša kīma Gī-Sîn amtu ša Sîn ešriši tūlidu lūlid*	61 her whole body. Just as Gī-Sîn, the maidservant of Sîn, gave birth normally, may
62 *ardatu multapšiqtu* ÉN É.NU.RU	62 (also) this young woman in difficult labour [61] give birth!" [62] Enuru-incantation.

Notes

Lines 1–3: Scurlock and Andersen (2005, 282 with 12.122) interpret the symptom description as "uterine atony". For discussion, see also Scurlock 2005, 311. The scribe omitted the expected *šumma* "if" at the beginning of line 1.

Line 1: The reading *šit-t[u]-š[a]* in line 1 tentatively follows Scurlock 2014a, 605. Note, however, that the word *šittu* "excrement" is rare (CAD Š/3, 142 s.v. *šittu* C). Note also Geller 2005a, No. 29: 6', 8'; No. 30: 14'.

Lines 2–3: The restoration of line 2 follows Scurlock (2014a, 607; 2014b, 113) who translates: "her waters and [her] blood have gone back [inside her]". I suggest analysing the verb GUR.MEŠ-*ru* in line 3 as *turrū*, i.e. as a D-stem 3rd person masc. plur. stative form. This is in accordance with the other verbal forms referring to symptoms in lines 1–2 (which are also statives), and also in accordance with all other instances of "blocked fluids", see the *Introduction* of this volume, with BM 38624+ obv. i 24'–25', 30'–31', ii 19'ff.; K.8678+ rev. 3' (written A.MEŠ GUR-*át* or *tur-rat*, see texts A.2.1 and A.1.4). A variant phrase referring to "blocked fluids" (*mê turrēti/turrūti*) is encountered in BAM 240: 67' (text D.2.1). For the meaning of the verb *târu* "to return; to make turn back" (D-stem) in the sense of "to be blocked, closed (from the inside)" in connection with doors or gates, see CAD T, 273b sub 11d; CAD S, 143 sub 11; Steinert 2013, *JMC* 22, 7–8. The "fluids" (*mû*) are understood here as the discharges emitted by woman during and after delivery rather than amniotic fluid (to which *mû* can also refer in some contexts).

The passage *emrat . . . ana šupšurīša* is translated in CAD P, 243 s.v. *pašāru* sub 12a as "(if a woman giving birth) has colic . . . to effect her release (from pain)". The verb *emēru* may refer to distention or bloating (of the intestines, following AHw 214, s.v. *emēru* II "aufgetrieben sein/werden") or to a state associated with pain (as proposed in CAD E, 148 "to have intestinal trouble (colic or the like)"); see also Schmidtchen 2021, 549–550; Scurlock 1991, *Incognita* 2, 177 note 141. The verb *pašāru* occurs again at the end of line 26, in the prognosis DU$_8$-*ma* (= *ippaššar*?) "she will find relief / release". The phrase *ana šupšurīša* "to cause her release" in line 3 presumably refers to the aim of inducing the expulsion of the postpartum fluids here (in other healing texts it can also refer more generally to undoing of witchcraft or release from sickness). See also Scurlock 1991, 178 note 154 (for the similar use of du$_8$ in reference to releasing the amniotic fluids in delivery).

Lines 7–9: A similar procedure for a fumigation is described in a Neo-Assyrian text on rectal diseases from Assur (BM 103386 rev. 9–12; Heeßel 2018, 322, 328, 335):

> 8 *šammē*(Ú.ḪI.A) *annûte*(ŠEŠ) *ištēniš*(DIŠ-*niš*) *tasâk*(SÚD) <<*ina*>> *pēnti*(DÈ) *ašāgi*(KIŠI$_{16}$) *ina kirri*(^{dug}KÍR) *tašakkan*(GAR-*an*) [11] *šammē*(Ú.ḪI.A) *šá-šu-nu ana pāni*(IGI) *tanaddi*(ŠUB) *amēla*(NA) *šu-a-tu ina muḫḫi*(UGU) *tušeššebšu*(TUŠ-*šú*) *tuqattaršu*(SAR-*šú*) *adi pit*$^{?}$*-ri-šú* [12] *i-lab-bi-ku u zu'ta*(IR) *inaddû*(ŠUB-*ú*) *illak*(DU-*ak*) *ina šāri*(TU$_{15}$) *zunni*(IM.A.BI) *u ṣēti*(UD.DA) *tu-ser-šú-ma iballuṭ*(TI)

> "(List of ingredients) – these eight plants you pound together, you place coals from *ašāgu*-thorn in a *kirru*-vessel. [11] These plants you put onto it. You have that man sit above sit, you fumigate him, until his . . . [12] *become soaking (wet)* and he exudes sweat. (When) it (the sweat) flows, you should shield(?) him from wind, rain and heat of the sun. Then he will recover."

Incidentally, the fumigation recipes in ms. A lines 3–9 and BM 103386 rev. 9–12 share three ingredients (*kukru*, *atā'išu* and resin of *baluḫḫu*-aromatic). Interestingly, BM 103386 obv. 16'–18' (Heeßel 2018, 319, 325) mentions a barber's stool (*litti gallābi*), on which the patient had to sit during the fumigation; also found in BAM 104: 62 and dupl. (Geller 2005a, No. 28), referring to a stool (^{giš}ŠÚ.A). In our ms. A, a stool is not mentioned, but perhaps this instruction was simply omitted. This stool presumably had a hole in the middle of the seat. Hippocratic texts for women's diseases describe a comparable apparatus and practice of fumigation from below.[242]

Line 8: Scurlock 2014a, 607 and 2014b, 113 translates ^{dug}KÍR (= *kirru*) as "(an overturned) pottery drum", presumably because KÍR can also be read ÙB = *uppu* "drum". The sign KÍR (LIBIŠ) is written in a defective form (it should consist of the signs ÁBxŠÀ, but the scribe wrote ÁBxSA). However, the *kirru*-vessel is attested in other prescriptions for fumigation (see previous note); it refers to a (storage) vessel of ovoid or *pithos* shape made clay, metal or stone; it is also a container for beer of a standardized size, see CAD K, 408–410 s.v. *kirru* A; SAD Vol. 3, 85 *kirru* I; Gaspa 2014, *Contenitori*, 123–125,

242 See e.g. *Diseases of Women* II, 5 (Potter 2018, 277): "Use a stool with an opening (sc. in its seat) and clothe the woman (var. set the woman upon it) by wrapping her in garments such that no air will be admitted." Similarly, *Diseases of Women* II, 94 (Potter 2018, 435). Hippocratic recipes, for fumigations/fomentations sometimes required digging a hole in the ground, in which a fire was lit for burning the fumigants; or the latter were filled into a vessel sealed with a lid in which a tube was fixed (which was then inserted in the woman's orifice). See Steinert 2014a; 2014b for discussion.

Fig. 16. In ritual texts, it served as a recipient for libated liquids. For the verb *esēpu* "to gather/collect" substances, such as coals, liquids, see CAD E, s.v. *esēpu* sub 1b-3'.

Line 9: The phrase *ina* TÚG.ḪI.A *tu*-ŠIR-*ši* is also found in line 15 in a parallel procedure for a fumigation. For the spelling TÚG.ḪI.A (= *lubaru* "a piece of cloth, rag") in medical texts, see CAD L, 230 sub 3a. The verbal form has been interpreted in different ways. CAD Š/2, 336a s.v. *šêru* B transliterates *tu-šer-ši* and books the present passage under a verb *šêru* B, as the only attestations for a verb *šêru* "to wrap, to envelop" (this reading is followed by Scurlock 2014a, 605). AHw 1219b assumes that the verb belonged to *šêru* A "to rise early" (D-stem). Lambert (1969, 29–30, 37), transliterated *tu*-ŠER-*ši* and tentatively translated "you rub her down(?) with a woolen cloth". He commented that the sign ŠIR can have the phonetic value sir_4 in Late Babylonian texts and suggested a relation with the verb *sêru/sâru*, which occurs in medical texts in the meaning "to rub (the body with medication)" (G- and D-stem; AHw 1038; CAD S, 227–229 s.v. *sêru*). Other examples of D-stem forms of *sêru* (from first millennium BCE texts) are spelled *tu-sa-'a-ar*, however, see CAD S, 229 sub 3.

Heeßel (2018, 335) commented on a few medical passages, in which the verb *tu-ser*(SUD)-*šú-ma* occurs in a comparable context, in a prescription for a fumigation, as ms. A. He proposed that *tu-ser*(SUD)-*šú-ma* may have to be analysed as a D-stem form of *esēru* "to enclose, to imprison". In the passages, he suggests *tu-ser*(SUD)-*šú-ma* rather has the meaning "to shield", in an instruction to protect the patient from "wind, rain and the heat of the sun", see BM 103386 rev. 12 (Heeßel 2018, 322 *ina šāri*(TU_{15}) *zunni*(IM.A.BI) *u ṣēti*(UD.DA) *tu-ser-šú-ma* TI; also BAM 549 i 6' (*ina zunni*(IM.A.BI) *u ṣēti*(UD.DA) *tu-s*[*er-šú-ma* TI]). In light of the similar context, it is likely that the expression *ina* TÚG.ḪI.A *tu*-ŠIR-*ši* in ms. A is the same verb (reading *tu*-sir_4-*ši*). Since however a durative form *tussaršu/-ši* would be expected, the signs SUD and ŠIR may have had a phonetic value /*sar*/ in these instances (cf. Borger 2004, MZL, No. 115, 584; AHw 249b; CAD E, 335b sub 4). De Ridder (2018, 55–56 § 84) discusses similar spellings in Middle Assyrian texts, where a CvC-sign with a fixed phonetic value containing /u/ or /i/ as the vowel are used to indicate an /a/, e.g. *i*-DIN for *iddan*, *e*-MUR for *emmar* and *ik-ta-ṣir* for *iktaṣar*.

Line 11: The sign after Ì looks like AMAR (which corresponds to *būru* "calf"), cf. Scurlock 2014a, 605). The context requires an emendation to ÁB! KÙ.GA "pure cow" (the signs AMAR and ÁB are very similar). The ingredient "fat from a pure cow", referring to cream or butter, is found in many other texts, see CAD Š/1, 329 sub n. See also the bilingual Old Babylonian birth incantation AUAM 73.3094 rev. 6'–7' (Wasserman and Zomer 2022, No. 10 lines 44–45); Farber 1977, 59: 52, also ibid., 61: 62, 66.

Line 13: CAD Ṭ, 117 sub b interprets the verb DÙ.MEŠ-*uš-ma* as a G-stem instead of a Gtn-stem of *epēšu*, translating: "do this (*teppušma*) day and night and you will see (*tammar*) good results".

Lines 14–16: The word E_{11}-*la-ma* in line 14 is interpreted differently in Scurlock (2014a, 607; 2014b, 114), translating "After she comes out (of the bath)". However, bathing/washing the patient has not been part of the treatment instructions up to this point. Only in the following prescription in line 25, the verb *elû* is found following the verb *raḫāṣu* "to wash/bath": RA-*si* E_{11}-*ma* "you wash her (with a lotion); (when she comes out (of the bath), . . .)". Thus, I understand the phrase E_{11}-*la-ma* in line 14 differently, as part of the preparation procedure (*tušellâ-ma* "you take (it) out (of the oven/fire)"), see also Lambert 1969, *Iraq* 31, 29–30. An unidentified substance was first boiled in an oven, then taken out and beer was sprinkled on the hot contents to produce vapours which were led to the woman's body openings. The patient sat down over the vessel containing the hot substance and her head and body was covered with cloth not to let the fumes or vapour escape. This treatment is very similar to other Babylonian as well as Hippocratic gynaecological recipes for fumigation from below (Steinert 2014a; 2014b).

The reading of the damaged term for a *materia medica* in line 14 is uncertain. I interpret the term before *tu-sa-làḫ* "you sprinkle" in line 16 as ⸢*qut*-PA$^{?}$⸣^{ri} for *qutārī* "fumigants" (following the restoration [*qutā*]*rī* in CAD Š/2, 336 s.v. *šêru* B; for the pseudo-logographic spelling *qut*-PA = *qut-āru*, see Reiner 1959–1960, 150b); Scurlock (2014a, 605) reads ⸢*qí*⸣-*ri* "hot bitumen" instead (as proposed in CAD S, 87b s.v. *salāḫu* sub 5b [*q*]*í*(?)-*ri*). At the end of line 16, I propose to restore ⸢*qú-ut*⸣-*ru* "smoke". Scurlock (2014a, 605) emends to ⸢*qut*!⸣-*ru*, following CAD Q, 326b s.v. *qutru* sub 1c.

Line 17: The plural KA.MEŠ-*šá* in *ana* KA.MEŠ-*šá u na-ḫi-ri-ša e-ru-ub* "(the smoke) should enter her mouth (lit. mouths) and nostrils" could indicate that not only the mouth is meant here, but "body openings" (specifically those of the lower body). However, in line 60, one also finds a logographic writing with a plural SAG.KI.MEŠ-*sa*, although the pronominal suffix indicates a singular noun (*pūssa* "her forehead"). Therefore, the fumigation in the prescription may have been administered via mouth and nostrils rather than the patient's genitals, either to treat the gastro-intestinal complaints mentioned before, or because ancient healers assumed an internal connection between the mouth and the uterus (for this notion, see e.g. Steinert 2021a, *Byzantinische Forschungen* 33, 48; Pommerening 2023).

Lines 18 and 26: The expression *še-ḫa* NU IGI-(*mar-ma*) is interpreted here in the sense of "she should not catch a draft", following CAD Š/2, s.v. *šēḫu* sub 1. For a different interpretation of *šēḫu* "wind" as "flatulence", see Fales 1989, 196; also Scurlock (1991, 151), translating "she will not experience gas but will release (it)". Scurlock (2014a, 607; 2014b, 114) translates more freely: "If she does not experience delirium" (i.e. from the treatment?), presumably because *šēḫu* "wind" can also refer to a spirit possessing a person (cf. CAD Š/2, s.v. *šēḫu* sub 2b).

The recommendation given in lines 18 and 26 reminds us of similar instructions in other medical texts to protect the patient from wind and other adverse weather influences following specific treatments, for example, in the case of treatments during which the patient was exposed to heat and sweating was induced.[243] For example, in a prescription for a fumigation against rectal disease discussed earlier (BM 103386 rev. 12; Heeßel 2018, 322) we find the instruction: *ina šāri*(TU$_{15}$) *zunni*(?, IM.A.BI) *u ṣēti*(UD.DA) *tu-ser-šú-ma* TI "(When the sweat flows,) you should shield(?) him from wind, rain(?) and the heat of the sun; then he will recover". See also BAM 549 obv. i 6' (in a prescription for some respiratory disease): *ina šāri*(TU$_{15}$) *zunni*(?, IM.A.BI) *u ṣēti*(UD.DA) *tu-s*[*er-šú-ma* TI]). The reading of the logogram IM.A.BI in these passages as *zunnu* "rain" is not certain; it follows a suggestion by Thompson 1934, *RA* 31, 7 fn. 3. The logogram for *zunnu* is usually IM.ŠÈG(=A.AN). An alternative solution for IM.A.BI may be to read it syllabically (or pseudo-logographically) as *šar*$_5$(IM)-*a-bi*, for *šarbu* (also *sar*(*a*)*bu*) "cold/rainy season", cf. CAD Š/2, 60 s.v. *šarbu*.

Lines 19–26: This prescription for the bath/wash shares similarities with BAM 240: 58', a recipe for a wash to treat retention of the lochia and postpartum fever (see text D.2.1 with lines 39'–40' for the symptom description). The latter recipe is shorter and uses fewer ingredients, but several of them are identical.

For *ṭūba amāru* "to experience improvement" (lines 13 and 19), see also CAD Ṭ, 117a, s.v. *ṭūbu* sub b. At the end of a remedy: e.g. BAM 566 i 15: DU$_{10}$.GA *immar*(IGI-*mar*) "he will improve". As introduction to a remedy: e.g. BAM 558 iv 15: *šumma ṭūba*(DU$_{10}$) *lā*(NU) *īmur*(IGI.DU$_8$) "if (his condition) has not improved"; Arnaud 1992, *SMEA* 30, 226: 10': [*šum*]-*ma ṭú-ú-ba i-ta-mar* (medical text from Emar).

For the *tangussu*-vessel (line 19), denoting a metal pot or kettle often used in medical procedures to boil or decoct ingredients, see Gaspa 2014, *Contenitori*, 95. The text BAM 240: 28 associates the use of a *tangussu*-vessel with the physician (*asû*), see text D.2.1.

Lines 25–26: The expression *bīt pagri* is interpreted in CAD P, 14b s.v. *pagru* sub 3a-1' as "burial chamber", (lit. "house of the corpse"), following Lambert 1969, *Iraq* 31, 30 "mausoleum". Scurlock (2014a, 607; 2014b, 114) proposes that *bīt pagri* means "slaughterhouse". Both interpretations seem implausible. I follow a different and much more straightforward idea (courtesy of M. Geller) and regard *bīt pagri*(*ša*) as a term meaning "(her) *own* room/house" (with omitted possessive pronominal suffix -*ša*), meaning that the patient returns to her quarters after coming out of the bath. The word *pagru* "body; self" is often used as an equivalent for *ramānu* "self" in idiomatic expressions. In the present passage, *pagru* exceptionally appears to replace *ramānu*, which is common in genitive expressions where it is used instead of the possessive suffix or pronoun (CAD R, 120–122 sub c-1').

Lines 27–29: For similar prescriptions (bandages) for postpartum complaints, compare e.g. BAM 240: 62'–63' (text D.2.1); BAM 408 ii 4'–10' (text A.2.9). For *šuḫḫu* "buttock(s)", see CAD Š/3, 206 sub mng. 1. Since no other liquid is mentioned in these lines, the term *billatu*, which designates a dry substance used to make a kind of instant beer, presumably refers to the finished *billatu*-beer here (i.e. *billatu* mixed with water), cf. Stol 1971, *BiOr* 28, 161b; 1994, 165.

Line 32: The emendation *up*$^!$-*pu-ša-ta* was proposed by Fales 1989, 196; cf. CAD E, 232b *uppušu* "to copy a tablet"; "to execute properly" (CDA^2, 75); Hunger 1968, 3–4. Scurlock (2014a, 606–607) reads *ša-bu-ša-ta* "(that tablet) is collected", from *šabāšu* "to collect, to gather" (cf. CAD Š/1, 6–8 s.v. *šabāšu*). The latter verb is so far unattested with reference to collecting texts. The scribal note in this line may indicate that the preceding text has been copied in full (from a given original?), but that the text to be assembled on the tablet is not yet completed. Presumably the scribe used at least two different sources for

243 For the same precaution taken by the Hippocratic physicians in connection with the fomentation of a female patient, see Potter 2018, 319 (*Diseases of Women* II Chapter 24): "You should carry out the fomentation during good weather and in a protected location where no cooling will take place, and cover the patient all around with cloths."

assembling ms. A. The verb *gamāru* "to come to an end; to finish" is also unusual here; in similar statements in colophons *qatû* "to finish" ((AL).TIL) is used, see Hunger 1968, 2; Wee 2019a, 318.

Lines 33–50: This incantation has a close parallel to a birth incantation in the Neo-Assyrian Birth Compendium (BAM 248 obv. ii 1–iii 5 = text D.1.1 lines 56–130). The latter composition is much longer than its Middle Assyrian precursor, but several lines seem to have been taken over almost verbatim, see *infra*, text D.1.1 especially lines 77–84, 99–101, 109–111, which are parallel to lines 37–49 here.

Line 33: In accordance with the rubric *šiptu ša multapšiqte* "incantation for a woman in difficult labour" in line 50, the logogram ^{munus}LA.<RA>.AḪ is understood here as *multapšiqtu*, cf. also CAD M/2, s.v. *mušapšiqtu* and *muštapšiqtu*.

Lines 34–35: CAD Q 178b s.v. *qatû* sub 2a interprets the feminine stative *ku-na-at* as *kunnât* "she is too (tenderly) attached (to the child)", as a D-stem of *kanû* "to care (for)"; I assume a D-stem of *kânu* "to fix, to make firm", see also CAD Š/2, 320 s.v. *šerru* sub d-2'. Some translations assume *šerru* in *še-er-ra ku-na-at* is the subject of the feminine stative *kunnat* ("the baby is stuck"), cf. Foster 2005, 1006; Scurlock 2014a, 608, 618 n. 59; Zomer (2018, 254): "she is attached to the baby".

Line 35: Lambert (1969, *Iraq* 31, 31) and Zomer (2018, 254–255) interpret ŠU.RA in lines 35 and 52 as a logogram for *maḫiṣ* "(the bolt) is secure", which is followed here. CAD S, 140a, 258b s.v. *sikkūru* instead assumes a scribal error for *aš-ru* (or *ašra*, a stative of *(w)ašāru*); this interpretation is inspired by an Old Babylonian prayer to the Gods of the Night (von Soden 1936, *ZA* 43, 306: 2: *wašrū* (var. *áš-ru*) *sikkūrū* "the bolts have been lowered" (replaced in the first millennium BCE version by *nadû šigarū ḫargullū*, see Mayer 1976, 533 K. 10659: 5); CAD A/2, 422b *ašāru* D.

Line 36: The emendation of this line follows Stol 2000a, 130 n. 127; Albertz 1978, 230 n. 256; differently CAD T, 344a s.v. *tēnūqu* sub 3 emending the sign sequence *ana ti-nu-qí la-lu-ú* to *ana* NU TI-*qí* (for *lā leqê*) *la-ku*$^{!}$*-ú* "(the door is made fast), not to receive(?) the child". Almost the same sequence is found again in line 53, which seems to repeat lines 35–36 almost verbatim. In the latter passage, however, the scribe wrote NU TI-*qí la-lu-ú* (for which see the note below). Veldhuis (1991, 12, 32, 64) accepts the reading *ana ti-nu-qí la-lu-ú* "for the suckling babe" in line 53, taking *lalû* "kid" (i.e. the young of a goat) as a term referring to a human baby (otherwise uncommon). Still another reading is proposed by Fales (1989, 196), reading (*ti-nu-qí*) *la-lu-ú* as a sandhi-spelling standing for *lā elû* "per non fare uscire il lattante". It is difficult to decide which emendation is to be preferred. I have opted to emend both passages in syntactically different ways. In line 36, I suggest emending *la-lu-ú* to *ka*$^{!}$*-lu-ú*, interpreting this as an irregular stative form of *kalû* "to detain; to keep in confinement; to prevent, hinder (progress); to block", with *pīt rēmi* "opening of the womb" as the subject. This emendation regards line 36 as parallel to the structure of lines 34–35, both of which consist of two phrases with statives. For discussion of the passage (lines 35–36), see also Durand 2012, in *Studies Fales*, 260–261 n. 25.

For the stative of *sanāqu* "to reach (a destination), to check, control", in *saniq bābu* "the door is *closed* (lit. fastened)", with a rare, special meaning "to be fastened" (in reference to doors or gates), see CAD S, 140 sub 5b; Mayer 2022, *OrNS* 91, 346 s.v. *tēnīqu* (translating "kontrolliert (d.h. festgemacht/verschlossen) ist die Tür für den Säugling").

Line 39: Different emendations have been proposed for the phrase SAḪAR$^{!}$.MEŠ ^{giš}TIR.MEŠ, "dust of the woods", which does not yield very good sense. The emendation SAḪAR$^{!}$.MEŠ ^{giš}NIR$^{!}$.MEŠ "the dust of the yoke(s)" (rather than "the dust of the woods") was proposed by Stol 2000a, 130 n. 127. For ^{giš}NIR = *nīru*, cf. also giš-nir-ra = *iṣ nīri* in Ḫh. Tablet V 308 (MSL 6, 32). Foster (*NABU* 2019/2, no. 47) suggests emending to SAḪAR$^{!}$(BA).MEŠ <<^{giš}>>ÙR$^{!}$(TIR).MEŠ "(she is covered) with the dust of constant chafing on the ground, (like a plow)". Sumerian ùr "to drag; to wipe clean; to beat; to sweep away" and ĝiš ùr "to harrow" correspond to *šakāku* "to harrow" in Akkadian, see CAD Š/1, 113–114 s.v. *šakāku* lex. section. Foster suggests that the MEŠ in ÙR.MEŠ indicates a tan-stem in the Akkadian correspondence. However, since the meaning "to harrow" is only attested for the G- and D-stem of *šakāku*, a D-stem infinitive is assumed here.

Line 41: I follow AHw 1555b and Zomer (2018, 254–255) in reading *ú-ta-a* from *etû* (D-stem) "to become dark", rather than *šam-ta-a*, interpreted as an adjective *šumṭû/šamṭû* derived from *maṭû* "to be(come) little" (CAD Š/3, 284a s.v. **šumṭû* "diminished"); Lambert 1969, 31; Scurlock (2014a, 606) translates "her eyes are diminished/weakened").

Line 42: The form *ša-pa-a* in this line (stative third person fem. pl.) is booked under the verb *šapû* which means "to be dense, thick" (usually said of clouds, light, flames, smoke, voices) in CAD Š/1, 489b s.v. *šapû* A sub 1e and in AHw 1177a *šapû* B "dick, dicht, laut sein/werden" sub 5; see also Zomer 2018, 255), together with three attestations from the *Diagnostic Handbook* Tablet 9 (Schmidtchen 2021, 409–410, 41415–416, 420), where this verb describes a symptom of the face (perhaps in the meaning "to be swollen; to swell"). However, since IGI.MEŠ-*šá* "her eyes" is the subject of *ša-pa-a*, Mayer (2016, *OrNS* 85, 189) assumes a derivation from *apû* B "to become dim, clouded" (said of the eyes) in the Š-stem here (*šāpâ* would be an Assyrian form instead of Babylonian *šūpâ*, cf. CAD A/2, 204b; AHw 62b s.v. *apû* III).

The phrase *ši-mat mu-te u ši-ma-ta* is booked under the noun *šimtu* "paint; mark(ing)" in CAD Š/3, 11a s.v. *šimtu* sub 2b-3', translating: "her eyes are clouded(?) with the mark of death and marks(?)". Zomer (2018, 254–255) understands the word *ši-ma-ta* as a genitive form *šīmāte* of *šīmtu* "(bad) fate" (emending *ši-ma-te*!), here denoting (premature) death as a bad fate (cf. CAD Š/3, 16–17 s.v. *šīmtu* sub mng. 2b and 3), forming a pair with the preceding noun *mūtu* "death". See also Scurlock 2014a, 608 and 618 n. 60, who believes that the word *šīmāte* signals the potential death of both mother and baby. My rendering follows Mayer (2016, *OrNS* 85, 189) who interprets *ši-ma-ta* as *šimmatu* "paralysis", translating the passage "vom Mal des Todes und von Lähmung sind ihre Augen verdüstert/verschleiert(?)".

Line 43: For reading *ik-ta-na-at-tam* instead of *ig-ta-na-lut*, see Albertz 1978, 230, n. 260; Stol 2000a, 130. AHw 982b reads the sign KA in *ú-ia* KA-*ša* as *rigmu* "cry" instead of *pû* "mouth".

Line 44: CAD S, 169b derives the form *sa-qa-at* from *sâqu* "to be(come) narrow, tight" translating "her breast (or: pectoral) is not restrained"; also Zomer 2018, 255 (with an Assyrian form *PāS* instead of Babylonian *PīS*). The phrase *ul sāqat irassa* "her breast is not restrained" stands in parallelism to *sappuḫū kulūlūša* "her headbands are loosened" (CAD K, 528b sub 1c; CAD S, 154a sub 5a).

Line 45: Stol (2016b, *BiOr* 73, 422, in his review of Steinert 2012a, *Aspekte*) thinks that *būltu* "shame" in the present passage is used synonymously to *bāštu* "dignity", arguing that the translation "she has no dignity" fits the context of the present passage better (thus also Zomer 2018, 255). However, in my view, the word *būštu* "shame" in the sentence "she wears no veil, she feels no shame (anymore)" marks the reversal of normative, expected behaviour (wearing a veil as a sign of modesty, decency = "shame"), see Steinert 2012a, 462–463; similarly Foster 2005, 1006; also Scurlock 2014a, 608: "she is not covered with a cloak, (yet) she is not ashamed".

Line 46: This line invokes Marduk to act on behalf of the woman in labour. The address has a parallel in BAM 248 obv. ii 44: *ina kittabrīšu iziza Marduk* "Stand by her side, oh Marduk". The verb DUG_4.GA.MEŠ-*si* in line 46 could be interpreted as an Gtn-stem imperative of *šasû* (i.e., "Stand by and speak/keep calling out (*šitassi*), merciful Marduk!", see Stol 2000a, 130; Foster 2005, 1006. Scurlock (2014a, 607–608) erroneously reads DUG_4.GA.MEŠ-*ši* "say something to her". Zomer (2018, 254–256) emends to DUG_4.GA.MEŠ-*ia*!? "(listen to) my utterance", proposing the verb *šime* has been omitted by mistake by the scribe. Zomer (2018, 256) quotes the parallel sentence in KAR 66: 23: *i-zi-za-am-ma ši-mi qa-ba-a-a* "Stand by and listen to my utterance!"

However, it may not be a coincidence that the verb *šasû* "to shout, to cry, to scream" is often found with reference to women in labour. This suggests the patient as the subject of *šasû* here. For instance, a goddess (presumably the mother goddess) is said to "scream like a woman in childbirth" (*išassi kīma ālitti*) in *Gilgamesh Epic* XI 117 (George 2003, 710–711, 886). Furthermore, *šasû* is used in the sense of "to invoke, to appeal to (a deity)", see CAD Š/2, 156–157 s.v. *šasû* sub 4b. The following line 47 may then be the speech of the patient rather than the baby.

Lines 46–47: This line has a parallel in BAM 248 obv. ii 46: *an-nu-ú me-ḫu-ú la-*⌜*ma-ku*⌝ *kul-dan-ni* "This is a storm (that) I am surrounded (with) – reach for me!". This exclamation is generally interpreted as speech uttered by the baby from inside the womb, while the preceding line would represent the midwife's/healer's voice, see Lambert 1969, 36; Finkel 1980, *AfO* 27, 45; Foster 2005, 1006 note 2; Zomer 2018, 256; Scurlock 2014a, 618 n. 62. However, the speech could equally be interpreted as the woman's voice (see BAM 248 (text D.1.1) note on line 101 for comments and the preceding note on line 46).

Line 48: *Šēli* is the Assyrian form of the Š-stem imperative singular of *elû*.

Lines 51–62: The birth incantation is a variant version of the spell "A Cow of Sîn" attested in multiple differing versions from the second and first millennium BCE (see Röllig 1985 and Veldhuis 1991 for in-depth studies of the different versions as well as BAM 248 (text D.1.1) for the synoptic edition of the incantation incorporating the other parallels). The Middle Assyrian version preserved in ms. A differs from the other known versions of the spell in the beginning (lines 51–53) which does not introduce the main character of the narrative as a cow beloved by Sîn, but rather frames the following narrative ambiguously as being concerned with "Gī-Sîn, the maidservant of Sîn" who has difficulty in delivery, which could refer to a woman rather than a cow (see also Veldhuis 1991, 32). In lines 53ff., the text then turns to the story of the cow who is cared for by the moon god acting as her shepherd. This version of the spell also omits the cow's impregnation by the bull but immediately turns to her suffering in labour. The intervention of the protective spirits (here called "the daughters of Anu") sent down from heaven to help the cow deliver is likewise abbreviated compared with the other versions of "A Cow of Sîn". The direct comparison of "Gī-Sîn, the maidservant of Sîn" with any woman in hard labour heightens the ambiguity of the main protagonist of the spell apparent already in the first lines.

Line 53: For the emendation of this line, see Stol 2000a, 130 n. 127 and the note on line 36 above, which also features this line almost in a verbatim manner. The passage is emended differently in CAD T, 344 s.v. *tēnīqu* sub 3, as *lā*(NU) TI-*qí la-ku*$^{!}$-*ú* "not to receive(?) the child". Veldhuis (1991, 12, 32, 64) accepts the reading *ana ti-nu-qí la-lu-ú* "for the suckling babe" in line 53, taking *lalû* "kid" (i.e. the young of a goat) as a term referring to a human baby. It is possible that the sequence *ana* NU ti qí is meant to stand for *ana lā etēqi/šūtuqi* (*lakû*) "not to let the infant pass", since the verb *leqû* "to take" assumed in the reading *ana lā*(NU) *leqê*(TI-*qí*) *lakû* "not to receive(?) the child" is unexpected.

Line 54: For discussion, see also text D.1.1 line 137.

Lines 59–61: Line 59 introduces two protective spirits sent from heaven to help the cow to deliver her calf. Differing from the other versions of "A Cow of Sîn" (see BAM 248 (text D.1.1) and parallels), our ms. A does not refer to them as *lamassu*-spirits but introduces them as 2 *ši-na* DUMU.MUNUS ^{d}*a-nim* "two are they, the daughters of Anu, (they descended from heaven)". For a parallel passage, see e.g. *Maqlû* III 31–33 (Abusch 2016, 306): *šittā šina mārāt Ani ša šamê . . . ultu šamê urradāni* "Two are they, the heavenly Daughters of Anu, . . ., they descend to me from heaven".

The different manuscripts of "A Cow of Sîn" present several textual variations for the lines describing the actions of the divine helpers assisting the cow, which have been re-analysed by Marquéz Rowe 2015, *AuOr* 33, 51–62. As one crucial divergence of ms. A lines 59–60, this text speaks of *mê ḫīlī* "water of (easy) labour" and *šaman pūri* "oil-from-the-jar" as the birth-promoting substances administered to the cow by the daughters of Anu. In the other manuscripts of "A Cow of Sîn", we find *me-e ḫa-li/ḫal-li*, which is now (following Marquéz Rowe 2015, 58–59) understood as "water-from-the bowl" (*ḫallu*), see *infra*, BAM 248 (notes on lines 150–152).

Line 60: Veldhuis (1991, 12–13) accepts the verb *lilput* and translates "he must touch (her forehead)". An emendation to *ilput* "she touched" (= smeared), already proposed by Lambert (1969, 31), is preferred here. The emendation *ú-<šap>-pi-<ḫa>* in line 60 (a D-stem form of *šapāḫu* "to sprinkle") follows Marquéz Rowe 2015, 54, which is in line with the other parallel manuscripts. Arnaud (2007, 76 note on line 8') proposed a differing emendation, reading *uk*$^{!}$*-tana-par*$_{5}$ (from *kapāru* Dtn-stem "to wipe (clean)"). The plural logographic spellings SAG.KI.MEŠ-*sa* and ^{munus}LA.RA.AḪ.MEŠ in lines 60–61 are misleading, since they in fact stand for singular nouns, as the phonetic complement -*sa* and the singular verbal form *lūlid* "may she give birth" in line 61 indicate. See also line 17 for the same phenomenon (in KA.MEŠ-*šá*).

II.2 Texts from the First Millennium BCE

Chapter A
Collections and Handbooks of Remedies for Women for Various Purposes

The texts edited in this chapter are found on tablets from first millennium BCE Assyria and Babylonia that represent shorter and longer collections or handbooks of remedies for women's health covering multiple topics and problems (such as fertility, bleeding, delivery, postpartum problems). In a few exceptional cases, the collected materials also include therapies for medical problems beyond women's health proper (texts A.1.4, A.2.6; cf. also text D.1.3). One of the texts combines prescriptions for rectal disease and an affection of the hips with treatments for women (text A.1.4); a second text combines love magic and prescriptions focusing both on women as targets/patients (text A.2.6).

The remedy collections in chapter A were assembled by ancient scribes both on large two-column tablets (texts A.2.1, A.2.4, A.2.5, A.2.9) and on single-column tablets (texts A.1.1, A.1.4, A.2.2, A.2.3, A.2.6–A.2.8). The latter group may often be characterized as excerpts for different purposes. In one case (text A.2.2), it can be shown that a longer handbook on women's health served as a teaching source, since a few of the prescriptions were copied by a student or apprentice on a small exercise tablet that was found in the same archival context as the longer handbook. Only one of the texts, however, is explicitly defined by the scribe as an extract/excerpt (*nisḫu*) of remedies (text A.2.7). This text most likely formed part of a longer medical series/compendium. Only one text (A.2.6) preserves a colophon.

Three of the texts in Chapter A date to the Neo-Assyrian period and stem from Assur and Sultantepe (text A.1.1–A.1.3). One tablet in a Neo-Babylonian script was excavated at Nineveh (A.1.4). The other texts (A.2.1–A.2.9) come from various sites in Babylonia (e.g. Babylon, Sippar, Uruk) and date to the Neo- and Late Babylonian period. Several of these texts contain loanwords from Aramaic and recipe formats typical for medical material from the Late Babylonian period, including scribal notes referring to oral lore (e.g. text A.2.5). Notable is further that the great majority of the texts treated here does not include any incantations, although occasional healing rituals can be found beside medical prescriptions proper (e.g. texts A.2.1, A. 2.7).

The texts in Chapter A offer many new insights and hitherto unknown materials. Remarkably, some of the prescriptions in these remedy collections are not concerned with gynaecological or obstetric problems but include healing procedures for medical problems such as skin diseases or fevers, i.e. ailments that are not gender-specific *per se*, the treatments for which were usually collected in separate medical compendia or thematic handbooks (e.g. texts A.2.3, A.2.6). One important tablet (text A.2.7) offers the first attestation for recipes for contraception known to date; a second recipe collection also deals with topics such as improving body odour and lack of female sexual desire (text A.2.2). The textual parallels or duplicating prescriptions identified for several of the source texts reflect many continuities in medical concepts and practices related to women's health through the first and second half of the first millennium BCE.

A.1 Texts Found in Assyria

A.1.1 STT 98 and STT 284: Prescriptions for Women's Health

The text STT 98 (ms. A_1) consists of five badly preserved fragments of a single-column tablet with a collection of prescriptions for women. The fragmentary lines belonging to the obverse of the tablet are concerned with promoting conception and fertility (A_1 obv. 2'–9', 16'–21'); two sections (A_1 obv. 10'–15' and obv. 22'–25') feature very fragmentary tests to determine whether a woman was able to conceive (for similar tests see also texts A.2.2 and B.2.2 in this volume). One fragment of STT 98 preserving part of the reverse of the tablet offers a few lines belonging to recipes mostly for speeding up delivery (A_1 rev. 1'–9').

The small fragment STT 284 (ms. A_2) likewise contains remnants of prescriptions for delivery (rev. 1–9). It belonged to the lower left corner of the obverse and upper left corner of the reverse of a tablet and as noted by Gurney and Hulin (STT II, 14), is probably a fragment of the same tablet as STT 98. The present edition follows this suggestion, which is also encouraged by the overlap of topics on the reverse.

https://doi.org/10.1515/9781501506475-004

List of Manuscripts

Siglum	Museum Number	Copy	Collation	Format; Ductus	Provenience
A_1 (+)	SU 52/83 (+) 52/83A (+) 52/111 (+) 52/130 (+) 52/130A	STT 98	Coll.	Fragments of a single-column tablet; Neo-Assyrian script; 7th cent. BCE	Sultantepe
A_2	SU 52/137	STT 284	Coll.	Fragment; Neo-Assyrian script; 7th cent. BCE	Sultantepe
B	VAT 13972	BAM 249	Coll.	Fragment of a two-column tablet; Neo-Assyrian script; ca. 8th/7th cent. BCE	Assur; N4 library

Overview

i'	Fragmentary prescription A_1 obv. 1'	...]1'
ii'	Prescription to enable a woman to get pregnant (potion) A_1 obv. 2'–3'	2'–3'
iii'	Prescription to enable a woman to get pregnant A_1 obv. 4'–5'	4'–5'
iv'	Prescription to enable a woman to get pregnant (potion?) A_1 obv. 6'–9'	6'–9'
v'	Test (for determining a woman's fertility or pregnancy) A_1 obv. 10'–15'	10'–15'
vi'	Fragmentary prescription to enable a woman to get pregnant A_1 obv. 16'	16'
vii'	Fragmentary prescription to enable a woman to get pregnant (potion?) A_1 obv. 17'–18'	17'–18'
viii'	Fragmentary prescription to enable a woman to get pregnant (potion?) A_1 obv. 19'–20'	19'–20'
ix'	Fragmentary prescription to enable a woman to get pregnant (tampon) A_1 obv. 21'	21'
x'	Test (for determining fertility or pregnancy) A_1 obv. 22'–25'	22'–25'[...
xi''	Fragmentary A_2 obv. 1'–5'	...]26''–30''
xii''	Fragmentary procedure (DÙ.DÙ.BI) A_2 obv. 6'–9'	31''–34''
xiii''	Fragmentary prescription A_2 rev. 1	35''
xiv''	Fragmentary prescription (for delivery) A_2 rev. 2–6	36''–40''
xv''	Fragmentary prescription (for delivery) A_2 rev. 7–9	41''–43''[...
xvi'''	Fragmentary prescription (for difficult delivery) A_1 rev. 1'–3' // B obv.$^?$ i' 1'–2'	...]44'''–46'''
xvii'''	Fragmentary prescription (for difficult delivery) A_1 rev. 4'–6' // B obv.$^?$ i' 3'–5'	47'''–49'''
xviii'''	Fragmentary prescription (for delivery) A_1 rev. 7'–9'	50'''–52'''[...

Previous Edition and Discussion

Reiner 1982a, *ZA* 72, 137–138 (transliteration of STT 98)
Volk 2004, in: V. Dasen (ed.), *Naissance et petite enfance*, 80 n. 52 (A_1 rev. 1'ff.)
Infra text D.1.3 (edition of BAM 249)

Transliteration

Beginning of A_1 obv. lost

1' A_1 obv. 1' [x] x-⸢*su*$^{?}$⸣ Š[EG$_6$-*šal*$^{?}$ ....]

2' A_1 obv. 2' [DIŠ] ⸢MUNUS⸣ NU PEŠ$_4$ *ana* ⸢PEŠ$_4$⸣ ⸢^{ú}⸣[.................]

3' A_1 obv. 3' [ŠE]G$_6$-*šal* ⸢NAG$^{?}$⸣-*ši* [NI]TA-*š*[*a* TE-*ši*$^{?}$ (...) PEŠ$_4$]

4' A_1 obv. 4' [DIŠ$^{?}$ MUNUS] ⸢NU⸣ PEŠ$_4$ *ana* PEŠ$_4$ ⸢$^{šim?}$⸣[............] x [x]

5' A_1 obv. 5' ⸢*ù*$^{?}$⸣ ⸢*ša*⸣-*gu-šá* DU-⸢*ku*$^{?}$⸣ [..................] P[EŠ$_4$]

6' A_1 obv. 6' DIŠ KI.MIN ^{ú}IGI-*lim* ⸢^{ú}⸣[IGI]-20 GAZ [... ... ^{ú}Ḫ]UR.SAG

7' A_1 obv. 7' ^{ú}A.ZAL.LÁ ^{ú}DILI$^{?}$ [x]x *raq-qat*$_7$(KÀD) ^{ú}[...] DIŠ-*niš* SÚD *ina* KAŠ ⸢ŠUB$^{?}$⸣

8' A_1 obv. 8' ⸢*ana*⸣ IGI ^{d}*g*[*u-l*]*a t*[*uš-bat*$^{?}$ *ina* A.GÚ].ZI.GA [*lam* GÌR-*šá ana* KI$^{?}$] GAR-*nu*

9' A_1 obv. 9' [NA]G$^{?}$-*ši* NITA-*š*[*a*$^{?}$ TE-*ši*$^{?}$] ([...]) PEŠ$_4$

10' A_1 obv. 10' [(*ana*) *maš-t*]*ak*-⸢*tu*$_4$$^{?}$⸣ [MUNUS ....] SAG [.... NA$_4$ *g*]*a-bi*-⸢*i*⸣

11' A_1 obv. 11' [.................. N]U *pa-tan* [..................] ⸢x x⸣

12' A_1 obv. 12' [..]

13' A_1 obv. 13' [x x] ⸢UL$^{?}$ x⸣ [...]

14' A_1 obv. 14' [*šum*]-*ma* ^{síg}ÀKA BI S[A$_5$ MUNUS BI PEŠ$_4$ *šum-ma* ^{síg}ÀKA SIG$_7$]

15' A_1 obv. 15' [MUNUS] BI [NU PEŠ$_4$]

16' A_1 obv. 16' [DIŠ K]I.MIN ^{ú}*ak-tam* Ú.NAM.T[I.LA .... NAG]-*ši*$^{?}$

17' A_1 obv. 17' DIŠ KI.MIN ^{ú}*tar-muš*$_8$ ^{ú}IGI-*lim* ⸢^{ú}⸣[.......... S]ÚD$^{?}$ *ina* KAŠ *tara-bak*

18' A_1 obv. 18' *ina* MUL$_4$ *tuš-bat ina še-rim* NU *pa-t*[*an*] ⸢*lam*$^{?}$⸣ IGI x [...... NAG-*m*]*a*$^{?}$ PEŠ$_4$

19' A_1 obv. 19' DIŠ KI.MIN ⸢SAḪAR$^{?}$⸣ SI[LA.LÍM.MA$^{?}$] ⸢^{ú}⸣[IGI-*li*]*m*$^{?}$ ^{ú}IGI-20 ⸢^{ú}⸣[x ^{ú}*a*]*n-nu-ḫa-ra*

20' A_1 obv. 20' ⸢NA$_4$⸣ *g*[*a-bi-i* x x x *ana*] KAŠ ŠUB$^{!}$-*di ina* [*še-rim* NAG(?)] KI.MIN$^{!}$

21' A_1 obv. 21' [DIŠ KI.MIN$^{?}$ x x x MUŠ.DÍM].GURUN.NA EDIN.NA *ina* ^{síg}[ÀKA *ana* ŠÀ].TÙR-<*šá*> GAR-*ma* PEŠ$_4$

22' A_1 obv. 22' [DIŠ KI.MIN$^{?}$ x x x ILL]U ^{šim}BULUḪ ILLU LI.TA[R x x]x DIDA ⸢SIG$_5$/SIG$^{?}$⸣

23' A_1 obv. 23' [SÚD$^{?}$ *ina* ^{síg}ÀKA NIGIN$^{?}$ *ana*] <<ŠÀ>> ŠÀ.T[ÙR]-⸢*šá*⸣ GAR-*an* [*šumma* ^{síg}ÀKA] ⸢BI⸣ ⸢SA$_5$$^{?}$⸣ [PEŠ$_4$]

24'	A_1 obv. 24'	[....................] ⸢x⸣ [..]
25'	A_1 obv. 25'	[....................] ⸢x⸣ [..]

Ms. A_1 obv. breaks
Gap of unknown length

26"	A_2 obv. 1'	[x x x] ⸢x⸣ [..]
27"	A_2 obv. 2'	[x] x-*at* TUKU *u* [..]
28"	A_2 obv. 3'	[x]-*ta-nu-ma šu*[*m*-..]
29"	A_2 obv. 4'	x x šu$^?$ a$^?$(or: MIN) ma *ina* x x ⸢^{giš}GAM⸣.[MA$^?$ ....]
30"	A_2 obv. 5'	⸢tab$^?$ zu$^?$⸣ *lip-pa* KAL *it*-x[......................................]

31"	A_2 obv. 6'	DÙ.DÙ.BI NA_4 *ga-bi-i mi-*[*ṣir-a-a*$^?$ ....]
32"	A_2 obv. 7'	⸢^{na4}PA$^?$⸣ ⸢^{na4}⸣*šu-u* ^{na4} [..]
33"	A_2 obv. 8'	⸢^{na4}⸣[*šu-u* MU]NUS$^?$ [..]
34"	A_2 obv. 9'	[x x] x [...]

Bottom of ms. A_2 obv.

35"	A_2 rev. 1	DIŠ KI.MIN [..]

36"	A_2 rev. 2	DIŠ MUNUS ⸢Ù⸣.[TU-*ma* ....]
37"	A_2 rev. 3	MUNUS B[I ....]
38"	A_2 rev. 4	⸢x⸣ [.......] ⸢x⸣ [..]
39"	A_2 rev. 5	[x x] *ina* ur ⸢x x⸣ [..]
40"	A_2 rev. 6	[$PIŠ_{10}$.^{d}Í]D$^?$ ^{ú}MAN$^?$.D[U$^?$....................................]

41"	A_2 obv. 7	[DIŠ] ⸢MUNUS⸣ ⸢Ù⸣.TU-*ma* [..............................]
42"	A_2 obv. 8	x ⸢^{giš}⸣ŠUR.MIN ⸢x⸣ [..]
43"	A_2 obv. 9	[x x] ⸢GAR⸣-*an-ma* [..]

Ms. A_2 obv. breaks; gap of unknown length

44'''	A_1 rev. 1'	DIŠ ^{munus}$PEŠ_4$ ⸢*ina*⸣ [Ù.TU *uš-tap-šiq* ....]
45'''	A_1 rev. 2'	^{giš}GEŠTIN.KA_5.A [.......................................]
	B obv.$^?$ i' 1'–2'	[.........] an [x x] ⸢x x x⸣ [x x x x] / [...............] x
46'''	A_1 rev. 3'	*ul uš-tap-pa-*⸢*áš*⸣*-ša*[*q* ....]
	B obv.$^?$ i' 2'$^{cont.}$	⸢*ul*⸣ ⸢*uš*$^?$*-tap*⸣$^!$*-áš-šaq ár-ḫiš* <<*ḫiš*>> *ul-lad*

47'''	A_1 rev. 4'	^{giš}⸢GEŠTIN.$KA_5$$^?$⸣.A ḪÁD.DA S[ÚD ....]
	B obv.$^?$ i' 3'–4'	[^{giš}GEŠTIN.K]A_5.A Ḫ[ÁD].⸢A⸣ ⸢SÚD$^?$⸣ ⸢*ina*⸣ ⸢Ì$^?$⸣ *pa-pa-an* ŠÀ-*šá* / [x x] x [ŠÉŠ$^?$-*m*]*a*$^?$

48'''	A_1 rev. 5'	*ár-ḫiš ul-lad šá* Š[À-*šá*? ....]
	B obv.? i' 4'cont.-5'	*ár-ḫiš ul-lad šá*?! ŠÀ-*šá* ⸢SILIM?!(BA)⸣ / [*bul-ṭu*? *lat*]-⸢*ku*?⸣ ⸢*mim*?-*ma*?⸣ *lem*?-⸢*nim*⸣
49'''	A_1 rev. 6'	*be-en-nu* [..]
	B obv.? i' 5'cont.	*be-en-nu u* DÙ GIG-*te*
50'''	A_1 rev. 7'	ᵘGEŠTIN.KA$_5$.⸢A⸣ [..]
51'''	A_1 rev. 8'	*ina* Ì+GIŠ EŠ [..]
52'''	A_1 rev. 9'	*Traces*

Ms. A_1 rev. breaks; remainder lost

Bound Transcription and Translation

Beginning lost

1' [...] ... *tu*[*šabšal*(?) ... ...]	1' [...], you bo[il(?)] ... [...].
2' [*šumma*] ⸢*sinništu*⸣ *lā irri ana šūrî* ...[... ...] 3' [*tuša*]*bšal* ⸢*tašaqqīši*⸣ *zik*[*ar*]*ša* [*iṭeḫḫēši*(?) (...) *irri*]	2' [If] a woman does not get pregnant, to enable her to get pregnant: [...]-plant, [... ...] 3' [you bo]il, you have her drink it. (Then) h[er m]ale (consort) [shall have intercourse with (lit. approach) her (...) (and) she will get pregnant].
4' [*šumma sinništu*] *lā irri ana šūrî* ...[... ...] ... 5' *u šagûša illakū* [... ...] *ir*[*ri*]	4' [If a woman] does not get pregnant, to enable her to get pregnant: [...]-aromatic, [... ...] ... 5' but (if?) her *menses* flow, [... ...], she will get pr[egnant(?)].
6' DIŠ KI.MIN *imḫur-līm* [*imḫur*]-*ešrā taḫaššal* [... ...] *azupīru* 7' *azallâ ēdu* [...] *raqqat*(*u*) ...[...] *ištēniš tasâk ina šikari* ⸢*tanaddi*(?)⸣ 8' *ana pān Gula t*[*ušbât ina šē*]*ri* [*lām šēpša ana erṣeti*] *išakkanu* 9' [*tašaq*]*qīši zikarš*[*a iṭeḫḫēši*(?)] [(...)] *irri*	6' Alternatively: you crush 'heals thousand'-plant (and) ['heals] twenty'-plant, 7' you pound together 6' [... ...], *azupīru*-plant, 7' *azallû*-plant, *ēdu*(?)-plant, thin(?) [...], [...]-plant. You pour(?) (all this) into beer. 8' You [let it stand outside overnight(?)] before the goddess Gula. [In the mor]ning, [before] she sets [her foot on the ground (getting out of bed)], 9' [you have] her [dr]ink (this). H[er] male (consort) [shall have intercourse with (lit. approach) her], [(...)], (then) she will get pregnant.
10' [(*ana*) *mašt*]*akti* [*sinništi*(?) ...] ... [... *aban g*]*abî* 11' [... ... *l*]*ā patān* [... ...] ... 12' [... ...] 13' [...] ... [... ...] 14' [*šum*]*ma itqu šī s*[*āmat sinništu šī irri šumma itqu arqat*] 15' [*sinništu*] *šī* [*ul irri*]	10' [(For) a te]st (determining) [a woman(?) ...: ...] ... [... al]um, 11' [... ... on an em]pty stomach [... ...], 12' [... ...], 13' [...] ... [...]. 14' [I]f that wad of wool is r[ed, this woman will get pregnant. If the wad of wool is yellow-green], 15' that [woman will not get pregnant].
16' [DIŠ K]I.MIN? *aktam šammi balā*[*ṭi* ... ... *tašaqqī*]*ši*(?)	16' [Alter]natively(?): *aktam*-plant, plant of lif[e, ...], [you have] her [drink it(?)].

17' DIŠ KI.MIN *tarmuš imḫur-līm* ...[... ... *tas*]*âk ina šikari tarabbak* 18' *ina kakkabi tušbāt ina šēri lā pat*[*ān*] *lām amāri*(?) [... ... *išattī-m*]*a*(?) *irri*

17' Alternatively: you [cr]ush *tarmuš*-plant, 'heals thousand'-plant, [...]-plant, [...], you steep (it) in beer. 18' You let it stand outside overnight under the star(s). [She shall drink (it)] in the morning, on an empty stomach, before seeing (the sun?) [...]. Then she will get pregnant.

19' DIŠ KI.MIN *eper s*[*ūq erbetti*(?) *imḫur-lī*]*m*(?) *imḫur-ešrā* [...] *annuḫara* 20' *aban g*[*abî* ... *ana*] *šikari tanaddi ina* [*šēri išatti*(?)] KI.MIN

19' Alternatively: dust(?) from a cr[ossroads(?), 'heals thousand']-plant, 'heals twenty'-plant, [...]-plant, (white) *annuḫaru*-pigment, 20' al[um, ...] you pour [into] beer. [She shall drink (it?)] in [the morning(?)], ditto (i.e. she will get pregnant).

21' [DIŠ KI.MIN(?)... *pizal*]*lurti ṣēri ina it*[*qi ana šas*]*sūrī*<*ša*> *tašakkan-ma irri*

21' [Alternatively(?)]: [...] gecko of the steppe you insert in a [wad of] wool into (her) womb (i.e. her vagina). Then she will get pregnant.

22' [DIŠ KI.MIN? ... *ḫī*]*l baluḫḫi ḫīl abukkati* [...] *billat našpi* 23' [*tasâk*(?) *ina itqi talammi*(?) *ana*] *šassūrīša tašakkan* [*šumma itqu*] *šī sāmat*(?) [*irri*]

24'–25' *traces*

22' [Alternatively(?)]: 23' [you crush(?)] 22' [...] resin of *baluḫḫu*-aromatic, resin of *abukkatu*-plant, [...], beerwort for making *našpu*-beer, 23' [you wrap it into a wad of wool(?)], you insert (it) [into] her womb (i.e. vagina). [If] that [wad] is red (after removing it), [she will get pregnant].

24'–25' *traces*

Ms. A_1 obv. breaks; gap of unknown length

26"–28" *too fragmentary for transcription*
29" [...] ... *ṣum*[*lalû*(?) ...] 30" [...] ... *lippa* ... [...]

26"–28" *too fragmentary for translation*
29" [...] ... *ṣum*[*lalû-plant*(?) ...] 30" [...] ... a wad ...[...]

31" DÙ.DÙ.BI *aban gabî mi*[*ṣrāya* ... ...] 32" *ayyartu*(?) *šû* ...[... ...] 33" [*šû sin*]*niš* [... ...] 34" [...] ... [... ...]

31" The procedure for it: Egy[ptian] alum, [... ...] 32" *ayyartu*-shell, *šû*-stone, [...]-stone, [... ...], 33" [fem]ale [*šû*-stone, ...] 34" [...] ... [... ...].

Bottom of Ms. A_2 obv.

35" DIŠ KI.MIN [... ...]

35" Alternatively: [... ...].

36" *šumma sinništu ūl*[*id-ma* ... ...] 37" *sinništu š*[*ī*(?) ... ...] 38"-39" *fragmentary* 40" [*kibrī*]*tu suā*[*du* ... ...]

36" If a woman gives bi[rth and ... ...] 37" th[at] woman [... ...] 38"–39" *fragmentary* 40" [*kibrī*]*tu*-sulphur, *suādu*-plant(?), [... ...].

41" [*šumma*] *sinništu ūlid-ma* [... ...] 42"... *šurmēnu*(?) ...[... ...] 43" [...] *tašakkan-ma* [... ...]

41" [If] a woman gives birth, and [... ...] 42" ... *šurmēnu*-cypress(?) ...[... ...] 43" [...] you put it. Then [... ...].

Ms. A_2 rev. breaks; gap of unknown length

44"' *šumma erītu ina* [*alādi uštapšiq* ... ...] 45"' *karān šēlebi* [... ...] 46"' *ul uštapaššaq* [*arḫiš ullad*]

44"' If a pregnant woman [suffers severely during (her) delivery ... ...] 45"' 'fox grape', [... ...], 46"' she will not have an agonizing labour, [(but) deliver quickly].

47''' *karān šēlebi tubbal tas[âk ina šamni(?) papān libbi ... tapaššaš-ma(?)]* 48''' *arḫiš ullad ša l[ibbīša(?) išallim(?) bulṭu lat]ku(?) mimma lemnu* 49''' *bennu [u kal marušte]*	47''' You dry (and) crush 'fox grape', [(mix it?) with oil(?), you rub(?) the area of her belly (with it) ... . Then] 48''' she will deliver quickly. [Her baby will be healthy(?). *A pro*]*ven* [*remedy against*(?)] anything evil, 49''' *bennu*-epilepsy [and all trouble].
50''' *karān šēlebi* [... ...] 51''' *ina šamni tapaššaš* [... ...] 52''' *traces*	50''' 'Fox grape'-plant, [... ...], 51''' you apply (it) as an ointment with oil [... ...]. 52''' *traces*

Ms. A_1 rev. breaks; remainder lost

Notes

Lines 2'–5': I have opted for reading NU PEŠ$_4$ as *lā irri*, "she does not get pregnant", rather than assuming a stative form *erât* "(If a woman is (not) pregnant". The purpose statement / introductory phrase in lines 2' and 4', seems to correspond to BM 42313+ obv. 8 and rev. 33 // BM 42333+: 5 (text A.2.2): DIŠ MUNUS NU PEŠ$_4$ *a-na šu-ri-i* "If a woman does not get pregnant, to enable (her) to get pregnant". Other passages use slightly varying syntactic formulations: BM 59710: 1 (text B.2.5): *ana* ^{munus}NU.PEŠ$_4$ *šu-r[i-'i]* "to enable a woman (who is) not pregnant to get pregnant"; BM 79061: 1 (text A.2.8): ^{munus}*la e-ri-tu$_4$ a-na šu-ri-'-[i]* "to enable a woman (who is) not pregnant to get pregnant"; BAM 250 rev. 3 (text B.1.4): (a total of 21 beads) ^{munus}NU.PEŠ$_4$ *ana* PEŠ$_4$ "to enable a woman (who is) not pregnant (*lā erītu*) to become pregnant (*ana šūrî*)".

The reconstruction of line 3' follows the parallel formulation below in line 9'. The text apparently recommends sexual intercourse after application of the treatment. Such recommendations are rarely found in other texts for promoting female fertility. However, they sometimes occur in Hippocratic texts, see e.g. *Diseases of Women* I, § 19, Potter 2018, 61; Reiner 1982a, 138. Note for a similar context also UET 7, No. 123 rev. 5' (text B.2.2), which gives a negative recommendation however (NITA-*šú* NU TE-*šú* "her male (consort) shall not approach her (sexually)".

Lines 4'–5': The occurrence of the term *šagû* (variant spelling for *sagû* "menses") in line 5' and reference to the flow of *šagû* in the context of a prescription to promote fertility is highly interesting and it is unfortunate that the passage is so fragmentary. The present passage confirms the form *šagû* in Assyrian texts, whereas Babylonian texts use *sagû* instead. For further discussion and references, see the section on bleeding in this volume, especially BAM 235–236, BM 47578, BM 54587 + 73802, BM 61975 (texts C.1.1–C.1.2, C.2.2–C.2.4) and the notes on *Diagnostic Handbook* Tablet 36: 100–102 and SpTU 1, No. 59: lines 6'–7' (see *infra*).

Lines 6'–9': The Akkadian reading and interpretation of DIŠ KI.MIN (as "if ditto" (i.e. *šumma ašar/ašri šanîm-(ma)*) or "alternatively/additionally" (*ana ašar/ašri šanîm-(ma)*) is still debated. See Köcher 1971, xxxii (on BAM 417); Kinnier Wilson 2011, *JMC* 17, 12; Geller and Panayotov 2020, 255–256; Johnson and Simkó 2024, 60 n. 124 for discussion. No decision is made here in favour of either reading. Attestations of (DIŠ) KI.MIN are collected under KI.MIN in the Akkadian glossary of the book. For a partially syllabic spelling, see text A.2.1 line 4' below.

At the end of line 7', one expects *ina* KAŠ *tara-bak* "you steep in beer", parallel to obv. 17', but the sign traces are not unequivocal. The interpretation of the signs *raq-qat$_7$*(KÀD) as the feminine adjective *raqqatu* "thin" is provisional, but it might be an attribute to the preceding broken ingredient.

In line 8', the phrase "before Gula (you let it spend the night)" should probably mean before Lyra, the star associated with the healing goddess. In the gap in line 8', one expects the phrase "before she sets her foot on the ground" from parallel passages; thus, the restoration [*lām* GÌR-*šú/šá ana* KI] before GAR-*nu*. Accordingly, the spacing of the fragments in the copy of STT 98 needs to be adjusted.

Lines 10'–15': The reconstruction at the beginning of line 10' is inspired by BM 42313+ rev. 29 // UET 7, No. 123 obv. 1, which may perhaps be restored as *ana maštakti* MUNUS NU [*e-r*]*i$^?$-i$^?$* "for a test (determining) a woman (who will) ⌜not conceive/get pregnant⌝" (see texts A.2.2, B.2.2). The test described in the two Babylonian parallels also uses alum (*gabû*), but the other ingredients which are applied in a tampon, do not appear to correspond to the traces in STT 98. However, as was already pointed out by Reiner (1982a, 138), lines 14'–15' in the Sultantepe text seem to follow the interpretation of colour changes of the tampon given in UET 7, No. 123 obv. 3–4 (text B.2.2; Reiner 1972, 134) and the duplicate BM 42313+ rev.

31–32 (text A.2.2). The Sultantepe text appears to present an abbreviated variant of the type of test procedure found in the two Babylonian parallels. The mention of an "empty stomach" in line 11' may indicate that the patient first had to drink a potion, before the test was applied in the form of a tampon inserted in her vagina. Compare also UET 7, No. 123 obv. 6–7 for a test using a potion: if the woman vomited after drinking the potion, she was believed to be fertile or pregnant.

Line 16': Interestingly, *aktam*-plant is also referred to as a "plant to get offspring (seed)" in drug compendia, see e.g. BAM 1 i 19–20 (Attia and Buisson 2012, *JMC* 19, 26; Geller 2020, *JMC* 35, 20; there inserted in the vagina); BAM 380 rev. 25 // BAM 381 iii 17–18 (Stol 2000a, 52–53).

Lines 17'–18': A procedure to make a barren woman conceive in N. 4001 obv. 14ff. (text B.2.1) uses two identical ingredients (*tarmuš* and *imḫur-līm*). 'It heals thousand'-plant is known as a plant for a barren woman (^{munus}NU.Ù.TU) in drug compendia, e.g. in BAM 380 rev. 27 /// BAM 381 iii 20 (Stol 2000a, 52–53, likewise prescribed in a potion as is the case in lines 17'–18'). For *imḫur-līm* as an emetic drug, cf. Böck 2023, 126. This effect may also have been intended in the present procedure (removing harmful matter from the body hindering conception?).

For line 18', compare also BAM 408 (= LKU 55) obv. 4'–5' (in a prescription for fertility): [...] *ina*$^{?}$ MUL$_4$ *tuš-bat ina še-rim* NU *pa-tan* / [(...)] NAG "you let it stand outside overnight under the star(s); she drinks it in the morning, on an empty stomach (...)" (see text A.2.9).

Lines 19'–20': The reading of the first ingredient in line 19' is very tentative. Perhaps, instead of "dust from a crossroads" (SAḪAR SI[LA.LÍM.MA]), read rather $^{giš!}$x[x x x] "[...]-tree".

Line 21': For gecko of the steppe (MUŠ.DÍM.GURUN.NA (*ša*) EDIN.NA) in prescriptions, see CAD P, 451–452 sub 1b. It is of interest that this ingredient is also found in treatments to stimulate sexual desire, see now Zisa 2021, 285, 290 (D prescr. 6: 51); 295–396, 408, 447 (K prescr. 31: 136 = N prescr. 8 ii 4); 442, 448–449 (N prescr. 17 iii 32). In the latter case, "copulating" (*ritkubu*) geckos were prescribed as first choice. In the context of promoting female fertility, the use of gecko may also be influenced by associations of the sexual organs with animals such as mice, lizards and geckos in love literature (see e.g., K. 7924 ii 10–11; Lambert 1975: 112, which speaks of "the lizard (*ṣurārû*) of [your] *vulva* (*rēmu*, lit. womb), the gecko (*pizalluru*) of [your] *vulva*").

Lines 26"–30": It is uncertain whether these lines belong to a prescription or perhaps to an incantation. The latter is even more likely since the next section begins with DÙ.DÙ.BI "the procedure for it", often marking procedural sections after recitations in ritual texts.

Lines 31"–34": Egyptian alum is also attested in UET 7, 123 obv. 13 (text B.2.2), in the context of fertility tests and prescriptions to treat infertility (^{na4}*gab-u mi-ṣir-a-a*). The present prescription may consist in an amulet or a tampon, since a variety of minerals appear to have been used.

Line 42": ⸢^{giš}⸣ŠUR.MIN is an irregular spelling for ^{giš}ŠUR.MÌN "cypress".

Lines 44'''–46''': The purpose of this and the following prescriptions was not yet recognized by Volk 2004, 80 n. 52, but the restoration of the passage could be confirmed by the duplicating prescription in BAM 249 obv.$^{?}$ i' 1'–2' (ms. B), which is, however, likewise fragmentary. The form ⸢*ul*⸣ ⸢*uš*$^{?}$-*tap*$^{!}$⸣-*áš-šaq* "she will [not] have an agonizing delivery" in line 2' is a Št-stem verbal form of *pašāqu* "to be narrow, difficult" (the spelling *ul uš-tap-pa-*⸢*áš*⸣-*ša*[*q*] in ms. A$_1$ rev. 3' is defective). The corresponding preterite *uštapšiq* occurs within the phrase *šumma sinništu/erītu ina alādi uštapšiq*(*šu*) "if a woman suffers severely during delivery", which is attested several times in parallel passages in the Neo-Assyrian Birth Compendium (BAM 248 //, text D.1.1) and similar texts (BAM 249 obv.$^{?}$ i' 8', 11' (text D.1.3)). Similar phrases using a Š-stem stative form of *pašāqu* (with the same meaning) are found in other sources (see K. 11956 + 14200 obv. 1 (text D.1.2); Assur Medical Catalogue lines 115 and 117 (Steinert et al. 2018, 218, 272–274 with discussion). In other contexts, the verb *pašāqu* (Št-stem) is used in the meaning "to suffer a serious crisis during one's illness" (see CAD P, 236a sub c-2'; AHw 842a; for the form *uštapaššaq* in omen apodoses, see e.g. George 1991, *RA* 85, 142 *Diagnostic Handbook* Tablet 1 line 6; Heeßel 2000, 233, 245 *Diagnostic Handbook* Tablet 19/20 lines 118'–119'). For the context of childbirth, note also CT 39, 44: 5: *sinništu šī uštapaššaq* "that woman will suffer severely during delivery" (*Šumma Ālu* Tablet 104). See further AMT 66/4 rev.$^{?}$ i' 3'–6' (text D.1.4).

Lines 47'''–49''': The rare expression *papān libbīša* "the area of her belly" in line 47''' occurs also in one prescription of the Neo-Assyrian Birth Compendium (BAM 248 rev. iv 19–20 and dupl., see text D.1.1 lines 211–212), in which the woman's belly is massaged downwards to promote delivery.

The phrase *arḫiš ullad* "she will give birth quickly" occurs several times in texts for speeding up a difficult delivery, often concluding a prescription: see, e.g., BAM 248 rev. iv 5 and 15 and dupl. (see text D.1.1 lines 197, 207). The prescription in BAM 248 rev. iv 13–15 // (potion) has one ingredient in common with line 47''' (as well as with lines 45''' and 50'''): 'fox grape' (*karān šēlebi*). See also BAM 248 iv 21 (text D.1.1 line 213) and *passim*. Note that compendia of *materia medica* know 'fox grape' as a plant of a woman in difficult labour (^{munus}LA.RA.AḪ, see BAM 380 rev. 33ff. // BAM 381 iii 27–30; Stol 2000a, 52–53).

Interestingly, lines 48'''–49''' appear to be a comment that explains alternative uses of the remedy. If this interpretation is correct, line 47''' may have contained an ointment that could be used as a panacea (or prophylactic remedy) to ward off anything evil (*mimma lemnu*), *bennu*-epilepsy and illness and to protect the newborn in particular. For plants/drugs against *bennu*-epilepsy, cf. Stol 1993, 103–104. For similar remedies to protect the newborn included in women's health-care texts related to delivery, see also BAM 248 rev. iv 39–43 and duplicates (text D.1.1). See also the discussion on the duplicate passage to lines 47'''–49''' in BAM 249 (text D.1.2) lines 3'–6'. A similar sequence of purposes (to ward off anything evil (*mimma lemnu*), *bennu*-epilepsy and illness (GIG)) is also attested in collections with prescriptions for amulet necklaces (e.g. BAM 358 ii 14', 17'–18'; with similar sequences in Schuster-Brandis 2008, 191, 199).

A.1.2 A. 3461: A Neo-Assyrian Fragment on Postpartum Complaints

This Neo-Assyrian fragment probably belonged to a single-column tablet that may have come from Assur. The fragment was purchased for the collection of the Oriental Institute of the University of Chicago (now Institute for the Study of Ancient Cultures) by J. H. Breasted (in 1919–1920) from the antiquities dealer Georges Khayat in Baghdad. The acquisition group to which A. 3461 belongs, contains 17 other tablets/fragments written in (Middle/Neo-)Assyrian script. Among them, one fragment (A. 3445), according to W. G. Lambert, joins to BM 103385 and LKA 107, the latter of which was excavated in Assur (the Neo-Assyrian fragments belong to a large collective tablet containing spells and rituals for "Entering the palace" (É.GAL.KU$_4$.RA).[244] It is therefore likely that other Assyrian fragments in the acquisition group stem from Assur. Three other Neo-Assyrian fragments in the group contain medical prescriptions, A. 3450 (= BAM 412, against intestinal ailments), A. 3468 (= BAM 414, against urinary tract diseases) and A. 3488 (= BAM 415, against *sagallu*-disease).[245]

A. 3461 seems to have contained incantations and remedies for different female health problems. The obverse begins with a fragmentary unknown *abracadabra*-spell (lines 1'–3') that mentions the Elamite sun god Naḫḫunte (who is otherwise invoked in birth incantations) and may have contained other Elamite divine names. The remainder of the obverse contains prescriptions for women, two of which are duplicated in another Neo-Assyrian tablet from Assur (ms. B = BAM 240, found in the N4 library). The latter text focuses on prescriptions for conditions affecting women during pregnancy and after delivery, e.g. gastrointestinal problems, diarrhoea, infection). The prescriptions duplicated in A. 3461 revolve around the key symptom of swelling/inflammation and bloating, caused in one case by wind in the patient's body. The last prescription on the obverse appears to have dealt with vaginal discharges or haemorrhage.

The reverse of A. 3461 preserves remnants of a prescription, followed by a fragmentary *abracadabra*-incantation featuring some Sumerian words or phrases, which, following parallels, probably starts with the opening words tuḫul tuḫul "thigh, thigh". Varying versions of this spell are attested in Nineveh medical texts: in therapies for hair loss in women (BAM 498–500(+), see also *infra* text H.1), and from a Nineveh text treating nosebleed (ms. C = BAM 526). The version in BAM 526 may duplicate the spell in A. 3461 (see below).

244 I would like to thank Susanne Paulus and Ryan Winters from the Institute for the Study of Ancient Cultures (ISAC) of the University of Chicago for detailed information on the acquisition group. See also the collection website for further information on the fragments (https://isac-idb.uchicago.edu/). The join between BM 103385, LKA 107 and A. 3445 has not been confirmed. For LKA 107, see Klan 2007, 43ff. Nos. 2, 5–8, 11–12, 17–19, 32, 37. For a photo of BM 103385, see https://www.britishmuseum.org/collection/object/W_1911-0408-75.

245 See Köcher 1971, BAM IV, xxxi. For BAM 412, 414 and 415, see also *BabMed Corpora* and CDLI.

List of Manuscripts

Siglum	Museum Number	Copy	Collation	Format; Ductus	Provenience
A	A. 3461	Pl. 9	Coll.	Fragment of a single-column(?) tablet; Neo-Assyrian script; 8th/7th cent. BCE[246]	Assur(?)
B	VAT 8881	BAM 240	Coll.	Single-column tablet in portrait format; Neo-Assyrian script; 8th/7th cent. BCE	Assur; N4 library
C	K. 13366	BAM 526	Coll.	Fragment of a two-column(?) tablet; Neo-Assyrian script; 7th cent. BCE	Nineveh; Ashurbanipal's library

Overview

i'	Fragmentary incantation A obv. 1'–3'	...]1'–3'
ii'	Fragmentary prescription (for a postpartum problem?) A obv. 4'–6'	4'–6'
iii'	Rubric (incantation) A obv. 7'	7'
iv'	Prescription against bloating (from 'wind') A obv. 8'–11' // B obv. 20'–22'	8'–11'
v'	Prescription (tampon) A obv. 12'–13' // B obv. 23'–24'	12'–13'
vi'	Fragmentary prescription A obv. 14'–15'	14'–15'[...
vii''	Fragmentary prescription A rev. 1'–3'	...]16''–18''
viii'	Fragmentary pseudo-Sumerian(?) incantation A rev. 4'–8' // // C 8'–11' (?)	19''–23''[...

Previous Edition and Discussion

Köcher 1980, BAM Vol. 6, xv, pl. 46 (copy; discussion of ms. C)
The Nineveh Medical Project (http://oracc.museum.upenn.edu/asbp/ninmed/pager; edition of ms. C)
Scurlock 2014a, 608–616, esp. 610 (edition of ms. B)
Infra text D.2.1 (edition of ms. B)

Transliteration

Beginning of ms. A obv. lost

1'	A obv. 1'	[x (x)]x [x x x x x] ab x[........................]
2'	A obv. 2'	[x u]g$^{?}$ ga ⌈ab nu u⌉ ⌈^{d}⌉sú-uk-ku x[.............]
3'	A obv. 3'	[im]-ḫu-ḫu im-ḫu ^{d}na-ḫu-un-d[i ... (TU$_{6}$) ÉN]

4'	A obv. 4'	[*ana šá-n*]*im*$^{?}$*-ma šum-ma* MUNUS$^{!}$ *ut-ta-tap-pi-iḫ* S[U-*šá*$^{?}$ ....]

246 Measurements: 5.2 x 4 x 2 cm.

5' A obv. 5' [(x) *q*]*a*$^{?}$*-lu-tu*$_{4}$ *ip-pa-ra-ḫu* Ì Š[EG$_{6}$ ....]

6' A obv. 6' [ÉN] ⸢7⸣-*šú* ŠID-*nu la pa-tan* NAG$^{?}$-*ši ina* x[..............]

7' A obv. 7' [(x)] KA.INIM.MA MUNUS x[......................]

A, B

8' A obv. 8' [DIŠ MUNUS T]U$_{15}$ *iš-biṭ-ma ma-lit ù* [....................]
B obv. 20' DIŠ MUNUS TU$_{15}$ *iš-biṭ-ma ma-lit ù* SU-*šá* KÚR.KÚR *ana* TI-*šá*

9' A obv. 9' [^{šim}GÚR.G]ÚR GAZI^{sar} ^{ú}KUR.RA ^{š}[^{im}LI ....]
B obv. 20'$^{\text{cont.}}$–21' ^{giš}GÚR.GÚR GAZI^{sar} ^{ú}KUR.RA / ^{šim}LI ^{ú}ḪAR.ḪAR ^{ú}NU.LUḪ.ḪA

10' A obv. 10' [*saḫ-l*]*é-e* NUMUN GADA Ú ⸢*a*⸣-*ši*-⸢*i*⸣ [.....................]
B obv. 21'$^{\text{cont.}}$–22' *saḫ-lé-e* NUMUN GADA Ú *a-ši-e* ^{šim}ḪAB / Ú BABBAR

11' A obv. 11' [x Ú].ḪI.A ŠEŠ *ina* KAŠ.SAG *u* Ì [.......................]
B obv. 22' 11 Ú.ḪI.A ŠEŠ *ina* KAŠ.SAG *u* Ì ŠEG$_{6}$-*šal* ÍL-*ma ina-eš*

A, B

12' A obv. 12' DIŠ KI.MIN ^{giš}*ḫa-šu-u* ^{ú}NU.LUḪ.ḪA [.....................]
B obv. 23' DIŠ KI.MIN ^{giš}*ḫa-šu-u* ^{ú}NU.LUH.HA ^{giš}ŠE.NÁ.A ZÚ.LUM.MA ^{ú}*a-ṣú-ṣi-im-tú*

13' A obv. 13' ⸢Ú⸣ BABBAR 6 Ú.ḪI.A ŠEŠ *ina* KA[Š.SAG ....]
B obv. 24' 5 Ú *an-nu-ti ina* KAŠ.SAG ŠEG$_{6}$-*šal ana* ŠÀ.TÙR-*šá* DUB

A, B

14' A obv. 14' [DIŠ MUNUS$^{?}$ x]-*šá* DU-⸢*ku*⸣ ⸢MUNUS$^{?}$⸣ ⸢BI$^{?}$⸣ [..........]

15' A obv. 15' [x x] x x [...]

Ms. A obv. breaks; gap of unknown length

16" A rev. 1' [...............] x x x x[...................................]

17" A rev. 2' [............ Ú$^{?}$].MEŠ *an-nu-ti ana* ŠÀ [..................]

18" A rev. 3' [......... ÉN ...] ŠID-*nu* SAR-*ši* x[.....................]

A, B

19" A rev. 4' [ÉN tu-ḫul tu-ḫul$^{?}$ ma-da ḫ]ul ma-da ḫ[ul-ḫul$^{?}$ ....]
C 7'-8' [ÉN (...)] tu-ḫul tu-ḫul ma-da [.........] / [...... ma]-da ma-da su-x[........]

20" A rev. 5' [......... k]i$^{?}$-še [d]iri$^{?}$-eš mu-ur-x[..........................]
C 9' [.................. dir]i$^{?}$ mu-ur-k[i$^{?}$...........................]

21" A rev. 6' [................] še$^{?}$ ki du-du $^{\textit{erasure?}}$ x[........................]
C 10' [...... š]e-da-a še-da-a še-da-a [.............................]

22" A rev. 7' [................]x-di nu-ur si-ip-p[a$^{?}$ ....]
C 11' [...............] x [...]

23" A rev. 8' [..............................] x [................................]

Ms. A rev. and C break; remainder lost

Bound Transcription and Translation

Beginning of ms. A obv. lost

1' *only traces preserved*
2' [x u]g$^{?}$ ga ⌜ab⌝ ⌜nu⌝ ⌜u⌝ ⌜^{d}⌝sú-uk-ku x[......]
3' [im]-ḫu-ḫu im-ḫu ^{d}na-ḫu-un-d[i ... (TU$_6$) ÉN]

1' *only traces preserved*
2' [...]... Sukku [... ...]
3' [im]ḫuḫu imḫu Naḫḫunte [... . Incantation (formula)].

4' *[ana šan]îm-ma(?) šumma sinništu uttatappiḫ zum[urša* ... ...] 5' [... *q]alûtu ipparraḫū šamnu ba[šlu(?)* ... ...] 6' *[šipta] sebîšu tamannu lā patān tašaqqīši ina* ...[... ...]

4' [Alternati]vely(?), and if the woman (also) becomes increasingly bloated and [her] body [...], 5' [roa]sted [...] (which) *are beginning to ferment*(?), boi[led(?)] oil [... ...]. 6' You recite the [incantation] seven times. (Then) you give (it) to her to drink on an empty stomach. With/in [... ...].

7' [(x)] KA.INIM.MA MUNUS ...[... ...]

7' Wording (of an incantation) for a woman [... ...].

8' *šumma sinništu šāra išbiṭ-ma malît u zumur[ša ittanakker ana bulluṭīša]* 9' *kukru kasû nīnû bur[āšu ḫašû nuḫurtu]* 10' *saḫlê zēr kitê šammi ašî [ṭūru šammu peṣû]* 11' *išteššer šammī annûti ina šikari u šamni [tušabšal inaššī-ma ina"eš]*

8' If wind has 'blown' (into) a woman so that she is filled up (with it), but [her body keeps changing (for the worse), to cure her]: 9' *kukru*-plant, *kasû*-plant, *nīnû*-plant, jun[iper, *ḫašû*-plant, *nuḫurtu*-plant], 10' *saḫlû*-plant, linseed, '*ašû*-disease'-plant, [*ṭūru*-aromatic, (and) 'white drug'] – 11' these [eleven drug]s [you boil] in beer and oil, [she applies (it) and she will get well.]

12' DIŠ KI.MIN *ḫašû nuḫurtu šunû suluppū aṣuṣimtu* 13' *šammu peṣû* 6 (var. 5) *šammī annûti ina šikari [tušabšal ana šassūrīša tašappak/tatabbak]*

12' Alternatively: *ḫašû*-plant, *nuḫurtu*-plant, *šunû*-plant, date(s), *aṣuṣimtu*-plant, 13' (ms. A adds) 'white drug' – these six (var. five) plants [you boil] in beer, [you pour (it) into her womb].

14' *[šumma sinništu ...]-ša illakū šinništu šī* [... ...] 15' *only traces preserved*

14' [If a woman]'s [...] flow(s), *that woman* [... ...] 15' *too fragmentary for translation*

Ms. A obv. breaks; gap of unknown length

16'' *only traces preserved*
17'' [... ...] *šammī annûti ina libbi* [... ...] 18'' [... ... *šipta* ...] *tamannu tuqattarši* [... ...]

16'' *too fragmentary for translation*
17'' [... ...] these [drug]s [you ...] into [...]. 18'' [...] you recite [the incantation ...], you fumigate her (with it) [... ...].

19'' [ÉN tu-ḫul tu-ḫul ma-da ḫ]ul ma-da ḫ[ul-ḫul ... ...]
20''–23'' *too fragmentary for transcription*

19'' [Incantation. tuḫul tuḫul mada ḫ]ul mada ḫ[ulḫul ... ...]
20''–23'' *too fragmentary for translation*

Ms. A rev. breaks; remainder lost

Notes

Lines 1'–3': For ^{d}*Sú/Zu-uk-ku*, compare the Elamite loanword *sukkû* in Akkadian, derived from *sunki-/sukkir* "king" (CAD S 362a; Hinz and Koch 1987, *Elamisches Wörterbuch*, Teil 2, 1106).

Naḫḫunte, the Elamite sun god, occurs in Mesopotamian birth incantations from the second and first millennium BCE (see *infra*, text D.1.1 BAM 248 i 58; iii 36, 40, etc.), often together with the goddess Narunde. Naḫḫunte is erroneously equated with the moon god Sîn and Narunde with Šamaš in two first millennium commentaries (in 11N-T3: 27 (Civil 1974) and U. 30654 (= UET 6/3, 897): 9', see *infra*, Chapter G). See also An = *Anum* VI 181 and 184 for both deities as siblings; further Stolper 1998–2001, "Nahhunte", *RlA* 9, 82–84; Koch 1998–2001, "Narunde", *RlA* 9, 180).

Lines 4'–7': The restoration at the beginning of line 4' is not entirely certain, but presumably it represents a partially syllabic spelling for DIŠ (KI).MIN, conventionally rendered as "if ditto" or "alternatively", which in medical texts introduces alternative remedies for the same purpose. The Akkadian reading of DIŠ KI.MIN is not entirely confirmed (CAD Š/1, 397a; Borger 2004, MZL, No. 742), but usually interpreted as *šumma ašar šanîm* or *ana* (*ašri*) *šanîm*, for "if ditto" (lit. "if (in) a second place/entry") or "alternatively" (see Geller and Panayotov 2020, 255–256; Johnson and Simkó 2024, 60 n. 124). The restoration *ana šanîm-ma* "alternatively" for the damaged beginning of line 4' in A. 3461 is preferred here, since the space at the beginning of the line seems too small for [DIŠ KI *šá-n*]*im-ma*. It seems that the phrase [*ana šan*]*îm-ma* at the beginning of line 4' in A. 3461 resumes the topic (protasis) of a previous entry (symptom description) and expands on it by adding additional symptoms, which are introduced by the following *šumma sinništu* "(and) if the woman ...". This implies that the incantation in lines 1'–3' does not form the beginning of the tablet but was preceded by at least one more prescription.

Line 4': Compare a similar passage in BAM 240: 45' (see text D.2.1), which also features the verb *napāḫu*, but in the Ntn-stem, not in the Dtn-stem as in A. 3461. That passage describes a further complication of the woman's initial symptoms (internal fever, blocked postpartum blood) after the administration of a vaginal suppository. The present passage in A. 3461 may describe a similar complication.

The verb *napāḫu* in the G- or D- or Ntn-stem (often written MÚ, MÚ.MÚ or MÚ.MEŠ) can mean "to be swollen/bloated" (cf. CAD N/1, 265 sub 3b, 268 sub 7; AHw 732 instead translates "(krankhaft) entzünden"; (G mng. 3, D mng. 5); Scurlock and Andersen 2005, 123–124, 286). It is difficult to grasp the exact nuance of this verb, since it occurs in medical texts very often in the context of other terms referring both to intestinal distention as well as colic and fever (Cadelli 2000, 348–349, 2019, 40–41; Bácskay 2018a, e.g. Nos. 18: 13, 19: 1, 40: 1; 64: 17; 79: 12; 80: 1; 81: 4; Johnson and Simkó 2024, 12, 18, 62 with n. 138 *passim*). The Dtn perfect form *ut-ta-tap-pi-iḫ* in A. 3461 obv. 4' may have the meaning "she becomes *increasingly* bloated/inflamed".

Line 5': The form *ip-pa-ra-ḫu* can be understood as an N-stem form of a verb *parāḫu*. The verb *parāḫu* means "to sprout" in the G-stem (said e.g. of trees) and "to ferment" in the D-stem (said of beer, cf. AHw, 827b sub *parāḫu* I; CAD P, 145). This verb is the same as *parā'u* B "to sprout, to flourish" (see Streck 2018, SAD, Vol. 1, 68; under separate lemmas in CAD P, 182; AHw, 833 s.v. *parā'u* II). However, for this verb, the dictionaries do not offer any attestations in the N-stem yet; it may have an ingressive meaning. A second attested verb *parā'u* A (also *parāḫu*) "to cut (through), to slit" is attested in the N-stem in a passive meaning but does not suit the present context well (cf. CAD P, 181).

In the gap before the restored adjective *qalûtu* "roasted", one expects a plant name in the plural such as *kasû*-plant or *saḫlû* "cress", to which the verb *ip-pa-ra-ḫu* refers. Both plants are used in a roasted state, for example in BAM 240 rev. 41', 43'–44', 50' (text D.2.1), concerned with similar (postpartum) conditions (infection, childbed fever).

Line 7': The text registers an incantation rubric here (and the recitation of a spell is mentioned in the previous prescription in line 6'), but the text of the spell was omitted by the copyist. The rubric thus seems to function as a place holder for the actual incantation.

Lines 8'–11': For the symptom description and discussion, cf. Scurlock and Andersen 2005, 92 4.15; Scurlock 2014a, 614; CAD N/1, 164a sub 2g and the notes to BAM 240 (text D.2.1 lines 20'–22'). I interpret the prescription as dealing with (postpartum) bloating due to 'wind'.

Lines 19''–23'': Some of the phrases and words in this fragmentary spell may be interpreted as Sumerian (tuḫul/tugul "thigh, hip(bone), mada "land, plain", ḫul "bad, evil"), although the formula can be classified as garbled mumbo-jumbo phrases (cf. Veldhuis 1999, 47–48). The restoration of the beginning of the spell in ms. A line 19'' follows BAM 498–500+ rev. iii 7–8 (see *infra*, text H.1 for discussion). The spell in A. 3461 rev. 4'–7' is much longer than BAM 498–500+ rev. iii 7–8, and the latter spell may represent an abbreviated version. The parallel BAM 526 lines 7'–11' (ms. C) may be a duplicate to the text of ms. A, but unfortunately is likewise too fragmentary to tell with certainty. Another Sumerian spell in BAM 498–500+ iii 26'–30' which was used with a remedy to counter hair loss in women (see *infra*, text H.1, see also ibid. iii 7–8) likewise uses a variant of the opening tuḫul-formula. But it is much better preserved to see that it does not form a proper duplicate to the spell in ms. A. For alternative readings of line 20'' in ms. C see the *Nineveh Medical Project* website.

A.1.3 BAM 245: Women and Epilepsy

This small Neo-Assyrian fragment from Assur contains only a few damaged lines of text. It can be assigned to the medical texts dealing with a female patient because of the feminine pronominal suffixes attached to verbal forms in the text that refer to instructions performed by the healer on the patient. Remarkably, the only section preserving a symptom description or a reference to an illness, does not deal with a specific "gynaecological" problem, but mentions *bennu*-epilepsy and refers to symptoms typical for demonic afflictions that are known from sections of the *Diagnostic Handbook* dealing with epilepsy-related ailments (which would be classified in the realm of neurological and psychiatric disorders in modern biomedicine). At present, no parallels from the tablets of the *Diagnostic Handbook* concerned with women or from therapeutic women's healthcare texts are known. But it is possible that Tablets 37–39 of the *Diagnostic Handbook* dealing with sick women were concerned similar subject matters as the prescriptions in BAM 245.

List of Manuscripts

Siglum	Museum Number	Copy	Collation	Format; Ductus	Provenience
A	VAT 11415	BAM 245	Coll.	Fragment of a tablet; Neo-Assyrian script; ca. 8th cent. BCE)	Assur

Overview

i' Fragmentary prescription ...]1'–4'
A obv.$^{?}$ 1'–4'

ii' Fragmentary prescription 5'–12'[...
A obv.$^{?}$ 5'–12'

Previous Edition and Discussion

Köcher 1964, BAM Vol. 3, xviii, pl. 48 (discussion; copy)
BabMed Corpora (https://www.geschkult.fu-berlin.de/e/babmed/Corpora/BAM-3/BAM-3_-245; transliteration)
CDLI P281822 (photo and transliteration)

Transliteration

Beginning of ms. A obv.(?) lost

1' A obv.$^{?}$ 1' [............]x *ak-tam* ma-x-[...]

2' A obv.$^{?}$ 2' [..............]x KI ZÌ ŠE.SA.A *ina* KA[Š ....]

3' A obv.$^{?}$ 3' [..............]x Ì.GIŠ ŠÀ ⌜*ú*$^{?}$*áš*$^{?}$⌝-*lam* [................................]

4' A obv.$^{?}$ 4' [...................] NAG-*ši-ma la ul-ta-a*[*p-pat*$^{?}$ ....]

5' A obv.$^{?}$ 5' [DIŠ MUNUS$^{?}$ ...] *iṣ-ṣe-né-eḫ ši-kín pa-ni-*[*šá* ....]

6' A obv.$^{?}$ 6' [................ *be-e*]*n-nu* DAB-*ši i-re-eḫ-ḫi-*[*ši*$^{?}$ ....]

7' A obv.$^{?}$ 7' [... IM.SAḪ]AR.BABBAR.KUR.RA IM.SAḪAR.GI$_{6}$.KUR.RA [......]

8' A obv.$^{?}$ 8' [...... ^{n}]^{a4}*it-te-mir* NA$_{4}$ *a-la*$^{?}$-<*di*> ^{na4}U[GU.AŠ.GÌ.GÌ$^{?}$ ....]

9' A obv.$^{?}$ 9' [................]x *ina* KUŠ DÙ.DÙ-*p*[*í* ....]

10' A obv.? 10' [........... DID]A SIG$_5$.GA ^{ši}[m ....]

11' A obv.? 11' [..................]x *tul-ta-nap-[pat*? ....]

12' A obv.? 12' [...........]x *ana* ŠÀ GAL$_4$.[LA-*šá* GAR-*an* ....]

Ms. A breaks; remainder lost

Bound Transcription and Translation

Beginning of ms. A obv.(?) lost

1' [... ...]... *aktam* ...[... ...] 2' [... ...] *itti qēm labti ina šikari* [... ...] 3' [... ...] *šaman libbi ašlam*(?) [... ...] 4' [... ...] *tašaqqīši-ma lā ulta*[*ppat*(?) ... ...]

1' [.....]..., *aktam*-plant, ...[... ...], 2' [... you ...] with flour of roasted barley in beer [.....], 3' [...]... fat(?) from the belly, *aš-lu*-rush(?), [......]. 4' [....] you give (it) to her to drink. But *she should not be* [*smeared*(?) (with it), ...].

5' [*šumma sinništu*(?) ...] *iṣṣenēḫ šikin pānī*[*ša* ... ...] 6' [... ... *be*]*nnu iṣbatuši ireḫḫī*[*ši*(?) ...] 7 [... ... *annu*]*ḫara qitmu* [... ...] 8' [... *it*]*temir aban alādi*(?) *ag*[*usīgu*(?) ... ...] 9' [... ...] *ina maški tašappi* [*ina kišādīša tašakkan* ...] 10' [... ... *bil*]*lat našpi* [... ...] 11' [... ...] ... *tultanap*[*pat*(?) ...] 12' [... ...] *ina ūr*[*īša tašakkan*(?) ... ...]

5' [If a woman(?) ...] laughs constantly, the appearance of [her] face [....], 6' [... *when ben*]*nu*-epilepsy afflicts her, it 'pours over' [her, ...], 7' [... (white) *ann*]*uḫaru*-pigment, (black) *qitmu*-mineral, [... ...], 8' *ittemir*-stone, the stone of giving birth(?), tur[quoise(?), ...], 9' [....] you wrap up in a piece of leather, [*you place (this) around her neck.* ...], 10' [... ..., beer] wort for *našpu*-beer, [...]-aromatic, [... ...], 11' [....], ... you smear repeatedly (?), [....], 12' [....], [you insert(?) (it)] into [her vagina, [... ...].

Ms. A breaks; remainder lost

Notes

Line 3': For *šaman libbi*, the fat from the inside (stomach, belly) of an animal, see CAD Š/1, 329 s.v. *šamnu* sub m.

Line 4': The restoration of the verb after NAG-*ši-ma* is not certain, but the form *ultap*[*pat*] may be a Dt-stem durative form of *lapātu* "to touch", which has the special meaning "to be delayed". However, a passive meaning to the D-stem *lupputu* "to touch, to anoint, to rub" would be better suited in the present passage; cf. CAD L, 91–92 s.v. *lapātu* sub 4i and line 11' below (*tultanappat* "you smear repeatedly").

Line 5': For abnormal laughter (*ṣiāḫu* G- or Gtn-stem) as part of the symptomology, see e.g. BAM 30: 54' (catchline): DIŠ NA *ina* KI.NÁ-*šú* GÙ.GÙ-*si iṣ-ṣe-né-eḫ* "If a man keeps repeatedly cries out (and) laughs in his sleep" (Scurlock 2014a, 673; text against gnashing the teeth in one's sleep). In the *Diagnostic Handbook*, abnormal laughter is mentioned in Tablet 15: 77' (Heeßel 2000, 155; Scurlock 2014a, 143). In Tablet 22: 6–7, laughing for no apparent reason (*ṣūh lā pakki iṣṣenēḫ*) is listed among the symptoms of "love sickness" (*muruṣ râmi*), affecting both men and women in the same way (Heeßel 2000, 251; Scurlock 2014a, 185; Couto-Ferreira 2010, 34). In Tablet 22: 62, continuous laughter (*iṣṣenēḫ*) is attributed to the Hand of *mukīl-rēš-lemutti*, "the Supporter of evil", or alternatively to the Hand of the goddess Ištar (Heeßel 2000, 256; Scurlock 2014a, 188). In Tablet 26: 14', laughter during a falling spell (*magal iṣīḫ* "he laughs much") is attributed to the *lilû*-demon (Heeßel 2000, 279; Scurlock 2014a, 196). In Tablet 40: 62, laughing very much (*mādiš iṣṣenēḫ*) is found among the symptoms of a lethal illness affecting an infant (Scurlock 2014a, 260).

After *iṣṣenēḫ*, restore perhaps *šikin pānīša* [KÚR.KÚR-*er*] "the appearance of [her] face [keeps changing (for the worse)]", cf. CAD Š/2, 437 sub 1d. Compare further *Diagnostic Handbook* Tablet 36: 77: DIŠ TU IGI.MEŠ-*šá ik-ki-ru* "if a childbearing woman's face changes (for the worse)"; BAM 240: 20' (text D.2.1): SU-*šá* KÚR.KÚR "her body keeps changing (for the worse)".

Line: 6': For the restoration of *bennu*-epilepsy, see also Stol 1993, 6. Two other fragments (BAM 249 obv.? i 5' from Assur and STT 98 rev. 6') mention *bennu* in the context of prescriptions for promoting delivery, where they may concern the protection of the newborn (see texts D.1.2 and A.1.1). The spelling *bennu* DAB-*ši* (not DAB-*si*) indicates that the verbal form of *ṣabātu* behind the logogram DAB ended in a vowel, which may be a subjunctive.

The following verb *ireḫḫi*, from *reḫû* "to pour (over); to inseminate" is found in the context of epilepsy-related symptom descriptions in the *Diagnostic Handbook* Tablet 26, which confirms the reading *bennu* in line 6' of the present text. See Tablet 26: 22' (Heeßel 2000, 280; Scurlock 2014a, 197): *ireḫḫišum-ma* "it flows over him and (he forgets himself)". Similarly, Tablet 26: 48' (*ireḫḫišum-ma*), 69' (*ireḫḫûšu*); Tablet 27: 18 (*irteneḫḫīšu*). For discussion, see also Stol 1993, 61–62 (who understands this expression as referring to the patient losing consciousness) and Steinert 2022.

Line 8': The *ittamir*-stone (here in the variant spelling *ittemir*) is designated as "the stone of giving birth" (*aban alādi*) in the commentary section in Hg. B IV 74 (MSL 10, 31); Stol 2000a, 49–50. The emendation proposed here is based on this qualification of the *ittamir*-stone. Cf. further Schuster-Brandis 2008, 420 and TCL 6, 49 (AO 6374: 8–12, see text C.3.9) for the use of this stone in an amulet to protect a pregnant woman from witchcraft.

Line 11': For *lapātu* "to touch" in the meaning "to smear (on)" (attested for the G- and D-stem), also "to moisten" (Gt-stem), see CAD L, 86 sub 1h, 89 sub 2a, 90 sub 4b.

A.1.4 K. 8678 +: Prescriptions for Rectal Diseases and Women's Health

This fragmentary single-column tablet in Neo-Babylonian script excavated at Nineveh presents one of the rare examples for a medical cuneiform text containing a mixture of gynaecological and non-gynaecological material. The text preserved on the obverse deals with recipes for rectal disease (DÚR.GIG "sick anus") and for a problem affecting the hips, while the reverse contains prescriptions for women. According to M. J. Geller (2005a, No. 44), the top edge of the tablet is partially preserved, however, the first line of the obverse is very eroded.

Two of the tablet fragments, AMT 58/9 (K. 13901) and AMT 81/9 (K. 10567), had been recognized as part of the same tablet as early as 1929 by R. C. Thompson, and were edited by Geller (2005a, No. 44) in his treatment of cuneiform texts on renal and rectal diseases. Subsequently, J. Fincke (2006-, *Nineveh Tablet Collection*) identified K. 8678, K. 16461 (AMT 62/5) and K. 19344 as new joins. The text was discussed together with an edition of the tablet's obverse by K. Simkó (2018), who also commented on the rationale that may have led the scribe of K. 8678+ to assemble treatments for rectal diseases and women's conditions on the same tablet. He concluded that the similarity of the treatments employed for both types of conditions (in particular, suppositories/tampons inserted into the anus or vagina, respectively) could stand behind the combination of prescriptions. Other reasons that may have played a role could have been the anatomical proximity of the treated conditions as well as perceived similarities in the physiological processes and disease conditions affecting the gastrointestinal tract and women's reproductive system. Another possibility might be that the prescriptions on the obverse of the tablet were compiled together with gynaecological material for use in the context of the medical treatment of women, e.g. in the context of pregnancy and birth.

Simkó (2018) also noticed that the structure and format of the section on the obverse and reverse differ. The text sections on the obverse mostly consist of lists of drug ingredients that briefly state the treatment form and ailment for which they could be used, while omitting most instructions for preparation and application. The preserved sections on the obverse are basically lists of ingredients for acorn-shaped suppositories (*allānu*), of which two sections make ample use of measurements.

While the format of the prescriptions on the obverse is telegraphic and resembles the structural components encountered in drug handbooks (therapeutic *Vademecums*), the format of the prescriptions for women on the reverse is more detailed, including two more elaborate procedures dealing with the problem of "blocked fluids", referring to the retention of the lochia, the postpartum discharges (cf. Steinert 2013). In the second of these two prescriptions (lines 30''–33'') the practitioner is instructed to dig a shallow hole in the ground, in which he put several ingredients (part of which are aromatics) on burning charcoals. Then the woman had to sit down (or squat) over the hole so that the fumes could reach her pubic region. The procedure shares essential features with descriptions of fumigation from below found in Hippocratic texts on women's diseases (see Steinert 2014a and 2014b for discussion).

The first remedy for "blocked fluids" (lines 24''–29'') is fragmentary, but it appears to describe essentially a form of heat treatment. This new interpretation proposed here for the first time suggests that a brick was heated, wrapped in cloth and placed on a movable(?) oven that was lowered into the ground. Then the patient sat down on the oven/brick and was covered with cloth, so as not to let the heat and fumes (of ingredients sprinkled on the oven) escape. Presumably, the applied local heat was supposed to trigger the movement of the lochia.

The remaining portions on the reverse (lines 34''–41'') offer rare examples of recipes to obtain an abortion. Such recipes were hitherto exclusively known from a small Neo-Assyrian tablet from Assur (BAM 246, text B.1.6). The recipes for abortion on the reverse of K. 8678+ employ tampons, i.e. drugs enveloped in a wad of wool (and inserted into the woman's vagina), while the suppositories on the obverse are mixture of pounded drugs mixed with a carrier substance (fat, wax).

The left tablet edge seems to have been inscribed with three lines of text, which may have contained a colophon; unfortunately, only traces remain which are barely readable. Since there has not been a complete edition of the five fragments, both the obverse and reverse are edited here for the convenience of the reader.

List of Manuscripts

Siglum	Museum Number	Copy	Collation	Format; Ductus	Provenience
a	K. 8678 + K. 10567 + K. 13901 + K. 16461 + K. 19344	AMT 81/9 + AMT 58/9 + AMT 62/5 Geller 2005a, pl. 28 (= AMT 58/9 + AMT 81/9)[247] Pl. 10–11	Coll.	Fragment of a single-column tablet; Neo-Babylonian script; 7th cent. BCE[248]	Nineveh; Ashurbanipal's Library

Overview

i'	Fragmentary list of ingredients (suppository) a obv. 1'–4'	...]1'–4'
ii'	List of ingredients for a suppository for rectal disease a obv. 5'–7'	5'–7'
iii'	List of ingredients for a suppository for rectal disease a obv. 8'–9'	8'–9'
iv'	List of ingredients for a suppository for a condition of the hips a obv. 10'–18'	10'–18'
v'	Fragmentary list of ingredients a obv. 19'–21'	19'–21'[...
vi''	Fragmentary prescription (suppository) a rev. 1'–2'	...]22''–23''
vii''	Prescription for a woman suffering from "blocked fluids" (lochia) a rev. 3'–8'	24''–29''
viii''	Prescription for a woman suffering from "blocked fluids" (fumigation) a rev. 9'–12'	30''–33''
ix''	Prescription to induce an abortion (suppository) a rev. 13'–15'	34''–36''
x''	Prescription to induce an abortion (suppository) a rev. 16'–17'	37''–38''

247 The join of AMT 58/9 (K. 13901) + AMT 81/9 (K. 10567) was identified by Thompson 1929, 85. Geers made an unpublished copy of K. 8678 (Folio A21; see https://www.ebl.lmu.de/library/K.8678).

248 Measurements: ca. 6.5 x 9.5 x 3 cm.

xi''	Prescription to induce an abortion (suppository) a rev. 18'–19'	39''-40''
xii''	Fragmentary prescription to induce an abortion a rev. 20'	41''[...
xiii'''	Colophon(?) a l. e. 1–3	42'''–44'''

Previous Edition and Discussion

Geller 2005a, *BAM* 7, 234–235 No. 44 (transliteration and translation of K. 10567 (AMT 81/9) + K. 13901 (AMT 58/9))
Lambert Folio 9538 (transliteration of K. 8678)
Steinert 2014a (discussion)
Steinert 2014b (discussion)
Simkó 2018, *FS Geller*, 537–555 (transliteration and translation of ms. a obv.; discussion)
CDLI P238756 (transliteration ms. a obv.; photo)
Electronic Babylonian Library (eBL) (https://www.ebl.lmu.de/library/K.8678; transliteration; photo)

Transliteration

Beginning of ms. a obv. lost

1' a obv. 1' [...] ⸢NUMUN⸣ ^{ú}[..........................]

2' a obv. 2' [.............. *saḫ*]-*le-e as*-⸢*né-e*⸣ x[x x x]

3' a obv. 3' [.............. DU]Ḫ.LÀL Ú.NAM.TI.L[A]

4' a obv. 4' [......] ⸢PAP$^{?}$⸣ x+3 Ú.MEŠ *al-la-nu* ⸢DÚR.GIG⸣

5' a obv. 5' [Ì].⸢UDU$^{?}$⸣ DUḪ.LÀ[L ^{š}]^{im}GÚR.GÚR ^{šim}LI

6' a obv. 6' [x x] ^{na4}*ga-bu-u* [MU]N$^{?}$ ^{ú}NAGA.SI Ú.NAM.TI.LA

7' a obv. 7' [ŠE.SA].⸢A$^{?}$⸣ DUḪ KAŠ ⸢*damaged gloss*⸣ PAP 10 ⸢Ú⸣.[ME]Š *al*-⸢*la-nu*⸣ DÚR.GIG

8' a obv. 8' [^{ú}*n*]*i-nu-ú* Ú.NAM.TI.⸢LA⸣ ⸢x⸣ [x] *dan-nu-ti*

9' a obv. 9' [NAG]A.⸢SI⸣ Ì.UDU DUḪ.LÀL PAP 6 *a*[*l-la*]-*nu* DÚR.GIG

10' a obv. 10' [1 G]ÍN *ḫi-li* ^{šim}BULUḪ 1 GÍN ^{šim}ḪAB 1[/2$^{?}$ GÍN x x x]

11' a obv. 11' [4]-*tú* DUḪ.LÀL 4 ZÚ.LUM.MA 4 ^{šim}[x x x (x)]

12' a obv. 12' ⸢1/2 SÌLA$^{?}$⸣ NAGA.SI 4-*tú* Ú BABBAR 4-*tú* U_5ARK[AB^{mušen}]

13' a obv. 13' ⸢2$^{?}$⸣ *gi-re-e* ^{šim}GIG 4 ^{giš}EREN.BAD [x x x]

14' a obv. 14' 4 ^{ú}KUR.KUR 2 *gi-re-e* Ú.ḪUR.SAG.GÁ [x] ⸢$^{ú?}$x⸣

15' a obv. 15' 2 *gi-re-e qut-ra-nu* 5-*aš rit-tú* ⸢$^{ú?}$⸣*pi-i*[*n-ze-er*]

16' a obv. 16' 2 *gi-re-e* ^{šim}MUG 2 *gi-re*-⸢*e*⸣ *saḫ-l*[*e-e*]

17' a obv. 17' [Ì *ḫ*]*al*$^{?}$-<*ṣa*> Ú.NAM.TI.LA ⸢*ina lìb-bi*$^{?}$⸣ Ú.ḪI.A *ta-n*[*a-ad-di*$^{?}$]

18' a obv. 18' [PAP 2]2$^{?}$ Ú.MEŠ ALLA DIŠ MURUB$_4$-⸢*šú*⸣ TU$_{15}$ G[IG$^{?}$]

19' a obv. 19' [x GÍN] ⸢Ì⸣.UDU 1 GÍN DUḪ.LÀ[L] 1/2 GÍN *as-né-*[*e*]

20' a obv. 20' [...............]x 1 GÍN [IL]LU ^{šim}BULUḪ [x x]

21' a obv. 21' [................] ⸢zag?⸣ [x] ⸢giš?⸣ ⸢x x⸣ [x]

Ms. a obv. breaks; gap of unknown length
Beginning of reverse lost

22'' a rev. 1' *ra-šum-*[x x] ⸢x⸣ [.........................]

23'' a rev. 2' ḪI.ḪI *maš-š*[*i*?*-t*]*a*? *u m*[*a-gal*? ....]

24'' a rev. 3' DIŠ MUNUS A.MEŠ GUR-*át* x[x x x x] ⸢SIG$_4$?⸣ [x x x]

25'' a rev. 4' [x x] x ⸢GAR⸣-*an* TINUR ⸢GAR-*an*⸣ ⸢BAR?⸣ ^{giš}[NU].⸢ÚR⸣.M[A?]

26'' a rev. 5' [*nam-ru*]*q*?*-qa ni-nu-ú* MAR K[I? BA]D?*-ma* T[INUR GAR?]

27'' a rev. 6' [*kan-na*?]*-tú šá* TÚG *ta-kan-na-an i*[*na lìb-bi*?] ⸢SIG$_4$?⸣ [NIGIN?]

28'' a rev. 7' [*ina* UG]U? TUŠ-*šeb-ši-ma* TÚG.ḪI.A [............]

29'' a rev. 8' ⸢DUL?⸣ *ta-pa-as-sà-am* [......]

30'' a rev. 9' DIŠ KI.MIN PÚ BAD-*ma* 2 ŠU.SI *tu-ša*[*p*?*-pal*]

31'' a rev. 10' [SI]G$_4$? DUL?-*ma* ZÌ *ina lìb-bi* ŠUB-*di* 1 NINDA *k*[*a*?*-mu-nu*]

32'' a rev. 11' [x NINDA] *ḫu-ṣab ḫi-li* 3-*šú* NINDA ^{šim}ḪAB x[x (x)]

33'' a rev. 12' [x x *ana*] UGU UDUB(LAGABxNE) DUB-*aq* MUNUS BI *ina* U[GU] ⸢TUŠ⸣-[(*šeb-ši*?)]

34'' a rev. 13' [*ana* ^{munus}PEŠ$_4$ *šà* Š]À-*šà* ŠUB-*e* ^{ú}NU.LUḪ.ḪA ^{ú}[GAZ]I^{sar}

35'' a rev. 14' [x x x ^{síg}]ZA.GÌN *šá ni-i*[*p*]*-še mit-ḫar* SÚ[D *ina*?] DUḪ.ŠE.GIŠ.Ì

36'' a rev. 15' [ḪI.ḪI? *ana* ŠÀ.T]ÙR-*šú* [GAR]-*an*

37'' a rev. 16' [DIŠ KI.MIN IM.SAḪAR.N]A$_4$.⸢KUR⸣.RA ^{ú}*nam-ruq-qu*

38'' a rev. 17' [x x x x x Ḫ]I.ḪI KI.MIN

39'' a rev. 18' [DIŠ KI.MIN? x x x x x *m*]*a-gal* NU GAZ *ina* KÀŠ 3 *u*$_4$*-me* GAR-*an*

40'' a rev. 19' [........... ḪI.Ḫ]I? *ina*? ^{síg}ZA.GÌN.NA KI.MIN

41'' a rev. 20' [DIŠ KI.MIN ....] ⸢x x x⸣ [^{munus}]⸢PEŠ$_4$?⸣ ⸢*šà*⸣ ŠÀ-*šà* ŠUB-*di*

Ms. a rev. breaks; gap of unknown length

42''' a l. e. 1 [.......] U[GU ....] ši [...................]

43''' a l. e. 2 [.....................] ⸢uk?⸣ [...................]

44''' a l. e. 3 [....... DU]B? 3.⸢KÁM?⸣ [...................]

Bound Transcription and Translation

Beginning of ms. a obv. lost

1' [... ...] *zēr* ...[... ...] 2' [... ... *saḫ*]*lê asnê* [...] 3' [... ... *iš*]*kūru šammi balāṭi* 4' [... ...] *napḫar* x+3 *šammū allān durugiqqi*	1' [... ...] seed of [...]-plant, [... ...], 2' [... of *sa*]*ḫlû*-plant (and) Dilmun date palm, [... ...], 3' [... ... w]ax, 'plant of life', [... ...], 4' [... ...] a total of x+3 drugs for a suppository (to cure) rectal disease ('sick anus').
5' [*li*]*pû*(?) *iškūru kukru burāšu* 6' [...] *gabû* [*ṭāb*]*tu*(?) *uḫūlu qarnānû šammi balāṭi* 7' [*lab*]*tu*(?) *tuḫḫī šikari*(?) *napḫar ešeret šammī allān durugiqqi*	5' [Tal]low(?), wax, *kukru*-plant, *burāšu*-juniper, 6' [...], alum, [sa]lt(?), 'horned' alkali (salicornia), 'plant of life', 7' [roasted gra]in(?), draff of beer(?) – a total of ten drugs for a suppository (to cure) rectal disease ('sick anus').
8' [*n*]*īnû šammi balāṭi* ...[...] *dannūti*(?) 9' [*uḫū*]*lu qarnānu lipû iškūru napḫar šeššet allān durugiqqi*	8' [*N*]*īnû*-plant, 'plant of life', strong(?) [...], 9' 'horned' [alka]li, tallow, wax – a total of six (ingredients) for a suppository (to cure) rectal disease ('sick anus').
10' [*ištēn ši*]*qil ḫīl baluḫḫi ištēn šiqil ṭūru z*[*ūz* ...] 11' [*reb*]*ūtu iškūru rebūtu*(?) *suluppū rebūtu*(?) [...] 12' *mišil qa*(?) *uḫūlu qarnānû rebūtu šammu peṣû rebūtu rikibti ark*[*abi*] 13' *šina girê kanaktu erbet šupuḫru* 14' *erbet atā'išu šina girê šammi ḫursāni*(?) ... 15' *šina girê qutrānu ḫamaš rittu pi*[*nzer*(?)] 16' *šina girê ballukku šina girê saḫlê* 17' [*šamna ḫa*]*l*<*ṣa*>(?) *šammi balāṭi ina libbi šammī tan*[*addi*(?)] 18' [*napḫar* 2]2(?) *šammū allānu šumma qabalšu šāra m*[*aruṣ*]	10' [One shek]el resin of *baluḫḫu*-aromatic, one shekel *ṭūru*-aromatic, ha[lf a shekel ...], 11' [a quart]er (of a shekel of) wax, a quarter (of a shekel of?) dates, a quarter (of a shekel of?) [....]-aromatic, 12' half a litre(?) 'horned' alkali, a quarter (of a shekel of) 'white drug', a quarter (of a shekel) of '*spur* of b[at]', 13' 1/12 of a shekel of *kanaktu*-aromatic, a sixth of a shekel of *šupuḫru*-cedar, [...], 14' a sixth (of a shekel) *atā'išu*-plant, 1/12 of a shekel of 'mountain-plant', ... of ...-plant, 15' 1/12 of a shekel of *qutrānu*, one fifth of a handful(?) of 'cob[web'(?)], 16' 1/12 of a shekel of *ballukku*-aromatic, 1/12 of a shekel of *saḫlû*-plant. 17' You a[dd(?)] [pr]essed(?) [oil], 'plant of life' to (these) drugs. 18' [A total of twenty]-two(?) drugs (for) a suppository for the case that his hip is [stricken] with wind(?).
19' [... *šiqil*] *lipû ištēn šiqil iškūru zūz asnû* 20' [... ...] *ištēn šiqil ḫīl baluḫḫi* [...] 21' *only traces preserved*	19' [x shekels of] tallow, one shekel of wax, half a shekel of Dilmun-date, 20' [... ...], one shekel resin of *baluḫḫu*-aromatic, 21' *too fragmentary for translation*

Ms. a obv. breaks; gap of unknown length
Beginning of ms. a rev. lost

22'' *too fragmentary for transcription* 23'' *tuballal maššīta u ma*[*gal*(?) ...]	22'' ... ...[... ... ...] 23'' you mix. The *suppository* and mu[ch(?) ... ...].
24'' *šumma sinništu mê turrat-ma* [... ...] *libittu*(?) [...] 25'' [...]... *tašakkan*(?) *tinūra tašakkan qilip*(?) *lur*[*mê*] 26'' [*namru*]*qqa*(?) *nīnû tazarru qaq*[*qara*(?) *tepe*]*ttē-ma*(?) *ti*[*nūra tašakkan*(?)] 27'' [*kannā*]*ti ša lubāri takannan in*[*a libbi*(?)] *libitta*(?) [*talammi*(?)] 28'' [*ina mu*]*ḫḫi tušeššebšī-ma lubārī* [.... ...] *kutma*(?) *tapassam* [...]	24'' If a woman is blocked with fluids and [... ...], a mudbrick(?) [... ...], 25'' [... ...] you set up(?). You set up an oven. 26'' You scatter 25'' pome[granate] rind(?), 26'' [*namru*]*qqu*-plant(?), *nīnû*-plant. You [op]en(?) (a hole in) the gro[und(?)] and [position(?)] the ov[en] (in it). 27'' You roll up together [ban]ds(?) of cloth. [You wrap(?)] the brick(?) wi[th it(?)]. 28'' You let her sit down [on] top (of it). With cloth [... ...] 29'' as a covering(?) you (should) cover (her?) [...].

30'' DIŠ KI.MIN *būrta tepettē-ma šina ubānāti tušap[pal]* 31'' *[libit]ta(?) takattam(?)-ma qēma(?) ina libbi tanaddi ištēn akal(?) k[amūna]* 32'' *[... akal] ḫuṣāb ḫīli šalšu akal ṭūra ... [...]* 33'' *[... ana] muḫḫi pēmti tasarraq sinništu šuāti ina mu[ḫḫi] tuš[eššeb(ši)?]*

30'' Alternatively (i.e. for a woman blocked with fluids), you dig a hole, you make it two fingers [deep]. 31'' You cover (it) with a [bri]ck(?), then you pour flour(?) into it. A tenth litre of cu[min(?)], 32'' [... tenth of a litre of] small (pieces of solid?) resin, one thirtieth of a litre of *ṭūru*-aromatic [...], 33'' [...] you strew (this) onto charcoals (in the hole). You let that woman s[it down(?)] above it.

34'' *[ana erīti ša lib]bīša šuddê(?) nuḫurta k[as]â* 35'' *[...] uqnâti(?) ša nipše mitḫār tasâk [ina] kupsi* 36'' *[tuballal(?) ana šas]sūrīšu [tašakk]an*

34'' [To] cause [a pregnant woman] to have a miscarriage (lit. expel her [foe]tus): 35'' You crush 34'' *nuḫurtu*-plant, *kasû*-plant, 35'' (and) combed [bl]ue wool(?) in equal quantities. 36'' [You mix (it)] 35'' [with] sesame pomace. 36'' You insert it [into] her womb (viz. vagina).

37'' [DIŠ KI.MIN *gab]û namruqqu* 38'' [... ... *tu]ballal* KI.MIN

37'' [Alternatively, 38'' you mix 37'' [al]um, *namruqqu*-plant, 38'' [... ...], ditto (i.e. you insert it into her womb (viz. vagina)).

39'' [DIŠ. KIMIN(?) ...] *magal(?) lā taḫaššal ina šīnāti šalāšat ūmē tašakkan* 40'' [... ...... *tubal]lal(?) ina uqnâti* KI.MIN

39'' [Alternatively(?), ...], you do not crush (it) very much(?). You put (it) in urine for three days. 40'' [... ... you m]ix(?), (you wrap it) in blue wool, ditto (i.e. insert it into her womb).

41'' [DIŠ KI.MIN(?) ... ...] ... *erītu ša libbīša inaddi*

41'' [Alternatively(?): ... ...] a pregnant woman will have a miscarriage.

Ms. a rev. breaks; gap of unknown length

42'''–43''' *only traces preserved* 44''' [... ... *tu]ppu šalšu(?)* [... ...]

42'''–43''' *only traces preserved* 44''' [... ...] third [tab]let(?) [... ...].

Notes

Lines 4', 7', 9': The disease name DÚR.GIG is often rendered as Akkadian *muruṣ šuburri* "disease of the rectum". However, the logogram may have to be read as a Sumerian loanword *durugiqqu*, see Heeßel 2018, *FS Geller*, 334 comment on rev. 3', with Köcher 1957–1958, *AfO* 18, 86 (quoting the lexical text VAT 14274 left col. line 6: DÚR.GIG = *du-ru-gi-iq-qu*).

Line 4': It looks as if there are traces of one sign for the number 10 (U) before the number 3 in line 4'. The total of ingredients may have consisted of 13 or 23 drugs.

Line 5': At the beginning of the line, Simkó (2018, 540) reads [(x x x) ᵘSUMUN]. ⌜DAR⌝ = *šumuttu* "beetroot(?)" instead of [Ì]. UDU "tallow; suet". Note however the repeated occurrence of tallow (*lipû*) beside wax as basic ingredient (carrier substance) for making a suppository in K. 8678+ (see also lines 9', 19').

Line 6': The reading [MU]N in line 6' follows eBL.

Line 7': The reading [ŠE.SA].⌜A?⌝ at the beginning of the line is tentative. The sign before DUḪ ends in a vertical or in a double vertical wedge. Another possible restoration could be [ŠE.NÁ].A = "*šunû*-plant".

The final ingredient listed in line 7' consists of the signs DUḪ KAŠ. The logogram DUḪ can be read as Akkadian *tuḫḫū* "draff, bran" (resulting from beer brewing), which is a solid commodity that is used e.g. as animal fodder (CAD T, 453–454 sub 2; Stol 1971, *BiOr* 28, 167–171). The texts often speak of DUḪ.DURU$_5$/ ḪÁD.DU, "moist bran" and "dry bran". However, the sequence DUḪ KAŠ is not attested in any other medical prescription or other textual source. The reading *tuḫḫī šikari* "draff of beer" is therefore tentative. Beside signs of damage, there are also traces of a cuneiform sign written in smaller script below the sign KAŠ, perhaps a gloss (I owe this observation to Henry Stadhouders, personal communication). Less likely, read *gab-bi* "all" (suggestion by M. J. Geller).

Line 8': The last drug ingredient in this line still defies identification. A solid ingredient is expected here, which throws doubt on the reading *dannūti* "strong" (masc. pl. adjective). In medical texts, *dannu* "strong" is usually found as attribute to alcoholic liquids, e.g. vinegar, wine or beer (CAD D, 93–94 sub 1a), but these nouns are not construed with a masculine plural complement. Otherwise, *dannu* can also mean "thick, hard, solid". Another possibility is to interpret *dannūti* as a genitive plural form of the noun *dannu*, which refers to large storage vessels for liquids and other commodities (see CAD D, 98–99; AHw 161b s.v. *dannu* II, with a plural form *dannūtu* in Neo-Babylonian). As a different alternative, eBL suggests to restore ᵘ[KI].KAL NU TI, "[...]-plant, not fresh". However, the opposite of "fresh" (*balṭu*) is usually expressed by HÁD.DU (*ablu*) "dried", not *lā balṭu*. M. J. Geller (personal communication) tentatively restores Ú.[MEŠ] *dan-nu-ti* "strong plants/ drugs".

Line 9': For the beginning of the line, Simkó (2018, 541, 542) proposes a different ingredient, ⸢Ì.GIŠ⸣ "oil" or [*saḫ-l*]*é*-⸢*e*⸣ "*saḫlû*-plant".

Lines 13'–16': The unit of measurement *girû* stands for 1/24 of a shekel or "one carat" (0.347g), cf. Borger 2004, MZL, p. 604; AHw 291b; CAD G, 96–97; Powell 1987–1990, "Masse und Gewichte", *RlA* 7, 511–513 § VA.1c. The word *girû* is related to Aramaic *gērā*, the (weight corresponding to a) seed of the carob tree. In lines 13'–16', small drug amounts of two and four *girû* (1/12 and 1/6 of a shekel) are prescribed. The numeral 4-*tú* in lines 11' and 12' can be understood as *rebūtu* "one-fourth of a shekel" or 6 *girû* (Powell 1987–1990, 512–513). The same numeral seems to be repeated in abbreviated form without phonetic complement twice in line 11'.

Line 14': Since the plant name *azupīru* is usually written ᵘḪUR.SAG or ᵘḪUR.SAG^{sar}, it seems better to understand Ú.ḪUR.SAG.GÁ as a Sumerian genitive construction "plant of the mountain" or "mountain plant" (*šammi ḫursāni*), similar to Ú.NAM.TI.LA = *šammi balāṭi* "plant of life" (following Simkó 2018, 541, 543).

Line 15': A drug called *qutrānu* is not attested elsewhere (see also Simkó 2018, 543). The name might be related to *qutrīnu/ qutrēnu* "incense" or to the medicinal plant *qud/tru/ qud/tratu* (CAD Q, 323–325, 327; AHw 926, 930–931). Perhaps the ending -*ānu* means "similar to *qutru*".

The following signs in line 15' might be read 5-*aš rit-tú* (*ḫamaš rittu*) "one fifth of a hand(ful)", with Stadhouders, *NABU* 2018/3, 127 No. 81. There are only rare examples for such a measurement (AHw 318b, s.v. *ḫamšu* sub 3; CAD R, 386b sub 3), for example in a Middle Assyrian text (VAT 9542 obv. 5; Ebeling 1951, 20), which is phrased a bit differently: Ú.MEŠ *ma-l*[*a*] *ri-te* "a handful of hay". Simkó (2018, 541) reads the sequence 5-*aš* LAG BABBAR, and translates "one-fifth (of a shekel) of *a white lump* (*of salt*)".

The reconstruction ᵘ*pi*[*nzer*] "cobweb" at the end of the line follows Stadhouders, *NABU* 2018/3, 127 No. 81 and eBL. This drug is attested repeatedly in rectal disease texts (see e.g., Heeßel 2018, *FS Geller*, 320 obv. 16', 31'; CAD P, 452–453 for different syllabic spellings). An alternative reading ᵘ*pi-l*[*e-e*] is also not excluded (cf. CAD P, 377a sub 2').

Line 17': The reconstruction of this line follows a suggestion by M. J. Geller (personal communication).

Line 18': The medical problem specified at the end of the line has been rendered MURUB$_4$-*šú* TU$_{15}$ G[IG] "his hip s[uffers] from wind". This reading seems highly plausible, since "wind" (*šāru*) as pathogenic entity is mentioned frequently as a symptom in connection with rectal disease, also explicitly with DÚR.GIG (see Simkó 2018, 544). Thus, there are many descriptions of a patient bloated with wind that is trapped in the body or that is butting out of the anus.[249] But there does not seem to be a single occurrence of "wind" that is said to befall the hip(s) (*qablu*, MURUB$_4$). "Wind" is usually localised either in the belly (*libbu*; ŠÀ) or anus (DÚR, *šuburru*), see e.g. BAM 159 v 48–49 (Scurlock 2014a, 499–501).[250] Alternatively, the sign traces at the end of line 18' also allow a reading MURUB$_4$-*šú im-š*[*i-id*] "his hip is affected by stroke". The hips are often described in medical texts as "hurting" (*akālu*) or being "stiff" (*ašṭu*). But again, a literal parallel for the expression *qabalšu imšid* is not known from other texts either, although stroke (*mišittu*) affecting the hips is mentioned, for example, in BAM 136 ii 3' // AMT 79/1 iv 11: *šumma amēlu mišitti qabli*(MURUB$_4$) *maruṣ*(GIG) "if a man suffers from stroke affecting the hip (and he cannot walk)" (Scurlock and Andersen 2005, 13.238). Nonetheless, the method of treatment applied in the

249 See e.g. BAM 95: 4, 7, 8–9 (Geller 2005a, *BAM* 7, No. 21, suppositories to stop 'wind' or to release trapped 'wind', inserted into the anus); AMT 47/1+ and dupl. ii 1–3 (Geller 2005, *BAM* 7, No. 24); STT 100: 3'–5' (Geller 2005a, *BAM* 7, No. 43).

250 Perhaps MURUB$_4$ "hip" here is meant to indicate the rectum or anus, cf. similarly the sign MÚRUB can stand for "buttocks" (*šuḫḫu*), see Jiménez 2023, in: *Synopses and Lists*, 16 (Ur$_5$-ra XV 24).

present section – a suppository (likely inserted into the anus) – does not speak for stroke as the treated problem, since the latter is more often treated with bandages.

Lines 22''–23'': The term *maššītu* occurs often in women's healthcare texts in the meaning of "suppository", see e.g. BM 38624+: 5', 10', 11', 52''', 90'''' (text A.2.1); SpTU 4, No. 153 obv. 2, 5, 6, 10, 15 (text C.1.10); FLP 1306: 20 (text C.1.9) and the *Introduction* for discussion.

Lines 24''–33'': These two sections deal with the condition of "blocked fluids", introduced in line 24'' as *šumma sinništu mê turrat* "if a woman is blocked with fluids". The text BM 38624+: 24'–29', 30'–33' (*infra* text A.2.1) offers additional pieces of information on this ailment, elucidating that blocked fluids refer to the postpartum discharges which are normally emitted after delivery (for a discussion of this condition, see also the *Introduction* of this volume). The retention of the "blood of a woman in childbed" was recognized as a serious problem often associated with symptoms of puerperal fever or infection, see *Iraq* 31, 29–30: 1ff. (text II.1.4); BAM 240: 39'ff. (text D.2.1). In the latter text, the verb *sekēru* "to enclose" is used rather than *turru* "to block". The condition "blocked fluids" is often treated with fumigations from below (e.g. *Iraq* 31, 29–30: 3–9, 14–17, see text II.1.4), as also seems to be the case in the latter of the two fragmentary instructions in ms. a lines 24''–33''.

Lines 24''–29'': The interpretation and restoration of the procedure described in this passage rests on a parallel in AMT 61/2 ii 2'–4' // BAM 559: 1'–6', a prescription treating an affliction of the pelvis and lower back (cf. BAM 559: 14'–15' referring to paralysis of the hips/thighs and to the affliction *niḫis narkabti*):

> DIŠ NA MURUB$_4$ *u* ^{uzu}Ú[R GIG ... ...] ... ... [... *t*]*u-šaḫ-ḫ*[*a-an* ... ...] *ta-ḫap-ša ina* ŠÀ *ta-ṣab-bu ta-šaḫ-*[*ḫaṭ*$^?$ ... ...] ... ⌜GAR-*an*⌝ *ina* KÀŠ.MEŠ Ì.GIŠ *u* [... ... *a-gur*]*-ra* SUD *a-gur-a ina* UGU *ta-ḫap-še* ...[... ... *ana* UG]U$^?$ MURUB$_4$.MIN-*šú* DIŠ-*nu* GAR.GAR-*an* EN DU$_{10}$.GA-*šú* ...
>
> "If a man [suffers] from the hip and thigh [... ...] ... [...] you heat [... ...], you soak a felt (blanket?) in it, (then) you rinse(?) (it) [... ...] you put, with urine, oil and [... ...] you sprinkle [the baked bri]ck (with it), you [...] the baked brick on top of the felt (blanket?), [... ...] you *repeatedly place it* on(?) each of(?) his hips, until he improves ..."[251]

In this very fragmentary passage, it appears that a baked brick (*agurru*) was heated (*šaḫānu* D-stem) and then wrapped(?) into a piece of felt (*taḫapšu*) that was previously soaked in a liquid, to be applied to the patient's hips (as a kind of heating treatment?). I believe that in the present passage in K. 8678+, a similar procedure is described. Thus, I propose that here a brick was heated, then wrapped in cloth and placed on an oven (*tinūru*) which was safely positioned in a pit dug into the ground. Then the patient had to sit down on the brick placed on the oven, while being totally covered with cloth. The application of heat to the patient's body was thus intended to trigger the flow of the lochia.

Line 25'': For the logogram TINUR/DILINA(LAGABxIM) = *tinūru* "oven", cf. CAD T, 420–421 s.v. *tinūru*.

Line 26'': After the word *ni-nu-ú* (*nīnû*-plant), it would be possible to read MAR-*q*[*í*] (*teqqi*) "you daub", but this seems less likely in the present context. Compare line 31'' in the next prescription, where flour(?) is similarly thrown into the hole dug into the ground, presumably to serve as part of the applied fumigants. Perhaps a similar procedure is described here, with the verb *zarû*(MAR) "to sprinkle, to scatter". After the sign MAR, the restoration K[I B]AD-*ma* "you open (a hole in) the ground" is proposed here (for a similar instruction see also line 30'' below). In that hole, I think the oven was lowered down, in order to position it in a way that it stood firmly and was in the right height for the patient to sit down on it.

Line 27'': The restoration [*kan-na*]*-tú* is inspired by a passage in the *Lamaštu* ritual series (Tablet II 118; Tablet III 36, 41, 43; Farber 2014, 112–113, 132, 174–175, 188–189, spelled *kan-na-a-ti/tú*). In the latter prescription for an amulet, *kannātu*-bands made from strands of dyed wool are used to wrap materials that were later attached to a necklace. Here we find the parallel instruction *šalaš kannāti* (*ša sebet ṣirpāni*) *takannan* "you twist together three band (from seven (strands of) dyed wool)" (see further CAD K, 142–143 s.v. *kanānu* "to twist, to wrap up" (sub 1b), 156–157 s.v. *kannu* B; AHw 435 s.v. *kanānu*; AHw 437–438 s.v. *kannu* II). The word *kannu* (pl. *kannātu*) also means "(menstrual) bandage" and occurs in this meaning in several women's healthcare texts (see *infra*, e.g. AO 6473: 40 (text C.3.9); BM 79061: 9, 13 (text A.2.8)). However, in the present prescription, the bands of cloth mentioned in line 27'' were used, I believe, to wrap the hot brick into them, on which the patient had to sit.

251 The transliteration presented is a composite of both sources.

Lines 28''–29'': In the expression *ina muḫḫi tušeššebši* "you let her sit down above it" in line 28'', the logogram TUŠ is complemented by two phonetic complements here, which is unusual. Similar procedures applying a fumigation from below with the patient sitting down above the installation are described in other medical texts. Within the women's health corpus, for example in BAM 237(+) obv. i 26'–27', abnormal haemorrhage during pregnancy is treated with a fumigation, containing the same expression *ina muḫḫi tušeššebši* (see further note on line 33'' below).

The first sign in line 29'' before *tapassam* "you cover" is not entirely certain. CAD P, s.v. *pasāmu* "to cover" sub 1, reads ⸢ù⸣; cf. AHw 841b s.v. *paṣāmu*. However, the sign looks more like DUL or KI. Therefore, I prefer reading DUL for Akkadian *kutmu* "covering". EBL proposes reading [D]È? "charcoals" instead. It is tentatively suggested from similarities to the following instruction in lines 30''ff. that the patient had to sit down on the hot oven/brick, while being covered with a cloth. Covering or wrapping the patient with a cloth is also mentioned in the Middle Assyrian text *Iraq* 31, 29–30 and pl. V, lines 9 and 15 in the context of fumigation (likewise in the context of treating retained lochia), which states: "you let the woman sit down over it (a vessel with fumigants), you *wrap* her with cloth" (MUNUS (*šá-ši*) *ina* UGU [*t*]*u-še-ša-ab ina* TÚG.ḪI.A *tu*-ŠIR-*ši*). See text II.1.4 for discussion.

At the end of line 29'', eBL suggests restoring [KI.MIN]. However, it is not entirely clear what the "ditto" would refer to (therefore one should perhaps better restore *iballuṭ* "she will recover").

Line 30'': In this line, the practitioner is instructed to dig (*šapālu* D-stem) a hole (PÚ). For *šapālu* in the D-stem in the meaning "to excavate, to dig down", see CAD Š/1, 425 sub 3b. The reading PÚ BAD-*ma* "you open a hole" improves the preliminary reading *ḫáp-pát-ma* proposed in Steinert 2013, *JMC* 22, 9 n. 17. The sign PÚ can be read *būrtu* or *būru*, both meaning "hole" (cf. CAD B, 338b s.v. *būrtu* A sub 4 and discussion). For similar instructions with the verb *petû* "to open", see e.g. BAM 323: 61 (Scurlock 2006, No. 218): "on the third day, when the sun is setting, you dig a hole in the steppe (*būrta*(PÚ) *tepettē*(BAD)-*ma*)". See also *Maqlû* IV 34–35 (Abusch 2016, 118–119, 247, 319): *būrta*(PÚ) *tap-ta-a* "you have made a hole (in a fuller's mat/in a gardener's channel)".

For *ubānu*(ŠU.SI) "finger" as a unit of length, see Powell 1987–1990, *RlA* 7, 458–459, 469–472. In Neo- and Late Babylonian times, one finger corresponds to 2.08 cm; in the Neo-Assyrian period to 1.66 cm (= 6 barleycorns, ŠE). Perhaps in the present case, the hole was dug as deep as twice the length of a finger, not twice the breadth of a finger.

Line 31'': Inspired by the use of a brick in lines 24''–29'', I propose restoring [SI]G$_4$ DUL-*ma* "you cover (the hole) with a [bri]ck" at the beginning of the line. The verb *katāmu* (DUL) "to cover" is often construed with garments as covering devices, but this makes little sense at this point of the procedure. In other attestations, the objects covered can be containers or openings (CAD K, 299 s.v. *katāmu* sub 1a).

Line 32'': The ingredient *ḫu-ṣab ḫi-li*(ILLU) is also attested in BM 42587+: 5' (text B.2.4): 1 GÍN *ḫuṣāb* ILLU "one shekel of small (pieces of solid, dried?) resin"; and in BM 38624+ line 64''' (text A.2.1): 3 GÍN *ḫu-ṣa-bu* ILLU, likewise with a measurement. The latter prescription has a similar purpose as the present remedy in K. 8678+ (to induce the menses (*sagû*)). In all three instances of *ḫuṣāb ḫīli*, the plant source of the resin or gum is not specified. The word *ḫuṣābu* refers to a cut piece, twig or (small) chip/splinter of wood, sometimes to a small quantity or to a thing of little value (see CAD Ḫ, 258–259; AHw 360–361; Heeßel 2007, *KAL 1*, no. 18 ii 6 "eine Kleinigkeit").

Line 33'': The different fumigants enumerated in the preceding lines were poured on charcoals (UDUB = *pēmtu*), over which the patient had to sit or squat. A similar therapy is applied in BAM 237(+) obv. i 26'–27' to stop bleeding (*naḫšātu*) during pregnancy, without describing the digging of a hole in the ground (see text C.1.4). Closer to the context of the present procedure in K. 8678+ are the prescriptions for fumigation (to trigger the lochia) in the Middle Assyrian text *Iraq* 31, 29–30 and pl. V lines 3–9 and 14–18 mentioned earlier, in which the fumigants were spread on charcoals in a vessel on which the patient had to sit or squat. During the treatment the patient had to be covered with a cloth (for full discussion see text II.1.4).

A Neo-Assyrian text from Assur dealing with rectal diseases (BM 103386), containing parallels to Tablet 2 of the tractate ANUS, contains a passage indicating that Mesopotamian healers may have used a chair or stool, on which the patient sat during fumigation.[252] BM 103386 contains two prescriptions for fumigation to treat rectal disease (DÚR.GIG). The first

252 As did their colleagues in ancient Greece who applied fumigation for problems such as the 'wandering womb' (see Steinert 2014a, 2014b for a comparison Hippocratic and Mesopotamian recipes for fumigation). The Hippocratic texts mention that this chair had a hole, through which the fumes could reach the patient's groin.

of them explicitly refers to a "barber's stool" or chair (*litti gallābi*, ^{giš}ŠÚ.A ŠU.I) on which the patient sat (BM 103386 obv. 16'–18' (Heeßel 2018, *FS Geller*, 319, 325, 331).[253] A second prescription for a fumigation in BM 103386 rev. 9–12; Heeßel 2018, 322, 328, 335) reveals that an important intended effect of the fumigation was to induce sweating (a similar process to inducing the flow of the lochia in the fumigations for women).[254] Covering the patient with a cloth also served as a precautionary measure to protect them from negative environmental influences (draft, wind, cold, heat). For further discussion, see also the edition of *Iraq* 31, 29–30 and pl. V in this volume (text II.1.4 lines 1–9, 14–18).

At the end of line 33'' in ms. a, instead of the verb TUŠ-[*šeb-ši*], eBL proposes restoring *ina* U[GU K]I.MIN "over it ditto", where the "ditto" would replace the phrase "you let her sit down (over it)" in any case.

Lines 34''–41'': For abortive drugs, see previously Stol 2000a, 41–42, 55; Biggs 2000, *FS Lambert*, 11–12; Böck 2013, 36–40. The recipes for abortive remedies in K. 8678+ employ suppositories inserted into the vagina, while those in BAM 246, the only other text on abortion, prescribes potions. The only common drug encountered within the sections on abortion in K. 8678+ and BAM 246 is the *namruqqu/nabruqqu*-plant (see text B.1.6). This drug is known from other texts as a plant for a woman who is *šalputtu* (see Stol 2000a, 53–55 for discussion), referring to a major complication during delivery (perhaps connected to foetal death due to prolonged labour and malpresentation). The *namruqqu*-plant thus seems to have had abortive properties, i.e. causing contractions of the uterus (Biggs 2000, *FS Lambert*, 11). However, *namruqqu*-plant is also used in prescriptions to promote conception (e.g., BAM 244 obv. 31, 33, text B.1.1) and in prescriptions to induce the flow of postpartum blood (lochia) which had stopped prematurely (see BM 38624+ rev. iv 5', text A.2.1).

Line 34'': The reading of ŠUB-*e* in the introductory phrase [*ana* ^{munus}PEŠ$_4$ *šà* Š]À-*šà* ŠUB-*e* in line 34'' is not entirely certain. ŠUB-*e* could be the genitive infinitive of the G- or Š-stem of *nadû* "to abort". Compare BAM 246: 1 (text B.1.6), where we may have to analyse the verb ŠUB-*di* as a Š-stem infinitive (*šuddî*): [^{munus}P]EŠ$_4$ *šà* ŠÀ-*šà ana* ŠUB-*di* "to cause a woman to have a miscarriage". Cf. CAD N/1, 79, 97 s.v. *nadû* sub 1d-2', 8h. Cf. also the comment on line 41''.

Line 35'': I owe the improved reading of this line to eBL; cf. Geller 2005a, *BAM* 7, No. 44. A spelling ^{giš}*še-nu-'u* for the *šunû*-plant, as read by Geller, is not attested elsewhere and therefore unlikely. For *nipšu* "combed wool; tuft of wool", see CAD N/2, 248–249. For *mitḫāru* "of the same amount", see CAD M/2, 163 sub 1-1'b'; AHw 662. I do not know any other examples for syllabic *mit-ḫar* from medical prescriptions, which usually use the word *malmališ* in such instances (with *sâku* "to pound"). For *mitḫār(u)*, the dictionaries exclusively list references from the diagnostic texts. One would expect an adverbial form here (*mitḫāriš*).

The prescription in lines 34''–36'' is unusual, because one of the ingredients which is to be pounded to produce a suppository is apparently blue, combed wool (*uqnâtu ša nipše*). More common in recipes for tampons is a procedure where the drug ingredients are first crushed and then wrapped into wool. The word *uqnâtu* (^{ú}ZA.GÌN.(NA)) also refers to a plant (used in medical prescriptions for ointments) and to the pigment derived from this plant that was used to make blue dyes (e.g., for blue wool, see Thavapalan 2020, 314–322.). The plant is probably to be identified with woad (*Isatis tinctoria*, yielding indigotin), see Thompson 1949, 171; CAD U/W, 195 sub 3 and discussion section; Thavapalan 2020, 319–320. Blue wool occurs occasionally in women's healthcare texts, primarily in prescriptions for amulets and for tampons; for the latter, see line 40'' in the present text; BAM 237(+) rev. iv 2 (text C.1.4) (tampon to stop abnormal bleeding during pregnancy, ingredients wrapped in blue wool); BM 42450 + 43809 rev. 11' (a tampon to promote pregnancy) (see text B.2.3; Finkel 2000, *FS Lambert*, 170). For the use of *uqnâtu*-plant, see further BM 38624+ lines 6'–9' (text A.2.1).

Line 36'' exceptionally uses the masculine pronominal suffix -*šú* in reference to the patient; in all other occurrences on the reverse of ms. a, the feminine suffixes -*šá* or -*ši* are used.

Line 37'': Other restorations are possible for the first fragmentary ingredient, e.g. [IM.SAḪAR.BAB]BAR.KUR.RA (*alluḫaru*), a mineral pigment and mordant (lit. "white dust of the mountains").

---

253 Interestingly, in contrast to the prescriptions in BM 103386, parallel women's healthcare texts such as BAM 237, *Iraq* 31, 29–30 and K. 8678+ do not explicitly mention that the patient is fumigated (*qutturu*) and thus seem to be abbreviated in their instructions.

254 Sweating appears to have been seen as having a positive therapeutic effect here. A similar procedure is preserved in BAM 174 obv. 14' // BAM 558 iv 9–10, in a prescription for a severe lung disease: "(you cover him with (hot) dregs (*bitru* or *piṭru*) of *billatu*-substance) until his ... *become soaking (wet)* and he exudes sweat and it flows" (EN *piṭ-ru-šú i-lab-bi-ku u* IR ŠUB *u* DU. Note that Scurlock (2014a, 481, 483) reads the passage differently, translating "until his chest and abdomen are lubricated and the bowels move" (*ir-ru-u* DU).

Line 39'': The instruction [*m*]*a-gal* NU GAZ "you do not crush (it) much" found here is unusual.

Line 41'': A phrase with an infinitive *nadû* "to abort" should be written ŠUB-*e* or ŠUB-*i*, see e.g., line 34'' above; or in negative forms, e.g. Assur Medical Catalogue 110: *ana šà* ŠÀ-*šà* NU! ŠUB-*e* "to prevent her from having a miscarriage" (Steinert et al. 2018, 217). Since the expression [munus]⸢PEŠ$_4$?⸣ ⸢*šà*⸣ ŠÀ-*šà* ŠUB-*di* occurs at the end of the line, it is probably to be interpreted as a prognosis ("the pregnant woman will have a miscarriage (*ša libbīša inaddi*)"). See also BAM 246: 7, 10 (text B.1.6): [*šà libbi*(Š]À)-*šà inaddâ*(ŠUB-*a*) "she will have a miscarriage".

A.2 Texts from Babylonia

A.2.1 BM 38624+: A Medical Compendium on Women's Diseases

The joined fragments of this large two-column tablet offer a notable example of a first millennium BCE medical compendium from Babylonia dedicated to women's health. The preserved text passages consist solely of therapeutic prescriptions for female health problems: remedies for fertility and conception, prescriptions to stop haemorrhage and to induce the menstrual flow (*sagû*), medicines for difficult delivery, for expelling the afterbirth and for treating postpartum complaints. In its mixture of topics, the tablet thus evokes the impression of a gynaecological handbook covering all major women's health problems. Since neither an incipit nor a colophon is preserved, it is unclear whether the text may have been related to a serialised therapeutic compendium (cf. the discussion in Steinert et al. 2018, especially on the section BIRTH). At least a few diagnostic formulations and remedies in BM 38624+ have parallels in the Neo-Assyrian texts BAM 240 and BAM 248 from Assur, but a true duplicate is not extant. Thus, the tablet may have formed a local practical textbook, similar to BM 42313+ (see text A.2.2).

List of Manuscripts

Siglum	Museum Number	Copy	Collation	Format; Ductus	Provenience
a	BM 38624 (80-11-12, 508) + BM 38828 (80-11-12, 713) + BM 45414 (81-7-1, 3175)	Pl. 12–13	Coll.	Fragments of a two-column tablet; Late Babylonian script; ca. 6th/5th cent. BCE(?)	probably Babylon[255]
B	VAT 8869	KAR 196 BAM 248	Coll.	Two-column tablet; Neo-Assyrian script; 8th/7th cent. BCE	Assur; N4 library
C_1 + C_5 + C_4	K. 2413 + K. 16363 + K. 18482	AMT 67/1 (only K. 2413)	Coll.	Fragments of a two-column tablet; Neo-Assyrian script; 7th cent. BCE	Nineveh
d	FLP 1306	Pl. 30	Coll.	Single-column tablet in portrait format; Neo/Late-Babylonian script; ca. 6th cent. BCE(?)	unknown (Babylonia)

Overview

i'	Prescription to promote conception (suppository?) a obv. i 1'–5'	...]1'–5'
ii'	Fragmentary prescription a obv. i 6'–9'	6'–9'
iii'	Fragmentary prescription (suppository?) a obv. i 10'	10'

255 See Leichty, Finkel and Walker 2019, *CBT* IV–V, 397. Measurements: 9.0 x 13.4 x 2.8 cm.

iv'	Prescription to stop bleeding (suppository)	11'–13'
	a obv. i 11'–13' // d rev. 1–5	
v'	Prescription to expel the retained afterbirth (potion)	14'–15'
	a obv. i 14'–15'	
vi'	Prescription to stop bleeding (tampon)	16'–17'
	a obv. i 16'–17'	
vii'	Prescription to stop bleeding (tampon)	18'–19'
	a obv. i 18'–19'	
viii'	Fragmentary prescription to stop bleeding	20'–21'
	a obv. i 20'–21'	
ix'	Fragmentary prescription to stop bleeding	22'–23'
	a obv. i 22'–23'	
x'	Prescription for "blocked fluids" (bandage?)	24'–29'
	a obv. i 24'–29'	
xi'	Prescription for "blocked fluids" (bandage)	30'–33'
	a obv. i 30'-33'	
xii'	Prescription for postpartum complaint (supple navel; sweating)	34'–37'[...
	a obv. i 34'–37' (cf. BAM 240 obv. 30'ff.)	
xiii''	Fragmentary prescription	...]38''–43''
	a obv. ii 1'–6'	
xiv''	Fragmentary prescription	44''–45''
	a obv. ii 7'–8'	
xv''	Fragmentary prescription	46''
	a obv. ii 9'	
xvi''	Fragmentary prescription	47''–48''
	a obv. ii 10'–11'	
xvii''	Fragmentary prescription	49''[...
	a obv. ii 12'–??	
xviii'''	Prescription to promote menstrual flow (suppository)	...]50'''–55'''
	a obv. ii 17'–22'	
xix'''	Prescription to expel retained afterbirth	56'''–57'''
	a obv. ii 23'–24'	
xx'''	Prescription to ease difficult delivery (potion)	58'''
	a obv. ii 25' // B rev. iv 29 // C_1 rev. iv 22	
xxi'''	Prescription to ease difficult delivery (potion)	59'''
	a obv. ii 26' // B rev. iv 23 // C_1 rev. iv 16	
xxii'''	Prescription to ease difficult delivery (potion)	60'''
	a obv. ii 27'	
xxiii'''	Prescription to promote the menstrual flow (*sagû*)	61'''–63'''
	a obv. ii 28'–30'	
xxiv'''	Prescription to promote the menstrual flow	64'''–66'''[...
	a obv. ii 31'–33'	
xxv''''	Fragmentary prescription and test	...]67''''–71''''
	a rev. iii 1'–5'	
xxvi''''	Fragmentary prescription	72''''–77''''[...
	a rev. iii 6'–11'	
xxvii'''''	Fragmentary	...]78''''
	a rev. iii 17'	
xxviii'''''	Fragmentary prescription	79''''–82''''
	a rev. iii 18'–21'	

xxix'''''	Fragmentary prescription a rev. iii 22'–23'	83'''''–84'''''[...
xxx'''''	Fragmentary prescription a rev. iv 1'	...]85'''''
xxxi'''''	Prescription a rev. iv 2'–3'	86'''''–87'''''
xxxii'''''	Prescription (suppository) a rev. iv 4'–8'	88'''''–92'''''
xxxiii'''''	Fragmentary prescription a rev. iv 9'–10'	93'''''–94'''''[...
xxxiv''''''	Fragmentary prescription a rev. iv 16'–21'	...]95''''''–100''''''
xxxv''''''	Fragmentary prescription a rev. iv 28'	...]101''''''
xxxvi'''''''	Fragmentary prescription a rev. iv 29'–31'	102'''''''–104'''''''
xxxvii'''''''	Fragmentary prescription a rev. iv 32'	105'''''''[...

Previous Edition and Discussion

Steinert 2021, *Byzantinische Forschungen* 33, 48 n. 37 (ms. a lines 1'–5')
Electronic Babylonian Library (eBL) (https://www.ebl.lmu.de/library/BM.38624; photo)
Infra text D.1.1 (mss. B and C), text C.1.9 (ms. d)

Transliteration

Beginning of ms. a obv. i lost

1'	a obv. i 1'	[x x x x x x x x 1 G]ÍN SU[ḪUŠ] ^{giš}GI.Z[Ú.LUM.MA]
2'	a obv. i 2'	[x x x x x 1 GÍ]N Ú BABBAR 1/2 GÍN ^{na4}*gab-b*[*u-u*]
3'	a obv. i 3'	[x x x x 1 GÍN ^{ú}]KU.NU.LUḪ.ḪA 1 GÍN NAGA.SI ⸢1/2 GÍN$^{?}$⸣
4'	a obv. i 4'	[x x x PAP$^{?}$] 12 Ú.ḪI.A *ina* ILLU ^{šim}BULUḪ Ì.UDU
5'	a obv. i 5'	[ḪI.ḪI ḪI]-*tú*$^{?}$ *šá* ^{munus}NU.PEŠ$_4$ *ana šu-ri-i*

6'	a obv. i 6'	[DIŠ KI.MIN$^{?}$] 1/2 GÍN ILLU LI.DUR 1/2 GÍN ^{šim}ḪAB
7'	a obv. i 7'	[x x]x 1/2 ⸢GÍN⸣ NAGA.SI 1/2 GÍN *ze-e šik-ke-e*
8'	a obv. i 8'	[x x] x ⸢GÍN⸣ ⸢^{na4}*gab-bu-u*⸣ ⸢^{ú}⸣ZA.GÌN ⸢ŠE.Ì.GIŠ$^{?}$⸣ ⸢EREN⸣
9'	a obv. i 9'	[..................................] *ina* UD-*šá* ŠUB-*di*

10'	a obv. i 10'	[.................. *ana*] IGI *ta-az-za-ru* ḪI-*tú šá lu-ub-bu-ku* :

11'	a obv. i 11' d rev. 1–2	[x x x x x x]x 1/2 NINDA ⸢^{ú}⸣*sim-bir-ri* 1 GÍN [^{šim}G]IG 1/2 GÍN ^{ú}KUR.KUR / 1 GÍN ⸢^{ú}⸣[NAGA.S]I$^{?}$ 1/2 NINDA *sim-bir-ri*
12'	a obv. i 12' d rev. 3–4	[x x x x x x] ⸢1/2 GÍN$^{?!}$⸣ ^{na4}*gab-bu-u ina* ILLU ^{šim}BULUḪ *šal-šú* ^{ši}[^{m}x] 1/2 GÍN ^{na4}*gab-bu-ú* / *ina* ILLU BULUḪ

13' a obv. i 13' [x x x x ḪI.ḪI$^{?}$] *maš-ši-ti šá* MÚD KUD-*as*
d rev. 4$^{\text{cont.}}$–5 GÚR.GÚR ^{g}[^{iš}E]REN ḪI.ḪI-*ma* / *maš-šit-tu*$_4$ MÚD KUD-*si*

14' a obv. i 14' [DIŠ MUNUS (Ù.TU-*ma*) *s*]*i-li-is-su ina lìb-bi-šú i-ku-uš*

15' a obv. i 15' [x x x x] gam$^{?}$ lu *šá* KA ^{dug}*nam-zi-tú* NAG-*ma*$^{?}$ ŠUB-*a*

16' a obv. i 16' [MÚD MUNUS *ana* KUD-*si*$^{?}$ x GÍN ^{ši}]^{m}GIG 1 1/2 GÍN ^{giš}EREN.BAD KUM SIM

17' a obv. i 17' [*ina* ^{síg}ÀKA NIGIN-*mi*$^{?}$] *ana* ŠÀ.TÙR-*šá* GAR-*ma* MÚD ⸢KUD-*is*$^{?}$⸣

18' a obv. i 18' [DIŠ KI.MIN ^{giš}KI]ŠI$_{16}$$^{?}$ ŠIKA-*tú* NUNUZ *lu-ur-mu* KA *tam-tim*

19' a obv. i 19' [SÚD *ina* ^{síg}ÀKA NIG]IN-*mi ana* ŠÀ.TÙR-*šá* GAR-*an-ma* KI.MIN

20' a obv. i 20' [..................] ⸢*ana*$^{?}$⸣ ⸢KUD⸣-*as* MÚD $^{\text{na4}}$KUR-*nu* DAB

21' a obv. i 21' [.................................]-⸢*i*⸣ [*ana*] ⸢MÚD⸣ KUD-*si*

22' a obv. i 22' [.......................................] ⸢x⸣

23' a obv. i 23' [.....................] ⸢MÚD⸣ [KUD-*si*$^{?}$]

24' a obv. i 24' [DIŠ MUNUS$^{?}$ *ina em*]-*ši-šú* ⸢*di*$^{?}$⸣-*ik-šú il-ta-nap-p*[*at*$^{?}$-*su-ma*]

25' a obv. i 25' [x x-*š*]*ú* GU$_7$.MEŠ-*šú* MUNUS BI A.MEŠ *tur-rat* Š[E.GIG$^{?}$]

26' a obv. i 26' [KU GA]ZI$^{\text{?sar}}$ *qa-lu-tu* KU ^{giš}*šu-ni-i* KU *ú*[*r-né-e*]

27' a obv. i 27' [KU ^{ši}]^{m}MUG ZÌ ŠE SIG KU *ku-us-pu* ZÌ G[Ú.GA]L

28' a obv. i 28' [K]U *ḫa-ru-bu* NUMUN GADA *ina* $^{\text{na4}}$*ma-suk-tu*$_4$ ⸢KUM⸣

29' a obv. i 29' [*má*]*l-ma-liš* SÚD *ina* KAŠ *tara-bak ina* TÚG SUR.RA L[Á$^{?}$-*i*]*d*$^{?}$-*ma* TIN-*uṭ*

30' a obv. i 30' [DIŠ MUNUS$^{?}$ A.MEŠ *tur*]-*rat u šap-la-a-nu a-b*[*u-u*]*n-na-ti-šú*

31' a obv. i 31' [x x x x x]-*ma ku*-⸢*pu-ut*⸣ *ru-t*[*a*$^{?}$(-)[x]-*šá*$^{?}$ TI.MEŠ

32' a obv. i 32' [x x x x x]x *ina* KUŠ SUR.RA MU[RUB$_4$.M]EŠ-*šá*$^{?}$ *u šap-la-a-nu*

33' a obv. i 33' [*a-bu-un-na-ti-šá*$^{?}$] [*t*]*a-aṣ-ṣa-mid*

34' a obv. i 34' [DIŠ MUNUS Ù.TU-*ma* LI.DUR-*sa* D]U$_8$-⸢*ma*$^{?}$⸣ *zu-'u-tú a-la-ka*

35' a obv. i 35' [*la i-kal-la* x x x x] ⸢^{ú}⸣*ga-ši-ru-u* ^{ú}EME-UR.GI$_7$

36' a obv. i 36' [.......................................]x x x *sík-te*

37' a obv. i 37' [...............................]x LÁ-*id-ma ina-aḫ*

Ms. a obv. i breaks; gap of unknown length

38'' a obv. ii 1' 1/2 GÍ[N ....]

39'' a obv. ii 2' ^{ši}[^{m} ....]

40'' a obv. ii 3' *ina* KAŠ [...................................]

41'' a obv. ii 4' *ina* ⸢A$^{?}$⸣ ⸢*ta*$^{?}$⸣-[..............................]

42'' a obv. ii 5' ⸢Ú.ḪI.A⸣ Š[EŠ ....]

43'' a obv. ii 6' PA x[..]

***

44'' a obv. ii 7' DIŠ KI.MIN *mi-šil* ⸢$^{ú/giš}$⸣[.....................]

45'' a obv. ii 8' *mi-šil* ^{ú}IGI-20 [...............................]

***

46'' a obv. ii 9' DIŠ KI.MIN GA x[............................]

***

47'' a obv. ii 10' DIŠ KI.MIN Ù[Z$^{?}$..............................]

48'' a obv. ii 11' *šá* ^{giš}x[..]

49'' a obv. ii 12' ⸢DIŠ⸣ ⸢KI.MIN⸣ [...............................]

four lines lost

50''' a obv. ii 17' [x x x x] ⸢x x x⸣ [....................................]

51''' a obv. ii 18' [1/2] NINDA ⸢^{ú}ḪAB⸣ 1/2 NINDA ^{giš}ḪAB 1/2 G[ÍN ....]

52''' a obv. ii 19' [*ina*] ⸢Ì.UDU⸣ SUMUN ḪI.ḪI *maš-ši-tú šá* MU[NUS x x x x x x]

53''' a obv. ii 20' ⸢*lu-u*⸣ MUNUS *šá me-e tur-ra-tú l*[*u-u* MUNUS *šá sa-gu-šá*$^{?}$]

54''' a obv. ii 21' *la im-ma-ru ana kul-lu-mu* DÙ-*uš* [x x x x x]

55''' a obv. ii 22' *áš-šú* ^{ú}*a-zu-pi-*⸢*ra*⸣*-nu* NU ZU-*ú* x x[x x x x]

***

56''' a obv. ii 23' DIŠ MUNUS *ina a-lad* ^{uzu}*si-lit-su ina lib-bi* ⸢*uš*⸣-[*ta-kiš*$^{?}$]

57''' a obv. ii 24' NUMUN ^{ú}*a-zu-pi-ra-nu* SÚD *ina* A.GEŠTIN.N[A NAG$^{?}$]

a

***

58''' a obv. ii 25' DIŠ MUNUS *a-lad uš-tap-šiq* ^{im}KAL.GU[G SÚD *ina* KAŠ NAG]

B rev. iv 29 DIŠ KI.MIN ^{im}KAL.GUG SÚD *ina* KAŠ NAG-*ma* KI.MIN

C_1 rev. iv 22 DIŠ KI.MIN ^{im}KAL.GUG SÚD *ina* KAŠ NAG-*ma* KI.MIN

a

***

59''' a obv. ii 26' DIŠ KI.MIN U_5 ARKAB^{mušen} S[ÚD x]

B rev. iv 23 DIŠ KI.MIN U_5 ARKAB^{mušen} SÚD KI.MIN

C_1 rev. iv 16 DIŠ KI.MIN U_5 ARKAB^{mušen} SÚD KI.MIN

a, B, C

***

60''' a obv. ii 27' DIŠ KI.MIN ^{ú}AN.DAḪ.ŠUM ^{šim}LI ^{im}KAL ^{š}[$^{im?}$x SÚD KI.MIN$^{?}$]

***

61''' a obv. ii 28' DIŠ MUNUS *sa-gu-šá ana kul-lu-mu šal-šú* ^{ú}KU.NU.[LUḪ.ḪA (x x)]

62''' a obv. ii 29' SUḪUŠ ^{giš}NAM.TAR NITA *ina* ⸢ILLU⸣ ⸢^{šim}⸣BULUḪ ḪI.ḪI [x x x x]

63''' a obv. ii 30' *sa-gu-šá im-mar ṭu-ub-tú šá mur-ṣ*[*i*$^{?}$ x x x]

***

64''' a obv. ii 31' 3 GÍN *ḫu-ṣa-bu* ILLU 3 GÍN ^{giš}LI [x x x x]

65''' a obv. ii 32' 3 [GÍN] ^{ú}KU.NU.LUḪ.ḪA 3 GÍN $^{\text{ú?}}$G[I.ZÚ.LUM.MA$^{?}$]

66''' a obv. ii 33' [.................................] ⸢3⸣ GÍN Ì.U[DU$^{?}$ x x x x x]

Ms. a obv. ii breaks; gap of unknown length

67'''' a rev. iii 1' Ú.ḪI.A ŠEŠ.MEŠ x[.................................]

68'''' a rev. iii 2' ILLU ^{šim}BULUḪ [...................................]

69'''' a rev. iii 3' [MUNUS *šá ina*] *a-lad me-e* [*tur-ra-tú* ....]

70'''' a rev. iii 4' ⸢^{munus}PEŠ$_4$$^{?}$⸣-*ti u šu*[*p-šuq-ti*$^{?}$ ....]

71'''' a rev. iii 5' ⸢*mál*⸣-*tak-tú šá* x[.....................................]

72'''' a rev. iii 6' 4-*tú* ^{šim}GÚR.GÚR 4-*tú* ⸢KÀŠ$^{?}$⸣ x[...................]

73'''' a rev. iii 7' 4-*tú* ^{ú}ḪAB 4-*tú* ^{ú}NU.LUḪ.ḪA [.....................]

74'''' a rev. iii 8' 4-*tú* NUMUN GADA 4-*tú* ^{šim}ḪAB 4-*tú* [...........]

75'''' a rev. iii 9' [x]x Ú.ḪI.A GAZ SIM *ina* ŠÀ$^{?}$ KAŠ [ŠUB$^{?}$ ......]

76'''' a rev. iii 10' [x x x x x] ⸢IGI⸣-*šú-ma*$^{?}$ [..............................]

77'''' a rev. iii 11' [x x x x x x]x.⸢MEŠ$^{?}$⸣ [.................................]

Break of ca. 5 lines

78''''' a rev. iii 17' ⸢x⸣ [...]

79''''' a rev. iii 18' DIŠ MUNUS *i*[*t-*..................................]

80''''' a rev. iii 19' NUNUZ TU$^{\text{m[ušen}}$ ....]

81''''' a rev. iii 20' ^{ú}DILI NITA x[....................................]

82''''' a rev. iii 21' *lu-lu-ú* [...]

83''''' a rev. iii 22' DIŠ KI.MIN ^{ú}LAG.[A.ŠÀ .... *ina* MUL]

84''''' a rev. iii 23' *tuš-bat ina še-rim* [...............................]

---

traces of a few lines before ms. a rev. iii breaks; gap of unknown length

85'''''' a rev. iv 1' ⸢x x x⸣ [...]

86'''''' a rev. iv 2' [$^{\text{(ú)}}$*šib-bur*]-*rat* ^{šim}ŠEŠ *ma-a-du* $^{\text{na4}}$*ga-*⸢*bu*⸣-[*u*] ⸢x x⸣

87'''''' a rev. iv 3' [*mu-u*]*t-tap-pi-iḫ-tú* GAR-*ma i-tar-ra-aṣ šu-ut* KA

88'''''' a rev. iv 4' [1/2 NINDA NAGA].SI 1/2 NINDA ^{ú}NU.LUḪ.ḪA 1 GÍN Ú BABBAR

89'''''' a rev. iv 5' [x x x x] 1/2 NINDA ^{ú}*nam-ruq-qu* 4-*tú si-ḫu* TI.LA

90'''''' a rev. iv 6' [x x ILL]U ^{šim}BULUḪ [x] GÍN DUḪ.LÀL ḪI.ḪI *maš-ši-tú*

91'''''	a rev. iv 7'	[*šá* x x x] ⸢*lu-u*⸣ ⸢MUNUS⸣ *šá ina a-lad me-e tur-ra-tú*
92'''''	a rev. iv 8'	[*lu-u*$^{?}$ ....] x ⸢GAR$^{?}$-*ma*⸣ *i-šal-lim*

93'''''	a rev. iv 9'	[...] x
94'''''	a rev. iv 10'	[.............................. ^{šim}]⸢GÚR.GÚR$^{?}$⸣

Break of ca. 5 lines

95''''''	a rev. iv 16'	[.................................... NAGA].⸢SI$^{?}$⸣
96''''''	a rev. iv 17'	[.................................... Ú] BABBAR
97''''''	a rev. iv 18'	[............................... ^{giš}KI]ŠI$_{16}$$^{?}$ ^{ú}*si-ḫu*
98''''''	a rev. iv 19'	[.................................... DID]A$^{?}$ SIG$_{5}$$^{?}$
99''''''	a rev. iv 20'	[..] x x
100''''''	a rev. iv 21'	[... ER]EN$^{?}$

Traces of ca. 5 lines

101'''''''	a rev. iv 28'	[................ ^{šim}]⸢GÚR.GÚR$^{?}$⸣ x [............]

102'''''''	a rev. iv 29'	[.............. 4]-*tú* ^{ú}ḪAB$^{?}$ 4-*tú* ^{š}[^{im} ....]
103'''''''	a rev. iv 30'	[......... 4-*tú* ^{šim}]⸢LI$^{?}$⸣ 4-*tú* $^{ú?}$G[I.ZÚ.LUM.MA$^{?}$ ....]
104'''''''	a rev. iv 31'	[........... ^{giš}ER]EN$^{?}$.BAD ḪI.ḪI x[.........................]

105'''''''	a rev. iv 32'	[...................] ⸢x⸣ nu$^{?}$ [...................]

Ms. a rev. iv breaks; remainder lost

Bound Transcription and Translation

Beginning of ms. a obv. i lost

$^{1'}$ [... ... *ištēn ši*]*qil šur*[*uš*] GI.Z[Ú.LUM.MA] $^{2'}$ [... ... *ištēn šiq*]*il šammu peṣû zūz gab*[*û*] $^{3'}$ [... ... *ištēn šiqil tīyatu ištēn šiqil uḫūlu qarnānû zūz* $^{4'}$ [... *napḫar*(?)] 12 *šammī ina ḫīl baluḫḫi lipî* [*tuballal maššī*]*tu ša lā erīti ana šūrî*	$^{1'}$ [... ..., one she]kel of the ro[ot of] GI.Z[Ú.LUM.MA-plant(?)], $^{2'}$ [... ..., one shekel 'white drug', half a shekel of al[um], $^{3'}$ [... ..., one shekel] *tīyatu*-[plant], one shekel of 'horned' alkali, half a shekel of $^{4'}$ [... – a total of(?)] twelve drugs: $^{5'}$ you [mix (them)] $^{4'}$ with resin of *baluḫḫu*-aromatic and fat. $^{5'}$ [(This is) a sup-p]ository (*maššītu*) to enable a woman who is not pregnant to get pregnant.
$^{6'}$ [DIŠ KI.MIN(?)] *zūz ḫīl abukkati zūz ṭūru* $^{7'}$ [...] *zūz uḫūlu qarnānû zūz zê šikkê* $^{8'}$ [...] ... *šiqil gabû uqnâtu šamaššammū*(?) *erēnu* $^{9'}$ [... ...] *ina* ...-*ša tanaddi*	$^{6'}$ [Alternatively(?), $^{9'}$ you(?) ...] $^{6'}$ half a shekel of *abukkatu*-resin, half a shekel of *ṭūru*-aromatic, $^{7'}$ [...], half a shekel(?) of 'horned' alkali, half a shekel of mongoose excrement, $^{8'}$ [...], ... shekel of alum, *uqnâtu*-plant (woad), sesame(?), cedar, $^{9'}$ [...], you *apply* (the medicine) to her ... .

10' [... ... *ana*] *pāni tazarru maššītu ša lubbuku*

10' [... ...] you sprinkle [...] on it. A suppository for *absorbing*.

11' [*ištēn šiqil kanakta zūz atā'iša ištēn šiqil uḫūla qarnānâ*] *mišil akal*(?) *simbirri* 12' [*šalšu* ...] *zūz gabâ ina ḫīl baluḫḫi* 13' [*kukri erēni tuballal*(?)] *maššītu ša dāma iparras* (var. *parāsi*)

13' [You mix] 11' [one shekel of *kanaktu*-aromatic, half a shekel of *atā'išu*-plant, one shekel of 'horned alkali'], half of a tenth of a litre *simbirru*-plant, 12' [one third (of a shekel) of ...-aromatic], half a shekel of alum in resin of *baluḫḫu*-aromatic, 13' [*kukru*-aromatic (and) cedar]. A suppository for stopping the blood.

14' [*šumma sinništu* (*ūlid-ma*) *s*]*ilīssu ina libbišu ikūš* 15' [... ...] ... *ša pī namzīti išattī-ma inaddâ*

14' [If a woman (gives birth and)] her afterbirth is delayed in her belly, 15' she shall drink [... ...] ... from the mouth of a brewing vessel. Then she will expel (the afterbirth).

16' [*dām sinništi ana parāsi*(?) ... *šiqil*] *kanakta ištēn šiqil zūz šupuḫra taḫaššal tanappi* 17' [*ina itqi talammi*(?)] *ana šassūrīša tašakkan-ma dāmu paris*

16' [To stop a woman's blood(?)]: you crush and sift [x shekels of] *kanaktu*-aromatic and one and a half shekels of *šupuḫru*-cedar, 17' [you wrap it in a wad of wool(?)], you insert it into her womb (viz. vagina). Then the blood will stop.

18' [DIŠ KI.MIN *ašā*]*gu ḫaṣabti pel lurmi imbu' tâmti* 19' [*tasâk ina itqi tal*]*ammi ana šassūrīša tašakkan-ma* KI.MIN

18' [Alternatively(?)], 19' [you crush 18' *aš*]*āgu*-thorn(?), ostrich eggshell, (and) *imbu' tâmti*-mineral, 19' you wrap [(it) in a wad of wool], insert it in her womb (viz. vagina), and ditto (i.e. the blood will stop).

20' [... ...] *ana*(?) *parās dāmi šadânu ṣābitu* 21' [... ...]... [*ana*(?)] *dāmi parāsi*

20' [... ...] for(?) stopping of the blood: magnetite, 21' [... ...], [for] stopping the blood.

22' [... ... ...]... 23' [... ...] *dāma* [*parāsi*(?)]

22' [... ... ...]... 23' [... ... (for) stopping(?)] the blood.

24' [*šumma sinništu*(?) *ina em*]*šīšu dikšu iltanappa*[*ssu-ma*] 25' [...-*š*]*u ītanakkalšu sinništu šī mê turrat ki*[*btu*] 26' [*sīkti*(?) *ka*]*sî qalûtu sīkti*(?) *šunî sīkti*(?) *u*[*rnê*] 27' [*sīkti*(?)] *ballukki qēm še'i uppuli sīkti kuspi qēm ḫa*[*llūri*] 28' [*q*]*ēm ḫarūbi zēr kitê ina masūkti taḫaššal* 29' [*ma*]*lmališ tasâk ina šikari tarabbak ina lubāri teṭerri taṣ*[*ammi*]*d-ma*(?) *iballuṭ*

24' [If a woman] keeps fee[ling] a pressing pain [in] her [lower] abdomen [and] 25' [her ...] continually hurt(s) [her], that woman is blocked (with) fluids. 28' You crush 25' wh[eat], 26' [powder] of roasted *kasû*-plant, powder of *šunû*-plant, powder of *u*[*rnû*-plant], 27' [powder of] *ballukku*-aromatic, flour of late barley, powder of sesame pomace, p[ea] flour, 28' carob flour (and) linseed in a mortar, 29' you pound (them) in equal quantities. You stir (it) into a paste with beer, you *smear* (it) on a (piece of) cloth, you [bandage(?)] (her with it). Then she will recover.

30' [*šumma sinništu*(?) *mê tur*]*rat u šaplānu abunnatīšu* 31' [... ...]-*ma kupput*(?) ... ... *bulluṭi*(?) 32' [... ...]... *ina maški teṭerri qablīša*(?) *u šaplānu* 33' [*abunnatīša*] *taṣammid*

30' [If a woman is bloc]ked [with fluids] and the area below her navel 31' [... ...], and it is compacted(?), (*to*) *treat*(?) *her*(?) ...: 32' [... ...], you *smear* (it) on a piece of leather, you bandage her hips(?) and the area below 33' [her navel (with it)].

34' [*šumma sinništu ūlid-ma abunnassa paṭ*]*rat-ma zu'tu alāka* 35' [*lā ikalla* ... ...] *gašīrû lišān kalbi* 36' [... ...] ... *sīkte*(?) 37' [... ...]... *taṣammid-ma inâḫ*

34' [If a woman gives birth and subsequently her navel feels su]pple(?), and 35' [she cannot hold back] 34' the sweat from flowing: 35' [... ...], *gašīrû*-plant, dog's tongue-plant, 36' [... ...]..., powder(?) of [...]. 37' You bandage (her with it), and she will find relief.

Ms. a obv. i breaks; gap of unknown length

38'' *zūz* [... ...] 39'' [... ... ...] 40'' *ina šikari* [... ...] 41'' *ina mê ta*-[... ...] 42'' *šammī annûti* [... ...] 43'' ...[... ... ...]	38'' Half a [shekel of ... ...], 39'' [...]-aromatic, [... ...] 40'' with beer [... ...]. 41'' You [...] in water [... ...]. 42'' These drugs [... ...]. 43'' ... [... ...]
44'' DIŠ KI.MIN *mišil* ...[... ...] 45'' *mišil imḫur-ešrā* [... ...]	44'' Alternatively, half (a shekel?) of [...]-plant, [... ...], 45'' half (a shekel?) of 'heals-twenty'-plant, [... ...].
46'' DIŠ KI.MIN *šizbu*(?) [... ...]	46'' Alternatively, milk(?) [... ...].
47'' DIŠ KI.MIN *en*[*zu*(?) ... ...] 48'' *ša* ...[... ...]	47'' Alternatively, [you ...] a go[at(?) ..., ...] 48'' of [...]-wood [... ...].
49'' DIŠ KI.MIN [... ...]	49'' Alternatively, [... ...].

Four lines lost

50''' [...] ... [... ...], 51''' [*mišil*] *akal būšāna mišil akal ḫûrata zūz* [... ...] 52''' [*ina*] *lipî labiri tuballal maššītu ša sinn*[*išti*(?) ... ...] 53''' *lū sinništi ša mê turratu l*[*ū sinništi ša sagûša*] 54''' *lā immaru ana kullumu teppuš* [... ...] 55''' *aššu azupīrānu lā tīdû*(?) ...[... ...]	50''' [...] ... [... ...], 52''' you mix 51''' [half] of a tenth of a litre *būšānu*-plant, half of a tenth of a litre *ḫûratu*-plant (madder), half a she[kel of ... ...] 52''' [with] old fat. You prepare (this) suppository for a wo[man ...] or for a woman who is blocked with fluids [or for a woman who] does not see her [menses], to make (them) appear. [...]. 55''' Since you(?) do not know the *azupīrānu*-plant, [...].
56''' *šumma sinništu ina alādi silīssu ina libbi uš*[*takīš*(?)] 57''' *zēr azupīrāni tasâk ina ṭābāti* [*išatti*(?)]	56''' If during delivery a woman's afterbirth is de[layed(?)] in the belly, 57''' you crush seeds of *azupīrānu*-plant, [she shall drink(?) (it)] in vinegar.
58''' *šumma sinništu alād*(*a*) *uštapšiq* (var. DIŠ KI.MIN) *kalgukka* [*tasâk ina šikari išatti*] (var. *išattī-ma* KI.MIN)	58''' If a woman suffers severely during delivery (var. Alternatively), [you crush] (reddish) *kalgukku*-mineral (pigment), [she shall drink (it) in beer] (var. adds: Then ditto (i.e., she will give birth quickly)).
59''' DIŠ KI.MIN *rikibti arkabi ta*[*sâk* KI.MIN]	59''' Alternatively, you cr[ush] 'spur(?) of a bat', [ditto].
60'' DIŠ KI.MIN *andaḫšu burāšu kalû* ...[... ...]	60'' Alternatively, [you ...] *andaḫšu*-plant, *burāšu*-juniper, *kalû*-pigment, [...]-aromatic, [... ...].
61''' *šumma sinništu sagûša ana kullumu šalšu tīyatu* [...] 62''' *šuruš pillê zikari ina ḫīl baluḫḫi tuballal* [... ...] 63''' *sagûša immar ṭūbtu ša murṣ*[*i* ...]	61''' To make a woman's menses appear: 62''' you mix 61''' one third (of a shekel?) *tīy*[*atu*-plant, ...], 62''' (and) root of male *pillû*-plant with resin of *baluḫḫu*-aromatic, [... ...]. 63'' She will see her menses. A *remedy* for the disease(s) [of(?) ...].
64''' *šalāšat šiqil ḫuṣābū ḫīli šalāšat šiqil burāšu* [...] 65''' *šalāšat šiqil tīyatu šalāšat šiqil* GI.[ZÚ.LUM.MA] 66''' [... ...] *šalāšat šiqil lip*[*û*(?) ... ...]	64''' Three shekels small (pieces of solid?) resin, three shekels of *burāšu*-juniper, [...], 65''' three shekels of *tīyatu*-plant, three shekels of GI.[ZÚ.LUM.MA-plant, ...], 66''' (with) three shekels of fa[t(?), ...].

Ms. a obv. ii breaks; gap of unknown length

67'''' *šammī annûti* ...[... ...] 68'''' *ḫīl baluḫḫi* [... ...] 69'''' [*sinništu ša ina*] *alādi mê* [*turratu*(?) ... ...] 70'''' *erīti u šu*[*pšuqti*(?) ... ...] 71'''' *maltaktu ša* ...[... ...]

67'''' these drugs ...[...], 68'''' resin of *baluḫḫu*-aromatic, [... *a remedy*] 69'''' [(for) a woman whose fluids [are blocked *following* (her)] delivery [...], 70'''' for a pregnant woman or for a woman having [a difficult delivery(?) ... ...]. 71'''' A test for ...[...].

72'''' *rebūtu kukru rebūtu šīnātu*(?) ...[... ...] 73'''' *rebūtu būšānu rebūtu nuḫurtu* [... ...] 74'''' *rebūtu zēr kitê rebūtu ṭūru rebūtu* [... ...] 75'''' ... *šammī taḫaššal tanappi ina libbi šikari* [*tanaddi*(?) ... ...] 76'''' *tammaršū-ma*(?) [... ...] 77'''' [... ...] ... [... ...]

72'''' One fourth (of a shekel?) *kukru*-aromatic, one fourth of urine(?) [... ...], 73'''' one fourth of *būšānu*-plant, one fourth of *nuḫurtu*-plant, [... ...], 74'''' one fourth of linseed, one fourth of *ṭūru*-aromatic, one fourth of [... ...], 75'''' (these) ... plants you crush, sift, [put (them)] into beer [...], 76'''' [...] you examine her(?) and [... ...] 77'''' [... ...] ... [...].

Break of ca. 5 lines

78'''' *traces*

78'''' *too fragmentary for translation*

79''''' *šumma sinništu* ...[... ...] 80''''' *pel summati* [... ...] 81''''' (*šammu*) *ēdu zikar* ...[... ...] 82''''' *lulû*(?) [... ...]

79''''' If a woman [... ...], 80''''' dove's egg (shell), [... ...], 81''''' male *ēdu*-plant, [... ...], 82''''' antimony(?), [... ...].

83''''' DIŠ KI.MIN *kirbān* [*eqli* ... ... *ina kakkabi*] 84''''' *tušbāt ina šēri* [... ...]

83''''' Alternatively, [field]-clod-[plant, ...], 84''''' you let (it) stay overnight 83''''' [under the star(s)]. 84''''' In the morning [... ...].

---

traces of a few lines before ms. a rev. iii breaks; gap of unknown length

85'''''' *traces*

85'''''' *too fragmentary for translation*

86'''''' [*šibbur*]*ratu murru mādu gabû* [...] 87'''''' [*mut*]*tapiḫtu išakkan*(?)-*ma itarraṣ šūt pî*

86'''''' [*šibbur*]*ratu*-aromatic, a large (amount) of *murru*-aromatic, alum, (and) [...]. 87'''''' She(?) shall apply (it) *as a muttapiḫtu*, then *it will be effective*. (This is) according to oral (tradition).

88'''''' [*mišil akal uḫūla*] *qarnānâ mišil akal nuḫurta ištēn šiqil šamma peṣâ* 89'''''' [...] *mišil akal namruqqu rebūtu sīḫu balṭu* 90'''''' [... *ḫī*]*l baluḫḫi* [...] *šiqil iškūra tuballal maššītu* 91'''''' [*ša* ...] *lū sinništi ša ina alādi mê turratu* 92'''''' [*lū* ...]... *išakkan-ma išallim*

88'''''' You mix [half of a tenth litre of] 'horned [alkali'], half of a tenth litre of *nuḫurtu*-plant, one shekel of 'white drug', 89'''''' [...], half of a tenth litre of *namruqqu*-plant, a quarter (of a litre?) of fresh *sīḫu*-plant, 90'''''' [... res]in of *baluḫḫu*-aromatic, (and) [x] shekels of wax. A suppository 91'''''' [for ... or for a woman] whose fluids are blocked *following* delivery 92'''''' [or for(?) ...]. She inserts (it?) [...]. Then she will be alright.

93'''''' [... ... ...] ... 94'''''' [... ... ... *ku*]*kru*

93''''''[... ... ...]...,94'''''' [... ... ...] *kukru*-[aromatic],

Break of ca. 5 lines

95''''''' [... ... ...] *uḫūlu qarnānû* 96''''''' [... ... ... *šammu*] *peṣû* 97''''''' [... ... ...] *ašāgu*(?) *sīḫu* 98''''''' [... ... ...] *billat našpi*(?) 99''''''' [... ...]... 100''''''' [... ... ...] *erēnu*(?)

95'''''''[... ... ...] horned [alkali], 96''''''' [... ...] 'white [drug'], 97''''''' [... ...] *ašāgu*-plant(?), *sīḫu*-plant, 98''''''' [... ...], *billatu*-substance for (making) *našpu*-beer(?), 99''''''' [... ...]..., 100''''''' [... ...] cedar(?)

Traces of ca. 5 fragmentary lines

[101''''''''] [... ...] *kukru* [... ...]	[101''''''''] [... ...], *kukru*-aromatic, [... ...].
[102''''''''] [... ... *rebū*]*tu būšāna rebūtu* ...[... ...] [103''''''''] [... ... *rebū-tu*] *burāša rebūtu* GI.[ZÚ.LUM.MA ... ...] [104''''''''] [... ... *šup*]*uḫra tuballal* ...[... ...]	[104''''''''] You mix [102''''''''] [... ... a qua]rter (shekel?) of *būšānu*-plant, a quarter of [...]-aromatic, [... ...], [103''''''''] [... ... a quarter of] juniper, a quarter of GI.[ZÚ.LUM.MA-plant, ...], [104''''''''] [... ...] (and) *šupuḫru*-cedar, [... ...].
[105''''''''] *traces*	[105''''''''] *too fragmentary for translation*

Ms. a rev. iv breaks; remainder lost

Notes

Lines 1'–5': For *maššītu* "suppository" (also written ḪI-*tú*, derived from the verb *našû* "to carry; to apply") in other women's healthcare texts, see e.g., SpTU 4, No. 153: 2; FLP 1306 rev. 20 (for stopping haemorrhage); BM 42313+ obv. 8–9, rev. 22 (for promoting conception/pregnancy); BM 50700: 11', 12', 28''' (for treating 'wind'); UET 7, No. 123 rev. 11' (for treating infertility). The word occurs several times in ms. a in connection with a purpose statement (see also lines 10', 13', 52'''–53''', 90''''). In the present remedy, the *maššītu* is applied to promote conception; in the other prescriptions in ms. a, it is applied for stopping or provoking bleeding (see below for discussion).

For purpose statements such as "to enable a woman who is not pregnant to get pregnant" and similar expressions in women's healthcare texts, see, e.g., STT 98 obv. 2'; BM 42313+ obv. 9, rev. 33 // BM 42333+: 5; BM 59710: 1; BM 79061: 1; BAM 250: 15 (see *infra*).

Lines 6'–9': For *uqnâtu* (ᵘZA.GÌN.(NA)), a plant and blue dye (probably woad, *isatis tinctoria*), see Thompson 1949, 171; CAD U/W, 195 sub 3 and discussion section; Thavapalan 2020, 319–320. Plant or drugs lists also attest to alternative Akkadian renderings and spellings: *šammi uqnâti* and *šammu qunātu* (the latter perhaps being a variant related to Aramaic *qān'ā* "woad"), which may suggest a reading Ú.ZA.GÌN.NA of the logogram instead of ᵘZA.GÌN.NA. For further references, see CAD U/W, 193 lex. section; BM 42450 + 43809 rev. 2', 11' (where it stands for "blue wool"), see *infra*; Finkel 2000, *FS Lambert*, 170); BM 59607 obv. 6' (Frazer 2017, CCP 4.2.Q with n. 5); Abusch and Schwemer 2016, text 7.24 line 12.

It is uncertain whether *zê šikkê* "mongoose excrement" is an alias name for a plant (cf. the designation "mongoose tail" (KUN ᵈNIN.KILIM) as an alias name for *šūšu*-plant (liquorice) in Uruanna III 1, CAD Š/2, 434 s.v. *šikkû* sub c).

For *nadû* (ŠUB) "to throw; to pour; to place; to insert" in the meaning "to apply, put (medication inside a patient's body)", see CAD N/1, 82b sub 2a-11'. The meaning and reading of the sign UD in line 9' is difficult to establish, but it should stand for a body part. Perhaps the puzzling sequence *ina* UD-*šá* is an error for *ina* ŠÀ.(TÙR)-*šá* "(you insert) into her womb".

Line 10': The spelling of the G stem durative form of *zarû* "to sprinkle, to scatter" in line 10' should be *ta-za-ar-ru* rather than *ta-az-za-ru*; see also below l. 33' *ta-aṣ-ṣa-mid* (instead of *ta-ṣa-am-mid*).

For *maššītu ša lubbuki* "suppository for absorbing" (the blood), see the *Introduction* sub 4.2 with further references and discussion. Note, for a similar phrasing as in line 10', BAM 303: 19–20 (Arbøll 2021, 286; cf. note on text A.2.3 line 28'''): Ú.ḪI.A *an-nu-ti ana* IGI *ta-za-ru maš-ši-ti šá* [x] "you scatter these drugs over it. A suppository for [...]". In this text, *maššītu* is also written ḪI-*tú* (lines 7' and 13': ḪI-*tú šá lu-ub-*[*bu*]-*ki*).

Lines 11'–13': While the parallel text FLP 1306 rev. 20 reads *maššīti ša dāma parāsi* (KUD-*si*), ms. a obv. i 13' writes KUD-*as*, which perhaps may have to be interpreted as the form *iparras*(*u*) "(which) stops (the blood)" rather than the infinitive (cf. text C.1.9). For *simbirru*-plant and 'horned alkali' (salt plant) as haemostatic drugs, see also K. 20254 obv. 7'–8', 9' (text C.1.7). SpTU 4, No. 153 obv. 5, 7 (text C.1.10) from Uruk recommends *simbirru*-plant as a cooling, haemostatic drug ("for damming up the blood").

Lines 14'–15': This prescription presents one rare example of a remedy to expel the afterbirth or placenta (*silītu*), for the case it is delayed in coming out after delivery. The text uses the verb *kâšu* (*kuāšu*) "to delay, to tarry" (CAD K, 294–295). A second prescription for this purpose occurs in ms. a ii 23'–24' (likewise a potion). See below.

Other prescriptions instruct the healer to use substances "from the mouth/opening of the *namzītu*-vessel". For example, SpTU 4, No. 153 obv. 30 (text D.1.11 line 12) prescribes a liquid substance from the mouth of a *namzītu*-vessel for a potion to promote difficult labour (perhaps *kasû*-juice); BM 42313+ rev. 35 // BM 42333+ obv. 9 (text A.2.2) uses a fatty substance from the mouth (opening) of a *dannu*-vat (for a tampon to promote fertility). Often, brewing vessels are involved, and the substance used may be some residue such as yeast, see e.g. CAD S, s.v. *saḫindu* and *sikkatu*. The brewing vessel bears a metaphorical connection to the womb/female body and to gestation, but it may also have other symbolic associations (e.g. a substance sticking to the inside of the brewing vessel's opening may signify the afterbirth held back in the womb). For discussion see also Steinert 2013, *JMC* 22, 10–14 with n. 34 as well as texts C.1.4 (BAM 237 obv. ii 1'ff. // SpTU 4, No. 129 i 21') and D.1.11 in this volume. For the *namzītu*-vessel, see also Maul 1994, 101–105; Stol 1994, 170–171; Gaspa 2014, *Contenitori*, 135–138 (*nazzītu*).

Lines 16'–17': The ingredients *kanaktu*-aromatic and *šupuḫru*-cedar are both recommended together to stop bleeding in SpTU 4, No. 153 obv. 10–11 (text C.1.10). For *kanaktu* to stop bleeding, see also the edition of FLP 1306 in this volume.

Lines 18'–19': Ostrich eggshell and *imbu' tâmti*-mineral are prescribed together in a compound remedy to staunch bleeding with roasted sheep bone and the wood from an old log, in SpTU 4, No. 153 obv. 11–12, FLP 1306: 11–15, and K. 20254 obv. 3'–5'. See further K. 8893 obv. 2', BAM 237 rev. iv 23; K. 263 + 10934 obv. 7 and 11 (for these texts see chapter C), Steinert 2012b and the *Introduction* of this book. The substance *imbu'* (*imbû*) *tâmti* is interpreted as a mineral collected at the seashore (perhaps coral or coral limestone) in CAD I/J, 108–109; Heeßel 2016, in: A. Imhausen (ed.), *Translating Writings*, 56 on obv. 6'; AHw 375b regards *imbû tâmti* as algae, followed by Schuster-Brandis 2008, 421–422.

Lines 24'–29': The symptom description in lines 24'–25' partially resembles that of BAM 240: 17'–18' (text D.2.1), but the diagnosis differs in both texts. The Assur text reads: DIŠ MUNUS Ù.TU-*ma elān ūrīša usaḫḫalši emšaša* TAG.MEŠ-*ši* / MUNUS BI NI.RA DAB-*si* "If a woman gives birth and subsequently feels a piercing pain (in) her pubic region (and) her lower abdomen continually hurts her, that woman is afflicted by NI.RA-disease". For *dikšu* "pressing pain" rather than "piercing pain" (CAD D, 137–138), see Johnson and Simkó 2024, 111 n. 307, 144 (STOMACH line 200, with *lapātu* "to afflict" in the Gtn-stem).

Similar remedies (bandages) against retention of the lochia ("blocked fluids") likewise prepared from several powdered ingredients (many of them identical to those in ms. a lines 25'–28') can be found in BAM 240: 41'–42', 50'–51' (text D.2.1). The Assyrian text describes the problem as "the blood of a woman in childbed, which has been locked in her womb" (line 40' *dām ḫarišti ša ina libbīša itteskiru*).

Lines 30'–33': The first preserved word in the difficult line 31' may be read as *kubbut* or *kupput*, i.e. D-stem stative forms. The latter word would be linked to the verb *kupputu* "to form a ball; to compress(?), to compact(?)", or the related verbal adjective *kupputu* "lump-shaped, in a block; compressed(?), compacted(?), conglomerated" (CAD K, 552–552 s.v. *kupputu* A, esp. sub 2). For the stative in the meaning "compacted", the dictionaries offer only references from omen texts describing internal organs or other body features. However, a reading *kubbut*, as D stem stative of *kabātu* "to be(come) heavy, burdensome, aggravating, serious" (e.g., in reference to illness) is likewise possible (however, usually the G-stem is used in such instances and not the D-stem, see CAD K, 15–16 sub 2). The reading and sense of the remaining text in line 31' has been difficult to establish. Perhaps, TI.MEŠ does not mean (*ana*) *bulluṭu* "to heal, to treat" here, but stands for *balṭūtu* "living, live, fresh" qualifying a medical ingredient preceding it.

Lines 34'–37': Lines 34'–35' have been reconstructed after BAM 240: 30' (text D.2.1), which features the same symptom description; but with a different recipe: DIŠ MUNUS MIN-*ma* LI.DUR-*sa* DU_8-*at* IR *a-la-ka la i-kal-la* ^{na4}PEŠ$_4$ *tur-ár* SÚD *ana* IGI ŠUB "If a woman gives birth and subsequently her navel is 'loose' (feels supple) (and) she cannot hold back the sweat from flowing: you desiccate and pound an *išqillatu*-shell (and) sprinkle it onto (the navel)." The following prescription in lines 35'–37' shares similarities with the recipe in BAM 240: 31'–32' (for the same purpose). Due to the fragmentary preservation of ms. a, it cannot be ascertained whether both prescriptions can be regarded as duplicates or close variants. The plant *ga-ši-ru-ú* is regarded as a variant form and spelling for the *šakirû*-plant (henbane), cf. also the spelling ^{ú}*ka-ši-ru-*[*ú*] attested in BAM 225: 13; CAD Š/1, 167–168; Böck 2022, 128–129.

Lines 50'''–55''': The Akkadian reading of the measurement NÍG or NINDA, in Neo-/Late Babylonian times standing for a tenth of a litre, which is found in line 51''' and *passim* is not certain (perhaps *akalu*, cf. Borger 2004, MZL, 442 No. 859; Powell 1987–1990, *RlA* 7, 498 §IV.7).

Several sections in ms. a exhibit a special structure, in which the prescription precedes the description of the conditions for which it could be used (see also lines 10', 13', 69'''–71''', 90''''–92''''). Often, several conditions or purposes are enumerated. In line 52''', this enumeration begins with *maššītu ša* MU[NUS … …], which M.J. Geller (personal communication) suggests restoring as ^{mu}[^{nus}NU.PEŠ$_4$ *ana* PEŠ$_4$] "(a mixture/suppository) [to enable] a woman [who is not pregnant to get pregnant]"; other restorations are not excluded.

Ms. a line 53''' has been restored after line 61''' below, which begins DIŠ MUNUS *sa-gu-šá ana kul-lu-mu* "to make a woman's menses appear". For other attestations of *sagû* discussed in this volume, see BM 54587 + 73802 line 6' (and *passim*); BM 61975 obv. 5'; BAM 235 obv. 7. The texts BM 47578: 2 and SpTU 1, No. 59: 14' replace *sagû* with *dāmu* "blood": "If a woman's blood is cut off so that she does not see her blood" (or, "so that her blood is not seen"; DIŠ MUNUS MÚD-*šá* KUD-*ma*$^?$ MÚD-*šá* NU IGI). Indeed, a commentary on *Diagnostic Handbook* Tablet 36 quotes the word *sagû* and equates it with *dām ardati* "the blood of a young woman" (SpTU 1, No. 39: 6'; see *infra* text I.1.2).

The phrase "if/since you do not know …" (*šumma/aššu* X *lā tīdû*) encountered in line 55''' usually occurs in commentaries, where it introduces explanations, see CAD I/J, 27 s.v. *idû* sub 1d; Gabbay 2016, 36–38. E.g., CT 39, 5: 56 (*Šumma ālu* commentary): *aššu* MUŠEN *lā tīdû ittidû šumšu* "since you do not know that bird, its name is *ittidû*." It is remarkable to find such an inserted explanation in a medical text, appended to a medical prescription. Unfortunately, the explanation of the *azupīrānu*-plant is not preserved. The plant must have been regarded as significant with regard to the treated condition (amenorrhoea). Interestingly, it is also used in the following prescription to induce the expulsion of the afterbirth.

Lines 56'''–57''': At the end of line 56''', I have restored a Št-stem form of *kâšu*, meaning "to be held up, delayed", since this verb (however in the G-stem) is also encountered in the same context (retained afterbirth) in line 14' above (cf. CAD K, 295b sub 3; AHw 463a). Note that the *azupīrānu*-plant is used here as a simple drug (in a potion with vinegar) to expel the afterbirth.

Lines 58''', 59''': While ms. a line 58''' begins with DIŠ MUNUS *a-lad uš-tap-šiq* (where *a-lad* may be a shortened *alāda*), the parallel texts (ms. B and C$_1$) read DIŠ KI.MIN, which refers back to an earlier line, in which the purpose statement reads DIŠ MUNUS *ina alādi*(Ù.TU) *uš-tap-šiq* (cf. the edition of BAM 248 (text D.1.1)).

Lines 61'''–63''': The restoration at the end of line 63''' *ṭūbtu ša mur-ṣ*[*i* …] "a *remedy* for the disease(s) [of …]" is courtesy of a suggestion by M.J. Geller (personal communication). Concerning "remedy", CAD Ṭ, 116 does not offer a translation for the word *ṭūbtu* (derived from *ṭâbu* "to be(come) pleasant, good"); AHw 1392–1393 sub 2 translates "med. Sedativum" (thus also CDA, 415). The term appears in a few other medical texts. In AMT 98/2: 8, a list of drugs is summarized as *annû ṭūbtu* "this is a *ṭubṭu*"; in line 11, another list of ingredients is designated as *napḫar* 16 Ú.ḪI.A *ṭūbtu* "total of sixteen drugs (for) a *ṭūbtu*". Note further the similar reference in BAM 40 obv. 6, where a recipe for a bandage is qualified as *annītu ṭūbtu*(DU$_{10}$.GA-*tu*$_4$) *ša* GIG […] "this (is) a *ṭūbtu* for […]-disease(s)". A lexical passage in MSL 13, 192 (Izi E): 250h equates Sumerian ú "plant, drug" with Akkadian *ṭūbtu*. There is certainly a link to the expression *ṭūba immar* (DU$_{10}$.GA IGI) "he will see/experience recovery/improvement" (cf. CAD Ṭ, 117 s.v. *ṭūbu* sub mng. b).

Line 64''': For *ḫuṣāb ḫīli* (small (solid) pieces of resin?), see also K. 8678+ rev. 11' (*ḫu-ṣab ḫi-li*) and in BM 42587+ obv. 5' (1 GÍN *ḫu-ṣab* ILLU), see texts A.1.4, B.2.4). In all these instances, *ḫuṣāb ḫīli* is not followed by a plant name. For *ḫuṣābu*, see CAD Ḫ, 258–259; AHw 360–361; Heeßel 2007, *KAL 1*, no. 18 ii 6 ("eine Kleinigkeit"). Perhaps a small quantity is meant here.

Lines 67''''–71'''': The enumeration in this fragmentary passage indicating different uses for *materia medica* listed before (unfortunately lost in the gap) is remarkable. Not only does the text mention suitability for a range of different contexts and conditions: during pregnancy, difficult delivery, retention of the lochia (when the "fluids are blocked *following* delivery"). It also mentions the possibility of applying certain drugs for a test. For *šupšuqtu*, "woman in difficult delivery" (used interchangeably with *muš(t)apšiqtu*, both derived from the same verb *pašāqu*), see also BAM 248 obv. i 36, rev. iv 6 and the commentary 11N-T3 lines 14–15 (see texts D.1.11, G.1).

In line 71'''', the sign traces do not support the reading *maltaktu ša* P[EŠ$_4$ NU PEŠ$_4$] "a test for (determining a woman's ability for) becoming pregnant or not becoming pregnant". However, *maltaktu* is repeatedly found in connection with fertility tests / birth prognoses. See especially BM 42313+ rev. 29 // UET 7, No. 123 obv. 1, the former of which may perhaps be restored as *ana maštakti* MUNUS NU [*e-r*]*i*$^?$-*i*$^?$ "for a test (determining) a woman (who will) not conceive/get pregnant" (see *infra* texts A.2.2, B.2.2). See further N. 4001 (text B.2.1) and STT 98 obv. 10' (text A.1.1). For *maltaktu* (also *maštaktu*) and the notion of "testing, trying" (*latāku*) in Mesopotamian medical texts, see also the discussion in Steinert 2015.

Lines 72''''–75'''': In this section, the measurements following the numeral *rebūtu* "one fourth, a quarter" are lacking. I suppose that the word "shekel" was simply left out in these instances. See also line 61''' above, where the measurement is likewise missing following *šalšu* "one third".

Lines 78''''–82'''': Instead of *lu-lu-ú* at the beginning of line 82'''', one could also read DAB.DAB-*ú* (e.g., a Gtn- or D-form of the verb *ṣabātu*, "to grasp repeatedly" or "to fasten, to bind"). Lack of context makes it difficult to decide.

Lines 86'''''–87''''': A word *muttappiḫtu*, as restored in line 87''''', is not attested in the dictionaries yet. The term appears to be related to the verb *napāḫu* "to blow; to ignite; to rise". In line 87''''', the term seems to designate a specific type of treatment or application form for the *materia medica*. Possibly, the word refers to an intended effect (perhaps a "heating treatment" aimed at producing sweat?). See the Introduction, section 4.2 for discussion.

The use of *itarraṣ* "it will succeed, prosper" concluding the prescription in line 87''''' is unusual for a medical text. One would expect a verb such as *šalāmu*, *balāṭu* "to be(come) alright, healthy" instead of *tarāṣu*. CAD T, 216b sub 2 lists a few references for the form stemming from omen apodoses, under *tarāṣu* B (cf. AHw 1326–1327).

A.2.2 BM 42313+: A Late Babylonian Recipe Collection on Women's Health

The Late Babylonian compendium with prescriptions for women (ms. a) was reconstructed from numerous fragments by I. L. Finkel and identified by him as a teaching source that was used in the context medical training carried out by the family of Bēl-rēmanni, a wealthy scribe associated with the Ebabbar temple at Sippar. That the compendium must have belonged to the archives associated with this family is indicated by the context of the fragments: they belong to the 81-7-1 collection of the British Museum, of which numerous tablets have been identified as part of these archives (see Jursa 1999; Finkel 2000, 171–173).[256] Moreover, several prescriptions of ms. a are duplicated in a small student's tablet stemming from the same context (ms. b), recognizable as such by the numerous haphazard stylus imprint marks left by the scribe on the reverse of the tablet. Ms. b duplicates a recipe against miscarriage and two recipes to promote pregnancy in a barren woman, which are included in ms. a among prescriptions for various women's health problems.

A few other prescriptions in ms. a find close parallels or duplicates in other women's healthcare texts from Assyria and Babylonia. In one case (ms. g), the parallel comes from a Middle Babylonian manuscript, pointing to the long continuity of some of the medical lore associated with treating women.

The topics treated in ms. a are diverse. The obverse of the tablet appears to begin with remedies to promote fertility (see line 8) and a prescription to protect a woman from miscarriage caused by sorcery (line 10). The purpose of the following recipes (between lines 11 and 27) is not entirely clear, but they may be concerned with provoking menstrual bleeding (other texts such as SpTU 1, No. 59 (text C.2.1) or compendia such as BM 38624+ (text A.2.1) deal with this topic or contain passages treating the absence of the menses). The remainder of the obverse (lines 28–41) features prescriptions to stop (abnormal) vaginal haemorrhage.

The reverse of ms. a (lines 42–46) begins with treatments for the enigmatic female condition NI.NE (or Ì.KÚM), which is attested in a text from Assur (BAM 237 = ms. F) dealing mainly with abnormal vaginal discharges, and which has previously been interpreted as puerperal fever (Scurlock and Andersen 2005, 281 12.119). However, details in the symptom descriptions given for NI.NE in ms. a, and the fact that the following section (lines 47–49) deals with treatments for problems with urination (retention of urine, uncontrolled release of urine, bed-wetting), may signal that NI.NE was likewise associated with urinary complaints (see the discussion below and the *Introduction* sub 4.2).

The following prescriptions in ms. a (lines 50–63) are concerned with pregnancy: preventing miscarriage, stopping bleeding or loss of amniotic fluid, preserving or promoting pregnancy. The next recipes (lines 64–69) are unusual and unparalleled in the women's health corpus: they consist in a prescription to improve a woman's body odour (if her sweat smells unpleasant) and in two prescriptions for the case that "a woman does not do (or: does not like to do) the 'work of women' (*šumma sinništu šipir šinnišāti lā ippuš*)", apparently a euphemistic expression that may refer to a woman's lack

256 Contrary to Finkel 2008, 200, mss. a and b most likely stem from Sippar, not from Babylon. See also Leichty, Finkel and Walker 2019, *CBT* IV–V, 509, 510 and Reade, in: *CBT* VI, xxxi on the 81-7-1 collection of the British Museum.

of pleasure or interest in engaging in sexual intercourse. The tablet concludes with a fertility test (lines 70–73) and prescription to promote fertility (lines 74–84).

In general, it should be emphasized that in contrast to many other healing texts from the first millennium BCE, ms. a exclusively contains medical prescriptions, but no incantations or rituals. The text displays several noteworthy features, such as the use of the masculine pronominal suffix *-šú* (instead of the feminine suffix *-šá*, when referring to the patient). While this is a typical feature of women's healthcare texts from the late periods, others are rarer, e.g., unusual spellings or forms such as *šá* ŠÀ-ŠÀ-ŠÀ-*šú* (for *ša liblibbīša*) instead of *šá* ŠÀ-*šá* or *šà* ŠÀ-*šà* (for *ša libbīša*) "her foetus" (lit. "that of her womb").

List of Manuscripts

Siglum	Museum Number	Copy	Collation	Format; Ductus	Provenience
a	BM 42313 (81-7-1, 73) + BM 42427 (81-7-1, 187) + BM 42585 (81-7-1, 345) + without No. (81-7-1, 353) + BM 43174 (81-7-1, 938) + BM 43215 (81-7-1, 979) + BM 43274 (81-7-1, 1038) + BM 43279 (81-7-1, 1043) + BM 43281 (81-7-1, 1045) + BM 43439 (81-7-1, 1203) + BM 43483 (81-7-1, 1247) + BM 43595 (81-7-1, 1359) + BM 43766 (81-7-1, 1527) + BM 43803 (81-7-1, 1564)	Pl. 14–15	Coll.	Single-column tablet in portrait format; Late Babylonian script; ca. 500 BCE	Sippar
b	BM 42333 (81-7-1, 93) + BM 42453 (81-7-1, 213) + BM 43602 (81-7-1, 1366)	Finkel, *FS Lambert*, Fig. 24	Coll.	Single-column tablet in landscape format; Late Babylonian script; ca. 500 BCE	Sippar
c	-	UET 7, No. 123	-	Single-column tablet; Neo-Babylonian script; ca. 7th/6th cent. BCE	Ur
d	K. 20254	Pl. 34	Coll.	Fragment of a tablet in Neo-Babylonian script; 7th cent. BCE	Nineveh; Ashurbanipal's library
e	FLP 1306	Pl. 30	Coll.	Single-column tablet; Late Babylonian script; ca. 6th–3rd cent. BCE(?)	Unknown (Babylonia)
F	VAT 8577 + 13655 + 13671 + 13706 + 13707 + 13708 + 13828 + 14177 + 14185 (+)	KAR 194 (only VAT 8577) BAM 237 (all fragments)	Coll.	Two-column tablet; Neo-Assyrian script; ca. 8th/7th cent. BCE	Assur; N4 library
g	VAT 10575 (+) VAT 9543	BAM 241 Pl. 7–8	Coll.	Fragments of a two-column tablet; Middle Babylonian script; 13th cent. BCE	Assur

Overview

i	Fragmentary prescription a obv. 1–4	1–4
ii	Fragmentary prescription (potion) a obv. 5	5
iii	Fragmentary prescription (potion) a obv. 6	6
iv	Fragmentary prescription a obv. 7	7
v	Prescription to promote conception (suppository) a obv. 8–9	8–9

vi	Prescription to protect a woman from miscarriage caused by sorcery a obv. 10 (cf. BM 42327+ obv. 1–4 //)	10
vii	Fragmentary prescription to stop bleeding during pregnancy(?) (potion) a obv. 11–12	11–12
viii	Prescription to induce the menses(?) a obv. 13–14	13–14
ix	Prescription to induce the menses(?) (potion?) a obv. 15	15
x	Prescription to induce the menses(?) (potion?) a obv. 16	16
xi	Prescription to induce the menses(?) (potion?) a obv. 17	17
xii	Prescription to induce the menses(?) a obv. 18	18
xiii	Prescription to induce the menses(?) a obv. 19	19
xiv	Prescription to induce the menses(?) (bandage) a obv. 20	20
xv	Prescription to induce the menses(?) (poultice) a obv. 21	21
xvi	Prescription to induce the menses(?) a obv. 22	22
xvii	Prescription to induce the menses(?) (suppository) a obv. 23	23
xviii	Prescription to induce the menses(?) (suppository) a obv. 24–25	24–25
xix	Prescription to induce the menses(?) (suppository) a obv. 26–27	26–27
xx	Prescription to stop haemorrhage (suppository) a obv. 28–29 // d obv.$^{?}$ 3'–5' // e obv. 11–15	28–29
xxi	Prescription to stop haemorrhage (suppository) a obv. 30	30
xxii	Prescription to stop haemorrhage (suppository) a obv. 31	31
xxiii	Prescription to stop haemorrhage (suppository) a obv. 32	32
xxiv	Prescription to stop haemorrhage (tampon?) a obv. 33	33
xxv	Prescription to stop haemorrhage (poultice) a obv. 34	34
xxvi	Prescription to stop haemorrhage (poultice) a obv. 35	35
xxvii	Prescription to stop haemorrhage (poultice) a obv. 36	36
xxviii	Two prescriptions to stop haemorrhage (bandage applied to the genitals) a obv. 37–41	37–41
xxix	Prescription for NI.NE-disease (suppository) a rev. 1–2 // F rev. 9–10	42–43
xxx	Prescription for NI.NE-disease (potion) a rev. 3	44

xxxi	Prescription for NI.NE-disease (injection into the urethra) a rev. 4 // g obv. ii 9'–10'	45
xxxii	Positive prognosis a rev. 5	46
xxxiii	Prescription for incontinence and urinary retention (tampon) a rev. 6	47
xxxiv	Symptom description concerning bed-wetting and painful urination (without prescription) a rev. 7–8	48–49
xxxv	Prescription to prevent miscarriage (potion) a rev. 9–11 // b obv. 1–4	50–52
xxxvi	Prescription to stop bleeding during pregnancy and to prevent miscarriage a rev. 12–14	53–55
xxxvii	Fragmentary prescription a rev. 15	56
xxxviii	Prescription to stop loss of amniotic fluid during pregnancy (tampon) a rev. 16	57
xxxix	Prescription to stop loss of amniotic fluid during pregnancy (tampon) a rev. 17	58
xl	Prescription to stop diarrhoea in a pregnant woman(?) (potion) a rev. 18–19	59–60
xli	Prescription to stop bleeding during pregnancy (ointment) a rev. 20–21	61–62
xlii	Prescription to promote conception/pregnancy (suppository) a rev. 22	63
xliii	Prescription to improve a woman's body odour (ointment) a rev. 23–25	64–66
xliv	Prescription to promote female sexual desire (tampon) a rev. 26–27	67–68
xlv	Prescription to promote female sexual desire (tampon) a rev. 28	69
xlvi	Pregnancy/fertility test a rev. 29–32 // c obv. 1–4	70–73
xlvii	Prescription against infertility (tampon) a rev. 33–36 // b obv. 5–11	74–77
xlviii	Prescription against infertility (tampon) a rev. 37–38 // b rev. 1–5	78–79
xlix	Prescription against infertility(?) (tampon) a rev. 39–41	80–82
l	Fragmentary prescription against infertility(?) a rev. 42–43	83–84

Previous Edition and Discussion

Finkel 2000, *FS Lambert*, 171–173 Text 17 (transliteration and translation of ms. b and duplicating passages in ms. a)[257]
Böck 2013, 32–33 (lines 74–77, 78–79)
Scurlock and Andersen 2005, 12.18, 12.49, 12.50, 12.119 (transliteration of lines 42–43, 50, 70–73, 77)
Steinert 2015, 109 (lines 70–73)
Steinert 2017a, 307 (lines 74–77)

257 For a photo of mss. a and b, see also Finkel 2008, 200 Fig. 189 and 190.

Electronic Babylonian Library (eBL) (https://www.ebl.lmu.de/library/BM.42333, edition of ms. b; photo), (https://www.ebl.lmu.de/library/BM.42313, photo ms. a)
Infra text B.2.2 (edition of ms. c), text C.1.7 (ms. d), text C.1.9 (ms. e), text C.1.4 (ms. F), text II.1.3 (ms. g)

Transliteration

1	a obv. 1	[DIŠ MUNUS$^{?}$ ....] x [...........................]
2	a obv. 2	[...........................] x x [.......................................]
3	a obv. 3	[.........................] ⸢ši/ḫa$^{?}$ ti a an$^{?}$⸣ [..............................]
4	a obv. 4	x [.......................] [.......................................]
5	a obv. 5	DIŠ [KI.MIN$^{?}$ ....]x *ina* KAŠ NAG-*šú ana* x[................]
6	a obv. 6	DIŠ K[I.MIN ......] ⸢x⸣ [......] *ina* KAŠ NAG-⸢*šú*⸣-*ma* [.........]
7	a obv. 7	DIŠ KI.MIN [*k*]*a-mu-nu* 10 ⸢NUMUN⸣ ⸢*kur*$^{?}$⸣-<*ka*>-*nam mál-ma-liš ina* Ì.UDU ḪI.ḪI [.......]
8	a obv. 8	DIŠ MUNUS NU ⸢PEŠ$_{4}$⸣ *ana šu-ri-i* ⸢^{šim}GÚR.GÚR⸣ ^{šim}LI ⸢$^{šim?}$⸣BULUḪ ^{šim}ḪA[B x x]
9	a obv. 9	*ina* KÀŠ NAM.LÚ.U$_{18}$.LU ŠE[G$_{6}$$^{?}$-*šal*] ⸢ḪI⸣-*tú* ^{munus}NU.⸢PEŠ$_{4}$$^{?}$⸣ *ana* [PEŠ$_{4}$]
10	a obv. 10	BE *ana* ^{munus}PE[Š$_{4}$] ⸢*kiš*⸣-*pi* NU ⸢TE$^{?}$-*e*$^{?}$⸣ [x x]x ⸢$^{giš?}$GEŠTIN.KA$_{5}$⸣.A SIG$_{7}$-*su* ⸢SÚD⸣ K[I Ì.GIŠ$^{?}$] \ ŠÉŠ-*šú* T[I-*uṭ*$^{?}$]
11	a obv. 11	^{KÚR} | DIŠ MUNUS *šá k*[*a$_{4}$-an-ni-šú* x x x x x *k*]*a-mu-nu* GA *šá* ^{munus}⸢*ú*⸣-[*suk-k*]*at šá* NITA ⸢*ú*$^{?}$⸣-[*li*]*d*
12	a obv. 12	NU *pa-t*[*an* NAG$^{?}$ *ú*]-*šal*-[*lam*]
13	a obv. 13	[DIŠ MUNU]S MIN$^{?}$ *ana* MÚD$^{?}$-[*šú* IGI$^{?}$ ...... ^{giš}*tas-k*]*a*$^{?}$-*rin-na šá* KUR SUMUN ḪI$^{?}$.[ḪI x x x x]-⸢*ú*$^{?}$⸣ ⸢$^{KÚR?}$⸣
14	a obv. 14	⸢*lu*⸣-*ú*$^{?}$-ʾ-*at-ma* [x x x x] x-*bat* MUNUS [MÚD-*šú* I]GI$^{?}$
15	a obv. 15	DIŠ KI.MIN 1/2 GÍN ^{šim}x[x x] x ⸢*ina*⸣ ⸢KAŠ⸣ ⸢KALA.GA$^{?}$⸣ [NAG$^{?}$ K]I.MIN$^{?}$
16	a obv. 16	DIŠ KI.MIN EME.ŠID.Z[I.DA ḪÁ]D.A GAZ SIM *ina* GEŠ[TIN$^{?}$ (...) NAG$^{?}$ KI].MIN
17	a obv. 17	DIŠ KI.MIN ⸢LÀL⸣ ⸢*ḫi-li*⸣ [(x) ŠEG$_{6}$-*š*]*al*$^{?}$ NAGA.SI *ana* ŠÀ ŠUB-*di* [x x x KI].MIN$^{?}$
18	a obv. 18	DIŠ KI.MIN *pap-pa-su šá* [MUN]U$_{5}$$^{?}$ *ina* KÀŠ$^{?}$ ŠEG$_{6}$-*šal ana* ⸢MÚD$^{?}$⸣ MUNUS IGI [SI]G$_{5}$$^{?}$
19	a obv. 19	[DIŠ K]I.MIN ⸢^{ú}⸣x[x x x x G]I$^{?}$ *kab*$^{?!}$(EN)-*ri* 4-*tú* BU[RU$_{5}$$^{?}$] ⸢4⸣-*tú* ^{š}[$^{im?}$x x x]
20	a obv. 20	D[IŠ KI.MIN$^{?}$ x x x x x] ⸢*tu*⸣-*pa-ṣa ina* KAŠ *tara-bak* [*ina* TÚG$^{?}$] *nàr-bi* KÉŠ-*ma*$^{?}$ *i*[*na-e*]*š*$^{?}$
21	a obv. 21	DIŠ ⸢KI.MIN⸣ 1$^{?}$ x[x x x x x *ana*] Ì.UDU ŠUB *ina* SÍG NIGIN-*m*[*i*] ⸢Ì⸣.GIŠ *ba-ḫír*$^{?}$ *t*[*a*-[*ṭ*]*e*$_{4}$$^{?}$-*pi*
22	a obv. 22	*šum*$_{4}$-*ma* NINDA$^{?}$ MU[NU$_{5}$$^{?}$ x x x x x]x x-⸢*ma*⸣ ⸢KÀŠ$^{?}$⸣ ⸢*ru*⸣-*ḫu-uṣ*
23	a obv. 23	*maš-šit šá* MUNUS MÚD$^{?}$-*š*[*ú*$^{?}$ KUD-*su*$^{?}$ x GÍN M]UN.ḪI.A 3 GÍN ⸢$^{šim?}$⸣[x x] ⸢*ina*⸣ ⸢MÚD$^{?}$⸣ ⸢ÉLLAG⸣ GU$_{4}$ [x]x *tara-ku*

24	a obv. 24	DIŠ KI.MIN <1> GÍN *ḫi-l*[*i*$^?$ 1 GÍN ^{š}]^{im}ḪAB 1 GÍN ^{šim}ŠEŠ 1 GÍN ⸢$^{\text{šim?}}$⸣[x 1 GÍN L]ÀL$^?$ BABBAR
25	a obv. 25	1 GÍN *ti-ia-a-t*[*i* (x) *t*]*a-sa-ku ina* Ì.UDU ÉLLAG GU$_4$ ⸢*tara-ku*⸣
26	a obv. 26	1 GÍN ^{šim}ḪAB 1 G[ÍN x] UZU MUŠEN$^?$ 2 GÍN MÚD ^{giš}EREN 1 GÍN ^{šim}⸢ŠEŠ⸣
27	a obv. 27	1 GÍN MUN.ḪI.A *ina* Ì.UD[U ÉLL]AG$^?$ *tara-ku al-la-nu la-ab-ku* TAG-*šú*
28	a obv. 28	*ana* MÚD MUNUS KUD-*si* 1 *kak-ka* ⸢GÌR.PAD⸣.DU UDU.NÍTA *ina* IZI *tur*-⸢*ár*⸣ ŠIKA NUNUZ GA.NU$_{11}$^{mušen}
	d obv.$^?$ 3'–4'	[....... .... GÌR.PAD.DU UDU$^?$].NÍTA *ina* IZI *tur*-⸢*ár*⸣ / [.........]
	e obv. 11–12	*e-ṣe-et* UDU.NÍTA *ina* IZI *tur*-<*ár*> SÚD$^?$ / ŠIKA NUNUZ *lu-ur-mu*
29	a obv. 29	KA A.AB.BA ⸢KU$^?$⸣ [^{giš}ÙR SUM]UN$^?$ *ina* ^{síg}ÀKA NIGIN-*mi ana* ŠÀ.TÙR-*šú* GAR-*ma šá* MÚD MUNUS KUD-*si*
	d obv.$^?$ 4'$^{\text{cont.}}$–5'	[.....................ŠU.Ù]R SUMUN *ina* ^{síg}ÀKA / [NIGIN-*mi ana* ŠÀ.TÙR-*šá*] GAR-*an*
	e obv. 12$^{\text{cont.}}$–15	KA *tam-tim* / ŠU.ÙR SUMUN *mál-ma-liš*$^!$(tar) *ina* ÀKA / NIGIN-*mi ina* ŠÀ.TÙR-*šú* GAR-*ma* / MÚD KUD-*si*
30	a obv. 30	DIŠ KI.MIN ^{šim}⸢ŠEŠ⸣ ⸢$^{\text{šim?}}$⸣*la-ba*-⸢*na*$^!$(*du*)-*tú*$^?$⸣ *ir-re-e*$^{!?}$(ir) ŠIKA$^?$ SÁḪAR *šá* KA UDUN *ta-mar-raq* [*ina*] ⸢Ì$^?$⸣ ḪI.ḪI KI.MIN
31	a obv. 31	*ana* MÚD MUNUS KUD-*si* ^{ú}*gu-ú-du ina* IZI [*tu-b*]*al*$^?$ LUḪ$^?$ ZÌ *ḫa-ru-bu* ŠUR.MÌN ḪI.ḪI. KI.MIN
32	a obv. 32	DIŠ KI.MIN MUN KÚM TI-*q*[*é*$^?$ x x] ⸢Ì$^?$⸣.ḪUL ḪI.ḪI KI.MIN
33	a obv. 33	[DIŠ K]I.MIN ^{ú}IN$_6$.ÚŠ EN NUMUN-*šú ina* ÍD LUḪ-*si* ⸢*ina*⸣ ⸢ÀKA$^?$⸣ [NIGIN-*mi*$^?$]
34	a obv. 34	[DIŠ KI.M]IN ^{ú}*šu-un-ḫu* ḪÁD.DU *ina* IZI *tu-bal* LUḪ [*te*]-*ṭe-pi*
35	a obv. 35	DIŠ KI.MIN *na-gab ṭi-pi* ^{ú}*gu-ú-du* [*te*$^?$]-*ṭe-pi*
36	a obv. 36	DIŠ KI.MIN ^{túg}KI.TA MAR-*ru* [*te*$^?$]-*ṭe-pi*
37	a obv. 37	DIŠ KI.MIN $^{\text{na4}}$*gab-bu-ú* ŠIKA SILA.LÍM.MA $^{\text{na4}}$ÉLLAG-*tu*$_4$ *a-ḫu-us-su ma-la* ⸢KAM-*ti*$^?$⸣-*šú-nu*
38	a obv. 38	$^{\text{na4}}$KUR-*nu* DAB *ina* MÚD ^{giš}EREN ḪI.ḪI *ina* ^{síg}ÀKA NIGIN-*mi ina sun* BAR-*šá* GAR ⸢*ka*$_4$⸣-*an-nu*
39	a obv. 39	*ana* KUD-*si u se-kìr-ši* ŠUB-*ú* SIG$_5$
40	a obv. 40	DIŠ KI.MIN ŠIKA $^{\text{na4}}$ZA.GÌN *šá tíq-nu* SAḪAR.GI$_6$$^?$ ^{ú}⸢SAḪAR$^?$⸣ x x NU$^?$.LUḪ$^?$ TI ŠEG$_6$$^?$ *lu ina* ^{síg}À[KA$^?$ *lu*$^?$]
41	a obv. 41	GADA$^?$ NIGIN$^?$-*ma* MAN <*ina*> ^{giš}ZU$^?$ ⸢IN$^?$⸣.[SAR$^?$]
42	a rev. 1	DIŠ MUNUS NI.NE *ki-is*$^!$(ma) KÀŠ GIG-*at* MÚD.MEŠ-*šú ana* x x x [x x x x]
	F rev. iv 9	DIŠ MUNUS NI.NE GIG -------------------------------------*omits*
43	a rev. 2	*šá-kín* MUNUS BI NI.NE GIG-*at* DÈ *ur-bat* DÈ *ṣar-bat* 14 KEŠDA K[ÉŠ$^?$ x x x x]
	F rev. iv 9$^{\text{cont.}}$–10	-------------------------------------*omits* 1 SÌLA DÈ ^{giš}ÁSAL 1 SÌLA DÈ ^{ú}*am-ḫa-ra* ḪI.⸢ḪI⸣ / 14 KEŠDA.MEŠ *šá* TÚG KÉŠ 1.TA.ÀM *ana* ŠÀ.TÙR-*šá* GAR-*an*
44	a rev. 3	DIŠ KI.MIN Ú BABBAR *ina* GEŠTIN SUR.RA ⸢NAG⸣ [x x x]
45	a rev. 4	DIŠ KI.MIN ^{šim}ŠEŠ *ina* Ì SÚD *ina* MUD ZABAR *ana múš-tin-ni-šú* DUB-[*ak*$^?$]
	g obv. ii 9'–10'	KI.MIN *mur-ra ta-ḫaš-šal ina* Ì *t*[*a-bal-lal*$^?$] / *ina up-pí ina šà-su-ri-šá i-ta-b*[*a-ak* (x x)]

46	a rev. 5	*šal-miš* É KÀŠ *i-kab-ba-*[*as*$^{?}$]
47	a rev. 6	DIŠ MUNUS ŠUB DAB KÀŠ$^{!}$(UŠ) GIG-*at* KA *tam-tim ina* ^{síg}ÀKA NIGIN-*mi ana* ŠÀ.TÙR-⸢*šú*⸣ ⸢GAR-*an*⸣
48	a rev. 7	DIŠ MUNUS *ina ṣal-lu-ti-šú* KÀŠ-*šú ina* ^{giš}NÁ-*šú iš-tin* ŠÀ KÀŠ$^{!}$.MEŠ *ma-a-*⸢*da*$^{?!}$*-ti*⸣ ⸢GAL$_{4}$$^{?}$⸣.<LA-*šú*>
49	a rev. 8	GU$_{7}$-*šú-ma* MUNUS BI KÀŠ *ši-*<*ta*>*-tu* ⸢BÚR⸣ [TI-*uṭ*$^{?}$]
50	a rev. 9	⸢DIŠ⸣ ⸢MUNUS⸣ *lu šá* ITI *lu šá* 2 ITI *lu šá* 3 ITI *šá* ŠÀ-ŠÀ-*š*[*à* ŠU]B.ŠUB-*a ḫ*[*u-*……]
	b obv. 1–3	DIŠ MUNUS *lu* [IT]I *lu* 2 ITI [*l*]*u* 3 ITI / *šà* ŠÀ-*šà* ŠUB.ŠUB-*a ḫu-la-a* ḪÁD.A / SÚD ÀR
51	a rev. 10	*ana* ŠÀ A 3-*šú ana* ŠÀ Ì 3-*šú ta-bal-lal an-nu-ḫa-r*[*a*] ⸢*ana*⸣ ⸢ŠÀ⸣ [x x (x)-*š*]*ú-*[*ma*]
	b obv. 3$^{cont.}$–4	*ana* ŠÀ A 3-*šú ana* ŠÀ Ì 3-*šú ta-bal-lal* / *a-nu-ḫa-ri ana* ŠÀ ŠUB NAG-*šú-ma*
52	a rev. 11	*šá* ŠÀ-ŠÀ-ŠÀ-*šú* [NU ŠUB.ŠUB]-*a*
	b obv. 4$^{cont.}$	*šà* ŠÀ-*šà* NU ŠUB.ŠUB
53	a rev. 12	DIŠ MUNUS *šá* 3 ITI MÚD-*šú* DU-*ak ana šà* ŠÀ-*šà* [NU ŠUB x x x x] SI ÁB
54	a rev. 13	*ták-pít* 14 ŠE$^{?}$ $^{šim.d}$MAŠ Ì.UDU ÚKUŠ.LAGAB [x x x x x x] ⸢x x⸣
55	a rev. 14	ŠIM$^{?!}$.ḪI.A DÙ.A.BI *ina di-di* GADA$^{?}$ GAR-*an* x[x x x x x x x x x]
56	a rev. 15	DIŠ MUNUS *i-par*$^{?}$*-ra-aḫ* ^{na4}KUR-*nu* DAB *ina* Ì [x x x x x x x x x]
57	a rev. 16	DIŠ ^{munus}PEŠ$_{4}$ A.MEŠ DU-*ku* GUB x[x x x x x x *ina* x NIGIN]-*mi* ⸢*ana*⸣ ⸢ŠÀ.TÙR-*šú*⸣ ⸢GAR-*an*$^{?}$⸣
58	a rev. 17	DIŠ KI.MIN ^{ú}ŠAKIRA *ina* ⸢Ì⸣ [SÚ]D *ina* ^{s}[^{íg}ÀKA NIGIN *ana* ŠÀ.TÙ]R-*šú* GAR-*an*
59	a rev. 18	⸢DIŠ⸣ ⸢^{munus}PEŠ$_{4}$$^{?}$⸣ ⸢x x⸣-*lit*$^{?}$ *šá ri-du-u*[*t ir-ri* TUKU$^{?}$ x x x] *pu-qut-ti nu-ḫur-ti*
60	a rev. 19	*ina* KAŠ SÚD *ina* MUL$_{4}$ *tuš-bat ina še-rim* [NU *pa-tan*$^{?}$] NAG-*šú*
61	a rev. 20	DIŠ ^{munus}⸢PEŠ$_{4}$⸣ MÚD.MEŠ U$_{4}$.1.KAM DU-*ku* U$_{4}$.1.KAM N[U DU-*ku u* U]ZU-⸢*šú*⸣ SIG$_{7}$ *a-na* TIN-*šú*
62	a rev. 21	*ka-mu-nu* SÚD *ina* Ì IGI ŠÀ-*šú* ŠÉŠ
63	a rev. 22	1 GÍN ^{ú}*tar-muš ta-mar-raq bul-*[x x x x x]x *ina* ŠÀ$^{?}$ ḪI.ḪI ḪI-*tú šá* PEŠ$_{4}$
64	a rev. 23	DIŠ MUNUS ⸢IR$^{?}$⸣-*sú* NU DU$_{10}$-*ta* DÈ ^{ú}[x x x x]x ḪI.Ḫ[I *t*]*u*$^{?}$-⸢*kaṣ-ṣa*⸣-[*a*$^{?}$]
65	a rev. 24	⸢MUNU$_{6}$$^{?}$⸣ ^{lú}KURUN.NAM *na-pi*$_{5}$*-tim* [x x x x x] ^{ú}⸢EME$^{?}$⸣-U[R.GI$_{7}$ *ma-la*$^{?}$] *ib-ba-šu*$^{?}$
66	a rev. 25	[x x x]x du ši ma za [………………………]x [ŠÉ]Š-*su*
67	a rev. 26	DIŠ MUNUS *ši-pir* ⸢MUNUS.MEŠ$^{?}$⸣ N[U DÙ$^{?}$] ⸢x⸣ [x x x x GÌR.PAD.D]U$^{?}$ UDU.⸢NÍTA⸣ [*t*]*ur-ár* SÚD
68	a rev. 27	*ina* TÚG KÉŠ [(x x x x)] *ana* ⸢ŠÀ.TÙR⸣-[*šú*] GAR-⸢*an*⸣-*ma*$^{!}$ *ina-eš*
69	a rev. 28	DIŠ MUNUS *ši-pir* MUNUS.MEŠ [NU DÙ *ši*]-*bir-ti*$^{?}$ ^{síg}ÀKA NIGIN-*m*[*i ana* Š]À.⸢TÙR⸣-*šú* GAR-*an*
70	a rev. 29	*ana maš-tak-ti* ⸢MUNUS⸣ ⸢NU⸣ [*e-r*]*i*$^{?}$*-i*$^{?}$ 1 GÍN ^{ú}*tar-muš* 1/2 [GÍN Ú BABBAR] 1 GÍN ^{na4}*gab-bu-ú*
	c obv. 1	[*mal-tak-ti* (MUNUS) *ki-i* PEŠ$_{4}$ *u ki-i* NU PEŠ$_{4}$$^{?}$ 1 GÍN ^{ú}*tar-muš*] 1/2 GÍN Ú BABBAR 4-*tú* ^{na4}*gab-u*
71	a rev. 30	*ina* ^{síg}ÀKA NIGIN-*mi* [*ana* ŠÀ.TÙR-*šú*] ⸢GAR-*ma*⸣ *kal u*$_{4}$*-mu ú-*⸢*kal*⸣ ⸢*uš*$^{?}$⸣-[*e*]*l*$^{?}$*-lam-ma*
	c obv. 2–3	[*mi-ṣir-a-a ina* ^{síg}ÀKA NIGIN-*mi ana* ŠÀ.TÙ]R-*šá* GAR-*an mu-šú gab-bi* / [*ú-kal* E$_{11}$-*ma*$^{?}$]

72	a rev. 31	*ina* A LUḪ-*si šum*$_4$-*ma* [^{síg}ÀKA SIG$_7$] ⌜MUNUS⌝ ⌜BI⌝ N[U] ⌜PEŠ$_4$$^?$⌝
	c obv. 3$^{cont.}$–4	[*ina* GEŠ]TIN$^?$-*nu* BABBAR LUḪ-*si ki-i* ^{síg}ÀKA *ši-i* SA$_5$-*at lu* MÚD *ul-lu-ḫa-tú* / [MUNUS BI PEŠ$_4$]
73	a rev. 32	*šum*$_4$-*ma* ^{síg}ÀKA SA$_5$-*at* [*lu* MÚD *ul*]-⌜*lu*⌝-*ḫat u* ŠÀ.TÙR-*šú* BABBAR-*ma* [MUN]US BI *ir-ri*
	c obv. 4$^{cont.}$	*vki-i* ^{síg}ÀKA SIG$_7$-*at* MUNUS BI NU PEŠ$_4$
74	a rev. 33	DIŠ MUNUS NU PEŠ$_4$ *a-na šu-r*[*i-i* 4] Ú 4 NINDA.ḪI.A ^{šim}GÚR.GÚR 1/2 G[ÍN ^{š}]^{im}LI
	b obv. 5–6	DIŠ MUNUS NU PEŠ$_4$ *a-na šu-ri-i* 4 Ú 4 NINDA.ḪI.A / ^{šim}GÚR.GÚR 1/2 GÍN ^{šim}LI
75	a rev. 34	1 GÍN *šam-ba-lil-*[*tu*$_4$ 1] GÍN ŠE.GIŠ.Ì *bu-'u-ú-š*[*u-tu*$_4$]
	b obv. 7–8	1 GÍN *šam-ba-*<*li*>-*il-tu*$_4$ 1 GÍN ŠE.GIŠ.Ì / *bu-'u-ú-šu-tú*
76	a rev. 35	1 GÍN *ši-qit-tú* [x x *i*]*na ḫu*$^{?!}$-*li-bi šá* KÁ *dan-nu* ḪI.ḪI *a*[*lla*-x x x]
	b obv. 8$^{cont.}$–10	1 GÍN *ši-qit-tú* / *ina ḫu-li-bi šá* KÁ *dan-nu* ḪI.ḪI / *alla-an* DÙ-*uš*
77	a rev. 36	*ana* ŠÀ.TÙR-*šú* GAR-[*an-ma* BAD-*m*]*a ir-ri u* A.MEŠ ŠUB.ŠUB-[*a*]
	b obv. 10$^{cont.}$–11	*ana* ŠÀ.TÙR GAR-*ma* / BAD-*ma ir-ri u* A.MEŠ ŠUB.ŠUB-*ma*
78	a rev. 37	^{munus}*la a-lit-ti* [*ana*] *šu-ri-*⌜*i*⌝ ⌜PÉŠ⌝.GIŠ.GI *ta-ka-ṣi* ŠÀ-*šú* ⌜BAD⌝-*m*[*a* x x x]
	b rev. 1–3	^{munus}*la a-lit-ti ana šu-ri-i* / PÉŠ.GIŠ$^!$.GI *ta-ka-aṣ* / ŠÀ-*šú* BAD-*ma* ^{šim}ŠEŠ DIRI
79	a rev. 38	⌜*ina*⌝ ⌜*ṣil-lu*⌝ ⌜ḪÁD⌝.[A] SÚD ÀR Ì.UDU ḪI.ḪI *ana* ŠÀ.⌜TÙR⌝-[*šú* x x x x x]
	b rev. 4–5	*ina ṣil-lu* ḪÁD.A SÚD ÀR Ì.UDU ḪI.ḪI / *ana* ŠÀ.TÙR-*šú* GAR-*ma ir-ri*
80	a rev. 39	[DIŠ KI.MIN$^?$ ^{ú}*tar-m*]*uš ina* LÀL SÚD *ana* ŠÀ.TÙR-*š*[*ú* GAR-*an-ma* KI.MIN$^?$]
81	a rev. 40	[DIŠ KI.MIN$^?$ x x ^{ú}*tar-m*]*uš* Ú BABBAR 1/2 GÍN [x x x x x]
82	a rev. 41	[x x x x x x S]ÚD *ana* ŠÀ.TÙR-*šú* [GAR-*an* x x x x]
83	a rev. 42	[DIŠ KI.MIN$^?$ x x x x x ^{ši}]^{m}LI *u*$_5$-*r*[*a-nu*$^?$ x x x x x x]
84	a rev. 43	[...............]x *šá* GIŠ Ú 1-*e*[*n*$^?$ x x x x x x]

Probably nothing missing to the bottom of the tablet

Bound Transcription and Translation

1 [*šumma sinništu* ... ...] ...[... ...] 2–4 *only traces preserved*	1 [If a woman ... ...] ...[... ...] 2–4 *too fragmentary for translation*
5 DIŠ [KI.MIN(?) ... ...]... *ina šikari tašaqqīšu ana* ...[... ...]	5 Alt[ernatively(?), ...], you have her drink (it) in beer, [you ... (it)] into [... ...].
6 DIŠ K[I.MIN ... ...] ... [...] *ina šikari tašaqqīšu-ma* [... ...]	6 Alter[natively, ...], ... you have her drink (it) in beer and [...].
7 DIŠ KI.MIN *kamūnu* 10 *zēr kurkānâm malmališ ina lipî tuballal* [... ...]	7 Alternatively, you mix *kamūnu*-plant (and) ten seeds of *kurkānû*-plant in equal quantities with fat, [... ...].

8 *šumma sinništu lā irri ana šūrî kukra baluḫḫa ṭūr[a ... ...]* 9 *ina šīnāti amēlūti tušab[šal(?)] maššītu lā erīti ana šūrî*	8 If a woman does not get pregnant, to enable (her) to get pregnant: 9 you [boil(?)] 8 *kukru*-aromatic, *burāšu*-juniper, *baluḫḫu*-aromatic, *ṭūru*-aromatic, [...] 9 in human urine. A suppository (*maššītu*) to enable a woman who does not get pregnant to [get pregnant].
10 *šumma ana erīti kišpī lā ṭeḫê [...] karān šēlebi arqūssu tasâk it[ti šamni(?)] tapaššassu ib[alluṭ(?)]*	10 For the case that sorcery should not come near a pregnant woman: you crush [...] (and) fresh 'fox grape', you rub her (with it mixed) with [oil]. (Then) she will get [well].
11 *šumma sinništu ša k[annīšu ... ... k]amūnu šizba ša (m)u[sukk]ati ša zikara ūlid(u)* 12 *lā pat[ān išatti(?) u]šal[lam]*	11 If a woman's men[strual bandage ... ...], 12 [she shall drink(?)] 11 *kamūnu*-plant 12 on an empty stomach 11 (with) milk of an "impure woman" who has given birth to a male (child). 12 (Then) she will stay healthy/bring pregnancy to term.
13 *[šumma sinn]ištu* MIN(?) *ana dāmī[ša amāri(?) ... ... tas-k]arinna ša šadî labira tuba[llal ... ...]...* 14 *lu''ât-ma [... ...]... sinništu [dāmāša im]mar(?)*	13 [If a wom]an ditto(?), so that [she may see(?) her] blood(?): you mix(?), [... ... (and) old [box]wood from the mountains. [... ...], 14 she is defiled and [...]. ... The woman [will s]ee [her blood(?)].
15 DIŠ KI.MIN *zūz (šiqil) ...[...] ... ina šikari danni [išatti* K]I.MIN	15 Alternatively, [she drinks(?)] half a shekel of [...]-aromatic, [...] in strong beer, ditto (i.e. she will see her blood(?)).
16 DIŠ KI.MIN *anduḫallata [tub]bal taḫaššal tanappi ina kar[āni (...) išatti(?)* KI].MIN	16 Alternatively, you dry, crush (and) sift *anduḫallatu*-lizard, [she drinks(?)] (it) in (...) wi[ne, di]tto.
17 DIŠ KI.MIN *dišpa ḫīl [(...) tušabš]al*? *uḫūla qarnānâ ana libbi tanaddi [...]* MIN?	17 Alternatively, [boil] syrup (and) resin(?) [(of ...)]. You add horned alkali to it, [...], ditto.
18 DIŠ KI.MIN *pappāsu ša [buq]li*? *ina šikari tušabšal ana dām sinništi amāri(?) [da]miq*	18 Alternatively, you boil [mal]t porridge in urine. (This is) [go]od for seeing a woman's blood.
19 [DIŠ K]I.MIN *...[... ... qan]î kabri(?) rebūtu er[bu(?)] rebūtu ...[...]*	19 [Alt]ernatively, [...]-plant, [...] of a *thick* reed(?), a quarter of lo[cust(?)], a quarter of [...-arom]atic [...].
20 D[IŠ KI.MIN(?) ... ...] *tupâṣa ina šikari tarabbak [ina lubāri(?)] narbi tarakkas-ma i[na''e]š*	20 A[lternatively(?)], you crush [... ...], steep (it) in beer. You make a bandage (with the mixture spread) [on a] moist [rag(?)]. Then she will [get we]ll(?).
21 DIŠ KI.MIN *...[... ana] lipî tanaddi ina šīpāti talammi šamna baḫir taṭeppi*	21 Alternatively, you put [... into] fat, wrap (it) in wool. You apply (it) as a poultice with oil, while hot (steaming).
22 *šumma akal buq[lu(?) ... ...] ...-ma šīnāti ruḫuṣ*	22 If [*you are using*(?)] a tenth of a litre of ma[lt(?), ...]. Then wash (it) in urine.
23 *maššītu ša sinništi dāmš[u parsu(?) ... šiqil ṭā]btu šalāšat šiqil ...[...]... ina dām(?) kalīt alpi [...] tarâk*	23 A suppository for a woman whose blood [has stopped(?): ... shekels] of salt, three shekels of [...]-aromatic, [...] you smear/blend (it) in blood(?) from the kidney of an [...] ox.

24 DIŠ KI.MIN *<ištēn> šiqil ḫīl[i(?) ištēn šiqil] ṭūra ištēn šiqil murra ištēn šiqil …[… ištēn šiqil] dišpa peṣâ* 25 *ištēn šiqil tīyat[a t]asâk ina lipî kalīt alpi tarâk*	24 Alternatively 25 you crush 24 <one> shekel of re[sin(?), one shekel of] *ṭūru*-aromatic, one shekel of *murru*-aromatic, one shekel of […]-aromatic, [one shekel of] white honey, 25 (and) one shekel of *tīyatu*-plant. You smear/blend (it) in fat from the kidney of an ox.
26 *ištēn šiqil ṭūra ištēn šiq[il …] šīr iṣṣūri*(?) *šina šiqil dām erēni ištēn šiqil murra* 27 *ištēn šiqil ṭābta ina šam[an kalī] ti*(?) *tarâk allānu labku talappassu*(?)	27 You smear/blend 26 one shekel of *ṭūru*-aromatic, one shekel of […] bird meat(?), two shekels of cedar 'blood', one shekel of *murru*-aromatic, 27 (and) one shekel of salt with kidney fat. You *apply it*(?) as a soft acorn-shaped suppository.
28 *ana dām sinništi parāsi ištēn kakka eṣemti immeri ina išāti turrar* (var. adds: *tasâk*) *ḫaṣab pel lurmi* 29 *imbu' tâmti sīkti [gušūri labi]ri* (var. adds: *malmališ*) *ina itqi talammi ana šassūrīšu tašakkan-ma ša dām sinništi parāsi*	28 To stop a woman's blood: you desiccate (var. adds: (and) crush) one shaft(?) of the bone of a sheep over the fire. 29 You wrap (it) up in a wad of wool 28 (with) (var. adds: an equal amount of) ostrich eggshell, 29 *imbu' tâmti*-mineral, (and) powder [of an] old [log]. You insert (it) into her womb (viz. vagina). (It is) for stopping a woman's blood.
30 DIŠ KI.MIN *murra labanātu errê*(?) *ḫaṣba šaḫarra ša pī utūni tamarraq [ina] šamni tuballal* KI.MIN	30 Alternatively, you crush finely *murru*-aromatic, frankincense, colocynth(?), (and) a porous sherd from the opening of an oven. You mix (it) with oil, ditto (i.e. you insert it into her womb).
31 *ana dām sinništi parāsi gūdu ina išāti [tub]bal temessi qēm ḫarūbi šurmēni tuballal* KI.MIN	31 To stop a woman's blood: you dry *gūdu*-plant(?) over a fire. You wash (and) mix (it) with carob flour and *šurmēnu*-cypress, ditto (i.e. you insert it into her womb).
32 DIŠ KI.MIN *ṭābta emmeta*(?) *tel[eqqe*(?) …] *napṭa tuballal* KI.MIN	32 Alternatively, you take hot(?) salt, mix it with [… (and)] naphtha, ditto (i.e. you insert it into her womb).
33 [DIŠ K]I.MIN *maštakal adi zērīšu ina nāri temessi ina itqi*(?) [*talammi*(?)]	33 [Alter]natively, you wash *maštakal*-soapwort with its seed in river (water), [you wrap(?) (it)] in a wad of wool(?).
34 [DIŠ KI.M]IN *šunḫu tubbal ina išāti tubbal temessi [te]ṭeppi*	34 [Altern]atively, you dry *šunḫu*-plant, desiccate it over a fire. You wash (it) (and) apply (it) as a poultice.
35 DIŠ KI.MIN *nagab ṭīpī gūdu [te]ṭeppi*	35 Alternatively, [you] apply *gūdu*-plant(?) with all(?) poultices.
36 DIŠ KI.MIN *šupālīta tazarru [te]ṭeppi*	36 Alternatively, you sprinkle an undergarment (with oil?), (and) apply as a poultice.
37 DIŠ KI.MIN *gabû ḫaṣab sūq erbetti takpītu aḫussu mala erištīšunu* 38 *šadânu ṣābitu ina dām erēni tuballal ina itqi talammi ina sun-*BAR*-ša tašakkan kannu* 39 *ana parāsi u sekērši nadû damiq* 40 DIŠ KI.MIN *ḫaṣab uqnê ša tiqnu qit-ma*(?) … NU.LUḪ *teleqqe tušabšal*(?) *lū ina it[qi lū] (ina)* 41 *kitê talammī-ma*(?) *šanû*(?) *<ina> lē'i [šaṭer*(?)]	37 Alternatively, 38 you mix 37 alum, a potsherd from a crossroads, a *takpītu*-pearl(?), *aḫussu*-mineral (soda ash), as much as you wish of them, 38 (and) magnetic haematite with cedar 'blood'. You wrap (this) in a wad of wool, you place (it) on her *loincloth*. (This) bandage (*kannu*) 39 is good (when) applied for stopping (the blood) and for damming her up. 40 Alternatively, you take a small piece(?) of lapis lazuli used as a jewellery ornament(?), *qitmu*-paste(?), …-plant (and) NU.LUḪ-plant. You boil(?) (these ingredients and then) wrap (them) in a wad of wool [or] 41 (in) linen. A variant(?), [copied(?)] (from) a wooden writing board(?).

42 *šumma sinništu* NI.NE *kīs šīnāti marṣat dāmūša ana* ... [...] 43 *šakin sinništu šī* NI.NE *marṣat diqmēn urbati* (var. *ištēn qa diqmēn ṣarbati*) *diqmēn ṣarbati* (var. *ištēn qa diqmēn amḫara tuballal*) 14 *riksī ša lubāri tarakkas* [(var.) *ištēnâ ana šassūrīša tašakkan*]	42 If a woman suffers from NI.NE (and) 'binding of the urine', (and) her blood [...] into/for [...] (and) 43 there is 42 [...], 43 this woman suffers from NI.NE-disease. You tie ashes of *urbatu*-rush, ashes of poplar (var. you mix one litre ashes of poplar (and) one litre of *amḫara*-plant) (into) fourteen knots of cloth. [(var.) You insert (them) one by one into her womb (i.e. vagina)].
44 DIŠ KI.MIN *šamma peṣâ ina karāni ṣaḫti išatti* [...]	44 Alternatively, she drinks 'white drug' in grape juice [...].
45 DIŠ KI.MIN *murra ina šamni tasâk* (var. *taḫaššal ina šamni t*[*aballal*$^{?}$]) *ina uppi siparri ana muštinnīšu* (var. *ina šassūrīša*) *tatabbak* (var. *itabbak*)	45 Alternatively, you pound *murru*-aromatic (var. adds: mix (it)) with oil. You pour (var. one pours) (it) into her urethra (var. her womb) with a bronze tube.
46 *šalmiš bīt šīnāti ikabba*[*s*]	46 She will be able to step into the 'house of urine' (i.e. the lavatory) in safety.
47 *šumma sinništu nadî ṣabāt*(?) *šīnāti marṣat imbu' tâmti ina itqi talammi ana šassūrīšu tašakkan*	47 If a woman suffers from (uncontrollable) discharging (and) 'seizing' of urine, you wrap *imbu' tâmti*-mineral in a wad of wool, insert it in her womb (viz. vagina).
48 *šumma sinništu ina ṣallūtīšu šīnātīšu ina eršīšu ištin libbi šīnāti mādāti ūr*<*šu*>(?) 49 *ikkalšū-ma sinništu šī šīnāti šītātu ipaššar*(?) [*iballuṭ*$^{?}$]	48 If during her sleep a woman urinates in her bed, (and) during (the urination of) large amounts of urine (her) crotch(?) 49 hurts her, this woman releases(?) *escaping* urine. [She will get well (again)$^{?}$].
50 *šumma sinništu lū ša arḫi lū ša sitta arḫī lū ša šalāšat arḫī ša liblibbīša* (var. *ša libbīša*) *ittanaddâ ḫ*[*ulâ tubbal tasâk teṭên*] 51 *ana libbi mê šalāšīšu ana libbi šamni šalāšīšu taballal annuḫara ana libbi tanaddi tašaqqīšu-ma* 52 *ša liblibbīša* (var. *ša libbīša*) *ul ittanaddâ*	50 If a woman, (being) either one month or two months or three months (pregnant) keeps having a miscarriage (lit. keeps aborting her foetus), you dry a *ḫulû*-rodent, crush it, grind it up, 51 you mix (it) three times with water, (and) three times with oil. You add *alluḫaru*-mineral. You have her drink (it). Then 52 she will not have miscarriages (anymore).
53 *šumma sinništu ša šalāšat arḫī dāmšu illak ana ša libbīša* [*lā nadê* ... ...] *qaran litti* 54 *takpītu* 14 *uṭṭat nikiptu lipî errî* [... ...] ... 55 *riqqī kalāma ina dīdī kitê tašakkan* ...[... ...]	53 If (in) a woman three months (pregnant) her blood flows, so that [she does not have] a miscarriage: [...], cow's horn(?), 54 a *takpītu*-pearl(?), fourteen grains of *nikiptu*-aromatic, pith of *errû*-colocynth, [... ...] — 55 all (these) *drugs* you put into a linen *dīdū*-cloth (a piece of underwear worn by women), [... ...].
56 *šumma sinništu ipparraḫ šadānû ṣābitu ina šamni* [... ...]	56 If a woman *is torn*(?), [you ...] magnetic haematite in oil, [... ...].
57 *šumma erītu mû illakū* ...[... ... *ina* ... *talam*]*mi ana šassūrīšu tašakkan*	57 If a pregnant woman's (amniotic) fluid flows, ...[... you wr]ap [in ...], you insert it into her womb (viz. vagina).
58 DIŠ KI.MIN *šakirâ ina šamni* [*tas*]*âk ina* [*itqi talammi ana šassū*]*rīšu tašakkan*	58 Alternatively, you pound *šakirû*-plant in oil, [wrap] (it) in a w[ad of wool], insert (it) [into her womb (viz. vagina)].

59 *šumma erītu ... ša ridû[t irrī iraššû(?) ...] puqutti nuḫurti* 60 *ina šikari tasâk ina kakkabi tušbāt ina šēri [lā patān(?)] tašaqqīšu*	59 If a pregnant woman(?) ... [gets] diarrhoea(?), 60 you crush 59 [...] of *puquttu* (and) *nuḫurtu*-plant 60 in beer, you let (it) stand outside overnight under the star(s). In the morning, you have her drink (it) [on an empty stomach(?)].
61 *šumma erītu dāmū ūmakkal illakū umākkal l[ā illakū u š]īršu aruq ana bulluṭīšu* 62 *kamūna tasâk ina šamni pān libbīšu tapaššaš*	61 If a pregnant woman's blood flows for one day, (but) does [not flow] the (next) day [and her bo]dy is yellow, in order to cure her: 62 you pound *kamūnu*-plant (cumin), you rub the surface of her belly (with it mixed) with oil.
63 *ištēn šiqil tarmuš tamarraq ...[... ...] ina libbi tuballal maššītu ša erî(?)*	63 You crush finely one shekel of *tarmuš*-plant, ...[...] you mix with it. A suppository for getting pregnant(?).
64 *šumma sinništu zu'ssu lā ṭābat diqmēn ...[... ...] tubal[lal t]ukaṣṣ[â]* 65 *buqli sābî napīti [... ...] lišān k[albi(?) mala] ibbaššû(?)* 66 *[...]... [... ...]... tapaššassu*	64 If a woman's sweat (smells) unpleasant: you mix ashes of [...]-plant, [...]. You let (it) cool down. 65 Sifted malt from the innkeeper [...], [dog's] tongue-plant(?), [as much as] is available(?) (of these ingredients?), 66 [...] ...[... ...], you rub her (with it).
67 *šumma sinništu šipir sinnišāti l[ā ippuš(?)] ... [... eṣem]ti immeri [t]urrar tasâk* 68 *ina lubāri tarakkas [... ...] ana šassūrī[šu] tašakkan-ma ina''eš*	67 If a woman does no[t do] the 'work of women' (i.e. does not (desire to) have intercourse), you dry out (and) crush [... (and)] a sheep bone. 68 You bind it in (a piece of) cloth, [(...)], you insert it into [her] womb (viz. vagina), and she will improve.
69 *šumma sinništu šipir sinnišāti [lā ippuš ši]birti(?) itqa talammi [ana ša]ssūrīšu tašakkan*	69 If a woman [does not do] the 'work of women', you wrap a *lump* (of malt?) with a wad of wool, you insert (it) [into] her womb (viz. vagina).
70 *ana maštakti sinništi [lā e]rî(?)* (var. *[maštakti sinništi kī irrû u kī lā irrû(?)]*) *ištēn šiqil tarmuš zūz šamma peṣâ ištēn šiqil* (var. *rebūtu*) *gabû* (var. *[miṣrāya]* 71 *ina itqi talammi [ana šass]ūrīša tašakkan-ma kal ūmi* (var. *mūšu gabbi*) *ukâl ušellâm-ma* 72 *ina mê* (var. *[ina kar]āni(?) peṣî*) *temessi šumma* (var. *kī*) *itqu [arqat]* (var. *sāmat lū dāma ulluḫatu*) *sinništu šī ul irri* (var. *sinništu šī irri*) 73 *šumma itqu sāmat [lū dāma ul]luḫat u šassūršu peṣât-ma [sinn]ištu šī irri* (var. *kī itqu arqat sinništu šī ul irri*)	70 For a test (to determine) a woman (who will) [not] [con]ceive(?) (var. [A test whether a woman will conceive or not conceive(?)]: 71 you wrap 70 one shekel of *tarmuš*-plant, half a shekel 'white drug', and a shekel (var. a fourth of a shekel) of (var. adds [Egyptian]) alum 71 in a wad of wool. You insert it [into her womb (viz. vagina)]. She keeps it there all day long (var. all night long). (Then) she removes (it) and 72 you wash (it) with water (var. with white [wi]ne?). If the wad is [yellow-green, that woman will not con]ceive. 73 If the wad is red [or strea]ked [with blood] and her womb is white/shiny(?), [that wom]an will conceive (ms. c: If that wad is red or streaked with blood, that woman will conceive. If the wad is yellow-green, that woman will not conceive).
74 *šumma sinništu lā irri ana šūrî erbet šammī erbet akal kukru zūz (šiqil) burāšu* 75 *ištēn šiqil šambaliltu ištēn šiqil šamaššammū bu''ušūtu* 76 *ištēn šiqil šiqittu [...] ina ḫulibi ša bāb danni tuballal allāna teppuš* 77 *ana šassūrīšu tašakkan-ma ipettē-ma irri u mê ittanaddī-ma*	74 If a woman does not get pregnant, to enable (her) to get pregnant: you mix four(sic!) drugs: four tenths of a litre(?) of *kukru*-aromatic, half a shekel of *burāšu*-juniper, 75 one shekel of fenugreek, one shekel of smelly sesame, 76 one shekel of [...] almonds with fatty material from the opening of a *dannu*-vat. You make an acorn-shaped suppository. 77 You insert (it) into her womb (viz. vagina). She will open up and become pregnant and she will repeatedly discharge (her) fluids.

78 *lā ālitta ana šūrî ušumma takâṣ libbašu tepettē-ma murra tumalla* 79 *ina ṣilli tubbal tasâk teṭên ina lipî tuballal ana šassūrīšu tašakkan-ma irri*	78 To enable a barren woman to get pregnant: you flay an *ušummu*-dormouse, open its interior, fill it with *murru*-aromatic. 79 You dry it in the shade, crush, grind (it). You mix (it) with tallow. You insert it into her womb (viz. vagina). Then she will get pregnant.
80 [DIŠ KI.MIN$^{?}$ *tarm*]*uš ina dišpi tasâk ana šassūrīš*[*u tašakkan-ma* KI.MIN(?)]	80 [Alternatively (?)], you pound [*tarm*]*uš*-plant with syrup, [you insert (it)] into her womb (viz. vagina). [Then ditto(?) (i.e., she will get pregnant)].
81 [DIŠ KI.MIN(?) ... *tarm*]*uš šammu peṣû zūz* (*šiqil*) [... ...] 82 [... ...] *tasâk ana šassūrīšu* [*tašakkan* ... ...]	81 [Alternatively (?)], 82 you pound 81 [..., *tarm*]*uš*-plant, 'white drug', half a shekel of [...], 82 [... ...], [you insert (it)] into her womb (viz. vagina), [... ...].
83 [DIŠ KI.MIN(?) ... ...] *burāšu ur*[*ânu*(?) ... ...] 84 [... ...] *ša iṣi šammu ištēn*(?) [... ...]	83 [Alternatively (?), ...] *burāšu*-juniper, *ur*[*ânu*-plant(?), ...], 84 [... ...] of wood(?), one(?) drug(?) [... ...].

Probably nothing missing to the bottom of the tablet

Notes

Line 7: The *kurkānû*-plant is recommended in other texts to promote female fertility, see e.g., N. 4001 obv. 15 // BM 51246+ obv. 11 (see *infra* texts A.2.7, B.2.1).

Lines 8–9: Alternatively in line 9, read KÀŠ K[ÚM ḪI.ḪI] "[you mix] with h[ot] urine". Note also BM 59710 obv. 6 (text B.2.5) for another prescription promoting conception that uses urine as a fluid ingredient. For the label *maššītu* (*ša*) *lā erīti ana šūrî* "suppository to enable a woman who is not pregnant to get pregnant" concluding a prescription, see also BM 38624+ line 4' (with a different recipe). For prescriptions promoting conception bearing a parallel purpose label as in ms. a lines 8–9, see also BAM 250 rev. 2–3; STT 98 obv. 2', 4'; BM 59710 obv. 1; BM 79061 obv. 1–2. See also below ms. a line 74 and duplicate.

Line 10: A similar, but more complex version of this prescription can be found in BM 42327+ obv. 1–4 // BM 51246+ obv. 1–3 // SpTU 3, No. 84 rev. 3–4 (see *infra* texts C.3.3, C.3.4). In the latter texts, dried "fox grape-plant" (*karān šēlebi*) is listed among other ingredients, while in ms. a, it is applied as a simple and used fresh. The latter manuscripts introduce the recipe with the clause *ana* ^{munus}PEŠ$_{4}$ UŠ$_{11}$.ZU NU TE-*ma ša* ŠÀ-*šá* NU ŠUB-*e* (var. *na*$^{!}$*-de-e*) "so that witchcraft not come near a pregnant woman and she not [have] a miscarriage". In this light, the first sign BE (usually understood as *šumma* "if") in ms. a seems superfluous. It remains unclear whether there was enough room in ms. a for restoring *šà* ŠÀ-*šà* NU ŠUB in the gap, according to the parallel from the other texts.

Lines 11–12: The sign KÚR inscribed on the left margin of the tablet, before the first sign of line 11, probably marks a scribal error of some kind. J. Fincke (2021, 61–68) gives a recent overview of KÚR and other similar correction marks made, as she surmises, by a collator or proof-reader, after the scribe had written the text. The correction marks highlight lines which contain mistakes, and Mesopotamian scribes usually position them on the margin or transitional area towards the left edge of the tablet. Beside the sign KÚR, the signs NU, AŠ, TAB, MIN and MAN are encountered as correction marks as well. W. G. Lambert (1982, 216) first recognized the use of the sign KÚR as a corrector's mark and suggested possible Akkadian equivalents could be *aḫû/aḫītu* "strange, abnormal" or an adjective derived from *nakāru* that stands for "strange, foreign" (see also Borger 2004, MZL, 264); the sign probably simply means "wrong" or "mistake" (George 2013, CUSAS 18, 107a; Fincke 2021, 64b). It remains unclear what specific textual error the KÚR mark signalled in line 11, because so much of the line is lost. For other examples of KÚR or similar signs as correction marks, see e.g., Cooper 1988, *FS Sachs*, 90; Maul 1994, *Zukunftsbewältigung*, 440 n. 13; Wiggermann 1992, *Mesopotamian Protective Spirits*, 129–130. Within the women's healthcare texts, see also LKA 9 rev. r. col. 13' for another instance of KÚR as a correction mark (see Abusch et al. 2020, Text 5.3 = text C.3.5 in the present volume).

The introductory label in line 11 is unfortunately incomplete, hampering the identification of the exact purpose of the prescription. The word *kannu* "textile band; menstrual bandage" is attested in similar contexts, in BM 79061 obv. 9–10, which speaks of the blood on a woman's menstrual bandage being "little and black". The text AO 6374 line 40 (text C.3.9), features an expression that may perhaps best suit lines 11–12 in ms. a. The former Late Babylonian text speaks of "the day for her (menstrual) bandage was late" (*u_4-mu šá ka_4-ni-šú* DIB-*iq-šú*), probably referring to the moment when a woman became aware that she had missed her menstrual period, as the first sign of a pregnancy (see *infra* for discussion). Incidentally, LKA 9 rev. r. col. 13' (text C.3.5) also uses the word *kannu* in a treatment to protect a pregnant woman from miscarriage caused by witchcraft, and the verb *ušallam* "she will stay healthy/bring (her pregnancy) to term" in ms. a line 12 points in a similar direction, i.e. that the prescription dealt with irregular bleeding during pregnancy. In LKA 9, *kannu* refers to a textile band or red wool which is tied on the woman's genitalia. A similar usage of a *kannu*-bandage is encountered in ms. a line 38 below. For *kannu*, see further Wasserman 2019, 1133, 1138.

On *musukkatu* (also *usukkatu*) "impure woman", referring to a ritually unclean woman during the postpartum period when she had just given birth, see e.g., Stol 2016, 439–440; Feder 2016, 112ff. Interestingly, milk of a *musukkatu* is often used as a potent medical ingredient, for example in prescriptions for eye ailments (e.g. Geller and Panayotov 2020, 66 (IGI 1 37'), 69–70 (IGI I 47'), 141–142 (IGI 2 148', 155'), 148 (IGI 2 205'), 163–164 (IGI 3 39'), 195 (line 5'). In a few prescriptions, milk of a *musukkatu* who has given birth to a male is recommended, see e.g., CTN 4, No. 72 i 6'–7' (Stadhouders 2011, *JMC* 18, 40, prescription against epilepsy): KI$^{!}$ GA$^{!}$ ^{munus}<Ú>.ZÚG-*ti šá ma-*[*ra*] Ù.TU ḪI.ḪI "you mix (the ingredients) with milk(!) of an impure woman who has given birth to a male child". Note further BAM 476: 11': KÀŠ ^{munus}Ú.ZÚG *šá* NITA Ù.TU "urine of an impure woman who has given birth to a male (child)". For discussion of the evidence and parallels in Egyptian medical papyri, see also Pommerening 2015; Steinert 2023, 278–280.

Lines 13–14: At the end of line 13, restore perhaps [^{munus}PEŠ$_4$ *šá* MÚD-*šú* IGI]-*ú*$^{?}$ "[A pregnant woman who sees her blood(?)], (is impure)"? For the association of pregnant women suffering from haemorrhage with ritual impurity, see also KAR 423 i 15 (omen apodosis): "If blood drips on the *isru* on the right and left, a woman who suffers from *nahšātu* (haemorrhage) will perform/has performed an impure offering" (*šumma*(BE) *ina isri imitta*(15) *u šumēla*(150) *damu*(MÚD) *usalliḫ* / *sinništu*(MUNUS) *ša nahšātu marṣat*(GIG-*at*) *nīqa*(SISKUR) *lu"â ireddi/irdi*(UŠ)). The text is a Neo-Assyrian excerpt from the *Bārûtu*-series, see Heeßel 2012: 35, 43, 53 comments to col. i 8–15. For the feminine stative *lu"ât* "she is impure" (from *lu"û* "to defile"), referring to a woman during childbirth (a notion that is presumably also linked to the loss of blood during delivery), see also the commentary 11N-T3 lines 2–3 (see text G.1).

Following the sign *ú* at the end of line 13, it almost looks as if a damaged smaller KÚR-sign was inscribed. However, it is hard to decide whether these traces are merely scratches or remnants of an inscribed correction mark, since Mesopotamian scribed usually position correction marks before and not at the end or after the corrected line in question, i.e. they are usually to be found on the left margin of a tablet's obverse or reverse (see Fincke 2021, 61–62, 63–65).

Line 16: For *anduḫallatu*, a kind of lizard, see AHw 50b; CAD A/2, 114 (for an attestation in a medical prescription, see e.g., in BAM 77: 37 boiled in a potion). Cf. Landsberger, *Fauna* 117. Lizards (especially "wall lizard", EME.DIR IZ.ZI) also occur in recipes to induce abortion and to ease difficult delivery (see BAM 246: 2, 8 (text B.1.6); BAM 249 obv.$^{?}$ i' 11' (text D.1.3); for discussion, cf. Böck 2013, 37–38). The similarity in the choice of this type of ingredient in the present passage may be due to a similar use or intended purpose here, perhaps to induce bleeding (i.e. to expel something from the body?).

Line 17: The reading of line 17 is tentative. The signs *ḫi-li* may stand for the word *ḫīlu* "resin", followed by a plant name in the gap. However, if the word continued in the gap, a possible reconstruction may be *ḫi-li-*[*mu*] (*ḫilimmu, ḫilammu*), a type of locust (CAD Ḫ, 184, equated with *ergilu*-locust). The plant name *ḫilabānu* "milkweed" (from Aramaic, equated with and corresponding to *šizbānu*) may be a further option, cf. CAD Ḫ, 184a; AHw 345a.

Line 18: For malt porridge (*pappas buqli*), see CAD P, 112 sub 1d. It is used, for example, as an ingredient in poultices wrapped around the head, against throbbing, painful temples (BAM 482 ii 25, 27 // BAM 3 iii 29 (Attia and Buisson 2003, 6; Scurlock 2006, No. 73, 78); see also BAM 6: 5 (Scurlock 2006, No. 94)).

Line 19: A thick reed (*qanû kabbaru*, written logographically GI.NÍG.GAL.GAL.LA; cf. Hh. VIII 82) is also encountered in the context of treatments to speed up delivery, see BAM 248 iii 48, 52 (*infra* text D.1.1). In line 19, probably a specific part of a reed was used (cf. CAD Q, 88a sub 1d for different parts of reed mentioned in medical-therapeutic texts).

For locusts in women's healthcare texts, see e.g. BM 51246+ // (text A.2.7) lines 12 (prescription to promote fertility), 24', 26' (contraceptives). The fraction "one quarter" appears without a measurement in line 19, but probably the amounts given refer to fractions of a shekel.

Line 20: The word *narbu* "soft" or "moist" (cf. CAD N/1, 350) is attested in other medical texts as an attribute to *lubāru* "cloth", as the material for bandages, see e.g. AMT 74 ii 35' (= ii 71): TÚG *nar-ba* Ì SUD "you sprinkle a moist cloth with oil" (Eypper 2016, *JMC* 27, 34–35 used as bandaging material).

Line 21: For the variant *taṭeppi* instead of *teṭeppi/tuṭeppi* "you apply as a poultice", see also BAM 513 ii 5' (Geller and Panayotov 2020, 71 ms. NB) and BAM 159 iv 21, quoted in CAD Ṭ, 101 s.v. *ṭepû* sub 1c. Instead of the stative form *baḫir* in line 21, the adjective/adverb *baḫ-ru* or *baḫ-ra* "steaming hot" would be expected. Otherwise, a phrase *lū baḫir* "it should be hot/while it is hot" is attested in prescriptions, cf. CAD B, 29 s.v. *baḫru* sub a. For *buḫḫuru* "to steam", see also Stol 2000b, *BiOr* 57, 627 with further references.

Line 22: This fragmentary line is a sort of comment or note perhaps explaining procedural details, with the unusual occurrence of an imperative form *ruḫuṣ* "soak/bathe!" rather than a present tense form. Note also that usually, the liquid with which someone (e.g. the patient) or something is bathed is constructed with *ina* rather than with a direct object as is done in line 22, cf. CAD R, s.v. *raḫāṣu* sub 1a.

Lines 23, 25, 27: The form *ta-ra-ku* is regarded as a form of *râku* "to smear; to knead(?)", see CAD R, 110–111 sub a. It is a recurring feature of ms. a to spell forms of middle weak verbs with an overhanging vowel. See also line 25 *ta-sa-ku* for *tasâk*, line 78 *ta-ka-ṣi* in ms. a vs. *ta-ka-aṣ* in ms. b.

Lines 26–27: For *labku* "soft" or "moist, fresh", cf. CAD L, 33–34 (*labku* is found as synonym to *narbu* "moist" in lexical texts). In connection with *allānu labku* "moist acorn-shaped suppository" in line 27, compare the expression (*māššītu*) *ša lubbuki* "(suppository) for absorbing", found in the context of prescriptions for stopping female bleeding. See e.g. SpTU 4, No. 153 obv. 2 (text C.1.10); BM 38624+ line 10' (text A.2.1) and the *Introduction* for discussion.

The verb form TAG-*šú* at the end of line 27 is irregular if one assumes a form of the Akkadian verb *lapātu* as underlying the logogram. One rather expects TAG-*su* (= *talappassu*) instead. The verb *lapātu* means "to touch", and in medical prescriptions, "to smear on". In the present instance referring to the application of a suppository (*allānu*), these meanings seem to be excluded. Perhaps, the intended meaning is "to prepare" or "to apply". An alternative reading *šum-šú* "(is) its name" instead of TAG-*šú* does not appear as very likely.

Lines 28–29: Similar ingredients as in lines 28–29 are also encountered in SpTU 4, No. 153 obv. 11–12 (text C.1.10), likewise in a treatment to stop bleeding.

The word *kakku* "weapon" is used here in a special meaning. In exceptional cases, *kakku* can refer to the shaft of a tool, the barb of a fish or the thorn of a plant (cf. CAD K, 56 s.v. *kakku* sub 4). Note that GAG/KAK stands for *eṣemtu* "bone" in MSL 14, 268: 6'. This word is not found in the parallel manuscripts d and e, as far as preserved.

Line 30: For *labanātu* "frankincense", cf. CAD L, 8; AHw 522a; Finkel 2000, 153–154, Text 3 line 1: 3 GÍN ^{šim}*la-ban-na-tu*$_4$. The word is probably a loan from Aramaic (cf. also Greek *libanos* "frankincense"), see Jursa 2009, *FS Sima*, 162.

Presumably, the sequence *ir-ri-ir* in line 30 is a mistake for *ir-re-e* (*irrû/errû*) "wild melon" (for this identification of *irrû*, against the translation "colocynth" proposed in the dictionaries, see Stol 1987b, *BSA* 3, 84; Powell 2003–2005, "Obst und Gemüse A.1", *RlA* 10, 20 §4.2). Compare further *erēru* "to be parched(?)" and *erru* "parched" (AHw 238b, 244a; CAD E, 280, 307b translate the latter with "(to be) mouldy"). However, the latter terms do not appear to fit the present passage, in terms of form, meaning and context.

The ingredient "porous potsherd from the opening of an oven" is found several times in prescriptions to stop bleeding, see also SpTU 4, No. 153 obv. 14 (*infra* text C.1.10).

Line 31: The reading ^{ú}*gu-ú-du* here and in line 35 below follows H. Stadhouders' (*NABU* 2018/3, 126–127 no. 81) interpretation of the same ingredient/sign sequence in another Late Babylonian medical text (BM 59626 obv. 4), which Stadhouders interprets as "bottle-gourd(?)". Note, however, that in the only other attestation of the word *gūdu* (likewise from Late Babylonian times), the term is preceded by the classifier kuš "leather" and refers to a "waterskin, flask" (cf. CAD G, 120). The word stems from Aramaic *gūdā'* (also *gūd*), which also means "leather bottle/bag", but does not refer to a plant (Sokoloff 2002, *A Dictionary of Jewish Babylonian Aramaic*, 266; Jastrow 1903, *A Dictionary of the Targumim*, 218). In this light, one could suggest an alternative reading of the sign sequence in question, namely *ú-qù šam-ṭù*. The former term could be linked to an unknown drug *ḫūqu/ūqu* explained in Uruanna as "green frog" (Ú *ḫu-qu* : AŠ BIL.ZA.ZA SIG_7, cited in CAD Ḫ, s.v. *hūqu* D, see KADP 2 iv 8'). The word *šamṭu* (*samṭu*) is attested as a foreign (probably Egyptian) name for acacia (CAD Š/1, 339 s.v. *šamṭu*, drawing a link to Egyptian *šndt*, Arabic *š/sanṭ*, Hebrew *šiṭṭā* "acacia"). Uruanna I 182 explains *šamṭu* as the name for the *ašāgu*-plant (a thorny shrub), in the language of the land Meluḫḫa (which refers to Egypt in first millennium BCE cuneiform texts), presumably referring to *Acacia nilotica*. Thompson (1949, DAB, 184, 338) identifies both the "resin of the *ašāgu*-plant" (*ḫīl ašāgi*) and the *š/samṭu*-plant with "gum Arabic".

It may seem unusual that the ingredients are first dried over the fire and then washed (i.e. moistened again), but the same order of instructions is found again in line 34 below. In line 31, the medicament is applied as a suppository, in line 34 as a poultice.

For *ḫarūbu* "carob", see Borger 2001, *Zeitschrift für Althebraistik* 14, 1–19; Böck, Ghazanfar and Nesbitt 2023, 100–104 (identifying *ḫarūbu* with the fruit pod of "false carob").

Line 34: The ingredient *šunḫu*, a bulbous plant, is also used in BAM 240: 48, but for a vaginal suppository (*infra* text D.2.1).

Line 36: The term ^{túg}KI.TA corresponds to Akkadian *šupālītu* which refers to a shirt- or tunic-like "undergarment", cf. CAD Š/1, 314a–b; AHw 1287b s.v. *šupālû* sub 3; Wasserman 2019, *FS Charpin*, 1136–1137.

Line 37: Because of its logogram ^{na4}ÉLLAG-tu_4 (Sumerian ÉLLAG means "kidney"), the Akkadian word *takpītu* (also *tukpītu*) has been interpreted as a kidney-shaped stone (bead), see CAD T, 459; AHw 1308; Beaulieu 1999, *RA* 93, 154–155; SAD, Vol. 2, 56. However, the Akkadian term *takpītu* derives from *takāpu* "to be covered with spots, dots" and may refer to the typical coloration associated with the *takpītu*-stone. Stol (2021, *BiOr* 78, 448b) suggests the translation "pearl". The term is also attested in a test to determine a woman's fertility in UET 7, No. 123 (line 9), where the coloration of the substance wrapped into a tampon looks "multicoloured like a *takpītu*-stone (bead)" (GIN_7 ⸢ÉLLAG⸣ *ibtarrum*)–after it had been inserted into the woman's vagina–signals her fertility (see text B.2.2). The word probably occurs once more in line 54 of ms. a, where it is spelled syllabically (*ták-pít*) and is used as an ingredient in a prescription to stop bleeding during pregnancy and prevent miscarriage (see the note below). In line 37, it is written logographically ^{na4}ÉLLAG-tu_4. In textual attestations, *takpītu* is often followed by a stone name (e.g., a *takpītu*-bead of *pappardilû*-stone), but this is not the case in the present text, which may signal that *takpītu* was regarded as a particular mineral rather than any stone bead of a particular shape or colour.

The word *aḫussu* is now recognized as a variant form of *uḫultu*, a soda-plant and the ash (alkaline mineral) produced from it, used in the production of glass and as a drug (CAD U/W, 48; AHw 23a, 1404b), The word is sometimes written with a classifier for minerals (e.g., KADP 27 rev. 18; KADP 36 iii 36 $^{(na4)}$*a-ḫu-su*). This mineral has to be distinguished from *aḫuššu* (*a'uššu, amuššu*), designating a bulbous plant (cf. AHw 89a; CAD A/2, 95b).

For the expression *mala erišti* "as much as desired", see also UET 7, No. 123 rev. 8'–9' (text B.2.2): *ma-la* $BURU_{14}$-*tú ta-máṣ-ṣi* "you may use as much as you wish"; cf. STT 96: 13 *mál-li-riš* (sandhi-writing for *mala lirīšu*) "as much as one should wish" (Scurlock 2014a, 493, 534 n. 8). The word *erištu* is more often written with the sign KAM (with phonetic complement), as in ms. a.

Line 38: The sign sequence *ina* BAD.BAR-*šá* GAR in line 38 appears to replace more common expressions such as *ana šassūrīša/ūrīša tašakkan* (*ana* ŠÀ.TÙR-*šá*/GAL_4.LA-*šá* GAR) "you insert it into her womb/vagina". However, the body part hiding behind the signs BAD BAR has been difficult to elucidate. To my knowledge, there is no logogram BAD.BAR standing for a body part. The sign BAD can be read as the syllable *sun*, which may be interpreted as *sūnu* "lap, crotch, genitals", or as *sūnu* "loincloth", i.e. a piece of clothing worn around the genitals (see CAD S, 386–390 s.v. *sūnu* A and B). The following word *kannu* "(menstrual) bandage" at the end of line 38 indicates that the treatment was not inserted as a tampon (as is usually the case with ingredients wrapped in a wad of wool) but applied to the outside of the patient's body. Presumably, the wad was placed on the genitals in the typical manner of a menstrual bandage. In fact, the word *sūnu* B is equated lexically with *ulāpu* "(menstrual) rag, bandage" (see Wasserman 2019, *FS Charpin*, 1133, 1135, for discussion). However, *sun*-BAR most likely represents one Akkadian word. It may be a learned writing for *sunābu* (*sunāpu*) "loincloth", which rarely occurs in lexical texts among terms for menstrual bandages (CAD S, 383).

Lines 38–39: The label *kannu ana parāsi u sekērši nadû*(ŠUB-*ú*) *damiq*(SIG_5) "(this) bandage is good (when) applied for stopping (the blood) and for damming her up" is unusual. The verb *parāsu* "to stop" is normally construed with *dāmu* "blood" as an object in similar formulations, but here it is found adjacent to *sekēru* "to dam up, to block" (often said of water courses and body parts). The latter is attested with reference to (postpartum) blood that is "locked" in the womb, as well as in reference to the infertile womb (which does not receive the male semen), see e.g. BAM 240: 40; BAM 244: 41, 49 (*infra* texts D.2.1, B.1.1), and CAD S, s.v. *sekēru* A sub 2 and 5b.

The prescription in lines 37–38 can be compared with a passage in a treatment to protect a pregnant woman from miscarriage in LKA 9 rev. r. col. 13'–14' (text C.3.5), where the patient is to tie a *kannu*-band of red wool, presumably around her crotch. As Abusch et al. (2020, CMAwR 3, 59 note on lines 13'–14') observe, the red *kannu*-band worn like a menstrual cloth can be regarded as a symbolic barrier intended to prevent bleeding or miscarriage of the foetus. The same logic seems to be at work in the present prescription as well.

Line 40: The Akkadian reading of the plant ${}^{\text{ú}}$NU.LUḪ is uncertain (Luukko and van Buylaere 2020, 89b). Thompson (1949, DAB, 357–359) identified the logogram NU.LUḪ with *tīyatu* and ${}^{\text{ú}}$NU.LUḪ.ḪA with *nuḫurtu*-plant and proposed both refer to kinds of asafoetida. For discussion see further van Soldt 1990, *UF* 22, 348–349; Stol (forthcoming), in: *PIHANS* 136, 313–330.

SAḪAR.GI$_6$ seems to be an abbreviation for ${}^{\text{(im)}}$SAḪAR.GI$_6$.KUR.RA, *qitmu*-mineral.

Line 41: This line close to the bottom edge, written in slightly smaller characters, is difficult to decipher and the readings proposed here are tentative. The first signs seem to present the continuation of the recipe which started in line 40. However, the rest of the line after NIGIN-*ma* "you wrap" should perhaps best be understood as an editorial note. The sign MAN can be read as *šanû* "another, something else", and perhaps indicates a textual variant or alternative remedy that was found in a source text, cf. CAD Š/1, 393b s.v. *šanû* A sub 1b-3'. The reference to a wooden writing board, if read correctly, seems telegraphic. An expression such as *kī pī/ina* ${}^{\text{giš}}$ZU "according to/on a wooden writing-board" would be expected. At the end of line 41, perhaps read ⌜IN⌝.[SAR] "he wrote" (usually corresponding to Akkadian *išṭur*, but perhaps better rendered with the stative *šaṭer* here). The whole passage could then mean "a variant (*šanû*), written (on) a wooden writing board". If interpreted correctly, this remark may refer specifically to the remedy in lines 40–41.

Line 42: The spelling *ki-ma* KÀŠ in ms. a is likely a mistake for *ki-is*! KÀŠ "binding of the urine", which is reminiscent of the ailment *kīs libbi* "binding of the belly". Other expressions describing difficulties with urination are formed with the verbs *sekēru* "to shut off, to block" and *ṣabātu* "to seize" (cf. CAD Š/3, 41 s.v. *šīnātu* sub b), while the more usual expression for urination found in comparable contexts is *enūma šīnātīšu išattinu* "when (the patient) urinates" (CAD Š/2, 192–193 s.v. *šatānu*). If the text is understood correctly, the disease term NI.NE may refer to a symptom occurring in connection with difficult urination. This seems to be indicated also by line 46, which consists of the positive prognosis "she will be able to step into the 'house of urine' safely" (*šalmiš bīt šīnāti ikabba*[*s*]), meaning the patient will not encounter the described problem anymore while urinating. To my knowledge, the expression "house of the urine" for the lavatory is not known from other texts. For the condition NI.NE (or Ì.KÚM "it burns"), perhaps referring to a painful, burning sensation during urination, see also BAM 237 rev. iv 9–10 (text C.1.4 lines 154'''–155''') and the *Introduction* sub 4.2.[258]

Unfortunately, the rest of the symptom description in line 42 is not preserved, but it mentioned something to do with blood or haemorrhage. The restoration proposed by Scurlock and Andersen (2005, 281 12.119) MÚD.MEŠ-*šú ana* ⌜ŠÀ.(-) TÙR-*šú*⌝ / *šá-ḫir* "(and) her blood has turned back into her womb", cannot be confirmed by collation; the gap at the end of line 42 is definitely longer (three to four more signs are completely missing from the right-hand corner of the tablet). Interestingly, the following three prescriptions in lines 43–45 treat the same condition with a suppository inserted into the vagina, a potion, and an injection of a pharmakon into the urethra.

Line 44: For 'white drug' (Ú BABBAR) as a simple against NI.NE-disease, see also BAM 237 rev. iv 12 (text C.1.4).

Line 47: The sign sequence ŠUB DAB KÀŠ is ambiguous, but most likely ŠUB stands for *nadû* "to discharge, to excrete (body fluids)" and DAB for *ṣabātu* "to seize". Both verbs are attested in expressions with *šīnātu* "urine" as a subject, describing contrasting complaints of urine retention and uncontrolled release of urine (perhaps incontinence). See, e.g., within the corpus of renal disease texts, BAM 104: 39 // (Geller 2005a, 176): [....]x *la* KÚM.KÚM *š*[*i-na*]*t-su*(?) ŠUB.ŠUB-*šú* "... is always hot, his *urine spatters* him, ..."; AMT 66/11+ i 6' (Geller 2005a, 118): [DIŠ NA ...] x *ù* KÀŠ-*šú it-ta-na-aṣ-ba-ta* "[If a man ...] and his urine has been constantly 'seized'". Instead of genitive constructions with the infinitive of *nadû* "to discharge, to

258 For the plant name Ú.NI.NE, occurring as a logogram for *šūšu* (liquorice), cf. Attia and Buisson 2012, *JMC* 19, 35 (on BAM 1 i 43); Stol 2007, 14, 39; CAD Š/3, 386b s.v. *šūšu* for discussion.

excrete (body fluids)" and *ṣabātu* "to seize", constructions with the derived nouns *nīdu* "laying/throwing down" and *ṣibtu* "seizure" (i.e., *nīd ṣibit šīnāti*) are also thinkable (cf. *nīd ru'ti* "spitting"), although not attested yet with *šīnātu*. On the other hand, there are attestations of disease designations with *ṣibtu*, such as *ṣibit pî* "seizure of the mouth", or *ṣibit libbi* "seizure of the inside/belly", beside *miqit libbi* "fall of the inside"; cf. also the expression *miqit irrī* "fall of the bowels" (= diarrhoea), cf. CAD N/1; CAD Ṣ, 163–164 sub 1c-1'. For *imbu' tâmti*, see e.g. BAM 237 rev. iv 15 (also used as a simple in a tampon, but against "crab disease", see text C.1.4).

Lines 48–49: Concerning the last fragmentary sign at the end of line 48 one expects here the subject to *ikkalšū-ma* "it hurts her" at the beginning of line 49, which is usually a body part. Therefore, I suggest emending the text to read GAL$_4$.<LA-*šú*> "her crotch (hurts her)" (cf. CAD U/W, 265 s.v. *ūru* B lex. section for occasional lexical equations of SAL = *ūru*). For the problem of urinating in one's sleep, compare BAM 115: 14', with a male patient (Geller 2005a, 76): [DIŠ N]A *ina* KI.NÁ-*šú* KÀŠ-*šú iš-*⌜*tin* ŠU⌝ ^{d}*be-let*-DINGIR.MEŠ T[I] "[If a m]an urinates in his sleep, it is the hand of the goddess Bēlet-ilī; he will recover." See also STT 238: 1, discussed in Verderame 2018, *FS Geller*, 779–800, where the condition is caused by the goddess Ninmaḫ.

Scurlock and Andersen (2005, 269 12.53) translate KÀŠ *ši-tu* in line 49 as "escaping urine". However, *šīnātu* "urine" is usually construed as a feminine plurale tantum, and thus a plural form of the verbal adjective *šītu/šētu* (from *šêtu* "to remain; to escape") is expected.

Lines 50, 52, 53: The restoration of ms. a line 50 follows the spelling *šá* ŠÀ-ŠÀ-ŠÀ-*šú* in line 52 (thus also Finkel 2000, 171), although there may be no room for -*šú* in the gap in line 50. The spelling *šá* ŠÀ-ŠÀ-ŠÀ-*šú* against *šà* ŠÀ-*šà* in ms. b is perhaps a mistake. Due to the gap in line 53, it cannot be confirmed whether the form *šá* ŠÀ-ŠÀ-ŠÀ-*šú* with the superfluous -*šú* was likewise used in the sequence *ana šà* ŠÀ-*šà* [NU ŠUB] in that line. Finkel (2000, 174) assumed that such redundant forms as *šá* ŠÀ-ŠÀ-ŠÀ-*šú* or *šá* ŠÀ-ŠÀ-*šú/šà* reflect a frozen, misunderstood logogram. It is possible that these spellings should be read as a variant expression *ša liblibbīša* replacing the more common phrase *ša libbīša* "her foetus". This may have been motivated by the similar expression *līp*(*i*) *līpi/libbi* "descendant", see also the discussion of BM 43110+ line 1' (text E.2.2).

The present prescription recommends the consumption of the edible animal *ḫulû* (perhaps a shrew). Another similar animal, the edible rodent *ušummu*-dormouse, is applied in lines 78–79 below to promote fertility and conception. See note on lines 78–79 for discussion.

Lines 53–55: For a different reading of the passage, see Scurlock and Andersen (2005, 266 12.33). Instead of the reading SI ÁB "cow's horn" at the end of line 53, a reading *si-lit* "placenta" is also thinkable, although rarely attested as a medical ingredient. For animal horns in treatments to stop bleeding, see e.g. K. 263+ line 30 (gazelle horn in beer); SpTU 4, No. 153 obv. 15–16 (cow's horn as ingredient of a suppository); BAM 237 obv. i 38' (goat's horn in beer against bleeding during pregnancy); rev. iii 6 (stag horn and goat's horn). See also Steinert 2012 and section C.1 for discussion.

Parallel to logographic ^{na4}ÉLLAG-*tu*$_4$ in line 37, the signs *ták-pít* at the beginning of line 54 may perhaps be interpreted as *tu/akpītu*-stone. For discussion of *tukpītu* (*takpītu*) as a type of stone bead, see note on line 37 above, where it occurs in a prescription to stop bleeding and is applied to the women's genitals with a bandage. The use of a stone or stone bead in the present treatment in ms. a may point to the external application of the remedy (presumably some form of amulet or bandage attached to the patient's body). This may be confirmed by the instruction to place the medication in a *dīdu*-cloth, which refers to an undergarment (perhaps a slip) worn by women, see also Wasserman 2019, 1132–1133.

For Ì.UDU = *lipû* "fat" in the sense of "pith, marrow (of a plant)", see CAD L, 204–205 s.v. *lipû* sub 2b with several attestations for *lipî errî* "pith of colocynth". An alias name for this substance is "human fat" (Ì.UDU NAM.LÚ.U$_{18}$.LU), according to Uruanna I 270 (also KADP 28 i 16; Fincke 2021, 280 Pl. CLXXXVI).

Line 56: The meaning of the verb *parā'u/parāḫu* "to cut through, to sever, to slit" (CAD P, 181) in line 56 could be "to be torn", referring perhaps to the tearing of the pelvic floor during delivery. Thus, the verb *parā'u* is found in reference to cut throats and slit veins (*dāmu* "blood", e.g. in *Enūma Eliš* IV 131, VI 32; Lambert 2013, 92, 110), but also with reference to severed body parts. Magnetic haematite employed in line 56 is often used in prescriptions to stop haemorrhage, which could point to a similar context of the present prescription. Thus, "to be cut" may alternatively be a euphemistic expression for bleeding, analogous to the expression "to be wounded by a weapon" (*ina kakki maḫṣat*), see e.g., BAM 235 line 4 (*infra* text C.1.1).

Line 57: For treatments to prevent the loss of amniotic fluid (and miscarriage), see also BM 51246+ lines 35'-40' (text A.2.7).

Line 58: Seeds of *šakirû*-plant are also prescribed in a potion to treat bleeding during pregnancy in BAM 237 rev. iv 8 (text C.1.4).

Lines 59–60: For a partial parallel of the symptom description, cf. BAM 240: 34': DIŠ MUNUS MIN-*ma ri-du-ut ir-ri* TUKU "If a woman ditto (i.e. gives birth), and subsequently she gets diarrhoea" (the prescription in BAM 240 differs, however). The traces at the beginning of ms. a line 59 may have to be read in accordance with BAM 240: 20' // : DIŠ MUNUS TU_{15} (*iš-biṭ-ma*) *ma-lit* "If wind (has 'blown' into) a woman so that she is filled up (with it)". See *infra* text D.2.1 for the parallels.

Line 61: Here and in a few other instances (lines 57, 77), ms. a omits the pronominal suffix referencing the patient that would usually be attached to terms for body fluids (such as *dāmu* "blood", *mû* "(amniotic) fluid").

Line 63: The *tarmuš*-plant is also attested in other prescriptions to promote fertility, see e.g., BM 51246+ obv. 11 // N. 4001 obv. 14 (*infra* text B.2.1). See also the fertility test in lines 70–73 as well as lines 80 and 81 in ms. a. The fragmentary word starting with the sign *b/pul-* may be another drug ingredient, e.g. *pulḫānu* (a plant) or *bulṭītu* (*bušṭītu*) "woodworm, termite(?)". Note also the parallel formulation in BM 38624+ obv. 5': [ḪI]-*tú šá* ^{munus}NU.$PEŠ_4$ *ana šu-ri-i* "suppository to enable a woman who is not pregnant to get pregnant". In the abbreviated expression *maššītu ša* $PEŠ_4$ in line 63 of ms. a $PEŠ_4$ could be a shorthand for $^{munus}PEŠ_4$, the infinitive *erû* "to get pregnant" or the derived noun *mērû* "pregnancy".

Lines 64–66: Since *zu'tu* (IR) "sweat" is a feminine noun, the spelling (NU) DU_{10}-*ta* in line 64 may indicate either the feminine adjective *ṭābta* "(un)pleasant" or the 3rd person fem. sg. stative form *ṭābat* "it is (un)pleasant". These lines offer the only example known to me of a prescription to improve a woman's body odour (or more specifically, the odour of her sweat).

The ingredient "malt from the innkeeper" at the beginning of line 65 is not attested elsewhere to my knowledge, although beer and other ingredients used by the innkeeper in beer brewing are mentioned as ingredients in medical texts. Instead of *napītu* "sifted" (from *napû*), a reference to "dried" malt (*buqlu na'pu*, from *na'āpu* "to whither, to dry (out)") is perhaps even more likely here (cf. Lambert 1960, BWL, 246 v 23 (bilingual proverb); Landsberger 1937, MSL 1, 111; Stol 1987–1990, *RlA* 7, 324). The feminine form of the adjective *na-*pi_5*-tim* with *buqlu* is extraordinary, although fem. plural forms of *buqlu* are attested (cf. CAD B, 323–325; SAD, Vol. 1, 45). Cf. also Stol 1987a, *BSA* 3, 65 (for *buqlu* in the secondary meaning "green vegetables"). At the end of line 65, *ib-ba-šu* may perhaps stand for the N-stem (present) of *bašû* "to become available".

Lines 67–68: A similar treatment as the one encountered here is recommended in BAM 240 lines 71'–74' for the case that a woman cannot retain her partner's semen (which prevents her from getting pregnant). The remedy in BAM 240 using the bones of an unmated kid, however, not the bones of a ram. The choice of the animal in both treatments is probably of significance (see also next note and text D.2.1).

Lines 67 and 69: The purpose of the two treatments in lines 67–69 is so far unparalleled in other women's healthcare texts. The expression "if a woman does not do the 'work' of women" is apparently euphemistic. It can be compared with the slightly varying phrase *šipir sinništi epēšu* "to do the 'work' of a woman" for an active female role in intercourse, which is found in Tablet I of the Standard Babylonian *Gilgamesh Epic* 185 and 192. It describes Šamḫat's seduction of Enkidu in the wild: *epšīšuma/īpussuma lullâ šipir sinništi* "Treat him/She treated him to the (sensuous) work of a woman" (George 2003, 548–549). It is remarkable to find this collocation for the first time in a women's healthcare context. The expression may refer to a woman's lack of or reduced desire for sexual intercourse. It is noteworthy here that the *Gilgamesh Epic* is quoted in two commentaries on the Assyrian birth compendium BAM 248, see *infra* 11N-T3: 40–41; UET 6/3, 897 rev. 7'–8' (text G.1-G.2)).

For similar expressions, phrased from a male perspective, note also *attā ina sūn sinništika šipir lū tēpuš* "you shall be active in your woman's lap" in the *Cuthean Legend* (J. G. Westenholz 1997, 326ff. line 159). Cf. further the expression *epēš* NAM.MUNUS.A(*sinnišūti*?) "to have intercourse", literally "doing womanhood", which is likewise used from the male perspective. It is attested in the sex omens of *Šumma ālu*, see CT 39, pl. 44: 4: *šumma amēlu epēš* NAM.MUNUS.A MUNUS-*šú ḫašiḫ … epēš* NAM.MUNUS.A *muṣlāla damiq* "If a man wishes to have intercourse with his wife, … intercourse during midday is good" (cited CAD S, 293b). For women's lack of sexual desire, compare also the corpus of the ŠÀ.ZI.GA-texts discussed in Zisa 2021, 42–43, with Steinert et al. 2018, 217, 266 Assur Medical Catalogue line 106 and *passim*.

Line 69: If read correctly, *šibirtu* "lump" may be understood as a shortcut for *šibirti buqli* "lump of malt" (cf. CAD Š/2, 379 s.v. *šibirtu* lex section, esp. Hh. XXIII iv 18). There is an assonance between the words *šipru* "work" (of women) and *šibirtu* (also *šipirtu*) "lump", which supports the latter reading.

Lines 70–73: For slightly differing readings, cf. Scurlock 2014a, 582–585; Scurlock and Andersen 2005, 262 12.17 and 12.18; Reiner 1982a, *ZA* 72, 137 for UET 7, No. 123: 1–4. As has been noted previously, the exact meaning of the Mesopotamian tests for woman is often ambiguous, it cannot always be determined whether we are dealing with a test to determine a woman's fertility or an actual pregnancy (see Reiner 1982a, 127–128, 131; Stol 2000a, 37 with n. 78; Böck 2013, 41; Steinert 2015, 107–109). Note, however, that ms. a concludes the prescription with syllabic *ir-ri*, what may mean "she will get pregnant" rather than "she is pregnant" (for which the text would perhaps rather use the stative form *erât*).

At the end of line 71 in ms. a, the text appears to read *uš-*[*e*]*l-lam-ma* "she removes it" (rather than expected *tu-še-lam-ma* "you remove (it)"), cf. Scurlock and Andersen 2005, 262. In ms. b this passage is not preserved, but one may perhaps restore [*ukâl* E_{11}-*ma*] in the gap at the beginning of obv. 3.

The text of ms. c (UET 7, No. 123) presents a few variants in formulation. Ms. c reverses the order of the colours of the wad in comparison to ms. a, but their interpretation as well as the ingredients and general procedure (inserting a wad of wool prepared with different substances into the woman's vagina and leaving it there for several hours; removing and washing it, before observing colour changes) are identical. The comment "her womb is white/shiny" (*u* ŠÀ.TÙR-*šú* BAB-BAR-*ma*) in line 73 (only found in ms. a) appears to signal that not only the wad of wool was observed to determine the woman's fertility, but that also some kind of vaginal exam may have been performed.

Lines 74–77: In line 74, the numeral 4 in 4 Ú "four plants/drugs" occurring in mss. a and b is a mistake, since the prescription lists at least five ingredients plus a carrier substance (fatty material). The sequence 4 Ú "four plants/drugs" is too unspecific to be regarded as an ingredient by itself. The sequence 4 NINDA/NÍG.ḪI.A $^{\check{s}im}$GÚR.GÚR is rendered by Böck (2013, 32) as "four little bread roles of *kukru* plant". If we read the sequence as two ingredients, the text would lack the specific amount of *kukru*-aromatic needed, in contrast to all other ingredients, for which specific measurements are listed. I therefore prefer to regard NINDA.ḪI.A as an exceptional plural spelling of the measurement NINDA (a tenth of a litre). For a similar occurrence of NINDA.ḪI.A, see SpTU 4, No. 153 obv. 27 (text D.1.11 line 9 with discussion).

In line 76 in ms. a, there is space for ca. two signs in the gap following *šiqittu* "almonds". Perhaps an attribute was added here which is lacking in ms. b.

Following the suggestion by Finkel 2000, 172 n. 9, I regard the word *ḫulibu* in line 76 as a loan from Aramaic *ḥlb* (*ḥēleb, ḥlebā*) "fatty tissue" or "viscous substance" (Jastrow, *Dictionary*, 460; *The Comprehensive Aramaic Lexicon* (CAL, online)). For *dannu* as a large storage container for different consumables (bread, spice, dates, beer, wine), cf. CAD D, 98–99; SAD Vol. 2, 18 sub *dannu* II ("pithos"), AHw 161b; CDA, 56 "(large) vat, barrel"; Gaspa 2014, *Contenitori*, 105–107.

Line 77: My interpretation of the end of the prescription follows Finkel 2000, 171–172; Böck 2013, 32; Steinert 2017a, 307; differently Scurlock and Andersen (2005, 268 12.50). I read the sentence starting with BAD-*ma* as a positive prognosis, understanding BAD-*ma* as *ipettē-ma* (*irri u* A.MEŠ ŠUB.ŠUB-*ma*) "she will open up (and get pregnant, and moreover she will repeatedly discharge (her) fluids)". Following a suggestion by I. Finkel (2000, 172 n. 11), the "fluids/water" which the woman emits are perhaps to be understood as a reference to female semen or fluids contributing to conception. Although A.MEŠ "fluids" usually refers to "amniotic fluids" in women's healthcare texts, the present context suggests a different meaning of the term. The expression *šá* BAD *u* $PE\check{S}_4$, to be rendered as a purpose statement, i.e. "for opening and getting pregnant" is found at the end of a recipe in other texts, (e.g., BM 42587+: 27 (text B.2.4); see also BM 79061 obv. 4 (text A.2.8): *šá pa-te-e* [*ù* $PE\check{S}_4$(?)] "for opening up [and getting pregnant(?)]", concluding a prescription for promoting conception and fertility.

Lines 78–79: This treatment applies an edible rodent, *ušummu*-dormouse, to promote fertility and conception. For the association of mice with fertility, see also Finkel 2000, 171; Böck 2013, 33–34. Mice also play a role in Mesopotamian treatments to increase male sexual desire or potency (see also Zisa 2021, 98 n. 208, 119–120, 195–196 and *passim*; especially *arrabu*-mouse is used in the latter therapies). For a similar animal, *ḫulû* (shrew), in a prescription to prevent miscarriage, see above lines 50–52.

A.2.3 BM 50700: A Collection of Recipes for Women

This Late Babylonian tablet fragment was perhaps found at Dilbat.[259] According to the script it may roughly be dated to the Achaemenid period. It contains prescriptions for different purposes, some of which are explicitly marked as destined for a female patient. The technical and at times difficult jargon used in BM 50700 (ms. a) reflects some influence of the Aramaic language, as is suggested by the occurrence of rare terms that are apparently or very likely Aramaic loanwords. The format of the better-preserved recipes shows similarities with the recipe structure witnessed in other women's healthcare compendia from later first millennium BCE Babylonia such as BM 38624+ (text A.2.1), in which the purpose of a prescription is stated at the very end of the recipe, and in which prescriptions usually do not feature an introductory symptom description, but immediately start with listing ingredients.

The contents of ms. a, for which no duplicating passages have been identified so far, are likewise unusual in some respects. Thus, the text contains remedies that are not typically "gynaecological" but may still be relevant to women suffering from gynaecological problems. For example, it features prescriptions for women suffering from skin diseases (*ruṭibtu, sikkatu, rišûtu*), in addition to prescriptions for conditions that have parallels in other women's healthcare texts (e.g., remedies for women suffering from bloating by "wind"). Several of the prescriptions are classified as *maššītu*, a term usually denoting suppositories in prescriptions for women.

List of Manuscripts

Siglum	Museum Number	Copy	Collation	Format; Ductus	Provenience
a	BM 50700 (82-3-23, 1692)	Pl. 16	Coll.	Fragment of a single-column tablet; Late Babylonian script; ca. 5th/4th cent. BCE[260]	Dilbat(?)

Overview

i'	Fragmentary prescription a obv. 1'	...]1'
ii'	Prescription a obv. 2'–3'	2'–3'
iii'	Prescription for a woman in childbed given on the day of delivery a obv. 4'–5'	4'–5'
iv'	Prescription for a woman suffering from *ruṭibtu* or *sikkatu*-disease a obv. 6'	6'
v'	Prescription (suppository for "absorbing") a obv. 7'–11'	7'–11'
vi'	Prescription (suppository) for *rišûtu*-disease a obv. 12'	12'
vi'	Prescription (tampon) a obv. 13'–14'	13'–14'
vii'	Fragmentary prescription a obv. 15'–16'	15'–16'
viii'	Fragmentary prescription a obv. 17'–18'	17'–18'[...

259 As described by Reade (1986, in: *CBT* VI, xxxii, xxxvii), the provenience of BM 50700 was marked in the register books as Dilbat. However, the tablets in the 82-3-23-collection of the Babylonian collection in the BM are known to have originated from different sites (Babylon, Sippar, Borsippa), and there are some doubts whether a few tablets marked as stemming from Dilbat might not actually have been found at Babylon.
260 Measurements: 7.8 x 7 x 3 cm.

ix''	Fragmentary prescription a rev. 1'	...]19''
x''	Fragmentary prescription a rev. 2'–4'	20''–22''[...
xi'''	Fragmentary prescription (for "absorbing") a rev. 1''-4''	...]23'''–26'''
xii'''	Prescription (suppository) for a woman affected by "wind" a rev. 5''–6''	27'''–28'''
xiii'''	Fragmentary prescription a rev. 7''–8''	29'''–30'''[...

Previous Edition and Discussion

Electronic Babylonian Library (eBL) (https://www.ebl.lmu.de/library/BM.50700)

Transliteration

Beginning of ms. a obv. lost

1' a obv. 1' Ì [x x]x [..]

2' a obv. 2' 1 NINDA [x x x 1] NINDA *saḫ-lé-*⸢*e*⸣ 1$^{?}$ NI[NDA x x x x]x ⸢NUMUN$^{?}$⸣ 3 NINDA ⸢*qu*$^{?}$⸣-[x x (x)]

3' a obv. 3' 1 ⸢NINDA⸣ [LI$^{?}$].⸢TAR⸣ 1 NINDA x[x x 1 NINDA$^{?}$] *ak-tam šá ri-b*[*i-ki*$^{?}$]

4' a obv. 4' ⸢KU⸣ ^{š}[^{im}]⸢MUG⸣ ⸢*tu*⸣*-lab-bak* [*ina* KURUN].⸢NAM⸣ Ì.NUN ḪI.ḪI *ri-bi-ku*

5' a obv. 5' *šá ḫa-riš-ti* [GU$_7$$^{?}$]*-šú u*$_4$*-mu šá* Ù.TU

6' a obv. 6' ⸢ZÌ⸣ ⸢ŠE.GIG$^{?}$⸣ ZÌ ZÍZ.ÀM *ina* Ì$^{?}$ [ḪI.ḪI *ri-b*]*i-ku šá* MUNUS *šá ru-ṭib-tú u*$^{?}$ *sik-kà-at mar-ṣa-*⸢*at*⸣

7' a obv. 7' [x x ŠI]M.ŠAL GAZ SIM NU[MUN$^{?}$ GADA *šá i-n*]*a* KAŠ *ir-muk ta-sa-pan t*[*u*]*-na-aṭ-ṭap*

8' a obv. 8' [ŠE].⸢GIG$^{?}$⸣ ÀR*-en ta-*[*nap-pi*$^{?}$] ^{ú}SULLIM^{sar} *tasa-mud*$^{?}$ ⸢*ta*$^{?}$⸣*-hap-pap ta*$^{!}$*-na*$^{?}$*-áš-šip*

9' a obv. 9' [*saḫ*]*-lé-e tu-qal-l*[*ap* ŠIM.ŠAL]*-e*$^{?}$ NUMUN GADA SULLIM^{sar} *saḫ-lé-e ina* KAŠ ŠE SUMUN

10' a obv. 10' [*lu*] *ina* Ì ⸢*ḫal-ṣa*⸣ ⸢*lu*$^{?}$⸣ [*ina* A.MEŠ$^{?}$ *ta-ra*]*m-muk šá tas-pu-nu u t*[*u-n*]*a-aṭ-ṭì-pu*

11' a obv. 11' [x x x]-⸢*ma*$^{?}$⸣ x x [Ḫ]I.ḪI ḪI*-tú šá lu-ub-bu-ku* x[x x GA]R$^{?}$*-ma* : ZÌ$^{?!}$ GIG.BA$^{?}$ *i-ṣ*[*i*] *šu-ut* [KA]

12' a obv. 12' [x x x x *ina* D]UḪ.LÀL$^{?}$ ḪI.ḪI ŠEG$_6$*-šal* Ì *ḫal-ṣa lu-u* Ì.U[DU TA]G.TAG ḪI*-tú šá ri-šu-*[*tú*$^{?}$]

13' a obv. 13' [x x x x x]x MUNU$_4$$^{?}$.È.⸢A$^{?}$⸣ ḪÁD.DU x[x x x] x [x x x]

14' a obv. 14' [x x x x x]x TAG.TAG *ina* ^{síg}ÀKA ⸢NIGIN⸣*-m*[*i* x x x]

15' a obv. 15' [x x x x *saḫ-l*]*é-e* ŠE.GIŠ.Ì ŠE.x[x x R]A$^{?}$ *i-ṣ*[*i*$^{?}$ x x x]

16' a obv. 16' [x x x x x D]UḪ.LÀL *u* ^{šim}ḪAB ^{š}[^{im}]x $^{ú?}$x [x x x x]

17' a obv. 17' [x x x x x ^{šim}L]I *ina* Ì.UDU *u* KAŠ [.........................]

18' a obv. 18' [x x x x x x s]a$^{?}$ ^{šim}ḪAB [..]

Ms. a obv. breaks; gap of unknown length
Beginning of ms. a rev. lost

19'' a rev. 1' [...............................] ⸢Ì.UDU⸣ [.....................]

20'' a rev. 2' [............................ *i*]*na*$^{?}$ *ḫu-bu-ta u*[*l*(-) ....]

21'' a rev. 3' [.............................] GAR-*an* ⸢*ta-ra*⸣-*sà-a*[*n*$^{?}$ ....]

22'' a rev. 4' [.............................]x EN *in*-x[..]

Gap of approximately 8 lines

23''' a rev. 13' [...] ⸢GAR-*an*⸣

24''' a rev. 14' [..]

25''' a rev. 15' [...] x ^{ú}x[x x]

26''' a rev. 16' [.. ḪI-*tú šá l*]*u-ub*-[*b*]*u-k*[*u* x x]

27''' a rev. 17' x x x x x x x[x x]x TI-⸢*qé*⸣ GAZ ⸢SIM⸣ *sa-ra*$^{?}$-*'u*$^{?}$ *šá*$^{?}$ ⸢U$_{8}$$^{?}$⸣.[UDU.ḪI].⸢A$^{?!}$⸣

28''' a rev. 18' x ⸢UDU$^{?}$⸣ ḪI.⸢ḪI⸣$^{?}$ ⸢ILLU⸣ BULUḪ *ina* [Ì.UD]U$^{?}$ ŠEG$_{6}$-*šal ana* ŠÀ$^{?}$ ḪI.ḪI *maš-šit šá* MUNUS *šá* ⸢TU$_{15}$$^{?}$⸣ x[x x]

29''' a rev. 19' ⸢*saḫ*$^{?}$⸣-*lé-e* LUḪ$^{!}$(KAL-*ši*$^{!?}$) *ina* GA ÈME [*tu-la*]*b-bak* ZÌ *tu-ḫu*^{me} *ina* KAŠ ⸢*tu*$^{?}$⸣-x[-x-(x)]

30''' a rev. 20' [x]x x x ⸢*ina*⸣ ⸢*aḫ*⸣-[x x] ḪI.ḪI ILLU BULUḪ *u* Ì.UDU SUMUN [x x x x]

Ms. a rev. breaks; remainder lost

Bound Transcription and Translation

Beginning of ms. a obv. lost

1' *traces*	1' *too fragmentary for translation*
2' *ištēn akal* [... *ištēn*] *akal saḫlê ištēn*(?) *ak*[*al* ... ...] ... *šalāšat akal* ...[...] 3' *ištēn akal* [*abuk*]*katu ištēn akal* ...[... *ištēn akal*(?)] *aktam ša rib*[*īki*]	2' One tenth of a litre of [..., one] tenth of a litre of *saḫlû*-plant, one tenth of a litre of [..., ...]..., three tenths of a litre of ...[...], 3' one tenth of a litre of [*abuk*]*katu*-aromatic, one tenth of a litre of [..., one tenth of a litre(?) of] *aktam*-plant. (Ingredients) for a paste (*rabīku*).
4' *sīkti ballukki tulabbak* [*ina kurun*]*ni ḫimēti tuballal ribīku* 5' *ša ḫarišti* [*tušakkal*(?)]-*šu ūmu ša ulladu*	4' You soak powder of *ballukku*-aromatic, you mix it with [*kurun*]*nu*-beer (and) ghee. A paste 5' for a woman in childbed (which) [you have] her [eat(?)] on the day she gives birth.
6' *qēm kibti qēm kunāši ina šamni* [*tuballal rib*]*īku ša sinništi ša ruṭibta u sikkata marṣat*	6' [You mix] wheat flour (and) emmer flour with oil. [A pa]ste for a woman who is sick with *ruṭibtu* ("dampness") or *sikkatu*-disease.

7' [...] *šimeššalâ taḫaššal tanappi zē[r kitê ša(?) in]a šikari irmuk(u) tasappan t[u]naṭṭap* 8' *[ki]bta teṭên ta[nappi(?)] šambalilta tasammud taḫappap tanaššip* 9' *[saḫ]lê tuqal-l[ap šimeššal]ê(?) zēr kitê sambalilta saḫlê ina šikar še'i labiri* 10' *[lū] ina šamni ḫalṣi lū [ina mê(?) tara]mmuk ša taspunu u t[un]aṭṭipu* 11' [...]*-ma ... tuballal maššītu ša lub-buki* ...[... *tašakk]an-ma(?) : qēm kibti īṣi šūt pî*

7' You crush (and) sift [...] *šimeššalû*-plant. You *drain*(?) [lin]-seed [that(?)] has been washed in beer, you *remove* (all the liquid?). 8' You grind (and) si[ft] wheat. You grind fenugreek, you *pound it finely*(?) (and) *pulverise it*. 9' You pe[el *saḫ*]-*lû*-plant (i.e. free it from husks?). You wash the [*šimešša-l*]*û*-plant(?), linseed, fenugreek (and) *saḫlû*-plant either in old barley beer, 10' [or] in pressed oil or [in water(?)]. (These ingredients) which you have *drained* and (*all liquid*) *removed*, 11' [you ...] and [mix (it)] with(?) .... A suppository for *absorbing*, ...[... you ins]ert (it). (Use) a little wheat flour (with it). (This is according to) oral lore.

12' [... ... *ina iš*]*kūri tuballal tušabšal šamna ḫalṣa lū li[pâ tul]appat maššītu ša rišûti*

12' You mix [... ... with] wax, you boil (it), you blend (it) with pressed oil or with tal[low]. A suppository for *rišûtu*-disease ("itching").

13' [... ... ...] *(buqla) qarnānâ(?) tubbal* ...[...]...[...] 14' [... ... ...]... *tulappat ina itqi talammi* [...]

13' [.......], you dry sprouted malt(?), ...[... ...], 14' [... ...] you blend [(it) with ...], you wrap (it) in a wad of wool, [*you insert it into her womb*(?)].

15' [... ... *saḫ*]*lê šamaššammū* ...[...]... *īṣi* [...] 16' [... ...] *iškūru u ṭūru* ... ...[... ...]

15' [... ... *saḫ*]*lû*-plant, sesame, ..., a little ..., [... ...], 16' [... ...] wax and *ṭūru*-aromatic, ...-aromatic, ...-plant, [... ...].

17' [... ... *bur*]*āšu ina lipî u šikari* [... ... ...] 18' [... ...]... *ṭūru* [... ... ...]

17' [... ... you ...] *burāšu*-juniper with tallow and beer [... ...], 18' [... ...], *ṭūru*-aromatic, [.... ... ...].

Ms. a obv. breaks; gap of unknown length
Beginning of ms. a rev. lost

19'' [... ... ...] *lipû* [... ... ...]

19'' [... ... ...] tallow [... ... ...].

20'' [... ... ...] *ina(?) ḫubūta ul* [... ... ...] 21'' [... ... ...] *tašakkan tarassan* [... ... ...] 22'' [... ... ...] *adi(?)* ...[... ... ...]

20'' [.... ... ...] *in a thicket* ...[... ... ...], 21'' [... ... ...] you put, you steep, [... ...], 22'' [... ...] until(?) it [... ... ...]

Gap of approximately 8 lines

23''' [... ... ...] *tašakkan* 24''' [... ... ...] 25''' [... ... ...] ...[...] 26''' [... ... *maššītu ša l*]*ubbuk*[*i* ...]

23''' [... ... ...] you put. 24''' [... ... ...], 25''' [... ... ...] plant, 26''' [... ... A suppository] for *absorbing*.

27''' ... ...[...] *teleqqe taḫaššal tanappi sar'i ša ṣēni* 28''' ... *tubal-lal ḫīl baluḫḫi ina [lip]î tušabšal ana libbi tuballal maššītu ša sinništi ša šāra(?)* ...[...]

27''' You take.... ...[...], you crush (and) sift (it). 28''' You mix (it) 27''' with *sar'u* of sheep (and) 28''' sheep ... . You boil resin of *baluḫḫu*-aromatic with tallow, you mix it with (the other ingredients). A suppository for a woman who is ... with 'wind'.

29''' *saḫlê temessi ina sizib atāni [tula]bbak qēma tuḫḫī ina šikari tu-*[... ...] 30''' [...]... ...[...] *tuballal ḫīl baluḫḫi u lipâ labi-ra* [... ...]

29''' You wash *saḫlû*-cress, you soak (it) in donkey's milk. You [...] flour and bran with beer, [... ...], 30''' [...] ...[...], you mix. Resin of *baluḫḫu*-aromatic and old tallow [... ...] ...

Ms. a rev. breaks; remainder lost

Notes

Lines 3', 4', 6': The term *ribīku*, understood as a variant form of the words *rabīku* or *ribku*, which dictionaries render as "decoction" or "mash" (CAD R, 20 and 321; AHw 935a "ein Absud" and AHw 980b "ein (Drogen-) Absud"), is interpreted here as a paste that could be eaten or applied to the skin (e.g., in line 6, it is applied to treat skin conditions). For discussion, see the *Introduction*, section 4.2.

Line 6': The word *ruṭibtu* literally means "dampness" (derived from *raṭābu* "to be damp"), it is used in the meaning "damp ground, irrigated field" (logogram KI.DURU$_5$) and as a disease term (cf. CAD R, 437–438 s.v. *ruṭibtu*; Livingstone 2013, 264–265). This disease is mentioned in the context of conditions of the lower extremities and in the context of skin ailments, where it refers to a suppurating, itching skin sore, from which a fluid oozes (Eypper 2016, *JMC* 27, 2, 6–8 *passim*; Scurlock and Andersen 2005, 210; *Diagnostic Handbook* Tablet 33, lines 18–19).

The second disease treated with the prescription in line 6' is the skin disease *sikkatu* (UZU.GAG.MEŠ) "pock, pimple". The term literally means "peg" and refers to different types of "peg-shaped" lesions (cf. CAD S, 251 s.v. *sikkatu* (*šiggatu*); AHw 1042a s.v. *sikkatu* II; Scurlock and Andersen 2005, 235–236; Cadelli 2019, *JMC* 34, 52 n. 433; Charpin 2018, *RA* 112, 198 on CUSAS 29, No. 23: 6). The remedy was presumably applied to the skin, and thus the term *ribīku* may refer to a paste-like product in this case.

Line 7': The restoration of NUM[UN GADA] is based on line 9', where this ingredient occurs again. An alternative reading may be NU[MUN GADA *ta-n*]*a-pí* "you sift linseed".

The occurrence of a 3rd person preterite form *irmuk* as part of an instruction is unexpected and perhaps to be interpreted as a mistake for *tarammuk* "you wash". But the word may also be explained as the verbal form of a relative clause referring to a previous step in the procedure (i.e. "linseed which has been washed (in beer)"), see also line 10' for a similar relative clause with *ša* + two verbs in the preterite. In the case of *irmuk*, the subjunctive ending *-u* has been omitted. Instead of *ir-muk*, it is also possible to read the sign MUG with a different phonetic value, namely as *ir-buk* "it has been steeped".

Lines 7' and 10': The verbs *sapānu* and *naṭāpu* (D-stem) occur twice in the present prescription, in line 7' and again in line 10'. Their specific sense in the present passage is difficult to elucidate, as they seem to be used in a technical meaning that diverges from the basic senses given in the dictionaries. Since they immediately follow each other both times, *sapānu* and *naṭāpu* seem to describe two subsequent steps in the preparation procedure. In line 7', the ingredient linseed undergoes the processes of *sapānu* and *naṭāpu*, while in line 10', all ingredients are treated in this fashion. In both cases, the ingredients are washed prior to this treatment, which may suggest that *sapānu* and *naṭāpu* refer to something like a drying process. The verb *sapānu* usually means "to lay flat; to flatten" or "to pluck", but for some occurrences in medical texts, a special meaning "to dip(?) (in a liquid)" has been proposed (see CAD S, 158–161 esp. sub 3, in the references cited there, a liquid is specified, however). Guessing from the present context, *sapānu* may mean "to lay out flat to dry" or perhaps "to drain".

The verb *naṭāpu* "to tear out; to pluck" (e.g. plants) has not previously been attested in medical texts in connection with the preparation of drugs (AHw 767b s.v. *naṭ/tāpu*; CAD N/2, 128–128). A fitting translation is difficult to come by. However, it is possible that the verb in the present text is an Aramaic loanword. Thus, the Aramaic verb *nṭp* means "to drip", in the D-stem "to drip copiously" or "to make to drip" (see the *Comprehensive Aramaic Dictionary* (CAL); Jastrow 1903, 901; Sokoloff 2002, 745). Thus, the verb would indicate the removal of any superfluous liquid from the ingredients after they have been washed.

Line 8': The processing of the ingredient fenugreek (*šambaliltu*) in this line is described with three different verbs enumerated in a row: *tasammud taḫappap tanaššip*. The first form comes from Akkadian *samādu* "to grind (into groats)", said e.g. of barley or sesame, but also of plant ingredients in medical texts (CAD S, 107; AHw 1016b).

The form *taḫappap* most likely belongs to the verb *ḫapāpu*, which is a variant of *ḫepû* "to break up; to smash; to pound" (AHw 321 s.v. *ḫapāpu* I). AHw 321 s.v. *ḫapāpu* II lists a second verb *ḫapāpu*, derived from Aramaic, with the meaning "to wash; to clean" (see e.g. Fincke 2011, in: *The Empirical Dimension*, 190 BM 41282+ obv. ii 4', 11'; Geller 2007, *JMC* 10, 9–10 AO 11447: 28 (Dtn-stem), 38 (G-stem)). In the present context, the former verb seems more likely. For another attestation of *ḫapāpu* in Late Babylonian medical texts for women's health, see SpTU 5, No. 253: 4' (text E.2.6).

The form *tanaššip* could belong to the verb *našāpu* (also *našābu*), which means "to blow away; to winnow"; cf. CAD N/2, 56–57; AHw 758b "(Korn) durchblasen; (Sesam) enthülsen". However, the dictionaries suggest that the G-stem of *našāpu* has an *u/u* vocalization (i.e. *inaššup*, *iššup*), while ms. a spells the form *ta*[!]*-na-áš-šib/p*. Perhaps we are again dealing with an Aramaic loanword. Thus, the verbal root nšp means "to blow", but also "to pound; to pulverise" in Aramaic, which would suit the present context much better (see the *Comprehensive Aramaic Dictionary* (CAL)). Thus, we would be dealing with three verbs for grinding and pounding, perhaps indicating increasing grades of fineness.

Line 11': The term *maššītu* (written ḪI-*tú*) occurs also at the end of lines 12' and 28''' in similar labels stating the purpose of the treatment. For the expression *maššītu ša lubbuki* "suppository for absorbing (fluids/blood)" in the women's healthcare texts, see also BM 38624+: 10' (text A.2.1), SpTU 4, No. 153 obv. lines 2, 9, 14 (text C.1.10); Steinert 2020, *JMC* 36, 58–60 and the *Introduction*, sub 4.2 for discussion.

The understanding of the end of line 11' is difficult and the proposed reading tentative. The sign following [GA]R?-*ma* looks like a disjunction sign (*Trennungszeichen*) with three oblique wedges; it seems to mark a short comment added to the text of the prescription. This comment (or the prescription as a whole?) is marked as *šūt pî* "oral explanation/tradition". For *šūt pî* "oral lore/tradition", see Frahm 2011, 44–45, 51–52 *passim*; Gabbay 2016, 51–52 and, for other instances in the women's health corpus, see BM 38624+: 86''''' (text A.2.1); BM 45736 iv 12 (text A.2.5); cf. SpTU 5, No. 253: 3' (text E.2.6).

Line 12': The condition *rišûtu* is a skin disease; the term itself may refer to redness or itchiness. CAD R, 381–382 suggests the noun is derived from *rašû* B meaning "to itch" (because of the lexical equation SA.UMBIN.AK.AK "to scratch the muscle with the fingernail" and because of the association of *rišûtu* with other terms for itching skin conditions). AHw 889–890 interprets *rišûtu* as "eine Rötung" (reddening), proposing a meaning "to turn red" for the associated verb *rašû* (AHw 962b s.v. *rašû* II). Both meaning aspects may be interrelated, see Scurlock and Andersen 2005, 210–211. Mention of seasonal outbreaks of *rišûtu* in the astronomical diaries suggests an infectious or epidemic disease (see Sachs and Hunger 1996, *Astronomical Diaries* Vol. 3, 94–95 obv. 33'-34', 104–105 (A) 21', 386–387 A obv. 46'; Del Monte 1997, 100; van Soldt 1991, *ZA* 81, 155).

Line 13': The sign sequence MUNU$_4$?.È.⸢A?⸣, if the signs are read correctly, could perhaps be an abbreviated spelling for MUNU$_4$.SI.È (also MUNU$_4$.SI.MÚ.A) = (*buqlu*) *qarnānû* "sprouted (malt)" (lit. 'horned', in Sumerian "malt which has grown a horn"), cf. Hh. XXIII iv 6–7; MSL 11, 73.

Line 20': The term *ḫu-bu-ta* in this very fragmentary line could represent the word *ḫubūtu* "thicket; bushes" (an Aramaic or West Semitic loanword), see AHw 352b.

Line 27''': The word *sar'u* is encountered only a few times as an ingredient in first millennium Babylonian medical texts and is always complemented by *ṣēnu* (U$_8$.UDU.ḪI.A) "sheep" in the genitive (CAD S, 189b s.v. *sar'u*). Usually written syllabically *sa-ar/ár-'i* (see BAM 497 ii 9 and BAM 303: 15'), the word is spelled *sa-ra-'i* in ms. a. The exact meaning of this word is unknown, but *sar'u* may be a variant of *sarbu* "(sheep) fat, tallow" (cf. CAD S, 175b for discussion).

Line 28''': At the end of line, perhaps restore (*maššītu ša sinništi*) *ša šāra uddupat* "(a suppository for a woman) who is bloated with wind", parallel to formulations encountered in the women's health compendium BAM 240: 25', 26', 28' (text D.2.1), which discusses different cases of pregnant or postpartum women suffering from "wind" (perhaps referring to flatulence or intestinal bloating). For *edēpu* "to be inflated (with wind)", see also the prescription in BAM 303: 14'-22', which is described as a recipe for "a suppository (*maššītu*) for [a ...] inflated with wind and for making stiff (muscles?) supple" (lines 20'–22': *maš-ši-ti šá* [x] / *šá* TU$_{15}$ *ed-pe-t*[*u*?] / *ù šag-gi a-na lu-ub-bu-ki*). Arbøll (2021, 286) suggests restoring [GÌR^{II}] "[feet]" in the gap; however, the 3rd person fem. sg. stative *edpetu* suggests a feminine singular noun, either a body part or perhaps even MUNUS "a woman"? The remedy in BAM 303: 14'ff. shares a few similarities with the prescription in ms. a 27'''–28''' (e.g. the use of *sar'u/sarbu ša ṣēni* "sheep fat(?)").

Line 29''': The peculiar sign sequence *tu-ḫu*^{me} may stand for *tuḫḫū* "bran; draff" with ME serving as a plural marker (personal suggestion by M. J. Geller).

A.2.4 BM 45559 + 45574: Prescriptions for Delivery and Postpartum Conditions

This fragment of a two-column tablet perhaps dating to the 6th or 5th cent. BCE was perhaps found at Babylon (it is registered in the Babylonian Collection of the British Museum as coming from the excavations of Hormuzd Rassam in Babylonia).[261] The fragment contains prescriptions for women's health and may have been part of a larger compendium. The

261 Leichty, Finkel and Walker 2019, *CBT* IV–V, 596.

reverse is badly worn off and only a few damaged lines can be deciphered. The better-preserved sections deal mostly with birth-related topics. A longer ruled-off section in col. i contains several short prescriptions for promoting safe childbirth(?) and for treating problems after delivery, especially with potions and suppositories. This section is remarkable, since individual prescriptions are not separated by rulings and often do not start at the beginning of a new line. The section includes a damaged passage marked in an unusual manner as *taḫsistu* "memorandum".

List of Manuscripts

Siglum	Museum Number	Copy	Collation	Format; Ductus	Provenience
a	BM 45559 (81-7-1, 3320) + BM 45574 (81-7-1, 3335)	Pl. 17	Coll.	Fragment of a two-column tablet; Neo-/Late Babylonian script; ca. 6th/5th cent. BCE[262]	probably Babylon

Overview

i'	Fragmentary prescription a obv. i 1'–2'	...]1'–2'
ii'	Prescriptions for women (associated with birth or delivery: potions, suppositories) a obv. i 3'–21'	3'–21'[...
iii'	Fragmentary a obv. ii 1'–2'	...]22''–23''
iv'	Fragmentary prescription for a woman a obv. ii 3'–6'	24''–27''
v'	Fragmentary prescription for a woman a obv. ii 7'–8'	28''–29''[...
vi'	Fragmentary prescription a rev. iv 1'–10'	...]30'''–39'''
vii'	Prescription for a woman during or after delivery (enema) a rev. iv 11'-15'	40'''–44'''
viii'	Fragmentary prescription for a woman during or after delivery a rev. iv 16'-18'	45'''–47'''[...

Previous Edition and Discussion

Electronic Babylonian Library (eBL) (https://www.ebl.lmu.de/library/BM.45559; photo)

Transliteration

Beginning of ms. a obv. i lost

1' a obv. i 1' ⸢*ki*⸣-*ma še-er-*[*ru*? ....]

2' a obv. i 2' *u* GABA.LÀL x[.................................]

3' a obv. i 3' DIŠ MUNUS *šà* ŠÀ-*šà ana šu-š*[*u-ri*? x x x x x]

4' a obv. i 4' *šá* ^giš^GIŠIMMAR *ma-la tara-*x[x x x x x x x]

262 Measurements: 7 x 7.8 x 2 cm.

5'	a obv. i 5'	*tu-šak-kal* 12 ŠU.SI x[x x x x x x x]
6'	a obv. i 6'	*ta-nam-di-ma a-di-i* 3 Š[U.SI x x x x x x x]
7'	a obv. i 7'	*ib-bak i-ni-iq-ma* ^{erasure}-<<*ma*>> ⸢6$^{?}$⸣ ⸢U$_{4}$⸣.MEŠ$^{?}$ x x x x x]
8'	a obv. i 8'	*tu-ra-bu-ʾ-šú-ma bur-ki-šá* G[U$_{7}$.MEŠ-*ši*$^{?}$ x x x] ⸢x⸣
9'	a obv. i 9'	⸢1⸣ ⸢GÍN⸣ ^{na4}*gab-u šá ḫat-ti* 1 GÍN [$^{(ú)}$*a-zu*]-⸢*pi*⸣-*ra-nu*
10'	a obv. i 10'	[*an*]-*daḫ-šú i-na* ŠÀ *ma-la šá* [x] ⸢*i*⸣-*šal-la-mu-u*
11'	a obv. i 11'	[x-]x[263] *pa-ṣu-ú zuk-ku š*[*al-š*]*ú* ⸢NINDA$^{?}$⸣ LÀL *šal-šú* NINDA Ì$^{!}$(NÍG) *ḫal-ṣa*
12'	a obv. i 12'	[*ta-ḫa*]-*qú-ma* NAG-*šú* DIŠ [KI.MIN$^{?}$] BULUḪ$^{?}$ Ì.UDU GU$_{4}$ DUḪ.LÀL
13'	a obv. i 13'	[x SI]G$_{5}^{?}$ BURU$_{5}$ A.AB.BA *an-daḫ-šú* DIDA SIG$_{5}$
14'	a obv. i 14'	[x x x] ⸢x x⸣-[*t*]*i*$^{?}$ DIŠ-*niš* ḪI.ḪI SÚD ^{síg}À[KA NIGIN-*m*]*a*$^{?}$
15'	a obv. i 15'	[x x]x *ana* ŠÀ [ŠUB]-*di alla-nu* DÙ-*uš ana* Š[À.TÙR]-⸢*šú*⸣
16'	a obv. i 16'	[GAR$^{?}$ *t*]*aḫ-sis*$_{x}$(BAD)-*tu*$_{4}$ ⸢MUN⸣ *šum*$_{4}$-*ma ina* GIG.BA *ina* x[x]
17'	a obv. i 17'	[*ḫ*]*u-un-ṭu tu-ḫa-*[*a*]*m-maṭ kus-pú*$^{?}$ 1-*ú tu*-⸢*lam*$^{?}$-*ma*$^{?}$⸣
18'	a obv. i 18'	[x] *pe-en-du* MUNU$_{4}$ [x]-*tu*$_{4}$ *ana* ŠÀ ŠUB-*di* ⸢GÚR.GÚR⸣
19'	a obv. i 19'	[x x]x-*me* ILLU [x x] ⸢x x x x x x⸣
20'	a obv. i 20'	[x x]x-*du* [..........................]
21'	a obv. i 21'	[x x x *ta*]-⸢*šá-ḫal*⸣ [.................]

Bottom of ms. a col. i; beginning of col. ii lost; gap of unknown length

22''	a obv. ii 1'	⸢x⸣ [.................................]
23''	a obv. ii 2'	⸢*ina*⸣ [...............................]

24''	a obv. ii 3'	DIŠ MUNUS [.....................]
25''	a obv. ii 4'	^{na4}[...................................]
26''	a obv. ii 5'	*ina* ⸢Ì$^{?}$⸣ [.............................]
27''	a obv. ii 6'	lu/giš$^{?}$ [.............................]

28''	a obv. ii 7'	⸢KI.MIN⸣ [.........................]
29''	a obv. ii 8'	x[...................................]

Ms. a obv. ii breaks; three lines lost
Ms. a rev. iii too badly worn off for transliteration; traces of ten lines
Beginning of rev. iv lost

30'''	a rev. iv 1'	[x x] x x [x] x x x x x
31'''	a rev. iv 2'	[x x] x x x [x x] x x x x x

263 The traces of the first damaged sign at the beginning of line 11' look like the end of the sign NE.

32''' a rev. iv 3' [x x] x x [x x] x x *tu-*⸢*ša*?-*al*?⸣-[x x]

33''' a rev. iv 4' [x] x x x x x x-*šú*? *šá* ⸢IM⸣ [x]

34''' a rev. iv 5' x [...] x x x x x x x x x ⸢da?⸣

35''' a rev. iv 6' x [...] x x x ⸢${}^{\text{šim}}$KU$_6$?⸣ x x

36''' a rev. iv 7' 1 ⸢GÍN?⸣ [...]x x x x x x-⸢*ma*?⸣

37''' a rev. iv 8' x[.........................] 3-*šú* 4-*šú* ⸢x-*ma*?⸣

38''' a rev. iv 9' *tu-sa-[ma]ḫ* x [.......] x x x x

39''' a rev. iv 10' *i-šal-lim* x[..............] x [x x]

40''' a rev. iv 11' DIŠ MUNUS Ù.TU-*ma* x[............]

41''' a rev. iv 12' KÚM? 1/2 GÍN NAG[A?!.SI ....]

42''' a rev. iv 13' *ina* 4 SÌLA KAŠ ŠE.B[AR?............]

43''' a rev. iv 14' *ana* DÚR-*šú* DUB-*m*[*a* ....]

44''' a rev. iv 15' EGIR *šá* x[....................................]

45''' a rev. iv 16' 1 GÍN *ḫal-ṣa* NU.LUḪ.ḪA ⸢1/2?⸣ [GÍN ...]

46''' a rev. iv 17' EN *ana* x x x[.................................]

47''' a rev. iv 18' x[...]

Ms. a rev. iv breaks; remainder lost

Bound Transcription and Translation

Beginning of ms. a obv. i lost

$^{1'}$ *kīma šer[ru(?) ... ...]* $^{2'}$ *u iškūru [... ...]*

$^{1'}$ As soon as the ba[by(?) ... ...] $^{2'}$ and wax [... ... ...].

$^{3'}$ *šumma sinništu ša libbīša ana šūš[uri(?) ... ...]* $^{4'}$ *ša gišimmari mala ...[... ...]* $^{5'}$ *tušakkal 12 ubānātu ...[... ...]* $^{6'}$ *tanamdi(n)-ma adi šalāš ubā[nātu(?) ... ...]* $^{7'}$ *ibbak inniq-ma šeššet ūm[ē ... ...]* $^{8'}$ *turabbu'ušu-ma burkīša īt[anakkalūši(?) ...]* $^{9'}$ *ištēn šiqil gabû ša ḫatti ištēn šiqil azupīrānu* $^{10'}$ *andaḫšu ina libbi mala ša [...] išallamū* $^{11'}$ *[...]... paṣû zukkû š[alš]u akal dišpa šalšu akal šamna ḫalṣa* $^{12'}$ *[taḫâ]q-ma tašaqqīšu* DIŠ [KI.MIN] *baluḫḫa lipi alpi iškūra* $^{13'}$ *[... dam]qu(?) erib tâmti andaḫšu billat našpi* $^{14'}$ *[...] ... ištēniš tuballal tasâk it[qa talammī-m]a* $^{15'}$ *[...]... ana libbi [tanad]di allāna teppuš ina ša[ssūrī]šu* $^{16'}$ *[tašakkan t]aḫsisti ṭābti šumma ina kibti ina ...[...]* $^{17'}$ *[ḫ]unṭi tuḫammaṭ kuspu ištēnû tulām-ma* $^{18'}$ *[...] pēndu buqla [...]... ana libbi tanaddi kukru* $^{19'}$ *[...]... ḫīl [...] ... ...* $^{20'}$ *traces* $^{21'}$ *[... ta]šaḫḫal [... ...]*

$^{3'}$ So that a woman *gives [birth easily to*(?)] her baby: ... ...] $^{4'}$ of the date palm, as much as ...[...] $^{5'}$ you give (her) to eat. Twelve fingers (full of?) [...] $^{6'}$ you administer, up to three fin[gers(?) *at a time*(?) ...]. $^{7'}$ She (the mother/midwife?) will *bring* (the baby?), it will (then) suck, and (for) six da[ys(?) ... ...]. $^{8'}$ (When) she(?) has (already) reared it(?), but her loins [keep] hur[ting her(?), ...], $^{9'}$ one shekel of alum from Ḫatti, one shekel of *azupīrānu*-plant, $^{10'}$ *andaḫšu*-plant – with it, everyone who/anything that [...], will be well(?). $^{11'}$ [...] A cleansing(?) *paṣû-drink*: $^{12'}$ [You mi]x $^{11'}$ ⸢one third(?)⸣ of a tenth litre of (date) syrup, one third of a tenth litre of pressed (oil), $^{12'}$ and you have her drink (it). Alt[ernatively(?)], *baluḫḫu*-aromatic, ox tallow, wax, $^{13'}$ good(?) [...], 'sea locust' (shrimp?), *andaḫšu*-plant, *billatu*-substance (for making) *našpu*-beer, $^{14'}$ [...] you mix together, crush, [wrap] (it) into a w[ad] of wool.

15' You [a]dd [...] to it, you make an acorn-shaped suppository, 16' [you insert (it)] 15' into he[r womb (viz. vagina)]. 16' Memorandum concerning salt: If 17' you heat/incinerate (it) 16' with wheat, with [...] 17' [(and) ri]pe (barley?), you *should soften* (it) first(?) with sesame pomace. 18' You add [...], charcoal, malt, [... ...] to it. *Kukru*-plant, 19' ..., resin of [...], 20' [...] ... [...] 21' [... you] filter, [... ...].

Bottom of obv. i; beginning of obv. ii lost

22''–23'' *traces*

22''–23'' *too fragmentary for translation*

24'' *šumma sinništu* [... ...] 25'' ...[... ...] 26'' *ina šamni* [... ...] 27'' ...[... ...]

24'' If a woman [... ...], 25'' [...]-stone, [... ....] 26'' with oil [... ...] 27'' ...[... ...].

28'' KI.MIN [... ...] 29'' [... ...]

28'' Alternatively, [... ...] 29'' [... ...]

Ms. a obv. ii breaks; three lines lost
Ms. a rev. iii too badly worn off for transliteration; traces of ten lines
Beginning of rev. iv lost

30'''–34''' *traces* 35''' [... ...] ${}^{\check{s}im}$KU$_6$ ...[...] 36''' *ištēn šiq[il(?)* ...] ... ...*-ma* 37''' ...[...] *šalāšīšu erbîšu* ...*-ma*(?) 38''' *tusa[mma]ḫ* ... [...] 39''' *išallim* [... ...] ...

30'''–34''' *too damaged for translation* 35''' [... ...] ${}^{\check{s}im}$KU$_6$-aromatic ... [...] 36''' one sh[ekel ...] ... . Then 37''' ...[... you ...] three times, four times and(?) 38''' you [mi]x [... ...] .... 39''' (Then) she will be all right, [... ....].

40''' *šumma sinništu ūlid-ma* [... ...] ... 41''' *ēm*(?) *zūz* (*šiqil*) *uḫū[lu qarnānû*(?) ... ...]... 42''' *ina erbet qa šikar uṭṭa[ti* ... ...] 43''' *ana šuburrīšu tatabbak-m[a* ... ...] 44''' *arka ša* ...[... ...]

40''' If a woman gives birth, and subsequently [... her ...]... 41''' is hot(?) [...], half a shekel of [horned(?)] alkali, [... ...], 42''' with four litres of barley beer, [... ...], 43''' you pour it into her anus, and [... ...]. 44''' Afterwards ...[... ...].

45''' *ištēn šiqil* (*šamna*) *ḫalṣa nuḫurta zūz* [... ...] 46''' *adi ana* ... [*iturru* ... ...] 47''' ...[... ...]

45''' One shekel of pressed (oil), *nuḫurtu*-plant, half a [shekel of ... *you boil*], 46'' until [*it is reduced*(?)] to [... ...], 47''' ...[... ...]

Ms. a rev. iv breaks; remainder lost

Notes

Line 1': Possibly restore ⸢*ki*⸣*-ma še-er-*[*ru* ...] "when the ba[by ...]", given the mention of the foetus (*ša libbiša*, *šà* ŠÀ-*šà*) in line 3', but since the context is lost, this remains uncertain.

Line 3': Other possible restorations could be *ana šullumi* "(for a woman) to bring (her foetus) to term", *ana šūludi* "to enable (her) to give birth", or even *ana šuddî* "to have (her) abort". A context of delivery seems to be the most probable guess here.

Lines 5' and 6': The term ŠU.SI = *ubānu* "finger" refers to a finger-shaped suppository, often applied to the rectum in medical treatments (CAD U/W, 6 s.v. *ubānu* sub 1c-2'). However, the expression "12 fingers" here could also refer to a measure of length, a "fingerbreadth" (CAD U/W, 6–8 sub 3), although the latter occurs only rarely in medical contexts.

The verb *nadānu* (SUM) "to give; to administer" is also used in Late Babylonian gynaecological texts from Uruk such as SpTU 4, No. 153, where it appears to refer to the application of vaginal suppositories (see text C.1.10).

Line 7': The understanding of the two verbs *ib-bak* and *i-ni-iq-ma* at the beginning of the line are difficult. The form *i-ni-iq-ma* can be connected with *enēqu* "to suck" (preferably the G-stem durative form *inniqma*), the subject should be the newborn sucking breast milk. Concerning the form *ibbak*, there are two homonymous verbs with this G present tense form: *abāku* A "to send; to dispatch, to bring along" (frequently used in Neo-Babylonian texts) and *abāku* B "to turn (something/someone) upside down/face down; to upset". The latter verb may be more probable in the present context (cf. CAD A/1, 3–8, 8–10). Thus, *ibbak* could refer to the activity of a birth helper (midwife) turning the newborn upside down, to encourage it to breathe. In this case, a term for "baby" (e.g. *šerru*) is expected as the direct object of *ibbak* at the end of line 6'. The turning of the baby with its belly pointing to the ground and with its head pointing upside down, may be mentioned as one of the actions of the divine midwife in the Sumerian hymn *Ninisina A* (lines 77–79; Römer 2001, 113; see Böck 2014a, 30, with adopted readings and slightly different interpretation in Steinkeller 2022, 26–27).

Line 8': If we consider *tu-ra-bu-ʾu-šú-ma* to be derived from the D-stem of *rabû* "to become large in size, to increase", the meaning "to rear, to raise" (children) for the D-stem (*rubbû*) first comes to mind. The spelling implies a subjunctive ending (subordinate clause). In this case, the prefix *tu-* in Late Babylonian texts could potentially be used for the 3rd person feminine singular (referring to the female patient). However, the form could also be a second person singular form, in which case we have to consider other meanings of the D-stem, such as "to enlarge; to increase" and "to make (sth.) swell up", which occurs in medical texts with reference to medical preparations, mixed ingredients or dough, less often to bodily symptoms (see CAD R, 45 s.v. *rabû* A sub 5c). Notably, some references listed there are listed in AHw 940 under the verb *rabû* IV, *rabāʾu* II "to set" instead, for the D-stem (sub mng. 2), giving the meaning "to make wet" ("feucht machen"), said of medical ingredients; other meanings of the D-stem of *rabû* IV are "to submerge under water", "to extinguish", "to douse" (see AHw 940b; also CDA² 294).

Line 9': Alum from the land of Hatti occurs in other texts; in a first millennium BCE context the geographical term denotes Syria rather than Asia Minor (cf. CAD G, 7 sub c-1'; Stol 1980–1983, "Leder(industrie)", *RlA* 6, 534 §20; Thavapalan 2020, 188).

Lines 11'–16': Here we find the rare case in which the prescription does not conclude at the end of the line, and in which the new recipe does not start at the beginning of a line or is set apart by a ruling. The same phenomenon of can be observed in lines 11' and 12', with an alternative prescription beginning in the middle of the line.

The phrase *pa-ṣu-ú zuk-ku* in line 11' is interpreted as a "cleansing/purifying *paṣû-drink*" (with *zukkû*, D-stem verbal adjective of *zakû*, understood here in the sense of "cleansing, purifying" rather than "purified"). The expression introduces the following prescription of a potion made with (date) syrup and oil. The term *paṣû* also occurs in a similar context in BM 45736 line 4' (text A.2.5): *pa-ṣu-ú šá ana maš-qut šá sa-ge-*⸢*e*⸣ [*kul-lu-mu* SIG_5/SUM? …] "a *paṣû-drink*, which (is) [good/prescribed(?)] as a potion for [provoking?] the menstrual flow" (also in BM 45736 line 24''). The notion of purification or cleansing in ms. a may be linked with promoting the lochial flow after a woman's delivery, a period during which women were regarded as impure (*musukkatu*). For further discussion, see the *Introduction*, section 4.2.

Line 12': For *ta-ḫa-qu* "you mix" (for *taḫâq*, from *ḫiāqu* "to mix (liquids)", see also BM 42507+ (and dupl.) line 7 (text E.2.1). The verb at the beginning of line 12' may alternatively be restored [*tu-za/zak*]-*ku-ma* "you clarify" (i.e. letting sediments sink down), occasionally attested in medical texts (cf. CAD Z 29 sub 4c; AHw 1506b, D-stem of *zakû* sub 3).

In the present line and in line 45''', *ḫalṣu* "pressed" appears to be used by itself for *šamnu ḫalṣu* "pressed oil". The sign NÍG bevor *ḫal-ṣa* in line 12' seems to be an error (dittography of NÍG following the measurement NINDA = *akalu*(?) "a tenth litre").

Line 16': For *taḫsistu*, see CAD T, 52–54 "memorandum; aide-mémoire" and the *Introduction*, section 4.2. The term is not common as a rubric in medical texts. The word is spelled *taḫ*-BAD-tu_4 in line 16', which suggests a phonetic value /*sis*/ for the sign BAD beside the values *ziz*, *zis* and *ṣiṣ* listed in Borger 2004, MZL, 270 No. 113.

Line 17': The word *ḫunṭu* (variant of *ḫunnuṭu*) means "ripe(ness)" and is used to qualify barley, see AHw 356a s.v. *ḫunnuṭu*; CAD Ḫ, 238a. The dictionaries exclusively list lexical attestations.

For the verb *lummu*, AHw 563b proposed a meaning "to dissolve"; CAD L, 246a suggests this verb is a variant of *lamāmu* A "to chew" (cf. ibid. mng. 2). Scurlock (2014a, 395 with n. 54 *passim*) interprets it in the sense of "to soften", e.g. in SpTU 2, 50: 11 (Scurlock 2014a, 362–363); SpTU 1, 44: 21, 22, 30, 36, 82 and dupl. (Scurlock 2014a, 391–398); BAM 159 v 12 // BAM 543 i 2 (Scurlock 2014a, 400–401). Compare UET 7, No. 123 rev. 8 (see text B.2.2 line 23'; here plant ashes are dissolved(?) in oil).

A.2.5 BM 45736: A Late Babylonian Collection of Prescriptions for Women's Health

This fragment of what must have been a two-column tablet is written in Late Babylonian script. It was purchased by the British Museum from the dealer Joseph Shemtob in 1881 (see Leichty, Finkel and Walker 2019, *CBT* IV–V, introduction and part 5) and may be dated roughly to the Achaemenid period. It preserves the lower portion of column i on the obverse (with bits of the column divider between col. i and ii visible), and the upper portion of column iv on the reverse.

The fragmentary passages in column i contain instructions for delivery mentioning the midwife (*šabsūtu*), followed by prescriptions for abnormal haemorrhage and for regulating *sagû*, the menstrual flow. The passages on the reverse (col. iv) appear to focus on ritual purification and on remedies bringing about release from impurity and providing happiness (*ṭūb libbi*). The latter remedies appear to concern the attainment of fertility and successful conception.

Of interest is the occurrence of the phrase (*šá/mala*) *iq-bak-k*[*a*] "(of which/as much as) one has told you" (lines 7' and 10'), which is also used in a Late Babylonian medical text on women's health from Uruk (SpTU 4, No. 153 obv. 4), and which may refer to information transmitted orally (see also line 26'', *ša pî* "oral lore"). Another feature that BM 45736 shares with SpTU 4, No. 153 from Uruk (and other Late Babylonian medical texts) is the regular occurrence of the verb *nadānu* (SUM) "to give; to prescribe; to administer", as a general term for the application of a remedy. Ms. a also shares several common ingredients used to stop abnormal female haemorrhage with other first millennium BCE texts from Babylonia (see e.g., SpTU 4, No. 153, FLP 1306, see section C.1 in this volume), pointing to elements of a common tradition of pharmaceutical lore.

List of Manuscripts

Siglum	Museum Number	Copy	Collation	Format; Ductus	Provenience
a	BM 45736 (81-7-6, 146 + 81-7-6, 379 + 81-7-6, 408)	Strassmaier, Folio 595c–d Pl. 18	Coll.	Fragment of a two-column tablet; Late Babylonian script; ca. 5th/4th cent. BCE[264]	probably Babylon

Overview

i'	Fragmentary instruction a obv. i 1'–3'	...]1'–3'
ii'	Instruction concerning a potion for the menstrual flow (*sagû*) a obv. i 4'	4'
iii'	Instruction concerning a potion for the menstrual flow (*sagû*) a obv. i 5'	5'
iv'	Prescriptions (for stopping bleeding) a obv. i 6'–12'	6'–12'
v'	Instruction concerning abnormally heavy bleeding a obv. i 13'–14'	13'–14'[...
vi''	Fragmentary instruction (ritual to restore purity?) a rev. iv 1–3	15''–17''
vii''	Prescription (for 'happiness' and fertility(?)) a rev. iv 4–11	18''–25''
viii''	Fragmentary prescription (poultice) a rev. iv 12–14	26''–28''[...

Previous Edition and Discussion

Electronic Babylonian Library (eBL) (https://www.ebl.lmu.de/library/BM.45736, partial transliteration; copy)
Lambert, Folio 09251 (transliteration)

264 Measurements: ca. 8.8 x 7.7 x 1.9 cm.

Transliteration

Beginning of ms. a obv. i lost

1' a obv. i 1' ^{munus}ŠÀ.ZU *i-ta-[nam-mar*$^{?}$ ....]

2' a obv. i 2' *i-šal-lim ki-i* LÚ.TU[R ....]

3' a obv. i 3' *i-qát-tu-nim-ma* ⸢LÚ.TUR⸣ [................................]

4' a obv. i 4' *pa-ṣu-ú šá ana maš-qut šá sa-ge-*⸢*e*⸣ [*kul-lu-mu* SUM/SIG$_5$$^{?}$ ......]

5' a obv. i 5' GA ÈME *šá ana sa-ge-e* [*kul-lu-mu* SUM/SIG$_5$$^{?}$ ....]

6' a obv. i 6' ^{giš}ḪAB KU.NU.LUḪ.ḪA Ú.NA[M].⸢TIN⸣ [x x x x x] *lu šá* K[A$^{?}$ x]

7' a obv. i 7' *ina* SISKUR$^{!}$(AMARxḪI) *ina* U$_4$ DINGIR-*šá* ⸢DU$_{10}$⸣ ⸢SUM⸣-*in* ŠIKA G[A.N]U$_{11}$⸢$^{mušen?}$⸣ [*l*]*u*$^{?}$ A.⸢MEŠ$^{?}$⸣ *šá iq-bak-k*[*a*]

8' a obv. i 8' *šá i-ṣi giš-ma-ru u te-e*[*l-la*]*-tú*$^{?}$ *lu* A.M[EŠ] ⸢*lu*$^{?}$⸣ *gír-u*$^{?}$ ŠIKA *gul-g*[*ul-li*]

9' a obv. i 9' *lu* KUŠ *giš-šú* UDU.NITA *kab*$^{?}$*-ri*$^{?}$ K[U$^{?}$.K]U$^{?}$ *ṣar-bat* ŠIKA NUNUZ ⸢*lu*⸣*-ur-mu*$^{?}$ KA *tam-tim*

10' a obv. i 10' [*m*]*a-*⸢*la*$^{?}$⸣ *iq-bak-ka* 1.⸢TA⸣.ÀM SUM-*in gab-bi* [1]-*en-šú la* SUM-*in*

11' a obv. i 11' [x x x t]*ú*$^{?}$ SIM ⸢GAZ⸣ *qa-lu-ú u* MAR-*qú i-din* [Ì].UDU BABBAR SIG$_{15}$

12' a obv. i 12' [x x x NU]MUN$^{?}$ MUNU$_5$$^{?}$ NUMUN ^{ú}IN$_6$.UŠ KI *an-n*[*i-t*]*i*$^{?}$ SUM-*in*

13' a obv. i 13' [x x *e-nu*]*-ma* MUNUS MÚD.ME-*šú at-ru-ma nak-da-a*[*t*] *iq-bak-ka*

14' a obv. i 14' [x x x ^{ú}*š*]*á-ki-ru-ú ina ku-ṣu* SIG$_{15}$ *ina* IM NU SAR :

Bottom of ms. a obv. i
Ms. a obv. ii and rev. iii not preserved

15'' a rev. iv 1 [x x x x]-*te* DU$_8$ *u* BAL UDU [... ...]

16'' a rev. iv 2 [x x x x *p*]*u-ḫu-šá* GAR-*m*[*a* ... ...]

17'' a rev. iv 3 *a-di*$^{?}$ *i-zak-ku-ú* [*i*$^{?}$]*-bal-lu-ṭu ṭ*[*u-ub lìb-bi*$^{?}$ (NU) GAR$^{?}$ (...)]

18'' a rev. iv 4 *e-nu-ma* ŠÀ.ḪÚL.LA [*ana* x x] ⸢ZÌ$^{?}$⸣ ZÍZ GEŠTIN DU$_{10}$.[GA x x x x x]

19'' a rev. iv 5 *tu-ban-ni* 3 SÌLA ^{giš}x[x x x ^{gi}]$^{š?}$ZÚ.LUM.MA [x x x x]

20'' a rev. iv 6 *ina* KAŠ ZÚ.LUM.MA ⸢LUḪ⸣-*s*[*i* x x x]x⸢$^{sar?}$⸣ 2 G[ÍN$^{?}$ x x]

21'' a rev. iv 7 2 GÍN GÍR 2 GÍN ŠAL 5 GI [DU$_{10}$.GA$^{?}$ x G]ÍN$^{?}$ MUG 1 GÍN x[x x]

22'' a rev. iv 8 2 GÍN *ia-a-ru-tú* 3 GÍN GAM.M[A x]x ḪÁD.D[A$^{?}$ x x]

23'' a rev. iv 9 *tu-pa-ʾ-ṣú a-na a-ḫa-meš* ḪI.[ḪI ....]

24'' a rev. iv 10 *pa-ṣu-ú ana* UGU ŠUB-*di* U$_4$.3.K[AM ....]

25'' a rev. iv 11 *šum$_4$-ma* BAL *ina* U$_4$.4.KAM SAR [.....................]

26'' a rev. iv 12 *ṭi-pi šá* KA *ma-la ta-*x[.....................................]

27'' a rev. iv 13 SÚD-*ma tu-kàṣ-ṣa* EN A.[MEŠ? ....]

28'' a rev. iv 14 ⸢*tu-ṣap*⸣*-p*[*a*? ....]

Ms. a rev. iv breaks; remainder lost

Bound Transcription and Translation

Beginning of ms. a obv. i lost

1' *šabsūtu īta*[*nammar*(?) ... ...] 2' *išallim kī šer*[*ru* ... ...] 3' *iqattûnim-ma šerru* [... ...]	1' the midwife shall ins[pect (her) regularly(?), ...], 2' she will be well. When the ba[by ...], 3' they (the birth pangs?) come to an end, and the baby [...].
4' *paṣû ša ana mašqût ša sagê* [... *nadnu/damqu*(?) ... ...]	4' A *paṣû*-drink, which [is prescribed/good?] as a potion for [...] the (menstrual) flow: [... ...].
5' *šizib atāni ša ana sagê* [... *nadnu/damqu*(?) ... ...]	5' The donkey's milk, which [is prescribed/good(?)] for [...] the menstrual flow [... ...].
6' *ḫûratu tīyatu šammi balāṭi* [... ...] *lū ša* ...[...] 7' *ina nīqi/ikribi*(?) *ina ūmi ša ilīša*(?) *ṭābi*(?) *tanamdin ḫaṣab lu*[*r*-*m*]*i*(?) *lū mê*(?) *ša iqbâkk*[*a*] 8' *ša īṣi giš*(*im*)*maru til*[*la*]*tu lū mû lū girû ḫaṣab gulgu*[*ulli*] 9' *lū mašak gišši immeri kabri sī*[*kt*]*i*(?) *ṣarbati ḫaṣab pel lurmi imbu' tâmti* 10' [*m*]*ala iqbâkka ištēnâ tanamdin gabbi* [*išt*]*iššu lā tanamdin* 11' [...]... *tanappi taḫaššal qalû u eqû idin lipû peṣû damqu*(?) 12' [... ...]... *buqli*(?) *zēr maštakal itti ann*[* īt*]*i tanamdin*	6' *Ḫûratu*-plant (madder), *tīyatu*-(plant), 'plant of life', [...] or of [...] 7' you administer (this) during sacrifice/prayer(?) on the auspicious(?) day *of her god*(?). (Or you apply) os[tri]ch (egg)shell or the sap, as one has told you to, 8' from the wood of date palm or grapevine, or (take) water, or a carat of a sherd from a sk[ull(?)], 9' or the skin from the hip of a fat sheep; ⸢powder(?)⸣ of poplar (wood), ostrich eggshell, *imbu' tâmti*-mineral, 10' (apply of them) as much as one has told you to. You administer (these ingredients) one by one/separately, you should not administer (them) all at once. 11' [...]... you sift (and) crush. Roast and administer (by) daubing on. 12' You (can also) give 11' good(?) white(?) tallow, 12' [...]... of malt(?) (and) seed of *maštakal*-plant together with this (i.e. the aforementioned drugs?).
13' [... *e*]*nūma sinništu dāmūšu atrū-ma nakdat iqbâkka* 14' [...] *šakirû ina kuṣṣi damiq ina ṭuppi ul šaṭer*	13' [... whe]n a woman's (menstrual) blood is excessive in quantity so that she is in a worrying state, (as) one has told you (to prescribe). 14' [...] *šakirû*-plant is good in winter. – (This treatment) is not copied on (this) tablet.

Bottom of ms. a col. i
Obv. col. ii and rev. col. iii not preserved

15'' [...]... *tapaṭṭar u tanaqqi immera*(?) [... ...] 16'' [... ... *p*]*ūḫša tašakkan-ma* [... ...] 17'' *adi izakkû* [*i*]*balluṭu ṭ*[*ūb libbi* (*ul*) *šakin/iššakkan*(?) (...)]	15'' [...]... you remove(?) and you pour a libation(?). A sheep(?) [...], 16'' [...] you provide as her substitute [...]. 17'' Until she becomes pure (and) healthy, h[appiness(?) *will* (*not*) *be established* (*for her*?) (...)].

18'' *enūma ḫūd libbi* [(*lā šaknu*?) *ana*(?) ...] *qēm kunāši karāna ṭāba* [... ...] 19'' *tubanni šalāšat qa* ...[...] *suluppī* [... ...] 20'' *ina šikar suluppi temessi* [...] ... *šina šiq*[*il* ...] 21'' *šina šiqil asu šina šiqil šimeššalû*(?) *ḫamšat qanû* [*ṭābu*(?) ... *šiq*]*il ballukku ištēn šiqil* ...[...] 22'' *šina šiqil yaruttu šalāšat šiqil ṣumlal*[*û* ...]... *tubbal*(?) [...] 23'' *tupâṣ ana aḫāmiš tubal*[*lal* ... ...] 24'' *paṣû ana muḫḫi tanaddi šalāšat ūm*[*ī* ... ...] 25'' *šumma ītetqū ina rebî ūmi tuqattar*(?) [... ...]

18'' When happiness [(*could not be established*?), *to* ... (?)]: emmer flour, good wine, [...] 19'' you *should prepare carefully*. Three litres of ...-wood, [... of] dates [...]. 20'' You wash (it/her) with date beer. ..., two shek[els of ...], 21'' two shekels of myrtle, two shekels of *šimeššalû*-aromatic(?), five (shekels of) ['sweet(?)] reed', [x] shekel(s) of *ballukku*-aromatic, one shekel of [...], 22'' two shekels of *yaruttu*-spice, three shekels *ṣumlalû*-plant, [...] you dry(?), [...], 23'' you crush, you mix together, [...] 24'' you add *paṣû*-beer to it. For three days [... ...]. 25'' When (the three days) have passed by: on the fourth day you fumigate(?) [...].

26'' *ṭīpi ša pî mala* ...[... ...] 27'' *tasâk-ma tukaṣṣâ adi mû*(?) [... ...] 28'' *tuṣapp*[*a*(?) ... ...]

26'' A poultice, according to oral lore(?): as much as ...[...], 27'' you crush and let it cool down, until the fluid(?) [...], 28'' you soak [... ...]

Ms. a rev. iv breaks; remainder lost

Notes

Lines 1'–3': The mention of the midwife and the baby (LÚ.TUR) in these lines makes it likely that the present section dealt with the topic of delivery. In a similar context, the inspection of the patient by the midwife monitoring the progress of labour is mentioned (see SpTU 4, No. 153: 24 from Uruk (text D.1.11): ^{munus}ŠÀ.ZU *tam-mar-ú-ma i-qab-bak-ka um-ma* Ù.TU.DA *qé-ru-ub* "you will (have) the midwife inspect (the woman), and she will tell you thus: 'Birth is near!'"). In the present text, we would have a 3rd person sg. form of *amāru*. The verb in line 1' could be restored as a Gtn-stem durative form *ītanammar*, as a G-stem perfect form or as or a Gt-stem form, (*ītamar* or *ītammar*). A Gtn-stem form could imply the continuous monitoring of the woman during the process of delivery.

Lines 2'–3' may have described a positive and a negative scenario, an easy and a difficult birth situation. The plural G-stem form of the verb *qatû* "to come to an end" in line 3' may perhaps refer back to birth pangs (*ḫīlū*, a plurale tantum) diminishing during a protracted labour process, which would signal a complication. Otherwise, the patient's life (*napištu*; *balāṭu*) may be in danger of coming to an end, cf. the birth incantation on a Middle Assyrian tablet (Lambert 1969, *Iraq* 31, 31: 35; see *infra* text II.1.4): *še-er-ra ku-na-at ana qa-tu-ú* ZI-*te* "she is stuck with the baby to the point to ending (her) life".

Lines 4' and 5': For discussion of the term *sagû*, see the *Introduction*, the texts in section C.2 of this volume as well as BAM 235–236 (texts C.1.2) and SpTU 1, No. 39: 6'–7', commenting on *Diagnostic Handbook* Tablet 36 (TDP 210: 100ff.; see text I.1.2; Wee 2017, *ZA* 107, 240). Both fragmentary lines 4' and 5' in ms. a comment on potions for the menstrual flow (*sagû*). It is not entirely certain, whether the instructions aimed at stopping or provoking the discharge of *sagû*; the reconstruction in the gap is therefore uncertain. There are attestations of prescriptions for either option; in the latter case, the texts speak of making the menstrual flow appear (*kullumu*), see BM 61975: 5' (text C.2.4): MUNUS *sa-gu-šá ana kul-lu-mu* "to make a woman's (menstrual) flow appear"; also BM 38624+ lines 53'''-54''', 61''' (text A.2.1); BM 54587+73802: 21' (text C.2.3; the latter text also includes recipes to stop *sagû*).

The word *paṣû* in line 4' appears to refer to a type of potion, not to a type of beer made from dates (lit. "white/light beer") known from the Neo-/Late Babylonian texts; see the *Introduction*, section 4.2 for discussion. This potion *paṣû* is also encountered in BM 45559+ line 11'–12' (text A.2.4). The latter passage contains a recipe for a *paṣû zukkû* "a cleansing/purifying *paṣû-drink*", which is probably given to the patient to drink after delivery. In the prescription in ms. a line 24'' (see below), however, it is more likely that *paṣû* refers to *paṣû*-beer", since it is added to a preparation as an ingredient. For *mašqûtu* "potion", cf. CAD M/1, 385a sub 2; AHw 629a, for other references of *mašqût* + treated disease/entity in the genitive.

Lines 6'–12': A few ingredients in lines 6'–12' are identical or similar to a passage in SpTU 4, No. 153 obv. 10–17, which deals with *materia medica* to stop female haemorrhage (e.g. during pregnancy or after birth). Identical substances found in SpTU 4, No. 153 obv. 11–12 are ostrich eggshell, sheep bone or other body parts of this animal, *imbû tâmti* (a mineral collected from the seashore, perhaps coral or coral limestone) and powder of poplar wood. For more parallels, see the texts BM 42313+: 28–29 (text A.2.2), K. 20254+ obv. 3'–5' (text C.1.6), FLP 1306: 11–15 (text C.1.8) in this volume.

For *ḫûratu*-plant "madder" (ms. a line 6'), a plant used as a red dyestuff (Thavapalan 2020, 331–338), which is likewise attested in remedies (amulets) to stop bleeding, see BAM 236 line 28' (text C.1.2) and dupl. and well as text F.1 lines 20, 29, 31 and text F.2. line 30' with discussion. For *tīyatu*-plant in prescriptions to stop bleeding, see also K. 8893 obv.(?) 5' (text C.1.6).

Another feature of ms. a is the repeated occurrence of the verb *nadānu* "to give" (in lines 7', 10', 12', written SUM-*in* for *tanaddin/tanamdin* "you give"), in the general sense of "to administer, apply (a drug or remedy)". This usage is also found in SpTU 4, No. 153 and UET 7, No. 123 (see text B.2.2).

Lines 7'–8': At the beginning of line 7', the sign SISKUR is defectively written AMARxḪI, not AMARxŠE. The interpretation of the passage is tentative. The phrase *ina* SISKUR *ina* U_4 DINGIR-*šá* DU_{10} could refer to a specific auspicious ritual timing of the therapeutic action, on the day when the sacrifice to the patient's personal god was performed (the sign SISKUR can be read as Akkadian *nīqu* "sacrifice" or *ikribu* "prayer"). For propitious days (referred to as *ūmu ṭābu* and with similar adjectives) in connection with performing rituals and religious offerings, see CAD U/W, 148–149 sub mng. 1c.

In line 8', we encounter a funny syllabic spelling of *gišimmaru* "date palm" (*giš-ma-ru*). The passage at the beginning of line 8' appears to recommend using the juice(?) (cf. line 7') extracted from the wood of date palm or grapevine (*tillatu*). This remarkable instruction shares similarities with a passage in another Late Babylonian women's healthcare text, SpTU 4, No. 153 obv. 13, which instructs to use powder of a specific type of wood (*ṣarbatu*, poplar), see text C.1.10.

For the expressions *ša iqbâkka* "which one has told you" (line 7') and *mala iqbâkka* "as much as one has told you (to use)" (line 10'), see also SpTU 4, No. 153 obv. 4 (text C.1.10). For similar uses of the expression *ša iqbû* "which is said/prescribed", see SpTU 4, No. 153 lines 5, 7, 13, 17.

Line 12': The ingredient "seed (i.e. kernels?) of malt" (*zēr buqli*) is only rarely attested, and the reading [NU]MUN $MUNU_5$ in this line is tentative at best (cf. CAD B, 323–324, sub a-1'). I am not aware of other references for this ingredient from first millennium BCE medical texts.

On the margin between col. i and ii, on the height of col. i 12', the scribe or collator wrote the correction mark KÚR in a slightly smaller script, marking a passage with textual corruptions or errors. Since such correction marks are usually positioned on the margin or transitional area towards the left edge of the tablet, the marker here belongs to a passage in column ii of the tablet, which is not preserved. For other occurrences in the women's health corpus, see also BM 42313+ line 11 (text A.2.2) and LKA 9 rev. r. col. 13' (text C.3.5).

Lines 13'–14': At the beginning of line 13', one could also think of restoring [KA.INIM].MA "Wording (of an incantation)". The suggested reconstruction of [*enū*]*ma* "when" follows line 18'', where another section starts with *enūma* (see below). At the beginning of line 13' in the gap may have stood a term of a specific type of remedy (such as "potion" or the like) used for the purpose of stopping the haemorrhage. For a similar formulation with *nakādu* "to be in a critical, worrisome state", referring to abnormally heavy vaginal bleeding, see also FLP 1306: 26–27 (text C.1.9): [MUNUS M]ÚD.ME-*šú sa-ad-ru-ma* / [*na-ak-d*]*a-at* "(If) a woman's blood is flowing all the time, so that she is [in a critical state]". See also Mayer 2019, *OrNS* 88, 302 s.v. *nakdu* "(ein Kranker), um den man (nicht) besorgt ist / um den man sich (keine) Sorgen machen muß".

The scribal note in line 14' (at the bottom of col. i) *ina tuppi ul šaṭer* "it has not been copied/written down on (this) tablet" signals that the copyist left out a passage of the source text in his copy. Depending on the restoration of line 13', this means the copyist did not write down the complete prescription or the text of an incantation against abnormal bleeding. For similar scribal notes pointing out that the scribe did not copy part of his *Vorlage*, but left out a section or passage, see CAD Š/2, 229a s.v. *šaṭāru* sub 1b–2'b', e.g. BAM 538 iv 49', a rubric in a Nineveh manuscript of the treatise on ailments of the teeth (TEETH Tablet 1), just before the colophon, which follows an Akkadian incantation, states that the preceding section is a spell for sick teeth" (KA.INIM.MA ZÚ.GIG.GA.KÁM) and that "the ritual procedure for it has not been copied (from the *Vorlage*)" (DÙ.DÙ.BI NU SAR).

Lines 15''–17'': The first passage in column iv of ms. a seems to describe ritual actions that concern the restoration of female purity, physical health and creation of 'happiness' (*ṭūb libbi*). From the contextual hints that can be gleaned from following two passages (lines 18''–25'' and lines 26''–28'') we surmise that *ṭūb libbi* 'happiness' is linked here with the successful conception of a child (and a woman's unfulfilled desire to have offspring). Compare especially BAM 240: 70' (text D.2.1) for (*lā*) *ṭūb libbi* "(un)happiness" in connection with a woman's inability to conceive/infertility.

Line 15'': Several possible readings could be suggested for the traces preserved in line 15''. The sign DUḪ may be read *tuḫḫū* "bran; draff", or as DU_8 = *paṭāru* "to loosen; to release (a person), undo (evil, sin, illness); to remove (an offering)", also "to depart; to stop" (intransitive), cf. CAD P, 286–298. The following *-u* may be a phonetic complement or *u* "and; or". The next sign BAL can likewise be interpreted in different ways: as a logogram, it may stand for *ballukku*-aromatic (written without the classifier šim) or for the verb *naqû* "to libate; to sacrifice". Because of the mention of a ritual substitute (*pūḫu*) I have opted to read the passage as ritual actions (cf. CAD P, 290a sub 1h).

Line 17'' and 18'': Following the tentative restoration of these lines, we expect here an expression with *ṭūb libbi* "happiness" and statements that refer to the patient's current situation (lack of "happiness") and the aim of the ritual/healing procedure (to establish "happiness"). Several expressions with such a meaning are attested, e.g. *ṭūb libbi* + *šakānu* "to provide", *amāru* "to see, experience" and *rašû* "to get", see CAD Ṭ, 118–119 s.v. *ṭūbu* sub mng. g.

Lines 18''–25'' and 26''–28'': The nature of the prescriptions and their ingredients point to their purpose of purification and attainment of fertility. Lines 18''–25'' focus on a bath/ablution performed on three consecutive days, followed in lines 26''–28'' by a fragmentary recipe for a poultice (*ṭīpu*). These two sections in ms. a share several similarities with a section in BAM 244: 10–30 from Assur (text B.1.1), a text likewise concerned with promoting female fertility and removing impurity. The latter passage likewise consists of instructions for preparing a medicinal bath (lines 10–21) in which the woman bathes three days in a row, as in ms. a. This procedure is also followed by a bandage (lines 21–30, *naṣmattu*). The sections of BM 45736 and BAM 244 under discussion also share a few parallel ingredients (such as *ballukku*-aromatic, *ṣumlalû*). Furthermore, the ingredient *šimeššalû* is used in a remedy for a woman who has stopped to bear (children) in BAM 243 obv.$^?$ 6' (text B.1.2).

Line 19'': The verb form *tu-ban-ni* at the beginning of line 19'' is understood here as a D-stem of *banû* B "to grow; to be pleasant", with the meaning "to prepare (foodstuffs) carefully; to adorn, beautify". However, a durative form (*tubanna*) rather than a preterite would be expected here. It is therefore possible that *tubanni* marks a preceding step in the procedure in line 18'' ("(when) you have carefully prepared (this), ..."). I am not aware of similar attestations of this verb from medical texts.

Line 20'': For KAŠ ZÚ.LUM.MA (*šikar suluppī*) "date beer", a fermented alcoholic beverage produced from dates, see Landsberger 1967, 56; Stol 1994, 157, 161 n. 58, 166–167 with n. 129; CAD Š/2, 428 s.v. *šikaru* sub 2a; SpTU 2, No. 23: 8 (drunk in a ritual); BAM 159 ii 15' (drunk against intestinal bloating). Note, in economic documents, e.g. YOS 6, No. 66: 16: 10 GUR ZÚ.LUM.MA *ana* KAŠ.ḪI.A "10 gur (= 1800 litres) of dates for beer"; TCL 12, No. 1: 1, 17–18 (Moore 1935, 2–3; Brinkman 2007), mentioning KAŠ *pa-ṣu-ú*, lit. "white beer" beside KAŠ ZÚ.LUM.MA "date beer". For *paṣû* as a kind of beverage in prescriptions for women, see text BM 45559+ line 11' (text A.2.4); BM 45736 line 4', 24'' (text A.2.5) and the Introduction, section 4.2.

Line 21'': Instead of GI [DU_{10}.GA] "sweet reed", one may alternatively restore GI.[ZU.LÚM.MA], the latter of which is perhaps to be read as Akkadian *kūru*-plant or *buṣinnu* "wick".

Lines 21''–22'': Several logograms for plant names in these lines are written without classifiers, e.g. ŠAL for ^{šim}ŠAL; similarly, $^{(\text{šim})}$MUG and $^{(\text{šim})}$GAM.MA. For *yaruttu*, an aromatic, see also Finkel 2000, *FS Lambert*, 188 Text 31: 8'.

Line 25'': For the passing of time, expressed with *etēqu* "to pass by", see CAD E, 387–388 sub 1f; AHw 261b sub 5.

Line 26'': For the expression *ṭīpu ša pî*(KA), compare SpTU 1, No. 44: 79; Scurlock 2014a, 394, 398, where a remedy against the *bu'šānu*-disease affecting the mouth and nose is classified as such (*ṭì-pu ša* KA "poultice/plaster for the mouth", followed by the explanation *naṣmat*(LÁ) *pî*(KA) "a bandage for the mouth"). The sign KA is ambiguous and could also be read *šá* $KIRI_4$ "for the nose". In the present context, I wonder whether *ša pî* means "according to oral lore" (lit. of the mouth; cf. CAD P, 466 s.v. *pû* sub 6; Gabbay 2016, 20–21, 51–52), unless *pû* "mouth" would be used euphemistically for the vulva.

Line 28'': For the verb *ṣapû* (D-stem) "to soak, to drench" (medical ingredients with a liquid substance), see AHw 1082 s.v. *ṣapû* II, e.g. BAM 160 obv. 6' // BAM 159 ii 15' (Parys 2014, *JMC* 23, 15; Scurlock 2014a, 529–530).

A.2.6 BM 47491: Love Magic and Women's Health

This Late Babylonian tablet has an almost cushion shaped form and is burned black on the reverse. It is registered in the Babylonian Collection of the British Museum as coming from the excavations of Hormuzd Rassam in Babylonia; it may have originated from Babylon or Borsippa.[265] According to the colophon, the tablet was owned and written by Iprā'ya, a member of the Ēṭiru family and known from colophons of scholarly texts (especially commentaries and texts of medical, astrological and divinatory content). According to the information gleaned from other colophons of tablets owned by Iprā'ya, he may have lived in the fifth or fourth century BCE during the Achaemenid period. A second tablet written by Iprā'ya that contains a text related to women's health is BM 47459 (see text D.3.1 ms. f in this volume).

While Finkel (1988, *FS Sachs*, 154) classified BM 47491 as gynaecological, not all contents of the tablet are strictly medical in nature or concerned with women's diseases. Thus, the sections on the obverse bear the rubric *ša šudbubi* "to make (someone) talk". This is probably to be understood as an abbreviation for a genre of love magic known under the designation (*ana*) MUNUS *šudbubu* "(for) making a woman agree (to have sexual intercourse)". Attestations for this genre are sparse, and therefore the three prescriptions in BM 47491 form interesting additions to this genre. Thus, a prescription introduced by *ana sinništi šudbubi*, in a Neo-Assyrian tablet from Assur with incantations, rituals and prescriptions for attracting a woman (cf. Biggs 1967, 71 KAR 61: 22–25), is the only attestation for this type of magic procedure (other sections in KAR 61 are rituals "for making a woman come (to have intercourse)", (*ana*) MUNUS GIN.NA). While the ritual "for making a woman talk" in KAR 61: 22–25 is a list of ingredients which are wrapped into sheep wool and placed at the performer's bed, the three sections on BM 47491 consist of lists of ingredients with only sparse instructions; only the last section explicitly states that the drugs had to be daubed on the eyes.

The genre MUNUS *šudbubu* is further mentioned from the so-called "Exorcist's Almanac" BRM 4, 20 (lines 17 and 53), a list of various types of magic or healing rituals, paired with the corresponding zodiac sign (or month), during which the rituals should be performed to be particularly effective (Reiner 1990; Geller 2002, 131–132; Geller 2014, 29, 32). This tablet from the 4th cent. BCE was owned by the scholar Iqīšâ. In the Almanac, which lists several other types of love magic, rituals "for making a woman 'talk'" are scheduled for the zodiac sign Aries (KI ^{mul}LÚ.ḪUN.[GÁ] = *agru* "Hireling"). A commentary in the latter part of BRM 4, 20 (line 53) explains the expression MUNUS *šudbubu* (see Geller 2005b for discussion). Erika Reiner (1995), drawing on parallels in Greco-Roman texts and on Mesopotamian necromantic rituals in which a dead person is invoked to utter an oral message, suggested a different interpretation for the phrase MUNUS *šudbubu*, in the sense of "to make (a woman) speak" in her sleep to reveal whether she has a lover or has been unfaithful (for similar forms of magic in Medieval Jewish tractates, see e.g. Caballero-Navas 2004, 142–143 with n. 14).[266] Although the exact meaning of *šudbubu* in BM 47491 alludes us, the association with prescriptions for a female patient on the reverse suggests a connection with the genre MUNUS *šudbubu*.[267]

The reverse of BM 47491 contains three prescriptions for salves (EŠ = *napšaltu*) for "a woman with fever/heat" (MUNUS *ša* KÚM). The purpose statement is somewhat ambiguous. Most likely, the sign KÚM stands for Akkadian *ummu* "heat, fever", designating a febrile condition. Since two types of this "heat" (*ummu*) are differentiated (KÚM *šalšu* "tertian fever(?)" and KÚM *lemnu* "bad fever"), this interpretation is most likely. Less likely the sign KÚM may stand for IZI, corresponding to Akkadian *išātu* "fire". In a few healing texts, *išātu* "fire" is a term for a skin sore as well as a metaphorical term for fever (see below). Moreover, it is not totally excluded that "heat" or "fire" is meant in a sexual way. Thus, in love incantations, fire and burning are metaphors for passionate emotions of love, desire as well as jealousy, witnessed, for example, in the similar rubric "(incantation to calm) the fire of the heart" (IZI ŠÀ.GA = *išāt libbim*) known from Old Babylonian love incantations (Wasserman 2016, 42, 248–250, with No. 24: 8 and also No. 23: note on line 9).

265 Leichty, Finkel and Walker 2019, *CBT* IV–V, 662.

266 The prescriptions for this kind of magic are not ointments, as is the case with the *šudbubu*-remedies discussed here, but objects brought close to the targeted person. An example from *The Book of Women's Love* edited by Caballero-Navas (ibid.) reads: "To discover all that a woman has done, and also a man: Take the tongue of a goose and put it on their breasts while they are sleeping, and they will tell you all they have done. ... The sages of Greece said (fol. 75v): Also if you put lodestone, that is called magnet, under her head and if she has committed adultery, she will be afraid and fall out of the bed; if not, she will embrace her husband tight."

267 For a parallel to *šudbubu* in Talmudic culture, see Boyarin 1993, *Carnal Israel*, 121–125, 129–131. The Talmud uses the term "talking" as a pun for sexual intercourse, and in the sense of talking about one's desire for intercourse to rouse the partner (in the context of marriage). Talmudic discourses on this topic usually prefer the husband in the active role (who however needs his wife's consent to have sex), although some positions approve to the wife speaking about her desire.

List of Manuscripts

Siglum	Museum Number	Copy	Collation	Format; Ductus	Provenience
a	BM 47491 (81-11-3, 196)	Pl. 19	Coll.	Single-column tablet in portrait format; Late Babylonian script; 5th or 4th cent. BCE[25]	Babylon or Borsippa

Overview

i Ingredients for "making (someone) talk" 1–11
a obv. 1–11
ii Ingredients for "making (someone) talk" 12–13
a obv. 12–13
iii Rubric 14
a obv. 14
iv Prescription for an eye salve to "make (someone) talk" 15–17
a obv. 15–17
v Prescription for a woman suffering from fever (salve) 18–20
a rev. 1–3
vi Prescription for a woman suffering from fever (salve) 21–23
a rev. 4–6
vii Prescription for a woman suffering from fever (salve) 24–26
a rev. 7–9
viii Colophon 27–29
a rev. 10–12

Previous Edition and Discussion

Electronic Babylonian Library (eBL) (https://www.ebl.lmu.de/library/BM.47491; photo)

Transliteration

1 a obv. 1 *ka-ar-ka pa-šú* ḪUL.⸢*A*⸣.MEŠ-*šú šá* x[x x]

2 a obv. 2 *ana* IGI-*šú* DU-*ak* SAG.DU *a-ri-bi*$^{\text{mu[šen]}}$

3 a obv. 3 KUŠ GU$_4$ GI$_6$ ^{ú}KUR.KUR *šá ina* IZI *ku-ub-bu-ub-*[*bu*$^?$]

4 a obv. 4 SUḪUŠ *u*$_5$*-ra-nu* ^{ú}*an-ki-nu-te* ^{ú}*ra-pad-du*

5 a obv. 5 <Ú> GIŠ.⸢GI$^?$⸣ ZÌ ŠE.MUŠ$_5$ ^{ú}*bu-up-pa-nu* ^{giš}ŠUR.MÌN-*ni*

6 a obv. 6 ⸢$^{\text{giš?}}$⸣[x] x x 7 NUMUN *iṣ piš-ri* SUḪUŠ ^{giš}DÌḪ

7 a obv. 7 $^{\text{g[iš}}$x x] ^{ú}⸢x.x.x⸣ ^{giš}NAM.TAR NITA ^{šim}LI

8 a obv. 8 [x x x x Ì].⸢UDU⸣ UR.BAR.RA ^{ú}*ka-si-bi*

9 a obv. 9 [x x] x x ⸢$^{\text{na4}}$⸣*ú-ru-ut-tu*$_4$

10 a obv. 10 $^{\text{n[a4]}}$⸢*im-ma-an*⸣*-na-ku* [$^{\text{na4}}$D]ÚR.MI.NA.BÀN.DA

---

268 Measurements: ca. 5 x 8 x 1.8 cm.

11 a obv. 11 [x Ú].⸢ḪI.A⸣ ⸢*an-nu*⸣*-tu šá šu-ud-bu-bu*

---

12 a obv. 12 [x x] ⸢SAG.DU⸣ *a-ri-bi*^{mušen} ^{šim}LI x x ⸢*bur*⸣*-ru-mu*

13 a obv. 13 [^{ú}KU]R.KUR$^{?}$ *šá ina* IZI ⸢*ku-ub*⸣*-bu-ub-bu* KUM

---

14 a obv. 14 ⸢*šá*⸣ *šu-ud-bu-bu*

---

15 a obv. 15 $^{\text{na4}}$PA $^{\text{na4}}$ZÚ KALA $^{\text{na4}}$ZÚ SIG$_7$

16 a obv. 16 *ina* MÚD *an-ze-e* IGI.MIN-*šú*

17 a obv. 17 *te-qu šá šu-ud-bu-bu*

Remainder of ms. a obv. left blank

18 a rev. 1 EŠ MUNUS *šá* KÚM *šal-šú* Ú A.ŠÀ ^{giš}*šu-*⸢*šum*⸣

19 a rev. 2 GA ÁB *ma-suk-ka-tu*$_4$ Ì.UDU ÉLLAG GU$_4$ GI$_6$

20 a rev. 3 *ina* Ì.GIŠ ^{giš}ŠUR.MÌN-*ni* ŠÉŠ-*aš*

---

21 a rev. 4 EŠ MUNUS *šá* KÚM *lem-nu* ^{šim}⸢ŠEŠ⸣ ^{šim}GÚR.GÚR

22 a rev. 5 ^{šim}LI *bi-iš-*<*šú*>$^{?}$ *ina* IZI ⸢*tur*⸣*-ár*

23 a rev. 6 *ina* Ì.GIŠ *pi-iṭ-ri-šú ta*[*l-t*]*a-nap-pat*

---

24 a rev. 7 EŠ MUNUS *šá* ⸢KÚM⸣ ⸢$^{\text{giš?}}$⸣GE[ŠTIN.KA$_5$.A$^{?}$] ⸢*e*⸣*-lap-pu-ú*

25 a rev. 8 <SAḪAR> *šá*$^{!}$(*ana*) *šap-la-nu*$^{?!}$ MUNUS *šá a-*⸢*la*⸣*-*⸢*du*$^{?}$⸣ *u kib-su*

26 a rev. 9 *tap-ru-su* ^{ú}IGI-*lim ina* Ì.GIŠ ⸢ŠÉŠ$^{?}$⸣-*su*

Colophon:

27 a rev. 10 ZU.A *ana* ZU.A$^{!}$ *li-*⸢*kal-lim*⸣ ⸢NU⸣ ⸢ZU⸣ ⸢NU⸣ I[GI.LÁ$^{?}$]

28 a rev. 11 IM AŠ ŠE.BA-*ʾ-ia* DUMU *šá* ^{md}*za-ba*$_4$*-ba*$_4$-NUNUZ-ÙRU

29 a rev. 12 A ^{m}*e-ṭi-ru* ^{iti}AB U$_4$.27.KAM

Remainder of ms. a rev. left blank

Bound Transcription and Translation

[1] *karkā pāšu lemnētūšu*(?) *ša* … [...] [2] *ana pānīšu tallak qaqqad āribi* [3] *mašak alpi ṣalmi atāʾišu ša ina išāti kubbubu* [4] *šuruš urâni ankinūtu rapaddu* [5] *šammi api*(?) *qēm šegušši buppānu šurmēnu* [6] … *sebet zēr iṣ pišri šuruš balti* [7] … … *pillû zikaru burāšu* [8] [...] *lipi barbari kassibu* [9] … *uruttu* [10] *immanakku turminabandû* [...] [11] [... *šam*]*mū annûtu ša šudbubi*

[1] Her(?) two mouths are blocked(?), her(?) wicked ones which [...] – [2] you will (be able to) approach her(?): a raven's head, [3] the hide of a black ox, *atāʾišu*-plant which has been charred over a fire, [4] root of *urânu*-plant, *ankinūtu*-plant, *rapādu*-plant, [5] canebrake-plant(?), flour of *šegušš̌u*-millet, *buppānu*-plant, cypress, [6] …, seven seeds(?) of "wood of release", root of *baltu*-plant, [7] …, …-plant, male *pillû*-plant, *burāšu*-juniper, [8] [...], 'wolf's tallow' (tamarisk?), *kassibu*-plant, [9] …, *uruttu*-stone, [10] *immanakku*-stone, *turminabandû*-stone – [11] these [...] drugs are for making (a woman?) agree (to have intercourse).

[12] [...] *qaqqad āribi burāšu ... burrumu* [13] *[atā]'išu ša ina išāti kubbubu taḫaššal*	[12] You crush [...], a raven's head, *burāšu*-juniper, multicoloured ..., [13] *atā'išu*-plant which has been charred over a fire.
[14] *ša šudbubi*	[14] (These are drugs) for making (a woman?) agree (to have intercourse).
[15] *ayyartu ṣurru dannu(?) ṣurru arqu* [16] *ina dām Anzê īnīšu* [17] *teqqi ša šudbubi*	[17] You daub [16] her(?) eyes [15] with *ayyartu*-shell, hard *ṣurru*-stone (obsidian?) (and) yellow-green *ṣurru*-stone [16] (mixed) with 'blood of the Anzû-bird'. [17] (It is) for making (a woman) agree (to have intercourse).
[18] *napšalti sinništi ša ummi šalši šammi eqli šūšu* [19] *šizib litti masukkati šaman kalīt alpi ṣalmi* [20] *ina šaman šurmēni tapaššaš*	[18] A salve for a woman with tertian(?) fever ("heat"): You rub (her) with 'field (clod) plant', liquorice, [19] milk of an 'impure' cow (i.e. one that has recently given birth), fat from the kidney of a black ox [20] (mixed) with cypress oil.
[21] *napšalti sinništi ša ummi lemni murra kukra* [22] *burāša biššu(?) ina išāti turrar* [23] *ina šamni piṭrīšu ta[lt]anappat*	[21] A salve for a woman with bad fever ("heat"): you desiccate *murru*-aromatic, *kukru*-aromatic, [22] *burāšu*-juniper (and) *biššu*-plant(?) over the fire. [23] You repeatedly smear her *piṭru* with (these plants mixed with) oil.
[24] *napšalti sinništi ša ummi kar[ān šēlebi(?)] elappû* [25] *<eperu> ša šaplān sinništi ša alāda u kibsa* [26] *taprusu imḫur-līm ina šamni tapaššassu*	[24] A salve for a woman with fever ("heat"): you rub her with [fox] gr[ape(?)], algae, [25] <dust> from *the lower extremities* (lit. below) of a woman [26] who has ceased [25] to bear and (to experience) the (normal) *course* (of women's menses), [26] (and) 'heals thousand'-plant (mixed) with oil.

Colophon:

[27] *mūdû ana mūdê likallim lā mūdû lā im[mar(?)]* [28] *tuppi Iprā'ya māru ša Zababa-pir'u-uṣur* [29] *mār Ēṭiru Abu* U_4.27.(-)KAM	[27] A knowledgeable person shall (only) show it to a knowledgeable person. An ignorant person shall not s[ee it(?)]. [28] Tablet of Iprā'ya, son of Zababa-pir'u-uṣur, [29] a descendant of (the) Ēṭiru (family), (written on) the 27th day of Abu (V).

Notes

Lines 1–2: The introduction to the first section on the obverse of the tablet is highly unusual and almost reminds us of an incantation incipit, although the text does not make this explicit. However, the usual *šumma* "if" introducing a description of the treated problem in medical texts is lacking. On the other hand, line 1 as well as the beginning of line 2 do not appear to list names of *materia magica*.

I have opted to link the first word *ka-ar-ka* in line 1 with the verb *karāku*, which means "to obstruct, to dam" (a waterway), but is occasionally found with body parts terms, in the meaning "to bind; to gag" (cf. CAD K, 199; AHw 446 "aufwickeln, zusammenfassen"). The form *ka-ar-ka* may indicate a feminine plural form of the stative; thus, *pa-šú* may in fact be a dual of *pû* (i.e. "her(?) two mouths are bound"). Given a likely connection of the prescription with love magic, the "two mouths" could allude to the aim of the prescription, i.e. to make a woman "speak" and consent to intercourse. "Her mouths are blocked" would mean the woman is not accessible, she does not agree verbally to grant a man access to her vulva. If this interpretation is correct, the masculine pronominal suffix -*šú* would consistently be used to refer to a feminine target or patient in BM 47491 (see also lines 16 and 23).

The following fragmentary passage in line 1 is difficult to restore. The plural form ḪUL.MEŠ-*šú* "her(?) bad ones(?)" may resume the "mouths". The phrase *ana* IGI-*šú* DU-*ak* at the beginning of line 2 appears to belong to the introductory statement in line 1. The expression *ana pānī*+pronominal suffix *alāku* can have the meanings "to go to meet someone, to visit", "to approach someone" or "to improve, to prosper" (CAD A/1, 318 s.v. *alāku* sub 4c-1'). Assuming a relation of *šudbubu* to the genre MUNUS *šudbubu* "to make a woman consent (to have intercourse)", a contextually fitting rendering for the expression may be *ana pānīšu tallak* "(so that) you can approach her", addressing a male. Note in this connection the related expression *ana sinništi alāku* "to go to a woman = to have intercourse with a woman" (CAD A/1, 321 sub 4c-7'; Zisa 2021, 46–47, 57, 64, 73–74 *passim*).

Line 2: Several of the animal ingredients in lines 2–11 are reminiscent of substances encountered in Late Babylonian astro-medical / astro-magical calendar texts, which systematically correlate days and months throughout the year with zodiac signs and micro-zodiacal correspondences and list specific substances associated with each sign, often following the schema of the name of a stone, a tree/wood, and a plant corresponding with a given sign/star name (see e.g., Heeßel 2000, 111–127; Heeßel 2005; 2008; Schreiber 2018a; 2018b). The substances are used predominantly for amulets, ointments or fumigations.

As can further be shown, in astro-medical texts associating animal substances with stars, the listed substances often relate to animals that symbolise sections of the zodiac or allude to the names of stars in the vicinity of the indicated zodiac sign (Wee 2006, 178–181; Schreiber 2018a, 511–514). For example, in the astro-magical calendar texts, the head of a raven is listed beside its blood and wings as substances used on days associated with the zodiac sign Virgo (^{mul}AB.SÍN "Furrow"), because the constellation Corvus (^{mul}UGA^{mušen} "Raven-star") is found in the vicinity of Virgo (Weidner 1967, 9–10; Reiner 1995, 117; Wee 2006, 179–180; Schreiber 2018a, 513–514; 2018b, 420, 423, 424).

Some of the animal ingredients listed in the obverse of BM 47491 are known from drug compendia as alias names for plants. Notably, "head of a black raven" (SAG.DU BURU$_5$ GI$_6$) is listed as an alias name for the *ṣaṣumtu*-plant in Uruanna III 103 (Rumor 2017, *JMC* 29, 19). On the other hand, the mention of a "raven's head" in line 3 (see also line 12 below) reminds us of the actual use of birds (e.g. blood, heads) in treatments for promoting sexual desire (ŠÀ.ZI.GA), where the use of a raven's head or heart are occasionally attested for the use in an ointment (Zisa 2021, 165–166, 169, 180–181 *passim*). For the head or skull of a raven in medical texts, see further CAD A/2, 265–267 s.v. *āribu* esp. sub 1c; AHw 68; Salonen 1973, 124–131. Note, in a women's healthcare text: BAM 237 rev. iv. 34 (as an ingredient in a potion to treat a discharge of fluids from the vagina).

Line 3: "*Atā'išu*-plant, which has been charred over a fire" (^{ú}KUR.KUR *šá ina* IZI *ku-ub-bu-ub-bu*) is found again as an ingredient in line 13. The scribe erroneously doubled the third consonant in *kubbubu* (stative of the D-stem of *kabābu* "to char, to burn"). Cf. CAD K, 2 s.v. *kabābu* sub 2b.

Line 4: On *rapādu* (*rapaddu*), a psychoactive, intoxicating plant growing in the steppe that causes insanity or delirium and is associated with witchcraft, see Heeßel 2002, *FS Walker*, 100 BM 59634: 10 (given in beer to make someone drunk); Abusch and Schwemer 2016, CMAwR 2, text 7.24; Stol 2017, *BiOr* 74, 374; Stol 2022, *BiOr* 79, 326–327. In the anti-witchcraft incantation edited by Abusch and Schwemer (a tablet of the scholar and exorcist Iqīšâ, 4th cent. BCE), the *rapādu*-plant (described as having a blue or purple colour) is assigned to the goddess Ištar, which fits its use in the present text associated with love magic. The prescription appended to that incantation (Abusch and Schwemer 2016, CMAwR 2, text 7.24 lines 25–26) prescribes *rapādu*-plant in *našpu*-beer, which when given to drink has the following effect: *mimma mala tašallūšu idabbub-ma* "whatever you ask him, he will say (*dabābu*)". The meaning of this passage is unclear, but the reference to talking and *šudbubu* in BM 47491 may not be incidental.

Line 5: The emendation of the first ingredient name in this line, to <Ú> GIŠ.GI, *šammi api* "canebrake plant", is tentative (this plant occurs in Uruanna II 327, cited in CAD A/2, 199 s.v. *apu* A lex. section).

A plant with the name *buppānu* is not yet attested in the dictionaries. The word *buppānu* literally means "face" or "on (its) face", which may point to a plant that creeps close to the ground (cf. AHw 139 s.v. *buppānī-*; CAD B, 322 *buppāni*; SAD Vol. 1, 45).

The drug name "head of a raven" (*qaqqad āribi*), which already occurred in line 2, is listed beside *šegušsu*-flour, one of the ingredients of line 5, in a Neo-Babylonian list of substances (stones and plants), in this case for use against different disease demons (CT 14, 16 (= BM 93084) rev. 4). In SpTU 4, No. 104 and 105, two astro-medical calendar texts from Late Babylonian Uruk owned by the scholar Iqīšâ, different drug ingredients are listed for ointments prepared on different days of the months Du'ūzu and Araḫsamna. The listed ingredients bear relations with the zodiac signs to which they correspond (Reiner 1995, 116–117; Wee 2006, 178–181; Schreiber 2018a, 511–514; 2018b, 417–425). Interestingly, similar to ms. a, flour of *šegušsu*-millet is likewise found beside "head and feathers of a raven" in SpTU 3, No. 104: 12 and 25; No. 105: 5, 18, 31, as a *materia medica* corresponding to the zodiac sign Virgo – an association that is based on the constellation

Spica ("Ear of Grain") which is found in the vicinity of Virgo (Wee 2006, 179–180; Schreiber 2018b, 525; see also note on line 2 above). For *šeguššu*, see Stol 1993–1997a, "Mohrhirse", *RlA* 8, 348–349; Dornauer 2018, 29, 87 (interpreted as a variety of proso millet).

Line 8: The drug "wolf's fat" is listed as an alias name for tamarisk in Uruanna III 512 (Ú Ì.[UDU] UR.BAR.RA = Ú ^{giš}*bi-nu*; see KADP 27 rev. 25', cited in CAD B, 109 s.v. *barbaru* sub 1e, variant Ú *ga-bi-id* UR.BAR.RA = Ú ^{giš} *bi-nu* "wolf's liver" = tamarisk" (cf. CAD B, 259 s.v. *bīnu* lex. section).

Note in connection with the listing of "wolf's fat" and *kassibu*-plant in line 8, the similar use of "wolf hair" beside *kassibu*-plant and fat from the kidney of a black ox (in a medicine bag) in BAM 311: 44' (against epilepsy). In BAM 469 rev. 28–29 // BAM 471 iv 12'–13', "wolf excrement" is found beside *kassibu*-plant, "lion fat" and fat from the kidney of an ox (for a fumigation against Hand of the ghost), see Scurlock 2006, No. 283; further CAD K, 247 s.v. *kassibu*.

Line 9: According to the dictionaries, the *uruttu*-stone seems to have been attested only in lexical lists and in the mythological text Lugale so far, cf. CAD U/W, 272 s.v. *uruttu* A; AHw 1437a.

Line 12: I am unable to decipher the last ingredient in this line qualified by the adjective *burrumu* "multicoloured; polychrome". This adjective (beside *barmu* "multicoloured") is often found as a characterization of various animals such as lizards, ants, scorpions and mammals, but also of minerals and wool (see AHw 107, 140; CAD B, 112–113, 331–332; Thavapalan 2020, 79–89 "multihued; versicoloured"). In medical prescriptions, "multicoloured lizard" (EME.DIR/EME.ŠID GÙN.A, *ṣurārû barmu*) is attested a number of times, for example, in texts for promoting sexual desire (ŠÀ.ZI.GA), but it is also attested in women's healthcare texts (cf. BAM 246: 2, 8 (text B.1.6) for "multicoloured wall-lizard" in recipes for abortion). See Zisa 2021, 167 *passim*.

Line 15: A mineral ^{na4}ZÚ KALAG (*ṣurru dannu*) "hard *ṣurru*-stone" is not attested elsewhere (Schuster-Brandis 2008, 457–458; CAD Ṣ, 258–259; AHw 1114). Since ^{na4}ZÚ SIG$_7$ "yellow-green *ṣurru*-stone" follows, perhaps one should read ^{na4}ZÚ SA$_5^!$ "red *ṣurru*-stone" instead of ^{na4}ZÚ KALA. So far only light (ZALAG), black/dark (GI$_6$) and yellow-green varieties of *ṣurru* are attested. M. Stol (personal communication) suggests KALAG may be an error for ZALAG.

Line 16: "Blood of the Anzû-bird", the famous mythical bird who stole the tablet of destinies, is attested as a drug name in Late Babylonian astro-medical calendar texts that equate the days of different months with a zodiac sign and recommend corresponding drug ingredients to be used on each day (SpTU 3, No. 104–105; Reiner 1995, 116–177; Wee 2006, 178–181; Schreiber 2018a, 515; 2018b, 417–425). In SpTU 3, No. 104–105, specific days of months Du'ūzu and Araḫsamna are correlated with the zodiac sign Sagitarrius (^{mul}PA.BIL.SAG) and with the ingredients "head, wings, and blood of Anzû-bird" (see SpTU 3, No. 104: 11, 24; No. 105: 8, 21; also head, wings and fat of Anzû-bird in BM 35072 + 47755 iii 10'; Schreiber 2028b, 483, 489). Because of the mythological nature of the Anzû-bird, the ingredient "blood of Anzû-bird" may have to be interpreted as alias name for a plant or other drug, perhaps an oil or resin (note the equation of "blood of the Anzû-bird with *qutru*-plant in BM 35072 + 47755 iii 23' (Schreiber 2018b, 484, 490). It is also possible that the mythological bird was replaced by an animal existing in nature (e.g. a bat or an eagle; see Wee 2006, 180–181; Schreiber 2018b, 500, 522, 526). The medical commentary BAM 307: 19 and 25 attests to other alias drug names of the same format, referencing a body part of the Anzû-bird: "talon (*ṣupru*) of Anzû-bird" seems to be equated with *amurdinnu*-bramble, and "wing (*rittu*) of Anzû-bird" with an unknown stone (CAD A/2, 155 sub d-3'; https://www.geschkult.fu-berlin.de/e/babmed/Corpora/BAM-3/BAM-3_-307). Note further the cult commentary CBS 6060 and duplicates, which contains the equation *dām erēni šaman anzî* "cedar 'blood' is the fat of the Anzû-bird" (Livingstone 1986, 178–179: 59; also ibid., 60–61, further equating *dišpu* "honey" with the "pus (LUGUD, *šarku*) of Anzû", and naphtha (Ì.ḪUL, *napṭu*) with "his (= Anzû's) tallow/fat").

Lines 18, 21 and 24: The references to specific types of fever or "heat" (KÚM = *ummu*) that affect women in these lines are not familiar from other texts on women's health or from texts dealing with fevers, although symptoms of puerperal fever are treated in other prescriptions for women, see e.g. BAM 240: 39–66 (text D.2.1).

The expression *ummu šalšu* "tertian (lit. third) fever (lit. heat)" in line 18 is totally unique for Mesopotamian medical texts; however, tertian fever (*tritaios pyretos*; Latin *febris tertiana*, i.e. fever recurring every third day) is a common type of fever in Graeco-Roman medicine, beginning with the Hippocratic texts (see, for example, *Affections* Chapter 18; Potter 1988, 31–33). In modern medicine, tertian fever is a type of intermittent fever, i.e. a pattern of fever in which the patient manifests intervals or phases of an elevated and normal temperature following each other. Such fever patterns are common in infectious diseases caused by specific microorganisms, such as malaria and tuberculosis. Tertian fever is an intermittent fever in which bouts of high temperature re-occur after an interval of two days (i.e. with a 48-hour periodicity). Interestingly, although the expression *ummu šalšu* is not attested elsewhere in cuneiform medical texts, there are descriptions of fevers with a pattern that is comparable to tertian fever. Notably, the "*li'bu*-fever of the mountain" and "seizure of the mountain" (*ṣibit šadî*) are described in these terms (Scurlock and Andersen 2005, 29, 482–483 19.218–19.220; Stol 2007, 12–14; Bácskay 2018a, No. 55: lines 158–164):

> "[If] *li'bu*-disease, seizure of the mountain, has seized (a man) and [then it leaves him but] on the third day seizes him (again and) [...] continually pursues him, he has a burning fever, severe *li'bu*-fever, and much sweat, his illness has been prolonged and has knocked him down ..." (Meier 1939, *ZA* 45, 208–209 col. v 15–21)
>
> *Diagnostic Handbook* Tablet 16: 25–27 (Heeßel 2000, 174–175; Scurlock 2014a, 152):
>
> "If it falls upon him for two days and then seizes him on the third day, and when it seizes him, he continually becomes rigid, and after he continually becomes rigid, he has a trembling, his limbs continually hurt him, his hands and feet are cold (and) afterwards fever rides him (var. flows over him) everywhere at once and sweat falls upon him and then it calms down: seizure of the mountain has seized him."
>
> *Diagnostic Handbook* Tablet 16: 28 (Heeßel 2000, 175; Scurlock 2014a, 152):
>
> "If it afflicts him for two days and flows (*ireḫḫīšu*) over him on the third day: (it is) seizure of the mountain; var. he will die."

The expression *ummu lemnu* "bad fever" in line 21 as a quality or category of fever is not attested elsewhere to my knowledge. Instead, one rather finds "strong fever" (*ummu dannu*), "constant fever" (*ummu kayyamānu*), "burning fever" (*ummu ṣarḫu*) or "lingering (chronic) fever" (*ummu lazzu*) in the fever texts (Bácskay 2018a, 276–277 *passim*). References to fevers that are specific to women are also rare. An Old Babylonian text contains a short prescription for a fever(?) affecting a woman, perhaps in childbed (George 2016, CUSAS 32, No. 73 obv. 14: *išātum* MUNUS *mu-us*-x x x; Bácskay 2018a, No. 0). In that text, the term *išātu* "fire" seems to be used instead of *ummu* "fever, heat"; however, the word *išātu* also occurs in the context of skin disease (designating or an abscess or inflammation), see Steinert et al. 2018, 245 note on line 61 with further references. For *išātu* in the metaphorical meaning "fever", see Stol 2007, 1–3; Bácskay 2018a, 7–8, No 51: 68.

Line 18: A *šammi eqli* "field plant" is attested as an alternative name for *kirbān eqli* "field-clod plant" in Uruanna I 481ff. (Ú *šá-mi* A.ŠÀ/GÁN : Ú LAG A.ŠÀ/GÁN (CAD K, 404 sub 3a). In that passage, *šammi eqli* is also associated with *kamme eqli*, a fungus (cf. CAD K, 125 s.v. *kammu* A sub c).

Line 19: The ingredient "milk of an 'impure' cow" (GA ÁB *ma-suk-ka-tu*$_4$) seems to be variant replacing "milk of an impure woman" (*šizib musukkati*), since prescriptions specify "cow's milk" or "milk of an impure woman". The term *musukkatu* (^{munus}Ú.ZÚG) refers to a woman who has recently given birth and is regarded as temporarily impure due to the postpartum discharges (lochia) that she emits, see Steinert 2023 for discussion. Breast milk of a *musukkatu* occurs, for example, in treatments for eye ailments, fever and epilepsy (Finkel 2018, 261–263 BM 64526+ lines 10–17; Geller and Panayotov 2020; Steinert 2023, 277–280 with fn. 170). The Egyptian medical papyri attribute to women's breast milk anti-inflammatory properties (Pommerening 2015), which also Mesopotamian healers may have been aware of. The cooling properties of the milk of a *musukkatu* may perhaps be seen as a contrast to the hot, impure discharges associated with women in their postpartum period.

Cow's milk is encountered a few times in prescriptions against fevers (see e.g., Bácskay 2018a, No. 39: 4 (= BAM 174 rev. 32), No. 71: 19 (= BAM 228 obv. 19 and dupl.), written GA GU$_4$.ÁB.(ḪI.A)). It is possible that "'impure' cow" is a scribal error for "impure woman". Yet, note another attestation of in a prescription against fever in the Late Babylonian text BM 55516+ (Bácskay 2023, *JCS* 75, 158–160 obv. 9'): ^{giš}TASKARIN ⸢SIG$_7$⸣ *ina* GA GU$_4$.ÁB.LU (for GU$_4$.ÁB.ḪI.A?) *ma-suk-ka-tu*$_4$ EŠ-*su* EŠ-*tu*$_4$ *šá* KÚM "(You mix) fresh boxwood with milk of impure cows(!?), you rub him. A salve for fever."

"Fat from the kidney of a black ox" (Ì.UDU ÉLLAG GU$_4$ GI$_6$) is a common ingredient in Mesopotamian medicine, although rarely attested in prescriptions against fever (Bácskay 2018a, No. 48: 33 (= BM 42272 rev. 20 and dupl.), a prescription for a fumigant).

Line 22: The signs following ^{šim}LI "*burāšu*-juniper" in line 22 can be read as *bi-iš* or ŠIM. However, the sign form of ŠIM used elsewhere in the present text differs. Different interpretations may be proposed. If *bi-iš* is to be read as an Akkadian word, it could stand for *bīšu* "stinking" or for *biššu*, a garden plant ("rue"(?); Thompson 1949, 76). For this plant, see also BM 46226 (= CT 14, 50) ii 16 *biš-šú*^{sar} (Finkel 2008, 110; Böck 2021, *Byzantinische Forschungen* 33, 5, 11); BM 30918 obv. 5:

^{ú}⸢*biš*⸣-*šá* (Bácskay and Simkó 2021, *Iraq* 83, 10, 12–13); 83-1-18, 727: 2' *biš-ši* (CCP 7.2.u8). If to be read as a variant form of ŠIM, a logographic sign for another aromatic following *burāšu* has been omitted by the scribe by mistake. Less likely, ŠIM may stand for an unspecific *riqqu* "aromatic plant" (however, in prescriptions, usually the plural ŠIM.ḪI.A or ŠIM.MEŠ is used); cf. CAD R, 369 s.v. *riqqu* sub c.

Line 23: The meaning of *piṭru* "split, fissure" as a body part is uncertain, for discussion cf. CAD P, 450 s.v. *piṭru*; SAD Vol. 1, 91a; Schmidtchen 2021, 621 (proposing an association with the joints and limbs of the body, since it is often mentioned beside *šer'ānu* "sinews, muscles"); see also Finkel 1976, 177–181 (line 153). Maul (2019, 301, 304 No. 79: 14') translates "Bauchdecke" (i.e. abdominal wall), following AHw 780b s.v. *pitru* sub 2; cf. AHw 762a s.v. *nâšu* D sub 2b, where the term is alternatively translated as "Zwerchfell" (i.e. diaphragm, midriff).

Line 24: For *alapû* (also *elapû*) "freshwater algae, seaweed" in medical texts, see CAD A/1, 336 sub b; Kinner Wilson 2005, *JMC* 6, 7, 11–12. For use in medical texts, see e.g. BAM 494 i 42', 45' (Bácskay and Simkó 2017, *JMC* 30, 9–10: "algae from the surface of the water" (*a-la-pa-a šá* IGI A.MEŠ). The application of an aquatic plant against fever in ms. a may be motivated by the association of water and therefore substances from this domain with coolness and thus, with a cooling effect. Compare in this connection the use of *ḫammu*, another aquatic plant synonymous with *alapû*, in prescriptions against fever, see Bácskay 2018a, text No. 1: 2 (= BAM 171 rev. 7): *ḫammu ša mê miṭrate* "*ḫammu*-plant from the water of a small canal"; ibid., No. 78: 13 (= BAM 66 rev. 16'): *ḫammu ša* (*pān*) *mê* "*ḫammu*-plant which (is found on the surface of) water" (ointment).

Lines 25–26: The expression *ša šaplān sinništi ša alāda u kibsa taprusu* "<dust> from the lower extremities (lit. below) of a woman who has ceased to bear and (to experience) the (normal) *course* (of women's menses?)" in lines 25–26 is unusual. Supposedly the text is corrupt and the word SAḪAR (*eperu*) "dust" should be restored at the beginning of line 25. For this ingredient, most of the time referred to as "dust from below a woman who has ceased giving birth", in rituals and prescriptions against fever, see BM 42272 rev. 11 and duplicates (Bácskay 2018a, No. 48: 24): SAḪAR KI.TA MUNUS *šá* Ù.TU KUD-*si*; and in a second prescription for an ointment/amulet in rev. 22 (= No. 48: 35); BM 55516+ obv. 10'–11' (Bácskay 2023, *JCS* 75, 160): "(You take) 'dog-fly', it heals thousand-(plant), dust from underneath a woman who has <ceased to?> give birth (SAḪAR KI.TA-*nu* MUNUŠ *šá* Ù.TU <KUD>) and (dust from) a mongoose-lair(?) [...]. You wrap (this) in a tuft of wool, put it around his neck. (You can also use this as) an ointment for a patient who has been seized by fever (*ummu*)."

As a slight variant, we also find dust from the house of a post-menopausal woman (BAM 476: 8: SAḪAR É MUNUS *šá* Ù.TU KUD-*at*) in a prescription for a medicine bag protecting from attacks of epilepsy. In other texts, a post-menopausal woman has to perform certain ritual acts such as spinning threads for amulets (cf. AMT 20,1 obv.(!) 30: red wool spun by a woman *ša alāda*(MUD) AL.KUD). In a few texts, a post-menopausal woman is designated alternatively as *sinništu parištu* "cut-off woman", the latter term is likewise derived from *parāsu* "to cut off, to stop" (e.g., BAM 237 obv. i 22, see text C.1.4). See also Finkel 2018, *FS* Geller, 261–263, 265 (BM 64526 line 15) and CT 17, 20: 75–76 munus mud-da gi$_4$-a = *sin-niš-tu pa-riš-tu* (quoted in CAD P, 187a).

In ms. a, the usual formulation is expanded by the noun *kibsu*, the stopping of which characterizes the woman in addition to the ceasing of fertility. The term *kibsu* usually means "step, track, access" (CAD K, 338a s.v. *kibsu* sub 1f). But here the word is used in a euphemistic manner to refer to the menses (or the usual course of the menstrual cycle) which have stopped (note other metaphorical meanings of *kibsu* as "way of acting, behaviour", CAD K, 338–339 sub 2). For another occurrence of *kibsu* + *parāsu* "to stop" to describe the ceasing of the menses, see BM 47578 line 13 (text C.2.2); cf. further BM 48557 obv. 2' (text A.2.10).

The reason for using a substance that was in touch with a post-menopausal woman in a salve to treat fever or heat may not primarily be found in notions of ritual purity and avoidance of impurity (the loss and discharge of bodily fluids associated with childbirth and menstruation is often linked with notions of impurity). Childbirth and loss of menstrual blood may have been regarded as "hot" states, and postmenopausal women therefore may have been seen as "cooler" than women in their reproductively active years (cf. Steinert 2020, *JMC* 36, 59).

For menopause and the ceasing of fertility, including treatments for "a woman who has ceased to bear", see further BAM 241 rev. iii 3 and BAM 243: 5' (DIŠ MUNUS *alāda* KUD-*sà-at*), edited in this volume (text II.1.3 and B.1.2). Instead of the usual feminine stative form *parsat*, ms. a uses the preterite form *taprusu* she has stopped" with the *ta-* infix for the 3rd person fem. sg.

Line 27: For similar secrecy formulae in colophons of scholarly texts, see Hunger 1968, 13–14; Lenzi 2008, 168–215; George and Taniguchi 2010, 110 K. 2596 iii 26'–30'. Note, within the women's healthcare texts, N. 4001: 27–28 (text B.2.1).

Line 28: The sign AŠ before the name of the tablet owner is understood here as a variant for DIŠ as a personal name marker (already proposed by Finkel 1988, 154 with n. 83 for additional attestations). The colophon identifies Iprā'ya, son of Zababa-pir'u-uṣur, descendant of Ēṭiru as the tablet owner. Iprā'ya is known as a scribe of several tablets of scientific content in the 81-11-03 collection of the British Museum, including hemerological, medical and astrological compilations (for the tablet collection of Iprā'ya and his family, see Finkel 1988, 153–155, 158–159; Jiménez 2016, 218). Iprā'ya also wrote several commentaries (Frahm 2011, 307). He probably was the scribe of a commentary on the exorcistic text *Marduk's Address to the Demons* (BM 47529+47685; http://ccp.yale.edu/P461231), and of a commentary on *Enūma Anu Enlil* (BM 47447; http://ccp.yale.edu/P461229), the latter of which is dated to the 19th year of one of the three Achaemenid rulers with the name Artaxerxes (either 445, 385 or 339 BCE); for other astrological commentaries attributed to him, see Ossendrijver 2019, 66 n. 49. For astrological texts written by Iprā'ya, see e.g. BM 47494 (Hunger 2004; Ossendrijver 2019, 66–68), a tablet with astrological predictions and correlations between constellations, cities and geographical regions, some of which contain elements of zodiacal astrology.

The name Iprā'ya was formerly read Šemā'ya or Šebā'ya, see Livingstone 1986, 259–260; Finkel 1988, 154 n. 83; Rochberg-Halton 1988, 284–290. For the reading ŠE.BA-'-*ia* = Iprā'ya (as a variant of the name Iprīya "my subsistence"), see Schwemer 2009, 58. For the Ēṭiru family, see also Wunsch 2014b.

A.2.7 BM 51246+: An Extract Tablet with Remedies for Women

The fragments of BM 51246+ (ms. a) preserve the upper part of the obverse and the lower part of the reverse of a single-column tablet in Late Babylonian script belonging to the Sippar collection of the British Museum.[269] The text was compiled from at least two different sources, as indicated in a rubric marking the first four lines of the obverse as stemming from an "old original" (ms. a line 5). The bottom line of the tablet's reverse however bears a colophon designating the contents as the "34th *nisḫu*-tablet of remedies [...]" (ms. a line 41'), indicating that the copied text belonged to a series or larger compendium. The mixture of topics dealt with in the preserved lines of ms. a (protecting from miscarriage, therapies for infertility, postpartum complaints, contraceptives, treatments to stop loss of amniotic fluid) suggest that the contents may form selections of therapies taken from a larger medical-therapeutic treatise (such as witnessed in the Assur Medical Catalogue (Steinert et al. 2018)) or from collections of material related to women's health compiled on multiple tablets each having a specific topic.

The first four lines on the obverse contain two prescriptions (ointment and amulet) to protect a pregnant woman from miscarriage caused by witchcraft. The prescriptions are known from two other Late Babylonian manuscripts (mss. b, c), with the difference that ms. a omits the text of the incantations recited over the remedies, and also omits a short ritual preserved in mss. b and c (texts C.3.3 and C.3.4). It is noteworthy that ms. a shares its incipit with ms. b, both of which are identical with the incipit of the third tablet of the treatise PREGNANCY in the Assur Medical Catalogue (Steinert et al. 2018, 217 line 110).

The next thematic section (lines 5–17) is a therapy to make an infertile woman conceive, consisting of a short spell and a prescription / ritual instruction. This section is duplicated in a Neo- Babylonian tablet from Nippur that also contained statements resembling prognoses in fertility tests and an unusual colophon (ms. d, see text B.2.1 for a complete edition).

The last lines preserved on the obverse (lines 18–22) deal with a postpartum condition hitherto unknown from gynaecological texts and associated with a bad body odour (*nipšu*). However, the beginning of line 18 in ms. a introducing the topic is also known as the tablet incipit of a chapter within the medical treatise BIRTH in the Assur Medical Catalogue (Steinert et al. 2018, 218 line 117).

The remedies on the reverse of the tablet offer a collection of prescriptions (mostly potions using simple drugs) for contraception (preventing that a woman gets pregnant), a rare topic within Mesopotamian women's healthcare texts. In fact, ms. a is the first text with prescriptions for this purpose known so far. The last two sections on the reverse (lines

269 CBT VI, 55 and xxxii on the proveniences of the 82-2-23 collection.

35'–40') are concerned with stopping the loss of amniotic fluid and preventing miscarriage. The final lines (lines 37'–40') contain a remarkable ritual involving the 'dog's tongue'-plant (*lišān kalbi*), which is associated with the sun god in the present text. The power attributed to the 'dog's tongue'-plant, in particular to its root, to preserve pregnancy adds a new facet to the plant's uses in women's healthcare, since 'dog's tongue'-plant was more renowned among Mesopotamian healers as a plant to facilitate difficult delivery. However, its embedding in a particular ritual framework (e.g. the precautions taken when procuring the plant, pulling out the plant in the morning), the use of the root (maybe symbolising the foetus in the uterus, because both exist in the dark, i.e. in the earth and in utero) and its connection with Šamaš (who takes care of the living, the dead as well as the unborn, helping the latter to come out from the darkness and see the sunlight, when the time of birth has come) may offer glimpses into the rationale underlying the choice of the 'dog's tongue'-plant in this specific ritual.

List of Manuscripts

Siglum	Museum Number	Copy	Collation	Format; Ductus	Provenience
a	BM 51246 + BM 53217 + BM 53744 (82-3-23, 2242 + 4251 + 4784)	Pl. 20	Coll.	Fragment of a single-column tablet, Late Babylonian script, 6th-3rd cent. BCE[270]	probably Sippar
b	BM 42327 + BM 42410 + BM 42604 + BM 42628 + BM 43474 + BM 43523 (81-7-1, 87 + 170 + 365 + 389 + 1238 + 1287)	Farber 1989 (*MC* 2), pl. 14–15	Coll.	Single-column tablet, Late Babylonian script, 6th-3rd cent.	Babylonia, exact provenience unknown
c	W. 23287	SpTU 3, No. 84	Photo coll.	Single-column tablet, Late Babylonian period, 4th cent. BCE	Uruk, library of Anu-ikṣur
d	N. 4001	Pl. 23	Coll.	Single-column tablet; Neo-Babylonian script, ca. 7th(?) cent. BCE	Nippur

Overview

i	Prescription (ointment) to protect a woman from miscarriage caused by witchcraft: a obv. 1–3 // b obv. 1–4 // c rev. 3–4	1–3
ii	Prescription (amulet) to protect a woman from miscarriage caused by witchcraft: Instructions (a obv. 4 // b obv. 7–9 // c rev. 6)	4
iii	Rubric (a obv. 5)	5
iv	Remedy to enable a woman to get pregnant: – Incantation (a obv. 6–9 // d obv. 1–12) – Rubric (a obv. 10 // d obv. 13) – Prescription (a obv. 11–17 // d obv. 14-rev. 2)	6–17
v	Prescription for a postpartum woman against *nipšu*-disease ("stench") a obv. 18–20	18–20
vi	Fragmentary prescription a obv. 21–22	21–22[...
vii'	Fragmentary prescription (a rev. 1')	...]23'
viii'	Fragmentary prescription (potion) (a rev. 2')	24'
ix'	Fragmentary prescription (a rev. 3')	25'
x'	Prescription for contraception(?) (a rev. 4')	26'
xi'	Prescription for contraception(?) (a rev. 5')	27'
xii'	Prescription (potion) for contraception(?) (a rev. 6')	28'
xiii'	Prescription (potion) for contraception(?) (a rev. 7'–8')	29'–30'
xiv'	Prescription (potion) for contraception(?) (a rev. 9')	31'

270 Measurements: ca. 9 x 8.5 x 2.7 cm.

xv'	Fragmentary Sumerian incantation (a rev. 10')	32'
xvi'	Prescription (potion) for contraception (a rev. 11')	33'
xvii'	Prescription (potion) for contraception (a rev. 12')	34'
xviii'	Prescription for stopping the loss of amniotic fluid and for preventing miscarriage (potion) a rev. 13'–14'	35'–36'
xix'	Ritual for stopping the loss of amniotic fluid and for preventing miscarriage a rev. 15'–18'	37'–40'
xx'	Colophon a rev. 19'	41'

Previous Edition and Discussion

Farber 1989, 26–27, 112ff. §§ 39A–40 (ms. a and b, lines 1–4)
Von Weiher 1988, *SpTU* 3, 116–123, No. 84 (edition of ms. c)
Volk 1999, *OrNS* 68, 4 fn. 11 (mss. a and b line 1)
Scurlock and Andersen 2005, 261 12.12, 268 12.50, 269 12.52 (ms. a obv. 1, rev. 12', 13'–14')
Steinert 2017a, 316–318 (ms. d, lines 7–13)
Abusch et al. 2020 (CMAwR 3), 60–63 text 5.4 (mss. a, b, c, lines 1–4)
Steinert 2021, *Byzantinische Forschungen* 33, 57–58 n. 84 (line 33' = a rev. 11')
Electronic Babylonian Library (eBL) (https://www.ebl.lmu.de/library/BM.51246)
Infra text C.3.3 (edition ms. b), text C.3.4 (ms. c), text B.2.1 (ms. d)

Transliteration

1	a obv. 1	*ana* ⸢^{munus}⸣PEŠ$_4$ UŠ$_{11}$.ZU NU TE-*ma ša* ŠÀ-*šá* NU [ŠUB-*e* ....]
	b obv. 1–2	[*ana*] ^{munus}PEŠ$_4$ UŠ$_{11}$.ZU NU TE-*ma šá* Š[À]-*šá* NU ŠUB-[*e*] / ^{na4}KUR-*nu* DAB KÙ.GA[N] ^{na4}ŠUBA ⸢SAḪAR⸣-*ru*
	c rev. 3	*ana* ^{munus}PEŠ$_4$ UŠ$_{11}$.ZU NU TE-*ma ša* ŠÀ-*šá* NU *na*$^!$-*de-e* [...]
2	a obv. 2	*ù* ^{giš}GEŠ.TIM.KA$_5$.A ḪÁD.DU SÚD *ina* MÚD BURU$_5$.Ḫ[ABRUD.DA^{mušen} ....]
	b obv. 2$^{cont.}$–3	GEŠTIN.KA$_5$.A ḪÁD.⸢A⸣ / SÚD *ina* MÚD BURU$_5$.ḪABRUD^{RU}.DA^{mušen} NÍTA *ina* Ì.GIŠ ^{giš}ŠUR.MÌN ḪI.ḪI
	c rev. 3$^{cont.}$–4	[...] *ina* MÚD BURU$_5$.ḪABRUD.DA NÍTA *ina* Ì ^{giš}ŠUR.MÌN ḪI.ḪI-*ma*
3	a obv. 3	ÉN *ez-ze-et šam-rat ana* ŠÀ ŠID-*nu*-[*ma*$^?$ ....]
	b obv. 4	ÉN *ez-ze-et šam-rat ana* ŠÀ ŠID-*nu-ma* ŠÉŠ-*ma* TIN-*uṭ*
	c rev. 4$^{cont.}$	É[N x x x x x x x x x x x x x]
a, b, c		
4	a obv. 4	---- -------- ^{na4}*šu-u* NÍTA ^{na4}*šu-u* MUNUS *ina* ŠU 15-*šá* KÉ[Š ....]
	b obv. 7–9	DIŠ KI.MIN ^{na4}ŠU.U NÍTA *u* MUNUS *ina* ŠU 15-*šá* KÉ[Š]-*as* / ÉN *a-šib ek-le-ti* 3-*šú ana* UGU ŠID-⸢*nu*⸣-*ma* / *kiš-pi* NU TE.⸢MEŠ⸣-*šú*
	c rev. 6	DIŠ KI.MIN ^{na4}ŠU.U NÍTA *u* MUNUS *ina* ŠU.MIN 15-*šú* KÉŠ ÉN *a-šib ek-let* [x x x x x x x x x x x]
a, b, c		
5	a obv. 5	GIN$_7$ KA *la-bi-ri-šú*$^!$(ŠÁ) [*šaṭer* (...)]
a		
6	a obv. 6	⸢ÉN⸣ ⸢munus$^?$⸣ pi$^?$-rat tup$^?$-pi$^?$ ⸢numun$^?$⸣ x x x (x) ⸢tup$^?$⸣-p[i$^?$ x x x x x x x x x x]
	d obv. 1–3	[...................] / [...................] / [la-aḫ-t]e-⸢eš⸣ ^{d}*iš-tar* ⸢la-aḫ-te-eš⸣

7	a obv. 7	[x x x] x x-⸢up$^{?}$⸣-pa ma$^{?}$-an-⸢sag-x⸣ ki-⸢tu⸣-$^{he\text{-}pí}$: g[u-x x x x x x x x x x]
	d obv. 4–6	[ma-an-sa]g$^{?}$-sa⸣ ki-tu-up-pa / [ma-an$^{?}$]-⸢sag-sa⸣ ki-tu-up-pa / gu-⸢ru⸣-um-ta ar-ra-ru-sa ki-tu-up-pa
8	a obv. 8	[x x x x] ⸢*i*⸣-*ri-iš* : ⸢^{munus}⸣*la a-lit-tu*$_{4}$ NUMUN *ú-še-ṣi* : ⸢*a*⸣-[*na* x x x x x x x x x x x]
	d obv. 7–10	^{d}⸢x⸣ A.ŠÀ *i*-⸢*ri*⸣-*iš* / *la a*-⸢*lit*⸣-*tu*$_{4}$ NUMUN *ú-še-ṣi* / ⸢*a-na*⸣ AB.SÍN *li-in-na-di-ma* / [M]U *li-ib-ni*
9	a obv. 9	[ÉN ^{d}*é-a*] ⸢*ù*⸣ ⸢^{d}⸣*asal-lú-ḫi* ^{erasure} 3-*šú ad*-⸢*di*$^{?}$⸣ [TU$_{6}$ ÉN]
	d obv. 11–12	⸢*ši-ip*⸣-*tu*$_{4}$ *ša* ^{d}*é-a ù* ^{d}*asal-lú-ḫi* / [3-*šú a*]*d-di* TU$_{6}$ ⸢ÉN⸣
a, d		________________
10	a obv. 10	[KA.INIM.MA ^{mun}]^{us}NU.⸢Ù⸣.TU ⸢*a*⸣-[*na ur-ri-i*]
	d obv. 13	⸢KA⸣.[INIM].MA ^{munus}NU.Ù.TU *a-na ur*-⸢*ri*⸣-*i*
a, d		________________
11	a obv. 11	[KÌD.KÌD.BI ^{ú}]IGI-*lim* ^{ú}IGI-20 ^{ú}⸢*tar-muš*⸣ x ⸢GÍN⸣ ⸢^{ú}⸣[KUR.RA^{sar} ....]
	d obv. 14–15	KÌD.KÌD.BI ^{ú}*tar-muš* ^{ú}*im-ḫur-lim* ^{ú}*im-hur*-20 / ⸢2$^{?}$ GÍN⸣ ^{ú}KUR.RA^{sar} ^{ú}*kur-ka-*^{erasure}*-nam ša* KUR
12	a obv. 12	[x x x x] ⸢6⸣ Ú.ḪI.A *an-nu-ti* ⸢TI⸣-[*qé*] *ina* K[AŠ] x x x [.................................]
	d obv. 16–18	7 BURU$_{5}$.⸢SAḪAR.RA⸣ 6 Ú.ḪI.A *an-nu-ti* TI-*qé* / *i-na* ⸢KAŠ⸣.[SA]G *i-na* ^{urudu}ŠEN.TUR *ina* IZI / ŠEG$_{6}$-*al*
13	a obv. 13	[x x x]x ⸢*ta*$^{?}$-*tab-bak*⸣ *ina* Ù[R ....]
	d obv. 18$^{cont.}$–19	[*i-n*]*a* ^{dug}BUR.ZI.GAL SÁḪAR *ta*-⸢*tab-bak*⸣ / *i-na* Ù[R] *a-na* IGI ⸢^{d}EN⸣.ZU NÍG.NA ⸢^{šim}⸣[LI GAR-*an*]
14	a obv. 14	[x x x]x ŠID$^{!}$(SI) *ina q*[*á-qá-ri*$^{?}$ ....]
	d obv. 20–22	ÉN ⸢3⸣-[*šú*] *a-na* ŠÀ$^{?}$ Š[ID-*nu*] / ⸢*i*$^{?}$-*na*⸣ ⸢*qá*⸣-*qá-ri*$^{?}$ *la i*$^{?}$-[x x x x] / [*ina* Ù]R/[MU]L$^{?}$ *tuš*$^{!}$-*bat* U$_{4}$.3.KA[M x x x x x]
15	a obv. 15	[x x x]x *ta*-⸢x-x⸣ [............................]
	d rev. 1–2	U$_{4}$.3.KAM *a-di ta*-x[x x x x x x] / ⸢^{ú}*kur*⸣-*ka-nam t*[*u-šak-kal-ši*$^{?}$ x]x x[x x]
16	a obv. 16	[x x x MUN]US *ši-i ut*-⸢*ta*⸣-x-x[................]
	d	*Omits*
17	a obv. 17	[x x x x] *ta*$^{!}$-*tar-ma* [...............................]
	d	*Omits*
a, d		________________
18	a obv. 18	[DIŠ MUNUS Ù.T]U-*ma ni-ip-šú* <<*šá*>> ⸢*ina*⸣ ⸢*kir*⸣-*r*[*i*$^{?}$-*šá* ....]
19	a obv. 19	[x x x] *ina* ^{urudu}⸢ŠEN.TUR⸣ ŠEG$_{6}$-⸢*al*⸣ x[............................]
20	a obv. 20	[x x x]x kal$^{?}$ *ta-sàk ina* KAŠ.S[AG ḪI.ḪI$^{?}$ ....]
a		________________
21	a obv. 21	[DIŠ KI.MIN(?) x x]x ⸢*ta*$^{?}$⸣-*sàk* [............................]
22	a obv. 22	[x x x x x] ⸢x⸣ [..............................]

Ms. a obv. breaks; gap of unknown length
Beginning of rev. lost

23'	a rev. 1'	[x x x x x x] ⸢PÉŠ.ÙR$^{!}$(SAR)⸣.R[A$^{?}$ x x x x x x x x x x]
		________________
24'	a rev. 2'	[x x x x *gul-g*]*ul*$^{?}$ BURU$_{5}$.IR.GI.L[UM x x x x x x x x x]
		________________

25'	a rev. 3'	[x x x]x GA.⸢RAŠ$^{?}$⸣ *ina* KAŠ NAG-*ma* [… …]
26'	a rev. 4'	⸢DIŠ⸣ ⸢KI.MIN$^{?}$⸣ ⸢BURU$_{5}$$^{?!}$⸣.GEŠTIN.NA *šá* PA.MEŠ-*šú* ^{na4}DUḪ.ŠI.A ḪÁD.⸢A$^{?}$⸣ [x x x x x x x x]
27'	a rev. 5'	DIŠ KI.MIN KÙ.SI$_{22}$ *li-<iq>-ti*$^{?}$ *ma-da* TI ŠEG$_{6}$-*šal e*-[x x x x x x x]
28'	a rev. 6'	DIŠ KI.MIN ^{ú}*im-ḫur-lim ta-sàk ina* KAŠ AZ *u*$_{4}$-*ma* NÍG.GIG-[*šá* IGI NAG-(*ma*) NU PEŠ$_{4}$$^{?}$]
29'	a rev. 7'	DIŠ KI.MIN SUḪUŠ ^{giš}NAM.TAR NÍTA ZI SUḪUŠ-*su* TI-*qé* x[x x x x x x]
30'	a rev. 8'	NAG-*ši ana* KAŠ ŠUB-*di ina* MUL$_{4}$ *tuš-bat ina še-rim* NU *pa*-[*tan* NAG-*ma* NU PEŠ$_{4}$$^{?}$]
31'	a rev. 9'	[DIŠ KI.MIN$^{?}$ x]x *ša* KA.GI.<NA> SIG.GI *ina* KAŠ NU *pa*-[*tan* NAG-*ma* NU PEŠ$_{4}$$^{?}$]
32'	a rev. 10'	[ÉN x x nam-ba$^{?}$]-⸢ra-an⸣-gi sig$_{4}$ é gi-li-ib gi-l[i$^{?}$-ib *ina* ŠÀ ŠID-*nu*$^{?}$]
33'	a rev. 11'	[DIŠ KI.MIN] ^{ú}⸢*an-ki*⸣-[*nu*]-⸢*te*⸣ ⸢*ta-sàk*⸣ *ina* KAŠ NU *pa-tan* NAG-*ma* [NU PEŠ$_{4}$]
34'	a rev. 12'	[DIŠ KI.MIN] ⸢^{ú}⸣LAL$^{?}$ *ta-sàk ina* K[AŠ] NU *pa-tan* NAG-*ma* NU PEŠ$_{4}$
35'	a rev. 13'	⸢DIŠ⸣ ⸢PEŠ$_{4}$⸣ A.A-*šá* DU-*ku ù* [*šà* ŠÀ]-⸢*šá*$^{?}$⸣ [ŠU]B-*a* 1 GÍN Ì.UDU ÚKUŠ.LAGAB KUR ^{ú}*im-ḫur-lim ina* KAŠ NAG-*ma* ⸢PEŠ$_{4}$⸣
36'	a rev. 14'	A-*šá* DU-*ku*$^{?}$ *ik-kal-lu-ú* [*šà* Š]À-*šá* *ú-šal-lam*
37'	a rev. 15'	DIŠ PEŠ$_{4}$ A-*šá* DU-*ku* ⸢*šà*⸣ ŠÀ-*šá a-n*[*a*] ⸢*la*$^{?}$⸣ [*na*]-*de*$^{?}$-*e* GIN$_{7}$ ^{d}UTU.ŠÚ.⸢A⸣ [*ana* ED]IN DU-*ak u* SUḪUŠ ^{ú}EME-UR.GI$_{7}$
38'	a rev. 16'	⸢*ḫe*⸣-*pí* SUR.RA NIGIN *ina še-rim ina* NU ZABAR$^{?}$ [T]A *šur-ši-šu ta-n*[*ap-p*]*al*$^{?}$ *e-nu-ma* ⸢*ta*$^{?}$⸣-[*nap-pa-lu* (*ana* ^{d}UTU$^{?}$)]
39'	a rev. 17'	*kam* DU$_{11}$.GA ^{d}UTU *an-nu-ú* Ú-⸢*ka*⸣ ⸢*ana*$^{?}$⸣ *ni-i*[*d*$^{?}$] x x x [x x] x x du [KI LÚ.NA.ME]
40'	a rev. 18'	NU DU$_{11}$.DU$_{11}$ *ana* É KU$_{4}$-*ub* Ú *ša*$^{?}$ [x x x x x x x x x x x x x]

Colophon:

41'	a rev. 19'	*tup-pi* 34 *nis-ḫu bul-ṭu* x[… … … … … … …]

Bottom of ms. a rev.

Bound Transcription and Translation

1 *ana erīti kišpī lā ṭeḫê-ma ša libbīša lā na*[*dê šadânu ṣābitu lulû šubû eperu*] 2 *u karān šēlebi tubbal tasâk ina dām iṣṣūr* [*ḫurri zikari ina šaman šurmēni taballal-ma*] 3 ÉN *ezzet šamrat ana libbi tamannū-*[*ma tapaššaš-ma iballuṭ*]	1 So that witchcraft not come near a pregnant woman and she not [have] a miscarriage: 2 You dry (and) pound 1 [magnetite, antimony, *šubû*-stone, dust] 2 and 'fox grape']. [You mix (these ingredients)] with the blood of a [male *ḫurru*]-bird [(and) with cypress-scented oil] (and) 3 you recite the incantation "She is fierce, she is violent" over it. [Then you rub (the woman with it) and she will get well.]
4 (DIŠ KI.MIN) *šû zikar u šû sinniš ina qāt imittīša tarak*[*kas* ÉN *āšib eklēti šalāšī-šu ana muḫḫi tamannū-ma kišpī ul iṭeḫḫûšu*]	4 (Var. adds: Alternatively,) you tie male *šû*-stone and female *šû*-stone on her right hand. [You recite the incantation "(O you) inhabitant of the dark" three times over it. Then witchcraft will not approach her.]

5 *kīma pî labirīšu* [*šaṭer* (…)]	5 [Written] according to the wording of its original [(…)].
6 ÉN *fragmentary* [la-aḫ-te-eš ^{d}*iš-tar* la-aḫ-te-eš] 7 [ma-an-sag$^{?}$-sa ki-tu]-up-pa ma-an-sa[g-sa] ki-tu-[up-pa] g[u-ru-um-ta ar-ra-ru-sa ki-tu-up-pa] 8 […] *eqla īriš lā ālittu zēra ušēṣi a*[*na absinni linnadī-ma šuma libni*] 9 [*šiptu ša Ea*] *u Asalluḫi šalāšīšu addi* [*tê šipti*]	6 Incantation: *fragmentary 'abracadabra' words* [Lahteš Ištar laḫteš], 7 [mansagsa kitu]ppa, mansa[gsa] kitu[ppa], g[urumta ar-rarusa kituppa]. 8 [(The god) NN] cultivated the field (by means of a seed-er-plough). The infertile woman made the seed sprout. Let it (the seed) be deposited in[to the furrow, let her create off-spring!] 9 I have cast [the spell of Ea] and Asalluḫi three times." [Incantation formula.]
10 [KA.INIM.MA] *lā ālittu a*[*na urrî*]	10 [Recitation] to make a barren woman [get pregnant].
11 [KÌD.KÌD.BI] *imḫur-līm imḫur-ešrā tarmuš šina*(?) *šiqil nīnê kurkānâ ša šadî* 12 [*sebet erib turbu'ti*] *šeššet šammī annûti teleq*[*qe*] *ina šikari* [*ina tangussi ina išāti tušabšal*] 13 [*ana burzigalli šaḫarri*] *tatabbak ina ūri* [*ana pān Sîn nignak burāši tašakkan*] 14 [*šipta šalāšīšu ana libbi*] *tamannu ina q*[*aqqari lā* … … *ina ūri/kakkab*]*i*(?) *tušbât šalāšat ūmī* … …] 15 [*šalāšat ūmī adi*] *ta*-[… *kurkānâm tušakkalši*(?) …] 16 [… *sinni*]*štu šī* …[… …] 17 [… …] *tatâr-ma* [… …]	11 [The procedure for it]: 'heals thousand'-plant, 'heals twenty'-plant, *tarmuš*-plant, two(?) shekels of *nīnû*-plant, *kurkānû*-plant of the mountains 12 (and) [seven 'dust locusts'] – you take these six drugs, [boil (them)] in beer [in a *tangussu*-vessel over the fire]. 13 You pour (the liquid) [into a porous *burzigallu*-vessel]. On the roof, [in front of (the moon god) Sîn you set up a censer with *burāšu*-juniper]. 14 You recite [the incantation three times over it (the *burzigallu*-vessel)]. [*It*(?) should not …] on the gr[ound, … . You let (it) stay overnight on the roof/under the stars(?). For three days … …]. 15 [Until the three days] … [… you have her eat(?) *kurkānû*-plant …]. 16 […] that wo[man] …[… …]. 17 [… …] you repeat (it), and [… …].
18 [*šumma sinništu ū*]*lid-ma nipšu* <<*ša*>> *ina kirr*[*ī-ša* … …] 19 […] *ina tangussi tušabšal* …[… …] 20 […] … *tasâk ina šikari* [*tuballal*(?) … …]	18 [If a woman gives] birth and then a smell […] in her throat [… …]. 19 You boil […] in a *tangussu*-vessel, …[… …] 20 […] … you crush (it), [mix(?)] with beer [… …].
21 [DIŠ KI.MIN(?) …]… *tasâk* …[… …] 22 *traces*	21 [Alternatively (?):] You crush [… …] 22 *too fragmentary for translation*
Ms. a obv. breaks	
23' […] *arrabu*(?) …[… …]	23' […] a dormouse, …[… …].
24' [… *gulg*]*ul*(?) *ergil*[*i* … …]	24' [… the he]ad(?) of an *ergilu*-locust [… …].
25' […]… *karašu ina šikari išattī-ma* [… …]	25' […]… she shall drink […] leek in beer, and [… …].
26' DIŠ KI.MIN(?) *erib karāni*(?) *ša kappūšu dušû tubbal* [… …]	26' Alternatively(?), you dry a grapevine locust(?) whose wings are (the colour of) *dušû*-stone, …[…].
27' DIŠ KI.MIN *ḫurāṣu liqti*(?) *māda teleqqe tušabšal e*-[… …]	27' Alternatively, you take much gold of fine quality(?), you boil it, … [… … …].

28' DIŠ KI.MIN *imḫur-līm tasâk ina šikari asi*(?) *ūma maruštā*[*ša immaru*(?) *išattī*-(*ma*) *ul irri*(?)]	28' Alternatively, you crush 'heals thousand'-plant, [she shall drink(?) (it)] in beer (and) myrtle (oil?), on the same day that [she sees her?] 'trouble' (menses). [Then she will not get pregnant(?)].
29' DIŠ KI.MIN *šuruš pillê zikari tanassaḫ šurussu teleqqe* ...[... ...] 30' *tašaqqīši ana šikari tanaddi ina kakkabi tušbât ina šērim lā pa*[*tān išattī-ma ul irri*(?)]	29' Alternatively, you pull out the root of a male *pillû*-plant, you take its root, [... ...], 30' you have her drink it. (Or) you put it into beer, you let it stand outside overnight. In the morning, [she shall drink (it)] on an empty sto[mach. Then she will not get pregnant(?)].
31' [DIŠ KI.MIN(?) ...] *ša šadânu damqi*(?) *ina šikari lā pa*[*tān išattī-ma ul irri*(?)]	31' [Alternatively, she shall drink ...] of good(?) *šadânu*-stone in beer on an empty stomach. [Then she will not get pregnant(?).]
32' [ÉN ... nam-ba?]-⸢ra-an⸣-gi sig_4 é gi-li-ib gi-l[i-ib *ina libbi tamannu*(?)]	32' [Incantation: "May [...] not return to her! House brick, block, bl[ock!" You recite (this) over (the remedy?)].
33' [DIŠ KI.MIN] *ankinūte tasâk ina šikari lā patān išattī-ma* [*ul irri*]	33' [Alternatively,] you crush *ankinūtu*-plant, she shall drink (it) in beer on an empty stomach. Then [she will not get pregnant.]
34' [DIŠ KI.MIN] *ašqulāla tasâk ina šik*[*ari*] *lā patān išattī-ma ul irri*	34' [Alternatively,] you crush *ašqulālu*-pant, she shall drink (it) in be[er] on an empty stomach. Then she will not get pregnant.
35' *šumma erītu mûša illakū u* [*ša libbī*]*ša* [*ina*]*ddâ ištēn šiqil lipî errî šadî imḫur-līm ina šikari išattī-ma erītu* 36' *mûša illakū ikkallû* [*ša lib*]*bīša ušallam*	35' If a pregnant woman's (amniotic) fluid flows and she (is in danger of) having a [mis]carriage, she shall drink one shekel pith of mountain colocynth(?) (and) 'heals thousand'-plant in beer. Then 36' the flowing (amniotic) fluid 35' of the pregnant woman 36' will be held back (and) she will bring her [foetus] to term.
37' *šumma erītu mûša illakū ša libbīša an*[*a*] *lā* [*na*]*dê kīma ereb Šamši* [*ana ṣē*]*ri tallak u šuruš lišān kalbi* 38' *ḫepi* (*zi*)*surrâ talammi ina šēri ina lā namāri*(?) [*iš*]*ti šuršīšu tan*[*ap*-*p*]*al enūma ta*[*nappalu* (*ana Šamaš*)?] 39' *kâm taqabbi Šamaš annû šammūka ana*(?) ...[...] ... [*itti mamma*] 40' *lā tadabbub ana bīti terrub šammu ša*(?) [... ...]	37' If a pregnant woman's (amniotic) fluid flows, so that she not [ha]ve a miscarriage: At sunset you go to the steppe. 37' The root of 'dog's tongue'-plant – 38' *broken* with a circle (of flour) you surround (the plant). In the (early) morning, when it is not (yet) light(?), you d[ig] out (the plant) with its root. When you [dig (it) out?], 39' you shall say 38' [(to Šamaš?)] 39' as follows: "Šamaš, this is your plant! *For* ...[..." ...] ... . 40' You(?) must not speak 39' [with anyone], 40' you(?) should go (straight back) home. The plant *which* [... ...].

Colophon:

41' *tuppi* 34 *nisḫu bulṭū* ...[... ...]	41' Thirty-fourth extract tablet. Remedies ...[... ...].

Notes

Lines 1–4: Farber (1989, 114) comments on use of the 3rd person sg. masc. suffix *-šú* instead of the feminine suffix *-šá* in reference to the patient, which can be seen e.g. in line 4 in mss. b and c, while ms. a appears to use *-šá* consistently. He suggests that the occurrence of *-šú* could be due to the fact that the text passage may have been taken over from a different context (baby incantation).

Lines 1–2: For the reading ⸢SAḪAR⸣*-ru* in ms. b, see the collations by Abusch et al. 2020 (CMAwR 3), pl. 62.

I owe the reading GEŠ.TIM in ms. a, representing a syllabic spelling of the logogram GEŠTIN, to Abusch et al. 2020. As they note (ibid., 63 comment on line 2), such spellings indicate that the logograms of common drug names may have been read in Sumerian rather than Akkadian.

Line 3: For the text of the Lamaštu incantation *ezzet šamrat* not included in ms. a, see the editions of mss. b and c in this volume (text C.3.4 and B.2.1).

Line 4: For the baby incantation *āšib eklēti* not included in ms. a, see the editions of mss. b and c in this volume (texts C.3.3–C.3.4).

Line 5: The suffix *-šá* in GIN$_7$ KA *la-bi-ri-šá* [*šá-ṭir* (...)] is uncommon. Note, however, the colophon of SpTU 5, No. 248 u. e. 1 (text C.3.10): GIN$_7$ LIBIR.RA*-ša ša-ṭ*[*è-er* ...]. Usually, the pronominal suffix is *-šú* (see Hunger 1968, s.v. *pû* and *labiru*).

Lines 6–9: For discussion of the spell, see also Steinert 2017a, 316–318. The incantation is better preserved in ms. d, but the beginning of the spell (a formula in an unknown language) may have differed in both manuscripts, although it is possible that both mss. simply do not overlap. Only starting from line 7, both mss. a and d begin to present overlapping text, duplicating each other. For the variant presented in ms. d, see the edition of N. 4001 in this volume (text B.2.1).

The Akkadian part of the incantation envisages a prototypical situation in which an infertile woman was able to bear with the help of an unidentified god, which should repeat itself in the patient. The respective male and female roles in procreation are described in the text via agricultural metaphors: the male role is to "inseminate" the earth by means of the "seeder plough" (expressed with the verb *erēšu*) and to deposit (*nadû*) the seed in the "furrow" (*absinnu*), the female role is "to make the seed sprout", i.e. to bring the foetus into being. For the analogy between the seeder plough and insemination, see also Lambert (1960, 178 obv. 32 *Disputation between Ox and Horse*), referring to the plough poetically as *rāḫ* [*kīdi*] "inseminator of [the steppe]". See also this comparison known, in multiple variants from other healing spells, e.g. *Maqlû* VII 22ff. (Abusch 2016, 263, 350; see also Cooper 1996; Cavigneaux 1999; Steinert 2012a, 241–242; CAD R, 253 sub 2b): *araḫḫēka ramānī ... kīma ... epinnu erṣeta irḫû erṣetu imḫuru zēraša* "I am impregnating you, my self, ... just as ... the plough impregnated the earth, and the earth received its seed". For Sumerian ab-sín "furrow" as a poetic term for *šassūru* "womb", see also CAD S, 145 sub lex. sect., Antagal B 88.

Line 10: For the reading of *ana ur-ri-i* as D-stem infinitive of *erû* "to get pregnant", with a factitive meaning "to make pregnant", see also the similar rubric concerned with infertility or promoting conception in BAM 241 rev. iii 7' (text II.1.3): [MUNUS N]U *a-li-da-at ana ur-re-*⸢*e*⸣ [...] "to make an infertile woman get pregnant ..." (with Reiner 1982a, *ZA* 72, 128; Stol 2000a, 35 n. 65; Volk 2004, 74 n. 17). In other instances, the Š-stem *šūrû* is encountered with a causative meaning.

H. Stadhouders (personal communication) suggests that *urrû* in line 10 represents the verb (*w/m*)*urrû* "to cut off, to severe", which is used to refer to the activity of cutting the umbilical cord or to the act of separation between mother and child (AHw 1497; Stol 2000a, 116 with n. 35). He proposes that the spell described with the rubric may be concerned with delivery instead. However, the fact that ms. d includes a set of sentences resembling birth prognoses found in fertility/pregnancy tests beside the spell and treatment duplicated in ms. a lines 1–17, rather speaks for a link with *erû* and promotion of female fertility.

Lines 11–17: Again, ms. d is better preserved than ms. a, and part of the instructions can be restored from the former manuscript. However, toward the end of the prescription, both manuscripts are very damaged, and the text does not overlap anymore, which poses difficulties for the reconstruction. It appears that the instructions in ms. d are abbreviated in comparison with ms. a, which adds text in lines 16–17 that is not found in ms. d.

As far as can be guessed from the preserved text, the treatment found in these lines involved the preparation of a potion consisting of six drugs (boiled in beer): *imḫur-līm*-plant, *imḫur-ešrā*-plant, *tarmuš*-plant, *nīnû*-plant, *kurkānû*-plant of the mountain(s) and "dust locusts" (BURU$_5$.SAḪAR.RA, *erib turbu'ti*). Of these drugs, at least *imḫur-līm*-plant and *kurkānû* are also recommended to promote fertility in other sources. The former is characterised as "a plant for a woman who does not bear" (Ú ^{munus}NU.Ù.TU / *šammi lā ālitti*) (to be drunk in beer) in the herbals BAM 380 rev. 27 // BAM 381 iii 20 (Stol 2000a, 52–53). The medical uses of the *kurkānû*-plant have lately been discussed by Scurlock (2020, *JMC* 35), suggesting an identification with turmeric (cf. the objections concerning this identification raised by Jursa 2009, 162 n. 74). Three prescriptions for infertility in BAM 244: 31, 33, 37 (two salves and one potion) employ a compound which included *kurkānû* (text B.1.1). The present prescription requires the use of "*kurkānû* of the mountain" (*kurkānû* (*ša*) *šadî*), which occurs in contrast to *kurkānû ša māti* "*kurkānû* of the land" (i.e. the cultivated plant variety) in the Late Babylonian medical commentary TCL 6, 34: 16–17 (see Scurlock 2014a, 342). In ms. a, the *kurkānû*-plant is mentioned once more by itself, and it is possible that it was additionally ingested by the woman as a simple remedy. For *kurkānû* as fertility enhancer see also the BM 79061 obv. 11 (text A.2.8); BM 42313+ obv. 7 (text A.2.2), BAM 247: 8 (text B.1.3).

The use of "dust locust" (*erib turbu'ti*) as a medical ingredient is rare, see AHw s.v. *erbû* sub 2e, e.g. AMT 74 iii 14 (Eypper 2016, *JMC* 27, 38, used for a salve against *sagbānu*-disease associated with festering lesions on the feet). The term *turbu'tu* "dust (heap), sand dune" points to a desert habitat of the animal (cf. Landsberger 1934, *Fauna*, 123). For discussion of animals classified as locusts (including shrimp, "sea-locust"), see also Heimpel 1976–1980, "Insekten", *RlA* 5, 105–109 (especially §5 for uses in medicine and magic); Heimpel 1996, *RA* 90, 101–120; Lion and Michel 1997, *MARI* 8, 707–724; Lion, Michel and Noël 2000, *JCS* 52, 55–60. The Sumerogram $BURU_5$.SAḪAR.RA is equated with *kirbān* (*kurbān*) *eqli* "field clod" in the Practical Vocabulary from Assur 422d, a term that usually refers to a medicinal plant (Landsberger and Gurney 1957–1958, *AfO* 18, 332; CAD K, 401–404 lex. section and sub 3; AHw 483–484 sub 8). Animals classified as "locusts" ($BURU_5$) may have been associated with fertility, because locusts were known to occur in large swarms as field pests. Another type of "locust", "sea-locust" (*erib tâmti*), perhaps shrimp or crayfish, occurs in another treatment (tampon) for fertility (BM 42450+: 17''–20'' (text B.2.3). For locust (*erbu*) in a recipe to induce menstrual bleeding, see also BM 42313+: 19 (text A.2.2).

The preparation of the present remedy for fertility further required that the prepared potion was left on the roof under the stars for three days in a porous vessel. Furthermore, an incense-offering had to be presented to the moon god Sîn. For the role of the moon god as a provider of offspring in another ritual in the case when a woman is "delayed in bearing (children)", see AO 4425A+B (*infra* text B.2.6).

Line 14: M. Stol (personal communication) suggests that the verb at the end of the line in ms. d may be *i*-[*ka-ab-ba-as*] "she shall (not) step (on the ground)". Alternatively, the subject of the verb may be the *burzigallu*-vessel, which is left outside under the stars in line 22.

Lines 18–20: The beginning of line 18 is emended following the Assur Medical Catalogue (Steinert et al. 2018, 218 line 117), which is the only other attestation for this formula so far and cited there as the incipit of a tablet belonging to a treatise concerned with birth and gynaecological conditions (BIRTH). The catalogue incipit is unfortunately also fragmentary, reading: [DIŠ MUNUS Ù.TU-*m*]*a ni-ip-šá ina kir-ri-š*[*á*$^?$ x x (x)]. The term *nipšu* "breathing; odour, (bad) smell" as an ailment is elsewhere attested in connection with skin sores and with conditions associated with a bad smell emitted from the body (see Steinert et al. 2018, 274–275 commentary on line 117 for discussion; Abusch et al. 2020, CMAwR 3, text 3.11, esp. lines 19, 21). The word *nipšu* is also found in reference to the smell of plants (e.g. SpTU 5, No. 272: 21, 26, 29). The exact meaning of *nipšu* in the present context remains unclear, but it is described here as a postpartum problem.

Line 23': Probably, PÉŠ.SAR.R[A] is a mistake for PÉŠ.ÙR.RA = *arrabu* "dormouse".

Line 24': For $BURU_5$.IR.GI.LUM = *ergilu*, a type of locust, see Landsberger, *Fauna*, 40, 44, 123; Militarev and Kogan 2005, 142–143 No. 103 (for Semitic cognates, e.g. Hebrew *ḥargōl*). The ingredient is also attested in a collection of rituals for "purifying the horse stables" and protection of the animals from epidemics, known from manuscripts found at Assur and Nineveh (KAR 91 rev. 12 and dupl.; Maul 2013, *ZA* 103, 26: 49'). Note also BAM 297: 15 (fragmentary context). For other varieties of locusts as an ingredient in ms. a, see also lines 12' and 26' (with notes). Terms for different "types" of locusts may also refer to different stages in the life cycle of adult locusts (cf. Müller 1995, 140–142).

Lines 26'–34': As much as can be guessed from the fragmentarily preserved text, the short prescriptions in this section could all be used for the purpose of contraception, and possibly, also the prescriptions in the preceding lines 23'–25' shared the same purpose. The concluding statement NU $PEŠ_4$ = *ul irri* "she will not get pregnant" is only preserved in line 34'. However, the entries preceding line 34' share the same general format of a catalogue of short, mostly one-line prescriptions, starting with DIŠ KI.MIN "alternatively". All these remedies appear to have been potions using mostly one drug (plant, mineral or animal (substance)) given in beer. One may compare the present recipes with entries in the gynaecological sections of drug lists described as Ú MUNUS NU PEŠ$_4$. So far this expression has been understood in a contrasting sense, as "drugs for a woman who does not get pregnant", referring to a (fertile) woman who has difficulties conceiving a(nother) child (Stol 2000a, 53–54; Couto-Ferreira 2014, 309). Yet, given the section of contraceptives in BM 51246+ and the similarity between the formulations it seems more likely that Ú MUNUS NU PEŠ$_4$ has to be understood as a "drug for (the purpose that) a woman not get pregnant/for not letting a woman get pregnant" (*šammi sinništi lā erî/šūrî*); see also Steinert 2021, *Byzantinische Forschungen* 33, 57–58 for discussion.

Drugs designated as Ú MUNUS NU PEŠ$_4$ are attested in BAM 380 rev. 25–41 (esp. 28–29) // BAM 381 iii 17–36 (esp. iii 21–22) and appear together with drugs for conception and to treat infertility. One may also compare the reference to a "plant for not getting pregnant / not bearing (children)" (*šammi lā erî/lā alādi*) in Hh. XVII 209–212; MSL 10, 90), beside a "plant for getting pregnant / bearing (children)". One of the plants listed as Ú MUNUS NU PEŠ$_4$ in BAM 380 and BAM 381 is *ankinūtu*-plant, which is also prescribed in the present section of BM 51246+ (ms. a line 33'). Significantly, the *ankinūtu*-plant is often associated with *ašqulālu*-plant (Stol 2000a, 54 with n. 35), as is also the case in BM 51246+ (ms. a), where *ašqulālu* is used in the prescription in line 34', directly following the recipe with *ankinūtu*-plant. The *ankinūtu*-plant is used among the drugs in a compound recipe to induce abortion in BAM 246 (text B.1.6). The *ašqulālu*-plant is otherwise also found as a "drug for (inducing?) labour pains" (*šammi ḫâli*) in Uruanna II 39 (see CAD Ḫ, 55). The use of these plants both as a contraceptive and abortifacient may indicate that the healers saw these purposes as related (e.g., for ejecting the male semen after intercourse, or the foetus, when conception had already occurred).

Line 26': The reading *erib karāni* "locust of the grapevine" for BURU$_5$(?).GEŠTIN.NA is not certain, as this logogram or expression is not attested so far. There are, however, other types of 'locusts' designated with such genitive phrases, e.g. *erib nāri* "river locust", *erib tâmti* "sea locust" (shellfish) and *erib turbu'ti* "dust locust", the latter of which was recommended earlier in the text (see above line 12). Note also the use of *ergilu*, another type of locust, in line 24. The *dušû*-stone (suggested identifications: chlorite or calcite) was of yellow or green colour (cf. Schuster-Brandis 2008, 407–409; Thavapalan 2020, 244–264). The typical colour of the locust's wings is compared here with the colour of this stone. For a very similar comparison working in the opposite direction, note that in *abnu šikinšu* (STT 108: 84; Schuster-Brandis 2008, 30: 84), the appearance of a stone (*turminabandû*) is compared with the wings of a dragonfly (*kīma kappī kallat Šamaš*).

Line 27': I have opted for emending the text and reading KÙ.SI$_{22}$ *li-<iq>-ti ma-da* TI "you take much gold of high quality". Although a word *litu* exists, it is not a highly plausible reading, since it designates a quality of silver and is only attested in Old Assyrian texts (cf. CAD L, 221a; AHw 556b "eine Silberlegierung"). However, *liqtu* is attested in reference to gold of high quality (CAD L, 207 sub 4a; differently AHw 555 sub 1 "Goldklumpen"). The use of gold and of a large quantity of it (*māda*) is unexpected, but a better reading of the passage escapes me. Possibly, restore *e-*[*nu-ma* ...] "when ..." in the gap.

Line 28': The more usual logogram in for *asu* "myrtle" medical texts is ^{šim}GÍR. For occasional writings $^{\text{(giš/šim)}}$AZ instead of ^{šim}GÍR, cf. CAD A/2, 342. After the sign AZ, the reading and restoration *u$_4$-ma* NÍG.GIG-[*šá* IGI NAG-*ši-*(*ma*) NU PEŠ$_4$$^?$] is inspired by SpTU 1, No. 59: 12' (text C.2.1), in which (NÍG).GIG = *maruštu* "trouble" is used as a euphemistic expression for the menses (see *infra*). The Uruk text SpTU 1, No. 59 contains prescriptions for the case that a woman does not "see" (*amāru*) her menses, to make them appear. If the restoration is correct, the present prescription in BM 51246+ would have to be taken on the day of the onset of the menses. To my knowledge, such a specific recommendation for the date of administering medicine in connection with the patient's menstrual cycle is not attested in any other gynaecological recipe in the corpus, but it may in fact be significant with a regard to the special context of the prescription (contraception). Alternatively, one may consider reading *u$_4$-ma* NÍG.GIG$^?$-[*šá* DIB], "on the day that [her] *menses* [have passed by]" (*ītiqu*), which could refer to the end of the menstrual discharge or to a missed period.

Lines 29'–30': This recipe compounds two prescriptions applying the root of male *pillû*-plant as a potion, probably each prepared with a different carrier substance / liquid. That this plant (the suggested identification with mandrake is not certain) is chosen as a contraceptive is particularly interesting. As M. Stol (2000a, 70) points out, root of male *pillû*-plant also occurs as the main ingredient in a salve in BAM 248 rev. iv 19–20 //, where it is used to speed up difficult labour (see text D.1.1). In the latter text, in particular, *pillû* growing on the north side is required. As Stol concludes, the male *pillû*-plant is associated with the characteristic that it does not bear fruit, which makes it a suitable drug in a prescription for ending a pregnancy, but also even more in a prescription for contraception encountered in BM 51246+. Stol (2000a, 57–58) further points out that *pillû*-plant is not encountered as an aphrodisiac or fertility-enhancing plant in Mesopotamian sources. Note, however, its use in a fragmentary remedy in BAM 244 obv. 4, a tablet concerned with promoting female fertility / treating infertility (text B.1.1).

Line 31': The sequence KA.GI SIG.GI is assumed to be a mistake for ^{na4}KA.GI.NA SIG$_5$.GA, *šadânu damqu* "good haematite". This stone designation is attested in stone lists and (rarely) in amulet prescriptions, see Schuster-Brandis 2008, 426 and "Kette 56"; Hh. XVI 5 (MSL 10, 5); MSL 10, 64 ii 36 (written KUR-*nu* SIG$_5$.GA). The use of SIG instead of SIG$_5$ (for *damqu*) is found in other texts, see e.g. Abusch and Schwemer 2011, CMAwR 1, 219: 100'''; Stadhouders 2011, *JMC* 18, 18 § 11, 23 n. 104, 26–28 §§ 3–5, 7, 11–13; Stol 2013, *BiOr* 70, 128 (12). If this interpretation is correct, maybe "powder" (KU.KU, *supantu* or KU, *sīktu*) of the stone was recommended in the present prescription. An alternative, but less likely reading may be GI.SIG = *kikkišu* "reed fence, reed hut".

Line 32': nam-ba-ra-an-gi is interpreted as a phonetic spelling for Sumerian nam-ba-ra-an-gi$_4$. The word gi-li-ib should probably be understood as gilib = *parāku* "to lie across; to block". Since this spell was used in connection with a remedy for contraception, the "house brick" (sig$_4$; šeg$_{12}$) could be understood metaphorically as a barrier blocking the woman's womb off against the semen. It is likely that line 32' ended with an instruction to recite the spell over the preceding or following remedy.

Lines 33'–34': For *ankinūtu*-plant and *ašqulālu*-plant in the present context (contraception), see the comments on lines 26'–34' above.

Lines 35'–36': For other prescriptions against the loss of amniotic fluid (A.MEŠ, *mû* lit. "water"), see also BM 42313+ lines 57–58 (text A.2.2); cf. Böck 2013, 46–47. The introductory formula in line 35' reads DIŠ MUNUS A.A-*šá* DU-*ku*, in which A.A appears to indicate the plurality of *mû* "water" or may simply be a mistake for the common spelling A.(MEŠ) (see e.g., BAM 237 rev. iv 29, 33, 38 = text C.1.4). The second part of the case description continues with the formulation *ù* [*šá* ŠÀ]-⸢*šá*$^?$⸣ ŠUB-*a*, which should be understood as "she is in danger of miscarrying/about to miscarry", since the following prescription aims at preserving pregnancy. The formula varies from line 37', which preserves the more common form: DIŠ PEŠ$_4$ A-*šá* DU-*ku* ⸢*šà*⸣ ŠÀ-*šá a-n*[*a*] ⸢*la*$^?$⸣ [*na*]-*de*$^?$-*e* "If a pregnant woman's (amniotic) fluid flows, so that she not have a miscarriage".

The ingredient ÚKUŠ.LAGAB KUR "mountain colocynth(?)" (*errî šadî*?) in line 35' of the recipe is not attested elsewhere to my knowledge. Note, however, similar (wild-growing) plants with this specification, especially ÚKUŠ.TI.GI.LUM KUR.RA and ÚKUŠ.LI.LI.GI KUR.RA, both equated with *tigilû šadî* "mountain *tigilû*-colocynth" (see e.g. MSL 10, 98; CAD T, 397). Stol (1987b, *BSA* 4, 84, 85) suggests identifying *irrû* (*errû*), translated as colocynth in the dictionaries, with the wild melon, and *tigilû* with the colocynth.

Lines 37'–40': A similar passage to lines 37'–40' invoking the sun god Šamaš is found in BM 40152 rev. iii 17–26 (text C.1.8), a ritual to stop female bleeding, in which the "shepherd's staff-plant" (*ḫaṭṭi rēʾî*) plays the central role (see text C.1.8 for discussion). The ritual procedure requiring that the root of a plant should be removed from the earth at a time when it did not "see the sun" (usually in the early morning before sunrise) is attested in other healing texts (and in connection with other medicinal plants).[271] Although such instructions have been linked with the propitious influence of the stars (Reiner 1995, 36–37), Böck (2014, 158) argues that such instructions may reflect empirical knowledge that some plants should not be exposed to direct sunlight, so that its properties would not diminish.

Line 38': Instead of *ina šēri ina* NU ZABAR, one would expect a phrase such as *ina šēri lām namāri* "in the morning/dawn, before it is light" (see e.g., Maul 1994, 130: 27; 134: 89). For this reason, it is suggested that ZABAR in our text replaces ZALAG/ZÁLAG = *namāru*. Sumerian zabar is equated with *namru* "bright, light" (and with *ebbu* and *ellu* "pure") in lexical texts, e.g. A III/3: 197–199 (MSL 14, 337); Diri I 128–130 (MSL 15, 108); cf. also Ḫg. II 225 (MSL 7, 171 with *namru* given as a synonym for *siparru* "bronze").

271 A similar (bilingual) ritual passage involving harvesting the *tigilû*-colocynth for healing purposes is found in SAG.GIG.GA.MEŠ Tablet 9 (CT 17, 19 i 17–24 and dupl.; SpTU 2, No. 2 i 29–40 etc.; Reiner 1995, 36). Medical prescriptions mentioning the procedure are: BAM 396 rev. iii 7 (Geller 2005a, No. 1); BAM 575 iii 25 (STOMACH 2; Cadelli 2000, 137; Johnson and Simkó 2024, 135: 160), requesting to use "(the root of a) 'dog's tongue' plant, which when you pull it up, has not seen the sun" (*šuruš* (SUḪUŠ) *lišān kalbi*(^{ú}EME-UR.GI$_7$) *ša ina nasāḫī*(ZI)-*ka Šamaš*(^{d}UTU) *lā*(NU) *īmuru*(IGI.(DU$_8$)). A variant formulation is *ša ina napāli* ^{d}UTU NU IGI.BAR "(the root of *pillû*-plant) which was not exposed to the sun when it was dug out" (Tsukimoto 1999, *Priests and Officials*, 193 line 46, in a medical text from Emar).

The other possibility would be to understand ZABAR in its usual reading *siparru* as a bronze tool, which would mean that the practitioner was not allowed to dig out the plant with a bronze instrument (*ina lā siparri* [*iš*]*tu šuršīšu tan*[*ap-p*]*al* "you dig up (the plant) with its root, without (using a) bronze (tool)"). A similar phrasing, to take the plant "with its root", without reference to a tool, occurs within an incantation, using the verb *šarāḫu* "to pluck" (BAM 215: 54 and dupl.; Köcher 1966, *AfO* 21, 18; Scurlock 1988, MMDG, No. 82; Böck 2007, *Muššu'u*, 74), in reference to the *anamiru*-plant: [ú] *a-na-mi-ru šam-mu ul-tu šur-ši-šú iš-ru-ḫu-ma* "they (the gods) pulled out the *anamiru*-plant with its root". For a passage, in which *siparru* "bronze" by itself perhaps indicates a bronze tool, cf. BAM 482 i 64: *ina si-pa-ri* / SI *pa-ri* 1-*šú* 2-*šú* 3-*šú ta-tak-*[*kip*] "you punct[ure] (the patient's temple) with a bronze (lancet) / with the horn of a lamb" (cf. Attia and Buisson 2003, *JMC* 1, 5, 16). For a similar treatment using a bronze instrument / lancet (KIN.TUR ZABAR), see also Stol 1993, 95 (STT 89: 156).

Line 39': For other healing plants referred to as "your (Šamaš's) plant", see AMT 74 ii 62 (K. 67+), see Eypper 2016, *JMC* 27, 34–35; here sunflower is used against sores on the feet. The legendary "belly plant" (*šammi libbi*), occurring as a remedy for a gastrointestinal disease (*kīs libbi*), is also associated with Šamaš in healing spells (e.g. STT 252: 11; Collins 1999, 148–151; BAM 576 ii 12' and dupl., Collins 1999, 145–148 line 11; Cadelli 2000, 83; Johnson and Simkó 2024, 92 line 169). One may expect a reference to the sun god's power to preserve the foetus in the womb in the gap in line 39'.

Line 41': Since the rubric in rev. 19' reaches the bottom of the tablet, it should be understood as a short colophon. Perhaps, restore *bulṭū l*[*at-ku-tu*] "proven remedies", or MU[NUS ...] "(remedies for) a wo[man ...]". The text is designated as the 34th *nisḫu*-tablet in a series. Unfortunately, it remains unclear whether this series comprised only medical-therapeutic material related to women's health or was part of a more comprehensive series.

A.2.8 BM 79061: A Short Collection of Remedies for Women

This fragment of a single-column tablet in Late Babylonian script was among the tablets purchased by E. A. Wallis Budge for the British Museum's Babylonian collection in Baghdad in 1889. The provenience of BM 79061 was simply registered as "Babylonia" in the museum register, but many of the texts in the 89-4-26 collection in fact stem from Sippar (Walker 1988, *CBT* VIII/3, xviii–xix).

The tablet fragment contains a small collection of recipes for women's conditions, focusing on prescriptions to promote fertility and on treatments for problems after delivery. The text displays remarkable features, such as the occurrence of hitherto unattested drug names. Besides its few peculiarities, the tablet shares similarities in vocabulary and recipe structure with tablets from the medical archive from Sippar published by I. L. Finkel (2000). Other features, however, for example some of the numerous syllabic spellings, may point to an older tradition, possibly even to a Middle or Old Babylonian origin of some of the prescriptions on the tablet.

List of Manuscripts

Siglum	Museum Number	Copy	Collation	Format; Ductus	Provenience
a	BM 79061 (Bu 89-4-26, 358)	Pl. 21–22	Coll.	Fragment of a single-column tablet in portrait format; Late Babylonian period; ca. 6th/5th cent. BCE	Babylonia

Overview

i	Prescription for fertility (ointment) a obv. 1–4	1–4
ii	Prescription for fertility (for ingestion) a obv. 5–8	5–8
iii	Prescription for fertility (potion) a obv. 9–12	9–12

iv	Prescription for fertility a obv. 13–14	13–14
v	Prescription for a problem after delivery (potion) a obv. 15–17	15–17
vi	Fragmentary prescription for fertility(?) a obv. 18–19	18–19[…
vii'	Prescription for a problem after delivery a rev. 1'–3'	…]20'–22'
viii'	Prescription for a problem after delivery (suppository) a rev. 4'–5'	23'–24'
ix'	Prescription for a problem after delivery a rev. 6'–8'	25'–27'
x'	Prescription for a problem after delivery a rev. 9'–13'	28'–32'
xi'	Prescription for fertility a rev. 14'–17'	33'–36'
xii'	Prescription a rev. 17'–u. e. 3	36'–40'

Previous Edition and Discussion

Steinert 2021, *Byzantinische Forschungen* 33, 68 (ms. a obv. 5–8)
Electronic Babylonian Library (eBL) (https://www.ebl.lmu.de/library/BM.79061)

Transliteration

1	a obv. 1	^{munus}*la e-ri-tu*$_4$ *a-*na* šu-ri-ʾ-*[*i*]
2	a obv. 2	^{ú}*kal-da-mi-iq* ^{ú}*nam-ru-qu* x[x]
3	a obv. 3	*ù* ŠIM *ḫi-i-li ta-bal-lal* Š[ÉŠ-*su*]
4	a obv. 4	*šá pa-te-e* [(*u* PEŠ$_4^?$)]
5	a obv. 5	DIŠ KI.MIN ^{ú}*tar-muš* ŠIM *ḫi-i-l*[*i* x x]
6	a obv. 6	^{šim}ḪAB *ḫa-me-di-ra-an-ni ri-*[x (x)]
7	a obv. 7	^{šim}x[x x x x x]-⸢x-*tu*⸣ [x x x]
8	a obv. 8	⸢ZÚ.LUM.MA⸣ *ta-s*[*a-ka*$^?$ x]x-⸢*ú*⸣ ⸢*tu-šá*⸣-[*kal-ši*]
9	a obv. 9	MUNUS [*da*$^?$]-*mi-šú ina* <<*šá*>> *ka*$_4$*-an-ni-*⸢*šú*⸣ ⸢GI$_6$⸣ ⸢*i-ṣi*⸣
10	a obv. 10	*la* [*ir*]-*ri* $^{\textit{erasure}}$ *a-na šu-ri-ʾ-*⸢*i*⸣
11	a obv. 11	^{ú}*k*[*u*]-*ur-ru-ka-nu* ^{ú}ZA.GÌN-*tu*$_4$ *za-aʾ-it*
12	a obv. 12	*nam-ru-qu u*$_4$*-mu-us-sú ta-*⸢*šaq*⸣-*qí-iš*
13	a obv. 13	MUNUS *šá* ⸢*ka*$_4^?$⸣-*an-ni-šú* 5-*šú* ^{ú}A.Z[AL.LÁ]
14	a obv. 14	*gír-*⸢*e*⸣ ⸢*gu*⸣-*uḫ-lu* [x x (x)]
15	a obv. 15	⸢MUNUS⸣ ⸢*ú*⸣-*lid-ma zu-ur-šú bi*$^!$-*ir*$^!$-*da*$^{?!}$ (bi da ir) *m*[*a-li*$^?$]

16 a obv. 16 [x x]x *šú-šá-na* NUMUM x x x[x x x x]

17 a obv. 17 [*ina* x x]x *u*$^{?}$ KAŠ.⸢SAG⸣ *ta-š[aq*$^{?}$*-qí-iš]*

---

18 a obv. 18 [...] ⸢x⸣ [x x] ⸢*a*⸣*-na pa-t[e-e*$^{?}$ ...]

19 a obv. 19 [...] šu$^{?}$ pa$^{?}$ x[...]

Ms. a obv. breaks; gap of unknown length
Beginning of ms. a rev. lost

20' a rev. 1' [MUNUS *ú*]-⸢*lid*⸣-[*ma* x] ⸢x⸣ [x x x x x x]

21' a rev. 2' [x x]-*nu ú-ta-ak-*⸢*kàr*⸣ x x[x x x]

22' a rev. 3' *ki ba-*⸢*ḫír*$^{?}$⸣ x ^{erasure} [x]

23' a rev. 4' *an-da*$^{?}$-[*aḫ*]-*šú*$^{?}$ *bi-il-le-tu*$_{4}$ ⸢SIG$_{5}$⸣ ⸢*te*⸣-[*ṭe*$_{4}$*-en*$^{?}$]

24' a rev. 5' *ta-b[al-la]l ina šá-su-*⸢*ri-šú*⸣ *ta-šak-k[an]*

25' a rev. 6' 1 GÍN ^{ši}[$^{m?}$ x x⸣ [x x x] ⸢gi$^{?}$⸣ ⸢ḫa⸣ x [x x]

26' a rev. 7' 2 GÍN ⸢$^{šim?}$⸣[x] ⸢x x⸣ [x x x] ú$^{?}$/šid [x x]

27' a rev. 8' *ina maš-ku* ⸢*te-ṭe*$^{?}$⸣-[*ri* ....]

28' a rev. 9' ⸢MUNUS⸣ *ú-lid-ma ana*$^{?}$ [...........]

29' a rev. 10' *ti-ia-a-t[i* ....]

30' a rev. 11' 5-*aš mi-ni-*[*ti*$^{?}$] ⸢^{ú}x x⸣ [x x x x]

31' a rev. 12' *ma-la ta-*[x x] x ⸢*ta-sa*⸣-[*ka ina* Ì.GIŠ$^{?}$]

32' a rev. 13' *ta-bal-lal* ⸢ŠÉŠ⸣-*áš-ši-ma*$^{?}$ *ip-p[a*$^{?}$*-áš-šar]*

33' a rev. 14' 1 GÍN *ka-*⸢*mu*⸣*-nu* [x] GÍN ⸢x (x)⸣ IL[LU x x]

34' a rev. 15' ŠIM *ḫi-i-li* MUNU$_{4}^{?}$ ⸢ZÌ$^{?}$⸣ *ta-bal-lal* [x x x x]

35' a rev. 16' *si-im-bir-ri nu-ḫur-tu*$_{4}$ *ina qú-pu-ú ta*$^{?}$-[x x x]

36' a rev. 17' *šá pa-te-e* | *si-im-bir-ri nu-ḫur-tu*$_{4}$ [x x x]

37' a rev. 18' *el-le-tu*$_{4}$ *ši-ki-in ti-nu-ú-ru* ⸢x⸣ [x (x)]

38' a u. e. 1 *qaq-qa-da*^{meš} *šá ka-ma-ru iš-te*$^{?}$ [(x)]

39' a u. e. 2 *ḫal-dap-pu-ú ta-sa-ka*

40' a u. e. 3 *šá tu-uš-tu*$_{4}$ ⸢*me*⸣*-e*

Bound Transcription and Translation

1 *lā erītu ana šūrî* 2 *kal-damiq namruqqu* [...] 3 *u riqqi ḫīlī taballal tapa*[*ššassu*] 4 *ša patê* [*u erî*(?)]	1 To enable a woman who is not pregnant to get pregnant: 2 You mix 'good-for-everything-plant', *namruqqu*-plant, [...] 3 and aromatic plant for the birth pangs and ru[b(?) her (with them)]. 4 (This is good) for opening up [and getting pregnant(?)].
5 DIŠ KI.MIN *tarmuš riqqi ḫīl*[*ī* ...] 6 *ṭūra ḫamedīrāni* ...[...] 7 ...[...] ...[...] 8 *suluppī tas*[*âk* ...]... *tuša*[*kkalši*]	5 Alternatively, 8 you po[und] 5 *tarmuš*-plant, aromatic plant for the birth p[angs, ...], 6 *ṭūru*-aromatic, *hamedīrānu*-plant(?), [...], 7 [...]-aromatic, ...[...], 8 dates, [...], you have [her eat (the mixture)].
9 *sinništu* [*dā*]*mšu ina kannīšu ṣalim īṣ*(*i*) 10 *lā* [*ir*]*ri*(?) *ana šūrî* 11 [*ku*]*rkānû*(?) *uqnâtu za'itu* 12 *namruqqu ūmussu tašaqqīši*	9 (If) a woman's blood on her menstrual bandage is black (and only) a little, 10 (and) she does not get pregnant(?), to enable (her) to get pregnant: 11 You give her *kurkānû*-plant(?), *uqnâtu*-plant, olive (oil), 12 (and) *namruqqu*-plant to drink daily.
13 *sinništu ša kannīšu* <...> *ḫummuš aza*[*llû*] 14 *girû guḫlu* [...]	13 (For) a woman whose menstrual bandage <...>: one fifth of a shekel of *azallû*-plant, 14 one carat (1/24 of a shekel) of antimony [...].
15 *sinništu ūlid-ma zu*(*mu*)*ršu birda*(?) *m*[*ali*(?)] 16 [...]-*šu šuššān zēr* ...[...] 17 [*ina* ...]... *u šikari taš*[*aqqīši*]	15 (If) a woman gives birth and subsequently h[er] body [is full of(?)] *birdu*-spots(?), 16 [...] her. A third (of a shekel?) of seed of ..., [...]. 17 You have [her drink (it) in ...] and beer.
18 [...] *ana pa*[*tê* ... ...] 19 [...] ... [... ...]	18 [...] for open[ing up ...] 19 *too fragmentary for translation*

Ms. a obv. breaks; gap of unknown length
Beginning of ms. a rev. lost

20' [*sinništu ū*]*lid-*[*ma* ...]...[... ...] 21' [...]... *uttakkar* ...[...] 22' *kī baḫir* ... [...]	20' [(If) a woman gives] birth and subsequently [...] 21' [...] it/she becomes changed (for the worse), ... [...] 22' when it is (still) hot ... [...].
23' *andaḫšu billat našpi te*[*ṭên*(?)] 24' *taballal ina šassūrīšu tašakk*[*an*]	23' You gr[ind] (and) 24' mix 23' *andaḫšu*-vegetable (and) *billatu*-substance (used for making) *našpu*-beer. 24' You insert (it) into her womb (viz. vagina).
25' *ištēn šiqil* ...[...] ... [...] 26' *šina šiqil* ... [...] ...[...] 27' *ina maški teṭe*[*rri* ......]	25' One shekel of [...]-aromatic, [... shekel(s) of ...], 26' two shekels of [...], ...[...] 27' you spr[ead (it)] on a (piece of) leather [...].
28' *sinništu ūlid-ma ana*(?) [... ...] 29' *tīyati* [... ... ...] 30' *ḫamaš minī*[*ti*(?)] ... [...] 31' *mala ta-*[...] ... *tasâ*[*k ina šamni*(?)] 32' *taballal tapaššašší-ma ipp*[*aššar*]	28' (If) a woman gives birth and subsequently [...], 31' you pound 29' *tīyatu*-plant, [...], 30' a fifth *of the norm*[*al amount of*(?) ...]-plant, [...], 31' as much as you [...], 32' you mix (it) 31' [with oil(?)], 32' you rub her (with it) and it/she will be rele[ased].

33' *ištēn šiqil kamūnu* [...] *šiqil* ... *ḫī*[*l* ...] 34' *riqqi ḫīlī buqlu qēmu*(?) *taballal* [...] 35' *simbirru nuḫurtu ina quppî*(?) *ta*-[...] 36' *ša patê* | *simbirru nuḫurtu* [...] 37' *elletu šikin tinūri* ... [...] 38' *qaqqadī ša kamāri ište* [(...)] 39' *ḫaltappî tasâk* 40' *ša tūšti mê*(?)

34' You mix 33' one shekel cumin, [...] shekel(s) ... res[in of ...], 34' aromatic plant for the birth pangs, malt, flour(?) [...]. 35' You [...] *simbirru*-plant (and) *nuḫurtu*-plant with a sharp knife. 36' (This is good) for opening (the womb). 39' You pound 36' *simbirru*-plant, *nuḫurtu*-plant, [...] 37' pure 36' [...], 37' soot(?) from an oven, [...], 38' heads(?) of *kamāru*-fish with 39' the rod of an incantation priest(?). 40' (This is good) for the *turning back* of the fluids(?).

Notes

Line 1: For the expression *lā erītu ana šūrî* "to enable a woman who is not pregnant to get pregnant" and similar formulations introducing prescriptions, see also BM 59710: 1 (text B.2.5): *ana* ^{munus}NU.PEŠ$_4$ *šu-r*[*i-'i*] "To enable a woman (who is) not pregnant to get pregnant"; BAM 250 rev. 3 (text B.1.4): (a total of 21 beads) ^{munus}NU.PEŠ$_4$ *ana* PEŠ$_4$ "to enable a woman (who is) not pregnant (*lā erītu*) to become pregnant" (*ana šūrî*). Sometimes, the diagnostic statement is introduced with *šumma* as a conditional clause, e.g. in STT 98: 2', 5': [DIŠ] ⌜MUNUS⌝ NU PEŠ$_4$ *ana* ⌜PEŠ$_4$ "[If] a woman does not get pregnant, to enable her to get pregnant"; BM 42313+ obv. 8, rev. 33 // BM 42333+: 5: DIŠ MUNUS NU PEŠ$_4$ *a-na šu-ri-i* "If a woman does not get pregnant, to enable (her) to get pregnant ...". See *infra* texts A.1.1, A.2.2.

Line 3: An aromatic plant with the name "aromatic for the birth pangs" (*riqqi ḫīlī*) is not known from other medical texts, neither a *ḫīlu*-plant. The form *ḫi-i-li* points to a genitive construction, as in analogous names with *šammu* "plant" (e.g., *šammi balāṭi* "plant of life"). The name *riqqi ḫīlī* would indicate that this unknown drug served to promote delivery (i.e. cause uterine contractions). This drug is found multiple times in ms. a (see also lines 5, 34'). It is noteworthy that the *namruqqu*-plant recommended beside *riqqi ḫīlī* in the present prescription is a recurring ingredient in recipes to provoke an abortion (BAM 246: 1–5) and is also a drug given in difficult labour (BAM 248 iv 13 and dupl.), see texts B.1.6, D.1.1. Drug compendia classify the *namruqqu*-plant as a drug to expel a foetus, when complications arise during delivery (cf. Stol 2000a, 52, 53–55). The application of "expelling" drugs for the purpose of "opening" the womb for conception in the present prescription is remarkable. Interesting is further the drug name *kal-damiq* in line 2 (written syllabically), meaning "it is good for all (diseases)", as in English "all-heal". Ms. a is again the first attestation for this name. Compare similar statements *ana* ... *damiq* (SIG$_5$) describing drugs that are useful for specific conditions, see e.g. CAD D, 73 s.v. *damqu* mng. 8 ("good" in the sense of "effective"); Stadhouders 2011, *JMC* 18, 16 ff. §§ 1, 3 6–8 *passim* (in *Šammu šikinšu*); Steinert 2015, 116–188 for discussion.

The spelling *ù* instead of *u* for "and" in line 3 is one of the features that may point to an older origin of the present text, cf. AHw 1397; von Soden and Röllig 1991, 47, 51; Aro 1955, 25.

Line 4: The restoration *šá pa-te-e* [*u* PEŠ$_4$] is suggested by the parallel label in BM 42587+: 27 *šá* BAD *u* PEŠ$_4$ "for opening up and getting pregnant" (text B.2.5). See also BM 42313+ line 77 and dupl. (Finkel 2000, *FS Lambert*, 172 Text 17: 11; text A.2.2 in this volume for discussion): BAD-*ma ir-ri* "she will open and become pregnant", in a prescription to promote female fertility. It is possible, however, that no text was written in the break at the end of this line and that the label was only *ša patê* "for opening" (note the variant spelling instead of *petê*). See also lines 18 and 36' for two more occurrences of this label *ša patê*.

Line 6: A drug with the name *ḫamedīrannu* or *ḫamedīrānu* ("*ḫamedīru*-like-plant") is not known from other texts. Perhaps this name is related to *ḫamadīru*, *ḫamadāru* "shrivelled, withered" (said of plants, grain), see AHw, 315, 1558; CAD Ḫ, 57–58; Mayer 2016, *OrNS* 85, 211–212; George 2016, 108–109 line 13 (*ḫamedīrūta alāku*). Otherwise, a connection to Aramaic *ḥmṭyry'* / *ḥwmṭry'*, a polygonum, is not excluded (Jastrow 1903, 435b; Sokoloff 2002, 468a). Compare further an unidentified insect *ḫamānīru* or *ḫamānirru*, which is exclusively attested in a disputation poem known in ancient times as *The Series of the Spider* (eSAD; Jiménez 2017, 304: 11, 29, 32 *passim*, 322–323). This animal is one of the contestants of this poem and is called "creation of the steppe, vagrant of the [city]".

At the end of line 6, perhaps restore *ripītu* (a fungus) or *riṭbu* (a plant), which however only occur rarely. Alternatively, one could read *taltallānu* (a medical plant) or *taltallu* "male inflorescence of the date palm".

Line 8: Note the syllabic spelling of *tušakkalši*, parallel to *ta-šaq-qí-iš* "you have her drink" in line 12 (the apocopated form of the pronominal suffix -*iš* instead of -*ši* occurs often in Late Babylonian texts. For the spelling *ta-sa-ka* for *tasâk* "you pound", see also below lines 31, 39. Such spellings with "overhanging" vowels are likewise typical for late texts.

Perhaps one may restore [u_4-*m*]*i-šam* "(your give it to her to eat) on a daily basis"? See similarly the next prescription.

Line 9: A remarkable feature of ms. a is that in most diagnostic labels introducing the prescriptions, the usual conditional *šumma*(DIŠ) "if" is omitted (see lines 9, 13, 15, 28).

The term *kannu* "menstrual bandage" encountered in lines 9 and 13 occurs in a few other women's healthcare texts (see BM 42313+ lines 38–39 (text A.2.2) and LKA 9 rev. r. col. 13'–14' (text C.3.5)). The present orthography (*ka*$_4$*-an-ni-šú*, also line 13) with the sign *ka*$_4$ is also attested in AO 6374 line 40 (text C.3.9, *ka*$_4$*-ni-šú*).

Line 10: An alternative restoration at the beginning of line 10 may be *la* [*e*]*-ri-*⌜*tu*$_4$⌝ *a-na šu-ri-ʾ-i*, which would indicate an alternative use of the prescription "to enable a woman (who is) not pregnant to get pregnant". The observation and treatment of scant, insufficient menstrual bleeding in the present prescription is unique in the corpus of Mesopotamian women's healthcare texts. The text seems to make a general statement (i.e. that a woman whose menses are scant does not get pregnant easily).

Line 11: Notably, ms. a uses the Aramaic loanword *zayt* "olive" (*zaytu, zāʾitu*) instead of the Akkadian equivalent *sirdu*. For other attestations in Late Babylonian medical texts, see eSAD; Finkel (2000), *FS Lambert*, 151 note to Text 1 obv. 11; see also ibid., 152 Text 2 rev. 12; 155 Text 4 obv. 1, 6. In these references, the ingredient is labelled explicitly as Ì.GIŠ *za-aʾ-it* "olive oil" and is used for salves.

The reading of the first drug in line 11 is ambiguous. It is suggested here that ^{ú}*k*[*u*]*-ur-ru-ka-nu* is an unusual spelling for *kurkānû*-plant, which is attested in other women's healthcare texts as a plan to promote female fertility (see e.g. N. 4001 obv. 15 // BM 51246+ obv. 11; N. 4001 rev. 2 (text A.2.7, B.2.1); BM 42313+ obv. 7 (text A.2.2), BAM 244: 31, 33, 37 (text B.1.1); BAM 247: 8 (text B.1.3), attested in two varieties, domesticated and wild). Syllabic spellings of that plant name usually do not have a reduplicated /r/ (usual spellings are *kur-ka-nu-u* or *kur-ka-nam*). Alternatively, one could read the signs as two words, i.e. ^{ú}*ku-ur-ru qà-nu*, i.e. "a thick piece of reed", cf. CAD K, 571–572 s.v. *kūru* C (also *kurru*) lex. section. However, all attestations for this expression appear to stem from lexical lists and not from medical contexts; furthermore, the classifier Ú before the word rather suggests a specific drug name.

Line 13: The introductory statement at the beginning of line 13, MUNUS *šá* ⌜*ka*$_4$$^?$⌝*-an-ni-šú*, appears to be abbreviated, since one expects at least a verb here to complete the sentence. Perhaps, the text AO 6374 line 40 offers a parallel and suitable expression for restoring the present prescription (see text C.3.9). This Late Babylonian text speaks of "the day that her (menstrual) bandage(s) have passed her by" (*u*$_4$*-mu šá ka*$_4$*-ni-šú* DIB-*iq-šú*), probably referring to the moment when a woman became aware that she had missed her menstrual period, as the first sign of a pregnancy. Thus, one may perhaps tentatively restore MUNUS *šá ka*$_4$*-an-ni-šú* <DIB-*iq-šú*> "(for) a woman who has missed her period" in ms. a line 13. If this is correct, the present prescription would have been concerned with inducing bleeding (and interrupting an early-term pregnancy). For a similar context, cf. also BM 42313+ lines 11–12 (see text A.2.2 for discussion).

The number 5-*šú* in line 13 should probably be understood as "one-fifth" or "a fifth (part of)". The numeral could be read as *ḫamšu* or *ḫanšu* "one-fifth" (often written *ḫa-an-šú*); it also stands for "one-fifth of a shekel" (= 1.66g), Akkadian *ḫummušu*, often written *ḫu-um-mu-šú* in Late Babylonian (Powell 1987–1990, *RlA* 7, 512 § VA.1f). For numbers referring to fractions in Late Babylonian texts, see also Streck 1995, 63–64, 66–68. For *girû* "carat" (1/24 of a shekel = 0.347g), see Powell 1989–1990, *RlA* 7, 512 § VA.1c.

Line 15: Spellings of *zumru* "body" without the middle consonant /m/ are occasionally attested, cf. CAD Z, 157; von Soden 1995, GAG, § 31d; Mayer 1992, *OrNS* 61, 51; 2014, *OrNS* 83, 391. After *zu-ur-šú*, the sequence BI DA IR is possibly an error for *birdu* (*bi-ir-da*) "pustule". Note for a tentative parallel, BAM 240: 29' (text D.2.1): DIŠ MUNUS Ù.TU-*ma* SU-*šá bir-di* DIRI DÚR-*šá ma-qit* "If a woman gives birth and subsequently her body is full of *birdu*-spots(?), (and) she has a prolapse of the rectum (lit. her anus has fallen)."

Line 16: The reading of the preserved signs in this line are uncertain due to lacking context. The sequence *šú-šá-na* may stand for *šuššān* "one third", followed by NUMUN "seed (of ...)". A measurement would be lacking, but a similar case may be presented in line 13.

Lines 20'–21': For the diagnostic passage, compare BAM 240: 20' (text D.2.1): DIŠ MUNUS TU$_{15}$ *iš-biṭ-ma ma-lit ù* SU-*šá* KÚR.(-)KÚR *ana* TI-*šá* "If 'wind' has 'blown' (into) a woman so that she is filled up (with it), but her body keeps changing (for the worse), to cure her ...". The form *uttakkar* in line 21' can be analysed as a Dt-stem durative form, which usually has a passive meaning ("to be changed; to be (physically) removed").

Lines 23'–24': Incidentally, a parallel for the ingredients *andaḫšu*-vegetable and *billatu*-substance used for a tampon to cure a postpartum complaint is found in BAM 240: 47'–49' (text D.2.1). In the latter text, a wad (*lippu*) inserted into the vagina containing a compound of several drugs is used for detained lochia causing "intestinal fever" and vomiting (among other symptoms), see BAM 240: 39'–40' for the symptom description.

Line 27': Instead of *ina maš-ku* "on (a piece of) leather" at the beginning of the line, one could also read *ina kusīti*(BAR. DUL$_5$) "on a *kusītu*-garment". For similar prescriptions of bandages in the context of postpartum ailments, using a piece of cloth (instead of leather), see also BAM 240: 61'–63' (text D.2.1); *Iraq* 31, 30: 29 (text II.1.4); BAM 408 line 16'' (text A.2.9).

Line 29': Incidentally, *tīyatu*-plant is also found as an ingredient in BAM 240: 47' (a prescription treating symptoms of puerperal fever including retained lochia). See *infra* text D.2.1.

Line 30': The word following the numeral 5-*aš* is uncertain, but perhaps it may be *minītu* "(normal/usual) amount/measure" or *mīnu* "amount" (cf. CAD M/2, 86–87 sub 1, 96–97; AHw 655, 656). Note for a similar passage, K. 8678+ obv. 15' (see *infra*): 5-*aš rit-tú* "a fifth of a handful" (5-*aš* would be *ḫamaš*, the bound form of *ḫamšu* "one fifth").

Line 32': The form *tapaššašši-ma* (⸢ŠÉŠ⸣-*áš-ši-ma*$^{?}$) "you rub her" is irregular (one does expect *tapaššassī-ma*). For the N-stem of *pašāru* ("to be undone, loosened, annulled"), cf. CAD P, 244 s.v. *pašāru* sub 13b. Compare, the Š-stem *šupšuru* "to bring about release (of the illness or the lochia)" in the context of postpartum conditions, in *Iraq* 31, 30: 3: (DIŠ) MUNUS Ù.TU-*ma em-rat šit-*⸢*te*⸣-*š*[*a*$^{?}$ x (x)] / ŠÀ.MEŠ-*ša es-lu* A.MEŠ-*ša u* MÚD.M[EŠ-*ša ina* ŠÀ-*bi-ša*$^{?}$] / GUR.MEŠ-*ru ana šup-šu-ri-ša* "(If) a woman gives birth and subsequently she has intestinal trouble, her excrement$^{?}$ [...], her intestines are blocked, her fluids and [her] blood are blocked [in her belly$^{?}$], to make her release (it)". Cf. also line 26 in the same text for *ippaššar*(DU$_8$-*ma*) "she will be released" concluding a prescription for the same purpose.

Lines 33'–40': The last section in ms. a is highly unusual and at times difficult to understand. It consists of two prescriptions, which are not separated by a ruling. Instead, we find a rare case in which the beginning of the second recipe does not start with a new line, but in the middle of line 36', after a little vertical line made by the scribe as a separating marker, to indicate the end of the first prescription and the beginning of the second one.

Line 35': In line 35', a reading *quppû* "sharp knife, scalpel" seems more likely than *kupû* "canebrake". After *ina qú-pu-ú* we expect a verb with a meaning such as "to cut; to chop" (e.g. *ta-par-ra-am*).

Lines 35' and 36': The *simbirru*-plant (a variant of *šibburratu*, presumably rue) and the *nuḫurtu*-plant (a type of asafoetida) are attested in several other prescriptions to stop bleeding, but they seem to be applied here for different purposes. See BAM 237 i 32', ii 17', iv 4 (text C.1.4); K. 263 + 10934 rev. 25 (text C.1.5); BAM 235 obv. 5 (text C.1.1); BAM 236 obv. 12 (text C.1.2) for *nuḫurtu*; BM 38624+ i 11'–13' (text A.2.1); SpTU 4, No. 153 obv. 5, 7 (text C.1.10); FLP 1306 rev. 17 (text C.1.9) for *simbirru*; K. 20254 obv.(?) 7' (text C.1.7). Note that *nuḫurtu* is also among the ingredients to treat symptoms of puerperal fever (including retention of the lochia) in BAM 240: 43', 47' and 52' (text D.2.1). For both plants, see Stol (forthcoming), in: *Gedenkschrift van Soldt*.

Line 37': The expression *šikin tinūri*, "deposited material from an oven" is not attested elsewhere to my knowledge. CAD Š/2, 439b s.v. *šiknu* C, lists similar expressions formed with terms for rivers and canals and renders the term *šiknu* as "sediment, deposit" in these contexts. Beside river silt, *šiknu* can also refer to a layer of cloud or accretions of substances in body parts. In the present case, the expression *šikin tinūri* may refer to soot from the interior of an oven.

Line 39': The word *ḫal-dap-pu-ú* may most likely refer to *ḫaltappû/ḫultuppû*, the rod of the incantation priest. We would then have a phrase *ište ḫaltappî tasâk* "you pound (the ingredients) with a *ḫaltappû*-rod (of the healer)". The preposition *išti* (also *ište, ištu*) "(together) with" is unusual here, but it occurs rarely instead of *ina*, see e.g. BAM 124 i 35–36: *iš-tu* ZÌ.DA ḪI.ḪI "you mix (drugs) with flour" (also i 49). Note, however, that there is also a plant name *ḫaltappānu*, of which *ḫal-dap-pu-ú* may be a variant form (CAD Ḫ, 52–53; AHw 314a). A reading *ḫal-lu-pu-ú* is neither excluded. Note further an aromatic *ḫallapunu* (written *ḫal-la-pu-un-na*) in a list of aromatics (Finkel 2000, *FS Lambert*, 188, Text 31: 9').

Line 40': The purpose of the last prescription on the tablet is interpreted as *tūrti mê* and that *tu-uš-tu*$_4$ stands for *tūrtu* "turning back (of the fluids)" (CAD T, 491 s.v. *tūrtu* A). This noun (derived from *târu* "to (re)turn") could be linked with the phrase *mê turru* "to be blocked with regard to the fluids", attested in a few women's healthcare texts and referring to the lochia that are retained in the uterus. See *infra*, for the texts *Iraq* 31, 29: 1–3 (text II.1.4); BM 38624+ i 24'–25', 30'–31', ii 19'–21' (text A.2.1); BAM 240: 67' (text D.2.1); K. 8678+ rev. 3' (text A.1.4) and the *Introduction* for discussion. For the shift /r/ → /š/ before /t/ in Neo- and Late Babylonian texts, see von Soden 1995, GAG §35c.

A.2.9 BAM 408: A Fragment with Prescriptions for Women

This fragment of a two-column tablet in a Late Babylonian script was found at Uruk in a secondary context. It preserves a few fragmentary recipes for fertility and for a postpartum problem.

List of Manuscripts

Siglum	Museum Number	Copy	Collation	Format; Ductus	Provenience
a	VAT 14528	LKU 55 BAM 408	Coll.	Fragment of a two-column tablet; Late Babylonian script; ca. 6th/5th cent. BCE	Uruk; secondary context

Overview

i'	Fragmentary prescriptions to promote female fertility (potion, tampon) a obv.$^?$ i' 1'–4'	...]1'–4'
ii'	Fragmentary prescription (against "wind blasting") a obv.$^?$ i' 5'–8'	5'–8'[...
iii'	Fragmentary prescription a obv.$^?$ ii' 1'–3'	...]9"–11"
iv'	Fragmentary prescription (for a postpartum problem?) a obv.$^?$ ii' 4'–10'	12"–18"[...

Previous Edition and Discussion

Falkenstein 1931, 22 and pl. XIX (No. 55) (copy; discussion)
Köcher 1971, BAM IV, xxxi, pl. 102 (copy; discussion)
CDLI P285479 (photo; transliteration)
BabMed Corpora (https://www.geschkult.fu-berlin.de/e/babmed/Corpora/BAM-4/BAM-4_-408/index.html; transliteration)
Electronic Babylonian Library (eBL) (https://www.ebl.lmu.de/library/VAT.14528; photo, copy)
Steinert 2021, *Byzantinische Forschungen* 33, 65 (lines 2'–3')

Transliteration

Beginning lost

1' a obv.$^?$ i' 1' [............ Ḫ]I.ḪI MUNUS BI ÍL-*ma*

2' a obv.$^?$ i' 2' [........... ^{giš}]NU.ÚR.MA ^{šim}ḪAB

3' a obv.$^?$ i' 3' [...............-*m*]*a*$^?$ *ir-ri*

4' a obv.$^?$ i' 4' [.................] *ina* MUL$_4$ *tuš-bat ina še-rim* NU *pa-tan* \ NAG

5' a obv.$^?$ i' 5' [DIŠ MUNUS$^?$ ....]x TU$_{15}$ *iš*$^?$*-biṭ*

6' a obv.$^?$ i' 6' [........ ZÀ.ḪI.LI^{sar} *ṭ*]*e*$_4$*-né-e-tì* NUMUN GADA

7'	a obv.$^{?}$ i' 7'	[............. Í]L$^{?}$-*ši-ma ina-eš*
8'	a obv.$^{?}$ i' 8'	[.............................] ⸢x⸣

Ms. a col. i' breaks; remainder lost

9''	a obv.$^{?}$ ii' 1'	⸢DIŠ⸣ [..]
10''	a obv.$^{?}$ ii' 2'	DIŠ KI.MIN KU [..................................]
11''	a obv.$^{?}$ ii' 3'	DIŠ-*niš* ḪI.ḪI *ina* K[AŠ NAG-*ši*$^{?}$ ....]
12''	a obv.$^{?}$ ii' 4'	DIŠ MUNUS Ù.TU-*ma* ⸢x⸣ [...................]
13''	a obv.$^{?}$ ii' 5'	ILLU ^{šim}BULUḪ IL[LU ....]
14''	a obv.$^{?}$ ii' 6'	TAG$^{?}$-*ma* Ì.UDU ḪI.Ḫ[I..........................]
15''	a obv.$^{?}$ ii' 7'	^{giš}EREN ^{šim}MUG [..................................]
16''	a obv.$^{?}$ ii' 8'	ŠEG$_6$-*šal ina* TÚG SUR-*r*[*i* ....]
17''	a obv.$^{?}$ ii' 9'	[^{síg}G]A.RÍG.AK.A [.................................]
18''	a obv.$^{?}$ ii' 10'	[...............]x man x ⸢x⸣ [..........................]

Ms. a col. ii' breaks; remainder lost

Bound Transcription and Translation

Beginning lost

1' [... ... *tu*]*ballal sinništu šī inaššī-ma* 2' [... ...] *lurmû ṭūru* 3' [... ...-*m*]*a irri* 4' [... ...] *ina kakkabi tušbât ina šēri lā patān išatti*

1' [... ... you] mix, the woman shall apply it. Then 2' [... ...], pomegranate, *ṭūru*-aromatic, 3' [... ...]. Then she will get pregnant. 4' [... ...] You let it stay outside overnight under the star(s). In the morning, she shall drink (it) on an empty stomach.

5' [*šumma sinništu*(?) ... ...] ... *šāru išbiṭ* 6' [... ... *saḫlê ṭ*]*ēnēti zēr kitê* 7' [... *inaš*]*šī-ma ina"eš* 8' *traces*

5' [If ... ...] ... wind has blown (into) [a woman(?)] 6' [... ...], finely ground [*saḫlû*-cress], linseed, 7' [... ... she shall ap]ply it, and she will get well. 8' *too fragmentary for translation*

Ms. a col. i' breaks; remainder lost

9'' DIŠ [... ...] 10'' DIŠ KI.MIN *sīkti* [... ...] 11'' *ištēniš tuballal ina šikari* [*tašaqqīši*(?) ... ...]

9'' If [... ...]. 10'' Alternatively, powder of [... ...] 11'' you mix together. [You *give it to her to drink*(?)] in beer [... ...].

12'' *šumma sinništu ūlid-ma* [... ...] 13'' *ḫīl baluḫḫi ḫīl* [... ...] 14'' *talappat-ma*(?) *ina lipî tuballal* [... ...] 15'' *erēna ballukka* [... ...] 16'' *tušabšal ina lubāri teṭerri* [... ...] 17'' *pušikku* [... ...] 18'' *traces*

12'' If a woman gives birth and [... ...], 13'' resin of *baluḫḫu*-aromatic, resin of [... ...] 14'' you *moisten* (lit. smear) and mix with tallow [... ...]. 16'' You boil 15'' cedar, *ballukku*-aromatic, [... ...], 16'' you *press* (the liquid) *through* (a piece of) cloth, [... ...] 17'' [co]mbed wool [... ...], 18'' *too fragmentary for translation*

Ms. a col. ii' breaks; remainder lost

Notes

Lines 1'–4': The verb *našû* "to wear; to apply" (ÍL) found in line 1' occurs in the context of tampons or suppositories inserted into the vagina, for treating different female complaints, including the promotion of fertility (cf. CAD N/2, 100a; Reiner 1982a, *ZA* 72, 131 n. 24, comparing this usage with ancient Greek terminology). For parallels, see BAM 240: 22, 45, 57 (text D.1.4). BAM 241 ii 3'–4' (text II.1.3 lines 27'''–30'''); UET 7, No. 123 obv. 8, 10 and rev. 11' (text B.2.2).

Lines 5'–8': The passage in lines 5'–7' appears to be a partial parallel to BAM 240: 20–22 // A. 3461 obv. 8'–11' (texts D.2.1, A.1.2). In line 5' of ms. a, a slightly different reading in comparison with the Neo-Assyrian parallel is possible: [... MUNUS B]I TU_{15} *ša-biṭ* "that [woman] is blown by wind". For the expression *šāru išbiṭ* and the condition of *šibiṭ šāri* "wind-blasting", see e.g. BAM 146 rev. 30 (Bácskay 2018a, 184; Schmidtchen 2021a, 40–41; Schmidtchen 2018b, 315 line 39; Steinert et al. 2018, 211, 231 line 31); Scurlock and Andersen 2005, 91–92, 203.

The adjective *ṭēnu* "(finely) ground" reconstructed in line 6' is a feminine plural form, which is usually encountered as an attribute of the ingredient *saḫlû* "cress(?)" (fem. pl.) in medical texts, see CAD Ṭ, 97–98 sub b for references. The parallel in BAM 240: 21' omits the adjective *ṭēnu*, but also prescribes *saḫlû* and linseed. Line 7' is restored after BAM 240: 22, which reads ÍL-*ma ina-eš* "she shall apply (it), then she will get well."

Lines 12''–18'': A parallel procedure in the corpus of women's healthcare texts (also in the context of postpartum problems, especially retention of the lochia) is described e.g. the Middle Assyrian text *Iraq* 31, 30: 29–31 (text II.1.4). Note also BAM 240: 63 (text D.2.1). Both these texts deal with postpartum complaints, and the present passage in BAM 408 may have been concerned with a comparable context. See also BM 79061: 25'–27' (text A.2.8).

The ingredients cedar, *ballukku* and *baluḫḫu*-aromatic (and resin of these plants) are likewise encountered in *Iraq* 31, 30: 5, 6 and 20 to treat a postpartum condition (retention of the lochia).

In ms. a line 17'' perhaps restore *pušikka* [*talammi*(NIGIN) ...] "you wrap (ingredients) with combed wool" or *pušikka* [*taṭammi*(NU.NU)] "you spin (a thread of) combed wool".

A.2.10 BM 48557: A Fragment on Women's Health from Babylon

This small fragment, which may have belonged to a large two-column tablet with a compendium on women's health, was excavated by Hormuzd Rassam at Babylon (Leichty, Finkel and Walker 2019, 619). It contains remnants of medical prescriptions for women, three of which appear to deal with stopping haemorrhage and inducing the menses.[272] Two of the prescriptions display a format that becomes more common in the Late Babylonian texts, in which the purpose of the remedies is briefly stated at the end of the prescription. One prescription uses the rare term *kibsu* "step, track" for the regular course of the menses, which is only attested in two other Late Babylonian texts so far (BM 47491 (text A.2.6) and BM 47578 (text C.2.2)).

List of Manuscripts

Siglum	Museum Number	Copy	Collation	Format; Ductus	Provenience
a	BM 48557 (81-11-3, 1268)	–	Photo Coll.	Fragment of a tablet; Neo-/Late Babylonian script; ca. 6th/5th cent. BCE	Babylon

272 The fragment was kindly brought to my attention by Henry Stadhouders and the eBL Project who identified its relation to the women's healthcare texts.

Overview

i'	Fragmentary prescription (for inducing the menses?) a obv. 1'–2'	...]1'–2'
ii'	Fragmentary prescription (to stop bleeding?) a obv. 3'–5'	3'–5'
iii'	Fragmentary prescription (to stop bleeding?) a obv. 6'–9'	6'–9'[...
iv'	Fragmentary prescription a rev. 1'–5'	...]10"–14"[...

Previous Edition and Discussion

Electronic Babylonian Library (eBL) (https://www.ebl.lmu.de/library/BM.48557; photos; transliteration)

Transliteration

Beginning of ms. a obv. lost

1' a obv. 1' [......... *ina* ^{síg}ÀKA] ⸢*ta*$^{?}$⸣-⸢*lam*$^{?}$⸣-[*mi* ....] ⸢x⸣

2' a obv. 2' [.........] ⸢*lu*⸣-*ú šá kib-su* [KUD$^{?}$ ....]

3' a obv. 3' [.........ŠIKA NU]NUZ *lu-ur-mu* KU ^{giš}Ù[R SUMUN$^{?}$ ......]

4' a obv. 4' [......... *ki*]*b*$^{?}$-*ri-tu*$_{4}$ *šá* IZI$^{?}$ [.........]

5' a obv. 5' [......... *ta-b*]*al-lal* MÚD MUNUS *a*[*na*$^{?}$ KUD-*si*$^{?}$]

6' a obv. 6' [......... 1/2$^{?}$ GÍN Ú.NAM.T]I.LA 1/2 GÍN *n*[*u*$^{?}$-*ḫur-tu*$_{4}$$^{?}$ ....]

7' a obv. 7' [.............]-*tu*$_{4}$ 1/2 GÍN ^{n}[^{a4}*ga-bu-u*$^{?}$ ....]

8' a obv. 8' [.............]x 1/2 GÍN *mur*-[*ru*$^{?}$ ....]

9' a obv. 9' [............ Ì.UD]U$^{?}$ *u* DUḪ.LÀL [.............]

Ms. a obv. breaks; gap of unknown length
Beginning of ms. a rev. lost

10" a rev. 1' [............. K]ASKAL.A$^{?}$ *ana* ⸢ŠÀ⸣ ⸢*rab*$^{?}$⸣-[.........]

11" a rev. 2' [............] ⸢*šá*$^{?}$⸣ ⸢KÁ⸣-*šá ina* ŠÀ [..............]

12" a rev. 3' [............]x x[x^{s}]$^{ar?}$ Ú BABBAR$^{?}$ [...........]

13" a rev. 4' [............] x ŠÀ(-)x[x MU]RUB$_{4}$$^{?}$.⸢MEŠ-*šú*$^{?}$⸣ ⸢TU$_{15}$⸣ [GIG$^{?}$]

14" a rev. 5' [............] x [................................]

Ms. a rev. breaks; remainder lost

Bound Transcription and Translation

Beginning of ms. a obv. lost

1' [... ... *ina itqi*] *talam*[*mi*(?) ... ...] 2' [... ...] *lū ša kibsu* [*parsu*(?) ...]

1' [... ...] you wrap(?) (it) [in a wad of wool, ...] 2' [(a remedy for) ... ...] or (for a woman?) whose (normal) *course* [has stopped(?) ...].

3' [... ... *ḫaṣab*] *pel lurmî sīkti gušūri* [*labiri* ... ...] 4' [... ... *ki*]*b-rītu*(?) *ša išāta*(?) [... ...] 5' [... ... *tab*]*allal dām sinništi a*[*na parāsi*(?)]

3' [... ... shell] of an ostrich egg, powder of an [old] beam [... ...], 4' [... ...] *kibrītu*-sulphur(?) that [*ignites*(?)] the fire(?) ... ...] 5' [... ... you] mix (together). (It is) for [stopping(?)] a woman's blood.

6' [... ... *zūz* (*šiqil*) *šammi*] *balāṭi zūz n*[*uḫurtu*(?) ... ...] 7' [... ...]... *zūz g*[*abû*(?) ...] 8' [... ...]... *zūz m*[*urru*(?) ...] 9' [... ... *li-p*]*û*(?) *u iškūru* [... ...]

6' [... ... half(?) a shekel 'plant] of life', half a shekel *n*[*uḫur-tu*-plant(?), ...] 7' [... ...]..., half a shekel of a[lum(?), ...], 8' [... ...]..., half a shekel *m*[*urru*-aromatic(?), ...], 9' [... ...] tallow and wax [... ...] ...

Ms. a obv. breaks; gap of unknown length
Beginning of ms. a rev. lost

10'' [... ...] *ḫarrāni*(?) *ana libbi* ...[...] 11'' [... ...] *ša bābīša ina libbi* [... ...] 12'' [... ...] ... *šammu peṣû*(?) [... ...] 13'' [... ...] ... *libbu*(?) ...[...] *qablātušu*(?) *šāra*(?) [*marṣā*(?)] 14'' [... ...] ... [... ...]

10'' [... ...] of the road into ...[...] 11'' [... ...] from her (i.e. the patient's?) door with(?) [...] 12'' [... ...] ... 'white drug'(?) [... ...] 13'' [... ...] ... (for a person whose(?)) belly(?) [... (and)] hips [are afflicted(?)] with wind(?). 14'' [... ...] ... [... ...]

Ms. a rev. breaks; remainder lost

Notes

Lines 1'–2': The term *kibsu* "step, track, access" (CAD K, 338a s.v. *kibsu* sub 1f) occurs also in BM 47491 lines 25–26 (text A.2.6) and in BM 47578 line 13 (text C.2.2), as a term for the menstrual period, when it has stopped (KUD, *parāsu*) to appear regularly. The expression alludes to the onset of menopause, as is made clear in BM 47491, where the ceasing of the menses is linked to the decline of fertility. Since *kibsu* also means "way of acting, behaviour" (CAD K, 338–339 sub 2), the word has to denote the "regular course (of the menses), period" in the context of the women's healthcare texts. The restoration proposed here follows BM 47578.

Line 3': Ostrich eggshells and powder of an old wooden beam occur repeatedly as ingredients in prescriptions to stop bleeding, see FLP 1306 obv. 11–15 // K. 20254 obv.? 3'-5' // BM 42313+ obv. 28–29 (see texts A.2.2, C.1.7, C.1.9); SpTU 4, No. 153: 11–12 (text C.1.10); K. 8893 obv.? 2' (text C.1.6). Ostrich eggshell is attested more regularly in this context (see BAM 237 iv 23 (text C.1.4 line 169'''); FLP 1306 line 23 (text C.1.9); K. 263 + 10934 obv. 7 and 11 (text C.1.5). See also Steinert 2012b, *Sudhoffs Archiv* 96, 83–84 for discussion.

Line 4': The restoration *kibrītu* "sulphur" is a guess, based on the occurrence of this ingredient in a prescription to stop irregular bleeding (during pregnancy) in BAM 237 obv. i 43'-44' (text C.1.4). The use of sulphur to ignite (*napāḫu*) a fire is attested in a Namburbi ritual (Maul 1994, 129: 6); see also Stol 2009–2011, "Schwefel", *RlA* 12, 318b §4.

Line 5': For texts giving the indication "to stop a woman's blood" at the end of the prescriptions, see e.g. FLP 1306 (text C.1.9); BM 38624+ (text A.2.1); BM 42313+ line 29 (text A.2.2); K. 20254 (text C.1.7).

Lines 6'–9': The ingredients *nuḫurtu*, *murru* and *gabû* ("alum") reconstructed in these lines are attested together as *materia medica* to stop bleeding (e.g. K. 8893 obv.(?) 7'–9' (text C.1.6). For *nuḫurtu*-plant (a form of asafoetida), see e.g. BAM 237 i 32', ii 17', iv 4 (text C.1.4); K. 263 + 10934 rev. 25 (text C.1.5); BAM 235 obv. 5 (text C.1.1); BAM 236 obv. 12 (text C.1.2). For *murru*-aromatic and *gabû* "alum" in the context of bleeding, see e.g. BAM 237 i 1', iii 7, iv 3; SpTU 4, No. 153: 1–6, 10; BM 38624+ obv. i' 11'–13'; FLP 1306 rev. 18, 22; BM 54587+ obv.(?) 4'.

"Plant of life" (*šammi balāṭi*) is encountered several times in K. 8678+ obv. 3', 6', 8', 17', (text A.1.4, in prescriptions for rectal disease). Note that Ú NAM.TI.LA is equated with *irrû* (*errû*) "wild melon; colocynth" in Uruanna I 257ff. (quoted in CAD I/J, 182 s.v. *irrû* lex. section); for the identification cf. Stol 1987b, *BSA* 3, 84.

Line 10'': For the lost element before KASKAL.A (or KASKAL.MIN?), compare perhaps *ḫallulāya ḫarrānāti*(KASKAL.MEŠ) "road centipede" as an ingredient in the context of treatments against Lamaštu (Farber 2014, 115, 139 Lam. II 115 and III 39).

Line 11'': The restoration is difficult due to the fragmentary context. If read correctly, *ša bābīša* "from her door" may refer to some substance taken from the entrance of the patient's house (e.g. dust).

Line 13'': The restoration follows K. 8678+ obv. 18' (text A.1.4), a prescription summarized as [PAP 2]2$^{?}$ Ú.MEŠ ALLA DIŠ MURUB$_4$-⸢*šú*⸣ TU$_{15}$ G[IG$^{?}$] "[a total of twenty]-two(?) drugs (for) a suppository for the case that his hip is [stricken] with wind(?)".

Chapter B
Fertility, Conception and Related Matters

The twelve texts and fragments edited in this section (stemming evenly from Assyria and Babylonia) focus predominantly on treatments for promoting fertility and conception, or, if formulated negatively, for overcoming a woman's inability to conceive. A few of the texts specify the aim to make a woman conceive who has "stopped" to bear children, signalling treatments for fertility beyond menopause. Apart from a few fragments of larger multi-column tablets, most texts in the present section are shorter extracts or collections on single-column tablets containing a group of treatments or, as is the case with two tablets, only a single recipe (texts B.1.4 and B.2.5).

The therapies for fertility consist predominantly of medical prescriptions, sometimes combined with a spell (as in texts B.1.1 and B.2.1). The most popular treatment method for promoting fertility are tampons or suppositories inserted into the vagina, but potions, ointments, lotions, bandages, as well as amulet necklaces were also prescribed. The prescriptions are usually only attested in one manuscript; there are relatively few duplicating passages. One Late Babylonian text preserves a ritual for the case that a woman failed to bear children, which was timed to take place on the 14th day of the month Nisannu (B.2.6). Uniquely, this ritual was performed by the healing specialist and the woman's husband, approaching the sun god and moon god with offerings and with a prayer (addressed to the moon god in particular); the woman does not appear to participate in the ritual at all.

The texts only rarely offer statements or contextual clues concerning causes or aetiologies of female infertility. One of the few preserved incantations recited over remedies to promote fertility attributes the cause of the patient's problem to witchcraft (text B.1.1), while in the case of the ritual performed when a woman was "delayed" in getting pregnant, help was sought from deities who were famed for granting offspring (in that case, the moon god Sîn and the sun god Šamaš). While the ultimate cause may often have been sought in an agent of disease (such as divine wrath or witches), Mesopotamian healers also looked for explanations on the level of physical impediments to conception. Like the Hippocratic doctors, they attributed infertility to a closure or deformation of the uterus (and its mouth). A closure of the uterus prevented that the woman received the male semen (see e.g., text B.1.1; BAM 240 (text D.2.1)); therefore, some prescriptions for fertility bear the rubric "for opening up and getting pregnant". Other texts mention infertility as a result of a womb that is "twisted" or "turned over", similarly resulting in a closure of the uterus' mouth (text B.1.1; B.2.2; SpTU 1, No. 43: 30, Geller 2014, 4; for discussion see also Steinert 2017a).

In addition to descriptions of therapies, two texts from Babylonia also contain test procedures or pregnancy prognoses with predictions whether a woman was able to conceive (texts B.2.1–B.2.2; cf. also text A.1.1 from Sultantepe). The exact meaning of these predictions remains debated, although they have often been interpreted as outright pregnancy tests. The test procedures mostly involve tampons filled with different plant and mineral ingredients, which the patient inserted into the vagina and kept there for a certain time. Predictions were then made based on different colorations of the tampon after its removal.

Beside the texts assembled here that have an exclusive thematic focus on matters of fertility, prescriptions for fertility and conception often were also included in longer collections of therapies for women (see Chapter A). Moreover, while most of the material edited here is pro-natalist in outlook, there also are a few rare texts attesting to recipes for contraception and for making a woman abort her foetus, i.e. for curbing fertility (text B.1.6, as well as BM 51246+ and K. 8678+, texts A.2.7, A.1.4). The prescribed abortive and contraceptive drugs were mostly taken by mouth (potions) or inserted into the vagina (tampons).

B.1 Texts from Assur and Nineveh

B.1.1 BAM 244: Treatments for Fertility and Conception

This Neo-Assyrian tablet from the "House of the incantation priest" at Assur focuses on treatments for fertility and conception, as is indicated by fragmentary statements in the prescriptions that take up the obverse and beginning of the reverse. One of these remedies begins with the purpose statement [^{munus}]*la a-lit-ta* <*ana*> *šu-*[*ri*]*-im-m*[*a* ...] "in order to enable an infertile woman to get pregnant" (line 8). Another prescription concludes with MUNUS BI [PEŠ$_4^?$-*m*]*a* MU TUKU-*ši* "this woman will [get pregnant(?)] and will get offspring (lit. a name)" (line 40; see also Stol 2000a, 35, 53–54).

https://doi.org/10.1515/9781501506475-005

The purpose of the following Akkadian incantation (lines 41–70) has been interpreted as being linked to facilitating birth or protecting a pregnant woman from the malicious effects of sorcery (Köcher 1964 (BAM III), xviii; Böck 2013, 47 with note 73 on lines 41, 48–49; cf. also Stol 2000a, 72 with n. 148 who believes the spell is for a woman in difficult labour). However, the rubric in line 71 can tentatively be restored as ⸢KA.INIM⸣.MA ÉN ^{munus}*la* ⸢*e*$^{?}$⸣-[*ri-tu ana šu-ri-i*] "wording of an incantation [to enable] a woman who is not [pregnant to get pregnant]". Stol (2000a, 53) proposes that the latter formulation refers not necessarily to a barren woman, but to a woman who had previously born a child and now wished to become pregnant again. The incantation refers to sorcery as the main cause of the woman's inability to conceive (Steinert 2020, 62; 2021, 59–60). Sorcery was apparently believed to cause bodily impurities that hindered conception, which were countered with the help of purifying plants addressed in the spell, some of which are also known as drugs to counter witchcraft. The composition thus shows that sorcery was not only believed to cause miscarriage (a problem often addressed in women's healthcare texts) but was also deemed responsible for female infertility. This belief finds a parallel in the view that sorcery could also cause loss of male sexual desire (cf. Zisa 2021).

The fragmentary abracadabra-spell in lines 72–75 appears to resemble the beginning of a spell for promoting fertility encountered in two Babylonian manuscripts (N. 4001 and BM 51246+, see text B.2.1).

List of Manuscripts

Siglum	Museum Number	Copy	Collation	Format; Ductus	Provenience
A	VAT 8007 + 13875 + 14099 (+) 16457	KAR 266 (VAT 8007) BAM 244	Coll.	Fragment of a single-column tablet in portrait format; Neo-Assyrian script; 7th cent. BCE	Assur, N4 library

Overview

i	Fragmentary prescription A obv. 1–5	1–5
ii	Fragmentary prescription A obv. 6–7	6–7
iii	Prescription to enable an infertile woman to get pregnant A obv. 8–9 (purpose statement) A obv. 10–30 (description of procedure (KÍD.KÍD.BI); compound remedy: lotion and bandage)	8–30
iv	Prescription to enable an infertile woman to get pregnant (ointment) A obv. 31–32	31–32
v	Prescription to enable an infertile woman to get pregnant (potion) A obv. 33	33
vi	Prescription to enable an infertile woman to get pregnant (potion) A obv. 34	34
vii	Prescription to enable an infertile woman to get pregnant (potion) A obv. 35	35
viii	Prescription to enable an infertile woman to get pregnant (potion) A obv. 36	36
ix	Prescription to enable an infertile woman to get pregnant (suppository) A obv. 37	37
x	Fragmentary prescription to enable an infertile woman to get pregnant (tampon) A rev. 1	38
	Instructions and prognosis A rev. 2–3	39–40

xi	Akkadian incantation A rev. 4–34	41–70
xii	Incantation rubric A rev. 35	71
xiii	Fragmentary instruction A rev. 36–39	72–75
xiv	Fragmentary incantation A rev. 40–42	76–78

Previous Edition and Discussion

Böck 2010a, *TUAT NF* 5, 109 (translation of ms. A obv. 8–30)
Böck 2013, 47 with n. 73 (ms. A lines 41, 47–48)
CDLI P285330 (photo; transliteration)
BabMed Corpora (https://www.geschkult.fu-berlin.de/e/babmed/Corpora/BAM-3/BAM-3_-244)
Steinert 2020, *JMC* 36, 62 (translation of ms. A obv. 8–10, 21–30)
Steinert 2021, 52–53, 59–61 (translation of ms. A obv. 8, 10–30, discussion)

Transliteration

1 A obv. 1 [.................] ⸢x x⸣ [...]

2 A obv. 2 [.................] ⸢x⸣ ŠE.S[AG$^?$ ....]

3 A obv. 3 [..................]x x x DU$_{10}$.GA ⸢^{ú}⸣[..............................]

4 A obv. 4 [GAZI^{sa}]$^{r?}$ BÍL-*ti* ^{ú}NAM.TAR [.......................................]

5 A obv. 5 [^{gi}]^{š}*ar-ga-nu* LAGAB MUNU$_6$ BÁRA.MUNU$_6$ [.............]

---

6 A obv. 6 [^{š}]^{im}KU$_6$ DIDA SIG.GA x[......................................]

7 A obv. 7 ⸢Ì.UDU⸣ GU$_4$.MEŠ EŠ *ana* $^{d?}$[*ba*]-*ba*$_6$$^?$ [........................]

---

8 A obv. 8 [^{munus}]*la a-lit-ta* <*ana*> *šu-*[*ri*]*-im-m*[*a* ....]

9 A obv. 9 [MU *šu-u*]*r-ši-im-ma* ⸢x x⸣.ḪI.A [............................]

---

10 A obv. 10 ⸢KÌD.KÌD.BI⸣ ⸢*a*⸣-*rat* ^{giš}KIRI$_6$.MEŠ *ma-la* [...................]

11 A obv. 11 [G]I *sug-bàn*$^!$-⸢*da*$^?$⸣ ⸢*šá*⸣ *eri*$^!$-*dù*$^!$-*ke*$_4$ ⸢*ma*⸣-x[.................]

12 A obv. 12 [S]UḪUŠ GI.ŠUL.ḪI ^{giš}DÌḪ ^{giš}KIŠI$_{16}$ [............................]

13 A obv. 13 Ú.BÍL.LÁ ^{giš}*si-ḫa* ^{giš}*ar-*[*ga-nu* ....]

14 A obv. 14 Ú ^{giš}TIR DÙ-*šú-nu* TI-*qé* x[...................................]

15 A obv. 15 ⸢*ina*⸣ A LUḪ-*si ana* DUG *te-sip* [*ina* NINDU ÚŠ-*er*$^?$ ....]

16 A obv. 16 ⸢*ina*⸣ *še-rim tu-še-il-la-a ana qer-*[*bi*$^?$ ....]

17 A obv. 17 [K]AŠ.SAG *ana lìb-bi* A.MEŠ *šá-tu-nu t*[*u-tab-bak* MUNUS *ša-ši ana mar-ḫa-ṣi*$^?$]

18 A obv. 18 *tu-še-ri-sa* EN A.MEŠ SED *tu-maš-šá-a'-ši* x[x x x x x x x]

19 A obv. 19 [T]A *mar-ḫa-ṣi* E$_{11}$-*ši-ma nap-šal-ta* ŠÉŠ-*s*[*i* x x x x x x x]

20 A obv. 20 MUNUS *ša-ši* 3 *u*$_4$-*me ana mar-ḫa-ṣi* [*tu-še-ri-sa*$^?$ x x x]

21 A obv. 21 [G]IN$_7$ U$_4$.MEŠ-*šá im-ta-lu-ú na-aṣ-ma-a*[*t-ta* DÙ-*uš*$^?$ x x x]

22 A obv. 22 [*š*]*a na-aṣ-ma-te šá-a-ši mé-re-eš-ta* [x x x x x x]

23 A obv. 23 ZÌ ŠE.BAR SIG$_5$ ZÌ GIG$^!$(NÁ) ZÌ ZÍZ.ÀM ZÌ *in-ni-ni* [ZÌ x x x (x)]

24 A obv. 24 ZÌ GÚ.GAL ZÌ GÚ.TUR ZÌ *kiš-še-ni* KU *ba-ri-ra-te* [KU x x x]

25 A obv. 25 KU ^{ú}KUR.RA KU ^{ú}ḪUR.SAG KU GAZI^{sar} KU ^{ši}[^{m}x x x]

26 A obv. 26 KU $^{\text{šim.d}}$MAŠ KU ^{šim}GIG KU ^{giš}⸢*e*⸣-*re-ni* K[U x x x]

27 A obv. 27 [K]U ^{šim}GÍR KU ^{šim}GAM.MA KU ⸢^{šim}⸣BAL ŠU.NIGIN 21 Z[Ì.DA.ḪI.A$^?$]

28 A obv. 28 [1].TA.ÀM TI-*qé* DIŠ-*niš* ḪI.ḪI *ina* ŠEN.TUR GIN$_7$ ŠU A.Z[U *tara-bak*$^?$]

29 A obv. 29 1/2 SÌLA Ì.GIŠ *tal-tap-pat ina* ⸢MURUB$_4$⸣-*šá pe-ni-šá u ra-pa*[*l-ti-šá*]

30 A obv. 30 [*t*]*u-ṣa-ab-ba-ma* ⸢KÉŠ$^{?!}$⸣ GUR.GUR-*ši-ma ina-*[*eš*]

---

31 A obv. 31 ^{ú}*kur-ka-nam šá* KUR-*e* ^{ú}*nab-rú-qi* ^{šim}GÚR.GÚR ^{šim}[x x]

32 A obv. 32 *ina* Ì.GI[Š]$^!$ ^{ši}[^{m}BULUḪ$^?$ ḪI].ḪI ŠÉŠ-*si-ma ina-*[*eš*]

---

33 A obv. 33 ^{ú}*kur-ka-*[*na*]-*a* ^{ú}*nab-rú-qi ta-sàk ina* GEŠTIN NAG *mim-ma* x[x] ⸢MIN⸣

---

34 A obv. 34 $^{\text{ú.d}}$MAŠ ⸢^{ú}⸣IGI-20 *ta-sàk ina* GEŠTIN NAG MIN

---

35 A obv. 35 ⸢Ú⸣ *ṣa-a*[*l-m*]*u*$^?$ ^{ú}*ṣa-ṣu-un-tu* DIŠ-*niš ta-sàk ina* GEŠTIN N[AG] MIN

---

36 A obv. 36 [^{ú}IG]I-*lim* ^{ú}IGI-20 DIŠ-*niš ta-sàk ina* <GEŠTIN> N[AG] MIN

---

37 A obv. 37 [^{ú}*kur-ka-na* (*šá*)$^?$] KUR-⸢*e*⸣ ⸢^{ú}⸣ḪAR.ḪUM.BA.ŠIR SÚD *ina* ARḪUŠ-*š*[*á* GAR-*ma*] *ina-eš*

---

38 A rev. 1 [x x x x x x x] *ina* ^{síg}ÀKA *ta-la-*[*am-mi ana*] GAL$_4$.LA-*šá* GAR-*ma ina-eš*

---

39 A rev. 2 [x x x x x x *maš-q*]*í-ti nap-šal-t*[*i u nà*]*r-ma-ak-ti*

40 A rev. 3 [x x x x x x]-*pi-iḫ* MUNUS BI [PEŠ$_4$$^?$-*m*]*a* MU TUKU-*ši*

---

41 A rev. 4 [ÉN *it-te*]-*en-né-e*[*s*$^?$-*k*]*er ú-ga-ri* [*ni-il*$^?$] A.MEŠ *ú-mal-l*[*i*]

42 A rev. 5 [LÚ-*la da*]*m-qa na-*[*as-qa*] *ina qer-bi* ⸢*ú*$^?$⸣-*še-*[*li*$^?$]

43 A rev. 6 [(x x)] ⸢*i*$^?$⸣-*ṣa-nu bur-i-ṣa-n*[*u*] *re-*[*mi*$^?$]

44 A rev. 7 [*re*$^?$]-*mi a-la-ap a-su-ri ni-k*[*i-ip*$^?$]-⸢*ti*⸣ *i*[*t*$^?$-*ta-kip*$^?$]

45 A rev. 8 [*á*]*r-nu ḫi-ṭu gíl-la-a-ti ma-t*[*u/li* x x] ⸢x⸣ [x]

46 A rev. 9 [*š*]*ib*$^!$-*sa-at* DINGIR ^{d}*iš-tar* [x x] x[x x]

47 A rev. 10 [*š*]*e-er-tu*$_4$ *tur-tu*$_4$ *pu-qu-du-u* x[x x x x]

48 A rev. 11 [*r*]*i-in-zu kiš-pu ru-ḫu-ú up-šá-*[*šu-ú* x x x]

49 A rev. 13 ⸢*i*$^{!}$⸣-*te*$^{!}$-*en-né-es-ker ú-g*[*a-r*]*i ni-i*[*l*$^{?}$ A.MEŠ *ú-mal-li*]

50 A rev. 14 LÚ-*la dam-qa na-as-qa ina qer-bi* [*ú-še-li*$^{?}$]

51 A rev. 15 *e-mur-ši-ma* ^{d}*asal-lú-ḫi* DUMU ^{d}⸢*é*⸣-[*a* (x x)]

52 A rev. 16 *e-ru-um-ma a-na* ^{d}*é-a* AD-*šú* ⸢*i*⸣-[*šá-as-si*$^{?}$]

53 A rev. 17 ⸢*a*⸣-*bi* MUNUS *ša i-k*[*u*$^{?}$]-*šá s*[*ik*$^{?}$-*ru*]

54 A rev. 18 *ina mi-ni-i i-še*[*m*$^{?}$]-*me-ma* [x x x]

55 A rev. 19 ^{d}*é-a* DUMU-*šú* ^{d}*asal-lú-ḫi i-*[*ip-pal*]

56 A rev. 20 UR$_{5}$.GIM DU$_{11}$.GA-*šu a-lik ma-ri* ^{d}[*asal-lú-ḫi*]

57 A rev. 21 ⸢*li*$^{?}$⸣-*qa-am-ma* Ú.MEŠ *a-d*[*a*$^{?}$-x]x x[x x x x]

58 A rev. 22 [^{gi}]^{š}ŠINIG ⸢*e*⸣-*da bi-nu-*⸢*ut*$^{?}$⸣ [DINGIR-*ti-ka*$^{?}$ x x]

59 A rev. 23 ^{šim}LI ⸢*šá*$^{?}$⸣ *ub-ba-bu* x[x x x x]

60 A rev. 24 [^{gi}]^{š}GIŠIMMAR *ma-ḫi-r*[*u*] *ka-*[*la ša-a-ri*]

61 A rev. 25 ⸢^{ú}⸣*tu-lal mu-lil tu-šá-r*[*i*$^{?}$] x[x x x x x]

62 A rev. 26 ⸢^{ú}⸣IGI-*lim* Ú *pi-riš-ti* ^{ú}IGI-⸢20$^{?}$⸣ [x x x x x]

63 A rev. 27 ⸢^{ú}⸣AN.ḪÚL.LA *ma-ḫi-ir kiš-pi* [x x x x x x]

64 A rev. 28 [DIŠ]-*niš* ḪI.ḪI-*ma ina* GEŠTIN TU$_{6}$-*ka* KÙ.GA [x x x x x x]

65 A rev. 29 [*ina*] KAŠ.SAG TU$_{6}$-*ka* KÙ.GA [x x x x x x]

66 A rev. 30 [*ina*] GA TU$_{6}$-*ka* KÙ.GA [x x x x x x]

67 A rev. 31 ⸢ÉN⸣ *ul iu-*⸢*ut*$^{?}$⸣-*tu* ÉN ^{d}⸢*é*⸣-[*a u* ^{d}*asal-lú-ḫi*]

68 A rev. 32 [ÉN] ^{d}*da-mu* ^{d}*nin-kar-ra-a*[*k* ^{d}x x x x x x]

69 A rev. 33 [ÉN ^{d}NIN.ŠU]BUR$^{?}$ AN-*e* ⸢^{d}⸣[x x x x x x]

70 A rev. 34 ⸢ÉN⸣ ^{d}*gu-la* GAŠAN TI.LA ^{d}*gu-la* DINGIR x[x x x x x x]

---

71 A rev. 35 ⸢KA.INIM⸣.MA ÉN ^{munus}*la* ⸢*e*$^{?}$⸣-[*ri-tu ana šu-ri-i*$^{?}$]

---

72 A rev. 36 [É]N *an-ni-tu ana mar-ḫa-ṣi na*[*p-šal-ti* x x ŠID-*nu*$^{?}$]

73 A rev. 37 [*ana*] *maš-qí-ti* ÉN *an-ni-tu ma-*x[x x x x x x]

74 A rev. 38 [*ṣ*]*i-im-*⸢*du*⸣ *nap*$^{?}$-*ša-šu maš-q*[*í-tu*$^{?}$ x x x x x x]

75 A rev. 39 [*l*]*u ka-a-ma-na-at-ma l*[*a*$^{?}$ *e-ri-tu* PEŠ$_{4}$$^{?}$]

---

76 A rev. 40 [ÉN] É.NU.RU aḫ-⸢sa-x x⸣ [............]

77 A rev. 41 [x]x-aḫ -x[..................................]

78 A rev. 42 [x l]a-aḫ-te-e[š$^{?}$ ...... TU$_{6}$ ÉN É.NU.RU$^{?}$]

Bottom of the tablet

Bound Transcription and Translation

1 *traces* 2 [... ...]... *yara[ḫḫu(?)* ... ...] 3 [... ...]... *ṭābu* [... ...] 4 [*kas*]*î qalûti pillû* [... ...] 5 *argānu šibirti buqli titāpū* [... ...]

1 ... ... 2 [... ...], fine qu[ality barley(?), ...], 3 [.........] sweet-smelling [..., ...]-plant, [... ...], 4 roasted [*kasû*-plant(?)], *pillû*-plant, [... ...], 5 *argānu*-conifer, a lump of malt, beer mash, [... ...].

---

6 ^{šim}KU$_6$ *billat našpi* ...[... ...] 7 *šaman alpi tapaššaš ana* [*Ba*]-*ba* [... ...]

6 ^{šim}KU$_6$-fennel, beerwort (used) for (making) *našpu*-beer, [... ...]. 7 You apply (this) as an ointment (mixed) with ox fat. To the goddess [Ba]ba(?) [... ...].

---

8 *lā ālitta* <*ana*> *šūrîm-m*[*a* ... ...] 9 [*šuma* (*ana*) *šu*]*ršîm-ma* ...[... ...].

8 <To> enable an infertile [woman to get] pregnant [... ...], 9 [to let (her)] get [offspring] ... [... ...].

KÌD.KÌD.BI *arat kirî mala* [... ...] 11 *qan sugbanda ša Eridu* ... [... ...] 12 *šuruš qan šalāli baltu ašāgu* [... ...] 13 Ú.BÍL.LÁ *sīḫa ar*[*gānu* ... ...] 14 *šammi qišti*(?) *kalâšunu teleqqe* [... ...] 15 *ina mê temessi ana karpati tessip* [*ina tinūri tesekker*(?) ...] 16 *ina šēri tušellâ ana qer*[*bi*(?) ...] 17 *šikara ana libbi mê šātunu t*[*utabbak*(?) *sinništa šâši ana marḫaṣi*(?)] 18 *tušerrissa adi mû iktaṣû tumašša'ši* [... ...] 19 *ištu marḫaṣi tušellešī-ma napšalta tapaššassi* [... ...] 20 *sinništa šâši šalāšat ūmē ana marḫaṣi* [*tušerrissa* ... ...] 21 [*kī*]*ma ūmūša imtalû naṣmat*[*ta teppuš*(?) ...] 22 [*š*]*a naṣmatte šâši mērešta* [... ...] 23 *qēm uṭṭati damqu qēm kibti*(!) *qēm kunāši qēm inninni* [*qēm* ...] 24 *qēm ḫallūri qēm kakkî qēm kiššēni sīkti*(?) *barīrāte* [*sīkti* ...] 25 *sīkti*(?) *nīnê sīkti*(?) *azupīri sīkti kasî sīkti*(?) [...] 26 *sīkti*(?) *nikipti sīkti*(?) *kanakti sīkti*(?) *erēni sīkti*(?) [...] 27 *sīkti*(?) *asi sīkti*(?) *ṣumlalê sīkti*(?) *ballukki napḫar* 21 *qē*[*mī*(?)] 28 [1].(-)TA.ÀM *teleqqe ištēniš tuballal ina tangussi kīma qāt as*[*î tarabbak*(?)] 29 *mišil qa šamni taltappat ina qablīša pēnīša u rap*[*altīša*] 30 *tuṣabbâ-ma tarakkas*(?) *tutâršī-ma ina''eš*

10 The procedure for this: leaves from garden (plants), as much as [... ...], 11 reed from the small marsh of Eridu, ...[... ...], 12 root of *šalālu*-reed, *baltu*-thorn, *ašāgu*-acacia, [... ...], 13 Ú.BÍL.LÁ, *sīḫu*-tree, *ar*[*gānu*-conifer, ...], 14 'forest-plant'(?) – you take all these (plants), [... ...], 15 you wash (them) with water, collect (the liquid) in a vessel. [*You heat (the liquid) in an oven*(?) ...]. 16 In the morning you take it out, [you ... ...] in[to(?)] (it). 17 You [pour(?)] beer into the liquid. 18 You let 17 [that woman] 18 descend 17 [into the ablution(?)], you rub her down (with it) until the water has become cold. [... ...]. 19 (Then) you let her come out from the ablution and you rub her with a salve. [... ...]. 20 [You let] that woman [descend(?)] into the ablution on three days, [... ...]. 21 When her (three) days are complete, [you *prepare the following*] poultice – [... ...], 22 of this poultice (one says that?) [*it is good for having*] a request [*fulfilled* (?): flour of ...(?)], 23 good barley flour, wheat(!) flour, emmer flour, flour of *ennēnu*-cereal, [powder of ...], 24 pea flour, lentil flour, *kiššēnu* (vetch)-flour, powder of *barīrātu*-plant, [powder of ...], 25 powder of *nīnû*-plant, powder of *azupīru*-plant, powder of *kasû*-plant, flour of [...], 26 powder of *nikiptu*-plant, powder of *kanaktu*-plant, cedar powder, [....]-powder, 27 powder of *asu*-plant, powder of *ṣumlalû*-plant, powder of *ballukku*-plant – in sum 21 (sorts of) flour/powder 28 you take one by one, you mix (them) together, [you make a paste] in a metal *tangussu*-pot like (one) used by (lit. from the hand of) a physician, 29 moistening (the *materia medica*) with half a litre of oil. 30 You soak 29 her hip(s), her (upper) thigh and [her] lo[wer back] (with it) 30 by applying it as a bandage(?). You keep doing (this, lit. you repeat it) for her, then she will get well.

---

31 *kurkānâ ša šadê nabruqqi kukra* [...] 32 *ina šaman* [*baluḫḫi*(?) *tu*]*ballal tapaššassī-ma ina''eš*

32 You m[ix] 31 *kurkānû*-plant of the mountains, *namruqqu*-plant, *kukru*-aromatic (and) [...]-aromatic 32 with oil of [*baluḫḫu*]-aromatic(?). You rub her (with it), and she will get [well].

---

33 *kurkānâ nabruqqi tasâk ina karāni išatti mimma* [...] MIN

33 You crush *kurkānû*-plant (and) *namruqqu*-plant. She shall drink (it) in wine. Whatever [...], ditto (i.e., she will get well).

34 *nikipta imḫur-ešrā tasâk ina karāni išatti* MIN	34 You pound *nikiptu*-plant (and) 'heals twenty'-plant. She shall drink (it) in wine, ditto (i.e., she will get well).
35 *šammu* ⸢*ṣalmu*(?)⸣ *ṣaṣumtu ištēniš tasâk ina karāni iš*[*at-ti*] MIN	35 You pound ⸢'black⸣(?) plant/drug' (and) *ṣaṣumtu*-plant together. She shall drink (it) in wine, ditto (i.e., she will get well).
36 [*imḫ*]*ur-līm imḫur-ešrā ištēniš tasâk ina* <*karāni*> *išatti* MIN	36 You pound 'heals-thousand'-plant and 'heals twenty'-plant together. She shall drink (it) in wine, ditto (i.e., she will get well).
37 [*kurkānâm* (*ša*)] *šadê ḫarmuna tasâk ina rēmīš*[*a tašak-kan-ma*] *ina"eš*	37 You pound [*kurkānû*-plant(?) of] the mountains (and) *ḫarmunu*-plant (together). [You insert (it)] into h[er] womb (viz. vagina). [Then] she will get well.
38 [... ...] *ina itqi ta*[*lammi ana*] *ūrīša tašakkan-ma ina"eš*	38 You wr[ap] [... ...] in a wad of wool, insert (it) [into] her vagina. Then she will get well.
39 [... ... *mašq*]*īti napšal*[*ti u na*]*rmakti* 40 [... ...]... *sinništu šī* [*irrī*(?)-*m*]*a šuma iraššī*	39 [... ... pot]ion, ointme[nt and b]ath/lotion, 40 [... ...]... . That woman will [get pregnant(?)] and get offspring (lit. "a name").
41 [ÉN *itte*]*ne*[*ske*]*r ugārī* [*nīl*] *mê umalli*	41 [Incantation:] "My meadow becomes blocked again and again, (although) I(?) filled [(it) with a flood] of water,
42 [*lullâ da*]*mqa na*[*sqa*] *ina qerbi ušē*[*li*(?)]	42 (although) I(?) was letting a pleasant, pre[cious] person em[erge] (lit. rise) in it.
43 [...] *iṣānū burriṣān*[*ū*] *rē*[*mī*(?)]	43 (But) the *burriṣānu filled up* [*my*] *wo*[*mb with*(?) ...].
44 [*rē*]*mī*(?) *alap asurrî nik*[*ip*]*ti i*[*ttakip*(?)]	44 The 'ox of the sewer' [*dealt out*] a bl[ow](?) *against* my [wo]mb(?).
45 [*a*]*rnu ḫīṭu gillāti* ...[...]	45 Misdeed(s), wrongdoing(s), crimes, ...[...],
46 [*š*]*ibsāt ili ištari* [...] ... [...]	46 [wr]ath of god (and) goddess, [... ...],
47 [*š*]*ērtu tūrtu puquddû* ...[...]	47 punishment, retribution, *charge*, [... ...],
48 [*r*]*inzu kišpū ruḫû upšā*[*šû* ...]	48 *sorcery*, witchcraft, spittle-magic, (evil) machin[ations, ...].
49 *ittenesker ug*[*ār*]*ī nī*[*l mê umalli*(?)]	49 My meadow becomes blocked again and again, [(although) I(?) filled (it)] with a flo[od of water],
50 *lullâ damqa nasqa ina qerbi* [*ušēli*(?)]	50 [(although) I was letting(?)] a pleasant, precious person [emerge] inside (it).
51 *ēmuršī-ma Asalluḫi mār E*[*a* (...)]	51 Asalluḫi, the son of Ea, saw her [(...)].
52 *ērum-ma ana Ea abīšu i*[*šassi*(?)]	52 He went inside and [cried out] to Ea, his father:
53 *abī sinništu ša īkūša se*[*kru*(?)]	53 'My father! The woman whose plot (of land) is bl[ocked(?)],
54 *ina mīnî išemmē-ma*(?) [...]	54 With what will *it listen*(?) and [...]?'
55 *Ea māršu Asalluḫi i*[*ppal-ma*(?)]	55 Ea [*answer*]*ed* his son Asalluḫi,
56 *kīam iqabbīšu alik mārī* [*Asalluḫi*]	56 saying to him as follows: 'Go, my son [Asalluḫi],
57 *liqâm-ma šammī* ...[... ...]	57 and take (these) plants: ...[... ...],
58 *bīna ēda binût* [*ilūtīka*(?) ...]	58 the free-standing tamarisk, the creation of [your divinity(?)...],
59 *burāšu ša*(?) *ubbabu* ...[...]	59 the juniper which(?) purifies [...],
60 *gišimmaru māḫiru ka*[*la šārī*]	60 the date palm, who withstands a[ll winds],
61 *tullal mullil tušār*[*i*(?)] ...[... ...]	61 the *tullal*-plant, the purifier of the battlefi[eld(?) ... ...],

62 *imḫur-līm šammi pirišti imḫur-ešrā*(?) [...]	62 'heals thousand'-plant, the plant of mystery, 'heals twenty'-plant(?), [... ...]
63 *anhullû māḫir kišpī* [... ...]	63 *anḫullû*-plant, the adversary of (lit. who withstands) witchcraft, [... ...] –
64 [*ištē*]*niš bullil/tuballal-ma ina karāni tû-ka ellu* [... ...]	64 mix (them) together. Then with wine (*after reciting*) your pure incantation, [*give them to her to drink*(?)],
65 [*ina*] *šikari tû-ka ellu* [... ...]	65 [with] beer (*after reciting*) your pure incantation [*give them to her to drink*(?)],
66 [*ina*] *šizbi tû-ka ellu* [... ...]	66 [with] milk (*after reciting*) your pure incantation [*give them to her to drink*(?)]!'
67 ⸢*šiptu*⸣ *ul yuttu šipat E*[*a u Asalluḫi*]	67 The spell is not mine, it is the incantation of E[a and Asalluhi],
68 [*šipat*] *Damu Ninkarra*[*k* ... ...]	68 (it is) [the incantation] of Damu (and) Ninkarr[ak, ...],
69 [*šipat Ninšu*]*bur*(?) *šamê* [... ...]	69 [(it is) the incantation of Ninšu]bur of heaven(?), of [... ...],
70 ⸢*šipat*⸣ *Gula bēlet balāṭi Gula* ...[... ...]	70 (it is) the incantation of Gula, the lady of life, (of) Gula, *the goddess* [... ...]!"
71 ⸢KA.INIM⸣.MA ÉN *lā e*[*rītu ana šūrî*(?)]	71 Wording of an incantation [to enable] a woman who is not [pregnant to get pregnant(?)].
72 [*šip*]*tu annītu ana marḫaṣi na*[*pšalti ... tamannu*(?)] 73 [*ana*] *mašqīti šiptu annītu* ...[... ...] 74 [*ṣ*]*imdu napšaš(t)u mašq*[*ītu*(?) ... ...] 75 [*l*]*ū kayyamānat-ma l*[*ā ēritu irri*(?)]	72 [You shall recite(?)] this incantation for the lotion, sal[ve (and) ...]. 73 [For] the potion, this incantation ...[... ...]. 74 [The ba]ndage, the *ointment*(?), the pot[ion(?) ... ...] 75 shall be (administered) regular(ly). Then (*the woman*) *who is not* [*pregnant will get pregnant*(?)].
76 [ÉN] É.NU.RU aḫ-⸢sa-x x⸣ [... ...]	76 Enuru-incantation. *Too fragmentary for translation*
77 *traces*	77 *traces*
78 [... l]a-aḫ-te-e[š(?) ... ... TU$_6$ ÉN É.NU.RU(?)]	78 [...] laḫteš [... ... Wording of an Enuru-spell(?).]

Bottom of the reverse of ms. A

Notes

Lines 6–7: ^{šim}KU$_6$ in line 6' is probably to be understood as a variant writing for ^{ú}KU$_6$. The Akkadian reading of this logogram is uncertain; drug compendia equate ^{ú}KU$_6$ with *šimru* and *urânu*, both of which are presumably varieties of fennel, see CAD Š/3, 8–9; CAD U/W, 206–208. CAD glosses *urânu* with "anise" and *šimru* with "fennel". Cf. in addition to the references in the dictionaries, Civil 2008, ARET 4, 105 No. 223 (on $^{\text{šim/ú}}$TÁL.TÁL = *urânu*).

For roasted *kasû*-plant (GAZI^{sar} BÍL.MEŠ) as an ingredient, see also BAM 240: 41', 43' (text D.2.1).

The reading of DIDA SIG$_5$/SIG.(GA) is not entirely certain. The attestations collected in CAD N/2, 78 s.v. *našpu* suggest either *billat našpi* or *billatu našiptu*. For the translation "beerwort/*billatu*-substance used for the production of *našpu*-beer", see also Abusch and Schwemer 2011, 55 text 1.6, notes on lines 9'–10'; Abusch et al. 2020, text A.1 rev. 2'; ibid., text 7.25 line 25. Note further Civil 2005, CTMMA 2, 234 no. 56 ii 5', 236 iii 14', and 238 (discussion). *Billatu* is a dry substance used as an ingredient in beer brewing and as an "instant beer" produced by mixing it with water, see Stol 1971, *BiOr* 28, 169; 1994, 165; Maul 1994, *Zukunftsbewältigung*, 51.

For Bau/Baba, a goddess of healing and midwifery related to Gula, see Sibbing-Plantholt 2022, 139–143 for a recent overview.

Lines 8–9: The restoration [MU *šu-u*]*r-ši-im-ma* in line 9 was proposed by Reiner 1982a, *ZA* 72, 128, on the basis of line 40, which resumes the section introduced in lines 8–9 with the words MUNUS BI [PEŠ$_4$$^{?}$-*m*]*a* MU TUKU-*ši* "that woman [will get pregnant and] acquire offspring (lit. a name)". The predominant syllabic spelling of the text in lines 8–9 (and elsewhere in BAM 244) and the accusative *lā ālitta* are noteworthy.

Line 11: The signs copied by Köcher in BAM 244 are [G]I SUG SIKIL x si ni ke_4 "pure reed from the marsh ...". The emendation for GI *sug-bàn-da šá eri-*du_{10}*-*ke_4 rests on the occurrence of the "reed of the small marsh of Eridu" in the bilingual birth incantation AUAM 73.3094 rev. 4'–5' (Cohen 1976, *RA* 70, 133ff.; Wasserman and Zomer 2022, No. 10 lines 42–43), which reads: gi sú-ug-bàn-da eri-du_{10}-ga / *qá-na-a ša sú-ug-bàn-da ša eri-*du_{10}*-ga*. Beside this Old Babylonian text, reed is also used in the prescriptions of the Neo-Assyrian Birth Compendium (BAM 248 and dupl.), which like BAM 244, was found in the N4 library (see text D.1.1 with discussion).

Line 13: The reading of the logogram Ú.BÍL.LÁ is unknown in this context. The logogram BÍL.LÁ is usually read *emṣu* "sour", and found as qualification of beer, vinegar, fruit and bread made of sourdough (CAD E, 153). Lexical lists equate Sumerian ú-bíl-lá (also ^{giš}ú-bíl-lá and similar spellings) with *pillû* "mandrake" (then spelled ^{giš}ú-bil-lá or ^{giš}bíl-lum) and with the loanword *upillû*, meaning "charcoal" (see CAD P, 376 lex. section; CAD U/W, 179 lex. section; ePSD2, s.v. billum and ubila). The most likely interpretation of Ú.BÍL.LÁ in the present context would be to understand it as a rare logogram for *pillû* instead of the more common $^{giš/ú}$NAM.TAR. Compare further BAM 237 rev. iv 30 (text C.1.4), which lists as one ingredient DÈ.LÁ ^{ú}*ur-ba-te* "ashes of *urbatu*-rushes", in which DÈ.LÁ is perhaps a variant of DÈ = *pēntu* "charcoal" or, more likely in our context, *diqmēnu* "ashes" (following a suggestion by Stol 2020b, *BiOr* 77, 570).

Line 14: In Uruanna I 425, we find the equation Ú *šá-mi* ^{giš}TIR = *labubittu*, the latter of which is a medicinal plant usually written with the logogram ^{ú}TUR.A.NI (AHw 526b; CAD L, 36 s.v. *labubittu* lex. section). The logogram Ú ^{giš}TIR literally means "forest-plant", but the word "forest" may perhaps refer to the canebrake here, since the plant is listed together with reed plants in Uruanna (for discussion and references, see Stol 2011, *Hippologica Ugaritica*, 389–390).

Line 16: Böck (2010a, 109) restores "sie soll es ... tragen" in the gap in this line, suggesting the application of a tampon. However, a continuation of the preparation of the remedy is expected at this point rather than an application on the patient.

Line 18: Guessing from the context, one may perhaps restore "when the water has cooled off, (you let her come out of the ablution)" in the gap of line 18 (e.g., *kīma mû iktaṣû*, with the perfect form of *kaṣû*).

Line 19: The recipe for the ointment that is only mentioned in passing at this point is, by all likelihood, the prescription written down in lines 31–32, immediately following the present section. In this light, it is likely that text in the gap of line 19 consisted in an additional instruction to give the patient one of the potions found in lines 33–36 to drink (i.e., restore [*maš-qí-ta* NAG-*ši*]).

Line 20: For MUNUS *šâši*, see also the Middle Assyrian text *Iraq* 31, 29: 9 (text II.1.4): "you let that woman sit over (the fumigants in the pot)" (MUNUS *šâši ina muḫḫi tušeššab*). At the end of line 20, perhaps again restore [*nap-šal-ta* ŠÉŠ-*si*] "you rub her with the salve".

Lines 21–30: The Akkadian reading of ZÌ or KU (also KU.KU) before the names of herbs, aromatics or minerals is not entirely certain, although it is clear that it refers to powdered ingredients or, in the case of cereals, to flour (Akkadian *qēmu*). For discussion, see Borger 2004, MZL, 425 sub no. 808; CAD S, 259–260 s.v. *sīktu*; CAD Q, 208 s.v. *qēmu* discussion sections. The Akkadian reading of the logogram KU.KU has now been identified as *supandu* or *supantu* (Schwemer, *NABU* 2021/2, No. 48 with further references). In other cases, KU ($ŠE_{10}$) corresponds to Akkadian *zû*, as in *zê buqli* "refuse of malt" or *zê summati* (lit. "dove's dung", a type of false carob) (cf. CAD Z, s.v. *zû* with discussion). When powdered forms of cereals, plants or aromatics are summed up as a specific number of ZÌ.DA.MEŠ or ZÌ.DA.ḪI.A, the Akkadian reading might be *qēmū* "flours" (cf. CAD Q, 208). Note, for a similar poultice with a large amount of powders or flours, BAM 124 iii 54–55 // BAM 125: 22–23 (Scurlock 2014a, 456: 46), where the ingredients are summed up as ZÌ.DA.MEŠ [Ú.ḪI].A *u* [ŠI]M.ḪI.A *si-ku* GAL-*ú na-aṣ-[ma-t]i* (MAŠ.MAŠ-*ti*) A.ZU-*ti* "(a total of 46) flours. (These) plants and aromatics are a great powder for a bandage (used) by the crafts of (the conjurer and) the physician".

Lines 21–22: The sense of this fragmentary passage is difficult to elucidate. CAD M/2, 22b s.v. *mēreštu* A sub 1c suggests restoring "[if she makes(?)] a request (*mērešta*) for this bandage", probably thinking of the formulation *mērešta erēšu* "to make a request, to ask a wish". The word *mēreštu* "request, wish" is often found in the context of deities requesting votive offerings, but also often refers to human wishes and desires. Perhaps our passage contained a laudatory qualification of the remedy. "Having a wish fulfilled/granted" (e.g. the phrase *mērešta nadānu*) could refer to the wish for a child being fulfilled with the help of the remedy. My tentative guess is thus to restore *mērešta* [*ana nadāni damiq*] or the like in the gap, but this remains highly conjectural. M. Stol (personal communication) pointed out an alternative reading as *mēreštu* B, meaning "cultivated field, cultivation" (CAD M/2, 23–24), and proposes that the fragmentary passage may specify the use of cultivated plants (in contrast to wild ingredients, i.e. coming "from the mountain(s)", such as *kurkānû*-plant).

Line 23: The sign sequence ZÌ NÁ is understood here as an error for ZÌ GIG "wheat flour", although it is also possible to emend the text to read ZÌ <ŠE>.NÁ.<A> "powder of chaste tree (*šunû*)". Cf. BAM 240: 41, 50 (text D.2.1), where this ingredient also occurs together with various other flours.

Line 24: The leguminous plant *kiššānu* (*kiššēnu*), identified as the Common vetch (*Vicia sativa*) based on cognate terms in modern dialects of Arabic, was also used as animal fodder according to Akkadian texts, see Stol 1985a, *BSA* 2, 130–132.

Line 28: Other restorations are possible at the end of line 28 (e.g. *tubaḫḫar* "you heat/steam", *tušabšal* "you boil"). Instead of *kīma qāt asî*, one would have expected *ša qāt asî* "from the hand of an *asû*". The expression *ina tangussi kīma qāt asî* "in a metal *tangussu*-vessel (that is) like (one) used by a physician" is not attested elsewhere to my knowledge. The term *tangussu* (*tamgussu*) denotes a metal pot or kettle (the logogram (ŠEN.TUR) is written with the classifier URUDU "copper"), which is often used to boil medical ingredients (see e.g. *Iraq* 31, 29: 19–25 (text II.1.4) for discussion, see also Gaspa 2014, *Contenitori*, 95). Instructions in medical texts for processing of materials in *tangussu*-vessels are often followed by *kīma rabīki tarabbak* "you make a decoction/mash" (CAD R, 9 sub d; CAD T, 150 sub b); perhaps our text passage is corrupt or has become abbreviated. But is not impossible that the *tangussu*-vessel was a trade-mark object used by physicians.

A similar phrase *ina qāt(ī) asî* "in the care (lit. hand(s) of a physician" referring to the treatments applied by the *asû* is found in a few other texts: see CAD A/2 345 sub a; Ritter 1968, 316a. Note in particular phrases referring to the failure of the physician's treatments in BAM 22 obv. 22 (eye diseases); AMT 2/7: 4' (= Geller 2005a, No. 15 Ms. P, renal diseases); AMT 101/3: 15 (= Geller 2005a, No. 38: 15'; rectal diseases). The treatise on EYES mentions specific treatments (lead spoon-salve) by the physician (Geller and Panayotov 2020, IGI 3: 105').

Line 30: An instruction for binding the preparation on the body is expected here, since lines 21–22 introduce the recipe for a bandage (*naṣmattu*), which ends here in line 30. Thus, the expected Akkadian verb in the instruction in line 30 would be *ṣamādu* "to bind, bandage", which is usually written with the logogram LÁ. However, the text seems to use the logogram KÉŠ, which corresponds to Akkadian *rakāsu* "to tie on; to bandage". For *ṣabû* (*ṣapû*) "to soak; to drench; to irrigate (a field)", in the D-stem also "to bathe", see CAD Ṣ, 45–46; Steinert 2020, *JMC* 36, 61, 62.

For the repetition of the treatment, expressed with the verb *turru* (*târu* D-stem), see also CAD T, 278 sub 13b. Compare, for example, GUR.GUR-*šum-ma* in BAM 503 iii 60', 63', 67', 74', 78' (Scurlock 2014a, 376–377); AMT 80/1 i 13 // BAM 548 i 13 (Scurlock 2014a, 466); further BAM 3 iv 27; BAM 506 obv. 8', 9'. Usually the number of days for which the treatment is to be continued is mentioned.

Lines 31–32: In line 32, the restoration *šaman baluḫḫi* "oil of *baluḫḫu*-aromatic" would fit the limited space in the gap (cf. CAD B, 75b for other attestations).

Line 33: Perhaps restore "she drinks it in wine, (with) whatever [she eats(?)]" in the gap.

Line 35: To my knowledge, the drug *šammu ṣalmu*, lit. "black/dark plant/drug", is not attested in other medical prescriptions. However, it is equated with the likewise unidentified *aktam*-plant in pharmaceutical lists, see, e.g., Uruanna I 203ff. (CT 14, 22 v–vi 43ff.), CT 41, 43 BM 59596 rev. 2 (CAD A/1, 282–283; AHw 30). *Aktam* is also known as a plant "to get seed (= offspring)", see BAM 1 i 19–20; BAM 380 rev. 25 // BAM 381 iii 17–18; see Stol 2000a, 52–53. For Ú GI_6 among other plants that are recommended for use on the third day of month Kislīmu (IX) and associated with the god Pabilsag (and the zodiac sign Sagittarius), see also VAT 7815: 5, rev. 5 (Weidner 1967, *Gestirndarstellungen*, 17ff., 45–46; Schreiber 2018b, 388–394).

Line 37: The uncertain restoration [^{ú}*kur-ka-na* (*šá*)] KUR "*kurkānû*-plant of the mountains" follows Scurlock (2020, *JMC* 35, 57). This plant name may be a variant of the term *kurrukummu*, which von Weiher (1983, 196) and Jursa (2009, *FS Sima*, 162 with note 74) identify with curcuma (attested e.g., in SpTU 2, No. 50: 5, corresponding to Aramaic *kūrkemā*). The present text uses both the wild and cultivated variety of *kurkānû*-plant: both are also encountered in initial position in lines 31 and 33 above. For further attestations in the women's healthcare texts as a fertility-enhancing plant, see N. 4001:

14–26 // (*kurkānû* of the mountains); BAM 247: 8 and *passim* (texts B.2.1 and B.1.3); BM 42313+ obv. 7 (text A.2.2); BM 79061 obv. 11 (text A.2.8, in the latter attestation, the plant is spelled ^{ú}*k*[*u*]-*ur-ru-ka-nu*). See further CAD K, 560–561; CAD S, 258a sub 1e.

Lines 39–40: The word *narmaktu* also occurs in another medical fragment from Assur (BAM 276: 3'), but that text is very damaged. For *narmaktu* following a total of ingredients, see also BAM 67 obv. 18 (Maul 2019, *Bannlösung*, 290 no. 77: 18) seven plants (for) "a lotion/bath against the ban" (*nàr-ma-ak-tú* NAM.RIM); note further ADD 1042: 11 (list of drugs for use); Goltz 1974, 91–92. While the enumeration of treatments here in line 39 uses the word *narmaktu* "bath", the prescription in lines 19–20 speaks of *marḫaṣu* "lotion, ablution" instead of *narmaktu*. However, it is likewise possible that the synonymous terms *narmaktu* and *marḫaṣu* refer to the same treatment that is described in lines 10–20. In this line of thought, in the gap at the beginning of lines 39–40, reference could have been made to reciting the following incantation (lines 41–70) over all the remedies and treatments described in the preceding lines. The similar instructions in lines 72–75 could then have explained the use of the short spell found in lines 76–78, or they may have modified the instructions given in lines 39–40.

For the prediction *šuma irašši* "she will get offspring (lit. a name)" in omen texts, see also Jiménez 2016, *JCS* 68, 215 with note 44 with further references.

Lines 41–70: Stol's comments (2000a, 72 with n. 148) on common elements of the present incantation with SpTU 2, No. 25, an anti-witchcraft spell (see now Abusch et al. 2020, *CMAwR* 3, text 7.35 for this text), do not seem warranted except for the similarity that the present spell also alludes to witchcraft. SpTU 2, No. 25 is not concerned with a problem concerning female fertility, pregnancy or birth; but it uses landscape metaphors speaking of rivers and meadows, as the present spell. According to the collations of Abusch et al. (2020, text 7.35), in SpTU 2, No. 25, a "porcupine" (*būrmayānu*) and not the *buriṣānu*-animal is mentioned (as suggested, among others, by Farber 1987b, *WdO* 18, 40 n. 55; cf. Stol 2020b, *BiOr* 77, 570), and this animal is made responsible for breaching the river (by destroying reed-made dams), causing the channel to overflow and thereby allowing the river meadows (*saḫḫātu*) to be carried away (see Abusch et al. 2020, *CMAwR* 3, text 7.35 comments on line 3). In the present incantation, the problem revolves around a blockage of the *ugāru*-land (see below), not a breach of the river. Cf. for the imagery of floods and broken dikes in connection with bleeding and diarrhoea, Steinert 2013; Stol 2020b, *BiOr* 77, 570.

The spell in lines 41–70 begins with a description of the problem from the first-person perspective of the patient (lines 41–50; a similar pattern is also found in SpTU 2, No. 25). Then the text turns to a dialogue between Ea and Asalluḫi (a traditional element of many healing incantations, which goes back to Sumerian formulae), in which Asalluḫi observes the woman's problem and goes to ask his father Ea, how he shall deal with the problem. Ea then instructs his son to take several potent and purifying healing plants and to administer them to the patient in a potion (lines 51–67). The fragmentary text of the spell presents many difficulties, and the interpretation offered here is in many respects tentative.

Lines 41–42: I owe part of my reconstruction of the opening line of the spell to Böck 2013, 47 with n. 73. However, my understanding of the identical lines 41 and 49 differs slightly. In lines 41 and 49, Böck (ibid.) suggests to read: [ŠÀ *it-te*]-*en-ni*-⌜*is-kir*⌝ u_2-*ga-ri*-[*in-ni*] A.MEŠ u_2-*mal-li* ... ⌜*i*⌝-*te*!-*en-ni-is-kir* u_2-*g*[*a-r*]*i-ni* ⌜A⌝.[MEŠ u_2-*mal-li*] and translates both lines "The womb is locked again and again, her womb is filled with amniotic fluid. ...". This rendering seems to understand u_2-*ga-ri*-(*in*)-*ni* as a variant spelling for the word *agarinnu* "crucible, mould; beer bread; fertile soil", which occurs as a poetic word for the womb (Steinert 2017a, 300–301 for discussion). The form *ugarinnu* is, however, not attested elsewhere. The interpretation offered here proposes to read *ú-ga-ri* "my meadow" (or irrigated land, spoken from the patient's perspective), which is used here as a metaphorical term for the womb (cf. CAD U/W, 27–33 s.v. *ugāru* "grassland, meadow, arable land"). The meadow/irrigated land which becomes blocked is thus a description of the woman's problem (i.e. infertility). The verb *sekēru* is both used in the meaning "to dam up, close, clog" (e.g., a canal, watercourse) and "to block (parts of the body)" (CAD S, 210–213) and thus lends itself perfectly to this kind of metaphor. Similar agricultural metaphors describing the female body in terms of a riverine landscape with a plot of irrigated land (*tamirtu*) are encountered elsewhere, e.g. in an incantation in BAM 235: 10–13 // BAM 236 rev. 1'–5' (see *infra* texts C.1.1–C.1.2), this time in the context of gynaecological bleeding. For a discussion of the landscape metaphors relating to the womb and to the processes of reproduction in Mesopotamian literary and healing texts, see further Couto-Ferreira 2017, 2018; Steinert 2013, 2017a, 2020.

The verbal form *umalli* at the end of line 41 is a D-stem form of *malû* "to become full", which is usually transitive, i.e., to fill something (with water/fluid). Therefore, the subject of the clause in the second half of the line cannot be the womb or arable land, which becomes full (one would expect a G-stem form of *malû*). I therefore propose to read [*ni-il*?] A.MEŠ *ú-mal-l[i]* "I filled it with a [flood(?)] of water" (the word *nīlu* is partially preserved in the identical line 49), understanding this as a poetic expression for the male semen filling the womb, resembling a flood of water flooding a meadow. The term *nīlu* "flooding" also means "semen" (CAD N/2, 234). It is also possible that *umalli* had a third person sg. subject ("he filled it"), referring to the woman's partner. For *ugāru*-plots being irrigated or flooded for cultivation, cf. CAD U/W, 30 sub 1c-1'c'.

Line 42: This line can partly be restored following line 50, which repeats the same text and refers to a "good, precious person" (*lullâ damqa nasqa*) as direct object of the sentence (for *nasqu* "selected, precious, choice, preeminent", cf. CAD N/2, 31 sub a-4'). My guess is that this refers to the foetus which is brought forth in the womb/meadow.

The restoration *ušēli* "I brought forth/let emerge" at the end line 42 is uncertain; this portion of the tablet is now completely deteriorated. M. Stol (personal communication) suggests reading *[p]a-še-[ru]* instead, guided by the sign traces on F. Köcher's copy. The term *pāširu*, lit. "releaser" is used as an attribute (adjective) to *mû* "water", but it can also refer to a part of the river (*pāšir nāri*); AHw 845a sub 4 suggests "Flußfilter(?)", based on an assumed meaning "clarifying, purifying" (cf. Maul 1994, *Zukunftsbewältigung*, 88 with n. 45, translating "lösende Wasser"). The alternative restoration *ú-še-li* (Š-stem *elû*) proposed here may be compared with the Š-stem of *aṣû* occurring in the sense of "to bring forth, to let (seed) sprout" in another spell against infertility (N. 4001 line 9 and dupl.; see text B.2.1, and Steinert 2017a, 317), where it refers to conception and foetal growth in metaphorical terms as the woman (field) letting the "seed" sprout. The text in line 42 similarly seems to say that the woman became pregnant successfully, i.e. the foetus was brought forth in the woman's womb. The following lines 43–44 then appear to describe the damaging action of two other agents, which are blamed as being responsible for the woman's problem (see the next note). This could suggest an allusion to the woman's inability to bring a conceived foetus to term, in addition to her inability to conceive.

Lines 43–44: According to the rare references collected in the dictionaries, the word *aburriṣānu* (or *burriṣānu*, as in line 43 of the present text) is an animal (insect or rodent(?), used as *materia medica*) and a demon (known from lexical lists). In the Lú Excerpt (MSL 12, 109: 173, *a-bur-ri-ṣa-nu* (Sumerian equation [x]-šub-ba) is listed beside *Kūbu* (the demon of premature foetuses) and other demonic figures and animals such as *paraštinnu*, *ḫallulāya* "centipede", Šulak, *lilû*, and Kilili (CAD A/1, 90; CAD K, 487 sub lex. section; CAD P, 179). In the present text, *burriṣānu* may be a negative demonic being rather than an animal, but this is mere guess.

The verb *i-ṣa-nu* in line 43 looks like a plural form. I would tentatively assign it to *ṣânu/ṣênu* "to fill up, to bloat", which usually occurs with liquids (e.g. filling up someone's body with bile or poison), see AHw 1081–1082 sub *ṣânu* I (note that CAD books the references for *ṣânu* under the verbs *za'ānu* "to adorn" and *ṣênu* "to load, to heap up"). The last word in line 43 may be *re-[mi]* "my womb", i.e. the *burriṣānu* filled up the woman's womb with a substance causing infertility (and which should then have been mentioned at the beginning of line 43).

The first word in line 44 may perhaps again be restored as *rēmī* "my womb". The expression *alap asurrî* "ox of the sewer" appears to be a metaphorical designation for the scorpion (I owe this insight to Stol 2020b, *BiOr* 77, 570 and personal communication). Thus, in an Old Babylonian incantation against scorpions (Cavigneaux 1994, *RA* 88, 155–157, 161; SEAL no. 7168), the animal is called "ox of the earth" (*alap erṣetim*, line 1), to whom the sewer gave birth (*ūldaššu asurrûm*, line 6); see also George 2010b, *NABU* 2010/1, 5–6 no. 5. For a discussion of the word *asurrû* as "sewer" (usually translated as damp course or lower course of a wall in the dictionaries), see George 2015, *Iraq* 77, 90–102, who notes that *asurrû* is frequently described as the habitat of animals and vermin such as snakes, mongooses and as a stinking place associated with demons.

The remainder of line 44 is difficult. The traces may suggest the word *nikimtu* "accumulation, bloating", which occurs as an internal illness (e.g., *nikmāt šāri*) and may be suggested by the context of the preceding lines of the spell. On the other hand, one could think of *nikiptu* "hit, blow" (from *nakāpu* "to gore, to butt" (said of horned animals) and "to pierce, to stab"). Cf. CAD N/1, 157–158 lex. section and sub 2b, where the verb *nakāpu* (Gt-stem) is used with reference to the aggressive and overwhelming action of animals, storms and demons. It is therefore tempting to restore *nikipti it[takip]* "it dealt out a blow", since the scorpion is also called "constantly goring one" (*munakkipu*) in the Old Babylonian incantation cited above (Cavigneaux 1994, *RA* 88, 155–157 line 2). The scorpion, an animal feared for its sting, but also associated with fertility, plays a negative, even demonic role in the present incantation as well, and seems to be partly responsible for the woman's health problem. Perhaps it acts as an instrument of the witch, like the *aburriṣānu*-animal (or demon).

Line 47: The word *tūrtu* "turning, reversion" often occurs in enumerations of wrongdoings and of causes of misfortune, as found for example in *Šurpu*, where *tūrtu* is frequently found beside *māmītu* "ban (due to a broken oath)" and may be translated as "retribution" (for breaking an oath) (see CAD T, 491 sub 2b for references). Note, for example, Lambert 1974, *JNES* 33, 280: 113 (DINGIR.ŠÀ.DAB.BA-incantation): *māmātīya pušur tūrti lumnīya u[suḫ] maruštī duppir* "Undo my oaths, remove the retribution for my misdeeds, drive away my trouble!". Abusch and Schwemer (2011, CMAwR 1, text 7.2 line 36) suggest that in more specific contexts the term may refer to the magical undoing of a ban (i.e. to escape the impending consequences of swearing a false oath) or more generally to the requital of sorcerous magic. Note further *Šurpu* III 96 (Reiner 1958, 22): *māmīt tūrta ana amēli turri* "the ban (as a consequence of) retaliating against someone". Note that *tūrtu* is also attested as a disease term in medical texts (e.g. in drug compendia), see CAD T, 491 sub 2b for references.

The word *puquddû*, derived from *paqādu* "to entrust", means "(formal) delivery, legal consignment" (CDA², 278) or "deposit; entrusted goods" (CAD, P 515a). Why this word occurs in the present enumeration of negative phenomena is difficult to understand; perhaps it refers to some obligation or legal charge afflicting the patient.

Line 48: The word *rinzu* in line 48 is a hapax and presumably another word for witchcraft or sorcery (see AHw 987a; CAD R, 365a). M. J. Geller (personal communication) suggests this term could be related to Aram. *rymz'*, "hand gesture", which could indicate some kind of sign of sorcerous magic.

Lines 49–50: For these two lines, which appear to resume the wording of lines 41–42, see the notes above.

Line 52 and 55: The reconstructions *išassi* "he cries" and *ippal* "he answers" in these two lines follow the wording of similar incantations featuring the Marduk-Ea-dialogue, see e.g. bilingual examples in *Šurpu* V–VI 20, 28, also VII 39, 46 (Reiner 1958, 30, 37).

Lines 53–54: These two lines with the direct speech of Asalluḫi are problematic. Line 53 summarizes the patient's problem in a way that does not exactly correspond to the description given earlier. The restoration *sinništu ša īkūša*(?) *se*[*kru*] "the woman whose plot (bounded by a dyke) is blocked(?)" differs from line 41 and 49 speaking of a meadow being blocked.

The phrase *ina mīnî iše*[*m*]*mē-ma* "with what will it *listen* ...?" in line 54 is unusual, as one would expect a phrase such as "with what will she calm down" (*ina mīnî ipaššaḫ*), known from similar incantations (see e.g., *Šurpu* V–VI 26, VII 44; Reiner 1958, 30, 37). If the reading *i-šem-me* is not mistaken, the subject of the verb is unlikely the patient, but rather the illness.

Lines 58–63: In this enumeration of drugs, each species is invoked by a standard epithet describing their respective powers/uses.

Line 58: The tentative restoration in this line is based on a parallel formulation in an anti-witchcraft incantation (SpTU 2, No. 25 and dupl.; Abusch et al. 2020 (CMAwR 3), text 7.35 line 7: *li-še-bi-la* ŠINIG *bi-nu-ut* DINGIR-*ti*-[*ka*] "May he send me the tamarisk, the creation of [your] (i.e. Marduk's) divinity!"

Line 59: For the formulation qualifying *burāšu*-juniper, compare a passage with a similar sense, but in a divine epithet, in *Ashurbanipal's Acrostic Hymn to Marduk* (Livingstone 1989, *SAA* 3, No. 2: 34–35): *dipāru namru ša ... ubbabu aršūti ušaḫlû* [...] "(Marduk,) shining torch, who ... purifies the unclean, makes the [...] shine". For the qualification of *burāšu* as a cleansing agent, note similar epithets given to other healing plants, discussed in the note on line 61 below.

Line 60: This line is restored following parallels for this epithet of the date palm, e.g. in *Maqlû* I 22 (Abusch 2016, 29): *gišimmaru māḫirat* (var. *māḫiru*) *kalu* (var. *kala*) *šārī*. See also SpTU 5, No. 248 line 33 (Abusch et al. 2020, CMAwR 3, text 5.5; *infra*), an incantation which begins with the words *gišimmaru māḫirat kal šārī* "date palm who withstands all winds".

Line 61: An exact parallel for the epithet *tullal mullil tušār*[*i*(?)] "*tullal*-plant, purifier of the battlefield(?)" is unknown to me. But similar laudatory epithets are given to other healing plants in incantations, e.g. Abusch et al. 2020, CMAwR 3, text 7.35 line 8: *maštakal mullilat ilī* (var. *ilūtīka*) "*maštakal*-soapwort, purifier of the gods"; ibid., text 8.49 line 2: *mullil zum*[*ur ša ilī*] "(oil,) the purifier of the body [of the gods]"; Abusch and Schwemer 2011, CMAwR 1, text 7–8, lines 37'–38': (the *gamlu*-staff) *mullila/i ša ilī rabûti* "the purifier of the great gods". The *tullal*-plant is a purificatory plant *per se* due to its name, which was associated with the verb *elēlu* "to become pure" (see CAD T, 464).

Line 63: The *anḫullû*-plant was believed to be particularly effective against witchcraft. For the epithet, compare Abusch and Schwemer 2011, CMAwR 1, text 7.8, 1 line 22': *anḫullû lā māḫir kišpī* (var. *šipti*) "*anḫullû*-plant which is immune to witchcraft (var. a spell)". For the *anḫullû*-plant, note further CMAwR 1, text 7.8, 4 lines 54'–55', 58'–60'; Abusch and Schwemer 2016, CMAwR 2, text 8.28 lines 105–106 (with additions in Abusch at el. 2020, CMAwR 3, text A.29); Abusch and Schwemer 2016, CMAwR 2, text 7.23.

Line 70: At the end of the line, one expects either an epithet of Gula or another divine name.

Line 71: In view of the introductory phrase *lā ālitta* <*ana*> *šūrîm-m*[*a*] "<To> enable an infertile woman to get pregnant" in line 8, the reading ⸢KA.INIM⸣.MA ÉN *lā e*[*rītu ana šūrî*] "wording of a spell [to enable] a woman who is not preg[nant to get pregnant]" as incantation rubric seems more plausible than the restoration ^{munus}LA.R[A.AḪ] "(recitation for) a woman in difficult childbirth" (cf. Stol 2000a, 72 with n. 148; note also Böck 2013, 73 who similarly speaks of the spell in lines 41–70 as an incantation "recited during a ritual to facilitate birth").

Lines 72–75: These lines appear to resemble lines 39–40, giving additional instructions on how the incantation(s) on the tablet had to be recited over the different remedies administered to the patient.

The form *nap-ša-šu* in line 74 is most likely a mistake for *napšaltu/napšaštu* "salve"; a derived noun based on the form *naprās* (i.e. **napšāšu*) is not attested so far for the root PŠŠ "to anoint". Similarly, the word *ṣimdu* "bandage" in line 74 is apparently used instead of the cognate term *naṣmattu* "bandage" found earlier in the text (lines 21 and 22).

Lines 76–78: A similar *abracadabra*-formula is preserved in N. 4001: 1ff. and dupl., as part of a different Akkadian incantation against infertility (see text B.2.1).

B.1.2 BAM 243: Recipes for Fertility beyond Menopause

This small Neo-Assyrian fragment from Assur (N4 library, see Pedersén 1986, 67 No. 322) in the collection of the Istanbul Archaeological Museum preserves a few fragmentary lines belonging to recipes to prolong fertility for a menopausal woman. The tablet has been collated from an old photo (Ph. Ass. 4193) made available by the Vorderasiatisches Museum.

List of Manuscripts

Siglum	Museum Number	Copy	Collation	Format; Ductus	Provenience
A	A 2732 (Ass. 13956/bu)	BAM 243	Photo coll.	Fragment of a tablet; Neo-Assyrian period; ca. 7th cent. BCE	Assur, N4 library

Overview

i' Fragmentary prescription against barrenness — 1'–4'
A obv.$^{?}$ 1'–4'

ii' Fragmentary prescription for fertility after menopause — 5'–6'[...
A obv.$^{?}$ 5'–6'

Previous Edition and Discussion

Kirsch 1996, *Die Behandlung von Frauenkrankheiten*, 111
Scurlock and Andersen 2005, 260 (12.9)
Böck 2010a, *TUAT NF* 5, 114 (translation of lines 5'–6')
Böck 2013, 35 with n. 30 (lines 5'–6')
CDLI P285329
BabMed Corpora (https://www.geschkult.fu-berlin.de/e/babmed/Corpora/BAM-3/BAM-3_-243; transliteration)

Transliteration

Beginning of ms. A lost

1' A obv.$^{?}$ 1' DIŠ MUNUS NU Ù.TU ⸢*ana*⸣ *š*[*u-ri-i* ....]

2' A obv.$^{?}$ 2' ^{šim}MAN.DU NUMUN GADA *sa*$^{!}$(IR)-*ḫ*[*i-in-du*$^{?}$ ....]

3' A obv.$^{?}$ 3' *sík-ka-tú* NÍG.ÀR.RA GI[G ....]

4' A obv.$^{?}$ 4' *ina* ^{urudu}ŠEN.TUR *ina* IZI ŠEG$_6$-*š*[*al* ....]

5' A obv.$^{?}$ 5' DIŠ MUNUS *a-la-da* ⸢KUD⸣-*at* ^{giš}*š*[*u-šum* ....]

6' A obv.$^{?}$ 6' ŠIM.ŠAL ^{giš}*dap-ra-nu* ^{ši}[^{m} ....]

Ms. A breaks; remainder lost

Bound Transcription and Translation

Beginning of ms. A lost

1' *šumma sinništu lā ullad ana š*[*ūrî* ... ...] 2' *suādu zēr kitê saḫi*[*ndu*(?) ... ...] 3' *sikkatu mundu kib*[*tu* ... ...] 4' *ina tamgussi ina išāti tušabš*[*al* ... ...]	1' If a woman does not bear, to en[able her to get pregnant: ...] 2' *suādu*-plant, linseed, *saḫ*[*indu*(?), ...], 3' *sikkatu*-beer ingredient, *mundu*-groats, whea[t ... ...], 4' you bo[il] (it) on the fire in a *tamgussu*-vessel [... ...].
5' *šumma sinništu alāda parsat šū*[*šu* ... ...] 6' *šimeššalû daprānu* ...[... ...]	5' If a woman has stopped bearing (children): lico[rice, ...], 6' *šimeššalû*-plant, *daprānu*-juniper, [....]-aromatic, [......].

Ms. A breaks; remainder lost

Notes

Lines 1'–4': Interestingly, the *suādu*-plant (possibly *cyperus esculentus* (chufa)) is designated in Uruanna as a plant for treating internal fever. In Uruanna III 101 (cited in CAD S, 338b sub a), we find: Ú *su-a-di* : AŠ KÚM ŠÀ-*bi* ZI-*ḫi* "the *suādu*-plant: a (plant) to remove fever of the belly/inside" (see KADP 12 ii 4, partially preserved). In a second entry, in Uruanna II 99 (CAD S, 338b sub a; cf. KADP 19 ii 20), the same plant is found as a plant for KÚM ŠÀ.SUR, "fever/heat of ŠÀ.SUR", where ŠÀ.SUR may be a variant for ŠÀ.TÙR "womb" (Ú *su-a-di*: Ú KÚM ŠÀ.SUR$^{!}$(text: GAR) (see CAD Š/2 145b, sub *šassūru* A, lex. section).

For *sikkatu*, an ingredient in beer production, see also BAM 240 rev. 56, prescribed in a different context (postpartum complaints). Landsberger (1962, MSL 8/2, 108) proposed that *sikkatu* may refer to yeast, which was rejected by Stol 1971, *BiOr* 28, 168. The term *sikkatu* itself is explained as "brewer's crushings" (*pa'ṣānu ša sirāšî*) in the commentary BRM 4, 32: 21 (Scurlock 2014a, 343; CDA^2, 268b).

The reading *sa*$^{!}$-*ḫi*-[*in-du*] is provisional and inspired by the fact that *sikkatu* and *saḫindu* are closely associated. In Uruanna III 468, *saḫindu* is explained as "*sikkatu* from the mouth of a beer mash-vessel" (*sikkatu ša pî agarinnu*). Being a Sumerian loanword from ^{šim}saḫ$_7$-ḫi-in, *saḫindu* is glossed with "yeast(?)" in CAD S, 57. Stol (1987–1990, "Malz", *RlA* 7, 326 §7) translates "Sauerteig" (sourdough). The ingredient *saḫindu* is prescribed a few times together with crushed malt (*ṭappīṣ buqli*) in medical texts (likewise in prescriptions for bandages, see e.g. BAM 3 iv 36 // AMT 96/1: 2 // BAM 217: 6 (in a bandage for stinging pain or swelling, *naṣmat dikši*); BAM 269 rev. 2 (bandage).

Lines 5'–6': For the same introductory purpose statement, see also BAM 241 rev. iii 3' (a text in Middle Babylonian script; *infra* text II.1.3).

B.1.3 BAM 247: A Fragment with Prescriptions for Fertility

This small fragment in the collection of the Vorderasiatisches Museum, Berlin constitutes the upper hand corner of a tablet, preserving prescriptions for suppositories to promote fertility and conception (cf. Köcher 1964, BAM III, p. xviii). In the case of two prescriptions, the therapeutic method of choice are tampons inserted into the woman's vagina.

List of Manuscripts

Siglum	Museum Number	Copy	Collation	Format; Ductus	Provenience
A	VAT 10476	BAM 247	Coll.	Fragment of a single-column tablet; Neo-Assyrian script; $8^{th}/7^{th}$ cent. BCE	Assur

Overview

i	Fragmentary prescription for fertility and conception A obv.$^{?}$ 1–5	1–5
ii	Fragmentary prescription for fertility (tampon) A obv.$^{?}$ 6–7	6–7
iii	Fragmentary prescription for fertility (tampon) A obv.$^{?}$ 8–11	8–11[...

Previous Edition and Discussion

Böck 2013, 32 with n. 15 (transliteration, translation)
CDLI P285332 (transliteration)
BabMed Corpora (transliteration)

Transliteration

1	A obv.$^{?}$ 1	[DIŠ MUNUS NU Ù].TU-*m*[*a ana*$^{?}$] Ù.TU [.........]
2	A obv.$^{?}$ 2	[x x] x ⸢ṣab$^{?}$ ba$^{?}$⸣ *ša* x[...................................]
3	A obv.$^{?}$ 3	[x x] x x.MEŠ NU x[...................................]
4	A obv.$^{?}$ 4	[x] ⸢li⸣ ⸢*la*$^{?}$⸣ *ip-pa-á*[*r-ra-as* ....]
5	A obv.$^{?}$ 5	⸢*i*⸣-*sa*-⸢*niq*⸣-*ši* x[..]
6	A obv.$^{?}$ 6	[PA] ^{giš}EREN [P]A ^{ú}*tar*-[*muš* ....]
7	A obv.$^{?}$ 7	[*ina*] Ì.GIŠ ḪI.ḪI ^{síg}[ÀK]A NIGIN-*mi* [*ana* ŠÀ.TÙR-*šá* GAR-*an* (...)]
8	A obv.$^{?}$ 8	[^{giš}]Ù.<SUḪ$_5$>$^{?}$ ^{ú}*kur-ka-nam* SUḪ[UŠ ....]
9	A obv.$^{?}$ 9	*lu ina* Ì.GIŠ *lu ina* ⸢A⸣ *lu ina* [... ḪI.ḪI ....]
10	A obv.$^{?}$ 10	^{síg}ÀKA NIGIN-*mi ana* Š[À.TÙR-*šá* GAR-*an* (...)]
11	A obv.$^{?}$ 11	x[...]

Ms. A obv. breaks; illegible sign traces on the reverse; rest left blank

Bound Transcription and Translation

[1] *[šumma sinništu lā ull]ad-m[a ana] šūludi(?) [… …]* [2–3] *traces* [4] *[…] … [l]ā ippa[rras(?) … …]* [5] *isanniqši [… …]*	[1] [If a woman does not be]ar (children), to enable (her) [to] give birth: [….], [2–3] *too fragmentary for translation* [4] [….]… should [*no*]*t* be stopped(?) [… … *Her husband*(?)] [5] […] shall approach her (for intercourse), […].
[6] *[arat] erēni arat tar[muš … …]* [7] *[ina] šamni tuballal it[qa] talammi [ana šassūrīša tašakkan (…)]*	[7] You mix [6] [twig(s)] of cedar, twig(s) of *tar*[*muš*]-plant, [….] [7] [with] oil. You wrap (the mixture)] into a wad of wool. [You insert (it) into her womb (viz. vagina). (…)]
[8] *ašūḫa(?) kurkānâ šuruš [… …]* [9] *lū ina šamni lū ina mê lū ina [… tuballal … …]* [10] *itqa talammi ana [šassūrīša tašak-kan (…)]* [11] *traces*	[9] [You mix] [8] *ašūḫu*-pine(?), *kurkānû*-plant, root of [… …] [9] either with oil or with water or with […]. [10] You wrap (the mixture) into a wad of wool, [(then) you insert (it)] into [her] wo[mb] (i.e. vagina). [(…)] [11] *traces*

Ms. A breaks; remainder lost

Notes

Line 1: Böck (2013, 32 n. 15) restores the beginning of this line differently: [DIŠ MUNUS *a-lit*]-*tu* [NU] Ù.TU […], translating "If a fertile woman is barren". However, there are traces of an additional sign following the first legible sign TU on the tablet, which were not copied by Köcher in BAM 247, but could represent the sign M[A]. Between this sign and the following Ù.TU is room for [*ana*]. Textual parallels for similar purpose statements let us propose a slightly differing restoration. For similar passages, see BAM 244: 8 (see text B.1.1): [^{munus}]*la a-lit-ta* <*ana*> *šu-*[*ri*]*-im-m*[*a* …] "in order to enable an infertile woman to get pregnant"; BAM 243 obv.$^{?}$ 1': DIŠ MUNUS NU Ù.TU ⌜*ana*⌝ *š*[*u-ri-i*] "if a woman does not bear, to enable (her) to get [pregnant]" (with Š-stem of *erû* instead of the Š-stem of *alādu*). See text B.1.2.

Line 4: Böck (2013, 76 n. 15) restores [*l*]*a ip-pa-á*[*r-ra-su*] "she should not stop doing it" (i.e. the treatment). The verb *parāsu* in the N-stem can mean "to be stopped; to be interrupted" (said of supplies, or messengers and of haemorrhage, the latter of which is often attested in women's healthcare texts but does not fit the present context too well). The N-stem is also found in connection with illness and evil; it often means "to be removed" (from a person; see CAD P 176–177 sub 11a-1'–2').

Line 5: Marten Stol (personal communication) suggests that the verb *sanāqu* "to check; to approach" at the beginning of this line refers to the recommendation to the woman's husband to have intercourse with her. The *Diagnostic Handbook* Tablet 36 instead uses the verb *qerēbu* "to approach" in reference to sexual intercourse in different months of pregnancy (see text A.1.1). Note for similar recommendations STT 98 obv. 3', 9' (text A.1.1, in treatments to enable a woman who does not get pregnant to conceive), where after application of the treatment, the woman's husband is to have intercourse with her (NITA-*šá* [TE-*ši*]). The restoration follows UET 7, No. 123 rev. 5', which gives a negative recommendation whatsoever (NITA-*šú* NU TE-*šú* "her man (i.e. consort, partner) shall not approach (*ṭeḫû*) her (sexually)". See text B.2.2 for discussion.

Böck (2013, 76) interprets the verb *sanāqu* differently, translating "you have to examine her", although *isanniqši* is a 3rd person sg. form (cf. CAD S, 134ff. s.v. *sanāqu* sub 1 and 3, with the meanings "to approach, to come near" and "to check; to supervise; to control"). Note for comparison UET 7, No. 123 rev. 6' (text B.2.2), which uses the verb *ḫâṭu* (written LÁ) "to watch (over), explore, to examine" with reference to the midwife examining the patient (LÁ can also be read *sanāqu*, see CAD S, 134a lex. section).

Line 8: Böck (2013) restores [DIŠ] *ù* "or" at the beginning of the line, apparently as an alternative formulation for DIŠ KI.MIN "alternatively". However, since other examples in which a prescription begins with *u* are unknown to me, I have opted to emend the text to [^{giš}]Ù. <SUḪ$_5$>, for *ašūḫu* "pine tree"; cf. CAD A/2, 478 sub b (with the translation "fir").

The *kurkānû*-plant is a plant recommended for its fertility-enhancing properties in other prescriptions. See e.g. BAM 244: 31, 33, 37; N. 4001: 14ff.; BM 79061 obv. 11 (see texts B.1.1, B.2.1; A.2.8).

B.1.4 BAM 250: An Amulet Necklace to Promote Conception

This small Neo-Assyrian tablet found in the tablet collection of the "House of the incantation priest" (library N4) at Assur contains only one remedy, consisting in an amulet with stones and metal beads to enable a woman to get pregnant. BAM 250 is one of the few attestations for an amulet necklace to promote female fertility currently known from Mesopotamian tablets (see also text B.1.5 from Nineveh). Thus, one finds more numerous examples for the use of necklaces in related contexts, especially to preserve pregnancy and protect women from having miscarriages (see Chapter F in this volume). It is nonetheless remarkable that in matters concerned with women's fertility, Mesopotamian healers appear to have relied to a greater extent on other types of prescriptions using herbs (as well as spells and rituals addressing deities) than on amulets.

The fact that BAM 250 contains only a single remedy may indicate that it was perhaps extracted from a larger collection (for practical application), or that it was an exercise written by an apprentice healer (thus Finkel 2000, *FS Lambert*, 144 Table 1).

The eleven lines of text on the obverse of the tablet, which must have contained seventeen of the twenty-one beads used for the necklace, is badly worn off. For this reason, Franz Köcher copied only the reverse of the tablet in *BAM* III. However, collation of the tablet allowed to identify a few traces on the obverse.

List of Manuscripts

Siglum	Museum Number	Copy	Collation	Format; Ductus	Provenience
A	A 218	BAM 250	Coll.	Small single-column tablet in portrait format; Neo-Assyrian script; 7th cent. BCE	Assur; N4 library

Overview

i	Amulet necklace of 21 stone beads to promote conception A obv. 1–rev. 5	1–17

Previous Edition and Discussion

Stol 2000a, 35 with n. 64
Biggs 2000, *FS Lambert*, 5
Scurlock and Andersen 2005, 261 (12.11)
Böck 2010a, *TUAT* NF 5, 109 (translation)
Böck 2013, *Journal Asiatique* 301, 36 with n. 32
Minen 2018, 181
CDLI P285335
BabMed Corpora (https://www.geschkult.fu-berlin.de/e/babmed/Corpora/BAM-3/BAM-3_-250)

Transliteration

1	A obv. 1	[x (x)] ⸢im$^{?}$⸣ x x x
2	A obv. 2	[^{na4}]ŠU[BA] ⸢Á.ZI⸣.DA
3	A obv. 3	ZA x x x x x
4	A obv. 4	PA$^{?}$ x x x x
5	A obv. 5	x x x x GI$_{6}^{?}$
6–11	A obv. 6–11	*Traces*

12	A lo. e. 1	[K]Ù.BABBAR K[Ù.S]I$_{22}$
13	A rev. 1	AN.BAR URUDU
14	A rev. 2	PAP 21 NA$_4$.MEŠ
15	A rev. 3	^{munus}NU.PEŠ$_4$ *ana* PEŠ$_4$
16	A rev. 4	*ina* DUR GADA È
17	A rev. 5	*ina* GÚ-*šá* GAR-*an*

Remainder of ms. A rev. left blank

Bound Transcription and Translation

[1] … … [2] *šubû imittu* [3–11] *traces*
[12] *kaspu ḫurāṣu* [13] *parzillu erû* [14] *napḫar 21 abnē* [15] *lā erītu ana šūrî* [16] *ana ṭurri kitê tašakkak* [17] *ina kišādīša tašakkan*

[1] … …, [2] 'right' *šubû*-'stone', [3–11] *traces*
[12] a silver (bead), a gold (bead), [13] an iron (bead), a copper (bead) – [14] a total of 21 stones (beads) [15] to enable a woman (who is) not pregnant to get pregnant. [16] You thread (them) on a linen thread. [17] (Then) you put (it) around her neck.

Remainder of ms. A rev. left blank

Notes

Line 15: Note for similar purpose statements STT 98 obv. 2'; BM 42313+ rev. 33 // BM 42333+: 5; BM 59710: 1; BM 79061: 1 (see *infra*). Böck (2013, 36) translates more freely "(in total 21 items) to make a barren woman fertile". Note, however, that the purpose statements of Mesopotamian prescriptions differentiate treatments for barrenness from prescriptions that promote conception in a non-barren woman, even if the ultimate goal of both types of prescriptions was the same (pregnancy). In other words, a woman who is not pregnant (*lā erītu*) was not necessarily regarded as barren (*lā ālittu*).

B.1.5 K. 14032 (AMT 66/9): Prescriptions for Fertility from Ashurbanipal's Library

This small Nineveh fragment probably belonged to a large (perhaps two-column) tablet. It preserves eight fragmentary lines of text indicating that they represented prescriptions to promote a woman's fertility after menopause. This purpose is suggested by the statement that the treatments can be used "for a woman who has stopped giving birth", which may refer to a menopausal woman or to a woman who has given birth before but does not get pregnant anymore. The applied treatments appear to have consisted of amulets (or leather bags).

List of Manuscripts

Siglum	Museum Number	Copy	Collation	Format; Ductus	Provenience
A	K. 14032	AMT 66/9[273]	Coll.	Fragment; Neo-Assyrian script; 7th cent. BCE	Nineveh; Ashurbanipal's library

Overview

i'	Fragmentary prescription (amulet?) A 1'	…]1'

273 Measurements: 2.5 x 3.3 x 0.4 cm.

ii'	Fragmentary prescription for women who has stopped to bear children (amulet) A 2'–3'	2'–3'
iii'	Fragmentary prescription (amulet) A 4'–5'	4'–5'
iv'	Fragmentary prescription (amulet?) A 6'–8'	6'–8'[...

Previous Edition and Discussion

CDLI P400593 (transliteration; photo)
BabMed Corpora (https://www.geschkult.fu-berlin.de/e/babmed/Corpora/AMT-2/AMT66-9/index.html) (transliteration)
Electronic Babylonian Library (eBL) (https://www.ebl.lmu.de/library/K.14032; transliteration)

Transliteration

Beginning lost

1' A 1' [...] ⸢*ina*?⸣ ⸢GÚ?-*šú*?⸣ [GAR-*an*? ....]

2' A 2' [...] *ana* MUNUS *šá* Ù.TU KUD-*á*[*t* SIG$_5$? ...]

3' A 3' [...] *ina* GÚ-*šú* [GAR? ...]

4' A 4' [... *ša* ...] ⸢*i*?⸣-*bar-ru* UB.PAD ⸢ú?⸣[...]

5' A 5' [... *ina* GÚ-*šú*?] ⸢GAR?⸣ TI [...]

6' A 6' [...] A.GAR.GAR MAŠ.DÀ SI [...]

7' A 7' [...]x NAGA.SI x[...]

8' A 8' [...]x ma? [...]

Ms. A breaks; remainder lost

Bound Transcription and Translation

Beginning lost

1' [...] *ina kišādīšu*(?) [*tašakkan*? ... ...]

1' [...you put (it)] around her neck(?) [... ...].

2' [... ...] *ana sinništi ša alāda parsa*[*t damiq*(?) ... ...] 3' [... ...] *ina kišādīšu* [*tašakkan*(?) ... ...]

2' [... ...], [it is good(?)] for a woman who has stopped bearing (children). [... ...] 3' [... you put(?) (it)] around her neck, [... ...].

4' [... *ša*? ...] *ibarru*(?) *ḫallulāya* ...[... ...] 5' [... ... *ina kišādīšu*(?)] *tašakkan*(?) *iballuṭ*(?) [... ...]

4' [a ... which ...] (*one*) *catches*(?) [...], *ḫallulāya*-insect (centipede), [...]-plant(?) [...], 5' [...], you put it around her neck(?), she will get well(?) [... ...].

6' [... ...] *piqanni ṣabīti qaran* [... ...] 7' [... ...] *uḫūlu qarnānû* [... ...] 8' *traces*

6' [...], dung pellets of a gazelle, horn of [...], 7'[... ...], salicornia, [...] 8' *too fragmentary for translation*

Ms. A breaks; remainder lost

Notes

Lines 1'–3': See also the following Assur texts containing a passage with this indication: BAM 243: 5' (text B.1.2): DIŠ MUNUS *a-la-da* [KUD]-*at* "If a woman has stopped bearing (children)"; BAM 241 iii 3' (text II.1.3): MUNUS *a-la-da* KUD-*sà*-[*at*...] "(If) a woman has stopped bearing".

Lines 4'–5': I tentatively follow the reading of eBL and read *i-bar-ru* at the beginning of line 4', interpreting it as a subjunctive durative form of *bâru* (*ba'āru*) "to catch (with a net)". This would necessitate the reference to an animal hunted by a net (a fish, bird or the like) which constituted an ingredient for an amulet. Such a reference is admittedly unusual for a medical text.

For the reading of UP.PAD as *ḫallulāja/ḫallulāya*, an insect, identified as centipede, see CAD Ḫ, 46–47; CAD U/W, 182b sub ***uppa/uttu*; Farber 1985, *ZA* 75, 215–216 1987c, *FS Reiner*, 102–104. AHw 1424 reads UP.PAD as *uppa/uttu*, translating "mole-cricket" instead. For amulet necklaces including 'centipede' as an ingredient, see Farber 2014, Lamaštu Tablet II 113–118; Tablet III 35–45; ibid., 278 BM 33399 ii 1–2 (syllabic spellings). See also an amulet for headache (SAG.KI.DAB.BA) using UP.PAD NÍTA *u* MUNUS "male and female centipede" in AMT 104 (K. 4023) iii 13'–16' // BAM 486 iii 3'-5' (CRANIUM Tablet 3, see *BabMed Corpora*; *NinMed Corpus* sub AMT 103/1+).

Lines 6'–8': For A.GAR.GAR MAŠ.DÀ, dung pellets (*piqannu*) of a gazelle, see e.g. CAD P, 385 sub b, used for instance in prescriptions for ghost-induced illnesses and epilepsy ('Lord of the roof'), see e.g. BAM 311: 37: DIŠ KI.MIN ^{na4}ZÁLAG ^{na4}*mu-ṣa* A.GAR.GAR MAŠ.DÀ SI DÀRA.MAŠ *ina* KUŠ "Alternatively, *zalāqu*-stone, *mūṣu*-stone, dung pellets from a gazelle, stag horn (to be worn around the neck) in a leather (bag)". Within the gynaecological texts, dung pellets (particularly those from the springtime, *ša pān šatti*) are used for a wash in BAM 240 rev. 61' (see text D.2.1). See also Steinert 2020, *JMC* 36.

B.1.6 BAM 246: Prescriptions for Abortion and Expelling the Afterbirth

This fragment of a small single-column tablet from Assur (in the possession of the Vorderasiatisches Museum, Berlin) is one of the few Mesopotamian texts that contain recipes to cause an abortion (see also K. 8678+ (text A.1.4) lines 34''–41'' for another text with abortive remedies). Because of the historical interest of the subject matter, BAM 246 has been repeatedly discussed in Assyriological literature. Despite the rareness of preserved prescriptions to procure an abortion in comparison with the large number of medical (and other) texts that have pro-natalist aims, texts such as BAM 246 show that abortion was not as taboo as one might think from the grave penalty (impaling and denial of burial) against a woman who procured an abortion on her own initiative, which is envisaged in the *Middle Assyrian Laws* § 53 (Pangas 1990; Roth 1997, 174; Stol 2000a, 41; 2016, 680; Peled 2020, 196). The three prescriptions preserved on the obverse of BAM 246 also show that knowledge about abortion was not restricted to midwives (or other female professionals assisting other women in matters of reproductive health), but also known to male healing specialists including conjurers at Assur (cf. Westenholz 1989, 258–259; Stol 2016, 612 and the *Introduction* for texts that accuse female professionals involved in childbirth of killing babies, perhaps an allusion to abortion). The laconic wording of the prescriptions (whose purpose is simply stated as "to cause a woman to abort her foetus") is vague concerning the actual contexts of use of the abortifacients, as these could also have been used to expel a dead full-term foetus rather than to interrupt an unwanted pregnancy (see also below).

All the recipes for abortion in BAM 246 are potions, while the abortive remedies in K. 8678+, a text from Nineveh in Neo-Babylonian script, prescribe tampons (see text A.1.4). The reverse of BAM 246 is badly worn off and almost illegible, and for this reason, Franz Köcher copied only the obverse of the tablet in *BAM* III. However, faint remnants of four ruled sections containing four recipes (4 + 2 + 6 + 5(?) lines) are still visible. Collation of these traces allowed to decipher parts of the first two ruled sections, which shows that these two prescriptions on the reverse are for expelling the afterbirth (*silītu*), another topic only rarely attested in texts on women's health (see BM 38624+ (text A.2.1) for other examples of prescriptions for this purpose). It is possible that the lost remainder of the text on the reverse of BAM 246 also focused on the same topic.

The combination of material on BAM 246 is also remarkable because all the preserved recipes appear to be potions. It has been shown that some of the ingredients in the prescriptions on the obverse were also used by Mesopotamian healers to speed up a difficult delivery. This indicates not only that some of the drugs recommended in BAM 246 caused contractions of the uterus, but that these active ingredients could be applied for different purposes with the same effect. It remains unknown whether the conspicuous ingredient (multicoloured) "wall lizard" mentioned in two of the prescriptions is an alias designation of an herbal drug or should be understood literally (see the notes below for discussion).

List of Manuscripts

Siglum	Museum Number	Copy	Collation	Format; Ductus	Provenience
A	VAT 13896	BAM 246 (obverse only)	Coll.	Fragment of a single-column tablet in portrait format; Neo-Assyrian script; $8^{th}/7^{th}$ cent. BCE	Assur, N4 library

Overview

i	Prescription to induce abortion (potion) A obv. 1–7	1–7
ii	Prescription to induce abortion (potion) A obv. 8–10	8–10
iii	Prescription to induce abortion (potion) A obv. 11–13	11–13[...
iv'	Fragmentary prescription to expel the afterbirth (potion) A rev. 1'–4'	...]14'–17'
v'	Fragmentary prescription to expel the afterbirth (potion) A rev. 5'–6'	18'–19'

Previous Edition and Discussion

Pangas 1990, *AuOr* 8, 215–216 (discussion)
Biggs 2000, *FS Lambert*, 11 (discussion)
Stol 2000a, 42 n. 100, 55 n. 46 (transliteration of obv. 1–5; discussion)
Kirsch 1996, 112
Volk 2004, in: V. Dasen (ed.), *Naissance*, 73 n. 12
Böck 2010a, *TUAT* NF 5, 110–111 (translation of ms. A obv.)
Böck 2013, 37 with nn. 37–39 (transliteration/translation of ms. A obv.)
CDLI P285331 (transliteration)
BabMed Corpora (transliteration)

Transliteration

1 A obv. 1 [^{munus}P]EŠ$_4$ *šà* ŠÀ-*šà ana* ŠUB-*di* ⸢a$^?$⸣ [x]

2 A obv. 2 [EME.D]IR IZ.ZI GÙN.A NUMUN ^{ú}DILI

3 A obv. 3 [^{ú}A]N.KI.NU.DI ^{ú}*a-zu-pi*$_4$*-ra-nu*

4 A obv. 4 ⸢^{ú}⸣*nab-ruq-qu* SUḪUŠ ^{ú}*bu-ṣi-ni*

5 A obv. 5 [KA]Š$^?$ ^{lú}KÚRUN.NA 8 Ú.ḪI.A ŠEŠ-*ti*

6 A obv. 6 [DIŠ-*niš* S]ÚD *ina* GEŠTIN NU *pa-tan* NAG-*ši-ma*

7 A obv. 7 [*šà* Š]À-*šà* ŠUB-*a*

---

8 A obv. 8 [DIŠ KI.MIN ŠE$_{10}$] EME.DIR IZ.ZI SÚD

9	A obv. 9	[*ina* KA]Š NU *pa-tan* NAG-*ma*
10	A obv. 10	[*šà* Š]À-*šà* ŠUB-*a*

11	A obv. 11	[DIŠ KI.MIN] ^{ú}*nab-ru-qu* SÚD
12	A obv. 12	[*ina* KA]Š ⸢NU⸣ ⸢*pa-tan*⸣ ⸢NAG-*ma*⸣
13	A obv. 13	[*šà* ŠÀ-*šà* ŠUB-*a*]

Ms. A obv. breaks; beginning of rev. lost

14'	A rev. 1'	*illegible traces*
15'	A rev. 2'	*illegible traces*
16'	A rev. 3'	[x] ra$^{?}$ KI Ì.GIŠ$^{?}$ x ši$^{?}$ x [x]
17'	A rev. 4'	⸢NAG$^{?}$⸣-*ma* ⸢ÙŠ⸣-*sa* ŠUB-⸢*a*⸣

18'	A rev. 5'	[DIŠ K]I.MIN ^{ú}x x x SÚD [x x]
19'	A rev. 6'	[NA]G-*ši-ma* ⸢ÙŠ⸣-*sa* [ŠUB-*a*]

A few illegible lines; remainder of ms. A rev. lost

Bound Transcription and Translation

[1] *[er]ītu ša libbīša ana šuddî …* [2] *[ṣur]ār igāri barmu zēr šammi ēdi* [3] *[ank]inūtu azupīrānu* [4] *nabruqqu šuruš buṣinni* [5] *[šik]ar(?) sābî samānat šammī annûti* [6] *[ištēniš ta]sâk ina karāni lā patān tašaqqīši-ma* [7] *[ša lib]bīša inaddâ*	[1] To cause a pregnant [woman] to expel her foetu): …, [2] multi-coloured wall-lizard, seed of 'solitary plant', [3] *ankinūtu*-plant, *azupīrānu*-plant, [4] *namruqqu*-plant, root of *buṣinnu*-plant, [5] [be] er(?) from the innkeeper – these eight drugs [6] you [po]und [together]. You give (it) to her to drink in wine on an empty stomach. Then [7] she will expel her foetus.
[8] [DIŠ KI.MIN *zê*] *ṣurār igāri tasâk* [9] *[ina šika]ri lā patān išattī-ma* [10] *[ša lib]bīša inaddâ*	[8] [Alternatively], you pound wall lizard [excrement]. [9] She shall drink (it) [with be]er on an empty stomach. [10] Then she will expel her foetus.
[11] [DIŠ KI.MIN] *nabruqqa tasâk* [12] *[ina šik]ari lā patān išattī-ma* [13] *[ša libbīša inaddâ]*	[11] [Alternatively,] you pound *namruqqu*-plant. [12] She shall drink (it) [with be]er on an empty stomach. [13] Then [she will expel her foetus.]
Ms. A obv. breaks; beginning of rev. lost [14'-15'] *traces* [16'] [...] *itti šamni*(?) ...[...] [17'] *išattī-ma silīssa inaddâ*	 [14'-15'] *illegible traces* [16'] [...] with oil(?) ...[...]. [17'] She shall drink it. Then she will expel her afterbirth.
[18'] [DIŠ K]I.MIN ... ... [19'] *tašaqqīši-ma silīssa [inaddâ]*	[18'] [Altern]atively, you crush [...]-plant, [...]. [19'] You have her drink (it). Then [she will expel] her afterbirth.

Remainder of ms. A rev. illegible

Notes

Line 1: Slightly differing restorations for line 1 have previously been suggested. At the end of line 1, Stol (2000a, 55 n. 46) reads ŠUB-*de-e*? (differently, ibid., 42 n. 100 *ana* ŠUB-*di*). Böck (2013, 37 n. 37) reconstructs [*ana* P]EŠ$_4$ *šà* ŠÀ-*šà ana* ŠUB-*di*-⸢*a*⸣. Volk (2004, 73 n. 12) suggests emending to ŠUB-*di*-⸢{*a*}⸣, because a restoration *ana* ŠUB-*di-a* would be ungrammatical. The verbal form may be analysed as an infinitive G- or Š-stem of *nadû* (the latter would have a causative meaning, i.e. "to cause (a pregnant woman) to abort (her foetus)." For assuming a Š-stem infinitive of *nadû* instead of a G-stem infinitive, see also CAD N/1, 97 sub 8h (ŠUB-*di* = *šuddî*); Mirelman 2015, *JCS* 67, 177, 181 on ms. A rev. 28, who understands the spelling ŠUB-*a* in BAM 246: 7, 10, 16' as *ušadda* "(the baby) is caused to drop (out)" instead of *inaddâ* "she will expel (her foetus)" (G durative + ventive). The end of line 1 has to contain the first ingredient of the recipe to match the total of 8 Ú.ḪI.A "eight drugs" summed up in line 5. Possible restorations for a logogram of a medicinal substance starting with the sign A might be (^{giš})A.AM = *adāru* (a kind of tree) or, less likely, ILLU(A.KAL) = *ḫīlu* "resin". However, the reading ⸢A⸣.[x] is not entirely certain.

Lines 1–5: Stol (2000a, 55) and Böck (2013, 37–39) have commented on the drugs encountered in this compound recipe and the two other recipes that follow; see also Garroway 2023. It is significant that of the eight ingredients listed in lines 1–5, two drugs are recommended as simples in the following two prescription to procure an abortion (lines 8 and 11). The *nabruqqu*-plant (also *namruqqu*) is known from other texts as a plant for a woman who is *šalputtu* (see Stol 2000a, 53–55 for discussion, with BAM 380 rev. 40 // BAM 381 iii 35), a term that is perhaps connected to foetal death due to prolonged labour and malpresentation. However, *nabruqqu*-plant was also used in prescriptions to promote conception (e.g., BAM 244 obv. 31, 33, text B.1.1) and in prescriptions to induce the flow of postpartum blood (lochia) which had stopped prematurely (see BM 38624+ rev. iv 5', text A.2.1). This herb was thus a versatile drug in texts on women's health. The "solitary plant" (*šammu* (*w*)*ēdu*), which is among the eight drugs in BAM 246 lines 1–5 is likewise recommended for a woman who is *šalputtu* in drug compendia (Stol 2000a, 53–55; cf. CAD E, 38; Thompson 1949, DAB, 353–354, 356–357 assumes an identification with asafoetida).

A drug occurring twice in BAM 246 is "wall lizard" (EME.DIR IZ.ZI, *ṣurār igāri*).[274] In line 8, this ingredient is applied as a simple; it is presumably identical with "multicoloured wall lizard" (EME.DIR IZ.ZI GÙN.A) in line 2. Again, it fits the picture that EME.DIR IZ.ZI, in this case "wall lizard excrement", is also encountered in a simple prescription to speed up a difficult delivery (BAM 248 rev. iv 16 and dupl., see text D.1.1). Böck (2013, 37–39) discusses the possibility that "wall lizard" or similar terms encountered here may be alternative designations for an herbal drug, used to keep the actual identity of the most efficacious ingredient to cause an abortion secret and inaccessible to non-specialists. This interpretation raises the question how to explain the occurrence of "uncoded" plant names such as *nabruqqu* side-by-side with bizarre or "coded" drug names such as "wall lizard" in the same context. For discussion of the issue of "secret" or "coded" drug names, see also Chalendar 2016, *Anthropozoologica* 51, 97–103; Rumor 2020, *JMC* 36, 37–53; 2024.

Remarkably, Pliny the Elder states in his *Natural History* (Book 28.29) that the Greek writer Democritus asserts the tongue of a chameleon worn as an amulet to be helpful against "the perils of childbirth", while the animal itself would facilitate parturition, if present in the house at the moment of childbirth. This provides an interesting parallel for the similar use of the drug "wall lizard" in the Mesopotamian texts.

For the abortive drugs *ankinūtu*, *azupīrānu* and root of *buṣinnu*-plant in BAM 246, Stol (2000a, 42) remarks that the identification of *azupīrānu* with saffron is tempting, since it was known as an abortifacient in other ancient traditions (see also Pangas 1990, 216 with n. 29; Riddle 1992, 244, Index). He further proposes a link of *buṣinnu*-plant (usually believed to be mullein, *Verbascum Thapsus*) with poplar or willow, both of which were likewise known as contraceptives in antiquity (Steinert 2021, *Byzantinische Forschungen* 33, 57–58, 61 for discussion). The *ankinūtu*-plant was also known as a contraceptive drug in Mesopotamia, see BM 51246+ rev. 11' (text A.2.7).

Line 5: The traces of the first sign in line 5 are interpreted here as [KA]Š, following collation of the tablet. "Beer of the brewer/innkeeper" (*šikar sābî*) is mentioned several times in medical and other texts (Stol 1994, 164–165; CAD S, 7–8 s.v.

274 Cf. Landsberger 1934, 114–115; CAD Ṣ, 254–255.

sābû sub a 3'-a'). Instead of [KA]Š lúDIN.NA, Böck (2013, 37 n. 37) restores [*mi-ḫ*]*at* lúDIN.NA and translates it as "distiller's wash", following the traces copied by Köcher in BAM 246.[275]

Lines 8–10: The same prescription with "wall lizard excrement" is also prescribed in the Neo-Assyrian Birth Compendium BAM 248 rev. iv 16 (and dupl.; text D.1.1) to speed up a difficult delivery and has been restored accordingly.

Lines 11–13: Note that the same simple recipe is also used in BAM 578 i 19 and dupl. (Tablet 3 of the treatise STOMACH), where it is prescribed for "bile disease" (or an ailment of the gall bladder; see Cadelli 2000, 189: 19 (ms. C); Johnson and Simkó 2024, 164).

Lines 14'–19': As mentioned above, these lines on the reverse of BAM 246 were not copied by F. Köcher; they are edited here for the first time based on the collation of the tablet. For other prescriptions (likewise potions) to expel the afterbirth (ÙŠ (ARḪUŠ) = *silītu*) that is delayed, see e.g. BM 38624 i 14'–15', ii 23'–24' (text A.2.1). The pharmaceutical list BAM 422 iii 5 listed a drug for expelling the afterbirth (Ú *šá-mi* ÙŠ ŠUB-*e*), whose name is unfortunately lost in the gap (cf. Scurlock and Andersen 2005, 261 12.13). For *silītu* "afterbirth", see further CAD S, 264b; Steinert and Paoletti 2014–2016, "Uterus", *RlA* 14, 513 §1.1.

B.2 Texts from Babylonia

B.2.1 N. 4001: A Treatment with Tests for Conception and Fertility

This tablet written in a Neo-Babylonian script, housed in the collection of the Museum of Archaeology and Anthropology of the University of Pennsylvania at Philadelphia, originates from Nippur. It contains an incantation and a therapeutic ritual to enable a barren woman to become pregnant (lines 1–12 and 14–26, with the incantation rubric KA.INIM.MA munusNU.Ù.TU *a-na ur-*⌜*ri*⌝*-i* in line 13). A close parallel to the spell and treatment is found in BM 51246+ (ms. b), a Late Babylonian collection of gynaecological material probably stemming from Sippar (see text A.2.7 for a complete edition).

Following the therapeutic procedure, on the reverse of N. 4001 (lines 27–33), the text continues with another fragmentary section consisting of injunctions concerning secrecy and the guarding of the knowledge related to a woman's fertility or pregnancy. These injunctions are followed by three lines beginning with *šumma* "if" and ending with (*ul*) *irri* "she will (not) get pregnant", resembling the format of the predictions of the so-called pregnancy tests or birth prognoses. Such procedures to determine whether a woman could conceive are attested in a text from Ur, like N. 4001 presumably dating to the Neo-Babylonian period (UET 7, No. 123, see text B.2.2).

The tablet closes with a highly unusual and detailed colophon (lines 34–43), referring to an older original that had belonged to Sîn-multēšir, son of Gaḫul-Tutu, grandson of Gula-balāssu-iqbi. Interestingly, this Sîn-multēšir is mentioned as the copyist of an older *Vorlage* in the colophon of another remarkable tablet, BM 78158 (Stadhouders 2018a, 169–170; see notes below).

List of Manuscripts

Siglum	Museum Number	Copy	Collation	Format; Ductus	Provenience
a	N. 4001[276]	Pl. 23	Coll.	Single-column tablet in portrait format; Neo-Babylonian script, ca. 7th(?) cent. BCE	Nippur

275 For *miḫḫatu*, a type of beer, see CAD M/2, 49b s.v. *miḫḫatu*; CAD S, 8 s.v. *sābû* sub a-1'-b'. The ingredient *miḫḫat sābî* is further attested in BAM 579 iv 20 (and dupl.) in a prescription for intestinal ailments (STOMACH Tablet 5; Cadelli 2000, 267, 287; Johnson and Simkó 2024, 248: 212').
276 Measurements: 8.0 cm x 5.5 cm x 1.5 cm.

(continued)

b	BM 51246 (82-3-23, 2242) + BM 53217 (82-3-23, 4251) + BM 53744 (82-3-23, 4784)	Pl. 20	coll.	Fragment of a single-column tablet, Late Babylonian script, 6th-3rd cent. BCE	probably Sippar

Overview

i	Remedy to enable a woman to get pregnant:	1–26
	– Incantation (a obv. 1–12 // b obv. 6–9)	
	– Rubric (a obv. 13 // b obv. 10)	
	– Prescription (a obv. 14–rev. 2 // b obv. 11–17)	
ii	Injunctions regarding secrecy and predictions concerning a woman's fertility a rev. 3–9	27–33
iii	Colophon a rev. 10–19	34–43

Previous Edition and Discussion

Steinert 2017a, 316–318 (ms. a, lines 7–13)
CDLI P278943 (photo ms. a)
Infra text A.2.7 (edition of ms. b)

Transliteration

1	a obv. 1	[.....................................]
	b obv. 6	⌈ÉN⌉ ⌈MUNUS$^{?}$⌉ pi$^{?}$-rat tup$^{?}$-pi$^{?}$
2	a obv. 2	[.....................................]
	b obv. 6$^{cont.}$	⌈numun$^{?}$⌉ x x x (x) ⌈tup$^{?}$⌉-p[i$^{?}$]
3	a obv. 3	[la-aḫ-t]e-⌈eš⌉ ^{d}*iš-tar* ⌈la-aḫ-te-eš⌉
	b obv. 6$^{cont.}$	[.....................................]
4	a obv. 4	[ma-an-sa]g$^{?}$-⌈sa⌉ ki-tu-up-pa
	b obv. 7	[x x x] x x-⌈up⌉-pa
5	a obv. 5	[ma-an$^{?}$]-⌈sag-sa⌉ ki-tu-up-pa
	b obv. 7$^{cont.}$	ma$^{?}$-an-s[ag]-⌈x⌉ ki$^{?}$-⌈tu$^{?}$⌉- $^{\textit{ḫe-pí}}$:
6	a obv. 6	gu-⌈ru⌉-um-ta ar-ra-ru-sa ki-tu-up-pa
	b obv. 7$^{cont.}$	g[u-.......................................]
7	a obv. 7	^{d}⌈x⌉ A.ŠÀ *i*-⌈*ri*⌉-*iš*
	b obv. 8	[.............] ⌈*i*⌉-*ri-iš* :
8	a obv. 8	*la a*-⌈*lit*⌉-*tu*$_4$ NUMUN *ú-še-ṣi*
	b obv. 8$^{cont.}$	⌈^{munus}⌉*la a-lit-tu*$_4$ NUMUN *ú-še-ṣi* :
9	a obv. 9	⌈*a-na*⌉ AB.SÍN *li-in-na-di-ma*
	b obv. 8$^{cont.}$	⌈*a*⌉-[*na*...........................]

10	a obv. 10	[M]U *li-ib-ni*
	b obv. 8$^{cont.}$	[................]
11	a obv. 11	[*ši*]-⸢*ip*⸣-*tu*$_4$ *ša* ^{d}*é-a ù* ^{d}*asal-lú-ḫi*
	b obv. 9	[ÉN ^{d}*é-a*] ⸢*ù*$^{?}$⸣ ⸢^{d}⸣*asal-lú-ḫi*
12	a obv. 12	[3-*šú a*]*d-di* TU$_6$ ⸢ÉN⸣
	b obv. 9$^{cont.}$	^{erasure} 3-*šú ad-*⸢*di*$^{?}$⸣ [TU$_6$ ÉN]
a, b		———
13	a obv. 13	⸢KA⸣.[INIM].MA ^{munus}NU.Ù.TU *a-na ur-*⸢*ri*⸣*-i*
	b obv. 10	[KA.INIM.MA ^{mun}]^{us}NU.⸢Ù⸣.TU ⸢*a*⸣-[*na ur-ri-i*]
a, b		———
14	a obv. 14	KÌD.KÌD.BI ^{ú}*tar-*⸢*muš*⸣ ^{ú}*im-ḫur-lim* ^{ú}*im-ḫur*-20
	b rev. 11	[KÌD.KÌD.BI ^{ú}]IGI-*lim* ^{ú}⸢IGI-20 ^{ú}⸢*tar-muš*⸣
15	a obv. 15	⸢2$^{?}$⸣ ⸢GÍN⸣ ^{ú}KUR.RA^{sar} ^{ú}*kur-ka-*^{erasure}*-nam ša* KUR
	b obv. 11$^{cont.}$	x GÍN ⸢^{ú}⸣[KUR.RA^{sar} ....]
16	a obv. 16	7 BU[RU$_5$].⸢SAḪAR.RA⸣ 6 Ú.⸢ḪI⸣.A *an-nu-ti* TI-*qé*
	b obv. 12	[......................] ⸢6⸣ Ú.ḪI.A *an-nu-ti* ⸢TI⸣-[*qé*]
17	a obv. 17	*i-na* ⸢KAŠ⸣.[SA]G *i-na* ^{urudu}ŠEN.TUR *ina* IZI
	b obv. 12$^{cont.}$	*ina* ⸢KAŠ⸣ x *ina* x x[..............................]
18	a obv. 18	ŠEG$_6$-*al* ⸢*a*⸣-[*n*]*a* ^{dug}BUR.ZI.GAL SÁḪAR *ta-t*[*ab-bak*]
	b obv. 12–13	[............................] / [x x x]x ⸢*ta*$^{?}$*-tab-bak*⸣
19	a obv. 19	*i-na* Ù[R] *a-na* IGI ⸢^{d}EN⸣.ZU NÍG.NA ⸢^{šim}⸣[LI GAR-*an*]
	b obv. 13$^{cont.}$	*ina* Ù[R$^{?}$..]
20	a obv. 20	ÉN ⸢3⸣-[*šú*] *a-na* ⸢ŠÀ⸣ Š[ID-*nu*]
	b obv. 14	[x x x]x ŠID$^{?!}$(SI)
21	a obv. 21	⸢*i*$^{?}$*-na*⸣ [*q*]*á*$^{?}$*-qá-ri la i-*x[x x x x]
	b obv. 14$^{cont.}$	*ina q*[*á-qá-ri*$^{?}$ ....]
22	a obv. 22	[*i-na* MU]L$^{?}$ *tuš*$^{!}$*-bat* U$_4$.3.KA[M x x x x x]
	b obv. 14$^{cont.}$	[....................................]
23	a rev. 1	U$_4$.3.KAM *a-di ta-*x[x x x x x x]
	b obv. 15	[x x x]x *ta-*⸢x-x⸣ [.................]
24	a rev. 2	⸢^{ú}*kur*⸣*-ka-nam t*[*u-šak-kal-ši*$^{?}$ x]x x[x x]
	b obv. 15$^{cont.}$	[...]
25	a	*Omits*
	b obv. 16	[x x x MUN]US *ši-i ut*$^{?}$-⸢*ta*$^{?}$⸣-x-x[.....................]
26	a	*omits*
	b obv. 17	[x x x x] *ta-tar-ma* [....................................]
a, b		———
27	a rev. 3	*ú-ṣur ma-am-m*[*a la mu-du-ú*$^{?}$] *la t*[*u-kal-lam*]

28 a rev. 4 ⌈*a-na*⌉ *ma-a*[*m-ma la mu-du-ú*$^{?}$] *ul* [*na-ṭu-ú*$^{?}$]

29 a rev. 5 [*a-n*]*a*$^{?}$ ⌈*ka*$^{?}$⌉-*š*[*a-di*$^{?}$ x x x x x x x]

30 a rev. 6 MUNUS *ša* PEŠ$_4$ *l*[*a* PEŠ$_4^{?}$ x x x x x x x]

31 a rev. 7 *šum-ma* MUNUS ⌈*ši*⌉-[*i*$^{?}$ x x x x x x x]x

32 a rev. 8 ⌈*šum*⌉-*ma* MU[NUS x x x x x x x *ir-r*]*i*

33 a rev. 9 [*šum-ma* x x x x x] ⌈MUNUS⌉ *ši-i* [*ul*] ⌈*ir-ri*⌉

a ____

Colophon:

34 a rev. 10 *ša p*[*i-i* SUMUN$^{?}$ *ša-ṭi-ir-m*]*a*$^{!?}$ *la-a-ti-ik ba-a-ri*

35 a rev. 11 *ù* [*up-pu-uš* ZU-*ú*] ZU-*a* ⌈IGI.LÁ$^{!}$(MIN)⌉.MEŠ ⌈2⌉ DUB$^{?}$.ḪI.A

36 a rev. 12 ⌈ITI$^{!}$⌉(MURUB$_4$) ⌈TU$^{?}$⌉ *ú-ṣ*[*ur*] ⌈*ma*⌉-*am-ma* ⌈*la*⌉ *tu-kal-la-am*

37 a rev. 13 *a*$^{?!}$(MIN)-*i-ba-am ana* KA IM.GÍD.DA *ṣe-er-pi*

38 a rev. 14 *ša* ^{md}30-*mu-ul-te-ši-ir* MAŠ ^{m}GA.ḪÚL-^{d}*tu-tu*

39 a rev. 15 MAŠ MAŠ ^{md}*g*[*u*]-*la*-⌈TI⌉-*su-iq-bi*

40 a rev. 16 [$^{m?}$ x]x [x x]x ^{lú}A.ZU ⌈*a-na*$^{?}$⌉ ⌈*la*⌉-*ma-di-šu*

41 a rev. 17 [*iš-ṭ*]*ù-ur* IGI.KÁR ^{m}ÌR-⌈*nu*$^{!}$-*ba*⌉-*at-ti*

42 a rev. 18 [DUMU$^{?}$ ^{m}TÉŠ$^{?}$]-⌈TIN⌉.TIR^{ki} GIN$_7$ SUMUN-*šú* ^{md}MAŠ-PAP-MU

43 a rev. 19 [IGI.KÁR *ḫi-i-ṭu*$^{?}$] ⌈*la*$^{?}$⌉ GÁL-*ši*

Remainder of the reverse probably left blank

Bound Transcription and Translation

1–2 [ÉN *fragmentary*]	1–2 [Incantation: *fragmentary abracadabra*-words]
3 [la-aḫ-t]e-⌈eš⌉ ^{d}*iš-tar* ⌈la-aḫ-te-eš⌉	3 "[Laht]eš Ištar laḫteš,
4 [ma-an-sa]g$^{?}$-⌈sa⌉ ki-tu-up-pa	4 [mansa]gsa kituppa,
5 [ma-an]-⌈sag-sa⌉ ki-tu-up-pa	5 [man]sagsa kituppa,
6 gu-⌈ru⌉-um-ta ar-ra-ru-sa ki-tu-up-pa	6 gurumta arrarusa kituppa.
7 ⌈x⌉ *eqla īriš*	7 ⌈(The god) NN⌉ has cultivated the field with a seeder-plough.
8 *lā ālittu zēra ušēṣi*	8 The barren woman made the seed sprout.
9 *ana absinni linnadī-ma*	9 Let (the seed) be deposited into the 'furrow',
10 [*šu*]*ma libni*	10 let her create [offspr]ing!
11 [*ši*]*ptu ša Ea u Asalluḫi*	12 I have cast 11 the [sp]ell of Ea and Asalluḫi 12 [three times]!"
12 [*šalāšīšu*] *addi tê šipti*	Incantation formula.

---

13 KA.INIM.MA *lā ālittu ana urrî*	13 Recitation to make a barren woman get pregnant.

---

14 KÌD.KÌD.BI *tarmuš imḫur-līm imḫur-ešrā* 15 *šina*(?) *šiqil nīnê kurkānâm ša šadî* 16 *sebet erib turbu'ti šeššet šammī annûti teleqqe* 17 *ina šikari ina tangussi ina išāti tušabšal* 18 *ana burzigalli šaḫarri tat*[*abbak*] 19 *ina ū*[*ri*] *ana pān Sîn nignak* [*burāši tašakkan*] 20 *šipta šalāšī*[*šu*] *ana libbi ta*[*mannu*] 21 *ina qaqqari lā* [... ...] 22 [*ina kakkab*]*i*(?) *tušbât šalāšat ūmī* [... ...] 23 *šalāšat ūmī adi ta*-[...] 24 *kurkānâm tu*[*šakkalši*(?) ...] 25 [... *sinni*]*štu šī* ...[... ...] 26 [... ...] *tatâr-ma* [... ...]

14 The procedure for it: *tarmuš*-plant, 'heals thousand'-plant, 'heals twenty'-plant, 15 two(?) shekels of *nīnû*-plant, *kurkānû*-plant of the mountains (and) 16 seven 'dust locusts' – you take these six drugs, 17 boil (them) in beer in a *tangussu*-vessel over the fire. 18 (Then) you pour (the liquid) into a porous *burzigallu*-vessel. 19 On the ro[of], in front of the moon god Sîn [you set up] a censer with [juniper]. 20 You rec[ite] the incantation three times over (the *burzigallu*-vessel). 21 It(?) should not [...] on the ground, [...]. 22 You let it stay overnight [under the sta]rs(?). (For) three days [... ...]. 23 Until the three days ... [...], 24 you [have her eat(?)] *kurkānû*-plant. 25 [...] that woman ...[...], 26 [...] you repeat (it) and [... ...].

---

27 *uṣur-ma mamm*[*a lā mūdâ*(?)] *lā t*[*ukallam*] 28 *ana ma*[*mma lā mūdû*(?) *ul* [*naṭû*(?)] 29 [*an*]*a kaš*[*ādi*(?) ... ...] 30 *sinništu ša irrû l*[*ā irrû*(?) ... ...] 31 *šumma sinništu šī*(?) [... ...] 32 *šumma sinni*[*štu* ... *ir*]*ri* 33 [*šumma* ... ...] *sinništu šī* [*ul*] *irri*

27 Take care! Do not s[how] (it) to some[one who is not knowledgeable(?)]! 28 [It is] not [suitable(?)] for someone [who is not knowledgeable(?)]. 29 *To fi*[*nd/discover whether*? ... ...]. 30 A woman who will get pregnant (or who will) no[t get pregnant(?) ... ...]. 31 If that(?) woman [... ...]. 32 If the wo[man ..., she will get pre]gnant. 33 [If ...], that woman will [not] get pregnant.

Colophon:

34 *ša p*[*î labiri*(?) *šaṭer-m*]*a latik bari* 35 *u* [*uppuš*(?) *mūdû*] *mūdâ likallim šina tuppāni*(?) 36 *araḫ*(?) *alādi/ālitti*(?) *uṣur-ma mamma lā tukallam* 37 *ay ibâm ana pī imgiddû ṣerpi* 38 *ša Sîn-multēšir mār Gaḫul-Tutu* 39 *mār māri Gula-balāssu-iqbi* 40 [... ...] ... *asû ana lamādīšu* 41 [*išṭ*]*ur bari Arad-nubatti* 42 [*mār Bāštī*(?)]-*Bābili kīma labirīšu Ninurta-nāṣir-šumi* 43 [*ibri ḫīṭu*(?)] *lā*(?) *ibašši*

34 [Written] after the word[ing of an old original(?)]. Tested, checked 35 and [made (properly/ready for use)]. [A knowledgeable person] may always show it to a knowledgeable person. (Belonging to?) two tablets(?) 36 (concerning) the month(?) of conception/the fertile woman(?). Take care! Don't show (it) to anyone! 37 One must not transgress (this injunction)! According to the wording of a fired oblong tablet 38 belonging to Sîn-multēšir, son of Gaḫul-Tutu, 39 grandson of Gula-balāssu-iqbi, 40 [(which) NN(?) ...] ..., the physician, 41 [has cop]ied 40 for his learning. 41 Collated by Arad-nubatti, 42 [son of Bāštū]-Bābili(?). (It is copied) according to its original – Ninurta-nāṣir-šumi 43 [*collated it* (*again*?).] There should not be [*any mistake* (in the copied text?)].

Notes

Lines 1–6: At the top of the tablet in ms. a, probably two lines from the beginning of the incantation are missing. There is some blank space preserved in the middle of the lost lines at the top of the tablet, which means that only beginning and end of lines 1–2 bore text. The beginning of the incantation is likewise only fragmentarily preserved on BM 51246+ (ms. b). It is possible that the first part of the chain of *abracadabra*-words (lines 1–3) differed between mss. a and b and thus present two variants of the opening lines of the composition. However, it is also possible that the preserved bits in both texts simply do not overlap. The Akkadian part of the incantation, from line 4 onward, runs parallel in mss. a and b. There is another short *abracadabra*-spell for removing infertility in BAM 244: 76–78 (text B.1.1), likewise fragmentary, which seems to share similarities with ms. a lines 1–3.

Lines 7–12: For discussion, see also text A.2.7 note on lines 6–9. The Akkadian part of the incantation envisages a prototypical situation in which an infertile woman was able to conceive with the help of an unidentified god, which should repeat itself in the patient. Unfortunately, the reading of the divine name at the beginning of line 7 is difficult. Based on the sign traces in ms. a, possible readings may be *šēdu*(dÁLAD) "protective spirit" or DINGIR É "the god of the house".

The traces at the beginning of line 10 in ms. a could be [M]U "name, offspring" or [NUM]UN "seed". Since *zēru* "seed" was already mentioned in the parallel sentence in the preceding lines 8–9, *šumu* "name, offspring" seems to be a more likely synonym here. For MU = *šumu* "offspring", see also BAM 244 rev. 3: MUNUS BI [PEŠ$_4$-*m*]*a* MU TUKU-*ši* "that woman [will get pregnant] and will get offspring" (see text B.1.1).

Line 13: For the reading of *ana ur-ri-i* as D-stem infinitive of *arû/erû* "to get pregnant", see text A.2.7 note on line 10. In other instances, the Š-stem *šūrû* is encountered with a causative meaning in synonymous purpose statements, see e.g. BM 42313+ obv. 5'; BM 42313+ rev. 37 // BM 42333+ rev. 1; BM 79061 obv. 1; probably also in BAM 243: 1' and BAM 244 obv. 8 (see *infra* for these texts).

Lines 14–26: For discussion of the procedure and the fertility-enhancing drugs in this passage, see text A.2.7 note on lines 11–17. The last lines of the instruction, which are badly preserved in both manuscripts, do not present any overlapping text. Given the fact that ca. two lines of text in ms. a correspond to one line in ms. b in this section, it seems likely that ms. b presented some textual variants and added instructions that are not included in ms. a.

Lines 23–26: Perhaps line 23 contained instructions to give the woman the prepared potion to drink; however, the text is too fragmentary to know. At the end of line 24, traces do not support the reading [MUN]US B[I *ir-rī*] "that woman will get pregnant", although this would be an expected logical conclusion of the prescription in ms. a, which ends in line 24. In lines 25–26, ms. b appears to present text that is not contained in ms. a. The instructions in ms. b thus must have been more elaborate than in ms. a.

Lines 27–33: My reconstruction of the interdictions or "secrecy phrases" in lines 27–28, warning to reveal the information on the tablet to an outsider, an uninitiated, unknowledgeable person, partially follows the standard expressions known from other colophons (cf. Hunger 1968, 13–14; Lenzi 2008, 168–215). However, the phrases found in the present text diverge from the more common expressions found elsewhere in scholarly texts, such as: *mūdû mūdâ likallim mūdû lā mūdâ lā ukallam* "the knowledgeable person may show it to an(other) knowledgeable person, (but) a knowledgeable person must not show it to an unknowledgeable person" and *lā mūdû lā immar/ay īmur* "someone who is not knowledgeable must not see it". Line 36 repeats the very strict interdiction *uṣur mamma lā tukallam* "Take care! Don't show (the tablet) to anybody!". However, there is room for the restoration *mamma* [*lā mūdâ*] *lā tu*[*kallam*] in line 27.

The following lines 29–33 are unfortunately very fragmentary, but the last three lines of the present section beginning with *šumma sinništu* "if a woman" and ending with (*ul*) *irri* "she will (not) get pregnant" resemble statements found in pregnancy prognoses (tests), such as UET 7, No. 123 obv. 1–4 // BM 42313+ rev. 29–32 (see *infra*, texts A.2.2, B.2.2).

Lines 35–36: I have restored [ZU-*ú*] ZU-*a* ⌜IGI.LÁ!(MIN)⌝.MEŠ, read as [*mūdû*] *mūdâ likallim* "[a knowledgeable person] may show it to a knowledgeable person".

The reading 2 DUB?.ḪI.A "two tablets" at the end of line 35 is not entirely certain and convincing, unless N. 4001 was the second of a set of two tablets, the first of which is not known to us. A second possibility would be that the "two tablets" refer to two sources from which the text on ms. a was compiled. However, the colophon only seems to refer to one *Vorlage*, a fired oblong tablet that belonged to Sîn-multēšir. The beginning of line 36 is likewise difficult. I have opted to emend the first sign and read (2 DUB?.ḪI.A) ITI! TU, which may be understood as "(two tablets concerning) the month of conception" (*araḫ alādi*) or possibly "two tablets concerning the month of the fertile woman" (*araḫ ālitti*). This expression could refer to the monthly menstrual cycle and to the healers' knowledge of a period in this cycle when conception was regarded as more likely to occur. However, until more proof is found that Mesopotamian healers possessed such detailed knowledge, this suggestion remains speculative.

Line 37: At the beginning of line 37 we may have a vetitive form, *a*(*y*) *i-ba-am* "one must not transgress", from *bâ'u* "to pass, walk along; to transgress" (i.e. *ay ibā'* + vent., where the aleph has not been realized in the script). I do not know of another occurrence of *bâ'u* in this meaning from colophons. But it would fit in with the interdiction "do not show (the tablet) to anyone" at the end of line 36.

For *ṣerpu* "fired (clay) object" (CAD Ṣ, 209 s.v. *ṣirpu* B sub 1; AHw 1092 s.v. *ṣerpu* II) in other colophons of Neo-Babylonian texts, see Hunger 1968, No. 151: 2: *kī pī tuppi gabari ṣerpi sāmi ša Nabû-eṭel-ilāni mār Dābibī āšipu* "according to the wording of a tablet, a copy of a red fired (clay tablet) belonging to Nabû-eṭel-ilāni, son of Dābibī, the conjurer" (from

Babylon); No. 157: 1 *kī pī gabari ṣerpi* "according to the wording of the copy of a fired (clay tablet)"; No. 427: 2: *kī pī ṭuppi gabari Ezida ṣerpi sāmi* "according to the wording of a tablet, a copy from the Ezida, a red fired (clay tablet)".

Line 38: According to Tallquist (1918, 79), the name ^{m}GA.ḪÚL-^{d}*Tu-tu* has to be read Gaḫul-Marduk. PNA, Vol. 1/II, 418–419 regards the element *ga-ḫúl* (also *ga-ḫal*) as perhaps of West-Semitic origin. However, Hunger (1968) proposed that the name should be understood as Sumerian (^{m}GA.ḪÚL-^{d}TU.TU) and be read as Luḫdu-Nabû in Akkadian, literally meaning "Let me be happy, o Nabû!". The divine name ^{d}*Tu-tu* (probably to be read syllabically) is more commonly known as one of the names of Marduk (see Richter 2014–2016, "Tutu", *RlA* 14, 241–242; Lambert 2013, 124 VII 9ff., 159; Tutu was a local god of Borsippa).

The fragmentary colophon of another Neo-Babylonian tablet with fertility or pregnancy tests found at Ur (UET 7, No. 123 rev. 15'; see text B.2.2) may have mentioned a person with this name ([... ^{m}GA.ḪÚL-^{d}]*Tu-tu*). One may thus wonder whether the Gaḫul-Tutu in N. 4001 and UET 7, No. 123 refer to the same person. The name occurs as a patronymic in other Neo-Babylonian texts, see e.g., Hunger 1968, No. 151; No. 467; No. 468; Abusch and Schwemer 2016, text 7.11 (Ms. h) = Maul 2019, *Bannlösung*, 248 No. 53 rev. 7 (from Babylon) = Hunger 1968, No. 467. For Gaḫul-Tutu as a family name, see Wunsch 2014a, 305; Frame and George 2005, 274–276 line 11.

The colophon of N. 4001 acknowledges Sîn-multēšir (= Sîn-muštēšir), son of Gaḫul-Tutu, as the owner of an original from which N. 4001 was copied. Another text of medical content, BM 78158 (88-4-19, 11), the late copy of an old tablet (the copied ductus of the original displays an archaizing script) also mentions a Sîn-multēšir, son of Gaḫul-Tutu, as the copyist of an "old, fired tablet". Sîn-multēšir's copy had served as the *Vorlage* for another tablet that was re-copied by the scribe of BM 78158. The anonymous scribe of BM 78158 integrated the colophon of the older original together with his own colophon (information courtesy of I.L. Finkel; Stadhouders 2018a, 169–170; see also CBT VIII, 139):[277]

BM 78158 rev.
20) *ki pí-i* DUB *ṣar-pa* LIBIR.RA *ša* GABA.RI ^{m}30-MU-MU DUMU ^{m}TUKU-DINGIR ^{lú}KA.TU$_{6}$.GÁL
21) [*š*]*a* ^{d}30-*mul-te-šir* DUMU ^{m}GA.ḪÚL-^{d}*Tu-tu*
22) *iš-ṭu-ru* SAR-*ma ba-ár*

---

23) *ki pí-i* DUB *ṣar-pa* LIBIR.RA *ša* TÉŠ-TIN.TIR^{ki} AN.GUB
24) SAR-*ma ba-ár*

[22] "Copied and checked [20] according to an old, fired tablet [22] that had been copied [21] by Sîn-multēšir, son of Gaḫul-Tutu, [20] from an older original written by Sîn-nādin-šumi, son of Ibašši-ilu, the *āšipu*.[278]

---

[24] Copied and checked [23] according to the wording of an old, fired tablet written by Bāštī-Bābili."[279]

Interestingly, the second colophon of BM 78158 mentions a certain Bāštī-Bābili, to whom the anonymous scribe of BM 78158 attributes the *Vorlage* that he used for his own copy. Although the name is damaged, it is possible that the colophon of N. 4001 mentions a man with the same name as the father of a certain Arad-nubatti. Whether BM 78158 and N. 4001 both refer to the same person remains uncertain.

Line 40: The interpretation of the beginning of the line is not entirely certain, but because [*iš-ṭ*]*u-ur* at the beginning of line 41 is not in the subjunctive (as would be expected if the clause starting with *ša* in line 39 continues to line 41), it is more likely that the name of the copyist of N. 4001 must be found in the gap at the beginning of line 40 and that *asû* "physician" is his profession. The phrase *ana lamādīšu* "for his study/learning" could point to someone still not fully trained in his profession. The mention of a physician in connection with the contents of the tablet is of course remarkable.

Line 41: The name (W)arad-nubatti is well-attested in Middle Babylonian texts, e.g. from Nippur (see Sassmannshausen 2001, 469; Hölscher 1996, 36–37).

---

277 The scribe of BM 78158 copied a text that was largely lost in the course of transmission, as it only preserves scattered remnants of cuneiform characters in an archaizing script that must have been copied from a very damaged *Vorlage*. The few textual remnants suggest that the copied text was also medical in nature, probably a medicinal plant list.

278 The end of the line is written around the margin and over part of the obverse. For a diverging reading of the line cf. Stadhouders 2018a, 169–170.

279 The reading of this line follows Stadhouders 2018a, 169–170 with note 34.

Lines 41–43: The interpretation of the final lines of the colophon is tentative. It seems that Arad-nubatti served as a collator. For the phrase IGI.KÁR PN "collated by PN" in colophons, see also Hunger 1968, No. 9: 5, 43: 7, 44: 7; 230: 5; 231: 4.

In line 42, the occurrence of the phrase *kīma labirīšu* "according to its original", followed by another personal name, is unexpected, but probably marks the beginning of the last sentence on the tablet. The name in line 42 may have to be read Ninurta-nāṣir-zēri(NUMUN) instead of Ninurta-nāṣir-šumi(MU). My tentative proposition is that this person served as a second collator. I do not know any parallels for the phrase *lā ibašši* "there is not/should not be ..." in a final position in colophons, which could provide a restoration. There does not seem to be room for a longer sentence (e.g. for the usual statements that the tablet should not be removed, be treated with care etc.).

B.2.2 UET 7, No. 123: Tests with Birth Prognoses and Treatments for Infertility

This Neo- or Late Babylonian fragment from Ur now kept at the Iraq Museum at Baghdad contains several test procedures as well as treatments ultimately aimed at enabling a woman to conceive. Whether the tests served to determine a woman's ability to conceive (or a physical state in which she was likely to get pregnant) or whether they served to confirm that a woman was indeed pregnant, is a matter of debate (see Reiner 1982a, 127–128; Böck 2013, 41; Steinert 2015, 107–109; Geller 2023, 5–6).[280] It is striking, however, that the tests with prognoses usually occur together with treatments to promote fertility and conception.

Most of the tests in ms. a (UET 7, No. 123) consist in a mixture of drugs that are wrapped into a wad of wool (*itqu*), which the woman inserted and kept in her vagina for some time. After removal of the tampon, the healer drew predictions based on different colorations the tampon could have. The interpretation of the predictions of the tests is ambiguous in cases where the verb in question, *arû/erû* "to get/to be pregnant", is written logographically. There are two possibilities to render the logographic sign PEŠ$_4$ in this context, as *erât* "she is pregnant" or as *irri* "she will get pregnant". Remarkably both ancient Egyptian and Hippocratic texts offer similar tests that usually focus on predicting whether a woman *can* or *cannot* conceive (although external physical signs of pregnancy are referred to on occasion).[281]

The present discussion tends toward the view that most, if not all, of the Mesopotamian tests in question may have been concerned with women who had problems conceiving and received treatments for improving their ability to get pregnant. This also finds support by the final part of the instructions on the reverse of ms. a, which contains a long passage that appears to connect therapies (potions, suppositories (*maššītu*)) for certain conditions of the uterus which hindered conception (such as deformation or malposition) with repeated testing of the woman. The aim of some of these tests may have been to determine not only a woman's physical condition, but also the effect of treatments previously performed to regulate and improve the state of a woman's uterus.

The test opening the obverse of ms. a, interestingly, finds a parallel in a Late Babylonian compendium on women's healthcare from Sippar (BM 42313+, see notes below and text A.2.2 in this volume). At times, ms. a uses a highly unusual technical vocabulary. Ms. a displays other textual peculiarities. For example, most of the classifiers for plants, aromatics or minerals before drug names are omitted. The use of the 3rd person fem. sg. pronominal suffix is inconsistent (both *-šá* and *šú* are used interchangeably, as in other Neo-/Late Babylonian texts). The text also uses *i-* and *ta-* interchangeably as prefixes for the 3rd person fem. sg. verbal forms. Another recurrent feature is the use of the verb *nadānu* (SUM) "to give; to administer" (a treatment), which is also common in Late Babylonian women's healthcare texts from Uruk (see e.g. SpTU 4, No. 153). Moreover, both SpTU 4, No. 153 and UET 7, No. 123 use discursive statements that resemble the terminology of commentaries (see below for discussion).

280 For example, Scurlock and Andersen (2005, 262) understand the tests as pregnancy tests, noting "changes in the vaginal secretions of pregnant women" that could have been the basis for the ancient tests, such as changes in vaginal acidity and salt, as well as changes in the levels of oestrogen and progesterone. Such an interpretation could only be confirmed by modern biochemical analysis of the recipes, impossible because most of the ingredients remain unknown.

281 For Egyptian tests with pregnancy prognoses, see Westendorf 1999, 432–439; for the transmissions of Egyptian tests to Greek (Hippocratic) authors, see Pommerening 2015. For similarities between Hippocratic and Mesopotamian prognoses, see also Steinert 2015, 107–109.

List of Manuscripts

Siglum	Museum Number	Copy	Collation	Format; Ductus	Provenience
a	– (no field number given)	UET 7, No. 123	–	Fragment of a single-column tablet; Neo- or Late Babylonian script; ca. 6th-4th cent. BCE?	Ur

Overview

i	Test procedure (a obv. 1–4) Therapeutic instruction and test (a obv. 5–7)	1–7
ii	Test a obv. 8–9	8–9
iii	Test a obv. 10–12	10–12
iv	Test a obv. 13–16	13–15[...
v'	Treatments and test a rev. 1'–14'	...]16'–29'
vi'	Colophon a rev. 15'	30'

Previous Edition and Discussion

Reiner 1982a, *ZA* 72, 124–138 (transliteration; translation; discussion)
Scurlock and Andersen 2005, 12.17 (transliteration / translation of obv. 1–4)
Böck 2010a, *TUAT NF* 5, 110 (translation of obv. 1–12)
Böck 2013, 41 (translation of obv. 8–9)
Scurlock 2014a *Sourcebook*, 582–585 (transliteration; translation; discussion)
Scurlock 2014b, 119–120 (translation of obv. 1–rev. 14')
CDLI P347082 (copy)
Steinert 2015, 109 (translation of obv. 1–4)
Geller 2021, *AfO* 54, 343–347 (obv. 1–4, 10–14, rev. 4'–9')
Geller 2023, *JMC* 41, 1–15

Transliteration

1	a obv. 1	[*mal-tak-ti* (MUNUS) *ki-i* PEŠ$_4$ *u ki-i* NU PEŠ$_4^?$ 1 GÍN ^{ú}*tar-muš*] 1/2 GÍN Ú BABBAR 4-*tú* $^{\text{na4}}$*gab-u*
2	a obv. 2	[*mi-ṣir-a-a ina* ^{síg}ÀKA NIGIN-*mi ana* ŠÀ.T]ÙR-*šá* GAR-*an mu-šu gab-bi*
3	a obv. 3	[*ú-kal* E$_{11}$-*ma*$^?$ *ina* GEŠ]TIN$^?$-*nu* BABBAR LUḪ-*si ki-i* ^{síg}ÀKA SA$_5$-*at lu* MÚD *ul-lu-ḫa-tú*
4	a obv. 4	[MUNUS BI PEŠ$_4$] *ki-i* ^{síg}ÀKA *ši-i* SIG$_7$-*at* MUNUS BI NU PEŠ$_4$ *ki-i lìb-bi* ŠÀ$^!$(PEŠ$_4$).TÙR-*šú*

5 a obv. 5 [TA GAL$_4$.LA$^?$]-*šú*$^?$ *ki pi-it* GÌR *u-ṣi* GUR$^{?!}$-*ma dul-la-šá e-pu-uš šip-ru-šú*

6 a obv. 6 [*ki* DÙ-*šú*$^?$] *maš-qit* NAG-*šú ki*$^?$ LÍL$^?$ *iṣ-b*[*a*$^?$-*a*]*s*$^?$-*su lam*$_5$(IGI) *maš-šit in-na-áš-šú* GÚR.GÚR

7 a obv. 7 LI ḪAR.ḪAR NU.LUḪ.ḪA *u* ILLU ⸢LI$^?$⸣.<TAR> [1]-*šú* 2-*šú* 3-*šú* NAG *ù* BURU$_8$-*šú* PEŠ$_4$

---

8 a obv. 8 DIŠ KI.MIN SULLIM^{sar} *ina* ^{síg}ÀKA NIGIN-*mi ana* [ŠÀ].TÙR-*šá* GAR 3 U$_4$ ÍL-⸢*ši*⸣-*ma*

9 a obv. 9 *šum*$_4$-*ma* SULLIM^{sar} GIN$_7$ ⸢ÉLLAG$^?$⸣ *ib-tar-rum* MUNUS BI PEŠ$_4$

---

10 a obv. 10 DIŠ KI.MIN Ú BABBAR NAGA.SI *ina* ^{síg}ÀKA NIGIN-*mi ana* ŠÀ.TÙR-*šá* GAR 3 U$_4$ ÍL-*ma*

11 a obv. 11 *ina šal-šú u*$_4$-*me* ^{síg}ÀKA *ina* A LUḪ-*si šum*$_4$-*ma* ^{síg}ÀKA [SA$_5$ MUNUS BI PEŠ$_4^?$]

12 a obv. 12 *šum*$_4$-*ma* ^{síg}ÀKA SIG$_7$ DIRI$^{?!}$-*tú* MUNUS BI [NU PEŠ$_4^?$ (...)]

---

13 a obv. 13 DIŠ KI.MIN ^{na4}*gab-u mi-ṣir-a-a* x[........... *šumma*$^?$ ....]

14 a obv. 14 [G]IN$_7^?$ *a-lap me* IGI.IGI MUNUS BI [....................]

15 a obv. 15 [L]I NAGA.SI$^{?!}$ PÈŠ [.......................................]

Ms. a obv. breaks; gap of unknown length

16' a rev. 1' [DIŠ$^?$ x x x x]x-⸢*šú*⸣ ⸢SA$_5$⸣ ⸢SU-*šú*⸣ x[.................]

17' a rev. 2' [x x x *ku*$^?$]-*un-gi is-sa-nu* [........................]

18' a rev. 3' [x *mim-m*]*a* NU SUM-*su* 1 NINDA GÚR.GÚR SIG$_7$ *k*[*ab-ba-r*]*a* ⸢x⸣ NINDA *saḫ-lé-*[*e* x x x x]

19' a rev. 4' 2.TA.ÀM BÍL(NExPAP) *ina* A SILA$_{11}$ *tu-kap-par*$_5$ DUḪ.LÀL Ì *ḫal-ṣa ta-sal-làḫ-ma ma*$^?$-⸢*áš*$^!$-*ši*$^!$-*tu*$^!$⸣

20' a rev. 5' 1-*šú* 2-*šú* 3-*šú ana* ŠÀ.TÙR-*šá* GAR-*an* NITA-*šú* NU TE-*šú a-di* U$_4$.2.KAM EGIR-*šá iz-zi-zu*

21' a rev. 6' *mim-ma gáb-bi* NU SUM-*su šá qer-bit-si* ZI-*ḫu u* ^{munus}ŠÀ.ZU LÁ-*šú mál-tak-ta-šú*

22' a rev. 7' *ki-i* PEŠ$_4$ *u ki-i* NU PEŠ$_4$ ^{ú}*ú-sa-bu ina* IZI BÍL *a-na di-iq-me-en-na* GUR.RU

23' a rev. 8' *ina* Ì *ḫal-ṣa* KÚM$^!$(NExPAP) SÚD *tu-lam lu ina* A *tu-kap-par*$_5$ 1 *maš-šit* DÙ-*uš ma-la* URU$_4^!$(BURU$_{14}$)-*tú*

24' a rev. 9' *ta-máṣ-ṣi ki-i* ŠURUN-*su saḫ-pu-ma ta-at-tar-ṣu-uš u maš-šit šá* GÚR.GÚR SIG$_7$

25' a rev. 10' *kab-ba-ra šá id-bu-bu ta-ad-da-áš-šum-ma iz-zi-zu maš-šit an-*<*ni*>*-ta*

26' a rev. 11' SUM-*šum-ma* ÍL-*ši ki-i* ŠURUN-*su maš-šit i-man-za-qu u ina* IGI A.MEŠ *ta-at-tam-ḫa-ḫu*

27' a rev. 12' [MUNUS B]I PEŠ$_4$ *ki-i maš-šit bal-ṭa-tú u ru-bu-us-su la* <*i*>-*man-za-qu ul* PEŠ$_4$

28' a rev. 13' [*ru-bu-u*]*s-su na-di* ÚŠ E *ki-i la saḫ-pa maš-šit šá* GÚR.GÚR SIG$_7$ *kab-ba-ra*

29' a rev. 14' [x x x *š*]*u*$^?$-*a-tú* SUM-*su u* [*mal-t*]*ak-tú ta-lat-tak* GABA.RI 1-*en* ^{giš}DA

Colophon:

30' a rev. 15' [GABA.RI DUB$^?$ .... ^{m}GA.ḪÚL$^?$-^{d}]*tu-tu* ZI-*ḫi*

Bound Transcription and Translation

1 *[maštakti sinništi kī irrû u kī lā irrû(?) ištēn šiqil tarmuš] zūz šamma peṣâ rebūtu gabû* 2 *[miṣirāya ina itqi talammi ana šass]ūrīša tašakkan-ma mūšu gabbi* 3 *[ukâl ušellâm-ma ina kar]āni peṣî(?) temessi kī itqu šī sāmat lū dāma ulluḫatu* 4 *[sinništu šī irri] kī itqu arqat sinništu šī ul irri kī libbi šassūrīšu* 5 *[ištu ūrī]šu(?) kī pīt šēpi(?) ūṣi tutār-ma dullaša epuš šiprušu* 6 *[kī tēpušu(?)] mašqīta tašaqqīšu kī šāru(?) iṣbassu(?) lām maššītu innaššû kukra* 7 *burāša ḫašâ nuḫurta u ḫīl abukkati [ištiš]šu šinīšu šalāšīšu išatti u uša'rāšu irri(?)*

1 [A test whether a woman will conceive or not conceive(?)]: 2 [you wrap] 1 one shekel of *tarmuš*-plant], half a shekel 'white drug', (and) a quarter of a shekel of [Egyptian] alum 2 [in a wad of wool]. You insert it into her womb (viz. vagina). 3 [She shall keep (it) (there)] 2 all night long. 3 (Then) she removes (it)] and you wash (it) [with] white [wi]ne(?). If the wad is red or spotted with blood, 4 [that woman will conceive]. If the wad is green-yellow, that woman will not conceive. If the inside of her womb (viz. vagina) 5 *protrudes [from]* her [*vulva*(?)] during *walking*(?), make it turn back(?) and perform the (necessary) procedure(?) for her/it! 6 [*When you have performed*] 5 the treatment(s) for her, 6 give her the (following) potion to drink. (Also) if 'wind'(?) afflicts(?) her, before a suppository is *applied*, 7 she should drink 6 *kukru*-aromatic, 7 *burāšu*-juniper, *ḫašû*-plant, *nuḫurtu*-plant and resin of *abukkatu*-aromatic [one], two, three times. And (if then) it causes her to vomit, she *will conceive*.

---

8 DIŠ KI.MIN *šambalilta ina itqi talammi ana [šas]sūrīša tašakkan šalāšat ūmī inaššī-ma* 9 *šumma šambaliltu kīma takpīti(?) ibtarrum sinništu šī irri*

8 Alternatively, you wrap *šambaliltu*-fenugreek in a wad of wool, (and) insert it into her womb. She wears it for three days, 9 and if then the fenugreek (looks) speckled/multi-coloured like a *takpītu*-pearl(?), then that woman *will conceive*.

---

10 DIŠ KI.MIN *šamma peṣâ uḫūla qarnānâ ina itqi talammi ana šassūrīša tašakkan šalāšat ūmī inaššī-ma* 11 *ina šalšu ūme itqa ina mê temessi šumma itqu [sāmat sinništu šī irri(?)]* 12 *šumma itqu urqa malât(?) sinništu šī [ul irri(?)]*

10 Alternatively, you wrap 'white drug' and salicornia in a wad of wool, you insert it into her womb (viz. vagina). She wears it for three days. 11 On the third day you wash the wad with water. If the wad [is red, that woman will conceive(?)]. 12 If the wad is full of green-yellow (spots?), that woman [will not conceive(?)].

---

13 DIŠ KI.MIN *gabû miṣirāya ...[... ... šumma(?) ... ...]* 14 *kīma alap(pû) mê ītanammar sinništu šī [... ...]* 15 *[bur]āšu uḫūlu qarnānû(?) tittu(?) [... ...]*

13 Alternatively, [you ...] Egyptian alum, [... ... If ... ...], 14 she keeps seeing (a discharge looking?) like seaweed (on the surface) of water, that woman [... ...] 15 [*burāšu*-juni]per, salicornia(?), fig(?) [... ...]

Ms. a obv. breaks; gap of unknown length

16' [*šumma*(?) … …]-*šu sām zumuršu* [… …] 17' [… *ku*]*n*-*gu*(?) *issanu* [… …] 18' [… *mimm*]*a lā innaddissu ištēn akal kukra arqa ka*[*bbar*]*a … akal saḫlê* [……] 19' 2.TA.ÀM *taqallu ina mê talâš tukappar iškūra šamna ḫalṣa tasallaḫ-ma maššītu*(?) 20' *ištiššu šinīšu šalāšīšu ana šassūrīša tašakkan zikaršu ul iṭeḫḫēšu adi šina ūmū arkīša izzizū* 21' *mimma gabbi ul innaddissu ša qerbīssa*(!) *innassaḫu u šabsūtu iḫâṭāšu maltaktāšu* 22' *kī irrû kī lā irrû usābu ina išāti taqallu ana diqmenni tutār* 23' *ina šamni ḫalṣi baḫri*(!) *tasâk tulām lū ina mê tukappar ištēn maššīta teppuš mala erišti*(?) 24' *tamaṣṣi kī rubussu saḫpu-ma tattarṣuš*(*u*) *u maššīt kukri arqi* 25' *kabbara ša idbubu taddaššum-ma izzizu maššīta annīta* 26' *taddaššum-ma inašši kī rubussu maššīta imanzaqu u ina pān mê tattamḫaḫu* 27' [*sinništu š*]*ī irri kī maššītu balṭatu u rubussu lā* (*i*)*manzaqu ul irri* 28' [*rubu*]*ssu nadi peḫi taqabbi*(?) *kī lā saḫpa maššīta ša kukri arqi kabbara* 29' [… *š*]*uātu tanaddissu u* [*malt*]*akta talattak gabari ištēn lēʾi*

16' [If(?) … …] her […] is red, her body [… …], 17' […] [*ku*]*ngu*-rush(?), Dilmun date, [… …], 18' [nothi]ng should be administered to her […]. (You take) one tenth of a litre of fresh ⸢thick(?)⸣ *kukru*-plant, (and one?) tenth of a litre of *saḫlû*-plant […]. 19' You roast each (of the drugs) twice. (Then) you knead (them together) with water, you make a thick paste/dough (out of it). You sprinkle (it) with wax and pressed oil, and then 20' you insert (this as a) 19' suppository 20' once, twice, three times into her womb (viz. vagina). Her man shall not approach her (sexually). For two days after that (lit. "until two days have stood behind her") 21' nothing at all should be given to her. (When) that which is (in) her womb is removed, then the midwife should examine her. (This is) *her* test (or: the test *for(?) her* to see) 22' whether she will conceive or whether she will not conceive: you roast *usābu*-plant in the fire, you turn it into ashes. 23' You crush (them) with hot(!) pressed oil, you *dissolve* (the ashes). Or you smear (the ashes into a paste/compound) with water. You make one suppository (*maššītu*), you take as much as 24' (you) wish(?). If her womb is *turned over* and you *want to straighten it*, then you should give her the suppository of fresh thick *kukru*, 25' which *was discussed* (before). And (when) it (the womb) has become upright (straight again), you give her that (other) suppository (for the test) and 26' she wears it. If her womb *absorbs* (lit. sucks up) the suppository and it (the suppository, after removing it and putting it in water?) *dissolves* on the surface of the water, 27' th[at woman] will conceive. If the suppository stays fresh and her womb does not *absorb* it, she will not conceive. 28' [Her womb] is barren; it is closed/sealed off (*peḫi*), (thus) *you shall say*. If it (her womb) is not *turned over*, you can (still) give her the [afore]mentioned suppository of fresh thick *kukru* 29' […] and then you perform the [te]st. (This text is) a copy of a writing board.

Colophon:

30' [*gabari tuppi … Gaḫul*(?)]-*Tutu nasḫi*

30' [Copy of an] excerpted [tablet(?) … of Gaḫul]-Tutu(?).

Notes

Lines 1–4: The tentative restoration at the beginning of line 1 is partially based on the traces in the parallel BM 42313+ rev. 29–32 (see text A.2.2 lines 70–73). In BM 42313+ rev. 29, the deciphered phrase *maštakti sinništi lā erî*(?) would literally mean "a test of a woman of not conceiving/getting pregnant", i.e. a test to determine a woman who is unable to conceive a child. It remains uncertain whether ms. a also began with the same introductory purpose statement. Geller (2021, 345) restores the beginning of line 1 in ms. a: [*mal-tak-ta-šú ki-i* PEŠ$_4$ *u ki-i* NU PEŠ$_4$] "its test if (a woman is) pregnant or not pregnant". I am following Geller's suggestion but have slightly modified the phrasing.

The wording of the test in ms. a lines 1–4 and in BM 42313+ shows some variation, although the general procedure and interpretation of the observed colourations of the wad of wool are identical. Ms. a uses *kī* and BM 42313+ *šumma* as conditional subjunction (the use of *kī* instead of *šumma* recurs in several lines of ms. a, see lines 3, 4, 5, 6, 22'. 24'. 26', 27', 28'). In the long continuous passage on the reverse of ms. a, *kī* appears to function as a key element structuring the text (cf. below). Notably, *kī* in the sense of "if, in case of, when" is prominent in Neo- and Late Babylonian texts and may be a sign of colloquial language (cf. CAD K, 318 sub 2'-a'). The wording of both manuscripts also differs at other places: instead of *kal ūmi ukâl* "she keeps it (there) all day long" in BM 42313+, ms. a reads *mūšu gabbu* "all night long"; the quantity of one ingredient differs (alum), and the wad appears to be washed in a different liquid in ms. a, not in water as in BM 42313+. Moreover, the order of the predictive conditional clauses is reversed in both manuscripts. Ms. a first gives the clause with the positive predicition (the woman will conceive), then the clause with the negative one (the woman will not conceive), while in BM 42313+ the order of the clauses is reversed.

Line 2: There restoration follows BM 42313+ obv. 29–30 quoted above, with the addition of *mi-ṣir-a-a* "Egyptian (alum)", an ingredient that recurs in line 13 of ms. a. This restoration agrees with the size of the gap at the beginning of line 2 and with the estimated number of missing signs.

Line 3: The restoration at the beginning of the line is tentative and based on the parallel passage in BM 42313+ rev. 29–30. The sign traces before LUḪ-*si* are not entirely clear, but in light of *ina* A LUḪ-*si* "you wash (the wad) in water" in BM 42313+ rev. 30, I propose reading [*ina* GEŠT]IN-*nu* BABBAR "in white [wi]ne".

Lines 4–5: A new sentence / passage begins at the end of line 4, starting with *ki-i* ŠÀ-*bi* ŠÀ$^{!}$.TÙR-*šú* "if (something from) the inside of her womb ...". The interpretation of the healer's observations in this line and the following line 5 are difficult to understand. The reading and interpretation of the phrase *kī pīt šēpi*(GÌR) in line 5, in the sense of "when walking", follows a suggestion by Scurlock 2014a, 582, 583; 2014b, 119; differently Böck 2010a, 110 as well as Geller 2023, 4, 8. An expression *pīt šēpi* lit. "opening of the foot" (i.e. walking, stepping) is so far unattested, but there is a parallel idiomatic expression *pīt purīdi* "stride, step" (lit. "opening of the leg"), cf. CAD P, 446 s.v. *pītu* A sub 1c-3'. Interpreting the verb *u-ṣi* "it emerges" in line 5 in the sense of "to protrude" (cf. CAD A/2, 366–367 sub mng. g, 368–369 sub mng. j), the passage could refer to uterine prolapse. Why this phenomenon is discussed in the present context, is difficult to know. However, uterine prolapse would certainly pose a serious hindrance for a woman's conception. The following instructions in ms. a with the verb *turru*(GUR, often also GUR.GUR) is interpreted here as "to make (the womb) turn back". Since the next phrase uses a verb in the imperative, perhaps one should restore a D-stem imperative form *tīr-ma* "make (it) turn back" instead of a durative form. Manual procedures for pressing a prolapsed uterus back inside as well as a range of other treatments for making it move back to its normal position are discussed, for example, in the Hippocratic text *Diseases of Women* II, 33–44, see Potter 2018, 353–367.

The specific meaning "(medical) treatment" for *dullu* "work" appears to be attested predominantly in Middle Babylonian texts, s. CAD D, s.v. *dullu* sub 5. I have chosen the translation "perform the (necessary) procedure for her/it" for *dullašu epuš* in line 5.

The word ME-*ru-šú* at the end of line 5 has been read *mērûšu* "her pregnancy" by Reiner 1982a, 134–135 and Scurlock 2014a, 582. Following Geller (2023, 2, 8), I have adopted the alternative reading *šip-ru-šú* "the treatment(s) for her" (although one would expect the form *šipiršu*). Like its synonym *dullu*, the word *šipru* is used in the sense of "treatment, therapy" (see CAD Š/3, 83–84 mng. 7).

Line 6: Decipherment of this line remains provisional. For other interpretations, cf. Reiner 1982a, 134–136; Scurlock 2014a, 582–583. Possibly, the present passage (lines 6–7) gives an alternative procedure for testing the patient, namely a potion instead of a tampon. If the text is interpreted correctly, this potion could also be prescribed as a treatment before applying a suppository, in the case that the patient suffered from 'wind' (reading *ki šāru*(LÍL$^{?}$) *iṣ-b*[*a*$^{?}$-*a*]*s*$^{?}$-*su*). The damaged signs copied by O. Gurney in UET 7, 123 are not entirely clear here. M. Geller (2023, 2, 4) proposes a different reading for this passage: *ki-*<*i*> É ^{giš}⸢NÁ⸣-*su* IGI "*when she sees her bedroom*" (as a euphemistic reference to sexual intercourse (but one expects É ^{giš}NÁ-*šú*). I have instead opted to read the following as *lām*(IGI) *maššītu innaššû* "before a suppository is applied" as a subordinate clause with the verb *našû* (N-stem) in the subjunctive.

Lines 6–7: In the prescription for the potion in line 7, Scurlock 2014a, 582 reads ILLU ⸢LI.TAR⸣ 2-*šú* 3-*šú* NAG, translating "(you have her drink ...) *abukkatu*-resin <once>, twice (or) three times". I prefer reading ILLU LI.<TAR> followed by [1]-*šú* "once" instead.

For reading BURU$_8$-*šú* in line 7 as a Š-stem of *arû* "to vomit", see also Reiner 1982a, 135–136, who notes that the sense of the verb should be factitive (i.e. to induce the patient to vomit, also practiced in other medical texts with a feather moved about in the patient's throat). However, I understand the patient as the object of the sentence (indicated by the pronominal suffix -*šú*), i.e. "if it (the potion) causes her to vomit", and not as the subject (cf. Scurlock 2014a, 583). Böck (2010a, 110) understands the healer addressed in the second person as the subject and translates: "[du] läßt sie sich erbrechen, dann wird sie schwanger werden". This translation assumes that the aim of the potion was therapeutic rather than a mere test. In this case, the potion used as an emetic may have been intended to remove some substance from the body, which was seen as an obstruction or hindrance to pregnancy or conception.[282]

Similar reaction tests are found in the Egyptian medical papyri and in Hippocratic texts. For Egyptian prognoses in which a woman's reaction (vomiting) is tested after the application of a substance to her body, see e.g. Westendorf 1999, 433 (Papyrus Kahun 27), 435 (Papyrus Berlin 193–195), 438 (Papyrus Carlsberg V 2,1–3 and VII 2,3–6). Notably, all the Egyptian tests aim at knowing whether a woman was able to conceive/get pregnant. The most similar of these examples (Berlin Papyrus 193; ca. 1250 BCE) was transmitted to Greek medical authors and adapted in the Hippocratic treatise *De sterilibus* 214 almost verbatim (see Pommerening 2015, esp. 2090): "[Recognizing] a woman who will give birth in comparison with a woman who will not give birth: Bottle gourd shall be pounded, shall be enclosed in milk of a woman who has given birth to a male child, shall be made into a remedy to be swallowed, shall be swallowed by the woman. If she vomits, she will give birth. If she breaks wind, she will not give birth." For a similar reaction test in Hippocratic sources that was used to confirm a woman's pregnancy, see e.g. *Aphorisms* V 41 (Jones 1959, 168–169): "If you wish to know whether a woman is with child, give her hydromel to drink [without supper] when she is going to sleep. If she has colic in the stomach she is with child, otherwise she is not".

Lines 8–9: The sign $^{(\text{ú})}$SULLIM$^{(\text{sar})}$ (= *šambaliltu*, "fenugreek") in lines 8 and 9 can alternatively be read as $^{(\text{ú})}$BAR$_8$$^{(\text{sar})}$, corresponding to the *dīšu*-plant in Akkadian, a type of grass or wild-growing cereal, cf. CAD Š/1, 311 s.v. *šambaliltu* sub b; CAD D, 164 s.v. *dīšu* sub 3; Borger 2004, MZL, Nos. 165 and 490.

The reading ÉLLAG (BIR) = *ta/ukpītu*-stone in line 9 was suggested by Böck 2013, 41 n. 52; see also Stol 2021, *BiOr* 78, 448. Scurlock (2014a, 582; 2014b, 120) and Geller (2023, 2, 4) read the sign in question as ŠEŠ instead, which can have the Akkadian readings *murru* ("*murru*-aromatic") or *šeguššu* (a type of millet). The word *takpītu* (also *tukpītu*), often written with the determinative na$_4$, has been interpreted as the designation of a stone bead of kidney-shape, since the logogram can literally be rendered as "kidney-(shaped) stone (bead)", see CAD T, 459 s.v. *tukpītu*; AHw 1308 s.v. *takpītu*; SAD, Vol. 2, 56 "a bead". Stol (2021, *BiOr* 78, 448) suggests translating the present passage as "(becomes(?) multicoloured like a) pearl". For discussion cf. also Beaulieu 1999, *RA* 93, 154–155; Arkhipov 2018, *Chaga Bazar VI*, 52–53, 59, 64. The word *takpītu* also occurs as an ingredient in BM 42313+, lines 37 and 54 (in prescriptions to stop bleeding, see text A.2.2).

The verbal form *ib-tar-rum* in line 9 is a Gt-stem of *barāmu* "to be multicoloured, speckled". For discussion of this colour term, see also Thavapalan 2020, 79–89.

Line 10: The substance Ú BABBAR (Akkadian *šammu peṣû*), lit. "white drug", is explained as ILLU *ṣar-bi-te* (^{giš}ÁSAL) "resin of *ṣarbatu*-poplar" in Uruanna I 225–227, in the Practical Vocabulary from Assur (line 108) and in AMT 40/5 iv 23' (Geller 2005a, *BAM* 7, No. 23). It is further equated with Ì.UDU BABBAR-*ú* "white tallow" in Uruanna III 61 (CAD P, 329b s.v. *peṣû* lex. section; CAD Ṣ, 108a, 109b s.v. *ṣarbatu* sub lex. section and f). It is a recurring ingredient in women's healthcare texts.

Line 11–12: For an alternative reading, see Geller 2023, 2–3.

Lines 13–15: The reading *a-lap me* (for *alapî* (*ša*) *mê*) "(if it looks like) seaweed (from the surface) of the water" in line 14 follows a suggestion of Geller (2021, 346). Cf. CAD A/1, 336 s.v. *alapû*, perhaps meaning "seaweed; algae". If correct, the expression seems abbreviated (the construct state of *alapû* should have a final vowel), compare BAM 494 i 45' (Bácskay and Simkó 2017, *JMC* 30, 10): *a-la-pa-a šá* IGI A.M[EŠ] "algae from the surface of the water" (as an ingredient). Nonetheless, that interpretation seems preferable to reading *a-lap me* "water ox (*alpu*)" (cf. CAD A/1, 335a; Butz 1977, *BiOr* 34, 290).

Lines 16'–29': The structure of this lengthy passage is complex and difficult to follow, consisting of several units that are interlinked with each other. In the following, I am proposing a new analysis of the structure of lines 16'–29'. Two different recipes for two different suppositories can be identified in lines 18'–20' and 21'–24', indicating two separate steps in the treatment, which involved a therapeutic **suppository made with fresh *kukru*-plant** which was supposed to have positive

282 An alternative interpretation may be that the woman's reaction to the potion confirmed that she was indeed pregnant. As proposed in Steinert (2015, 109 n. 23), the conclusion drawn here may have been based on analogy: vomiting may have been seen as analogous to miscarriage (in both cases, something is expelled from the body), and therefore the vomiting was seen as a sign for the woman's pregnancy or ability to conceive.

effects on the state of the uterus, and then a **suppository made with *usābu*-plant used as a test** indicating the woman's fertility and success of the treatment:

Lines 16'–17'	Fragmentary
Lines 18'–20'	Instruction for preparing a **suppository made with fresh *kukru*-plant** (for treating the uterus)
Lines 20'–21'	Instructions for applying the suppository with fresh *kukru*-plant
Lines 21'–24'	Instructions for preparing a **suppository made with *usābu*-plant used as a test** (for recognizing the state of the uterus / ability to conceive)
Lines 24'–26'	Further instructions for applying the suppository of *kukru*-plant (for straightening the womb)
Lines 26'–29'	Description how to interpret the test described in lines 21'–24' (suppository with *usābu*-plant) and concluding instructions

Line 17': The restoration of the preserved signs in this line is tentative. The form *issanu* is a variant spelling of *asnû* "Dilmun date" found in Late Babylonian texts (see also AHw 75; CAD A/2, 338). The preceding word should also refer to a medical substance. The term *kungu* refers to a kind of rush; it is equated with *zēr urbati* "seed of *urbatu*-rush", see CAD K, 539a. Alternatively, one could read [*mu*]-*un-gi* as a variant spelling for *mangu*, which refers to a type of alkali (AHw 602; CAD M/1, 211; Thompson DAB, 31, 35). Geller (2023, 3) restores [^{ú}nu.mu].un.gi as a syllabic rendering of ^{ú}NUMUN.GI, which is a rare Sumerian correspondence for *baltu*-thorn.

Line 18': The phrase GÚR.GÚR SIG$_7$ *k*[*ab-ba-r*]*a* "thick fresh *kukru*-plant" is restored following lines 24'–25', where the same expression occurs again.

Line 19': For numerals with the element TA.ÀM attached to them having the meaning "x times (each)", see e.g. SpTU 5, No. 248 rev. 23': *ana* ŠÀ GEŠTU.MIN.MEŠ *ki-lal-*⌜*le*⌝*-e* 3.TA.ÀM ŠID-*nu* "she (the pregnant woman) recites (the spell) over both (of the pregnant ewe's) ears, (over) each one three times" (Scurlock 2014a, 687; see also *infra* text C.3.10). Cf. also Streck 1995, *Zahl und Zeit*, 69.

The sign occurring here and in line 23' below appears to be a variant form of the sign BÍL (NExPAB) (cf. Borger 2004, MZL 104 No. 312).

The verb *kapāru* "to smear; to wipe off" in the D-stem often appears in medical or ritual contexts, where the patient's body is wiped off with a paste or dough, for cleansing purposes (CAD K 178–180). But since the pronominal suffix is missing here, the verb may refer to another action that is part of the preparation of the suppository. I tentatively suggest that *tukappar* could have the sense "to smear", "to make a thick paste/dough" or compound from the ingredients in the present passage. The emendation *ma*$^{?}$-⌜*áš*$^{!}$-*ši*$^{!}$-*tu*$^{!}$⌝ "suppository" at the end of line 19' follows Geller 2023, 3.

Line 20': The idiomatic expression *a-di* U$_4$ 2.KAM EGIR-*šá iz-zi-zu* "until two days have passed" (lit. "until two days have stood behind her") is unusual (cf. CAD A/2, 279 sub 1b-2'; AHw 1468–1469). Geller (2023, 5) connects this phrase with the preceding sentence and translates: "Her man should not have sex with her until two days after that (the tampon) has been in place". I connect the expression with the following statement that during the stipulated period of two days, nothing (i.e. no other treatment) should be given to the patient. Differently Geller (2021, 344), who assumes that the patient had to fast. In any case, the present line indicates that the woman should not have sexual intercourse while the treatment with the suppository of fresh *kukru* was ongoing.

Line 21': The phrase *šá qer-bit-si* ZI-*ḫu* is difficult. In addition to the erroneous pronominal suffix *qerbīt-si* instead of *qerbīt-sa/-su* "her womb", the preposition *ina* seems to be missing, since *qerbītu* by itself is not used as a preposition for "within, inside" (cf. CAD Q, 214). The correct expression would have been *ša ina qerbītīša* "that which is in her womb". The following verb ZI-*ḫu* may be a plural form of *nasāḫu* (i.e. "they shall remove" what is in her womb), although one rather expects a passive (N-stem) form ("it will/should be removed"; see also Geller 2021, 344). The statement may indicate that the procedure for the suppository made with *kukru*-plant described in the preceding lines 18'–20', which is followed by the instruction for another fertility test (in lines 22'–28'), could have aimed at removing some "matter" from the womb that was considered as a hindrance to conception, and thus aimed at preparing the womb for conception. Similar notions and treatments for removing harmful matter from the womb that impede conception are encountered in Hippocratic treatises on women's health such as *Diseases of Women* I and II (Potter 2018). For discussion of these similarities, see below notes on line 24'. Alternatively, "that which is (in) her womb" in line 21' may have referred to the applied suppository, although this seems less likely.

Lines 21'–22': This passage requires the midwife to examine the patient, presumably to check the effect of the ongoing treatment. Unfortunately, the details of this examination or the reason why the midwife was required to do it (and not the male healer), remain unclear. Was a manual examination of the patient's womb required, and this close-up inspection was not appropriate or allowed to a male healer? The following text passage is likewise ambiguous in its formulation: "*Her* test" (*maltaktašu*) could refer to the patient (i.e. the test for her) or to a test used and communicated (to the male healer) by the midwife, which is then reported in the following lines of the text.

Line 23': For *tu-lam* "you *dissolve*", cf. CAD L, 246a s.v. *lummu*; AHw 563b "auflösen?"; Scurlock (2014a, 395 with n. 54 *passim*) translates this verb as "to soften" (assuming a relation of *lummu* to *lamāmu* "to chew"). For this line, cf. also CAD Ṭ, 111b s.v. *ṭikmennu* sub 1b; CAD U/W, 274 s.v. *usābu* sub 3. See also BM 45559+ obv. i 17' (text A.2.4 line 17'). For arguments that the Akkadian word for "ashes" should be rendered as *diqmēnu* (or *diqmennu*) rather than *ṭikmennu*, see SAD, Vol. 2, 35. The present passage is the only attestation for the word *usāb/pu* as a plant (written with the classifier Ú). Geller (2023, 5, 10) interprets it as a rendering of Greek *hyssop.*

Geller (2021, 346) translates *ina* Ì *ḫal-ṣa* BÍL in line 23' as "roast it in pressed oil". I prefer to emend the BÍL to KÚM[!] = *baḫru* "hot" instead because of the following verb SÚD "you crush" (i.e. you crush in hot pressed oil"). For the form of the sign BÍL in this text (with the sign PAB inscribed into the sign NE), see also above line 19'.

For the expression *mala erišti maṣû* "to take as much as desired", cf. CAD M/1, 347 sub 2 *mala libbi maṣû* "to do what one wants; to have full discretion". The word *erištu* "wish; request" in line 23' is spelled in an unusual fashion: as $BURU_{14}$ (ENxKÁR)-*tú* instead of *eriš*$_4$(URU$_4$)-*tú* (or KAM-*tú*). Geller (2021, 346 n. 22) regards the spelling *ta-máṣ*(MÁŠ)-*ṣi* as an indication for a late date of the text.

Line 24': The sign ŠURUN corresponds to Akkadian *rubṣu* "lair, shelter; womb" (cf. CAD R 395, sub 3), which is a rare, metaphorical term for the womb (see the commentary ḪAR-gud B IV 30 (MSL 9, 34), which gives *rubṣu* and *rēmu* as equations of Sumerian [uzu]a-sila-ĝar-ra "afterbirth", see also Steinert 2014–2016, "Uterus", *RlA* 14, 513–514 §1.1–1.2). The word is spelled syllabically below in line 27'. For other Semitic (e.g. Syriac, Mandaic) cognates with the same meaning "womb", see Militarev and Kogan, *Semitic Etymological Dictionary* I, 200 no. 226.

The verbal form *ta-at-tar-ṣu-uš* may be analysed as a G-stem perfect form or as a Gt-stem preterite form of *tarāṣu*, (2nd person masc. sg.). From the homonymous verbs listed under *tarāṣu* in the dictionaries, *tarāṣu* "to stretch out, to point, to straighten (a limb), to erect", is often attested with body parts (e.g. hands, feet) and therefore most likely indicated here (cf. CAD T, 208–215 s.v. *tarāṣu* A; AHw 1326–1327, s.v. *tarāṣu* I). A Gt-form may perhaps signal a change of direction or movement. I also assume that the pronominal suffix (-*š*(*u*)), in which the form ends, refers to the uterus, which needs straightening or bringing back into the correct position. The verb *tarāṣu* "to straighten" thus contrasts with the preceding verb *saḫāpu* "to turn over" and indicates the aim of the therapy. For different interpretations, see Scurlock 2014a, 584; Geller 2023, 5, 11.

I suggest that *saḫāpu* "to cover, to overwhelm" and *tarāṣu* "to stretch out; to set in place" in line 24' (and below in line 28', where *saḫpu* is negated and *tarāṣu* not mentioned) refer respectively to the uterus being in an abnormal position and to the correction of this position back to normal. The verb *saḫāpu* can mean "to turn over, upside down" (said of capsized boats or wagons falling over), and "to lie flat/face down" (CAD S, 30ff. s.v. *saḫāpu*, especially sub 3a–b). In the latter meaning, *saḫāpu* occurs a few times in medical texts, in references to the patient lying on his belly or being turned face down. More closely to UET 7, No. 123, *saḫāpu* in the stative occurs with reference to other internal organs. In the incantations BAM 574 iv 20–22 and iv 26–27 for indigestion (*kīs libbi* "binding of the belly"), it is likewise found in contrast with the verb *tarāṣu*, as well as *ešēru* "to be straight". The verbs *saḫāpu*, parallel to *zâru* "to twist, to turn around" and *saḫāru* "to turn (around)", here describe the digestive tract as being in an abnormal state of obstruction or constriction:

BAM 574 iv 26–27 (STOMACH 1):
[ir]rū suḫḫurū zîr karšu u šī riqītu buppāniša saḫpat / [li]truṣ karšu riqītu litruṣ
"The intestines are tangled up, the stomach is twisted and the *large intestine* itself lies flat face down. [May] the stomach stretch out, may the *large intestine* stretch out!" (cf. Collins 1999, 153–154 Belly 17; Cadelli 2000, 88 *passim*; Johnson and Simkó 2024, 101)

BAM 574 iv 20–22 (STOMACH 1):
irrū suḫḫurū zîr karšu u šī riqītu buppāniša saḫpat / lišlim karšu irrū lištēširūma / riqītu litruṣ
"The intestines are tangled up, the stomach is twisted, and the *large intestine* itself lies flat face down. May the stomach become better, may the intestines straighten themselves out, may the *large intestine* stretch out!" (cf. Collins 1999, 155–157 Belly 19; Cadelli 2000, 87 *passim*; Johnson and Simkó 2024, 100 with n. 274)

The condition of the womb described as *saḫāpu* ("turned over"), as an abnormal uterine position hindering conception, may be compared with the "womb that is twisted" (*rēmu ša zîri*), which is mentioned in the disease taxonomy SpTU 1, No. 43, beside barrenness (*lā ālidūti*, see Geller 2014, 4). The aim of the treatment in ms. a is to bring it back into a straight position, so that it "stands up" again (see line 25': *izzizu*). These abnormal states ascribed to internal organs such as the intestines and the womb seem to be based on inferences (drawing on observed external symptoms) and analogical reasoning, although in the case of the woman's womb, the conclusion may have been drawn from a manual vaginal examination – as in the case of the Hippocratic physicians who observed through examination with a finger whether the mouth of the uterus was closed or whether it had shifted in an abnormal position, etc.).[283]

Interestingly, the Hippocratic texts describe similar views regarding the causes of a woman's infertility or inability to conceive. Thus, the treatise *Diseases of Women* I discusses and treats cases in which the mouth of the woman's uterus is not straight but folded over, and therefore the uterus is unable to take up the semen:

"Women who cohabit but are still unable to become pregnant you must question as to whether ... the seed is immediately discharged (sc. after intercourse), or on the next day, or on the third, sixth or seventh day. Now if she says the seed is discharged immediately after intercourse, the mouth (sc. of the uterus) is not straight, but folded over and it fails to take up the seed. If she says this happens on the second or third day, then her uterus is full of moisture and the seed gets washed away. If it is on the sixth or seventh day, the seed is decomposing and being discharged in that state.

Now if the seed is not being taken up at the beginning, first the mouth of the uterus must be treated so that it will be straight. Then, if the seed is being washed away on the second or third day, the uterus and the head (sc. require treatment). Finally, when the seed is decomposing and being discharged, the uterus itself and the whole body (sc. require treatment), being full of moisture. ..." (Potter 2018, *Hippocrates*, Volume XI, 43 Chapter 10).

The following Chapter 11 contains tests for determining whether phlegm or bile was the responsible body humour that led to an excess of moisture in the woman's body or womb. These tests share a few similarities with the Mesopotamian fertility tests using tampons, but the Hippocratic tests analyse the colour and consistency of the woman's menstrual discharges which are collected on pieces of cloth and then exposed to heat, sunlight and water (Potter 2018, 43ff. (Chapter 11), 65 (Chapter 22)). The treatments applied to the patient depend on the diagnosis previously made: "If the mouth (of the uterus) is occluded, dilate it, if the uterus is lying at an angle, straighten it, if it is moist, dry it, and similarly by applying opposite measures." (Potter 2018, 45). If the mouth of the uterus was not straight or had bent towards the side, the Hippocratic physicians recommended measures such as fumigations (using lead sounds) or manual procedures to straighten the uterus (Potter 2018, 48–49 (*Diseases of Women* I Chapter 11), 53 (Chapter 13)).[284] Alternatively, suppositories inserted into the vagina are prescribed to open the uterus and to clean out fluids, similar to the treatments in UET 7, No. 123 (e.g. Potter 2018, 177 (Chapter 75 [15], 215 (Chapter 81 [1]), 219 (Chapter 84 [1]). The removal of excessive moisture from the uterus or

283 Alternatively, the patient was supposed to examine herself in this manner; in some cases, the physician or the patient were supposed to manipulate and correct the position of the mouth of the uterus manually. See e.g. *Diseases of Women* I Chapter 13, 20, 60 (Potter 2018, 53, 63, 125; *Diseases of Women* II Chapter 23, 24 (Potter 2018, 313, 321, 339).

284 Note, for example, the following passage (Potter 2018, 53, Chapter 13): "If the mouth (of the uterus) is tightly closed, open it with pine dilators and lead sounds. Apply a mild fomentation made from fennel, and clean the uterus with suppositories that will make it thinner and set it in a straight position. ... In women whose cervix has turned to the side and is leaning against a hip—for this too may occur and prevent the uterus from receiving the seed: now when something like this has happened, you should foment with fragrant substances; after the fomentation, have the patient draw (sc. her cervix) aside with a finger, and push it away from the hip. When she has done this, straighten (sc. the uterus) with pine twigs and a lead sound in the way described above. After the uterus has been straightened and dilated, clean it with mild suppositories, and attend to the rest according to established practice." For similar passages on an inclination of the uterus towards the hip, see Potter 2018, 313ff. *Diseases of Women* II Chapters 22–26, 37.

the elimination of harmful humours are often referred to as purification or cleaning (*katharsis*) in the Hippocratic texts (e.g., Potter 2018, 45, 47 (Chapter 11), 215 (Chapter 81 [1], 219 (Chapter 84 [1])). While there are also significant differences between the Mesopotamian and the Hippocratic procedures to promote fertility, we can nonetheless recognize similar elements and ideas, such as notions of a closed or bent uterus or ideas of harmful matter in the womb hindering conception (see above note on line 21').

Line 25': Instead of *šá id-bu-bu*, the reading *šá iṭ-pu-pu* from the verb *ṭapāpu* "to become saturated" was proposed by Reiner 1982a, 135, followed by Scurlock 2014a, 584 and Geller 2023, 5. I have opted instead for a simpler solution and read *ša id-bu-bu* "which has been discussed (before)", as a discursive statement referring back to the prescription for the suppository of *kukru* a few lines earlier (lines 18'–21'). In commentaries as well as in the text SpTU 4, No. 153 from Uruk with prescriptions for women, similar statements are found with the verb *qabû* "to say" (e.g. *šá iqbû* (E-*ú*)), see Gabbay 2016, 201ff. and *infra* texts C.1.10 and D.1.11 for discussion).

The 2nd person sg. form *ta-ad-da-áš-šum-ma* "you give (it) to her" in line 25', from *nadānu* "to give; to administer", reflects the Assyrian G-stem durative form (i.e. < *taddan+-šum+-ma*. The Babylonian form should be *tanaddiššum-ma*. The latter form probably stands behind the spelling SUM-*su* in lines 18' and 29' (cf. also line 21'), but here the suffix -*šu*(*m*) has been assimilated to -*su* (*n+š* > *ss*), as is often the case in Neo- or Late Babylonian texts (see von Soden, GAG § 102l).

Lines 26'–27': The verb *mazāqu* means "to suck" is said, for example, of the 'tooth worm' sucking the blood of the gums, of a baby sucking at the breast, or of a patient sucking a medication. I have chosen the rendering "to absorb" for the present, rather technical context. The following verb *maḫāḫu* means "to soak; to steep in a liquid; to dissolve (in liquid)" (AHw 577b; CAD M/1, 49–50). The form *tattamḫaḫu* is interpreted here as a rare Nt-stem form with a reflexive meaning "to dissolve" (cf. von Soden GAG § 95d). I interpret the prefix *ta-* as the 3rd person fem. sg. prefix, with *maššītu* "suppository" as the indicated subject of the verb. Thus, the present test procedure checked whether the patient's womb absorbed (something of?) the applied as a suppository (which is here not a woollen tampon, but a mixture of drugs mixed with a fatty substance!), or whether it stayed "fresh" and was not absorbed by the womb. The phrase *ina pān mê tattamḫaḫu* "(if) it dissolves on the surface of water" may refer to a further test mechanism, where the suppository, after it had been removed and put into water, dissolved on the surface (see thus Reiner 1982a, 132; Scurlock 2014a, 584 translates the phrase as "it is softened by the water"; for a completely different interpretation cf. Geller 2023, 5, 11–12). For the meaning "to dissolve" (in water) of *maḫāḫu*, see also Guichard 2014, 15, 43–44 col. ii 6: *littamḫaḫ nakrum kī* [*ṭīdim ina mê*(?)] "may the enemy dissolve like [clay in water]" (likewise Nt-stem?); Parpola and Watanabe 1988, SAA 2, 55: *ki-i šá ṣal-mu šá* DUḪ.LÀL *ina* IZI *iš-šar-rap-u-ni šá ṭi-ṭi ina* A.MEŠ *i-maḫ-ḫa-ḫu-u-ni* [*k*]*i-i ḫa-an-né-e la-an-ku-nu ina* GIŠ.BAR *liq-mu-u ina* A.MEŠ *lu-ṭa-bu-u* "Just as an image of wax is burnt in the fire and one of clay dissolved in water, (so) may your figure be burned in the fire and sunk in water".[285]

In short, the ability of the womb to "absorb" the suppository is interpreted as a positive sign that the woman was able to conceive; the inability to absorb it is understood as a sign of the woman's continued inability to conceive. The logic applied here appears to resemble another explanation for infertility, namely based on the sign whether the woman's womb was able to receive and retain the male semen or not, see BAM 240: 67–69 (*infra* text D.2.1) for discussion.

Line 28': In line 28', Scurlock 2014a, 583 reads *na-ṭi-pè-e* "([the fruit of] her ⌜womb⌝) has been plucked out", from *naṭāpu* "to tear out"; however, the form should be *naṭip* in this case. I propose to read *na-di* "it (the womb) is barren", followed by two logographic signs. The sign BAD can be read as a form of *peḫû* "to bar, to block, to seal" (corresponding to Sumerian úš). Parallel to *nadi*, I have chosen the stative (*peḫi*), which often occurs in reference to body openings that are closed off (see CAD P, 316 sub 1c). The following sign E, which is probably not to be understood as a phonetic complement, may be interpreted as a logogram for *qabû* "to speak; to say". A second person sg. form *taqabbi* "you (shall) say" could indicate the verdict or interpretation given by the healer about the woman's state of fertility.

285 A comparable passage in the Hippocratic treatise *Diseases of Women* II Chapter 24 says about a suppository of resin and oil inserted in the case that a woman's uterus falls against her hip: "Apply one of these and wait until it melts, and then apply the second one" (Potter 2018, 327).

Line 30': The fragmentary colophon may be compared with the colophon of N. 4001, a Neo-Babylonian tablet, which is said to have been copied from an original owned by Sîn-multēšir, son of Gaḫul-Tutu (see *infra* text B.2.1). It is probably not a coincidence that N. 4001 (found at Nippur) contains not only an incantation and ritual for infertility, but also tests. Therefore, the Gaḫul-Tutu mentioned in N. 4001 and perhaps also in ms. a may refer to the same person.

B.2.3 BM 42450 + 43809: Prescriptions for Female Fertility

This fragmentary tablet belongs to a group of Late Babylonian medical and magico-medical texts within the 81-7-1 collection of the British Museum's Department of Western Asiatic Antiquities. Studies by Jursa (1999, 3, 12–13, 19–22) and Finkel (2000) elucidate that this group of magico-medical texts within the 81-7-1 collection shares many graphic, physical and textual characteristics with the texts from the business archives of the Bēl-rēmanni family from Sippar dating to the Achaemenid period. These similarities, together with acquisition details, support the conclusion that the magico-medical texts and the Bēl-rēmanni texts belonged to a larger archive or text ensemble, which reflects activities of advanced scribal training in the areas of law and medicine/healing offered by the family of Bēl-rēmanni.

The "medical archive" published by Finkel (2000), a group of ca. 90 tablets and fragments, to which BM 42450 + 43809 belongs, offers distinctive features pointing to the character of these texts as school tablets. Although there are several larger or multi-column tablets within this group, a greater number of the texts from this archive consist in small tablets of various formats, whose shape and physical features (e.g., careless moulding, use of recycled clay, clumsy erasures), script and orthographical peculiarities often point to an inexperienced scribe. Furthermore, multiple copyists with a distinctive hand could be identified within the group. Among the texts, Finkel (2000, Texts 5, 15–18), identified several tablets duplicating the same text (e.g., prescriptions).

From the medical texts of the 81-7-1 collection, eight tablets and fragments are concerned with prescriptions for women's health (see also texts A.2.2, B.2.4, E.2.1, E.2.2 in this volume). The present text is a small school tablet that preserves part of two prescriptions, both of which may have had the purpose of promoting female fertility. One of the prescriptions is explicitly labelled as being "good for pregnancy" (*ana mērê damiq*). This label corresponds to similar purpose statements found in the women's healthcare corpus, such as "to enable a woman who is not pregnant to get pregnant".

List of Manuscripts

Siglum	Museum Number	Copy	Collation	Format; Ductus	Provenience
a	BM 42450 + 43809 (81-7-1, 210 + 1570)[286]	Finkel, *FS Lambert*, fig. 23	Coll.	Fragment of a single-column tablet in portrait format; Late Babylonian script; 6th/5th cent. BCE	Sippar

Overview

i'	Prescription for female fertility / conception (tampon) a obv. 1'–rev. 6'(?)	...]1'–10' [...], 11''–16''(?)
ii'	Prescription (tampon) a rev. 7'–10'	17''–20'' [...

Previous Edition and Discussion

Finkel 2000, *FS Lambert*, 169–170, No. 16 (edition)
Electronic Babylonian Library (eBL) (https://www.ebl.lmu.de/library/BM.42450; transliteration)

286 Measurements: 4.5 cm x 4.9 cm x 2.2 cm.

Transliteration

ca. two lines at the beginning of ms. a obv. lost

1'	a obv. 1'	[x (x)] x x [x x x x]
2'	a obv. 2'	[1 G]ÍN Ú x[x x x x]
3'	a obv. 3'	⸢*ta*⸣-*ṣáḫ*-⸢*ḫat*⸣ x[x x x]
4'	a obv. 4'	*ina* KAŠ.ḪI.A SUMUN *t*[*u-lab-bak*$^{?}$]
5'	a obv. 5'	1 GÍN ^{šim}MUG ⸢*sa*⸣-[*pan*]
6'	a obv. 6'	*ta-par-ra-am*
7'	a obv. 7'	⸢1$^{?}$⸣ <GÍN$^{?}$> *saḫ*$^{!}$-*le-e šá la n*[*a-pu-ú*$^{?}$]
8'	a obv. 8'	[*tu*]-*lab-bak*
9'	a obv. 9'	[1 GÍN *i*]*n-za-ru-ú*
10'	a obv. 10'	[x x x x]x [x x]

Ms. a obv. breaks; gap of a few lines

11''	a rev. 1'	[x x x *t*]*a*-⸢*šak-kan*⸣
12''	a rev. 2'	⸢*ina*⸣ ⸢SÍG⸣ *qu-na-a-ta*
13''	a rev. 3'	*ta-lam-mu a-na* MUNUS [BI]
14''	a rev. 4'	*tu-šá-zaz*$_{x}$(ÁŠ) 1+*et ma*[*š-ši-tú*$^{?}$]
15''	a rev. 5'	*šá* SÍG.ḪI.A EGIR-*šú ta-na-á*[*š-ši*$^{?}$]
16''	a rev. 6'	*a-na me-re-e* SIG$_{5}$
17''	a rev. 7'	*ka-da-nu šá e-da-šú* [x x]
18''	a rev. 8'	*e-ri-bi ti-amtu*(GÉME) [x x (x)]
19''	a rev. 9'	MÚD EREN *in*-⸢*za-ru*⸣-[*ú*]
20''	a rev. 10'	*ina* SÍG *qu-na*-⸢*a*⸣-[*ta*]

Ms. a rev. breaks; ca. two lines lost

Bound Transcription and Translation

ca. two lines at the beginning of ms. a obv. lost

$^{1'}$ [...] ... [... ...] $^{2'}$ [*ištēn ši*]*qil* ... [... ...] $^{3'}$ [*t*]*aṣaḫḫat* ...[...] $^{4'}$ *ina šikari labiri t*[*ulabbak*(?)] $^{5'}$ *ištēn šiqil ballukka sapān* $^{6'}$ *taparram* $^{7'}$ *ištēn šiqil saḫlê ša lā n*[*apû*(?)] $^{8'}$ [*tu*]*labbak* $^{9'}$ [*ištēn šiqil i*]*nzarû* $^{10'}$ [...] ...[...]

$^{1'}$ ... [... ...], $^{2'}$ one shekel of [...]-plant, [... ...] $^{3'}$ you squeeze (it) out, [... ...] $^{4'}$ you [steep(?)] (it) in old beer (dregs). $^{6'}$ You chop $^{5'}$ one shekel of *ballukku*-soap. $^{8'}$ You steep $^{7'}$ one (shekel of?) *saḫlû*-plant which is not [sifted(?)]. $^{10'}$ [You ...] $^{9'}$ one shekel of *inzarû*-aromatic, (...)

Ms. a obv. breaks; gap of a few lines

11'' [...] *tašakkan* 12'' *ina šīpāti qunātā* 13'' *talammi ana sinniš-ti* [*šuāti*] 14'' *tušazzaz ištēt ma*[*ššītu*(?)] 15'' *ša šīpāti arkīšu tana*[*ššī*(?)] 16'' *ana mērê damiq*

11'' [...] you put/insert (it). 13'' You wrap (it) 12'' in woad-dyed wool. 14'' You *administer* (it) 13'' to [that] woman. 15'' Afterwards *you app*[*ly* (*it*) *as*(?)] 14'' a su[ppository] 15'' with (undyed) wool. 16'' It is good for pregnancy (i.e. getting pregnant).

17'' *kadānu ša* ... [...] 18'' *erib tâmti* [...] 19'' *dām erēni inzarû* 20'' *ina šīpāti qunā*[*tā*]

17'' (*You wrap*) *kadānu*-plant whose ... is [...], 18'' 'sea locust' (shrimp?), [...] 19'' cedar 'blood', (and) *inzarû*-aromatic 20'' in woad-dyed wool.

Ms. a rev. breaks; ca. two lines lost

Notes

Lines 5'–6': For the verb *parāmu* "to rend, to slice through" (probably an Aramaic loan), see CAD P, 161a. CAD (ibid.) quotes our present passage, but reads 1 *šiqil ballukka* [(x)] in line 5', not accepting Finkel's restoration ⸢*sa*⸣-[*pan*] at the end of the line. There are traces of one more sign following ^{šim}MUG, however, which fit the sign SA. There are other attestations of the sequence ^{šim}MUG *sa-pan/pa-an* (see Finkel (2000, 154 Text 3, note on line 3, as well as Texts 5, 8, 10). Following a suggestion by F. Köcher, Finkel (ibid., 154) identifies the term *sapān*(*u*) as a loanword from Aramaic *s'pwn*, corresponding to Greek *sapōn* and Latin *sapo* "soap" (also SAD S, s.v. *sapān(u)* "soap(plant)"; differently CAD S, 158 s.v. *sapannu* sub c, marked as "obscure"). The term may itself refer to an alkaline plant, but in all instances known to me, *sapān* is used to qualify a preceding ingredient. In most cases, this is *ballukku*-aromatic, an unidentified shrub or tree yielding a resinous substance used in medicine. However, *sa-pan* similarly follows the *maštakal*-plant (soapwort) in Text 5 obv. 1' edited by Finkel (2000, 161). For *ballukku sapān*, see also BM 42507 obv. 4 and duplicates (text E.2.1); SpTU 5, No. 253 rev. 6 (text E.2.6); Finkel 2000, 163 Text 10 rev. 26; UET 4, Nos. 146: 3, 147: 11. Perhaps, *ballukku sapān* refers to a compound of a soapwort plant and the resin of *ballukku*-plant, or the substance yielded by this plant was "soap-like".

Line 7': Finkel (2000, 170) proposed a differing reading for this line: *ana*? *saḫ*!*-le-e šá-at-t*[*ì* ...] "[you ... (it)] in that *saḫlû*", presuming that the lost beginning of the obverse already mentioned the processing of the *saḫlû*-plant. However, *saḫlû*-plant as an ingredient in medical recipes is sometimes followed and qualified by adjectives in the fem. plural, such as *pāṣāti* "crushed", *ṭēnēti* "milled, ground", *sīkāti* "pulverized", *qalâti* "roasted" or *lā napâti* "not sifted", see CAD S, 64b sub 2c. Usually, *saḫlû*-seeds are meant in such cases. Moreover, the word *ša* following *saḫlû* in line 7' suggests that a relative clause follows. Therefore, a stative form of *napû* may have stood in the gap. The sign DIŠ at the beginning of line 7' most likely stands for the numeral 1, but by mistake the scribe omitted the measurement GÍN "shekel" after the number.

Line 12'': The word *qunātu* (or *qunātā*; eSAD) is an Aramaic loanword (related to *qān'ā* / *qanā'* "woad", referring to the blue dye *Isatis tinctoria*). The apparently occurs as a variant of the corresponding Akkadian term *uqnâtu*, which designates a plant and the pigment it yields (woad) as well as the wool dyed with the pigment, see von Soden 1968, *OrNS* 37, 264: 123; Finkel 2000, 170 n. rev. 2', 11'; see also the commentary BM 59607 obv. 6' (Frazer 2017, CCP 4.2.Q), equating Ú.ZA.GÌN.NA with *šam-mu qu-na-a-tú*, which points to the equation of *qunātu* with *uqnâtu*. For the association of *qunātu*-woad with the colour of the *rapādu*-plant, see also Abusch and Schwemer 2016, CMAwR 2, text 7.24 line 12, with note on line 4.

Lines 14''–15'': At the beginning of line 14'', I propose to read the sign sequence *tu-šá*-ÁŠ as *tu-šá-zíz/zaz*$_{x}$ as a Š-stem form of the verb *i/uzuzzu*, which can have the meaning "to provide, to make available (for someone)" (CAD U/W, 391 s.v. *uzuzzu* sub 27). However, a durative form *tu-šá-zaz*$_{x}$ would be expected rather than a preterite form *tu-šá-zíz*. Cf. Finkel 2000, 170 note on rev. 4'.

The following restoration 1-*et ma*[*š-ši-tú*] "one sup[pository]" seems plausible given the mention of wool in line 15". The verbal form *tana*[*ššī*] from *našû* "to wear, to apply" corresponds well with the cognate word *maššītu*. In similar passages, however, the patient is usually the subject/agent, so we may have to interpret the verb as a 3rd person sg. form with the prefix *ta-*.

Line 16'': I interpret the concluding purpose label in line 16'' as *ana mērê damiq* "it is good (i.e. useful, effective) for (promoting) pregnancy" (i.e. getting pregnant) rather than *ana mērê dummuqi* "to make pregnancy easier", as proposed by Finkel

2000, 169, 171. For the label *ana* ... *damiq*(SIG_5) "it (a drug, prescription) is useful/good for ..." in medical texts and beyond, see also Steinert 2015, 116–118.

Line 17'': CDA^2, 140 and eSAD list a word *kadānu* referring to a rush-like plant. This plant is attested once more in BAM 379 iv 13 // SpTU 3, No. 106 rev. 2 (manuscripts of the plant description text *Šammu šikinšu* where the plant is recommended for rectal disease; see Stadhouders 2011, *JMC* 18, 37; 2012, *JMC* 19, 17). The entry in question reads: "The wool-bearing *pappānu*-plant: its name is *kadānu*-plant" (^{ú}*pap-pa*$^!$*-a-nu* SÍG.MEŠ ÍL ^{ú}*ka-da-nu šum-šu*). The plant *pappānu* is otherwise unknown. It is probably not identical with the plant name PA-PA-*a-nu* that was read as *papānu* in AHw 823b. The latter is now usually understood as a pseudo-logographic writing for the plant *arariānu* (cf. CAD A/2, 232–233; CAD P, 106a discussion).

The following sequence *šá e-da*(-)*šú* is difficult to elucidate. Perhaps it should be understood as an infinite *e/idû* "(the *kadānu*-plant), knowledge of which is [...]." But alternatively, *e-da* relates to *ēdu* "solitary", which sometimes forms an attribute to plant names. Otherwise, one might expect a descriptive phrase referring to a specific feature or part of the *kadānu*-plant.

B.2.4 BM 42587+: Tampons for Promoting Fertility and Other Purposes

This fragmentary tablet with a small collection of prescriptions belonging to the 81-7-1 collection of cuneiform texts in the Babylonian collection of the British Museum was first edited by Finkel (2000, Text 15), together with a group of medical and magico-medical texts (a "medical archive") which belonged together with the business archive of the Bēl-rēmanni family from Sippar (dating to the Achaemenid period) (see Jursa 1999). However, Finkel regarded the present text as atypical among the 81-7-1 medical texts and judged the script as of a later, perhaps Seleucid date. The exact provenience of the text therefore remains uncertain.

The prescriptions on the tablet appear to focus exclusively on tampons or suppositories. While the exact purpose of some of the prescriptions remains elusive, at least two of them can be shown to concern female health: one tampon could be used to stop bleeding, others for promoting fertility/conception (the purpose of the latter is specified once as "for opening up and getting pregnant").

The present text displays several distinctive features. Firstly, almost all the prescriptions use exact measurements of ingredients (shekels, grains). Secondly, the scribe used several playful or rare spellings and logographic writings (e.g., ^{na4}E-*ú* for ^{na4}*gab-ú* "alum"; NÍNDA for *aṣû/šūṣî* "to (make semen) sprout"). The prescriptions follow a structure common in other Late Babylonian texts, in which the purpose of the remedy is stated at the very end of the prescription instead of the beginning, and in which the remedies begin without any introductory statement. Typical features of recipes in medical compendia such as the label DIŠ KI.MIN "alternatively" highlighting alternative remedies for the same condition or purpose, or symptom descriptions beginning with DIŠ MUNUS/NA "If a woman/man" are missing in the preserved sections of ms. a. Moreover, several of the prescriptions seem to have been written down in an abbreviated form, in which most of the verbs providing instructions for preparation and application are omitted. In some of the prescriptions we find only a skeleton list of ingredients and a purpose statement. This may indicate that the text was written down from oral dictation rather than by copying a *Vorlage*.

List of Manuscripts

Siglum	Museum Number	Copy	Collation	Format; Ductus	Provenience
a	BM 42587 + BM 42640 + BM 43217 + BM 43287 + BM 43475 + BM 43812 (81-7-1, 347 + 401 + 981 + 1051 + 1239 + 1573)[287]	Finkel, *FS Lambert*, Fig. 22	Coll.	Single-column tablet in portrait format; Late Babylonian script; ca. 4th–3rd cent. BCE	Babylonia

287 Measurements: 5 cm x 7.5 cm x 2 cm.

Overview

i'	Prescription for stopping bleeding (tampon) a obv. 1'–4'	...]1'–4'
ii'	Prescription for promoting pregnancy(?) (suppository) a obv. 5'–8'	5'–8'
iii'	Prescription for promoting pregnancy(?) (tampon) a obv. 9'–10'	9'–10'
iv'	Prescription for promoting pregnancy(?) (tampon) a obv. 11'–lo. e. 3	11'–18'
v'	Prescription for promoting conception (tampon) a rev. 1–8	19'–26'
vi'	Prescription (tampon) a rev. 9–13	27'–31'
vii'	Fragmentary prescription a rev. 14–15	32'–33'[...

Previous Edition and Discussion

Finkel 2000, *FS Lambert*, 168–169 Text 15 (transliteration)
Electronic Babylonian Library (eBL) (https://www.ebl.lmu.de/library/BM.42587)

Transliteration

Beginning of ms. a obv. (about one line) lost

1' a obv. 1' ⸢1⸣ GÍN ⸢^{ú}⸣[x x x x x x x x x x x]

2' a obv. 2' 1 GÍN ^{ú}[x x x x x x x x x x]

3' a obv. 3' SUR-*at* [K]I$^{?}$ ⸢Ì.GIŠ⸣ ⸢UD.DU⸣ ⸢2⸣ ⸢1/2$^{?}$⸣ ⸢GÍN⸣ ⸢ILLU⸣ x[(x)]

4' a obv. 4' 1 GÍN ⸢Ì⸣.[UD]U SUMUN 1/2 NINDA KURUN$^{!}$.NAM *ina* ^{síg}ÀKA *šá* MÚD KUD-*s*[*i*]

5' a obv. 5' 1 GÍN *ḫu-ṣab* ILLU 2 GÍN EŠ$_{22}$ 2 GÍN *ni-nu-ú*

6' a obv. 6' 2 GÍN KU.NU.LUḪ 2 NINDA ^{ú}*zi-bu-ú*

7' a obv. 7' 2 NINDA *ka-mu-nu ina* 3 GÍN ILLU 3 GÍN Ì.UDU SUMUN

8' a obv. 8' ḪI.ḪI *šá* NÍNDA ⸢NUMUN$^{?}$⸣-*rù*

9' a obv. 9' ^{ú}*qut-ri* Ú BABBAR ^{na4}E-*ú mál-ma-liš*

1' a obv. 10' *ina* ^{síg}ÀKA *šá* NÍNDA

11' a obv. 11' 1 GÍN ⸢^{šim}⸣GÚR.GÚR 1 GÍN ^{ú}MAŠ.TAB.BA

12' a obv. 12' 1 GÍN ⸢^{ú}⸣KUR.KUR 1 GÍN NAGA.SI 1 GÍN MUN

13' a obv. 13' 1 GÍN [^{ú}KUR].RA 1 GÍN ⸢*zi*⸣-*bu-ú* 1 GÍN LI

14' a obv. 14' ⸢1⸣ ⸢GÍN⸣ [x x x 1 GÍN] ⸢^{ú}⸣*ak-tam* 1 GÍN ^{na4}*gab-u*

15' a obv. 15' [1 GÍN x x x 1 GÍ]N URUDU SUMUN *ša-ḫi-it-tu*$_4$

16' a lo. e. 1 [1 GÍN x x x 1 GÍN MÚD] ^{giš}EREN 1 GÍN Ì.UDU SUMUN

17' a lo. e. 2 [x x x x x x x DIŠ-*n*]*iš* ḪI.ḪI *ina* ^{síg}ÀKA

18' a lo. e. 3 [NIGIN-*mi* x x x x x x]x

19' a rev. 1 [..........................] ⸢30?⸣ ^{giš}LI

20' a rev. 2 [................. ^{g}]^{iš}ḪAB 30 *ak-tam*

21' a rev. 3 15 Š[E.................. 3]0? *ka-lab* DINGIR.MAḪ$^{!?}$

22' a rev. 4 30 ^{ši}[^{m} ....] 15 ŠE NAGA.SI

23' a rev. 5 20 ILL[U x] ⸢x x⸣ 30 ^{ú}*zi-bu-ú*

24' a rev. 6 25 ŠE Ú.NAM.TIN 3-*aš* ÀKA *uq-né-e*

25' a rev. 7 30 DIDA SIG$_5$ 3 GÍN ILLU

26' a rev. 8 30 Ì.UDU ⸢SUMUN⸣ 15 DUḪ.LÀL *šá* BAD *u* PEŠ$_4$

27' a rev. 9 2 GÍN KU.NU.LUḪ.HA 1 GÍN ^{ú}*zi-bu-ú*

28' a rev. 10 30 ^{ú}KUR.RA 30 ^{ú}*ka-*⸢*mu*⸣*-nu* 30 NAGA.SI

29' a rev. 11 15 ŠE $^{\text{na4}}$[*ga*]*b-*⸢*ú*⸣ ⸢15⸣ ⸢ŠE⸣ Ú.NAM.TIN

30' a rev. 12 3-*aš* À[KA x x x x x *ina* MÚD] ^{giš}EREN

31' a rev. 13 ḪI.ḪI [............ *šá* ....]

32' a rev. 14 1 GÍN ^{ú}[......................]

33' a rev. 15 x x [...........................]

Ms. a rev. breaks; remainder (one or two lines) lost

Bound Transcription and Translation

Beginning of ms. a obv. (about one line) lost

$^{1'}$ *ištēn šiqil* ...[... ...] $^{2'}$ *ištēn šiqil* ...[... ...] $^{3'}$ *taṣaḫḫat* [*itt*]*i*(?) *šamni elli*(?) *šina zūz* (*šiqil*) *ḫīl* ...[...] $^{4'}$ *ištēn šiqil lipî labiri mišil akal*(?) *kurunni ina itqi ša dāmi parāsi*

$^{1'}$ a shekel of [...]-plant, [... ...], $^{2'}$ a shekel of [...]-plant, [... ...] $^{3'}$ you press (it) out. [(You mix it) wit]h(?) pure(?) oil, two and a half(?) shekels of [...]-resin, $^{4'}$ a shekel of old tallow (and) half of a tenth litre of beer. (You administer it) in a wad of wool. (It is good) for stopping the blood.

$^{5'}$ *ištēn šiqil ḫuṣāb ḫīli šina šiqil šiqdu šina šiqil nīnû* $^{6'}$ *šina šiqil tīyatu šina šiqil zibû* $^{7'}$ *šina akal*(?) *kamūnu ina šalāšat šiqil ḫīli šalāšat šiqil lipî labiri* $^{8'}$ *tuballal ša šūṣî*(?) *zēri*

$^{8'}$ You mix $^{5'}$ one shekel of small (pieces of solid?) resin, two shekels of almonds, two shekels of *nīnû*-plant, $^{6'}$ two shekels of *tīyatu*-plant, two shekels of black cumin, $^{7'}$ (and) a fifth of a litre of *kamūnu* (cumin) with three shekels of resin(?) (and) three shekels of old tallow. $^{8'}$ (It is good) for *letting the seed sprout*(?) [i.e. promoting the growth of the foetus from semen?].

9' *qutri šammu peṣû gabû malmališ* 10' *ina itqi ša šūṣî(?)*

9' (You wrap and administer) *qutru*-plant, 'white drug', (and) alum in equal amounts 10' in a wad of wool. (It is good) for *letting (the seed) sprout(?)*.

11' *ištēn šiqil kukru ištēn šiqil maštu(?)* 12' *ištēn šiqil atā'išu ištēn šiqil uḫūlu qarnānû ištēn šiqil ṭābtu* 13' *ištēn šiqil [nī]-nû ištēn šiqil zibû ištēn šiqil burāšu* 14' *ištēn šiqil [... ištēn šiqil] aktam ištēn šiqil gabû* 15' *[ištēn šiqil ... ištēn ši]qil erû labiru šaḫittu* 16' *[ištēn šiqil ... ištēn šiqil dām] erēni ištēn šiqil lipû labiru* 17' [... ... *ištē*]*niš tuballal ina itqi* 18' *[talammi ... ...]*...

17' You mix [toget]her 11' one shekel of *kukru*-plant, one shekel of *maštu*-plant, 12' one shekel of *atā'išu*-plant, one shekel of salicornia, one shekel salt, 13' one shekel of *nīnû*-plant, one shekel of black cumin, one shekel of juniper, 14' [one shekel of ..., one shekel] of *aktam*-plant, one shekel of alum, 15' [one shekel of ..., one shek]el of old copper (having) a *patina*, 16' [one shekel ..., one shekel] of cedar ['blood'], one shekel of old fat, 17' [... ...], 18' [you wrap (it)] 17' in a wad of wool. 18' [... ...].

19' [... ...] 30(?) *burāšu* 20' [... ...] *ḫûratu* 30 *aktam* 21' 15 *uṭṭat* [... ...] 30 *kalab Bēlet-ilī(?)* 22' 30 [... ...] 15 *uṭṭat uḫūlu qarnānû* 23' 20 *ḫīl* [...] ... 30 *zibû* 24' 25 *uṭṭat šammi balāṭi šalāš itqāti(?) uqnê* 25' 30 *billat našpi šalāšat šiqil ḫīlu* 26' 30 *lipû labiru* 15 *iškūru ša petî u erî*

19' [... ...], thirty(?) (grains of) *burāšu*-juniper, 20' [... ... (grains of)] *ḫûratu*-plant (madder), thirty (grains of) *aktam*-plant, 21' fifteen grai[ns of ..., ...], thirty (grains of) 'dog of Bēlet-ilī'-*plant*(?),22' thirty (grains of) [...-aromatic, ...] fifteen grains of salicornia, 23' twenty (grains) resin(?) of [...], thirty (grains of) black cumin, 24' twenty-five grains of 'plant of life', three wads(?) of blue (wool), 25' thirty (grains) of *billatu*-substance for (making) *našpu*-beer, three shekels of resin(?), 26' thirty (grains of) old tallow, fifteen of wax. (A suppository) for opening and getting pregnant.

27' *šina šiqil tīyatu ištēn šiqil zibû* 28' 30 *nīnû* 30 *kamūnu* 30 *uḫūlu qarnānû* 29' 15 *uṭṭat gabû* 15 *uṭṭat šammi balāṭi* 30' *šalāš itq[āti(?) ... ina dām] erēni* 31' *tuballal [... ša ...]*

27' Two shekels of *tīyatu*-plant, one shekel of black cumin, 28' thirty (grains?) of *nīnû*-plant, thirty of *kamūnu*-plant, thirty of salicornia, 29' fifteen grains of ... alum, fifteen grains of 'plant of life' – 30' (ingredients for) three wa[ds of ... ...]. 31' You mix (the ingredients) 30' [with] cedar ['blood']. 31' [...]. (It is good) for ... ...].

32' *ištēn šiqil* [... ...] 33' ... [... ...]

32' One shekel of [...]-plant, [... ...], 33' ... [... ...]

Ms. a rev. breaks; remainder (one or two lines) lost

Notes

Line 3': At the end of the line, perhaps restore ILLU B[ULUḪ], "resin of *baluḫḫu*-aromatic" (^{šim}BULUḪ), which is often used in prescriptions for suppositories. For the signs preceding ILLU, Finkel (2000, 168) read ⌈*a*?-*na*?⌉ 1 GÍN ILLU (corresponding to his copy on p. 169). But collation of the tablet as well as context leads me to suggest a different reading (2 1/2 GÍN ILLU).

The logogram UD.DU following Ì.GIŠ "oil" in line 3' only makes senses as an attribute to Ì.GIŠ (i.e. an adjective rather than a verb). However, the more common reading as ḪÁD.DU (for *ablu* "dried") seems to be excluded here. The Sumerogram UD.DU is also attested in lexical lists as an equivalent for the Akkadian terms *ellu*, *ebbu*, *namru* "pure, shining" (MSL 15, 40; Diri I 188, cited CAD E, s.v. *ellu* lex. section), which are common attributes of *šamnu* "oil", albeit usually written with more common logograms (KÙ, SIKIL, etc.). See CAD Š/1, 328 s.v. *šamnu* sub j; CAD E, 103 s.v. *ellu* sub 1a-2'.

Before Ì.GIŠ, the restoration of KI (for *itti* "with") is tentative. Alternatively, there might be enough room for restoring [1 GÍ]N "[one shek]el (pure oil)".

Line 4': The sign NÍG before KURUN.NAM was omitted in Finkel's transliteration (2000, 168: line 5) but copied correctly on p. 169 Fig. 22. The Akkadian reading of the measurement NÍG (or NINDA), probably standing for a 1/10 of a litre, is uncertain; the rendering as *akalu* is therefore given here with a question mark.

Line 5': The meaning of the first ingredient *ḫuṣāb* ILLU (never followed by a plant name) is uncertain. Perhaps small pieces of solid (rather than liquid) resin or gum are meant. The expression is also attested with a measurement in BM 38624+ line 64''' (text A.2.1, *ḫu-ṣa-bu* ILLU, prescription to induce the menses) and in K. 8678+ rev. 11' (text A.1.4 line 32'', remedy to induce the lochia), in a fully syllabic rendering (*ḫu-ṣab ḫi-li*). In lines 7' and 25' of ms. a, the logogram ILLU "resin" is likewise not followed by the name of a specific resinous plant. The text seems to be abbreviated here.

Finkel (2000, 168) reads the second ingredient in line 5' as ŠAKIRA (URU/KAxGU) for the *šakirû*-plant, but the sign in question looks like LAMxKUR = $EŠ_{22}$ for *šiqdu* / *šiqittu* "almond (tree)".

Lines 8' and 10': The reading of the signs following *šá* at the end of lines 8' and 10', both times indicating the purpose of the prescription, is tentative since it is without parallel so far. In line 8', we read NÍNDA ⌜NUMUN?⌝-*rù*; in line 10' only the sign NÍNDA seems to be repeated as the purpose statement of the next prescription, which suggests that the same purpose as in line 8' is repeated, albeit abbreviated. The Sumerogram NÍNDA occurs as a rare lexical equivalent for Akkadian *aṣû* "to come out" in the meaning "to sprout; to grow", said of seed (*zēru*) and plants (see, e.g., MSL 16, 236: 189 for the lexical equation; for this meaning of *aṣû* see CAD A/2, 356, 369 s.v. *aṣû* lex. section and sub 2j-2'). My interpretation of the expression is inspired by the metaphorical language of an incantation to treat infertility, in which "letting the seed" sprout refers to the woman's ability to let a foetus develop from the received male semen (see N. 4001: 8 and duplicate; text B.2.1). In this passage, it is said that *lā ālittu zēra ušēṣi* "the infertile woman let the seed sprout" (Š-stem of *aṣû*), which was previously poured into the "furrow" (another agricultural metaphor for the womb). In other words, the prescriptions in lines 5'–8' and 9'–10' would be concerned with treating infertility, expressed in metaphorical terms, reminiscent of the imagery found in incantations. See also Steinert 2017a, 316–318 for discussion.

Line 9': Since the logogram E stands for Akkadian *qabû* "to speak", the spelling ^{na4}E-*ú* is a playful orthography for ^{na4}*gab-ú* (*gabû*) "alum".

Lines 11'–18': The present prescription shares several ingredients with BM 48710 obv. 1'–9' (text E.2.4), and lines 11'–18' in ms. a may present a variant of the latter text. Both manuscripts mention *nīnû*-plant, *burāšu*-juniper, black cumin, cedar 'blood' and possibly old copper as ingredients. The purpose of the prescription is lost in both texts, but in both cases the remedy is inserted into the vagina.

Line 11': In BAM V p. xxix, F. Köcher proposed that MAŠ.TAB.BA is the logogram for the Akkadian disease name *ašû*, which has been accepted by later scholars (Scurlock and Andersen 2005, 720 n. 72; Bácskay and Simkó 2017, *JMC* 30, 40 note on BAM 494 obv. ii 30, see also ibid., ii 35, 39, 55). If this is correct, Ú.MAŠ.TAB.BA can be understood as "plant for *ašû*-disease", contra CAD M/1, s.v. *māštu* sub 3, reading Ú.MAŠ.TAB.BA as *šammi māšti* "herb for *māštu*-disease", or literally "twin plant". However, in Uruanna II 168 (cited in CAD M/1, 395b s.v. *māštu* lex. sect.), the drug Ú *maš-tú/te* is equated with "seed of the *ašû*-disease plant" (NUMUN *šammi ašî*), which may suggest that Ú.MAŠ.TAB.BA could also be read *māštu*. The drug name *šammi ašî* is known from other texts, see CAD A/2, 477 sub 2; BAM 494 ii 36. For other attestations of Ú.MAŠ.TAB.(BA), see further BAM 379 iv 9 and BAM 240: 48' (text D.2.1).

Line 15': The word *ša-ḫi-it-tu*$_4$ qualifying URUDU SUMUN "old copper" at the end of the line is difficult. AHw 1232a, s.v. *šiḫittu* II (also *šaḫittu*) sees in the word *šiḫittu* a garden plant, while CAD Š/2, 415a s.v. *šiḫittu* tentatively regards the term as a feminine adjective, because it also serves as an attribute of (usually feminine) plant names such as *šambaliltu* (most attestations stem from lexical texts and from Uruanna). Its Sumerian correspondence is sur (also sur-sur or sur-ra), which may suggest an underlying meaning "pressed, to squeezed out" (Akkadian *ṣaḫātu*, *ṣaḫtu*, often said of oil, wine) or "to drip" (liquid) (Akkadian *ṣarāru*). However, since *erû* "copper" is a masculine noun, *šaḫittu* may mean something else in this context.

"Old copper" is attested as an ingredient in other medical texts (e.g. BAM 515 ii 27 (EYES), see Geller and Panayotov 2020, 131: 99' with note on p. 278. "Old copper" is also listed in Uruanna (III 476b), where mention is made of the technique of leaving it in the ground to erode: *epri* URUDU, SAḪAR.URUDU Ì.GU_7.E : URUDU SUMUN *šá qaq-qa-ru* GU_7-*šú* "copper dust, eroded 'copper dust': old copper which the soil has eroded". See also Uruanna III 514: KU URUDU Ì.GU_7.E URUDU SUMUN *šá qaq-qa-ru* GU_7-*šú*. Thus, one wonders whether *šaḫittu* is perhaps related to *šuḫtu* (SAḪAR.URUDU) "verdigris; patina (lit.

"copper dust)".[288] This may possibly be confirmed by BM 48710 obv.? i' 5' where the word *šaḫittu* occurs once more (written *šá-ḫi-tú*) in a remedy (for a tampon) that may form a variant of the present remedy (see text E.2.4 for discussion). There one can restore the passage in question as [URUDU SUMUN *šá*?] ⌜*šá*?⌝-*ḫi-tú* ŠUB "[old copper which] has produced *patina*".

Line 16': For old (= rancid) ox fat in the medical prescriptions, see e.g. Bácskay 2021a, *RA* 115, 166 §12b (used for a wad (*lippu*) for the ears); AMT 103 ii 20 (Ì.UDU GU_4 LIBIR.RA), cited in CAD L, 204a.

Line 21': Finkel (2000, 169) reads the last ingredient in this line *ka-lab* ᵈKIN.SIG, which is hitherto unattested. Furthermore, a deity ᵈKIN.SIG is likewise unknown. The term KIN.SIG usually corresponds to *kinsigu* "late afternoon; afternoon meal" (also *naptanu* and *naptan līlâti*, see CAD K, 387–388). For this reason, I tentatively suggest that the divine name should in fact be read DINGIR.MAḪ!. The whole expression is not attested elsewhere to my knowledge, but it seems reminiscent of parallel designations such as *kalab Šamaš* (lit. "hound of Šamaš"), or *kalab urṣi*, referring to insects or other animals. Note also the drug *kalab Gula* "dog of Gula" (Ú UR.GI_7 ᵈME.ME/ᵈ*Gu-la*, which is another name for the *būšānu*-plant (see CAD K, 61–62; Böck 2014, 131–132).

The measurement ŠE = *uṭṭatu* "grain" (= 1/20 g or 1/180 of a shekel) which occurs several times in the present and the following prescription of ms. a indicates the use of very small and exact quantities of ingredients, which is unusual.

Line 24': The reading 3-*aš* ÀKA *uq-né-e* improves Finkel (2000, 169), reading 3 *ina* ÀKA *uq-né-e* "three in a wad of lapis lazuli (wool)". The word *uqnû* "lapis lazuli" needs to stand for "blue wool" (*uqnâtu*, *qunātu*). This means that the ingredients listed in the prescriptions were distributed over three wads of wool, applied in three doses. Alternatively, one could read 3-*aš šibirti*(LAG) *uqnê* "three lumps of lapis lazuli", but this seems less likely in the present context.

Line 26': Finkel (2000, 169) reads the purpose statement concluding the prescription as *šá* ÚŠ *u* $PEŠ_4$ "for bleeding and pregnancy". But the reading BAD = *petû* "to open", referring to the removal of a blockage or closure of the womb hindering it from receiving the male semen, seems more likely in connection with $PEŠ_4$ "to become pregnant". The expression is paralleled in another treatment (suppository) to promote conception found in BM 42313+: 36 // BM 42333+ obv. 11 (Finkel 2000, 172 Text 17 and *infra* text A.2.2), which concludes: BAD-*ma ir-ri* "she will open up and become pregnant". See further BM 79061 obv. 3 (text A.2.8): *šá pa-te-e* [(*u* $PEŠ_4$?)], concluding a remedy to enable conception (also in obv. 18 and rev. 17'). For discussion, see also Böck 2013, 32; Steinert 2017a, 306–307.

Line 30': For the reading 3-*aš* ÀKA, see line 24' above.

B.2.5 BM 59710: A Remedy to Promote Conception

This fragment of a small tablet in landscape format preserves only the left side (presumably about half of the tablet is missing). It belongs to the Sippar collection of the British Museum's Babylonian Collection and was excavated there by Hormuzd Rassam. The physical features of the fragment and the form of the script resemble those of the medical archive from Sippar published by Finkel (2000) dating to the Achaemenid period, which includes several of such smaller tablets containing only one or a few prescriptions that can often be identified as student tablets. The present text however belongs to a different sub-collection (82-7-14) than the archive associated with Bēl-rēmanni identified by Jursa (1999) and Finkel (2000), which mostly belong to the 81-7-1-group. The present text offers a fragmentary recipe for conception, presumably for an ointment.

288 Another possibility is the noun *šaḫittu* (also *šiḫittu*), which is listed as a separate lemma in the dictionaries (AHw 1232, *šiḫittum* A; CAD Š/2, 415 s.v. *šiḫittu* A) and which means "clearing of obligation" ("Schuldbereinigung"), from the verb *šaḫātu* "to wash, rinse; to clear". In this case, *šaḫittu* may refer to old, but cleaned copper. M. Stol (personal communication) further suggests *šaḫittu* may refer to an exudation(?) of copper, with a connection to *šiḫṭu* "discard(ed)" (cf. CAD Š/2, 418a).

List of Manuscripts

Siglum	Museum Number	Copy	Collation	Format; Ductus	Provenience
a	BM 59710 (82-7-14, 4120)[289]	Pl. 26	Coll.	Fragment of a single-column tablet; Late Babylonian script; ca. 6th/5th cent. BCE(?)	Sippar

Overview

i	Fragmentary prescription for conception a obv. 1–rev. 1	1–8

Previous Edition and Discussion

–

Transliteration

1 a obv. 1 *ana* munusNU.PEŠ$_4$ *šu-r*[*i-i* ....]

2 a obv. 2 *šá* 1-*en* ITI *ina* x[..........................]

3 a obv. 3 *ù ku-ub-bu-*[*bu*? ....]

4 a obv. 4 1/2 GÍN KU *ni-i*[*p-ṣi*? ....]

5 a obv. 5 1/2 GÍN KU šiₗ[m ....]

6 a obv. 6 *ina* KÀŠ.ḪI.A [..............................]

7 a lo. e. 1 *šá* KA *ma*-x[................................]

8 a rev. 1 *ina* Ì.GIŠ ḪI.[ḪI ....]

Remainder of ms. a rev. left blank

Bound Transcription and Translation

[1] *ana lā erīti šūr*[*î* ... ...] [2] *ša ištēn arḫu ina* ...[... ...] [3] *u kubbu-*[*bu*(?) ... ...] [4] *zūz* (*šiqil*) *sīkti nip*[*ṣi*(?) ... ...] [5] *zūz sīkti* [... ...] [6] *ina šīnāti* [... ...] [7] *ša pî*(?) ...[... ...] [8] *ina šamni tubal*[*lal* ... ...]

[1] To enable a woman (who is) not pregnant to get preg[nant: ... ...] [2] which [...] for one month in [... ...] [3] and has been burn[ed(?) ... ...], [4] half a shekel powder of [*metal*] *fil*[*ings*(?), ...], [5] half a shekel powder of [...]-aromatic, [... ...] [6] in urine [... ...] [7] from the mouth(?) of [... ...] [8] you mix with oil, [... ...].

Notes

Line 1: For the same or similar purpose statements introducing remedies, see also BM 79061: 1; BAM 250 rev. 3; BM 42313+ obv. 8 and rev. 33 // BM 42333+: 5; STT 98: 2', 4' edited in this volume.

---

289 Measurements: 2.2 cm x 2.3 cm x 1.4 cm.

Lines 1–3: The passage following the purpose statement ("to let a woman who is not pregnant get pregnant") is difficult to interpret, but it is assumed here that this passage forms part of the prescription. Possibly, specific instructions for processing an ingredient are given in line 2, e.g. that this ingredient underwent a one-month preparation process (e.g. that it was put into a liquid for extraction).

Several restorations of the word following *ù* in line 3 are possible, e.g. *kubburu* "very thick" or *kubbutu* "very heavy" or *kubbubu* "burned, charred". For the latter word, see also BM 47491: 3, 13 (*infra* text A.2.6): "*atā'išu*-plant, which has been charred over a fire" (^{ú}KUR.KUR *šá ina* IZI *ku-ub-bu-ub-bu*).

Line 4: Possibly, the word *nipṣu* "(metal) filings, powder" should be restored here, cf. AHw 792a; CAD N/2, 247–248 esp. sub 2 for attestations in medical texts. Often the expression *nipiṣ erî* "copper powder" is encountered, see e.g., AMT 13/5 + AMT 14/5 obv. ii 7' (CRANIUM Tablet 3, see *NinMed Corpus*). Such particles were also ground into finer powder (KU, *sīktu*). As another possible reading, the word *nipšu* "combed wool" is neither excluded here.

Line 6: For urine in prescriptions for women's health matters, see e.g. BM 42313+: 18, 22 (text A.2.2); K. 8678+: 39'' (text A.1.4).

Line 7: If *šá* KA stands for *ša pî* "from the mouth", a reference to a vessel may have followed.

Line 8: The instruction points to the application of the remedy in the form of an ointment, as is elsewhere attested in treatments for fertility, see e.g. BM 79061: 1–4 (text A.2.8).

B.2.6 AO 4425A+B: A Ritual for Acquiring Offspring with a Prayer to the Moon God

This small single-column tablet in Late Babylonian script (consisting of two joined fragments A and B) was bought by the Musée du Louvre in 1909 from the Parisian antiquities dealer I. Elias Géjou. Its provenience is unknown. The reverse is partially left blank, and the text is not followed by a colophon.

The tablet contains a ritual to be performed if a woman is "delayed" (*ūtappil*, from *uppulu* "to make late; to delay") in "giving birth" (i.e. bearing children). No duplicate or parallel is currently known to the text. The ritual combined with a prayer to the moon god Sîn is performed by the specialist for the household head (i.e. the woman's husband) who beseeches the deity to grant him a son/heir (*aplu*). The text provides another source attesting to the central role of the moon god (beside the sun god Šamaš) in connection with childbearing. Thus, several birth incantations from the second and first millennium BCE invoke Sîn and Šamaš; there are also more formal prayers addressed to Šamaš from Nineveh, which ask for protection from the hazards of pregnancy and delivery (see *infra*, Chapter D). Remarkably, the woman or wife delayed in bearing children is not involved at all in the present ritual, in contrast to other rituals concerned with matters of pregnancy and other aspects of female reproductive life.

List of Manuscripts

Siglum	Museum Number	Copy	Collation	Format; Ductus	Provenience
a	AO 4425A+B[290]	Pl. 24–25	Coll.	Single-column tablet; Late Babylonian script	unknown (Babylonia)

Overview

i Ritual instructions 1–16
a obv. 1–16

290 Measurements: 6.5 cm x 10 cm x 1.5 cm.

ii Prayer to Sîn and closing instructions 17–27
a obv. 17–rev. 7

Previous Edition and Discussion

–

Transliteration

1 a obv. 1 BAD MUNUS *ina* Ù.TU *ú-tap-pi-il*

2 a obv. 2 ^{iti}BÁRA.ZAG.GAR U$_{4}$.14.KAM *i-na u*$_{4}$*-um* ^{d}30 *u* ^{d}UTU

3 a obv. 3 TÉŠ.BI IGI.DU$_{8}$.MEŠ-*ma di-in* KUR *i-din-nu*

4 a obv. 4 LÚ BI ⸢KA⸣.PÌRIG *ina* ÙR É KAŠ NINDA KURUM$_{6}$-*su*

5 a obv. 5 *ana* ^{d}30 *u* ^{d}UTU ⸢KÁDRA⸣(NÍG.ŠÀ) GIN$^{!?}$(KÁD) BÁḪAR *ina bi-ri*$^{?}$*-it*$^{!}$(šu)

6 a obv. 6 ^{d}30 *u* ^{d}UTU ⸢KURUN.NAM⸣ 3-*šú i-sar-raq*

7 a obv. 7 4 KEŠDA LI GAR-*an* ⸢1⸣ ⸢^{dug}⸣LA.ḪA.AN GA

8 a obv. 8 1 ^{dug}LA.ḪA.AN A ⸢DIRI$^{?}$⸣-*ma tu-ka-an*

9 a obv. 9 ^{dug}LA.ḪA.AN A ⸢Á$^{?}$⸣ ^{dug}LA.ḪA.AN GA

10 a obv. 10 *i-na* 150-*šú* G[IN]-*ma* LÚ BI *ina bi-ri-it*

11 a obv. 11 ⸢*ki-lal*⸣-[*la-an*$^{?}$ x *i*$^{?}$]-*za-ra-ma*

12 a obv. 12 7-*šú* ^{d}[^{ug}LA.ḪA.AN] ⸢A⸣ ⸢*tu*⸣-*šá-aq-qá-a-šú*

13 a obv. 13 ^{dug}L[A.ḪA.AN A GA D]Ù$^{?}$.A.BI

14 a obv. 14 ⸢*ta*$^{?}$⸣-[*tab-ba-ak*$^{?}$ LÚ BI KÁDR]A$^{?}$-*šú* SUM$^{?}$

15 a obv. 15 k[a$^{?}$ x x x x (x)]-*su-ma ana* IGI ^{d}30

16 a obv. 16 *t*[*a-az-za-az*$^{?}$ *ki-a-am* D]U$_{11}$$^{?}$.[GA$^{?}$]-*šú*

---

17 a obv. 17 ^{d}⸢30⸣ ⸢*na-an-na-ar*⸣ AN-*e at-ta*

18 a obv. 18 ⸢*e*$^{?}$*-da*$^{?}$*-na*$^{?}$⸣ ⸢*tap-pá*⸣-*a-am tu-šár-ša*

19 a obv. 19 *ana* ⸢*ša*$^{?}$-x-x⸣ *šu*$^{?}$*-šu-ri*

20 a obv. 20 ⸢*ta-nam-din*⸣ [(x) x] ⸢*tu*$^{?}$*-maš*$^{?}$⸣-*šar*

21 a rev. 1 *a-n*[*a-k*]*u an-ḫu šu-nu-ḫu* ÌR-*ka*

22 a rev. 2 *aš-šum* ⸢*ap-li*⸣-*ia u šu-mi-ia am-ḫu-ur-ka*

23 a rev. 3 *ina* IGI-*ka el-lim li-iz-za-ki-ir-ma*

24 a rev. 4 *šá ki-ni li-iz-zi-iz lu-ur-ši ap-la u šu-ma*

25 a rev. 5 *da-li-li-ka lu-ud-lul*

26 a rev. 6 3-*šú an-ni-a-am* DU$_{11}$.GA-*ma*

27 a rev. 7 *uš-ke-en ta-pa-ṭú-ra-nim*$^{?}$ KEŠDA DU$_{8}$-*ár*

Remainder of ms. a rev. left blank

Bound Transcription and Translation

1 *šumma sinništu ina alādi ūtappil* 2 *nisannu* U_4.14.KAM *ina ūm Sîn u Šamaš* 3 *ištēniš innammarū-ma dīn māti idinnū* 4 *amēlu šū āšipu ina ūr bīti šikara akla kurummassu* 5 *ana Sîn u Šamaš kadrâ ukannū(?!) paḫāru ina birīt(?)* 6 *Sîn u Šamaš kurunna šalāšīšu isarraq* 7 *erbet riksī burāši tašakkan ištēn laḫanna šizba* 8 *ištēn laḫanna mê tumallā(?)-ma tukân* 9 *laḫan mê idi(?) laḫan šizbi* 10 *ina šumēlīšu tu[kân]-ma amēlu šū ina birīt* 11 *kilal[lān ... i]zarrū!?-ma* 12 *sebîšu [laḫan] mê tušaqqāšu* 13 *l[aḫannī mê šizbi ka]lāma* 14 *ta[tabbak(?) amēlu šū kad]râšu inaddin* 15 *...[... ...]-ma ana maḫar Sîn* 16 *t[azzaz(?) kīam tu]šaqbāšu*

1 If a woman is delayed in bearing (offspring): 2 On the 14th day of the month Nisannu, when Sîn and Šamaš are seen together 3 and perform judgement for the land, 4 that man (whose wife is delayed in bearing) (and) the ritual specialist 5 *set up*(?!) 4 on the roof of the house beer (and) bread as his (the man's) food offering 5 (and) a greeting gift for Sîn and Šamaš. A potter 6 shall sprinkle *kurunnu*-beer three times 5 in between 6 Sîn and Šamaš. 7 You set down four bundles of juniper. You ⌜fill(?)⌝ one bottle with milk (and) 8 one bottle with water and set them down (on the ground). 9 You place the bottle with milk beside the bottle with water 10 on his (= the client's) left. Then that man 11 [st]rews(!?) [...] (in the area) between bo[th (bottles)]. Then 12 you lift up the b[ottle with] water for him(?) seven times. 13 (Then) you [pour out] all the b[ottle(s) with milk and water(?)], 14 (and) he gives his [gif]t(?). 15 [... you ...] him and facing Sîn 16 yo[u will stand(?) and have] him [spe]ak [as follows]:

---

17 *Sîn nannār šamê attā*
18 *ēdāna(?) tappâm tušarša*
19 *ana ... šūšuri*
20 *tanamdin [...] tumaššar(?)*
21 *an[āk]u anḫu šūnuḫu aradka*
22 *aššum aplīya u šumīya amḫurka*

23 *ina maḫrīka ellim lizzakir-ma*
24 *ša kīni lizziz lurši apla u šuma*

25 *dalīlīka ludlul*
26 *šalāšīšu anniam iqabbī-ma* 27 *uškên tapaṭṭurānim riksa tapaṭṭar*

17 "O Sîn, you are the light of heaven,
18 you let a lonely person acquire a companion,
19 to a ... 20 you give 19 *prosperity*(?),
20 you release(?) the [...].
21 I, your weary and exhausted servant,
22 have approached you because of my heir and offspring (lit. "name").
23 In your brilliant presence it shall be pronounced:
24 may (one) who is legitimate take up (his) position! Let me acquire an heir and offspring,
25 (then) I will praise your glory!"
26 He shall say thus three times. Then 27 he shall bow down. (Then) you (pl.) shall withdraw, (as) you (sg.) remove the ritual arrangement.

Notes

Line 1: The incipit was previously cited by R. Labat in his short article "Geburt" in *RlA* 3 (1957–1971), 178b; see also CAD U/W, 187a. In contrast to other interpreters who have understood the incipit in line 1 (*šumma sinništu ina alādi ūtappil* "if a woman is delayed in 'giving birth'") as referring to protracted delivery (e.g., Labat ibid., Scurlock 1991, 144 with n. 70), the present ritual is understood here as a response to a couple's prolonged childlessness, which in Mesopotamian medical texts is usually attributed to the woman's failure to conceive (since the verb *alādu* does not only mean "to give birth", but also "to bear (children)"). However, apart from or in addition to medical treatments promoting a woman's fertility, childless couples often sought divine help and intervention, because it could not be excluded that a man was punished for some wrongdoing by the gods (especially by his personal god) denying him offspring (see e.g. Steinert 2012a, 238, 398–399). Certain deities were known to possess the power to grant offspring and promote fertility, such as the moon god Sîn, the sun god Šamaš and the goddess Ištar (responsible for sexuality and fertility). See e.g. two rituals with prayers to Ištar, presumably performed for a woman who asks the goddess for offspring (Zgoll 2003, *Die Kunst des Betens*, 156–157

"Ištar 23", with line 9: *šu-ut-li-[mi-(in)-ni-m]a zēra*(NUMUN) *per'a*(NUNUZ) *lu-bé-li* "Grant me offspring, a descendant I want to *call my own* (*bêlu*)!"; ibid., 185 "Ištar 4", with line 19': *šur-ki-im-ma šuma*(MU) *u zēra*(NUMUN) *lu rēmu*(ARḪUŠ) *si-li-ti* "Grant me an heir (lit. name) and offspring, may my womb be a (fertile) womb!"). The requests share similarities with ms. a lines 22 and 24.

Lines 2–3: While the prayer in lines 17–27 is addressed only to Sîn, the offering is for the sun and moon god together (*ina ūm Sîn u Šamaš ištēniš innammarū-ma dīn māti idinnū* "on the day Sîn and Šamaš are seen together and perform judgement for the land"). The date on which the ritual is performed (the 14th day of Nisannu), is well-suited, as both celestial bodies can be seen in opposition on this day on the horizon (the full moon rises in the east when the sun sets in the evening, and it sets in the west when the sun rises the next morning). Since this is a monthly occurrence, the timing of the "judgement" in Nisannu must be related to the events of the New Year's Festival (the gods making decisions concerning things to come in the new year). For other healing rituals scheduled for the middle of the month when the full moon and sun are present together (often the 15th day is specified), see Reiner 1995, *Astral Magic*, 136–138; Stol 1992, 256; Schwemer 2010, *OrNS* 79, 498–499 ad lines 2–3; Abusch and Schwemer 2016, CMAwR 2, 289, 293 text 8.36 line 2 (also referring to Sîn and Šamaš deciding the fate of the population during their joint visibility); BAM 323: 93 (and dupl.; Scurlock 2006, No. 91: 5).

Both Sîn and Šamaš have a connection to childbirth and granting offspring and are addressed in other prayers relating to this matter. See e.g. a bilingual prayer to Utu/Šamaš from Nineveh requesting his aid in saving a woman in difficult childbirth (caused by witchcraft), see Abusch et al. 2020, CMAwR 3, text 5.6 and *infra* text D.1.8. Already in 2nd millennium BCE texts, we find the connection of Utu to the birth of the child, see e.g. Geller 1995, *ASJ* 17, 110: 112 for an incantation to Utu referring either to the mother in childbirth or the newborn child. In second and first millennium BCE birth incantations, the baby is often prompted to come out and see the light of the sun. In one Old Babylonian birth incantation (VS 17, 34; Wasserman and Zomer 2022, No. 12), both Šamaš and Sîn shed tears out of compassion for the woman/cow in difficult labour. The connection of the moon god to pregnant women is best reflected in the incantation and *historiola* about the Cow of Sîn (BAM 248 etc., see Veldhuis 1991 and *infra* text D.1.1); for discussion see also Steinert 2017b. Among first millennium BCE prayers, a close parallel to AO 4425A+B can be found in the prayer "Sîn 3", edited by Mayer 1976, 495ff. (cf. below).

Line 3: It is unclear whether the phrase "they perform judgement over the land" refers to a specific event in Nisannu; it might mean that sun and moon god, being visible together, can be approached by anyone who needs their help. Thus, Sîn and Šamaš are also said to make decisions for the people each month during the time of the full moon (see previous note for references). In the hemerological tradition, the 14th of Nisannu is indeed a favourable day for addressing both deities. See e.g. hemerologies for the 14th of Nisannu (KAR 178 ii 8–10 // KAR 176 ii 23ff.): KI.MIN *amēlu ana Sîn u Šamaš pāšu* [*ippuš*] / .../ KI.MIN *kurummatsu ana Sîn u Šamaš u Nin*[*gal ukânma maḫir*] "Ditto: a man should address Sîn and Šamaš ... Ditto, he shall set up his offering to Sîn, Šamaš and Ningal" (Labat 1939, 58). In the light of AO 4425, the sentence about approaching the deities should be positive; cf. KAR 177 rev. iv 40–45, iii 1–7.

There are also references to sun and moon god on the 14th day of Nisannu in the astrological reports of Assyrian court scholars. For instance, in Hunger 1992, SAA 8, No. 108–110, the Assyrian court scholar Akkullānu comments on the sign of sun and (full) moon seen together on the 14th day of the month, which is interpreted as a positive sign for the king and the land of Akkad, including divine favour. The same omen can be found in the reports SAA 8, No. 15 (report of Issar-šumu-ereš). In contrast, if sun and moon are not seen together on the 14th or 15th of Nisannu, it is a negative sign (forecasting a razzia of the enemy in the land and an uprising, see SAA 8, No. 25 (Issar-šumu-ereš); also ibid., No. 499). Cf. further SAA 8, No. 267, 378, 464.

Line 4: The use of the logogram KA.PÌRIG instead of lúMAŠ.MAŠ for the ritual specialist in a ritual text is a very rare occurrence. KA.PÌRIG is mostly attested in lexical lists as a learned term equated with Akkadian *āšipu*, and in the *Diagnostic Handbook* (see Labat 1951, 2; Heeßel 2001–2002, *AfO* 48–49, 28 (line 1 ms. D); Geller 2007b, *JMC* 9, 2–3; Geller 2010, 45ff.; Schmidtchen 2018b, 313 lines 2 and 5; Arbøll 2021, 129 fn. 6; Wasserman 2020, *BiOr* 77, 448, 451 ad line 26, possibly in the subscript of an Old Babylonian magical text). Geller (2018b, 38) regards the KA.PÌRIG as an archaizing title for a type of exorcist specifically concerned with the diagnostic-prognostic arts. It is further remarkable that in this ritual, client and specialist appear almost as equals in terms of their division of labour in the ritual.

Line 5: The signs look more like NÍG.ŠÀ (KÁDRA) than NÍG.PEŠ$_4$ (KÀDRA), which corresponds to Akkadian *kadrû* "gift" or *ṭātu* (*ṭa'tu*) "gift, payment; bribe", cf. CAD K, 32–33 lex. section; CAD Ṭ, 62–66. The writing NÍG.ŠÀ for KÁDRA is rare (cf. Borger 2004, MZL 446 No. 859).

The following sign KÁD in line 5 is tentatively interpreted as an error for GIN = *kânu* D ("to set up offerings, ritual arrangements"). For the Late Babylonian sign form of KÁD, cf. Figulla 1951, *Iraq* 13, 97 line 23). The logogram KÁD can stand for *kaṣāru* "to tie together; to collect; to assemble", but this usage of the logogram is only found in personal names. M. Stol (personal communication) proposed that the sign may be a faulty A that should have formed part of KÀDRA (NÍG.PEŠ$_4$), but we rather expect a verb such as "to set up" or "to place" here.

The participation of a potter ($^{(lú)}$BÁḪAR) in the ritual is unusual, but this profession may have been associated with birth and offspring since traditionally in Babylonian anthropogonic myths, gods shape human beings from clay (like a potter making vessels).

Lines 5–6: The emendation of *bi-ri-šu* to *bi-ri-it* is not entirely certain. The former could also be rendered "in between him(self), (Sîn and Šamaš)". Note though the occurrence of *ina bi-ri-it* below in line 10.

Lines 7–8: The bottles with milk and water used here as part of the offering may allude to the baby and to birth more generally (as suggested to me by M. Stol, personal communication).

Line 11: One expects a third person singular verbal form at the end of the line of which the client is the subject. The reconstructed form *[i]-za-ra-ma*, from *zarû* "to scatter, sprinkle", is problematic however, since *zarû* has a *u/u*-vocalization and is generally not used with the ventive. One may assume that the form *[i]-za-ra-ma* is an error for *izarrū-ma* "he sprinkles"; or alternatively, one could reconstruct a second person plural form *[ta]-za-ra-ma* referring to the client and the ritual specialist together. The object of the verb (perhaps flour or a similar substance given as an offering) is unfortunately lost in the gap.

Line 12: Since *šaqû* "to give to drink" is not attested in the D-stem, the verb here should be a D-stem of *šaqû* "to be high, elevated" (with the meaning "to lift up").

Line 18: See also STT 60: 10 (and dupls.); Mayer 1976, 503ff. "Šamaš 1" line 106: *eṭla*(GURUŠ) *ēda*(DILI) *tap-pa-a tu-šar-ši* "you (Šamaš) provide the lonely young man with a companion". Cf. CAD E, 27 s.v. *ēdēnu/ēdānu* "isolated, unattached, lone person" and *ēdēnû/ēdānû* (adj.) "single, solitary" (ibid., 27–28).

Line 19: From parallel prayers, we expect a reference to the bestowing of offspring by the deity, see e.g. "Šamaš 1" line 107 (Mayer 1976, 505): *ana la i-šá-ri ta-nam-din ap-lu* "to an impotent(?) one you give a son". The verb *šūšuru* (Š-stem of *ešēru*) also occurs in connection with easy childbirth in similar contexts, see e.g. "Sîn 3", edited by Mayer 1976, 495ff. (BMS 6: 37–70 // K. 16342 // LKA 52 // STT 57: 57–84 // STT 58: 2--52 // STT 59: 1–29), which mirror the purpose of the present prayer (to get offspring):

> [43] *a-šar at-ta ta-qab-bu-ú na-di-tum uš-⸢téš-šèr⸣* … [46] *šá ap-la la i-šu-ú tu-šar-šá-a* IBILA [47] *la a-lit-tum ina ba-li-ka* NUMUN *u me-re-e ul iṣ-ṣab-bat*
>
> [43] "Where you order it, a barren woman will give birth easily, … . [46] The one who has no heir, you let (him) get an heir; [47] without you, a barren woman will not take hold of semen and pregnancy."

Possibly, the form *šu-šu-ri* in line 19 should be analysed as the adjective *šūšuru* "righteous; straight", cf. BMS 2: 20; BMS 3: 16: *tuštešše**r** lā šūšura* "you set the unsuccessful one on a straight course"; cf. CAD E, s.v. *ešēru* sub 12c-3'. The verb *tanamdin* "you give" which follows in line 20 however suggests *šu-šu-ri* functions as the direct object. Thus, *šušūru* may here be a nominalized infinitive in the meaning "prosperity" or "success", in accordance with the meanings of *ešēru* Š ("to give success, put in order, set on a straight course").

Line 20: In prayers, the verb *(w)uššuru* "to release; to set free" occurs often with *ṣabtu* "captured one", *šallu* "prisoner/deported one" or *kasû* "bound one", see e.g. CAD U/W, 316 sub f.

Line 21: See CAD A/2, 119a; Mayer 1976, 70ff. for parallels and study of this formula.

Line 24: Compare for the phrase *ša kīni lizziz* the personal name *Kīnum-lizziz* "may an honest/correct/legitimate one stand up" (MDP 22, 84 rev. 10), referring to the name bearer (cf. CAD K, s.v. *kīnu* sub 2c and 3c). In the present line, *kīnu* refers to the hoped-for offspring (preferably a male heir). For personal names with *kīnu* "legitimate" (heir, son) see further Stamm 1939, *Namengebung*, 295ff.

Line 26: Note the Old Babylonian form *an-ni-a-am*.

Line 27: The form *ta-pa-ṭú-ra-nim* is a second person plural form with a ventive ending, which is unexpected. The form is irregular (the verb *paṭāru* "to untie, remove" normally has a *a/u*-vocalization, but G-stem durative forms such as *ipaṭṭur* are attested in Nuzi texts, cf. CAD P, 287a). In the present context, the plural form should address the client and the ritual specialist withdrawing from the scene of the ritual. Similar expressions with *paṭāru* in the meaning "to leave, withdraw, depart" are attested in ritual texts, see e.g. Maul 1994, 318: 41; 487: 44 (Namburbi rituals): TA IGI ^{d}UTU DU$_{8}$-*ma* "(when you have said this), you disengage from the presence of Šamaš (and depart)". See also CAD P, 297 s.v. *paṭāru* sub 9a-1'c'. For the form cf. YOS 10, 47: 61 (Old Babylonian omens): *bi-ra-at ālim*(URU) *i-pa-ṭa-ra-nim* "the fortified outposts of the city will desert". For removing (*paṭāru*) the ritual arrangement (*riksu*), see also CAD P, 290 sub 1h.

Chapter C
Bleeding, Menstruation and Pregnancy

C.1 Remedies to Stop Gynaecological Bleeding

The texts edited in this chapter attest to the continued importance of the topic of irregular haemorrhage and discharges in the gynaecological corpus of the first millennium BCE, as a continuation and extension of older textual traditions and magico-medical practices, especially incantations and different types of remedies (such as tampons/suppositories, amulets) devoted to this problem (e.g. Krebernik 1984, no. 37; Finkel 1980; Scurlock 1991; Rudik 2011: 332–336). From the mention of incipits concerned with gynaecological haemorrhage in the Assur Medical Catalogue (AMC), we know that in the Neo-Assyrian period remedies for this purpose had been collected within the gynaecological sections of a serialized medical compendium (see Steinert et al. 2018 for discussion, especially on AMC lines 112 and 118; cf. the Introduction in this book). Thus, AMC line 112 mentions treatments "for the case that a pregnant woman's blood flows" (DIŠ ^{munus}PEŠ$_4$ MÚD.MEŠ-*šá* DU-*ku*), which are listed as a topic of a treatise concerned with PREGNANCY/OFFSPRING (AMC lines 109–110, see especially section C.3 for texts associated with this treatise). The next section in AMC line 118 concerned with the topic BIRTH lists as the incipit of a tablet belonging to this section a phrase that resembles a line encountered in the Assur text BAM 235 (text C.1.1) edited here, concerned with stopping vaginal discharges (*šagû/sagû*) that are described as bright red (*pelû*); the term *sagû* is also encountered in Late Babylonian texts that deal with regulation the menses (see section C.2 of this book).

The texts dealing with abnormal bleeding during or outside of pregnancy are represented by tablets from Assur (BAM 235–236, BAM 237–239, KAL 7, No. 16), from Ashurbanipal's library at Nineveh (K. 263 + 10934, K. 8893, K. 20254, all of them written in Babylonian script and possibly imported from Babylonia), and by texts from Babylonia (BM 40152, FLP 1306, SpTU 4, No. 153). Of these texts, SpTU 4, No. 153 from Late Babylonian Uruk contained not only prescriptions for stopping bleeding, but another section concerned with difficult delivery (and may have been a collection of prescriptions for women), while the other texts focus, more or less, on the specific topic of stopping bleeding. BAM 237(+) from Assur is concerned with *naḫšātu* (bleeding during pregnancy) in particular, but it includes in its final column treatments for similar ailments characterised by abnormal discharges. Remedies to stop abnormal bleeding or recipes for related conditions, such as the loss of amniotic fluid, were also included in multi-thematic handbooks on women's diseases and in smaller extract tablets, which are edited in other sections of this book (e.g. BM 38624+, BM 42313+, BM 51246+, BM 42587+). Remedies to induce (menstrual) bleeding are discussed in section C.2.

The prescriptions to stop gynaecological bleeding reflect both continuity and variation in the applied ingredients and practices. The most prominent type of remedy consists in tampons (wads of wool or less often, pieces of linen) filled with different substances and inserted into the vagina, but also potions, ointments and amulets are found repeatedly in the prescriptions. The ingredients of remedies against bleeding stem from plants, minerals as well as animals, and some of these ingredients are known to have haemostatic or astringent properties. Several of the ingredients used in context of stopping gynaecological bleeding in Mesopotamian texts are also encountered as remedies for similar purposes in other ancient medical traditions (Steinert 2012b; 2021a, 62ff.). Some recurring conspicuous ingredients in the prescriptions edited in section C.1 are shells (or cowrie snails), which were classified as "stones" rather than animals in Mesopotamian texts (the terms are usually written with the classifier for minerals, na$_4$), eggshells (of birds such as ostrich and dove), animal horn (of cow, goat, gazelle, stag, billy goat) as well as animal blood (of *ḫurru*-bird, billy goat). Several of the ingredients to stop gynaecological bleeding are also recommended in texts dealing with renal and rectal diseases for similar conditions (blood in the urine, bleeding from the anus, discharge), such as ostrich eggshells or shells (Geller 2005a). Some of these ingredients may have been effective. It is significant here that shells, eggshells and animal horns contain as main component calcium carbonate, which in modern trials has been shown to have haemostatic properties that improve wound healing (e.g. He et al. 2021).

In addition to empirical knowledge of specific pharmaceutical properties, the uses of some ingredients to stop gynaecological bleeding may have been bolstered by other perceivable properties (e.g., colours) as well as by analogical reasoning and cultural associations (such as the association of shells with female genitals and fertility). Moreover, the preparation procedures of the remedies against bleeding give us important hints about the assumed effect the remedies were expected to unfold (Steinert 2020). Thus, ingredients in Mesopotamian remedies against bleeding regularly had to be

https://doi.org/10.1515/9781501506475-006

roasted or desiccated, so as if to enact their hoped-for effect of "drying out" excessive moisture inherent in the blood flow. These logics underlying the uses of specific ingredients and their properties are also occasionally hinted at in the text themselves (see e.g. text C.1.10).

C.1.1–1.2 BAM 235 and BAM 236: Irregular Bleeding

BAM 235 and 236 are Neo-Assyrian fragments of two one-column tablets from Assur, which contain recipes and rituals for women suffering from haemorrhage. Both BAM 235 and 236 start with medical recipes for suppositories and potions, followed by the incantation "Her blood is a red river" (*nār sāmti dāmša*), which is to be recited over knots that are part of an amulet of coloured wool and *ḫûratu*-plant (a plant used also for dyeing, probably madder), to be worn by the woman around her hips. BAM 236 closes with another incantation. The recently published fragment KAL 7, No. 16 offers a third related Assur fragment, which may have formed part of BAM 235 (see text C.1.3).

C.1.1 BAM 235: Treatments to Stop a Woman's Blood from Assur

The fragment begins with prescriptions to stop haemorrhage, designated here as *šagû* or *šugû* (lines 1, 7). It is proposed here is that the word *šugû* qualified by *pelû* "bright red" designates a kind of bloody discharge and is a variant of the word *šagû*. The term *šagû* (in Assyrian texts) must be identical with the word *sagû* found in Babylonian medical texts and in a Late Babylonian medical commentary from Uruk (SpTU 1, No. 39: 6′ff.) as a word for female blood (equated with *dām ardati* "the blood of a young woman") and probably a term for the menses in this period (see the Introduction for further discussion).

A further parallel to BAM 235 obv. 1 and 7 is found in the Assur Medical Catalogue line 118, which lists as the title of a tablet belonging to a section within a therapeutic series concerned with women (BIRTH) the phrase: [DIŠ MUN]US *šá-gu-šá p*[*e-lu-ú*?] "[If a woman]'s *menstrual discharges* [are bright]-red(?)". This passage could alternatively be reconstructed according to the beginning of BAM 235: 1 and 7 (see Steinert et al. 2018, 218, 275 and below). The meaning "menses" or menstrual blood for *sagû* is also indicated by a few first millennium BCE texts with recipes to induce *sagû* that has stopped to occur (see e.g. BM 54587 + 73802 rev.(?) 9′; text C.2.3).

List of Manuscripts

Siglum	Museum Number	Copy	Collation	Format; Ductus	Provenience
A	VAT 13724	BAM 235	Coll.	Fragment of a single-column tablet; Neo-Assyrian script; 8th/7th cent. BCE	Assur, N4 library[291]
B	A 203	BAM 236	Coll.	Fragment of a single-column tablet; Neo-Assyrian script; 8th/7th cent. BCE	Assur, N4 library

Overview

i	Prescription to stop bleeding (*sagû/šagû*) (tampon) A obv. 1–3	1–3
ii	Ritual and prescription to stop bleeding (potion) A obv. 4–6	4–6
iii	Prescription to stop bleeding (*sagû/šagû*) (suppositories/tampons) A obv. 7–9	7–9

291 Pedersén 1986, 67 No. 314.

iv	Akkadian incantation to stop bleeding: *nār sāmti dāmša* A obv. 10–13 // B rev. 1′–5′	10–13
v	Incantation rubric A obv. 14 // B rev. 6′	14
vi	Prescriptions for a knotted string, tampon and amulet to stop bleeding A obv. 15–18 // B rev. 7′–9′	15–18
vii	Fragmentary A obv. 19–20	19–20[...

Previous Edition and Discussion

Kirsch 1996, 94–96
Collins 1999, 181–182 (edition of BAM 235: 10–13 // BAM 236 rev. 1′–5′)
Scurlock 2014a, 585–587
Scurlock 2014b, 110 (translation of BAM 235: 10–16 // BAM 236 rev. 1′–9′)
Steinert 2012b, 72 n. 33
Steinert 2013, *JMC* 22, 5ff. (discussion)
CDLI P285321 (photo and transliteration)
BabMed Corpora (https://www.geschkult.fu-berlin.de/e/babmed/Corpora/BAM-3/BAM-3_-235) (transliteration)
Infra text C.1.2 (edition of ms. B)

Transliteration

1	A obv. 1	[DIŠ MUNU]S$^{?}$ *šu*$^{?}$*-gu-šá pe-lu-*[*ti* DU-*ku-ma* NU KUD-*su ana* KUD-*si*$^{?}$]
2	A obv. 2	[^{n}]^{a4}KUR-*nu* DAB SÚD *ina* ^{síg}ÀKA NIGIN-*mi ana* ŠÀ G[AL$_4$$^{!}$.LA-*šá* GAR-*an-ma*]
3	A obv. 3	[M]ÚD$^{!}$(PAP).MEŠ-*šá* K[UD-*su* (...)]
4	A obv. 4	[DIŠ] MUNUS ^{giš}TUKUL *ma*[*ḫ-ṣ*]*a-at* MÚD BURU$_5$.[ḪABRUD.DA^{mušen} ...]
5	A obv. 5	⸢^{ú}⸣NU.LUḪ.ḪA DIŠ-*niš* SÚD *ina* KAŠ NAG-*ši* [... *ana* ^{d}...]
6	A obv. 6	[NÍG].BA GAR-*an še-gu-ú i-šá-si-m*[*a* ....]
7	A obv. 7	[DIŠ MUNUS] ⸢*šá*$^{?}$⸣*-gu-šá pe-lu-ti* DU-*ku ni-iḫ-*[..........]
8	A obv. 8	[AN].ZAḪ ^{ú}NÚMUN 14 *rik-si* [...........................]
9	A obv. 9	[1.T]A.ÀM *ana* ŠÀ GAL$_4$.LA-*šá* GAR-*an* [.....................]
10	A obv. 10 B rev. 1′	[ÉN Í]D ^{na4}GUG MÚD-*šá a-tap* ^{na4}G[UG (...)] [........ ^{na4}G]UG MÚD-⸢*ša*$^{?}$⸣ *a-*⸢*tap*⸣ ⸢^{na4}⸣G[UG]
11	A obv. 11 B rev. 2′	[*ta*$^{?}$]*-mir-ti* ^{na4}GUG A.MEŠ [............] [.....................] ⸢A⸣.MEŠ *ub-ba-lu*
12	A obv. 12 B rev. 2′$^{cont.}$–3′	[*man*]*-nu liq-bi ana re-mi-ni-i* ^{d}A[MAR.UTU] *man-nu liq-b*[*i / ana r*]*e-mi-ni-i* ^{d}AMAR.UTU
13	A obv. 13 B rev. 4′–5′	[*t*]*a-mir-ti* ^{na4}GUG [...] [......... ^{n}]^{a4}GUG *li-is-ki-ru* ÍLDAG ^{na4}ZA.GÌ[N] / [^{ú}]*aš-la ub-bal*

A, B

14	A obv. 14	[K]A.INIM.MA MÚD MUNUS [KUD-*si*]
	B rev. 6′	[KA].INIM.MA MÚD MUNUS KUD-*si*

A, B ____

15	A obv. 15	[DÙ.D]Ù.BI SÍG BABBAR SÍG SA$_5$ DIŠ-*niš* NU.NU 7 KÉ[Š (...) KÉŠ]
	B rev. 7′-8′	[DÙ].DÙ.BI SÍG BABBAR SÍG SA$_5$ DIŠ-*niš* NU.NU / [7 K]A.KÉŠ ^{giš}ḪAB KÉŠ
16	A obv. 16	[*e-m*]*a* KÉŠ(“SAR”)-*ru* ÉN 7-*šú* ŠID-*n*[*u*] *ina* MUR[UB$_4$-*šá* KÉŠ-*ma ina-aš*]
	B rev. 8′$^{\text{cont.}}$-9′	*e-ma* KA.KÉŠ / [ÉN 7-*šú*] ŠID-*nu ina* MURUB$_4$-*šá* KÉŠ-*ma ina-aš*
17	A obv. 17	[x]x *ina* ^{síg}ÀKA *t*[*a-lam-mi*$^{?}$] x x[................................]
	B *omits*	
18	A obv. 18	[......] $^{\text{na4}}$KA.G[I.NA ....] x [...............]
	B *omits*	

A, B ____

19	A obv. 19	[x (x)]-ur/lik-ma MÚD x[.......................................]
20	A obv. 20	[x x]x DIŠ$^{?}$-*niš*$^{?}$ x[...]

Ms. A obv. breaks; remainder lost
Only traces of signs preserved on the reverse

Bound Transcription and Translation

[1] [*šumma sinništ*]*u šugûša*(?) *pelû*[*ti illakū-ma lā ipparrasū ana parāsi*(?)] [2] *šadânu ṣābitu tasâk ina itqi talammi ana libbi ū*[*rīša tašakkan-ma*] [3] *dāmūša ip*[*arrasū* (...)]	[1] [If a woman's] (*menstrual*) *discharges* [flow] with a bright red (colour) [and they cannot be stopped, in order to stop them(?)]: [2] you pound magnetic haematite, you wrap it in a wad of wool, [you insert it] into [her] va[gina. Then] [3] her [bl]ood will st[op ...].
[4] [*šumma*] *sinništu kakka ma*[*ḫṣ*]*at dām iṣṣūr* [*ḫurri* ...] [5] *nuḫurta ištēniš tasâk ina šikari tašaqqīši* [... *ana* ...] [6] *qīšta tašakkan šegû išassī-m*[*a* ... ...]	[4] If a woman is 'hit by a weapon' (i.e. has a haemorrhage), you crush blood of a par[tridge(?), ...], [5] (and) *nuḫurtu*-plant together, you give it to her to drink in beer, [... ...], [6] you present a gift [to deity ...], she utters a *šegû*-prayer an[d ... ...].
[7] [*šumma sinništu*] *šagûša pelûti illakū niḫ*-[... ...] [8] [*an*]-*zaḫḫu urbatu* 14 *riksī* [... ...] [9] *ištēnâ ana libbi ūrīša tašakkan* [... ...]	[7] [If a woman's] (*menstrual*) *discharges* flow with a bright red (colour), ...[... ...] [8] *anzaḫḫu*-frit(?), *urbatu*-rushes, [*you make*(?)] fourteen bundles [...], [9] you insert (them) [one] by one into her vagina [...].
[10] [ÉN *n*]*ār sāmti dāmša atap sā*[*mti*]	[10] [Incantation]: Her blood is a red (lit. carnelian-coloured) [riv]er, a red canal!
[11] [*ta*]*mirti sāmti mû ubbalū*	[11] The waters are carrying (away) the red [mea]dow!
[12] [*man*]*nu liqbi ana rēmēnî Marduk*	[12] Who shall speak to merciful Marduk?
[13] *tamirti sāmti liskirū adāra uqnâ ašla ubbal*	[13] Let them dam up the red meadow with *adāru*-wood(?), lapis lazuli (and) *ašlu*-rush, (so that) it (the meadow) will (then) dry up.
[14] KA.INIM.MA *dām sinništi parāsi*	[14] An [inc]antation for stopping a woman's blood.

15 DÙ.DÙ.BI *šīpāti peṣâti šīpāti sāmāti ištēniš taṭammi sebet kiṣrī ḫûrati takaṣṣar* 16 *ēma taktaṣru šiptu sebīšu tamannu ina qablīša tarakkas-ma inâš* 17 [...]... *ina itqi ta*[*lammi*(?)] ... [... ...] 18 [... ...] *šadâ*[*nu* ... ...] ...[... ...]

15 The procedure for it: you twine together white wool (and) red wool, you tie seven knots (of) *ḫûratu*-plant (into the string). 16 Wherever you have tied (a knot), you recite the incantation seven times. You bind (it) around her waist. Then she will get well. 17 Yo[u wrap ...] in a wad of wool [....], 18 [... ...] haema[tite(?) ... ...].

---

19 [...]... *dām* [... ...] 20 [...]... *ištēniš*(?) ...[... ...]

19 [...] ..., blood of [... ...] 20 [... you] ... together, [... ...]

Ms. A obv. breaks; remainder lost

Notes

Line 1: The upper edge of the tablet still indicated in Köcher's copy is slightly deteriorated today. The reconstruction of line 1 follows line 7, which seems to be parallel in wording, as well as the traces preserved on the old photo of BAM 235 in the possession of the Vorderasiatisches Museum (Ph.Ass. 4201). The colour term *pelû* "bright red" characterises the colour of blood beside *da'mu* "maroon, brown", cf. CAD P, s.v. *pelû* "red-hued"; Thavapalan 2020, 128–133. "Bright red" blood flowing from the nose occurs as a symptom in the *Diagnostic Handbook* (e.g. Tablet 16: 10, 55′, 77–78, Heeßel 2000, 172, 177, 179).

In BAM 235 obv. 3, MÚD.MEŠ "blood" is apparently used instead of *šugû* in the symptom description (for *dāmu* used in the plural, see also Stol 2021, *BiOr* 78, 437. In the present context, plurality may denote the intensity of the blood flow; for discussion see below text C.1.3 and *passim* in this chapter).

For interpretations of line 1 differing from the one suggested here, cf. AHw 853, reading logographic GU as *qû* ("Fäden")-*šá* ("von Gebärender"). In this vein, cf. also van Dijk 1975, *OrNS* 44, 59 n. 18, referring to a possible parallel for gu in BAM 235: 1, in a Sumerian birth incantation (JRL 24 E6+24: 4′), which speaks of the symptom gu-lá (threads hanging down?), in the context of a complication during delivery. Similarly, Scurlock 2014a, 586–587, who understands GU as "veins" (and translates the line "[If ...] her vein(s) [let flow] bright red (blood)").

Line 4: For the blood of *ḫurru*-bird (*iṣṣūr ḫurri*, "partridge(?)") in a similar potion to stop bleeding, see also K. 263+ obv. 8–10 (text C.1.5); SpTU 3, No. 84: 56–57 (text C.3.3). In the context of blood loss, the prescription of animal blood implies analogical reasoning (like cures like) or a restorative treatment. Compare also Geller 2005a, No. 35 (BAM 99): 30–32; BAM 152 iii 11–12 for bull's blood given to drink in a prescription against bleeding from the rectum. For blood as a remedy in Mesopotamian healing texts, see also Steinert 2023.

Line 6: Compare BAM 237 obv. i 9′ff., 12′, and 15′-16′ (text C.1.4), where a *šigû*-prayer (Assyrian *šegû*) is addressed to Ištar; CAD Š/2, 413b. For gifts to deities in connection with *šigû*-prayers see CAD Q, 276b, e.g. RAcc. 38 rev. 24; IVR Add. p. 10 to pl. 54 No. 2 obv.(!) 21, 36; cf. van der Toorn 1985, *Sin and Sanction*, 118; for references in prayers to gifts given to the deity, see also Mayer 1976, 153. Scurlock (2014a, 586) reads [NÍG].NA "censer" instead of [NÍG].BA (*qīštu*) "gift".

Line 7: The first sign ŠÁ copied by Köcher is not entirely certain, but the context clearly suggests *šá-gu-šá* (for *sagû*). The spelling *šu-gu-šá* in obv. line 1 appears to be a variant (cf. the discussion above). The form *pelûti* shows that *šagû* is constructed as a plural noun here.

Line 8: The reconstructed [AN].ZAḪ may have to be read [x] DÈ "[...] ashes" instead, followed by ^{ú}NÚMUN, i.e. "[x] ashes of *urbatu*-rush". Note the similar recipe in BAM 236 obv. 13 (see below). The logogram ^{ú}NÚMUN (or ^{ú}GUG$_4$) can be read *elpetu* or *urbatu* in Akkadian, both referring to a kind of rush or grass, cf. CAD U/W, 211–212; Borger 2004, MZL, 267 No. 102.

Lines 10–13: For the imagery, compare also SpTU 2, 130 No. 25 (Abusch et al. 2020, CMAwR 3, text 7.35), BAM 244: 41ff. (*infra* text B.1.1) and BAM 237 and dupl. lines 48″ff. (text C.1.4). At the beginning of line 10, Scurlock (2014a, 586; 2014b, 110) reads [T]U$_6^!$ ÉN "[Sp]ell (and) recitation". However, the tablet seems to show a clear [Í]D, and only one sign seems to be missing at the beginning of the line. The term *tamirtu* (here translated as "meadow") refers to a kind of irrigated agricultural land.

My translation of line 11 follows Collins 1999, 181–182. For varying translations of the spell, cf. Scurlock 2014a, 587 and 2014b, 110. In line 13, I partially follow the translation of Scurlock 2014a, 587. It remains unclear who "they" refers to in the incantation (cf. Farber 1990 for discussion of similar formulas of the *mannam lušpur* type). Possibly, "they" are the agents *adāru*-wood, lapis lazuli and *ašlu*-rush in this spell rather than divine helpers. For a parallel imagery of damming up a canal, see also the incantation *urbatu urbatu* (BAM 480 iii 65–68) in the context of an abscess on the head (Worthington 2005, *JMC* 5, 13, 21 lines 198′–201′; Scurlock 2014a, 441, 443).

Lines 15–16: A differing reconstruction and translation is suggested by Scurlock 2014a, 586–587; 2014b, 110, especially for the beginning of line 16: [^{giš}ḪA]B^{sar} ŠUB "you dribble *ḫûratu* (on the knots)". However, *ḫûratu* is usually not written with the classifier SAR, which rather invites the reading KÉŠ("SAR")-*ru* instead. The traces of assumed [^{giš}ḪA]B on Köcher's copy of BAM 235 favour a reconstruction similar to the duplicate BAM 236 rev. 8, which reads [7$^{?}$ K]A.KÉŠ ^{giš}ḪAB KÉŠ *e-ma* KA.KÉŠ(= *kiṣru*) <KÉŠ> "you tie [seven(?)] knots of *ḫûratu*-plant. Wherever <you have tied> a knot (you recite the incantation)." Thus, at the beginning of BAM 235 obv. 16, I prefer to restore [*e-m*]*a* KÉŠ("SAR")-*ru* "whenever you have made a knot (*taktaṣru*)", with a perfect form of the verb *kaṣāru* for KÉŠ("SAR")-*ru*. For "knots" of the *ḫûratu*-plant (madder), which contained a red dye, see also *infra*, text F.1 lines 20, 29, 31 and text F.2. line 30′ with discussion.

Line 19: Perhaps restore *dām* [*erēni*] "[cedar] blood" in the gap. For this drug, see Böck 2023, 121–125.

C.1.2 BAM 236: Another Tablet with Treatments to Stop a Woman's Blood from Assur

List of Manuscripts

Siglum	Museum Number	Copy	Collation	Format; Ductus	Provenience
A	A 203	BAM 236	Coll.	Fragment of a single-column tablet; Neo-Assyrian script; 8th/7th cent. BCE	Assur, N4 library[292]
B	VAT 13724	BAM 235	Coll.	Fragment of a single-column tablet; Neo-Assyrian script; 8th/7th cent. BCE	Assur, N4 library
c	BM 40152 (81-3-24, 17)	Pl. 28–29	Coll.	Fragment of a two-column tablet; Late Babylonian script; ca. 6th/5th cent. BCE	Babylon

Overview

i	Fragmentary A obv. 1–4	1–4
ii	Fragmentary A obv. 5	5
iii	Fragmentary prescription A obv. 6	6
iv	Fragmentary prescription A obv. 7–8	7–8
v	Fragmentary prescription to stop bleeding (potion) A obv. 9–11	9–11
vi	Fragmentary prescription to stop bleeding (potion) A obv. 12	12
vii	Prescription to stop bleeding (suppository) A obv. 13	13

292 Pedersén 1986, 67 No. 334. The fragment belongs to the collection of the Istanbul Archaeological Museum.

viii	Prescription to stop bleeding (suppository) A obv. 14	14
ix	Prescription to stop bleeding (tampon) A obv. 15–17 // c obv. ii 9′–11′	15–17
x	Prescription to stop bleeding A obv. 18–20	18–20[...
xi′	Akkadian incantation to stop bleeding: *nār sāmti dāmša* A rev. 1′–5′ // B obv. 10–13	...]21′–25′
xii′	Incantation rubric A rev. 6′ / B obv. 14	26′
xiii′	Procedure: prescription to stop bleeding (knotted strings to be tied around the hips) A rev. 7′–9′ // B obv. 15–16	27′–29′
xiv′	Fragmentary Sumerian incantation A rev. 10′–12′	30′–32′

Previous Edition and Discussion

Kirsch 1996, 94–96
Collins 1999, 181–182 (BAM 235: 10–13 // BAM 236 rev. 1′–5′)
Böck 2013, 29 note 6 (transliteration and translations of lines 15–17)
Scurlock 2014a, 585–587
Scurlock 2014b, 110 (translation of BAM 235: 10–16 // BAM 236 rev. 1′–9′)
CDLI P285322 (transliteration)
BabMed Corpora (https://www.geschkult.fu-berlin.de/e/babmed/Corpora/BAM-3/BAM-3_-236/index.html) (transliteration)
Infra text C.1.1 (ms. B), text C.1.8 (ms. c)

Transliteration

1	A obv. 1	[DIŠ MUNUS MÚD.MEŠ-*šá* DU$^{?}$]-⸢*ku*$^{?}$⸣ [...................]
2	A obv. 2	*not preserved*
3	A obv. 3	*not preserved*
4	A obv. 4	[.....................] x MI$^{?}$ x [...................]
5	A obv. 5	[.....................] x bad i [...................]
6	A obv. 6	[.....................] ⸢^{ú}⸣IGI-*lim* [...............]
7	A obv. 7	[..................] ^{ú}[.............................]
8	A obv. 8	[...........................] x [...................]
9	A obv. 9	[..............................] SÚD [............]
10	A obv. 10	[.............] x [.................................]
11	A obv. 11	[........................... *ina*] KAŠ NAG-*šú*
12	A obv. 12	DIŠ KI.MIN ⸢^{ú}⸣NU.[LUḪ.ḪA SÚD$^{?}$] *ina* KAŠ NAG
13	A obv. 13	DIŠ KI.MIN DÈ *ur-ba-te i-na-áš-ši* MIN

14 A obv. 14 DIŠ KI.MIN NUMUN ^{ú}IN$_{6}$.ÚŠ ḪÁD.DU SÚD *i-na-á*[*š-ši*]

A, c ______________________________

15 A obv. 15 [DIŠ KI.MI]N IM.[SAḪAR].BABBAR.KUR.RA IM.SAḪAR.GI$_{6}$.KUR.RA
c obv. ii 9′ [DIŠ] KI.MIN ⸢IM⸣.SAḪ[AR.NA$_{4}$].KUR.RA IM.SAḪAR.GI$_{6}$.KUR.RA

16 A obv. 16 [IM.SAḪA]R.N[A$_{4}$$^{!}$].KUR.RA DIŠ-*niš ina* ^{síg}ÀKA NIGIN-[*m*]*a*$^{?}$
c obv. ii 10′ [IM].SAḪAR.BABBAR.KUR.RA DIŠ-*niš ina* $^{síg?}$ÀKA ⸢NIGIN-*mi*⸣

17 A obv. 17 [*ana* ŠÀ].⸢TÙR⸣$^{!}$-*šá* GAR-*an-ma* MÚD.MEŠ-*šá* KUD-*su*$^{!}$
c obv. ii 11′ [*ana* ŠÀ].TÙR-*šá* GAR-*ma* MÚD.MEŠ-*ša* KUD-⸢*si*⸣

A, c ______________________________

18 A obv. 18 [DIŠ KI.MIN$^{?}$ ^{ú}]IN$_{6}$.ÚŠ SÚD *ina* ^{síg}Ḫ[É.M]E.DA N[IGIN$^{!}$]

19 A obv. 19 [x x *ana* ŠÀ.TÙ]R$^{!}$-*šá* GAR-*a*[*n* MIN$^{?}$]

20 A obv. 20 [x x x]x e (or: *ina* A$^{?}$) nu$^{?}$ [x x x x]

Ms. A obv. breaks; gap of unknown length

21′ A rev. 1′ [x x ^{na4}G]UG MÚD-⸢*ša*$^{?}$⸣ *a*-⸢*tap*⸣ ⸢^{na4}⸣G[UG]
B obv. 10 [ÉN Í]D ^{na4}GUG MÚD-*šá a-tap* ^{na4}G[UG (…)]

22′ A rev. 2′ [x x x] ⸢A⸣.MEŠ *ub-ba-lu man-nu liq-b*[*i*]
B obv. 11–12 [*ta*$^{?}$]-*mir-ti* ^{na4}GUG A.MEŠ [............] / [*man*]-*nu liq-bi*

23′ A rev. 3′ [*ana r*]*e-mi-ni-i* ^{d}AMAR.UTU
B obv. 12$^{cont.}$ *ana re-mi-ni-i* ^{d}A[MAR.UTU]

24′ A rev. 4′ [x x ^{n}]^{a4}GUG *li-is-ki-ru* ÍLDAG ^{na4}ZA.GÌ[N]
B obv. 13 [*t*]*a-mir-ti* ^{na4}GUG [................................]

25′ A rev. 5′ [^{ú}]*aš-la ub-bal*
B obv. 13$^{cont.}$ [...............]

A, B ______________________________

26′ A rev. 6′ [KA].INIM.MA MÚD MUNUS KUD-*si*
B obv. 14 [K]A.INIM.MA MÚD MUNUS [KUD-*si*]

A, B ______________________________

27′ A rev. 7′ [DÙ].DÙ.BI SÍG BABBAR SÍG SA$_{5}$ DIŠ-*niš* NU.NU
B obv. 15 [DÙ.D]Ù.BI SÍG BABBAR SÍG SA$_{5}$ DIŠ-*niš* NU.NU

28′ A rev. 8′ [7 K]A.KÉŠ ^{giš}ḪAB KÉŠ *e-ma* KA.KÉŠ <KÉŠ>
B obv. 15–16 7 KÉ[Š (…) KÉŠ] / [*e-m*]*a* KÉŠ(“SAR”)-*ru*

29′ A rev. 9′ [ÉN 7-*šú*] ŠID-*nu ina* MURUB$_{4}$-*šá* KÉŠ-*ma ina-aš*
B obv. 16$^{cont.}$ ÉN 7-*šú* ŠID-*n*[*u*] *ina* MUR[UB$_{4}$-*šá* KÉŠ-*ma ina-aš*]

Afor continuation of ms. B see edition of BAM 235 in this volume (text C.1.1)

30′ A rev. 10′ [É]N ⸢ka$^{?}$⸣ ⸢kud$^{?}$⸣ ú ^{gi}ḫal šú tum íb-dè

31′ A rev. 11′ [x k]i$^{?}$-tum ḫu [l]ú dili ú-bil-lá de$_{6}$ zi-ìl íb-dè

32′ A rev. 12′ [x gi]g$^{?}$ igi ^{giš}ká$^{?!}$ lú sìg al-ti x

Bound Transcription and Translation

1 [*šumma sinništu dāmūša illa*]*kū* [... ...] 2–4 *too fragmentary for transcription*	1 [*If a woman's blood*(?)] flows, [... ...] 2–4 *too fragmentary for translation*
5 *too fragmentary for transcription*	5 *too fragmentary for translation*
6 [... ...] *imḫur-līm* [... ...]	6 [... ...], 'heals thousand'-plant, [... ...].
7–8 *fragmentary*	7–8 *fragmentary*
9 [... ...] *tasâk* [... ...] 10 [... ...] 11 [... ... *ina*] *šikari tašaqqīši* 12 DIŠ KI.MIN *nu*[*ḫurta tasâk*(?)] *ina šikari išatti*	9 [... ...] you pound, [... ...] 10 [... ...], 11 [... ...] you have her drink (it) [in] beer. 12 Alternatively, [you pound] *nuḫurtu*-plant, she shall drink (it) in beer.
13 DIŠ KI.MIN *diqmēni urbate inašši* MIN	13 Alternatively, she shall apply ashes of *urbatu*-rushes, ditto (i.e. her bleeding will stop).
14 DIŠ KI.MIN *zēr maštakal tubbal tasâk ina*[*šši*]	14 Alternatively, you dry (and) pound the seeds of *maštakal*-soapwort (and) she shall apply it.
15 [DIŠ KI.MIN] *alluḫara qitma* 16 [*ga*]*bâ ištēniš ina itqi talammī-ma* 17 [*ana ša*]*ssūrīša tašakkan-ma dāmūša iparrasū*	15 [Alternatively,] you wrap (white) *alluḫaru*-pigment, (black) *qitmu*-pigment 16 [(and) al]um together in a wad of wool. 17 You insert (it) [into] her womb and her bleeding will stop.
18 [DIŠ KI.MIN(?)] *maštakal tasâk ina tabarri tal*[*ammi*] 19 [... *ana šass*]*ūrīša tašakkan* [MIN(?)] 20 *fragmentary* *Ms. A obv. breaks; gap of unknown length* 21' [ÉN *nār sā*]*mti dāmša atap sā*[*mti*] 22' *tamirti sāmti mû ubbalū mannu liqbi* 23' *ana rēmēnî Marduk* 24' [*tamirti*] *sāmti liskirū adāra uqnâ* 25' *ašla ubbal*	18 [Alternatively(?), you pound *maštakal*-soapwort, you w[rap] (it) in red wool. 19 You insert (it) [... into] her [wo]mb, [ditto(?)]. 20 *too fragmentary for translation* 21' [Incantation]: Her blood is a [re]d [river], a r[ed] canal! 22' The waters are carrying (away) [the red meadow]! Who shall speak 23' to merciful Marduk? 24' Let them dam up the red [meadow] with *adāru*-wood(?), lapis lazuli 25' (and) *ašlu*-rush, (so that) it (the meadow) will (then) dry up.
26' KA.INIM.MA *dām sinništi parāsi*	26' An [inc]antation for stopping a woman's blood.
27' DÙ.DÙ.BI *šīpāti peṣâti šīpāti sāmāti ištēniš taṭammi* 28' [*sebet ki*]*ṣrī ḫûrati takaṣṣar ēma kiṣra* <*taktaṣru*> 29' *šiptu sebīšu tamannu ina qablīša tarakkas-ma inâš*	27' The procedure for it: you twine together white wool (and) red wool. 28' You tie seven knots (of) *ḫûratu*-plant (into the string). [When]ever <you have tied> a knot, 29' you recite [the incantation seven times]. You bind (it) around her waist. Then she will get well.

30′ [É]N ⸢ka$^{?}$⸣ ⸢kud$^{?}$⸣ ú ^{gi}ḫal šú tum íb-dè	30′ [Spe]ll: The 'mouth' is *blocked*(?) (lit. cut off). Plants brought(?) in a reed basket have been heaped up(?).
31′ [x k]i$^{?}$-tum ḫu [l]ú dili ú-bil-lá de$_6$ zi-ìl íb-dè	31′ ... ... a single human being(?), ú-bil-lá-plant(?) has been brought(?) ... has been heaped up.
32′ [x gi]g$^{?}$ igi ^{ĝiš}ká lú sìg al-ti ⸢x⸣	32′ [...]... ... has approached the front (of the) gate of the stricken human being ... .

Bottom of ms. A rev.

Notes

Lines 1–20: The preserved ingredients of the prescriptions in these lines are well known from other texts to stop bleeding. For *nuḫurtu*-plant (line 12), see e.g. the following texts edited in this volume: K. 263 + 10394 rev. 25 (potion); BAM 237 i 32′; ii 17′, iii 20′ (potion), iv 13. Dried seed of *maštakal*-soapwort (line 14) are used, for example, in FLP 1306 obv. 4–6; the plant is also prescribed in K. 263 + 10934 obv. 2, 19 (potion); BAM 237 i 39′ (suppository); ii 34′–35′ (potion) and *passim*; SpTU 4, No. 153: 7, 11; FLP 1306 rev. 28; BM 40152 rev. iii 27, 29. For *urbatu*-rushes (line 13), see e.g. BAM 237 iv 30 (for vaginal discharges other than blood).

In line 1, it is also possible to restore *šagûša* instead of MÚD.MEŠ-*šá* "her blood" (see above BAM 235, text C.1.1).

Lines 30′–32′: The text of this short spell has been inscribed with large blank spaces in between, resembling a colophon, presumably in the intention to fill all the remaining of space on the reverse of the tablet. The text of the spell looks like a mixture of rudimentary Sumerian words and abracadabra syllables. The first two words in line 30′ can be read as Sumerian ka "mouth; opening" and kud "cut off (water); to block; to staunch (the flow of fluids)", which may refer to stopping the haemorrhage from the vagina. The rest of the line as well as the latter part of line 31′ appear to speak of objects that are brought (šú tum perhaps standing for šu túm/de$_6$ "to carry") and heaped up(?) (dè, for dé "to pour"), presumably to staunch the blood flow. The term ^{gi}ḫal refers to a basket for keeping fish or birds in Ur III texts from Umma, see Englund 1990, 149–155; Borelli 2021, *NABU* 2021/1, no. 7. In line 31′, the Sumerian word ú-bil-lá can be recognized, which usually means "charcoal" (Akkadian *upillû*). However, in lexical texts from Emar, u$_5$-bíl-lá is equated with Akkadian *illūru*, a plant with a distinct red flower and fruit (Arnaud 1985, Emar 6/2, 508–515, 730 Msk 74209a+ rev. iii 54). This plant occurs as an ingredient in potions to stop *naḫšātu*-discharge in BAM 237 obv. i 28, 30 (*infra* text C.1.4). See also BAM 237 rev. iv 11 (against NI.NE).

In line 32′, ti in al-ti may stand for te(ĝ) "to approach, come near" (i.e. he/she/it/they approached").

C.1.3 KAL 7, No. 16: A Fragment from Assur with Amulets to Stop Female Bleeding

This fragment from the library N4 at Assur ("House of the incantation priest") and dating to the 7th cent. BCE presumably belonged to a single-column tablet. The fragment preserves the lower left corner of a tablet; only the beginning of a few lines written on the bottom edge, the reverse and left edge are preserved. Because the content matter is related to gynaecological haemorrhage, W. Meinhold (2017, 51) suggests that the fragment may belong to BAM 235 (text C.1.1), although no direct join is possible. On this account, I offer a slightly diverging interpretation of the fragment as preserving remedies for "stopping the blood" (MÚD KUD-*si*) instead of *naḫšātu*-disease (as suggested by Meinhold).

List of Manuscripts

Siglum	Museum Number	Copy	Collation	Format; Ductus	Provenience
A	VAT 20785 (Ass. 13956 co*)	KAL 7, No. 16	–	Fragment of a single-column tablet; Neo-Assyrian script; 7th cent. BCE	Assur, N4 library

Overview

i′	Fragmentary prescription to stop bleeding (amulet tied around the hips) A lo. e. 1–rev. 2	...]1′–4′
ii′	Fragmentary prescription to stop bleeding (amulet tied around the hips) A rev. 3–7	5′–9′
iii′	Fragmentary prescription to stop bleeding (amulet) A rev. 8–9	10′–11′
iv′	Fragmentary prescription to stop bleeding A rev. 10–12	12′–14′[...
v″	Rubric(?) A l. e. 1	...]15″

Previous Edition and Discussion

Meinhold 2017, 51–52, 159 No. 16

Transliteration

Ms. A obv. lost

1′	A lo. e. 1	⸢*šá*$^{?}$⸣ x [.............................]
2′	A lo. e. 2	PA *šá* 7 [GÙN.MEŠ-*šá* ....]
3′	A rev. 1	*ina* MURU[B$_4$-*šá* KÉŠ ....]
4′	A rev. 2	[....................]

5′	A rev. 3	ŠUBA G[UG$^{?}$ ....]
6′	A rev. 4	*ina* ^{síg}HÉ.[ME.DA ....]
7′	A rev. 5	SA MAŠ.DÀ [.....................]
8′	A rev. 6	È-*a*[*k* ....]
9′	A rev. 7	*ina* M[URUB$_4$-*šá* KÉŠ ...]

10′	A rev. 8	SÍG BABBAR [.........................]
11′	A rev. 9	[.....................................]

12′	A rev. 10	*ana* MUNUS *šá* MÚD.[MEŠ-*šá* DU-*ku*$^{?}$ NU KUD-*su*]
13′	A rev. 11	*ana* KUD-*si* [...]
14′	A rev. 12	MÚD.ME[Š-*šá* KUD-*su* (...)]

Ms. A rev. breaks; gap of unknown length

15″	A l. e. 1	MÚD.MEŠ [*šá* MUNUS *ana* KUD-*si*$^{?}$]

Bound Transcription and Translation

Ms. A obv. lost

1′ *ša* ...[... ...] 2′ *ayyartu ša sebet* [*tikpūša* ... ...] 3′ *ina qabl*[*īša tarakkas* ...] 4′ [... ...]	1′ *which* [... ...], 2′ an *ayyartu*-shell with seven dots, [... ...] 3′ [you tie] around her hips [... ...]. 4′ [... ...].
5′ *šubû sā*[*mtu* ... ...] 6′ *ina tab*[*arri* ... ...] 7′ *šer'ān ṣabī*[*ti* ... ...] 8′ *tašakkak* [... ...] 9′ *ina qab*[*līša tarakkas* ...]	5′ *Šubû*-'stone', car[nelian, ...] 6′ on red wool [... ...] 7′ (and) the tendon of a gazelle [...] 8′ you thread [(the stones), ...]. 9′ [You tie (the amulet)] around [her] hip[s ...].
10′ *šīpāti peṣâti* [... ...] 11′ [... ...]	10′ White wool, [... ...] 11′ [... ...].
12′ *ana sinništi ša dāmūša* [*illakū lā ipparrasū*] 13′ *ana parāsi* [... ...] 14′ *dāmū*[*ša iparrasū* ... ...]	12′ For a woman whose blood [flows (and) cannot be stopped], 13′ to stop it: [... ...]. 14′ (Then) [her] blood will stop ... ...].

Ms. A rev. breaks; gap of unknown length

15″ *dāmī* [*ša sinništi ana parāsi*(?)]	15″ [(Remedies) to stop a woman's(?)] blood.

Notes

Lines 1′–4′: *Ayyartu*-shell (or coral) with seven dots (*tikpu*; cf. Schuster-Brandis 2008, 438; CAD T, 403b) is used in BAM 237(+) in similar prescriptions for amulets against *naḫšātu*-disease, see BAM 237 obv. i 47′–48′ (also Schuster-Brandis 2008, 140 Kette 135) and iii 28 (*infra* text C.1.4).

Lines 5′–9′: A similar amulet featuring the ingredients (although in different order) in these lines can be found, for example, in BAM 237 i 4′–8′ (especially the sinew from a male and female gazelle), used to treat *naḫšātu*-disease.

Lines 10′–11′: A similar prescription for an amulet string to stop a woman's blood (MÚD MUNUS *ana* KUD-*si*) starting with white wool is found in BAM 235: 15′–16′ // BAM 236 rev. 7′–9′, see above texts C.1.1–C.1.2).

Lines 12′–14′ and 15″: I suggest a restoration differing from Meinhold (2017, 51–52), following parallel formulations in other texts concerning stopping abnormal gynaecological bleeding (see Steinert 2012b and 2013a). The main argument against Meinhold's restoration is that there are no parallels for diagnostic passages introducing a recipe with the phrase "If a woman suffers from *naḫšātu*-disease" (thus, in BAM 237, reference to *naḫšātu* as a diagnosis is only made via incantation rubrics (KA.INIM.MA MUNUS *ša naḫšāte* GIG-(*at*)). However, there are numerous instances for diagnostic sections referring to stopping (*parāsu*) a woman's blood (*dāmu*), e.g. K. 263 + 10934: 1, BM 40152 iii 6; FLP 1306: 21–22; BAM 236 obv. 17′, BAM 235: 14 // BAM 236 rev. 6′ etc. (all edited in section C.1 of this volume).

The beginning of line 12′, with the relative pronoun *ša* after MUNUS introducing a relative clause, displays a slightly different syntax, i.e. "for (*ana*) a woman whose blood [flows (and) cannot be stopped] ...", rather than the more usual phrase "If (*šumma*) a woman ...". For *dāmu* "blood" in the plural, see also Stol 2021, *BiOr* 78, 437. In the present text corpus, the spelling MÚD.MEŠ indicating plurality seems to dominate (see also BAM 237 obv. ii 1′ // (text C.1.4); BM 42313+ rev. 1 (text A.2.2); *Iraq* 31, 31: 40 (text II.1.4) and *passim* in this book).

Line 15″: The phrase written on the left edge of VAT 20785 may have been a topical heading or title for the contents on the tablet, functioning like the title on the spine of books, assisting the user of the library, in which the tablet was kept (if standing on a shelf). For another instance of this phenomenon, see e.g. *infra* text C.3.1.

C.1.4 BAM 237 (+) BAM 238 (+) BAM 239: An Assur Compendium with Treatments Concerning Bleeding during Pregnancy (*naḫšātu*) and Related Conditions

BAM 237(+) (ms. A_1) is a large two-column tablet in Neo-Assyrian script from the "House of the incantation priest" (N4 library) at Assur, containing recipes and rituals, mostly to treat irregular bleeding during pregnancy (*naḫšātu*). The final sections on the reverse (col. iv 9–44) also assemble medical treatments for other, related women's ailments characterised by abnormal discharges. Because of its thematic focus, and because its format corresponds to the format of Nineveh tablets belonging to serialised compendia, it is possible that BAM 237(+) forms a manuscript belonging to a section of a serialised medical compendium dealing with women's ailments, which are listed in the so-called Assur Medical Catalogue (Steinert et al. 2018). However, since no incipit or colophon/catchline is preserved on BAM 237 confirming this suggestion, this connection remains hypothetical, since the ailment *naḫšātu* itself is not mentioned in the AMC (cf. Steinert et al. 2018, 272 for discussion and possible connection to Tablet 3 of the section PREGNANCY, which included thematic sections for the case that "a pregnant woman's blood flows", mentioned in AMC line 112).

Column i of BAM 237 begins with a complex treatment (lines 1′–20′) involving a potion, an ointment and amulet stones, combined with a ritual performed over three days, involving *šigû* "lamentation prayers" (one of them addressed at the goddess Ištar), offerings and the deposition of a potsherd found standing in the street, in a secluded place within the patient's house. This procedure apparently alludes to the desired blocking of her leaking body opening. Column i continues with various treatments against *naḫšātu*, including amulets, potions, tampons containing drugs, fumigations.

The fragmentary columns ii and iii contain several short spells (Akkadian as well as *abracadabra* or pseudo-Sumerian) combined with shorter prescriptions. The first preserved lines of column ii contain the end of the incantation *mimmû ilū ibnû amēlūtu* "All that the gods created of mankind" (if column ii started with this incantation, about seven lines from the top of the tablet are missing), whose use in the corpus of women's diseases is so far unique. This spell is otherwise solely known from first millennium BCE compendia of amulet stones from Nineveh and Babylonia, where it was recited to stop nosebleed (mss. b–d).[293] The Nineveh fragment K. 4782: 10′ (ms. e), belonging to a list of amulet stones, cites the incipit of this incantation, as well to be recited over an amulet against nosebleed. A comparable phenomenon can be observed in the text BM 40152 from Babylon concerned with female bleeding, which contains a section with a ritual introduced with the statement that it could be used alternatively "for stopping nosebleed or a woman's blood" (rev. iii 17, see text C.1.8).

The incantation *mimmû ilū ibnû amēlūtu* uses poetic metaphors comparing bleeding with a meadow flooded with water, with a fermenting vessel whose stopper is leaking, and with a waterskin whose knot is not strong. Interestingly, the text begins by alluding to the creation of humankind by the gods and to the role of the mother goddess Bēlet-ilī in this process, known from Babylonian mythological texts such as *Atramḫasīs* and *Enki and Ninmaḫ*. However, in the incantation *mimmû ilū ibnû amēlūtu*, Bēlet-ilī is said to have "created" the blood of her creatures, i.e. made their bodies of flesh and blood. Thus, the text portrays bleeding as an inherent feature of the human body tied to the way it was created by divine action. Interestingly, the incantation describes bleeding in men and women through reference to contrasting body openings, implying gender polarity: men bleed from the nose, women from the vagina. The gods, taking pity on their creatures, then send an anonymous deity up to heaven in order to bring down "the seal of Anu" to "seal up" the leaking body openings, alluding to the use of stones and minerals in amulets and as haemostatic, astringent or "drying" substances applied in tampons or potions. Unfortunately, the identity of the deity who is sent to heaven is unclear; he or she is addressed as a deity who can stop the flow of blood.

Of interest are the deities mentioned by name in the incantation *mimmû ilū ibnû amēlūtu*. Notably, Ea and Bēlet-ilī appear as main agents in the first lines of the composition, clearly referring to the central roles of Enki/Ea and the mother goddess (Ninmah, Bēlet-ilī, Mami) in anthropogonic myths such as found in *Atramḫasīs* Tablet I and in *Enki and Ninmaḫ*. Especially in *Atramḫasīs*, flesh and blood are mentioned (beside clay) as materials, from which the mother goddess shaped the first human being; blood, as befitting the purpose of the incantation, plays the central role in the spell and is said to have been created (*banû*) by the goddess. The consequence of this is that human beings bleed, about which Ea and Belēt-ilī (Mami) are greatly upset and start to cry. This motif is remarkable, and one can ask whether it was meant to emphasise the emotional attachment of the gods to their creatures (as in an incantation in BAM 248 (obv. i 40, text D.1.1) resembling the birth incantation "A Cow of Sîn", in which the moon god cries for his cow in birth pangs). The tears of Ea and Bēlet-ilī

293 According to Schuster-Brandis (2008, 193), mss. b and d belong to the series *kunuk ḫalti* "cylindrical *ḫaltu*-stone".

may also signal remorse or a realisation of failure on their part. In any case, the urgency of the problem is expressed in the fact that all the gods are assembled for a solution (ms. c i 16′ mentions Ištar, Šamaš, Gula, all of which play a central role in healing texts).

Two small fragments, VAT 14123 and VAT 14145, published by Köcher as BAM 238 and BAM 239, most likely belong to BAM 237. However, since their exact placement in relation to BAM 237 is uncertain, these two fragments are edited separately below as mss. A_2 and A_3.

List of Manuscripts

Siglum	Museum Number	Copy	Collation	Format; Ductus	Provenience
A_1	VAT 8577 + VAT 13655 + VAT 13671 + VAT 13706 + VAT 13707 + VAT 13708 + VAT 13828 + VAT 14177 + VAT 14185 (+)	KAR 194 (only VAT 8577) BAM 237 (all fragments)	Coll.	Two-column tablet, Neo-Assyrian script, 8th–7th cent. BCE	Assur, N4 library
a	BM 42313 (81-7-1, 73) + BM 42427 (81-7-1, 187) + BM 42585 (81-7-1, 345) + without No. (81-7-1, 353) + BM 43174 (81-7-1, 938) + BM 43215 (81-7-1, 979) + BM 43274 (81-7-1, 1038) + BM 43279 (81-7-1, 1043) + BM 43281 (81-7-1, 1045) + 43439 (81-7-1, 1203) + BM 43483 (81-7-1, 1247) + BM 43595 (81-7-1, 1359) + BM 43766 (81-7-1, 1527) + BM 43803 (81-7-1, 1564)	Pl. 14–15	Coll.	Single-column tablet in portrait format; Late Babylonian script; ca. 500 BCE	Sippar
b	VAT 16446	BAM 386	Coll.	Fragment of a two- or three-column tablet; Neo-Babylonian script; ca. 6th cent. BCE(?)	Babylon
c	W. 23279	SpTU 4, No. 129	–	Three-column tablet; Late Babylonian script; 5th–4th cent. BCE	Uruk; library of the Šangû-Ninurta family
d	K. 3304 + K. 7698 + K. 8785 + K. 9217	–	Coll.	Fragments of a two-column tablet; Neo-Babylonian script; 7th cent. BCE	Nineveh; library of Ashurbanipal

Overview

i′	Prescription for an ointment for a woman suffering from *naḫšātu*-discharge (abnormal bleeding) A_1 obv. i 1′–3′	...]1′–3′
ii′	Prescription for an amulet for a woman suffering from *naḫšātu*-discharge A_1 obv. i 4′–8′	4′–8′
iii′	Instruction for a ritual to be performed in the house of a woman suffering from *naḫšātu*-discharge, to be repeated on three consecutive days (depositing of a potsherd; recitation of *šigû*-prayers), accompanied by aforementioned potion, ointment (lines 1′–3′) and amulet (lines 4′–8′); continuation of the ritual on the fourth day at the door of the woman's house, recitation of a *šigû*-prayer before Ištar, recitation of incantation) A_1 obv. i 9′–16′	9′–16′
iv′	Rubric: incantation for a woman suffering from *naḫšātu*-discharge; with label *bulṭu latku* "proven remedy" A_1 obv. i 17′	17′
v′	Incantation: ^{d}INNIN an-ki-bi-da-ke$_4$ *Ištar šugallītu* (recited on the fourth day of the ritual described in lines 9′–16′?) A_1 obv. i 18′–20′	18′–20′

vi′	Rubric: incantation for a woman suffering from *naḫšātu*-discharge A_1 obv. i 21′	21′
vii′	Procedure (KÌD.KÌD.BI) for an amulet tied around the woman's hips A_1 obv. i 22′–24′	22′–24′
viii′	Prescription for a suppository inserted in the vagina against *naḫšātu*-discharge A_1 obv. i 25′	25′
ix′	Prescription for a fumigation from below against *naḫšātu*-discharge A_1 obv. i 26′–27′	26′–27′
x′	Prescription for a potion against *naḫšātu*-discharge A_1 obv. i 28′–29′	28′–29′
xi′	Prescription for a potion against *naḫšātu*-discharge A_1 obv. i 30′	30′
xii′	Prescription for an amulet tied around the woman's hips against *naḫšātu*-discharge A_1 obv. i 31′	31′
xiii′	Prescription for a potion against *naḫšātu*-discharge A_1 obv. i 32′	32′
xiv′	Prescription for a vaginal suppository against *naḫšātu*-discharge A_1 obv. i 33′	33′
xv′	Prescription for a vaginal suppository against *naḫšātu*-discharge A_1 obv. i 34′	34′
xvi′	Prescription for a vaginal suppository against *naḫšātu*-discharge A_1 obv. i 35′	35′
xvii′	Prescription for a vaginal suppository against *naḫšātu*-discharge A_1 obv. i 36′	36′
xviii′	Prescription for a potion against *naḫšātu*-discharge A_1 obv. i 37′	37′
xix′	Prescription for a potion against *naḫšātu*-discharge A_1 obv. i 38′	38′
xx′	Prescription for a vaginal suppository against *naḫšātu*-discharge A_1 obv. i 39′	39′
xxi′	Prescription for a potion, an amulet and a vaginal suppository against *naḫšātu*-discharge A_1 obv. i 40′–42′	40′–41′
xxii′	Prescription for a vaginal suppository against *naḫšātu*-discharge A_1 obv. i 43′–44′	42′–43′
xxiii′	Prescription for a vaginal suppository against *naḫšātu*-discharge A_1 obv. i 45′–46′	44′–45′
xxiv′	Prescription for an amulet tied around the woman's hips against *naḫšātu*-discharge A_1 obv. i 47′–48′	46′–47′[…
xxv″	Incantation: *mimmû ilū ibnû amēlūtu* A_1 obv. ii 1′–6′ // b obv. $i^!$ 1′–6′ // c obv. $i^!$ 11′–27′ // d obv. i 1′–7′	…]48″–64″
xxvi″	Rubric: incantation for a woman suffering from *naḫšātu*-discharge (var. against nosebleed) A_1 obv. ii 7′ (var. b obv. $i^!$ 7′ // c obv. $i^!$ 28′)	65″
xxvii″	Fragmentary treatment instruction (KÌD.KÌD.BI) (amulet?) A_1 obv. ii 8′–10′	66″–68″
xviii″	Incantation: [ÉN ^{d}inni]$n^?$ ⸢munus⸣ mu-du A_1 obv. ii 11′–14′	69″–72″
xxix″	Rubric: incantation for a woman suffering from *naḫšātu*-discharge A_1 obv. ii 15′	73″
xxx″	Procedure (KÌD.KÌD.BI) for a potion against *naḫšātu* A_1 obv. ii 16′	74″

xxxi″	Alternative prescription for a potion against *naḫšātu* A_1 obv. ii 17′	75″
xxxii″	Enuru-incantation: kiri$_6$ ur-zé kéš A_1 obv. ii 18′–21′	76″–79″
xxxiii″	Rubric: incantation for a woman suffering from *naḫšātu* A_1 obv. ii 22′	80″
xxxiv″	Procedure (KÌD.KÌD.BI) for a potion against *naḫšātu* A_1 obv. ii 23′-24′	81″–82″
xxxv″	Incantaton: [z]i$^?$ ḫab-lu-ur-zé kéš A_1 obv. ii 25′–27′	83″–85″
xxxvi″	Rubric: Incantation for a woman suffering from *naḫšātu* A_1 obv. ii 28′	86″
xxxvii″	Procedure (KÌD.KÌD.BI) for a potion against *naḫšātu* A_1 obv. ii 29′	87″
xxxviii″	Enuru-incantation: an-ma-ma-na-še ki-ma-ma-na-še A_1 obv. ii 30′–32′	88″–90″
xxxix″	Rubric: Incantation for a woman suffering from *naḫšātu* A obv. ii 33′	91″
xl″	Procedure (KÌD.KÌD.BI) for a potion against *naḫšātu* A_1 obv. ii 34′–35′	92″–93″
xli″	Alternative prescription for an amulet against *naḫšātu* A obv. ii 36′	94″
xlii″	Fragmentary Enuru-incantation A_1 obv. ii 37′–39′	95″–97″
xliii″	Rubric: Incantation for a woman suffering from *naḫšātu* A_1 obv. ii 40′	98″
xliv″	Procedure (KÌD.KÌD.BI) for an amulet against *naḫšātu* tied around the woman's hips A_1 obv. ii 41′–42′	99″–100″
xlv″	Alternative prescription for an amulet against *naḫšātu* tied around the woman's hips A_1 obv. 43′–44′	101″–102″
xlvi″	Prescription for an amulet against *naḫšātu* tied around the woman's hands A_1 obv. ii 45′–46′	103″–104″
xlvii″	Prescription for an amulet against *naḫšātu* tied around the left hand A_1 obv. ii 47′	105″
xlviii″	Fragmentary prescription for an amulet against *naḫšātu* A_1 rev. iii 1–3	106″–108″
xlix″	Fragmentary prescription for an amulet against *naḫšātu* A_1 rev. iii 4–5	109″–110″
l″	Fragmentary prescription for an amulet(?) against *naḫšātu* A_1 rev. iii 6–7	111″–112″
li″	Fragmentary prescription for an amulet(?)against *naḫšātu* A_1 rev. iii 8	113″
lii″	Enuru-incantation: dím-dím an-na dím-dím an-na A_1 rev. iii 9–18	114″–123″
liii″	Rubric: incantation for a woman suffering from *naḫšātu* A_1 rev. iii 19	124″
liv″	Procedure (KÌD.KÌD.BI) for a potion against *naḫšātu* A_1 rev. iii 20–21	125″–126″
lv″	Enuru-incantation: i-g[i-da ba]-túm i-gi-da ba-túm A_1 rev. iii 22–25	127″–130″

lvi″	Rubric: incantation for a woman suffering from *naḫšātu* A_1 rev. iii 26	131″
lvii″	Prescription for a potion and an amulet against *naḫšātu* A_1 rev. iii 27–29	132″–134″
lviii″	Fragmentary Enuru-incantation A_1 rev. iii 30–31	135″–136″
lix″	Rubric: incantation for a woman suffering from *naḫšātu* A_1 rev. iii 32	137″
lx″	Procedure (KÌD.KÌD.BI) for a vaginal suppository against *naḫšātu* A_1 rev. iii 33	138″
lxi″	Enuru-incantation: ú-du zag ḫuš ú-du zag A_1 rev. iii 34–35	139″–140″
lxii″	Rubric: incantation for a woman suffering from *naḫšātu* A_1 rev. iii 36	141″
lxiii″	Fragmentary prescription against *naḫšātu* A_1 rev. iii 37	142″
lxiv″	Fragmentary Enuru-incantation A_1 rev. iii 38–40	143″–145″ [...
lxv‴	Prescription for a potion A_1 rev. iv 1	146‴
lxvi‴	Prescription for a vaginal suppository A_1 rev. iv 2	147‴
lxvii‴	Prescription for a potion A_1 rev. iv 3	148‴
lxviii‴	Prescription for a potion A_1 rev. iv 4	149‴
lxix‴	Prescription for a potion A_1 rev. iv 5	150‴
lxx‴	Prescription for a vaginal suppository A_1 rev. iv 6–7	151‴–152‴
lxxi‴	Prescription for a potion A_1 rev. iv 8	153‴
lxxii‴	Prescription for a vaginal suppository against NI.NE-disease A_1 rev. iv 9–10 // a rev. 1–2	154‴–155‴
lxxiii‴	Alternative prescription for a remedy against NI.NE-disease injected into the urethra A_1 rev. iv 11	156‴
lxxiv‴	Alternative prescription for a remedy against NI.NE-disease injected into the urethra A_1 rev. iv 12	157‴
lxxv‴	Alternative prescription for a potion against NI.NE-disease A_1 rev. iv 13	158‴
lxxvi‴	Alternative prescription for a potion against NI.NE-disease A_1 rev. iv 14	159‴
lxxvii‴	Prescriptions for vaginal suppositories and potions against ‘crab’-disease (*alluttu*) A_1 rev. iv 15–28	160‴–173‴
lxxviii‴	Prescription for a woman suffering from vaginal discharge by ‘drugs of hatred’ (suppository) A_1 rev. iv 29–33	174‴–178‴
lxxix‴	Alternative prescription for a potion against vaginal discharge A_1 rev. iv 34–38	179‴–183‴
lxxx‴	Alternative prescription (amulet) with incantation šal-lu-ur-za kéš dam-gal-la kur A_1 rev. iv 39–43	184‴–188‴

lxxxi‴	Rubric: incantation for a woman suffering from vaginal discharges A_1 rev. iv 44	189‴
lxxxii‴	Fragmentary A_1 rev. iv 45	190‴[...

Previous Editions and Discussion

Scurlock 2014a, 571–581 (ms. A_1 rev. i and iv)
Abusch et al. 2020, CMAwR 3, 90–93 text 5.10 (overview and edition of ms. A_1 rev. iv 29–45)
Collins 1999, 177–180 (edition of the incantation *mimmû ilū ibnû amēlūtu*, ms. A_1 obv. ii 1′–6′ and duplicates)
Finkel 1980, *AfO* 27, 41ff., 50–51 (discussion of ms. A_1 obv. i 1′–12′)
Thomsen 1987, *Zauberdiagnose*, 48, 82 note 112 (ms. A_1 obv. i 5′–7′)
Scurlock 1991, 138–140 (discussion)
Schuster-Brandis 2008, 109–110 Kette 62; ibid., 322ff. Text 11 (edition of ms. c, SpTU 4, No. 129), ibid., 140 Kette 134a (ms. A_1 rev. iv 29, 39–41), ibid., 45 (ms. A_1 obv. i 5′), ibid., 54 (ms. A_1 iv 33), ibid., 55 (ms. A_1 i 40′–42′, iv 33), ibid., 415 (ms. A_1 iv 10)
Böck 2013, 43–46 (discussion of ms. A_1 obv. i 9′–20′, rev. iv 15, 17–18, 21–22, 29–30)
Steinert 2017a, 318–320 (discussion)
Steinert et al. 2018, 226, 272 (discussion)
Steinert 2020, *JMC* 36, 58 (discussion)
Steinert 2021a, *Byzantinische Forschungen* 33, 48, 51, 64–65, 67 (discussion)
CDLI P285323 (photo and transliteration ms. A_1); P285457 (ms. b); P348723 (ms. c); P238268, P238698 (ms. d)
BabMed Corpora (transliteration ms. A_1)
Electronic Babylonian Library (eBL) (https://www.ebl.lmu.de/library/K.3304) (ms. d)

Transliteration

Beginning of ms. A_1 obv. i lost

1′	A_1 obv. i 1′	[x x x x x x x x ^im^]KAL ^im^KAL.⌜GUG⌝ ⌜IM.SAḪAR⌝.[NA₄.KUR.RA x x x x]
2′	A_1 obv. i 2′	^na4^KA.GI.NA ⌜DAB.BA⌝ [NA₄ KÙ.BABBAR NA₄] KÙ.SI₂₂ ^na4^AN.ZAḪ.GI₆ EME-PÉŠ.A.ŠÀ.GA 20 Ú.⌜ḪI.A⌝ ⌜*an*⌝-*nu-ti*
3′	A_1 obv. i 3′	TÉŠ.BI SÚD *ina* LÀL Ì.NUN *u* Ì AMAR ḪI.ḪI ÉN 3-*šú ana* ŠÀ ŠID-*nu-ma* LI.DUR-*sa* KÁ GAL₄.LA-*šá* ŠÉŠ-*aš*
4′	A_1 obv. i 4′	^na4^*ḫal-ta* ^na4^ŠUBA Á.ZI.DA ^na4^ŠUBA Á.GÙB.BA ^na4^*šu-u* NITA *u* MUNUS
5′	A_1 obv. i 5′	^na4^GUG MÚD.MEŠ ^na4^*ka-pa-ṣa* ^na4^*ía-ni-ba* ^na4^*zib-tu₄* 9 NA₄.MEŠ *an-nu-ti*
6′	A_1 obv. i 6′	*ina* ^síg^ḪÉ.ME.DA ^síg^ZA.GÌN.NA ^síg^GA.RÍG.AK.A SA ÁB RI.RI.GA SA MAŠ.DÀ *šá* NITA *u* MUNUS
7′	A_1 obv. i 7′	^ú^*aš-lam* NITA MUNUS.MUD TÉŠ.BI NU.NU È-*ak* 7 *u* 7 KA.KÉŠ KÉŠ ^ú^DILI NUMUN ^ú^*tu-lal*
8′	A_1 obv. i 8′	*ina* ^síg^ḪÉ.ME.DA *ina bi-rit* KA.KÉŠ *u* NA₄.MEŠ *tála-pap* ÉN 3-*šú ana* UGU ŠID-*ma ina* MURUB₄-*šá* KÉŠ
9′	A_1 obv. i 9′	ŠIKA E.SÍR.KA.LÍMMU GUB.BA TI-*qé* A TU₅ Ì ŠÉŠ ^síg^ḪÉ.ME.DA NIGIN-*mi*
10′	A_1 obv. i 10′	*ina* É *ina* EGIR ^giš^IG *ina* KI *par-si* GAR-*an-ši* KI *ta-ša-biṭ* A *ta-sa-laḫ-ši* NÍG.NA ^šim^LI
11′	A_1 obv. i 11′	^ú^KUR.KUR GAR-*an-ši* MUNUS BI *i-kam-mis-ma* Á-*šá ana* EGIR-*šá ú-tar* ÉN 3-*šú* ŠID-*nu*
12′	A_1 obv. i 12′	3-*šú še-gu-ú i-šá-si* NU *uš-kìn* GIN₇ *an-na-a tuš-tál-li-mu* NINDA.Ì.⌜DÉ.A⌝ LÀL Ì.NUN.NA
13′	A_1 obv. i 13′	GAR-*an* BAL-*tú* BAL-*qí uš-kìn* 3 U₄ GUR.GUR-*ár* GIN₇ *an-nam* DÙ.DÙ-*šu* [*maš-q*]*u-tu*^?^ NAG-*ši*

14′	A$_1$ obv. i 14′	*nap*-ŠIL-*tu* ŠÉŠ-*si* NA$_4$.MEŠ KÉŠ-*si ina* 4 *u*$_4$*-me* ^{giš}*si-ḫa* ^{giš}*ár-ga-n*[*u* ^{ú}*b*]*a-ri-ra-t*[*u*][294]
15′	A$_1$ obv. i 15′	*ana* IGI ^{giš}IG *ta-sa-raq* MUNUS BI *ana* IGI ^{giš}IG *še-gu-u i-ša-si ana* IGI ⸢^{d}*iš*⸣-[*tar*]
16′	A$_1$ obv. i 16′	*še-gu-u i-ša-si* ÉN 3-*šú* ŠID-*nu-ma i*-[*di-šá* DU$_8^?$]
17′	A$_1$ obv. i 17′	KA.INIM.MA MUNUS *ša na-aḫ-šá-te* GIG *bul-ṭu* [*lat-ku*]
18′	A$_1$ obv. i 18′	ÉN ^{d}INANNA an-ki-bi-da-ke$_4$ ^{d}INANNA *šu*$^{!}$*-gal-l*[*i-tu*$_4$]
19′	A$_1$ obv. i 19′	*ka-ad-ra-a-a-i-tu*$_4$ *šu-gal-li-tu*$_4$: *ka-ad-ra-a-a-i-tu*$_4$ *te-li-t*[*u*$_4$ x x]
20′	A$_1$ obv. i 20′	^{d}*iš-ta-ri-tu*$_4$ *ù an-ki-bi-i-tu*$_4$ *ki-ṣi-ru ša* AN-*e* TU$_6$ [ÉN]
21′	A$_1$ obv. i 21′	KA.INIM.MA MUNUS *ša na-aḫ-šá-te* GIG-[*at*]
22′	A$_1$ obv. i 22′	DÙ.DÙ.BI ^{ú}NINNI$_5$ NITA ^{síg}ḪÉ.ME.DA SA ÁB RI.RI.GA MUNUS KUD-*tu*$_4$ NU.NU 14 KA.KÉŠ K[ÉŠ x (x)]
23′	A$_1$ obv. i 23′	^{na4}AD.BAR *ina* MURUB$_4$ KA.KÉŠ *ina* ^{síg}ḪÉ.ME.DA NIGIN-*mi* KA.KÉŠ *ina* KI.TA ḪÁŠ-*šá* GAR-*a*[*n-ma*]
24′	A$_1$ obv. i 24′	*ina* MURUB$_4$-*šá* KÉŠ-*ma na-aḫ-šá-tú* KUD-*sa*
25′	A$_1$ obv. i 25′	NA$_4$ ZÚ.LUM *tur-ár* SÚD ^{síg}ÀKA NIGIN *ana* ŠÀ.TÙR-*šá* GAR-*an*
26′	A$_1$ obv. i 26′	GÌR.PAD.DU NAM.LÚ.U$_{19}$.LU *ina* DÈ *ta-sár-raq* MUNUS BI *ina* UGU TUŠ-*ši* A.MEŠ-*šá ana* UGU DU-*ku*
27′	A$_1$ obv. i 27′	*šum-ma* NU KUD-*su* GUR-*ma* TUŠ-*ši* MIN
28′	A$_1$ obv. i 28′	^{ú}*el-lu-ra* SAḪAR *ḫe-re-eṣ ma-gar-ri* ^{giš}GIGIR-*ti ana* KAŠ.SAG ŠUB *ina* MUL$_4$ *tuš-bat*
29′	A$_1$ obv. i 29′	*ina še-rim la pa-tan* NAG ⸢*na*⸣-*aḫ-šá-tu* KUD-*sa*
30′	A$_1$ obv. i 30′	^{ú}*el*-⸢*lu-ra*⸣ SÚD *ina* KAŠ NAG MIN
31′	A$_1$ obv. i 31′	^{síg}ḪÉ.ME.DA SA ÁB RI.RI.GA NU.NU AN.BAR ^{na4}AD.BAR *tála-pap ina* MURUB$_4$-*šá* [KÉŠ] ⸢MIN⸣
32′	A$_1$ obv. i 32′	^{ú}NU.LUḪ.ḪA SÚD *ina* KAŠ NAG MIN
33′	A$_1$ obv. i 33′	IM.SAḪAR.BABBAR.KUR.RA SÚD ^{síg}ÀKA NIGIN *ana* ŠÀ.TÙR-*šá* GAR-*an* MIN
34′	A$_1$ obv. i 34′	NUNUZ TU^{mušen} SÚD ^{síg}ÀKA NIGIN *ana* ŠÀ.TÙR-*šá* GAR MIN
35′	A$_1$ obv. i 35′	NUNUZ TU.KUR$_4^{mušen}$ SÚD ^{síg}ÀKA NIGIN *ana* ŠÀ.TÙR-*šá* GAR MIN
36′	A$_1$ obv. i 36′	IM.SAḪAR.GI$_6$.KUR IM.SAḪAR.BABBAR.KUR SÚD ^{síg}ÀKA NIGIN *ana* ŠÀ.TÙR-*šá* GAR MIN
37′	A$_1$ obv. i 37′	^{ú}*im-ḫur*-20 : ^{ú}IGI-*lim* SÚD *ina* KAŠ NAG MIN

294 In Köcher's copy, there are traces of a sign in front of *ba*, which look like the end of Ú or possibly GIŠ. They are now not visible anymore on the tablet.

38′ A$_1$ obv. i 38′ SI ÙZ *ša* NIGIN BIL ^{ú}NÚMUN *tur-ár ina* KAŠ NAG MIN

39′ A$_1$ obv. i 39′ ^{ú}IN.NU.UŠ A.GAR.GAR-^{d}ÍD ^{síg}ḪÉ.ME.DA SÍG BABBAR *ta-lá-pap si-ik-ti* ^{na4}AD.BAR SUD *ana* ŠA.TÙR-*šá* GAR MIN

40′ A$_1$ obv. i 40′-41′ ^{na4}GUG.ZÚ (gloss) : ^{na4}gug ^{na4}*ka-pa-ṣa* *ta-sàk ina* KAŠ.SAG NAG MIN ^{na4}AD.BAR NUMUN ^{ú}IN.NU.UŠ SÚD ^{síg}ḪÉ.ME.DA

41′ A$_1$ obv. i 42′ SA ÁB RI.RI.GA NIGIN *ina* MURUB$_4$-*šá* KÉŠ : *ana* ŠÀ.TÙR-*šá* GAR-*an* MIN

42′ A$_1$ obv. i 43′ PIŠ$_{10}$.^{d}ÍD IM.SAḪAR.BABBAR.KUR.RA IM.SAḪAR.GE$_6$.KUR.RA IM.SAḪAR.NA$_4$.KUR.RA AN.ZAḪ.GI$_6$ (gloss) : AN.ZAḪ SÚD

43′ A$_1$ obv. i 44′ ^{síg}ÀKA NIGIN *ana* ŠÀ.TÙR-*šá* GAR MIN

44′ A$_1$ obv. i 45′ ^{na4}KA.GI.NA DAB.BA AN.BAR KÙ.GAN ^{na4}*u$_5$-ri-za* ^{na4}*ka-pa-ṣu* ^{na4}*šu-a*

45′ A$_1$ obv. i 46′ ^{na4}*ía-ár-tú* SÚD ^{síg}ÀKA NIGIN *ana* ŠÀ.TÙR-*šá* GAR MIN

46′ A$_1$ obv. i 47′ ^{na4}*ía-ár-tú šá* 7 GÙN-*šá* ^{na4}AN.BAR ^{na4}*zíb-tu$_4$* ^{na4}SAG.LI.MUD NUMUN ^{ú}IN.NU.UŠ

47′ A$_1$ obv. i 48′ *ina* SA ÁB RI.RI.GA SA U$_8$ RI.RI.<GA> È-*ak* 14 KA.KÉŠ KÉŠ *ina* MURUB$_4$-*šá tara-kás* MIN

Bottom of ms. A$_1$ obv. i, beginning of obv. ii lost; gap of unknown length

48″ c obv. i$^!$ 11′ [É]N *mim-mu-ú* DINGIR.MEŠ DÙ-*ú a-me-lu-tu*

49″ c obv. i$^!$ 12′ [DINGIR.M]AḪ MÚD-*ši-na ib-ni*

50″ c obv. i$^!$ 13′ [*i-mu*]*r-ši-na-ti-ma* ^{d}IDIM *i-bak-ki*

51″ c obv. i$^!$ 14′ [*eli le-t*]*i* ^{d}*ma-mi il-la-ku di-ma-šá*

52″ c obv. i$^!$ 15′ [x x *i*]*l*$^?$-*su-ni* DINGIR.MEŠ *ka-la-ma*

53″ c obv. i$^!$ 16′ [x x] x ^{d}15 DINGIR.MAḪ ^{d}UTU *u* ^{d}*gu-la*

54″ c obv. i$^!$ 17′ [MÚD.MEŠ$^?$ *šá*] GURUŠ *ina ap-pi-šú u šá* KI.SIKIL *ina* GAL$_4$.LA-*šá*

55″ A$_1$ obv. ii 1′ *it-t*[*a-* ....]
c obv. i$^!$ 18′ [*it-t*]*a-*[*na-tu-k*]*u* [*u* D]U.DU-*ku* MÚD.MEŠ-*šú di-ma-šú*

56″ A$_1$ obv. ii 2′ *it-ta-na-at-t*[*uk* ....]
c obv. i$^!$ 19′ [*i*]*t-ta-na-tuk u* DU.DU-*ak*

57″ A$_1$ *Omits*
c obv. i$^!$ 20′ GI[N$_7$] ⸢*ta-mir-ti*⸣ *ša la kul-lu-u ka-lu-ú-šá*

58″ A$_1$ *Omits*
c obv. i$^!$ 21′ ⸢GIN$_7$⸣ ^{dug}NÍG.DÚR.BÙR *šá* ⸢*pu*⸣-*ru*-⸢*sa-šá*⸣ *la pár-súm*
d obv. i 1′ [x x x x] x x x [x x x x x x]

59″ A$_1$ *Omits*
b obv. i$^!$ 1′ [..] ⸢SA⸣
c obv. i$^!$ 22′ [G]IN$_7$ *na-a-a-du šá la* ⸢*dun*⸣-*nu-nu* KEŠDA *la tak-lu* SA
d obv. i 2′ ⸢GIN$_7$⸣ ⸢$^{kuš?}$⸣*na-a-di šá* NU *dun-n*[*u-nu* x x x x x]

60″	A$_1$ obv. ii 3′	*at-ta* DINGIR *š[a* ....]
	b obv. i$^!$ 2′	[x x x x x x x x x x NAM].LÚ.U$_{18}$.LU
	c obv. i$^!$ 23′	*[a]t-ta*$^!$ DINGIR *šá ta-ku-lu sa-ʾ-mat* NAM.LÚ.U$_{18}$.LU
	d obv. i 3′	*at-ta* DINGIR *šá ta-ku-lu*$^!$(ma) *sa-ʾ-[mat* x x x x x]
61″	A$_1$ obv. ii 4′	*e-li-ma a-[na* ....]
	b obv. i$^!$ 3′	[x x x x x x x x x ^{na4}KI]ŠIB ^{d}*a-num*
	c obv. i$^!$ 24′	⸢*e*⸣*-li-ma ana* AN-*e šu-ri-da* ^{na4}KIŠIB ^{d}*a-nu*
	d obv. i 4′	*e-li-ma ana* AN-*e šu-ri-di* ^{n}[^{a4}KIŠIB x x x]
62″	A$_1$ obv. ii 5′	*ša* GURUŠ *ru-ku-us* SAG.D[U-x]
	b obv. i$^!$ 4′	[x x x x x] SAG.DU-*su*
	c obv. i$^!$ 25′	*ša* NITA *ru-ku-us* ⸢SAG⸣.DU-*su*
	d obv. i 5′	*ša* NITA *ru-kus* SAG.DU-*su* :
63″	A$_1$ obv. ii 5′	[...]
	b obv. i$^!$ 5′	[x x x x x x] ⸢GAL$_4$⸣.LA-*šá* ŠUB-*a ši-pat-su*
	c obv. i$^!$ 26′	*šá* MUNUS UGU NU *du-muq* GAL$_4$.LA-*šá* ŠUB-*a ši-pat-su*
	d obv. i 5′-6′	*ša* MUNUS U[GU x x x] \ GAL$_4$.LA-*šá* ŠUB-[x x x (x)]
64″	A$_1$ obv. ii 6′	*mim-mu ma-la il-la-*[...................................]
	b obv. i$^!$ 6′	[x x x x (x) *da-mi]-iq-ta-šá liq-bi* TU$_6$ ÉN.É.NU.RU
	c obv. i$^!$ 27′	⸢*mim*⸣*-ma ša*$^!$(ta) DU-*ku da-mi-iq-ta-šá liq-bi te* ÉN
	d obv. i 7′	*mim-mu-ú šá*$^!$(uš) DU-*ku da-me-iq-ta-šá l[iq-bi te* É]N

A, b, c, d ______________________________

65″	A$_1$ obv. ii 7′	KA.INIM.MA MUN[US *ša na-aḫ-šá-a-ti* GIG-*at*]
	b obv. i$^!$ 7′	[.......................] KIR$_4$-*šú šur-du-ma* DU-*ku*
	c obv. i$^!$ 28′	KA.INIM.<MA> MÚD *ina* KIR$_4$-*šú šur-du-ma* DU-*ku*$^!$(GUB.BA)

A, b, c ______________________________

66″	A$_1$ obv. ii 8′	KÌD.KÌD.B[I ....]
67″	A$_1$ obv. ii 9′	^{na4}*š[u-u* ....]
68″	A$_1$ obv. ii 10′	⸢x⸣ [...]

69″	A$_1$ obv. ii 11′	[ÉN ^{d}inan]na$^?$ ⸢munus⸣ mu-du x [x x x x x x x x]
70″	A$_1$ obv. ii 12′	[x (x)] ⸢^{d}⸣inanna munus ná [x x x x x x x x x]
71″	A$_1$ obv. ii 13′	[x x]x mu-un-ù-tu-ud [x x x x x x x] ⸢x x⸣
72″	A$_1$ obv. ii 14′	[x x ú]r-ma *lim-ḫur* x[x x x x munus$^?$] nu si-s[á]

73″	A$_1$ obv. ii 15′	[KA.INI]M.MA MUNUS *ša na-aḫ-[šá-a-ti]* GIG-*at*

74″	A$_1$ obv. ii 16′	⸢KÌD.KÌD.BI⸣ [AN.Z]AḪ SÚD *ina* KAŠ.SAG NAG-*ši-ma [na]-aḫ-šá-tu* KUD-*sa*

75″	A$_1$ obv. ii 17′	DIŠ KI.MIN ^{ú}NU.LUḪ.ḪA SÚD *ana* ŠÀ KAŠ.SAG ŠUB-*di ina* MU[L$_4$ *tu*]*š-bat ina še-rim* NU *pa-tan* NAG-*ši-ma* MIN

76″ A$_1$ obv. ii 18′ ÉN É.NU.RU kiri$_6$ ur-zé kéš *ta-k*[*al-l*]*a* kur *ta-kal-la*

77″ A$_1$ obv. ii 19′ a-šà gal-zu abzu-ke$_4$ piriĝ ḫuš *ina* ki [p]iriĝ ḫuš GUB-*zu*

78″ A$_1$ obv. ii 20′ piriĝ sa *ḫuš-sa-a* ⸢*tu*$^?$-*še*$^?$⸣-*du-ši*

79″ A$_1$ obv. ii 21′ šà-tùr ^{d}inanna ba-du$_{10}$-ga T[U$_6$ É]N É.NU.RU

80″ A$_1$ obv. ii 22′ KA.INIM.MA MUNUS *ša na-aḫ-šá-a-*[*ti*] GIG-*at*

81″ A$_1$ obv. ii 23′ KÌD.KÌD.BI ^{giš}KIŠI$_{16}$-*ḫa-*[*a*]*ḫ* SÚD *ana* KAŠ.SA[G ŠUB-*di*$^?$ *ina* ^{urud}]^{u}GAG.U$_4$.TAG.GA

82″ A$_1$ obv. ii 24′ [*ina* IGI] ^{d}UTU *tu-ma-ḫ*[*aṣ-m*]*a* [NAG-*m*]*a* MIN

83″ A$_1$ obv. ii 25′ [ÉN z]i$^?$ ḫab-lu-ur-zé ké[š x x x k]al [x x x ab]zu-ta-a

84″ A$_1$ obv. ii 26′ [piriĝ ḫur-r]a piriĝ ḫur-ra d[u$^?$ x x x x ḫur-r]a$^?$ za-tu

85″ A$_1$ obv. ii 27′ ku x[x x] ⸢^{d}⸣šà-zu ⸢^{d}⸣[x x x d]u$_{10}$-ga [x] ⸢x⸣ [x x]

86″ A$_1$ obv. ii 28′ KA.I[NIM.M]A MUNUS *š*[*a na-aḫ-š*]*a-a-ti* G[IG-*at*]

87″ A$_1$ obv. ii 29′ KÌD.KÌD.B[I] ⸢^{ú}⸣ÚKUŠ.[TI.GI.LI$^?$ *ina* KAŠ].SAG *u* Ì.NUN TAG.GA-*at ana* IGI ^{d}UTU GAZ N[AG-*ma* MIN]

88″ A$_1$ obv. ii 30′ ÉN É.NU.R[U an-ma-ma-na-še ki-ma-ma-na-še a]n-ma-ma-na-še ki-ma-ma-na-še

89″ A$_1$ obv. ii 31′ pa ḫul-gin$_7$ [x x x x] pa zi-zi pa zi-zi

90″ A$_1$ obv. ii 32′ pa-še gam zi-z[i x x x x ḫu]l$^?$ šu u-ne-ni-ta TU$_6$ ÉN É.NU.RU

91″ A$_1$ obv. ii 33′ KA.INIM.MA [MUNUS *š*]*a na-aḫ-šá-a-ti* GIG-*a*[*t*]

92″ A$_1$ obv. ii 34′ KÌD.KÌD.BI NUMUN ^{ú}I[N.NU.U]Š ḪÁD.DU SÚD *ina* A SED *ta-ma-*[*ḫa-aṣ*]

93″ A$_1$ obv. ii 35′ ÉN 7-*šú* ŠID-*nu la pa-tan* NAG-*ši-ma* [MIN]

94″ A$_1$ obv. ii 36′ ^{na4}AD.BAR *ša* 7 *pil-š*[*u p*]*al-*⸢*šu*⸣ ⸢TI-*qe*⸣ SÍG SA$_5$ NIGIN *ina* ḪÁŠ-[*šá* KÉŠ-*ma* MIN]

95″ A$_1$ obv. ii 37′ ÉN É.NU.RU MUL [x x] pa$^?$-zu ní-zu [x x x x]

96″ A$_1$ obv. ii 38′ *si-i'*-x [.........] *a-na* ŠUB *ḫur-*[x x x x]

97″ A$_1$ obv. ii 39′ *ši*-x[...........]x *šu-ul-pu* x[x x x]

98″ A$_1$ obv. ii 40′ K[A.INIM.MA MUNUS *ša na-a*]*ḫ-šá-a-ti* G[IG-*at*]

99″ A$_1$ obv. ii 41′ KÌ[D.KÌD.BI SÍG$^?$ x G]ÌŠ.NU.ZU [SÍG$^?$ x x x] NU.NU ŠIKA E.SÍR.K[A.LÍMMU *za-qip-tu* TI-*qé*(?)]

100″ A$_1$ obv. ii 42′ [*ina* SÍG (x) NÍGIN$^?$ x] KA.KÉŠ KÉŠ É[N$^!$ 7-*šú*$^?$ ŠID-*nu ina* Í]B-*šá* KÉ[Š-*ma* MIN]

101″ A$_1$ obv. ii 43′ [DIŠ KI.MIN$^?$ SA Á]B RI.RI.GA NU.NU [x x x x x] x [x x x]

102″ A$_1$ obv. ii 44′ [ŠIKA E.SÍR.KA.LÍM]MU *za-qip-tu ina* MURUB$_4$ *ina* x [x x x KÉŠ-*ma* MIN]

103″ A$_1$ obv. ii 45′ [x x x] NU.NU 4 GIG ^{giš}MA.NU [x x x x x x x x]

104″	A_1 obv. ii 46′	[ÉN *ina* U]GU ŠID-*nu ina* ŠU.MEŠ-*šá* K[ÉŠ$^?$ x x x x x x]
105″	A_1 obv. ii 47′	[x x x]x *ina* ŠU-*šá ša* GÙB KÉ[Š x x x x x x x]
106″	A_1 rev. iii 1	[x] ⸢x x zu$^?$ x⸣ ^{s}[^{íg}ḪÉ.M]E.DA [NU.NU$^?$ x x x x x x x x x x]
107″	A_1 rev. iii 2	^{na4}AD.BAR *ša* 7 G[ÙN.MEŠ *ta*]*k-pu* x [x x x x x x x x x]
108″	A_1 rev. iii 3	^{na4}AD.BAR *ina šap-*[*la*]*-an* ḪÁŠ-*šá ana* IGI [x x x x x x KÉŠ-*ma* MIN$^?$]
109″	A_1 rev. iii 4	^{síg}ḪÉ.ME.DA SÍG BAB[BAR] SÍG GI_6 NU.NU 14 KA.KÉ[Š KÉŠ x x x x x ^{na4}AD.BAR$^?$]
110″	A_1 rev. iii 5	^{síg}ḪÉ.ME.DA NIGIN ^{na4}AD.BAR *ù* KA.KÉŠ *ana* I[GI$^?$ x x x x x x KÉŠ-*ma* MIN$^?$]
111″	A_1 rev. iii 6	*sap-pár-ti* SI DÀRA.MAŠ *sap-pár-ti* SI UDU.MÁŠ [x x x x x x x x x]
112″	A_1 rev. iii 7	IM.SAḪAR.NA_4.KUR.RA IM.SAḪAR.BABBAR.KUR ŠIKA SÁḪAR-*ra* [x x x x x x x x x x]
113″	A_1 rev. iii 8	KU.KU ^{giš}EREN ^{giš}ÁSAL SI [DÀRA.MAŠ$^?$ x x x x x x x x x x]
114″	A_1 rev. iii 9	ÉN É.NU.RU dím-[dím an-na dím-dím an-na x x x x x x]
115″	A_1 rev. iii 10	dím-[dím] ^{d}en-ki dím-dím ^{d}en-ki-k[e_4 x x x x x x x x]
116″	A_1 rev. iii 11	dím-dím ^{d}en-ki-ke_4 [x x x x x x]
117″	A_1 rev. iii 12	áš-bala$^!$ ⸢du_{11}⸣-du_{11}-ga ⸢^{d}⸣en-ki-[ke_4]
118″	A_1 rev. iii 13	inim ḫul [lú(?)] du-du ḫul-a [x x x]
119″	A_1 rev. iii 14	ka ad še-g[a$^?$ x] ḫul-a zu-ba nam-ba-ti-⸢x⸣ [x x]
120″	A_1 rev. iii 15	egir-bi [x x] nu-du-du egir-bi nu-k[éš-x]
121″	A_1 rev. iii 16	[x] ⸢x⸣ [x x x x] ^{d}asal-lú-ḫi ^{d}en-bi-lù-l[ù]
122″	A_1 rev. iii 17	[x x x x x] zi-z[i]
123″	A_1 rev. iii 18	[x x x x x x D]U pa-è ḫé-im-mi-íb-⸢$du_{11}$$^?$⸣ TU_6 ÉN É.NU.RU
124″	A_1 rev. iii 19	[KA.INIM.MA M]UNUS *ša na-aḫ-šá-a-ti* GIG-*at*
125″	A_1 rev. iii 20	⸢KÌD⸣.KÌD.BI [SUḪUŠ$^?$ ^{ú}NU.LUḪ].ḪA $ŠEG_6$-*šal* ḪÁD.DU *ta-sàk*
126″	A_1 rev. iii 21	ZÌ GÚ.GAL *qa-la-t*[*i*$^?$ *ina* x x]x *u* KAŠ TÉŠ.BI ḪI.ḪI NAG MIN-*ma* MIN
127″	A_1 rev. iii 22	ÉN É.NU.RU i-g[i-da ba]-du i-gi-da ba-du
128″	A_1 rev. iii 23	[a]l-ma-na še-g[a (x x)] al-ma-na še-ga
129″	A_1 rev. iii 24	⸢e⸣-du-ub an$^{?!}$-du-[ub a]n zi-ga an zi-ga
130″	A_1 rev. iii 25	[x]-⸢x⸣-dab-e-da [x x x x x]x-le-e TU_6 ÉN É.NU.RU
131″	A_1 rev. iii 26	[KA.INIM].MA [MUNUS *ša n*]*a-aḫ-*[*š*]*á-a-ti* GIG-*at*
132″	A_1 rev. iii 27	KÌD.KÌD.[BI x x x *ina* KAŠ.S]AG NAG ^{na4}[x] ⸢x x⸣ [x x] ⸢^{na4}MUŠ.GÍR⸣

133″ A_1 rev. iii 28 ^{na4}BABBAR.DI[LI x x x x x x]x ^{na4}*ía-ár-[t]ú š[a*$^{?}$ 7 GÙN]-*šá*$^{?!}$

134″ A_1 rev. iii 29 <*ina*> SÍG BABBAR [x x x È-*ak*$^{?}$ ÉN] ⸢7$^{?}$⸣-*šú* ŠID-*nu-[ma in]a* ÍB-*šá* KÉŠ [MIN$^{?}$]

135″ A_1 rev. iii 30 ÉN É.NU.[RU x x x]-*šim/rig me-[e-šá a-a*$^{?}$] *it-tu-ku*

136″ A_1 rev. iii 31 *ina a-mat* AN.ŠÁR *lu-[ú*$^{?}$ x-x]-x *a-a it*-<*tal*>-*l[u-ku*$^{?}$ T]U_6 ÉN É.NU.R[U]

137″ A_1 rev. iii 32 KA.INIM.MA MUNUS *ša na-[aḫ-šá-a-t]i* GIG-[*at*]

138″ A_1 rev. iii 33 KÌD.KÌD.BI ^{na4}KA.GI.NA DAB.BA *ina* A SÚD NAG ^{s}[^{íg}ÀKA NIGIN$^{?}$] *ana* ŠÀ.TÙR-*šá* GAR-*an*

139″ A_1 rev. iii 34 ÉN É.NU.RU ⸢ú-du⸣ zag ḫuš [ú-d]u zag ḫuš [(x)]

140″ A_1 rev. iii 35 ú-du u_4-ma dub zag [(x)] ḫuš [(x)]

141″ A_1 rev. iii 36 KA.INIM.MA MUNUS *ša na-*⸢*aḫ*⸣-[*šá-a-ti* GIG-*at*]

142″ A_1 rev. iii 37 [K]ÌD.KÌD.BI ^{ú}*tar-muš* SÚD [x x x x x x x] x [x x]

143″ A_1 rev. iii 38 ÉN É.NU.RU ḫu-x[..]

144″ A_1 rev. iii 39 [na]m$^{?}$-ri pa nam-[ri..]

145″ A_1 rev. iii 40 [x] x li tu [...]

Ms. A_1 rev. iii breaks; gap of unknown length

146‴ A_1 rev. iv 1 NUMUN ^{ú}*a-zal-le-e* ^{ú}KUR.RA ^{ú}ḪUR.SAG SÚD *ina* KAŠ [NAG]

147‴ A_1 rev. iv 2 SUḪUŠ ^{giš}GIŠIMMAR SUḪUŠ ^{giš}ŠINIG SUḪUŠ ^{giš}KIŠI$_{16}$ *tur-ár* SÚD *ina* ^{síg}ZA.GÌN.NA NIGIN *ana* ŠÀ.TÙR-*šá* GAR-*an*

148‴ A_1 rev. iv 3 IM.SIG$_7$.SIG$_7$ IM.KÙ.SI$_{22}$ ^{im}KAL.LA IM.SAḪAR.NA$_4$.KUR.RA *ina* KAŠ NAG

149‴ A_1 rev. iv 4 NUMUN ^{giš}*šu-šum* NU.LUḪ.ḪA ^{šim}LI SÚD *ina* KAŠ NAG

150‴ A_1 rev. iv 5 NUMUN ^{giš}KIŠI$_{16}$ NUMUN ^{giš}DÌḪ SUḪUŠ ^{giš}NAM.TAL NÍTA *ta-sàk ina* KAŠ NAG

151‴ A_1 rev. iv 6 *ka-mun* ^{giš}ŠINIG NIM.UR$_4$.UR$_4$ MUŠ.DÍM.GUR$_4$.RU.NU ŠE$_{10}$ EME.DIR

152‴ A_1 rev. iv 7 *tur-ár* SÚD *ina* ^{síg}ḪÉ.ME.DA NIGIN-*mi ana* ŠÀ.TÙR-*šá* GAR-*an*

153‴ A_1 rev. iv 8 NUMUN ^{giš}MA.NU NUMUN ^{ú}*pu-qut-te* NUMUN ^{ú}ŠAKIRA SÚD *ina* KAŠ NAG

154‴ A_1 rev. iv 9 DIŠ MUNUS NI.NE GIG -- 1 SÌLA DÈ ^{giš}ÁSAL 1 SÌLA DÈ ^{ú}*am-ḫa-ra* ḪI.⸢ḪI⸣

a rev. 1–2 DIŠ MUNUS NI.NE *ki-is*$^{!}$ KAŠ GIG-*at* MÚD.MEŠ-*šú ana* ⸢x x x⸣ [x x x x] / *šá-kín* MUNUS BI NI.NE GIG-*at* DÈ *ur-bat* DÈ *ṣar-bat*

155‴ A_1 rev. iv 10 14 KEŠDA.MEŠ *šá* TÚG KÉŠ 1.TA.ÀM *ana* ŠÀ.TÙR-*šá* GAR-*an*

a rev. 2$^{cont.}$ 14 KEŠDA K[ÉŠ$^{?}$ x x x x]

A, a ______________________________

156‴	A$_1$ rev. iv 11	NUMUN ^{ú}EME-UR.GI$_7$ ^{ú}NÍNDA ^{na4}PEŠ$_4$.ANŠE *ta-sàk ana muš-tin-ni-ša* DUB-*ak*
157‴	A$_1$ rev. iv 12	Ú BABBAR *ta-sàk ina* Ì.GIŠ ḪI.ḪI *ina* MUD ZABAR *ina muš-tin-ni-ša* DUB-*ak*
158‴	A$_1$ rev. iv 13	^{ú}IN.NU.UŠ ḪÁD.DU SÚD *ina* KAŠ NAG NU.LUḪ.ḪA ḪÁD.DU SÚD *ina* KAŠ NAG
159‴	A$_1$ rev. iv 14	NUMUN *pú-qut-te* ḪÁD.DU SÚD *ina* KAŠ NAG SI DÀRA.MAŠ ḪÁD.DU SÚD *ina* KAŠ NAG
160‴	A$_1$ rev. iv 15	[DIŠ MUNUS *a*]*l-lu-tú* GIG KA A.AB.BA *ta-sàk* ^{síg}ÀKA NIGIN *ana* ŠÀ.TÙR-*šá* GAR-*an*
161‴	A$_1$ rev. iv 16	[DIŠ KI.MIN$^{?}$ x x]x [*t*]*a-sàk* ^{síg}ÀKA NIGIN *ana* ŠÀ.TÙR-*šá* GAR-*an*
162‴	A$_1$ rev. iv 17	[IM.SAḪAR.BABBAR.K]UR.RA SÚD ^{síg}ÀKA NIGIN IM.SAḪAR.NA$_4$.KUR.RA SÚD ^{síg}ÀKA NIGIN
163‴	A$_1$ rev. iv 18	[B]AR ^{giš}NU.ÚR.MA SÚD ^{síg}ÀKA NIGIN BAR ^{giš}AL.LA.AN SÚD ^{síg}ÀKA NIGIN
164‴	A$_1$ rev. iv 19	ZÚ NAM$^{!}$(GEME).LÚ.U$_{18}$.LU SÚD ^{síg}ÀKA NIGIN ZÌ GI$_6$ *tur-ár* ^{síg}ÀKA NIGIN PA-<*àri*>-*a-n*[*u*] *tur-ár* SÚD
165‴	A$_1$ rev. iv 20	^{síg}ÀKA NIGIN ^{giš}ŠINIG *tur-ár* SÚD ^{síg}ÀKA NIGIN NUMUN ^{ú}KI.^{d}IŠKUR *tur-ár* SÚD
166‴	A$_1$ rev. iv 21	^{síg}ÀKA NIGIN NUMUN ^{giš}ŠE.NU *tur-ár* SÚD ^{síg}ÀKA NIGIN DÈ ^{giš}ÁS[AL] *ta-sàk*
167‴	A$_1$ rev. iv 22	^{síg}ÀKA NIGIN DÈ ^{giš}EREN SÚD ^{síg}ÀKA NIGIN DÈ ^{ú}NÚMUN [SÚ]D ^{síg}ÀKA NIG[IN]
168‴	A$_1$ rev. iv 23	DÈ ^{ú}*a-la-me-e ta-sàk* ^{síg}ÀKA NIGIN ŠIKA SÁḪAR SÚD ^{síg}ÀKA NIGIN NU[NUZ$^{?}$ G]A.NU$_{11}$[^{mušen}]
169‴	A$_1$ rev. iv 24	SÚD ^{síg}ÀKA NIGIN NUMUN ^{giš}ESI *ta-qàl-lu* SÚD ^{síg}ÀKA NIGIN *ga-bi-*[*e* (x) SÚD]
170‴	A$_1$ rev. iv 25	^{síg}ÀKA NIGIN BI.RI GU$_4$ IZI *qal-liš tu-kal-lam* ^{ú}ḪAR.ḪAR ^{giš}[x x x]
171‴	A$_1$ rev. iv 26	DIŠ-*niš* SÚD *ina* KAŠ NAG ILLU *a-bu-ka-tu$_4$* SÚD *ina* KAŠ NAG ^{ú}*im-ḫur-lim* ⸢^{ú}⸣[*im-ḫur*-20$^{?}$]
172‴	A$_1$ rev. iv 27	SÚD *ina* KAŠ NAG NUMUN GI.ZÚ.LUM SÚD ^{síg}ÀKA NIGIN Ì.UDU [x x x]
173‴	A$_1$ rev. iv 28	^{síg}ÀKA NIGIN *ana* ŠÀ.TÙR-*šá* <GAR> *ina-*[*i*]*š*
174‴	A$_1$ rev. iv 29	DIŠ MUNUS Ú.ḪI.A *ze-ru-te šu-ku-ul* A.MEŠ *ina* ŠÀ GAL$_4$.LA-*šá ma-gal* DU-*ku-m*[*a*$^{?}$ x x] TUKU-*ú*
175‴	A$_1$ rev. iv 30	*ana* NÍG.GIG-*ša* NU GÍD.DA DÈ.LÁ ^{ú}*ur-ba-te* GÌR.PAD.DU *tur-ár* N[A$_4$ x x x]x *ta-qa-lu*
176‴	A$_1$ rev. iv 31	GURUN ^{giš}*ṣa-da-ni* LAG-A.ŠÀ.GA SUḪUŠ ^{ú}*qúl-qúl-li-a-ni* 6 Ú.[ḪI.A *an-n*]*u-ti*
177‴	A$_1$ rev. iv 32	TÉŠ.BI *tuš-te-mid ana* 15-*šú* Ì.BA *ina* TÚG.ḪI.A *ḫal-li tu-*[*rak*]*-kas*
178‴	A$_1$ rev. iv 33	1.TA.ÀM *ana* GAL$_4$.LA-*šá* GAR-*an-ma* A.[MEŠ-*šá* KU]D-*su*
179‴	A$_1$ rev. iv 34	DIŠ KI.MIN *ma-áš-qi-sa* UGU *ku-pi-ti* UGU UGA^{mušen} U[GU$^{?}$ x x (x)] BAR GIŠ.KÍN
180‴	A$_1$ rev. iv 35	NUNUZ KIŠI$_9$ SA$_5$ Ì.UDU BAR.GÙN.<GÙN>.NA KUR-*i ša* ZAG.LU ŠIKA SILA.LÍMMU ⸢Ì⸣.[UDU x x G]ÌŠ BA.AL.GI
181‴	A$_1$ rev. iv 36	^{šim}LI ^{ú}IGI-*lim* KA A.AB.BA ^{ú}AN.KI.NU.DI SUḪUŠ ^{giš}x[x S]UḪUŠ ^{ú}ḪAR.ḪAR
182‴	A$_1$ rev. iv 37	SUḪUŠ ^{giš}GI.ZÚ.LUM.MA *pa-pa-si-*^{d}ÍD SUḪUŠ Ú.KU$_6$ *ku-li-l*[*i* x (x)] Ì.UDU ^{šim}GIG
183‴	A$_1$ rev. iv 38	25 Ú.ḪI.A *an-nu-ti* TÉŠ.BI SÚD *ina* KAŠ NU *pa-tan* NAG-*ši-m*[*a* A].MEŠ-*šá* KUD-*s*[*u*]
184‴	A$_1$ rev. iv 39	DIŠ KI.MIN *tu-ka-ṣar-ši* ^{na4}*ḫal-ta* ^{na4}ŠUBA Á.ZI.DA ^{na4}ŠU[BA] ⸢Á⸣.[GÙB.BA]
185‴	A$_1$ rev. iv 40	⸢^{na4}⸣GUG *ša* MÚD *la-tik-ta* 7 *ḫe-er-ṣi šá* ^{giš}MA.NU *tu-pa-la-áš i*[*na*$^{?}$ x x x x]
186‴	A$_1$ rev. iv 41	[KÉ]Š KÉŠ-*ma* ^{síg}ḪÉ.ME.DA SÍG BABBAR *tu-šá-kak* 7 KÉŠ.MEŠ *ta-ka-ṣa-ar* ⸢*e*⸣-[*ma tak-ta-aṣ-ru*]

187''' A_1 rev. iv 42 [ÉN *k*]*i-a-am* ŠID-*nu* ÉN šal-lu-ur-za kéš dam-gal-la kur š[al-lu-ur-za kéš]

188''' A_1 rev. iv 43 [ḫar-ra g]i-ri ḫar-ra gi-ri har-ra gi-ri šá-ḫi-ma-za-a-te x[x x x x]

189''' A_1 rev. iv 44 [KA.INIM.MA DIŠ MUNUS A.M]EŠ *ina* ŠÀ GAL_4.LA-*šá* DU-[*ku* (...)]

190''' A_1 rev. iv 45 [.........................] *traces* [...............................]

(Ms. A_1 rev. iv breaks)

Bound Transcription and Translation

Beginning of ms. A_1 obv. i lost; gap of unknown length

1'–3' (A_1 obv. i 1'–3')

[1'] [.... *ka*]*lû kalgukku ga*[*bû* ...] [2'] *šadânu ṣābitu* [*aban kaspi aban*] *ḫurāṣi kutpû lišān ḫarriri ešrā šammī annûti* [3'] *ištēniš tasâk ina dišpi ḫimēti u šaman būri tuballal šipta šalāšīšu ana libbi tamannū-ma abunnassu bāb ūrīša tapaššaš*

[1'] [...], yellow *kalû*-ochre, *kalgukku*-pigment, al[um, ...], [2'] magnetite, [a silver 'stone'], a gold ['stone'], *kutpû*-glass, 'field mouse-tongue' – these twenty drugs [3'] you crush together. You mix (the resulting powder) with syrup, ghee and calf fat. You recite the incantation three times over it. Then you rub her navel (and) the opening of her vagina (with it).

4'–8' (A_1 obv. i 4'–8')

[4'] *ḫalta šubû imittu šubû šumēlu šû zikar u sinniš* [5'] *sāmtu* (*ša*) *dāmī kapāṣa yāniba zibtu* 9 *abnī annûti* [6'] *ina tabarri uqnâti pušikki šer'ān litti miqitti šer'ān ṣabīti ša zikar u sinniš* [7'] *ašla zikar ālittu ištēniš iṭammi tašakkak sebet u sebet kiṣrī takaṣṣar šamma ēda zēr tullal* [8'] *ina tabarri ina birīt kiṣrī u abnī talappap šipta šalāšīšu ana muḫḫi tamannū-ma ina qablīša tarakkas*

[4'] *Ḫaltu*-stone, 'right' *šubû*-'stone', 'left' *šubû*-'stone', male and female *šû*-'stone', [5'] blood-red carnelian, *kapāṣu*-shell, *yānibu*-'stone', *zibtu*-'stone' – these nine stones [6'] you thread on (a cord consisting of) red wool, blue-coloured wool, combed wool, tendon(s) from the cadaver of a cow, tendon(s) from a male and a female gazelle and [7'] male *ašlu*-rush spun (together) by a fertile woman (*ālittu*). You tie seven and seven knots (in the cord). [8'] You attach wads of [7'] 'solitary plant' (and) seed of *tullal*-plant [8'] (wrapped) in red wool between the knots and (amulet) stones. You recite the incantation three times over it, and then you tie (it) around her waist.

9'–16' (A_1 obv. i 9'–16')

[9'] *ḫaṣabti sūq erbetti zaqiptu teleqqe mê tarammuk šamna tapaššaš tabarra talammi* [10'] *ina bīti ina arki dalti ina ašri parsi tašakkanši qaqqara tašabbiṭ mê tasallaḫši nignak burāši* [11'] *atā'iši tašakkanši sinništu šī ikammis-ma idaša ana arkīša utâr šipta šalāšīšu tamannu* [12'] *šalāšīšu šegû išassi ul uškên kīma annâ tuštallimu miris dišpi ḫimēti* [13'] *tašakkan maqqītu tanaqqi uškên šalāšat ūmē tutâr kīma annâ ītete ppušu* [*mašq*]*ûtu tašaqqīši* [14'] *napšaltu tapaššas-si abnē tarakkassi ina rebī ūme sīḫa argān*[*u b*]*ārīrat*[*u*] [15'] *ana pān dalti tasarraq sinništu šī ana pān dalti šegû išassi ana pān Iš*[*tar*] [16'] *šegû išassi šipta šalāšīšu tamannū-ma i*[*dīša ipaṭṭar*(?)]

[9'] You take a potsherd standing upright at a crossroads. You wash (it) with water, you anoint (it) with oil. You wrap (it) in red-coloured wool. [10'] You put it in a secluded place in the house, behind the door. You sweep the floor, sprinkle water on it (the potsherd). [11'] You set up for it(?) [10'] a censer with *burāšu*-juniper [11'] (and) *atā'išu*-plant. That woman kneels down, putting her arm(s) behind her (back). You recite the incantation three times. [12'] (Then) she utters a *šegû*-prayer (lamentation) three times, (but) she does not prostrate herself (yet). When you have completed this, [13'] you place [12'] *mersu*-confection (made with) syrup (and) ghee (as an offering). [13'] You pour out a libation. (Then) she prostrates herself. You repeat (the ritual) for three days. When you have done this repeatedly, you have her drink (the aforementioned) [potion], [14'] you rub her with the (aforementioned) salve, you tie the

---

(aforementioned) amulet stones on her. On the fourth day, 15′ you scatter 14′ *sīḫu*-wood, *argānu*-conifer, *barīrātu*-plant 15′ in front of the door. That woman performs a *šegû*-prayer in front of the door, 16′ (then) she performs a *šegû*-prayer 15′ in front of the goddess Ištar. 16′ You recite the incantation (again) three times. Then she [may loosen her arms (again)(?)].

17′ (A_1 obv. i 17′)

17′ KA.INIM.MA *sinništi ša naḫšāte marṣat bulṭu [latku]*

17′ Wording (of an incantation) for a woman who suffers from *naḫšātu*-discharge. (This is) a [tried] remedy.

18′–20′ (A_1 obv. i 18′–20′)

18′ ÉN *Ištar* an-ki-bi-da-ke_4 *Ištar šugall[ītu]* 19′ *kadrayītu šugallītu kadrayītu telīt[u ...]* 20′ *ištarītu u ankibītu kiṣru ša šamê tê [šipti]*

18′ Incantation: "Ištar, goddess of heaven and earth, Ištar, generous (lit. "big-handed") one, 19′ impetuous/aggressive one, generous one, impetuous/aggressive one, capable o[ne, ...], 20′ divine one, and one of heaven and earth, meteorite/bond of heaven!" [Incantation formula].

21′ (A_1 obv. i 21′)

21′ KA.INIM.MA *sinništi ša naḫšāte marṣat*

21′ Wording of an incantation for a woman who suffers from *naḫšātu*-discharge.

22′–24′ (A_1 obv. i 22′–24′)

22′ DÙ.DÙ.BI *ašla zikar tabarra šer'ān litti miqitti sinništu parištu iṭammi* 14 *kiṣrī ta[kaṣṣar (...)]* 23′ *atbaru ina qabal kiṣrī ina tabarri talammi kiṣrī ina šaplān emšīša tašakka[n-ma]* 24′ *ina qablīša tarakkas-ma naḫšātu iparrasā*

22′ The procedure for it: You k[not] fourteen knots (into a cord of) male *ašlu*-rush, red wool (and) sinews from the cadaver of a cow (which) a post-menopausal woman twines (together) [(...)]. 23′ You wrap *atbaru*-stone with red wool (and attach it) in the middle of the knots. You place the knots below her abdomen [and] 24′ you tie (the cord) around her waist. Then the *naḫšātu*-discharge will stop.

25′ (A_1 obv. i 25′)

25′ *aban suluppī turrar tasâk itqa talammi ana šassūrīša tašakkan*

25′ You desiccate date stone, pound (it), wrap (it) in a wad of wool, insert (it) into her womb (viz. vagina).

26′–27′ (A_1 obv. i 26′–27′)

26′ *eṣemti amēlūti ina pēmti tasarraq sinništu šuātu ina muḫḫi tušeššebši mûša ana muḫḫi illakū* 27′ *šumma lā iparrasū tatâr-ma tušeššebši* MIN

26′ You scatter 'human bone' over charcoal. (Then) you have that woman sit down (squat) above it. Her discharges ('fluids') should flow on it. 27′ If (the haemorrhage) does not stop, you repeat (it), and have her sit down (again), ditto (i.e. the haemorrhage will stop).

28′–29′ (A_1 obv. i 28′–29′)

28′ *ellūra eper ḫereṣ magarri narkabti ana šikari tanaddi ina kakkabi tušbât* 29′ *ina šēri lā patān išatti naḫšātu iparrasā*

28′ You put *illūru*-plant (and) dust from the track of a wagon wheel into beer, you let it stay out overnight under the star(s). 29′ In the morning she shall drink (it) on an empty stomach. (Then) the *naḫšātu*-discharge will stop.

30′ (A_1 obv. i 30′)

30′ *ellūra tasâk ina šikari išatti* MIN

30′ You pound *illūru*-plant. She shall drink (it) in beer, ditto (i.e. then the *naḫšātu*-discharge will stop).

31′ (A_1 obv. i 31′)

31′ *tabarra šer'ān litti miqitti taṭammi parzilla atbara talappap ina qablīša* [*tarakkas*] MIN

31′ You twine red wool (and) sinew(s) from a cow carcass. You wrap (it around) iron (and) *atbaru*-stone (beads), you [tie] (it) around her waist, ditto (i.e. the *naḫšātu*-discharge will stop).

32′ (A_1 obv. i 32′)

32′ *nuḫurta tasâk ina šikari išatti* MIN

32′ You pound *nuḫurtu*-plant, she shall drink (it) in beer, ditto (i.e. the *naḫšātu*-discharge will stop).

33′ (A_1 obv. i 33′)

33′ *alluḫara tasâk itqa talammi ana šassūrīša tašakkan* MIN

33′ You pound (white) *alluḫaru*-mineral (pigment), you wrap (it) in a wad of wool, you insert (it) in her womb (viz. vagina), ditto (i.e. the *naḫšātu*-discharge will stop).

34′ (A_1 obv. i 34′)

34′ *pel summati tasâk itqa talammi ana šassūrīša tašakkan* MIN

34′ You pound a dove egg (shell), wrap (it) in a wad of wool, insert (it) into her womb (viz. vagina), ditto.

35′ (A_1 obv. i 35′)

35′ *pel sukannini tasâk itqa talammi ana šassūrīša tašakkan* MIN

35′ You pound a turtledove egg (shell), wrap (it) in a wad of wool, insert (it) into her womb (viz. vagina), ditto.

36′ (A_1 obv. i 36′)

36′ *qitma alluḫara tasâk itqa talammi ana šassūrīša tašakkan* MIN

36′ You pound (black) *qitmu*-mineral pigment (and) (white) *alluḫaru*-mineral (pigment), wrap (it) in a wad of wool, insert (it) into her womb (viz. vagina), ditto.

37′ (A_1 obv. i 37′)

37′ *imḫur-ešrā* : *imḫur-līm tasâk ina šikari išatti* MIN

37′ You pound 'heals twenty'-plant, (alternatively) 'heals thousand'-plant. She shall drink (it) in beer, ditto.

38′ (A_1 obv. i 38′)

38′ *qaran enzi ša saḫratu taqallu urbatu*(?) *turrar ina šikari išatti* MIN

38′ You roast horn of a goat that is *curved* (and) you desiccate *urbatu*-rush(?). She shall drink (this) in beer, ditto.

39′ (A_1 obv. i 39′)

39′ *maštakal agargarītu tabarra šīpāti peṣâti talappap sīkti atbari tasallaḫ ana šassūrīša tašakkan* MIN

39′ You wrap *maštakal*-plant (and) black sulphur with red and white wool, you sprinkle (it) with powder of *atbaru*-stone (basalt), you insert it into her womb (viz. vagina), ditto.

40′–41′ (A_1 obv. i 40′–41′)

40′ *ṣurrānītu* : ^(gloss)^ *sāmta kapāṣa tasâk ina šikari išatti* MIN *atbara zēr maštakal tasâk tabarra* 41′ *šer'ān litti miqitti talammi ina qablīša tarakkas* : ^(variant)^ *ana šassūrīša tašakkan* MIN

40′ You pound *ṣurrānītu*-stone (lit. *ṣurru*-carnelian), *gloss:* (alternatively) carnelian (or) *kapāṣu*-shell, she shall drink (it) in beer, ditto. You pound *atbaru*-stone (basalt) (and) seed of *maštakal*-plant, 41′ you wrap (it) 40′ with red wool 41′ (and) tendons from a cow carcass, you bind it around her waist; (alternatively) you insert (it) into her womb (viz. vagina), ditto.

42′–43′ (A_1 obv. i 43′–44′)

42′ *kibrītu alluḫara qitma gabâ kutpâ* : (gloss) *anzaḫḫa tasâk* 43′ *itqa talammi ana šassūrīša tašakkan* MIN

42′ You pound *kibrītu*-sulphur, *alluḫaru*-mineral, *qitmu*-mineral (black pigment), alum, *kutpû*-mineral ('black frit'), gloss: (alternatively) *anzaḫḫu*-mineral. 43′ You wrap (it) in a wad of wool, insert (it) into her womb (viz. vagina), ditto.

44′–45′ (A_1 obv. i 45′–46′)

45′ *šadânu ṣābitu parzilla lulâ urīza kapāṣu šua* 46′ *ayyartu tasâk itqa talammi ana šassūrīša tašakkan* MIN

46′ You pound 45′ magnetite, iron, antimony, *urīzu*-stone, *kapāṣu*-shell, *šû*-stone 46′ (and) *ayyartu*-shell, you wrap (it) in a wad of wool, insert (it) into her womb, ditto.

46′–47′ (A_1 obv. i 47′–48′)

46′ *ayyartu ša sebet tikpūša parzilla zibtu saggilmud zēr maštakal* 47′ *ina šer'ān litti miqitti šer'ān laḫri miqitti tašakkak* 14 *kiṣrī takaṣṣar ina qablīša tarakkas* MIN

47′ You string 46′ *ayyartu*-shell with seven dots, iron (beads), *zibtu*-stone, *saggilmud*-stone, (and) seed of *maštakal*-plant 47′ on tendons from a cow carcass (and) tendons from an ewe carcass. You knot fourteen knots, tie (the cord) around her waist, ditto.

(Ms. A_1 bottom of obv. i; beginning of obv. ii broken; gap of unkown length)

48″–64″ (A_1 obv. ii 1′–6′ // b i! 1′–6′ // c i 11′–27′ // d i 1′–7′)

48″ [É]N *mimmû ilū ibnû amēlūtu*

49″ [*Bēlet-i*]*lī dāmšina ibni*

50″ [*īmu*]*ršinātī-ma Ea ibakki*

51″ [*ana lēt*]*i Mami illakū dimāša*

52″ [... *i*]*lsûni ilī kalāma*

53″ [...]... *Ištar Bēlet-ilī Šamaš u Gula*

54″ [*dāmū ša*(?)] *eṭli* (var. *zikari*) *ina appīšu u ša ardati ina ūrīša*

55″ *ittanattukū u ittanallakū dāmūšu dimāšu*

56″ *ittanattuk u ittanallak*

57″ *kīma tamerti ša lā kullū kālûša*

58″ *kīma namzīti ša purussaša lā parsu*

59″ *kīma nādi ša lā dunnunu riksu lā taklu šer'ānu*

60″ *attā ilu ša takullû sa'mat amēlūti*

61″ *elī-ma ana šamê šūrida kunuk Anu*

62″ *ša eṭli* (var.: *zikari*) *rukus qaqqassu*

63″ *ša sinništi eli lā dumuq ūrīša idâ šipassu*

64″ *mimma ša illaku* (var. A: *mimmu mala illaku*) *damiqtaša liqbi tê šipti* (var. A: *tê* ÉN É.NU.RU)

48″ Incantation: "(For) all (that) the gods created (of) mankind,

49″ [Bēlet-i]lī created their blood.

50″ Ea [sa]w them and began to cry.

51″ Tears came to Mami's ch[eeks].

52″ [... they ca]lled(?) all the gods,

53″ [...], Ištar, Bēlet-ilī, Šamaš, and Gula (saying):

54″ '[Blood(?)] 55″ continually drips 54″ [from] the (young) man's nose and from the young woman's vagina,

55″ and his (i.e. their) blood flows continually. His (i.e. their) tears

56″ continually drip and flow –

57″ li[ke] a (waterlogged) meadow whose dikes are not holding back (the water),

58″ ⌜like⌝ a fermenting vessel whose stopper does not stop (the outflow),

59″ like a waterskin whose knot is not strong, whose drawstring is untrustworthy.

60″ (But) you are the god who stops(?) the *redness*(?) (i.e. blood) of humankind!

61″ Go up to heaven and bring down the seal of Anu!

62″ Bind the (young) man's head (with it)!

63″ Put a sealing upon the unpleasantness of the woman's vagina!

64″ Let him put in a good word for her, whatever is *appropriate*!'" Wording of an (Enuru)-incantation.

65″ (A_1 obv. ii 7′, var. b i 7′ // c i 28′)

65″ KA.INIM.MA *sinniš[ti ša naḫšāti marṣat]* (var.: KA.INIM.(-)MA (*šumma*) *dāmū ina appīšu šurdû-ma illlakū*)

65″ Incantation for a wom[an who suffers from *naḫšātu*-discharge]. (var. mss. b and c: Incantation (for the case that) blood is copiously flowing from his (the patient's) nose.)

66″–68″ (A_1 obv. ii 8′–10′)

66″ KÌD.KÌD.B[I ....] 67″ *šû* [....] 68″ ...[...]

66″ The procedure for it: [.......], 67″ *šû*-stone, [......], 68″ ...[....].

69″–72″ (A_1 obv. ii 11′–14′)

69″ [ÉN ^{d}inan]na$^{?}$ ⸢munus⸣ mu-du [...]
70″ [...] ⸢^{d}⸣inanna munus ná [...]
71″ [...]... mu-un-ù-tu-ud [...]
72″ [... ú]r-ma *limḫur* ...[... munus(?)] nu si-s[á]

69″ [Incantation: "Inann]a, the woman goes, [.....].
70″ [...] Inanna, the woman lying down [....].
71″ [....], she has given birth, [....].
72″ [...]... *let her receive*(?) [... the woman who(?)] does not have a normal pregnancy."

73″ (A_1 obv. ii 15′)

73″ [KA.INI]M.MA *sinništi ša naḫ[šāti] marṣat*

73″ [Word]ing (of an incantation) for a woman who suffers from *naḫ[šātu]*-discharge.

74″ (A_1 obv. ii 16′)

74″ KÌD.KÌD.BI *[anz]aḫḫa tasâk ina šikari išattī-ma [na]ḫšātu iparrasā*

74″ The procedure for it: You pound *[anz]aḫḫu*-frit, she shall drink (it) in beer and the *[na]ḫšātu*-discharge will stop.

75″ (A_1 obv. ii 17′)

75″ DIŠ KI.MIN *nuḫurta tasâk ana libbi šikari tanaddi ina kakka[bi tu]šbât ina šēri lā patān tašaqqīši-ma* MIN

75″ Alternatively, you pound *nuḫurtu*-plant, you put (it) into beer. You let (it) stand outside overnight. In the morning you give (it) to her to drink on empty stomach. Then ditto (i.e. the *naḫšātu*-discharge will stop).

76″–79″ (A_1 obv. ii 18′–21′)

76″ ÉN É.NU.RU kiri$_6$ ur-zé kéš *tak[all]a* kur *takalla*
77″ a-šà gal-zu abzu-ke$_4$ piriĝ ḫuš *ina* ki [p]iriĝ ḫuš *tazzazu*
78″ piriĝ sa *ḫuššâ*(?) *tušeddûši*(?) 79″ šà-tùr ^{d}inanna ba-du$_{10}$-ga *t[ê* É]N É.NU.RU

76″ Enuru-incantation: "The garden plot(?) ... is bound(?). *You will block it*(?), mountain, *you will block it*(?) (i.e. the blood?).
77″ (In) the field, o wise one of the Abzu, red conjurer(?), in the netherworld/on earth, o red conjurer(?), you are standing(?).
78″ Conjurer(?), *you should assign for her a red string*(?).
79″ The womb, Inanna, is pleasant." Wor[ding] of the Enu-ru-[inc]antation.

80″ (A_1 obv. ii 22′)

80″ KA.INIM.MA *sinništi ša naḫšā[ti] marṣat*

80″ Wording (of an incantation) for a woman who suffers from *naḫšā[tu]*-discharge.

81″–82″ (A_1 obv. ii 23′–24′)

81″ KÌD.KÌD.BI *ulḫaḫ tasâk ana šikari [tanaddi(?) ina] šiltāḫi*
82″ *[ina pān] Šamaš tumaḫ[ḫaṣ-m]a [išattī-m]a* MIN

81″ The procedure for it: You pound *ulḫaḫ*-acacia, [you throw it] into beer. 82″ (Then) you sti[r (it) intensely 81″ with an] arrow 82″ [in front of] the sun god. Then [she shall drink it], and ditto (i.e. the *naḫšātu*-discharge will stop).

83″–85″ (A_1 obv. ii 25′–27′)

83″ [ÉN] *fragmentary abracadabra-spell*

83″–85″ [Incantation]: *fragmentary abracadabra-spell*

86″ (A_1 obv. ii 28′)

86″ KA.I[NIM.M]A *sinništi š[a naḫš]āti ma[rṣa]t*

86″ Wor[ding] (of an incantation) for a woman who suf[fers from *naḫš]ātu*-discharge.

87″ (A_1 obv. ii 29′)

87″ KÌD.KÌD.B[I] [*tigilû*(?) *ina šikari*] *u ḫimēti tulappat ina pān Šamaš taḫaššal i*[*šattī-ma* MIN]

87″ The procedure for it: You smear [colocynth/squash(?) with beer] and ghee. You crush it in front of Šamaš. She shall [drink it. Then ditto] (i.e. the *naḫšātu*-discharge will stop).

88″–90″ (A_1 obv. ii 30′–32′)

88″ ÉN É.NU.R[U an-ma-ma-na-še ki-ma-ma-na-še a]n-ma-ma-na-še ki-ma-ma-na-še 89″ pa ḫul-gin$_7$ [x x x x] pa zi-zi pa zi-zi 90″ pa-še gam zi-z[i x x x x ḫu]l$^?$ šu u-ne-ni-ta *tê* ÉN É.NU.RU

88″–89″ Enuru-incantation: *fragmentary abracadabra-spell*

90″ ... Wording of the Enuru-incantation.

91″ (A_1 obv. ii 33′)

91″ KA.INIM.MA [*sinništi š*]*a naḫšāti marṣa*[*t*]

91″ Wording (of an incantation) for [a woman w]ho suffers from *naḫšātu*-discharge.

92″–93″ (A_1 obv. ii 34′–35′)

92″ KÌD.KÌD.BI *zēr ma*[*štaka*]*l tubbal tasâk ina mê kaṣûti tama*[*ḫḫaṣ*(?)] 93″ *šipta sebîšu tamannu lā patān tašaqqīši-ma* [MIN]

92″ The procedure for it: You dry (and) pound seed of *maštakal*-soapwort. [You stir(?)] it into cold water, 93″ you recite the incantation seven times (over it). (Then) you give it to her to drink on empty stomach and [ditto] (i.e. the *naḫšātu*-discharge will stop).

94″ (A_1 obv. ii 36′)

94″ *atbaru ša sebet pilš*[*ū pa*]*lšū teleqqe šīpāti sāmāti talammi ina emšī*[*ša tarakkas-ma* MIN]

94″ You take an *atbaru*-stone that has seven holes in it, wrap it with red wool. [You tie it] around [her] lower abdomen [and ditto] (i.e. the *naḫšātu*-discharge will stop).

95″–97″ (A_1 obv. ii 37′–39′)

95″–97″ ÉN É.NU.RU *fragmentary incantation*

95″–97″ Enuru-incantation: *text too fragmentary for translation*

98″ (A_1 obv. ii 40′)

98″ K[A.INIM.MA *sinništi ša na*]*ḫšāti m*[*arṣat*]

98″ Wo[rding (of an incantation) for a woman who] su[ffers] from [*na*]*ḫšātu*-discharge.

99″–100″ (A_1 obv. ii 41′–42′)

99″ KÌ[D.KÌD.BI *šīpāti*(?) ...] *lā petīti* [*šīpāti*(?) ...] *taṭammi ḫaṣabti sūq er*[*betti zaqiptu teleqqe*(?)] 100″ [*ina šīpāti* (...) *talammi* ...] *kiṣrī takaṣṣar ši*[*pta sebîšu*(?) *tamannu ina qab*]*līša tarakk*[*as-ma* MIN]

99″ The pro[cedure for it]: You twine [wool(?) of an] unmated [... (and) ... wool]. [You take] a potsherd [standing upright on] a crossroads, 100″ [you wrap it with (...) wool$^?$]. (Then) you knot [...] knots (into the cord). [You recite] the incantation [seven(?) times, y]ou bind it [around] her [wa]ist, and ditto (i.e. the *naḫšātu*-discharge will stop).

101″–102″ (A_1 obv. ii 43′–44′)

101″ [DIŠ KI.MIN? *šer'ān lit*]*ti miqitti taṭammi* [....] ... [...] 102″ [*ḫaṣabti sūq erbet*]*ti zaqiptu ina qabli ina* ...[... *ina* ... *tarakkas-ma* MIN(?)]

101″ [Alternatively(?), you twine [tendons from] a cow carcass [...] ...[...]. 102″ [*You attach* a potsherd] standing upright on a cr[ossroads] in the middle *with* ...[...], [... you tie (it) (around her ...), ditto(?)].

103″–104″ (A_1 obv. ii 45′–46′)

103″ [...] *taṭammi erbet ḫereṣ e'ri* [...] 104″ [*šipta ina mu*]*ḫḫi tamannu ina qātīša t*[*arakkas*(?) ...]

103″ [...] you twine together, four pieces of *e'ru*-wood [you ....], 104″ you recite [the incantation ov]er (it), you t[ie] it around her hands [...].

105″ (A_1 obv. ii 47′)

105″ [...]... *ina qātīša ša šumēli tarak*[*kas* ...]

105″ [...]... You tie [...] around her left hand, [...].

106″–108″ (A_1 rev. iii 1–3)

106″ [...] ... *t*[*abar*]*ra* [*taṭammi*(?) ......] 107″ *atbaru ša sebet t*[*ikpū ta*]*kpū* ...[.....] 108″ *atbara ina šap*[*l*]*ān emšīša ana pān* [... *tarakkas-ma* MIN(?)]

106″ [...] ... [you twine(?)] r[ed wo]ol, [...]. 107″ An *atbaru*-stone dotted with seven dots, ... [...]. 108″ [You *attach*(?)] the *atbaru*-stone bel[ow] her abdomen, *in front of* [..., ditto(?)].

109″–110″ (A_1 rev. iii 4–5)

109″ *tabarra šīpāti peṣ*[*âti*] *šīpāti ṣalmāti taṭammi* 14 *kiṣr*[*ī takaṣṣar* .... *atbara*(?)] 110″ *tabarra talammi atbara u kiṣrī ana p*[*ān*(?) ... *tarakkas-ma* MIN(?)]

109″ You twine (together) red wool, wh[ite] wool (and) black wool, [you knot] fourteen knots (into the cord). [...]. 110″ You wrap 109″ [*atbaru*-stone(?)] 110″ with red wool, [you *attach*] the *atbaru*-stone and the knot(s) *in fr*[*ont of* ..., and ditto(?)].

111″–112″ (A_1 rev. iii 6–7)

111″ *sapparti qaran ayyali sapparti qaran urīṣi* [... ...] 112″ *gabû alluḫara ḫaṣba šaḫarra* [... ...]

111″ *The substance from the bottom of* a stag horn, *substance from the bottom* of a billy goat's horn, [...], 112″ alum, *alluḫaru*-mineral, a porous potsherd [...].

113″ (A_1 rev. iii 8)

113″ *supanti erēni ṣarbati qaran* [*ayyali*(?) ... ...]

113″ Powder of cedar wood, poplar, [stag(?)] horn, [... ...].

114″–123″ (A_1 rev. iii 9–18)

114″ ÉN É.NU.RU dím-[dím an-na dím-dím an-na ...]

114″ Enuru incantation: "Crea[tions of heaven, creations of heaven, ...],

115″ dím-[dím] ^{d}en-ki dím-dím ^{d}en-ki-k[e$_4$ ...]

115″ creati[ons] of Enki, creations of Enki, [...],

116″ dím-dím ^{d}en-ki-ke$_4$ [...]

116″ creations of Enki, [...].

117″ áš-bala! ⌜du$_{11}$⌝-du$_{11}$-ga ⌜^{d}⌝en-ki-[ke$_4$]

117″ Bad curse spoken by Enki.

118″ inim ḫul [lú(?)] du-du ḫul-a [...]

118″ Bad word(s) [(that) a human being(?)] uttered(?), evil [...].

119″ ka ad še-g[a? x] ḫul-a zu-ba nam-ba-ti ⌜x⌝ [x x]

119″ Utterance(?), (be) favour[able]! [...] evil, ..., shall not come near ... [...]!

120″ egir-bi [...] nu-du-du egir-bi nu-k[éš-x]

120″ It shall not go [...] after him(?), it shall not be bound on his(?) back!

121″ [...] ... [...] ^{d}asal-lú-ḫi ^{d}en-bi-lù-l[ù]

121″ [*By the command of*(?) ...], Asalluḫi, Enbilulu

122″ [...] zi-z[i]

122″ [...] be removed!

123″ [... D]U pa-è ḫé-im-mi-íb-⌜du$_{11}$?⌝ TU$_6$ ÉN É.NU.RU

123″ [...]... become apparent, let it (the spell?) be spoken for him(?)!" Wording of the Enuru-incantation.

124″ (A_1 rev. iii 19)

124″ [KA.INIM.MA *si*]*nništi ša naḫšāti marṣat*

124″ [Wording (of an incantation) for a wo]man who suffers from *naḫšātu*-discharge.

125″–126″ (A_1 rev. iii 20–21)

125″ KÌD.KÌD.BI [*šuruš*(?) *nuḫur*]*ti tušabšal tubbal tasâk* 126″ *qēm ḫallūrī qalât*[*i ina* ...] ... *u šikari ištēniš tuballal išatti* MIN-*ma* MIN

125″ The procedure for it: You boil, dry and pound [root of(?) *nuḫur*]*tu*-plant. 126″ you mix (it) together (with) roast[ed] chickpea flour [in ...] and beer. She shall drink (it), *a second time* (she shall drink it?), and ditto (i.e. the *naḫšātu*-discharge will stop).

127″-130″ (A_1 rev. iii 22–25)

127″ ÉN É.NU.RU i-g[i-da ba]-du i-gi-da ba-du 128″ [a]l-ma-na še-g[a (x x)] al-ma-na še-ga 129″ ⸢e⸣-du-ub an[?!]-du-[ub a]n zi-ga an zi-ga 130″ *(fragmentary)* TU_6 ÉN É.NU.RU

127″–129″ Enuru-incantation: *text of pseudo-Sumerian spell*

130″ *(fragmentary)* Wording of the Enuru-incantation.

131″ (A_1 rev. iii 26)

131″ [KA.INIM].MA [*sinništi ša n*]*aḫ*[*š*]*āti marṣat*

131″ [Word]ing (of an incantation) [for a woman who] suffers from *naḫšātu*-discharge.

132″–134″ (A_1 rev. iii 27–29)

132″ KÌD.KÌD.[BI ... *ina šikar*]*i tašaqqī*[*ši* ...] ... [...] *muššaru* 133″ *pappardil*[*lû* ...] *ayyartu š*[*a sebet tikpū*]-*ša*(?) 134″ <*ina*> *šīpāti peṣâti* [... *tašakkak*(?) *šipta se*]*bîšu*(?) *tamannū*-[*ma in*]*a qablīša tarakkas* [MIN(?)]

132″ The procedure for [it]: You have [her] drink [... in beer]. 134″ [You thread(?)] 133″ [...]-stone, [...], *muššaru*-stone, *pappardilû*-stone, [...], (and) an *ayyartu*-shell with [seven dots] 134″ on white wool [....]. You recite [the incantation] seven(?) times. Then] you tie it around her waist, [ditto(?)] (i.e. the *naḫšātu*-discharge will stop).

135″–136″ (A_1 rev. iii 30–31)

135″ ÉN É.NU.[RU ...]... *mû*[*ša ay*(?)] *ittukū* 136″ *ina amāt Aššur lū* [...]... *ay it*<*tal*>*l*[*ukū*] *tê* ÉN É.NU.RU

135″ Enuru-incantation: "[...]... [her(?)] flu[ids(?) must not] drip down. 136″ By the command of Aššur, [they(?)] shall [...], [they] must not keep fl[owing off]!" Wording of the Enuru-incantation.

137″ (A_1 rev. iii 32)

137″ KA.INIM.MA *sinništi ša* [*naḫšāt*]*i marṣat*

137″ Wording (of an incantation) for a woman who suffers from [*naḫšāt*]*u*-discharge.

138″ (A_1 rev. iii 33)

138″ KÌD.KÌD.BI *šadânu ṣābitu ina mê tasâk išatti* [*itqa talammi*(?)] *ana šassūrīša tašakkan*

138″ The procedure for it: You pound magnetite in water, she shall drink (it). [(Alternatively), you wrap (it) in a wad of wool], you insert it into her womb (viz. vagina).

139″–140″ (A_1 rev. iii 34–35)

139″ ÉN É.NU.RU ⸢ú-du⸣ zag ḫuš [ú-d]u zag ḫuš [(x)] 140″ ú-du u_4-ma dub zag [(x)] ḫuš [(x)]

139″–140″ Enuru-incantation: *text of an abracadabra-spell*

141″ (A_1 rev. iii 36)

141″ KA.INIM.MA *sinništi ša naḫ*[*šāti marṣat*]

141″ Wording (of an incantation) for a woman who suffers from *naḫ*[*šātu*-discharge].

142″ (A_1 rev. iii 37)

[142″] [K]ÌD.KÌD.BI *tarmuš tasâk* [...]

[142″] The procedure for it: You crush *tarmuš*-plant, [...].

143″–145″ (A_1 rev. iii 38–40)

[143″–145″] ÉN.É.NU.RU *(too fragmentary for transcription)*

[143″–145″] Enuru-incantation: *text of fragmentary spell*

(Ms. A_1 rev. iii breaks; gap of unkown length)

146‴ (A_1 rev. iv 1)

[146‴] *zēr azallê nīnâ azupīra tasâk ina šikari* [*išatti*]

[146‴] You pound seed of *azallû*-plant, *nīnû*-plant, *azupīru*-plant, [she shall drink] (it) in beer.

147‴ (A_1 rev. iv 2)

[147‴] *šuruš gišimmari šuruš bīni šuruš ašāgi turrar tasâk ina uqnâti talammi ana šassūrīša tašakkan*

[147‴] You desiccate date palm root, tamarisk root (and) *ašāgu*-acacia root. You pound it, wrap it in blue wool (and) insert it into her womb (viz. vagina).

148‴ (A_1 rev. iv 3)

[148‴] *da'mātu illūr pānī kalû gabû ina šikari išatti*

[148‴] She shall drink (dark yellow) *da'mātu*-pigment, (reddish) *illūr pānī*-pigment, (yellow) *kalû*-ochre (and) alum in beer.

149‴ (A_1 rev. iv 4)

[149‴] *zēr šūši nuḫurta burāša tasâk ina šikari išatti*

[149‴] You pound seed of the *šūšu*-plant (liquorice), *nuḫurtu*-plant (and) *burāšu*-juniper, she shall drink (it) in beer.

150‴ (A_1 rev. iv 5)

[150‴] *zēr ašāgi zēr balti šuruš pillê zikar tasâk ina šikari išatti*

[150‴] You pound seed of *ašāgu*-thorn, seed of *baltu*-thorn (and) root of male *pillû*-plant, (and) she shall drink (it) in beer.

151‴–152‴ (A_1 rev. iv 6–7)

[151‴] *kamūn bīni ḫāmītu pizallurtu zê ṣurāri* [152‴] *turrar tasâk ina tabarri talammi ana šassūrīša tašakkan*

[152‴] You desiccate and pound [151‴] tamarisk galls, *ḫāmītu*-wasp, gecko (and) lizard excrement. [152‴] You wrap (it) in red wool, insert (it) into her womb (viz. vagina).

153‴ (A_1 rev. iv 8)

[153‴] *zēr e'ri zēr puqutte zēr šakirî tasâk ina šikari išatti*

[153‴] You pound seed of *e'ru*-tree, seed of *puquttu*-thorn, seed of *šakirû*-plant. She shall drink (it) in beer.

154‴–155‴ (A_1 rev. iv 9–10)

[154‴] *šumma sinništu* NI.NE (var. adds: *kīs šīnāti*) *marṣat* (var. adds: *dāmūša ana* ...[...] *šakin sinništu šī* NI.NE *marṣat*) *ištēn qa diqmēn ṣarbati ištēn qa diqmēn amḫara* (var. *diqmēn urbati diqmēn ṣarbati*) *tuballal* [155‴] *14 riksī ša lubāri tarakkas ištēnâ ana šassūrīša tašakkan*

[154‴] If a woman suffers from NI.NE (var. adds: (and) 'binding of the urine'), (and) her blood [...] into/for [...] (and) there is [...], this woman suffers from NI.NE.), you mix one litre ashes of *ṣarbatu*-poplar (and) one litre ashes of *amḫara*-plant (var.: ashes of *urbatu*-rush (and) ashes of poplar). [155‴] You tie (this into) fourteen knots of cloth (and) you insert (them) one by one into her womb (viz. vagina).

156‴ (A_1 rev. iv 11)

[156‴] *zēr lišān kalbi illūra biṣṣūr atāni tasâk ana muštinnīša tašappak*

[156‴] You pound seed of 'dog's tongue'-plant, *illūru*-plant (and) 'donkey-vulva'-shell, you pour (it) into her urethra.

157''' (A_1 rev. iv 12)

[157'''] *šamma peṣâ tasâk ina šamni tuballal ina uppi sippari ina muštinnīša tašappak*

[157'''] You pound 'white drug', mix it with oil (and) pour (it) into her urethra with a bronze tube.

158''' (A_1 rev. iv 13)

[158'''] *maštakal tubbal tasâk ina šikari išatti nuḫurta tubbal tasâk ina šikari išatti*

[158'''] You dry (and) pound *maštakal*-plant, she shall drink (it) in beer; you dry (and) pound *nuḫurtu*-plant, she shall drink (it) in beer.

159''' (A_1 rev. iv 14)

[159'''] *zēr puqutte tubbal tasâk ina šikari išatti qaran ayyali tubbal tasâk ina šikari išatti*

[159'''] You dry (and) pound seeds of *puquttu*-thorn, she shall drink (it) in beer. You dry (and) pound stag horn, she shall drink (it) in beer.

160'''–173''' (A_1 rev. iv 15–28)

[160'''] *šumma sinništu allu(t)tu marṣat imbu' tâmti tasâk itqa talammi ana šassūrīša tašakkan* [161'''] [DIŠ KI.MIN(?) ... *t*]*a-sâk itqa talammi ana šassūrīša tašakkan* [162'''] [*alluḫ*]*ara tasâk itqa talammi gabû tasâk itqa talammi* [163'''] [*qi*]*lip lur-mî tasâk itqa talammi qilip allāni tasâk itqa talammi* [164'''] *šinni amēlūti tasâk itqa talammi qēma*(?) *ṣalma turrar itqa talammi ar<ari>ānu turrar tasâk* [165'''] *itqa talammi bīna turrar tasâk itqa talammi zēr qutri turrar tasâk* [166'''] *itqa talammi zēr šunî turrar itqa talammi diqmēn ṣarbati tasâk* [167'''] *itqa talammi diqmēn erēni tasâk itqa talammi diqmēn urbati* [*tas*]*âk itqa talam*[*mi*] [168'''] *diqmēn alamê tasâk itqa talammi haṣba šaḫarra tasâk itqa talammi pe*[*l*] *lur*[*mi*] [169'''] *tasâk itqa talammi zēr ušî taqallu tasâk itqa talammi gab*[*ê* (...) *tasâk*] [170'''] *itqa talammi ṭulīm alpi išāta qalliš tukallam ḫašâ* [...] [171'''] *ištēniš tasâk ina šikari išatti ḫīl abukkata tasâk ina šikari išatti imḫur-līm* [*imḫur-ešrā*(?)] [172'''] *tasâk ina šikari išatti zēr* GI.ZÚ.LUM *tasâk itqa talammi lipâ* [...] [173'''] *itqa talammi ana šassūrīša* <*tašakkan*> *ina''eš*

[160'''] [If a woman] suffers from 'crab-(disease)', you pound *imbu' tâmti*-mineral, wrap (it) in a wad of wool, insert it into her womb. [161'''] [Alternatively(?), y]ou pound [...], wrap (it) with a wad of wool, put it into her womb. [162'''] You pound [*alluḫ*]*aru*-mineral, wrap (it) in a wad of wool. You pound alum, wrap (it) in a wad of wool. [163'''] You pound pomegranate [ri]nd, wrap (it) in a wad of wool. You pound oak bark, wrap (it) in a wad of wool. [164'''] You pound a human tooth, wrap (it) in a wad of wool. You desiccate black flour(?), wrap (it) in a wad of wool. You desiccate (and) pound *arariānu*-(plant), [165'''] you wrap (it) in a wad of wool. You desiccate (and) pound tamarisk, wrap (it) in a wad of wool. You desiccate and pound seed of *qutru*-plant, [166'''] you wrap (it) in a wad of wool. You desiccate (and) pound *šunû* (chaste tree?) seed, you wrap (it) in a wad of wool. You pound ashes of poplar, [167'''] you wrap (it) in a wad of wool. You pound ashes of cedar, wrap (it) in a wad of wool. You pound ashes of *urbatu*-rush, wr[ap] (it) in a wad of wool. [168'''] You pound ashes of *alamû*-plant, you wrap (it) in a wad of wool. You pound a porous potsherd, you wrap (it) in a wad of wool. [169'''] You pound [168'''] ostrich e[gg (shell)], [169'''] you wrap (it) in a wad of wool. You roast and pound seed of *ušû*-tree, you wrap (it) in a wad of wool. [You pound] al[um], [170'''] you wrap (it) in a wad of wool. You expose the spleen of an ox slightly to a fire. [171'''] You pound (it) together [170'''] (with) *ḫašû*-plant (thyme), [...]. [171'''] She shall drink (it) in beer. You pound *abukkatu*-resin, she shall drink (it) in beer. [172'''] You pound [171'''] 'heals thousand'-plant, ['heals twenty'?]-plant, [172'''] she shall drink (it) in beer. You pound seed of GI.ZÚ.LUM-plant, you wrap (it) in a wad of wool. [You ...] tallow, [...], [173'''] you wrap (it) in a wad of wool, <you insert> (it) into her womb. (Then) she will get well.

174‴–178‴ (A_1 rev. iv 29–33)

174‴ *šumma sinništu šammī zērūte šūkul<at> mû ina libbi ūrīša magal illakū* ...[...] *iraššû* 175‴ *ana murṣīša lā arāki diqmēn(?) urbate eṣemta turrar ab*[*an* ...] ... *taqallu* 176‴ *inib ṣadāni kirbān-eqli šuruš qulqulliāni šeššet šamm*[*ī an-n*]*ûti* 177‴ *ištēniš tuštemmed ana* 15-*šu tazâz ina lubār ḫalli tu*[*rak*]*kas* 178‴ 1.TA.ÀM *ana libbi ūrīša tašakkan-ma m*[*ûša ipar*]*rasū*

174‴ If a woman has been given herbs/drugs of hate-magic to eat (and because of this) watery discharge flows excessively from her vagina, a[nd] she develops [...] – 175‴ so that her illness will not be prolonged: You roast ashes(?) of *urbatu*-rush and bone (over a fire), you desiccate ...-'stone(s)', 176‴ fruit of *ṣadānu*-tree, *kirbān eqli* ('field clod')-plant, root of *qulqulliānu*-plant, [the]se six drugs 177‴ you mix together. You divide (the mixture) into fifteen (portions), you [bi]nd (these) into (pieces of) loin cloth. 178‴ You insert (the pieces of cloth) one by one into her vagina and [her] watery discharg[e will s]top.

179‴–183‴ (A_1 rev. iv 34–38)

179‴ DIŠ KI.MIN *mašqīssa muḫḫi kupīti muḫḫi erēbi m*[*uḫḫi*(?) ...] *qilip kiškanî* 180‴ *pel kulbābi sāmi lipî ḫurbabil šadî ša imitti ḫaṣab sūq erbetti l*[*ipî* ...*uš*]*ar raqqi* 181‴ *burāšu imḫur-līm imbu' tâmti ankinūtu šuruš* ... [... *š*]*uruš ḫašî* 182‴ *šuruš* GI.ZÚ.LUM.MA *pappasītu šuruš* Ú.KU$_6$ *kulī*[*li* ...] *lipî kanakti* 183‴ 25 *šammī annûti ištēniš tasâk ina šikari lā patān tašaqqīši-m*[*a m*]*ûša iparras*[*ū*]

179‴ Alternatively, a potion for her: the skull of a *kupītu*-bird, the skull of a crow, the *sk*[*ull of* ...], bark of the *kiškanû*-tree, 180‴ egg(s) of red ant(s), tallow from the right shoulder of a mountain-chameleon, a potsherd from a crossroads, f[at of ..., the pe]nis of a turtle, 181‴ *burāšu*-juniper, 'heals thousand'-plant, *imbu' tâmti*-mineral, *ankinūtu*-plant, root of [...] tree, root of *ḫašû*-plant, 182‴ root of GI.ZÚ.LUM.MA-plant, *pappasītu*-mineral, Ú.KU$_6$-fennel root, may[fly], 'fat' (pith) of *kanaktu*-plant. 183‴ These twenty-five drugs you pound together, you give (them) to her to drink in beer on empty stomach. [Th]en her [watery] discharge will stop.

184‴–188‴ (A_1 rev. iv 39–43)

184‴ DIŠ KI.MIN *tukaṣṣarši ḫalta šubâ imitta šu*[*bâ*] *š*[*umēla*] 185‴ *sāmta ša dāmi latikta sebet ḫerṣī ša e'ri tupallaš i*[*na*(?) ...] 186‴ [*kiṣ*]*ra takaṣṣar-ma ina tabarri šīpāti peṣêti tušakkak sebet kiṣrī takaṣṣar ē*[*ma taktaṣru*] 187‴ [*šipta k*]*iam tamannu* ÉN šal-lu-ur-za kéš dam-gal-la kur šal-l[u-ur-za kéš] 188‴ [ḫar-ra-g]i-ri ḫar-ra-gi-ri ḫar-ra-gi-ri šá-ḫi-ma-za-a-te ... [...]

184‴ Alternatively, you make knots for her: 185‴ you pierce 184‴ *ḫaltu*-stone, right *šubû*-'stone', l[eft] *šubû*-'stone,' 185‴ *genuine* (lit. 'tested') blood-red carnelian (and) seven pieces of *e'ru*-wood. *I*[*n/with* ...] 186‴ you tie a [kn]ot. Then you string (everything) on (a cord of) red and white wool. You tie seven knots (into the string). When[ever you have tied (a knot)], 187‴ you recite [the incantation] as follows. Incantation: Šallurza, bind! Wide mountain, Ša[llurza, bind!] 188‴ [Ḫarra g]iri ḫarra giri ḫarra giri šaḫimazate ... [...].

189‴ (A_1 rev. iv 44)

189‴ [KA.INIM.MA *šumma sinništu m*]*û ina libbi ūrīša illakū*

189‴ [Wording (of an incantation) for the case that watery disch]arges flow from a [woman's] vagina.

190‴ (A_1 rev. iv 45) *traces*

too fragmentary for translation

Ms. A_1 rev. iv breaks; remainder lost

Notes

Lines 1′–3′ (A_1 obv. i 1′–3′): The mineral pigments *kalû* and *kalgukku* often occur together. The former has been identified as yellow ochre, see Stol 1998, *FS Borger*, 347; Thavapalan 2020, 197, 346–350. The pigment *kalgukku* (IM.KAL.GUG) is identified by some Assyriologists with red ochre, supported by the element GUG in the Sumerogram, which means red/carnelian (Stol 1998, *FS Borger*, 347, with Charpin 1984, *MARI* 3, 258 note 2; Joannès 1984, ARM 23, 144); Thavapalan (2020,

197, 342–346) provides arguments for *kalgukku* as a "lead-based yellow colorant" ("lead yellow") and describes the colour spectrum of both pigments as ranging between yellow to red.

The ingredient "calf fat" (*šaman būri*, written Ì AMAR) in line 3′ is unexpected; the dictionaries do not offer parallels (CAD B, 340–342; CAD Š/1, 392). Could this be a scribal error for *šaman pūri* (Ì BUR) "oil from the jar"?

Lines 4′–8′ (A_1 col. i 4′–8′): The mineral ingredients listed here repeatedly occur together in amulet prescriptions for pregnant women, see chapters C.3 and F in this volume. Most of the minerals listed here are in fact shells or cowrie snails (*kapāṣu, yānibu, zibtu*, perhaps also *šubû, šû*), which have strong connotations with female genitals and with pregnancy (Oppenheim 1963, *OrNS* 32, 411; Schuster-Brandis 2008, 446, 449; Stol 2000a, 51–52; Scurlock 1991; Steinert 2012b, 82; Steinert 2017a). For *ḫaltu*-stone, which is often encountered in amulets, especially in the form of cylindrical beads (*kunuk ḫalti*), cf. CAD Ḫ, 53 s.v. *ḫaltu*; cf. Schuster-Brandis 2008, 193ff., 416 *passim*) and chapter F in this volume. For "blood-(red) carnelian," *sāmtu (ša) dāmi/ī*, here written ^{na4}GUG MÚD.MEŠ, see also below rev. iv 40 (line 185‴), where we find a varying spelling and formulation: ^{na4}GUG *šá* MÚD *latikta* "genuine(?) (lit. 'tested') blood-red carnelian". Cf. CAD S, 122 sub 3; Schuster-Brandis 2008, 415 and the note below.

For MUNUS.MUD "fertile" woman" (*ālittu*) in line 7′, compare the lexical equations of Sumerian mud with *(w)alādu* "to bear" and *banû* "to create", see CAD A/1 s.v. *alādu*; CAD B s.v. *banû* A. The present passage has not found an entry in the dictionaries under the lemma *(w)ālittu* (AHw 1458–1459; CAD A/1, 341–342 sub b). The syntax is admittedly somewhat unusual. The specification of having a "fertile woman" spin a thread for an amulet is in contrast with the activity of a post-menopausal woman in this role in line 22′ (obv. i 22′). Scurlock (2014a, 578 with n. 2) understands the logogram MUNUS.MUD differently, as a rendering of *da'mātu* "a dark-yellow mineral paste/pigment" (cf. CAD D 75a sub c, AHw 156–157, usually written IM.SIG$_7$.SIG$_7$ however).

Lines 9′–16′ (A_1 obv. i 9′–16′): For discussion of this ritual, see also Scurlock 1991; Scurlock 2014a, 572; Böck 2013, 45–46. The potsherd put in a secluded place (or room) in the woman's house, behind a door, signals obstruction and the desired effect of the treatment (stopping of bleeding). On the other hand, the sherd can also be seen as symbolising the woman's foetus (thus Böck 2013, 46; for the connection between potsherds and offspring, see also George 1991, *RA* 85, 146–147, 152–154 on a relevant commentary passage).

The goddess Ištar serves as divine helper in this ritual who is addressed with a *šigû*-prayer (Assyrian *šegû*). For *šigû*-prayers, cf. CAD Š/2, 413–414 (interpreted as "a lamentation" or "a type of prayer"); van der Toorn 1985, 117–121, 125–139; 1994, 54 (suggesting the woman's haemorrhage signalled some kind of guilt that was confessed in the prayer); Oshima 2011, 296–304 (likewise classifying *šigû* as a penitential prayer). For another ritual for a woman with a haemorrhage in which she utters a *šigû*-prayer, see also BAM 235 obv. 5 (text C.1.1). A (porous) potsherd, often found standing upright in the street or on a crossroads, is used in other prescriptions in BAM 237 (ii 41′–42′, ii 43′–44′, iii 6–7, iv 23, iv 35).

Lines 10′–11′ (A_1 obv. i 10′–11′): The reading KI *ta-ša-biṭ* "you sweep the ground" in line 10′ is preferred here over the reconstruction proposed in CAD Š/2, 431 s.v. *šikittu* A, discussion and Scurlock (2014a, 573): KI.TA *ša* É A *ta-sal-laḫ-ši*, translated by Scurlock (2014a, 578): "Below the house you sprinkle her with (some of the wash) water". The feminine suffix in GAR-*an-ši* and *tasallaḫši* could refer to the patient ("you set down/sprinkle (for) her"), but here it is more likely a reference to the potsherd (ŠIKA = *ḫaṣabtu* is likewise feminine); cf. CAD S, s.v. *salāḫu* A sub 1b; Scurlock 2014a, 573, 578 (with a differing reading); Böck 2013, 45. As pointed out in the previous note, the potsherd could symbolise an aborted foetus (that the woman has previously(?) lost). Before it is deposited, the potsherd is washed, anointed with oil and wrapped in red wool, resembling actions of first care given to a newborn baby (washing, anointing, clothing). The *šigû*-prayers (lamentations) uttered by the woman (in front of the door) on four consecutive days may have been concerned with the loss of a foetus. Another possibility proposed to me by Marten Stol (personal communication) is that the door (*daltu*) behind which the potsherd is deposited is indicated by the feminine pronominal suffix.

Lines 13′–14′ (A_1 obv. i 13′–14′): The potion, amulet and salve mentioned refer to the prescriptions in the preceding sections. The recipe for the potion is lost in the lacuna at the beginning of the tablet; the salve refers to the recipe in obv. i 1′–3′, the stone amulet refers to obv. i 4′–8′.

Line 16′ (A_1 obv. i 16′): The restoration *i-[di-šá* DU$_8$] "[she may loosen] her arms" at the end of the line follows a proposition by Henry Stadhouders in Abusch and Schwemer 2016, CMAwR 2, 454–455 and Abusch et al 2020, CMAwR 3, 389 (correction of CMAwR 1, 138 text 7.6.7 lines 28, 33), offering further textual parallels. This ritual gesture is the reversal of the patient kneeling down and putting her arms behind her back in line 11′.

Line 17′ (A_1 col. i 17′): For *bulṭu latku*, "tested/proven remedy", see Steinert 2015.

Lines 18′–20′ (A_1 obv. i 18′–20′): The goddess Inanna/Ištar is also encountered or invoked in the spells in obv. ii 11′–14′ and ii 18′–21′ (cf. below). The word *šugallītu* is a loanword from Sumerian šu-gal, "the one with big hands", and attested as a profession and divine epithet (cf. CAD Š/3, s.v. *šugallû*; Powell 1973, *ZA* 63, 105; Michalowski 1986, *JCS* 38, 167: 7, 169–170). The expression may be metaphorical here (i.e. "generous"). For *kiṣru ša šamê*, "bond/meteor of heaven", cf. CAD K, s.v. *kiṣru* sub 11b.

Line 22′ (A_1 obv. i 22′): For MUNUS KUD-tu_4 as a post-menopausal woman, see CAD P, 187. The term is apparently derived from *parāsu* "to cut off; to stop", which is often used with reference to stopping haemorrhage in gynaecological texts. The bilingual text CT 17, 20: 75–76 (SAG.GIG) offers the equation munus mud-da-gi_4-a = *sin-niš-tu pa-riš-tu* (similar to BAM 237 i 22′, the woman is to spin and twine threads in this passage). Postmenopausal and old women (*pa/uršumtu*) were employed to prepare substances for healing rituals (such as grinding grain or twisting/spinning threads), because they could not be a source of potential defilement through menstrual discharges (see CAD P, 525 s.v. *puršumu* sub lex. section). See also Finkel 2018, *FS Geller*, 261, 263, 265 BM 64526 obv. 15.

Line 24′ (A_1 obv. i 24′): The spelling KUD-*sa* (also in line 29′ and 74″) is ambiguous. It could stand for a present tense form of the G- or N-stem or for a stative form (3rd person fem. plural in each case, corresponding to the feminine plural of *naḫšātu*). Line 27′ alternatively spells KUD-*su* (corresponding to the masculine plural of A.MEŠ (*mû*) "fluids". CAD P, 177a s.v. *parāsu* sub 11a-3′ lists the present attestations in BAM 237 under the N-stem (cf. CAD P, 167–168 sub 1d), while a G-stem is tentatively assumed here.

Lines 26′–27′ (A_1 obv. i 26′–27′): B. Böck (2010a, *TUAT NF* 5, 112 n. 232) interprets DÚR-*ši* as *qinnatu* "bottom, anus" ("mit ihrem Gesäß soll sie ihr Wasser darüber fließen lassen"). I prefer to read it as a verbal form of (*w*)*ašābu* (Š-stem, *tušeššebši*), see CAD A/2, s.v. *ašābu* sub 4a for parallels of such formulas in medical texts. The text describes the procedure for a fumigation "from below", cf. Steinert 2014a; 2014b for discussion. Cf. for a similar instruction KAR 247 rev.(?) left col. 3′ (text C.3.6): [MUNUS *ina m*]*uḫ-ḫi* TUŠ-*ab* "the woman sits (down) above it".

Lines 28′–30′ (A_1 obv. i 28′–30′): *Illūru* is a plant with red flower and fruit, befitting its application against bleeding (cf. CAD I/J, 87–88). The blood of a sacrificial lamb can be compared with the colour of this flower/berry (cited CAD I/J, 87 b sub a). See also ms. A_1 iv 11 (line 156‴).

Line 33′ (A_1 obv. i 33′): For the mineral *alluḫaru* (IM.SAḪAR.BABBAR.KUR.RA, lit. "white dust of the mountains"), which, similar to alum (*gabû*), was used as a mordant in the leather industry, see Stol 1980–1983, "Leder(industrie)", *RlA* 6, 533 §18; Waetzoldt 2011, in: *Garšana Studies* (*CUSAS* 6), 435–436; Thavapalan 2020, 186–187, 336; Morgan and Richardson 2020, *Iraq* 82, 186–189.

Line 37′ (A_1 obv. i 37′): On the embedded gloss, in which the scribe added a (formerly omitted) drug (*imḫur-līm*) as an alternative to *imḫur-ešrā*, see Bácskay 2021b, 122; Scurlock 2014a, 57s.

Line 38′ (A_1 obv. i 38′): The sign $^{(ú)}$NÚMUN can be read *elpetu*, but also as *urbatu*/$^{(ú)}$$GUG_4$, both of which are rushes (cf. Borger 2004, MZL, 65–66, 267 sub no. 102; CAD E, 108–109 with discussion). CAD U/W, 212b sub b books this line under *urbatu*.

Scurlock (2014, 579) translates *ša* NIGIN in this line as "(a goat horn) that curls". The phrase is quoted but left untranslated in CAD U/W, 212b sub b. Most likely, NIGIN stands for *saḫāru* "to turn; to curve, curl" (said of hair and other body parts), cf. CAD S, 44–45 sub 3b-1′–2′. Marten Stol (personal communication) suggests that the phrase *ša* NIGIN may specify the goat rather than the horn and draws a connection to the term *sāḫirtu* A "heifer" (literally "free-roaming, i.e. not tethered"), a term, which however refers exclusively to cows (CAD S, 59, written ÁB.NIGIN or GUD.(ÁB).NIGIN).

Line 41′ (A_1 obv. i 41′): For the gloss in line 41′, cf. the discussion in Schuster-Brandis 2008, 396ff.; Bácskay 2021b, 123–124; Scurlock 2014a, 616 *ad* 4. Bácskay (2021b, 123–124) notes that the passage contains two glosses, the former of which presents a variant(?) ingredient for *ṣurrānītu* (i.e. *sāmtu*-carnelian), while the latter presents an alternative *materia medica* (*kapāṣu*-shell), to which presumably belongs the complementary treatment instruction (insertion into the vagina instead of application via an amulet). For *ṣurrānītu* (^{na4}GUG.ZÚ lit. "*ṣurru*-carnelian", a red stone or type of carnelian having dots in the colour of *ṣurru*-stone), cf. CAD Ṣ, 257 s.v. **ṣurrānû*; Schuster-Brandis 2008, 415–416; for seals made of *ṣurrānītu*, see Charpin 2017, *RA* 111, 171 (note 71); Cavigneaux 1996, AUWE 23, no. 53: 6.

Line 42′ (A_1 obv. i 43′): For the gloss embedding a variant ingredient – *anzaḫḫu*-mineral (a "primary glass") instead of *kutpû*-mineral (AN.ZAḪ.GI$_6$, 'black frit'), cf. Scurlock 2014a, 579; Bácskay 2021b, 124. For *anzaḫḫu*, see also Thavapalan 2020, 146–148 *passim*.

Lines 44′–45′ (A_1 obv. i 45′–46′): According to CAD Š/3, 162 discussion, ^{na4}*šu-a* in our passage might not stand for the *šû*-stone, but for a shell ^{na4}šu-ḫu-um listed beside the shells *ayyartu* and *kapāṣu* in a forerunner to ḪAR-ra *ḫubullu*. However, some references to *šû*-stone ('male' and 'female' *šû*-stone) may have stood for a shell or cowrie snail, cf. Schuster-Brandis 2008, 448–449. For *urīzu*-stone, see also K. 263+10934 (*infra* text C.1.9).

Lines 46′–47′ (A_1 obv. i 47′–48′): Instead of ^{na4}*zíb-tu*$_4$, Stol (2000a, 49 n. 7) proposes to read ^{na4}*ḫáš-tum* (a stone attested in the Old Babylonian version of Lugale 603–611, which Stol regards as a variant for the *ḫaltu*-stone, cf. Schuster-Brandis 2008, 416; Joannès 1989, *RA* 83, 122–123). For *ḫaltu*-stone used in BAM 237, see above obv. i 4′. More often, a cylindrical bead of *ḫaltu*-stone (^{na4}KIŠIB *ḫalti*) is used in amulets, cf. AHw 1558b; SpTU 2, no. 22 iii 40; BAM 376 i 17, iii 20; Schuster-Brandis 2008, 193ff. *passim*. The *zibtu*-stone may refer to a shell, as it is elsewhere mentioned among "stones of the sea" (cf. Oppenheim 1963, *OrNS* 32, 411; Schuster-Brandis 2008, 456; Arkhipov 2012, 39, 58; 2018, 50). See further BAM 498–500 rev. iii 33; ^{na4}*zíb-tú gu-ti-tú* as an ingredient in an amulet against hair loss in a female patient (see *infra*, Chapter H Appendix). For *ayyartu* with seven dots, referring to a shell or perhaps coral, see also ms. A rev. iii 2, 28; CAD T, 403b sub a).

For "tendon of a cow cadaver" (SA ÁB RI.RI.GA), see also lines 41′ and 101″ in the present text; CAD M/2, 101–102 s.v. *miqittu* sub 3a; CAD L, 217 s.v. *littu* sub a-2′.

Lines 48″–64″, 65″ and 66″–68″ (A_1 obv. ii 1′–6′ //, ii 7′, ii 8′–10′): The incantation can be almost completely restored with the help of the duplicates from Nineveh, Babylon and Uruk, all of which use it for amulets to stop nosebleed. Mss. b-d preserve only the wording of the spell; the accompanying instructions and ingredients for the amulet employed in conjunction with the spell are partially preserved on the Neo-Assyrian fragment K. 4782: 7′–10′ (amulets, CDLI photo P395714), which only cites the incipit of the incantation in line 10′: ÉN *mim-mu-ú* DINGIR.MEŠ DÙ-*ú a-me-lu-t*[*u* ... ŠID-*nu*]. According to this fragment, the amulet consisted of six stones, of which only three are fully preserved (*mūṣu*-stone, carnelian, *šubû*-stone; cf. line 8′: 6 NA$_4$.MEŠ MÚD *ina* KIR$_4$-*šú* DU-*ku* "six stones (when) blood is flowing from his nose"; see also K. 4782: 13′; Schuster-Brandis 2008, 109f. Kette 62). The fragmentary fourth ingredient, a plant name, in K. 4782: 7′ is probably to be restored as ^{ú}AŠ.TÁ[L.TÁL] (*ardadillu*). As far as can be told from the few traces in ms. A_1 ii 8′–10′, the treatment accompanying the spell in BAM 237 may differ from the one in K. 4782, but it probably consisted of an amulet as well (the beginning of ms. A_1 ii 9′ is most likely *šû*-stone).

In ms. c i 21′, *ša purussaša lā parsu*, is interpreted here as a stative form of *parāsu* parallel to *ša lā kullū kālûša* in c i 20′ (cf. CAD P 529b, reading BAR-*ṣu*, without translation). The metaphors encountered in mss. b–d (meadow, waterskin, fermenting vessel) are very similar to those in incantations against diarrhoea and other digestive ailments, see Steinert 2013, *JMC* 22, 11; Steinert and Vacín 2018). Ms. A_1 omits these three lines (59–61).

Line 61″ (ms. c i 23′ and d i 3′) addresses a deity who is sent up to heaven to bring down the seal of Anu. The title given to him is taken here as a performative statement highlighting the deity's expertise and power to stop the blood. The phrase *sa'mat amēlūti* "the redness of humankind" would be a poetic expression for blood (cf. CAD S 126ff. s.v. *sāmu* (also *sa'mu*) "red"; cf. CAD S 124–125 s.v. *sāmtu* B (*sāntu*, *sā'tu*) "redness"). The form (*ša*) *takullû* (Assyrian form instead of *takallû*) is probably best interpreted here as *kalû* "to hold back, to cut off (water), to stop, to block". The word *ši-pat-su* is ambiguous and could be read either as *šiptu* with pronominal suffix, "(his) incantation", or as *šipassu* (also written *šipatsu*) "clay sealing" (CAD Š/3, 57, often with the verb *nadû*). It is possible that the deity responsible for bringing the blood-staunching remedy was already addressed by name in the gap at the beginning of line 54″; however, I have opted to restore [MÚD.MEŠ *šá*] at the beginning of this line, following Mayer 2022b, *OrNS* 91, 337 s.v. *damu*.

Line 64″ (A_1 obv. ii 6′ //): For *mimma/mimmu ša illaku*, with *alāku* in the meaning "to be suitable; to fit", see CAD A/1, 312–313 sub 3l. Mss. c and d both present a scribal error in this passage.

Line 65″ (A_1 obv. ii 7′ //): For the combination of *redû* Š-stem ("to make a fluid flow away; to sweep away (in a flood)") and *alāku*, with the meaning "to flow copiously", used in the rubric in mss. b-d with reference to nosebleed, cf. also BAM 580 iii 21, in a different context (skin diseases): "pus flows copiously (from an open sore)" (MÚD.[BABBAR] *šur-du-ma* DU-*ak*; Scurlock and Andersen 2005, 229 10.113; CAD R, 243–244 sub 14). Ms. c appears to present a variant GUB.BA = *šuzuzzu* at the end of the rubric, which is emended here to DU-*ku*! following ms. b. The Š-stem of *izuzzu* "to stand" is not used elsewhere in the sense of "to stop" (bleeding), cf. Mayer 2022b, *OrNS* 91, 337 translating it as "zum Stehen zu bringen".

Lines 69″–72″ (A_1 obv. ii 11′–14′): The reading of this fragmentary spell featuring Inanna remains tentative; possibly, the goddess is described as a female model for the human patient (cf. line 13′). Most passages look Sumerian, others could also be read as Akkadian (e.g. *limḫur*(?) in line 14′).

Lines 76″–79″ (A_1 obv. ii 18′–21′): The reading and interpretation of the incantation is very tentative. The text seems to resemble the following incantation in col. ii 25′–27′, which repeats certain words or phrases. The first sign SAR in col. ii 18′ may be read as Sumerian $kiri_6$ "orchard; garden", parallel to a-šà "field" at the beginning of col. ii 19′. These two words may be agricultural metaphors referring to the "womb" (šà-tùr) mentioned in col. ii 21′. The text in ii 21′ may be understood as a Sumerian sentence: šà-tùr ^{d}inanna ba-du_{10}-ga "the womb, oh Inanna (or possibly "the womb of Inanna"), is good/sweet". In contrast, lines ii 18′–20′ may present a mixture of Sumerian (or logographic writings) and Akkadian. Thus, I tentatively take *ta-kal-la* occurring twice in ii 18′ as a second person verbal form (G-stem present) of Akkadian *kalû* "to hold back". It remains unclear who the masculine subject of this verb is, but a deity would be expected (maybe Ea or Asalluḫi?). The verb may refer to the power of a deity to hold back water from flooding the "garden" (i.e. to hold back or stop haemorrhage). The sequence $kiri_6$ ur-zé kéš in line 18′ is difficult, but understanding kéš as "bound" (or possibly an imperative) with reference to the garden would fit the context. Maybe, ur-zé stands for Sumerian ur-zu "your servant", but this is mere guess (Sumerian zé usually means "gall, bile"; ur may also stand for úr "loin, lap").

In ii 19′–20′, we find the sign PIRIG three times, which could be read as Sumerian piriĝ "lion". Since ^{lú}(KA).PIRIG/PÌRIG is encountered in first millennium BCE texts and lexical sources as a word corresponding to *āšipu* "conjurer", the present text may be a reflection of this tradition (cf. Geller 2010, 45–48 for discussion; see also *infra* text B.2.6 line 4). The Sumerian phrase gal-zu abzu-ke_4 "the wise one of the Abzu" preceding the signs piriĝ ḫuš in ii 19′ might thus refer either to the Enki/Ea or Asalluḫi, the divine exorcists par excellence. Sumerian ḫuš can mean "fierce, terrible, furious" or possibly stand for ḫuš-(a) "red", and thus piriĝ ḫuš "fierce/red lion/exorcist" could be another divine epithet. Notably, ^{d}ḫuš is an epithet of Marduk, and ^{d}ḫuš-ki-a "fierce god of the netherworld" a title of Nergal (Lambert 1972–1975, *RlA* 4, 522–523). In ii 20′, *ḫuš-sa-a* could be an error for *ḫuš-ša-a* "red" (often said of garments), and SA *ḫuš-sa-a* would be "a red string/tendon/sinew". If the signs ⸢*tu-še*⸣-*du-ši* are correctly read as an Akkadian verbal form, it may be a Š-stem of *edû* "to know", used in the meanings "to make something known; to announce, proclaim; to mark".

Lines 81″–82″ (A_1 obv. ii 23′–24′): For $KIŠI_{16}$-*ḫa-aḫ* as *ulḫaḫ*, referring to a type of *ašāgu*-acacia, see CAD U/W, 72b s.v. *ulḫaḫ*; Hallo and van Dijk 1968, *The Exaltation of Inanna*, 75. For stirring a medical liquid with an arrow, see also BAM 248 obv. i 68–69, where oil, with which the woman is rubbed to ease delivery, is stirred with an arrow (see text D.1.1). In the present prescription in BAM 237, the ingredients stirred with an arrow are used for a potion. For the use of an arrow, see also the ritual to stop bleeding in BM 40152 iii 17–26 (*infra* text C.1.8). The therapeutic instructions in obv. ii 24′ and ii 29′ to prepare the remedy "in front of Šamaš" may be linked to the sun god's role in several rituals for women (also in connection with birth). See BM 40152 rev. iii 17–26 (text C.1.8) and *passim*.

Lines 83″–85″ (A_1 obv. ii 25′–27′): This incantation appears to resemble obv. ii 18′–21′. Interestingly, it mentions the god Marduk (^{d}ŠÀ.ZU). However, Sumerian šà-zu (lit. "knowing the inside (of the body)") also means "midwife", and ^{d}šà-zu diĝir-re-e-ne "midwife of the gods" is a title of the mother goddess (Krebernik 1993–1997, *RlA* 8, 507).

Line 87″ (A_1 obv. ii 29′): Possibly ÚKUŠ.TI.GI.LI (*tigilû*) "colocynth, squash" is to be restored in the gap. For various logographic writings of this word, see CAD T, s.v. *tigilû*.

Lines 88″–90″ (A_1 obv. ii 30′–32′): The formula in ii 30′ is of uncertain meaning. It is attested in variant spellings in several older incantations (in Early Dynastic, Ur III, Old Babylonian and first millennium BCE texts), see N. Rudik 2011, 66ff. *passim* for discussion. It is the opening formula in a number of Sumerian incantations from the Old Babylonian period to stop haemorrhage during pregnancy (ka-inim-ma munus kéš-da-kam "spell(s) for binding a woman"), which appear to preserve older versions of the text encountered in BAM 237 ii 30′–32′: CBS 10489 + 10756, YOS 11, No. 40 and CBS 1509 (previously edited by Finkel 1980, *AfO* 27, 1980, 41ff. texts A–C).

Lines 89″–90″ (A_1 obv. ii 31′–32′): Compared with parallels in Old Babylonian spells to stop haemorrhage, pa in ii 31′ and 32′ may stand for or pa_5 "canal". Cf. Finkel 1980, 42 CBS 10489 + 10756: 4: a-idim úš-e-dè pa_5-a-dug_4-ga de-de-dè "in order to dam up the water of the source flowing into the irrigation canal" (pa_5-a-dug_4-ga, Akk. *namkaru*). See also CBS 1509 col. iv 3–4 (Finkel 1980, 39–40 text C col. iv). Thus, pa zi-zi in BAM 237 ii 31′ could mean "the rising canal" (referring to a rising flood describing the haemorrhage in metaphorical terms). See also CBS 1509 col. iii 4 (Finkel 1980, 39–40 text C col. iii): pa_5 z[i-zi-dam(?) pa_5 z]i-zi-dam i-zi gá-g[á] "At the rising of the canal, at the rising of the canal, a flood being set(?), …".

Line 90″ (A_1 obv. ii 32′): The sign še in BAM ii 30′ and 32′ appears to replace the morpheme -šè in the Old Babylonian parallels. Thus, pa-še in BAM 237 ii 32′ could stand for pa_5-šè. The sign gam in BAM ii 32′ in the phrase pa-še gam zi-zi could stand for gaba zi-zi in the Old Babylonian sources. In lexical sources, Sumerian gaba zi-(zi) is equated with *nêʾu ša irti* "to turn back (the breast)", meaning "to remove; turn someone back; to make someone depart" (CAD N/2, 198). However, for the context of the Sumerian spells, Finkel (1980, 43–44) suggested a meaning of "to calm down". The phrase šu u-ne-ni-ta may possibly be understood as a corrupt spelling of a form such as šu ù-me-ni-ti (šu ti "to take; to receive").

Line 92″ (A_1 obv. ii 34′): For *maštakal*-soapwort in remedies to stop bleeding, which was prescribed in potions, tampons and amulets, see also K. 263+10934 obv. 2, 19; BAM 236 obv. 14 (dried seed), 18; FLP 1306 obv. 4–6 (dried seed), rev. 28; BM 40152 rev. iii 27, 29 and further texts in this chapter. *Maštakal* is also found in BAM 237 i 39′–42′, i 47′–48′ and iv 13.

For *maḫāṣu* "to stir" (powder, medication) into a liquid, restored here (*ta-ma-*[*ḫa-aṣ*]), see also line 82″ (*tu-ma-ḫ*[*aṣ-ma*] in the D-stem); CAD M/1, 78–79 sub 3e.

Line 94″ (A_1 obv. ii 36′): For *atbaru*-stone, a dark, grey basalt, cf. Schuster-Brandis 2008, 393. Instead of *atbaru*-stone with seven holes (*pilšu*), a second prescription in BAM 237 rev. iii 2 uses *atbaru*-stone with seven dots (*tikpu*). For *atbaru*, see also Stol 1979, *On Trees*, 85–86; Ramez 2019, 849.

Lines 95″–97″ (A_1 obv. ii 37′–39′): Due to the fragmentary preservation of the text, the reading of the spell is uncertain.

Lines 99″–100″ (A_1 obv. ii 41′–42′): Cf. CAD Q, s.v. *qablu* sub 2a-1′; ÍB occurs in lexical and bilingual texts for *qablu* "hip, waist", see e.g. Vokabular Sb 157 (MSL 3, 141); Ḫh. XIII 42, 339b (MSL 8, 10 and 48).

Lines 103″–104″ (A_1 obv. ii 45′–46′): For GIG, read as Akkadian *ḫerṣu* "block", derived from *ḫarāṣu* "to cut off", see CAD Ḫ, s.v. *ḫirṣu*; CAD E, s.v. *eʾru* sub b 3 c′. The word also occurs in col. iv 40 in syllabic spelling (seven *ḫerṣu* of *eʾru*-wood are pierced and strung on white and red wool). See further KAR 223: 4 //: 14 GIG ^{giš}MA.NU *ina* SÍG SA_5 *tušakkak* "you string 14 pieces of *eʾru*-wood on red wool" (see *infra* text D.3.1).

Lines 111″–112″ (A_1 rev. iii 6–7): The term *sappartu* is rendered as "tip of an animal's horn" in CAD S, 165–166; differently AHw 1027a: "Fell an Hornwurzel", similarly also Durand 1983, *ARM* 21, 281–283. Compare the use of this ingredient in BAM 503 i 16′ in the context of ear diseases caused by a ghost, specifying KA *sapparti qaran alpi* "the point(?) of the *sappartu* of an ox's horn" (Scurlock 2014a, 369). It remains unclear whether hair or a substance from the bottom part of the horn is meant here. The ingredients in the present remedy include minerals and may have been used for a leather bag or for a tampon (if the ingredients were crushed).

Lines 114″–123″ (A_1 rev. iii 9–18): The beginning of this Sumerian incantation is identical with the beginning of a spell known from Nineveh tablets of the series ŠÀ.ZI.GA, see K. 9451 + 1167 6+ Sm 818 + Sm 961 i 15′–16′, Biggs 1967, 45–46 No. 26: 15′–16′: ÉN dím-[dím an-n]a [dím-dí]m an-na (the remainder is unfortunately lost). Cf. Zisa 2021, 389, 399 No. K.1 IV (ms. B o. i 15′–16′) reads GIM [dím-an-n]a GIM d[ím-an-na] "Like crea[tion? of heav]en?, like cr[eation of heaven]" instead. The incipit of this incantation is also cited in the ŠÀ.ZI.GA incantation catalogue LKA 94 i 14 (see Biggs 1967, 12: dím-dím an-na; Zisa 2021, 218 reading GIM dím-an-na).

In line 118″ (A_1 iii 13), du-du might stand for du_{11}-du_{11} "speaking", in rev. iii 14 nam-ba-ti, ti may stand for te(ĝ) "to approach, come near".

Lines 125″–126″ (A_1 rev. iii 20–21): For roasted chickpeas (GÚ.GAL *qa-la-a-te*), see e.g. BAM 431 rev. ii 8′ (CAD Ḫ, s.v. *ḫallūru*). *Nuḫurtu*-plant is often found in remedies to stop bleeding, see also K. 263 + 10934 rev. 25; BAM 235 obv. 5; BAM 236 obv. 12 and *passim* in this chapter. See also BAM 237 i 32′, ii 17′, iv 4 and 13.

In the gap in line 126″ (iii 21), one expects the name of a fluid that is used in addition to beer. Possibly, restore [*ina* A GA]ZI$^{(sar)}$, "[with juice of *ka*]*sû*-plant".

The repetition of MIN-*ma* MIN at the end of iii 21 is somewhat unexpected. It is thus assumed here that MIN-*ma* stands for "a second time (you give to drink)" (*šanîš*?), and that the final MIN refers to the phrase *naḫšātu iparrasā* "the *naḫšātu*-discharge will stop".

Lines 127″–130″ (A_1 rev. iii 22–25): This looks like a pseudo-Sumerian spell. In line iii 22, i-gi may stand for igi "eye"; igi gub/du$_{(8)}$ means "to see". Alternatively, one could also read i-gi-da ba-túm as "with the eye(s) it was brought (there)" (as an allusion to the evil eye or to sorcery). In iii 23, še-ga means "favourable"; zi-ga in iii 24 "to rise; to be removed".

Lines 135″–136″ (A_1 rev. iii 30–31): At the beginning of iii 31, perhaps restore [*an-nu*]-*rig* "now". In iii 31, emendation to *ay it*<*tal*>*l*[*ukū*] (Gtn-stem preterite of *alāku*) "they shall not keep flowing off" (i.e. the fluids, *mû*) is proposed here as a suitable form with the vetitive.

Line 138″ (A_1 rev. iii 33): *šadânu ṣābitu* "magnetite" is often encountered in remedies to stop bleeding, see also BAM 237 i 45′; SpTU 4, No. 153 obv. 17 (potion) and in K. 263 + 10934 rev. 38 (tampon) and 33 (potion); BAM 235 obv. 2 (tampon); BM 40152 iii 6–8, iii 9–13. See *infra* texts C.1.5, C.1.1, C.1.8 and *passim*).

Line 142″ (A_1 rev. iii 37): For *tarmuš*-plant in remedies to staunch bleeding, see also K. 263 + 10934 obv. 14 (text C.1.5).

Line 148‴ (A_1 rev. iv 3): For mineral pigments such as *dāmātu/da'mātu* (IM.SIG$_7$.SIG$_7$), a dark yellow to brownish earth, *illūr pānī* (also *lurpânu*; IM.KÙ.SI$_{22}$, lit. "gold earth") "rouge" (red-coloured cosmetic pigment, perhaps lead-based) and *kalû* "yellow ochre", see Thavapalan 2020, 194–199, 341–354; Frahm 2011, *Commentaries*, 397 obv. 10, 398 obv. 6, 401 n. 1881. For the use of clays or mineral earths such as *kalû* "yellow ochre" in the context of bleeding, cf. Steinert 2012b, 76–77. Alum (*gabû*) is well known as a haemostatic drug and occurs very often in the Mesopotamian recipes, see the other texts edited in this chapter.

Lines 151‴–152‴ (A_1 rev. iv 6–7): For the identification of *kamūn bīni* as the galls growing on tamarisk, see Streck 2004, *ZA* 94, 285–286. The term *kamūnu* B refers to a fungus or mushroom, which resembles galls as the swelling growths on plants.

The logographic spelling MUŠ.DÍM.GUR$_4$.RU.NU for *pizallurtu* (or *pizallūru*) "gecko" in iv 6 is a variant for MUŠ.DÍM. GURUN.NA; other attested spellings include MUŠ.DA.GUR$_4$.RA and MUŠ.DÍM.KUR.RA. Beside the animal, the word *pizallurtu* also designates a medicinal plant, but the latter is written with a different logogram (^{ú}AM.SI.ḪAR.RA.NA, lit. "elephant of the road"), cf. CAD P 451–452 s.v. *pizallūru*. Several other prescriptions attest to the use of the animal, either whole or in part, e.g. the blood of a gecko to treat scorpion sting, or "copulating geckos of the steppe" (for sexual desire and jaundice), see CAD P 451–452 sub 1b; Zisa 2021, 408–409 Text K Prescription 31: 135–140 = Text N Prescription 8 (ii 3–8). The latter use of geckos mirrors its occurrence as an ingredient in a text to promote conception (STT 98: 21′, see text A.1.1). For associations of geckos and lizards with fertility, see also Zisa 2021, 167 *passim*.

In the present prescription not only gecko, but also "sand wasp" (NIM.UR$_4$.UR$_4$ = *ḫāmītu*, cf. Landsberger 1934, *Fauna*, 133) and "excrement of *ṣurāru*-lizard" make an appearance as ingredients for a tampon to stop bleeding. It is unknown whether "lizard excrement" (*zê ṣurāri*) is an alias name for a plant substance. For "excrement of multicoloured wall lizard" (*ṣurār igāri barmu*) in prescriptions to cause an abortion and to speed up difficult labour, see BAM 246 (text B.1.6) and BAM 248 (text D.1.1).

Lines 154‴–155‴ (A_1 rev. iv 9–10): For discussion of the disease term NI.NE (or Ì.KÚM), see the *Introduction*, section 4.2. The disease name appears beside the symptom *kīs šīnāti*(KÀŠ) "binding of the urine" (i.e. difficulty of emptying the bladder) in BM 42313+ rev. 1–2 (text A.2.2). BM 42313+ rev. 2 offers basically the same treatment as BAM 237 iv 10, a tampon of drugs bound up in pieces of cloth, but it uses one alternative plant ingredient (*urbatu*-rush instead of *amḫara*-plant). Böck (2010a, *TUAT NF* 5, 112) translates the instruction in BAM 237 iv 10 differently: "verknüpfst es mit 14 Knoten in einem Tuch und führst es mit einem Mal in ihren Mutterleib ein". The choice of ashes, i.e. charred plant materials, could be linked with the intended drying effect of the treatment, cf. SpTU 4, No. 153: 1–4, 11, 15 (*infra* text C.1.10 and *passim*), which refers to the drying effect of certain drugs recommended to stop bleeding. See also below A_1 iv 21–23, CAD Ṭ, 111b s.v. *ṭikmennu*.

Line 157‴ (A_1 rev. iv 12): Note that BM 42313+ rev. 3 recommends "white drug" (Ú BABBAR) for NI.NE-disease, but here in a potion (see text A.2.2). BM 42313+ rev. 4 uses the same application form, introducing the medicine into the urethra with a bronze tube, but the recipe applies a different ingredient, *murru*-aromatic, instead of "white drug" (Ú BABBAR, explained in drug lists as resin of *ṣarbatu*-poplar) in BAM 237 iv 12. For Ú BABBAR, see also texts B.2.2 (UET 7, No. 123 obv. 1, 10), B.2.4 (BM 42587 obv. 9′) and *passim*.

Lines 160‴–173‴ (A_1 rev. iv 15–28): At the beginning of line 160‴, collation of the tablet did not confirm the reading [^{munus}P]EŠ$_4$, which has been proposed by Böck 2013, 43–44 with n. 60. Böck suggests reading the following word as *lūtu/lu'tu* (*lu-tam*) "dirt", regarding it as a term for an abnormal discharge regarded as impure and caused by witchcraft (i.e. "if a pregnant woman suffers from 'dirt' (i.e. dirty discharge)". However, the traces of the first visible sign in line 15 are clearly AL, not PEŠ$_4$, confirming the reading *al-lu-tú* (for this reading, see also Labat 1957–1971a, "Frauenkrankheiten", *RlA* 3, 109; Finkel 1980, *AfO* 27, 45 n. 13). Scurlock (2014a, 580; also Scurlock and Andersen 2005, 2.25) understands the word *alluttu* "crab" as a reference to body parasites. The term is otherwise not attested in the gynaecological corpus as a disease name, but its similarity with ancient Greek *karkinos* "crab" is striking. *Karkinos* was not only the term for the zodiac sign Cancer, but also for malign tumours in Greek medical texts (and incidentally the word from which English "cancer" stems). Because of this similar semantic pattern, it is tempting to regard *alluttu* "crab"-disease as the Akkadian counterpart to *karkinos* (for discussion, see Steinert 2021a, *Byzantinische Forschungen* 33, 64–65; Stol 2016, 448). Ancient physicians would have recognised uterine tumours first in symptoms of abnormal bloody discharges and severe pain in the lower belly, which would explain the discussion of this disease in a text dealing with abnormal vaginal discharges and haemorrhage.

The remedies collected in this section of BAM 237 are remarkable, since they consist mostly of simples (each recipe has only one drug wrapped up in a tampon or given in a potion).

At the beginning of line 163‴ (iv 18), instead of [B]AR ^{giš}NU.ÚR.MA "pomegranate [ri]nd", a reading [*ar*]*ti* ([P]A) "[tw]ig (of pomegranate tree)" is not excluded.

At the beginning of line 164‴ (iv 19), ZÚ GEME.LÚ.U$_{18}$.LU is probably a mistake for ZÚ NAM.LÚ.U$_{18}$.LU "human tooth". Scurlock (2014a, 576) reads KA.MÚRGU$^{!}$ "(human) vertebra" instead. Human tooth is also used in a prescription against toothache, see AMT 24/3: 11: ZÚ NAM.LÚ.U$_{18}$.LU *tur-ár* SÚD$^{!}$(MAR) "you char and pound human tooth". The application of tooth is comparable to the use of animal bones or eggshells in haemostatic remedies (all these materials contain calcium). The ingredient "black flour" (KU/ZÌ GI$_6$) is unusual, but compare for black grain, Cooper 1972, *ZA* 62, 73: 18. Scurlock 2014a, 576 reads TÚG GI$_6$ "black cloth" instead.

In line 169‴ (iv 24), it would also be possible to read GA.RA[Š^{sar}] instead of *ga-bi-*[*e*], since *gabû* is usually preceded by NA$_4$.

Line 170‴ (A_1 rev. iv 25): For *ḫašû* (^{ú}ḪAR.ḪAR) "thyme", see Stol 2011–2013, "Thymian", *RlA* 13, 641.

Line 172‴ (A_1 rev. iv 27): The plant term GI.ZÚ.LUM.MA is equated with the Akkadian terms *buṣinnu* "wick", *kūru* and *kurṣiptu*, see CAD K, 572 s.v. *kūru* C; AHw 143a, 512a, 515b; Abusch et al. 2020, CMAwR 3, 472. Geller and Panayotov (2020, 273 on lines 19–20) understand GI.ZÚ.LUM.MA literally as "date reed", "the small brances holding the dates". The plant list Uruanna equates Ú GI.ZÚ.LUM.MA with GI.MEŠ *ḫaṣṣuṣūti* "snapped-off reeds" (quoted in CAD Q, 86a s.v. *qanû* lex. section; Rumor 2017, *JMC* 29, 7: 18).

Lines 174‴–178‴ (A_1 rev. iv 29–33): The diagnostic phrase in col. iv 29, *šumma sinništu šammē zērūte šūkul* "if a woman has been given drugs of hatred to eat", features a frozen masculine stative form instead of feminine *šūkulat*, see Abusch and Schwemer 2011, CMAwR 1, 36 for discussion. The word *ze-ru-te* can be understood either as a masc. plural form of the verbal adjective *zīru* "hated; hateful(?)" or as the noun *zērūtu* "hatred". The belief that sorcery could lead to serious health problems, through the ingestion of bewitched food or drink, is widespread in Mesopotamia and often dealt with in healing texts. For a parallel passage from the corpus of anti-witchcraft literature, see e.g. Abusch and Schwemer 2011, 36 Text 1.1.1: 21′: [*ana pi*]*šerti kišpī ša ina šūmī šūkul*(*u*) "For undoing witchcraft that (the patient) was given to eat with garlic (beside witchcraft that he was given to drink in beer in line 13′; see also ibid. lines 74⁗–75⁗).

It is assumed here that the watery discharges (A.MEŠ, *mû*, lit. "water") which are flowing from the woman's vagina refer to an abnormal genital discharge differentiated from blood. The text does not explicitly speak of a pregnant patient. If one assumes that all prescriptions on the tablet deal with ailments of pregnant women, the word *mû* can alternatively be understood as amniotic fluid. Cf. also lines 178‴, 183‴ and 189‴. Scurlock and Andersen 2005, nos. 4.21 and 4.22 discuss the present prescriptions as cases of vaginitis; Labat 1957–1971a, "Frauenkrankheiten", *RlA* 3, 109 suggested leukorrhoea.

In line 175‴ (iv 30), I read *ana* NÍG.GIG-*ša* NU GÍD.DA, with NÍG.GIG as a variant logogram for GIG = *murṣu* "illness" (cf. CAD M/2, 224 and 225 sub 1b; Abusch et al. 2020, 91) The interpretation of the logogram DÈ.LÁ as a variant spelling for DÈ = *pēntu* "charcoal" or *diqmēnu* "ashes" follows a suggestion by Stol (2020b, *BiOr* 77, 570b), since DÈ *urbate* "ashes of *urbatu*-rushes" is found more often in BAM 237 (see e.g. rev. iv 10). Other interpreters read the logogram BÍL.LÁ, which is equated with Akkadian *emṣu* "sour", cf. CAD E, s.v. *emṣu*. Scurlock (2014a, 581) translates BÍL.LÁ as sourdough; CAD U/W 212 offers no translation. Since BÍL.LÁ and ^{ú}*ur-ba-te* also occur side by side in BAM 12: 30′ (where both ingredients are sifted and then knead into a dough with *kasû*-juice), Abusch et al. (2020, text 5.10 line 2) consider BÍL.LÁ ^{ú}*ur-ba-te* as the name of one drug, a part or product of *urbatu*-rush. For the meaning "sourdough, yeast" and discussion of *emṣu* "cheese", cf. Fritzsche 2011.

At the end of the line, Abusch et al. (2020, text 5.10 notes on line 2) suggest to restore N[A_4 ^{giš}*nu-úr-me*]-⸢*e*⸣ "pomegranate seeds".

Line 177‴ (A_1 rev. iv 32): The phrase *ana* 15-*šú* NI BA is ambiguous and has been interpreted in differing ways. That *ni-ba* is an abbreviation for the shell *yānibu* (cf. Oppenheim 1963, *OrNS* 32, 411; Schuster-Brandis 2008, 421 with. N. 783; Deller, Mayer and Sommerfeld 1987, *OrNS* 56, 217) is unlikely here, since the determinative na_4 is missing. In their recent treatment of the passage, Abusch et al. (2020, CMAwR 3, 90, 92 text 5.10 note to line 4) read *ni-ba* and understand *nību* as a "small portion of the medication, which is applied fifteen times". They relate the passage with *nību* B, referring to a small piece of stone or metal, see CAD N/2 206a s.v. *nību* B; Abusch and Schwemer 2011, CMAwR 1, 409: 30 ("small pieces"). For a differing interpretation, cf. Scurlock 2014a, 581, 617 with n. 6, 15, connecting the term with *nību* A "name; amount; number" (CAD N/2 204–206 s.v *nību* A; AHw 785b). Scurlock translates: "You tie fifteen-count (knots) in a loincloth (and sprinkle them with the mixture)." Compare Schuster-Brandis 2008, 239 on 231: 118; CTMMA 2, 170 no. 32 iv 21 where *nību* indicates the number (of stones needed) for one necklace (*kišādu*). The present edition follows CAD Z, 78a s.v. *zâzu* sub 2b-1′ and AHw 1518a mng. II, 4, regarding Ì.BA as a logogram for *tazâz* (from *zâzu*) "you divide". There are syllabic attestations of the phrase *ana* X-*šu tazâz* "you divide into X parts" from other medical texts, see e.g. Geller 2005a, *BAM* 7, no. 34 (BAM 68: 49): A.MEŠ *ana* 3-*šú ta-za-az-ma* "you divide the liquid into three parts" (followed by instruction for application).

After the mixture of ingredients is divided into fifteen portions, these are, I suggest, wrapped into pieces of cloth, here exceptionally referred to as *ṣubāt* or *lubār*(TÚG.ḪI.A) *ḫalli* "loincloth", lit. "cloth of the crotch"; cf. CAD Ṣ, 225b discussion. Abusch et al. (2020, 92 note on line 4) think the term designates "a kind of (menstrual) cloth, usually designated as *kannu*". Rather than restoring the verb *tu-*[*rak*]*-kas* "you tie/bind" (D-stem of *rakāsu*) as proposed here (see CAD R, 102 sub 8a for similar uses), Abusch et al. (2020, 90 text 5.10 line 4) suggest restoring *tu-*[*par*]*-ras* (D-stem of *parāsu*), translating the passage "(Fifteen times) you [divi]de up a portion (of the mixture) on a loin cloth". Scurlock (2014a, 581) reconstructs *tu-*[*šar*]*-kas* (Š-stem of *rakāsu*), which is semantically problematic.

Lines 179‴–183‴ (A_1 rev. iv 34–38): For collations of individual passages in these lines, see Abusch et al. 2020, CMAwR 3, pl. 63. This prescription for a potion to stop watery discharge uses several peculiar "animal" ingredients, some of which may be alias names for plants. For *kupītu*-bird, see AHw 508. Instead of *muḫḫu* (UGU) "skull, brain", one usually encounters SAG.(DU) in references to birds' heads as ingredients in recipes (see CAD A/2, 266 sub 1c). It is likely that *muḫḫu* is used here as a synonym for *qaqqadu* or *rēšu*, but it is also possible that it refers specifically to the brain or skull. For these meanings of *muḫḫu* see Militarev and Kogan 2000, No. 187; Westenholz and Sigrist 2006; 2008, 227–228; Stol 2007, *BiOr* 64, 334 ("brain" or "marrow"); Steinert 2012a, *Aspekte*, 386 with n. 6. For the ritual use of *kupītu*-bird and raven in anti-witchcraft procedures, see Rutz 2016, *ZA* 106, 55–56 N 11′ with comments on our passage on p. 59. See also Abusch and Schwemer 2011, CMAwR 1, text 1.1, 1: 98‴‴, where the "head of a white crow" (SAG.DU *erēbi peṣê*) is part of an ointment appearing in a collection of prescriptions for the case that a man has been given bewitched foodstuffs to eat, similar to the present prescription in BAM 237. A second parallel is a catalogue of ointments against various forms of witchcraft, each combining a different bird's head with a medicinal plant and oil (Abusch and Schwemer 2016, CMAwR 2, text 10.6.1: 14 and 18; Abusch et al. 2020, CMAwR 3, text A.23 additions). In the light of the plant name "crow's foot", it remains to be seen whether "crow's head" is likewise an alias name for a plant.

Probably, (Ì.UDU) BAR.GÙN.<GÙN>.NA KUR-*i* in line 180‴ (iv 35) stands for BAR.GÙN.GÙN.NU KUR.RA, known from lexical texts as a logogram for *ayar ili* and *ḫurbabillu*, both of which are presumably alternative names for the chameleon (CAD A/1, 227–228, sub 1b and lex. section; in favour of the identification of these terms with the chameleon, see CAD Ḫ, 248 s.v. *ḫurbabillu* lex. section; Militarev and Kogan 2005, 140–141). However, the orthography BAR.GÙN.NA KUR-*i* in BAM 237 indicates that the scribe understood the element KUR-*i* as Akkadian *šadû* in the genitive (i.e. *ḫurbabil šadî* "mountain chameleon"). Abusch et al. 2020, CMAwR 3, 92 note to line 7 note that *lipî*(Ì.UDU) *ḫurbabilli* "chameleon fat/tallow" is also attested in Uruanna III (Rumor 2017, *JMC* 29, 15: 71), as an alias name for the plant *ada/umatu* (a plant with a red blossom?). Note also, presumably the same ingredient, in BAM 217: 2: Ì.UDU *a-a-ar* DINGIR (among ingredients for an ointment); also BAM 476 rev. 10 (ingredient for a leather bag worn as an amulet). Scurlock (2014a, 581) translates "'fat' of a wild multicolored snake(?!)", understanding this as an exotic name for a plant.

Other medical texts use "penis of a *raqqu*-turtle" (GÌŠ BAL.GI^{ku6}), possibly an alias name for a plant, see e.g. BAM 311: 68 (among ingredients for a leather bag against *bennu*-epilepsy); *Diagnostic Handbook* Tablet 28: 17–18 (a leather bag against AN.TA.ŠUB.BA-epilepsy); BM 56605 obv. right column 43 (Heeßel 2000, 119, 121, 310, 313, 316; CAD R 173 sub c).

In line 182''' (iv 37), the logogram Ú.KU$_6$ can be read as Akkadian *šimru* or *urânu* (the latter usually written ^{ú}TÁL.TÁL), both being types of fennel, cf. CAD U/W, 206ff. ("anise"); CAD Š/3, 8–9; AHw 1228 and 1230; Civil 2008, 105 no. 223 "fennel".

The sum of 25 drugs in line 183''' (iv 38) is probably erroneous; the preceding list of ingredients may only have comprised 22 or 23 items, see also Abusch et al. 2020, CMAwR 3, 92 note on line 10.

Lines 184'''–188''' (A$_1$ rev. iv 39–43): For lines 184'''–186''' (iv 39–41), see also Abusch and Schwemer 2011 (CMAwR 1), 50f. commentary on text 1.5.1: 4'-8'. The reference to specific ingredients as *latku* "tested" is rare; usually this qualification is assigned to complete remedies. "Tested" carnelian (*sāmtu latiktu*) probably means "true/genuine" carnelian (i.e. the stone). Cuneiform texts not only differentiate several varieties of carnelian, but the term *sāmtu* (^{na4}GUG) was also used for types of red (and yellow) glass (Thavapalan 2020, 144–148). Genuine *sāmtu* may have meant carnelian from regions associated with the stone (i.e. Meluḫḫa or Marḫaši). It is unknown how the genuineness of *sāmtu* would be determined or tested, but texts from the Greco-Roman world similarly mention the possibility of recognising "fake" medical ingredients (cf. Steinert 2015, 119).

The translation of the incantation in lines 187'''–188''' (iv 42–43) partially follows Scurlock 2014a, 577, 581. The word šallurza looks like a foreign term, but it may be related to *šallūru* "plum". For šá-ḫi-ma-za-a-te, one could also suggest the reading *ša ḫimṣāte* "of the profits/plundered goods", although the latter part of the spell in iv 43 appear to be mumbo-jumbo phrases or words of a foreign tongue.

Line 189''' (A$_1$ rev. iv 44): The "fluids" or watery discharge (*mû*, A.MEŠ) flowing from the woman's vagina could refer to an abnormal discharge resembling a clear fluid or to amniotic fluid (for discussion cf. Böck 2013; Steinert 2013, 4–5; 2017 and the comments on lines 174'''–178''' above).

C.1.4.1 BAM 238

This small fragment which belongs to BAM 237 but cannot be placed with certainty, is edited here for convenience as ms. A$_2$.

List of Manuscripts

Siglum	Museum Number	Copy	Collation	Format; Ductus	Provenience
A$_2$	VAT 14123 (+)	BAM 238	Coll.	Small tablet fragment; Neo-Assyrian script, 8th/7th cent. BCE	Assur, N4 library[295]

Overview

i' Fragmentary (incantation?) 1'–2'
A$_2$ obv.$^?$ 1'–2'

ii' Rubric 3'
A$_2$ obv.$^?$ 3'

iii' Fragmentary (ritual?) 4'–5'[...
A$_2$ obv.$^?$ 4'–5'

Previous Edition and Discussion

CDLI P285324 (photo together with BAM 237; transliteration)

295 Pedersén 1986, 71 No. 495.

Transliteration

Beginning lost

1′ A_2 obv.? 1′ [.................] ÉN k[a ....]

2′ A_2 obv.? 2′ [.................]-*bu-uk*? [.......................]

3′ A_2 obv.? 3′ [KA.INIM.MA] MUNUS [*šá na-aḫ-ša-te* GIG?]

4′ A_2 obv.? 4′ [KÌD.KÌD.BI? ....] ⸢x x x⸣ [...................]
5′ A_2 obv.? 5′ [..........................] x 14 [.....................]

Ms. A_2 breaks; remainder lost

Bound Transcription and Translation

Beginning lost

1′–2′ *fragmentary*	1′–2′ *too fragmentary for translation*
3′ [KA.INIM.MA] *sinništi* [*ša naḫšāti marṣat*]	3′ [Wording (of an incantation)] for a woman [who suffers from *naḫšātu*-discharge].
4′–5′ [KÌD.KÌD.BI] *fragmentary*	4′–5′ [The procedure for it(?)]: *too fragmentary for translation*

Ms. A_2 breaks

C.1.4.2 BAM 239

Like BAM 238 (ms. A_2), this tiny fragment edited here as ms. A_3 belongs to BAM 237 but cannot be placed with certainty. Because the preserved rulings do not fit any of the known sections of BAM 237 and offer varying line endings, BAM 239 may belong either to the beginning of col. i or to the end of col. iv.

List of Manuscripts

Siglum	Museum Number	Copy	Collation	Format; Ductus	Provenience
A_3	VAT 14145 (+)	BAM 239	Coll.	Small tablet fragment; Neo-Assyrian script; 8th–7th cent. BCE	Assur, N4 library[296]

Overview

i′	Fragmentary A_3 obv.? 1′	...]1′
ii′	Fragmentary prescription A_3 obv.? 2′	2′
iii′	Fragmentary prescription (bandage) A_3 obv.? 3′	3′

---

296 Pedersén 1986, 71 No. 495.

iv′	Fragmentary prescription (bandage) A_3 obv.? 4′	4′
v′	Fragmentary prescription A_3 obv.? 5′	5′
vi′	Fragmentary prescription A_3 obv.? 6′	6′
vii′	Fragmentary prescription A_3 obv.? 7′	7′
viii′	Fragmentary prescription A_3 obv.? 8′	8′[...

Previous Edition and Discussion

CDLI P288325 (photo)

Transliteration

Beginning lost

1′ A_3 obv.? 1′ [.................] x [x x]

2′ A_3 obv.? 2′ [................ *na-aḫ-šá-tu*?] KU[D-*sa*]

3′ A_3 obv.? 3′ [................ *ana*? ...]-*šá* LÁ KU[D-*sa*]

4′ A_3 obv.? 4′ [............ *ana na-aṣ-m*]*at*?-*te-šá* LÁ KUD-*s*[*a*]

5′ A_3 obv.? 5′ [................]x ⸢*ú-kal*⸣-*ši-ma* MIN

6′ A_3 obv.? 6′ [.................................]x-*ši*

7′ A_3 obv.? 7′ [........................-*š*]*ú*? KU_4-*eb*

8′ A_3 obv.? 8′ [.......................]x ⸢KU_4?⸣-⸢*eb*⸣

Ms. A_3 breaks; remainder lost

Bound Transcription and Translation

Beginning lost

1′ *traces*	1′ *too fragmentary for translation*
2′ [... *naḫšātu*] *iparra*[*sā*]	2′ [... (then) the *naḫšātu*-discharge(?)] will st[op].
3′ [... *ana* ...]-*ša taṣammid ipar*[*rasā*]	3′ [...] you bind [on] her [...]. (Then) it (i.e. the *naḫšātu*-discharge) will st[op].

4′ [... *ana naṣma*]*ttēša taṣammid iparras*[*ā*]	4′ [.........] you bind (it) on as a [band]age for her. (Then) it (the *naḫšātu*-discharge) will st[op].
5′ [...]... *ukâlšī-ma* MIN	5′ [.....................] *she wears/applies it*(?). Then ditto (i.e. the *naḫšātu*-discharge will stop).
6′ [...]-*ši*	6′[... ..., *you* ....] her.
7′ [...]... *tušerreb*	7′ [... ...]... you let (it) enter(?).
8′ [...]... *tušerreb*	8′ [... ...]... you let (it) enter(?).

Text breaks

Notes

Line 4′: For *naṣmattu* "bandage" in women's healthcare texts, see e.g. BAM 244 obv. 21, 22, in a treatment for fertility and conception. Line 3′ may have presented the same ending as line 4′ (see further *infra* text B.1.1). The quotation of the present passage in CAD K, 525b s.v. *kullumūtu* is misleading.

Line 5′: It is also possible to read *ú-kal-lim-ma* (from *kullumu* "to show, to reveal") instead of *ukâlšī-ma*. However, since the present tense form *ukallam* would be expected, this reading seems less likely than *ú-kal-ši-ma*. The present reading understands this as a form of *kullu*. In comparable instructions in medical texts, one finds *ukâl* "he/she wears (it)", often referring to suppositories applied to the vagina or the rectum (cf. for other references, CAD K, 150 sub 2d). The feminine pronominal suffix -*ši* could refer to the applied medication, which would need to be a feminine noun (such as *maššītu* "suppository", *lubuštu* or *ṣubātu* "(piece of) cloth" (into which the medication was wrapped), or *naṣmattu* "bandage", mentioned in the previous line 4′). However, *naṣmattu* is usually applied externally, to the skin, not internally. Alternatively, *kullu* could be used here in the meaning "to provide somebody with something" (CAD K, 516 s.v. *kullu* sub 4c), in that case *ukâlši* would mean "he/she provides (it) for her".

Lines 7′ and 8′: KU$_4$-*eb* is interpreted here as a Š-stem form of *erēbu* "to enter". Perhaps the instruction concerns the introduction of *materia medica* into the patient's body. Cf. possibly a parallel recipe for a vaginal fumigation in Lambert 1969, *Iraq* 31, 28ff. obv. 16–17 (see *infra* text II.1.4): ⸢*qú-ut*⸣-*ru ana* KA.MEŠ-*ša u na-ḫi-ri-ša e-ru-ub* "the fume(s) should enter her mouth and nostrils".

C.1.5 K. 263 + 10934: A Tablet with Treatments to Stop Female Bleeding

The tablet K. 263 + 10934 contains medical recipes and a ritual against the abnormal flow of a woman's blood (in rev. 37, it offers the rubric [KA.INI]M.MA MÚD MUNUS *ana* KUD-*su*). It is a single-column tablet in Neo-Babylonian script from the Nineveh collection, possibly dating to the early Neo-Babylonian period and later brought from Babylonia to Nineveh during Ashurbanipal's reign.[297] Its top left-hand corner and bottom right-hand corner are still missing. The joined fragment K. 10934 forms the top right-hand corner. The handwriting is rather large, adding together with a few missing signs to the impression that this tablet could form an excerpt collecting recipes exclusively dealing with gynaecological haemorrhage.[298]

The obverse of K. 263 + 10934 contains three sections of recipes for tampons, using plant and mineral ingredients respectively. The second section (lines 6–10) describes the preparation of a potion consisting of the blood of a bird, probably a male partridge (*iṣṣūr hurri*). All the recipes of the third section (lines 11–23) apply a drug containing only a single component (*simplicium*) which consists of one plant, mineral or animal substance to be drunk in beer. This is remarkable given the tendency in Mesopotamian medical texts of the first millennium BCE for compound recipes.

297 I. L. Finkel, personal communication.

298 See for a similar suggestion J. Fincke, http://fincke.uni-hd.de/nineveh/babylonian/index.htm. The two then unjoined fragments were mentioned by Fincke (2003–2004, 143; both fragments were joined by her in 2005).

The reverse of K. 263+ (lines 24–41) continues with recipes for potions with various drugs (mineral, plants and animal substances) and for suppositories (line 32). The ruled-off line 37 contains the rubric [KA.INI]M.MA MÚD MUNUS *ana* KUD-*su* "spell for stopping a woman's blood", which should follow an incantation as a subscript, but here the incantation was omitted. Possibly, this rubric was meant as a reminder for the specialist that an incantation had to be recited in conjunction with the preceding or following prescription(s).[299]

The last section on the reverse of K. 263+ (lines 42–48) is interesting but damaged, consisting of a ritual instruction and a short incantation addressed to a plural object and invoking the gods Asalluḫi and Ea. However, the damaged beginning of line 42 probably consists of a short two-word sentence and is set off by a 'ditto'-sign from the ritual instruction. This seems to be the incipit of an incantation. Before the preserved PA_5.MEŠ-*šú* "her canals" (*atappātu* or *palgū*) a verbal form is expected, e.g. "May her canals be dammed up!" (i.e. a form of *sekēru*) or the like. The motif of the flooded canal is also encountered in an incantation for stopping a woman's blood in BAM 235: 10–16 // BAM 236 rev. 1′–9′ (texts C.1.1–C.1.2), which speaks of the woman's blood as a "red river, a red canal (*atappu*)", and of the inside of the woman's body as a meadow, which is to be dammed up (*sekēru*).

The ritual instructions in lines 42–45 are unique within the gynaecological corpus, although partial parallels can be found in other medical and ritual texts (see the notes below). The ritual actions employ symbolic and metaphorical associations relating to the woman's body and her disorder. An object, presumably a waterskin in which something was deposited or which was filled with a liquid, is to be closed with a mixture of clay and chaff and to be sealed with a carnelian seal. The sealed waterskin then had to be buried in a hole dug at a canal. The waterskin alludes to the female body and its open canal (or more specifically the womb and its neck), which is to be sealed off, while the use of a carnelian seal employs a colour symbolism entailing the colour of blood.

The metaphorical motifs of water and irrigation canal that is sealed off with a seal is already encountered in Old Babylonian Sumerian incantations probably composed for a similar purpose (irregular bleeding, see Finkel 1980, 37ff. 47f. A 15ff., B 15ff., C i 9–15, ii 9–18). Another first millennium parallel to the metaphor of sealing a body opening with a seal is presented by BAM 237 ii 1′–6′ (// BAM 386 i! 1′–6′ // SpTU 4, No. 129 vi 11′–27′), an incantation which was used against *naḫšātu* (abnormal flow of blood during pregnancy) and against nosebleed. In this incantation, a deity is asked to bring down from heaven "the seal of Anu" and to seal with it the "disorder of her (the woman's) vagina" (*lā dumuq ūrīša*, see *infra* text C.1.4).

Several close parallels for prescriptions and ingredients in K. 263+ are known from other Mesopotamian gynaecological texts (for parallel ingredients in ancient Egyptian, Graeco-Roman and Medieval Jewish gynaecological remedies, see Steinert 2012b, 75–85). These parallels encountered in texts from Assyrian and Babylonia (see especially BAM 237; BM 40152; FLP 1306; SpTU 4, No. 153 edited in this chapter), suggest a common inventory of substances in first millennium BCE texts recommended for stopping haemorrhages because their haemostatic, astringent or drying qualities.

List of Manuscripts

Siglum	Museum Number	Copy	Collation	Format; Ductus	Provenience
a	K. 263 + K. 10934	Geers, Folio A116 (K. 10934), Folio G15 (K. 263) *Sudhoffs Archiv* 96, 93–94	Coll.	Single-column tablet; Neo-Babylonian script; 7th cent. BCE	Nineveh; Ashurbanipal's library

Overview

i	Prescriptions to stop bleeding (tampons) a obv. 1–5	1–5
ii	Prescriptions to stop bleeding (tampons, potion) a obv. 6–10	6–10
iii	Prescriptions to stop bleeding (potions) a obv. 11–rev. 8	11–31

299 Note a similar occurrence of a KA.INIM.MA-rubric with the incantation missing after ritual instructions in BAM 237 i 17′ (see Finkel 1980, 50–51 and *infra* text C.1.4).

iv	Prescription to stop bleeding (tampon) a rev. 9	32
v	Prescription to stop bleeding (potion) a rev. 10–13	33–36
vi	Rubric a rev. 14	37
vii	Prescription to stop bleeding (potion, tampon) a rev. 15–16	38–39
viii	Prescription to stop bleeding (tampon) a rev. 17	40
ix	Prescription to stop bleeding (potion) a rev. 18	41
x	Ritual and spell to stop bleeding a rev. 19–u. e. 1	42–48

Previous Edition and Discussion

Geers, Folio A116 (copy of K. 10934); Folio G15 (copy of K. 263)
Fincke 2003–2004, 143 (discussion)
Steinert 2012b, *Sudhoffs Archiv* 96, 65–68 (edition)
CDLI P237802 (photo)
Electronic Babylonian Library (eBL) (https://www.ebl.lmu.de/library/K.263)

Transliteration

1 a obv. 1 [DIŠ MUNUS MÚD-*šá* DU-*k*]*u*$^?$ NU KUD-*su a-na* KUD-*si*

2 a obv. 2 [x x x x] *ta-sàk ina* MÚD ^{giš}EREN ḪI.ḪI

3 a obv. 3 [*ina* ^{síg}ḪÉ.ME.DA[300]] NIGIN-*mi ana* ŠÀ.TÙR-*šá* GAR-*ma* KUD-*is*

4 a obv. 4 [(DIŠ$^?$) KI.MIN ^{im}KA]L ^{im}KAL.GUG DIŠ-*niš* SÚD

5 a obv. 5 [*ina* ^{síg}ḪÉ.ME.DA NIG]IN-*mi* KI.MIN

---

6 a obv. 6 [KI.MIN x x x SÚ]D$^?$ KI.MIN

7 a obv. 7 [KI.MIN NUNUZ TU$^{?\text{m}}$]^{ušen}[301] SÚD KI.MIN

8 a obv. 8 [KI.MIN BURU$_5$.ḪABRUD⸣]^{u}.DA NITA SAG.DU-*su* KUD-*is*

9 a obv. 9 [MÚD-*šú ina* ^{dug}BUR.Z]I *ta-maḫ-ḫar ana* IGI ^{mul}ÙZ

10 a obv. 10 ⸢*tuš-bat*⸣ ⸢*ina*⸣ *še-rim la pa-tan* NAG-*ma* MÚD-*šú* KUD-*is*

---

11 a obv. 11 KI.MIN NUNUZ TU^{mušen} SÚD *ina* KAŠ *la pa-tan* NAG-*m*[*a* MÚD] ⸢KUD$^?$⸣

12 a obv. 12 KI.MIN NA$_4$ *ga-bi-i* SÚD KI[.MIN]

13 a obv. 13 KI.MIN ^{ú}IGI-*lim* SÚD K[I.MIN]

---

300 See also rev. 32.
301 Another possible restoration would be [^{ú}*tar-m*]*uš*$_8$.

14	a obv. 14	KI.MIN ^{ú}*tar-muš*$_{8}$ SÚD	[KI.MIN]
15	a obv. 15	KI.MIN ^{ú}KUR.RA SÚD	[KI.MIN]
16	a obv. 16	KI.MIN ^{ú}<GEŠTIN>.KA$_{5}$.A SÚD	[KI.MIN]
17	a obv. 17	KI.MIN NUMUN ^{ú}*pu-qut-ti* SÚD	[KI.MIN]
18	a obv. 18	KI.MIN ⸢NUMUN⸣ ŠINIG SÚD	[KI.MIN]
19	a obv. 19	KI.MIN ^{ú}IN$_{6}$.ÚŠ SÚD	[KI.MIN]
20	a obv. 20	KI.MIN PEŠ$_{4}$.ANŠE SÚD	[KI.MIN]
21	a obv. 21	KI.MIN $^{\text{na4}}$*ka-pa-ṣu* SÚD	[KI.MIN]
22	a obv. 22	KI.MIN $^{\text{na4}}$*ḫu-rí-zu* SÚD	[KI.MIN]
23	a obv. 23	KI.MIN $^{\text{na4}}$ŠUBA Á.ZI.DA S[ÚD	KI.MIN]
24	a rev. 1	[KI.MIN $^{\text{n]a4}}$⸢*kak-ku*⸣*-sak-ku* S[ÚD	KI.MIN]
25	a rev. 2	[KI.MIN x $^{\text{gi}]\text{š}}$MÁ$^{?}$ MÚD MÁ[Š$^{?}$ x x x]	
26	a rev. 3	[x x x ^{ú}NÍN]DA$^{?}$[302] SÚD *i*[*na* KAŠ NAG-*ma* KI.MIN$^{?}$]	
27	a rev. 4	⸢KI.MIN⸣ ⸢^{ú}*nu-ḫur*⸣*-tú*$^{?}$ *ina* [KAŠ NAG-*ma*	KI.MIN$^{?}$]
28	a rev. 5	KI.MIN ^{ú}LAG-A.ŠÀ UGU x x x [...]	
29	a rev. 6	TI-*qé ina* KAŠ *tara-muk ina* $^{\text{mul4}}$Ù[Z$^{?}$ *tu*]*š-bat ina* [*še-rim*$^{?}$]	
30	a rev. 7	NAG-*ma* MÚD-*šá* KUD-*su* KI.MIN LAG-A.ŠÀ SI M[AŠ.DÀ]	
31	a rev. 8	*ina* KAŠ *tara-muk* K[I.MIN$^{?}$]	
32	a rev. 9	$^{\text{na4}}$KUR-*nu* DAB SÚD *ina* ^{síg}ḪÉ.ME.DA NIGIN-*mi* ⸢*ana*⸣ ⸢ŠÀ⸣.[TÙR-*šú* GAR-*an*]	
33	a rev. 10	KU.KU $^{\text{na4}}$KUR-*nu* DAB KU.KU $^{\text{na4}}$*u*$_{5}^{!}$*-ri-zu*	
34	a rev. 11	KU.KU $^{\text{na4}}$ŠUBA Á.ZI.DA DIŠ-*niš* ḪI.[ḪI]	
35	a rev. 12	*ina* KAŠ *ta*$_{5}$*-maḫ-aṣ ina še-rim la pa-tan la-*<*am*> GÌR-[*šú*]	
36	a rev. 13	[*ana q*]*aq-qàr* GAR-*an* NAG-*ma* MÚD-*šú* KUD-*si*	
37	a rev. 14	[KA.INI]M.MA MÚD MUNUS *ana* KUD-*su*	
38	a rev. 15	[KI.MIN$^{?}$ $^{\text{na4}}$KU]R-*nu* DAB SÚD <*ina*> SÍG NIGIN-*mi ana* ŠÀ.TÙR-*šú* GAR-*an*	
39	a rev. 16	[*ina* KAŠ *la*] *pa-tan* NAG-*šú*	
40	a rev. 17	[KI.MIN$^{?}$ $^{\text{na4}}$AN].BAR$^{?}$ *ina* ^{síg}ḪÉ.<ME>.DA NIGIN-*mi ana* ŠÀ.TÙR-*šú* GAR-*an*	
41	a rev. 18	[KI.MIN$^{?}$ x x x] *ina* A.MEŠ NU *pa-tan* NAG-*šú*	

302 The trace of the first visible sign could also be the end of MI/GI$_{6}$, e.g. AN.ZAḪ.GI$_{6}$ (*kutpû*) "black frit" or ^{ú}GAMUN.GI$_{6}$ (*zibû*) "black cumin".

42	a rev. 19	[ÉN *lu-ú se-ek*$^?$*-r*]*a* PA$_5$.MEŠ-*šú* : DÙ.DÙ.[B]I *ina pal*$^?$*-ki*$^?$ ⸢*ḫur*⸣*-ri*
43	a rev. 20	[*ana* ^{d}UTU.ŠÚ.A BAD$^?$ x-*š*]*ap/ep-pu* A.EDIN.⸢LÁ$^?$⸣ ⸢*ina*⸣ IM *pe-e* KÁ-*šú* ÚŠ$^!$*-ḫi*
44	a rev. 21	[(x x) UR$_5$.GIM DU$_{11}$.GA$^?$ *a-l*]*ak-tu*$_4$ *par-sa-a-a*[*t ina*] ^{na4}KIŠIB ^{na4}GUG KÁ-*šú*
45	a rev. 22	[*ta-bar-ram ina ḫur-ri* GAR-*an*$^?$ K]Á-<*šú*> *ina*$^!$(PAP) IGI ⸢KUR⸣ ⸢*ta*⸣*-bar-ram* ÉN ⸢3⸣*-šú* ŠID-*nu*
46	a rev. 23	[ÉN .... *utammi*$^?$]*-ku-nu-š*[*i*]
47	a rev. 24	[...................... UR]UDU$^?$ ⸢*ak-nu-uk*$^?$⸣ *pi*$^?$*-ku-nu*
48	a u. e. 1	[x x x *ina qibīt* ^{d}]⸢40⸣ *u* ^{d}*asal-lú-ḫi* ⸢TU$_6$⸣ ⸢ÉN⸣

Bound Transcription and Translation

[1] [*šumma sinništu dāmūša illak*]*ū lā ipparrasū ana parāsi* [2] [... ...] *tasâk ina dām erēni tuballal* [3] [*ina tabarri*] *talammi ana šassūrīša tašakkan paris* [4] [(DIŠ) KI.MIN *kal*]*â kalgukka ištēniš tasâk* [5] [*ina tabarri tala*]*mmi* KI.MIN	[1] [If a woman's blood flow]s (and) cannot be stopped, to stop it: [2] You crush [...], mix it with cedar 'blood', [3] you wrap it [in red wool], you insert it into her womb (viz. vagina) and it will stop. [4] [Alternatively], you pound [*kal*]*û* (yellow ochre) and *kalgukku* (reddish pigment) together, [5] you [wr]ap it [in red wool], ditto (i.e. you insert it into her womb and (her blood) will stop).
[6] [KI.MIN ... ... *ta*]*sâk* KI.MIN [7] [KI.MIN *pel summa*]*ti*(?) *tasâk* KI.MIN [8] [KI.MIN *iṣṣūr ḫur*]*ri zikaru qaqqassu tanakkis* [9] [*dāmšu ina purs*]*īti tamaḫḫar ana pān enzi* [10] *tušbât ina šēri lā patān išattī-ma dāmšu paris*	[6] [Alternatively,] [you po]und [...], ditto (i.e. you insert it into her vagina (lit. womb) and (her blood) will stop). [7] [Alternatively], you pound do[ve's egg (shell)], ditto. [8] [Alternatively], you cut off the head of a male [partr]idge. [9] You collect [its blood in a *purs*]*ītu*-vessel, underneath the Goat star [10] ⸢you let it stand⸣ outside overnight. She shall drink (it) in the morning on an empty stomach. Then her blood will stop.
[11] KI.MIN *pel summati ina šikari lā patān išattī-m*[*a dām*(*ša*)] *paris*(?) [12] KI.MIN *aban gabî tasâk* KI.MIN [13] KI.MIN *imḫur-līm tasâk* KI.MIN [14] KI.MIN *tarmuš tasâk* K[I.MIN] [15] KI.MIN *nīnâ tasâk* [KI.MIN] [16] KI.MIN <*karān*> *šēlebi tasâk* [KI.MIN] [17] KI.MIN *zēr puqutti tasâk* [KI.MIN] [18] KI.MIN *zēr bīni tasâk* [KI.MIN] [19] KI.MIN *maštakal tasâk* [KI.MIN] [20] KI.MIN *biṣṣūr atāni tasâk* [KI.MIN] [21] KI.MIN *kapāṣa tasâk* [KI.MIN] [22] KI.MIN *ḫurīza tasâk* [KI.MIN] [23] KI.MIN *šubû imittu ta*[*sâk* KI.MIN] [24] [KI.MIN] *kakkusakku ta*[*sâk* KI.MIN] [25] [KI.MIN ...] *eleppi*(?) *dām ur*[*īṣi*(?) ...] [26] [... *ill*]*ūru*(?) *tasâk ina* [*šikari išattī-ma* KI.MIN(?)] [27] KI.MIN *nuḫurta ina š*[*ikari išattī-ma* KI.MIN(?)] [28] KI.MIN *kirbān eqli eli*[*kulla*(?) ...] [29] *teleqqe ina šikari tarammuk ina en*[*zi tušb*]*āt ina* [*šēri*] [30] *išattī-ma dāmūša iparrasū* KI.MIN *kirbān eqli qaran ṣa*[*bīti*] [31] *ina šikari tarammuk* K[I.MIN]	[11] Alternatively, she shall drink (the shell of) a dove's egg in beer. Th[en (her) blood] will stop. [12] Alternatively, you pound alum, ditto (i.e. she shall drink (it) in beer. Then her blood will stop). [13] Alternatively, you pound 'heals thousand'-plant, d[itto]. [14] Alternatively, you pound *tarmuš*-plant, [ditto]. [15] Alternatively, you pound *nīnû*-plant, [ditto]. [16] Alternatively, you pound fox <grape>, [ditto]. [17] Alternatively, you pound seed of *puquttu*-plant, [ditto]. [18] Alternatively, you pound tamarisk seed, [ditto]. [19] Alternatively, you pound *maštakal*-plant, [ditto]. [20] Alternatively, you pound (the shell called) 'donkey mare's genitals'-shell, [ditto]. [21] Alternatively, you pound *kapāṣu*-shell, [ditto]. [22] Alternatively, you pound *urīzu*-stone, [ditto]. [23] Alternatively you po[und] 'right' *šubû*-stone, [ditto]. [24] [Alternatively, you pou]nd, *kakkusakku*-sto[ne, ditto]. [25] [Alternatively,] [26] you pound [25] [...] of a boat(?), blood of a billy go[at(?), ...], [26] [..., (and) *illū*]*ru*-plant(?). [She shall drink (it)] in [beer, and ditto(?)]. [27] Alternatively, [she shall drink] *nuḫurtu*-plant(?) in b[eer, and ditto(?)]. [28] Alternatively, [29] you take [28] *kirbān eqli*-plant, *eli*[*kulla*-plant(?), ...], [29] you soak (it) in beer, you let it stay out overnight under the G[oat(?)]-star. In [the morning] [30] she shall drink it, and her blood will stop. Alternatively, [31] you soak [30] *kirbān eqli*-plant (and) ga[zelle] horn [31] in beer, d[itto].

32 *šadânu ṣābitu tasâk ina tabarri talammi ana ša[ssūrīša tašakkan]*	32 You crush magnetite, wrap (it) in red wool, [insert it] into [her] wo[mb (viz. vagina)].
33 *supanti šadâni ṣābiti supanti urīzi* 34 *supanti šubî imitti tub[allal]* 35 *ina šikari tamaḫḫaṣ ina šēri lā patān lā<m> šēp[šu]* 36 *[ana q]aqqari išakkan(u) išattī-ma dāmšu paris*(!)	33 You mix powder of magnetite, powder of *urīzu*-stone, 34 (and) powder of 'right' *šubû*-stone together, 35 you stir (these ingredients) in beer. In the morning, be<fore> 36 she gets up (lit. before she sets her foot on the ground), she shall drink it, and her blood will stop.
37 KA.INIM.MA *dām sinništi parāsi*	37 Wording (of a spell) to stop a woman's blood.
38 [KI.MIN(?) *šadâ]nu ṣābitu tasâk* <*ina*> *šīpāti talammi ana šassūrīšu tašakkan* 39 [*ina šikari*(?) *lā*] *patān tašaqqīšu*	38 [Alternatively(?)], you crush [magn]etite, wrap it <in> wool, insert it into her womb (viz. vagina).39 [(Or) you have her drink it (i.e. crushed magnetite) [in beer(?)] on an empty stomach.
40 [KI.MIN(?) *par*]*zilla ina tabarri talammi ana šassūrīšu tašakkan*	40 [Alternatively(?)], you wrap ['ir]on-[stone'(?)] in red wool, insert (it) into her womb.
41 [KI.MIN(?) ...] *ina mê lā patān tašaqqīšu*	41 [Alternatively(?)], you have her drink [...] in water on an empty stomach.
42 [ÉN *lū sek*]*rā*(?) *atappātūšu* DÙ.DÙ.BI *ina palgi*(?) *ḫurra* 43 [*ana ereb šamši tepetti*(?)[303] ...]... *nādu ina ṭīdi pê pâšu tepeḫḫi* 44 [(...) *kīam taqabbi*(?) *al*]*aktu parsat* [*ina*] *kunuk sāmti pâšu* 45 [*tabarram ina ḫurri tašakkan*(?) *bā*]*bšu ina pān napāḫi tabarram šipta šalāšīšu tamannu*	42 [Incantation: "[May] her canals [be blocked]!" The procedure for [it]: By a canal[304] [*you open*(?)] a hole 43 [*toward the west*(?), ...] ... a waterskin, you lute its opening with clay (mixed with) chaff. 44 [... *you say as follows*(?): "The ro]ad is blocked." [You seal] its opening [with] a seal of carnelian, 45 [you put it in the hole], you seal [(its) open]ing before (sun) rise, you recite the incantation three times.
46 [ÉN ... ... *utammī*]*kunūši*(?)	46 [Incantation: "... I have conjured] you (masc. pl.),
47 [... ... *e*]*râ aknuk pīkunu*	47 [... .... with a ... of co]pper I have sealed your (masc. pl.) mouth.
48 [... *ina qibīt*] *Ea u Asalluḫi tê šipti*	48 [... .... by the command of(?) E]a and Asalluḫi!" Incantation formula.

Notes

General remarks

The variation between the feminine vs. masculine pronominal suffix *–šá* (in lines 3, 30) and *–šú* (in lines 10, 36, 38–42, common in other first millennium BCE texts) may hint at the use of more than one textual source to assemble this tablet (cf. also the variant writings of *urīzu* in lines 22 and 33).

Instead of the common phrase DIŠ KI.MIN "alternatively" to begin entries for the same purpose as before, the text seems to use throughout only KI.MIN "another (prescription)", with the possible exception of lines 6–10, which could have started with DIŠ KI.MIN instead, confirming that the ruled sections of lines 1–5 and 6–10 were possibly taken from a different source than the following sections starting with line 11. Moreover, the scribe wrote the KI.MIN signs in an abbreviated

303 Instead of [*ana ereb šamši tepetti*] "you open a hole toward sunset", one may alternatively restore the verb *teḫerri* "you dig".
304 Due to the context, I interpret the spelling *pal-ki* as a variant for *palgu* "canal".

fashion, with only one vertical wedge for the sign MIN, and the KI-sign with only three horizontal wedges, except for the first time in line 5 where he wrote it with four horizontals.

Since as a rule a recipe always starts at the beginning at a new line, it seems that the section starting with KI.MIN in the middle of line 30 is an alternative recipe with *kirbān eqli*-plant (possibly from a different textual source) for lines 28–30.

Line 2: Within prescriptions for women, cedar (wood) is applied e.g. in BAM 237 iii 8′ (as powder), while K. 263+ uses the resin for a suppository. For cedar "blood" to staunch bleeding, see also FLP 1306 obv. 8 (text C.1.9).

Lines 8–10: The Goat-Star ("She-goat") is identified with the constellation Lyra and associated with the healing goddess Gula. For parallels of the instructions, see CAD M/1, s.v. *maḫāru* sub 1d "to collect liquid in a container", CAD P, s.v. *pursītu* sub b. Of related interest here is the use of the blood of a male bird, probably a partridge (*iṣṣūr ḫurri*). Its head is cut off and its blood collected and later drunk by the patient.[305] Very close parallels to this recipe can be found in the ritual series ŠÀ.ZI.GA used to arouse male sexual desire (e.g. KUB 4, 48 i 12ff. (Biggs 1967, 54; Zisa 2021, 165, 439–440); BAM 272: 12′–14′ (Biggs 1967, 54; Zisa 2021, 312 lines 65–67)). There are further parallels for this treatment in first millennium BCE texts from Assur against the abnormal flow of a woman's blood (BAM 235: 4–5 (text C.1.1)) and against rectal haemorrhage (Geller 2005a, 214–215 No. 35: 30ff.; using bull blood). In the last prescription, half of the blood is used for an ointment (mixed with oil), the other half is "crushed" in water and given as a potion.[306]

Line 11: For the application of dove's egg (shell), compare the prescription of ostrich eggshells, which is attested several times in other first millennium texts to stop female bleeding (see e.g. FLP 1306 obv. 12, rev. 23; SpTU 4, No. 153 obv. 11–12, *infra* texts C.1.9–C.1.10).

Line 12: For alum (*gabû*; *aban gabî*) as an astringent drug to stop haemorrhage, see e.g. BAM 237 i 1′ (as part of an ointment applied to the vulva); SpTU 4, No. 153: 1–6; BM 38624+ obv. i' 11′–13′; FLP 1306 rev. 18, 22 (tampons). See *infra*.

Line 19: For the soapwort plant *maštakal* in other gynaecological recipes to stop bleeding, especially in tampons, see e.g. in BAM 237 i 39′ against *naḫšātu*.

Line 23 (and line 34): The texts often mention two varieties of *šubû*-'stone': right/left *šubû*. Schuster-Brandis (2008, 446–447) suggests that *šubû* could be a kind of shell or cowry snail and that the designation "left/right" could describe the form of the shell.[307] Note a parallel recipe to K. 263+ rev. 34ff. in BM 40152 rev. iii 9–13 (text C.1.8), which also uses powder of magnetite and *šubû*-stone in a potion to stop bleeding.

Line 25: For billy goat's blood (MÚD MÁŠ.ZU) in a medical text, see also AMT 97/6: 11 (Scurlock 2006, no. 329, to treat a ghost-induced affliction). Pitch (*kupru*) from a boat is used, for example, in a prescription for an ointment in the series against the demoness Lamaštu (Tablet I 32, Farber 2014, 74, 146). In the present context (a potion), one could also think of dust (*eperu*) from a boat.

Line 28: Probably two more plants follow *kirbān eqli* (^{ú}LAG-A.ŠÀ) "field clod-plant". The only plant known to me beginning with the sign UGU is *elikulla*. The name is written in various spellings such as *eli*(UGU)-*kul-la*, *el-kul-la*, *el-kúl-la*, *i-li-kul-la*, *e-li-kul-*(*la*), note also *er-gu-la*, *er-kul/kúl-la* (see Luukko and van Buylaere 2020, CMAwR 4, 33 s.v. *elkulla*). However, the beginning of the sign after UGU in line 28 does not look like KUL (NUMUN), KÚL (GUL) or KU, but it could possibly be the beginning of GÚ, presenting a hitherto unattested spelling UGU-*g*[*ú-*(*ul*)-*la*].

Line 32 (also lines 33, 38): For *šadânu ṣābitu* "magnetite, lodestone", cf. CAD Š/1, 37 sub 2; Borger 2004, MZL, 256 sub No. 24 $^{\text{na4}}$KA.GI.NA "magnetischer Hämatit"; Schuster-Brandis 2008, 425. The identification of *šadânu ṣābitu* as magnetite/magnetic iron or loadstone has been established through its name, lit. "seizing *šadânu* (haematite)", and through its description in the explanatory stone list *abnu šikinšu* where it is said to have a black colour with red dots.[308] This mineral is often applied to stop bleeding (in potions and tampons), e.g. in BAM 237 i 45′–46′ (compound remedy against *naḫšātu*, text

305 It is likely that goat blood formed an ingredient of another recipe in ms. a, in lines 25–26. See below.

306 See further a ritual against physical and psychological problems caused by witchcraft (AMT 35/3 rev. iv 4′ff. // BAM 434 obv. iii 7ff. // BAM 445+ obv. 36ff. (Abusch/Schwemer 2011, 155, 157 Text 7.7: 73–75), using bird blood for a protective ointment.

307 Cf. CAD Š/3, s.v. *šubû* A, where an identification with agate is proposed.

308 See Schuster-Brandis 2008, 425. Both haematite and magnetite belong to the group of the iron oxides.

C.1.4). Note also a similar recipe in BM 40152 rev. iii 6–8 (text C.1.8) using magnetite and *urīzu*-stone.[309] That magnetite was considered as a general haemostatic can be inferred from its use outside gynaecology. Thus, powder of magnetite is also inserted in an anal suppository against haemorrhage from the rectum and diarrhoea (Geller 2005a, 140–141 No. 22 rev. iii 16′; ibid., 214–215 No. 35 rev. 45–46).

Line 33: In the stone description text *abnu šikinšu*, the *urīzu*-stone is described as having the appearance of a lion hide (BAM 378 iii' 7′, dupl. STT 108: 39, Schuster-Brandis 2008, 28: 39). Cf. the similar description of yellow jasper in Greek and Arabic lapidaries mentioned by Michel 1995, 385.

Lines 35–36: From parallels one would expect the phrase *lām šēpša ana qaqqari išakkanu* "(she drinks it in the morning) before she sets her foot on the ground", see e.g. BAM 403: 7; AMT 34/3: 4; Geller 2005a, No. 2 line 8. The orthography of the form *tamaḫḫaṣ* found here is unusual (cf. CAD M/1, 78f. sub 3e); *maḫāṣu* is normally written SÌG-*aṣ* or syllabically.

Line 40: For iron (*aban parzilli; parzillu*), cf. CAD P, 215f. s.v. *parzillu* sub 2; AHw 838a sub 3; Schuster-Brandis (2008, 394–395) for its use in amulets. See also recipes against *naḫšātu* in BAM 237 i 47′ (^{na4}AN.BAR in a prescription for an amulet), beside AN.BAR "iron" in BAM 237 i 31′ (also for an amulet), see text C.1.4. As suggested by Abusch and Schwemer (2011, CMAwR 1, 471), ^{na4}AN.BAR could designate an iron bead or a stone bead whose appearance resembles iron. Colour symbolism might be implied in the use of this mineral, highlighted by its combination with red wool.

Lines 42–48: The restoration in the gap at the beginning of line 42 is tentative. The incipit of an incantation metaphorically referring to the bleeding through imagery of canals seems to be quoted here. From the context, I suggest restoring the precative particle *lū* plus a fem. pl. stative form of *sekēru* "to block". If this is correct, the following logogram PA$_5$.MEŠ should stand for a feminine noun, i.e. *atappu* "(small) canal". The logogram PA$_5$ is attested for Akkadian *palgu* and *atappu*, both standing for types of canals. It remains uncertain whether the very fragmentary Akkadian spell in lines 46–48 which follows the ritual instruction and concludes the tablet is actually the incantation quoted in line 42.

Similar rituals as encountered in lines 42–48, where something (e.g. dough with which the patient has been wiped off, or a figurine) is deposited in a hole which is sealed off (with a seal of *šubû*-stone and *šadânu*-stone) can be found elsewhere in the medical texts, yet unfortunately they do not offer a real duplicate for the instructions in K. 263+.[310]

Unfortunately, the spell in lines 46–48 is so damaged. It remains unclear who is addressed and conjured with the masculine plural "you" (see the pronominal suffixes -*kunūši* and -*kunu*). It is possible that the "canals" are addressed here.

C.1.6 K. 8893: Tampons for Treating Female Conditions

This fragment of a single-column tablet in Neo-Babylonian script from Nineveh partially preserves four recipes for vaginal suppositories and tampons (*allānu, itqu*) for the treatment of women, as is indicated by the instruction "(you insert it) into her womb" (viz. vagina) in two of the prescriptions. The exact purpose of the remedies remains unclear, as no purpose statements or diagnostic sections are preserved. However, the occurrence of drugs such as alum or ostrich eggshell may indicate that the treatments dealt with stopping haemorrhage or a kind of vaginal discharge (cf. Steinert 2012b).

List of Manuscripts

Siglum	Museum Number	Copy	Collation	Format; Ductus	Provenience
a	K. 8893	Geers, Folio A32 Pl. 27	Coll.	Fragment of a single-column tablet; Neo-Babylonian script, 7th cent. BCE[311]	Nineveh, Ashurbanipal's library

309 Magnetite is also used beside other minerals (e.g. alum) in a suppository for the same purpose in BM 42313+: 34′–35′ (text A.2.2).

310 E.g. CT 23, 1: 9ff.; series against the disease *sagallu*. Cf. also PBS 1/1, 15 rev. 30–35 (Laessøe 1955, 30–31); BAM 542 iii 8–12 (K. 2450, cited in CAD B, s.v. *barāmu* sub 1b), where the sealed object is a clay model of the gums); PBS 1/2, 120 rev. 11–14 (Abusch and Schwemer 2011, 168, 186: 42′–45′).

311 Measurements: 4.3 x 4.3 x 1.1 cm.

Overview

i′	Fragmentary prescription (suppository/tampon) a obv.? 1′–4′	…]1′–4′
ii′	Fragmentary prescription (suppository) a obv.? 5′–6′	5′–6′
iii′	Fragmentary prescription (suppository) a obv.? 7′–9′	7′–9′
iv′	Fragmentary prescription a obv.? 10′–12′	10′–12′[…

Previous Edition and Discussion

CDLI P238816 (photo)
Electronic Babylonian Library (eBL) (https://www.ebl.lmu.de/library/K.8893; transliteration)
Fincke 2003–2004, 142.

Transliteration

Beginning lost

1′ a obv.? 1′ [………….] ⌜x⌝ […………..]

2′ a obv.? 2′ […… NUN]UZ? GA.⌜NU11^mušen?⌝ KU ^giš^Ù[R SUMUN ……]

3′ a obv.? 3′ […… *ana*] ŠÀ.TÙR-*šá* [GAR-*an* ……]

4′ a obv.? 4′ [……]x *ina* Ì.UDU ḪI.ḪI *ina* ^síg^À[KA? NIGIN *ana* ŠÀ.TÙR-*šá* GAR-*an*?]

5′ a obv.? 5′ [… ŠIM].ŠAL ^šim^ŠEŠ ^ú^*ti-iá*!?-*t*[*u*4? ………]

6′ a obv.? 6′ [… *ina* Ì].UDU SUMUN ḪI.ḪI *alla-nu* DÙ-*u*[*š ana* ŠÀ.TÙR-*šá* GAR- *an* (…)]

7′ a obv.? 7′ […]x ^ú^*nu-ḫur-ti* ^šim^ŠEŠ ^ú^[……..]

8′ a obv.? 8′ […] MUN *eme-sal-lim* ^na4^*ga-bu-*[*u* ……..]

9′ a obv.? 9′ […] *alla-nu* DÙ-*uš ana* ŠÀ.TÙR-*šá* [GAR-*an* …]

10′ a obv.? 10′ […] *saḫ-lé-e mi-šil*!(ZA) ^na4^*ga-bu-*[*u* ………]

11′ a obv.? 11′ […^ši^]^m⌜^GÚR.GÚR?⌝ MUN *eme-sal-lim mi-šil* [……….]

12′ a obv.? 12′ [………]x x[…]

Ms. a obv.? breaks; remainder lost
Reverse not preserved

Bound Transcription and Translation

Beginning lost

1′ *only traces preserved*
2′ [... ...] *pel lurmi sīkti gu[šūri labiri ... ...]* 3′ [... *ana*] *šassūrīša* [*tašakkan* ... ...] 4′ [... ...] *ina lipî tuballal ina it[qi talammi ana šassūrīša tašakkan*]

1′ *too fragmentary for translation*
2′ [...] ostrich egg (shell), powder of [an old] be[am, ...], [...], 3′ [... you insert (it) into] her womb (viz. vagina) [...]. 4′ [...] you mix (it) with fat, [you wrap (it)] into a wad of wool, [you insert it into her womb (viz. vagina)].

5′ [... *šime*]*ššalû murru tīyatu* [...] 6′ [... *ina*] *lipî labiri tuballal allāna teppuš* [*ana šassūrīša tašakkan*]

5′ [... *šime*]*ššalû*-tree, *murru*-plant, *tīyatu*-plant, [...], 6′ [...] you mix [with] old fat, make an acorn-shaped suppository, [you insert (it) into her womb (viz. vagina)].

7′ [...] *nuḫurtu murru* ...[... ...] 8′ [...] *ṭābat emesalli gabû* [... ...] 9′ [... ...] *allāna teppuš ana šassūrīša* [*tašakkan* (...)]

7′ [...], *nuḫurtu*-plant, *murru*-plant, [...]-plant, [...], 8′ [...], *emesallu*-salt, alum, [...], 9′ [...] you make an acorn-shaped suppository, [you insert (it)] into her womb (viz. vagina) [(...)].

10′ [...] *saḫlê mišil*(?) *gabû* [... ...] 11′ [... ...] *kukru ṭābat emesalli mišil* [.. ...] 12′ *only traces preserved*

10′ [...], *saḫlû*-plant (cress?), half(?) (a shekel?) alum, [...], 11′ [...] *kukru*-aromatic, *emesallu*-salt, half (a shekel?) of [...], 12′ *too fragmentary for translation*

Ms. a obv.? breaks; remainder lost
Reverse not preserved

Notes

Line 2′: For ostrich eggshell or dove eggshell in remedies for stopping haemorrhage, see also K. 263 + 10934 obv. 7 and 11; FLP 1306 obv. 12, rev. 23; SpTU 4, No. 153 obv. 11–12 (texts C.1.5, C.1.9–C.1.10); Steinert 2012b, 83–84 and the *Introduction*.

Line 5′: The ingredients mentioned here (*šimeššalû*, *murru*, *tīyatu*) are also used for treatments (e.g. suppositories) in other gynaecological remedies, see e.g. BAM 243: 6′ (text B.1.2); BAM 240 rev. 47′ (text D.2.1); BAM 241 ii 9′ (text II.1.3).

Lines 10′-11′: I owe the reading *mi-šil* "half" (a unit, measurement) in both lines to eBL. The unit of measurement is unfortunately lost in the lacuna. Instead of *saḫ-lé-e* "cress" in line 10′, eBL suggest reading *ur-né-e* (*urnû*-plant).

C.1.7 K. 20254: A Fragment from Nineveh

This is another fragment from Nineveh in Neo-Babylonian script with medical prescriptions for women. The piece preserves seven fragmentary lines from the right-hand side of a single-column tablet, the text being partially written over the edge. The exact purpose of the remedies (vaginal suppositories) remains uncertain; however, the preserved ingredients with parallels in other texts point to the use of the remedies to staunch bleeding.

List of Manuscripts

Siglum	Museum Number	Copy	Collation	Format; Ductus	Provenience
a	K. 20254[312]	Lambert, Folio 14148 Pl. 34	Coll.	Fragment of a single-column tablet; Neo-Babylonian script; 7th cent. BCE	Nineveh; Ashurbanipal's library

312 Measurements: 2.8 x 3.9 x 1.5 cm.

b	FLP 1306	Pl. 30	Coll.	Single-column tablet in Late Babylonian script; ca. 6th–3rd cent. BCE(?)	unknown (Babylonia)
c	BM 42313+ (81-7-1, 73) + 42427 (81-7-1, 187) + 42585 (81-7-1, 345) + o.N. (81-7-1, 353) + 43174 (81-7-1, 938) + 43215 (81-7-1, 979) + 43274 (81-7-1, 1038) + 43279 (81-7-1, 1043) + 43281 (81-7-1, 1045) + 43439 (81-7-1, 1203) + 43483 (81-7-1, 1247) + 43595 (81-7-1, 1359) + 43766 (81-7-1, 1527) + 43803 (81-7-1, 1564)	Pl. 14–15	Coll.	Single-column tablet in Late Babylonian script, ca. 500. BCE	Sippar

Overview

i′	Fragmentary a obv.$^{?}$ 1′	...]1′
ii′	Fragmentary a obv.$^{?}$ 2′	2′
iii′	Prescription(s) to stop bleeding (tampons) a obv.$^{?}$ 3′–6′ // b obv. 11–15 // c obv. 28–29	3′–6′
iv′	Fragmentary prescription (tampon) a obv.$^{?}$ 7′–8′	7′–8′
v′	Fragmentary prescription a obv.$^{?}$ 9′–10′	9′–10′[...

Previous Edition and Discussion

CDLI P239949 (no photo or transliteration avaible)
Electronic Babylonian Library (eBL) (https://www.ebl.lmu.de/library/K.20254; transliteration of ms. a)
Fincke 2003–2004, 143 (ms. a)
Infra text C.1.9 (edition of ms. b), text A.2.2 (edition of ms. c)

Transliteration

Beginning of ms. a obv.$^{?}$ lost

1′ a obv.$^{?}$ 1′ [..] x x [.......]

2′ a obv.$^{?}$ 2′ [..............................] *blank* [.......]

3′ a obv.$^{?}$ 3′ [.............................. GÌR.PAD.DU UDU$^{?}$].NÍTA *ina* IZI *tur-*⸢*ár*⸣
b obv. 11 ---------------------------- *e-ṣe-et* UDU.NÍTA *ina* IZI *tur-*<*ár*> SÚD$^{?}$
c obv. 28 *ana* MÚD MUNUS KUD-*si* 1 *kak-ka* ⸢GÌR.PAD⸣.DU UDU.NÍTA *ina* IZI TUR-⸢*ár*⸣

4′ a obv.$^{?}$ 4′ [.. ŠU.Ù]R SUMUN *ina* ^{síg}ÀKA
b obv. 12–13 ŠIKA NUNUZ *lu-ur-mu* KA *tam-tim* / ŠU.ÙR SUMUN *mál-ma-liš*$^{!}$(TAR) *ina* ÀKA
c obv. 28$^{cont.}$–29 ŠIKA NUNUZ GA.NU$_{11}$^{mušen} / KA A.AB.BA ⸢KU$^{?}$⸣ [^{giš}ÙR SUM]UN$^{?}$ *ina* ^{síg}ÀKA

5′ a obv.$^{?}$ 5′ [NIGIN-*mi ana* ŠÀ.TÙR-*šá*] GAR-*an*
b obv. 14–15 NIGIN-*mi ina* ŠÀ.TÙR-*šú* GAR-*ma* / MÚD KUD-*si*
c obv. 29$^{cont.}$ NIGIN-*mi ana* ŠÀ.TÙR-*šú* GAR-*ma šá* MÚD MUNUS KUD-*si*

6′	a obv.$^{?}$ 6′	[.............................. *ina* ^{síg}]ÀKA$^{?}$ NIGIN-*mi ana* ŠÀ.TÙR-*šá* GAR
7′	a obv.$^{?}$ 7′	[...]x NAGA.SI ^{ú}*sim-bi*[*r-ri*]
8′	a obv.$^{?}$ 8′	[...]x *ana* ŠÀ.TÙR-*šá* GA[R]
9′	a obv.$^{?}$ 9′	[..] ⸢ú⸣*sim-b*[*ir-ri* (x x x)]
10′	a obv.$^{?}$ 10′	[..] x [.....................]

Ms. a obv.? breaks; remainder lost
Reverse not preserved

Bound Transcription and Translation

Beginning lost

1′ *only traces preserved*	1′ *too fragmentary for translation*
2′ *not preserved*	2′ *not preserved*
3′ [*ana dām sinništi parāsi ištēn kakka*] *eṣemti immeri ina išāti turrar* (var. adds: *tasâk*) 4′ [*ḫaṣab pel lurmî imbu' tâmti sīkti*(?) *guš*]*ūri labiri* (var. adds *malmališ*) *ina itqi* 5′ [*talammi ana šassūrīša*] *tašakkan-*(*ma*) (var. adds: *ša dām* (*sinništi*) *parāsi*) 6′ [... ... *ina*] *itqi talammi ana šassūrīša tašakkan*	3′ [To stop a woman's blood:] you desiccate (var. adds: (and) crush) [one shaft of the bone of a] she[ep] over a fire. 5′ You [wrap (it)] up 4′ in a wad of wool [with (var. adds: an equal amount of) ostrich eggshell, *imbu' tâmti*-mineral] (and) powder of an old [be]am. 5′ You insert (it) [into her womb (viz. vagina)]. (Var. adds: (This is) for stopping (a woman's) blood). 6′ [... ...] you wrap in a wad [of wool], you insert (it) into her womb (viz. vagina).
7′ [... ...]... *uḫūlu qarnānû simbir*[*ru*] 8′ [... ...]... *ana šassūrīša tašakkan*	7′ [... ...], 'horned' alkali (salicornia), *simbi*[*rru*]-plant, 8′ [... ...], you insert (it) into her womb (viz. vagina).
9′ [... ...] *simb*[*irru* (...)]	9′ [... ...] *simbi*[*rru*]-plant, [(...)]

Ms. a obv.? breaks; remainder lost
Reverse not preserved

Notes

Lines 3′–5′: The variant 1 *kak-ka* GÌR.PAD.DU "one shaft(?) of a bone" (in ms. c) in line 3′ is uncertain. There are a few recipes for stopping gynaecological haemorrhage that use roasted sheep bone, eggshells and wood from an old log/beam. FLP 1306: 11–15 (ms. b) forms a close parallel or duplicating recipe to K. 20254: 3′–5′ (ms. a). The text of mss. a-c presents a few variations in wording; ms. a appears to be somewhat abbreviated compared with the parallels in mss. b and c. Furthermore, SpTU 4, No. 153 obv. 11–12 likewise prescribes roasted sheep bone in a compound remedy to staunch a woman's blood, with other partially similar ingredients (see text C.1.10). Compare also BM 45736: 6′–12′ (text A.2.5) and BAM 237 iv 30 (text C.1.4, using bone in a tampon to stop watery discharge from the vagina). For discussion of these ingredients, see the *Introduction*.

Line 6′: This line appears to contain a short one-line remedy appended to lines 3′–5′, which is not preserved in mss. b and c.

Lines 7′ and 9′: The *simbirru*-plant is also prescribed in a fragmentary recipe for a suppository to stop bleeding in BM 38624+ i 11′–13′ (text A.2.1). SpTU 4, No. 153 obv. 5, 7 recommends this plant as a cooling, haemostatic drug ("for blocking the blood"), as does FLP 1306 rev. 17 (see *infra* texts C.1.9–C.1.0). The *simbirru*-plant (also *sibbirru*) is identical with the *šibburratu*-plant (*sibburratu*), cf. CAD S, 230 sub lex. section; CAD Š/2, 376–377 with discussion; Attia and Buisson 2012, *JMC* 19, 33.

C.1.8 BM 40152: A Collection of Remedies to Stop a Woman's Blood

This two-column tablet in a Late Babylonian script containing a collection of recipes, incantations and rituals to stop gynaecological bleeding was excavated by Hormozd Rassam at Babylon.[313] The tablet was presumably assembled from different sources, as is indicated by the occurrence of a rubric identifying a section of remedies as copied from a wooden writing board (wax tablet) with remedies that belonged to the scholar Nūr-Marduk from Babylon (rev. iii 14–16). The text offers a few prescriptions (amulets, tampons, potions), for which parallels or variants can be identified in other texts edited in this chapter (e.g. BAM 236, BAM 237 and K. 263 + 10934). This points to some shared medical traditions in Babylonia and Assyria during the first millennium BCE, especially regarding the use of certain medicinal substances. On the other hand, BM 40152 rev. iii 17–26 preserves a ritual, which is so far unparalleled, and which could be used for stopping gynaecological bleeding and nosebleed. The application of the same treatment for two related conditions can be compared with BAM 237 ii 1′–6′ //, where a spell to stop nosebleed was used in the context of bleeding during pregnancy (see text C.1.4).

List of Manuscripts

Siglum	Museum Number	Copy	Collation	Format; Ductus	Provenience
a	BM 40152 (81-3-24, 17)[314]	Pl. 28–29	Coll.	Fragment of a two-column tablet; Late-Babylonian script; ca. 6th/5th cent. BCE	Babylon
B	A 203	BAM 236	Coll.	Fragment of a single-column tablet; Neo-Assyrian script; 8th/7th cent. BCE	Assur, N4 library

Overview

i′	Fragmentary prescription (amulet necklace) a obv. ii 1′–8′	...]1′–8′
ii′	Prescription to stop bleeding (tampon) a obv. ii 9′–11′ // B obv. 15–17	9′–11′
iii′	Incantation to stop bleeding a obv. ii 12′–14′	12′–14′
iv′	Incantation rubric a obv. ii 15′	15′
v′	Ritual instructions a rev. iii 1–5	16′–20′
vi′	Prescription (tampon) to stop bleeding a rev. iii 6–8	21′–23′
vii′	Prescription (potion) to stop bleeding a rev. iii 9–13	24′–28′

313 The British Museum register gives Babylon as the provenance of the 81-3-24 collection, see Leichty, Finkel and Walker 2019, *CBT* IV–V, 438.

314 Measurements: ca. 7 x 9 x 2 cm.

viii′	Subscript a rev. iii 14–16	29′–31′
ix′	Ritual instructions a rev. iii 17–26	32′–41′
x′	Fragmentary prescription a rev. iii 27–29	42′–44′
xi′	Fragmentary a rev. iii 30	45′–[...
xii″	Fragmentary prescriptions a rev. iv 1′–8′	...]46″–53″
xiii″	Fragmentary prescriptions a rev. iv 9′–13′	54″–58″
xiv″	Fragmentary a rev. iv 14′	59″–[....

Previous Edition and Discussion

Electronic Babylonian Library (eBL) (transliteration; https://www.ebl.lmu.de/library/BM.40152)
Infra text C.1.2 (edition of ms. B)

Transliteration

Ms. a obv. i not preserved
Beginning of obv. ii lost

1′	a obv. ii 1′	[.....................] ⸢x⸣ x [x]
2′	a obv. ii 2′	[.....................] NU.NU
3′	a obv. ii 3′	[.....................] È-*ak*
4′	a obv. ii 4′	[.......... *líp-pi*$^{?}$] *ta-lap-pap*
5′	a obv. ii 5′	[.................. KÉŠ] KÉŠ-*ár*
6′	a obv. ii 6′	[.......................] ⸢ÉN⸣ ⸢ŠID⸣-*nu*
7′	a obv. ii 7′	[............ ^{na4}ŠUB]A ⸢NITA⸣ *ina* SAG.KI-⸢*šá*⸣
8′	a obv. ii 8′	[KÉŠ$^{?}$ (...)] *ina-eš*
9′	a obv. ii 9′ B obv. 15	[DIŠ] KI.MIN ⸢IM⸣.SAḪ[AR.NA$_4$].KUR.RA IM.SAḪAR.GI$_6$.KUR.RA [DIŠ KI.MI]N IM.[SAḪAR].BABBAR.KUR.RA IM.SAḪAR.GI$_6$.KUR.RA
10′	a obv. ii 10′ B obv. 16	[IM].SAḪAR.BABBAR.KUR.RA DIŠ-*niš ina* $^{síg?}$ÀKA ⸢NIGIN-*mi*⸣ [IM.SAḪA]R.N[A$_4$$^{!}$].KUR.RA DIŠ-*niš ina* ^{síg}ÀKA NIGIN-[*m*]*a*$^{?}$
11′	a obv. ii 11′ B obv. 17	[*ana* ŠÀ].TÙR-*šá* GAR-*ma* MÚD.MEŠ-*ša* KUD-⸢*si*$^{?}$⸣ [*ana* ŠÀ].⸢TÙR⸣$^{!}$-*šá* GAR-*an-ma* MÚD.MEŠ-*šá* KUD-*su*$^{!}$

a, B
____

12′	a obv. ii 12′	[ÉN *se*]*k*$^{?}$-*re-et* ÍD *qut-tu-ú* A.MEŠ-*šá*
13′	a obv. ii 13′	[*mu-suk*$^{?}$]-*ka-tu* MUNUS KUD ⸢*pa*$^{?}$⸣-[*r*]*i-is* *ḫa-ni*-⸢*iq*$^{?}$-*ti*⸣

14′ a obv. ii 14′ [ÉN] ⸢^{d}⸣ *gu-la ma-ḫi-ra la* ⸢TUKU-*ú*⸣

15′ a obv. ii 15′ [KA.INIM.MA MÚD MUNU]S KUD-*si ša-gu*$_{5}$*-šá* NU S[I].⸢SÁ$^{?}$⸣

Bottom of ms. a obv. ii

16′ a rev. iii 1 [x x *ina* ḪABR]UD$^{?}$ *šá* ^{d}UTU.ŠÚ.A [ÚŠ-*ḫi*$^{?}$]

17′ a rev. iii 2 [(x) ŠIKA *šá*] SILA.LÍM.MA *za-qip-tú ina* IGI [ḪABRUD$^{?}$ GAR-*an*$^{?}$ (...)]

18′ a rev. iii 3 [*ina* N]ÍG.SILA$_{11}$.GÁ ZÍZ.AN.NA KÁ-[*šú* ÚŠ-*ḫi*$^{?}$ (...)]

19′ a rev. iii 4 x-⸢*tú*⸣ x x x *u i-na-*⸢*pal*$^{?}$⸣ ⸢*lu*$^{?}$⸣ [x x x x]

20′ a rev. iii 5 ⸢ÉN⸣ 3-*šú* ŠID-*ma* [x x x]

21′ a rev. iii 6 ⸢DIŠ⸣ ⸢MUNUS⸣ MÚD.MEŠ-*šá* DU-*ku-ma la* KUD-*su*

22′ a rev. iii 7 $^{[n]a4}$KUR-*nu* DAB SÚD ^{na4}*u*$_{5}$*-ri-zu*

23′ a rev. iii 8 [SÚ]D *ina* ⸢^{síg}ḪÉ.ME.DA⸣ ⸢NIGIN$^{?}$⸣ *ana* ŠÀ.TÙR$^{!}$-*šá* GAR-*an*

24′ a rev. iii 9 ⸢DIŠ⸣ ⸢KI.MIN⸣ KU.KU ^{na4}NÍR ^{na4}KUR-*nu* DAB

25′ a rev. iii 10 ⸢^{na4}⸣ŠUBA$^{!}$ NITA SIM$^{!}$(ZI)-*pí* DIŠ-*niš* ḪI.ḪI

26′ a rev. iii 11 *ina* KAŠ SÌG-⸢*aṣ*⸣ *ina še-rim ba-lu pa-tan*

27′ a rev. iii 12 *la-*⸢*am*⸣ GÌR-*šá ana* KI GAR-*nu* NAG-*ma*

28′ a rev. iii 13 ⸢MÚD.MEŠ⸣-*šá* KUD.MEŠ-*su*

29′ a rev. iii 14 [*b*]*u-ul-ṭú lat-*⸢*ku*⸣*-tu*$_{4}$ *šá ana* ŠU *šu-ṣu-ú*

30′ a rev. iii 15 [GAB]A.RI ^{giš}*le-u*$_{5}$*-um*

31′ a rev. iii 16 *ša* ^{m}*nu-úr-*^{d}AMAR.UTU UM.ME.⸢A⸣ KÁ.DINGIR.⸢RA^{ki}⸣

32′ a rev. iii 17 *ana* MÚD KIR$_{4}$ *u* MÚD MUNUS KUD-*si*

33′ a rev. iii 18 ^{giš}NÍG.GIDRU SIPA *e-de-na-a tu-qad-dáš*

34′ a rev. iii 19 GIN$_{7}$ ^{d}UTU.ŠÚ.A *zì-sur-ra-a* NIGIN

35′ a rev. iii 20 7 ŠE *ana* IGI ^{d}UTU *ta-na-suk*

36′ a rev. iii 21 ^{d}UTU *pa-ru-ka li-ku-lu* DU$_{11}$.GA

37′ a rev. iii 22 *ina še-rim la-am* ^{d}UTU.È *ina* ^{urudu}GAG.U$_{4}$.TAG.GA

38′ a rev. iii 23 SUḪUŠ-*su* TI-*qé* ⸢4⸣ ⸢ŠE$^{?}$⸣ *ana* SUḪUŠ-*šú* ŠUB-*di*

39′ a rev. iii 24 SAG.DU-*su ana* KI ⸢x x x x x⸣

40′ a rev. iii 25 SUḪUŠ-*su* TI-*qé-m*[*a* ....]

41′ a rev. iii 26 *šum*$_{4}$*-ma ta-aš-ša*[*k-* ....]

42′ a rev. iii 27 NUMUN ^{ú}IN.NU.U[Š ....]

43′ a rev. iii 28 *ana* ŠÀ.TÙR-[*šá* GAR ....]

44′ a rev. iii 29 NUMUN ^{ú}I[N.NU.UŠ ....]

45′ a rev. iii 30 ⸢x x x⸣ [..............................]

Ms. a rev. iii breaks; gap of unknown length
Beginning of rev. iv lost

46″ a rev. iv 1′ [............... NU] ⸢*pa-tan*⸣ ⸢*ina*⸣ ⸢KAŠ⸣ ⸢NAG⸣

47″ a rev. iv 2′ [....................................] *ina* KAŠ NAG

48″ a rev. iv 3′ [......... *u_5-r*]*a-an-na* SÚD$^{?}$ *ina* KAŠ NAG

49″ a rev. iv 4′ [....................................] *ina* KAŠ NAG

50″ a rev. iv 5′ [................................ S]ÚD *ina* KAŠ NAG

51″ a rev. iv 6′ [..........................]x-*ma* SÚD *ina* KAŠ NAG

52″ a rev. iv 7′ [....................... *ana* MÚD.MEŠ$^{?}$] KUD-*si*

53″ a rev. iv 8′ [.................... *ina* G]ÌR$^{?!}$.MIN$^{?}$-*šá*[315] KÉŠ

54″ a rev. iv 9′ [............................] ^{na4}*kak-ku-sak-ku*

55″ a rev. iv 10′ [...................... ^{na4}ŠUBA 2],30 *síḫ-ru*

56″ a rev. iv 11′ [..] NAG

57″ a rev. iv 12′ [......... *ina* KA]Š$^{?}$ KALA.GA NAG

58″ a rev. iv 13′ [..................] *ina* MUL$_4$ *tuš-bat* NAG

59″ a rev. iv 14′ [...........] ⸢x x⸣ ga

Ms. a rev. iv breaks; remainder lost

Bound Transcription and Translation

Ms. a obv. i not preserved
Beginning of obv. ii lost

1′ [... ...] ... 2′ [... ...] *taṭammi* 3′ [... ...] *tašakkak* 4′ [... ... *lippī*] *talappap* 5′ [... ... *kiṣrī*] *takaṣṣar* 6′ [... ...] *šipta tamannu* 7′ [... ... *šub*]*û zikaru ina pūtīša* 8′ [*tarakkas*(?) (...)] *ina*ʾ*eš*	1′ [... ...] ... 2′ [...] you spin [... (a thread of ...)], 3′ [...] you thread (stones on the cord), 4′ [... ...] you wrap [... with burls], 5′ [... knots] you knot (into the cord), 6′ [... ...] you recite the incantation, 7′ [...] male [*šu*]*bû*-stone] 8′ [you tie] 7′ on her forehead. 8′ [(...) Then] she will recover.
9′ [DIŠ K]I.MIN [*ga*]*bâ qitma* 10′ *alluḫara ištēniš ina itqi talammī*(-*ma*) 11′ [*ana ša*]*ssūrīša tašakkan-ma dāmūša iparrasū*	9′ [Alterna]tively, you wrap al[um], (black) *qitmu*-pigment, 10′ (white) *alluḫaru*-pigment together into a wad of wool. 11′ You insert it [into] her [wo]mb (viz. vagina). Then her blood will stop.

---

315 Apparently not MURUB$_4$ “waist”.

12' [ÉN *se*]*kret nāru quttû mûša*	12' [Incantation]: The river/canal is [dam]med up, its waters have ceased (to flow).
13' [*musuk*]*katu*(?) *sinništu parištu pāris ḫaniqti*(?)	13' [(For) the impure(?)] woman, the post-menopausal woman *is the stauncher*(?) of the … .
14' [*šipat*] *Gula māḫira lā išû*	14' It is an [incantation] of the goddess Gula (who) has no rival.
15' [KA.INIM.MA *dām sinniš*]*ti parāsi šagûša lā išarū*(?)	15' [A spell] for stopping [a woman's blood] whose menses are *not normal*(?).
16' [… *ina ḫur*]*ri ša ereb šamši* [*tepeḫḫi*(?)] 17' [(…) *ḫaṣabta ša*] *sūq erbetti zaqipta ina pān* [*ḫurri tašakkan*(?) (…)] 18' [*ina l*]*īš kunāši pâ*[*šu tepeḫḫi*(?) (…)] 19' … … *u inappal*(?) …[…] 20' *šipta šalāšīšu tamannū-ma* […]	16' [You enclose(?) … in] a hole towards the west (sunset), 17' [(…) you set up(?)] a potsherd from] a crossroads which is standing upright (in the street) in front of [the hole(?) (…)]. 18' [You seal its ope]ning [with] emmer dough. [(…)] 19' […] … *and she/he will dig up*(?) … […]. 20' You recite the spell three times. Then […].
21' *šumma sinništu dāmūša illakū-ma lā ipparrasū* 22' *šadâna ṣābita tasâk urīza* 23' *tasâk ina tabarri talammi ana šassūrīša tašakkan*	21' If a woman's blood flows and cannot be stopped: 22' You crush magnetite, 23' you crush 22' *urīzu*-stone, 23' you wrap it into red-coloured wool, insert it into her womb (viz. vagina).
24' DIŠ KI.MIN *supanti ḫulāli ṣadâna ṣābita* 25' *šubâ zikara tanappi ištēniš tuballal* 26' *ina šikari tamaḫḫaṣ ina šēri balu patān* 27' *lām šēpša ana qaqqari išakkanu išattī-ma* 28' *dāmūša iparrasū*	24' Alternatively, 25' you sift (and) mix 24' powder of *ḫulālu*-stone, magnetite 25' (and) male *šubû*-'stone' together. 26' You stir (them) into beer. In the morning, on an empty stomach, 27' before setting her foot on the ground (getting out of bed) she shall drink it. 28' Then her blood will stop.
29' [*b*]*ulṭū latkūtu ša ana qāti šūṣû* 30' [*ga*]*bari lē'i* 31' *ša Nūr-Marduk ummân Bābili*	29' Proven remedies, which are suitable for use. A copy of an original wooden writing board 31' of Nūr-Marduk, the *ummânu*-scholar of Babylon.
32' *ana dām appi u dām sinništi parāsi* 33' *ḫaṭṭi rē'î ēdēnâ tuqaddaš* 34' *kīma ereb šamši zisurrâ talammi* 35' *sebe uṭṭāti*(?) *ana maḫar Šamaš tanassuk* 36' *Šamaš parûka līkulū taqabbi* 37' *ina šēri lām ṣīt šamši ina šiltāḫi* 38' *šurussu teleqqe erbe uṭṭāti*(?) *ana šuršīšu tanaddi* 39' *qaqqassu ana qaqqari* … … 40' *šurussu teleqqē-m*[*a* … …] 41' *šumma tašša*[*k-*… …]	32' In order to stop nosebleed or a woman's blood: 33' You purify/clean a solitary shepherd's staff-plant. 34' When the sun sets, you surround it with a magic flour circle. 35' You scatter seven kernels of grain(?) in front of Šamaš. 36' You shall say (thus): "Šamaš, may your mules eat (this)!" 37' In the morning before sunrise 38' you take up its (the shepherd's staff-plant's) root with an arrow, you scatter four kernels of grain(?) over its root, 39' [you …] its top toward the ground(?), … . 40' You take up its root (again), and […]. 41' If you … […].
42' *zēr maštak*[*al* … …] 43' *ana šassūrī*[*ša tašakkan* … …] 44' *zēr ma*[*štakal* … …]	42' Seed of *maštakal*-soapwort, […], 43' [you insert] into [her] womb (viz. vagina) […]. 44' Seed of *maštakal*-soapwort, […].
45' *only traces preserved*	45' *too fragmentary for translation*

Ms. a rev. iii breaks; gap of unknown length
Beginning of rev. iv lost

46″ [... ... *lā*] *patān ina šikari išatti* 47″ [... ...] *ina šikari išatti* 48″ [... *urâ*]*nna tasâk ina šikari išatti* 49″ [... ...] *ina šikari išatti* 50″ [... ... *ta*]*sâk ina šikari išatti* 51″ [... ...]...-*ma tasâk ina šikari išatti* 52″ [... ... *ana dāmī*(?)] *parāsi* 53″ [... ... *ina šē*]-*pīša*(?) *tarakkas*

46″ [...] she drinks (it) in beer on an empty stomach. 47″ [...], she drinks (it) in beer. 48″ [... *ur*]*ânu*-fennel you crush, she drinks (it) in beer. 49″ [...] she drinks (it) in beer. 50″ [...], ... you crush, she drinks (it) in beer. 51″ [...] ... you crush, she drinks (it) in beer. 52″ [... for] stopping [the blood?]. 53″ [...] you tie (it) [around] her feet(?).

54″ [... ...] *kakkusakku* 55″ [... ... *šubû šum*]*ēlu seḫru* 56″ [... ...] *išatti* 57″ [... ... *ina šik*]*ari danni išatti* 58″ [... ...] *ina kakkabi tušbât išatti*

54″ [...] *kakkusakku*-stone, 55″ [... "le]ft" (and) *convoluted* [*šubû*-'stone'], 56″ [...] she shall drink. 57″ [...] she shall drink in strong [be]er. [...] 58″ you let (it) stay out overnight under the star(s), (then) she shall drink (it).

59″ *only traces preserved*

59″ *too fragmentary for translation*

Ms. a rev. iv breaks; remainder lost

Notes

General remark: In their transliteration, eBL proposes to reverse the obverse and reverse of the tablet, which is not followed here.

Lines 1′–8′: For a similar passage, see e.g. BAM 237 obv. i 4′–8′ (text C.1.4). For the variety of 'male' *šubû*-stone (probably a kind of shell), see also ms. a rev. iii 10 (line 25′), where it is used for a potion. Another stone with 'male' and 'female' variety often encountered in amulets is the *šû*-stone, see Chapter F; BAM 237 obv. i 4′–8′ (text C.1.4), BM 42327+ obv. 7–9 (text C.3.3) // SpTU 3, No. 84 rev. 6 (line 59 = text C.3.4) // BM 51246+ obv. 4 (text A.2.7); LKA 9 rev. r. col. 14′ (text C.3.5); KAR 247: 57″″ (text C.3.6); AO 6473 obv. 2 (text C.3.9).

Lines 9′–11′: Mss. a and B present very slight differences, e.g. in the order of the listed ingredients. For similar prescriptions to stop a vaginal discharge using these mineral ingredients, see e.g. BAM 237 i 33′, 36′, 43′–44′, iii 6–7, iv 17 (text C.1.4).

Lines 12′–14′: While the first line of this short spell employs the well-known metaphor of the overflowing canal that has been dammed up to describe the woman's haemorrhage, the following line 13′ presents problems for understanding, and the proposed reading is tentative. The word *musukkatu* "impure woman" restored at the beginning of line 13′ is a term for parturients, who were regarded to be in a period of (ritual) impurity due to their lochial discharges (cf. Feder 2016, 106–107, van der Toorn 1994; Stol 2000a; 2016; Steinert 2023). Its occurrence in this incantation may draw a link between abnormal bleeding and impurity in this text.

The second expression in line 13′, MUNUS KUD, read as *sinništu parištu*, occurs in a few ritual and healing texts, as a term for a post-menopausal woman, usually in instructions which specify that such a woman should spin or thread a cord used for an amulet (see CAD P, 187a s.v. *parištu*; e.g. BAM 237 obv. i 22′ (text C.1.4), written MUNUS KUD-tu_4). Since post-menopausal women were regarded as free of (potential) defilement by menstrual blood, the term *sinništu parištu* would stand in contrast to *musukkatu* preceding it.

The end of line 13′ remains likewise uncertain. The reconstructed word *pa-ri-is* may be the participle in the construct state with a following genitive noun. Since *parāsu* is typically used in the gynaecological texts with the meaning "to stop; to staunch (bleeding)", its meaning here probably alludes to this common usage, although the meaning "to (be) separated; to be set apart; to be cut off" is likewise possible. If the reading of the last word as *ḫaniqtu* is correct, it might mean "constricted (woman)", derived from *ḫanāqu* "to strangle; to constrict; to compress". Whether this also refers to a woman whose blood has stopped to flow (parallel to the post-menopausal woman mentioned before) is unclear.

Line 15′: The restoration of this rubric is tentative. The suggestion to read *ša-gu*$_5$*-šá* NU S[I].SÁ "whose menses" (*sagû*) are not normal" stems from a corresponding spelling *šá-gu*$_5$(KU)-*šá* in SpTU 1, No. 59 rev. 6′, 10′ (*sa-gu*$_5$*-šá*). Compare BAM 235: 4, 7 (*šá/šu-gu-šá*); cf. BM 38624+ ii 20′, 28′, 30′; BM 54587 + 73802 obv. 6′, 8′, 9′, rev. 3, 9; BM 61975 obv. 5′, 7′ (*sa-gu-šá*). See also SpTU 1, No. 39: 6′ and SpTU 1, No. 59 (text C.2.1) for discussion. A differing reading of line 15′ is proposed by eBL: *šá* TÚG-*šá* ⌜*mu*⌝-*s*[*uk*]-*ki*-MEŠ? "whose (menstrual) cloth(?) is ...(?)".

Lines 16′–20′: A similar procedure is encountered in BAM 237 i 9′ff., a ritual against *naḫšātu* (bleeding during pregnancy), in which a potsherd from a crossroads standing upright in the street is buried in a secluded place in the woman's house. Here, however, the potsherd served to seal a hole, in which something else was deposited (lost in the lacuna). In both rituals the potsherd symbolises blockage or closure. The reading of the verb form *inappal* in line 19′, perhaps from *napālu* "to dig up", is tentative. The verb also occurs in pharmaceutical handbooks in recommendations to dig up the root of a medicinal plant (in this case dog's tongue-plant, *lišān kalbi*) before sunrise (e.g. STT 92 ii 5 // BAM 1 ii 61, Attia and Buisson 2012, *JMC* 19, 28).

Lines 21′–23′: *Urīzu*-stone is also prescribed together with magnetite and other minerals in BAM 237 i 45′–46′, for a tampon (against *naḫšātu*, bleeding during pregnancy). It is likewise found in potions in K. 263 + 10934 (lines 22 and 33–36, likewise with magnetite). See texts C.1.4 and C.1.5.

Lines 24′–28′: This recipe corresponds to K. 263+10934 lines 33–36 (text C.1.5), with slightly different ingredients, replacing *ḫulālu*-stone with *urīzu*-stone, and "male" *šubû*-stone with "right" *šubû*-stone.

Lines 29′–31′: This remarkable rubric declares that the preceding prescriptions are "tested" or "well-proven" (*latku*) remedies copied from a tablet that belonged to the scholar (*ummânu*) Nūr-Marduk from Babylon. For remedies with the labels *latku* and *ana qāti šūṣû* and their relation to medical practice and experience, see Steinert 2015; Couto-Ferreira 2018b; Arbøll 2021, 194–195 *passim*.

Lines 32′–41′: This peculiar and in some respects unique ritual is unfortunately very fragmentary. The alternative usage of the same procedure for nosebleed or for gynaecological bleeding is also encountered in the case of the incantation *mimmû ilū ibnû amēlūtu* "All that the gods created of humankind" attested in BAM 237 ii 1′–6′ // BAM 386 i[!] 1′–6′ // SpTU 4, No. 129 i 11′–27′ // K. 3304 + 8785 + 9217 i 1′–7′ (text C.1.4).

In line 33′, *e-de-na-a* is probably better understood as the adjective *ēdēnû* "solitary; lonely" rather than the *ēdēnû*-plant (cf. CAD E, 27–28; AHw 186a s.v. *edēna* and *edēnû*). The verb *qadāšu* in the D-stem means "to make clean; to purify" (often in a ritual sense), "to dedicate, to consecrate". Here, it may refer to cleaning the "shepherd's staff-plant" (^{giš}NÍG.GIDRU SIPA, *ḫaṭṭi rē'î*), which has been uprooted from the ground (not mentioned in our text, but for similar ritual contexts see Reiner 1995, *Astral Magic*, 36–38) and which later seems to play a crucial role in the ritual (for the "shepherd's staff-plant" (*ḫaṭṭi rē'î*), cf. Böck 2014a, 141–142 (associating it with the *lišān kalbi*-plant); Geller 2015, 35, 38, 40 (KADP 4: 11, 29); Sibbing-Plantholt 2022, 294). The text instructs to pour out seven kernels of grain(?) in front of the setting sun (cf. CAD U/W, 355 s.v. *uṭṭatu* sub mng. 2). These grains, however, are given to the mules (*parû*) of Šamaš. The mules of Šamaš are mentioned elsewhere, for example in an incantation in the *Bīt rimki* ritual (BMS 60: 15 and dupl.; Laessøe 1955, 57: 63), as swift runners transporting the sun god (see also George 2003, 578–579, 814 *Gilgamesh Epic* III 96).

The ritual continues in the following morning before sunrise, with actions involving the shepherd staff-plant, especially its root and top. In particular, the ritual specialist uses an arrow (Akkadian *mulmullu* or *šiltāḫu*) to pick up the plant root, maybe so as not to touch the purified plant with the hands. An arrow also occurs in a recipe to speed up difficult labour in BAM 248 obv. i 68–69 (text D.1.1), where the arrow is used to stir oil, with which the patient was then massaged, playing on the notion of swiftness of movement, with which the (flying) arrow is associated. However, in the present context of a remedy to stop haemorrhage, the arrow may have an apotropaic meaning, since it serves to inflict wounds (see also BAM 237 ii 23′–24′ (text C.1.4), in a recipe for a potion to stop bleeding).

Line 34′: For similar instructions involving the uprooting of certain healing plants that grow alone in the wilderness, including the ritual action of surrounding the plant with a magic flour circle (*zisurrû*), see Reiner 1995, *Astral Magic*, 36–38, especially CT 17, 19 i 17–24 (quoted there); cf. Böck 2014a, 157–158 for a possible medical motivation underlying these nocturnal rituals.

Line 35′: The logogram ŠE may stand for *še'u* "barley, grain" or *uṭṭatu/uṭṭetu* "grain; kernel" (cf. CAD U/W, 355 sub mng. 2; CAD Š/2, 354; AHw 1446b, sub mng. 8 (plural).

Line 48″: For the restoration, cf. CAD U/W 207–208 s.v. *urânu* "fennel, anise".

Lines 54″–58″: *Kakkusakku*-stone is also attested in K. 263 + 10934: 24 (text C.1.5) in a potion to stop bleeding. The variety of *šubû*-stone encountered here designated as *siḫru* or *seḫru* may mean "convoluted" (Schuster-Brandis 2008, 447; CAD S, 239–240 sub 5).

C.1.9 FLP 1306: An Extract with Remedies to Stop Bleeding

This extract tablet in the collection of the Free Library Philadelphia contains recipes to stop irregular gynaecological bleeding during and outside pregnancy. The text was first identified by David I. Owen and was kindly brought to my attention by Marten Stol who shared with me his preliminary transliteration. The remedies in FLP 1306 (ms. a) offer several close parallels to other Neo- and Late Babylonian texts (mss. b-d). But similar prescriptions can likewise be found in K. 263 + 10934 from Nineveh and in SpTU 4, No. 153 from Uruk (see texts C.1.5, C.1.10 and discussion below), which use similar drug ingredients. Noteworthy features of the present text are the exclusive focus on tampons (*itqu*) and suppositories (*maššītu*) containing drugs inserted into the vagina and the inclusion of measurements for the ingredients in two sections of the tablet. Ms. a exclusively uses the masculine pronominal suffix to refer to the patient and it generally drops the conditional *šumma* "if" in the introductory phrases to the recipes. Moreover, ms. a several times inserts a reference to the remedies' purpose at the end of the prescriptions, which is a recurring feature of Late Babylonian medical texts. The text may therefore date to the Achaemenid period (6th/5th cent. BCE) rather than the earlier Neo-Babylonian period.

List of Manuscripts

Siglum	Museum Number	Copy	Collation	Format; Ductus	Provenience
a	FLP 1306[316]	Pl. 30	Coll.	Single-column tablet in portrait format; Late Babylonian script; ca. 6th–3rd cent. BCE(?)	Unknown (Babylonia)
b	K. 20254	Pl. 34	Coll.	Fragment of a tablet; Neo-Babylonian script; 7th cent. BCE	Nineveh, Ashurbanipal's library
c	BM 38624 (80-11-12, 508) + BM 38828 (80-11-12, 713) + BM 45414 (81-7-1, 3175)	Pl. 12–13	Coll.	Fragments of a two-column tablet; Late Babylonian script; ca. 6th/5th cent. BCE	probably Babylon
d	BM 42313+ (81-7-1, 73) + BM 42427 (81-7-1, 187) + BM 42585 (81-7-1, 345) + without No. (81-7-1, 353) + BM 43174 (81-7-1, 938) + BM 43215 (81-7-1, 979) + BM 43274 (81-7-1, 1038) + BM 43279 (81-7-1, 1043) + BM 43281 (81-7-1, 1045) + BM 43439 (81-7-1, 1203) + BM 43483 (81-7-1, 1247) + BM 43595 (81-7-1, 1359) + BM 43766 (81-7-1, 1527) + BM 43803 (81-7-1, 1564)	Pl. 14–15	Coll.	Single-column tablet in Late Babylonian script, ca. 500 BCE	Sippar

Overview

i	Prescription to stop bleeding (tampon) a obv. 1–3	1–3
ii	Prescription to stop bleeding (tampon) a obv. 4–6	4–6
iii	Prescription to stop bleeding (suppository) a obv. 7–10	7–10
iv	Prescription to stop bleeding (tampon) a obv. 11–15 // b obv.? 3′–5′ // d obv. 28–29	11–15

316 Measurements: 8 x 5 x 1.5 cm.

v	Prescription to stop bleeding (suppository) a rev. 1–5 // c obv. i 11′–13′	16–20
vi	Prescription to stop bleeding (tampon) a rev. 6–10	21–25
vii	Prescription to stop bleeding (suppository) a rev. 11–13	26–28
viii	Prescription to stop bleeding (suppository) a rev. 14–l. e. 1	29–32

Previous Edition and Discussion

CDLI P459867 (photo of ms. a)

Infra text C.1.7 (edition of ms. b), text A.2.1 (edition of ms. c), text A.2.2 (edition of ms. d)

Transliteration

1	a obv. 1	⸢^{munus}PEŠ$_4$$^{?}$⸣ *šá* MÚD ⸢*i*$^{?}$⸣-[*ta-nam-ma-ru*$^{?}$]
2	a obv. 2	[^{na4}]KUR$^{!}$-*nu* DAB *ina* ÀKA N[IGIN]
3	a obv. 3	[*ana* Š]À.TÙR-*šú* GAR *šá* MÚD KUD-⸢*si*⸣
4	a obv. 4	KI.MIN NUMUN ^{ú}IN.NU.UŠ *tu-ub-*⸢*bal*⸣
5	a obv. 5	GAZ SIM *ina* ÀKA NIGIN-*mi ina* ŠÀ.TÙR-*šú* GAR-*ma*
6	a obv. 6	MÚD KUD-*si*
7	a obv. 7	1 GÍN ^{na4}KUR-*nu* DAB 1 GÍN ^{šim}GIG
8	a obv. 8	1 1/2 GÍN MÚD ^{giš}EREN GAZ SIM
9	a obv. 9	*ina* ILLU BULUḪ ḪI.ḪI *ana* ŠÀ.TÙR<-*šú*> GAR-*ma*
10	a obv. 10	MÚD KUD-*si*
11	a obv. 11 b obv.$^{?}$ 3′ d obv. 28	*e-ṣe-et* UDU.NÍTA *ina* IZI *tur-*<*ár*> SÚD$^{?!}$ [....... .... GÌR.PAD.DU UDU$^{?}$].NÍTA *ina* IZI *tur-*⸢*ár*⸣ *ana* MÚD MUNUS KUD-*si* 1 *kak-ka* ⸢GÌR.PAD⸣.DU UDU.NÍTA *ina* IZI TUR-⸢*ár*⸣
12	a obv. 12 b obv.$^{?}$ 4′ d obv. 28–29	ŠIKA NUNUZ *lu-ur-mu* KA *tam-tim* [...] ŠIKA NUNUZ GA.NU$_{11}$^{mušen} / KA A.AB.BA
13	a obv. 13 b obv.$^{?}$ 4′$^{cont.}$ d obv. 29$^{cont.}$	ŠU.ÙR SUMUN *mál-ma-liš*$^{!}$(TAR) *ina* ÀKA [ŠU.Ù]R SUMUN *ina* ^{síg}ÀKA ⸢KU$^{?}$⸣ [^{giš}ÙR SUM]UN$^{?}$ *ina* ^{síg}ÀKA
14	a obv. 14 b obv.$^{?}$ 5′ d obv. 29$^{cont.}$	NIGIN-*mi ina* ŠÀ.TÙR-*šú* GAR-*ma* [NIGIN-*mi ana* ŠÀ.TÙR-*šá*] GAR-*an* NIGIN-*mi ana* ŠÀ.TÙR-*šú* GAR-*ma*
15	a obv. 15 b obv.$^{?}$ 5′ d obv. 29$^{cont.}$	MÚD KUD-*si* *Omits* *šá* MÚD MUNUS KUD-*si*

16	a rev. 1	1 GÍN [^{šim}G]IG 1/2 GÍN ^{ú}KUR.KUR
	c obv. i 11′	[...]
17	a rev. 2	1 GÍN $^{⸢\text{ú}⸣}$[NAGA.S]I$^{?}$ 1/2 NINDA *sim-bir-ri*
	c obv. i 11′$^{\text{cont.}}$	[...........................] 1/2 NINDA $^{⸢\text{ú}⸣}$*sim-bir-ri*
18	a rev. 3	*šal-šú* ^{ši}[^{m}x] 1/2 GÍN $^{\text{na4}}$*gab-bu-ú*
	c obv. i 12′	[x x x x x x] ⸢1/2 GÍN$^{?!}$⸣ $^{\text{na4}}$*gab-bu-u*
19	a rev. 4	*ina* ILLU BULUḪ GÚR.GÚR ^{g}[^{iš}E]REN ḪI.ḪI-*ma*
	c obv. i 12′$^{\text{cont.}}$–13′	*ina* ILLU ^{šim}BULUḪ / [x x x x ḪI.ḪI$^{?}$]
20	a rev. 5	*maš-šit-tu*$_4$ MÚD KUD-*si*
	c obv. i 13′$^{\text{cont.}}$	*maš-ši-ti šá* MÚD KUD-*as*
21	a rev. 6	MUNUS$^{?}$ MÚD.ME-*šú* DU-*ku* NU KUD-*si*
22	a rev. 7	*ana* KUD-*si* $^{\text{na4}}$*gab-bu-ú* KAL.GUG
23	a rev. 8	*zap*$^{!}$-*pi*[317] ANŠE ŠIKA NUNUZ *lu*$^{!}$-*ur-mu*
24	a rev. 9	[^{ši}]^{m}GÚR.<GÚR>[318] DIŠ-*niš* SÚD *ina* ^{síg}ḪE.ME.DA
25	a rev. 10	[NIGIN-*m*]*i ana* ŠÀ.TÙR-*šú* GAR-*ma* MÚD KUD-*si*
26	a rev. 11	[MUNUS M]ÚD.ME-*šú sa-ad-ru-ma*
27	a rev. 12	[*na-ak-d*]*a-at* ^{ú}IN.NU.UŠ SIG$_7$-*su*
28	a rev. 13	[DIŠ-*niš* SÚ]D$^{?}$ 1-*šú* 2-*šú* 3-*šú* ÍL-*šú*
29	a rev. 14	[KI.MIN$^{?}$ x GÍN ^{n}]$^{\text{a4}}$KUR-*nu* D[AB]
30	a u. e. 1	[x GÍN ^{šim}G]IG 1/2 GÍN [x (x)]
31	a u. e. 2	[x GÍN] ^{giš}⸢EREN⸣ ⸢GAZ⸣ S[IM]
32	a l. e. 1	*ina* ILLU BULUḪ ḪI.ḪI *ana* ŠÀ.TÙR-*š*[*ú* GAR-*ma* (MÚD KUD-*si*)]

Bound Transcription and Translation

[1] *erītu ša dāma ī*[*tanammaru*(?)] [2] *šadâna ṣābita ina itqi ta*[*lammi*] [3] [*ana ša*]*ssūrīšu tašakkan ša dāmi parāsi*	[1] (For) a pregnant woman who [keeps discovering(?)] blood: [2] you w[rap] magnetic hematite in a wad of wool, [3] you insert (it) into her womb (viz. vagina). (It is) for stopping the blood.
[4] KI.MIN *zēr maštakal tubbal* [5] *taḫaššal tanappi ina itqi ta-lammi ina šassūrīšu tašakkan-ma* [6] *dāma parāsi*	[4] Alternatively, you dry, [5] crush and sift [4] seed of *maš-takal*-soapwort. [5] You wrap (it) in a wad of wool, insert (it) into her womb (viz. vagina). [6] (It is for) stopping the blood.

317 The first sign looks a bit like ḪA and DIŠ.

318 Alternatively, read ^{šim}GAM.<MA> = *ṣumlalû*.

7 *ištēn šiqil šadâna ṣābitu ištēn šiqil kanakta* 8 *ištēn zūz (ši-qil) dām erēni taḫaššal tanappi* 9 *ina ḫīl baluḫḫi tuballal ana šassūrī<šu> tašakkan-ma* 10 *dāma parāsi*

8 You crush and sift 7 one shekel of magnetic hematite, one shekel of *kanaktu*-aromatic, 8 one and a half shekel of cedar 'blood'. 9 You mix (it) with resin of *baluḫḫu*-aromatic, insert (it) into (her) womb (viz. vagina). 10 (It is for) stopping the blood.

---

11 (var. adds: *ana dām sinništi parāsi*) *eṣet immeri ina išāti turr<ar> tasâk*(?) 12 *ḫaṣab pel lurmî imbu' tâmti* 13 (var. *sīk-ti*) *gušūri labiri malmališ ina itqi* 14 *talammi ina šassūrīšu tašakkan-ma* 15 *dāma parāsi* (var. *ša dām sinništi parāsi*)

11 (Var. adds: To stop a woman's blood:) You roast over a fire (and) bray the bone of a sheep. 14 You wrap (it) 13 in a wad of wool (with) an equal amount 12 of ostrich eggshell, *imbû tâmti*-mineral (and) 13 (var. powder of) an old beam. 14 You insert (it) into her womb (viz. vagina). 15 (It is for) stopping (var. adds: a woman's) blood.

---

16 *ištēn šiqil kanakta zūz (šiqil) atā'iša* 17 *ištēn šiqil [uḫūla qarnā]nâ zūz (šiqil) simbirri* 18 *šalšu* [...] *zūz (šiqil) gabâ* 19 *ina ḫīl baluḫḫi kukri erēni tuballal-ma* 20 *maššītu ša dāma parāsi* (var. *iparras*?)

19 You mix 16 one shekel of *kanaktu*-aromatic, half a shekel of *atā'išu*-plant, 17 one shekel of 'hor[ned alkali]', one half of a tenth of a litre of *simbirru*-plant, 18 one third (of a shekel) of [...]-aromatic (and) half a shekel of alum 19 with resin of *bal-uḫḫu*-aromatic, *kukru*-aromatic and ce[dar]. 20 A suppository for stopping the blood.

---

21 *sinništu dāmūšu illakū lā ipparrasū* 22 *ana parāsi gabâ kalgukka* 23 *zappi imēri ḫaṣab pel lurmî* 24 *kukra ištēniš tasâk ina tabarri* 25 *[talam]mi ana šassūrīšu tašakkan-ma dāma parāsi*

21 (For) a woman whose blood flows and cannot be stopped, 22 to stop it: 24 you pound together 22 alum, *kalgukku*-reddish pigment, 23 donkey bristle, ostrich eggshell (and) 24 *kukru*-aromatic, 25 [you wr]ap (it) 24 in red-coloured wool, 25 insert (it) into her womb (viz. vagina). (It is for) stopping the blood.

---

26 *[sinništu dā]mūšu sadrū-ma* 27 *[nakd]at maštakal arqūs-su* 28 *[ištēniš tas]âk ištīššu šinīšu šalāšīšu tušaššāšu*

26 (If) a woman's blood is flowing all the time, so that 27 she is [in a critical state]: 28 [you pou]nd [together] 27 fresh *maš-takal*-soapwort. 28 You have her apply (it) one, two, three times.

---

29 [KI.MIN(?) ... *šiqil*] *šadâna ṣā[bita]* 30 [... *šiqil kana*]*kta zūz (šiqil)* [...] 31 [... *šiqil*] *erēna taḫaššal ta[nappi]* 32 *ina ḫīl baluḫḫi tuballal ana šassūrīš[u tašakkan-ma (dāma parā-si)]*

29 [Alternatively(?)], 31 you crush (and) si[ft] 29 [x shekels] of magnetic haematite, 30 [x shekels of *kan*]*aktu*-aromatic, half a shekel of [...], 31 [x shekels] of cedar. 32 You mix (it) with *baluḫḫu*-resin, [insert (it)] into her womb (viz. vagina). (It is for stopping the blood)].

Notes

Lines 1–3: For the restoration of line 1, compare the Late Babylonian Uruk text SpTU 4, No. 153 obv. 8 (text C.1.10): *šá* ^{munus}PEŠ$_4$ *šá* 3 4 ITI.MEŠ-*šú u* MÚD *i-ta-nam-ma-ru* "for a pregnant woman who is three (or) four months (pregnant) and keeps seeing blood".

Lines 11–15: For the ingredients including bone, eggshell and old log or beam (*gušūru*), see also SpTU 4, No. 153 obv. 11–13 (text C.1.10); BM 45736: 6′–12′ (text A.2.5) and the *Introduction* for discussion.

Lines 16–20: *Atā'išu* is also recommended beside *simbirru*-plant in SpTU 4, No. 153 obv. 5 for "blocking" (the blood). See text C.1.10 below. For "horned alkali" (*uḫūlu qarnānû*) to stop female bleeding, see also K. 20254 obv. 7′ (text C.1.7). This ingredient occurs in related prescriptions in the renal and rectal disease texts: for haemorrhage from the penis (e.g. BAM 396 iv 3–5 // BAM 159 iv 3′–5′ (Geller 2005a, No. 1); BAM 112 ii 17′–19′ (Geller 2005a, No. 4); BAM 182 obv. 6′ // BAM 159 i 10 (Geller 2005a, No. 31)) and from the anus (in the form of suppositories, e.g. BAM 95: 29–30, 31–33 (Geller 2005a, No. 21)).

Lines 21–25: For bristle of a donkey, cf. CAD Z, 49f. s.v. *zappu* "bristle, animal hair" (more often in healing texts, bristle of a horse is encountered). Donkey hair (*zappi imēri*) as an ingredient is so far unique in the gynaecological prescriptions and not attested as a haemostatic drug in related texts. For the application of *kukru*-plant against bleeding in FLP 1306 (lines 19, 24), see also K. 8893: 11′ (text C.1.6).

Lines 26–29: For lines 26–27, compare BM 45736: 13′ (text A.2.5): [x x *e-nu*]-*ma*? MUNUS MÚD.ME-*šú at-ru-ma nak-da-a*[*t*] "[A ... wh]en a woman's blood (flows) in an excessive quantity so that she is in a critical condition". The verb *sadāru* "to occur regularly; to set in a row; to do little by little" used here to describe a constant blood flow is equated with *alāku* "to go; to flow" in the *Šumma izbu* Commentary line 544 (Leichty 1970, 228).

Lines 30–32: For a similar prescription, see SpTU 4, No. 153 obv. 10–11 (text C.1.10).

C.1.10 SpTU 4, No. 153: Prescriptions for Tampons to Stop Female Bleeding

This Late Babylonian text from Uruk in the collection of the Iraq Museum Baghdad, of which only the obverse is preserved, contains two thematic sections. The obverse begins with recipes to stop gynaecological haemorrhage (lines 1–18) and is followed by a section on treatments to speed up a contracted delivery (lines 19–31). The latter part of the fragment is edited in the section on birth (see text D.1.11). The text is remarkable for its inclusion of passages that provide contextual information and resemble commentaries, explaining specific text passages or giving the rationale for the use of specific therapeutic substances. These statements provide precious information about the pharmaceutical properties ascribed to drugs or observed by Babylonian healers (Steinert 2020, 58–60). Parallels for the use of specific ingredients and their applications in other texts edited in chapter C.1 (such as FLP 1306 and K. 263 + 10934) attest to continuities as well as variability of medical practices in the treatment of gynaecological bleeding during the first and second half of the first millennium BCE.

The text belonged to the collection of the descendants of Ekur-zakir, a family of *āšipus*, whose members lived in the 4th–3rd cent. BCE (cf. Clancier 2009, 53, 59–61, 396). Collations from photos kindly provided by Anmar Fadhil revealed that the preserved upper edge of the tablet contained one more line of text and a fragmentary colophon which was not previously copied by E. von Weiher in his *editio princeps* (see text D.1.11 for discussion). The tablet has deteriorated a bit further since von Weiher documented it; several signs copied by him are not visible anymore today. It is possible that SpTU 5, No. 253 (text E.2.6), another fragment on women's diseases from the Ekur-zakir archive, belongs to the same tablet as SpTU 4, No. 153 (see text E.2.6 for discussion).

List of Manuscripts

Siglum	Museum Number	Copy	Collation	Format; Ductus	Provenience
a	IM 76998 W. 22649	SpTU 4, No. 153 Pl. 26	Photo coll.	Fragment of a single-column tablet in portrait format; Late Babylonian script; 4th/3rd cent. BCE	Uruk; library of the descendants of Ekur-zakir

Overview

i	Prescription to stop bleeding (suppositories) a obv. 1–4	1–4
ii	Prescription to stop bleeding (suppositories) a obv. 5–6	5–6
iii	Prescription to stop bleeding a obv. 7–9	7–9
iv	Prescription to stop bleeding a obv. 10–13	10–13

v	Prescription to stop bleeding a obv. 14	14
vi	Prescription to stop bleeding (suppository) a obv. 15–16	15–16
vii	Prescription to stop bleeding (potion) a obv. 17	17
viii	Prescription to stop bleeding (tampon) a obv. 18	18

Previous Edition and Discussion

von Weiher 1993, SpTU 4, 89–91 (transliteration, translation), 181 (copy)
Finkel 1994, *NABU* 1994, No. 69 (discussion)
Geller 1995–1996, *AfO* 42–43, 246–247 (transliteration, translation of lines 21–31; discussion)
Böck 2010a, *TUAT NF* 5, 113 (translation of lines 21–31)
Steinert 2020, *JMC* 36, 58–60 (lines 1–4, 7–9, 10–11, 14–15)
CDLI P348746 (copy)
Infra text D.1.11

Transliteration

1 a obv. 1 DIŠ MUNUS MÚD.MEŠ-*šú* DU.MEŠ-*ma la ip-par-ra-su ana pa-ra-si* ^{na4}*gab-ú* ^{im}KAL.G[UG SUM-*ši* EGIR$^{?}$]

2 a obv. 2 *šá lu-ub-bu-ku* SUM-*ši* EGIR *šá lu-ub-bu-ku u* ÚŠ-*e* SUM-*su* EGIR *maš-šit an-n*[*it šá* ^{na4}*gab-ú*$^{?}$]

3 a obv. 3 *u* ^{im}KAL.GUG SUM-*su* ^{na4}*gab-ú tu-qal-la* ^{im}KAL.GUG *lìb-bu-u*$^{?}$ [x x x x]

4 a obv. 4 DÙ-*uš* Ú.MEŠ *an-nu-tu ma-la iq-bak-ka* 1.TA.ÀM *ina-aš-ši ki-i ru-ṭib-ti* {*i-b*[*a-lu*$^{?}$ x x]}

---

5 a obv. 5 ^{ú}KUR.KUR ^{ú}MAŠ.TAB.BA ^{ú}*sim-bir-ri* ^{šim}GAM.MA 4 Ú.MEŠ *šá ana maš-ši-ti* E-*ú šá* Ú{Š-*e ši-i* x[x]}

6 a obv. 6 EGIR *šá lu-ub-bu-ku* ÍL-*ú* EGIR *maš-šit an-nit* SUM-*su* EGIR *maš-šit šá* ^{na4}*gab-ú* {*u* ^{im}KAL.GU[G SUM-*su*]}

---

7 a obv. 7 ^{ú}IN$_{6}$.ÚŠ *sim-bar*[319] *ana tak-ṣa-a-tú šá* ^{munus}PEŠ$_{4}$ E-*ú* MUNUS *šá*$^{!}$ Ù.TU-*ma* MÚD.MEŠ-*šú la i*{*p-par-ra-su* SUM-*s*[*u* (...)]}

8 a obv. 8 *šá* ^{munus}PEŠ$_{4}$ *šá* 3 4 ITI.MEŠ-*šú u* MÚD *i-ta-nam-ma-ru* SUM-*su* : *ina u*$_{4}$-*mu* ŠE TIL-*šú* SU{M-*su ina u*$_{4}$-*m*[*u*] *l*[*a*$^{?}$ ŠE *la*$^{?}$]}

9 a obv. 9 SUM-*su ina* ŠÀ UZU-*šú* SED-*ú u* MÚD *ik-kal-lu-u* : Ú.MEŠ *šá ú-lab-ba*{*k-*[*ku*$^{?}$ x x x]}

---

10 a obv. 10 ⸢MAN$^{?}$⸣-*nu*$^{?}$ KU ^{šim}GIG *u* EREN.BAD *šá* EGIR *maš-šit i-ṣi ta-ta-nam-mar ana* ÚŠ-*e* SU[M$^{?}$-*su*] {*gab-*⸢*ú*⸣ [(...)]}

11 a obv. 11 ^{šim}GIG *ú-lab-bak* EREN.BAD *ub-bal* ILLU IN$_{6}$.ÚŠ GÌR.PAD.DU UDU.NÍTA *ina* IZI *tur-ár* ŠI{KA NUNUZ GA}.(-)[NU$_{11}$^{mušen}]

12 a obv. 12 KA *tam-tim* KU ^{giš}ÙR SUMUN 1.TA.ÀM SUM-*su ki-i* 1.TA.ÀM SUM-*šú ma-la i*{*l-te-ne*[*q*$^{?}$-*qé* (Ú.MEŠ)]}

13 a obv. 13 *gab-bi tu-sam-maḫ-ma* SUM-*su* KU ^{giš}ÙR *šá* E-*ú ul šá* ^{giš}GIŠIMMAR {(KU) *šá* ^{giš}ÁS[AL]}

---

14 a obv. 14 ⸢^{dug}⸣ÚTUL GIBIL$_{4}$ *u* ŠIKA SÁḪAR *šá* KA UDUN *ma-'-diš* DU$_{10}$.GA *ú-lab-bak ú-kàṣ-ṣa* {*u ub-*[*bal*$^{?}$ (x x)]}

---

319 An erroneous writing for the *simbirru*-plant?

15	a obv. 15	⌜IGI⌝ ⌜UDU⌝.NÍTA SI UDU.NÍTA *šá ina* IZI *iq-lu-ú ma-ʾ-diš* DU_{10}.GA *di-iq-me-en-na-šú-nu* $^{⌜síg!}$ÀKA$^{?⌝}$ [NIGIN$^{?}$] x x [x x]
16	a obv. 16	⌜*ki*$^{?}$-*ṣir*$^{?⌝}$ UDU SI UDU 1+*et maš-šit* NUMUN ŠINIG ^{na4}*gab-ú u* ^{im}KAL.⌜LA.GUG⌝ [x x (x)]
17	a obv. 17	$^{⌜na4}$KUR⌝-*nu* DAB *šá ana maš-qit šá* MÚD MUNUS KUD-*si* E-*ú šá* x x [x x x] DUB [x x x]
18	a obv. 18	$^{⌜síg⌝}$ÀKA SÍG$^{?}$ $^{ḫe\text{-}pí}$ <*me*>-⌜UGU$^{?⌝}$ NA_4 1.TA.ÀM SUM-*su* 1 1/6(ŠÚ) SÌLA x[x x x x x] x x [x x]

For the continuation of ms. a obv. see text D.1.11

Bound Transcription and Translation

[1] *šumma sinništu dāmūšu ītanallakū-ma lā ipparrasū ana parāsi gabâ kalg[ukka tanaddinši arki(?)]* [2] *ša lubbuku tanaddinši arki ša lubbuku u peḫê tanaddissu arki maššīt ann[īt ša gabî(?)]* [3] *u kalgukki tanaddissu gabâ tuqalla kalgukku libbū* [...] [4] *teppuš šammī annûti mala iqbâkka ištēnâ inašši kī ruṭibti ibb[alū(?) ...]*	[1] If a woman's blood keeps flowing all the time and cannot be stopped, to stop it: [you administer to her (lit. "give her")] alum, reddish *kalgukku*-pigment. [Thereafter(?)] [2] you give her (the suppository) for *absorbing* (lit. 'soaking'). Thereafter you give her (the suppository) for *absorbing* and for blocking (the flow). Thereafter you give her (again) thi[s] suppository (*maššītu*) [of alum(?)] [3] and (reddish) *kalgukku*-pigment. You should roast the alum; (and) the *kalgukku*-pigment – this means: [...], [4] you make [3] [*a suppository*(?)]. [4] Of these drugs, as much as one has told you (to be appropriate), she applies one unit (i.e. the same amount) of each. Like(?) moisture(?) it (i.e. the blood) will [*dry*(?) ...].
[5] *atāʾišu māštu simbirri ṣumlalû erbēt šammū ša ana maššīti iqbû ša peḫê šī* ...[...] [6] *arki ša lubbuku iššû arki maššīt annīt tanaddissu arki maššīt ša gabî u kalguk[ki tanaddisu]*	[5] *Atāʾišu*-plant, *māštu*-plant, *simbirru*-plant (and) *ṣumlalû*-plant: (these are) four plants which are prescribed (lit. "which it said") for a suppository (which) is for blocking. [...] [6] After she has applied the (suppository) for *absorbing*, thereafter you give her this suppository. Thereafter [you give her (again)] the suppository of alum and (reddish) *kalgukku*-pigment.
[7] *maštakal simbirru(?) ana takṣâti ša erīti iqbû sinništu ša uldu-ma dāmūšu lā ipparrasū tanaddiss[u (...)]* [8] *ša erīti ša šalāšat erbet arḫūšu u dāma ītanammaru tanaddissu : ina ūmi magri gamrīšu(?) tanaddissu ina ūm[i] l[ā magri lā]* [9] *tanaddissu ina libbi šīrūšu ikaṣṣû u dāmū ikkallû : šammū ša ulabbak[ū(?) ...]*	[7] *Maštakal* (and) *simbirru*-plant(?) are prescribed for cooling a pregnant woman. You can (also) administer (it to) a woman who has given birth and whose blood cannot be stopped. [(...)] [8] You can administer (it also) *to* a pregnant woman who is (in) her third or fourth month and keeps discovering blood: you administer (it) on a completely(?) auspicious (*magru*) day, (but) you [must not(?)] [9] administer (it) [8] on an in[auspicious(?)] day. [9] Through this her body will cool down and the blood will be held back. (These are) drugs that *absorb* [...].

10 šanû(?) sīkti kanakti šupuḫri ša arki maššīt iṣi tātanammar(u) ana peḫê tanad[dissu(?)] gabû [(...)] 11 kanaktu ulabbak šupuḫru ubbal ḫīl maštakal eṣemti immeri ina išāti turrar ḫaṣab pel lur[mî] 12 imbû tâmti sīkti gušūri labiri ištēnâ tanaddissu kī ištēnâ tanaddinušu mala iltene[qqe (šammī)] 13 gabbi tusammaḫ-ma tanaddissu sīkti gušūri ša iqbû ul ša gišimmari [(sīktu)] ša ṣarb[ati]

10 Another (remedy?): Powder of *kanaktu*-aromatic and *šupuḫru*-cedar, which, after a *suppository* of wood(?), you will always find (to be good) – you admi[nister (it) to her] for blocking. Alum [(... and?)] 11 *kanaktu*-aromatic will *absorb*, *šupuḫru*-cedar will dry (out). You (can also) desiccate resin of(?) *maštakal*-soapwort (and) sheep bone over a fire. You (can also) administer to her (lit. 'give her') the shell of an ostrich egg, 12 *imbû tâmti*-mineral (and) powder of an old beam, one unit (i.e. the same amount of) each (ingredient). When you administer to her (the substances), one unit (i.e. the same amount) of each, as much as she can ta[ke each time], 13 you should mix all 12 [(*the drugs*)] 13 and administer (them) to her. The powder of the beam that is prescribed (lit. 'that it (= the text) said (above)'), shall not be of date palm, (but) [(powder)] of poplar (wood).

---

14 diqāru eššu u ḫaṣbu šaḫarru ša pī utūni ma'diš ṭāb ulabbak ukaṣṣa u ub[bal (...)]

14 A new(?) pot or a porous potsherd from the opening of an oven is very good (as well): it *absorbs*, cools and dri[es out(?) (...)].

---

15 īn immeri qaran immeri ša ina išāti iqlû ma'diš ṭāb diqmennāšunu itqa [talammi(?)] ... [...] 16 kiṣir(?) immeri qaran immeri ištēt maššīt zēr bīni gabî u kalgukki [...]

15 A sheep's eye (and) sheep's horn, which have been roasted over a fire, are very good (as well). [You wrap] their ashes into a wad of wool, [...]. 16 The joint(?) of a sheep, sheep's horn, a suppository of *bīnu*-tamarisk seeds, alum and reddish *kalgukku*-pigment [...].

---

17 šadânu ṣābitu ša ana mašqīt ša dām sinništi parāsi iqbû ša ...[...] tasarraq(?) [...]

17 The magnetic haematite, which is prescribed (lit. said) for a potion for stopping a woman's blood, concerning (which) [...], you sprinkle(?) [...].

---

18 itqi šīpāti ḫepi mêli(?) abni ištēnâ tanaddissu ištēn šeššu qa ...[...] ...[...]

18 A wad of *broken* wool (and?) a leather bag(?) (filled with?) stone(s) you administer to her, one at a time(?). One and a sixth of a litre of ... [...].

For the continuation of ms. a obv. see text D.1.11

Notes

General remark: A remarkable feature in SpTU 4, No. 153 are the varying orthographies of SUM "to give" with the varying pronominal suffixes *-su* (lines 2–3, 6–9, 12–13, 25), *-šú* (line 12), *-ši* (lines 2, 26) referring to the (female) patient. The suffix *-su* in SUM-*su* points to an assimilated form of *nadānu* "to give, to administer", i.e. *tanaddissu* (> *tanaddin+-šu*); see GAG § 102l for irregular assimilated forms of *nadānu* + pronominal suffixes of the 3rd person in Late Babylonian texts. Note, for example, Cole 1996, 180 No. 84: 7 *ta-nam-di-˹su˺*; compare ibid., 94 No. 31: 13 *ta-nam-din-su* (with dissimilation). Geller (1995–1996, 246) suggested instead that the verb behind SUM (SÌ) in the present text may be *paqādu* "to take care of (person)", which seems less likely.

Line 1: For the purpose statement, see also K. 263 + 10934 obv. 1; FLP 1306 rev. 21–22.

Line 2: Here and in the following lines, the text states the expected therapeutic effects of the treatments or substances which are administered subsequently, especially *ša lubbuku u peḫê* "for *absorbing* (lit. soaking) and blocking". For these verbs, see the discussion in the *Introduction*. The treatments/drugs for *absorbing* and blocking alluded to in line 2 could refer to the substances recommended in the following sections, where drugs are repeatedly classified according to the effect of *lubbuku* and *peḫû*, in addition to drying and cooling properties.

Line 3: For *libbū* in commentaries, see CAD L, s.v. *libbu* sub 4a-2′b′; Gabbay 2016, 127–133, esp. 129–130. In the present passage, *libbū* probably introduces a "semantic equation" or "specification" explaining the preceding phrases referring to the preparation of alum and *kalgukku*-mineral pigment.

Line 4: The phrase *mala iqbâkka* presumably refers to information on drug dosages that are not written down in the text, but were communicated orally ("these drugs, as much as one has told you (to use)"). For another occurrence in a Late Babylonian women's healthcare text, see BM 45736 line 10′ (text A.2.5). For the similar expressions *mala/ša iqbû* "as much as/of which it (= the base text) said" in commentaries, which serve to introduce textual citations or explanations, see Gabbay 2016, 212–213 and similar uses in SpTU 4, No. 153 lines 5, 7, 13, 17 below.

The restoration of the end of line 4 is tentative. The word *ruṭibtu* "dampness/flooded ground" also occurs as a specific ailment associated with moistness (cf. CAD R, 437–438 especially sub 2 on *ruṭibtu*). However, in the present passage, the term *ruṭibtu* may express that the patient's haemorrhage is associated with an excess of moisture in the body (metaphorically compared with a watered field). Instead of a preposition, *kī* could also function here as a conjunction ("when (the moisture has dried)").

Lines 5–6: The *ṣumlalû*-plant (^{šim}GAM.MA, terebinth or turpentine, a kind of pistachio; the resin of which has medical uses) is not common in gynaecological prescriptions to stop bleeding, but it is used for instance in renal disease texts in the context of treating discharge (*mūṣu*) from the penis (see e.g. Geller 2005a, No. 2a ms. B5 = AMT 58/6: 7′). The *māštu*-plant (^{ú}MAŠ.TAB.BA) occurs only rarely in gynaecological material and is not known primarily as a haemostatic drug (see also texts B.2.4: 11′; text D.2.1: 48′).

Lines 5, 7, 13, 17: The phrase *ša* (…) *iqbû* often occurs in commentaries, where it can refer to a word or expression encountered in the base text commented upon (cf. Gabbay 2016, 201–260 for discussion, esp. 238–240). In SpTU 4, No. 153, the phrase (*ša*) *ana* … *iqbû* has a prescriptive and explanatory nuance, i.e. referring to drugs or treatments "which are prescribed (for a certain condition)" that are either found in the remedies included in SpTU 4, No. 153, or that were known to the scribe to be useful for a certain purpose. For discussion, see the *Introduction*.

Lines 7–9: For "cooling" (*takṣâtu*) in association with stopping haemorrhage. see also Steinert 2020, *JMC* 36, 59 and the *Introduction*. In the break at the end of line 7, one could suggest restoring [*ana tak-ṣa-a-tú*], since line 8 again begins with *ša erīti*. The repetition of the phrase *ana takṣâti ša erīti* "for the cooling of a pregnant woman" from the beginning of line 7 may be preferable, since one would otherwise expect *ana erīti* … *tanadissu* in line 8. However, *ana* is also omitted in line 7 in the corresponding construction with *nadānu*.

For the hemerological specification in line 8–9 to administer the treatment only on a completely auspicious day, compare similar patterns in the so-called *Babylonian Almanac* and in lists of lucky and unlucky days, which also specify days that are completely auspicious (*kalîš magir*) and days that are only auspicious during midday (see Livingstone 2013, 7 *passim*). The hemerological works also include interdictions for a physician (*asû*) to treat patients on specific days. Note that this passage in line 8–9 is separated from the rest of the text in the paragraph by disjunction signs (*Trennungszeichen*); it was thus marked by the scribe as an insertion or added commentary.

Line 9: The verbal endings in SED-*ú* and *ik-kal-lu-u* indicate masculine plural subjects, although neither of the logograms UZU nor MÚD are written with the plural marker MEŠ.

Line 13: The verbs *summuḫu* and *bullulu* "to mix", both used in medical texts, are difficult to distinguish semantically.

Line 14: NE could also be read as KÚM "hot" (*emmu*) instead of *eššu* "new". The use of a porous potsherd (probably applied crushed) to stop haemorrhage is also attested in BM 42313+ obv. 30 (text A.2.2). For discussion of this ingredient, see the *Introduction*.

Lines 15–16: The sheep's eye and horn (burned to ashes) contrast with the colour and liquid quality of blood. The roasting process of the ingredients implies that they were imbued with a drying quality what would stop the haemorrhage. See the *Introduction* for further discussion.

Lines 17–18: The text of this passage seems to be abbreviated. In line 17, magnetic haematite (*šadânu ṣābitu*) is referred to as an ingredient of a potion. The following line seems to refer to the application form of a tampon (*itqu*) and possibly a leather pouch filled with stones (if we emend the text, marked by *ḫepi* as already damaged in the ancient *Vorlage* copied by the scribe of SpTU 4 No. 153, to <*me*>-*elu*(UGU), for *mêlu* "leather bag").

In line 17 following the word *maš-qit*, von Weiher's copy suggests traces of an erased sign. Collation from photos suggests instead that the scribe left a blank space to the following phrase. The tablet's surface is slightly damaged here, causing the impression of an erasure. The scribe left another blank space in this line following the word E-*ú*. This either served to distribute the signs equally over the whole line or to highlight visually a key phrase of the text.

In line 18, the phrase 1.TA.ÀM "(you administer to her) one by one" or "separately" may specify that the tampon and *mêlu*-bag had to be applied separately from each other. The numeral 1.TA.ÀM is encountered in other prescriptions for suppositories, see e.g. BAM 237 iv 10; iv 32–33 (text C.1.4). However, in lines 4 and 12 of SpTU 4, No. 153, I understand 1.TA.(-)ÀM in a distributive meaning "one (unit) of each", indicating that the same amount of each ingredient had to be used; cf. Streck 1995, 69–70; Chalendar 2020, 63–64.

C.2 Treatments to Induce Female Bleeding and to Regulate the Menses

As far as their preserved contents allow us to judge, the four texts presented in this subsection share a certain interest in the topic of women's menstrual health, specifically in regulating the menses. They date at all likelihood to the Late Babylonian period and come from different places (Uruk, Babylon or Borsippa, and Sippar). The fragments are of particular interest not only because of their contents, but also because of their heterogenous formats and the hints to compendial contexts they provide. At least the fragment from Uruk (SpTU 1, No. 59, text C.2.1) belonged to the context of the Late Babylonian therapeutic compendium *šumma amēlu muḫḫašu umma ukâl*, as we know thanks to its colophon. Another one of the fragments could have belonged to a longer medical therapeutic series (BM 61975+, text C.2.4). Another text (BM 47578, text C.2.3) is marked as a short extract (*nisḫu*) of prescriptions and likely presents a school tablet, while the fourth text (BM 54587 + 73802, text C.2.3) represents a shorter collection of prescriptions.

In terms of contents, all four texts deal with "women's blood" (*dām sinništi*) or, more specifically, with the menses (*sagû*, *maruštu*), and contain references to inducing the menstrual flow when it has stopped (*parāsu*), sometimes expressed with the verb *kullumu* "to make (the menses/blood) appear". Another term for the menses occurring in one of the texts is *kibsu* "(regular) course" (see texts C.2.2, A.2.6, A.2.10). Beyond the texts edited here, other Late Babylonian collections of prescriptions for women's health contain remedies for the same purpose (e.g., BM 38624+, BM 42313+ edited in this volume, section A). We cannot be certain about the exact causes behind the amenorrhoea treated in the texts which are never mentioned (e.g. menopause, poor diet). But it is possible that the prescriptions could have served to interrupt an early-term pregnancy (see the *Introduction* for discussion).

C.2.1 SpTU 1, No. 59: Women's Menses in the Late Babylonian Therapeutic Compendium *šumma amēlu muḫḫašu umma ukâl*

This fragment from Uruk stemming from the library of the exorcist Anu-ikṣur (of the Šangû-Ninurta family active in the 5th–4th centuries BCE, Clancier 2009a, 52, 58–59) forms one of the rare cases, in which a women's healthcare text is identified as belonging to a serialised medical compendium. According to the tablet's colophon identifying Anu-ikṣur as the copyist, this text formed the 41st tablet of the medical therapeutic series *šumma amēlu muḫḫašu umma ukâl* "if a man's skull contains heat", which is known in several versions and recensions from the Neo-Assyrian and Late Babylonian period (see e.g., Heeßel 2010c, *TUAT NF* 5, 31–35; Panayotov 2018; Steinert 2018; Steinert et al. 2018 for overviews). The catchline preceding the colophon (line 14′) quotes the incipit of the following tablet in the series, entitled "if a woman's blood is cut off so that her blood is not [seen]" (or "so that she does not see her blood"). This line occurs as the incipit of a short extract tablet from the Late Babylonian period, designated, however, as the 40th *nisḫu*-extract (BM 47578, see text C.2.2, and below for discussion).

With the exception of lines 12′–13′, the other sections of SpTU 1, No. 59 preserving the lower part of the tablet's reverse do not feature any introductory purpose statements. But the references to a woman "who does not see her 'trouble' (*maruštu*)" and the purpose described as letting her "see her 'trouble'" (line 12′) may indicate that the preceding fragmentary sections were similarly concerned with inducing menstrual bleeding (see also Stol 2000a, 26, 199; Stol 2016a, 446). Böck (2010, *TUAT NF* 5, 110) understands the recipes as provoking menstruation in the context of contraception to prevent the nidation of a fertilized ovum (cf. Riddle 1992, 26). But other causes and contexts, in which amenorrhoea or absence of the menses could have occurred, are not excluded (e.g., late menarche, a woman entering menopause).

The prescriptions recommend an enema injected into the vagina, potions, and a tampon – therapeutic procedures that are also applied in other contexts (e.g., stopping the menstrual flow or other abnormal discharges).

List of Manuscripts

Siglum	Museum Number	Copy	Collation	Format; Ductus	Provenience
a	W. 22307/50 + 54 + 62 + 69 + 76	SpTU 1, No. 59	–	Fragment of a tablet; Late Babylonian script; 5th cent. BCE	Uruk; Library of Anu-ikṣur

Overview

i′	Fragmentary prescription a rev. 1′–2′	...]1′–2′
ii′	Prescription (enema introduced into vagina) a rev. 3′–6′	3′–6′
iii′	Prescription (potion) a rev. 7′	7′
iv′	Prescription (potion) a rev. 8′	8′
v′	Fragmentary prescription a rev. 9′–10′	9′–10′
vi′	Prescription (tampon) a rev. 11′	11′
vii′	Prescription to induce menstrual bleeding (potion?) a rev. 12′–13′	12′–13′
viii′	Catchline a rev. 14′	14′
ix′	Colophon a rev. 15′–18′	15′–18′

Previous Edition and Discussion

Hunger 1976, SpTU 1, 65–66 (transliteration; translation)
Böck 2010a, *TUAT NF* 5, 110 (translation lines 12′–13′)
Scurlock and Andersen 2005, 260 12.4 and 12.5 (lines 12′, 14′)
CDLI P348480 (copy; transliteration)

Transliteration

Ms. a obv. and beginning of rev. lost

1′	a rev. 1′	[x x x x x x] ^{š}[^{im} ....]
2′	a rev. 2′	[x x x x x x] x *ba-lu p*[*a-tan* ....]
3′	a rev. 3′	[x x x x x ^{šim}L]I ^{ú}ḪAR.ḪAR ⸢^{ú}⸣[x x x x x x]
4′	a rev. 4′	[x x x x x *ina*$^{?}$] IL[LU] ^{šim}BULUḪ *mál-ma-liš* [ḪI.ḪI$^{?}$ x x x]
5′	a rev. 5′	[x x x x x] *ina* KAŠ *ina* ^{urudu}ŠEN.TUR ŠEG$_6$-*šal* ⸢SED⸣ [x x x]
6′	a rev. 6′	[x x U$_5^{?}$ ARK]AB^{mušen} *ana* ŠÀ.TÙR-*šá* DUB-*ma šá-g*[*u*$_5$-*šá* x x]
7′	a rev. 7′	[x x x x x].AM$^{?}$ ^{ú}IGI-*lim* DIŠ-*niš ta-mar-raq ina* KAŠ *la pa-tan* NAG.M[EŠ$^{?}$ (x)]
8′	a rev. 8′	[x x x x x x] ^{ú}EME-UR.GI$_7$ DIŠ-*niš ta-mar-raq ina* KAŠ N[AG x]
9′	a rev. 9′	[x x x x x ^{ú}]⸢IGI-*lim*⸣ ⸢^{ú}IGI-20⸣ [^{ú}Ḫ]AR.ḪAR ^{ú}KUR.KUR ÚKUŠ.LAG[AB x x]
10′	a rev. 10′	[......................... *s*]*a*$^{?}$-*gu*$_5$-*šá ár-ḫiš* [x x]
11′	a rev. 11′	[x x x] maš/bar$^{?}$ *tu-pa-a*[*ṣ*$^{?}$ *ta*]*ra-sà-an* [*ina*] TÚG *tara-kás ana* ŠÀ.T[ÙR-*šá* GAR-*an*]
12′	a rev. 12′	[*ana* MUNUS$^{?}$] *ša* <NÍG>.GIG-*šá* NU *im-mar* NÍG.GIG-*šá i*[*m*]-*mar* ^{ú}IGI-20 SUḪU[Š x x x]
13′	a rev. 13′	^{ú}*ṣa-ṣu-un-tú* DIŠ-*niš ta-mar-*⸢*raq*⸣ *ina* Ì ⸢KAŠ⸣ *u* A.GEŠTIN.N[A ḪI.ḪI NAG$^{?}$]
14′	a rev. 14′	DIŠ MUNUS MÚD-*šá* KUD-*ma* MÚD-*šá* NU [IGI (...)]
15′	a rev. 15′	⸢DUB⸣ ⸢41⸣.KAM DIŠ NA UGU-[*šú* K]ÚM *ú-kal bul-ṭu* ⸢É$^{?}$⸣ [^{m}*Dà-bi*$_x$-*bi*$_x^{?}$]
16′	a rev. 16′	GABA.RI ⸢UNUG^{ki}⸣ [GIN$_7$ SUMUN]-*šú* ^{md}60-*ik-ṣur* A-*šú šá* ^{m}[^{d}UTU-MU-*na* (...)]
17′	a rev. 17′	IN.SAR-*ma ib-ri*$_{12}$ IM ^{md}UTU-MU-*n*[*a* x x x x x x x]
18′	a rev. 18′	*pa-liḫ* ^{d}*a-n*[*u u*] ^{d}15 NU *i*$_{11}$(ḪI)-*t*[*a*$_8$(ŠÁR)-*áb-bà-alla*$^{?}$]

Remainder of the rev. left blank(?)

Bound Transcription and Translation

Ms. a obv. and beginning of rev. lost

$^{1'}$ [... ...] ... [... ...] $^{2'}$ [... ...] *balu pa*[*tān* ... ...]	$^{1'}$ [... ...]-aromatic, [... ...] $^{2'}$ [... ... she ... (it)] on an empty sto[mach, ...].
$^{3'}$ [... ... *bu*]*rāšu ḫašû* ...[... ...] $^{4'}$ [... ... *ina*] *ḫ*[*īl*] *baluḫḫi mal-mališ* [*tuballal*(?) ...] $^{5'}$ [... ...] *ina šikari ina tamgussi tušabšal tukaṣṣa* [...] $^{6'}$ [... *rikibti ark*]*abi ana šassūrīša tatabbak-ma šag*[*ûša*(?) ...]	$^{3'}$ [... ...], *burāšu*-juniper, *ḫašû*-plant, [...]-plant, [... ...]. $^{4'}$ [... ...] (and) resin of the *baluḫḫu*-aromatic you [mix(?)] in equal quantities, [... ...]. $^{5'}$ [... ...] you boil with beer in a metal pot. You cool it down, [... ...] $^{6'}$ [... (with) *spur*(?) of a b]at you pour (it) into her womb. Then [her] men[ses(?) will ...].
$^{7'}$ [... ...]... *imḫur-līm ištēniš tamarraq ina šikari lā patān ištan*[*atti*(?) (...)]	$^{7'}$ You crush together [... ...] (and) 'heals thousand'-plant. She shall drink (it) re[peatedly(?)] in beer on an empty stomach, [(...)].

8′ [... ...] *lišān kalbi ištēniš tamarraq ina šikari iš*[*atti* ...]	8′ You crush together [... ...] (and) dog's tongue-plant. [She shall drink (it)] in beer [(...)].
9′ [... ...] *imḫur-līm imḫur-ešrā* [*ḫ*]*ašû atā'išu er*[*rû* ...] 10′ [... ...] *sagûša*(?) *arḫiš* [...]	9′ [... ...] 'heals thousand'-plant, 'heals twenty'-plant, *ḫašû*-plant, *atā'išu*-plant, coloc[ynth(?), ...], 10′ [... ...], her menses(?) [will ...] quickly.
11′ [...]... *tupâ*[*ṣ ta*]*rassan* [*ina*] *lubāri tarakkas ana šass*[*ūrīša tašakkan*]	11′ You crush (and) moisten [...]... . You bind it [in] a piece of cloth (and) [insert it] into [her wo]mb (viz. vagina).
12′ [*ana sinništi*(?)] *ša maruštāša lā immar maruštāša immar imḫur-ešrā šuruš* [...] 13′ *ṣaṣuntu ištēniš tamarraq ina šamni šikari u ṭābāti* [*tuballal išatti*(?)]	12′ [So that a woman(?)] who does not experience (lit. see) her 'trouble' (i.e. period), sees her 'trouble' (i.e. period): You crush 'heals twenty'-plant, root of [...], 13′ (and) *ṣaṣumtu*-plant together, [you mix(?) (it)] with oil, beer and/or vinegar, [she shall drink it(?)].
Catchline: 14′ *šumma sinništu dāmša paris-ma dāmša lā* [*innamir*(?)]	14′ 'If a woman's blood is cut off so that her blood [is not seen(?)].'
Colophon: 15′ *tuppu* 41.KAM *šumma amēlu muḫḫašu umma ukâl bulṭū b*[*īt Dābibī*$^{?}$] 16′ *gabari Uruk* [*kīma labirīšu*] *Anu-ikṣur mār* [*Šamaš-iddina* (...)] 17′ *išṭur-ma ibri tuppi Šamaš-iddina* [... ...] 18′ *pāliḫ Anu u Ištar lā it*[*abbala*]	15′ 41st tablet of (the series) 'If a man's skull contains heat'. Remedies from the house of [Dābibī(?)].16′ A copy (of an original) from Uruk. 17′ Written 16′ [according to its original] 17′ and collated 16′ by Anu-ikṣur, son of [Šamaš-iddina, (...)]. Tablet of Šamaš-iddina, [... ...]. 18′ Anyone who reveres Anu and Ištar must not carry (the tablet) off.

Notes

Lines 6′ and 10′: At the end of lines 6′ and 10′, perhaps restore [*s*]*a*$^{!}$-*gu*$_5$-*šá ár-ḫiš* [*im-mar*$^{?}$] "[she will] quickly [see] her menses(?)", given the topic of inducing menstrual bleeding explicitly referred to in lines 12′–14′ below. Alternative restorations for a verb at the end of the line are possible, however. Thus, the word *sagû* is also used in a contrasting context, in which the aim of a treatment is to stop abnormally strong menses (KUD-*su*, *ip*(*p*)*arrasū*). There are several different spellings of the term *sagû* in Babylonian and Assyrian medical texts, which point to alternating forms beginning with *s* or *š* (*s/šagû*), which may perhaps justify the heterogeneous spellings in the present text. See e.g., BM 40152 ii 15′ (*ša-gu*$_5$-*šá*); BAM 235: 4, 7 (*šá/šu-gu-šá*); the most common spelling is *sa-gu-šá* (see e.g., BM 38624 lines 61‴–63‴; BM 54587+73802 obv. 6′, 8′, 9′, rev. 3, 9; BM 61975 obv. 5′, 7′); *sa-gu-u* (SpTU 1, No. 39: 6′, a medical commentary from Uruk, where the term is equated with *dām ardati* "a young woman's blood"). See *infra* for these texts.

Perhaps in line 6′, restore [U$_5$ ARK]AB^{mušen} = *rikibti arkabi* "*spur*(?) of a bat" as ingredient name. This item is rare in women's healthcare texts, see especially BAM 248 rev. iv 23 //, where it is used as a simple ingredient in a potion to speed up difficult labour (text D.1.1 line 215). If the purpose of the present remedy in SpTU 1, No. 59 was to induce the menstrual flow, the ingredient *rikibti arkabi* may have had expellant properties. For discussion of *rikibti arkabi*, see Zisa 2021 with previous literature and the *Introduction* of this volume.

Lines 7′ and 9′: The plants *imḫur-līm* and *imḫur-ešrā* are also prescribed in BM 47578: 10, where they are listed as drugs to be drunk in beer to induce the menstrual flow (together with *tarmuš*-plant), see *infra* text C.2.2. However, these plants are also used for other purposes and ailments in women's healthcare texts. See the *Introduction* and Böck 2023 for discussion.

Line 11′: At the beginning of the line, perhaps restore [ŠIM.^{d}]MAŠ standing for *nikiptu*-aromatic. There may have been room for [DIŠ KI.MIN] before the plant name. If so, the prescription would present an example for prescribing a simple drug.

Lines 12′–13′: In line 12′, I have opted for emending the text to [DIŠ MUNUS$^{?}$] *ša* <NÍG>.GIG-*šá* NU *im-mar* NÍG.GIG-*šá i*[*m*]-*mar* rather than emending the second half of this sentence to <<*šá*>> GIG-*šá i*[*m*]-*mar*. Both GIG and NÍG.GIG can occur as variant logograms or Sumerian correspondences of Akkadian *maruštu* "trouble, hardship", but the latter is more common (see CAD M/1, 317; GIG usually stands for *murṣu* "disease"). Apparently, the term *maruštu* euphemistically refers to the menses (see Stol 2000a, 25–26, 199; Steinert 2023 for discussion). Thus, *maruštu* (written syllabically) is attested in Tablet 36 of the *Diagnostic Handbook* (line 94, see *infra* text I.1.1) in a context that similarly points to this meaning.

Line 14′: The catchline (and incipit of Tablet 42 of the series) quoted here is also attested as the incipit of the text BM 47578, a tablet designated as the 40th extract (*nisḫu*) (see text C.2.2, lines 1–2). The end of the catchline DIŠ MUNUS MÚD-*šá* KUD-*ma* MÚD-*šá* NU IGI may be read as *dāmūša lā innamir* (N-stem of *amāru*), "so that her blood is not seen", or as *dāmāša lā immar* "she does not see her menses (blood)", in accordance to parallel passages promising that after a specific treatment the woman "will see her period" (usually *sa-gu-šá im-mar*), see e.g., BM 38624+ line 63‴ (see the edition of this text (A.2.1) in this volume for further discussion). See also Köcher 1978, 33 note 20.

Line 15′: The restoration is based on a few other colophons of medical-therapeutic texts (and on commentaries on such texts) from the Late Babylonian period stemming from Uruk, Babylon, Nippur and Sippar. These texts refer most likely to several recensions of the therapeutic series "If a man's skull contains heat" (*šumma amēlu muḫḫašu umma ukâl*), composed of and ordered in numbered tablets (*tuppu*), sections (*pirsu*) or extracts (*nisḫu*) (see Panayotov 2018, 115; Steinert 2018, 176 with n. 105; Steinert et al. 2018 for discussion). In most of these colophons the title "remedies from the house of Dābibī" is appended to the series title. The most important attestations are the following:

The Uruk text SpTU 1, No. 48 is labelled as the 45th and final tablet of this series in rev. 7′ (DUB 45(?).⌜KAM⌝.MA? DIŠ NA UGU-*šú* KÚM *ú-kal bul-*[*ṭu* É] ᵐ*Dà*(DÙ)-*bi*ₓ(DÙ)-*bi*ₓ(DÙ) ZAG.TIL.LA.⌜BI.ŠÈ⌝ [...].

SpTU 1, No. 44: 85 identifies the text as the 9-*ú pir-su* DIŠ NA UGU-*šú* KÚM *ú-kal* [*bul-ṭu* É ᵐ*Dà*(DÙ)-*bi*ₓ(DÙ)-*bi*ₓ(DÙ)?].

BAM 403 (also from Uruk) rev. 7′–8′ is designated as the 19-*ú nis-ḫu* DIŠ NA U[GU- *šú* KÚM *ú-kal*] / [*bul-ṭu*] ⌜É⌝ ᵐ*Da-bi-bi*.

The colophon of BM 35512 rev. 20′ (from Babylon) calls the text the 34 *nis-ḫu* DIŠ NA UGU-*šú* KÚM *ú-kal*, but then continues with *bul-ṭu* GABA.RI É ᵐ*Dà-bi-*[*bi*] "remedies (according to) a copy (of an original tablet) from the house of Dā[bibī]" (see Bácskay 2018a, 30 with n. 91; Bácskay 2018c, *FS Geller*, 94, 105, 115).

The colophons of commentaries on the *pirsu*-recension of this series regularly appear to omit the series title "If a man's skull contains heat" but refer (in addition to the incipit of the commented text) only to "remedies from the house of Dābibī" (which is why Frahm 2011, 230, 232 regards the latter as a series title in itself; cf. Civil 1974, *JNES* 33, 336). This variant designation is attested in the following texts:

BAM 401 (from Sippar) is identified in the colophon as a commentary on the 22nd *pirsu* of "remedies from the house of Dābibī" (rev. 33: 22 *pir-su* DIN-*ṭi* É *Da-bi-bi*), presumably omitting the series title proper (Frahm, Frazer and Jiménez 2013c (*CCP* 4.2.P)).

SpTU 1, No. 51 from Uruk is identified as a commentary on the 2nd *pirsu* of "remedies from the house of Dābibī" (*bul-ṭu* É ᵐ*Dà-bi-bi 2-ú* [*pirsu*]; Jiménez 2015 (*CCP* 4.2.G); Clancier 2009b (*GKAB*)).

11N-T4 (rev. 28) from Nippur (Civil 1974, *JNES* 33, 336–338; Frazer 2015 (CCP 4.2.B); Scurlock 2017, 310–312) is identified as a commentary on the 24th *pirsu* of "remedies from the house of Dābibī" (24 *pir-su bul-ṭu* É *Da-bi-bi*).

The commentary BM 59607 presumably from Sippar (Frazer 2017, CCP 4.2.Q) does not give a specific section (*pirsu*) to which the commentary belongs. But it likewise marks the commented material as "remedies from the house of Dābibī" (rev. 10′ *bul-ṭu* É *Da-bi-bi*).

See further Köcher 1978, 33 n. 14 on the reading ᵐDÙ-DÙ-DÙ as *Dà-bi*ₓ*-bi*ₓ); as well as Leichty 1988 (*FS Sachs*); Panayotov 2018, 115 for discussion. Some scholars render the family name attested in the Neo- and Late Babylonian period as *Dābibī/u* (lit. "my plea", see AHw 148b; Wunsch 2014a, 304).

Line 16′: There is probably room for an extended genealogy in line 16′, adding "descendent of Šangû-Ninurta" (A-*šú šá* ˡᵘ́SANGA-ᵈ*Nin-urta* or similar renderings). For the colophons of texts from the library of the conjurer Anu-ikṣur and his family, the descendants of Šangû-Ninurta, see also Clancier 2009a, 49–50, 52, 389.

Line 17′: There is room for a professional title or genealogy of Šamaš-iddina in line 17′, as found, e.g. in SpTU 3, No. 84: 99–100, SpTU 4, Nos. 127, 128 (tablets written by Šamaš-iddina): ˡᵘ́MAŠ.MAŠ (DUMU *ša* ᵐ*Na-di-nu*) DUMU ˡᵘ́SANGA-ᵈ*Nin-urta*).

Line 18′: Hunger, SpTU 1, 65 reads *i*$_{11}$-*t*[*ab-bal*], but the copy of SpTU 1, No. 59 may also suggest *i*$_{11}$(ḪI)-*t*[*a*$_8$(ŠÁR)-*áb-bà-alla*]. The latter spelling is attested for example, in SpTU 5, No. 248 upper edge 2, in another colophon by Anu-ikṣur. See also Jiménez 2016b, 234 for discussion.

C.2.2 BM 47578: An Extract with Prescriptions to Induce the Menstrual Flow

This small Late Babylonian tablet in landscape format contains recipes (potions and vaginal suppositories) for a woman "whose blood is cut off" (*dāmša paris*), apparently aiming to induce menstrual bleeding when it stops to occur (perhaps due to the onset of menopause). The text starts with the note "fortieth *nisḫu*-extract", which suggests that the contents formed part of a series or longer compilation of material. The tablet, which may originate from Babylon or Borsippa, shows signs of re-use and its almost oval, irregular shape is extremely unusual.[320] Perhaps it is a school tablet.

List of Manuscripts

Siglum	Museum Number	Copy	Collation	Format; Ductus	Provenience
a	BM 47578 (81-11-3, 283)	Pl. 31	Coll.	Single-column tablet in landscape format; Late Babylonian script; ca. 5th–3rd cent. BCE	Babylonia; exact provenience unknown

Overview

i	Rubric and purpose statement (to induce the menses) a obv. 1–2	1–2
ii	Prescriptions (to induce the menses) a obv. 3–rev. 3	3–12
iii	Rubric, scribal remark(?) a rev. 4	13

Previous Edition and Discussion

–

Electronic Babylonian Library (eBL) (https://www.ebl.lmu.de/library/BM.47578; photos)

Transliteration

1	a obv. 1	40 *nis-ḫu*
2	a obv. 2	DIŠ MUNUS MÚD-*šá* KUD-*ma*? MÚD-*šá* NU IGI
3	a obv. 3	ú*šu-mut-tu*$_4$ *ina* KAŠ NAG LAL *ina* KAŠ NAG
4	a obv. 4	úKUR.RA NU.LUḪ.ḪA SÚD *ina* KAŠ NAG
5	a obv. 5	SI DÀRA.<MAŠ> SÚD *ina* sígÀKA KU gišÙR SUMUN
6	a obv. 6	GÌR.PAD.DU AMAR!?(UDUN) GAZ SIM *ina* sígÀKA

320 The tablets of the 1881-11-03 collection come from the excavations of Hormuzd Rassam in Babylonia. Cf. Reade 1986, in: CBT VI, p. xxxii, xxxiv; Leichty, Finkel and Walker 2019, *CBT* IV–V, 656, 665. Measurements: 5.2 cm x 3.7 cm x 1 cm.

7	a obv. 7	^{na4}*u*$_5$*-ri-ia-*<*ḫu*> SÚD *ina* KAŠ NAG ^{na4}GUG$^?$
8	a obv. 8	SÚD *ina* KAŠ NAG NA$_4$.SAḪAR.KUR.RA SÚD
9	a lo. e. 1	<*ina*> ^{síg}ÀKA$^?$ x x
10	a rev. 1	^{ú}IGI-*lim*$^?$ ^{ú}IGI-20 SÚD *tar-muš* SÚD *ina* KAŠ (NAG)
11	a rev. 2	^{giš}ḪAB SÚD *ina* KAŠ NAG ^{šim}ŠEŠ SÚD *ina* KAŠ (NAG)
12	a rev. 3	^{na4}KUR-*nu* DAB *ina* MURUB$_4$-*šú* KÉŠ GÚ.GAL GI$_6$ SÚD *ina* KAŠ NAG
13	a rev. 4	*šá kib-su* KUD-*su*$^?$ ⌜*za*⌝-<<*a*>>-*mar* \ ZI-*ḫi*

Bound Transcription and Translation

^{1}40 *nisḫu* ^{2}*šumma sinništu dāmša paris-ma dāmša lā immar*	^{1}Fortieth extract. ^{2}If a woman's blood is cut off so that she does not see her menses (lit. blood):
^{3}*šumuttu ina šikari išatti ašqulāla ina šikari išatti* ^{4}*nīnâ nuḫurta tasâk ina šikari išatti* ^{5}*qaran ayyali tasâk ina itqi sīkti gušūri labiri* ^{6}*eṣemti būri*(?) *taḫaššal tanappi ina itqi* ^{7}*uriyāḫu tasâk ina šikari išatti sāmta*(?) ^{8}*tasâk ina šikari išatti gabû tasâk* ^{9}*ina*(?) *itqi* ... ^{10}*imḫur-līm imḫur-ešrā tasâk tarmuš tasâk ina šikari* (*išatti*) ^{11}*ḫûrata tasâk ina šikari išatti murra tasâk ina šikari* (*išatti*) ^{12}*šadâna ṣābitu ina qablīšu tarakkas ḫallūrī ṣalmūti tasâk ina šikari išatti*	^{3}She shall drink *šumuttu*-plant in beer. She shall drink *ašqulālu*-(plant) in beer. ^{4}You pound *nīnû*-plant (and) *nuḫurtu*-plant and she shall drink (it) in beer. ^{5}You pound stag horn, (you apply it wrapped) in a wad of wool. ^{6}You crush (and) sift ^{5}powder from an old wooden beam ^{6}(and) calf(?) bone, (you apply it wrapped) in a wad of wool. ^{7}You pound *uriyāḫu*-stone, she shall drink (it) in beer. ^{8}You pound ^{7}carnelian(?), ^{8}she shall drink (it) in beer. You pound alum, ^{9}... in a wad of wool. ^{10}You pound 'heals thousand'-plant (and) 'heals twenty'-plant, you pound *tarmuš*-plant, (she drinks it) in beer. ^{11}You pound *ḫûratu*-plant (madder), she shall drink (it) in beer. You pound *murru*-aromatic, (she drinks it) in beer. ^{12}You pound black chickpeas, she shall drink (it) in beer.
^{13}*ša kibsu parsu*(?) *zamar nasḫi*	^{13}(For one?) whose (normal) *course* (has) ceased(?). Quickly excerpted.

Notes

Line 2: A few other texts use the same or similar statements referring to inducing a woman's menses that have stopped. Ms. a uses the expression DIŠ MUNUS MÚD-*šá* KUD-*ma*$^?$ MÚD-*šá* NU IGI "If a woman's blood has stopped so that she does not see(?) her blood". The logographic writing NU IGI is clearly *lā immar*, or a form of the N-stem of *amāru* (e.g., *dāmšā innamir* "her blood is not seen"). See also SpTU 1, No. 59: 14′ (text C.2.1), where this line or tablet incipit occurs as a tablet catchline.

Lines 3–4: The scribe omitted the classifier ú in front of LAL and NU.LUḪ.ḪA.

Lines 5–7: Instances of omitted signs in these lines reflect the hasty work of the scribe. The reading SI DÀRA.<MAŠ> "stag horn" seems more likely than SI DÀRA, *qaran turāḫi* "ibex horn" (CAD T, s.v. *turāḫu* does not offer any instances for the use of the latter in medical texts).

Line 5: "Powder of an old wooden beam" (KU ^{giš}ÙR SUMUN) is also encountered as a remedy in the Late Babylonian text SpTU 4, No. 153 obv. 10, 12, 13, but there the prescription is used to stop gynaecological bleeding (see *infra* text C.1.10). Different suggestions for the Akkadian reading of the sign KU in the present context include *si/īktu, sīku* "powder" and *qēmu* "flour"; cf. Borger 2004, MZL, 425 no. 808; CAD S, 259–260 s.v. *sīktu*; CAD Q, 208 s.v. *qēmu* discussion sections. The logogram KU interchanges with KU.KU in this context (followed different types of wood, plants, or stones, metals). There is now evidence that KU.KU corresponds to *supantu* (*supandu*) "powder; shavings", see Schwemer 2021, *NABU* 2021/2, 117 no. 48. Luukko and van Buylaere 2020, CMAwR 4, 109 (index) still list both spellings KU and KU.KU under the word *sīku/sīktu*. For the writing KU, see also Abusch and Schwemer 2016, CMAwR 2, text 8.28: 14 (with note on lines 14–15). For KU.KU, see CMAwR 2, text 3.4, 1: 26; text 3.4, 3: 11; text 3.5: 26; text 8.28: 101; text 9.8: 45. A syllabic spelling (*si-ik-ti, sik-ti*) in a comparable context is found in CMAwR 3, text 3.15: 9′. For powder of a beam, see also Maul 1994, *Zukunftsbewältigung*, 375: 7′: KU.KU ^{giš}ÙR.MEŠ (in a Namburbi ritual).

Line 6: I assume a scribal mistake in this line, emending to GÌR.PAD.DU AMAR$^{!}$ "calf bone" (the sign UDUN was confused with AMAR). For the use of animal bones in medical texts, see also Stol 2016–2018, *RlA* 15, 411–413 esp. § 6. Within the women's healthcare texts, bones of animals (she-goat, sheep, birds) as ingredients are further attested in BAM 237 iv 29–33, iv 34–38 (against watery discharges), BAM 240: 71′–74′; BM 42313+: 67–68 (for promoting fertility and desire for intercourse). See *infra* for these texts.

Line 7: For the *uriyāḫu*-stone, see CAD U/W, 225–226 s.v. *urijāḫu*. In Uruanna III 139 (quoted ibid.), this stone name is equated with red *šubû*-stone (^{na4}ŠUBA SA$_5$) and explained as "stone of birth/childbearing" (*aban alādi*).

Line 8: NA$_4$.SAḪAR.KUR.RA appears to be a mistake for IM.SAḪAR.NA$_4$.KUR.RA = *gabû* "alum".

Line 9: The signs written on the lower edge are squashed and partially damaged, but apparently the instruction is not *ina* KAŠ NAG.

Line 11: The identification of *murru* with myrrh (cf. AHw 676a; CAD M/2, 221a) is uncertain or at least doubtful, see Farber 1993–1997, "Myrrhe B. Philologisch", *RlA* 8, 536–537; Jursa (2009, *FS Sima*, 163 fn. 78). For alternative propositions to identify *murru*, see Stol (1980–1983, "Leder(industrie)", *RlA* 6, 533 § 16); cf. Kinnier Wilson 2011, *JMC* 17, 4–5.

Line 12: For black *ḫallūru*-peas (GÚ.GAL GI$_6$), see also Finkel 2000, *FS Lambert*, 165 Text 12: 15. The word is complemented by an adjective with a masculine plural form, e.g. in SpTU 1, No. 63: 9 GÚ.GAL *sa-an-du-tú*; in Old Babylonian texts, it is also found with feminine plural complements (e.g. AbB 9, No. 58: 6 GÚ.GAL *sà-am-da-a-tim*).

Line 13: The expression *ša kibsu parsu*, lit. "whose course is cut off", is understood here as a euphemistic reference to the absence of the woman's menstrual period. The noun *kibsu* can also mean "behaviour, course of life" and may thus be understood here as a euphemistic term for the regular occurrence of the menses. For another occurrence of *kibsu* + *parāsu* for the ceasing of the menses (related to the post-menopausal period), see BM 47491 lines 25–26 (text A.2.6) and BM 48557 line 2′ (text A.2.10).

There seem to be traces of an erased sign in the indented line before ZI-*ḫi*. The signs *za-a-mar* ZI-*ḫi* are probably best understood to represent the phrase *zamar nasḫa* "quickly excerpted".

C.2.3 BM 54587 + 73802: Regulating the Menses and Female Fertility

The two fragments (joined by the present author) belong to a Late Babylonian tablet, which presumably stems from Sippar.[321] The text has proven very difficult to decipher, but the preserved passages appear to contain treatments for stopping the (menstrual) flow (*sagû*) (perhaps in situations in which it is excessively heavy or long-lasting) and for provoking it. One section seems to refer also to the aim of enhancing female fertility after menopause, which is remarkable given the strong interest witnessed by the prescriptions to regulate women's menstrual periods. The combination of topics in the present text therefore imply that the ancient healer drew a connection between the ceasing of menstrual periods and fertility in menopausal women. As far as can be told, most of the prescriptions apply tampons introduced into the vagina and potions. Because the word *sagû* occurs only rarely and exclusively in first millennium BCE texts, the present text adds to our understanding of the development of the medical terminology related to women's discharges. Most texts speak of "a woman's blood" (*dām sinništi*) in very ambiguous terms, while the term *sagû* may indicate a growing specialisation in the terminology.

321 Reade 1986, in: CBT VI, xxxii–xxxiii.

List of Manuscripts

Siglum	Museum Number	Copy	Collation	Format; Ductus	Provenience
a	BM 54587 (82-5-22, 907) + BM 73802 (82-9-18, 13813)	Pl. 32	Coll.	Fragments of a single-column tablet; Late Babylonian script, ca. 5th–3rd cent. BCE(?)[322]	Sippar(?)

Overview

i′	Fragmentary prescription a obv.$^{?}$ 1′	...]–1′
ii′	Fragmentary prescription a obv.$^{?}$ 2′–3′	2′–3′
iii′	Prescription (tampon) to stop the menstrual flow (*sagû*) a obv.$^{?}$ 4′–6′	4′–6′
iv′	Prescription (tampon) to stop(?) the menstrual flow (*sagû*) and for fertility after menopause(?) a obv.$^{?}$ 7′–12′	7′–12′
v′	Prescription (potion) to stop(?) the menstrual flow (*sagû*) a rev.$^{?}$ 1–3	13′–15′
vi′	Prescription (potion) to stop(?) the menstrual flow (*sagû*) a rev.$^{?}$ 4–8	16′–20′
vii′	Prescription (tampon) to induce menstrual bleeding (*sagû*) a rev.$^{?}$ 9–13	21′–25′[...

Previous Edition and Discussion

–

Electronic Babylonian Library (https://www.ebl.lmu.de/library/BM.54587)

Transliteration

Beginning of ms. a obv.(?) lost

1′ a obv.$^{?}$ 1′ [.......... ^{šim}G]AM.M[A ... .]

2′ a obv.$^{?}$ 2′ [DIŠ KI.MIN$^{?}$ ...]x-*mu* NU ÍL MUNUS B[I ....]

3′ a obv.$^{?}$ 3′ [.............]x-*šú šum-ma šá* 15-*šú a-na* x[..........]

4′ a obv.$^{?}$ 4′ [DIŠ KI.MIN$^{?}$ ...] ⸢$^{\text{šim?}}$*ka*$^{?}$-*man*$^{?}$-*ti*$^{?}$⸣ PÈŠ$^{?}$ ⸢A⸣ G[AZI^{sar}] ⸢^{šim}⸣ŠEŠ ⸢^{rú}⸣[x x]

5′ a obv.$^{?}$ 5′ [... *lu* ^{síg}À]KA$^{?}$ *lu al-*⸢*la-na*$^{?}$⸣ x x-*nu* ⸢*ina*$^{?}$⸣ *i-mi-*⸢*it*$^{?}$⸣-*t*[*i*$^{?}$-*šú*$^{?}$]

6′ a obv.$^{?}$ 6′ [...... *ina*] ^{síg}ÀKA *ana* ŠÀ.TÙR-*šú* GAR-*ma* ⸢*sa*⸣-*gu-šú* KUD-*s*[*u*$^{?}$]

7′ a obv.$^{?}$ 7′ [......] ⸢*ina*⸣ ⸢A⸣ ⸢LUḪ⸣-*ma ina* ^{síg}⸢ÀKA⸣ ⸢NIGIN-*mi*⸣ *ana*$^{?}$ ŠÀ.SUR-*šá* GAR-*a*[*n*-(*ma*)]

8′ a obv.$^{?}$ 8′ [............]x x ⸢*sa*⸣-⸢*gu*⸣-⸢*šú*$^{?}$⸣ ⸢DIRI$^{?}$⸣.MEŠ-*šú* TI-*q*[*é*$^{?}$ x x]

---

322 Measurements: ca. 7 x 5 x 2 cm.

9′	a obv.$^{?}$ 9′	[.............]-*ma sa-gu-šú* [KUD-*su*$^{?}$]
10′	a obv.$^{?}$ 10′	[..................]-x-*ma i-šal-*[*lim*]
11′	a obv.$^{?}$ 11′	[..................] *ana* ⸢AK$^{?}$⸣ MUD AL.[KUD $SIG_5$$^{?}$]
12′	a obv.$^{?}$ 12′	[..................]x-*e te-ep-pu-šu*$^{?!}$ x[x x x]

(Bottom of the obv.)

13′	a rev.$^{?}$ 1	[DIŠ KI.MIN$^{?}$ ...... ^{ú}]⸢A.ZAL.LÁ$^{?}$⸣ *ina* 3 SÌLA A.MEŠ [x x (x)]
14′	a rev.$^{?}$ 2	[...........................]x ⸢*ana*⸣ ⸢ŠÀ⸣ ⸢ŠUB⸣-*d*[*i*$^{?}$ x x x]
15′	a rev.$^{?}$ 3	[... MUNUS BI U_4.1.KAM$^{?}$ *ú-b*]*ar-re-e-ma* NAG-*ma s*[*a-gu-šú* KUD-*su*$^{?}$ (x)]
16′	a rev.$^{?}$ 4	[..................]-⸢*ú*⸣ 1/2 GÍN KUŠ AM.S[I.ḪA.RA.NA$^{?}$]
17′	a rev.$^{?}$ 5	[.......] ⸢giš$^{?}$⸣ [*ta*]-⸢*šá*$^{?}$⸣-*ḫal ú-bar-re-e-ma* ⸢NAG⸣ x x x
18′	a rev.$^{?}$ 6	[....................] ⸢Ú⸣ [x] *it-ti* x-x [x]
19′	a rev.$^{?}$ 7	[...............]x *šu-tu-qu* 1/2 NINDA A.MEŠ *šú-nu-tu*
20′	a rev.$^{?}$ 8	[.......]x MUNUS BI U_4.1.KAM *ú-bar-re-e-ma* NAG
21′	a rev.$^{?}$ 9	[MUNUS *sa-gu-šá ana*] *kul-lu-mu* 3 ⸢MUN$^{?}$⸣-*tú* ⸢^{šim}MAN.DU⸣ *tur-á*[*r*$^{?}$]
22′	a rev.$^{?}$ 10	[x x x x x] *ina* ^{síg}ÀKA ⸢NIGIN$^{?}$⸣ 1-*en* TA.ÀM *ana* Š[À.TÙR-*šú* GAR-*an*]
23′	a rev.$^{?}$ 11	[x x x x x x 1.T]A.ÀM EGIR *a-ḫa-meš* [x x x x]
24′	a rev.$^{?}$ 12	[x x x x x x x] MUNUS BI ⸢*it-ta-na-šu*$^{?}$⸣ [x x x x]
25′	a rev.$^{?}$ 13	[..............] x x [..................]

Ms. a rev.(?) breaks; remainder lost

Bound Transcription and Translation

Beginning of ms. a obv.(?) lost

1′ [... ... *ṣum*]*lalû* [... ...]	1′ [... ... *ṣum*]*lalû*-plant [... ...].
2′ [DIŠ KI.MIN(?) ...]... *lā inašši*(?) *sinništu š*[*ī* ... ...] 3′ [... ...]... *šumma ša imittīšu*(?) *ana* ...[... ...]	2′ [Alternatively(?), ...] ... she cannot lift(?) [...], that woman [... ...] 3′ [... ...] ... If with(?) her right hand/side(?) towards [... ...].
4′ [DIŠ KI.MIN(?) ...] *kamanti tittu*(?) *mê* [*kasî*(?)] *murru* [...] 5′ [... *lū it*]*qa*(?) *lū allāna*(?) ... *ina imittī*[*šu*(?)] 6′ [... ... *ina*] *itqi ana šassūrīša tašakkan-ma sagûšu iparrasū*	4′ [Alternatively (?), ...] *kamantu*-plant, fig(?), [*kasû*]-juice(?), *murru*-plant, [...]-plant, 5′ [... (you make?) a w]ad(?) or an acorn-shaped suppository, ... On [(her?)] right hand(?) 6′ [... ...]. You insert (it) into her womb (viz. vagina) [in] a wad of wool. Then her *menses* will stop.

7′ [... ...] *ina mê temessī-ma ina itqi talammi ana šassūrīša tašakka*[*n-*(*ma*)] 8′ [... ...]... *sagûšu*(?) *atrūšu*(?) *ileqqe*(?) [...] 9′ [...]-*ma sagûšu* [*iparrasū*(?)] 10′ [... ...]-*ma išal*[*lim*] 11′ [... ...] *ana epēš* (*sinništi ša*) *alāda par*[*sat damiq*(?)] 12′ [... ...]... *tep-pušu* ...[...]

7′ [... ...] you wash with water. You wrap it into a wad of wool, insert it into her womb (viz. vagina). 8′ [... ...]... She takes(?) (it when) her menses are excessively (heavy?) [...]. 9′ [... ...] Then her menses [will stop(?).] 10′ [... ...] Then she will be all right. 11′ [... ... *it is good*?] for treating(?) (a woman for whom?) childbearing has [stopped]. 12′ [... ...]... (when) you perform (the treatment?), [...].

13′ [DIŠ KI.MIN? ... ...] *azallâ*(?) *ina šalāšat qa mê* [...] 14′ [... ....]... *ana libbi tanaddi* [...] 15′ [... *sinništu šī ištēn ūmu u-b*]*arrē-ma išattī-ma s*[*agûšu iparrasū*(?)]

13′ [Alternatively(?), you ... ...] (and) *azallû*-plant in three litres of water. 14′ [... ...]... you pour into it [...]. 15′ [... For one day the woman(?)] shall fast. Then she shall drink (it), and [her] men[ses *will stop*(?)].

16′ [... ...]... *mišil šiqil mašak piz*[*allurti*(?)] 17′ [... ...]... [*ta*]-*šaḫḫal*(?) *ubarrē-ma išatti* ... 18′ [... ...] ... ... 19′ [... ...]... *šūtuqu mišil akal*(?) *mû šunūtu* 20′ [... ...]... *sinništu šī ūmakkal ubar-rē-ma išatti*

16′ [... ...]... half a shekel of the skin of *piz*[*allurtu*-gecko?], 17′ [... ... you] crush(?). She shall fast (for some time) and then drink (it) ... . 18′ [... ...] ... ... 19′ [... ...]... (to) make (it) pass by(?), 20′ [you ...] 19′ half a tenth of a litre of this fluid, 20′ [... ...]... . That woman shall fast for one day and then drink (it).

21′ [*sinništu sagûša ana*] *kullumu šalāš ṭābtu*(?) *suādu tur-rar* 22′ [... ...] *ina itqi talammi ištēnâ*(?) *ana š*[*assūrīšu tašak-kan*] 23′ [... ... *iš*]*tēnâ arka aḫāmeš* [... ...] 24′ [... ...] *sinništu šī ittanaššu* [... ...] 25′ [... ...] ... [... ...]

21′ [For] making [a woman's menses] appear: you char three (shekels of?) salt(?) (and) *suādu*-plant, 22′ [... ...] you wrap (this) into wad(s) of wool. [You insert (them)] one by one(?) into [her womb (viz. vagina)]. 23′ [... *you administer them to her* (first) one] by one(?), afterwards together [...]. 24′ [... ...] That woman keeps wearing (it?) [... ...] 25′ *too fragmentary for translation*

Notes

Lines 2′–3′: The reading of the traces in these two lines is very tentative. The signs NU ÍL in line 2′, may be read *lā inašši* "she cannot lift/raise (a body part)", a usage of *našû* often found in medical texts. Alternatively, NU ÍL may stand for a stative form used in the sense of "it (a body part, most often the belly) is raised/tense/swollen" (see CAD N/2, 85–86 s.v. *našû* A sub 1d).

The sequence *šum-ma šá* 15-*šú a-na* [...] in line 3′ could be interpreted in different ways. The reading *ša imittīšu* "that on/from her (i.e. the patient's) right side" may be suggested in light of the possible occurrence of the word *imittu* in the next section. But a reading NINDA 15-*šú* is not excluded, i.e. "if (you/she ...) bread fifteen times onto [...]".

Lines 4′–6′: For *murru*-plant used against bleeding (in a suppository), see also K. 8893 obv.(?) 5′, 7′ (text C.1.6). The reading of the traces at the beginning of line 4′ as ^{šim}*ka-man-ti* is not certain; usually, *kamantu* is written with the classifier ú rather than šim. Note Labat 1960, *RA* 54, 175 rev. 4 *ka-man-tim* (in a Neo-Babylonian list of medical substances).

Line 6′: The expression *sagûša iparrasū*(KUD-*su*) "her menses will stop" in line 6′ replaces the more usual "her blood (*dām*(*ū*)*ša*) will stop" found in prescriptions countering an abnormal flow of blood. The present remedy may have been intended to treat an abnormally heavy or extended menstrual period. For discussion of the term *sagû* "flow of blood; menses", see the *Introduction*. The spelling of the verb KUD-*su* indicates that *sagû* is a plural noun, similar to *dāmu* "blood", which is used in the singular or plural.

Lines 7′–12′: For line 7′, compare perhaps the ritual instruction against *naḫšātu* (irregular bleeding in BAM 237 obv. i 9′, where a potsherd from a crossroads is washed, anointed and wrapped in wool, and then deposited in a secluded place (text C.1.4). Crushed potsherds were also used for tampons inserted into the vagina to stop bleeding, see e.g., SpTU 4, No. 153: 14 (text C.1.10); or tied to the woman's body as an amulet (e.g. BAM 237 obv. ii 41′–42′, 43′–44′; rev. iv 23, text C.1.4).

For the reading *šagûšu atrūšu* "her menses are excessively (heavy)" proposed in line 8′, compare BM 45736: 13′ (text A.2.5): [... *e-nu*]-*ma*? MUNUS MÚD.ME-*šú at-ru-ma nak-da-a*[*t*] "[... (a remedy?) *wh*]*en* a woman's blood is excessive in quantity so that she is in a critical condition". The verb (*w)atāru* "to exceed; to surpass" is otherwise unattested in medical texts, although it occurs in omen texts (including physiognomy), cf. CAD A/2, 487–489 sub mng. 1; AHw 1489–1490.

In line 9′, other restorations of a verb at the end of the line are possible. Instead of *sagûšu iparrasū* "her menses will stop", alternative restorations such as "she will see her menses" (*im-mar*) or "they will be normal" (SI.SÁ, *išārū*) are likewise thinkable. However, it seems more likely that the present passage concludes the treatment for stopping too excessive menstrual bleeding in lines 7′–8′ by giving a positive prognosis. The following lines 10′–12′ appear to list further uses to which the remedy could be applied.

For the tentative reading *ana* AK MUD AL.[KUD SIG$_5$] in line 11′, perhaps to be interpreted as *ana epēš (sinništi ša) alāda parsat damiq*(?) "it is good for treating (a woman for whom) childbearing has stopped", referring to treatments for women who had reached menopause but desired to bear another child (for the expression, see CAD P, 167 s.v. *parāsu* sub 1b; for the lexical equation mud = *alādu* "to engender, create, give birth", see e.g. CT 11, 29–32 obv. i 51). There is also a synonymous word *parištu* "post-menopausal woman" derived from the verb *parāsu*, but the few attestations of this term usually use the logographic spelling MUNUS KUD(-*tu*$_4$), for *sinništu parištu* "post-menopausal woman" (CAD P, 187 s.v. *parištu*; e.g., BAM 237 obv. i 22′). The expression *sinništu ša alāda parsat* "(a woman) who has stopped to bear (children)" occurs in a few other medical texts. The condition is treated e.g., in BAM 241 iii 3 (written MUNUS *a-la-da* KUD-*sà*-[*at*], see *infra* text II.1.3). In the instruction for an amulet charm in AMT 20/1 obv! i 30–31 (// "Jastrow tablet" (Scurlock 2003, *JMC* 2, 17) rev. 10), the phrase MUNUS *šá* MUD AL.KUD occurs in a similar context as *sinništu parištu* in BAM 237 i 22′, where a post-menopausal woman has to spin or twine threads used for the charm (Schuster-Brandis 2008, 135 fn. 352; with Reiner 1982, *ZA* 72, 129). Thus, it seems that in ms. a line 11′ the expression MUNUS *šá* MUD AL.KUD was written in an abbreviated fashion.

Lines 13′–15′: The interpretation of this remedy as another treatment for stopping the menses (e.g., when they are abnormally strong) comes from a related use of the unidentified *azallû*-plant to treat *naḫšātu*-discharge (bleeding during pregnancy) in BAM 237 rev. iv 1 (text C.1.4, where it is given in a potion with beer).

Line 15′ has been restored following ms. a line 20′ below, which likewise recommends that the patient should fast for one day before taking the medicine. This recommendation is apparently a variation of the practice often encountered in Mesopotamian medical prescriptions, namely that a remedy should be taken (in the morning) on an empty stomach (*lā / balu patān*), see the next note.

Lines 16′–20′: The reading KUŠ AM.SI.ḪA.RA.NA = *mašak piz/ṣallurti* "skin of a *pizallurtu*-gecko(?)" in line 16′ is provisional. The term *mašku* "skin" almost exclusively refers to animal hides, although it can exceptionally denote the rind of the pomegranate which resembles leather (see CAD M/1, 379 s.v. *mašku* sub 4; Stol 1980–1983, *RlA* 6, 532–533 § 14). The word *pizallurtu* can refer to a plant, in which case it is usually written úAM.SI.ḪA.RA.NA (lit. "elephant of the road-plant"). The plant is normally differentiated from the animal *pizallurtu* "gecko", for which the logogram MUŠ.DÍM.GURUN.NA is used, see CAD P, 451–452 lex. sect. and sub 2. Otherwise, the logogram AM.SI.ḪAR.RA.AN (= *ibilu*) denotes the Bactrian camel (with two humps). Within the women's healthcare texts, gecko (*pizallurtu*) as an animal ingredient is also attested in treatments for female fertility (STT 98: 21′) and to stop bleeding (*naḫšātu*, BAM 237 rev. iv 6–7). See *infra* for further comments.

I interpret the verb *ú-bar-re-e-ma* in lines 15′, 17′ and 20′, as a D-stem form of *barû* B (also *berû*), "to become/go hungry; to starve" (AHw 123a; CAD B, 119–120 s.v. *barû* B sub 2). For another attestation of *burrû* "to fast" in the medical compendium BM 78963 (ca. 6th/5th cent. BCE), see Stadhouders and Johnson 2018, *FS* Geller, 561, 580 § 15c (line 64: *ú-bar-re-e-ma* NAG "he should fast (for some time) and then drink it"), 582–583 § 18 line 78 (*ša lā burrê išatti* "he should drink (the potion) without fasting"), 603–604 (where the voluntary aspect of the D-stem (i.e. "to observe a period of fasting") is noted). In the present text, one day of fasting before taking medical potions is specified.

The form *šūtuqu* in line 19′ could be an infinitive or a stative plural of the Š-stem of *etēqu* "to pass by". There is an occurrence of *etēqu* within the women's healthcare texts, which may be related to the present passage in ms. a. Thus, AO 6473 rev. 12 speaks about the woman's menstrual bandage(s) (*kannu*) having passed her by (*ītiqšu*), referring to the last menses before her pregnancy or to the moment that a woman missed her period and noticed that she was pregnant (see text C.3.9 for discussion). Following this parallel, one could restore [*ana ka*$_4$-*ni*]-*šu šu-tu-qu* "(to) let/cause her menstrual bandage(s) (to) pass by", in line 19′. However, there are other meanings of the Š-stem of *etēqu* which would suit the present passage. For example, *šūtuqu* occurs in the meanings "to make (misfortune, evil portents) pass by; to avert", but also "to exceed, surpass" or "to cause delay" (CAD E, s.v. *etēqu* A sub 4, 5d and 6). Cf. also KAR 223 and dupl. rev. 6 (text D.3.1).

Lines 21′–25′: The same introductory statement as in line 21′ "to make a woman's menses (*sagû*) appear" (MUNUS *sa-gu-šá ana kul-lu-mu*) is also attested in BM 38624+ line 61‴ (text A.2.1) and in BM 61975 obv. 5′ (text C.2.3). The prescription in BM 38624 (line 63‴) concludes with *sa-gu-šá im-mar* "she will have (see) her menses". For discussion of the term *sagû* see also the notes on lines 4′–6′ and lines 7′–12′ above. The verb *kullumu* has the basic meanings "to show, to disclose" (e.g. ominous signs); "to reveal (something hidden)"; "to manifest (a certain behaviour or characteristic)" (CAD K, 519–525 mng. 1 and 3, 5). In the present context, the expression *sagûša ana kullumu* refers to provoking or releasing a flow of blood locked in the body (uterus), hence the translation "to make (the menses) appear". Elsewhere in medical texts, the verb *kullumu* occurs in the diagnostic passages describing bloody urine or similar body substances, see e.g. BAM 112: 3′: [KÀ]Š.MEŠ-*šú* MÚD *ú-kal-lam* "his urine shows blood" (Geller 2005a, No. 4); BAM 75: 6: MÚD GI_6 *ukallam* "(vomited-up material) shows dark blood" (*adamatu*).

The sequence 3 ⸢MUN?⸣-*tú* in line 21′ is difficult to explain, if read correctly. One would expect a measurement after the numeral (e.g. shekel), but perhaps it was omitted by mistake. Cf. CAD Ṭ, s.v. *ṭābtu* A for references to salt in medical texts.

In line 24′, the verbal form *ittanaššu* (as a Gtn-stem of *našû*) is somewhat irregular, as the expected form would have been *ittanašši* "she keeps wearing/applying (it)". For the verb *našû* "to carry, wear" in connection with the application of tampons and suppositories, see e.g., BAM 240: 44′–45′ (text D.2.1); UET 7, No. 123 obv. 8 and rev. 11 (text B.2.2): ÍL-*ši-(ma)* "she wears (it)".

C.2.4 BM 61975: An Extract from a Collection of Remedies

This fragment written in a Neo- or Late Babylonian script may have belonged to a single-column tablet with a collection of remedies against different diseases or to a large two-column collective tablet similar in format to tablets belonging to serialized medical compendia known from Ashurbanipal's library in Nineveh.

The contents of the fragment are somewhat unusual and puzzling. The remnants of nine lines on the obverse appear to be concerned with remedies for women's diseases and health problems. One of the remedies concerns provoking the menstrual flow (*sagû ana kullumu*). Other remedies for this purpose (but no duplicating passages) are attested also in a few other Babylonian tablets on women's health issues from the first millennium BCE (see especially BM 54587 + 73802 (text C.2.3), BM 38624+ (text A.2.1) and SpTU 1, No. 59 (text C.2.1)).

The reverse preserves three fragmentary prescriptions, which, however, seem to point to quite a different topic that is treated here, namely skin diseases of the head. Remarkably, these prescriptions are followed by a catchline (rev. 6′ = line 15″) citing the beginning of a treatment for the case that DIŠ NA *ku-ra-ru* GIG "If a man suffers from *kurāru*-disease". The quotation runs parallel to a remedy known from Assur medical texts that are related to the series CRANIUM (on the diseases of the head). Thus, the *kurāru*-disease is listed as a topic dealt with in the series CRANIUM in the Assur Medical Catalogue (see Steinert et al. 2018, 209 lines 1–7, mentioned there in line 6), and remedies for this condition are also attested on tablets from Nineveh that may represent witnesses to the series CRANIUM (see Bácskay and Simkó 2017, *JMC* 30, on BAM 494 rev. iii).

After the catchline and another blank line, the remainder of the reverse (line 16″) continues with what looks like the beginning of a colophon, but unfortunately the text breaks off here. It remains uncertain whether the present tablet may have belonged to a serialised medical compendium, in which sections on women's diseases preceded sections concerned with skin ailments (of the head). This ordering of topics would differ from the order of medical treatises in the Assur Medical Catalogue (AMC), our main source for a serialized compendium of therapeutic texts in the first half of the first millennium BCE (dating to the 8th/7th cent. BCE), where the sections dealing with skin diseases (CRANIUM and SKIN) precede sections concerned with women's health, the latter of which form almost the final sections within the whole compendium or medical corpus (cf. Steinert et al. 2018). Therefore, the combination of heterogeneous contents in ms. a could point to a *Sammeltafel* or to an extract of prescriptions for various diseases; but the possibility that BM 61975 presents a witness of a serialized medical compendium of therapeutic texts from Babylonia diverging from the evidence known from the Neo-Assyrian period is not excluded either.

List of Manuscripts

Siglum	Museum Number	Copy	Collation	Format; Ductus	Provenience
a	BM 61975 (AH 82-9-18, 1944)	Pl. 36	Coll.	Fragment of a single- or two-column tablet; Neo- or Late Babylonian script; ca. 6th/5th cent. BCE(?)	Sippar(?)[323]

Overview

i′	Prescriptions for women's health (to induce the menstrual flow) a obv. 1′–9′	...]1′–9′[...
ii′	Prescription (for a disease of the head?) a rev. 1′–2′	...]10″–11″
iii′	Prescription (for a disease of the head?) a rev. 3′–4′	12″–13″
iv′	Prescription (for a disease of the head?) a rev. 5′	14″
v′	Catchline(?) a rev. 6′	15″
vi″	Colophon(?) a rev. 7′	16″–[...

Previous Edition and Discussion

–

Electronic Babylonian Library (https://www.ebl.lmu.de/library/BM.61975)

Transliteration

Beginning of ms. a obv. lost

1′ a obv. 1′ ⌜x⌝ x x [...]

2′ a obv. 2′ ⌜1/2 GÍN?⌝ [x x] ⌜x⌝ 1/2 ⌜GÍN⌝ ⌜^{šim}⌝GIG [..............................]

3′ a obv. 3′ 1/2 ⌜GÍN⌝ KA x[x x x] GÍN EME-UR.GI$_7$ PAB 10[+x Ú.ḪI.A? ...]

4′ a obv. 4′ GAZ ⌜SIM⌝ MUNUS *šá* [x x G]IG *ina* KAŠ *lu-ú* [*ina* ... NAG? (...)]

5′ a obv. 5′ MUNUS ⌜*sa-gu*⌝-[*šá*] *ana kul-lu-mu ina* 2-*ta* ŠU.MIN x[.......]

6′ a obv. 6′ [x x x x]-*na-ṭu* Ú.ḪI.A ŠEŠ.MEŠ [..................................]

7′ a obv. 7′ [x x *sa-gu-šá*] *im-mar áš-šá* NAG-*ú* ^{ú}x[............................]

8′ a obv. 8′ [x x x x *mi-šil* ^{n}]$^{\text{a4}}$*ga-bu-ú mi-šil* ^{n}[$^{\text{a4?}}$................................]

9′ a obv. 9′ [x x x x x ^{ú}IGI]-20? *ba-áš-lu* [..]

Ms. a obv. breaks; gap of unknown length

323 See Reade 1986, *CBT* VI, xxxiii.

10″ a rev. 1′ DIŠ? [..]

11″ a rev. 2′ SAG.DU-*su* LUḪ-*si* ⸢x⸣ [................]

12″ a rev. 3′ DIŠ KI.MIN Ú BABBAR SÚD *ak-tam* SÚD ⸢x⸣ [.........]

13″ a rev. 4′ *ina* LÀL KUR-*i* [......]

14″ a rev. 5′ DIŠ ⸢KI.MIN⸣ ŠE$_{10}$? BURU$_5$.ḪABRUD.DA^{mušen} GAZ SIM G[I? ....]

15″ a rev. 6′ DIŠ NA ⸢*ku*⸣-*ra-ru* GIG Ì.NUN.NA E[Š? ....]

One line left blank

16″ a rev. 7′ D[UB?] ⸢x.KAM?⸣ [x x] x x [.........................]

Ms. a rev. breaks; remainder lost

Bound Transcription and Translation

Beginning of ms. a obv. lost

1′ ...[... ...] 2′ *zūz* (*šiqil*) *kanaktu* [... ...] 3′ *zūz* (*šiqil*) ...[... *zūz*(?)] (*šiqil*) *lišān kalbi napḫar* 10[+x *šammī* ...] 4′ *taḫaššal tanappi sinništu ša* [... *marṣ*]*at ina šikari lū* [*ina* ... *išatti*(?)] 5′ *sinništu sagû*[*ša*] *ana kullumu ina šitta qātī* ...[...] 6′ [... ...]... *šammī annûti* [... ...] 7′ [... *sagûša*] *immar ašša ištatû* ...[... ...] 8′ ... ... *mišil*] *gabû mišil* ...[... ...] 9′[... ... *imḫūr*]-*ešrā*(?) *bašlu* [... ...]

1′ ... [... ...] 2′ half a shekel of *kanaktu-aromatic*, [... ...] 3′ half a shekel of [..., half] a shekel dog's tongue-plant – a total of ten [+x drugs ...] 4′ you crush (and) sift. A woman who [suf]fers from [... drinks(?) (it)] in beer or [in ...]. 5′ In order to make a woman'[s] menses appear: in two handfuls (of?) ...[...] 6′ [... ...]... these drugs [... ...] 7′ [...] she will see [her menses]. As soon as she has drunk (the potion), [... ...] 8′ [... ... half (a shekel?)] alum, half [... ...] 9′ [... ...] boiled ['heals] twenty'-plant [... ...]

Ms. a obv. breaks; gap of unknown length

10″ DIŠ [... ... ...] 11″ *qaqqassu temessi* ...[... ...]

10″ If(?) [... ...] 11″ you wash his(?) head ...[... ...].

12″ DIŠ KI.MIN *šamma peṣâ tasâk aktam tasâk* [... ...] 13″ *ina dišip šadî* [... ...]

12″ Alternatively, you crush 'white drug', you crush *ak-tam*-plant, [... ...] 13″ with 'mountain honey' [... ...].

14″ DIŠ KI.MIN *zê*? *iṣṣūr ḫurri taḫaššal tanappi* ...[... ...]

14″ Alternatively, you pound (and) sift 'partridge excrement(?)' ...[... ...].

15″ *šumma amēlu kurāru maruṣ ḫimēṭa tapa*[*ššaš*(?) ... ...]

15″ (Catchline:) If a man suffers from *kurāru*-disease, you an[oint(?) (him)] with ghee, [... ...].

One line blank(?)

16″ *tu*[*ppu*?] x.KAM ...[... ...]

16″ [...]x-th tablet(?) (of) [... ...]

Ms. a rev. breaks; remainder lost

Notes

Lines 1′–9′: This section with several prescriptions mentions two different female health problems. The first condition remains unclear due to a textual gap. In lines 5′–7′, we find a prescription "for making a woman's menses appear" (*sinništu sagûša ana kullumu*) so that "she will see her menses" (*sagûša immar*). This very same problem is also treated in a few other Late Babylonian texts, see especially BM 54587 + 73802: 21′–25′ (text C.2.3); BM 38624+ lines 61‴–63‴ (text A.2.1); cf. also SpTU 1, No. 59: 12′–14′ (text C.2.1). For further discussion, see the *Introduction*.

The phrase *ina* 2-*ta* ŠU.MIN (*šitta qātī*) in line 5′ may stand for equal parts of a whole (i.e. "two parts") or for the fraction "two thirds", see CAD Q, 194–195 s.v. *qātu* sub 11; Michel 1992, 97; Streck 1995, 62 § 52. Perhaps the text referred to two parts or portions into which the medication in the following prescription needed to be divided (cf. Johnson and Simkó 2024, 252 (STOMACH 5) BAM 579 iv 40 for the similar expression *ana* 1-*et qa-ti*, translated there as "for each portion"). However, another interpretation of the expression is possible, namely as a quantity or measurement meaning "two handfuls of", cf. Herréro 1984, 49 (quoting AMT 55/4: 7, written 2 ŠU); note further Finkel 2000, 155 Text 5 (BAM 391) line 18: ŠU.MIN *ka-mu-nu* "two handfuls of cumin" (without numeral though); see also Chalendar 2020, 62–63, 65–66 for discussion.

The conjunction *ašša* "because of; as soon as" (written *áš-šá*) encountered in line 7′ occurs often in Neo- and Late Babylonian texts with a following verbal form in the perfect, cf. CAD A/2, 460; AHw 83b; Dietrich 1969, 72, 86.

Lines 10″–11″: Washing the patient's head with prepared concoctions is often recommended in therapies for skin diseases on the head, see e.g., BAM 494 ii 64, ii 68, ii 73 (Bácskay and Simkó 2017, *JMC* 30, 15, treatments of *ašû*-disease); BAM 480 iii 24 (Scurlock 2014a, 314; Bácskay 2018, 56, for fever of the head).

Lines 12″–13″: 'White drug' (*šammu peṣû*) and *aktam*-plant are prescribed side by side in BAM 494 rev. iii 5 against *guraš-tu*-disease (a skin condition similar to *kurāru*, see Bácskay and Simkó 2017, 16; Scurlock and Andersen 2005, 234). Likewise, "mountain honey" (*dišip šadî*; "wild honey") is used in the preparation of ointments against such conditions (*ašû*, *guraštu*), see e.g. BAM 494 obv. ii 71 (Bácskay and Simkó 2017, 15): "you mix (*kibrītu*-sulphur) with 'mountain honey', you rub (him) repeatedly (with it)" (*ina* LÀL KUR-*i* ḪI.ḪI EŠ.[MEŠ?]). See also BAM 494 rev. iii 4, rev. iii 8; BAM 480 i 47′ (Scurlock 2014a, 309).

Line 14″: A drug "excrement of *ḫurru*-bird (partridge?)" (*zê iṣṣūr ḫurri*) is only rarely attested in the women's healthcare texts (see SpTU 4, No. 153 obv. 22, 25 (text D.1.11) to promote delivery).

Line 15″: This entry is attested in AO 11447 obv. 42 // BAM 3 i 48, two excerpt tablets from Assur with material related to the therapeutic treatise CRANIUM concerned with diseases of the head and skin ailments on the head (Böck 2003, *AuOr* 21, 175 Text No. 19; Geller 2007, *JMC* 10, 5 and 10). The catchline quoted in BM 61975 line 15″ may present a slight variant of the remedy preserved in BAM 3 i 48 //. It is noteworthy that the entry is not known as a tablet incipit (of a serialised compendium) so far. The term *kurāru* refers to a skin lesion ("carbuncle; pustule") on the head or other areas of the body. For treatments against *kurāru*-disease, see e.g. Bácskay and Simkó 2017, *JMC* 30, BAM 494 iii 20′–iv 6 and dupl.; Böck 2003, *AuOr* 21, 168–180; Wasserman 1996–1997, *RA* 90–91, 1–5, 31–32. For discussion of the condition, see also Fincke 2011, 181–184 (on the related term *kuraštu*, *gura/ištu*).

Line 16″: Because the scribe seems to have left one line blank between lines 15″ and 16″, the latter line looks like the beginning of a colophon, which, if the remnants of the signs are read correctly, began with a reference to the title of the composition or compendium to which BM 61975 belonged as well as to the numbered position of the tablet within a series (i.e., whether it formed the first, second, third etc. tablet of a given compendium or series).

C.3 Texts Concerned with Protecting Pregnant Women from Miscarriage

The texts edited in this section share a common concern with protecting pregnant women and their foetuses. The sources stem from the Neo-Assyrian and the Late Babylonian period. The tablets and fragments from Nineveh, Assur and Sultantepe (texts C.3.1–C.3.2, C.3.5–C.3.7) provide textual evidence for the existence of collections of rituals and treatments in the Neo-Assyrian period, while the more extensive sources from Babylonia (especially from Uruk, Babylon, Sippar), for some of which duplicating Neo-Assyrian passages are extant, attest to the continuity of a long-standing shared tradition of texts and healing practices (texts C.3.3–C.3.4, C.3.8–C.3.10). Moreover, parallels between passages in some of the texts treated here with tablet incipits of serialized medical-therapeutic treatises listed in the Assur Medical Catalogue allow us to attribute the treatments dealt with here more concretely and specifically in a thematic compendial context (cf. Steinert et al. 2018, 217–218, 269–272 especially in the treatise PREGNANCY/OFFSPRING in lines 109–114).

From the incipits and topics outlined for the treatise PREGNANCY/OFFSPRING quoted in AMC 109–114 we learn that the treatise dealt not only with preventing miscarriage and protecting unborn children, but also with cases of repeated infant death in a family. These topics are also simultaneously reflected in some of the sources edited here (e.g., SpTU 3, No. 84 text C.3.4), and there are several attestations of verbatim parallels between lines in AMC 109–114 and the texts in the present section (e.g., texts C.3.3–C.3.5). Both the incipits of the section PREGNANCY/OFFSPRING and the textual sources emphasize witchcraft as the primary cause of miscarriage and infant death. Because of the associations with the anti-witchcraft texts, seven of the texts assembled in section C.3 have recently been edited by Abusch, Schwemer, Luukko and van Buylaere (Abusch et al. 2020, CMAwR 3, texts 5.1–5.5, 5.8–5.9) but often limited to certain text passages. In the present publication all the relevant first millennium BCE texts known to date are edited in toto, complemented by a few new fragments. Beside witchcraft, some of the texts in section C.3 associate miscarriage and infant death with other agents and causes, including the "Hand" of Lamaštu, other aggressive demons (such as the *šēdu*-demon), the "Hand" of the healing goddess(es) Gula/Ninkarrak and the Hand of the "Ban" (*māmītu*) inflicted by a broken oath, are mentioned and dealt with in the preserved ritual procedures.

The procedures described in the texts to protect pregnant women and their offspring fulfil both protective/apotropaic and exorcistic functions. Prescriptions for amulet necklaces (strings with stones and leather bags) make up a considerable portion of the procedures, as do (often quite complex) ritual procedures. The ritual procedures include, beside apotropaic incantations, several prayers/recitations to different deities, among whom are, unsurprisingly, goddesses concerned with childbirth or healing (and sometimes directly held responsible for the treated problems): especially recitations to the mother goddess Ninmaḫ, the healing goddesses Gula and Ninkarrak, and to the astral constellation "Wagon" (^{mul}MAR.GÍD.(-)DA, Akkadian *Ereqqu*, Ursa Major) associated with Venus/the goddess Ištar play a role in the texts (see texts C.3.4, C.3.6, C.3.8, C.3.10 lines 62, 64, 79, 96).

Lastly, a few text snippets quoted in AMC for the treatise PREGNANCY/OFFSPRING suggest that other related topics and healing procedures formed part of the text collections belonging to the treatise, especially procedures to stop bleeding and loss of amniotic fluid during pregnancy (AMC line 112). For texts focussing on anomalous bleeding/haemorrhage (including bleeding during pregnancy) and other discharges, see section C.1 and some of the collections of treatments for women edited in section A of this book.

C.3.1 STT 241: Amulet Stones and an Incantation for Protecting Pregnant Women

This single-column tablet belonged to an ensemble of scholarly tablets and fragments found together in the provincial town of Sultantepe (ancient Ḫuzirina, near Ḫarran) at the edge of the Neo-Assyrian empire, in a hoard close to the remains of a private house that may have belonged to a priestly family. Its scribe, a certain Sîn-iddina, is otherwise unknown. The tablet is inscribed with a complete procedure for a "woman who does not bring (her pregnancies) to term" (MUNUS NU SI.SÁ, Akkadian (*sinništu*) *lā muš(t)ēšertu*), consisting of instructions for making an ensemble of amulet strings with different stones that were worn by the patient on different body parts (head, hands, feet, waist and navel). These instructions are followed by the text of an Akkadian spell that was recited over the amulets before they were attached to the woman's body. The incantation which shares similarities with a few lines in a spell from the exorcistic incantation series Ḫulbazizi makes the attacks of a malicious *šēdu*-demon responsible for the patient's repeated miscarriages, an aetiology that is so far unique to the present text. The spell invokes the help of the sun god Šamaš and other deities to protect the (pregnant) patient from another miscarriage. A rubric which is added to the text on the left edge of the tablet extends the purpose of the text to other demonic agents: "to block the *šēdu*, the *rābiṣu* ('lurker'), the *ardat-lilî*-demon" from reaching any adolescent girl (line 32–33).

As is known from other first millennium BCE texts edited in section C.3 of this book as well as from older sources of Mesopotamian healing traditions, amulet necklaces and spells formed an important approach in the context of protecting pregnant women from miscarriage (e.g. Finkel 1980; Scurlock 1991; Steinert et al. 2018, 272 ad line 114 and the similar rubric ^{munus}PEŠ$_4$ KÉŠ.DA "to bind a pregnant woman").

List of Manuscripts

Siglum	Museum Number	Copy	Collation	Format; Ductus	Provenience
A	SU 52/99 + 149	STT 241	Coll.	single-column tablet in landscape format; Neo-Assyrian script; 7th cent. BCE	Sultantepe

Overview

i	Instruction for amulet stones against miscarriage to be placed around the temples, hands, feet, waist and navel A obv. 1–7	1–7
ii	Incantation *māḫiṣ muḫḫi mubbil liq pīya mubbil qaqqadi* A obv. 8–rev. 10	8–28
iii	Incantation rubric and instruction A rev. 11–12	29–30
iv	Colophon A rev. 13	31
v	Rubric(?) A l. e. 1–2	32–33

Previous Edition and Discussion

Schuster-Brandis 2008, 149–150 (transliteration, translation of lines 1–7)
Scurlock 1991, *Incognita* 2, 165 note 38
Stol 2000a, 132–133 (discussion)

Transliteration

1	A obv. 1	^{na4}AN.ZA.GUL.MEŠ [*ina* SAG].⸢KI$^{?}$⸣.MEŠ-*šá*
2	A obv. 2	^{na4}⸢*ḫal-tu*$^{?}$⸣ ⸢(x)⸣ ⸢^{na4}⸣[x x]x ^{na4}ZA.GÌN *ina* ŠU.MIN ZAG-*šá*
3	A obv. 3	^{na4}AŠ.GÌ.GÌ *ina* ŠU.MIN GÙB-*šá* ^{na4}⸢PA$^{?}$⸣ ^{na4}*zi*-É *ina* ⸢GÌR⸣.MIN ZAG-*šá*
4	A obv. 4	^{na4}*šu-bu-u* ^{na4}PA *ina* [G]ÌR.MIN GÙB-*šá*
5	A obv. 5	^{na4}*šu-bu-u* ^{na4}KUR-*nu* DAB.BA *ina* MURUB$_{4}$.MEŠ-*šá*
6	A obv. 6	^{na4}ŠIKA SILA.LÍMMU-*ti ina* LI$^{!}$.DUR-*šá*
7	A obv. 7	PAP 12 NA$_{4}$.MEŠ *ša* MUNUS NU SI.SÁ.KÁM

8	A obv. 8	ÉN ⸢*ma*⸣-*ḫi-ṣi muḫ-ḫi mu-bíl liq pi-ia*
9	A obv. 9	*mu-bíl* [SA]G.DU [*a*]-*kil* ^{uzu}SA-*ni*
10	A obv. 10	*ši-biṭ š*[*i*$^{?}$-*ḫi*]-*iṭ*$^{?!}$ GIN$_{7}$ G[U$_{4}$$^{?}$] ⸢*ek*$^{?}$⸣-[*di*$^{?}$] *ú-šá-*[*aḫ-ḫi-iṭ*$^{?}$]
11	A obv. 11	^{d}ALAD$^{?}$ [*l*]*a*$^{?}$ DU$_{10}$.G[A$^{?}$ ....]
12	A obv. 12	*ša*$^{?}$ x-[x]-*ṣa*$^{?}$ ŠU$^{?}$-*s*[*u*$^{?}$ ....]
13	A obv. 13	*ina ḫu*$^{?}$-x [x] x[.................................]
14	A lo. e. 1	^{d}*šá-maš be-*[*el* ....]
15	A lo. e. 2	*iṣ-bat-ka* x[.....................................]

16	A lo. e. 3	*ik*-[......................................]
17	A lo. e. 4	*ina pi-i* [......................................]
18	A lo. e. 5	*ina pi-i še*$^{?}$-[...................................]
19	A rev. 1	*ina* NU.ME DUR [............................]
20	A rev. 2	^{d}*lil-lum* ^{d}GAŠAN-*k*[*id-mu-ri*$^{?}$ ....]
21	A rev. 3	*a-di im-ma-lu-u* [..............................]
22	A rev. 4	*la* È-*ma* ^{d}[.....................................]
23	A rev. 5	*ki-ma im-tal-lu-*[*u* ....]
24	A rev. 6	^{d}*lil-lum* ^{d}GAŠAN$^{!}$-*k*[*id-mu-ri*$^{?}$...... *nūr*$^{?}$] ^{d}*šá-maš* IGI.LÁ
25	A rev. 7	AD-*šú* A[M]A-*šú ni*$^{?}$-*š*[*u-ti-šú*$^{?}$] IGI.LÁ
26	A rev. 8	ÉN *u*[*l*] ⸢*ia-a*⸣-*tú*-⸢*nu*⸣ É[N ^{d}*é*]-⸢*a*⸣ ^{d}*asal-lú-ḫi*
27	A rev. 9	⸢ÉN⸣ ^{d}*da-mu* ^{d}*g*[*u-la*] ⸢^{d}⸣*nin-gìrima*
28	A rev. 10	EN T[U$_{6}$$^{?}$] TU$_{6}$ ÉN
29	A rev. 11	KA.INIM.MA MUNUS NU S[I].SÁ.[KÁM É]N *an*-[*ni-tu*$_{4}$] 7-*šú*
30	A rev. 12	*ina* U[G]U NA$_{4}$.MEŠ [ŠID]-*nu*

Colophon:

31	A rev. 13	*šà-ṭír* ^{md}30—SUM-*n*[*a šá* TÙM NUMUN-*šú*$^{?}$] ZÁḪ

Rubric:

32	A l. e. 1	^{d}ALAD MÀŠK[IM$^{?}$] ⸢KI$^{?}$⸣.SIKIL.[L]ÍL.LÁ$^{?!}$(A) *ana* KUD
33	A l. e. 2	⸢*ana*$^{?}$⸣ *kal* MUNUS.GURUŠ.TUR

Bound Transcription and Translation

[1] AN.ZA.GUL.MEŠ [*ina nakkapā*]*tīša* [2] *ḫaltu* ... *uqnû ina qāt imittīša* [3] *ašgikû ina qāt šumēlīša ayyartu*(?) *zibītu ina šēp imittīša* [4] *šubû ayyartu ina* [*š*]*ēp šumēlīša* [5] *šubû šadânu ṣābitu ina qablīša* [6] *ḫaṣab sūq erbetti ina abunnatīša* [7] *napḫar* 12 *abnī ša sinništi lā muš*(*t*)*ēšerti*

[1] AN.ZA.GUL.MEŠ-stone [on her tem]ples, [2] *ḫaltu*-stone, ...-stone (and) lapis lazuli on her right hand, [3] *ašgikû*-stone (turquoise) on her left hand, *ayyartu*-shell(?) (and) *zibītu*-stone on her right foot, [4] *šubû*-stone (and) *ayyartu*-shell on her left foot, [5] *šubû*-stone (and) magnetite on her hips, [6] a potsherd from a cross-roads on her navel. [7] A total of twelve stones for a woman who has difficulty bringing her pregnancies to term.

8 ÉN *māḫiṣ muḫḫi mubbil liq pīya*	8 Incantation: "The one who hits (my) skull, who dries out my palate,
9 *mubbil qaqqadi* [*ā*]*kil* [*šer*]*'āni*	9 who dries out (my) head, [h]urts (my) [ten]dons –
10 *šibiṭ šiḫiṭ*(?) *kīma l*[*ê*] [*ek*]*di*(?) *uša*[*ḫḫiṭ*(?)]	10 it is a blow; it is an attack(?)! It at[tacks(?)] like a [wi]ld bu[ll].
11 *šēdu* [*lā*] *ṭābu*(?) [... ...]	11 O malevolent *šēdu*-demon [... ...],
12 *ša* ... *qāssu* [... ...]	12 whose hand(s) are ... [... ...],
13 *ina* ...[... ...]	13 with/in ...[... ...].
14 *Šamaš bē*[*l* ... ...]	14 Šamaš, the lo[rd of ... ...],
15 *iṣbatka* [... ...]	15 he has seized you, ...[.....],
16 ...[... ...]	16 ...[... ...].
17 *ina pî* [... ...]	17 *By the command of* [... ...],
18 *ina pî* ...[... ...]	18 *by the command of* ...[... ...],
19 *ina balu*(?) ...[... ...]	19 *without*(?) ...[... ...].
20 *Lillu Šarrat-ki*[*dmuri* ... ...]	20 (O) Lillu, Šarrat-k[idmuri(?), ...],
21 *adi immalû* [... ...]	21 before [...] have become full [... ...],
22 *lā uṣṣī-ma* ...[... ...]	22 may it (the baby?) not come out! ...[... ...].
23 *kīma imtalû* [... ...]	23 As soon as [...] have become full, [... ...].
24 *Lillu Šarg*[*az* ... ... *nūr*] *Šamaš līmur*	24 (O) Lillu, Šarrat-k[idmuri(?), ...] *may it see* [the light of(?)] the sun!
25 *abāšu ummāšu* ...[... ...] *līmur*	25 *May it see* its father (and) its mother ...[...]!
26 *šiptu ul yattun šip*[*ti E*]*a Asalluḫi*	26 The incantation is not mine. It is the incan[tation of E]a (and) Asalluḫi,
27 *šipti Damu G*[*ula*] *Ningirima*	27 (it is) the incantation of Damu, G[ula] (and) Ningirima,
28 *bēl šip*[*ti*] *tê šipti*	28 the lord(s) of spell(s)." Incantation formula.
29 KA.INIM.MA *sinništi lā muš*(*t*)*ēš*[*erti ši*]*pta annīta sebîšu* 30 *ina muḫḫi abnī* [*tamannū*]*-ma*	29 Wording (of an incantation) for a woman who has trouble bringing her pregnancies to term. You recite this incanta[tion] seven times 30 over the stones.
Colophon:	
31 *šāṭir Sîn-iddin*[*a ša itabbalu zēršu*(?)] *liḫliq*	31 The scribe (is) Sîn-iddin[a. *Who carries off* (*the tablet*?), may his descendants(?)] perish.
Rubric:	
32 *šēdu rābiṣu ardat-lilî ana parāsi* 33 *ana*(?) *kal batūlti*(?)	32 To block the *šēdu*, the *rābiṣu*, the *ardat-lilî*-demon. 33 *For every* young maiden(?).

Notes

Lines 1–7: For a similar list of stones applied in protective amulets for the same purpose, see also AO 6473 (TCL 6, 49; text C.3.9) and Chapter F on Amulet Texts.

Line 1: The Akkadian reading of $^{\text{na4}}$AN.ZA.GUL.MEŠ (more common spellings are $^{\text{na4}}$AN.ZA/ZU.GUL.ME; in Lugale 534 $^{\text{na4}}$an-zú-gul-me) is not entirely certain; see von Soden 1939, *ZA* 45, 47; Schuster-Brandis 2008, 396. The stone is listed in Ḫḫ. Tablet XVI, but only the version from Emar preserves an Akkadian correspondence (*zašk/qītu*), cf. MSL 10, 13: 344–347, ibid., 27 and 47; Arnaud 1987, Emar VI/4, 123 Text No. 533: 173′–176′.

Line 7: See also Stol 2000a, 132–133. For the rubric and term MUNUS NU SI.SÁ, see also KAR 223: 5 and dupl. (a ritual to avoid birth in the month Nisannu, Stadhouders and Steinert 2018, *JMC* 32, 65; *infra* text D.3.1), mentioning stones for the hips of a MUNUS NU SI.SÁ. The Akkadian correspondence of MUNUS NU SI.SÁ, *sinništu lā muš*(*t*)*ēšertu*, is attested in SpTU 5, No. 248: 1 (text C.3.10).

The term *lā mušēšertu*, a negated Š-stem participle of the verb *ešēru* ("to put in good condition", "to cause to prosper"), refers to a woman who has had repeated miscarriages. However, the Št-stem participle (*muštēšertu*) of the same verb is more commonly used in the same meaning, for example in omen apodoses. Thus, a liver omen reads: *la a-lit-ti ul-lad la muš-te-šir-tú uš-te-(eš)-šer/šìr* "an infertile woman will give birth, a woman who has difficulty bringing to term will bring to term" (DA 96, 25 // CT 30, 30a: 5; quoted in Stol 2000a, 103–104 with fn. 72; note the same apodosis written logographically in Böck 2000, 94–95: 97 (*Alamdimmû* Tablet III): NU Ù.TU Ù.TU NU SI.SÁ SI.SÁ).

However, durative forms of the Št-stem of *ešēru* elsewhere refer to a straightforward delivery. In BAM 248 iv 12 //, *uš-te-šir* "she will deliver with ease" ($Št^1$, see AHw 255b sub 5) interchanges with logographic (MUNUS BI) SI.SÁ (see *infra* text D.1.1). In BAM 248 i 53 //, *šerru ušteššer(a)* ($Št^2$, see AHw 256b sub 8c) refers to the foetus ("the baby will be born straightforwardly").

Lines 8–28: The incipit of the incantation *māḫiṣ muḫḫi mubbil liq pīya mubbil qaqqadi*, written out in full in ms. A, is also quoted in AO 6473 (TCL 6, 49) obv. 26, a Late Babylonian tablet from Uruk with amulets and incantations to prevent miscarriage (see *infra* text C.3.10). The same spell may be cited in DT 28 obv. i 1′ (see *infra* text F.1, K. 4727+ and duplicates). See further Stol 2000a, 132–133 n. 144; CAD L, s.v. *līq pî* sub b.

Lines 8–9: The text of these two lines is identical with two lines of the incantation *ēkim sūqi pārik ribīti* "He who snatches (people) away (from) the street, who blocks the thoroughfare", attested in the series Ḫulbazizi (STT 214–217 obv. iii 24–25 /// KAR 88 fr. 4 iii 4–5 // K. 2506+ obv. iii 3′–4′; see Ebeling 1953b, *ArOr* 21, 417, 419–420 note 203; cf. Finkel 1976, 108, 184–186 No. 31: 172–174 and pl. 11; Gurney, in: STT II, p. 11). Apart from these two lines of stock phrases, that incantation differs from STT 241: 8–28, however. Apparently, the parallel opening lines in STT 241 obv. 8–9 refer to or address the demonic agent attacking the woman and her foetus. Stol (2000a, 132–133 n. 72) wondered instead whether the opening lines referred to the newborn baby. Since the context of the spell is to protect pregnant women from miscarriage and keep the foetus alive, the speaker attacked by demonic threat may be either the woman or perhaps her foetus.

Line 10: The word *šibṭu* means "plague, epidemic" (CAD Š/2, 387–388 s.v. *šibṭu* A), and in a second meaning "gale; blast of wind" (cf. CAD Š/2, 387–389, who differentiate two separate lemmas, while AHw 1228a suggests one lemma with two different meanings). Since *šibṭu* occurs in both meanings in incantations, it is not entirely certain which nuance is intended here. For *šiḫṭu* "attack, strike, raid, razzia" (said e.g. of wild animals and demons), see CAD Š/2, 416b sub 1; cf. CAD Š/1, 92a sub 7 (*šaḫāṭu* "to attack" (D-stem)). The adjective *ekdu* "wild; furious" usually qualifies wild bulls (e.g., *rīmu*, GU_4.AM) or lions. The sign GU_4 can also be read *lû* "(wild) bull; lion" instead of *alpu* "ox".

Line 11: The mention of a malevolent *šēdu*-demon/spirit (*šēdu lā ṭābu*) as responsible agent is in line with the rubric written on the right edge of the tablet, "to keep away (cut off) the *šēdu*, *rābiṣu* (lurker) and *ardat-lilî* (wind-maiden) demons". These disease agents are well-known from other medical texts and incantations. However, the present text is unique in presenting these demonic agents as causing miscarriage. This misfortune is more frequently attributed to the demoness Lamaštu and to witchcraft. Note that usually *šēdu*-demons are designated either as "good" (*damqu*) acting as protective personal agents, or "bad" (*lemnu*), when they occur in incantations beside other disease demons (see CAD Š/2, 256–259). The term *šēdu* is also attested in reference to senders of disease that are "deputy powers/spirits" (*šēdu šanû*) of specific deities, see e.g. Arbøll 2019, *JMC* 33 (BAM 202 rev. 7′); Schmidtchen 2021b, *JMC* 37, 31ff.

Line 14: Different epithets of the sun god begin with *bēl*, e.g. *bēl kitti u mīšari* "lord of right and justice", *bēl dīni* "lord of judgment", but also *bēl šamê u erṣeti* "lord of heaven and earth", *bēl elâti u šaplâti* "lord of the upper and lower world", *bēl mātāti* "lord of the lands" or *bēl gimri* "lord of the universe" (see e.g. Mayer 1976, 410–422).

Line 15: Presumably, the demon is addressed here as "you" and the subject of *iṣbat* is the sun god, although this is mere conjecture. There are other possible readings, e.g. the sign KA could also belong to the following word or it may have to be read logographically. This remains uncertain until better-preserved sources for the spell are known.

Line 19: The logogram NU.ME.(A) can be read as Akkadian *balu* "without". The following sign DUR may be read *riksu* "bond", which could refer to cosmic bonds. Note also that *riksu ša amēli* "the bond of humankind" is an expression for the umbilical cord (see 11N-T3: 13; *infra* text G.1). Without context the passage remains unclear.

Line 20: It appears that here and in line 24 deities are invoked as supportive or protective agents. According to god lists, the god Lillu (^{d}Lil, *Lil-lu*) is a son of the mother goddess (sometimes equated with Ninurta). His name was also written ^{d}BÁḪAR, lit. "Potter" (Krebernik 1987–1990a, *RlA* 7, 19–20). Perhaps this association explains the occurrence of Lillu in the present incantation against miscarriage, since in Mesopotamian myths human beings are classically created by shaping them from clay. Furthermore, Lillu is equated with the dying god Lú-lîl (or Mulu-lîl) known from a Sumerian composition in which he is in the Netherworld and instructs his sister how to perform the funerary rites for him (Katz 2003, 205ff.).

The second divine name in line 20 is only partially preserved, but given the first sign GAŠAN after the divine determinative it may be restored as Šarrat-kidmuri, the "queen of the (Bīt)-Kidmuri", which is a manifestation of Ištar (also appearing as ^{d}15 *ša Bīt-Kidmuri*). The name Kidmuru refers to a temple in Nimrud built for Ištar. Šarrat-kidmuri occurs in the greeting formulas of Neo-Assyrian letters beside other forms of Ištar (Šarrat-Ninua, Šarrat-Arba'il), see Krebernik 2009–2011a, *RlA* 12, 75. For Ištar of Kidmuru's links to pregnancy and birth, see Arbøll 2023, 272–273, quoting SAA 10, No. 294, a letter of the court scholar Urad-Gula that mentions a banquet performed at the Kidmuru temple on behalf of Urad-Gula's wife so that she may be provided with offspring. See also Rm. 376 (discussed in chapter D.1.1, ms. C).

Lines 21–25: The present interpretation proposes that these fragmentary lines refer to the baby which should not be born before its term is completed. The subject of the verb *malû* "to be(come) full" in lines 21 and 23 should be the "days" or "months" (of pregnancy). For *malû* "to reach fullness", said of days or months, see e.g. BAM 244: 21 (referring to the patient): *kīma* U_4.MEŠ-*šá im-ta-lu-ú* "when her days (i.e. those of her treatment) are complete" (*infra* text B.1.1). See also CAD M/1, 180–181 s.v. *malû* sub 4.

Coming out and seeing the sunlight is a recurring phrase in birth incantations (and baby incantations), see e.g. BAM 248 ii 56, iv 1 //: *li/lit-ta-ṣa-am-ma li-ta-mar/li-mu-ra* ZÁLAG ^{d}UTU-*ši* "May it come out (quickly) and see the sunlight!" (text D.1.1). See also BAM 248 i 56, 66; KAR 223: 18 // (text D.2.1) for similar passages; Polonsky 2006, *FS Leichty*, 297–312, esp. 302 with fn. 24; Bosworth 2016, 33–53 for discussion. The foetus is called "inhabitant of the dark, who has not seen the sunlight" (*āšib eklēti lā āmir nūr Šamši*), see e.g. BM 42327+: 10–11 // SpTU 3, No. 84 rev. 7–8 (see Farber 1989a, 112; Polonsky 2006, 301 fn. 22; Abusch et al. 2022, text 5.4 and *infra* text C.3.4).

Line 24: This line appears to repeat the divine characters invoked in line 20. Thus, after ^{d}*Lil-lum*, we assume ^{d}GAŠAN$^{!}$-*k*[*id-mu-ri*$^{?}$], although the sign following the divine determinative looks like ḪI/ŠÁR rather than GAŠAN. Thus, one could think of ^{d}Šár-gaz, a mythical deified weapon of the god Ninurta. ^{d}Šár-gaz forms a pair with another weapon ^{d}Šár-ùr (a mace or throwing stick), see Krebernik 2009–2011b, *RlA* 12, 84–86.

Line 25: The sign following AMA-*šú* copied as NI in STT 241 may also be IR; there is a slight trace that may suggest a third vertical wedge. In the latter case one may suggest as an alternative restoration *ir-ḫ*[*u-šú*] "(may he see his father and his mother who) engen[dered him]".

Line 31: The restoration of the gap after the name of the scribe follows similar curse formulas in colophons, see e.g. Hunger 1968, No. 239: 5ff. Hunger himself (1968, 119 No. 401) suggested a patronymic in the gap; Baker (2002, *PNA* 3/1, 1134–1135 sub 11) follows Hunger in restoring "[son/descendant of ...]haia".

Lines 32–33: These two lines inscribed on the left edge of the tablet would have been visible when the tablet was deposited on the library shelf, similar to the printed spines of today's books.

Line 32: This line on the left edge of the tablet appears to serve as a kind of thematic rubric for the text on the tablet or purpose statement, namely to "block (cut off) the *šēdu*, the *rābiṣu*, the *ardat lilî*-demon". Among these demons, the "wind demons" (*lilû*, *ardat lilî*) are known to attack especially adolescent boys and girls, but occasionally also infants. See e.g. BAM 248 iv 41–43 and dupl. (against the *lilû*-demon, see Farber 1989a, 126–127 §45 and *infra*); Schmidtchen 2019, *JMC* 33, 33: 22 (*lilû* and *alû*-demon).

Line 33: Curiously, this line is written upside down in relation to the other line on the left edge, i.e. the scribe turned the tablet 180 degrees to inscribe the text. The tablet surface is damaged before the first visible sign KAL. Thus, one sign may be lost before KAL. The sense of the expression remains unclear to me, although one expects another statement of the text's purpose here. There are several possibilities of reading the preserved signs. One possibility is GURUŠ MUNUS GURUŠ. TUR "young man, woman, boy". This is somewhat unexpected, since the text on the tablet specifically focuses on pregnant women and their unborn babies. In line with the mention of *šēdu*, *rābiṣu*, the *ardat lilî*-demon in line 32, the enumeration in line 33 could refer to the human victims of these demons. Because of *ardat lilî*-demon in line 32, I suggest reading *ana*(?) *kal* MUNUS.GURUŠ.TUR "for every adolescent girl", because the wind-demons are specifically known to attack young people. An alternative reading of the line could be *ana* GURUŠ.<TUR> MUNUS GURUŠ.TUR "for the adolescent boy and girl".

C.3.2 K. 11647 (AMT 66/3): A Fragment of a Compendium with Treatments for Pregnant Women

This small fragment from Ashurbanipal's library at Nineveh written in a tiny Neo-Assyrian script must have belonged to a large two-column tablet. The piece preserves a portion of the centre of the tablet, with parts of two text columns and column divider visible. It may have contained a collection of therapeutic material for women's health matters, comparable to the Neo-Assyrian Birth Compendium (see *infra* text D.1.1, BAM 248 and duplicates from Nineveh). It is likewise possible that it even belonged to a serialised medical compendium comparable to the treatises concerned with women (PREGNANCY, BIRTH) that are listed in the Assur Medical Catalogue (Steinert et al. 2018), but this remains uncertain.

The present text has been placed in section C due to the contents of the eleven fragmentary lines in col. ii' on the obverse(?) which partially preserve a prescription followed by a rubric indicating that treatment was used for a pregnant woman, perhaps to protect her from miscarriage or (less likely) to induce an abortion. The recipe is followed by a fragmentary *abracadabra*-spell.

The eleven fragmentary lines preserved of column iii' on the reverse are likewise inscribed with an unknown incantation.

List of Manuscripts

Siglum	Museum Number	Copy	Collation	Format; Ductus	Provenience
A	K. 11647[324]	AMT 66/3	Coll.	Fragment of a two-column(?) tablet; Neo-Assyrian script; 7th cent. BCE	Nineveh, library of Ashurbanipal

Overview

i'	Fragmentary A obv.(?) i' 1'–2'	1'–2'[...
ii''	Fragmentary prescription A obv.(?) ii' 1'–4'	...]3''–6''
iii''	Rubric A obv.(?) ii' 5'	7''
iv''	Fragmentary incantation A obv.(?) ii' 6'–11'	8''–13''[...
v'''	Fragmentary incantation A rev.(?) iii' 1'–12'	...]14'''–25'''

Previous Edition and Discussion

Thompson 1934, "Assyrian prescriptions for diseases of the urinary tract etc.", *Babyloniaca* 14, 84 and 136
CDLI P399372 (transliteration; photo)
BabMed Corpora (https://www.geschkult.fu-berlin.de/e/babmed/Corpora/AMT-2/AMT66-3/index.html) (transliteration)
Electronic Babylonian Library (eBL) (https://www.ebl.lmu.de/library/K.11647; transliteration)

Transliteration

Beginning of ms. A obv.(?) i' lost

324 Measurements: 5.5 x 4 x 2.7 cm.

1′	A obv.(?) i′ 1′	[...] MIN$^{?}$
2′	A obv.(?) i′ 2′	[...] MIN$^{?}$

Ms. A obv.(?) i' breaks; gap of unknown length

3″	A obv.(?) ii′ 1′	[x x x x] x x x x [...................................]
4″	A obv.(?) ii′ 2′	[x x x] *a-na* AN-*e* [...................................]
5″	A obv.(?) ii′ 3′	[x (x)] ŠE$_{10}$$^{?!}$ MUNU$_4$ SUR 7-*š*[*ú*$^{?}$ ....]
6″	A obv.(?) ii′ 4′	[*t*]*a*$^{?}$-*rak-ma* x[.......................................]

7″	A obv.(?) ii′ 5′	^{munus}PEŠ$_4$ *šà* ŠÀ-*šà* [*ana* (NU) ŠUB-*di*$^{?}$ (...)]

8″	A obv.(?) ii′ 6′	ÉN sur-sur ki-ki [...................................]
9″	A obv.(?) ii′ 7′	ki-ki šár-r[a$^{?}$ ....]
10″	A obv.(?) ii′ 8′	ḫar-ḫa šár-[ra ....]
11″	A obv.(?) ii′ 9′	dab-ba [..]
12″	A obv.(?) ii′ 10′	g[i$^{?}$ ....]
13″	A obv.(?) ii′ 11′	u[r$^{?}$ ....]

Ms. A obv.(?) ii' breaks; gap of unknown length

14‴	A rev.(?) iii′ 1′	[x] ⸢ka$^{?}$⸣ x[...................................]
15‴	A rev.(?) iii′ 2′	⸢a$^{?}$⸣-la a-k[a$^{?}$ ....]
16‴	A rev.(?) iii′ 3′	ki-na ḫe-me-⸢e$^{?}$⸣ [...................................]
17‴	A rev.(?) iii′ 4′	*ú-ru-ru* [..]
18‴	A rev.(?) iii′ 5′	[*an*]*a*$^{?}$ *i-šip-pu* kur-kur [...........................]
19‴	A rev.(?) iii′ 6′	íd kur-ra gíd-gíd [...................................]
20‴	A rev.(?) iii′ 7′	ḫa-zí-in te-še igi [...................................]
21‴	A rev.(?) iii′ 8′	ḫa-zí-in te-še igi x[..................................]
22‴	A rev.(?) iii′ 9′	igi igi igi ú ḫul-a [...................................]
23‴	A rev.(?) iii′ 10′	i-te bar an x x x[.......................................]
24‴	A rev.(?) iii′ 11′	a ḫul ⸢x⸣ [...]
25‴	A rev.(?) iii′ 12′	⸢x x⸣ [...]

Ms. A rev.(?) iii' breaks; remainder lost

Bound Transcription and Translation

Beginning of ms. A obv.(?) i' lost

1′ [... ...] MIN	[... ...], ditto(?).
2′ [... ...] MIN	[... ...], ditto (?).

Ms. A obv. i' breaks; gap of unknown length

3″ *traces*	3″ *too fragmentary for translation*
4″ [...] *ana šamê* [... ...] 5″ [...] *zê buqli teṭerri*(?) *sebî*[*šu* ... ...] 6″ *tarâk-ma* [... ...]	4″ [...] towards heaven [... ...] 5″ [...] you *smear* (with?) refuse of malt, seven times [you ... ...], 6″ you knead/smear (it). Then [... ...].
7″ *erītu ša libbīša* [*ana* (*lā*) *šuddî*/*nadê*(?)]	7″ [So that] a pregnant woman [(not) abort(?)] her foetus.
8″ ÉN sur-sur ki-ki [... ...] 9″ ki-ki šár-r[a? ... ...] 10″ ḫar-ḫa šár-[ra ... ...] 11″ dab-ba [... ...]	8″ Incantation. “Sursur kiki [... ...], 9″ kiki šarr[a ... ...], 10″ ḫarḫa šar[ra ...], 11″ dabba [...],
12″–13″ *traces*	12″–13″ *too fragmentary for translation*

Ms. A obv.(?) ii' breaks; gap of unknown length

14‴ *traces*	14‴ *too fragmentary for translation*
15‴ ⸢a?⸣-la a-k[a? ... ...]	15‴ in(?) an abundance of water (?) [... ...],
16‴ ki-na ḫe-me-⸢e?⸣-[... ...]	16‴ In his/her place ...[... ...].
17‴ *urrurū*(?) [... ...]	17‴ *Dried out are* [... ...],
18‴ [*an*]*a išippu* kur-kur [... ...]	18‴ t[o] the conjurer of (all) the lands [... ...],
19‴ íd kur-ra gíd-gíd [... ...]	19‴ the long river of the netherworld [... ...].
20‴ ḫa-zí-in te-še igi [... ...]	20‴ an axe ...[... ...],
21‴ ḫa-zí-in te-še igi x[... ...]	21‴ an axe ... [... ...].
22‴ igi igi igi ú ḫul-a [... ...]	22‴ Eye, eye, eye! Plant *of destruction* [... ...],
23‴ i-te bar an x x x[... ...]	23‴ *it approached*(?) *the outskirts of heaven* [...],
24‴–25‴ *too fragmentary for transcription*	24‴–25‴ *too fragmentary for translation*

Ms. A rev.(?) iii' breaks; remainder lost

Notes

General remark: The identification of the obverse and reverse of the tablet is uncertain. The present edition follows Thompson’s assignment in AMT.

Lines 5″–6″: The reading ŠE$_{10}^{!?}$ MUNU$_4$ “refuse(?) of malt” in line 5″ is tentative and based on context; the sign before MUNU$_4$ rather resembles KI. The following logogram SUR is ambiguous. In medical texts, SUR usually stands for Akkadian *ṭerû* “to press out; to squeeze out”, or better “to smear”. The verb *ṭerû* occurs in the context of preparing bandages or poultices, where extracted compounds of drugs are smeared on a piece of cloth or leather before application, see CAD Ṭ, 103; cf. Goltz 1974, 54–55. Other possible readings of SUR are *ṣaḫātu* “to press; to process” (oil or wine) and *ṣarāru* “to pour out”, but these verbs usually involve liquids. In line 6″, the verbal form is read *ta-rak-ma* in CAD K, 110b sub a; the verb *râku* is rendered as “to smear” or “to knead” there, while AHw 948b translates *râku* with “ausschütten” (i.e., “to pour out”).

Line 7″: For the reconstructed rubric, compare e.g. the texts BM 42327+: 1ff.; TCL 6, 49 rev. 13ff., SpTU 3, No. 84: 56ff.; LKA 9 rev. r. col. 7′ff.; BM 51246+ obv. 1ff.; KAL 2, No. 41 obv. i' 10ff. (see *infra*). All these texts contain treatments for protecting pregnant women from miscarriage caused by sorcery (*ana* ^{munus}PEŠ$_4$ UŠ$_{11}$.ZU NU TE-*ma ša* ŠÀ-*šá* NU ŠUB-*e*). The present rubric in line 7″ may have been abbreviated.

A second option is to restore the passage in the contrasting sense, “to cause a pregnant woman to expel her foetus” (^{munus}PEŠ$_4$ *šà* ŠÀ-*šà ana* ŠUB-*di*, for which we find a parallel in BAM 246: 1: [^{munus}P]EŠ$_4$ *šà* ŠÀ-*šà ana* ŠUB-*di* (text B.1.6). Cf. also K. 8678+ rev. 13′ and 20′ (text A.1.4) for varying formulae. Recipes to procure an abortion are otherwise rare in the

Mesopotamian gynaecological corpus and have so far not been encountered in a longer compendium. The present text may perhaps form the first such case.

Lines 14‴–25‴: It is not always clear from the fragmentary traces, whether the text should be read as Sumerian or Akkadian, or a mixture of it. Most likely these lines belong to an incantation.

Line 15″: Sumerian a-la (or la-la) means "plenty, exuberance". Alternatively, one could read *a-la-a* as Akkadian *alû* "bull" or *alû*-demon (in the accusative). eBL suggest reading *a-la-a-k*[*a*] (i.e. an accusative infinitive form of *alāku* "to go").

Line 16‴: The reading of this line is only tentative. Perhaps, ki-na ("in his/her place(?)") is a phonetic spelling for Sumerian ki-ná "bedchamber". The sign sequence ḫi/e-me-e could also be read as an Akkadian word, *ḫimû*. This term designates reeds that were bound on the skin to soothe snake bite; elsewhere they are arranged around the bed for protection (cf. CAD Ḫ, 193–194).

Line 17‴: The provisional reading as Akkadian *urrurū* "they are dried out" is highly tentative. Alternatively, one could interpret the signs as Sumerian ú šub-šub, a "plant (that is) fallen/laid down" (on the ground)? In the present context, one could also think of a plant that causes miscarriage (i.e., "dropping (šub) of the foetus").

Line 18‴: eBL restore *ana* before the word *išippu*. In first millennium BCE texts, *išippu* is an antiquated word synonymous with *āšipu* "conjurer", derived from Sumerian išib, designating a type of purification priest. The "conjurer of (all) lands" may be an honorific title of a deity, e.g. Enki or Asalluḫi.

Lines 20‴–21‴: In Thompson's copy of the fragment in AMT, line 21‴, being a repetition of line 20‴, was omitted. The word ḫa-zí-in is a loanword from Akkadian *ḫaṣṣinnu* "axe", and it may even perhaps be interpreted as Akkadian text in the present passage. The following sign sequence te-še igi could also be read as Akkadian *te-še-ši*, a 2nd person singular form of *ešû* "to trouble, confuse", with the pronominal suffix *-ši* referring to *haṣṣinnu* (the word is constructed as feminine in the plural).

C.3.3 BM 42327+: Rituals for Protecting Pregnant Women from Miscarriage

The single-column tablet BM 42327+ (ms. a) contains three prescriptions and two associated incantations for protecting a pregnant woman from miscarriage caused by witchcraft. The tablet written in a Late-Babylonian script stems from Rassam's excavations in Babylonia, but its exact provenience is uncertain (possibly Babylon or Sippar). The prescriptions on BM 42327+ are also attested on two other Late-Babylonian tablets, BM 51246+ (ms. b, of uncertain provenience) and SpTU 3, No. 84 (ms. c, from Uruk), both of which present longer collections of material concerned with women's health and related matters. The text on BM 42327+ duplicates a continuous section of text on SpTU 3, No. 84 (rev. 3–25), the latter of which however includes further rituals to protect households from sickness and death befalling their offspring (see text C.3.4 for the complete edition). In contrast, only the first four lines of BM 51246+ obv. duplicate BM 42327+ (leaving out the second prescription and the text of the cited incantations), after which the text continues with gynaecological material on other topics (see text A.2.7). Interestingly, these first four lines in ms. b are identified as stemming from a different source than the following text.

It is crucial to point out that BM 42327+ and SpTU 3, No. 84 present textual evidence for a serialized section of therapeutic material, whose title is known from a passage in the Assur Medical Catalogue (AMC lines 109–114) and which has been dubbed PREGNANCY/OFFSPRING according to its main topic (Steinert et al. 2018, 217–218, 268–272). Thus, BM 42327+ begins with an incipit matching the incipit of Tablet 3 of this AMC section entitled *ana erīti kišpī lā ṭeḫê-ma ša libbīša lā nadê* "So that witchcraft not come near a pregnant woman and for her not to have a miscarriage (lit. drop her foetus)". Furthermore, BM 42327+ contains a catchline that may be mentioned in AMC line 113, followed by the series name corresponding to the title and first tablet of the section PREGNANCY/OFFSPRING in AMC (line 109 and 111): *šumma amēlu ana Ninkarrak paqid-ma* "If a man has been handed over to the goddess Ninkarrak" (see below ms. a, lines 40–41).

The first prescription of BM 42327+ (ms. a lines 1–4) is furthermore a variant of the recipe of a salve for a pregnant woman found on LKA 9, a Neo-Assyrian text from Assur (rev. r. col. 7′–13′, see text C.3.5). However, in BM 42327+, a Lamaštu incantation (*Ezzet šamrat ilat namurrat*) is recited over it (written out in full in ms. a, obv. 14–rev. 8), which is not referred to in LKA 9. This incantation is preserved as well in SpTU 3, No. 84, (ms. c), but also in another Late Babylonian collection of amulet charms for pregnant women (AO 6473, ms. d, see text C.3.9).

The second prescription is an instruction to bury a potsherd from a crossroads under the inner threshold of the house where the patient lives. This passage is missing from BM 51246+ (ms. b), but preserved in SpTU 3, No. 84 (ms. c).

The third prescription consists of an amulet of 'male' and 'female' *šû*-'stone' attached to the woman's right hand, accompanied by the baby incantation *Āšib ekleti lā āmir nūr Šamaš* (the text of which is not included in BM 51246+, ms. b). A variant of this amulet is again found in LKA 9 (using merely male *šû*-'stone' attached to the left hand, rev. r. col. 14′–15′), over which a different baby incantation was recited (LKA 9 rev. r. col. 16′–21′, see text C.3.5). The 'gendered' *šû*-stone is also common in the group of amulets for pregnant women associated with the series *kunuk ḫalti* (K. 4727+ // lines, 12, 15, 21, 29, 34; text F.1).

BM 42327+ concludes with the Lamaštu incantation *Ezzet šamrat ilat namurrat*, followed by a fragmentary colophon. It is interesting that in the present text(s) this incantation is prescribed to protect from miscarriage caused by witchcraft and not by the demoness Lamaštu. This can be compared with the use of a baby incantation for the related context of protecting from miscarriage in LKA 9. Lamaštu is included among the agents causing miscarriage mentioned in the rituals of SpTU 3, No. 84, however (see text C.3.4 for discussion).

List of Manuscripts

Siglum	Museum Number	Copy	Collation	Format; Ductus	Provenience
a	BM 42327 + BM 42410 + BM 42604 + BM 42628 + BM 43474 + BM 43523 (81-7-1, 87 + 170 + 365 + 389 + 1238 + 1287)	Farber 1989a, pl. 14–15	Coll.	Single-column tablet, Late Babylonian script, ca. 6th–3rd cent. BCE	Babylonia, exact provenience unknown
b	BM 51246 + 53217 + 53744 (82-3-23, 2242 + 4251 + 4784)	Pl. 20	Coll.	Fragment of a single-column tablet, Late Babylonian script, 6th–3rd cent. BCE	probably Sippar
c	W. 23287	SpTU 3, No. 84	-	Single column tablet; Late Babylonian period, 5th cent. BCE	Uruk, library of the descendants of Šangû-Ninurta
d	AO 6473	Thureau-Dangin, *RA* 18, 162–163 TCL 6, 49	Coll.	single-column tablet; Late Babylonian script; 3rd–2nd cent. BCE)	Uruk
e		Nougayrol, *Syria* 42, p. 228 (photo)	-	Amulet	modern forgery after lost original

Overview

i	Prescription (ointment) to protect a woman from miscarriage caused by witchcraft a obv. 1–4 // b obv. 1–3 // c rev. 3–4	1–4
ii	Ritual instruction to protect a woman from miscarriage caused by witchcraft a obv. 5–6 // c rev. 5	5–6
iii	Prescription (amulet) to protect a woman from miscarriage caused by witchcraft:	7–13
	– Instructions (a obv. 7–9 // b obv. 4 // c rev. 6)	7–9
	– Incantation: *Āšib ekleti lā āmir nūr Šamaš* (a obv. 10–13 // c rev. 7–8)	10–13
iv	Lamaštu incantation: *Ezzet šamrat ilat namurrat* (a obv. 14–rev. 7 // c rev. 9–24 // d rev. 13–29 // e 1–17)	14–38
	Instruction (a rev. 8 // c rev. 25) to recite spell over the ointment (lines 1–4)	39
v	Catchline and series title a rev. 9–10	40–41
vi	Colophon a rev. 11–14	42–45

Previous Edition and Discussion

Farber 1989a, *Schlaf*, 26f., 112ff. § 39A and §40 (ms. a and b, lines 1–13)
Von Weiher 1988, SpTU 3, 116–123, No. 84 (ms. c)
Farber 2014, *Lamaštu*, 268ff., 298f. (Lamaštu incantation *ezzet šamrat* [mss. a, c, d, e])
Scurlock 1991, *Incognita* 2, 140 (translation)
Polonsky 2006, *Studies Leichty*, 301 fn. 22 (lines 10–11, ms. a)
Besnier 2010, http://oracc.org/cams/gkab/P348688 (ms. c)
Scurlock 2014a, *Sourcebook*, 587–589 (ms. c)
Bosworth 2016, *Infant Weeping*, 51 (translation of lines 10–13, ms. a)
Abusch et al., 2020, CMAwR 3, 60–63 text 5.4 (edition of lines 1–13, mss. a, b, c) and pl. 62 (collations)
Infra text A.2.7 (edition of ms. b), text C.3.4 (edition of ms. c), text C.3.9 (edition of ms. d)

Transliteration

1	a obv. 1	[*ana*] ^{munus}PEŠ$_4$ UŠ$_{11}$.ZU NU TE-*ma šá* Š[À]-*šá* NU ŠUB-[*e*]
	b obv. 1	⸢*ana*⸣ ⸢^{munus}⸣PEŠ$_4$ UŠ$_{11}$.ZU NU TE-*ma ša* ŠÀ-*šá* N[U ŠUB-*e*]
	c rev. 3	*ana* ^{munus}PEŠ$_4$ UŠ$_{11}$.ZU NU TE-*ma ša* ŠÀ-*šá* NU *na*$^!$-*de-e*
2	a obv. 2	^{na4}KUR-*nu* DAB KÙ.GA[N] ^{na4}ŠUBA ⸢SAḪAR⸣-*ru* GEŠTIN.KA$_5$.A HÁD.⸢A⸣
	b obv. 1$^{cont.}$–2	[..] / *ù* ^{giš}GEŠ.TIM.KA$_5$.A ḪÁD.DU
	c rev. 3$^{cont.}$	[ ]
3	a obv. 3	SÚD *ina* MÚD BURU$_5$.ḪABRUD^{ru}.DA^{mušen} NÍTA *ina* Ì.GIŠ ^{giš}ŠUR.MÌN ḪI.ḪI
	b obv. 2$^{cont.}$	SÚD *ina* MÚD BURU$_5$.Ḫ[ABRUD.DA^{mušen} ....]
	c rev. 3$^{cont.}$–4	[...] / *ina* MÚD BURU$_5$.ḪABRUD.DA NÍTA *ina* Ì ^{giš}ŠUR.MÌN ḪI.ḪI-*ma*
4	a obv. 4	ÉN *ez-ze-et šam-rat ana* ŠÀ ŠID-*nu-ma* ŠÉŠ-*ma* TIN-*uṭ*
	b obv. 3	ÉN *ez-ze-et šam-rat ana* ŠÀ ŠID-*nu*-[*ma* ....]
	c rev. 4$^{cont.}$	É[N]
a, b, c		
5	a obv. 5	DIŠ KI.MIN ŠIKA SILA.LÍM.MA *za-qip-tu*$_4$ TI-*qé-ma ina* KUN$_4$ É-*a-ni-tú*
	b	*Omits*
	c rev. 5	DIŠ KI.MIN ŠIKA SILA.LÍM.MA *za-qip-ti* TI-*qé-ma* <*ina*> KUN$_4$ *b*[*i-ta-ni-tú*]
6	a obv. 6	*te-te-mer-ma* GABA *kiš-pi* ⸢*tur*⸣-*rat*
	b	*Omits*
	c rev. 5$^{cont.}$	[ ]
a, c		
7	a obv. 7	DIŠ KI.MIN ^{na4}*šu-u* NÍTA *u* MUNUS *ina* ŠU 15-*šá* KÉ[Š]-*as*
	b obv. 4	----- -------- ^{na4}*šu-u* NÍTA ^{na4}*šu-u* MUNUS *ina* ŠU 15-*šá* KÉ[Š]
	c rev. 6	DIŠ KI.MIN ^{na4}*šu-u* NÍTA *u* MUNUS *ina* ŠU.MIN 15-*šú* KÉŠ
8	a obv. 8	ÉN *a-šib ek-le-ti* 3-*šú ana* UGU ŠID-⸢*nu*⸣-*ma*
	b obv. 4$^{cont.}$	[...]
	c rev. 6$^{cont.}$	ÉN *a-šib ek-let* [..................................]
9	a obv. 9	*kiš-pi* NU TE.⸢MEŠ⸣-*šú*
	b obv. 4$^{cont.}$	[.................................]
	c rev. 6$^{cont.}$	[.................................]
a, b, c		

10	a obv. 10	ÉN *a-šib ek-le-ti la a-m*[*i*]-⸢*ri*⸣ ZÁLAG [^{d}U]TU-*ši*
	c rev. 7	ÉN *a-šib ek-let la a-mi-ru* ZÁLAG ^{d}UTU-*ši*
11	a obv. 11	È-*am-ma ta-*⸢*ta-mar*⸣ ⸢ZÁLAG⸣ ⸢^{d}UTU⸣-[*ši lu*] *né-ḫe-e-ti*
	c rev. 7$^{cont.}$–8	È-*am-ma* I[GI-*mar* ....] / *lu-u né-ḫe-e-ti*
12	a obv. 12	GIN$_7$ A.MEŠ *a-gam-mi lu* ⸢*ṣal-la*⸣-*a-t*[*a* G]IN$_7$ *á*[*r*]-*m*[*e*]-*e šá* MAŠ.DÀ
	c rev. 8$^{cont.}$	GIN$_7$ A.ME *a-gam-me lu-u ṣal-la-ta* GIN$_7$ *ár-*⸢*mé-e šá*⸣ [......]
13	a obv. 13	EN *i-nap-pa-*⸢*ḫu*⸣ ^{d}UTU *pa-šìr-*[*k*]*a* [É]N
	c rev. 8$^{cont.}$	[ ]
a, c		————————————
14	a obv. 14	É[N] ⸢*ez-ze*⸣-[*et*] *šam-rat i-lat na-mur-*[*rat*]
	c rev. 9	ÉN *ez-ze-et šam-rat* DINGIR-*at na-mur-rat*
	d rev. 13	ÉN *ez-ze-et šam-rat i-lat na-mur-rat*
	e 1	[É]N SAL.LA-*et šam-rat* DINGIR-*a*[*t*] ------
15	a obv. 15	[x x x *bar-ba*]*r-rat* DUMU.MUNUS ^{d}*a-n*[*u*]
	c rev. 9$^{cont.}$	*u ši-i bar-bar-rat* DU[MU.MUNUS ....]
	d rev. 13$^{cont.}$	*u ši-i bar-bar-rat* DUMU.MUNUS ^{d}*a-nu*
	e 2	----- [*bar-b*]*a-rat* DUMU.MUNUS ^{d}*a-*[*n*]*im*
16	a obv. 16	[....................]-⸢*ú*⸣ ŠU.MIN-*šá lu-ʾ-*[*tú*]
	c rev. 10	GÌR-*šá An-*[*zu*]-*ú* ŠU.MIN-*šá lu-ʾ-tú*
	d rev. 14	GÌR.MIN-*šú An-zu-ú* ŠU.MIN-*šá lu-ʾ-tú*
	e 2$^{cont.}$–3	G[ÌR- ....] ------- / ŠU.MIN-*šá mu-tum*
17	a obv. 17	[x x x x *da-p*]*i-ni pa-nu-šá šak-*[*nu*]
	c rev. 10$^{cont.}$	*pa-an* UR.MAḪ *da-pi-nu pa-n*[*u-*x x x]
	d rev. 14$^{cont.}$	IGI UR.MAḪ *da-pi-nu* IGI.ME-*šú* GAR-*an*
	e 3$^{cont.}$–4	*pa-a*[*n* ....] ----------------- / *ša-ak-nu*
18	a obv. 18	*i*[*š-tu a-pi i-l*]*am-ma uš-šu-rat pe-re*[*t-su*]
	c rev. 11	*iš-tu a-pi i-lam-ma uš-šu-rat pe-ret-su*
	d rev. 15	*iš-tu a-pi i-lam-ma uš-šú-rat pe-ret-su*
	e 4$^{cont.}$	TA GIŠ.[GI ......] --------- ---------
19	a obv. 19	*bu-*[x x x *di-d*]*a-a-šá ki-bís* GU$_4$ ⸢*il*⸣-[*lak*]
	c rev. 11$^{cont.}$–12	*bu-ut-tu-qa d*[*i-da-a-šú*] / *kib-si* GU$_4$ *il-lak*
	d rev. 15$^{cont.}$–16	*bu-ut-tu-qa di-da-a-šú* / *kib-su* GU$_4$ *il*$^{!}$(GEŠTIN)-*lak*
	e 5	KUD.MEŠ *di*$^{!}$-*da-šá* ------------------------(*omits*)
20	a obv. 20	*ki-bís* [x x *i-red-d*]*e ina* UZU *ù* MÚD ŠU.⸢MIN-*šá*⸣ [*šak-n*]*a*
	c rev. 12$^{cont.}$	*kib-si* UDU.NÍTA UŠ-*de ina* UZU *u* MÚD ŠU.MIN-[*šú* x x]
	d rev. 16$^{cont.}$	*kib-su* UDU.NÍTA *i-red-de i-na* UZU *u* MÚD ŠU.MIN-*šú* : *šak-nu*
	e 5$^{cont.}$–6	----------------------------- *i*[*na*$^{?}$ ......] -------------------- / GAR$^{?}$-*nu*$^{?}$
21	a obv. 21	*a-pa-niš* [...... *ṣ*]*e-ra-niš i-ḫal-lu-*⸢*up*⸣
	c rev. 13	*a-pa-niš* KU$_4$-*ub ṣe-ra-niš i-ḫal-lu-up*
	d rev. 17	*a-pa-niš i-ru-bu ṣe-ra-niš i-ḫal-lu-up*
	e 6$^{cont.}$	*a-pa-niš* KU$_4$-*b*[*u*$^{?}$ ....] -----------
22	a obv. 22	É *ir-r*[*u-ub* É *u*]*ṣ-ṣa bi-la-*⸢*a*⸣-*ni* DUMU.MEŠ-*ki-na*
	c rev. 13$^{cont.}$–14	É KU$_4$ É È *bi-*[x-x] / DUMU.MEŠ-*ki-na*

	d rev. 18–19	*bi-i-tú ir-ru-ub bi-i-tú uṣ-ṣu* / *bí-la-ni* DUMU.MEŠ-*ki-na*
	e 7	--------------- É È *bi-la-n*[*i*$^{?}$ ....]
23	a obv. 23	*lu-še-ni-i*[*q* ... DUMU.MUNUS].MEŠ-*ki-na lu-tar-ri*
	c rev. 14$^{\text{cont.}}$	*lu-še-niq u* DUMU.<MUNUS>.MEŠ-*ki-na lut-t*[*ar-ra*]
	d rev. 19$^{\text{cont.}}$	*lu-še-niq u* DUMU.MUNUS.MEŠ-*ki-na lu-ut-tar-ra*
	e 7$^{\text{cont.}}$–8	--------- / *ù* DUMU.MUNUS.MEŠ-*ki-na lu*$^{?}$*-ut-tar-ri*$^{?}$
24	a obv. 24	*ana pi-i* DUMU.[MUNUS.MEŠ-*ki-n*]*a lu-uš-ti-kan tu-la-a*
	c rev. 15	*a-na pi-i* DUMU.MUNUS.MEŠ-*ki-na lu-uš-tak-ka-na tu-la-a*
	d rev. 20	*a-na pi-i* DUMU.MUNUS.MEŠ-*ki-na lu-uš-tak-ka-na tu-la-a*
	e 8$^{\text{cont.}}$–9	---------------------------------- / *lu-uš*$^{!}$*-tak*$^{?}$*-na* UBUR.MIN-*a-a*
25	a obv. 25	*iš-mé-ši-m*[*a* x x x A]D-*šá am-ma-ku* DUMU.MUNUS ^{d}*a-nim*
	c rev. 15$^{\text{cont.}}$–16	*iš-me-ši-ma* ^{d}*é-*[*a* x x] / *am-ma-ki* DUMU.MUNUS ^{d}*a-nu*
	d rev. 21	*iš-me-ši-ma* ^{d}IDIM AD-*šú am-ma-ki* DUMU.MUNUS ^{d}*a-nim*
	e 9$^{\text{cont.}}$–10	*iš-me-ši-ma* ---- <*i*$^{?}$*-bak*$^{?}$>- / *ki am-ma-ku* DUMU.MUNUS ^{d}*a-nim*
26	a obv. 26	*mu-ut-tar-ra-ta* L[Ú-*t*]*u*$_4$ *tal-ma-di-ma*
	c rev. 16$^{\text{cont.}}$	*mu-ut-tar-ra-at* LÚ-*ut-tu*$_4$ *tal-ma-di-*[*ma*]
	d rev. 21$^{\text{cont.}}$	*mut*$^{!}$*-tar-ra-tú* LÚ-*tú tal-ma-*[*di*]*-ma*
	e 10$^{\text{cont.}}$–11	---------------- *a-mi-* / *lu* ----------
27	a obv. 27	*am-ma-ki ina* UZU [....................]-*ka šak-na*
	c rev. 17	*am-ma-ki ina* UZU *u* MÚD ŠU.MIN-*ki šak-na*
	d rev. 22	*am-ma-ki ina* UZU *u* MÚD ŠU.MIN-*ki šak-nu*
	e 11$^{\text{cont.}}$–12	KI.MIN *ina* UZU *ù* MÚD / ŠU --------------
28	a obv. 28	*am-ma-ki* É *ter-*[*ru-bi*] ⸢É⸣ *tu-ṣi-i*
	c rev. 17$^{\text{cont.}}$	*am-ma-ki* É KU$_4$-*bi* É È
	d rev. 23	*am-ma-ki* É *ter-ru-bu* É *tu-ṣi-i*
	e 12$^{\text{cont.}}$	KI.MIN É KU$_4$-*bi* É ⸢È$^{!}$⸣(UD.<DU>)
29	a obv. 29	*mu-úḫ-ri šá* ^{lú}DAM.[GÀ]R -------------- *ṣi-di-is-su*
	c rev. 18	*mu-uḫ-ri šá* ^{lú}DAM.GÀR *qa-an-na-šú u ṣi-di-is-*[*su*]
	d rev. 24	*mu-uḫ-ri šá* ^{lú}DAM.GÀR *qa-an-na-šú u ṣi-di-is*$^{!}$(*ṣi*)*-su*
	e 13	*mu-uḫ*$^{?}$*-ri šá* DAM.<GÀR> -----------------------
30	a obv. 30	[*m*]*u-úḫ-ri šá* ^{lú}⸢SIMUG⸣ *se-*mé*-ri si-mat* ŠU.MIN-*ki*
	c rev. 19	*mu-uḫ-ri šá* ^{lú}SIMUG *se-mer si-mat* ŠU.MIN-*ki*
	d rev. 25	*mu-uḫ-ri šá* ^{lú}SIMUG *se-me-ri si-mat* ŠU.MIN-*ki*
	e 13$^{\text{cont.}}$–14	KI.MIN *šá* / $^{\text{[l]ú}}$SIMUG$^{?}$ -----------------------------
31	a obv. 31	[*u*] GÌR.MIN-*ki mu-úḫ-ri šá* ^{lú}KÙ.DIM
	c rev. 19$^{\text{cont.}}$–20	*u* GÌR.MIN-*k*[*i*] / *mu-uḫ-ri šá* ^{lú}KÙ.DIM
	d rev. 25$^{\text{cont.}}$–26	*u* GÌR.MIN-*ki* / *mu-uḫ-ri šá* ^{lú}KÙ.DIM
	e 14$^{\text{cont.}}$	----------------- KI.<MIN> *šá* ^{lú}*ku*$^{?}$-<....>
32	a rev. 1	*in-ṣab-tu*$_4$ *si-mat* GEŠTU.MIN-*ki*
	c rev. 20$^{\text{cont.}}$	*in-ṣab-ti si-mat* GEŠTU.MIN-*k*[*i*]
	d rev. 26$^{\text{cont.}}$	*in-ṣa-ab-tú si-mat* GEŠTU.MIN-*ki*
	e 14$^{\text{cont.}}$–15	------------------------------ / [......]
33	a rev. 2	*mu-úḫ-ri šá* ^{lú}BUR.⸢GUL⸣ $^{\text{na4}}$GUG *si-mat* GÚ-*ki*
	c rev. 21	*mu-uḫ-ri šá* ^{lú}BUR.GUL $^{\text{na4}}$GUG *si-mat* GÚ-*ki*
	d rev. 27	*mu-uḫ-ri šá* ^{lú}BUR.GUL $^{\text{na4}}$GUG *si-mat* GÚ-*ki*

	e 15$^{cont.}$	[K]I.MIN *šá* ^{lú}BUR.GUL ------------------------
34	a rev. 3	*mu-úḫ-ri šá* ^{lú}NAGAR ^{giš}GA.RÍG ^{giš}*pi-laq-qu* --------------
	c rev. 22	[*mu-u*]*ḫ-ri šá* ^{lú}NAGAR ^{giš}GA.RÍG ^{giš}BAL *du-di-it-ti šid-di*
	d rev. 28	*mu-uḫ-ri šá* ^{lú}NAGAR ^{giš}GA.RÍG ^{giš}BAL
	e 15$^{cont.}$–16	KI.MIN / [*šá* ^{lú}NAGA]R$^{?}$ -------------------------------------
35	a rev. 4	*ù ki-ri-is-su si-*[*mat*] *qé-e-ki*
	c rev. 23	[*u ki-ri*]*s-su*$^{?}$ *si-mat qé-e-ki* :
	d rev. 28$^{cont.}$	*u du-di-it-ti* <*si-mat qé-e*>*-ki*
	e 16	--------------------------------
36	a rev. 5	*ú-tam-mi-ki* ^{d}*a-num* AD-*ki*
	c rev. 23	*ú-tam-mi-ki* ^{d}*a-nu* AD-*ki*
	d rev. 29	*ú-tam-mi-ki* ^{d}60 AD-*ka*
	e 16$^{cont.}$	*ú-tám-mi-k*[*i* ....]
37	a rev. 6	*ú-tam-mi-ki an-*[*tum*] AMA-*ki*
	c rev. 24	------------ [x x AM]A-*ki*
	d rev. 29$^{cont.}$	------------- *an-tum* AMA-⸢*ka*⸣
	e 16$^{cont.}$	--------------------------------
38	a rev. 7	*ú-tam-mi-ki* ^{d}[*é-a ba-nu-ú*]*-ki* ÉN
	c rev. 24$^{cont.}$	*ú-tam-mi-ki* ^{d}*é-a* DÙ-*ki* TU_6 ÉN
	d rev. 29$^{cont.}$	*ú-tam-mi-ki* ^{d}IDIM *ba-nu-ú* MU-*ki*
	e 17	[.....] (*traces*)

a, c ____

(*Ms. d: bottom of the tablet*)

39	a rev. 8	ÉN *an-n*[*i-*tu_4 x x *nap-šal-t*]*i* ŠID-*nu*
	c rev. 25	[ÉN *an-ni*]*-ti ana* UGU *nap-šal-ti* ŠID-*nu*

a, c ____

Catchline:

40	a rev. 9	DIŠ ^{munus}$PEŠ_4$ [x x x x x-*a*]*ḫ ú-šam-ṣu*
41	a rev. 10	DIŠ NA [*ana* ^{d}*nin-kar-ra-ak*] *pa-qid-m*[*a*]

Ms. a: one line left blank

Colophon:

42	a rev. 11	[*gaba-ri* x x^{k}]^{i} *ki-ma la-bi-*[*ri-šú šaṭer*]
43	a rev. 12	[x x x] *tup-pi* ^{m}*it-ti-*^{d}A[MAR.UTU-*balāṭu*]
44	a rev. 13	A-*šú* ⸢*šá*$^{?!}$⸣ ^{m}x x x x x x x x
45	a rev. 14	*pa-liḫ* ^{d}MUATI NU ⸢TÙM⸣ [x x x x x]

Ms. a: Rest of reverse left blank

Bound Transcription and Translation

[1] *ana erīti kišpī lā ṭeḫê-ma ša libbīša lā nadê* [2] *šadânu ṣābitu lulû šubû eperu (u) karān šēlebi tubbal* [3] *tasâk ina dām iṣṣūr ḫurri zikari ina šaman šurmēni taballal-(ma)* [4] ÉN *ezzet šamrat ana libbi tamannū-ma tapaššaš-ma iballuṭ*	[1] So that witchcraft not come near a pregnant woman and for her not to have a miscarriage (lit. expel her foetus): [2] You dry (and) [3] pound [2] magnetite, antimony, *šubû*-stone, dust (and) 'fox grape'. [3] You mix (these ingredients) with the blood of a male partridge(?) (and) with cypress-scented oil (and) [4] you recite the incantation "She is fierce, she is violent" over it. Then you rub (the woman with it) and she will get well.
[5] DIŠ KI.MIN *ḫaṣabti sūq erbetti zaqiptu teleqqē-ma ina askuppi bītānītu* [6] *tetemmer-ma irat kišpī turrat*	[5] Alternatively, you take an upright-standing potsherd from a crossroads and [6] bury (it) under an inner threshold. Then witchcraft (lit. the breast of witchcraft) will be turned away.
[7] DIŠ KI.MIN *šû zikar u* (var. *šû*) *sinniš ina qāt imittīša tarakkas* [8] ÉN *āšib eklēti šalāšīšu ana muḫḫi tamannū-ma* [9] *kišpī ul iṭeḫḫûšu*	[7] Alternatively, you tie male and female *šû*-'stone' to her right hand. [8] You recite the incantation "Inhabitant of the dark" three times over it. Then [9] witchcraft will not approach her.
[10] ÉN *āšib eklēti lā āmir nūr šamši*	[10] Incantation: "Inhabitant of the dark, who did not see the sunlight –
[11] *tattaṣâm-ma tātamar nūr šamši lū nēḫēti*	[11] you have come out and seen the sunlight. May you be calm
[12] *kīma mê agamme lū ṣallāta kīma armê ša ṣabīti*	[12] like the water of the marshes, may you sleep like the young of a gazelle,
[13] *adi inappaḫu Šamaš pāširk*[*a*] É[N]	[13] until Šamaš rises, the one who releases yo[u]." Incant[ation].
[14] ÉN *ezzet šamrat ilat namurrat*	[14] Incantation: "She is furious, she is violent, she is goddess, she is terrifying
[15] [*u šī*] *barbarat mārat Anu*	[15] [and she] is a she-wolf, the daughter of Anu!
[16] *šēpāša Anzû qātāša lu'tu* (var.: *mūtu*)	[16] Her feet are (those of) Anzû, her hands are decay (var.: death).
[17] *pān nēši dapīni pānūša šaknū*	[17] The face of a ferocious lion is (set as) her face.
[18] *ištu api īlâm-ma uššurat peressa*	[18] She came up from the canebrake, her hair hanging down,
[19] *buttuqā dīdāša kibis alpi illak*	[19] her underwear torn off. She walks in the tracks of the cattle,
[20] *kibis immeri iredde ina šīri u dāmi qātāša šaknā*	[20] she follows the tracks of sheep; her hands are steeped in flesh and blood.
[21] *apāniš irrub ṣerrāniš iḫallup*	[21] She enters through the window, glides in by the door pivot.
[22] *bīta irrub bīta uṣṣi bilāni mārīkina*	[22] She enters the house, she leaves the house (saying): 'Bring (fem. pl.) me your (fem. pl.) sons!
[23] *lušēniq u mārātīkina luttarri*	[23] I want to suckle (them), and of your daughters I want to take care!
[24] *ana pî mārātīkina luštakkana tulâ*	[24] In the mouth of your daughters I want to place my nipples!'
[25] *išmēšī-ma Ea abuša ammaki mārat Anu*	[25] Ea, her father, heard her and (said): 'Instead that you, O daughter of Anu,
[26] *muttarrâta amēlūta talmadī-ma*	[26] kept on acting as a nurse, you should have learned human behaviour, and
[27] *ammaki ina šīri u dāmi qātāki šaknā*	[27] instead of putting your hands in flesh and blood,
[28] *ammaki bīta terrubī bīta tuṣṣî*	[28] instead of entering the house (and) leaving the house,

29 *muḫrī ša tamkāri (qannašu u) ṣidīssu*	29 accept from the merchant his travel provisions (var.: his *purse* and his travel provisions)!
30 *muḫrī ša nappāḫi semerī simat qātīki* 31 *u šēpīki muḫrī ša kutimmi* 32 *inṣabtu simat uznīki*	30 Accept from the smith rings befitting your hands 31 and your feet! Accept from the goldsmith 32 earring(s) befitting your ears!
33 *muḫrī ša purkulli sāmta simat kišādīki*	33 Accept from stonecutter a carnelian befitting your neck!
34 *muḫrī ša naggāri muštâ pilaqqa* 35 *u kirissu* (var. ms. d: *u duditti*; ms. c: *duditti šiddi [u kiri]ssu) simat qêki*	34 Accept from the carpenter a comb, a spindle 35 and a needle (var. ms. d: and a pin; ms. c: a pin, a cloth bale [and a nee]dle) befitting your threads!
36 *utammīki Anu abāki*	36 I conjure you by Anu, your father,
37 *utammīki Antu ummāki*	37 I conjure you by Antu, your mother.
38 *utammīki Ea bānīki* (var.: *bānû šumīki*) (TU$_6$) ÉN	38 I conjure you by Ea, your creator (var.: who creates your name).'" Incantation (formula).
39 *šiptu annītu ana muḫḫi napšalti tamannu*	39 You recite this incantation over the ointment.
Catchline:	
40 *šumma erītu [... ...] ušamṣû*	40 "If a pregnant woman [...], one shall let (her) obtain (what she desires?)".
41 *šumma amēlu [ana Ninkarrak] paqid-m[a]*	41 (Series title): "If a man is handed over [to the goddess Ninkarrak]".
Colophon:	
42 *[gabari ...] kīma labi[rīšu šaṭer]* 43 *[...] tuppi Itti-Mar[duk-balāṭu]* 44 *māršu ša ...... (fragmentary)* 45 *pāliḫ Nabû lā itabbal [...]*	42 [A copy from ...]. [Written] according to its ori[ginal]. 43 [...]. Tablet of Itti-Mar[duk-balāṭu], 44 son/descendant of .... 45 Anyone who reveres Nabû must not carry off (the tablet) [...].

Notes

Line 2: For the reading ⸢SAḪAR⸣-*ru* in ms. a, see the collations by Abusch et al. 2020 (CMAwR 3), pl. 62. I owe the reading GEŠ.TIM in ms. b, representing a syllabic spelling of the logogram GEŠTIN, to Abusch et al. 2020. As they note (ibid., 63 comment on line 2), such spellings indicate that the logograms of common drug names may have been read in Sumerian rather than Akkadian.

Line 5: The ritual of burying an upright-standing potsherd from a crossroads under a threshold of the house symbolises a barrier that should hinder the witchcraft from entering the house. For a similar ritual use of a such a potsherd (in the context of stopping bleeding), see also BAM 237 i 9′–16′; BM 40152 iii 1–5 (texts C.1.4, C.1.8). Potsherds (from a crossroads) are a recurring ingredient in remedies to stop haemorrhage in the women's health texts (e.g. for amulets, tampons, potions), see e.g. STT 241: 6 (text C.3.1); BAM 237 ii 41′–44′, iii 6–7, iv 23, iv 35 (text C.1.4); SpTU 4, No. 153: 14 (text C.1.10).

Line 10: For the reading *a-m[i]-⸢ri⸣* in ms. a, see collation by Abusch et al. 2020 (CMAwR 3), pl. 62.

Line 11–12: The spelling *né-ḫe-e-ti* stands for the 2nd person masc. sg. *nēḫēta.* For the imagery of still water and sleeping gazelle fawns in baby incantations, see Farber 1989a, 155–158; Boswell 2016, *Infant Weeping*, 38, 40.

Lines 14–38: For comments on the incantation, see Farber 2014, 329–330 (text "RA") and the edition of AO 6473 lines 41–57 in the present publication (text C.3.9).

Line 40: For a possible restoration of this catchline, we may compare this entry in the so-called *adi*-section for the treatise PREGNANCY/OFFSPRING in the Assur Medical Catalogue (AMC line 113; Steinert et al. 2018, 218 and 271 commentary). The *adi*-section cites among the topics included in the treatise the following protasis: DIŠ ^{munus}PEŠ$_4$ *i-⸢sa-ap⸣-[pid-(ma) la i-na-a]ḫ*$^?$ "If a pregnant woman m[ourns (and) cannot not cal]m down(?)", which may correspond to the preserved traces of the fragmentary catchline cited here, in BM 42327+. However, the citation in AMC does not include the verb *ú-šam-ṣu*, which leaves the restoration inconclusive. So far, no matching protasis or diagnostic passage could be identified in the women's healthcare texts. For *maṣû* Š-stem in the sense of "to let (someone) obtain, to grant", cf. CAD M/1, 349 sub mng. 7, usually in the phrase *mala/ammar libbi šumṣû* "to let someone obtain his/her heart's desire". The other meanings of *maṣû* Š-stem, "to make equal; to make suffice; to use sufficient quantities of ingredients (in the preparation of a remedy)" do not fit the present context very well.

Line 41: For the title of the therapeutic sub-series or treatise cited here (dubbed PREGNANCY/OFFSPRING), see the Assur Medical Catalogue (AMC line 109 and 111, see Steinert et al. 2018, 217, 269–270), where it is listed together with apotropaic rituals to save a man's children from dying and a woman from miscarriage due to witchcraft. Although there are positive phrases with *paqādu* "to entrust, to hand over", e.g. *ana qāt ilišu p.* "to entrust somebody to the hand of his god", the incipit here has a negative meaning. Ninkarrak as a hypostasis of the healing goddess Ninisina/Gula is here associated with the sickness or death of offspring in a man's house. This link is underlined by the mention of Gula among the responsible agents of infant illness or death in SpTU 3, No. 84 rev. 26 (ms. c, line 79), a text certainly representing material from the section PREGNANCY and a partial duplicate to BM 42327+ (see *infra* text C.3.4). Moreover, Ninkarrak was an oath goddess, and the recurring infant deaths were also explained as punishment for swearing a false oath (since the "Ban" (*māmītu*) is among the causes listed in SpTU 3, No. 84). For Ninkarrak, see Westenholz 2010; Böck 2014, 11–12; Sibbing-Plantholt 2022, 106–123.

For similar uses of *paqādu* in healing texts, compare the following examples: LKA 89 rev. iv 4′ (catchline, Abusch and Schwemer 2016, CMAwR 2, text 8.25 ms. B): DIŠ NA NU.MEŠ-*šu ana* ^{lú}UG$_7$ *paqdū* "if figurines representing a person are handed over to a dead man"; Abusch and Schwemer 2011, CMAwR 1, text 8.1: 8–9: NU.MEŠ-*šú … ana Ereškigal paqdū* "figurines of him have been handed over to Ereškigal" (cf. ibid. text 8.3: 2). For a singular stative form see e.g. Biggs 1967, 68: 3′: [DIŠ KI.MI]N *ana* GIDIM *paqid* "Alternatively, he has been handed over to a ghost"; *Diagnostic Handbook* Tablet 16 line 10 (Heeßel 2000, 172; Scurlock 2014a, 151): *ana gallê mūti paqid* "he has been handed over to a *gallû*-demon of death"; also Köcher, Oppenheim and Güterbock 1957–1958, *AfO* 18, 65 VAT 7525 ii 13 (Old Babylonian physiognomic omens): *awīlum šû ana qātī mūtim paqid* "that man has been handed over into the hands of Death".

Lines 43–44: There are several scribes and scholars known from colophons with the name Itti-Marduk-balāṭu (see Hunger 1968, 150), but due to the badly damaged filiation in line 44, it is still not possible to identify the scribe/owner of BM 42327+ with certainty. For Neo-/ Late Babylonian attestations of the name, see https://prosobab.leidenuniv.nl/list.php.

Bácskay and Simkó (2021, *Iraq* 83, 183–203) recently published two medical tablets (BM 30918 and BM 31071) that mention Itti-Marduk-balāṭu, a member of the prominent Babylonian Egibi family, as their owner. This Itti-Marduk-balāṭu (whose father Nabû-aḫḫē-iddin also had received scribal training and served as a royal judge of Nabonidus in Babylon) was active in the second half of the 6th century BCE and was known so far mainly through his business activities. In the colophon of BM 30918, he is called an incantation priest (*mašmaššu*). For more information on his activities and relations to scholarship, see Wunsch 2000, 12–15; Spar and van Dassow 2000, CTMMA 3, LXXVII, Nos. 54, 56–63; Bácskay and Simkó (2021, *RA* 83, 184–186, 193–194). He might be identical with the Itti-Marduk-balāṭu of BM 42327+.

Note for a further namesake (but from a much later time), Itti-Marduk-balāṭu (II), son of Iddin-Bēl (II), a descendent of the Mušēzib family, who was an astrologer of the Esagil temple at Babylon active in the second century BCE. He wrote BM 33333B (dated to 177/176 BCE), a tablet with board game instructions (Finkel 2008b, 29–30; the name is spelled ^{m}KI-^{d}ŠÚ-TIN); Wee 2018, *FS Geller*, 842). For a reconstruction of the family tree and the career of Itti-Marduk-balāṭu (II), see Oelsner 2000, 802–811, 814; on the offices of Itti-Marduk-balāṭu, cf. Boiy 2004, 175–176, 211, 259–260, 273; Frahm 2011, 307; for a fragment of Tablet X of the *Gilgamesh Epic* tablet owned by Itti-Marduk-balāṭu (II), see George 2003, 740. See also Clancier 2009a, 174.

For Itti-Marduk-balāṭu, son of Mušallim-Marduk, an exorcist from Uruk and scribe of a copy of Tablet 37 of the *Diagnostic Handbook*, see *infra*, Chapter 2.1.

C.3.4 SpTU 3, No. 84: A Collection of Rituals for the Protection of Pregnant Women and their Offspring

This Late Babylonian tablet from Uruk was written by the exorcist Šamaš-iddina, a member of the Šangû-Ninurta family, and belonged to the library of his son Anu-ikṣur, who was active in the late fifth century BCE (Clancier 2009a, 58–59). It contains a collection of rituals and prescriptions to protect parents from losing their offspring, unborn or born. Two sections of the tablet are destined for the protection of pregnant women from miscarriage (lines 1–16 and 56–78), while the other sections concern rituals for a man or a household in which the children have either died, keep on dying or are often sick. The misfortune is attributed to different causes, especially to witchcraft, to punishment by the "Ban" (caused by a broken oath), to the demoness Lamaštu and the healing goddess Gula. The material contained in SpTU 3, No. 84 is related to a treatise (or sub-series) of therapeutic material known from the so-called Assur Medical Catalogue by the title *Šumma amēlu ana Ninkarrak paqid* "If a man is handed over to Ninkarrak" (Steinert et al. 2018, 217 *passim* PREGNANCY / OFF-SPRING), but also uses incantations thematically related to or drawn from other collections and genres of incantations/ rituals, such as rituals to calm a crying baby and rituals against Lamaštu.

The six rituals preserved on the tablet are either performed for the pregnant woman (lines 1–16 and 56–78), or for the head of the household and/or a child/baby (lines 17–23, 24–36, 37–55, 79–97). The first section (lines 1–16) of the tablet contains a ritual to protect a pregnant woman from miscarriage due to the attack of Lamaštu, in which a strangled lamb serves as the substitute for the future babies the woman will conceive and is given to a figurine of Lamaštu which is sent off to the netherworld by boat.

The second section (lines 17–23) is a ritual for a man whose children have died and who wants to avoid the same misfortune happening to the next child. The ritual shares similarities with practices attested in anti-witchcraft rituals: a bag is filled with different materials and placed in an abandoned street, to be picked up by unsuspecting passers-by. As the recitations in the ritual illustrate, the bag is used as a "substitute" for the child, while simultaneously playing the role of a vehicle carrying the evil that affects the unfortunate household head. Thus, it was hoped that the evil would be transferred to the person who picked up the bag.

The third section of SpTU 3, No. 84 (ms. a, lines 24–36) with a Sumerian incantation to the mother goddess Ninmaḫ has a parallel in a Neo-Assyrian tablet from Assur (LKA 142 associated with the library N4, ms. B). The latter tablet contains a second incantation prayer whose incipit is cited as the catchline of SpTU 3, No. 84 (line 98).

The fourth section of ms. a (lines 37–55) is duplicated in a Neo-Assyrian tablet from Sultantepe (STT 254, ms. C) and is concerned with undoing the "Ban" (due to a broken oath, *māmītu*) bound to a man with the effect that his children keep dying or are often sick. The text from Sultantepe preserves two more rituals not included in ms. a: another short ritual to protect a baby and a ritual against the evil effects of a "bag of sorceries" encountered in one's environment (Abusch and Schwemer 2011, CMAwR 1, text 11.2). The ritual dealing with the "Ban" uses figurines which represent the patient's family, to which the evil affecting the patient was transferred and which were then handed over to the river as substitutes for the patient and his living family members. One of the recitations uttered by the patient indicates that his ancestors were believed to be the cause of the patient's misfortune (i.e. a "ban" incurred by the parents and grandparents was inherited by the patient).

The fifth section of SpTU 3, No. 84 (lines 56–78) containing prescriptions and incantations for a pregnant woman to avoid miscarriage caused by witchcraft is duplicated in three other Late Babylonian texts (in part or whole). Ms. d (BM 42327+) and ms. f (AO 6473) focus entirely on the topic of protecting pregnant women, but the latter contains further prescriptions for amulets worn on the body. In ms. e (BM 51246+) only the prescriptions were written down, but the incantations (a baby-spell and a Lamaštu spell) recited with them are omitted. However, ms. e continues with an extract of other prescriptions for women's health issues not duplicated elsewhere (for mss. d, e and f see further texts C.3.3, A.2.7 and C.3.8).

The sixth and last section of SpTU 3, No. 84 contains another ritual to save a man's children, if they keep dying or are sick. The procedure involved making a figurine representing the "robber" of the offspring, which was to be buried at specific places (such as the city wall), thus being ritually banned to the Netherworld. The procedure included offerings to Ursa Major and the mother goddess Ninmaḫ who are seen as protective divine forces. Different possible causes for the treated problem are enumerated that could be addressed with the ritual: the Hand of Gula, the Hand of Lamaštu, the Hand of an opponent (i.e. witchcraft) or the "Ban".

List of Manuscripts

Siglum	Museum Number	Copy	Collation	Format; Ductus	Provenience
a	IM 76849 W. 23287	SpTU 3, No. 84	Photo coll.	Single-column tablet in portrait format; Late Babylonian script; 5th cent. BCE	Uruk, Library of Anu-ikṣur
B	A 177	LKA 142	Photo coll.	Single-column tablet; Neo-Assyrian script, 8th/7th cent. BCE	Assur, library N4
C	SU 51/13	STT 254	Photo coll.	Single-column tablet in landscape format; Neo-Assyrian script, 7th cent. BCE	Sultantepe
d	BM 42327 + 42410 + 42604 + 42628 + 43474 + 43523 (81-7-1, 87 + 170 + 365 + 389 + 1238 + 1287)	Farber 1989a, pl. 14–15	Coll.	Single-column tablet; Late Babylonian script, 6th–3rd cent. BCE	Babylonia, exact provenience unknown
e	BM 51246 + 53217 + 53744 (82-3-23, 2242 + 4251 + 4784)	Pl. 20	Coll.	Fragment of a single-column tablet; Late Babylonian script, 6th–3rd cent. BCE	probably Sippar
f	AO 6473	Thureau-Dangin, *RA* 18, 162–163 *TCL* 6, 49	Coll.	Single-column tablet; Late Babylonian script; 3rd–2nd cent. BCE)	Uruk
g		Nougayrol, *Syria* 42, p. 228 (photo)	-	Amulet	modern forgery after lost original

Overview

i Ritual for a woman who has had repeated miscarriages due to the attacks of Lamaštu, to help her give birth to healthy babies: 1–16
- Instructions to fashion a figurine of Lamaštu (a obv. 1–7)
- Recitation addressed to Šamaš (a obv. 8)
- Instructions for an offering (a obv. 9)
- Recitation (a obv. 10–11)
- Instructions for offering to Šamaš and disposal of the figurine (a obv. 12–14)
- Incantation (a obv. 15–16)

ii Ritual for a man whose children have died: 17–23
- Instructions for preparation of a bag filled with materials deposited in an abandoned street (a obv. 17–19, 22), with recitations by the man (a obv. 20–21, 23)

iii Ritual to protect a surviving son with Sumerian incantation to Ninmaḫ (a obv. 24–36 // B obv. 1–18): 24–36
- Instructions for preparation of an offering and for wiping the child off with dough (a obv. 24–26 // B obv. 1–5)
- Incantation to Ninmaḫ (a obv. 27–34 // B obv. 6–16)
- Instructions for ritual disposal and purification (a obv. 35–36 // B obv. 17–18)

iv Ritual to protect a family whose children keep dying or are often sick (caused by the ban due to a broken oath) (a obv. 37–rev. 2 // C obv.! 1–20): 37–55

- Instruction for making seven figurines (representing the patient's family) and for a ritual at a river meadow (including offerings on seven altars) (a obv. 37–43 // C obv.! 1–6)
- Recitation (introducing tamarisk as purifying agent) (a obv. 44–46 // C obv.! 7–9)
- Washing of the patient over the figurines and address to the river (a obv. 47–48 // C obv.! 10–12)
- Washing of the patient standing on tamarisk and soapwort with recitation; disposal of figurines (a obv. 49–51 // C obv.! 13–16)
- Recitation of incantation *addinka* <*ana*> *pūḫīya* with purification of the patient by washing with tamarisk water, anointing and fumigation with censer and torch; recitation of incantation a-ab-ba ama diĝir-re-e-ne (a obv. 52–rev. 2 // C obv.! 17–20)

v Prescription (ointment) to protect a woman from miscarriage caused by witchcraft: 56–57
a rev. 3–4 // d obv. 1–4 // e obv. 1–3

vi Prescription to protect a woman from miscarriage caused by witchcraft 58
a rev. 5 // d obv. 5–6

vii Prescription (amulet) to protect a woman from miscarriage caused by witchcraft: 59–61

- Instructions (a rev. 6 // d obv. 7–9 // e obv. 4)
- Incantation: *Āšib eklēti lā āmir nūr Šamaš* (a rev. 7–8 // d obv. 10–13)

viii Lamaštu incantation: *Ezzet šamrat ilat namurrat* 62–78
(a rev. 9–24 // d obv. 14–rev. 7 // f rev. 13–29 // g 1–17)
Instruction (a rev. 25 // d rev. 8) to recite spell over the ointment (in lines 56–57)

ix Ritual to save the children of a man whose children keep dying or are often sick (a rev. 26–44): 79–97

- Instructions for making a figurine of the evil attacking the children and for setting up an offering before the Wagon star and for Ninmaḫ (a rev. 26–37)
- Recitation and instructions for burying the figurine (a rev. 38–44)

x Catchline (a rev. 45 // B obv. 19) 98

xi Colophon of Šamaš-iddina, son of Nādinu, of the Šangû-Ninurta family (a rev. 46–47) 99–100

Previous Edition and Discussion

Reiner and Civil 1967, *JNES* 26, 192 (comments on ms. C)
Von Weiher 1988, SpTU 3, 116–123 (ms. a)
Farber 1989a, *Schlaf*, 26–27, 112ff. § 39A and §40 (mss. c and d, lines 56–61)
Farber 1989b, 224–232 (corrections and remarks on ms. a)
Foster 2005, 981–982 (translation of the incantation against Lamaštu, *ezzet šamrat ilat namurrat*, lines 62–78)
Farber 2014, *Lamaštu*, 35–36, 277, 308–309, 335–336 (edition of ms. a, lines 1–16) and 51, 268–270, 298–299 ("RA", edition of lines 62–77)
Scurlock 2014a, 587–589 (lines 56–78)
Scurlock 2014b, 127–128 (translation of lines 1–16)
Besnier 2010, http://oracc.org/cams/gkab/P348688 (edition of ms. a)
Abusch et al. 2020 (CMAwR 3), 59–63 text 5.4 (edition of lines 56–61; mss. a, c, d)
CDLI P348688 (copy ms. a); P414051 (ms. B)
Infra text C.3.3 (edition of ms. d), text A.2.7 (edition of ms. e), text C.3.9 (edition of ms. f)

Summary of the sections in ms. C (STT 254) not included in the transliteration:

Rev.! 1–5: Ritual against evil threatening a baby (see Reiner and Civil 1967, *JNES* 67, 192 for comments, and below)

Rev.! 6–21: Anti-witchcraft ritual against the evil induced by contact with "a sack of sorceries" (*narūq upšāšê*) (// A. 3471) (edited in Abusch and Schwemer 2011, CMAwR 1, text 11.2)

Rev.! 22: Catchline and colophon:
[DIŠ NA NU].MEŠ-*šú ana a-ra-le-e pa-*<*aq*>*-du* : D[UB *šá*? EG]IR-*šú* SAR "[If figurines representing a man] have been handed over to the Netherworld" – (this is) the tab[let that] is (to be) written [after]wards."

Transliteration

1	a obv. 1	[DIŠ MUNUS$^?$ x x x x x x x x x x] KAR.MEŠ *ana* KAR NITA *u* MUNUS ⸢*e*⸣-*nu-ma*
2	a obv. 2	[x x x x NU DUMU.MUNUS ^{d}*a-nim šá*] IM *ú-šal*$^!$-*li* ÍD DÙ-*u*[*š*]
3	a obv. 3	[x x x x x x x x x x] *ana* ŠU-*šá* GAR ^{dug}BUR.ZI.GAL I[M] DIRI-*ma* GAR-*an*
4	a obv. 4	[x x x x x x x x x x GAR]-*an-ši*$^!$ SILA$_4$ *ta-ḫa-naq-ma* SAG.DU-*su* NU KUD-*is*
5	a obv. 5	[x x x x x x x] x ⸢*ki*⸣-*ma* LÚ.TUR TÚG.ḪI.A *tu-kar-rak-šú* DIŠ-*niš ḫi-ši-iḫ-tú*
6	a obv. 6	[x x x x x x x] x-*ma ina* GÚ ÍD GAR-*an* NÍG.NA ^{šim}LI
7	a obv. 7	[GAR-*an* ... *ana* IGI ^{d}UTU] UR$_5$.GIM DU$_{11}$.GA
8	a obv. 8	[*mu-ša*]*p*-⸢*šir*$^{?!}$⸣ ⸢ŠÀ⸣.ḪUL *mu-paṭ-ṭir ár-ni at-ta am-me-ni* ŠÀ.ḪUL *ta-ba-an-ni am-me-ni la* DU$_8$.DU$_8$ *an-ni-ia*
9	a obv. 9	3-*šú* DU$_{11}$.GA-*ma* MUNUS BI KAŠ BAL-*qí* SILA$_4$ *a-na bi-rit tu-le-šú* ŠUB-*di* UR$_5$.GIM DU$_{11}$.GA
10	a obv. 10	*e-ri ul ú-šal-lim ú-lid ul ab-ni mu-šal-lim-tu lim-ḫu-ra-an-ni*
11	a obv. 11	*u ba-ni-ti li-iš-šu-ra* <*šá*> *e-li-ía ana-ku lu-ši-ir u lu-še-ši-ir ina* É *áš*$^!$-*ba*$^!$-*ku* (*ba áš ku*)
12	a obv. 12	3-*šú* DU$_{11}$.GA-*ma* KAŠ.SAG *ina* ZÌ ŠE.SA.A *ana* IGI ^{d}UTU BAL-*qí* SILA$_4$ UR$_4$-*šá i-maḫ-ḫar-ši-ma*
13	a obv. 13	*ana* ÚR-*šá* GAR-*an-ma ana* KU$_4$ *šam-ši* DU-*ma* NU DUMU.MUNUS ^{d}*a-nu u mim-ma ma-la taš-ku-nu*
14	a obv. 14	*ana* ŠÀ ^{giš}MÁ GAR-*an-ma ana e-ber-ti* ÍD *tu-še-ber* ZÌ.SUR.[R]A NIGIN-*ši u* ÉN *an-ni-ti* ŠID-*nu*
15	a obv. 15	KUR *u* ÍD [*t*]*a-ma-ti u* NA$_4$ *zaq-ra-ti* AN *u* KI ^{d}*a*-⸢*num*$^?$⸣ ⸢*ù*$^{?!}$⸣ *an*-⸢*tum*⸣ ⸢AMA$^?$⸣ AD-*šú* TU.UD.DA LÚ.⸢ÙLU⸣ BI
16	a obv. 16	[*i*]*š-tu i-na-an-ni ana* NENNI-*tu*$_4$ DUMU NENNI-*tu*$_4$ DU-*ki-ma ana* É *áš-ba-t*[*u*$_4$] ⸢*ter-ru-bi-ma*⸣ *an-nu-tì tum-ma-ta*
17	a obv. 17	[DIŠ] NA *mi-iḫ-ri ma-ḫi-ir* DUMU.MEŠ-*šú* UG$_7$-*tu*$_4$ *e-nu-ma* DUMU-*šú it*-⸢*ta*$^?$-'*i*$^?$-*id-ma*$^?$⸣
18	a obv. 18	[BU]R$^{?!}$ *ta-na-suk-ma ḫu-pa-a* TIL *ta-nap-pa-al-ma* ⸢NA⸣ ⸢BI⸣ *mim-mu* ŠUB ⸢*i*$^?$-*pa*$^?$-*aḫ*$^?$-*ḫar*$^?$⸣
19	a obv. 19	[*uk*$^?$]-*la-ti-šú it-ti-šú ana* ŠÀ ^{kuš}A.GÁ.LÁ GAR-*ma* ⸢x x x⸣ kud$^?$-*ma* NA$^?$ BI ⸢TA$^?$⸣ [É] ⸢*ana*⸣ ⸢SILA⸣ ⸢È$^?$⸣ \ GIN$_7$ DU-⸢*ku*$^?$⸣ *kam* D[U$_{11}$.GA$^?$]
20	a obv. 20	[*ki-mu*]-*ú mi-iḫ-ri am-ḫu-ru* ÍL-*ku* GI[N$_7$ *a*]*m-ḫu-ru lim-ḫu-ru-n*[*in-ni* x x x x]
21	a obv. 21	[*šá*$^?$] ÍL-*ú ina* ŠU.MIN-*ía lim-ḫu-ru-nin-ni* <*šá*$^?$> ÍL-*ú su-qu lim*-⸢*ḫur*⸣-⸢*šú*$^?$⸣ ⸢*lu-ú*$^?$⸣ x x x x
22	a obv. 22	[GI]N$_7$$^?$-⸢*ma*⸣ DU$_{11}$.GA *ina* SILA ŠUB-*i* GAR-*ma kam* DU$_{11}$.GA
23	a obv. 23	[*ana pu-uḫ*$^?$] *ma-ri-ia ad-din-ka* DU$_{11}$.GA-*ma ana* EGIR-*šú* NU IGI.BAR SILA ⸢DU$^!$⸣-*ku*$^!$ NU ⸢DU-*ak*$^!$⸣ KI MUNUS BAR-*t*[*ì*] NU DU$_{11}$-*ma ana* É-*šú* SI.SÁ
24	a obv. 24 B obv. 1–2	[DIŠ LÚ.TUR$^?$] *mi-ḫi-ir-šú i-te-ti-iq-šú ana* ḪUL NU TE-*e mim-ma* ḪUL NU DIM$_4$ [x x x x x] *mi-ḫi-ir-šú e-te*-⸢*te*⸣-*eq-š*[*u*] / [x x x x x] *mim-ma lem-ni la sa-na-qí-m*[*a*]
25	a obv. 25	[GIN$_7$ ^{d}UTU S]AR-*ḫa* ÙR SAR A KÙ SUD KEŠDA KÉŠ LÚ.TUR *šú-a-ti ana* IGI ⸢KEŠDA⸣

	B obv. 3–4	[x x x x x] *it-tap-ḫa* ÙR *ta-šá-bit* A KÙ SU[D] / [x x x x x] *šu-a-ti*$^{!}$ *ana* IGI *rík-si*
26	a obv. 26	[x x x x]-*šú* NÍG.SILA$_{11}$.GÁ *tu-kap-pa-<ar>-šú kam* DU$_{11}$.G[A]
	B obv. 4–5	*tul-ta-za-as-su-ma* / [x x x *tu*]-*kap-par-šu* UR$_5$.GIM DU$_{11}$.G[A]

27	a obv. 27	[x x x ^{d}n]in-maḫ an-na nin kur-kur-ra-k[e$_4$]
	B obv. 6	[x x x]x ^{d}nin-maḫ an-na gub-ba nin kur-kur-r[a-ke$_4$]
28	a obv. 28	[x x (x) ur$^{?}$]-saĝ ^{d}šul-pa-è-a an-na gub-ba
	B	(*omits*)
29	a obv. 29	[mul á zi-d]a gub-ba mul á gùb-bu gub-ba níĝ-nam ḫul-lu-bi
	B obv. 7–8	[x x x x] gub-ba mul á gùb-bu gub-b[a] / ⸢x x⸣ [x x]
30	a obv. 30	[ḫé-em-ma-ra]-è : gaba-ri gaba-ri-bi-šè ḫé-em-ma-ra-è
	B obv. 8$^{cont.}$–9	ḫé-em-ma-ra-⸢è⸣ / ⸢gaba⸣-r[i gaba-r]i$^{?}$-bi-šè ḫé-em-me-a-⸢è⸣
31	a obv. 31	[x x]-⸢ga⸣ ⸢kur-kur$^{?}$⸣-ra ḫé-em-ma-ra-è : ^{d}i-gi$_4$-gi$_4$ ga-ta gaba-ri ⸢ḫé-em-ma-ra-è⸣
	B obv. 10–12	x x ⸢du$_{11}$$^{?}$-ga$^{?}$⸣ kur-kur ḫé-em-ma-ra-è / ⸢lú-gig⸣ ⸢íb$^{?}$⸣ ⸢dumu$^{?}$-ga$^{?}$⸣ niĝin ḫé-em-ma-ra-⸢è⸣ / ⸢i$^{?}$-gi-gi⸣ <ga>-ta$^{?}$ gaba-ri ḫul$^{!}$ ḫé-em-ma-ra-è
32	a obv. 32	[^{d}ni]n$^{?}$-maḫ níĝ nam-lú-u$_{18}$-lu saĝ-gi$_6$-ga níĝ-dím-dím-[ma]
	B obv. 13	⸢diĝir-maḫ⸣ níĝ-dím nam-lú-u$_{18}$-lu-ka gig-ga níĝ-dím-dím-[ma]
33	a obv. 33	[x x d]u$_{11}$-ga-bi ḫé-em-ma-ra-è : níĝ-gig lú gur-⸢ra$^{?}$⸣ ⸢lú$^{?}$⸣-tur-bi ⸢im⸣-m[a$^{?}$-x x x]
	B obv. 14–15	ur$^{!}$-gin$_7$ du$_{11}$-ga-bi ḫé-em-ma-ra-[è] / ⸢sa⸣ ⸢ḫuĝ-ĝá⸣ ⸢lú-tur⸣ ḫé-ti mu-ni-in-ĝar [x (x)]
34	a obv. 34	[x x] in-nú : diĝir-maḫ ka-tar-zu ḫé-en-s[i-il-e-en]
	B obv. 16	⸢íl⸣ x ⸢ra$^{?}$⸣ ⸢diĝir$^{?}$⸣-maḫ ka-tar-zu ḫé-en-si-il-[e-en]

a, B

35	a obv. 35	[3-*šú*] DU$_{11}$.GA-*ma* A *u* KAŠ BAL-*qí ku-pi-ra-ti-šú* <*ana*> ÍD$^{!}$(AD) Š[UB$^{!}$-*di*$^{?}$]
	B obv. 17	3-*šú* ŠID-*nu-ma* A KAŠ BAL-*qí ku-pi-ra-ti-šú ana* ÍD Š[UB-*di*]
36	a obv. 36	[(x) *t*]*úl-lal-šú-ma mim-ma lem-nu ana* LÚ.TU[R NU TE]
	B obv. 18	[*tu-u*]*l-lal-ma mim-ma lem-nu* LÚ.TUR.ŠÈ NU TE.G[Á]

a, B (*single ruling in* B)

37	a obv. 37	[DIŠ NA] DUMU.MEŠ-*šú* UG$_7$.UG$_7$-*tu$_4$ lu* GIG.ME-*šú ma-a'-du lu* x[x x x]
	C obv.$^{!}$ 1	[DIŠ NA x x x U]G$_7$.UG$_7$-*tú* GIG.MEŠ-*š*[*ú m*]*a-a'-du* ZI.GA ÌR *u* GÉME GAR-*šú*
38	a obv. 38	[*lu*] *ḫu-lu-uq-šú ma-a'-du lu* NAM.ÉRIM x[x x x x]
	C obv.$^{!}$ 1–2	*lu ḫ*[*u*$^{?}$-x x x] *ma-a'-da* / [x x NAM.É]RIM DAB-⸢*su*⸣

a

39	a obv. 39	[^{lú}]MU$_7$$^{!}$.MU$_7$$^{!}$ *ina* GI$_6$ A.GÚB.BA GUB-*an ina še-rim* 7 NU Ì.[UDU x x x DÙ-*uš*]
	C obv.$^{!}$ 2$^{cont.}$	⸢$^{lú!}$MAŠ⸣.MAŠ *ina* GI$_6$ ^{dug}A.GÚB.BA GUB-*an* 7 N[U.(MEŠ) Ì.UDU x]x DUḪ.LÀL DÙ-*uš*
40	a obv. 40	[*ina*] *ú-šal-li* ÍD KI GÌR *pár-sat* KI SAR A KÙ SUD 7 GI.DU$_8$$^{!}$(DU).[MEŠ$^{?}$ x x x x x x]
	C obv.$^{!}$ 3	[x x x Í]D KI GÌR KUD-*at* K[I S]AR A KÙ.GA SUD 7 GI.DU$_8$ *ana* I[GI ÍD G]UB-*an*
41	a obv. 41	*ana* ^{d}DÌM.ME GAR-*an* ZÚ.LUM.MA ZÌ.EŠA DUB-*aq* NINDA.Ì.D[É.A LÀL Ì.NUN.NA GAR-*an*]
	C obv.$^{!}$ 4	[x x x] ⸢7⸣.TA$^{!}$.ÀM NINDA.DIM$_x$(RAB-GAM-KÁM) GAR-*an* ZÚ.LUM.MA ZÌ.EŠA-*a*$^{?}$ [x x NINDA.Ì.(-)D]É$^{!}$(MURUB$_4$).A ⸢LÀL⸣ Ì.NUN GAR-*an*
42	a obv. 42	7 NÍG.NA ^{šim}LI GAR-*an* 7 ^{dug}LA.ḪA.AN SÁḪAR.MEŠ KAŠ.S[AG DIRI-*ma* GUB-*an* x x x]
	C obv.$^{!}$ 5	[x x x ^{šim}L]I GAR-*an* 7 ^{dug}LA.ḪA.AN SÁḪAR.MEŠ KAŠ.⸢SAG$^{!}$⸣ ⸢DIRI-*ma*$^{?}$⸣ ⸢GUB⸣-[*an* (x) x x].DA

43 a obv. 43 ZÌ.DUB.DUB.BU ŠUB.ŠUB-*di* GIN$_7$ *an-nam ana* IGI ÍD KÉŠ-*su* B[AL$^?$ x x x x UR$_5$.GIM DU$_{11}$.GA]
C obv.$^!$ 6 [x x x x] ŠUB GIN$_7$ *an-nam ana* IGI ÍD KÉŠ-*su* BAL-*tú* BAL-*qí-ma* [x x x x] ⸢UR$_5$.GIM⸣ DU$_{11}$.GA

---

44 a obv. 44 *ana-ku* ŠINIG *a-ḫu-ú šá e-diš-ši-šú iz-za-az-zu ana-ku* x[x x x x x x x x x x]
C obv.$^!$ 7 [x x x x] ⸢*a-ḫu*⸣*-ú* <<Ú>> *ša e-diš-ši-šú* GUB$^{!?}$*-zu*$^{!?}$:$^?$ *ana-ku* ^{giš}ŠINIG *a-ḫu-u*

45 a obv. 45 *šá taṣ-bu-ru ú-ru-ú-a ša la-di-ni-ia la i-*[x x x x x x x x x x x]
C obv.$^!$ 7$^{cont.}$–8 *šá*$^{!?}$(A) *ta*$^?$-x[x x x x]-*ia ana-ku* / [x x x *šá*$^?$ *bu*]*-ul* ^{d}ŠÁKKAN *ig-mu-ru*$^{!?}$(RI) *la-ri-ia* <<*šá*>>

46 a obv. 46 *a-na-ku lu-ub-ki ana* BIR-*ti qim-ma-ti-ia* : GIN$_7^?$ [x x x x x x x x x x]
C obv.$^!$ 8$^{cont.}$–9 *ana-ku lu-ub-ki ana* BIR-*t*[*i qim-ma*]*-ti-ia* / [x x x x G]IN$_7$ *ir-re-e ma la at at*$^?$-x[x x]-*ri*

a, C

---

47 a obv. 47 *an-nam* DU$_{11}$.GA-*ma ana* UGU NU Ì.UDU A *i-r*[*a-am-muk* x x x x x UR$_5$.GIM DU$_{11}$.GA]
C obv.$^!$ 10 [x x x x]-*ma*$^?$ *ana* UGU NU Ì.UDU A.MEŠ TU$_5^!$ NU *šú-nu-ti ana a-aḫ* ÍD [x]-*ma* UR$_5$.GIM DU$_{11}$.GA

a, C

---

48 a obv. 48 *at-ta* ÍD *šá tab-ni-i a-me-lu-tú* 7 NU.MEŠ [x x x x x x x x x x x x x]
C obv.$^!$ 11 [x x x x x x *a-m*]*e-lu-tú* 7 NU *an-nu-ti šá kim-ti-ia*$_5$ NUMUN$^?$-*ia*$_5$ ⸢*u*$^?$⸣ ⸢*sa-la*⸣-[*ti-ia*$_5$] x x[x] x[x]
C obv.$^!$ 12 [x x x x x]x *mu-uḫ-ri-ni-ma* [x x]x x[x x]

a, C

---

49 a obv. 49 *an-nam* DU$_{11}$.GA-*ma ina* UGU ŠINIG ^{ú}IN$_6$.Ú[Š x x x x x x x x x x x UR$_5$.GIM DU$_{11}$.GA]
C obv.$^!$ 13 [x x x x x x x] ⸢$^{giš?!}$*bi*$^?$*-ni*$^?$⸣ ⸢$^{ú?}$IN$_6$.ÚŠ⸣ ⸢GAR$^?$-*an*⸣ [x x GU]B$^?$-*an ina* UGU-⸢*šú-nu*$^?$⸣ [GU]B-⸢*zu*⸣ A.MEŠ T[U$_5$-*m*]*a*$^?$ ⸢7⸣ *u*$^!$ 7-*šú* UR$_5$.GIM DU$_{11}$.GA

a, C

---

50 a obv. 50 *ma-mit a-bi-ía ma-mit a-bi a-bi-ia* [x x x x x x x x x x x x x x x x x]
C obv.$^!$ 14 [x x x x x x x *ma-mit*] ⸢AMA⸣-*ia*$_5$ AMA AMA-*ia*$_5$ *l*[*u* B]ÚR-⸢*ni*$^?$⸣ ⸢x x⸣ *ma-mit* ⸢x⸣ GAL-*tú lu* BÚR-[*n*]*i*$^?$

51a a obv. 51 *ana-ku at-mu-ú ma-mit* DINGIR.MEŠ GAL.MEŠ [x x x x x x x x x x x x x x x x x]
C obv.$^!$ 15 [x x x x *ma-mit*$^?$] ⸢*šá*$^?$⸣ *at*$^!$(LA)*-mu-u ma-mit* DINGIR.MEŠ GAL-*ti lu* BÚR-*ni*

a, C

51b C obv.$^!$ 16 [x x x x x *ana* ÍD ŠUB$^?$]-*di-ma* UR$_5$.GIM DU$_{11}$.GA

C

---

52 a obv. 52 [É]N *ad-din-ka* <*ana*> *pu-ḫi-ia* [x x x x x x x x x x x x x x x x x x x x x]
C obv.$^!$ 17 [x x x x x x x *š*]*á*$^?$ *kim-ti-ia*$_5$ NUMUN$^?$-*ia*$_5$

53 a obv. 53 [*u*] *sa-la-ti-ia* x[x x x x x x x x x x x x x x x x x x x x x]
C obv.$^!$ 17$^{cont.}$ *u sa-la-ti-ia* ---------------------------------- *(omits)*

C

---

54 a rev. 1 ⸢LÚ⸣ *šu-a-tim* A ŠINIG TU$_5$-*šú-ma* Ì.GI[Š x x x x x x x x x x]
C obv.$^!$ 18 [x x x x x x T]U$_5$-*šú* Ì+GIŠ IM.BABBAR ŠÉŠ-*šú* KEŠDA DU$_8$-*ma*

55 a rev. 2 NÍG.NA GI.IZI.LÁ *tuš-ba-a'-šú* ÉN a-ab-ba a[ma x x x x x x x x x]
C obv.$^!$ 19–20 [x x x x x] *tuš-ba-a'-*<*šú*> ÉN a-ab-ba ama diĝir-re-e-ne *ana* UGU ŠID-*nu* / [x x x x SILA DI]B$^?$ *la* DIB-*ma*$^{!?}$ *ana* EGIR-*šú* NU GUR *ana* É-*šú* KU$_4$ NAM.ÉRIM BÚR-[*i*]*r*$^{!?}$

a, *single ruling in ms.* C

---

56 a rev. 3 *ana* ^{munus}PEŠ$_4$ UŠ$_{11}$.ZU NU TE-*ma ša* ŠÀ-*šá* NU *na*$^!$*-de-e* [x x x x x x x x x x x x x x x x]

	d obv. 1–3	[*ana*] ^{munus}PEŠ$_4$ UŠ$_{11}$.ZU NU TE-*ma šá* Š[À]-*šá* NU ŠUB-[*e*] / ^{na4}KUR-*nu* DAB KÙ.GA[N] ^{na4}ŠUBA ⸢SAḪAR⸣-*ru* GEŠTIN.KA$_5$.A ḪÁD.⸢A⸣ / SÚD
	e obv. 1–2	⸢*ana*⸣ ⸢^{munus}⸣PEŠ$_4$ UŠ$_{11}$.ZU NU TE-*ma ša* ŠÀ-*šá* N[U ŠUB-*e*] [……………………………………………] / *ù* ^{giš}GEŠ.TIM.KA$_5$.A HÁD.DU SÚD
57	a rev. 4	*ina* MÚD BURU$_5$.ḪABRUD.DA NÍTA *ina* Ì ^{giš}ŠUR.MÌN ḪI.ḪI-*ma* É[N x x x x x x x x x x x x]
	d obv. 3–4	*ina* MÚD BURU$_5$.ḪABRUD^{RU}.DA^{mušen} NÍTA *ina* Ì.GIŠ ^{giš}ŠUR.MÌN ḪI.ḪI / ÉN *ez-ze-et šam-rat ana* ŠÀ ŠID-*nu-ma* ŠÉŠ-*ma* TIN-*uṭ*
	e obv. 2$^{cont.}$–3	*ina* MÚD BURU$_5$.Ḫ[ABRUD.DA^{mušen} ………………] / ÉN *ez-ze-et šam-rat ana* ŠÀ ŠID-*nu*-[*ma* ………………]
a, d, e		______________________________
58	a rev. 5	DIŠ KI.MIN ŠIKA SILA.LÍM.MA *za-qip-ti* TI-*qé-ma* <*ina*> KUN$_4$ *b*[*i-ta-ni-tú* x x x x x x x x x]
	d obv. 5–6	DIŠ KI.MIN ŠIKA SILA.LÍM.MA *za-qip-tu$_4$* TI-*qé-ma ina* KUN$_4$ É-*a-ni-tú* / *te-te-mer-ma* GABA *kiš-pi* ⸢*tur*⸣-*rat*
	e	(*omits*)
a, d		______________________________
59	a rev. 6	DIŠ KI.MIN ^{na4}*šu-u* NÍTA *u* MUNUS *ina* ŠU.MIN 15-*šú* KÉŠ ÉN *a-šib ek-let* [x x x x x x x x x x x]
	d obv. 7–9	DIŠ KI.MIN ^{na4}*šu-u* NÍTA *u* MUNUS *ina* ŠU 15-*šá* KÉ[Š]-*as* / ÉN *a-šib ek-le-ti* 3-*šú ana* UGU ŠID-⸢*nu*⸣-*ma* / *kiš-pi* NU TE.⸢MEŠ⸣-*šú*
	e obv. 4	----- -------- ^{na4}*šu-u* NÍTA ^{na4}ŠU.U MUNUS *ina* ŠU 15-*šá* KÉ[Š …………………………………………]
a, d, e		______________________________
60	a rev. 7	ÉN *a-šib ek-let la a-mi-ru* ZÁLAG ^{d}UTU-*ši* È-*am-ma* I[GI-*mar* x x x x]
	d obv. 10–11	ÉN *a-šib ek-le-ti la a-m*[*i*]-⸢*ri*⸣ ZÁLAG [^{d}U]TU-*ši* / È-*am-ma ta*-⸢*ta-mar* ZÁLAG ^{d}UTU⸣-[*ši*]
61	a rev. 8	*lu-u né-ḫe-e-ti* GIN$_7$ A.ME *a-gam-me lu-u ṣal-la-ta* GIN$_7$ *ár*-⸢*mé-e*⸣ ⸢*šá*⸣ [x x x x x x x x]
	d obv. 11$^{cont.}$–13	[*lu*] *né-ḫe-e-ti* / GIN$_7$ A.MEŠ *a-gam-mi lu* ⸢*ṣal-la*⸣-*a-t*[*a* G]IN$_7$ *á*[*r*]-*m*[*e*]-*e šá* MAŠ.DÀ / EN *i-nap-pa*-⸢*ḫu*⸣ ^{d}UTU *pa-šir*-[*k*]*a* [É]N
a, d		______________________________
62	a rev. 9	ÉN *ez-ze-et šam-rat* DINGIR-*at na-mur-rat u ši-i bar-bar-rat* DU[MU.MUNUS ^{d}*a-nu*][325]
63	a rev. 10	GÌR-*šá an*-[*zu*]-*ú* ŠU.MIN-*šá lu-ʾ-tú pa-an* UR.MAḪ *da-pi-nu pa-n*[*u-šá šak-nu*]
64	a rev. 11	*iš-tu a-pi i-lam-ma uš-šu-rat pe-ret-su bu-ut-tu-qa d*[*i-da-a-šú*]
65	a rev. 12	*kib-si* GU$_4$ *il-lak kib-si* UDU.NÍTA UŠ-*de ina* UZU *u* MÚD ŠU.MIN-[*šú šak-na*]
66	a rev. 13	*a-pa-niš* KU$_4$-*ub ṣe-ra-niš i-ḫal-lu-up* É KU$_4$ É È *bi*-[*la-a-ni*]
67	a rev. 14	DUMU.MEŠ-*ki-na lu-še-niq u* DUMU.<MUNUS>.MEŠ-*ki-na lut-t*[*ar-ri*]
68	a rev. 15	*a-na pi-i* DUMU.MUNUS.MEŠ-*ki-na lu-uš-tak-ka-na tu-la-a iš-me-ši-ma* ^{d}*é*-[*a* AD-*šá*]
69	a rev. 16	*am-ma-ki* DUMU.MUNUS ^{d}*a-nu mu-ut-tar-ra-at* LÚ-*ut-tu$_4$ tal-ma-di*-[*ma*]
70	a rev. 17	*am-ma-ki ina* UZU *u* MÚD ŠU.MIN-*ki šak-na am-ma-ki* É KU$_4$-*bi* É È
71	a rev. 18	*mu-uḫ-ri šá* ^{lú}DAM.GÀR *qa-an-na-šú u ṣi-di-is*-[*su*]
72	a rev. 19	*mu-uḫ-ri šá* ^{lú}SIMUG *se-mer si-mat* ŠU.MIN-*ki u* GÌR.MIN-*k*[*i*]

325 For a full edition of the incantation including all duplicates (d obv. 14–rev. 7 // f rev. 13–29 // g 1–17), see text C.3.3 lines 14–38.

73	a rev. 20	*mu-uḫ-ri šá* ^{lú}KÙ.DIM *in-ṣab-ti si-mat* GEŠTU.MIN-*k*[*i*]
74	a rev. 21	*mu-uḫ-ri šá* ^{lú}BUR.GUL $^{\text{na4}}$GUG *si-mat* GÚ-*ki*
75	a rev. 22	[*mu-u*]*ḫ-ri šá* ^{lú}NAGAR ^{giš}GA.RÍG ^{giš}BAL *du-di-it-ti šid-di*
76	a rev. 23	[*u ki-ri*]*s-su*$^{?!}$ *si-mat qé-e-ki* : *ú-tam-mi-ki* ^{d}*a-nu* AD-*ki*
77	a rev. 24	[*an-tum* AM]A-*ki ú-tam-mi-ki* ^{d}*é-a* DÙ-*ki* TU$_6$ ÉN

78	a rev. 25	[ÉN *an-ni*]*-ti ana* UGU *nap-šal-ti* ŠID-*nu*
	d rev. 8	ÉN *an-n*[*i-tu*$_4$ x x *nap-šal-t*]*i* ŠID-*nu*

a, d

(*Ms. d: colophon follows*)

79	a rev. 26	[DIŠ NA *lu ina* Š]U ^{d}*gu-la lu ina* ŠU ^{d}DÌM.ME *lu ina* ŠU GABA.RI *lu ina* ŠU NAM.ÉRIM
80	a rev. 27	[x x x x]x DUMU.MEŠ-<*šú*> UG$_7$-*tu*$_4$ *lu* GIG.MEŠ-*šú ma-a'-du* DUMU.MEŠ-*šú* <*ana*> *e-ṭe-ri*
81	a rev. 28	[x x x x]x IM PÚ IM KI.GAR IGI ^{d}UTU *tu-qa-da-áš* IM *ta-kar-ri-iṣ-ma*
82	a rev. 29	[NU (x) DÙ-*uš*$^{?}$ *i*]*na muḫ-ḫi-šú kam* SAR-*ár ek-ke-mu la eṭ-ṭe-ru ik-kil-lu*$_4$
83	a rev. 30	[*ša mamman lā*$^{?}$] ⌜*ú*$^{?}$⌝*-še-zi-bu ḫab-ba-tu ina* MAŠ.SÌL 150-*šú* SAR-*ár* ^{túg}GÚ.È
84	a rev. 31	[*tuḫallapšu* TÚG U$_4$.1.KAM$^{?}$] MU$_4$.MU$_4$-*su* ḪAR ZABAR *ina* ŠU.MIN-*šú u* GÌR.MIN-*šú* GAR-*an-šú* ^{kuš}E.ÍB
85	a rev. 32	[*ina* MURUB$_4$-*šú* GAR-*an*$^{?}$] *né-bè-eḫ* KÙ.SI$_{22}$ *ina* SAG.DU-*šú te-ret-ti lu* U$_4$ GI$_6$ *ina* SAG
86	a rev. 33	[DUMU-*šú* GAR-*an šum*$_4$*-ma* DUMU$^{?}$]-*šu ú-ta-naq* GA *ana* KA-*šú tu-sar-ra-aq*$^{!}$(AḪ) *šum*$_4$*-ma* DUMU-*šú*
87	a rev. 34	[*ip-ta-ras*$^{?}$ *mim*]*-ma ma-la ik-ka-lu ana* IGI-*šú* GAR-*an šum*$_4$*-ma* GENNA *šu-ú*
88	a rev. 35	[NU Ù.TU$^{?}$ *mim-ma m*]*a-la* ^{munus}PEŠ$_4$ *ik-ka-lu tu-ṭaḫ-ḫa-áš-šú ina* U$_4$ *tara*$^{!}$(šá)-⌜*kàs*⌝ ÙR SAR
89	a rev. 36	[A KÙ SUD *ana* IGI ^{mul}]MAR.GÍD.DA KEŠDA KÉŠ ZÚ.LUM.MA ZÌ.EŠA DUB-*aq* NINDA.Ì.DÉ.A
90	a rev. 37	[L]ÀL ⌜Ì.NUN.NA⌝ G[AR]-*a*[*n* S]ÍSKUR BAL-*qí* KURUM$_6$ *ana* ^{d}*nin-maḫ* GAR KAŠ BAL-*qí ki*-⌜*am*⌝ DU$_{11}$.GA

91	a rev. 38	*an-nu-ú ḫab-ba-ta* ⌜*šá*⌝ *iḫ-t*[*a-n*]*a-b-ba-tu* NUMUN *šá* ^{munus}NENNI DUMU.MUNUS NENNI *it-ta-nab-ba-lu*
92	a rev. 39	*šat-ti-šam-ma ú-šab-ku-ú ta-ri-ta ú-š*[*a*]*d-ma-mu mu-še-niq-t*[*a*] *šá i*-⌜*na*⌝*-an-na*
93	a rev. 40	*ina maḫ-ri-ki ma-ḫi-ir qí-ne-e-šú ki-ma ad-dú-ki* x x x x x x-*ki*
94	a rev. 41	*mam-ma la i-šem-mu-ú na-zaq* DUMU.MEŠ *šá* ^{munus}NENNI DUMU.MUNUS NENNI *mam-ma a-a iš-mé*
95	a rev. 42	7-*šú an-nam* DU$_{11}$.GA-*ma* NU BI *ana* ŠÀ ^{dug}LA.ḪA.AN SÁḪAR GAR-*ma* ⌜KÁ⌝-*šu* ÚŠ-*ḫi*
96	a rev. 43	*šum-ma* ŠU ^{d}*gu-la ina* UB BÀD *te-qeb-ber šum*$_4$*-ma* ŠU.MIN ^{d}⌜DÌM⌝.ME *ina* GISSU BÀD GAR-*an-šú*
97	a rev. 44	*šum*$_4$*-ma* ŠU.MIN NAM.ÉRIM *ina ku-tal* UDUN *te-qeb-ber-šú šum*$_4$*-ma* ŠU.MIN GABA.RI *ina* SILA.LÍM.MA \ *te-qeb-ber-ma* DUMU.MEŠ-*šú in-né-ṭe-ru*

Catchline:

98	a rev. 45	ÉN *be-lu ga-aš-rù šur-bu-ú e-tel-lu*$_4$ *a-li-id* AN-*e be-el šap-la-a-ti*
	B obv. 19–20	[ÉN x x]x *ga-aš-ru šur-bu-u e-tel-lu a-li-id* ⌜*e-la-a-te*⌝ / [EN$^{?}$ *š*]*ap-la-a-ti*

Colophon:

99	a rev. 46	GABA.RI ^{giš}DA SAR-*ma ba-ri tup-pi* ^{md}UTU-SUM-*na* ^{lú}MAŠ.MAŠ

100 a rev. 47 DUMU *šá* ^{m}*na-di-nu* DUMU ^{lú}SANGA-^{d}*nin-urta* ^{lú}*qaq-qar-*^{d}*anu*^{ki}*-ú* \ MUD ^{d}60 *u* ^{d}15 NU TÙM

For sake of interest, I am adding here a transliteration and translation of the ritual to protect a baby from evil in ms. C rev.$^{!}$ 1–6. For the reading of line 4, see Reiner and Civil 1967, *JNES* 26, 192.

C rev.$^{!}$ 1 [....... ZÚ].LUM.MA ZÌ.EŠA DUB-*aq* NINDA.Ì.DÉ.ÀM LÁL Ì.NUN GAR-*an*
C rev.$^{!}$ 2 [........] UDU.NÍTA SÍSKUR BAL NA BI *ina* UGU ^{giš}*bi-nu* GUB-*an*-[*ma*]
C rev.$^{!}$ 3 [........] UR$_5$.GIM DU$_{11}$.GA

C rev.$^{!}$ 4 [.......] ⸢7⸣-*šú* DU$_{11}$.GA EN U$_4$ ⸢*bal*⸣*-ṭú*$^{!}$ *šèr-ru la-ka-a*$^{!}$ ⸢TUK$^{?}$⸣*-ši*
C rev.$^{!}$ 5 [.......] NU TE-*šú*

---

[1] [... ...] you strew dates (and) *sasqû*-flour. You place *mersu*-confection made with syrup and ghee. [2] [... ...] you sacrifice a ram. You have that man stand on tamarisk (branches) [and] [3] [... ...]. You(?) speak as follows:

---

[4] [... ...] you(?) should say (this) seven times. For (all the) day(s) he is alive, a suckling baby (that) he will have(?) [5] [... ... *evil*] will not come close to him.

Bound Transcription and Translation

[1] [*šumma sinništu ... ...*] *īteneṭṭir*(?) *ana eṭēri zikar u sinniš enūma* [2] [*... ṣalam mārat Anu ša*] *ṭīd ušalli nāri teppuš* [3] [*... ...*] *ana qātīša tašakkan burzigalla ṭīda tumallā-ma tašakkan* [4] [*... ... tašakk*]*anši*(?) *puḫāda taḫannaq qaqqassu lā tanakkis* [5] [*... ... k*]*īma ṣeḫri lubāra tukarrakšu ištēniš ḫišiḫta* [6] [*... ...*]*-ma ina kišād nāri tašakkan nignak burāši* [7] [*tašakkan ... ana Šamaš*] *kīam taqabbi*

[1] [If a woman *has repeated miscarriages (or) Lamaštu*(?)] *keeps robbing*(?) [*her babies*], to save (the offspring), male or female: When [2] [... ...], you make [a figurine of the Daughter of Anu from] clay from an irrigated plot of agricultural land by the river. [3] [... ...] you put into her hand, you fill a *burzigallu*-bowl with clay and set it up. [4] [... *you set up*] for her(?). You strangle a lamb, but do not cut off its head. [5] [... ...] you wrap it in a piece of cloth like a baby. The required things, all together, [6] [you ... ...] and set (them) down by the riverbank. [7] [You set up] [6] a censer with juniper, [7] [... to Šamaš] you say as follows:

---

[8] [*muša*]*pšir lumun libbi mupaṭṭer arni ammēni lumun libbi tabanni ammēni lā tupaṭṭar annīya*

[8] "[You are the one who disp]els distress, the one who releases from sin. Why are you creating sorrow (for me)? Why do you not remove my sins?"

---

[9] *šalāšīšu taqabbī-ma sinništu šī šikara inaqqi puḫāda ana birīt tulêšu inaddi kīam iqabbi*

[9] You say thus three times. Then that woman libates beer. She puts the lamb down between her breasts (and) speaks as follows:

---

10 *ēri ul ušallim ūlid ul abni mušallimtu limḫuranni* 11 *u bānītu liššura <ša> eliya anāku lūšir u lušēšir ina bīt ašbāku*	10 "I became pregnant, (but) I did not bring (my foetus) to term. I gave birth, (but) I did not create (a living being). Let a woman who brings (her baby) to term receive (it) from me, 11 and may a woman who 'creates' (a living baby) *remove* <what is> on me! Let me be all right and *let me give birth soundly* in the house (where) I live!"
12 *šalāšīšu iqabbī-ma šikara ina qēm labti ana pān Šamaš inaqqi puḫādu ...-ša imaḫḫaršī-ma* 13 *ana sūnīša tašakkan-ma ana ereb šamši tallak-ma ṣalam mārat Anu u mimma mala taškunu* 14 *ana libbi eleppi tašakkan-ma ana ebirti nāri tušebber-ma zisurrâ talammīši u šipta annīta tamannu*	12 She says (this) three times. Then she libates fine beer (mixed) with flour of roasted grain before Šamaš. The lamb receives her ... from her, and then 13 you place (it) in her lap. Next you go towards sunset, and then 14 you put 13 the figurine of the Daughter of Anu and all the things that you have set up (for the ritual) 14 onto a boat and let it cross over to the other bank of the river. You surround her (the patient?) with a flour circle and recite this incantation:
15 *šadû u nāru tâmātu u abnātu zaqrātu šamû u erṣetu Anu u Antu(?) ummu abūšu ālidū amēli šuāti*	15 "Mountain(s) and river(s), seas and steep rock(s), heaven and earth, Anu and Antu(?) are his mother(s) (and) father(s) who engender that human being!"
16 *[i]štu inanna ana annannītu mārat annannīti tallakī-ma ana bīt ašbat(u) terrubī-ma annûti tummâta*	16 "[(If) fr]om now on you (fem.) go to Mrs. NN, daughter of Mrs. NN, and enter the house where she lives, then you are conjured by these (powers)!"
17 *[šumma] amēlu miḫrī maḫir mārūšu imtūtū enūma mārāšu itta'id-ma(?)* 18 *[pū]ra(?) tanassuk-ma ḫupâ gamra tanappal-ma amēlu šū mimmu nasku(?) ipaḫḫar(?)* 19 *[uk]-lātīšu(?) ittīšu ana libbi narūqi tašakkan-ma ...-ma amēlu šū ištu(?) [bīti] ana sūqi uṣṣi kīma illaku kâm iq[abbi]*	17 [If] a man faces (inflicted) *misfortunes* (in that) his children have died: when he becomes concerned (for?) his (other, surviving) child, 18 you discard a *[pū]ru*-vessel(?) and completely(?) *smash* the sherd(s). Then that man collects(?) everything that has been discarded(?). 19 You put his [prov]isions(?) with it into a bag, and .... Then that man goes out from [the house] to the street. As he is walking, he sa[ys] as follows:
20 *[kīm]ū miḫrī amḫuru našâku kīm[a a]mḫuru limḫurūn[inni ...]* 21 *[ša] anaššû ina qātēya limḫurūninni <ša> anaššû sūqu limḫuršu lū(?) [...]*	20 "[Instea]d of the (carriers of) misfortune that I received I am carrying (this). As I have received (it), may they receive it from [me! The ...] 21 [that] I am carrying: may they receive it from my hands! May the street receive <what> I am carrying! Be it [...]!"
22 *[kī]ma iqtabû ina sūqi nadî išakkan-ma kâm iqabbi*	22 [Wh]en he has said (this), he sets (the bag) down in an abandoned street and says as follows:
23 *[ana pūḫ(?)] mārīya addinka iqabbī-ma ana arkīšu lā ippallas sūq illiku lā illak itti sinništi aḫīti lā idabbub ana bītīšu iššer*	23 "I have given you (this) [as a substitute] for my child." He says (this), but he must not look behind him; on the street on which he came he shall not go (back). He should not speak to a strange woman; he should go straight home.

24 [*šumma ṣehru*$^?$] *miḫiršu ītetiqšu ana lumni lā ṭeḫê mimma lemnu lā sanāqi* 25 [*kīma Šamaš*] *ittapḫa ūra tašabbiṭ mê ellūti tasallaḫ riksa tarakkas ṣeḫra šuāti ana pān riksi* 26 *tultazassu-ma līša tukapparšu kâm taqabbi*	24 [In the case of a child(?)] whom his (i.e. his father's?) *misfortune* passed by, so that evil not approach (again), so that nothing evil come close: 25 [As soon as the sun] has risen, you sweep the roof, you sprinkle pure water, you set up an offering. 26 [You position] 25 that child in front of the offering arrangement, 26 you wipe him off with dough. (Then) you speak as follows:
27 [...] ^{d}nin-maḫ an-na (var. gub-ba) nin-kur-kur-r[a-ke$_4$]	27 "[...] Ninmaḫ of heaven (var. present in the sky), lady of the mountains,
28 [... ur$^?$]-saĝ ^{d}šul-pa-è-a an-na gub-ba	28 [... he]ro(?) Šulpa'ea present in the sky,
29 [mul á-zi-d]a gub-ba mul á-gùb-bu gub-ba níĝ-nam ḫul-lu-bi	29 [a star] that is present on [the right], a star that is present on the left – whatever evil there is
30 [ḫé-em-ma-ra]-è : gaba-ri gaba-ri-bi-šè ḫé-em-ma-ra-è	30 shall leave (go out). May the rival leave (go out to) his rival!
31 [...]-⸢ga⸣ ⸢kur-kur$^?$⸣-ra ḫé-em-ma-ra-è : (ms. B adds: ⸢lú-gig⸣ ⸢íb$^?$⸣ ⸢dumu$^?$-ga$^?$⸣ niĝin ḫé-em-ma-ra-⸢è⸣) ^{d}i-gi$_4$-gi$_4$ ga-ta gaba-ri (ms. B adds: ḫul) ḫé-em-ma-ra-è	31 May the [...] of(?) the mountains leave! (ms. B adds: "May it *all* leave the sick, accursed(?) person, a suckling!) O Igigi, may the (ms. B adds: evil) rival leave the suckling!
32 [^{d}ni]n-maḫ níĝ nam-lú-u$_{18}$-lu saĝ-gi$_6$-ga (ms. B: níĝ-dím nam-lú-u$_{18}$-lu-ka gig-ga gig-ga) níĝ-dím-dím-[ma]	32 [O Ni]nmaḫ (ms. B: Diĝirmaḫ), 33 by your(!?) command, may [those] 32 (ms. B: evil) machinations of the (ms. a: black-headed) people
33 [ur-gin$_7$$^?$ d]u$_{11}$-ga-bi ḫé-em-ma-ra-è : níĝ-gig lú gur-⸢ra$^?$⸣ ⸢lú$^?$⸣-tur-bi im-ma-[...] (ms. B: ⸢sa⸣ ⸢ḫuĝ-ĝá⸣ ⸢lú-tur⸣ ḫé-ti mu-ni-in-ĝar [x (x)]	33 leave! Turn away the evil (from that) man, (so that) this child may [*live*(?) ...] (ms. B: To pacify(?) the tendons, that the child may live, she has placed him [...]),
34 [...]-in-nú : diĝir-maḫ ka-tar-zu ḫé-en-s[i-il-e-en]	34 [...] lies down(?). O Diĝirmaḫ, (then) I will truly glorify you!"
35 *šalāšīšu taqabbī-ma mê u šikara tanaqqī-ma kupirātīšu ana nāri tan*[*addi*] 36 [(...) *t*]*ullalšu-ma mimma lemnu ana ṣeḫri ul iṭeḫḫi*	35 You say (this) three times. Then you make a libation of water and beer. You th[row] what has been wiped off him into the river. 36 [You] cleanse him [(with ...)]. Then anything evil will not appro[ach] the chi[ld].
37 [*šumma amēlu*] *mārūšu imtanuttū lū murṣānūšu ma'dū lū* [*ṣīt ardi u amti šakinšu*] 38 [*lū*] *ḫuluq*(*qû*)*šu ma'dū lū māmītu iṣ*[*bassu* (...)]	37 [If (either) a man]'s children die one after another or if his illnesses are many, or [loss(es) of slave(s) and servant girl(s) occur to him] 38 [or] his financial losses are many, or a ban has [seized him, (...)]:
39 *āšipu* (var. *mašmaššu*) *ina mūši agbubbâ ukân ina šēri sebet ṣalmī li*[*pî ... ippuš*] (var. *sebet ṣal*[*mī lipî* ...] *iškūri ippuš*]) 40 [*ina*] *ušalli nāri ašar šēpu parsat qaqqara išabbiṭ mê ellūti isallaḫ sebet paṭī*[*rī ana pān nāri ukân* ...] 41 *ana Lamaštu* (var. 7.TA.ÀM *pannigu*) *išakkan suluppī sasqâ isarraq mir*[*is dišpi ḫimēti išakkan*] 42 *sebet nignak burāši išakkan sebet laḫannī šaḫarrūti šikar*[*a umallā-ma ukân* ...] 43 *zidubdubbî ittanaddi kīma annâ ana pān nāri irtaksu* [*maqqītu inaqqī-ma ... kâm iqabbi*]	39 At night-time the exorcist sets up a holy water-vessel. In the morning [he fashions] seven figurines of tal[low ...] (var. he fashions seven figurines [of tallow ...] and(?) wax). 40 [At] a river meadow, at a secluded place he sweeps the ground, he sprinkles pure water. [Facing the river], he [sets up] seven portable al[tars. ...] 41 he sets down for Lamaštu (var. he sets down seven *bundles* of *pannigu*-bread). He scatters dates and *sasqû*-flour. [He places] *mersu*-[confection (made) of syrup and ghee]. 42 He sets up seven censers with juniper. [He fills] seven porous bottles with first-class beer [and sets (them) down, ...]. 43 He heaps up flour heaps. When he has arranged (all) this facing the river, [he makes a libation. Then ... he speaks as follows]:

44 *anāku bīnu aḫû ša ēdiššīšu izzazzu anāku [bīnu aḫû ša(?) ...]* 45 *ša taṣburu urûa ša ladin(n)īya lā i-[... ...]* (var. *anāku [... ša b]ūl Šakkan igmuru larîya)* 46 *anāku lubki ana naspuḫti(?) qimmatīya kīma(?)* [... ...] (var. [... *k]īma irrê* ...[...])	44 "I am an estranged tamarisk who stands all by itself. I am an [estranged tamarisk *who* ...], 45 whose branches you bent, which did not [...] my resin [...] (var.: I am [...] whose branches the wild animals of Šakkan have consumed completely). 46 Let me weep over the disintegration of my crown! *Like*(?) [...]. (var.: *Like* a colocynth(?) ...[...].)
47 *annâ iqabbī-ma ana muḫḫi ṣalam lipî mê ir[ammuk ṣalmī šunūti ana aḫ nāri ...-ma kâm iqabbi]*	47 He says this and then he (the patient) wa[shes himself] with water over the figurines of tallow. [He *brings* those figurines to the riverbank. Then he speaks as follows]:
48 *attā nāru ša tabnī amēlūtu sebet ṣalmū [annûti ša kimtīya zērīya u salātīya ... muḫrīnni-ma ...]*	48 "You are the river who created humankind – [these] seven figurines [of my kin, my offspring and my family ... receive (them) from me and ...]."
49 *annâ iqabbī-ma ina muḫḫi bīni maštakal iša[kkan(?) ... ukân(?) ina muḫḫišunu izzaz(zu) mê irammuk-ma sebe u sebîšu kâm iqabbi]*	49 He says this. Then he places (the figurines?)] on tamarisk (and) *maštakal*-soap[wort(?). He sets down(?) ... . He (the patient), *while standing on them* (the figurines), washes himself with water, speaking seven and seven times as follows]:
50 *māmīt abīya māmīt abi abīya māmīt ummīya ummi ummīya lū pašratāni(?) ... māmīt ... rabītu lū pašratāni(?) ... māmīt (ša?) ...* 51a *anāku atmû māmīt ilī rabûti lū pašratāni(?)* 51b [... ... *ana nāri(?) inad]dī-ma kâm iqabbi*	50 "The ban of my father, the ban of my grandfather, the ban of my mother (and) my grandmother shall be dispelled (for me). The great ban of ... shall be dispelled (for me). ... *the oath which* ...] 51a I have sworn, (and) the ban of the great gods, shall be dispelled (for me)." 51b [... he thro]ws [(the figurines) *into the river*(?)] and speaks as follows:
52 [É]N *addinka* <*ana*> *pūḫīya* [... ...] *kimtīya zērīya* 53 *u salātīya* ...[... ...] 54 *amēla šuātu mê bīni turammakšu-ma šamna gaṣṣa tapaššassu riksa tapaṭṭar-ma* (...) 55 *nignakka gizillâ tušbā'šu-ma šipta* a-ab-ba ama diĝir-re-e-ne *ana muḫḫi tamannu* [... *sūq īti*]*qu lā ittiq-ma ana arkīšu lā itâr ana bītīšu irrub māmītu pašir*(?)	52 Incantation: "I have given you (this as) my substitute, [...]. 53 [The *figurines*(?)] of my kin, my offspring and my family [...]." 54 You wash that man with tamarisk water. Then [you rub him] with oil and gypsum. (Then) you remove the offering arrangement and (...). 55 You move the censer and torch past him, you recite the incantation "Ocean, mother of the gods". [...] He must not go back [by the (same) street he ca]me (by), and he must not turn back. He shall go (back) home. The ban will be annulled(?).
56 *ana erīti kišpī lā ṭeḫê-ma ša libbīša lā nadê šadânu ṣābitu lulû šubû eperu (u) karān šēlebi tubbal tasâk* 57 *ina dām iṣṣūr ḫurri zikari ina šaman šurmēni taballal-ma* ÉN *ezzet šamrat ana libbi tamannū-ma tapaššaš-ma iballuṭ*	56 So that witchcraft not come near a pregnant woman and for her not to have a miscarriage: You dry (and) pound magnetite, antimony, *šubû*-stone, dust (and) 'fox grape'. 57 You mix (these ingredients) with the blood of a male partridge(?) (and) with cypress-scented oil (and) you recite the incantation "She is fierce, she is violent" over it. Then you rub (the woman with it) and she will get well.
58 DIŠ KI.MIN *ḫaṣabti sūq erbetti zaqiptu teleqqē-ma ina askuppi b[ītānītu tetemmer-ma irat kišpī turrat]*	58 Alternatively: you take an upright-standing potsherd from a crossroads and [bury (it)] under an in[ner threshold. Then witchcraft (lit. the breast of witchcraft) will be turned away].

59 DIŠ KI.MIN *šû zikar u* (var. *šû*) *sinniš ina qāt imittīša tarakkas* ÉN *āšib eklēti* [*šalāšī-šu ana muḫḫi tamannū-ma kišpī ul iṭeḫḫûšu*]	59 Alternatively: you tie male and female *šû*-stone to her right hand. [You recite] the incantation "Inhabitant of the dark" [three times over it. Then witchcraft will not approach her.]
60 ÉN *āšib eklēti lā āmir nūr Šamaš tattaṣâm-ma tāt*[*amar nūr Šamši*]	60 Incantation: "Inhabitant of the dark, who did not see the sunlight – you have come out and [seen the sunlight.]
61 *lū nēḫēti kīma mê agamme lū ṣallāta kīma ar*[*mê ša ṣabīti adi inappaḫu Šamaš pāširka* ÉN]	61 May you be calm like the water of the marshes, may you sleep like the yo[ung of a gazelle, until Šamaš rises, the one who releases you." Incantation].
62 ÉN *ezzet šamrat ilat namurrat u šī barbarat mār*[*at Anu*]	62 Incantation: "She is furious, she is violent, she is goddess, she is terrifying and she is a she-wolf, the daughter [of Anu]!
63 *šēpāša Anzû qātāša lu'tu pān nēši dapīni pānū*[*ša šaknū*]	63 Her feet are (those of) Anzû, her hands are decay. The face of a ferocious lion [is set as [her] face.
64 *ištu api īlâm-ma uššurat peressa buttuqā dī*[*dāša*]	64 She came up from the canebrake, her hair hanging down, [her] loin[cloths] torn off.
65 *kibis alpi illak kibis immeri iredde ina šīri u dāmi qātā*[*ša šaknā*]	65 She walks in the tracks of the cattle, she follows the tracks of sheep; her hands [are placed] in flesh and blood.
66 *apāniš irrub ṣerrāniš iḫallup bīta irrub bīta uṣṣi bi*[*lāni*]	66 She enters through the window, glides in by the door pivot. She enters the house, she leaves the house (saying): 'Br[ing (fem. pl.) me]
67 *mārīkina lušēniq u mārātīkina lut*[*tarri*]	67 your sons! I want to suckle (them), and of your daughters I want to take care!
68 *ana pî mārātīkina luštakkana tulâ išmēšī-ma E*[*a abūša*]	68 In the mouth of your daughters I want to place my nipples!' Ea, [her father], heard her and (said):
69 *ammaki mārat Anu muttarrâta amēlūta talmadī-*[*ma*]	69 'Instead that you, oh daughter of Anu, kept on acting as a nurse, you should have learned human behaviour, [and]
70 *ammaki ina šīri u dāmi qātāki šaknā ammaki bīta terrubī bīta tuṣṣî*	70 instead of putting your hands in flesh and blood, instead of entering the house (and) leaving the house,
71 *muḫrī ša tamkāri qannāšu u ṣidīs*[*su*]	71 accept from the merchant his *purse* and his travel provisions!
72 *muḫrī ša nappāḫi semērī simat qātīki u šēpī*[*ki*]	72 Accept from the smith rings befitting your hands and [your] feet!
73 *muḫrī ša kutimmi inṣabtu simat uznīk*[*i*]	73 Accept from the goldsmith earring(s) befitting your ears!
74 *muḫrī ša purkulli sāmta simat kišādīki*	74 Accept from stonecutter a carnelian befitting your neck!
75 [*muḫ*]*rī ša naggāri mušṭâ pilaqqa duditti šiddi*	75 Accept from the carpenter a comb, a spindle, a toggle pin, a cloth bale
76 [*u kiri*]*ssu simat qêki utammīki Anu abāki*	76 [and a nee]dle befitting your threads! I conjure you by Anu, your father,
77 [*Antu*] *ummāki utammīki Ea bānīki* TU_6 ÉN	77 [(and) by Antu], your mother. I conjure you by Ea, your creator!'" Incantation formula.
78 [*šiptu annī*]*tu ana muḫḫi napšalti tamanu*	78 You recite [th]is [incantation] over the ointment.

[79] *[šumma amēlu ina q]āt Gula ina qāt Lamaštu lū ina qāt māḫiri lū ina qāt māmīti* [80] *[... ...] mārū<šu> imuttū lū murṣānūšu ma'dū mārīšu <ana> eṭēri* [81] *[...]... ṭīd būrti ṭīd kullati maḫar Šamaš tuqaddaš ṭīda takarriṣ-ma* [82] *[ṣalma ṭeppuš] ina muḫḫīšu kâm tašaṭṭar ekkēmu lā eṭṭeru ikkillu* [83] *[ša mamman lā?] ušēzibu ḫabbātu ina naglab šumēlīšu tašaṭṭar naḫlapta* [84] *[tuḫallapšu ṣubāt ūmakkal?] tulabbassu semer siparri ina qātīšu u šēpīšu tašakkan miserra* [85] *[ina qablīšu tašakkan] nēbeḫ ḫurāṣi ina qaqqadīšu teretti lū urra mūša ina rēš* [86] *[mārīšu tašakkan šumma mār]šu ūtannaq šizba ana pīšu tasarraq(?) šumma māršu* [87] *[iptaras(?) mim]ma ikkalu ana pānīšu tašakkan šumma šerru šū* [88] *[lā i''aldu/aldu mimma ma]la ērītu ikkalu tuṭaḫḫâššu ina ūmi tarakkas(u) ūra tašabbiṭ* [89] *[mê ellūti tasallaḫ ana pān Er]eqqi riksa tarakkas suluppī sasqâ tasarraq miris* [90] *dišpi ḫimēti tašakkan niqâ tanaqqi kurummatu ana Ninmaḫ tašakkan šikara tanaqqi kīam taqabbi*

[79] [In the case of a man] [80] whose children die [79] because of the 'Ha]nd' of Gula, or because of the 'Hand' of Lamaštu, or because of the 'Hand' of a rival or because of the 'Hand' of the Ban [80] [...] or their (text: his) illnesses are many – to save his children: [81] [...] you purify clay from a well (and) clay from a potter's clay (pit) in front of Šamaš. You nip off clay and [82] [fashion a figurine.] You write on it as follows: "Merciless robber, clamour [83] [which] spares [nobody], bandit!" You write (this) on its left shoulder. [You cover it] with a cloak, [84] you dress it [in an everyday garment(?)]. You put bronze rings on its hands and feet, [85] [you put] [84] a belt [85] [around its hip]. You attach a band of gold to its head. Be it day (or) night, [86] [you place it] [85] at the head [86] [of his child's (bed). If] his [child] is still breastfed, you *sprinkle* milk into its (the figurine's) mouth. If his child [87] [*is already weaned*], you put [what] ever it (the child) eats in front of it. If that baby [88] [*has not been born* (*yet*?)], you supply it with [what]ever the pregnant woman eats. On the day (that) you set up (the arrangement) you sweep the roof, [89] [you sprinkle pure water.] You set up an offering [in front of the "Wa]gon [star]" (Ursa Major). You scatter dates and *sasqû*-flour, you set up *mersu*-confection [90] (made of) syrup (and) ghee. You perform a sacrifice, you set up a ration for Ninmaḫ, you libate beer. (Then) you speak as follows:

---

[91] *annû ḫabbātu ša iḫt[an]abbatu zēru ša annannīti mārat annanna ittanabbalu* [92] *šattišamma ušabkû tārīta ušadmamu mušēniqtaša inanna* [93] *ina maḫrīki maḫir qinêšu kīma addûki ... [... ...]-ki* [94] *mamma lā išemmû nazāq mārī ša annannīti mārat annanna mamma ay išme* [95] *sebîšu annâ taqabbī-ma ṣalma šuāti ina libbi laḫanni šaḫarri tašakkan-ma b[āb]šu tepeḫḫi* [96] *šumma qāt Gula ina tubuq dūri teqebber šumma qāt Lamaštu ina ṣilli dūri tašakkanšu* [97] *šumma qāt māmīti ina kutal utūni teqebberšu šumma qāt māḫiri ina sūq erbetti teqebber-ma mārūšu inneṭṭerū*

[91] "This is the robber who keeps robbing, who keeps carrying off the offspring of Mrs. NN, daughter of NN [92] (and who), year after year, makes the nursemaid cry, makes her wet-nurse mourn – now [93] in your (i.e. Ninmaḫ's) presence he has received *what he is envious of.* Just as I (now) set out for you ...[...] [94] (so that) nobody will hear your [93] [...], [94] may nobody hear (anymore) the distressed (cries) of the children of Mrs. NN, daughter of NN!" [95] You say this seven times. Then you put the figurine into a porous vessel and seal its opening. [96] If it is the 'Hand' of Gula, you bury (it) in the corner of the (city) wall. If it is the 'Hand' of Lamaštu, you deposit it in the shadow of the (city) wall. [97] If it is the 'Hand' of the Ban, you bury it behind an oven. If it is the 'Hand' of an opponent, you bury (it) at a crossroads. Then his children will be saved.

Catchline:

[98] ÉN *bēlu gašru šurbû etellu ālid šamê* (var. *elâte*) *bēl šaplāti*

[98] Incantation: "Strong lord, supreme one, prince, creator of heaven (var. the upper regions), lord of the lower regions".

Colophon:

[99] *gabari lē'i šaṭer-ma bari tuppi Šamaš-iddina mašmaššu* [100] *mār Nādinu mār Šangû-Ninurta qaqqaranû pāliḫ Anu u Ištar lā itabbal*

[99] Copy of a wooden writing board, written and collated. Tablet of Šamaš-iddina, the incantation priest, [100] son of Nādinu, descendent of (the) Šangû-Ninurta (family), the Urukean. He who reveres Anu and Ištar shall not take (the tablet) away.

Notes

Line 1: The introductory passage of this ritual is difficult to restore and interpret due to lacking duplicates or parallels for this damaged section. It seems reasonable to assume from the following lines, especially from the recitation spoken by the patient in lines 10–11 and from the mention of a figurine of Lamaštu in line 13, that the first ritual on SpTU 3, No. 84 is concerned with preventing further stillbirths from happening to a woman and that her miscarriages were attributed to the demoness Lamaštu. Several diverging interpretations of line 1 have been proposed by previous editors and translators, but it is reasonable to expect a reference to the woman's repeated miscarriages or loss of children at the beginning of the line (12–14 signs lost) and a reference to the demoness Lamaštu as the cause of the patient's previous miscarriages. Farber (2014, 277, 309) suggests emending [...] KAR.MEŠ to PEŠ$_4^?$.MEŠ (*ana* KAR), translating "to save [the ...] of pregnant women" (*erâti ana eṭēri*).

Scurlock (2014b, 127) restores freely from the context: "[If a woman's children] cannot be saved, to save (them) (and) [for her to bear] only well-formed male and female (children)", which suggests that she reads ⌜SILIM⌝.MA (*šalmūtu*) "healthy" at the end of line 1. Besnier (GKAB) translates: "[...] they take away, for the man's and woman's desolation ...", and suggests a reading ⌜GU⌝ MA at the end of the line, without offering an interpretation. The present tentative interpretation proposes to interpret the first two preserved signs KAR.MEŠ as a Gtn-stem of *eṭēru* (or *ekēmu*) in the meaning "to take away, to rob", with Lamaštu as the subject and children or babies as its object lost in the gap. Thus, we would have a reference to the demoness' repeated attacks in the past. The following *ana eṭēri*(KAR) is understood in the meaning "to save (them, i.e. the children)", with the expected pronominal suffix *-šunu* missing. The following NITA *ù* MUNUS could be an apposition to include offspring of either sex, but it is also possible that this phrase belongs syntactically to the following clause.

Line 2: For the reading *ú-šal*$^!$*-li* instead of the copy's *ú-šàl-li*, see already von Weiher 1988, 116. Von Weiher (ibid.) and Besnier (GKAB) propose an alternative reading at the end of the line: ^{id}⌜*i*⌝*-dig-*[*lat*] "(clay) from the Tigris (meadows)".

Line 6: According to the dictionaries, the verb *karāku* (here used in the D-stem with the meaning "to wrap") is not attested in texts from the Old or Middle Babylonian period (AHw 446; CAD K, 199), which provides a hint that the present text was not composed before the first millennium BCE.

Line 7: The restoration [*ana pān* ^{d}UTU] in the gap is conjectural, but suggested by the ritual actions in line 12, where the woman libates beer *ana pān Šamaš*. It is not entirely clear whether the short recitation in line 8 was spoken by the healer (on behalf of the patient). Given the content of the recitation in line 8, it is possible that these words had to be uttered by the patient rather than the ritual specialist, and that one should restore [MUNUS BI *ana pān* ^{d}UTU] *kīam iqabbi* "[facing Šamaš, the woman] speaks thus".

Line 8: The restoration [*mu-šap-ši-i*]*ḫ* suggested by Farber is not completely borne out by the sign traces. The reading [*mu-ša*]*p-šir* is proposed here as alternative based on the collation of photos of ms. a.

Lines 10–11: See Farber 2014, 335–336 for the idiomatic meanings of the words *šalāmu* and *ešēru* in these lines. Befitting the context of pregnancy and childbirth I understand *šalāmu* D as "to bring a pregnancy to term", *ešēru* G as "to have a normal pregnancy" and *ešēru* Š "to give birth easily/soundly". In accordance with these meanings, I render *mušallimtu* as "a woman who brings (her pregnancy) to term" and *bānītu* as "a woman who creates" (a normal baby), "creatrix". Stol 2000a, 129 translates the end of line 11 with a more general nuance: "Let me fare well and let me make fare well in the house where I live." For similar passages, see also SpTU 5, 248 obv. 29–32 and KAR 247 obv.$^?$ l. col. 4′ (*infra*). The latter features the exact expression *lūšir lušēšir ina bīt ašbāku* encountered here.

Line 11: I interpret the verb *li-iš-šu-ra* as a form of *našāru*, but not in the meaning "to diminish", as other translations of the text have done, but in the meaning "to remove" (see CAD N/2, 61b; AHw 759 mng. 3), a semantic nuance that creates a parallel with *limḫuranni* "may she receive from me" in line 10. Farber notes that the use of *liššura* suggests a word play with *lūšir and lušēšir* in the same line. For differing interpretations of the passage, compare Farber (2014, 309, with 336 note on line 11): "may a woman who can create (*bānīti*, lit. "creatrix") diminish my ...!". Stol (2000a, 129) offers a similar rendering ("let one who has borne, diminish (it) for me"). The phrase *e-li-iá* following *liššura* is problematic but may be explained as an appended subordinate clause of which the *ša* was omitted. In accordance with the context, I understand it as an elliptic reference to the trouble that is upon the patient. The translations offered by Scurlock (2014b, 127 "may one who brings to term) leave me my reward" (*banītu*)) and Besnier (op. cit.: "May the conciliable one intercede for me and may he bow down (to me with) favourable words!") do not seem to fit the context of the passage very well.

Line 12: The sign sequence SILA$_4$ UR$_4$ *šá* proves difficult to resolve. Von Weiher (1988), Besnier (op. cit.) and Scurlock (2014b, 127) opt for the reading ^{sila4}UR$_4$ = *buqāmu* "lamb ready for plucking; shorn sheep", followed by *ša* introducing a relative clause. Farber (2014, 336) gives convincing arguments against this interpretation: in line 4, the sheep is introduced as *puḫādu*(SILA$_4$) "lamb", not *buqāmu*. And the predicate following *šá* does not have a subjunctive ending. Farber (2014, 277, 309) suggests reading SILA$_4$ UR$_4$-*šá imaḫḫaršī-ma* "the lamb receives her ... from her", proposing that the sign UR$_4$ may be an error for SÍG "(her) hair". He suggests that with the hair the lamb received the woman's misfortune and was then disposed together with the other ritual paraphernalia that were loaded onto the boat with the Lamaštu figurine. Scurlock (op. cit.) renders the passage as "the shearling which is to receive (the evil) from her", also suggesting a ritual transfer. This ritual transfer was apparently acted out by placing the lamb in the woman's lap.

Line 13: The reading *ana* KU$_4$ *šam-ši* DU-*ma* follows Farber 2014, 277, 309. Besnier (op. cit.) reads the signs differently: *ana tu-ú-lì* DU-*ma "it goes to (her) breast"*; also Scurlock 2014b, 127: "you make it go to her breast". Letting the lamb "go to the breast" would underline the role of the sheep as a ritual replacement for the woman's babies, possibly signalling a gesture imitating breastfeeding. However, it is difficult to see how a dead lamb could make such a movement, and the expression "to go to the breast" is not attested elsewhere, to my knowledge. On the other hand, turning towards sunset in order to dispose of the figurine of Lamaštu and to send it to the netherworld makes perfect sense in this context. Thus, I have opted for this option.

Line 15: The improved and partially emended reading of this damaged line is tentative, although based on collation from tablet photos. Scurlock (2014b, 127) translates instead: "Mountains and rivers, seas and precious stones, heaven and earth (and) DN$_1$, whom DN$_2$ bore are her arraigners", but her reading of the last three signs escapes me. For the natural entities invoked in this line, such as mountains, rivers, sea, heaven and earth, see also oath formulae in political treaty documents, see e.g. Eidem 1991, 195, 203: 16–18; Fitzmeyer 1995, 42–43: 11–12; Beckman 2003–2005, *RlA* 10, 314 (Hittite treaties and prayers).

Line 16: The improved reading is based on collation from tablet photos. This rules out the earlier reading *ni-še* (Farber 1989b, 226–227 n. 11) and logographic ZI(?) as an irregular spelling for the plural *nīšū* "oaths" (Farber 2014, 336), as a reference to the entities and forces enumerated in line 15. Besnier (op. cit.) translates "you are adjured by these *lives*". Note that Farber (2014, 277, 309) restores [DIŠ] = *šumma* "if" at the beginning of the line, interpreting it as a conditional clause "(Woe to you), if, from now on, you go toward NN, ...", as an example for a "Drohfluch" or threatening curse.

Lines 17–23: This ritual is performed for a man whose children died in the past and who wishes to protect his living child from the same fate. The procedure uses a sack (*narūqu*) filled with different, largely unidentified materials, which is deposited in an abandoned street to be picked up by passers-by. The sack is given as a replacement for the man's child but also symbolises the misfortune that has befallen the man; it was hoped that the evil would be transferred to the one who picks up the sack and leave the man. This ritual shares elements with a ritual for a woman who has had previous miscarriages in another tablet from the library of Anu-ikṣur, SpTU 5, No. 248 (see text C.3.10, ritual 3, especially lines 75–82), where different foodstuffs and a mouse were wrapped up in wool deposited at a crossroads with the same intention. Parts of the recitations uttered by the patient in SpTU 3, No. 84: 17–23 and in SpTU 3, No. 248 lines 78 and 82 resemble each other. The procedure of ritual transfer by depositing contaminated substances in a bag to be picked by someone is also known from anti-witchcraft rituals (see below comment on line 19).

Line 17: For the beginning of the line, see Farber 1989b, 227 and 2014, 36. This introductory passage can be connected to a similar incipit quoted in the Assur Medical Catalogue (line 109) as the second tablet of the medical treatise OFFSPRING/PREGNANCY entitled "If a man is handed over to Ninkarrak" (Steinert et al. 2018, 217). The incipit in AMC reads: DIŠ NA *mi-iḫ-ra im-ḫur-ma* DUMU.MEŠ-*šú ana* ŠU-*šú* È.MEŠ "If a man has experienced misfortune so that his sons are lost for him" (*ana qātīšu ittaṣû*(?), but it would also be possible to interpret È.MEŠ as a Gtn-form of (*w*)*aṣû*). Note also ZI.GA = *ṣītu* "loss" in Maul 2019, 99 No. 3: (BAM 234 obv.) 2–3 (experiencing constant loss and cases of death). The somewhat euphemistic phrase "they are lost for him" is replaced in ms. a by DUMU.MEŠ-*šú* UG$_7$-*tu*$_4$ "his children have died" (*imtūtū*). The specific phrasing in AMC is not attested elsewhere. The restoration of the verbal form *it-ta-'i-id-ma* (G perfect of *na'ādu*) at the end of the line supposes that this passage referred to a child born after the death of older siblings whom the ritual aimed to protect.

For the expression *miḫra maḫāru* "to receive/be confronted with a *miḫru*", which also occurs in line 20 of the present text and is often found in rituals countering the "Ban" (NAM.ÉRIM, *māmītu*), cf. Maul 2019, 101, 104 Text 3 (BAM 234) obv. 1. Maul understands the term *miḫru* (*meḫru*) in a more specific, material manner, which diverges from the general translation "mishap, misfortune" given in the dictionaries, namely as "ein mit pathogenen Kräften aufgeladener 'Unheilsträger'", which "has been set against" (*imḫur, maḫir*) the person pursued by the "Ban". Maul (ibid., 104) comments: "Als *miḫru* (wörtlich: "Entgegennehmung") bezeichnete man einen 'Unheilsträger' stofflicher Natur, über den durch unmittelbaren Kontakt ... jene pathogenen Kräfte in den menschlichen Körper gelangten, welche das Leiden letztlich bewirkten". Such material carriers of the Ban affliction referred to by *miḫru* with which one could "infect" oneself through physical contact, could be, for example, body substances or dirty wash water of already infected persons (see Maul ibid. for discussion and references). Thus, the term occurs beside objects linked to evil magic (such as "bags of sorcery" containing charmed materials laid out to infect other people), see Maul 2019, Text 16–26 line 63. The recitation in line 20 of the present text (ms. a) similarly refers to the bag with substances laid out in the street, through which the patient's evil was to be transferred to another person, as a replacement for the *miḫru* that the patient received: [*kīm*]*ū miḫrī amḫuru našâku kīm*[*a a*]*mḫuru limḫurūn*[*inni*] "[Instea]d of the (carriers of) misfortune that I received, I am carrying (this). As I have received (it), may they receive it from [me]!" See also the comments on line 19 below. That *miḫru* is understood as something physical confronting the affected person, can also be seen in line 24 of the present text, where the *miḫru* is said to have "passed by" (*ītetiq*), i.e. left the child of the man pursued by the "Ban".

Line 18: At the beginning of the line, Farber 1989b, 227 restores [*ana me*]-*e* "(you throw) into water". An alternative reading [BU]R for *pūru* (a clay vessel or bowl) suggested here may better fit the following phrase, speaking of *smashing/demolishing* (*napālu*) a potsherd (*ḫupû*), but this restoration remains tentative. Besnier (op. cit.) understands *ḫu-pa-a* TIL as "(*you smash*) *the complete fragment*". The term *ḫupû*(^{dug}SÌLA.GAZ) can refer to a disposable "pot, vessel", often used in anti-witchcraft rituals to dispose and destroy figurines of the warlock and witch (see e.g., Abusch and Schwemer 2011, CMAwR 1, text 1.5 line 18′, text 8.4 line 58, text 8.12 line 11; Abusch and Schwemer 2016, CMAwR 2, text 8.18 line 12′, text 11.3, 1 line 42). But the word *ḫupû* in the plural can also refer to sherds or to wood shavings or cuttings. In the present context, the word stands in the singular, but the meaning "sherd" or "fragment" fits the context better. The following word *gamra*(TIL) can be understood as an adverbial accusative ("completely"), perhaps meaning that one of the potsherds of the *pūru*-vessel was further broken down into tinier pieces. Admittedly, the rendering of *napālu* as "to smash/demolish" here diverges from the meanings given in the dictionaries ("to dig up" (things from the ground); "to quarry (stones); "to tear down (buildings)", see CAD N/1, 272–275 s.v. *napālu* A). The potsherd(s) and pottery pieces, which were presumably filled into the sack (together with other materials?), may be a symbolic reference to the children that have died (alluding to the mythological theme of creating human beings from clay). For the reading *ḫupû* of ^{dug}SÌLA.GAZ, cf. Schwemer 2009, *OrNS* 78, 64, commentary on BM 40568 rev. 2.

Line 19: For the ritual action of disposing bags or sacks filled different materials as a substitute in anti-witchcraft rituals, see Schwemer 2007a, 218ff. with n. 115. In many instances, the bag is designated as *kīsu* "purse" (^{kuš}NÍG.NA$_4$). For example, in one such ritual (Abusch and Schwemer 2011, CMAwR 1, text 8.2 lines 26, 38, 82, 122), a *kīsu*-bag is filled with precious metals and stones and deposited as the patient's "replacement" or substitute (*pūḫu*, *dinānu*, ibid. line 82). Such bags, containing contaminated substances, were also used by the alleged witches; in that case they are called *narūq upšāšê* "sack of sorceries". One ritual against the effects of having come into contact with such a sack is edited in Abusch and Schwemer 2011, CMAwR 1, text 11.2 (esp. lines 2 and 12 with commentary). The restoration [*uk*]-*la-ti-šú* "his provisions" at the beginning of line 19 is a guess from the context; the word seems to refer to material(s) put into the leather bag together with the potsherds. In the second damaged passage in line 19 one expects an instruction such as "you tie up/seal" (the bag).

Lines 20–21: The reading [*ki-mu*]-*ú* "instead (of the misfortune)" at the beginning of line 20 follows Farber 1989b, 227. My interpretation of the end of line 21 follows Besnier (op. cit.); differently Farber 1989b, 227. See also the comments on line 17 above.

Line 22: At the beginning of this line, one expects the phrase *ēma iqtabû* "when he has said (this)", but the sign traces do not support the reading *e-ma*. An alternative reading may be [*e-n*]*u*!-*ma* (suggestion of M. J. Geller).

Line 23: The emendation of ms. a follows Farber 1989b, 227.

Line 24: For the reading of this line, see Farber 2014, 36. See also Farber 1989b, 227–228 for his comments on lines 24–26. Notably, for lines 24–26, ms. B offers several syllabic spellings, especially of verbal forms, in places where ms. a uses predominantly logographic writings. Note e.g., *i-te-ti-iq* in ms. a vs. the Assyrian form *e-te-te-eq* in ms. B. I follow Farber's interpretation and understand the expression *mi-ḫi-ir-šú i-te-ti-iq-šú* "*his* misfortune has passed him by" as referring to the father's misfortune which the child has escaped (i.e. the evil with which the household head was doomed in the past has been dispelled and the child has survived). For the word *miḫru* (*meḫru*), which is usually translated as mishap or misfortune, but can be described more concretely as a material carrier of pathogens transmitting the evil manifesting itself in sickness and misfortune, see the comments on line 17 above.

Lines 27–34: The text of this incantation to the mother goddess presented by mss. a and B diverges at several points. The goddess is addressed with the name Ninmaḫ and at times with Dingirmaḫ in the text. In the first lines, the goddess is invoked in her astral aspect, as a star or constellation "standing in the sky". The ^{mul}Nin-maḫ is known from the astrological-astronomical compendium MUL.APIN (Tablet I ii 21), where it is among the "stars of Ea" (referring to the Southern path of the sky) and is designated as "the star which stands at its right", i.e. at the right of the "Great Star" (^{mul}Gu-la), the star of Eridu (equated with Ea, see Hunger and Pingree 1989, MUL.APIN, 35–36; Watson and Horowitz 2011, 65, 189).

In line 28 of ms. a, Ninmaḫ's husband, the god Šulpa'ea is invoked with her, likewise as an astral deity (his name literally means "young one who comes forth shining", and as a star Šulpa'ea is associated with Jupiter), see e.g. Delnero 2011–2013, *RlA* 13, 285–286. This line is missing in ms. B.

Line 30: Ms. B appears to differ slightly from ms. a obv. 30, but I have not been able to decipher the traces at the beginning of ms. B obv. 9.

Line 31: The text in ms. a took up two lines of text in an older *Vorlage*, as indicated by the two sentences divided by a disjunction signs (*Trennungszeichen*). Ms. B obv. 10 corresponds to the first half of ms. a obv. 31, but the next two lines in ms. B (obv. 11–12) differ from ms. a. They may provisionally be read: ⸢lú-gig⸣ ⸢íb$^{?}$⸣ ⸢dumu$^{?}$-ga$^{?}$⸣ niĝin ḫé-em-ma-ra-⸢è⸣ / ⸢i$^{?}$-gi-gi⸣ <ga>-ta$^{?}$ gaba-ri ḫul$^{!}$ ḫé-em-ma-ra-è "May it *all* leave the sick, accursed (íb?) person, a suckling (dumu-ga, lit. "milk-child"). O Igigi, may the evil rival leave the <suckling>!" Following Besnier (op. cit.), I interpret ga "milk" in ms. a as an abbreviation of dumu-ga "suckling", corresponding to *ša šizbi* in Akkadian texts (written (DUMU).GA). Cf. CAD Š/3, 151 sub 2. Another Sumerian term for suckling is dumu-gaba "child of the breast". The emendation in line 12 in ms. B follows ms. a obv. 31: ^{d}i-gi$_4$-gi$_4$ ga-ta gaba-ri ḫé-em-ma-ra-è "O Igigi, may the opponent leave the *suckling*!"

Lines 32–33: The end of the incantation in ms. B obv. 13–15 again presents some differences in comparison with ms. a, but also textual difficulties. The readings at the line beginnings in line 33 are tentative.

Line 35: The emendation of ms. a at the end of the line follows von Weiher, based on ms. B, although it seems that ms. a preserved a text passage diverging from the Neo-Assyrian parallel.

Line 37: For the beginning of the line, see Farber 1989b, 228 with n. 16 and Farber 2014, 36. Ms. C obv.$^{!}$ 1 suggests a restoration Z[I$^{!}$.GA ...] for ms. a obv. 37. Ms. C has ZI.GA ÌR *u* GÉME GAR-*šú* instead of expected GAR-*su* (i.e., stative fem. + pron. suffix, *šaknassu*). Although *ṣītu* "loss" is usually feminine, masculine stative forms do occur, see e.g. Abusch and Schwemer 2016 (CMAwR 2), text 3.6 line 1: *ṣītu*(ZI.GA) *sa-dir-šú* "he repeatedly suffers loss(es)". For similar passages in texts concerned with the "Ban", referring to deaths in the household, see also Maul 2019, Text 3 (BAM 234) obv. 3–4; Text 11 obv. 3–4: DUMU.MEŠ-*šú lu* GAL.MEŠ *lu* TUR.MEŠ *in-da-nu-tu ṣi-it* ÌR *u* GÉME TUKU.TUKU-*ši* ÚŠ *ana* É-*šú sa-dir* "(If) his children – be they old or young – die one after another, (if) he repeatedly suffers losses of servants and maidservants, (if) death regular occurs in his household".

Line 38: In ms. C, at the beginning of obv.$^{!}$ 2, one may also restore [NA BI NAM. É]RIM DAB-*su* "[the B]an has seized [that man]". However, ms. a continues the enumeration with *lū* NAM.ÉRIM x[...], and there is room for two or three more signs in the gap at the end of line 38, after a probable D[AB-*su*]. For a discussion of the concept of the "Ban", representing the personified divine punishment inflicted on a person for swearing a false oath, see the discussion in Maul 2019, 33–40. To the first signs of Ban affliction which would manifest before the punished person became affected by symptoms of grave sickness, belong economic misfortune, death of family members (in our case especially the offspring), servants or livestock (see e.g., Maul 2019, Text 3 (BAM 234) obv. 1–4; Text 11 obv. 1–4). It is a typical element that the evil of the Ban is a punishment meted out among family members over several generations. Often, as in the incantation used in the present ritual, the misfortune caused by the Ban is depicted as a guilt inherited by one's family (see below).

Line 39: At the beginning of the line, von Weiher's copy shows $^{[\text{lú}]}$UŠ$_{11}$.UŠ$_{11}$(KAxBAD) instead of MU$_7$.MU$_7$(KAxLI). However, ms. C obv.$^{!}$ 2 preserves ⸢$^{\text{lú}!}$MAŠ⸣.MAŠ, *mašmaššu* "conjurer". The text in ms. C obv.(!) 2 appears to present a variant, which, however, is somewhat difficult to reconcile with what is preserved of the ritual procedure. Thus, ms. a obv. 39 breaks off after the mention of seven figurines of tallow before the verb DÙ-*uš*. But ms. C reads 7 N[U x x x N]U(?) DUḪ.LÀL DÙ-*uš*, which makes a restoration 7 N[U Ì.UDU (*u*) 7 N]U DUḪ.LÀL "(you make) seven fig[urines of tallow (and) seven fig]urines of wax" likely. The "figurines of tallow" (NU Ì.UDU) are mentioned explicitly in ms. C obv.$^{!}$ line 10, over which the patient washes himself. The following recitation of the patient refers to them as "these seven figurines of my kin" etc., and this number corresponds with seven altars, seven censers and seven bottles of beer that are presented as part of the offering arrangement. Figurines of wax, however, are not mentioned again in the preserved text. This leaves open different possible interpretations: ms. C obv.$^{!}$ 2 could be corrupt; or, ms. C obv.$^{!}$ 2 could speak of seven figurines made of a mixture of wax and tallow (7 N[U.(MEŠ) Ì.UDU] ⸢*u*$^{?}$⸣ DUḪ.LÀL).

Line 40: In ms. C obv.$^{!}$ 3, the restoration 7 GI.DU$_8$ *ana p*[*ān nāri*] *ukân* "he sets up seven portable altars facing [the river]" seems likely, although other options are possible (e.g. facing the rising sun).

Line 41: At the beginning of the line, ms. a presents a notable variant to ms. C obv.$^{!}$ 4, which is probably based on an error that has crept in during the course of textual transmission. Thus, instead of *ana* ^{d}DÌM.ME GAR-*an* "he sets up for Lamaštu" in the Uruk manuscript, ms. C reads [x x x] ⸢7⸣.TA$^{!}$.ÀM NINDA.DIM$_x$(RAB-GAM-KÁM) GAR-*an* "he sets down seven (loaves) each of *pannigu*-bread". In the gap at the beginning of this line, one may restore [7 ŠUKU.MEŠ] "[seven rations] (of seven *pannigu*-bread loaves each)". For similar attestations, see e.g. Maul 1994, 51, 279: 14′, 338: 10, 370: 25′ *passim* in Namburbi rituals. Following ZÚ.LUM.MA ZÌ.EŠA in ms. C, one expects D[UB-*aq*] as in ms. a, against the sign traces copied in STT 254.

Line 42: At the end of ms. C obv.$^{!}$ 5, perhaps restore [*ina* Á.ZI].DA "on the right side (of the bottles)".

Lines 44–46: This remarkable recitation is spoken from the first-person perspective of a free-standing tamarisk in the steppe who is distressed because its branches have been cut off and its twigs eaten up by the wild animals. The introductory phrase *anāku bīnu aḫû ša ēdiššīšu izzazzu* "I am an estranged tamarisk who stands all by itself" can be compared with other recitations recited in rituals, in which healing plants praise themselves and their powers (e.g., Abusch and Schwemer 2011, text 7.8, 4: 69′–78′ (about the 'wood of release') and 7.8, 6: 14′–24′ (about the *ašqulālu*-plant). However, the distress of the tamarisk about "the disintegration" of its crown in the present passage may have been seen as mirroring the disintegration of the patient's family. Elsewhere, the "ripped out" tamarisk (*bīnu nasḫu*) serves as a simile for the removal of the evil affecting the patient (Maul 1994, 65, also 304 K. 3365 obv. 11–12). In the present ritual, tamarisk is later used (beside *maštakal*-soapwort) as a purifying agent. In the course of the ritual, the patient had to step on these plants and wash himself. Towards the end of the ritual, he was further purified with "tamarisk water" which was probably prepared beforehand. It is likely that the tamarisk was already mentioned in the gap at the end of line 43, just before the recitation.

Both mss. a and B are unfortunately quite damaged at this point and only overlap at times, which makes textual reconstruction of the recitation difficult. In ms. C obv.$^{!}$ 7, the text seems to present some level of corruption. The beginning of ms. a obv. 44 appears to run parallel to ms. C obv.$^{!}$ 7, which after a break preserves ⸢*a-ḫu*⸣-*ú* <<Ú>> *ša e-diš-ši-šú ana-ku*$^{?!}$ GAM. Since ms. a read *ša ēdiššīšu izzazzu*, I have opted for an emendation of GUB$^{!?}$-*zu*$^{!?}$:$^{?}$ following *e-diš-ši-šú* in ms. C. Then ms. C repeats the phrase "I am an estranged tamarisk", followed by two signs which look like A and GÍR on the copy of STT 254, but which may have to be emended following the beginning line 45 in ms. a: *šá ta-*... (i.e. "whose ... you have ...-ed").

In line 45, I follow Farber 1989b, 228 and read *ladin(n)īya* "my resin" (cf. AHw 527a; CAD L, 36 s.v. *ladinnu* (also *lad(u)nu*, an expensive aromatic resin known to the Greeks as Ladanum; see Jursa 2009, in: *FS Sima*, 162–163 for discussion). Elsewhere, resin (*ḫīlu*) of the tamarisk is mentioned, which may refer to its salt exudate (Streck 2011–2013, "Tamariske", *RlA* 13, 429–430). For the text lost in the gap of ms. a obv. 45, ms. C offers the remarkable phrase [*ša bu*]-*ul Šakkan ig-mu-ru*$^{!}$(RI) *la-ri-ia* "(I am ...) [whose] branches the (wild) animals of Šakkan have consumed completely". The following *šá* appears to be superfluous.

In line 46, BIR-*ti* may be read as *sapiḫti* (the feminine form of the adjective *sapḫu* "dispersed") or as *naspuḫti* "disintegration, dispersal", cf. Farber 1989b, 229 fn. 20. I have opted for the latter option. Ms. C obv.$^{!}$ 8 presents the same phrase as ms. a, *anāku lubkī ana naspuḫti qimmatīya*, but the continuation of the text is lost in the break at the beginning of obv.! 9. Following this phrase in ms. a, it would also be possible to restore *qim-*[*ma-ti* ...] "my crown" or the like instead of *kīma* (see also Farber 1989b, 229). However, ms. C obv.! 9, after a gap continues with *kīma irrê* "like a colocynth". I am unable to make sense of the end of this line. The tamarisk, speaking in the first person, compares itself with a colocynth. Perhaps, a contrast between the high-growing tamarisk tree and the colocynth which grows near to the ground was expressed here.

Line 47: Ms. C obv.! 10 makes the restoration *ana aḫ nāri* [*illak*]*-ma* "he goes to the river" unlikely, since it introduces the figurines (NU *šunūti*) as object of the sentence. Thus, a verb like "to bring" most likely has to be restored here (e.g. (*w*)*abālu*, *našû*). The ritual use of figurines over which the patient washed himself in order to transfer the evil affecting him to the substitute, is very common, see e.g. Maul 1994, 74; 139: 134–140 (Namburbi ritual). In rituals against the Ban, figurines representing the ban or the patient were used as effigies, over which the patient had to wash to remove the pathogenic substance adhering to him, see e.g. Maul 2019, 43 and *passim*, Text 3 lines 13, 36–37; Text 12 obv. 2; Text 27–33 lines 77–78, 100–102; Text 48–51 lines 39–40. In the present ritual, the seven figurines seem to represent the patient's family members (see below).

Line 48: The parallel in ms. C obv.! 11–12 adds to the understanding of this recitation addressed to the river and to the understanding of the whole ritual procedure. Thus, it becomes clear that the seven figurines of tallow (and wax) represent the patient's family members endangered by the ban affecting the household head, including his offspring. The logogram NUMUN-*ia*$_5$ here may stand for *mār-mārīya* "my grandsons, descendants" (a correspondence, which is attested in the lexical list Antagal C 70 (MSL 17, 197), where NUMUN = *mar-ma-ru* appears in a group with *līp-līpi* "descendant"). In obv.! 12, ms. C offers the fem. imperative form *muḫrīnni-ma* "receive from me", which reminds one of comparable contexts in Namburbi rituals, where the river is asked to take the figurines representing the evil of the ominous sign that the patient has observed. In such passages, the river is further asked to take down with its waters the representation of the evil and transport it to the Apsû (*šūridī apsûkki* "take (it) down to the Apsû with you", see e.g., Maul 1994, 87 rev. 7–8, 406 line 41′).

Line 49: Once more, ms. C obv.! 13 adds to the understanding of this line but is likewise damaged. However, it seems clear that the patient had to step on tamarisk branches and *maštakal*-soapwort that had been spread on the ground (for this "carpet" of "garden plants", see Maul 1994, 62, 306: 6′, 325: 15, 330 obv. 5′–6′). This action was also part of the ritual in STT 254 (ms. C) rev.! 1–5: NA BI *ina* UGU ^{giš}*bi-nu* GUB-*an-*[*ma*] "you have that man stand on tamarisk" (rev.! 2). However, it is possible that the figurines representing the patient's family simultaneously had to be placed on the plants, and that the following washing of the patient on the plants served once more to release the evil of the ban bound to him and transfer it to the figurines.

Lines 50–51: This short recitation addressing the river (*Nāru*) must have been spoken by the patient (i.e. by the male head of the household affected by loss of offspring). In it, he requests that the "ban" of the gods and the "ban" of the patient's parents and grandparents (both are designated as *māmītu*) be removed from him. The reference to the "ban" of the patient's parents and grandparents means that the patient inherited his guilt from his relatives and that the crime of swearing a false oath (or breaking an oath) was committed by previous generations and is punished by the gods among the descendants. Similar statements can be found in other ritual texts concerned with the Ban, see e.g. Maul 2019, Text 3 obv. 11–12 (*arni* AD *u* AMA ŠEŠ *u* NIN$_9$ IM.RI.A IM.RI.A IM.RI.A DAB-*šú-ma* "the guilt of father and mother, of brother and sister, of the family, relatives and kin has seized him"; ibid., obv. 38; Text 45 rev. 3′–5′; Text 46–47 lines 22–24: *lū māmīt abīya lū māmīt ummīya lū māmīt aḫīya lū māmīt aḫātīya lū māmīt kimtīya nišūtīya salātīya* "be it the ban of my father, the ban of my mother, the ban of my brother, the ban of my sister, the ban of my family, relatives and kin"; also Text 48–51 lines 23–26; Text 54 obv. 6′–8′ *passim*.

Ms. C obv.! 14–15 feature a curious the form *lu* BÚR-*ni* (fully preserved only in obv.! 15), which should presumably be read as a stative form + pronominal suffix of the 1st person sg. or ventive (i.e., *lū pašratāni* "it shall be undone (for me)"; for this form in Assyrian, see Hämeen-Anttila 2000 (SAAS 13), 91). One would expect a feminine stative form, given the phrase *ma-mit* ⸢x⸣ GAL-*tú* "the great ban of ..." in ms. C obv.! 14 (the damaged sign may be KI = *erṣetu*, i.e. "the great ban of the Netherworld(?)"). In obv.! 20, the phonetic complement is slightly damaged, but here a reading BÚR-⸢*ir*⸣ is possible, which, however, would represent a 3rd person sg. masculine stative form (*pašir*). If that reading is correct, this would indicate that *māmītu* is exceptionally constructed with a masculine verbal form in this passage (both feminine and masculine verbal forms are attested with *māmītu*).

Ms. C differs from ms. a by adding another ruling between obv.! 15 and 16, separating the recitation from the following instruction, the latter of which has to be expected in the lost second half of lines 50–51 of ms. a. In a similar vein, the short recitation in ms. C obv.! 17 is written in a line of its own and separated from the concluding instructions in obv.! 18–20 by a ruling, which is again not the case in ms. a, where all this was written in one text block of three consecutive lines (52–55). In the gap at the beginning of ms. C obv.! 16, one expects an instruction to throw the figurines into the river, while the patient declared that he gives these figurines as a substitute for his family and children (obv.! 17).

Lines 52–55: In ms. C obv.! 17, possibly restore [... NU.MEŠ *š*]*á kimtīya* etc. "[the figurines o]f my kin". For figurines serving as substitute (*pūḫu*) for the patient, to which the evil affecting the patient is transferred and which are then disposed of by throwing them into the river, see also Maul 1994, 74, 139–140: lines 137–140, with the phrase *ana pūḫīya addinka* "I have given you (sg.) as my substitute", with which the recitation in ms. a starts (with emendation *addinka* <*ana*> *pūḫīya*). See also in rituals against the "Ban", e.g. Maul 2019, Text 3 lines 34–37; Text 48–41 lines 39–40 and *passim*. It is remarkable that the present recitation addresses the figurines with a second person sg. pronominal suffix instead of a plural suffix, but the context does not suggest another referent here than the figurines.

Comparing the long gap in ms. a obv. 53 and the overlap between both manuscripts, it appears that in ms. B the recitation by the patient was much shorter than in ms. a. On the other hand, it is likely that the final instructions in ms. a line 55 lost in the gap were abbreviated in comparison with the text preserved in ms. C obv.! 20, attesting to further variation between both manuscripts. The Sumerian incantation a-ab-ba ama diĝir-re-e-ne cited by incipit now restorable from ms. C obv.! 19 should be identical with the incantation a-a-ab-ba ama diĝir-re-e-ne whose full text is included in *Šurpu* Tablet IX 70ff. (cf. Reiner 1953, 47; corrected in Reiner and Civil 1967, *JNES* 26, 185 with STT 205 rev. 1).

Lines 56–78: For comments on the incantation, see Farber 1989b, 229–230; Farber 2014, 329–330, and the editions of mss. d (BM 42327+) and f (AO 6473) in this volume (texts C.3.3 and C.3.9). The beginning of line 56 is known from the Assur Medical Catalogue (line 110) as the third and final tablet of a medical treatise entitled "If a man is handed over to the goddess Ninkarrak" (*šumma amēlu ana Ninkarrak paqid*), the latter of which is also cited in ms. d (BM 42327+), see Steinert et al. 2018, 217 and *infra* (text C.3.3).

Line 71: For the word *qannu* in this text, cf. CAD Ṣ, s.v. *ṣidītu* sub f; Farber 1989b, *ZA* 79, 230; 2014, 330 "RA" line 17. Instead of the translation "garment fringe", Farber suggests the contextual meaning "purse", possibly derived from the custom of binding silver into the garment fringe (of the bride).

Lines 75–76: For textual variants and discussion of the female items related to spinning, sewing and female apparel enumerated here, see the comments in Farber 1989b, 229; 2014, 330 "RA" line 21. For discussion of these objects in Lamaštu texts and amulet depictions, see also Farber 1987c, in: *FS Reiner*, 96ff.

Lines 79–97: As pointed out by Farber (1989b, 230), this section containing an independent text unit and ritual (not a continuation of the preceding text section) is divided only by a single, not by a double ruling, as would be expected.

Lines 79–80: For the reading of these two lines, see Farber 2014, 36 fn. 90.

Line 83: The restoration and reading at the beginning of the line follows Farber 1989b, 231 n. 27. Besnier (op. cit.) reads ZI.ZI-*bu* "(the bandits) will keep attacking" instead.

Line 84: The restoration in the gap follows Farber 1989b, 231 fn. 28.

Line 85: Instead of reading *lū urra*(U_4) *mūša*(GI_6) "be it day (or) night", Farber (1989b, 231) suggests to emend the sign LU and read *kal*! u_4-*mi* "all day".

Line 86: For reconstruction cf. Farber 1989b, 231 with fn. 32. The erroneous form *tu-sar-ra-aḫ* appears to result from corruption and confusion between *salāḫu* "to sprinkle" and *sarāqu* "to strew, pour".

Line 87: The reconstruction at the beginning of the line follows the context. For *parāsu* "to cut off, to separate" in the sense "to wean", see CAD P, 171 sub 3c, and ibid., 412–413 sub *pirsu* B ("weaned child").

Line 89: The "Wagon Star" (*Ereqqu*, Ursa Major) is also invoked in a Late Babylonian ritual for a woman with childbirth difficulties (BM 48030, CMAwR 3, text 5.9 and *infra* text C.3.8). The constellation is designated as "mother of all the gods" in KAL 4, No. 53 rev. 10 (Maul and Strauß 2011, 105–106). Since the present ritual mentions an offering to Ursa Major beside bread portions offered to the goddess Ninmaḫ, both appear to be seen as related in this text. The "Wagon Star" is otherwise associated with Ninlil in MUL.APIN (Tablet I i 15), but mostly with Venus (i.e. the goddess Ištar) and with Antu (Reiner 1995, 57–58, 139). See also BAM 241 (+) VAT 9543 line 45‴ (*infra* text II.1.3).

Lines 91–94: See also Farber 1989b, 232 for comments on these lines. I have been unable to find a plausible reading for the damaged and seemingly corrupt passages in line 93. The translation largely follows Farber 1989b, 232.

Line 98: This incantation to an unknown god (presumably Šamaš, or alternatively Marduk) was written down in full on LKA 142 obv. 19ff., with the text continuing on the reverse of the tablet which is almost completely worn off, but preserves a colophon marking the tablet as a copy of Kiṣir-Aššur or Kiṣir-Nabû (information courtesy of Daniel Schwemer). The incipit in LKA 142 has a slightly variant wording in comparison to SpTU 3, No. 84, see also Mayer 1976, 426. *Ālid šamê* "creator of the heavens" in the Uruk manuscript replaces *ālid elâte* in LKA 142, which raises the possibility that in LKA 142, the incipit continued as *ālid elâte [u ša]plâti* "creator of the upper [and low]er regions" instead of *ālid elâti bēl šaplâti* "creator of the above, lord of the below" (cf. AHw 1457 sub mng. III 1). The epithet *bēl elâti u šaplâti* "lord of the upper and lower regions" is given to Marduk and Šamaš; the latter is also known as judge (*dayyānu*) of the upper and lower world and called "creator of the above and below" (*bānû* AN.TA.MEŠ KI.TA.MEŠ) in a Šamaš hymn known from copies stemming from Assur (KAR 361: 2 // KAR 105: 2; Foster 2005, 827–828). For references see CAD Š/1, 464–465 sub 2; CAD E, 77–78 sub 2.

Line 100: For *qaqqar-Anu* (*qaqqarān(u)*), see e.g. *qaq-qa-ra*-AN = *Uruk* (*Malku* = *šarru* I 218; Hrůša 2010, 209, 317), *qaq-qa-ra*-AN^{ki} = ŠU (Ḫḫ. XXI; MSL 11, 13: 20a); SpTU 1, No. 33 rev. 11′ (another colophon of a tablet written by Anu-ikṣur, with a commentary on the *Diagnostic Handbook Sakikkû*). Cryptographic spelling in SpTU 1, No. 48: 9′: ^{lú}KI-^{d}60-*u* (a medical therapeutic text copied by Šamaš-iddina).

C.3.5 LKA 9: Procedures to Avert Witchcraft-Induced Miscarriage on a *Sammeltafel* from Assur

LKA 9 presents part of a large multi-column *Sammeltafel* in Neo-Assyrian script from Assur. Its different sections are all concerned in some way with (magical) stones (see Farber 1989a, *Schlaf*, 22–23). The left column preserved on the obverse contains part of a longer list of stones for magic amulets. Their uses (as good luck charm, to ward off witchcraft, illness, and as help with psychological problems such as fear, anxiety) are indicated (for the edition of this part of the tablets, see Schuster-Brandis 2008, 346–350 "Kette Hammurapis" Frg. C and for a description of the context ibid., 167ff. Kette 206; Simkó 2017). The right column of the obverse (or col. ii) contains an extract from Tablet 2 of Lugale (van Dijk 1983, II 50ff. ll. 74–86 Fragment n).

The right column of the reverse re-edited here preserves prescriptions to protect pregnant women from witchcraft-induced miscarriage. The first remedies are for an amulet and for medicine bags to be worn around the neck (lines 1′–6′), the latter of which served to protect the woman from a special type of witchcraft connected to "showing" (*kullumu*) the victim an evil-portending or frightening object (see Reiner 1959–1960, *AfO* 19, 150; cf. Abusch 2008, *Studies Stol*, 53–68 for similar forms of witchcraft in which evil signs are "sent" to or "seen" by the victim). The next section (lines 7′–15′) preserves a prescription for an ointment, a bandage worn around the genitals and an amulet with stones. The incantation that was recited with this remedy, the baby incantation *Āšib eklēti binût amēlūti* "Inhabitant of the dark, human child", is partially preserved in lines 16′–21′, but recently a well-preserved duplicate to the incantation from the Middle Babylonian period has been published by W.H. van Soldt (2015, 524–525 No. 448), which is included here as ms. b. The latter tablet appends a rubric classifying the spell as KA.INIM.MA LÚ.TUR ḪUN.GÁ.KAM "incantation to calm a baby" (rev. 18) and a fragmentary prescription (rev. 19–20).

The prescription in ms. a lines 7′–15′ is known in a slightly differing wording and associated with a different incantation, from three Late Babylonian manuscripts (BM 42327+, BM 51246+ and SpTU 3, No. 84, see *infra* texts C.3.3, A.2.7 and C.3.4).

The left column of the reverse of LKA 9 partially preserves a ritual for the baby (see Farber 1989a, *Schlaf*, 78ff. § 21 ms. g).

List of Manuscripts

Siglum	Museum Number	Copy	Collation	Format; Ductus	Provenience
A	A 37	LKA 9	Coll.	Fragment of a three- or four-column tablet; Neo-Assyrian script, 8th/7th cent. BCE	Assur, N4 library
b	CUNES 52-15-029	CUSAS 30, No. 448	–	Single-column tablet in landscape format; Middle Babylonian period; ca. 13th/12th cent. BCE	unknown (Babylonia)

Overview

i Anti-witchcraft phylactery for a pregnant woman: ...]1′–4′
- Fragmentary instructions (A rev. r. col. 1′)
- Purpose statement (A rev. r. col. 2′–4′)

ii Alternative anti-witchcraft phylactery for a pregnant woman 5′–6′
A rev. r. col. 5′–6′

iii Anti-witchcraft ritual against miscarriage (ointment and protective bandage): 7′–21′[...
- Purpose clause (A rev. r. col. 7′–8′)
- Ritual instructions (A rev. r. col. 8′–15′)
- Incantation: *Āšib eklēti binût amēlūti* (A rev. r. col. 16′–21′ // b obv. 1–rev. 17)

Previous Edition and Discussion

Reiner 1959–1960, *AfO* 19, 150 (lines 2′–4′)
Reiner 1966, *Monde du sorcier*, 93 (lines 7′–19′)
Thomsen 1987, *Zauberdiagnose*, 53 with n. 129 (lines 2′–3′), 67 with nn. 167–168 (lines 7′–17′)
Farber 1989a, *Schlaf*, 26–27, 110ff. Text § 39 (lines 7′–21′)
Scurlock 1991, *Incognita* 2, 140–141 (translation)
Stol 2000a, 156 (lines 2′–4′)
Polonsky 2006, *Studies Leichty*, 301 n. 22 (lines 16′–20′)
Steinert 2012b, *Sudhoffs Archiv* 96, 83 (lines 8′–13′)
Bosworth 2016, *Infant Weeping*, 51 (translation of lines 16′–20′)
Abusch et al. 2020 (CMAwR 3), 56–59 (edition) and pl. 61–62 (collations)
van Soldt 2015, *CUSAS* 30, 524–525 No. 448 (edition of ms. b)

Transliteration

Beginning of the right col. on the reverse lost

1′ A rev. r. col. 1′ ^{na4}⸢AN.NA⸣ ⸢*ina*⸣ ⸢KUŠ⸣ ⸢*ina*⸣ ⸢GÚ-*šá*⸣ GAR-*an*-[*ši*]

2′ A rev. r. col. 2′ *me-e-lu šá* ^{munus}PEŠ$_4$ *u* ^{munus}*ḫa-riš-t*[*i*]

3′ A rev. r. col. 3′ *šá kul-lu-ma-tu*$_4$ *pa-šá-ri ina* GÚ-*šá* GAR-*an-m*[*a*]

4′ A rev. r. col. 4′ *ú-kal-la-mu-ši-ma* NU TE-*ši*

5′ A rev. r. col. 5′ DIŠ KI.MIN ^{na4}*ár-zal-la* ^{im}GÀ(gán).LI

6′ A rev. r. col. 6′ ^{im}GÀ(gán).LI.GUG *ina* KUŠ *ina* GÚ-*šá* GAR-*an-ši*

7′	A rev. r. col. 7′	*ana* ^{munus}*e-ri-ti kiš-pu* NU TE-*e*
8′	A rev. r. col. 8′	*ša* ŠÀ-*šá la* ŠUB-*e* ^{na4}KA.GI.NA DAB.B[A]
9′	A rev. r. col. 9′	KÙ.GAN SAḪAR ^{na4}ŠUBA *ù* GEŠTIN.KA$_5$.⸢E⸣
10′	A rev. r. col. 10′	ḪÁD.DU *ta*$^!$-*sàk i-na* MÚD BURU$_5$.ḪABRUD$^!$.DA MUNUS
11′	A rev. r. col. 11′	ḪI.ḪI-*ma ina* Ì+GIŠ ŠUR.MÌN ŠU.TI-*ma*
12′	A rev. r. col. 12′	UGU ŠÀ-*ša em-ši-ša ù* SAG.DU-*sa*
13′	A rev. r. col. 13′	^{KÚR} | ŠÉŠ-*ma ka-an-ni* TÚG *ša* ^{síg}ḪÉ.ME.D[A]
14′	A rev. r. col. 14′	*ta-ka-ṣar-ma* ^{na4}*šu-u* NÍTA *ina* ŠU GÙB-*šá* GAR-*an*-[*ši*$^?$]
15′	A rev. r. col. 15′	*ù* ÉN *an-ni-ta* ŠUB-*di-ma kiš-pu* NU T[E-*ši*]
16′	A rev. r. col. 16′	ÉN *a-šib ek-le-tim bi-nu-ut a-mi-lu*-[*ti*]
	b obv. 1–2	ÉN É.NU.[RU] / *a-ši-ib ek-le-ti bi-nu-ut a-wi-l*[*u-ti*]
17′	A rev. r. col. 17′	*am-mi-ni la tab-ki ina* ŠÀ AMA-[*ka*]
	b obv. 3	*am-mi-ni la ta-tab-ki i-na lìb-bi um-m*[*i-ka*]
18′	A rev. r. col. 18′	*a-di la tu-ṣa-am-ma tam-ma-ru ša-ru-ri* ^{d}[UTU]
	b obv. 4–5	*aš-šu tu-ṣa-am-ma-a ta-mu-r*[*u*] / *ša-ru-ru* ^{d}UTU-*š*[*i*]
19′	A rev. r. col. 19′	*tul-te-eb-ki ta-ri*-[*it-ka*]
	b obv. 6	*tu-uš-tab-ki ta-ra-ti-ka*
20′	A rev. r. col. 20′	*tul-te-e*ʾ-⸢*di-ir*⸣ [x x x]
	b obv. 7	*tu-uš-ta-dir mu-še-ni-qé-ti-ka*
21′	A rev. r. col. 21′	x x [................]
	b obv. 8	*i-na i-in a-bi-ka ù um-mi-ka*
22′	A rev. r. col.	*Breaks*
	b obv. 9	*di-ma-ta ta-aš-tak*-⸢*na*⸣
23′	b lo. e. 1	[*k*]*i-ma né-ḫu-ú-ti me-e bu-ú-ri*
24′	b rev. 1	⸢*ki*⸣-*ma ṣal-la-li-i im-mé-er ṣa-bi-tim*
25′	b rev. 2	⸢*ki-ma*⸣ *a-lik ur-ki al-pi ṭa-ri-du-ti*
26′	b rev. 3	*li-i*[*m*]-*taq-qú-ta-ak-ku ku-ú-rum*
27′	b rev. 4	ÉN *ul iu-ut-tu*
28′	b rev. 5	ÉN ^{d}*é-a ù* ^{d}*asal-lú-ḫi*
29′	b rev. 6	ÉN ^{d}*nin-gìrima* EN *ši-i*[*p*$^?$-*ti*]
30′	b rev. 7	^{d}*gu-la id-di-ma a-na-ku aš-ši* TU$_6$ É[N]

Bound Transcription and Translation

[...] 1′ *annaka ina maški ina kišādīša tašakkan*[*ši*]

[...], 1′ a tin (bead wrapped) in (a) leather (bag). You put (it) around her neck.

2′ *mêlu ša erīti u ḫarišt[i]* 3′ *ša kullumatu pašāri ina kišādīša tašakkan-m[a]* 4′ *ukallamūši-ma ul iṭeḫḫēši*	2′ A leather bag for releasing a pregnant woman or a woman in childbed, 3′ to whom (something) has been "shown". You put (it) around her neck and 4′ should they show (something) to her, it will not approach her.
5′ DIŠ KI.MIN *arzalla kalâ* 6′ *kalgukka ina maški ina kišādīša tašakkanši*	5′ Alternatively, you put *arzallu*-stone, *kalû*-mineral (yellow ochre) 6′ (and) reddish *kalgukku*-mineral (pigment) in leather (bag) around her neck.
7′ *ana erīti kišpū lā ṭeḫê* 8′ *ša libbīša lā nadê šadâna ṣābita* 9′ *lulâ epera šubâ u karān šēlebi* 10′ *tubbal tasâk ina dām iṣṣūr ḫurri sinništi* 11′ *taballal-ma ina šaman šurmēni teleqqē-ma* 12′ *muḫḫi libbīša emšīša u qaqqassa* 13′ *tapaššaš-ma kanni ṣubāti ša tabar[ri]* 14′ *takaṣṣar-ma šû zikar ina qāt šumēlīša tašakkan[ši]* 15′ *u šipta annīta tanaddī-ma kišpū ul iṭeḫ[ḫûši]*	7′ So that witchcraft not come near a pregnant woman 8′ (so that) she does not have a miscarriage: 10′ You dry (and) pound 8′ magnetite, 9′ antimony, dust, *šubû*-stone (and) 'fox grape'-plant. 11′ You mix (it) 10′ with the blood of a female partridge. 11′ Then you apply (lit. take) (it) in cypress oil: 13′ you smear (it) 12′ on her upper abdomen, her lower abdomen and her head. 13′ Then 14′ you tie a 13′ strap of cloth made of red wool (to her crotch) 14′ and put male *šû*-stone (on a cord) around her left hand. 15′ Finally, you cast this incantation, then witchcraft will not appro[ach her].
16′ ÉN *āšib eklēti binût amēlū[ti]*	16′ Incantation: "Inhabitant of the dark, creation of humanki[nd],
17′ *ammīni lā tabki* (var. *tatabkī*) *ina libbi ummī[ka]*	17′ why did you not cry in [your] mother's womb,
18′ *adi lā tūṣâm-ma tammaru* (var. *aššu tūṣâm-mā tāmuru*) *šarūrī Šamaš*	18′ before you came out and saw the rays of the sun? (var. (Is it) because you came out and saw the rays of the sun?)
19′ *tultebki tārī[tka]* (var. *tuštabki tārâtīka*)	19′ You have made [your] nurse[maid] (var. your nursemaids) cry,
20′ *tulteʾdir* (var. *tuštādir*) *mušēniqētīka*	20′ you have given your wet-nurse(s) a fright.
21′ *ina īn abīka u ummīka*	22′ You have made 21′ the eyes of your father and mother 22′ (wet) with tears.
22′ *dimāti taštak(a)na*	
23′ *kīma nēḫūti mê būri*	23′ Like quiet water in a well,
24′ *kīma ṣallālî immer ṣabīti*	24′ like a sleepy buck(?) (born) of a gazelle,
25′ *kīma ālik urki alpī ṭaridūti*	25′ like a driver of oxen that are driven out,
26′ *limtaqqutakku kūru*	26′ may a daze descend upon you!
27′ *šiptu ul yuttu*	27′ The incantation is not mine,
28′ *šipat Ea u Asalluḫi*	28′ (it is) an incantation of Ea and Asalluḫi,
29′ *šipat Ningirim bēl ši[pti]*	29′ an incantation of Ningirima, the master of incan[tation(s)].
30′ *Gula iddī-ma anāku aššī tê šipti*	30′ Gula cast (it) and I recited it." Incantation formula.

Notes

Lines 1′–6′: For a discussion of these prescriptions, see Scurlock 1991, 164–166; Stol 2000a, 156; Thomsen 1987, *Zauberdiagnose*, 53–54.

Line 1′: The reading ^{na4}AN.NA follows the collation of Abusch et al. 2020 (CMAwR 3), 57 and pl. 61, against Farber 1989a, *Schlaf*, 23 n. 26 (reading NA_4 $^{d⌜}$LAMMA⌝).

Line 2′: For *mêlu* as a leather pouch/bag, see Reiner 1959–1960, *AfO* 19, 151; Farber 1973, 64–66; Goltz 1974, 73; Schuster-Brandis 2008, 63, 66, against the interpretation of the term as a bandage or "poultice" (worn around the neck, as proposed in AHw 643b; CAD M/2, 14–15). Lambert (1980, 77) leaves the matter undecided.

Line 3′: The grammatical reading of *ša kullumatu* "(to release a pregnant woman) who has been shown (something)" as a feminine singular stative form (with a passive meaning) of *kullumu* "to show, reveal" with the subjunctive ending follows Stol 2000a, 156 and Stol 2020b, *BiOr* 77, 569a. A different interpretation has been advanced by Abusch et al. 2020, CMAwR 3, 58 with note on l. 3′, who regard the word as a feminine plural of the verbal adjective *kullumu* "shown (item)", signalling an "evil-portending or frightening object" (ibid. 56) contaminated by sorcerous practices and believed to inflict a miscarriage on a pregnant woman if witnessed by her (cf. also Abusch 2008, *Studies Stol*, 53–68 for such forms of witchcraft). Stol (2000a, 156; 2020b, *BiOr* 77, 569a) prefers to describe the passage as an illustration of "maternal imagination" instead. The concept of bewitchment behind the expression with *kullumu* shares certain similarities with the phrase *miḫra maḫāru* "to be confronted by a *miḫru*". The term *miḫru* (often translated more abstractly as "misfortune") seems to refer to a similarly evil-portending object that is regarded as the cause of infant death in SpTU 3, No. 84 (see text C.3.3 line 17, with note; for discussion see also Maul 2019, 101, 104 Text 3 (BAM 234) obv. 1).

Lines 5′–6′: For *arzallu*-stone, see Schuster-Brandis 2008, 399. It is equated with *sikillu*, *zalāqu* and *ittamir*-stone in Uruanna III. For *ittamir* used in amulets to protect from witchcraft-induced miscarriage, see also AO 6473 (see text C.3.10).

For *kalû* and *kalgukku* in the present context, compare also their use to stop bleeding, (see Scurlock 1991, *Incognita* 2, 166; Steinert 2012b, *Sudhoffs Archiv* 96, 76–77 and the texts edited in chapter C.1 of this volume).

Line 7′: This line is probably given as the incipit of the third and last tablet of the treatise PREGNANCY/OFFSPRING in the Assur Medical Catalogue line 110, cf. Steinert et al. 2018 (BAM 9), 217, 270–271.

Lines 13′–14′: The sign KÚR written on the margin beside line 13′ is interpreted as a correction mark indicating a scribal error or something unusual in the text of this line. Another KÚR, is written on the column dividing line in obv. ii 21′ of the tablet. For KÚR and other correction marks, see Fincke 2021, 58–72 with earlier literature. Abusch et al. 2020 (CMAwR 3), 59 suggest that the KÚR in line 13′ could refer to the unusual phrase *ka-an-ni* TÚG, which might be a mistake for ^{túg}*ka-an-ni*. The present reading follows the suggestion of Abusch et al. (ibid.) that the *kannu*-band made of red wool was attached to the woman's crotch and signalled "a symbolic barrier" against miscarriage; *kannu* stands for a menstrual bandage in other texts (see e.g. Scurlock 1991, 164 n. 34; AO 6473) rev. 12 (text C.3.10); CAD K, 156–157 s.v. *kannu* B mng. d; AHw 438 s.v. *kannu(m)* II).

For male *šû*-'stone' that is tied around the pregnant woman's left hand to prevent miscarriage, see also KAL 2, No. 41 rev.! iv' 13 (text C.3.8).

Lines 16′–21′: As Farber (1989a, 23, 112) notes, the use in ms. A of a baby incantation – a genre originally intended to calm a crying infant – does not seem to fit its use in the present context of a ritual to prevent miscarriage. However, another text intended for the same purpose uses a baby incantation (see *infra*, BM 42327+ obv. 10–13 // SpTU 3, No. 84 rev. 7–8 *āšib eklēti lā āmir nūr Šamaš*). Abusch et al. 2020 (CMAwR 3), 59 propose that these incantations signalled "the wish for a healthy baby by implicitly anticipating it". For the unusual features of the spell, see Abusch et al. (ibid.).

Line 18′: As noted by van Soldt (2015, *CUSAS* 30, 524 note on line 4), the long vowel at the end of *ṭūṣâm-mā* indicates a question.

Lines 19′–20′: Ms. A appears to have singular objects in these two lines, ms. b has plurals instead (nursemaids, wet nurses).

Line 22′: The form *di-ma-ta* may stand for the singular form *dimta* (van Soldt 2015, *CUSAS* 30, 524 note on line 9 suggests it could be an older form) or for the accusative plural *dimāti*.

Lines 23′–25′: For similar passages, see e.g. BM 42327+ obv. 10–13 // SpTU 4, No. 84 rev. 7–8 (texts C.3.3 and C.3.4): *lū nēḫēti kīma mê agamme lū ṣallāta kīma armê ša ṣabīti* "May you be calm like the water of the marshes, may you sleep like the *young* of a gazelle". The present text (line 24′) has *ṣal-la-li-i im-mé-er ṣa-bi-tim* "like a sleepy buck of a gazelle", in which *immeru* "(male) sheep" is used instead of the term *armû* (*arwû*) "male gazelle" (also translated as "young (of a gazelle)") in texts C.3.3 and C.3.4 and other passages (Farber 1989a, 36–37: 22; 38 note on lines 19–22; 42–43 §3 line 48; 46–47 §4 line 61; 156–157). The phrase *immer ṣabīti* may be a variant of *armû* (...) *mār ṣabīti* "male young of a gazelle" found in a few examples (cf. Farber ibid., 156–157 for examples and discussion). For calm waters and ox drivers, see Farber ibid., 42–43 §3 lines 49–50, 157–158.

Instead of the form *ṣallālû* "sleepy" in ms. b, a different incantation uses *ṣallalu* (Farber ibid., 46–47 §4: 61–62 and 157: *kī(ma) armê ṣallali* [*mār*] *ṣabīti ša ṣēri* "(may someone give him sleep) like (the sleep of) a sleepy male [young] of a gazelle of the steppe"); for these forms cf. von Soden 1995, GAG, §55m sub 19a, §56o sub 35a (both formations are used for adjectives referring to habitual activities or high intensity, but neither term is otherwise found in the Akkadian dictionaries).

The word *ṭaridūti* is understood here as a variant spelling of the verbal adjective *ṭardu* (in the plural).

Line 29′: Van Soldt (2015, CUSAS 30, 524 line 16) suggests restoring the plural of *šiptu* in EN *ši-p[a*?*-ti]* "master of incantations". For this epithet of the goddess Ningirim(a), see also SpTU 5, No. 248 obv. 18 (text C.3.10), there *be-let* ÉN "mistress of the incantation".

C.3.6 KAR 247: Rituals for Pregnant Women to Avert Miscarriage and Provide a Normal Pregnancy

This tablet fragment (ms. A) preserves rituals for women experiencing difficulties in bringing their pregnancies to term (cf. the mention of a *sinništu lā muš(t)ēšertu* in line 6′). The text shares thematic links with texts related to the treatise PREGNANCY/OFFSPRING in the Assur Medical Catalogue (Steinert et al. 2018, 217–218 AMC lines 109–114) which is concerned mainly with the protection of pregnant women (e.g. avoiding miscarriage). In at least two sections of KAR 247, the woman's inability to bring pregnancies to term is attributed to witchcraft. It is thus possible that the two-column tablet to which the fragment belonged, may have represented material related to the tablets of the treatise PREGNANCY listed in the AMC, e.g. Tablet 3 with the title "For witchcraft not to approach a pregnant woman and to prevent her from having a miscarriage" (AMC 110: [*ana* munusPEŠ$_4$ UŠ$_{11}$.ZU NU T]E-*ši-ma ana šá* ŠÀ-*šà* NU! ⸢ŠUB⸣-*e*). The ritual shares similarities with other rituals to protect from miscarriage edited in chapter C.3, which were often destined for women who had difficulties bringing their pregnancies to term (e.g., SpTU 5, No. 248; BM 42327+; SpTU 3, No. 84; texts C.3.10, C.3.3, C.3.4).

Since the edition of ms. A in CMAwR 3 (text 5.8), the present author identified a longer passage in CTN 4, No. 105 (ms. B) as a duplicate to one of the incantations in KAR 247. This allows us to identify the fragmentary incantation in the left column of the obverse of ms. A as a prayer to the goddess Ninmaḫ, and to restore a larger portion of its text. Ms. B preserves a fragment of a two-column tablet written in Neo-Assyrian script that was found during excavations of the library of the Nabû temple at Nimrud. While ms. A appears to contain solely treatments and rituals for women who suffered from repeated miscarriages, ms. B displays a differing combination of textual materials. Thus, column iii on the reverse of ms. B preserves rituals and incantations to pacify a crying baby, and some of these passages have duplicates in similar collections of LÚ.TUR.ḪUN.GÁ-texts (Farber 1989a, 20–21, 92–93 §28 (ll. 10′–21′), 48–50 §5 (ll. 22′–33′), 106–107 §35 (ll. 1′–9′)). A similar combination of related topics can be observed, for example, in the Neo-Assyrian Birth Compendium BAM 248 (and dupl.), which focuses on difficult delivery but concludes in the final lines with protective treatments for the baby related to the rituals of the LÚ.TUR.ḪUN.GÁ-texts (see text D.1.1).

List of Manuscripts

Siglum	Museum Number	Copy	Collation	Format; Ductus	Provenience
A	VAT 8809	KAR 247 CMAwR 3, pl. 9	–	Fragment of a two-column tablet; Neo-Assyrian script, 8th/7th cent. BCE	Assur, N4 library
B	ND 5590 IM 67636	CTN 4, pl. 66 No. 105	–	Fragment of a two-column tablet; Neo-Assyrian script, 8th/7th cent. BCE	Nimrud (Kalḫu); Temple of Nabû

Overview

i′ Fragmentary ritual against witchcraft for a pregnant woman ...]1′–5′
A obv.(?) l. col. 1′–5′

ii′ Fragmentary ritual for a woman who does not bring pregnancies to term ([*ana sinništi lā muš(t)ē*]*šerti šūšuri*): 6′–32′[...

- A obv.(?) l. col. 6′–9′: Ritual instructions
- A obv.(?) l. col. 10′–17′ // B obv. ii 6–26: Prayer addressed at the goddess Ninmaḫ
- B obv. ii 27–31: Fragmentary ritual instructions

iii′	Fragmentary ritual instructions A obv.(?) r. col. 1′-6′	...]33″–38″[...
iv′	Fragmentary ritual against witchcraft for a pregnant woman: – A rev.(?) r. col. 1′–5′: fragmentary prayer – A obv.(?) l. col. 6′–10′: ritual instructions	...]39‴–48‴[...
v′	Fragmentary ritual instructions A rev.(?) l. col. 1′–17′	...]49⁗–65⁗[...

Previous Edition and Discussion

Abusch et al. 2020, CMAwR 3, 84–87 text 5.8 (ms. A); pl. 9
CDLI P369211 (copy)

Transliteration

Beginning of ms. A obv.(?) lost

1′	A obv.$^{?}$ l. col. 1′	[x x x x x x] x x x x [x x x x x]
2′	A obv.$^{?}$ l. col. 2′	[x x x x x] *ina* É *áš-ba-ku ne-*[*mel*$^{?}$ x x x]
3′	A obv.$^{?}$ l. col. 3′	[x x x x *ze*]-*ru-ti muḫ-ri-i*[*n-ni* x x x]
4′	A obv.$^{?}$ l. col. 4′	[*lu-ši-ir lu-še*$^{?}$-*š*]*i-ir ina* É *áš-ba-ku* [x x x x]
5′	A obv.$^{?}$ l. col. 5′	[x x x x] x *ta-tab-bak* SILA DIB NU ⸢DIB⸣ [x x x]
6′	A obv.$^{?}$ l. col. 6′	[*ana sin-niš-ti* NU S]I.SÁ *šu-šu-ri* DÙ.DÙ.BI *ana* IGI ⸢^{d}⸣[x x]
7′	A obv.$^{?}$ l. col. 7′	[^{giš}BANŠUR$^{?}$ GU]B-*an* ZÚ.LUM.MA ZÌ.EŠA DU[B-*aq*]
8′	A obv.$^{?}$ l. col. 8′	[NINDA.Ì.DÉ.À]M LÀL Ì.NUN.NA GAR-*a*[*n*]
9′	A obv.$^{?}$ l. col. 9′	[NÍG.NA ^{šim}L]I GAR-*an* KAŠ BAL-*qí* ŠID-*tú an-ni-tú* 3-*šú* ŠID-[*nu*]
10′	A obv.$^{?}$ l. col. 10′ B obv. ii 6–7	[ÉN ^{d}x (x)] GAŠAN GAL-*tú at-ti-ma ša ba-lu-uk-ki* [^{d}*n*]*in-maḫ* GAŠAN *ra-bi-i-*[*tu*$_4$ x x x] / ⸢*ša*⸣ *ina ba-lu-uk-ki*
11′	A obv.$^{?}$ l. col. 11′ B obv. ii 7$^{cont.}$–8	[*ri-ḫu-tu*$_4^{?}$ *š*]*a a-me-lu-ti ana* ⸢*qer-bi-ti*⸣ ⸢*la*⸣ ⸢*i-ra*⸣-*ḫu-u* *ri-*[*ḫu-tu*$_4$] / ⸢*ša*⸣ *a-mi-lu-te a-na qer-b*[*i-ti* ....]
12′	A obv.$^{?}$ l. col. 12′ B obv. ii 9–10	[x x x x NU]MUN *a-me-lu-ti ta-ra-am-mì* ⸢GAŠAN⸣-*tu*$_4$ GAL-*tu*$_4$ [(*at-ti*$^{?}$)] / *ša* NUMUN *a-me-lu-te*$^{!}$(ŠU) *ta-ra-*⸢*am*⸣-*mi*
13′	A obv.$^{?}$ l. col. 13′ B obv. ii 10$^{cont.}$–11	[NENNI-*tu*$_4^{?}$ *šá* DINGI]R-*šá* NENNI ^{d}15-*šá* NENNI-*tu*$_4$ ⸢NENNI⸣-*t*[*u*$_4^{?}$] / *ša* DINGIR-*šú* NENNI ^{d}*iš*$_8$-*tár-šú* [NENNI-*tu*$_4$]
14′	A obv.$^{?}$ l. col. 14′ B obv. ii 12	[DUMU.MUNUS NENNI(?) *šá* DINGI]R-*šá* NENNI ^{d}15-*šá* ⸢NENNI⸣-*tu*$_4$ *šum* NENNI DUMU.MUNUS NENNI *ša* DINGIR-*šá* NEN[NI] ⸢^{d}⸣[*ištar-šá* NENNI-*tu*$_4$]
15′	A obv.$^{?}$ l. col. 15′ B obv. ii 13–14	[x x x x x *u*]*p-šá-še-e mim-ma lem-nu* NU DIM$_4$ *ana* IBILA *šur-še-e* NUMUN ⸢NENNI$^{?}$⸣ [*šub-ši-i*$^{?}$ ...] / *mim*$^{!}$(U)-*ma lem-nu* <*ana*> *la*$^{!}$(AD) *sa-na-*⸢*aq*⸣
16′	A obv.$^{?}$ l. col. 16′ B obv. ii 14$^{cont.}$–15	[x x x x x x x G]AL-*ti* Ì+GIŠ DU$_{10}$.GA *ina* ^{giš}DÍLIM EŠ-*aš* ⸢NENNI⸣ [x x] / *ana* IGI DINGIR-*ti-ka* GAL-*te* Ì DU$_{10}$.GA [..............]
17′	A obv.$^{?}$ l. col. 17′	[x x x x ^{ú}KUR.K]UR$^{?}$ ^{giš}GAN.U$_5$ x x x

B obv. ii 16 *ana* LÍL BAD ^{ú}ḪAR.ḪAR ^{ú}KUR.KUR [.........]

Ms. A obv. (?) left column breaks

18′ B obv. ii 17 ⸢SUḪUŠ⸣ ^{giš}*šu-šum* SUḪUŠ [..................]

19′ B obv. ii 18 ⸢SUḪUŠ⸣ ^{giš}*al-la-nu a-šar* [.....................]

20′ B obv. ii 19 *ana* IGI DINGIR-*ti-ki* GAL-*te* Ì DU$_{10}$!.GA [......]

21′ B obv. ii 20 ⸢x x x⸣ ⸢DI/KI? *ri*⸣-[..........................]

22′ B obv. ii 21 [x x l]uḫ? sa x x[..............................]

23′ B obv. ii 22 ⸢x⸣ [x] ⸢ḪUL?⸣ ⸢*ša*⸣ *tab*?-*ni*? [....................]

24′ B obv. ii 23 ši [x] la *i-sa-*[.....................................]

25′ B obv. ii 24 ⸢ba?⸣ [x (x)] *lib-ba-ši li-pu* x[..........]

26′ B obv. ii 25 x[-x-ṭ]*u li-mi-ra* [..............]

27′ B obv. ii 26 [*d*]*a*?-*li-li-ki ra-bu-*[*ti lid-lul*]

28′ B obv. ii 27 [(x) *m*]*i-nu-tú an-ni-tú* 3-*šú* [ŠID-*nu*?]

29′ B obv. ii 28 [x x x] ⸢KAŠ⸣ BAL!?(TI)-*qí* MUNUS ⸢BI⸣ [.........]

30′ B obv. ii 29 [x x x] ⸢x⸣ Ì DU$_{10}$.GA [.....................]

31′ B obv. ii 30 [x x MUNUS? ŠÉ]Š-*ma* x[.................]

32′ B obv. ii 31 [x x x x] x [...................................]

Ms. B obv. ii breaks; remainder lost

33″ A obv.? r. col. 1′ bi x [..............................]

34″ A obv.? r. col. 2′ *ša* SILA$_{4}$? x [....................]

35″ A obv.? r. col. 3′ *ù la* x [...................................]

36″ A obv.? r. col. 4′ *tu-ṣa-lam pi-*[...................]

37″ A obv.? r. col. 5′ GIN$_{7}$ ^{lú}⸢AZU?⸣ [....................]

38″ A obv.? r. col. 6′ TÉŠ.BI ḪE ⸢su?⸣ [.................]

Ms. A obv.(?) right column breaks

39‴ A rev.? r. col. 1′ x [...................................]

40‴ A rev.? r. col. 2′ *la* x [...............................]

41‴ A rev.? r. col. 3′ ^{d}⸢*gu*⸣-*la* x[.........................]

42‴ A rev.? r. col. 4′ ⸢*ša*⸣ ⸢*e-piš-ti*⸣ [....................]

43‴ A rev.? r. col. 5′ ŠE.NUMUN-*šú* [.....................]

44‴ A rev.? r. col. 6′ *an-nam* D[U$_{11}$.GA-*ma* ....]

45‴	A rev.$^?$ r. col. 7′	*a-na* x [.........................]
46‴	A rev.$^?$ r. col. 8′	^{giš}ŠI[NIG ....]
47‴	A rev.$^?$ r. col. 9′	KÉŠ [...................................]
48‴	A rev.$^?$ r. col. 10′	x [...............................]

Ms. A rev.(?) right column breaks

49⁗	A rev.$^?$ l. col. 1′	[x x (x) GAR]-*an* KAŠ BAL-*qí* ^{munus}ÁŠ.GÀR GÌŠ.NU.⸢ZU⸣ [*tanakkis*(?)]
50⁗	A rev.$^?$ l. col. 2′	[x (x)] pa$^?$ *ana* ŠÀ ^{giš}BÁN ŠUB-*di* ŠE.MUŠ$_5$ ^{giš}BÁN DIRI-⸢*ma*⸣
51⁗	A rev.$^?$ l. col. 3′	[MUNUS *ina mu*]*ḫ-ḫi* TUŠ-⸢*ab*⸣ ⸢SÍG⸣ ÙZ SÍG.MEŠ *ina* KI.TA GÌR.MEŠ-⸢*šá*⸣ GAR-*an*
52⁗	A rev.$^?$ l. col. 4′	[x x S]ÍG BABBAR SA MAŠ.DÀ SA KUR.GI^{mušen} DIŠ-*niš* NU.NU 7.TA.ÀM
53⁗	A rev.$^?$ l. col. 5′	[KA.KÉ]Š KÉŠ *e-ma* KÉŠ ÉN tu lu ba ḫa šu ⸢ši⸣ ⸢a-ga⸣ ši-ḫa
54⁗	A rev.$^?$ l. col. 6′	[a-ga-la-t]i-la ⸢ši-ḫa⸣ ⸢a-ga-ti-la⸣ ⸢ši-ḫa⸣ ⸢a-ga⸣-[l]a-⸢ti-la⸣ ⸢ši-ḫa⸣ ÉN
55⁗	A rev.$^?$ l. col. 7′	[ÉN *an-n*]*i-tú ina muḫ-ḫi* ŠID-*nu* MUNUS BI *tu-kàṣ-ṣar-ši*
56⁗	A rev.$^?$ l. col. 8′	[$^{\text{na4}}$(x)] x $^{\text{na4}}$ZA.GÌN $^{\text{na4}}$PA *šá* 7 GÙN.MEŠ-*šá* $^{\text{na4}}$*ka-pa-ṣu*
57⁗	A rev.$^?$ l. col. 9′	[$^{\text{na4}}$*z*]*i*-É $^{\text{<na4>}}$*šu-u* NÍTA *u* MUNUS *ina* SÍG GÙN.A È
58⁗	A rev.$^?$ l. col. 10′	[x x] ⸢Ì⸣ *ta-šab-bàḫ* BUR.ZI.SAL ^{giš}TASKARIN Ì DIRI-*ma* KI NA$_4$.MEŠ
59⁗	A rev.$^?$ l. col. 11′	[x x x *ina*] ⸢Ì⸣ GAR-*an* ⸢EN⸣ ⸢Ù.TU⸣ ⸢Ì.GIŠ⸣ BI ⸢*zi-mì*⸣-*šá u* ⸢ŠÀ⸣.MEŠ-*šá*
60⁗	A rev.$^?$ l. col. 12′	[ŠÉŠ.MEŠ$^?$ x] x x ⸢*ap*$^?$-*ti-šá*⸣ ⸢GAR⸣-*an* ŠE.MUŠ$_5$ ⸢ZÌ.EŠA⸣
61⁗	A rev.$^?$ l. col. 13′	[x x x x x x] x *tara-kás-ma ina* É KUD-⸢*si*⸣ *lu ina* <IGI> ^{d}UTU
62⁗	A rev.$^?$ l. col. 14′	[x x x x x x] x *a-di ul-la-du ina u*$_4$-*mi* 3-*šú* TAG.MEŠ
63⁗	A rev.$^?$ l. col. 15′	[x x x x x x x] x x-*ši u*$_4$-*um i'-al-du*
64⁗	A rev.$^?$ l. col. 16′	[x x x x x x] x [(x) ^{n}]$^{\text{a4}}$*en-gi*$^?$-⸢*su*$^?$⸣ *šá* k[a$^?$ x]
65⁗	A rev.$^?$ l. col. 17′	[........................] x ⸢LÚ.TUR-*šá*⸣ SILIM-[*im*$^?$]

Ms. A rev.(?) left column breaks

Bound Transcription and Translation

Beginning of ms. A obv.(?) lost

1′ [......] ... [.......]	1′ [......] ... [.......],
2′ [......] *ina bīt ašbāku nē*[*mel* ......]	2′ [......] succ[ess] in the house where I live!
3′ [...... *zē*]*rūti muḫrī*[*nni* ....]	3′ Receive from [me] the [hate]ful [...], [...].
4′ ([*lūšir lušēš*]*ir*(?) *ina bīt ašbāku* [.......]	4′ [*Let me be alright and let me bring*] *to term*(?) in the house where I live [.....]!"
5′ [......] ... *tatabbak sūq ītiqu lā ittiq* [....]	5′ [...] ... you pour. She must not go (back) by the (same) street by which she came [...].

6′ [*ana sinništi lā muš(t)ē*]*šerti šūšuri* DÙ.DÙ.BI *ana maḫar* [.....] 7′ [*paššūra*(?) *tuk*]*ān suluppī sasqâ tasa*[*rraq*] 8′ [*mi-r*]*is dišpi ḫimēti tašakkan* 9′ [*nignak burā*]*ši tašakkan šikara tanaqqi minûtu annītu šalāšīšu tamannu*

6′ [To make a woman who does not bring (pregnancies)] to term give birth successfully – the procedure for it: Before [...] 7′ [you arran]ge [*a table*]. You str[ew] dates (and) fine flour. 8′ You place [*mersu*-con]fection made of syrup (and) ghee (there). 9′ You set up a [censer with *burā*]*šu*-juniper. You pour a libation of beer (and) recite this incantation three times:

10′ [ÉN ᵈ*Ninmaḫ*] *bēltu rabītu attī-ma ša balukki*
11′ *ri*[*ḫûtu š*]*a amēlūti ana qerbīti lā iraḫḫû*
12′ *bēltu rabītu* [(*attī*)] *ša zēr amēlūti tarammī*
13′ *annannītu ša ilša annanna ištarša annannītu*
14′ (*šum annannīti*) *mārat annanna ša ilša annanna ištarša annannītu*
15′ *ana apli šuršê zēr annannīti*(?) [*šubšî*(?) *u*]*pšāšê mimma lemnu lā sanāqi*(?)
16′ *annannītu* [...] *ana pān ilūtīka rabīti šamna ṭāba ina itqūri ippaššaš*
17′ *ana silīti nesî*(?) *ḫašâ atā'iša* ᵍⁱˢGAN.U₅ ...

10′ [Incantation]: "O Ninmaḫ, you are the great lady, without whom
11′ man's se[men] cannot inseminate the womb,
12′ (you are the) great lady who loves human offspring.
13′ Mrs. So-and-so, whose [go]d is N.N., whose goddess is N.N.,
14′ (*concerning* Mrs. So-and-so), daughter of N.N., whose god is N.N., whose goddess is N.N.:
15′ to let (her) acquire an heir, (to) [create] progeny (lit. seed) for Mrs. So-and-so, (...) (so that) [so]rceries) (and) any evil not approach (her), –
16′ Mrs. So-and-so [...], in the presence of your great divinity she is rubbed with aromatic oil from a salve bowl.
17′ So that illness depart(?) – with *ḫašû*-plant, *atā'išu*-plant, GAN.U₅-wood, ...,

Ms. A obv.(?) left col. breaks

18′ *šuruš šūši šuruš* [... ...]
19′ *šuruš allāni ašar* [... ...]
20′ *ana pān ilūtīka rabīti šamna ṭāba* [*ippaššaš*?]

Lines 21′–24′ too fragmentary for transcription and translation

25′ [... ...] *libbaši līpu* [......]
26′ [... ...] *limmira* [... ...]
27′ [*d*]*alīlīki rabûti* [*lidlul*]
28′ [(...)] *minûtu annītu šalāšīšu* [*tamannu*]
29′ [...] *šikara tanaqqi*(?) *sinništu šī* [...]
30′ [... ...] *šamnu ṭābu* [... ...]
31′ [... ... *sinništu*(?) *ipta*]*ššaš-ma* [... ...]
32′ *traces*

18′ root of *šūšu*-plant, root of [... ...],
19′ root of *allānu*-oak from a place where [... ...],
20′ in the presence of your great divinity [she is rubbed(?)] (with) aromatic oil (mixed with these plants).

...

25′ [...] let a descendant come into being, [...]!
26′ [...] may she/it become bright, [...]!
27′ [May she sing] great praises of you!"
28′ [(...) You recite] this incantation three times].
29′ [...] you libate(?) beer. That woman [...]
30′ [... ...] aromatic oil [... ...]
31′ [... ... the woman(?) an]oints herself. Then [... ...]
32′ *too fragmentary for translation*

Ms. B obv. ii breaks

33″ [... ...]
34″ *ša puḫādi*(?) [... ...]
35″ *u lā* ...[... ...]
36″ *tuṣallam pi*-[... ...]
37″ *kīma bārî* [.......]
38″ *ištēniš* ...[... ...]

33″ [... ...]
34″ of a lamb(?) [... ...]
35″ and ...[... ....]
36″ you blacken(?), ...[... ...]
37″ like (that of) a diviner [... ...]
38″ together ...[... ...]

Ms. A obv.(?) right col. breaks

39'''–40''' *fragmentary*
41''' *Gula [... ...]* 42''' *ša ēpišti [... ...]* 43''' *zēršu [... ...]*

39'''–40''' *too fragmentary for translation*
41''' (O) Gula, [... ... *the machinations*(?)] 42''' of the sorceress [...] 43''' its seed [... ...].

44''' *annâ ta[qabbī-ma ... ...]* 45''' *ana [... ...]* 46''' *bī[nu ... ...]* 47'''–48''' *(too fragmentary for transcription)*

44''' You s[ay] this [and then ...] 45''' to[wards ... 46''' tamar[isk ...] ... 47'''–48''' (*too fragmentary for translation*)

Ms. A rev.(?) right col. breaks

49'''' *[... tašakk]an šikara tanaqqi unīqa lā petīta [tanakkis(?)]* 50'''' *[...] ... ana libbi sūti tanaddi šeguššа sūta tumallā-ma* 51'''' *[sinništu ina m]uḫḫi uššab šārat enzi šīpāti ina šapal šēpīša tašakkan* 52'''' *[...] šīpāti peṣêti šer'ān ṣabīti šer'ān kurkî ištēniš taṭammi* 7.TA.ÀM 53'''' *[kiš]ra takaṣṣar ēma taktaṣru* ÉN tu lu ba ḫa šu ši a-ga ši-ḫa 54'''' [a-ga-la-t]i-la ši-ḫa a-ga-ti-la ši-ḫa a-ga-l[a]-ti-la ši-ḫa ÉN 55'''' *[šiptu an-n]ītu ina muḫḫi tamannu sinništa šuāti tukaṣṣarši* 56'''' [...]... *uqnâ ayyarta ša sebet tikpūša kapāṣu* 57'''' *[z]ibīta šû zikar u sinniš ina šīpāti barmāti tašakkak* 58'''' *[...] šamna tašabbaḫ burzisal taskarinni šamna tumallā-ma itti abnī* 59'''' *[.... ina] šamni tašakkan adi ulladu šamna šuāti zīmīša u qerbīša* 60'''' *[iptanaššaš(?) ...] aptīša(?) tašakkan šeguššа sasqâ* 61'''' *[.....] ... tarakkas-ma ina bīti parsi lū(?) ina <maḫar> Šamaš* 62'''' *[....] ... adi ulladu ina ūmi šalāšīšu iltanappat* 63'''' *[....] ... ūm i''aldu* 64'''' *[....] ... [....] engisû ša(?) [...]* 65'''' *[.....] ... šerraša išallim*

49'''' You set up [...]; your pour a libation of beer. [You *slaughter*] a virgin kid. 50'''' You put [...] into a *sūtu*-vessel; you fill the *sūtu*-vessel with *šeguššu*-millet. Then 51'''' [the woman] sits (down) on/above (it). You place goat hair (and) wool under her feet. 52''''You twine together (a string) of [...], white wool, the tendon of a gazelle (and) the tendon of a goose. Seven times 53'''' you tie [a kno]t. Whenever you have tied (a knot), (you recite the) incantation: "tu lu ba ḫa šu ši a-ga ši-ḫa 54'''' [a-ga-la-t]i-la ši-ḫa a-ga-ti-la ši-ḫa a-ga-l[a]-ti-la ši-ḫa." Incantation formula. 55'''' [Th]is [incantation] you recite over it. You tie (knots for) that woman. 57'''' You string 56'''' [...-mineral], lapis lazuli, *ayyartu*-shell with seven dots, *kapāṣu*-shell, 57'''' [*z*]*ibītu*-stone, (as well as) male and female *šû*-stone on (a cord) of multi-coloured wool. 58'''' You sprinkle oil [...]. You fill a *burzisallu*-vessel of boxwood with oil. Together with the stones 59'''' you put [... into the] oil. Until she gives birth, 60'''' [*she shall keep rubbing*] 59'''' her *face and belly* with that oil. 60'''' You place [... *at*(?)] her *window*. 61'''' [You ...] 60'''' *šeguššu*-millet, fine flour 61'''' [...] you set up and in a secluded room or(?) be<fore> Šamaš [you ...]. 62'''' [...] ... Until she gives birth, *she shall touch* (*it*) three times a day. 63'''' [...] ... The day (the child) is born 64'''' [....] ... [....] *engisû*-stone which(?) [...] 65'''' [...] ... her baby will be well.

Ms. A rev.(?) l. col. breaks

Notes

Line 2′: The phrase *ina bīt ašbāk(u)* also occurs in other texts for women with childbirth difficulties: in BM 48030 obv. 9 (fragmentary), in SpTU 5, No. 248 obv. 32 (text C.3.10): *ina bīt ašbāk pānī lū maḫrat* "May my wish be granted in the house where I live!", and in SpTU 3, No. 84 obv. 11 (a ritual against repeated stillbirths caused by Lamaštu): *anāku lūšir lušēšir ina bīt āšbāku* "Let me be alright and let me have a normal pregnancy in the house where I live!" (text C.3.4). The phrase is also attested in other Akkadian prayers (e.g., a Dingiršadabba prayer, see Jaques 2015, *Mon dieu*, 85: 21). In BM 48030 obv. 9, *ina bīt ašbāku* also appears to be followed by the word *nēmelu* "success" and may thus be parallel to ms. A line 2′ (see text C.3.8). For *nēmelu* in a similar context, see also SpTU 5, No. 248 obv. 32 (text C.3.10): *anāku ša ina libbīya lišlim-ma nēmelšu lūmur* "(But as for) me, may the fruit of my womb be in good health, so that I may see it prosper!" (followed by *ina bīt ašbāk*).

Line 3′: Abusch et al. (2020: 87, note on line 3′) suggest restoring *kišpī ruḫê* at the beginning of the line, with reference to Abusch et a. 2016 (CMAwR 2), text 8.28: 106: *kišpī ruḫê zērūti* "witchcraft (and) hateful magic". Cf. also Abusch (2016), *Maqlû* VI 126″: *upšāšê muḫrīnni* "(O salt (*ṭābtu*),) take over/receive (fem.) from me the (sorcerous) machinations!" The addressed subject of the sentence in KAR 247 should thus also be feminine. For similar ritual transfers of impurities, expressed with the verb *maḫāru* in the female patient's prayers, cf. also SpTU 5, No. 248 obv. 13, 33 *passim* (text C.3.10).

Line 4′: The reconstruction follows SpTU 3, No. 84 obv. 11: *anāku lūšir lušēšir ina bīt āšbāku* "Let me be all right and let me have a normal pregnancy in the house where I live!" (see text C.3.4), as suggested by Abusch et al. (2020), text 5.8.

Line 5′: For this phrase, see also BM 48030 rev. 2′; SpTU 5, No 248 rev. 33, 35 (*infra*). It is also found often in other rituals not concerned with a female patient (see Abusch et al. 2020, 89 note on line 13′).

Line 6′: The restoration follows SpTU 5, No. 248 rev. 13 and 26, there written logographically: *ana* MUNUS NU SI.SÁ SI.SÁ DÙ.DÙ.BI (text C.3.10). See also Schwemer 2007a, *Abwehrzauber*, 37 fn. 46. Thanks to ms. B, the deity receiving an offering here and addressed in the prayer in lines 10′ff. can now be identified as Ninmaḫ. The goddess Gula is addressed in ms. A line 41‴. For MUNUS NU SI.SÁ, *sinništu lā muš(t)ēšertu* "a woman who does not bring to term", see also STT 241 (text C.3.1).

Line 7′: Possibly, restore GI.DU$_8$ "portable altar" instead of ^{giš}BANŠUR.

Line 8′: Instead of NINDA.Ì.DÉ.A, this text uses the more unusual spelling NINDA.Ì.DÉ.ÀM.

Line 10′: Abusch et al. (CMAwR 3, 87 note on line 10′) mention the fact that the incipit of the prayer "Ištar 22" (Farber 1977, *BID*, 68–69, Hauptritual 1a, lines 43–49) is similar to the present prayer. In ms. B, there is not enough space for ÉN, which is reconstructed at the beginning of ms. A.

Line 11′: For reconstruction, see CAD R, 253b sub 2b. Note the slight variant in ms. A *ša ina ba-lu-uk-ki* vs. ms. B *ša ba-lu-uk-ki*. For the connection of the mother goddess (or of goddesses associated with her functions) with semen, note especially the folk-etymological association of Zarpanītu (whose name was interpreted as Zēr-bānītu "semen creatrix") with semen and progeny (see Krebernik 1993–1997, *RlA* 8, 516 §7.13). Note K. 3371 + K. 232: 22 (ABRT 2, 16 and JRAS 1929, 10–11): *Zarpanītu ša kīma šumīša-ma bānât zēri* "Zarpanītu, who, according to her very name creates offspring (lit. seed)". Zarpanītu was also venerated under the title ^{d}E$_4$-ru$_6$, which alludes to Sumerian a-ri-a "semen". An astral constellation with this name (Erua) is associated with her, which receives the same interpretation *bānât riḫûti* "creatrix of semen" (see Wee 2016, *JNES* 75, 162–163, 166 5R 46 No. 1: 46).

Lines 13′–14′: The masculine suffixes in ms. B in line 13′ would also justify the restoration NENNI DU[MU NENNI] "Mr. So-and-so, so[n of Mr. So-and-So]", which would mean that the female patient's husband would be introduced first. However, ms. A displays feminine suffixes in the corresponding line, which suggests that only a female patient is introduced, although the same formula referring to her is repeated in line 14′, which is unusual. However, line 13′ appears to introduce the patient, while line 14′ beginning with *šum* "concerning" marks the beginning of the plea on the patient's behalf (as surmised already by Abusch et al. 2020, CMAwR 3, 87 note on lines 13′–14′).

For *šumu* "name" in similar uses denoting "concerning" or the like, cf. CAD Š/3, 394 sub 3. The phrase *ana šumi* "because of, as for" or the preposition/conjunction *aššu* "because (of)" would be expected rather than the form *šum* (perhaps the text is abbreviated here). Cf. Mayer 1976, 291–292 for expressions with *aššu* in prayers.

Line 15′: In this line, there is no apparent textual overlap between mss. A and B, and it is not excluded that the wording of both manuscripts in this line differed completely. The text of ms. A focuses on the patient's request for offspring. The remnants of obv. ii 13 in ms. B suggest two parallel expressions with the keywords *aplu* "heir, son" and *zēru* "descendent" (lit. seed). After *ana* IBILA *šur-še-e* "to let let (her) get an heir" (Böck 2013, *JA* 103, 42 n. 53; cf. CAD R, 204a sub 8a (Š-stem of *rašû*) for similar examples), a second expression followed, presumably with another infinitive in the genitive lost in gap. The restoration is only tentative (cf. CAD B, 156 s.v. *bašû* (Š-stem) sub 3a-2′, "to make sth. come into existence, to create sth."). Ms. A, however, appears to focus on witchcraft as the underlying cause of the problem threatening the patient. The parallel line preserves the keyword *upšāšû* "sorcerous machinations". The following passage runs parallel in both mss., but the text of ms. B (in obv. ii 14) appears to be corrupt. The emendation proposes another expression with a negated infinitive (*ana*) *mimma lemnu lā sanāqi* "so that any evil may not come near"; the logographic spelling in ms. A (NU DIM$_4$) is ambiguous.

Lines 16′–17′: Ms. B erroneously uses the masculine pronominal suffix in *ana maḫar/pān ilūtīka* in line 16′; however, in line 20′ the phrase is correctly repeated as *ana maḫar/pān ilūtīki*. For similar phrases in prayers, see also Mayer 1976, 293–294.

The sign sequence at the beginning of line 17′ in ms. A, *ana* LÍL BAD, is difficult to interpret; perhaps the text is corrupt. Since a syllabic reading of the signs does not yield a meaningful Akkadian word, I tentatively regard the signs LÍL and BAD as logograms yielding the phrase *ana silīti nesî* "so that the illness (affecting the patient) departs". The reconstruction of ms. A [... ^{ú}KUR.K]UR$^{?}$ follows ms. B. Abusch et al. 2020, text 5.8 restore ^{ú}*eli*$^{?}$-*k*]*ul* instead.

Line 25′: The form *lib-ba-ši* is presumably an N-stem precative of *bašû*: "may a descendant (*līpu*) come into being". Possibly, read *m*[*a-ru*] "son" after *li-pu*. For similar pleas concerning hoped-for offspring, see e.g. BMS 30: 14; Mayer 1976, 458; Zgoll 2003, 184–188 (Ištar prayer 4 line 18′): *šurkīm-ma šuma u zēra lū rēmu silītī* "grant me an heir and offspring; may my womb be fertile"; also Zgoll 2003, Ištar prayer 23. See further Mayer 1976, 289–290. Compare also AO 4425A (*infra* text B.2.6).

Line 26′: Perhaps restore *š*[*a e-ṭ*]*u* "(may) what is dark (become bright)" at the beginning. Compare a similar expression in Ebeling 1953, 134: 87–88; Foster 2005, 604: *eṭû qatru limmir kinūnī / belīti linnapiḫ dipārī* "May my dark (and) smoky brazier become bright, may my extinguished torch be kindled (again)!"

Line 28′: Judging from the copy of CTN 4, No. 105, there is hardly enough space for [DÙ.DÙ.BI] at the beginning of the line. The expression with *minûtu* "recitation (of an incantation)" in line 2′ also occurs in line 9′ (ms. A obv.(?) l. col. 9′, written logographically): ŠID-*tú an-ni-tú* 3-*šú* ŠID-[*nu*] "you recite this incantation three times".

Line 29′: The emendation to KAŠ BAL$^{!}$-*qí* "you libate beer" is suggested by the context, although it is of course possible to read TI-*qé* "you take".

Line 34″: Ebeling's copy in KAR 247 reads SILA$_4$, while the copy in CMAwR 3, pl. 9 has AMA.

Line 51″″: The instruction that the patient should sit down (or squat) above a vessel filled with *materia medica* is elsewhere known in the context of fumigation from below, but in the present text there seems to be no reference to glowing charcoals (perhaps it was omitted), which are filled into the fumigation vessel in the other examples (see e.g., BAM 237 i 26′–27′: GÌR.PAD.DU NAM.LÚ.U$_{19}$.LU *ina* DÈ *ta-sár-raq* MUNUS BI *ina* UGU TUŠ-*ši* "You scatter 'human bone' over coal, you make that woman sit down above it" (text C.1.4); cf. also K. 8678+ rev. 7′ and 12′ (text A.1.4). For fumigation from below, see also Steinert 2014a; 2014b.

Lines 53″″–54″″: This fragmentary *abracadabra*-spell is otherwise unknown. The reconstruction follows Abusch et al. 2020, CMAwR 3, text 5.8 with note on lines 38″″–39″″. They suggest that the word a-ga-la-ti-la (with variant a-ga-ti-la) could represent the word *agan(n)utillû* "dropsy". The word ši-ḫa could be *šēḫu* "wind", which also occurs as a medical problem.

Line 55″″: For the phrase *tukaṣṣarši* "you make knots for her", see also BAM 237 rev. iv 39 (text C.1.4), where this statement introduces an instruction for making an amulet necklace. In the present text, however, the phrase MUNUS BI *tukaṣṣarši* rather seems to conclude the preceding instruction to twist tendons and wool and to tie knots into the thread. It thus may refer to tying the resulting band to the woman's body.

Lines 56″″–60″″: The stones that are threaded on a string here are not attached to the woman's body but are placed in a *burzisallu*-vessel together with oil. Following the reconstruction of Abusch et al. (CMAwR 3, text 5.8 for line 59″″, it is suggested here that the woman had to rub herself (her face and belly) regularly with the prepared oil until she gave birth. Thus, I suggest restoring *iptanaššaš* (or *ipaššaš*, ŠÉŠ.(MEŠ)) at the beginning of line 60″″. The fragmentary instruction [...] ... *aptīša*(?) *tašakkan* may have said that the vessel with the oil should be placed in the vicinity of the woman's window (*aptu*), although this remains uncertain. Cf. for a similar instruction, SpTU 5, No. 248 rev. 39 quoted in the next note. For $^{(dug)}$BUR.ZI.SAL.(LA), see also Abusch and Schwemer 2011 (CMAwR 1), 80 with note on line 52″.

Lines 61″″–62″″: Note a parallel in the ritual of SpTU 5, No. 248 rev. 39 (text C.3.10): "You place a *sheaf* of *šeguššu*-cereal (millet) at a crossroads and hang (it) in a window. The pregnant woman shall touch (it) regularly until she gives birth (*adi ulladu iltanappat*)". Following this parallel, it is suggested here that TAG.MEŠ in line 62″″ could be read *iltanappat* or *ulappat* "she shall keep touching (it three times a day)" rather than *taltanappat* "you rub (her)" suggested by Abusch et al. (CMAwR 3, text 5.8). The preceding instructions in lines 60″″–61″″ do not seem to be concerned with the preparation of an ointment but may rather refer to the preparation of an offering mentioning Šamaš.

The phrase *ina bīti parsi* referring to the place of the offering in line 61″″ may be a "secluded room" in the woman's house rather than a "secluded house". The instruction *tarakkas-ma* in line 61″″ may mean "you arrange" (with reference to an offering arrangement) rather than "you bind" (referring to tying on an amulet), which would fit better with the reference to *šeguššu*-millet and fine flour at the end of line 60‴.

C.3.7 VAT 13629 + 13866 (KAL 2, No. 41): Amulet Charms and Spells against Witchcraft-Induced Miscarriage

This fragment of a two- or three-column tablet found at the so-called "House of the incantation priest" at Assur belonged to the library of the family of the healer Kiṣir-Aššur. It contains instructions for the preparation of protective amulets for pregnant women.

The longer passage preserved on the obverse of the tablet contains amulets for various parts of a pregnant woman's body (ordered "from head to feet"). The instructions for these amulets are known from several other first millennium BCE manuscripts from Nineveh, Assur, Sultantepe and Babylonia (K. 4727+ and duplicates, edited as text F.1), some of which may have belonged to the series *kunuk ḫalti* "cylindrical (bead of) *ḫaltu*-stone" (cf. Schuster-Brandis 2008, 148–149, 192–197).

The remaining text passages of KAL 2, No. 41 on the obverse and reverse re-edited here feature amulet prescriptions to protect a pregnant woman from witchcraft and to prevent a miscarriage. They are complemented by the wording of incantations that had to be recited during the manufacture of the amulets.

List of Manuscripts

Siglum	Museum Number	Copy	Collation	Format; Ductus	Provenience
A	VAT 13629 + VAT 13866	KAL 2, No. 41	–	Fragment of a two- or three-column tablet, Neo-Assyrian script, 8th/7th cent. BCE	Assur, library N4

Overview

i′	Fragmentary incantation(?) A obv.! ii′ 1′–7′	...]1′–7′[...
ii″	Fragmentary ritual to protect a pregnant woman from witchcraft (amulet) A rev.! iv′ 1–4	8″–11″
iii″	Fragmentary anti-witchcraft ritual for preventing miscarriage (amulet) A rev.! iv′ 5–9	12″–16″
iv″	Anti-witchcraft ritual for preventing miscarriage (amulet and incantation) A rev.! iv′ 10–16	17″–23″
v″	Fragmentary A rev.! iv′ 17–18	24″–25″[...

Previous Edition and Discussion

Schwemer 2007b, KAL 2, 100–102, No. 41; copy on p. 193
Abusch et al. 2020, CMAwR 3, 53–55 text 5.2 (edition of ms. A rev.! iv/vi 1–18)
CDLI P480934 (copy)

Summary of the sections in ms. A not included here (for an edition of these lines, see text F.1, K. 4727+ //):

Obv.! i′ 1′–5′: Instructions for an amulet for the navel and hips of a pregnant woman
Obv.! i′ 6′–11′: Instructions for an amulet for the right thigh of a pregnant woman
Obv.! i′ 12′–16′: Instructions for an amulet for the left thigh of a pregnant woman

Obv.$^{!}$ i′ 17′: Instructions for an amulet for the right foot of a pregnant woman

Transliteration

Beginning of ms. A obv.$^{!}$ ii′ lost

1′	A obv.$^{!}$ ii′ 1′	x [……………………………]
2′	A obv.$^{!}$ ii′ 2′	*i*$^{?}$-*mi*$^{?}$-[…………………………]
3′	A obv.$^{!}$ ii′ 3′	^{d}IDIM ^{d}*as*[*al-lú-ḫi*$^{?}$ ………………]
4′	A obv.$^{!}$ ii′ 4′	EN KALA *u* x[……………………]
5′	A obv.$^{!}$ ii′ 5′	*la ṣab*-x[…………………………]
6′	A obv.$^{!}$ ii′ 6′	*ki*-⸢*i*⸣ [……………………………]
7′	A obv.$^{!}$ ii′ 7′	x[…………………………………]

A obv.$^{!}$ ii′ breaks

A rev.$^{!}$ iii′: only traces preserved

8″	A rev.$^{!}$ iv′ 1	[ÉN$^{?}$ x x x x] x x [x x (x)]
9″	A rev.$^{!}$ iv′ 2	[x x x x x] ⸢*ina*⸣ *pa*-⸢*ni*$^{?}$⸣(-)[x-(x)]
10″	A rev.$^{!}$ iv′ 3	[x x x] *e* NIGIN-*ra*
11″	A rev.$^{!}$ iv′ 4	[*ana* ^{munus}PE]Š$_4$ *kiš-pi* NU TE-*e*
12″	A rev.$^{!}$ iv′ 5	[*ša* ŠÀ-*šá a*$^{?}$]-⸢*na*⸣ SILIM-*mi* ŠU.BI.AŠ.ÀM {x}
13″	A rev.$^{!}$ iv′ 6	[x x x x] *ina* ŠU GÙB-⸢*šá*⸣ GAR-*an-š*[*i*]
14″	A rev.$^{!}$ iv′ 7	*whole line erased*
15″	A rev.$^{!}$ iv′ 8	[ÉN x] x x ⸢mu$^{?}$⸣-ra-dab TU$_6$ ⸢ÉN⸣
16″	A rev.$^{!}$ iv′ 9	[ÉN *a*]*n-ni-tú* ŠID-*ma kiš-pi* NU TE-*ši*
17″	A rev.$^{!}$ iv′ 10	[(DIŠ) *ana* ^{munus}PE]Š$_4$ *ip-ši ep-šu-ši-ma*
18″	A rev.$^{!}$ iv′ 11	[*ana ša* Š]À-*šá* ŠUB.ŠUB-*e*
19″	A rev.$^{!}$ iv′ 12	[*ana š*]*a* ŠÀ-*šá* NU ŠUB-*e* ŠU.BI.AŠ.ÀM
20″	A rev.$^{!}$ iv′ 13	[x ^{n}]^{a4}⸢*šu*⸣-*u* NÍTA *ina* ŠU GÙB <<GÙB>>-*šá* GAR-*an*
21″	A rev.$^{!}$ iv′ 14	[ÉN] munus <<igi>> zú-kéš zú-kéš-da
22″	A rev.$^{!}$ iv′ 15	[z]ú-kéš zú-kéš-da TU$_6$ ÉN
23″	A rev.$^{!}$ iv′ 16	[É]N *an-ni-tú* ŠUB-*ma kiš-pi* NU TE-*ši*

24″ A rev.! iv′ 17 [x x x x x (x)]x x ta? SÚD

25″ A rev.! iv′ 18 [x x x x x x x x x] x x

Ms. A rev.! iv′ breaks; remainder lost

Bound Transcription and Translation

Beginning of ms. A obv.! ii′ lost

1′–7′ *Fragmentary*	1′–7′ *Too fragmentary for translation*
A obv.! ii′ breaks *A rev.! iii′: only traces preserved* 8″ [ÉN? ... ...] ... [... ...] 9″ [... ...] *ina pāni* [...](?) 10″ [... ...] *ē tasḫura*	 8″ [Incantation(?): "... ...] ... [... ...], 9″ [... ...] *before* [...], 10″ [... ...] do not seek me out!"
11″ [*ana erī*]*ti kišpī lā ṭeḫê*	11″ [So that] witchcraft not approach [a pregn]ant woman.
12″ [*ša libbīša a*]*na šullumi* ŠU.BI.AŠ.ÀM 13″ [... ...] *ina qāt šumēlīša tašakkanš*[*i*] 14″ (*line erased*) 15″ [ÉN ...] ... mu-ra-dab(?) *tê šipti*	12″ [So that (a pregnant woman)] bring [her foetus] to term, ditto. 13″ You put [...] on her left hand. 14″ (*line erased*) 15″ [Incantation: "...] ... ." Incantation formula.
16″ [*šiptu a*]*nnītu tamannū-ma kišpī ul iṭeḫḫû-ši*	16″ You recite [t]his incantation, and then witchcraft will not approach her.
17″ [(*šumma*) *ana e*]*rīti ipšī epšūši-ma* 18″ [*ana ša li*]*bbīša šuddê* 19″ [*ana š*]*a libbīša lā nadê* ŠU.BI.AŠ.ÀM 20″ [...] *šû zikar ina qāt šumēlīša tašakkan* 21″ [ÉN] munus munus <<igi>> zú-kéš zú-kéš-da 22″ [z]ú-kéš zú-kéš-da TU$_6$ ÉN	17″ [(If) sorceries have been performed [against a pre]gnant woman, so as 18″ [to] cause her to have a miscarriage, 19″ [so that] she not miscarry her foetus, ditto. 20″ You put [...] male *šû*-stone(s) on her left hand. 21″ [Incantation:] "Woman, woman, the knot is knotted, 22″ the knot is knotted." Incantation formula.
23″ [*ši*]*ptu annītu tanaddī-ma kišpī ul iṭeḫḫûši*	23″ You cast this [inc]antation, then witchcraft will not approach her.

(lines 24″–25″ too fragmentary for transcription / translation)
Ms. A rev.! iv′ breaks; remainder lost

Notes

Textual considerations lead to the conclusion that obverse and reverse of the tablet as identified by Schwemer's copy in KAL 2 need to be reversed (cf. Schwemer 2007b, KAL 2, p. 102; Abusch et al. 2020, 55; note, however, obv.! i and ii in their summary on p. 54 need to be reversed as well). Thus, the use of "ditto" in col. iv′ 5 and 12 would be difficult to explain if these lines had been placed at the beginning of the tablet.

Lines 1′–7′: The traces suggest that these lines are part of an incantation. In line 3′, the god Ea (dIDIM) and perhaps also his son Asalluḫi may be invoked. In line 4′, read perhaps *bēlu*(EN) *dannu*(KALA) "strong lord".

Line 10″: Alternatively, read *ē tasḫurā* (pl.).

Line 12″: The phrase *ša libbīša šullumu* is also attested in the *Diagnostic Handbook* Tablet 36: 43–44, 85 and in BM 51246+ rev. 14′ (= line 36′: *ša libbīša ušallam*) (for both texts, see *infra*). The latter prescription is for preventing miscarriage signalled by the loss of amniotic fluid. It is uncertain what exactly the "ditto" refers to here (e.g. whether it replaces a treatment instruction that was already described in the previous text section or part of the introductory formula ("so that witchcraft does not approach her")).

Line 13″: As the parallel prescription in line 20″ below, the instruction is abbreviated; the material (string) on which amulet ingredients (lost in the gap) were strung is not mentioned.

Lines 17″–19″: This purpose statement combining a conditional clause and two infinitive phrases is unusual. The interpretation of line 18″ follows Abusch et al. (2020 CMAwR 3, 54–55 with note on line 11), who interpret the reduplicated form ŠUB.ŠUB-*e* as a Š-stem infinitive (*šuddê*), although reduplicated forms usually stand for a Gtn-stem. They note that the scribe also superfluously wrote GÙB twice in line 20″. However, it is likewise possible that ŠUB.ŠUB-*e* is a mistake for ŠUB.ŠUB-*a* (*itaddâ* or *ittanaddâ*) and that the passage may have to be read slightly different: [DIŠ ^{munus}P]EŠ$_4$ *ip-ši ep-ši-šu-ma* / [*ša* Š]À-*šá* ŠUB.ŠUB-*a* / [*ana š*]*a* ŠÀ-*šá* NU ŠUB-*e* "[If] sorcery has been performed against a pregnant [woman], and (because of this) she had repeated miscarriages, [so that] she not have an(other) miscarriage". See also Steinert et al. 2018, 270.

Line 20″: Schwemer (2007b, KAL 2, 102 note on col. i$^?$ 13) suggests that a number is missing at the beginning of the line.

Lines 21–22″: For the incantation, see also AO 6473 obv. 15 (text C.3.9) used with a different amulet, but for the same purpose (preserving pregnancy). The deletion of igi follows the text in AO 6473.

C.3.8 BM 48030: A Ritual for a Pregnant Woman with Prayer to Ursa Major

This fragment in a Late Babylonian script preserves part of a ritual including an incantation or prayer to the constellation Ursa Major (^{mul}MAR.GÍD.DA, *Ereqqu* "Wagon") spoken by the patient, which shares phraseological similarities with similar recitations in KAR 247 and SpTU 5, No. 248 (texts C.3.6 and C.3.10). These similarities suggest that the present ritual, like the other two texts, was performed for pregnant women who had suffered previous miscarriages. In the latter two texts, the problem is attributed predominantly to witchcraft. Ursa Major was associated with Venus (i.e. the goddess Ištar) and with Antu (Reiner 1995, 57–58, 139), and several Akkadian prayers or incantations to Ursa Major are known (e.g. Mayer 1976, 429–430; Abusch and Schwemer 2011, CMAwR 1, text 10.2). In another incantation (KAL 4, No. 53 rev. 10; Maul and Strauß 2011, 105), Ursa Major is addressed as a benign female entity, as "mother of all the gods", befitting her role as a protector of childbearing women in the present text.

List of Manuscripts

Siglum	Museum Number	Copy	Collation	Format; Ductus	Provenience
a	BM 48030 (81-11-3, 739)	CMAwR 3, pl. 3	–	Fragment, Late Babylonian script, ca. 5th–3rd cent. BCE	Babylonia (exact provenience uncertain)

Overview

i	Fragmentary ritual with incantation addressed to Ursa Major a obv. 1–11, rev. 1′–2′	1–11 [...], 12′–13′
ii′	Fragmentary prescription a rev. 3′	14′[...

Previous Edition and Discussion

Lambert, *Nachlass*, Folio 9329 (transliteration)
Abusch et al. 2020, CMAwR 3, 88–89 text 5.9 (edition)
Electronic Babylonian Library (eBL) (transliteration; discussion; https://www.ebl.lmu.de/library/BM.48030)

Transliteration

1 a obv. 1 [x x] ša$^{?}$ ga si$^{?}$ [...........]

2 a obv. 2 ⸢^{mul}⸣MAR.GÍD.D[A ......]

3 a obv. 3 ^{mul}MAR.GÍD.D[A ....]

4 a obv. 4 ^{mul}MAR.GÍD.D[A ....]

5 a obv. 5 ^{d}+*en-líl i-la-ti* [...............]

6 a obv. 6 ^{d}*nin-líl i-la-t*[*i* ....]

7 a obv. 7 *ana-ku* NENNI-*tu*$_4$ DUMU.MUNUS NENNI-*t*[*u*$_4$ ...]

8 a obv. 8 *ana* MU-*ia ma-l*[*u-ú*$^{?}$ ......]

9 a obv. 9 ⸢*ina*⸣ É *áš-ba-ku n*[*e-mel*$^{?}$ ......]

10 a obv. 10 ⸢*ú-lid*⸣-*ma ul a-mur* x [...........]

11 a obv. 11 [x x] ⸢ú ma nu⸣ x x [...............]

Ms. a obv. breaks

12′ a rev. 1′ [x] x(-)⸢*an-ni*⸣(-)[................]

13′ a rev. 2′ ⸢SILA⸣ DIB NU DI[B ....]

14′ a rev. 3′ ^{ú}*tar-m*[*uš* ....]

Ms. a rev. breaks

Bound Transcription and Translation

1 [...] ... [...]	1 [...] ... [...]
2 *Ereqqu* [...]	2 Ursa Major, [....].
3 *Ereqqu* [...]	3 Ursa Major, [....].
4 *Ereqqu* [...]	4 Ursa Major, [....].
5 *Enlil ilāti* [....]	5 Enlil of the goddesses, [....],
6 *Ninlil ilāti* [....]	6 Ninlil of the goddesses, [....].
7 *anāku annannītu mārat annannīt*[*i* ...]	7 I, Mrs. So-and-so, daughter of Mrs. So-and-So, [....].
8 *ina šumīya-ma mal*[*û*(?) ....]	8 On my account ...[....].
9 *ina bīt ašbāku n*[*ēmel*(?) ....]	9 In the house where I live [...] suc[cess ....].
10 *ūlid-ma ul āmur* ...[...]	10 I gave birth, but I did not see [...].
11 (*too fragmentary for transcription*)	11 (*too fragmentary for translation*)

break

12′ (*too fragmentary for transcription*) 13′ *sūq ītiqu lā itt[iq* ...]	12′ (*too fragmentary for translation*) 13′ She must not go (back) by the (same) street by which she came. [...]
14′ *tarm[uš* ...]	14′ *Tarm[uš*-plant, ...]

Ms. a rev. breaks

Notes

Lines 2–6: For another association of Ursa Major with sexual reproduction, note the prohibition in KAR 178 rev. iv 61–62 to have intercourse with one's wife on the seventh day of the seventh month of the Babylonian calendar, because it was a taboo of the "Wagon star" and of the god Anu. The "Wagon" may have been believed to be of assistance to pregnant women not only because of her female character, but also because the patient's problem was believed to be caused by witchcraft (for other anti-witchcraft rituals that are performed in front of Ursa Major, see e.g., Abusch and Schwemer 2011, text 10.2, 10.5: 8′–16′; Abusch and Schwemer 2016, text 10.10).

Line 7: For parallels to this formula and the identification of female patients via the matronymic, see also Finkel 2018, *FS Geller*, 232–271, esp. 238ff. Finkel notes that in standard usage, both men and women are identified with their patronymic rather than the mother's name in Mesopotamia; however, exceptions can be found in the case of foundlings or persons whose mothers were unmarried. However, in Late Babylonian healing texts concerned with women, there are other cases in which the matronymic is used, e.g. in the incantations against fever inscribed on clay amulets for a woman named Baba-ēṭerat (from Nippur) discussed by Finkel 2018, 239–247. For examples within the corpus of women's healthcare texts, see e.g. SpTU 3, No. 84 obv. 16, 94 (text C.3.4).

For women identified by a matronymic in Neo-Babylonian documents, see further Wunsch 1993, No. 3: 2–3; Wunsch 2003, No. 12: 14, No. 28: 9′; Sandowicz (forthcoming), *Their Mothers' Children: Neo- and Late Babylonian Matronyms.* Note also BE 17/1, No. 31 rev. 27 and PBS 1/2, No. 71 rev. 8 (two medical letter reports from Middle Babylonian Nippur concerning the ailments of female musicians, referring to two unnamed women as "daughter of ᶠNN", see Waschow 1936, MAOG 10, 30–31, 34–35 nos. 1 and 5; https://build-oracc.museum.upenn.edu/akkec/midbab/corpus).

Line 9: The expression *ina bīt ašbāk(u)* occurs also in SpTU 5, No. 248 obv. 32, 34, in KAR 247 obv.(?) l. col. 2′, 4′, and further in SpTU 3, 84 obv. 11, all of which are rituals to protect pregnant women from miscarriage. KAR 247 obv.(?) l. col. 2′ probably used the same phrase as BM 48030 obv. 9: *ina* É *áš-ba-ku ne-[mel*? ...]. The phrase is not restricted to female patients, see Jaques, *Mon dieu*, 85: 21 (a fragmentary DINGIR.ŠÀ.DAB.BA-prayer). See texts C.3.4, C.3.6 and C.3.10.

Line 12′: As observed by Abusch et al. 2020, CMAwR 3, 89 note on line 12′, this could be the last line of the prayer (with the element *-anni* "me"), similar to KAR 247 obv.? l. col. 4′–5′, where the prayer and the following one-line instruction are not separated by a ruling either.

Line 13′: This expression is encountered in similar rituals for pregnant women (e.g. SpTU 5, No. 248 rev. 33, 35; KAR 247 obv.? l. col. 5′). But it is also found in other ritual texts, e.g. in Namburbi-rituals (see Maul 1994, 252: 55, 274: 47′, 285: 13, 286: 13′ *passim*); Abusch et al. 2020, CMAwR 3, 89 note on line 13′.

C.3.9 AO 6473 (TCL 6, 49): Amulet Charms for Pregnant Women Protecting from Miscarriage

This Late Babylonian tablet from Uruk (ms. a) contains rituals for amulet charms to protect a pregnant woman from miscarriage, accompanied by incantations. One of these rituals (ms. a obv. 8ff.) concerned the preparation of an amulet to protect a pregnant woman against witchcraft, which makes use of the Akkadian anti-witchcraft incantation *ittardāni ana māti* "They (the witches) have come down to the land" (obv. 16–25, see also CMAwR 1, text 7.8, 1) and the Sumerian spell munus zú-kéš zú-kéš-da, which was spoken over knots tied into the amulet cord.

The tablet continues in obv. 26–27 noting two further incantation incipits. The first one probably refers to the same incantation that was recited over an amulet for a pregnant woman partially preserved in STT 241 obv. 8–rev. 26 (text

C.3.1). The incipit in obv. 27 belongs to an unknown spell against the child-snatching demoness Lamaštu (Farber 2014, 35 *ezzēt(a) šam(ma)rāt(a) dannāt(a)*). These two lines are followed by fragmentary ritual instructions (obv. 28–rev. 1), mentioning among amulet ingredients placed around the neck of the pregnant woman a Pazuzu figurine – an element which likewise suggests that a ritual to counter Lamaštu was adapted to a related context, the protection of pregnant women.

The next two sections (ms. a rev. 2–8 and 9–11) contain further prescriptions for protective amulets. The tablet ends with a complete (non-canonical) Lamaštu incantation, *ezzet šamrat ilat namurrat* (Farber 2014, 268–270, 298–299), found also in two other texts concerned with pregnant women, in which this incantation is used to counter witchcraft-induced miscarriage (mss. c and d, see below). It is not explicitly stated for which of the amulets this incantation had to be recited.

The amulets consist of various stones, shells and plants, which are tied around different body parts of the pregnant woman. The key element is the tying of magic knots, which symbolise the desired closure of the womb during pregnancy, a very common magic ritual practise cross-culturally. One significant stone in this tablet is the *ittamir*-stone, known as a "stone for giving birth" (MSL 10, 31 Ḫg. B IV 74), but also as a stone against witchcraft (Abusch and Schwemer 2011, text 7.8., 1 l. 25′).

The amulet prescription in obv. 1–7 first of AO 6473 is attributed to an older original owned by an individual called Dāda or Dādi (obv. 7), while the remainder of the prescriptions is said to have been copied from an original from Babylon in rev. 11, while simultaneously presenting "oral lore" (*šūt pî*).

List of Manuscripts

Siglum	Museum Number	Copy	Collation	Format; Ductus	Provenience
a	AO 6473	Thureau-Dangin, *RA* 18, 162–163 TCL 6, 49	Coll.	single-column tablet; Late Babylonian script; 3rd–2nd cent. BCE)	Uruk
B	K. 8112 + K. 9666 (+)[326]	Abusch and Schwemer, CMAwR 1, pl. 31	Coll.	Fragments of a three-column(?) tablet; Neo-Assyrian script; 7th cent. BCE	Nineveh, Ashurbanipal's library
C_1 (+) C_2	VAT 14150 + VAT 14156 (+) VAT 14151 + VAT 14152 + VAT 14153 + VAT 13628	KAL 2, No. 36 KAL 7, No. 11	–	Fragments of a three-column tablet; Neo-Assyrian script; 7th cent. BCE	Assur, N4-library
d	W. 23287	SpTU 3, No. 84	Photo Coll.	Single-column tablet, Late Babylonian script, 5th cent. BCE	Uruk; library of Anu-ikṣur (Šangû-Ninurta family)
e	BM 42327+ BM 42410 + BM 42604 + BM 42628 + BM 43474 + BM 43523	Farber 1989a, pl. 14–15	Coll.	Single-column tablet, Late Babylonian script, 6th–3rd cent. BCE	Babylonia (exact provenience uncertain)
f	–	Nougayrol, *Syria* 42, p. 228 (photo)	–	Amulet	modern forgery after lost original

Overview

i	Instructions for an amulet to protect a pregnant woman from miscarriage, to be placed around the neck, hands and feet (a obv. 1–7)	1–7

326 Indirect joins with further fragments, edited by Abusch and Schwemer, *CMAwR* 1, text 7.8, as ms. A_1–A_7 (with pl. 31–33): K. 8079 (+) K. 8162 + 10357 (+) K. 8933 (+) K. 10358 (+) K. 11243 (+) K. 12936.

ii	Ritual for an amulet to protect a pregnant woman from witchcraft – Instructions: preparation of an amulet necklace (a obv. 8–14) – Recitation of the incantation: Munus zú-kéš zú-kéš-da zú-kéš zú-kéš-da (a obv. 15) – Incantation *Ittardāni ana māti* (a obv. 16–24 // B obv. i 13′–24′ // C$_2$ rev. v 31′–41′) – Ušburruda rubric (a obv. 25)	8–25
iii	Incantation incipit: *Māḫiṣ muhhi mubbil liq pî mubbil qaqqadi* (a obv. 26)	26
iv	Incantation incipit (Lamaštu spell): *ezzēta šam(ma)rāt(a) dannāt(a)* (a obv. 27)	27
v	Instruction for an amulet with a bronze (figurine or head of) Pazuzu to be placed around a pregnant woman's neck (a obv. 28–rev. 1)	28–29
vi	Instructions for amulets against miscarriage to be placed around the head, neck, hands, hips and feet of a pregnant woman (a rev. 2–8)	30–36
vii	Instruction to add figurines of frogs(?) to the stones placed around the woman's hands and feet (a rev. 9–11)	37–39
viii	Instruction not to handle the stones of the pregnant woman's amulets during the first hundred days (of pregnancy?) (a rev. 12)	40
ix	Incantation against Lamaštu, *ezzet šamrat ilat namurrat* (a rev. 13–29 // d rev. 9–24 // e obv. 14–rev. 7 // f 1–17)	41–57

Previous Edition and Discussion

Thureau-Dangin 1921, *RA* 18, 164–171 (copy; edition)
Scurlock 1991, *Incognita* 2, 141 (translation)
Foster 2005, 981–982 (translation of the incantation *ezzet šamrat ilat namurrat*, lines 41–57 = ms. a rev. 13–29 //)
Schuster-Brandis 2008, 147–148 (Kette 153, lines 13–14)
Farber 2014, 268–270, 298–299 (edition of the incantation *ezzet šamrat ilat namurrat*, lines 41–57 = ms. a rev. 13–29 //)
Abusch and Schwemer 2011, CMAwR 1, text 7.8, 1 lines 13′–27′ (= ms. a obv. 16–24, incantation *Ittardāni ana māti*)
Meinhold 2017, KAL 7, No. 11 rev. v 31′–41′ (= ms. C, incantation *Ittardāni ana māti*)
Abusch et al. 2020, CMAwR 3, text 5.1, 1 (= ms. a obv. 8–15, 25, the *ittamir*-stone amulet)
Infra text C.3.4 (edition of ms. d), text C.3.3 (edition of mss. e and f)

Transliteration

1	a obv. 1	$^{\text{NA4.⌜ME?⌝}}$ZÚ ZALAG.MEŠ *ina* DUR SÍG BABBAR È ^{síg}GA.RIG.AK.A
2	a obv. 2	5 ŠU.SI *ina bi-ri-šú-nu* | *tara-kás* $^{\text{na4}}$KIŠIB *ḫal-tú* $^{\text{na4}}$KIŠIB ŠUBA $^{\text{na4}}$*šu-u* NÍTA *u* MUNUS *ina* GÚ-*šú* GAR-*an*
3	a obv. 3	$^{\text{na4}}$ŠUBA Á.ZI.DA *ina* ŠU.MIN 15-*šú* KÉŠ $^{\text{na4}}$ŠUBA Á.GÙB.BU *ina* ŠU.MIN $^{\textit{erasure}}$150 KÉŠ
4	a obv. 4	NA$_4$ ZÚ.LUM $^{\text{na4}}$ZÁLAG $^{\text{na4}}$*mu-ṣa* $^{\text{na4}}$AŠ.GÌ.GÌ *ina* MURUB$_4$-*šú* KÉŠ $^{\text{na4}}$*ni-ba* $^{\text{na4}}$NÍR *ina* GÌR.MIN 15-*šú*
5	a obv. 5	$^{\text{na4}}$GUG $^{\text{na4}}$ZA.GÌN *ina* GÌR.MIN 150-*šú* MIN NA$_4$.MEŠ *an-nu-tú ina* ^{síg}*ba-ru-un-du*
6	a obv. 6	*šá* ^{síg}ZA.GÌN.NA È *líp-pi šá* SÍG SA$_5$ *tála-pap ina lìb-bi* NA$_4$ *šá* ŠU.MIN *u* GÌR.MIN
7	a obv. 7	*iz-ḫa* GEŠTIN DÙ-*uš tak-ṣir šá* ^{munus}PEŠ$_4$ *šà* ŠÀ-<*šà*> NU ŠUB *gaba-rì* U.U
8	a obv. 8	$^{\text{na4}}$*it-ta-mir* KIR$_4$ SUḪUŠ *u* MURUB$_4$ KÙ.SI$_{22}$ *tu-uḫ-ḫa-za* DUR SÍG GI$_6$ È-*ak*

9	a obv. 9	2 ^{na4}KUR-*nu* DAB *kup-pu-tú* 2 NA$_{4}$ <ZÚ>.LUM KI *bir-rat* KÙ.SI$_{22}$ *u* 2 *me-li* ^{ú}*ḫu-bur*
10	a obv. 10	GIŠ BÚR! *u* ^{ú}IGI-20 *ina* ŠÀ GAR-*an* Á *ana* Á *šá* ^{na4}*it-ta-mir* È-*ak*
11	a obv. 11	1.TA.ÀM *líp-pi ḫúp-pi šá* ^{síg}ZA.GÌN.NA Á *ana* Á *tála-pap* 7.TA.ÀM
12	a obv. 12	*ki-ṣir* Á *ana* Á *ta-kàṣ-ṣar* ÉN *it-tar-da-ni ana* KUR 3-*šú ana muḫ-ḫi* ŠID-*nu-ma*
13	a obv. 13	*ana* GÚ ^{munus}PEŠ$_{4}$-*tú ku-ri-nu-uš-šú* ŠUB-*m*[*a*] KI GÚ-*šú ta-ḫa-naq-ma*
14	a obv. 14	[IT]I-*us-su tu-še-re-du-šum-ma* 1+*en* ITI *šá* Ù.TU-*šú* NU IGI-*šú*
15	a obv. 15	ÉN munus zú-kéš zú-kéš-da zú-kéš!(sag) zú-kéš-da *te* ÉN *ana muḫ-ḫi ki-ṣir* | *šá ta-kaṣ-ṣàr* ŠID-*nu*
16	a obv. 16	ÉN *it-tar-da-ni ana* KUR *kaš-šá-pa-a-tú e-li-ia-na-ti*
	B obv. i 13′–14′	[................] *ana ma-a-ti* / [............] ⸢*e*⸣-*li-ia-na-a-tu*$_{4}$
	C$_{2}$ rev. v 31′	--- *it-tar-du-ni ana ma-a-ti kaš-šá-pa-a-tu*$_{4}$ ⸢*e*⸣-[*li-ia-na-a-tu*$_{4}$]
17	a obv. 17	*i-šá-as-sa-a il-lu*!-*ru i-saḫ-ḫa-ru za-ma-ru*
	B obv. i 15′	[........................ *isaḫḫa-r*]*a za-ma-ra*
	C$_{2}$ rev. v 32′	*i-šá-as-sa-a il-lu-ra i-saḫ-ḫu-r*[*a* ....]
18	a obv. 18	*na-šá-a me-e a-ab*!(ba)-*ba*!(ab) *tam-tim* DAGAL-*tim it-ta-nam-da-a ana* SILA.MEŠ
	B obv. i 16′–17′	[................................ *tam-t*]*im* DAGAL-*tim* / [.............] SILA
	C$_{2}$ rev. v 33′–34′	*na-šá-a* A.MEŠ *a-ab-ba ta-*<*am*>*-tim* D[AGAL-*ti*]*m* / *it-ta-*<*nam*>*-da-a* [..........]
19	a obv. 19	*i-kam-ma-a* GURUŠ.MEŠ *i-šag-gi-šú* KI.SIKIL.MEŠ *iš-ta-nak-ka-na qu-lat*
	B obv. i 18′–19′	[.. K]I.SIKIL.MEŠ / [.......... *qu-la*]-⸢*a*⸣-*tim*
	C$_{2}$ rev. v 35′–36′	*i-sak*$_{6}$-*ki-pa* GURUŠ.MEŠ *i-šag-gi-šá* ⸢KI⸣.SIK[IL.M]EŠ / *iš-ta-nak-ka-na qu-la-*⸢*a*⸣-[*t*]*im*
20	a obv. 20	*ana-ku áš-šak-ka-na-ki-na-šim-ma* ^{ú}*ti-is-kur mu-sak-ki-ru šá* KA-*ki-na*
	B obv. i 20′–21′	[.... *aššakkanakkināšim-m*]*a* / [................................ KA-*ki-n*]*a*
	C$_{2}$ rev. v 37′–38′	*ana-ku áš-šak-ka-na-ki-na-šim-ma* ^{ú}*ti-is-kur* / *mu-na-ki-ra šá* INIM.MEŠ-*ki-na*
21	a obv. 21	^{ú}AN.ḪÚL.LA *la ma-ḫir kiš-pi* GIŠ BÚR *šá ú-pa-áš-šá-ru kiš-pi*
	B obv. i 22′–23′	[........................... É]N / [.. *kiš-p*]*i*
	C$_{2}$ rev. v 39′–40′	^{ú}AN.ḪÚL *la ma-ḫir* ÉN / ^{giš}GAN.U$_{5}$ *šá ú-pa-áš-šá-ru kiš-pi*
22	a obv. 22	^{ú}IGI-20 *šá la ú-qar-ra-bu ru-ḫe-e ana zu-ru* ^{na4}*it-ta-mir*
	B obv. i 24′	[............................ *ru-ḫe*]-*e* --- ------ --------
	C$_{2}$ rev. v 41′	^{ú}⸢*im-ḫur*⸣-*aš*-⸢*ra*⸣ *ša* ⸢*la*⸣ *ú-qar-ra-bu ru-ḫe-e* ---- ---- ----

(*Ms. B breaks, ms. C$_{2}$ rev. v ends here; the beginning of rev. vi is not preserved*)

23	a obv. 23	⸢*šá*⸣ *mu-up-pi-šá-a-tú šá* 7 ^{munus}UŠ$_{11}$.ZU.MEŠ *ú-pa-áš-šá-ru*
24	a obv. 24	*kiš-pi-ki-na u ru-ḫe-e-ki-na ú-tar ana* TU$_{15}$ *te* ÉN
25	a obv. 25	KA.INIM.MA UŠ$_{11}$.BÚR.RU.D[A.KAM]
26	a obv. 26	ÉN *ma-ḫi-iṣ muḫ-ḫi mu-ub*!(bi)-*bil liq pi-i mu-u*[*b-bil* SAG.DU ŠID-*nu*?]
27	a obv. 27	[É]N *ez-ze-ta ša-am-ma-rat dan-na-a*[*t* x x x ŠID-*nu*?]

28	a obv. 28	$^{\text{ḫe-pí eš-šú}}$ *laḫ-mi u* 1 *pa-zu-zu* ZABAR *šá* x[x x x x x x x]
29	a rev. 1	[*líp-pi*$^{?}$] *ul tála-pap ina* GÚ-*šú* GAR-*an* NA$_4$.MEŠ ARḪUŠ *u* [x x x x x x]
30	a rev. 2	[x] ⸢$^{\text{na4}}$*it-ta-mir*$^{?}$⸣ *ina* ^{síg}*ba-ru-*<<DA>>*-un-du šá* SÍG BABBAR *u* SÍG S[A$_5$ È-*ma*]
31	a rev. 3	⸢*líp*⸣-[*pi*] ⸢*šá*⸣ ⸢SÍG⸣ ⸢SA$_5$⸣ *tála-pap* 1-*en ina* SÍG KI.MIN È-*ma líp-pi šá* SÍG S[A$_5$]
32	a rev. 4	Á *ana* Á *tála-pap* 4.TA.ÀM *ki-ṣir* Á *ana* Á *ta-kàṣ-*[*ṣar*]
33	a rev. 5	*ina* SAG.DU-*šú* KÉŠ 1 *ina* SÍG KI.MIN È-*ma líp-pi tála-pap ina* G[Ú-*šú* KÉŠ]
34	a rev. 6	2 *ina* SÍG KI.MIN 1.TA.ÀM È-*ma ina* ŠU.MIN.MEŠ-*šú* 15-*šú u* 150 KÉŠ
35	a rev. 7	1 *ina* SÍG KI.MIN È-*ma ina* MURUB$_4$-*šú* KÉŠ-*ma* EN Ù.TU *ul* DU$_8$-*šú*
36	a rev. 8	2 $^{\text{na4}}$BABBAR.DILI *ina* SÍG KI.MIN 1.TA.ÀM KÉŠ-*ma ina* GÌR.MIN.MEŠ 15 *u* 150 KÉŠ
37	a rev. 9	*šá* 30 U$_4$.MEŠ *šá* KUR-*du ina* SÍG KI.MIN È *ina lìb-bi* 2.TA.ÀM NA$_4$.MEŠ ⸢BIL.ZA$^{?}$⸣.ZA.MEŠ
38	a rev. 10	*šá* ŠU.MIN.MEŠ-*šú u* GÌR.MIN.MEŠ-*šú* DAB-*bat tak-ṣir šá* ^{munus}PEŠ$_4$-*tú šà* ŠÀ-*šú* NU ŠUB-*e*
39	a rev. 11	*šu-ut* KA *ana* ŠU.MIN È *gaba-rì* TIN.TIR^{ki}
40	a rev. 12	TA *u$_4$-mu šá ka$_4$-ni-šú* DIB-*iq-šú* EN 1 *me u$_4$-mu* NA$_4$.MEŠ *šá tak-ṣir šá* ^{munus}PEŠ$_4$ *ul* DAB-*bat*
41	a rev. 13	ÉN *ez-ze-et šam-rat i-lat na-mur-rat u ši-i bar-bar-rat* DUMU.MUNUS ^{d}*a-nu*[327]
42	a rev. 14	GÌR.MIN-*šú an-zu-ú* ŠU.MIN-*šá lu-'-tú* IGI UR.MAḪ *da-pi-nu* IGI.ME-*šú* GAR-*an*
43	a rev. 15	*iš-tu a-pi i-lam-ma uš-šú-rat pe-ret-su bu-ut-tu-qa di-da-a-šú*
44	a rev. 16	*kib-su* GU$_4$ *il*$^{!}$(GEŠTIN)-*lak kib-su* UDU.NÍTA *i-red-de i-na* UZU *u* MÚD ŠU.MIN-*šú* : *šak-nu*
45	a rev. 17	*a-pa-niš i-ru-bu ṣe-ra-niš i-ḫal-lu-up*
46	a rev. 18	*bi-i-tú ir-ru-ub bi-i-tú uṣ-ṣu*
47	a rev. 19	*bí-la-ni* DUMU.MEŠ-*ki-na lu-še-niq u* DUMU.MUNUS.MEŠ-*ki-na lu-ut-tar-ra*
48	a rev. 20	*a-na pi-i* DUMU.MUNUS.MEŠ-*ki-na lu-uš-tak-ka-na tu-la-a*
49	a rev. 21	*iš-me-ši-ma* ^{d}IDIM AD-*šú am-ma-ki* DUMU.MUNUS ^{d}*a-nim mut*$^{!}$*-tar-ra-tú* LÚ-*tú tal-ma-*[*di*]*-ma*
50	a rev. 22	*am-ma-ki ina* UZU *u* MÚD ŠU.MIN-*ki šak-nu*
51	a rev. 23	*am-ma-ki* É *ter-ru-bu* É *tu-ṣi-i*
52	a rev. 24	*mu-uḫ-ri šá* ^{lú}DAM.GÀR *qa-an-na-šú u ṣi-di-is*$^{!}$(ṣi)*-su*
53	a rev. 25	*mu-uḫ-ri šá* ^{lú}SIMUG *se-me-ri si-mat* ŠU.MIN-*ki u* GÌR.MIN-*ki*
54	a rev. 26	*mu-uḫ-ri šá* ^{lú}KÙ.DIM *in-ṣa-ab-tú si-mat* GEŠTU.MIN-*ki*

327 For a full edition of the incantation including all duplicates (d rev. 9–24 // e obv. 14–rev. 7 // f 1–17), see text C.3.3 lines 14–38.

55	a rev. 27	*mu-uḫ-ri šá* ^{lú}BUR.GUL $^{\text{na4}}$GUG *si-mat* GÚ-*ki*
56	a rev. 28	*mu-uḫ-ri šá* ^{lú}NAGAR ^{giš}GA.RÍG ^{giš}BAL *u du-di-it-ti* <*si-mat qé-e*>-*ki*
57	a rev. 29	*ú-tam-mi-ki* ^{d}60 AD-*ka an-tum* AMA-⸢*ka*⸣ *ú-tam-mi-ki* ^{d}IDIM *ba-nu-ú* MU-*ki*

Ms. a bottom of the reverse; for continuation of mss. d and e see texts C.3.3 and C.3.4

Bound Transcription and Translation

[1] *ṣurrī namrūti ina ṭurri šīpāti peṣâti tašakkak pušikka* [2] *ḫamiš ubānāti ina birīšunu tarakkas kunuk ḫalti kunuk šubî šû zikar u sinniš ina kišādīšu tašakkan* [3] *šubû imittu ina qāt imittīšu tarakkas šubû šumēlu ina qāt šumēlīšu tarakkas* [4] *aban suluppī zalāqu mūṣa ašgikû ina qablīšu tarakkas (yā)niba ḫulāla ina šēp imittīšu* [5] *sāmta uqnâ ina šēp šumēlīšu* MIN *abnē annûtu ina barundu* [6] *ša uqnâti tašakkak lippī ša šīpāti sāmāti talappap ina libbi abnī ša qātī u šēpī* [7] *izḫa karāni teppuš takṣiru ša erītu ša libbīša lā nadê gabari Dāda*

[1] You thread light-coloured *ṣurru*-stones on a cord of white wool. [2] You tie five 'fingers' of [1] combed wool [2] between them. You put (it with) a cylindrical *ḫaltu*-stone, a cylindrical *šubû*-'stone' (and) 'male' and 'female' *šû*-stones around her neck. [3] You tie 'right' *šubû*-stone around her right hand, you tie 'left' *šubû*-'stone' around (her) left hand, [4] you tie date-stone, *zalāqu*-stone, *mūṣu*-stone (and) *ašgikû*-stone (turquoise) around her hips, (*yā*)*nibu*-'stone' (and) *ḫulālu*-stone around her right foot, [5] carnelian (and) lapis lazuli around her left foot ditto (i.e. you tie). [6] You thread [5] these stones on a cord of multi-coloured wool (made) [6] with blue wool. You wind wads of red wool (around the cord). Among the stone(s) for the hands and feet [7] you fashion a string of grape(-shaped ornaments). An amulet charm for a pregnant woman (so that she does) not miscarry. A copy of (a tablet of) Dāda.

---

[8] *ittamir appa išda u qabla ḫurāṣa tuḫḫaza ina ṭurri šīpāti ṣalmāti tašakkak* [9] *šina šadânū ṣabītu kupputu šina aban suluppī itti birât ḫurāṣi u šina mêlī ḫubur* [10] *iṣ pišri imḫur-ešrā ina libbi tašakkan idi ana idi ša ittamir tašakkak* [11] *ištēnâ lippī ḫuppī ša uqnâti idi ana idi talappap* 7.TA.ÀM [12] *kiṣir idi ana idi takaṣṣar šiptu ittardāni ana māti šalāšīšu ana muḫḫi tamannū-ma* [13] *ina kišād erīti kurinnuššu tanaddī-ma ašar kišādīšu taḫannaq-ma* [14] *[arḫ]ussu tušered-duššum-ma ištēn arḫu ša alādīšu lā tammaršu*

[8] You coat the tip, bottom and middle of an *ittamir*-stone (bead) with gold (foil), you thread it on a cord of black wool. [9] Two magnetite stones in nugget form, two date-stones with clasps of gold and two leather bags – *ḫuburu*-plant, [10] 'wood of release' (*iṣ pišri*) and 'heals twenty'-plant you put inside (the bags). You thread (the stones and the bags) on each side of the *ittamir*-stone. [11] You wrap *ḫuppu*-burls of blue wool on each side (around the cord), one (on) each (side). [12] You knot seven knots on each side (of the burls). You recite the incantation "They have come down to the land" over (the amulet) three times. Then [13] you place (it) around the neck of the pregnant woman as her *kurinnu*-necklace and fasten (it) tightly around her neck. [14] Every [mon]th you let (the amulet) descend (a little from her neck), but (during) the one month (in which) she is to give birth you shall not see her.

---

[15] ÉN munus zú-kéš zú-kéš-da zú-kéš zú-kéš-da *tê šipti ana muḫḫi kiṣir ša takaṣṣar tamannu*

[15] Incantation: "Woman, the knot is knotted, the knot is knotted." Incantation formula. You recite (this) over the knot(s) that you knot.

16 ÉN *ittardāni ana māti kaššāpātu elīyanātu*	16 Incantation: "The witches, the 'mendacious ones', have come down to the land to me.
17 *išassâ illuru isaḫḫarā zamāra*	17 They call out '*illuru*', they *begin* to sing.
18 *našâ mê ayabba tâmti rapašti ittanamdâ ana sūqāti*	18 They carry water of the Ocean, from the wide sea, they keep spilling (it) onto the streets.
19 *ikammâ* (var. *isakkipā*) *eṭlūti išaggišā ardāti ištanakkanā qūlāti*	19 They bind (var.: push away) the young men, they murder the girls, they spread deadly silence everywhere.
20 *anāku aššakkanakkināšim-ma tiskur musakkiru ša pîkina* (var. *munakkira ša amātīkina*)	20 I have equipped myself against you with the *tiskur*-plant that blocks your mouth (var.: that changes your words),
21 *anḫullû lā māḫir kišpī* (var. *šiptī*) *iṣ pišri* (var. ^{giš}GAN.U$_5$) *ša upaššaru kišpī*	21 with the *anḫullû*-plant that is immune against witchcraft (var.: the spell), with the 'wood-of-release' (var.: with GAN.U$_5$-wood) that undoes witchcraft,
22 *imḫur-ešrā ša lā uqarrabu ruḫê ana zu(m)ru ittamir* 23 *ša muppišātu ša sebe kaššāpāti upaššaru*	22 with 'heals-twenty'-plant that does not allow magic to come near the body, with *ittamir*-stone 23 that undoes the machinations of the seven witches.
24 *kišpīkina u ruḫêkina utār ana šāri tê šipti*	24 I turn your witchcraft and your magic into wind!" Incantation formula.
25 KA.INIM.MA UŠ$_{11}$.BÚR.RU.D[A.KAM]	25 [It is] the wording (of the incantation) to undo witchcraft.
26 ÉN *māhiṣ muḫḫi mubbil liq pî mu[bbil qaqqadi tamannu*(?)]	26 [You recite(?)] the incantation "The one who hits (my) skull, dries (my) palate, dr[ies (my) head]".
27 ÉN *ezzēt(a) šammarāt(a) dannā[t(a)* … *tamannu*(?)]	27 [You recite(?)] the incantation "You are furious, you are impetuous, you are fierce" [… …].
28 *ḫepî eššu laḫmi*(?) *u ištēn Pazuzu siparri ša* …[……] 29 [*lippī*] *ul talappap ina kišādīšu tašakkan abnī rēmi u* […….]	28 (Gloss:) *new break* (…) of a 'hairy one'(?) and one Pazuzu (figurine) of bronze which [……], 29 you do not wrap [wads] (on it). You put (it) around her neck. Stones for *mercy* and […….].
30 […] *ittamir ina barundu ša šīpāti peṣâti u šīpāti sā[māti tašakkak-ma]* 31 *lip[pī] ša šīpāti sāmāti talappap ištēn ina šīpāti* KI.MIN *tašakkak lippī ša šīpāti sā[māti]* 32 *idi ana idi talappap* 4.TA.ÀM *kiṣir idi ana idi takaṣ[ṣar]* 33 *ina qaqqadīšu tarakkas ištēn ina šīpāti* KI.MIN *tašakkak-ma lippī talappap ina kiš[ādīšu tarakkas]* 34 *šina ina šīpāti* KI.MIN *ištēnâ tašakkak-ma ina qātīšu imittīšu u šumēlīšu tarakkas* 35 *ištēn ina šīpāti* KI.MIN *tašakkak-ma ina qablīšu tarakkas-ma adi ulladu ul tapaṭṭaršu* 36 *šina pappardilû ina šīpāti* KI.MIN *ištēnâ tarakkas-ma ina šēpi imitti u šumēli tarakkas*	30 [You thread …] *ittamir*-stone(s) on multicoloured wool (made) of white wool and r[ed] wool. [Then] 31 you wrap wads of red wool (around the cord): You thread one (of the *ittamir*-stones?) on the ditto (multicoloured) wool. Then you wrap wads of red wool 32 on each side (of the stone), on each side (of the cord) you knot four knots each. 33 You tie (this) around her head. You thread one (*ittamir*-stone?) on ditto wool, then you wrap wads (around the cord); you [tie (it)] around her ne[ck]. 34 You thread two (stones) separately on ditto wool and tie (one string each) around her right and left hand. 35 You thread one (stone) on ditto wool and tie (it) around her hips. You shall not remove it (the amulets) until she gives birth. 36 You tie two *pappardilû*-stones separately on ditto wool and tie (one string each) around the right and left foot.

37 *ša šalāšā ūmū ša ikšudū ina šīpāti* KI.MIN *taštakaku ina libbi* 2.TA.ÀM *abnī muṣa''irānī*(?) 38 *ša qātīšu u šēpīšu tuṣab-bat*(?) *takṣīr*(*u*) *ša erītu ša libbīšu lā nadê*	37 *When* thirty days have passed that you have strung (the stones) on ditto wool, you 38 attach 37 (figurines of) frogs with the two stones (that are tied around) 37 each of 38 her hands and feet. Amulet charm(s) for a pregnant woman (so that) she does not miscarry her foetus.
39 *šūt pî ana qātī šūṣû gabarī Bābili*	39 Oral lore, *well proven*, (according to) a copy (of a tablet) from Babylon.

---

40 *ištu ūmu ša kannīšu ītiqšu adi ištēn mē ūmī abnī ša takṣīr*(*i*) *ša erīti ul tuṣabbat*(?)	40 From the day that she missed(?) her period (lit. the day that her (menstrual) bandage(s) have passed her by) until one hundred days you should not attach the stones for the amulet charm(s) of the pregnant woman.

---

41 ÉN *ezzet šamrat ilat namurrat u šī barbarat mārat Anu*	41 Incantation: "She is furious, she is violent, she is goddess, she is terrifying, and she is a she-wolf, the daughter of Anu!
42 *šēpāša Anzû qātāša lu'tu pān nēši dapīni pānūša šaknū*	42 Her feet are (those of) Anzû, her hands are decay. The face of a ferocious lion is (set as) her face.
43 *ištu api īlâm-ma uššurat pēressa buttuqā dīdāša*	43 She came up from the canebrake, her hair hanging down, her loincloths torn off.
44 *kibis alpi illak kibis immeri iredde ina šīri u dāmi qātāša šaknā*	44 She walks in the tracks of the cattle, she follows the tracks of sheep; her hands are placed in flesh and blood.
45 *apāniš irrub ṣerrāniš iḫallup*	45 She enters through the window, glides in by the door pivot.
46 *bīta irrub bīta uṣṣi*	46 She enters the house, she leaves the house (saying):
47 *bilāni mārīkina lušēniq u mārātīkina luttarri*	47 'Bring (fem. pl.) me your sons! I want to suckle (them), and of your daughters I want to take care!
48 *ana pî mārātīkina luštakkana tulâ*	48 In the mouth of your daughters I want to place my nipples!'
49 *išmēšī-ma Ea abūša ammaki mārat Anu muttarrâta amēlūta talmadī-ma*	49 Ea, her father, heard her and (said): 'Instead that you, daughter of Anu, kept on acting as a nurse, you should have learned human behaviour, and
50 *ammaki ina šīri u dāmi qātāki šaknā*	50 instead of putting your hands in flesh and blood,
51 *ammaki bīta terrubī bīta tuṣṣî*	51 instead of entering the house (and) leaving the house,
52 *muḫrī ša tamkāri qannāšu u ṣidīssu*	52 accept from the merchant his *purse* and his travel provi-sions!
53 *muḫrī ša nappāḫi semērī simat qātīki u šēpīki*	53 Accept from the smith rings befitting your hands and your feet!
54 *muḫrī ša kutimmi inṣabtu simat uznīki*	54 Accept from the goldsmith earring(s) befitting your ears!
55 *muḫrī ša purkulli sāmta simat kišādīki*	55 Accept from the stonecutter a carnelian befitting your neck!
56 *muḫrī ša naggāri muštâ pilaqqa u duditti* <*simat qê*>*ki*	56 Accept from the carpenter a comb, a spindle and a pin <be-fitting> your <threads>!
57 *utammīki Anu abāki* (*utammīki*) *Antu ummāki utam-mīki Ea bānû šumīki*	57 I conjure you by Anu, your father, (var. adds: I conjure you) by Antu, your mother. I conjure you by Ea, who creates your name."

Notes

Line 1: The reading $^{\text{na4.⌜me⌝}}$ZÚ ZALAG.MEŠ at the beginning of the line follows Schuster-Brandis 2008, 147. Thureau-Dangin (1921, 164) suggested that the second damaged sign is a gloss but proposed no reading (that sign is indeed of smaller size). In lack of a better interpretation, the scribe perhaps intended to signal the plurality of *ṣurru* with the gloss. For $^{\text{na4}}$ZÚ ZALAG as a light-coloured variety of the *ṣurru*-stone, cf. CAD Ṣ, 258b; Schuster-Brandis 2008, 458. The reading *ṣurru namru* is confirmed by a syllabic spelling in LKA 114 rev. 18, parallel to $^{\text{na4}}$ZÚ ZALAG in the duplicate BM 64364 rev. 8 (Maul 1994,

341: 49). *Ṣurru* is usually regarded as obsidian or flint, being used not only for precious stones but also for knives that were used for surgical procedures.

Because two light-coloured *ṣurru*-stones are used for an amulet destined to be worn on the forehead in a similar group of amulets for pregnant women ordered from "head to feet" (Schuster-Brandis 2008, 148–149 "Ketten 154–162"; see K. 4727+ and duplicates edited as text F.1 in this volume), Schuster-Brandis (2008, 147) believes the *ṣurru*-stones in AO 6473: 1 were likewise applied to the forehead. Note, however, that the first instruction for application comes at the end of line 2, indicating that lines 1–2 are to be regarded as one prescription for an amulet necklace attached to the neck. The amulet for the forehead, whose main component likewise consisted of light-coloured *ṣurru*-stones, was either omitted from the group of amulets in the Uruk text, in comparison with "Ketten 154–162" (K. 4727+ //), or it was fused with the amulet for the neck. Apart from a few identical components, the ingredients (stone beads) of the different amulets in AO 6473 and K. 4727+ // differ from each other to a large extent.

Line 2: The "five fingers" of wool here and similarly in BAM 346: 2 (see text F.1) are understood as a unit of length in the dictionaries, see CAD U/W, 7 s.v. *ubānu* sub 3a; CAD P, 542 s.v. *pušikku*; AHw 1399 sub 2. But since text instructs to place the "fingers" "between" the stones (i.e. interchanging with the *ṣurru*-beads?), perhaps finger-shaped burls of wool are meant here, cf. the meaning "finger-shaped suppository" for *ubānu* (CAD U/W, 6 sub 1c-2'; Goltz 1974, 75, written ŠU.SI or U).

Line 4: The ingredient *aban suluppi* "date-stone" is usually understood as "date kernel", Schuster-Brandis 2008, 147, 458.

Line 5: For spellings using *CVC* signs to express *CCV* in Late Babylonian texts (such as *ki-ṣir* for *kiṣri*), see Schwemer 2017, *The Anti-Witchcraft Ritual Maqlû*, 79–80.

Line 7: Schuster-Brandis (2008, 147) emends *iz-ḫa* GEŠTIN "a string of grapes" to ^{giš}KIN$^{!}$.GEŠTIN = *isḫunnatu* "cluster of grapes". AHw 387a s.v. *isḫu* understands *is-ḫa* GEŠTIN as an "assignment of wine", which seems unexpected in the middle of instructions for making an amulet. Stone ornaments in the shape of grape clusters are attested elsewhere (cf. CAD I/J, 190 s.v. *isḫunnu*; AHw 387 s.v. *is/šḫunnatu* sub 2). I propose to read *iz-ḫa* GEŠTIN "a string of grapes" (the word *izḫu* "string" occurs in connection with food offerings in the cult, referring to strings of fish or birds (CAD I/J, 318). In either case, the text most likely indicates the use of (stone) ornaments in the shape of grapes or grape clusters here.

At the end of the line, Schuster-Brandis 2008, 147 reads DU$_8$-*rim* ("to loosen it") instead of *gaba-rì*. She speculates that the amulet was meant to reverse a preceding ritual against miscarriage to let the woman give birth when the expected time for delivery had arrived. This interpretation seems unlikely against ms. a rev. 11, which has the parallel formulation *gaba-rì* TIN.TIR^{ki} "copy (of an original) from Babylon".

For the reading of the personal name (or name element) $^{\text{(m)}}$U.U (and similar forms) as *Dāda* or *Dādi, Dadda, Daddi* (derived from *dādu* "darling" or from the divine name Dadi), see *PNA* 1/II, 358–364; Pedersén 1984–1986, 313–315; 1986, 88; Millard 1994, 92–93; Watanabe 1989, *ZA* 79, 272–273.

Lines 8–14: For this passage, see also Hirsch 1966, *OrNS* 35, 415.

Line 8: For the *ittamir*-stone as a "stone of giving birth", which plays a central role in the present text, see Ḫg. B IV 74 (MSL 10, 31), cf. Schuster-Brandis, 420, 449–450; Stol 2000a, 50. It also occurs as a "stone of "not giving birth" (MSL 10, 72 Recension D 8'), perhaps meaning a stone to prevent premature birth. The symbolism of the stone in the context of pregnancy and birth may not only be related to its name (as Stol 2000a, 50 has suggested), but also to its colour, which, according to Mesopotamian description texts, looks like "uncooked ox blood" dotted with specks of iron (Schuster-Brandis 2008, 420). Scurlock (1991, 141) proposed this appearance was seen as reminiscent of the appearance of a partially formed foetus. See also lines 22–23 and 30–36 for the *ittamir*-stone.

Line 9: For the interpretation of *kupputu* as "lump-shaped", see CAD K 552; differently Thureau-Dangin 1921, 164, 168 with fn. 10, who reads *kubbutu* "heavy" (thus also AHw 497b).

The emendation <ZÚ>.LUM follows Thureau-Dangin (1921, 164 fn. 5); see also ms. a obv. 4 for the mention of NA$_4$ ZÚ.LUM (*aban suluppi*) "date stone".

For the reading *bir-rat* as derived from *birītu* "clasp, fetter"; see CAD K, 330 s.v. *kibirru*; CAD B, s.v. 254 *birītu* sub 4. Schuster-Brandis (2008, 148 nn. 384, 386) reads the emended passage differently: *kús-si*$_8^{?!}$*-bir-rat* KÙ.SI$_{22}$ (or *kús*-<<KI>>-*bir-rat* KÙ.SI$_{22}$) "a coriander-shaped (bead) of gold", drawing on the mention of *kisibirrītu* "coriander-(shaped beads)" in parallel texts on amulets for women (cf. BAM 346: 4; BAM 363: 3 (texts F.1–F.2, there spelled *kús-bir-rat-tú*).

Line 10: For the "wood of release" (*iṣ pišri*) among plants against sorcery and used for amulets, see CAD P, 430; Luukko and van Buylaere 2020, CMAwR 4, index. *Iṣ pišri* and *imḫur-ešrā*-plant are mentioned side by side again below in ms. a obv. 21 within the incantation *Ittardāni ana māti*.

Line 11: For *lippu*-wrappings or wads made of wool in amulet texts, cf. Schuster-Brandis 2008, 62, 66–67. Like *mêlu* "leather pouches", *lippu*-wads (a noun derived from *lapāpu* "to wrap around") could be filled with different materials, before being attached as components to amulet strings. For the reading *ḫúp-pi* instead of *kap-pi*, see Farber 2014, *Lamaštu*, Tablet III 36, 48 with comments on p. 254. CAD K, 176 lists the present line under *kapāpu*, translating *lippī kap-pi* as "wads wrapped(?) with"; AHw 444b has the reference under *kappu* II "hand; paw", (with unclear meaning). Abusch et al. (2020, CMAwR 3, 51 and 52 note on line 4) accept *lippī ḫuppī* but leave the term *ḫuppu* untranslated. The present author interprets *lippu ḫuppu* as a type of wad or burl, see also Steinert 2016, *ZA* 106, 250 with fn. 59 and K. 4727+ and dupl., note on lines 7 and 35 (*infra* text F.1).

Line 13: For *kurinnu* "necklace, neck ornament", see Postgate 1994, *Studies Hrouda*, 244.

Lines 13–14: The meaning of the gradual loosening of the knots and lowering of the woman's necklace was already pointed out by R. Labat 1957–1971, "Geburt", *RlA* 3, 178b; see also Abusch et al., CMAwR 3, 52 notes on lines 6–7; differing interpretations are given by Scurlock 1991, *Incognita* 2, 141 and Schuster-Brandis 2008, 148. The gradual lowering of the necklace can be seen as parallel to the gradual downward movement of the foetus, while avoiding a miscarriage. Abusch et al. (ibid.) suggest that the amulet was probably prepared for the woman as soon as her pregnancy had become apparent, but that for the first hundred days of her pregnancy nothing was done with the amulet (cf. ms. a rev. 12). At one hundred days, the practitioner would then loosen one pair of knots and continue to do so every thirty days. And when all seven pairs were untied the woman had reached her due date. Following Labat, (*RlA* 3, 179) and Stol (2000a, 206) who interpret this passage as a reference that a postpartum woman was regarded impure for thirty days after her delivery, Abusch et al. (CMAwR 3, 51, 52) understand line 14 to mean "for one month after her delivery you must not see her". However, the instruction could also refer to the last month of pregnancy instead, meaning that the practitioner was not to do anything further with the necklace until with the woman's delivery, similar to the statement in ms. a rev. 7 (line 35) saying that the amulet should not be removed until she gives birth. In my view, the interpretation that lines 13–14 refer to a notion of impurity should be questioned, because the statement is not explicit at all. For the question of impurity and women's reproductive processes, cf. Steinert 2023.

Line 14: As pointed out by Abusch et al. (CMAwR 3), 52 ad line 7, the spelling *tu-še-re-du-šum-ma* represents a ventive form (*tušereddaššum-ma*).

Line 15: The same incantation is recited in VAT 13629 + 13866 (KAL 2, No. 41, CMAwR 3, text 5.2) rev.$^{!}$ iv' 14–15, a tablet with amulets for pregnant women from Assur (see text C.3.8). The emendation of saĝ to kéš in ms. a is based on the Assur text. The spell is explicitly used against witchcraft in the Assur text as well: [ÉN] munus <<igi>> zú-kéš zú-kéš-da / zú-kéš zú-kéš-da TU$_6$ ÉN / [É]N *an-ni-tú* ŠUB-*ma kiš-pi* NU TE-*ši*. In the Assur text, the spell is recited over a different amulet, to protect a pregnant woman from miscarriage, even if witchcraft had already been performed against her ([*šumma ana erī*] *ti ipšī epšūšima* "If sorceries have been performed against a pregnant woman").

Related to the imagery of knotting and binding, standing for the closure of the pregnant woman's womb keeping her safe from miscarriage, are also Sumerian incantations against bleeding during pregnancy with the rubric KA.INIM.MA MUNUS.KÉŠ.DA.KAM "recitation to bind a woman" (and similar rubrics), see Finkel 1980, 38–39, 42–43 text C (CBS 1509 i 20, iii 25); Steinert 2018, 183; Steinert et al. 2018, 272. Such spells are probably referred to with the rubric ^{munus}PEŠ$_4$.KÉŠ.DA "to bind a pregnant woman" that is listed in the Assur Medical Catalogue (Steinert et al. 2018, 218 line 114) and in the Exorcist's Manual (KAR 44: 15 and dupl., see Geller 2018a, 298; Heeßel 2023, 294, with the added gloss MUNUS *lā aldu* "woman not giving birth") as a genre of incantations for women.

Line 17: For *illuru* as an ill-boding song contrasting with the happy *alalu*-song, see Stol 2020b, *BiOr* 77, 571.

Line 22: For the variant *zu-ru* instead of *zumru*, see also BM 79061 obv. 15 (text A.2.8).

Line 26: The incantation incipit cited here probably refers to the same incantation that is written down in full in STT 241: obv. 8–rev. 26 and recited there over amulet stones for a woman who has difficulty bringing pregnancies to term (MUNUS NU SI.SÁ, *sinništu lā muš(t)ēšertu*). See *infra* text C.3.1 and Finkel 1976, *Hulbazizi*, 185–186.

Line 27: The incipit *ezzēt(a) šam(ma)rāt(a) dannāt(a)* belongs an otherwise unknown spell against the child-snatching demoness Lamaštu (Farber 2014, 35). The form *šá-am-ma-rat* (for *šammarāta*) is a variant of *šam-rat* (*šamrāta*), see CAD Š/1, 314, 332 s.v. *šammaru* "impetuous(?)" and *šamru* "fierce, violent" sub e-2' for similar incantation incipits.

Lines 28–29: At the beginning of line 28 after the gloss, Heeßel (2002a, *Pazuzu*, 74) reads *tam-mi* "(be)schwörst du", understanding this as the defective verbal form *tutammi* (of *tamû* D-stem; "to conjure; to adjure"). For *laḫmu*, the mythological figure identified in iconography as the naked hero with curls, who is attested as a protective being linked with Ea/Enki and often represented at temple gates, in palaces, on seals, and in the form of protective figurines, see Wiggermann 1992, 164–166 *passim*, with Wiggermann 1983, *JEOL* 27 90ff.; Rittig 1977, *Kleinpastik*, 51–58.

The interpretation of the end of line 29 is provisional. For NA_4.MEŠ ARḪUŠ, cf. Schuster-Brandis 2008, 399, discussing the "stone of mercy" (NA_4 ARḪUŠ, *aban rēmi*), which is only rarely attested in amulet texts, however. Alternatively, stones for the womb could be meant in the present text.

Lines 30–36: This passage contains instructions for another group of amulets tied around different body parts (ordered from head to toe). The beginning of line 30 is damaged, but I assume a number in the gap before ⸢^{na4}*it-ta-mir*⸣ (the reading follows collation of the tablet). If the reconstruction proposed here is correct, it should be seven *ittamir* stones, one for each of the amulets (for the head, neck, hands, hips and feet). The instructions in lines 31–36 are elliptical, but I assume that the numbers 1(*-en*) and 2 introducing each of the amulets stand for "one/two (*ittamir*)-stone(s)". The *ittamir*-stone is also part of the amulets in lines 8–14 and mentioned as a powerful stone against witchcraft in the incantation *Ittardāni ana māti* in lines 22–23.

Line 37: Abusch et al. 2020 (CMAwR 3), 51 understand the formulation at the beginning of the line as a reference to a period of one month after the placement of the preceding amulets (rev. 2–8?).

The present line presents a first concrete mention of a frog pendant as part of a protective amulet worn by a pregnant woman. However, such figurines of frogs (*muṣa''irānu, muṣârānu*) are mentioned outside the healing texts, e.g. in lexical lists and inventories, where they are made of stone, see Ḫḫ. XVI 80 (MSL 10, 7): ^{na4}BIL.ZA.ZA ZA.GÌN = *muṣa''irānu* "(lapis lazuli) frog (figurine)". An inventory from Qatna (Bottéro 1949, *RA* 43, 154: 179; 180: 13) mentions frogs made of lapis lazuli and carnelian which formed part of necklaces (*kišādu*). See further Bottéro 1949, *RA* 43, 16; Landsberger 1934, *Fauna*, 140–141. Visual representations of frogs, especially small figurines of frogs that could be used as amulet pendants (made of lapis lazuli, steatite, alabaster, haematite, gold, green quartz ceramics and other materials), are quite frequently attested, see e.g. van Buren 1939, 101–103 with figs. 103–105; Thavapalan 2020, 76 note 272; Dittrich and Götting-Martin 2021. Dittrich and Götting-Martin also discuss symbolic connotations associated with frogs in the Mesopotamian worldview. Notably, frog pendants are often found in graves (including children's graves), which together with their animal characteristics and both aquatic and terrestrial habitat suggests associations with rebirth and fertility. Frogs were also associated with the god Enki/Ea and his domain, the Apsû, as well as with Ištar. They occur in magico-medical contexts linked to promoting male potency (e.g. Wasserman 2016, 151 PRAK 1 B 472 i 12' (where the term *ḫudušsu* "frog" denotes the female genital organs); Zisa 2021, 168, 286–287 text D.I line 6). Parallels to the use of frog pendants worn by women in the contexts of childbirth and pregnancy can be found in Egyptian sources (Dittrich and Götting-Martin 2021, 100 with references).

Line 38: Abusch et al. (2020, CMAwR 3, 51) understand DAB-*bat* in a different sense, namely that two stones had to be removed from each of the amulets attached to the arms and feet of the woman. However, for this the scribe would have used DU_8 rather than *ṣabātu*, as above in line 7. For *ṣabātu* "to hold (in place)" in connection with amulets (with reference to mountings), see e.g. YOS 6, 216: 11: 118 *kurṣū ḫurāṣi ina 2 pingū ina guḫalṣa ḫurāṣi ṣabit* "118 golden links held on a gold wire by a knob" (also ibid. l. 8: *ina* DUR GADA.ḪI.A *ṣabit*). The form DAB-*bat* here could stand for the D-stem, which can have the meaning "to fasten; to tie; to link", see CAD Ṣ, 36f., sub 10i. See, for a similar context, MDP 4, 167–168, pl. 18 No. 3: 5 (inscription of Tepti-aḫar): *di-du-ší-na i-na tu-ur-re-e lu ṣú-ub-bu-tu*! "their (the female temple guardians') *dīdu*-garments should be fastened(!) with strings" (Reiner 1973, *AfO* 24, 95; Malbran-Labat 1995, 57). For this usage of DAB-*bat* in amulet prescriptions, see also K. 4727+ // (text F.1). For a parallel usage of DAB-*bat* in the Lamaštu rituals in connection with the manufacture of protective amulets, see Farber 2014, 186ff. Tablet III 30–43, esp. line 43. Farber (ibid., 254 comments on III 43) assumes a Š-stem of *ṣabātu* in this context. Cf. also below commentary to line 40.

Line 39: For this line see also Frahm 2011, 44–45 with n. 167. The expression *šūt pî* is usually understood as oral lore, as knowledge that was not enshrined in the texts. For *šūt pî* in medical texts, see also BM 42298 (Finkel 2000, 180–182) obv. 22; and in the present corpus BM 38624+ iv 3' (text A.2.1).

For *ana qātī šūṣû* as "well proven", see Abusch and Schwemer 2011, 63–64 with note on text 1.8.2: 10'. In BM 40152 rev. iii 14, the phrase occurs beside *bulṭū latkūtu* "tested remedies" (see text C.1.8). Usually, *ša ana qātī šūṣû* is understood to mean "what is at hand, available" (CAD A/2, 371; Black 1987, *BiOr* 44, 34 n. 7). Objections have been raised by Schwemer 2007b, KAL 2, 114 (note on BAM 190 obv. 19) and by Reiner 1961, *OrNS* 30, 10 n. 1: "which are suitable for use(?)". See also Steinert 2015; Arbøll 2019, 113, 133, 195 note 37.

Line 40: Abusch et al. 2020 (CMAwR 3, 52 note lines 6–7) understand the instruction to the practitioner not to "handle" (*ṣabātu*) the amulets of the pregnant woman during the first hundred days of pregnancy in connection with the untying of knots described in the instructions for the amulets in lines 8–15: the first knots would be untied one hundred days after the initial placement of the amulet. Cf. Farber 2014, 35 for a different suggestion. However, the time specification at the beginning of line 40 may point to another meaning of *ṣabātu* in this instance, namely "to prepare; to undertake", either in the G- or the Š-stem (CAD Ṣ, 21 sub 5 and 38–39 sub 11g, also "to set up, put in place" sub 11e; cf. also the phrase *ana ṣabāt epēši* in connection with the preparation of rituals). This could also mean that the amulets were prepared when hundred days had passed since she had her last menstrual period, after which it may have been certain that the woman was indeed pregnant. Abusch et al. 2020 understand the phrase *ištu ūmu ša kannīšu ītiqšu* here "from the day that she missed her period" (i.e. the day when the woman noticed she may be pregnant), since *etēqu* "to pass by" can have the meaning "to elapse, to delay, to be overdue". However, it is theoretically possible that the phrase refers to the day when the woman's last period was over (literally "when her menstrual bandages have passed her by"). For a different interpretation of the line, reading *qannu* "fringe" instead of *kannu* "bandage", see Mayer 2017, *OrNS* 86, 30.

Lines 41–57: For comments on the incantation, see Farber 1989b, *ZA* 79, 229–230; Farber 2014, 329–330 as well as texts C.3.3 and C.3.4 in the present volume.

Line 41: The incantation incipit *ezzet šamrat ilat namurrat* is identical with the incipits of two other incantations included in the canonical Lamaštu series (Tablet II 84 and 119), see Farber 2014, 238. Line 41b is identical with Tablet I 37(b) of the Lamaštu series, see Farber 2014, 74.

Line 42: This line is almost identical with Tablet I 106 of the Lamaštu series; for the translation see also Farber 1989b, 230. For the use of an identical phrase as in line 42b, see also "Lam. II" 36(b) (Farber 2014, 100).

Line 43: For the meaning of the term *dī/ādu/ū* as an item of female underwear, see Wasserman 2019, *FS Charpin*, 1131–1132, 1138 (with further literature), understood as a tunic- or skirt-like underclothing; cf. further CAD D 135f.; CAD R, 130a; Farber 2014, 329. A very similar line is found in an Old Assyrian Lamaštu incantation (Farber 2014, 280–281 "OA_2" ll. 16–17: *perassa waššarat dādūša šaḫṭū* "her hair is hanging loose, her underwear is stripped off".

Line 49: For *muttarrâta* as a Gtn-form of *tarû* "to (repeatedly) lift up (a child)" related to *tārītu* "nurse, nanny", see Farber 1989b, *ZA* 79, 230.

Line 52: For the word *qannu* in this text, cf. CAD Ṣ, s.v. *ṣidītu* sub f; Farber 1989b, *ZA* 79, 230. Instead of the translation "garment fringe" (*qannu*), CAD Q 138b suggests "horn (*qarnu*) filled with oil". Farber suggests the contextual meaning "purse", possibly derived from the custom of binding silver into the garment fringe (of the bride).

Line 56: The enumeration of items at the end of the line varies in all three manuscripts (see *infra* text C.3.3 and C.3.4). In ms. a, the phrase *simat qê* "befitting (your) thread(s)" (i.e. sewing needs) has been left out and has been emended following suggestions of Farber 1989b, 229 and 2014, 330. In mss. a, the older term *dudittu* interchanges with the younger *kirissu* in ms. e replacing *dudittu*. For these female items related to clothing, spinning and sewing, encountered in Lamaštu texts and amulet depictions, see also Farber 1987c, *FS Reiner*, 96ff.; H. Klein 1983, *ZA* 73, 255–284; Green 1998–2001, "Nadel", *RlA* 9, 69–73.

Line 57: The reading of ms. a *bānû šumīki* "the creator of your name" (or offspring?) is not entirely certain.

C.3.10 SpTU 5, No. 248: Ritual Procedures for Women Promoting a Normal Pregnancy

This Late Babylonian tablet (ms. a) from Uruk contains three ritual procedures (*nēpešu*) for women having trouble to bring their pregnancies to term (*sinništu lā muš(t)ēšertu*). The rituals were performed for a pregnant woman so that she would have a normal pregnancy, but the recitations to be spoken by the patient during the rituals make clear that she had suffered previous miscarriages or stillbirths. The tablet was copied by the exorcist Anu-ikṣur in the Achaemenid period (5th/4th cent. BCE; cf. Clancier 2009a, 58–59). The tiny fragment K. 19506 (ms. b) in Neo-Babylonian script from Ashurbanipal's library now offers a first duplicate passage to SpTU 5, No. 248, rev. 32'–39', showing that these rituals were already known in the seventh century BCE and probably originate in Babylonia. The text has been discussed and translated several times (e.g. Scurlock 2002, 2014a, 2014b; Couto-Ferreira 2013); the present discussion has profited much from the recent treatment of SpTU 5, No. 248 by Abusch et al. (2020, CMAwR 3), who had access to photos of the tablet and who have provided extensive collations and several improved readings, which have been amply adopted here.

Despite the many difficulties of interpretation, which the text still poses, the rituals in SpTU 5, No. 248, in their complexity and multiple stages taking place at different locations, offer many interesting details. The first and the third ritual in SpTU 5, No. 248 attribute the cause of the patient's stillbirths to witchcraft (as becomes clear from the recitations), while the second ritual does not mention witchcraft. In the first and third ritual, the patient's problem is seen as a state brought about by contamination with something bewitched, and these rituals employ several rites of transfer to remove the patient's contamination from her body, to transfer it to another carrier and to purify the patient. Several divine and ritual agents (the sun god Šamaš, the god Ea, the goddess Gula, the divine River, soapwort plant, a date palm, an oven, a pregnant ewe and a pregnant jenny) play a role in the multi-stage ritual processes.

The first ritual (lines 1–61) begins at sunset, when the patient is shaved, and her hair put into a leather bag that she places around the neck. The exorcist further attaches a charm to the pregnant woman's right hand and places loaves of bread, mutton and grain seeds at the head of her bed.

In the morning, before sunrise, the practitioner hangs something (probably the aforementioned leather bag) from the wall of the woman's house. Then he takes her to a secluded place in a blocked road. Abusch et al. (CMAwR 3, text 5.5) presume that the prayer to Šamaš (ms. a obv. 41–rev. 3, lines 41–52) had to be recited at this point, in which the exorcist asks the sun god to condemn the warlock and witch so that the woman can be released from the evil that causes her miscarriages. Then the bread, meat and grain seeds, which had spent the night near the woman's bed and are contaminated with her birthing difficulties are left behind in the street. The short recitation spoken by the woman in lines 8–9 implies that the contamination which she has received from the warlock and witch, will be transferred to "unnamed" persons (unsuspecting humans or animals) who would pick up the foodstuffs and consume them. After these words, the woman undresses, is washed, puts on a new garment and returns home without looking back.

The next stage of the ritual, the exorcist and the pregnant woman go to the river. At this point, the exorcist probably recited the prayer addressed to the god of the subterranean waters Ea (lines 53–61), with the plea to help the woman. The woman has to go into the river and direct water downward, while the practitioner recites an incantation to the river (lines 13–18) three times. It was hoped that the river would purify the woman and carry off her difficulties. Then the woman, still standing in the river, washes herself with potash made from soapwort-plant (*uḫūlu*), while addressing the soapwort-plant with a short invocation focused on being cleansed from the bewitchment (lines 20–25).

The following stage of the ritual takes place at a potter's oven, where another ritual transfer took place. The woman embraces the oven and asks it to receive her inability to produce healthy offspring. In exchange the woman hopes to receive the oven's ability to produce sound 'vessels', thereby metaphorically linking the female body with the pottery oven, and the embryo with a clay pot (this imagery alludes to the creation of humankind from clay in anthropogonic myths such as *Atramḫasīs*). Finally, the practitioner and the woman go to a garden, where she addresses a date palm in a short incantation asking the tree to give her its properties (health and fertility).

In the second ritual (ms. a rev. 13–25, lines 62–74), the woman's inability to bear healthy children is transferred to a pregnant ewe that has previously given birth to healthy lambs; the woman requests to receive the ewe's ability to have a normal pregnancy. The ritual begins with an offering to the healing goddess Gula (addressed as Ninkarrak in the prayer, another healing goddess equated with her) accompanied by the recitation of a short prayer. The rite of transfer in Ritual 2 resembles the procedure with the pregnant jenny in Ritual 3 (lines 85–87). The patient speaks into the ears of the ewe requesting to receive from it the ability to bring foetuses to term. Then she slips through underneath the animal seven times; in Ritual 3 the patient similarly passes three times underneath the jenny. While in Ritual 3, the woman's contamination is additionally transferred to the jenny by having the patient feed the animal, in Ritual 2 the woman spits into the ewe's mouth. Then the animal is brought out to the steppe and abandoned there.

The third ritual (ms. a rev. 26–42, lines 75–91) begins with depositing different foodstuffs and a dead female mouse wrapped up in wool at a crossroads; the woman speaks a similar recitation as in lines 8–9 of Ritual 1, which refers to anonymous passers-by who will receive the woman's misfortune by picking up the deposited objects, as a reversal of the acts of bewitchment that the patient had "received". These ritual actions are to be repeated several times. In the following part of the ritual, the patient slips underneath a pregnant donkey, again with the aim to get rid of her difficulties and to receive the jenny's ability to have a healthy pregnancy. In the latter part of the procedure, a sheaf(?) of *šegušsu*-millet is deposited at a crossroads as well as hung up in the window of the woman's house, the latter of which she was to touch regularly until the day of her delivery. A last sequence takes place on "the day of her labour", i.e. when the woman delivered. A young girl is to shape figurines of a man and a woman by mixing ground-up grain with the amniotic fluid of the patient. These figurines, presumably representing the warlock and witch, are disposed of in the street at midnight. Thereby any contamination by the witchcraft still lingering in the woman's body was removed from her and her baby; the warlock and witch were symbolically polluted with the amniotic fluid and condemned to death (the figurines would be eaten by animals or just decompose).

Recently, duplicating fragments to Rituals 2 and 3 of SpTU 5, No. 248 have been identified among texts in Neo-Babylonian script from Nineveh (mss. b and c) by the *Electronic Babylonian Library* (eBL) Project.[328] These fragments show that the rituals for a pregnant woman were known and in use already during the Neo-Assyrian period.[329]

List of Manuscripts

Siglum	Museum Number	Copy	Collation	Format; Ductus	Provenience
a	W. 23262 IM 76830	SpTU 5, No. 248	Photo coll.	Single-column tablet (portrait format); Late Babylonian script; 5th cent. BCE	Uruk, library of Anu-ikṣur
b	K. 19506	Pl. 27	Coll.	Fragment; Neo-Babylonian script; 7th cent. BCE	Nineveh, library of Ashurbanipal
c	Sm. 123 (+) Sm. 1138 (+) Sm. 1991	AMT 66/5 (Sm. 1991 only) Geers, Folio B140 (Sm. 1138) Geers, Folio D82 (Sm. 123)	Coll.	Fragments of a single-column(?) tablet; Neo-Babylonian script; 7th cent. BCE	Nineveh, library of Ashurbanipal

Overview

i Ritual for a woman who does not bring pregnancies to term — 1–61
- Ritual instructions (at sunset): — 1–6
  - Isolating and shaving of the patient and putting her hair in a leather bag around her neck (a obv. 1–3); putting an amulet necklace with stones around her hand (a obv. 3–5); placing foodstuffs at the patient's head (a obv. 5–6)
- Ritual instructions (in the morning): — 6–11
  - setting out foodstuffs in a blocked road; recitation (by the patient); patient is washed and dons a new garment (a obv. 6–11)

328 That the fragments of ms. c belong to the same tablet was recognized by Z. Földi (of the *Electronic Babylonian Library* Project). Whether K. 19506 (ms. b) likewise belongs to this tablet (as suggested by eBL) remains uncertain.

329 The text section of Ritual 2 finds another partial duplicate in an unpublished Neo-Assyrian text from Assur (A 492). I owe this information to Abusch et al. 2020, CMAwR 3, 68. I would like to thank Daniel Schwemer for providing me with a photo of A 492.

- Ritual instructions (at the river): 12–18
  - the patient goes to and descends into the river; practitioner recites incantation (a obv. 12)
- incantation <*Nāru*> *ešrētu* (a obv. 13–18)
- Ritual instructions: 19 –25
  - patient is given soapwort plant (*uḫūlu*) (a obv. 19)
- Incantation *Uḫūlu uḫūlu* (a obv. 20–25)
- Ritual instructions: 26–32
  - patient goes to potter's kiln and embraces it; patient recites incantation *Atūnu ellet mārat Ani rabītu* (a obv. 26–32)
- Ritual instructions:
  - patient goes to the garden, embraces a date palm; patient recites incantation *Gišimmaru māḫirat kal šāri* (a obv. 33–40) 33–40
- Incantation: *Šamaš attā-ma ša kališ kibrāt unammaru* (a obv. 41–rev. 3) 41–52
- Incantation: *E*[*a a*]*ttā-ma bānû kalāmu* (a rev. 4–12) 53–61

ii Ritual for a woman who does not bring pregnancies to term 62–74
- Ritual instructions (at night?): 62–67
  - offering to Gula (a rev. 13–14)
- patient recites prayer *Ninkarrak bēltu šurbūtu ummu rēmēnītu* (a rev. 15–18 // c obv. 1')
- Ritual instructions (in the morning): 68–74
  - burning a pile of brushwood on bricks before Šamaš (a rev. 19–20 // c obv. 2')
- rites with a pregnant ewe (patient speaks recitation into the ewe's ears, slips through underneath the animal, spits into the animal's mouth); disposal of the ewe in the steppe (a rev. 20–25 // c obv. 2'–9')

iii Ritual for a woman who does not give birth successfully 75–91
- Ritual instructions (at dawn): 75–84
  - foodstuffs are left at a crossroads; patient speaks recitation (a rev. 26–30 // c rev. 1–6)
  - a killed mouse is left at the crossroads; patient speaks recitation (a rev. 31–35 // b 1'–3' / c rev. 7–10)
- Ritual instructions: 85–91
  - rites with a pregnant jenny: patient feeds the jenny, speaks a recitation to it, slips through underneath animal (a rev. 36–38 // b 4'–6')
  - rites with *šegušš*u-millet (hung up in the window; patient touches it regularly until she delivers); making two figurines of a man and a woman from dough of *šegušš*u (on the day of the patient's delivery) and disposal of the figurines (a rev. 39–43 // b 7'–10')

iv Colophon (a u. e. 1–2) 92–93

Previous Edition and Discussion

von Weiher 1998, SpTU 5, 58–65 No. 248 (edition)
Hecker 2008, *TUAT NF* 4, 107–110 (translation)
Cunningham 2009, http://oracc.org/cams/gkab/P348835 (ms. a)
Scurlock 2002, 215–223 (translation and analysis)
Fincke 2003, *AfO* 50, 142, 143 (discussion of fragments of mss. b, c)
Foster 2005, *Before the Muses*, 979 (translation of obv. 26–32), 980 (translation of obv. 33–40)
Böck 2013, *Journal Asiatique* 103, 48–49 (translation of a rev. 13–25)
Couto-Ferreira 2013, 97–116 (discussion)
Scurlock 2014a, *Sourcebook*, 684–691 (edition)
Scurlock 2014b, 122–126 (translation)
Couto-Ferreira 2015, 187–200 (discussion)
Abusch et al. 2020, CMAwR 3, 64–76 text 5.5 (edition, without rev. 13–25) and collations, pl. 62–62, no. 25–46
Stol 2020b, *BiOr* 77, 569–570
BabMed Corpora (https://www.geschkult.fu-berlin.de/e/babmed/Corpora/AMT-2/AMT66-5/index.html) (transliteration of

Sm. 1991)
CDLI P239871 (photo, ms. b); P240436 (photo, transliteration of Sm. 1991); P240236 (photo of Sm. 123); P240343 (photo of Sm. 1138)
Electronic Babylonian Library (eBL) (https://www.ebl.lmu.de/library/K.19506; https://www.ebl.lmu.de/library/Sm.123) (transliteration of mss. b and c)

Transliteration
The first ritual

1	a obv. 1	[*ana*$^?$] ⸢*a*$^?$-*ri*$^?$-*ti*⸣ ⸢BÚR$^?$⸣ *sin-niš-tu*$_4$ *la mu-še-šèr-tu*$_4$ *it-ti ri-bi šá* ^{d}UTU-*ši*
2	a obv. 2	*ta-pa-ra-as ina* KUŠ *gal-la-bu-us te-ep-pu-ši-ma ina* ^{kuš}*na-áš-tu-qa*
3	a obv. 3	*eš-še-tu*$_4$ *ina* GÚ-*šú ta-šak-kan* ^{na4}URUDU ^{na4}ZA.GÌN ^{na4}AŠ *zi-ka-ri* ^{na4}*šá-da-nu* DAB.BA
4	a obv. 4	*u* ^{na4}*zi*!(iz)-*bi-tú ina sa-mu-tú ta-šak-kak* 3 *li-ip-pi ina* ^{síg}ḪÉ.ME.DA *ta-lap-pa-ap*
5	a obv. 5	*ina* ŠU.MIN 15-*šú ta-šak-kan u* NINDA *ku-ri-tú* UDU.NÍTA *a-di* UZU-*šú* 2 SÌLA ŠE.NUMUN
6	a obv. 6	*it-ti-i ta-nam-di-is-su ina re-ši-šú i-ba-a-tú ina še-e-ri la-ma* ^{d}UTU
7	a obv. 7	*na-pa-a-ḫu ul-tu* UGU *i-ga-ri tu-ša-qal-la-al-šú il-lak-ma ina a-šar pa-ar-su*
8	a obv. 8	*ina* UGU KASKAL.MIN *pa-rik-tu*$_4$ NINDA.ḪI.A UZU *u* ŠE.NUMUN *ta-šak-kan-ma na-bu-ú it-tan-nu-nu*
9	a obv. 9	*la na-bu-ú in-da-ḫar-ú-'i-in-ni* 5-*šú i-qab-bi e-ma-a' iq-ta-bu-ú*
10	a obv. 10	TÚG-*su i-šaḫ-ḫaṭ-ma* A.MEŠ *tu-ra-am-ma-ak-šú i-te-eb-*<*be*>*-e-ma*
11	a obv. 11	TÚG-*su* 2-*ú il-lab-ba-áš u le-es-su a-na ku-tal-li-šú ul i-na-an-di*
12	a obv. 12	*a-na* ÍD *il-lak-ma a-na* ÍD *ur-rad* A.MEŠ *a-na mu-qal-pi-tu*$_4$ 3-*šú ib-bak*
13	a obv. 13	*u* ÉN *ana muḫ-ḫi-šú ta-man-nu* ÉN <ÍD> *eš-re-tu*$_4$ *šu-šu-ru mu-kamuḫ-ra-an-ni-ma*
14	a obv. 14	*ár-nu šèr-tú gíl-lat ḫi-ṭi-tu*$_4$ *lum-nu mi-niš-tu*$_4$ *šá zu-um-ri-i-ia it-ti* A.MEŠ-*ka*
15	a obv. 15	*a-na qid-da-tu*$_4$ *ta-bal* ÍD.MEŠ *lim-la-a' a-gam-mu li-ṭe-e-pi a-da-ap-a-ta*
16	a obv. 16	⸢*li*⸣-*še-ṣa-a' ri-kis lum-ni-ia* ÍD *eš-re-tú šu-šu-ru mu-ka šu-ši-ra-an-ni-ma*
17	a obv. 17	*dà-lí-lí-ka lud-lul* TU$_6$ *ul ia-a-tu-un* ÉN ^{d}IDIM *u* ^{d}*asal-lú-ḫi*
18	a obv. 18	ÉN ^{d} *da-mu u* ^{d}*gu-la* ÉN ^{d}*nin-gìrima be-let* ÉN *te* ÉN
19	a obv. 19	3-*šú ta-qab-bi* [NAG]A *ta-nam-di-is-su ù* ÉN *a-na muḫ-ḫi-šú* ŠID-*nu*
20	a obv. 20	ÉN NAGA NAGA ^{d}30 *i*-⸢*ri*⸣-*ka* ^{d}UTU *ú-rab-bi-ka*
21	a obv. 21	^{d}*ad-da-a ina ur-pe-e-ti* A.MEŠ *iš-ta-qí-ka* ⸢*i-te-riš-ka-ma*⸣ ⸢*am-te*$^?$-*e*$^?$- *su*$^{?!}$⸣ ŠU.MIN-⸢*a-a*⸣
22	a obv. 22	*šá ka-šap* DÙ-⸢*šu*⸣ *uš-taḫ-ḫi-it šá kaš-šap-tu*$_4$ DÙ-*šu uš-taḫ-ḫi-it*
23	a obv. 23	*šá e-piš* DÙ-*šu uš-taḫ-ḫi-it šá e-piš-tu*$_4$ DÙ-*šu uš-taḫ-ḫi-it*
24	a obv. 24	*šá muš-te-pi-šú* DÙ-*šu uš-taḫ-ḫi-it ka-šap u kaš-šap-tu*$_4$ *e-piš u e-piš-tu*$_4$
25	a obv. 25	[*p*]*i*-⸢*i*⸣-[*ku*]-*nu lu-ú it-tu-um-ma lu-ú en-de-tu-nu i-gàr te* ÉN

26 a obv. 26 TA ÍD *il-lam-ma ana muḫ-ḫi a-tu-nu* BÁḪAR *il-lak-ma a-tu-nu i-ḫaṣ-ṣí-in-ma*

27 a obv. 27 *ki-a-am i-qab-bi* ⸢*a*⸣*-tu-nu el-let* DUMU.MUNUS ^{d}*a-nim ra-bi-tu*$_4$ *šá ina lìb-bi-šú na-an-ḫu-za-at*

28 a obv. 28 ⸢IZI⸣ MURUB$_4$ *ina lìb-bi-šú* ^{d}*gíra*(GIŠ.BAR) *qar-du ir-mu-ú šu-bat-su šal-ma-ti-ma*

29 a obv. 29 *ú-de-e-ka šal-mu šat* ⸢*ana*⸣ *šat ta-ma-al-le-*⸢*e*⸣ *u ta-ri-qa u a-na-ku er-re-e-ma*

30 a obv. 30 *šá ina lìb-bi-ia ul ú-[š]al-lam šal-ma-nu-ut-ka bi-in-nim-ma la šal-ma-nu-ta-ma*

31 a obv. 31 *li-qé-e ú-du-ú* ⸢*šal*⸣*-mu* TA ŠÀ*-ka la il-la-a' u ana-ku šá ina lìb-bi-ia*

32 a obv. 32 *liš-lim-ma* ⸢*né*⸣*-mel-šú lu-m[u-u]r ina* É *áš-bak pa-ni lu-ú maḫ-rat te* ÉN

---

33 a obv. 33 *ana* ^{giš}KIRI$_6$ *ur-rad-m[a]* ^{giš}GIŠIMMAR *i-ḫaṣ-ṣí-in-ma* ^{giš}GIŠIMMAR *ma-ḫi-rat kal šá-a-ri mu-uḫ-ra-an-ni-ma*

34 a obv. 34 *ár-nu šèr-tú gíl-lat ḫi-ṭi-ti u a-na-ku ina* É *áš-ba-ak u*$_8$*-ú-a a-a la ṣa-la-la*

35 a obv. 35 *di-'u di-lip-tu*$_4$ ⸢*ṣi*⸣*-it še-er-ra* ÌR *u* GÉME *ma-la ba-šu-ú ina* EDIN*-ia a-a-mu-ut*

36 a obv. 36 *la-i te-nu-ú i-ta-[r]i u ši-i qer-bé-et-ma ú-da la maḫ-rat*

37 a obv. 37 *a-šar ḫa[r-p]u up-ul tu-šab-šú a-šar up-ul tu-šab-šú ḫar-pu*

38 a obv. 38 *iṣ-ṣi [na]p-ṣu* <*in*>*-bi tu-šar-šú iṣ-ṣi la na-šu-ú tu-šar-šú in-bi*

39 a obv. 39 *la ṭu-ub* ŠÀ *la ṭu-ub* UZU *u ḫa-mu* DINGIR*-ía u* ^{d}15*-ia šá ina la e-de-e*

40 a obv. 40 *a-tam-ma-ru ú-kab-bi-s[u] ul i-di mu-ḫur mu-ḫur-an-ni-ma da-li-li-ka lud-lul te* ÉN

---

41 a obv. 41 ÉN ^{d}UTU *at-ta-ma šá ka-liš kib-rat* ZALAG *šá e-liš u šap-liš* EN*-šú-nu at-ta-ma*

42 a obv. 42 *šá e-piš u e-piš-tú di-ni*$_7$*-šú-n[u] ta-pa-ar-ra-as šá kaš-šap u kaš-šap-tú* EŠ.BAR*-šú-nu ta-*⸢*šak-kan*⸣

43 a obv. 43 *šá ḫe-bi-il*$_5$ *u ḫe-bil-ti ár-nu-šú [t]u-qát*(ŠU.MIN)*-ta*$_5$ *ub-be-ak-ka la mu-šal-in-d[u*$^{?}$]

44 a obv. 44 *šá en-de-et ár-nu šá e-piš u e-piš-tú ú-kal-lu-šú u qú-lum šá kaš-šap u k[aš-šap-tú]*

45 a obv. 45 *ú-šá-az-ba-lu-uš bil-tu*$_4$ *šá še-er-ri ul-la-du-ma* x[x x x x]

46 a obv. 46 *la ú-rab-bu-ú še-er-*<*ri*>*-šu-ma l[a] ú-rap-pa-šú kim-is-su* m[u$^{?}$ x x x x]

47 a obv. 47 *la ip-pal-la-su kim-is-su* ⸢*a*⸣*-bi u ba-an-ta* x[x x x x x x x x (x)]

48 a obv. 48 ⸢*at*⸣*-ta-ma* ^{d}UTU *šá ka-liš kib*$^{!}$*-ra[t]-*⸢*ta*⸣ <ZALAG> *šá* ^{munus}*sin-[niš-tu*$_4$ x x x x (x x)]

49 a obv. 49 *[e]-pu-uš di-in-šú šá kaš-šap [u kaš-ša]p-*⸢*tú*⸣ x[x x x x x x x x x (x)]

50 a rev. 1 [x x x x x] x [..]

51 a rev. 2 [x x x x x] *šu* ⸢*li*$^{?}$⸣ x [..]

52 a rev. 3 [x] x[x x x *š]e-er-ri ul-la-d[u* ....]

---

53 a rev. 4 [É]N ^{d}I[DIM *a]t-ta-ma ba-nu-ú ka-la-mu* ⸢*šá*$^{?}$⸣ [*kullat nišī*(?)]

54 a rev. 5 ⸢*ba-nu-šú*⸣*-nu at-ta-ma ub-be-ak-ka* ^{munus}*sin-niš-t[u*$_4$ *lā mušallimtu*(?)]

55 a rev. 6 *šá en-de-et ár-nu a-na ap-si-i a-na ma-ḫar-ka* x[x x (x)]

56 a rev. 7 ^{munus}*sin-niš-tú e-pu-uš di-ni*$_7$*-šu-ma pu-uṭ-ru* ⸢*ár*⸣*-nu-šú* ⸢*gíl-lat-su*⸣ [*še-ret-su*$^{?}$]

No.	MS	Text
57	a rev. 8	*u bil-lat-su* ÍD.MEŠ *liš-šá-aʾ a-gam-ma li-ṭe-pi a-da-ap-*⸢*a*⸣-[*ta*]
58	a rev. 9	*li-še-ṣa-aʾ ri-kis lu-um-*[*n*]*i-šú ár-nu e-piš e-piš-t*[*ú*]
59	a rev. 10	*kaš-šap kaš-šap-tú i-mid-da a-na* ^{munus}*sin-niš-tú šu-zu-bu*
60	a rev. 11	*pu-uṭ-ru ina zu-mur-ri-šú lu-rab-bi še-er-ri*
61	a rev. 12	*lu*$_4$*-rap-pí-iš kim-mit-su da-li-li-ka lid-lul te* ÉN

The second ritual

No.	MS	Text
62	a rev. 13	*ana* MUNUS NU SI.SÁ SI.SÁ DÙ.DÙ.BI *ana* ^{d}*gu-la* NÍG.NA ^{šim}LI GAR-*an*
63	a rev. 14	*mi-iḫ-ḫa* BAL-*qí-ma kam* DU$_{11}$.GA

No.	MS	Text
64	a rev. 15	^{d}*nin-kar-ra-ak-a* GAŠAN [*šu*]*r-bu-tu* AMA *reme-ni-*⸢*tu*$_4$$^{!}$(ka)⸣
65	a rev. 16	*im-mer-tú šá* ^{d}ŠÁKKAN *u* [^{d}]*dumu-zi mé-ra-a-a lim-ḫu-ra-an-ni-ma*
66	a rev. 17	*mé-ra-šú lid-di-na l*[*a*] *mu-še-ši-ru-ti lim-ḫu-ra-an-ni-ma*
	c obv. 1'	[.........................] x
67	a rev. 18	*mu-še-ši-ru-sa lid-di-na*
	c obv. 1'$^{cont.}$	⸢*mu-še*⸣*-š*[*i-ru-sa* ......]

a, c

No.	MS	Text
68	a rev. 19	3-*šú* DU$_{11}$.GA-*ma ina š*[*e-r*]*im ana* IGI ^{d}UTU *ina* UGU SIG$_4$.ḪI.A *ab-ra* SAR-*aḫ*
	c obv. 2'	[.. *ina*] ⸢UGU⸣ SIG$_4$ *ab-ra* S[AR-*aḫ*$^{?}$]
69	a rev. 20	$^{giš.šim}$LI DUB-*aq* ⸢U$_8$⸣ PEŠ$_4$ *mu-šal-lim-ti*
	c obv. 3'	[......................... P]EŠ$_4$ ⸢*mu*⸣*-š*[*al-lim-ti*]
70	a rev. 21	*ana* IGI ‹d›20 DU$_{10}$.GAM-*si-ma* 2 ⸢GURUŠ$^{?}$⸣.MEŠ *i-na-áš-šu ù* ^{munus}PEŠ$_4$ *ana* ŠÀ GEŠTU.MIN U$_8$ PEŠ$_4$ *kam* DU$_{11}$.GA
	c obv. 3'$^{cont.}$–4'	*ana* IGI ^{d}UTU DU$_{10}$.GAM-*si-ma* ⸢2$^{?}$⸣ [......] / [......................... ^{mu}]^{nus}PEŠ$_4$ *ana* ŠÀ G[EŠTU.MEŠ$^{?}$ U$_8$ P]EŠ$_4$ UR$_5$.GIM DU$_{11}$.[GA]

a, c

No.	MS	Text
71	a rev. 22	*im-mer-tú šá* ^{d}ŠÁKKAN [*u*] ⸢^{d}⸣*dumu-zi mé-ra-a-a tab-li-ma mi-ḫir-ki bi-la*
	c obv. 5'	[...............] ^{d}ŠÁKKAN *u* ^{d}*dum*[*u-zi m*]*é-ra-a-a tab-li-ma m*[*i-ḫir-ki* ......]
72	a rev. 23	*la mu-še-ši-ru-t*[*i*] *tab-li-ma mu-še-ši-ru-ut-ka bi-la*
	c obv. 6'	[*la mu-še-ši-r*]*u*$^{?}$*-ti tab-li-ma m*[*u-še-ši*]*-ru-ut-ki bi-*[*la*]

a, c

No.	MS	Text
73	a rev. 24	*ana* ŠÀ GEŠTU.MIN.MEŠ *ki-lal-*[*l*]*e-e* 3.TA.ÀM ŠID-*nu ki-ma* ŠID-*ú ina šap-la-an* U$_8$ *uṣ-ṣi*
	c obv. 7'–8'	*ana* Š[À GEŠT]U.MEŠ-*šú ki-lal-le-e* ⸢3⸣.[TA.À]M ŠID-*nu e-ma* Š[ID-*ú*] / *ina* [*šap-l*]*a-an* U$_8$ *uṣ-ṣi*
74	a rev. 25	*u ina* 7-*i* È-*šá ana* [UG]U$^{?}$ IGI.MEŠ-*šú* NIGIN-*ma* ÚḪ-*su ana* KA U$_8$ ŠUB-*ma ana* EDIN È-*ma* TAG$_4$-*šú*
	c obv. 8'$^{cont.}$–9'	⸢*ù*⸣ *i*[*na* x x È-*š*]*á*$^{?}$ *ana* UGU ⸢IGI⸣.M[EŠ-*šú* .....] / Ú[Ḫ-*s*]*a ana* KA U$_8$ ŠUB-*m*[*a*$^{?!}$ ....]

a

The third ritual

No.	MS	Text
75	a rev. 26	*ana* ⸢MUNUS⸣ x x [x] ⸢x x⸣ [x x x]x-⸢*tu*$^{?}$*-te*$^{?}$⸣ ⸢ŠIM⸣.MEŠ *ù* ZÌ DUB UDU.NÍTA
	c rev. 1	*ana* MUNUS Ù$^{!}$.T[U$^{?}$ ....]

76 a rev. 27 — *t[a-ṭa-ba-aḫ*$^{?}$]-⌜*ma*⌝ ⌜*ina*⌝ ⌜*še-rim*⌝ ⌜2⌝.TA.ÀM NINDA.MEŠ *ina* SILA.LÍM.MA GAR-*an ù ina bi-rit* SILA.LÍM.MA
c rev. 1$^{\text{cont.}}$–3 — [..] / 10 NINDA.MEŠ ⌜*ù*$^{?}$⌝ [......] / *ina* SILA.LÍM.M[A GAR-*an* ....]

77 a rev. 28 — *ku-*⌜*rit*⌝ ⌜UDU.NÍTA⌝ *u* NINDA GAR-*ma na-aq-bi-ta an-ni-ta* DU$_{11}$.GA
c rev. 3$^{\text{cont.}}$–4 — [..] / *an-ni-t*[*a*$^{?}$ DU$_{11}$.GA]

a ______________________________

78 a rev. 29 — *na-šu-ma am-ta-ḫar na-šá-ku-ma lim-ḫu-ru-in-ni* 3-*šú* ÉN *an-ni-tú* DU$_{11}$.GA
c rev. 4$^{\text{cont.}}$–5 — [..] 3-*šú* É[N *an-ni-tú* ....]

79 a rev. 30 — *u* 3-*šú* NINDA.MEŠ GAR-*an let-su a-na ku-tal-li-šú ul i-nam-di*
c rev. 5$^{\text{cont.}}$–6 — [..] / *ul i-*[*nam-di*$^{?}$]

a, c ______________________________

80 a rev. 31 — *ḫa-am-ṣi-ir-ta* GAZ-*ma* a te a tú TA ^{giš}EREN *ina* ŠU.MIN-*šú* DAB-*si* ^{šim}MUG SAG.DU-*su* KÉŠ-*ma*
c rev. 7–8 — *ḫa-a*[*m-ṣi-ir-ta* ....] / SAG.[DU-*su* KÉŠ-*ma*$^{?}$]

81 a rev. 32 — *ina* ^{síg}GA.RÍG.AK.A *ta-kar-rik ina* SILA.LÍM.MA GAR-*an na-aq-bi-ta an-ni-tú* DU$_{11}$.GA
c rev. 8$^{\text{cont.}}$–9 — [..] / *na-*[*aq-bi-ta* ....]

82 a rev. 33 — *na-šu-ma am-ta-ḫar na-šá-ku-ma lim-ḫu-ru-in-ni* DU$_{11}$.GA-*ma* SILA DIB NU DIB
b 1' — [.........................*na-šá*]-⌜*ku-ma*⌝ [...]
c rev. 9$^{\text{cont.}}$–10 — [...] / D[U$_{11}$.GA-*ma*$^{?}$ ....]

____

83 a rev. 34 — *an-nam u an-nam ina la-pat* AN-*e* DÙ.DÙ-*uš-ma ina* SILA.LÍM.MA GAR-*an-ma na-aq-bi-tú an-ni-tú* DU$_{11}$.GA
b 2' — [...] *ina* SILA.LÍM.MA [GAR-*an* ...]

84 a rev. 35 — *na-šu-ma am-ta-ḫar na-šá-ku-ma lim-ḫu-ru-in-ni* DU$_{11}$.GA-*ma* SILA DIB NU DIB
b 3' — [......................... *na-šá*]-*ku-ma lim-ḫur-i*[*n-ni*$^{?}$ ....]

a ______________________________

85 a rev. 36 — ÈME PEŠ$_{4}$ *tuš-zaz-ma* ŠE.BAR MUNUS *ina up-ni-šú* ÍL-*ma šu-*⌜*pal*⌝ ÈME PEŠ$_{4}$ *i-ḫal-lu-um-ma*
b 4' — [............... ŠE].⌜BAR$^{?}$⌝ MUNUS *ina up-*[*ni-šú* ÍL-*ma* ....]

86 a rev. 37 — ÈME 3-*šú ú-šá-kal-ma na-aq-bi-ta an-ni-ta a-na* ÈME D[U$_{11}$].GA *ša* ŠÀ-*ki li-mut-ma*
b 5' — [............ *ú*]-⌜*šá*⌝-*kal-ma na-a*[*q-bi-ta* ....]

87 a rev. 38 — *šá*$^{!}$(diš) ŠÀ-*ía lib-luṭ* 3-*šú ina šu-pal* ÈME *i-ḫal-lu-up*$^{!}$ *u* 3-*šú* ŠE.BAR ÈME *ú-šá-áš-šá*
b 6'–7' — [...] *šá* ŠÀ-*ia*$_{5}$ *lib-*[*luṭ* ....] / [.....................] ÈME *ú-š*[*á-áš-šá* ...]

88 a rev. 39 — *ṣab-bar* ŠE.MUŠ$_{5}$ *ina* SILA.LÍM.MA GAR-*an-ma ina ap-ti tal-lal-ma* ^{munus}PEŠ$_{4}$ ⌜EN⌝ Ù.⌜TU-*di*⌝ *ú-lap-pat-ma*
b 8' — [............................ *ina ap-ti ta*]*l-lal*$^{?}$ ^{munus}PEŠ$_{4}$ [..................]

89 a rev. 40 — *ina u*$_{4}$*-um ḫi-li-šá* MUNUS.TUR *i-ṭe*$_{4}$*-en-ma ina* A *ḫi-li-šá i-la-aš-šu-uš-ma* NU NITA DÙ-*uš*
b 9' — [...................... *i-ṭe*$_{4}$]-⌜*en*⌝-*ma ina* [A *ḫi-li-šá* ....]

90 a rev. 41 — ⌜*ù*⌝ NU MUNUS DÙ-*uš* EN *mi-šil* GI$_{6}$ *ina* <É> *te-ru-*⌜*ba*⌝ *ina mi-šil* GI$_{6}$ *ana* SILA ŠUB-*di lu ana* KASKAL ŠUB-*uš-šú*
b 10' — [........]x x [.........]

91 a rev. 42 — [x] x [x x] x-*ma*$^{?}$ ⌜^{giš}GAN$^{?}$⌝ x x x [x x] x-*ma ana* É-*šú* KU$_{4}$-*ub* 3 *ne-pe-šá* GABA.RI ^{uru}KAR-EN-KUR.KUR

____

Colophon:

92 a u. e. 1 [GI]N$_{7}$ LIBIR.RA-*ša ša-ṭ[è-er-ma bari tuppi* ^{m}AN.Š]ÁR-ZÚ.KÉŠ *bu*$_{12}$*-kúr* ^{md}*ša-máš*-SUM-*na*

93 a u. e. 2 ŠA.ÁB.BA$_{4}$.ALLA ^{lú}SANGA-^{d}[*nin-urta pāliḫ* AN.ŠÁ]R *u*
^{d}KI.ŠÁR NU *i*$_{11}$*-ta*$_{8}$*-áb-bà-alla* \ [*lū ina m*]*e-re-eš-ti* NU *u-*⌜*ša*⌝*-am-àš*[330]

Bound Transcription and Translation

The first ritual

[1] [*ana a*]*rīti pašāri*(?) *sinništu lā mušēšertu itti rībi ša šamši* [2] *taparras ina maški gallābūs(su) teppušī-ma ina naštuqa* [3] *eššetu ina kišādīšu tašakkan erû uqnû* $^{\mathrm{na4}}$AŠ *zikari šadânu ṣābitu* [4] *u zibītu*$^{!}$ *ina sāmūtu tašakkak šalāšat lippī ina tabarri talappap* [5] *ina qāt imittīšu tašakkan u akalu kurītu immeri adi šīrīšu šina qa zērī* [6] *ittî tanamdissu ina rēšīšu ibâtu ina šēri lāma šamši* [7] *napāḫi ultu muḫḫi igāri tušqallalšu illak-ma ina ašar parsu* [8] *ina muḫḫi ḫarrāni pariktu akalī šīru u zēru tašakkan-ma nabû ittannūnu* [9] *lā nabû indaḫ(a)rū'inni ḫamšīšu iqabbi ēma iqtabû* [10] *ṣubāssu išaḫḫaṭ-ma mê turammakšu itebbē-ma* [11] *ṣubāssu šanû illabbaš u lēssu ana kutallīšu ul inandi* [12] *ana nāri illak-ma ana nāri urrad mê ana muqqalpītu šalāšīšu ibbak* [13] *u šipta ana muḫḫīšu tamannu*	[1] [*In order to*] *release a pregnant woman*: At sunset [2] you isolate [1] the (pregnant) woman who cannot bring (her pregnancies) to term. On a piece of leather, she(!) submits(!) to a shaving. Then you put (the shaved hair) in a [3] new [2] leather bag [3] (and place it) around her neck. You thread (a) copper (bead), lapis lazuli, male AŠ-stone, magnetite, [4] and *zibītu*$^{!}$-stone on red (yarn); you wrap three wads of red wool (around it). [5] You put (it) on her right hand. In addition, [6] you give her [5] bread, the shin of a sheep with its meat, (and) [6] in addition, [5] two litres of grain seed. [6] It shall stand overnight at the head of her (bed). In the morning, before the sun [7] rises, you have her suspend it (the leather bag?) from a wall. She goes (with you), and [8] you lay down the bread (loaves), meat and barley [7] at a secluded place, [8] on a blocked road. [9] Then she says five times: [8] "The named ones have given me, [9] the ones not named have received from me." When she has said (this), [10] she takes off her garment and you wash her with water. (Then) she gets up and [11] she puts on another garment. And, without looking back, [12] she goes to the river and descends into the river. Three times she *brings* water downstream. [13] Meanwhile, you recite the (following) incantation over it.
ÉN <*nāru*> *ešrētu šūšurū mûka*	Incantation: "<River>, you are just, your waters put (things) in order.
muḫranni-ma [14] *arnu šērtu gillat ḫiṭītu lumnu mēneštu ša zumrīya*	Receive from me [14] the guilt, wrongdoing, sin, misdeed, evil (and) weakness of my body!
itti mêka [15] *ana qiddatu tabal nārātu limlâ agammu liṭēpi adappāta*	With your waters [15] carry (them) off downstream! May the rivers fill up, may the marshland become submerged!
[16] *lišēṣâ rikis lumnīya nāru ešrētu šūšurū mûka šūširanni-ma* [17] *dalīlīka ludlul*	[16] May [15] the channels [16] expel the knot of evil affecting me! River, you are righteous, your waters put (things) in order. Put me in order, then [17] I shall praise your glory!
šiptu ul yattun šipat Ea u Asalluḫi [18] *šipat Damu u Gula šipat Ningirima bēlet šipti tê* ÉN	The incantation is not mine. It is the incantation of Ea and Asalluḫi, [18] the incantation of Damu and Gula, the incantation of Ningirima, the mistress of the incantation." Incantation formula.

---

330 At the bottom of the upper edge, Abusch et al. (2020, CMAwR 3, 68) propose to read the signs *šá* ^{m}20-[MU?], written in smaller script, as "of Šamaš-[iddina]".

19 *šalāšīšu taqabbi uḫūla tanamdissu u šipta ana muḫḫīšu tamannu*	19 You say (this) three times. You give her (potash from) *uḫū-lu*-soapwort plant, and you recite the (following) incantation over it.

20 ÉN *uḫūlu uḫūlu Sîn īrīka Šamaš urabbīka*	20 Incantation: "Soapwort, soapwort! Sîn has engendered you, Šamaš has made you grow,
21 *Addâ ina urpēti mê ištaqīka īteriška-ma amtesu(?) qātāya*	21 Addâ has given you water from the clouds, he cultivated you so that I could *wash* my hands (with you).
22 *ša kaššāp īpušu uštaḫḫit ša kaššāptu īpušu uštaḫḫit*	22 I have washed off what the sorcerer did, I have washed off what the witch did.
23 *ša ēpiš īpušu uštaḫḫit ša ēpištu īpušu uštaḫḫit*	23 I have washed off what the sorcerer did, I have washed off what the sorceress did.
24 *ša muštēpišu īpušu uštaḫḫit kaššāpu u kaššāptu ēpišu u ēpištu*	24 I have washed off what the bewitcher did. Warlock and witch, sorcerer and sorceress:
25 *[p]ī[ku]nu lū ittûm-ma lū endētunu igār tê* ÉN	25 May your mouth be (as black as) bitumen, may you be *pressed* (against) the wall!" Incantation formula.

26 *ultu nāri illâm-ma ana muḫḫi atūn paḫāri illak-ma atūnu iḫaṣṣin-ma*	26 She comes up from the river. Then she walks to a potter's oven and embraces the oven.
27 *kīam iqabbi*	27 Then she speaks thus:
atūnu elletu mārat Ani rabītu	"Pure oven, great daughter of Anu,
ša ina libbīšu nanḫuzat 28 *išāt qabli*	in whose inside the 28 fire of battle 27 is kindled,
ina libbīšu Girra qardu irmû šubassu	in whose inside the heroic fire god has set up his residence.
šalmāti-ma 29 *udêka šalmū*	You are intact, and 29 your ware is intact.
šat ana šat tamallê u tarêqa	Year after year you become full and you become empty.
u anāku errē-ma 30 *ša ina libbīya ul u[ša]llam*	But I, I become pregnant, but 30 I cannot bring to term what is in my belly.
šalmānūtka binnim-ma lā šalmānūta-ma 31 *liqê*	Give me your sound condition and 31 take away (from me my) 30 unsound condition!
udû šalmu ultu libbīka lā illâ	31 A sound vessel shall not emerge from your interior.
anāku ša libbīya 32 *lišlim-ma nēmelšu lūmur*	(But as for) me, may the fruit of my womb 32 be in good health, so that I may see it thriving!
ina bīt ašbāk pānī lū maḫrat tê ÉN	In the house where I live, let me be acceptable!" Incantation formula.

33 *ana kirî urrad-ma gišimmara iḫaṣṣin-ma*	33 She goes down to a garden (orchard) an[d] embraces a date palm. Then (she says thus):
gišimmaru māḫirat kal šāri	"Date palm, who withstands all winds,
muḫranni-ma 34 *arnu šērtu gillat ḫiṭīti*	receive from me 34 the guilt, wrongdoing, sin, misdeed!
u anāku ina bīt ašbāk ū'a ayya lā ṣalāla	But as for me – in the house where I live: (receive from me) the woe, alas, sleeplessness,
35 *di'u diliptu ṣīt šerra ardi u amti mala bašû ina ṣērīya*	35 *di'u*-disease, trouble, the loss of a child, of a servant and a maid, as many (evils) as are (inflicted) on me!
ay (i)mūt 36 *lā'ī tēnû itâri*	May 36 my baby 35 not die, 36 a replacement shall return.
u šī qerbet-ma ūda lā maḫrat	Moreover, as for her, she is near (giving birth), may she not encounter difficulties.

37 *ašar ḫa[r]pu uppul tušabšu ašar uppul tušabšu ḫarpu*	37 Where there is an early (harvest), you provide a late (harvest); where there is a late (harvest), you provide an early (harvest).
38 *iṣṣi [na]pṣu <in>bī tušaršu iṣṣi lā nāšû tušaršu inbī*	38 You make a [dama]ged tree bear fruit, you make a barren tree bear fruit!
39 *lā ṭūb libbi lā ṭūb šīri u ḫāmū ilīya u ištarīya* *ša ina lā edê* 40 *ātammaru ukabbisu ul īde*	40 I do not know 39 (the cause of my) unhappiness, ill health and the rubbish (offensive to) my god and my goddess, which I, unwittingly, 40 may have encountered in various places (or) stepped upon.
muḫur muḫurannī-ma dalīlīka ludlul tê ÉN	Accept (my) prayer, then I will praise your glory!" Incantation formula.

---

41 ÉN *Šamaš attā-ma ša kališ kibrāt unammaru*	41 Incantation: "Šamaš, you are the one who illuminates the whole world,
ša eliš u šapliš bēlšunu attā-ma	you are the lord of the above and lower world!
42 *ša ēpiš u ēpištu dīn(i)šunu taparras*	42 You decide the case of sorcerer and sorceress,
ša kaššāp u kaššāptu purussêšunu tašakkan	you pronounce the verdict of warlock and witch.
43 *ša ḫēbil u ḫēbilti arnūšu[nu t]uqatta*	43 You bring the punishment of the man and woman who have done wrong to an end.
ube"âkka lā mušallint[u]	A woman who cannot bring (her baby) to term is seeking you,
44 *ša endet arnu ša ēpiš u ēpištu ukallûšu*	44 (a woman) on whom punishment was imposed with which sorcerer and sorceress keep a firm hold on her,
u qūlu ša kaššāp u k[aššāptu] 45 *ušazbalūš biltu*	and a silence which warlock and wit[ch] 45 have her carry as a burden,
ša šerrī ulladu-ma ...[......]	who bears babies, but then [... ...],
46 *lā urabbû šer<rī>šu-ma l[ā] urappašu kimissu* ...[......]	46 (who) does not raise her babies and does not expand her family ...[......],
47 *lā ipallasu kimissu abi u bānta* ...[......]	47 (who) does not see her family, father and mother ...[........].
48 *attā-ma Šamaš ša kališ kibrāt <unammaru> ša sin[ništu* ...]	48 It is you, Šamaš, who <illuminates> the whole world, who [....] a wo[man ...]!
49 *[e]puš dīnšu ša kaššāp [u kaššā]ptu* ... [.......]	49 [Re]nder judgement for her! [*Pronounce the verdict*] of warlock [and wit]ch [... ...]!
50 [.....] .... [......]	50 [......] ... [......],
51 [.....] .... [......]	51 [.....] ... [.....],
52 [.....] ... [... *š]erri ulladu* [......]	52 [.... the b]aby that she gives birth to [......]!"

---

53 [É]N *E[a a]ttā-ma bānû kalāmu* *ša [kullat nišī(?)]* 54 *bānûšunu attā-ma*	53 [Incan]tation: "E[a], it is [y]ou who creates everything, 54 you are the creator 53 of [*all people*]!
ube"âkka sinništu [lā mušallimtu]	54 A woman [who cannot bring (her babies) to term] is seeking you,
55 *ša endet arnu ana apsî ana maḫarka* ...[......]	55 (a woman) on whom punishment has been imposed. To the subterranean ocean, before you [... ...].
56 *sinništu epuš dīn(i)šu-ma puṭru arnušu gillassu [šēressu(?)]* 57 *u bilassu*	56 A woman: render a judgment for her and remove her guilt, her crime, [*her fault*], 57 and her burden.
nārātu liššâ agamma liṭēpi adappāta	May the rivers carry (their water), may the marshland become submerged!

[58] *lišēṣâ rikis lumnīšu* *arnu ēpiš ēpištu* [59] *kaššāp kaššāptu imidda* *ana sinništu šūzubu* [60] *puṭru ina zumrīšu* *lurabbi šerrī* [61] *lurappiš kimissu dalīlīka lidlul tê* ÉN	[58] May [57] the canals expel the knot of her evil! Impose the punishment on the sorcerer (and) sorceress, [59] the warlock and witch! In order to save the women: [60] remove (it) from her body! Let her raise babies, [61] let her expand her family! (Then) she will praise your glory!" Incantation formula.

The second ritual

[62] *ana sinništi lā mušēšerti šūšuri* DÙ.DÙ.BI *ana Gula nignak burāši tašakkan* [63] *miḫḫa tanaqqī-ma kâm iqabbi*	[62] To make a woman who has difficulty giving birth successfully give birth successfully – the procedure for it: You set up a censer of juniper for Gula, [63] you libate *miḫḫu*-beer. Then she speaks thus:
[64] *Ninkarrak bēltu* [*šu*]*rbūtu ummu rēmēnītu*! [65] *immertu ša Šakkan u Dumuzi mērā limḫuranni-ma* [66] *mērâšu liddina* *lā mušēšerūtī limḫuranni-ma* [67] *mušēšerūssa liddina*	[64] "Ninkarrak, supreme mistress, merciful mother! [65] Let the ewe of Šakkan and Dumuzi receive from me my pregnancy and [66] let it give me its pregnancy! Let it receive from me my inability *to bring to term* and [67] let it give me its ability *to bring to term*!"
[68] *šalāšīšu iqabbi-ma ina š*[*ēr*]*i ana maḫar Šamaš ina muḫḫi libnāti abra tanappaḫ* [69] *burāša tasarraq laḫru arītu mušallimti* [70] *ana maḫar Šamaš tušakmassī-ma šina e*[*ṭ*-*l*]*ū*(?) *inaššû u arītu ana libbi uznī laḫri arīti kâm iqabbi*	[68] She shall speak thus three times. In the morning, before Šamaš you ignite a pile of brushwood on top of bricks. [69] You strew juniper (on top of it). [70] You let [69] a pregnant ewe who delivers (her young) soundly [70] crouch down before Šamaš. Then two [young m]en(?) shall lift (it) up (from the ground), and the pregnant woman shall speak thus into the ears of the pregnant ewe:
[71] *immertu ša Šakkan* [*u*] *Dumuzi mērā tablī-ma miḫirki bilâ* [72] *lā mušēšerūt*[*ī*] *tablī-ma mušēšerūtka bilâ*	[71] "Ewe of Šakkan and Dumuzi! Take away my pregnancy and bring me your equivalent! [72] Take away my inability *to bring to term* and bring me your ability to *bring to term*!"
[73] *ana libbi uznī kilallē* 3.TA.ÀM *imannu kīma imtanû ina šaplān laḫri uṣṣi* [74] *u ina sebî aṣîša ana muḫḫi pānīšu isaḫḫar-ma ru'ussu ana pī laḫri inaddī-ma ana ṣēri tušeṣṣī-ma tezzibšu*	[73] She shall recite (this) three times into both its (the ewe's) ears. When she has recited (this), she comes out from below the ewe. [74] And when she comes out (from below the ewe) for the seventh (time), she turns her face towards (the ewe) and spits into the ewe's mouth. Then you bring (it) out into the steppe and abandon it (there).

The third ritual

[75] *ana sinništi šūludi(?)* [...] ... *riqqī u qēma tasarraq immera* [76] *t[aṭabbaḫ(?)]-ma ina šēri* 2.TA.ÀM (var. 10) *akalī ina sūq erbetti išakkan u ina birīt sūq erbetti* [77] *kurīt immeri u akala išakkan-ma naqbīta annīta iqabbi*	[75] To enable a woman to give birth (successfully) [... ...] ... You strew aromatic plants and flour. [76] *Y[ou slaughter]* [75] a sheep. [76] In the morning she places two (var. ten) bread loaves at a crossroads. Moreover, in *the middle* of (lit. between) the crossroads [77] she places the shin of the sheep and bread. Then she speaks this recitation:
[78] *našû-ma amtaḫar našâku-ma limḫurū'inni šalāšīšu šiptu annītu iqabbi* [79] *u šalāšīšu akalī išakkan lēssu ana kutallīšu ul inamdi*	[78] "I have received what they were carrying. May they receive from me what I am carrying!" She says this incantation three times, [79] and three times she places the bread loaves, without looking back.
[80] *ḫamṣirta tadâk-ma* ... *erēni ina qātīšu tušaṣbassi ballukka qaqqassu tarakkas-ma* [81] *ina pušikki takarrik ina sūq erbetti išakkan naqbīta annītu iqabbi*	[80] You kill a female mouse and you make it hold a ... of cedar in its paws; you tie *ballukku*-aromatic to its head and [81] wrap (it) in combed wool. She puts it at a crossroads (and) speaks this recitation:
[82] *našû-ma amtaḫar našâku-ma limḫurū'inni iqabbī-ma sūq ītiqu lā ittiq*	[82] "I have received what they were carrying. May they receive from me what I am carrying!" She says (this); then she must not go (back) by the (same) street by which she came.
[83] *annâ u annâ ina lapāt šamê īteneppuš-ma ina sūq erbetti išakkan-ma naqbītu annītu iqabbi*	[83] She performs these two (rites) repeatedly at dawn and places (items) at a crossroads and then speaks this recitation:
[84] *našû-ma amtaḫar našâku-ma limḫurū'inni*	[84] "I have received what they were carrying. May they receive from me what I am carrying!"
iqabbī-ma sūq ītiqu lā ittiq	She says (this); but she must not go (back) by the street by which she came.
[85] *atānu arītu tušzaz-ma uṭṭata šinništu ina upnīšu inaššī-ma šupāl atāni arīti iḫallum-ma* [86] *atāna šalāšīšu ušakkal-ma naqbīta annīta ana atāni iqabbi ša libbīki limūt-ma* [87] *ša libbīya libluṭ šalāšīšu ina šupāl atāni iḫallup u šalāšīšu uṭṭata atāna ušašša* [88] *ṣabbar(?) šegušši ina sūq erbetti tašakkan-ma ina apti tallal-ma arītu adi alādi ulappat-ma* [89] *ina ūm ḫīlīša ṣeḫertu iṭên-ma ina mê ḫīlīša ilaššuš-ma ṣalam zikari ippuš* [90] *u ṣalam sinništi ippuš adi mišil mūši ina* <*bīti*> *terruba ina mišil mūši ana sūqi tanaddi lū ana ḫarrāni ušamqatūšu* [91] ... [.....] ... [.....] ...*-ma ana bītīšu terrub*	[85] You make a pregnant jenny stand (still), and the woman slips through (underneath) the pregnant jenny, carrying barley in her hands. [86] Then she feeds the jenny three times and says this recitation to the jenny: "May your foetus die, [87] and may my baby live!" Three times she slips through underneath the jenny, and three times she *feeds* the jenny the barley. [88] You place a *sheaf*(?) of millet at a crossroads and hang (it) in a window. The pregnant woman shall touch (it) regularly until she gives birth. [89] On the day of her birth pangs, a young woman grinds up (the millet), kneads it with her amniotic fluid (lit. the waters of her labour) and fashions a figurine of a man. [90] And she (also) fashions a figurine of a woman. Just before midnight you enter <the house>. At midnight you throw (the figurines) into the street, or one disposes of them(!) on a road. [91] [...] ... [...] ... and you (may) enter her house.
šalāšat nēpeša gabari Kār-bēl-mātāti	Three rituals. A copy from Kār-bēl-mātāti.

Colophon:

92 *kīma labirīša šaṭe[r-ma bari ṭuppi An]u-ikṣur bukur Šamaš-iddina* 93 *[l]iblibbi Šangû-[Ninurta pāliḫ An]u u Antu lā itabbala [lū ina] mērešti lā ušam'aš*

92 Wri[tten] according to its original [and collated. Tablet of Anu]-ikṣur, son of Šamaš-iddina, 93 descendent of Šangû-[Ninurta. Anyone who reveres An]u and Antu must not carry (it) off [or int]entionally *withhold* it.

Notes

Line 1: Abusch et al. (2020, 66) suggest reading the damaged first signs as [*ana*] ⌜*šup*?-*šuq*?-*ti* BÚR⌝, with the tentative translation "[*In order to*] *release (a woman) who is having difficulties (in childbirth)*". They correctly note that the following rituals were performed for a pregnant woman who has suffered from miscarriages in the past, interpreted here as a problem caused by witchcraft, the dominant theme of the tablet. See also Scurlock 2014a, 688; Couto-Ferreira 2013, 100. However, the reading *šupšuqtu* remains somewhat doubtful, since this term appears to be used exclusively for women having a difficult delivery, as far as textual attestations suggest. Thus, this term occurs exclusively in the birth compendium BAM 248 iv 6–9 //, beside the word *muštapšiqtu* "woman in hard labour" (for ^{munus}LA.RA.AḪ, varying with *mušapšiqtu*, see text D.1.1). The term would thus not be adequate for the present context. An alternative restoration closer to the topic of the tablet is suggested here: [*ana a*]-⌜*ri-ti*⌝ ⌜BÚR⌝ "[*in order to*] *release a pregnant woman*".

Apart from the fragmentary rubric in SpTU 5, 248 obv. 1, the patient is exceptionally introduced as *sinništu lā mušēšertu* "a woman who does not bring (her pregnancies) to term" in the same line. This expression with a Š-stem participle of *ešēru* (instead of the more common Št-stem participle *lā muštēšertu*) is not attested in any other text so far, but is apparently used here as the Akkadian equivalent of the logographic MUNUS NU SI.SÁ encountered in line 62 (and possibly also in line 75), within the introductory rubric *ana* MUNUS NU SI.SÁ SI.SÁ, "to make a woman who does not bear successfully bear successfully". In addition to the unusual *mušēšertu*, SpTU 5, 248 also uses a derived abstract noun (*lā*) *mušēšerūtu* "(in)ability to bring (babies) to term" in lines 66, 67 and 72, likewise only known from the present text.

Treatments or rituals for a MUNUS NU SI.SÁ are not mentioned specifically in the Exorcist's Manual or in the Assur Medical Catalogue (AMC), although both catalogues mention a related type of rituals, ^{munus}PEŠ$_4$.KÉŠ.DA "to bind a pregnant woman" (cf. Steinert et al. 2018, 218, 272 line 114; Geller 2018a, 298, 305; Heeßel 2023, 294 line 15). A tablet with amulets and an incantation for a MUNUS NU SI.SÁ is known from STT 241 rev. 29 (text C.3.1), although the evil influences from which the pregnant woman was protected may not be witchcraft-related in this case (see *infra*). In the ritual preserved on KAR 223: 5 and dupl., stones that are put around the hips of a MUNUS NU SI.SÁ are used to delay delivery (see text D.3.1). Otherwise, the phrase is (MUNUS) NU SI.SÁ is sometimes encountered in omen apodoses, forecasting that a woman who has trouble bringing to term will bear successfully. For example, *Alamdimmû* Tablet III, offers the apodosis NU Ù.TU Ù.TU NU SI.SÁ SI.SÁ "an infertile woman will bear, a woman who does not bear successfully will bring to term" (Böck 2000, 94: 97). In the extispicy text Manzāzu (Tablet 4), we find this apodosis written syllabically: *la a-lit-tú ul-lad : la muš-te-šir/šìr-tú uš-te-(eš)-šir/šìr* (Koch 2000, Babylonian Liver Omens, 101 K. 1401a+ A 39; variant CT 30, 30 (K.1454): 5).

A similar variation between the Š-stem and the Št-stem as seen in *muš(t)ēšertu* is also found in the use of the verb *ešēru* in connection with delivery. Attestations of the Š-stem of *ešēru* with a connection to childbirth often refer to the unborn child and suggest a meaning "to let (the child) pass, to have a straightforward, normal childbirth)". See CAD E, s.v. *ešēru* sub 6a-2', e.g. SB *Atramḫasīs* (K. 3399+ = CT 15, 49 rev. iv 61) *rēmu kuṣṣurma ul ušēšir šerra* "the womb was knotted, it did not let the child pass through/come out straight" (Lambert and Millard 1969, 110–111). The Št-stem of *ešēru*, is further encountered in the meaning "to give birth easily", in connection with delivery (written syllabically and SI.SÁ, e.g. in the birth rituals of BAM 248 //, see text D.1.1).

Line 2: The expression *gallābūssu epēšu* means "to submit to a complete cleansing of the body by the *gallābu*", i.e. shaving of body hair (CAD G, 17–18). The subject of the verb should be the patient, i.e. a 3rd person sg., not a 2nd person sg. with a 3rd fem. sg. pronominal suffix (the text uses -*šu* as the 3rd sg. fem. suffix). The form *teppušī* (2nd fem. sg.) therefore seems to be a mistake for an expected 3rd person sg. form (*ippuš*). For shaving before delivery, cf. von Soden 1957–1958, 120 (assuming that only the genital area of a woman was shaved by the midwife prior to delivery); Stol 2000a, 172; Stol 2006–2008, "Rasieren", *RlA* 11, 261 §5.1; Scurlock 2002, 216.

For ^{kuš}*naštuq* or *naštuk* "leather bag", see CAD N/2 79b; AHw 1579b (a loanword from Greek, possibly introduced through Aramaic).

Line 3: ^{na4}AŠ (*zikari*) is only attested here. Scurlock interprets this spelling in analogy to ^{ú}DILI (*ēdu*-plant) as "lone stone". The Akkadian reading is uncertain. For stones having a 'male' and 'female' variety, see e.g. the *šû*-'stone' and *šubû*-'stone' (CAD Š/3 186 sub c-3'; Schuster-Brandis 2008, 449 *passim*; Thavapalan 2020, 158). Male *šû*-'stone' is attested in amulet prescriptions to protect women from miscarriage, see e.g. LKA 9 rev. r. col. 14'; SpTU 3, No. 84 rev. 6 (and dupl., see *infra* texts C.3.4 and C.3.5); K. 4727+ and duplicates (text F.1).

Line 4: Following Abusch et al. (2020, CMAwR, 72 note 4), ^{na4}*iz-bi-tú* is understood as an error for ^{na4}*zi-bi-tú*, a stone frequently attested in amulet texts. Differently, Scurlock (2014a, 684; 2014b, 122), reading *iṣbitu*-stone (from *ṣabātu* "to seize"); Couto-Ferreira 2013, 102 fn. 18: *isbitu*(?); Hecker 2008, *TUAT NF* 4, 107: ^{na4}GIŠ.BI BABBAR. None of these readings are otherwise attested. The word *sāmūtu* "(something) red" is noted by Stol (2020b, *BiOr* 77, 569) as a neologism. One would expect "on a red thread/yarn" or similar.

Line 6: For *tanamdissu* "you give her" (*nš* > *ss*), see von Soden 1995, GAG § 30i.

Line 7: The translation of *tušqallalšu* follows Abusch et al. (2020, CMAwR 3, 68, 72), who understand the pronominal suffix -*šu* as referring to the patient and assume a causative meaning of *šuqallulu* here ("you have her suspend (it from a wall)". The text does not specify the object that is to be hung up on a wall in the patient's house, but most likely it was the leather bag that was filled with the patient's hair rather than the bread, meat and grain that was set up at the patient's head the night before and is taken to the crossroads in line 8 (cf. Scurlock 2002, 217; Couto-Ferreira 2013, 102).

Lines 8–9: For this recitation, see Abusch et al 2020, CMAwR 3, 66. As discussed there, the term *nabû* "named" (ones) refers to the warlock and witch, whereas "the unnamed" are "the unsuspecting people (or animals) that will eat the foodstuffs and thus acquire the woman's inability to give birth to a living child."

In line 8, the form *ittannūnu* stands for *ittadnūni* "they have given (it) to me".

Line 9: For the irregular form *indaḫarū'inni* and the variant spelling *e-ma-a'* (for *ēma*) indicating a long final vowel, see Abusch et al. 2020, CMAwR 3, 73 n. 9.

Line 11: The form *inandi* stands for *inaddi* (for the dissimilation /dd/ > /nd/, von Soden GAG, § 32b). The expression *lēssu ana kutallīšu ul inandi* literally means "she does not cast her cheek backwards" (i.e., should not look back); cf. also BAM 248 rev. iii 45 (text D.1.1).

Lines 12–18: For similar purification rites at the river in which the patient descends into the river and *directs* water upstream and downstream as a symbolic action, with similar incantations addressed to the divine river, see e.g., Maul 1994, 85–89, 140–141 lines 136–147, 288–289 rev. 1–17; 360–361: 68–79; 405–406: 36–45; Abusch and Schwemer 2016, CMAwR 2, text 11.3 line 23. The expression *mê ana muqqalpītu šalāšīšu ibbak* "she brings/sends water downstream three times" is translated by Scurlock 2014b, 122: "she draws water three times in a downstream direction". The use of the verb *abāku* "to bring" is described as an indicator of the late date of the text by Stol (2020b, *BiOr* 77, 569). The word *muqqalpītu* "downstream" is replaced by *qiddatu* in the incantation in line 15.

Line 13: The form *ešrētu* is a Late Babylonian spelling for the 2nd person sg. fem. stative form *ešrēti* "you are just", see also Abusch et al. 2020, CMAwR 3, 72 n. 13, 16; cf. Scurlock (2014a, 688, 2014b, 122) translating differently "you flow in a straight line". The use of the pronominal suffix -*ka* instead of -*ki* with reference to the (feminine) river resembles the use of the masculine suffix -*šú* instead of feminine -*šá* (in reference to the patient) elsewhere in this text (e.g. line 10). Note also the masculine imperative form *tabal* in line 15.

Line 15: The form *li-ṭe-(e)-pi* in lines 15 and 57 has been derived from *ṭepû* "to attach, add" (e.g., Scurlock 2014a, 688; Scurlock 2014b, 122) or from an otherwise unknown verb *ṭêpu* (CAD Ṭ, s.v. *ṭêpu*). Abusch et al. (2020, CMAwR 3, 73 n. 15) suggest a connection to the verb *d/ṭâpu* attested in lexical texts an equivalent of Sumerian dun_5 "to churn" (CAD D, 106; cf. AHw 167 s.v. *dêpu* "stossen"), and regard *agammu* "marshland" as the subject of the precative *liṭēp*(*i*) (with an overhanging vowel). SAD Vol. 2, 115 s.v. *ṭebû* interpret the form *li-ṭe-(e)-pi* as a by-form of *ṭebû*/*ṭepû* "to sink" and quote our passage under the Dt-stem. They translate: "may the rivers become full, may the swamp become submerged (*liṭēpi*)"; their reading is followed here.

Like earlier editors, SAD Vol. 2, 115 read the sequence as *mû*(A) *ṭa-ab/p-a-ta* "(may) the water in which you have emerged yourself (remove the bond of evil)" and list the form *ṭab/p'āta* under *ṭebû/ṭepû* "to sink, submerge". Abusch et al. (2020, CMAwR 3, text 5.5 and 73 n. 15) interpret the sequence *a-da-ap-a-ta* as a spelling of *atappāti* "channels" (also *adappu* in first millennium BCE texts), a reading which is followed here. Abusch et al. assume a differing syntactical structure in lines 15–16: for them *agammu* "marshland" functions as object of the first sentence ("may the rivers fill the marshland") and simultaneously as subject of the second verb. Analogously, *atappāti* "channels" is seen as object of *liṭēpi* and simultaneously as subject of the following precative *lišēṣâ*. The environmental imagery evokes the idea of a "smooth and unhindered progress of the water" (from the rivers into the marshes forming smaller canals), which in their view may allude to the journey of the baby in the womb, but which is equally linked with the idea of the water as an unstoppable carrier for transporting off the patient's impurity.

Lines 17–18: For this common formula, see already Lambert 1962, *JCS* 16, 72–73; Lambert 1970, *AfO* 23, 41: 16–18, 34–36.

Lines 20–25: For another incantation presumably addressed to *uḫūlu* "soapwort-plant", cf. Abusch and Schwemer 2016, CMAwR 2, text 7.20.

Line 20: The form *i-ri-ka* is interpreted as a G-stem form of *erû* "to be(come) pregnant", which here appears in the meaning "to engender" (Abusch et al. 2020, CMAwR 3, 73 n. 20), similar to (*w*)*alādu* "to give birth" and "to engender". The verb expected here would have been *reḫû* "to beget, to inseminate", in analogy with the following *urabbīka* "he has made you grow" (from *rabû* D-stem "to bring up, to rear (children)", see CAD R, 48a sub b).

Line 21: For the improved reading and interpretation of this line, see Abusch et al. (2020, CMAwR 3, text 5.5, with 73 n. 21 and collations on pl. 62), which is adopted here.

Lines 24–25: The reading of this passage follows Abusch et al. (2020, CMAwR 3, text 5.5, with 73–74 nn. 24–25 for discussion. For the expression *lū endetūnu igār* in line 25, see also Stol 2020b, *BiOr* 77, 569.

Line 26: For the association of a woman's womb with an oven, see also Scurlock 2002, 219; Couto-Ferreira 2013; Steinert 2017a, 320–322. For lines 26–32 and for metaphors of birth and reproduction in connection with the glassmaking kiln, see also Thavapalan 2021, *JCS* 73, 166–169.

Lines 27–28: For the improved reading of the beginning of line 28 IZI MURUB$_4$ as *išāt qabli* "the fire of battle", see Abusch et al. 2020, CMAwR 3, text 5.5 with 74 note 27–28 and collations on pl. 62.

Line 30: For *šalmānūtu* as a neologism for *šalmūtu* "health, well-being", see Stol 2020b, *BiOr* 77, 569. The form *binnim-ma* "give (fem.) me!" (from *bīn* or *binna* "give!") is a witness to the late date of the text, cf. AHw 126b; CAD B, 216–217.

Line 31: For the reading ⸢*šal*⸣-*mu*, see Abusch et al. 2020, CMAwR 3, text 5.5, with collations on pl. 62.

Line 32: For the reading ⸢*ne*⸣-*mel-šú*, see Abusch et al. 2020, CMAwR 3, text 5.5, with collations on pl. 62. For *pānū* + *maḫāru*, "to be acceptable, pleasing", cf. CAD M/1 64–65 sub 4b-2'. Abusch et al. translate "may my wish be granted".

Line 35–36: For revised reading of this passage, which is followed here, see Abusch et al. 2020, text 5.5, 74 n. 35–36 and collation on pl. 62. Note the unusual switch from a first- to a third-person perspective in line 36. The form *a-a-mu-ut* is understood as a vetitive in the third person (*ay imūt*), with *lā'ī* "my baby" as subject. The phrase *tēnû itâri* "a replacement may return" is seen as a reference to the unborn baby, which is to replace a stillborn baby of the patient's previous pregnancy. The spelling of *itâr* with an overhanging vowel is a recurring feature of middle weak verbs in Neo- and Late Babylonian texts, see von Soden 1995, GAG §104g. See also line 15 (for a similar spelling of the verb *ṭêpu*). For *ḫaṣānu* "to embrace", see AHw 331b "in den Arm nehmen".

Lines 37–38: For the motif, see CAD U/W 186b s.v. *uppulu*; von Weiher 1988, SpTU 5, 64. The emendation [*na*]*p-ṣu* <*in*>-*bi* follows Abusch et al. 2020, text 5.5 with pl. 62 (collation).

Lines 39–40: See also *Maqlû* VII 121–122 (Abusch 2016, 185, 265, 357); Abusch and Schwemer 2016, CMAwR 2, text 8.21: 40‴–47‴. Abusch et al. 2020, text 5.5, with 74 note 40 understand the writing *mu-ḫur mu-ḫur-an-ni-ma* as standing for *muḫrī muḫranni-ma* "accept (my) prayer from me", with a G-stem imperative form of *maḫāru*. Note, however, that *muḫru* is usually constructed with a D-stem of *maḫāru* (CAD M/1, 67 s.v. *maḫāru* sub 7a; CAD M/2 177 s.v. *muḫru*).

Lines 41–52: Since the preceding text sections do not refer to the recitation of this prayer to the sun god, its function and placement within the ritual proceedings is uncertain. According to Scurlock (2002, 215 with fn. 37), the prayer was recited at sunset, in connection with shaving the patient and the preparation of the leather bag containing her hair (lines 2–3). Couto-Ferrreira (2013, 111) suggests the prayer was recited "in conjunction with the sunrise" and invoked Šamaš "in his role as judge". Abusch et al. (2020, 64, 74) believe the prayer was recited by the exorcist "early in the morning", at the secluded place in a blocked road where he takes the woman (lines 7–8) and leaves the foodstuffs that have absorbed the patient's contamination by having spent the night in her presence. Their proposition is adopted here.

Line 42: The reading at the end of the line follows Abusch et al. 2020, CMAwR 3, text 5.5 with collations on pl. 62.

Line 43: See Abusch et al. 2020, 75 note on line 43. The spellings *ḫe-bi-il*$_5$ and *ḫe-bil-ti* are assumed to be variant spellings of *ḫābilu* and *ḫābiltu* "man / woman who have done wrong"; *mu-šal-in-d[u]* is understood as *mušallimtu* "a woman who brings to term, delivers soundly". See also line 30 for the verb *šullumu* in the meaning "to bring to term". The spelling *ub-be-ak-ka* is also found in line 54 (for a 3rd sg. durative form of *bu''û*).

Line 44: For the reading *qú-lum* see the collations in Abusch et al. 2020, pl. 62.

Lines 46–47: The forms *kimissu* (instead of *kimassu* or *kimtašu*) and *še-er-šu* instead of *šerra/īšu* are irregular and a sign of the late date of the text. For the reading of line 47, see Abusch et al. 2020, text 5.5 with collations on pl. 63.

Line 48: For the emendation, see already von Weiher SpTU 5; Abusch et al. 2020, pl. 63. Scurlock (2014a, 686) restores ^{munus}*sin-[niš-tu la mu-šal-lim-tum]* at the end of the line, but as Abusch et al. (2020, 75) note, an additional verb is required here.

Line 49: For this line, see Abusch et al. 2020, 67, 75 and collations on pl. 63.

Lines 50–51: See Abusch et al. 2020, text 5.5 with collations on pl. 63.

Lines 53–61: As with the preceding prayer to Šamaš (lines 41–52), this prayer to Ea is not mentioned in the ritual instructions of the preceding text, and its placement in the ritual proceedings is not certain. Abusch et al. (2020, 64) propose the prayer was recited by the exorcist at the river, introducing the patient to Ea as the god of the subterranean waters as well as healing and magic. The imagery of the Apsû and the purifying river waters in the recitation fit well with this placement. After the prayer to Ea, the patient would have descended into the river, directing water downstream, while the exorcist spoke the prayer to the divine River.

Lines 53–54: For the new readings, see Abusch et al. 2020, pl. 63. The restoration of line 54 follows Scurlock 2014a, 686.

Line 56, 60: The text uses a variant form *puṭru* instead of correct *puṭur* for the masc. sg. imperative.

Lines 56–58: For the parallel passage in lines 15–16, see the discussion in the note above. The verb *liššâ* "may (the rivers) carry (their waters)" instead of *limlâ* "may (the rivers) fill" in line 15 appears to be a mistake. The translation follows Abusch et al. 2020, text 5.5.

Lines 60–61: For the spelling *zu-mur-ri-šú* see Abusch et al. 2020, 75 note on line 60. For *lurabbi* and *lurappiš* as Late Babylonian third person precatives, cf. Schwemer 2017, 77.

Line 64: The emendation follows the unpublished parallel A 492 obv. 6'. For the healing goddesses Gula and Ninkarrak, their associations with childbirth and midwifery and their close association, see now Sibbing-Plantholt 2022, 27–205, esp. 103–104, and 106–123. Note also that the title of the treatise PREGNANCY/OFFSPRING in the Assur Medical Catalogue (lines 109–114; Steinert et al. 2018, 217–218, 269–270) is "If a man is handed over to Ninkarrak" (*šumma amēlu ana Ninkarrak paqid*). This underlines the relations of the rituals in SpTU 5, No. 248 to the treatise PREGNANCY. Notably, Ninkarrak was also a deity associated with oath/ban (*māmītu*), and the infant deaths and miscarriages dealt with in the present text(s) belonging to the treatise PREGNANCY may have been attributed to divine punishment by Ninkarrak triggered a broken oath (see further Sibbing-Plantholt 2022, 110–114).

Line 70: Ms. c now allows to emend the slightly corrupt text of ms. a, and to improve previous readings. Instead of von Weiher's (1998, 62) reading *ana* IGI *nis-ḫi lis-si-ma*: "soll sie vor dem auserwählten rufen" (similarly Böck 2013, 49; cf. Scurlock 2014a, 687), the text of ms. c reads *ana* IGI ^{d}UTU DÙG.GAM-*si-ma* "you let (a pregnant ewe) crouch down before Šamaš", with a Š-stem of *kamāsu* "to kneel" followed by the feminine pronominal suffix (*tušakmassi*). Thus, following *ana* IGI ᵈUTU in ms. c, we can emend ms. a to *ana* IGI ‹ᵈ›20. The restoration 2 G[URU]Š.MEŠ *i-na-áš-šu* follows Scurlock (2014a, 687).

Lines 73–74: In the parallel sequence of the rite with the pregnant jenny in Ritual 3 (lines 85–87), the verb *ḫalāpu* "to slip through" is used instead of *aṣû* "to come out" found here, in the rite with the pregnant ewe. In line 74, ms. c allows us to restore the text of ms. a as *ana* [UG]U IGI.MEŠ-*šú* NIGIN "she turns her face towards (the ewe)" (*ana muḫḫi pānīšu isaḫḫar*). For *pānī saḫāru* "to turn the face towards someone", cf. the expression *pānīšu ana ṣērīya išḫuram-ma* "(as soon as) he directed his attention towards me" (ARM 2, 129: 21, quoted in CAD S, 41 sub 2a-2').

Lines 75–77: The new readings in these lines follow Abusch et al. 2020, text 5.5 with collations on pl. 63. One is tempted to restore at the beginning of line 75 *ana* MUNUS NU SI.SÁ SI.SÁ DÙ.DÙ.BI, following the beginning of Ritual 2 in line 62, but the traces in line 75 (ms. a rev. 26) are not unambiguous. Ms. c is fragmentary but begins with the phrase *ana* MUNUS Ù.TU "to enable a woman to give birth/bear (successfully)".

Line 80: As collations by Abusch et al. 2020 (CMAwR 3), pl. 63 show, the sign sequence is to be read a te a tú rather than a kar tú, see also the discussion ibid., 75 note on 2, line 6. Scurlock (2014a, 687) reads *a-qar-tú* TA ᵍⁱˢEREN and translates "jewellery(?) (made) from cedar". Although it is possible to emend the text to *a-qár*!*-tú* (for *uqurtu* "precious object, jewel", cf. CAD U/W, 204 sub a), such a spelling as well as the following TA (for *ultu* "from", "out of") instead of the genitive particle *šá* are highly unusual.

Scurlock (2002, 221) suggests that the killed female mouse wrapped in combed wool plays the role of a "foetus surrogate", representing the miscarried foetuses of the patient (because the mouse is treated in the same manner as a newborn who is swaddled).

Line 83: The phrase *annâ u annâ* (lit. "this and this") refers to the two rites (placing foodstuffs and a dead mouse at a crossroads) described in the preceding paragraphs (lines 75–82). The woman had to repeat them several times. For the expression *ina lapāt šamê* "at the touching of the sky" (i.e. at dawn), cf. CAD Š/1, 346 sub 5'; BE 17, 47: 14: *ina šamê lapāti*.

Line 87: The verb *ú-šá-áš-šá* (*našû* Š, lit. "she *lets* the jenny *pick up* the barley") is unusual (*ušakkal* "she feeds" would be expected, as in line 86).

Line 88: The two signs at the beginning of the line, ZÁLAG and BAR, are problematic. Abusch et al. (2020, text 5.5,2 line 14) suggest reading *ṣab-bar*, which they understand as a term for an item made of grain seeds or whole plants of *šeguššu*-cereal (millet), perhaps a plaited sheaf. A word *ṣabbaru* is presently unknown, but may be derived from *ṣabāru* "to bend, to twist, to spin" (see ibid., 75–75 for discussion). Stol (2020b, *BiOr* 77, 570) proposes a different reading of the signs as 2 (GUR) (or?) 2 (PI) 1 (BÁN). He notes the possible relevance of uses of millet against spirits of the dead and witchcraft in other texts and notes that one *sūtu* (BÁN) was the amount of a normal daily ration of grain. For *šeguššu* as a variety of proso millet, see Stol 1993–1997a, "Mohrhirse", *RlA* 8, 348–349; Dornauer 2018, 29, 87.

The reading ⌜EN⌝ ⌜Ù.TU-*di*⌝ follows collations by Abusch et al. (2020, pl. 63).

Line 89: Following Abusch et al. 2020, 76 (note on line 15), the form *i-la-aš-šu-uš-ma* instead of *ilâš-ma* is interpreted as an irregular form of *lâšu* with "overhanging vowel" (*ilaššu*), the final *-š* is interpreted as the suffixed pronoun *-šu*. Stol (2020b, *BiOr* 77, 569) assumes a verb *lašāsu* as a variant of *lâšu*. The male and female puppets formed here from a mixture of amniotic fluid and flour are regarded by Abusch et al. (2020, 65) as representations of warlock and witch (and their evil influence) which seems to fit the disposal of these figurines (they are thrown into the street). Stol (2020b, *BiOr* 77, 569) thinks the figurines represent the expected babies.

Line 90: Abusch et al. 2020, 76 (note on line 16) render the phrase *adi mišil mūši* as "just before midnight" instead of "until midnight", to fit *erēbu* "to enter" as a verb for a punctual action.

Line 91: The reading [ᵐᵈAN.Š]ÁR–ZÚ–KÉŠ for Anu-ikṣur follows Abusch et al. 2020, text 5.5 and pl. 63. For the colophon, see also Jiménez 2016b, *Babel und Bibel* 9, 237–239.

Line 93: ŠA.ÁB.BA$_4$.ALLA is an unusual orthography for ŠÀ.BAL.BAL (*liblibbi*) "offspring". The verbal form *u-*⌜*ša*⌝*-am-àš* in the expression *ina mērešti lā u-*⌜*ša*⌝*-am-àš* in ms. a appears to be a is a variant of the more common *umšamki/aš(šu)* "May he not withhold it (the tablet) intentionally!" (Š-stem of *makû* "to be lacking"), see Jiménez 2016, 228–235 for discussion.

For the spelling *i*$_{11}$(ḪI)-*ta*$_{8}$(ŠÁR)-*áb-bà-alla* in this colophon, see Jiménez 2016b, 234. Another colophon by Anu-ikṣur is preserved in SpTU 1, No. 59, a tablet with prescriptions for women identified as part of the therapeutic series *Šumma amēlu muḫḫašu umma ukâl*, see text C.2.1.

C.4 Embryology

C.4.1 BM 37014: Calculating the Growth of the Foetus

Theoretical discussions about human embryological development are absent from the cuneiform medical sources as are theoretical treatises in general.[331] Several omens in the teratological omen series *Šumma izbu* (Tablet 1) envisage a woman giving birth to a variety of material forms and objects including foetuses resembling animals or having strange features (de Zorzi 2014, 344–360). Some of these phenomena may relate to observed miscarriages in different stages of pregnancy and foetal formation. However, the omens are not concerned with portraying foetal development in a systematic manner but with interpreting the ominous significance of abnormal births and miscarriages.[332] Babylonian scholars nonetheless took a theoretical interest in describing the development of the foetus in utero. This is shown by a section in a Late Babylonian mathematical text from Uruk (SpTU 4, No. 173 ii 2–9 = ms. b), a tablet that belonged to the library of the descendants of Šangû-Ninurta (Clancier 2009a, 397). The significance of this passage was recognized and discussed by Hunger (1994), who later identified another parallel in SpTU 2, No. 43: 13–17 (Hunger 1996), a text (otherwise of astrological content) written by the scholar Iqīšâ of the Ekur-zakir family.[333]

The present discussion adds a second manuscript for the calculation scheme of the growth of the foetus found in SpTU 4, No. 173, which is preserved on a small fragment of a Late Babylonian cuneiform tablet presumably found at Babylon (BM 37014, ms. a).[334] Although the right half of ms. a is lost, it seems to run parallel to the fully preserved ms. b. Thus it can be surmised that both texts present the same scheme giving the size of the foetus in the first ten days of gestation, continuing with one month and ten months (after which birth is to take place). The contents of the text sections of ms. a that preceded and followed this calculation cannot be determined yet, but they could have been mathematical as well.

List of Manuscripts

Siglum	Museum Number	Copy	Collation	Format; Ductus	Provenience
a	BM 37014 (80-6-17, 758)[335]	Pl. 34	Coll.	fragment of a single-column(?) tablet; Late Babylonian script, ca. 4th/3rd cent. BCE	Babylon?
b	W. 23281	SpTU 4, No. 173	–	two-column tablet; Late Babylonian script; 5th/4th cent. BCE	Uruk; library of the descendants of Šangû-Ninurta

331 For an overview of Mesopotamian views on the subject and brief discussion of other, more detailed ancient traditions concerning embryology, see Stol 2000, 9–26; 2009b; Couto-Ferreira 2015–2016.

332 For the *kūbu*, the numinous or deified foetus of human shape, see Stol 2000, 29–32.

333 This source varies from mss. a and b presented here, describing the multiplications for computing the size of the foetus after one month and after ten months of gestation.

334 I owe knowledge of the fragment to Christopher Walker (personal communication). Leichty, Finkel and Walker 2019, *CBT* IV–V, 346, still classify the fragment as either medical or astrological (horoscope). The fragment comes from the excavations of Hormuzd Rassam. The register of the British Museum's Babylonian collection gives Babylon as the provenience of the 80-6-17 collection.

335 Measurements: 3.4 cm x 3.1 cm 2.2 cm.

Overview

i′	Fragmentary a obv. 1′	...]1′
ii′	Mathematical schema for the growth of the foetus a obv. 2′–rev. 6′ // b obv. ii 2–9	2′–13′
iii′	Fragmentary a rev. 7′	14′[...

Previous Edition and Discussion

Lambert, *Notebooks*, Folio 9315 (transliteration of ms. a)
Hunger 1994, *NABU* 1994/2, 32 No. 34 (ms. b)
Hunger 1996, *NABU* 1996/2, 35 No. 39 (discussion)
Stol 2000a, 12
Stol 2009b, 143–144 (discussion)
Electronic Babylonian Library (eBL) (transliteration; https://www.ebl.lmu.de/library/BM.37014)

Transliteration

Beginning of ms. a obv. lost

1′	a obv. 1′	⸢10⸣ ⸢GI.MEŠ$^{?}$⸣(blank)[.........]

a, b ____

2′	a obv. 2′	LÚ.TUR *u_4-mu šá ina* ŠÀ AM[A-*šú* ....]
	b obv. ii 2	LÚ.TUR *u_4-mu šá ina* ŠÀ AMA$^{!}$-*šú* DÙ-*ú* 1/2 ŠE *šú-ú*
3′	a obv. 3′	*i-na šá-ni-i u_4-m[u* ....]
	b obv. ii 3	*i-na* 2-*i u_4-mu* ŠE *šú-ú*
4′	a obv. 4′	*i-na šal-šú* ⸢*u_4*⸣-[*mu* ....]
	b obv. ii 4	*i-na šal-šú u_4-mu* ŠE 1/2 ŠE *šú-ú*
5′	a obv. 5′	*i-na* 4-⸢*i*⸣ [*u_4-mu* ....]
	b obv. ii 4$^{cont.}$	*i-na* 4-*i u_4-mu* 2 ŠE *šú-ú*
6′	a obv. 6′	*ina* ⸢5⸣-[*šú u_4-mu* ....]
	b obv. ii 5	*ina* 5-*šú u_4-mu* 2 1/2 ŠE *šú-ú*
7′	a obv. 7′	*ina* [6-*šú u_4-mu* ....]
	b obv. ii 5$^{cont.}$	*ina* 6$^{!}$-*šú u_4-mu* 3 ŠE *šú-ú*
8′	a rev. 1′	*i-na* 7-⸢*i*⸣ [*u_4-mu* ....]
	b obv. ii 6	*i-na* 7-*i u_4-mu* 3 1/2 ŠE *šú-ú*
9′	a rev. 2′	*i-na* 8-*i* [*u_4-mu* ....]
	b obv. ii 6$^{cont.}$	*i-na* 8-*i u_4-mu* 4 ŠE *šú-ú*
10′	a rev. 3′	*i-na* 9-*i u_4-mu* [...............]
	b obv. ii 7	*i-na* 9-*i u_4-mu* 4 1/2 ŠE *šú-ú*

11′	a rev. 4′	*i-na* 10-*i* *u*$_4$*-mu* [..........]
	b obv. ii $7^{\text{cont.}}$	*i-na* 10-*i* *u*$_4$*-mu* 5 ŠE *šú-ú* <<*šú-ú*>>
12′	a rev. 5′	*ina* ITI U$_4$.MEŠ [.............]
	b obv. ii 8	*ina* ITI U$_4$.MEŠ 3 ŠU.SI *šú-ú*
13′	a rev. 6′	[*ina*] 10-*i* ITI.[MEŠ 1 KÙŠ *šú-ú*]
	b obv. ii 9	*ina* 10-*i* ITI.MEŠ 1 KÙŠ *šú-ú*

a, b ____

14′	a rev. 7′	[x x] ⌜x x x⌝ [......................]

Ms. a rev. breaks; remainder lost

Bound Transcription and Translation

Beginning of ms. a obv. lost

1′ 10(?) *qanû* [... ...]	1′ ten(?) reeds [... ...].
2′ *ṣeḫru ūmu ša ina libbi ummīšu banû mišil uṭṭat šū*	2′ An (unborn) child – on the day it is created in his mother's womb – he is half a barleycorn (long).
3′ *ina šanî ūmu uṭṭat šū*	3′ On the second day, he is one barleycorn (long).
4′ *ina šalšu ūmu uṭṭat mišil uṭṭat šū*	4′ On the third day, he is one and a half barleycorns (long).
5′ *ina rebî ūmu šina uṭṭat šū*	5′ On the fourth day, he is two barleycorns (long).
6′ *ina ḫamšu ūmu šina uṭṭat mišil uṭṭat šū*	6′ On the fifth day, he is two and a half barleycorns (long).
7′ *ina šeššu ūmu šalaš uṭṭat šū*	7′ On the sixth day, he is three barleycorns (long).
8′ *ina sebî ūmu šalaš mišil uṭṭat šū*	8′ On the seventh day, he is three and a half barleycorns (long).
9′ *ina samānî ūmu erbe uṭṭat šū*	9′ On the eighth day, he is four barleycorns (long).
10′ *ina tešî ūmu erbe mišil uṭṭat šū*	10′ On the ninth day, he is four and a half barleycorns (long).
11′ *ina ešrî ūmu ḫamiš uṭṭat šū*	11′ On the tenth day, he is five barleycorns (long).
12′ *ina arḫi ūmī šalaš ubān šū*	12′ When one month's days (30 days) (are over), he is three fingers' breadth (long).
13′ *ina ešeret arḫī ištēn ammat šū*	13′ When ten months (are over and the baby is born), he is one cubit (long).
14′ *traces*	14′ *too fragmentary for translation*

Ms. a rev. breaks; remainder lost

Notes

Line 1′: The measure of length *qanû* (GI) "reed" stands for six cubits (3 m). In Neo- and Late Babylonian times it equals 7 cubits (3.5 m), Powell 1987–1990, *RlA* 7, 463 § I.2.g, 470, 471 § I.4.i. The lost section preceding lines 2′ff. may thus have been mathematical as well. The first sign U could be read as the number 10 or as *u* "and", which would indicate the continuation of a sentence from the preceding, lost line. Note here, specifically, a group of Late Babylonian metro-mathematical texts referred to as "seed and reeds", from the subscript ŠE.NUMUN *u* GI.MEŠ preserved in a colophon of one of these texts (Friberg, Hunger and al-Rawi 1990, *BaM* 21, 545, 556–557 W 23291-x, rev. iv colophon; also ibid. 542 BE 20/1 no. 30 subscript to col. iii). As the authors of that study explain, the subscript "characterizes the text as one that teaches the proper use of *seed measure* and *reed measure.* 'Seed measure' and 'reed measure' are convenient names for the two complementary methods for surface mensuration which replace the traditional *area measure* in Mesopotamia in the 1st millennium. Reed measure was used for house plots ..., seed measure for more substantial pieces of land" (ibid., 484).

Line 2′–13′: The parallel passage to line 2′ in SpTU 2, No. 43: 13 spells out 1/2 ŠE as [*mi*]-*šil uṭ-ṭa-at* (in the absolute state). In the Late Babylonian sources discussed here, the unit of length *uṭṭatu* (ŠE) "grain, barleycorn" equals 1/5 of a "finger(breadth)" (*ubānu*, ŠU.SI, one "finger" = 1.66 cm), while in a text from Assur representing an earlier tradition, one ŠE equals 1/6 of a "finger" (CAD U/W, 356–357 s.v. *uṭṭatu* sub 3b; Powell 1987–1990, *RlA* 7, 458–459). In turn, thirty "fingers" (or 150 "barleycorns") equals one cubit (50 cm), which is the size of the baby after ten months of gestation. The parallel text SpTU 2, No. 43: 17 adds that "upon this (the baby) will be born" (*i-na muḫ-ḫi im-mal-lad*).

Chapter D
Birth and the Postpartum Period

The texts edited in the present section deal specifically with problems arising around delivery and during the postpartum period, i.e. the first weeks after the delivery of a baby. The section is divided into healing texts with treatments to ease or speed up difficult or obstructed labour (section D.1), one text focusing on postpartum conditions (section D.2) and one text with rituals to prolong pregnancy and to delay or postpone a delivery that was due during an inauspicious month of the Babylonian calendar (section D.3).

The first millennium BCE texts edited in section D.1 consist of sources in Neo-Assyrian script stemming from Assur and from Ashurbanipal's library at Nineveh, as well as an equal number of sources in Neo-Babylonian and Late Babylonian script from Nineveh and Babylonia. Several of the text manuscripts in section D belonged to multi-column collective tablets that may have been part of a larger thematic medical treatise on women's health, while other sources (e.g. D.1.8, D.1.9) bear only one specific composition (usually a birth incantation). There are hints to such thematic treatises on women's health focussing on birth and the postpartum period from the Assur Medical Catalogue (AMC), which lists the incipits of a thematic treatise (dubbed BIRTH) that consisted of eight tablets, and whose first three tablets bear relations to passages in the texts edited in section D.1 (see Steinert et al. 2018, 218, 272–275 notes on lines 115–117). The most important sources for a magico-medical compendium on the topic of difficult birth comparable to tablets listed in the section BIRTH in the AMC belong to the so-called "Neo-Assyrian Birth Compendium" (BAM 248 and duplicates, edited as text D.1.1) attested in duplicating sources from Assur, Nineveh and Babylonia, a collection of texts (incantations and medical/ritual treatments) to speed up difficult labour. Some of the incantations and treatments in the "Neo-Assyrian Birth Compendium" go back to the second millennium BCE, as textual precursors from the Old Babylonian and Middle Babylonian/Assyrian period confirm (see *infra* for discussion).

Mesopotamian healers did not perform the role of a male birth helper (accoucheur) who was manually involved in the delivery process. However, they applied some treatments to support the woman in labour, e.g. through massages, ointments and through medicaments that induced contractions of the uterus. Many of the treatments consist in a combination of magico-medical procedures. Some of the texts (especially D.1.5–D.1.6 and D.1.11) also contain references to the involvement of a midwife during the delivery side by side with the male healer. These texts describe the midwife as having intimate knowledge of and direct access to the female body: she surveyed the progress of labour and intervened in the birth process through manual actions (e.g. reaching for the child stuck in the birth canal; cutting the umbilical cord, taking care for the newborn). The divine patrons of midwifery, especially various mother- and birth-goddesses, play a role in several of the incantations within texts edited in the present section (D.1.1, D.1.1, D.1.5, D.1.9)

Section D.2 presents merely one Neo-Assyrian tablet from Assur (BAM 240) that includes prescriptions for postpartum complaints (including childbed fever), some of which have precursors in a Middle Assyrian tablet (see text II.1.4) and parallels in first millennium BCE compendia from Babylonia (see section A in this volume).

Section D.3 deals with a group of texts with two rituals to delay the inauspicious birth of a child due for the first month of the Babylonian calendar (Nisannu) through divine intervention. These rituals are now attested in six duplicating millennium BCE manuscripts from Babylonia and Assyria.

D.1 Texts Concerned with Delivery

D.1.1 A Neo-Assyrian Compendium for a Woman Having a Difficult Delivery

This text referred to here as the "Neo-Assyrian Birth Compendium" has been edited and discussed repeatedly as a crucial source for the continuities of textual traditions and processes of long-term transmission of Sumerian and Akkadian birth incantations from earlier periods to the first millennium BCE. The name "Neo-Assyrian Birth Compendium" has been chosen in line with the date and provenience of the main manuscripts (ms. A from Assur and B_{1-5} from Nineveh), which form two-column tablets that contained ca. 250 lines of text. This format is well-known from tablets belonging to the therapeutic series *šumma amēlu muḫḫašu umma ukâl* and other medical treatises preserved in numerous tablets and fragments found at Nineveh and other sites in Assyria and Babylonia. Neither of the main manuscripts of the Birth Compendium can

https://doi.org/10.1515/9781501506475-007

be firmly attributed to the treatise BIRTH in the Assur Medical Catalogue (AMC) through a matching incipit (see note on line 1). Only ms. A from Assur preserves a catchline which, however, does not match any of the tablet incipits of the section BIRTH in the AMC (see note on line 236 below). However, two incipits of the eight tablets of BIRTH listed in the AMC recur in certain text lines and phrases within the manuscripts of the Birth Compendium or in texts with related content (see Steinert et al. 2018, 218, 272–274 on lines 115 and 117; note especially ms. A rev. iv 13 // B_1 rev. iv 6 // H i' 8' (line 205); ms. I (AMT 66/4) rev. i' 3ff.; ms. G (K. 11956 +) lines 1ff.; ms. d (BM 38624+) obv. ii 25ff.; K. 1930 + 11752: 12'; see also *infra* D.1.4, D.1.2, A.2.1, D.1.7 for these texts).

Many of the incantations in the Birth Compendium bear a rubric (KA.INIM.MA ^{munus}LA.RA.AḪ.A.KAM "wording (of a spell) for a woman in difficult labour") that is also found among other incantation genres concerned with women and babies in the Exorcist's Manual (KAR 44: 15 and dupl.; Geller 2018a, 298; Heeßel 2023, 294): namely spells to "bind a pregnant woman" (^{munus}PEŠ$_4$.KÉŠ.DA), spells against Lamaštu and spells to calm an infant (LÚ.TUR.ḪUN.GÁ), genres relating to textual materials presented in chapter C.3 of the present book. Thus, as their inclusion in the Exorcist's Manual shows, the genre of birth incantations identified as ^{munus}LA.RA.AḪ-incantations bears strong connections to the professional text corpus of the *āšipu.* The rubric ^{munus}LA.RA.AḪ, which corresponds to Akkadian *muš(t)apšiqtu* and *šupšuqtu* "woman in difficult labour", is known predominantly from first millennium BCE texts and replaces the rubric KA.INIM.MA MUNUS.Ù.TU.(-)DA.KAM "wording (of an incantation) for a woman in labour" that is current especially in Old Babylonian birth incantations.

The Birth Compendium as known from mss. A and B_{1-5} comprises to a larger part a collection of incantations (from column i to the beginning of column iv) interspersed with therapeutic instructions. The remainder of column iv is a collection of prescriptions to speed up difficult labour, many of which form short recipes using one or only few ingredients. This catalogue of prescriptions is concluded by an appendix of prescriptions to protect the newborn from harm caused by divine or demonic interference. The therapeutic strategies applied in the Birth Compendium focus on potions administered on an empty stomach, on ointments and massages applied to the woman's belly. Beside drugs of herbal and animal origin, the therapeutic/ritual instructions feature several substances and items that attest to analogical reasoning or to "sympathetic magic" alluding directly to the wording or aim of the incantations recited over the remedies.

Several first millennium BCE sources within the group of women's healthcare texts provide parallels to the prescriptions in the Birth Compendium. These parallels are encountered in shorter tablets with extracts of treatments for women in labour (ms. G) and in multi-thematic collections of prescriptions for women (esp. mss. H, I and d). The prophylactic prescriptions for the newborn at the end of the Birth Compendium were integrated from a different context of medical texts concerned with infants, since they also occur in a manuscript of a treatise with treatments for infants affected by epilepsy or seizures (ms. F). Notably, ms. a (presumably from Babylon) presents a fragment of a tablet that preserves extracts of incantations and treatments from the Birth Compendium that run parallel to sections in col. i and iii of ms. A. Thus, ms. a now provides direct evidence showing that the incantations and therapies of the Birth Compendium were also known and transmitted in first millennium BCE Babylonia.

Some of the incantations in the Birth Compendium have been shown to possess close precursors in second millennium BCE birth incantations, being a witness to a "stream of textual tradition" that continued to be developed and modified in the course of transmission. For example, the first very fragmentarily preserved incantation in the Compendium, a Sumerian spell with a partial interlinear Akkadian translation (lines 1–21), contains passages that resemble Old Babylonian birth incantations (see Veldhuis 1989 and notes below). Textual parallels for the Akkadian spells in the Birth Compendium stem predominantly from texts dating to the second half of the second millennium BCE. The second incantation of the Compendium (lines 22–36) bears resemblance to an incantation partially preserved on a fragment from Hattuša (ms. b 15'–21') and to an Old Babylonian Akkadian birth incantation (VS 17, 34; Wasserman and Zomer 2022, No. 12). But the highest number of earlier parallels is known for the famous incantation "A Cow of Sîn" (lines 135–160), see e.g. Röllig 1985; Veldhuis 1991; Marquéz Rowe 2015 for detailed studies), which must have been a very popular composition throughout the ages, since it is attested in several earlier versions preserved on Middle Assyrian/Babylonian sources that stem from Assyria (ms. C and D), as well as from Hattuša and Ugarit in the periphery (mss. b and c). The present edition integrates the earlier second millennium BCE versions of "A Cow of Sîn" beside the first millennium version preserved the Birth Compendium, to give an impression of the considerable textual changes and variations encountered in the different manuscripts beside the overt similarities in the structure and plot of the composition. Overall, the repeated recurrence of the same images and themes in different spells of the Birth Compendium (e.g. the woman in labour as a cow, the woman in labour as a boat travelling down a river, direct addresses to the baby and comparisons with the young of wild animals) shows that it was common to draw on well-established models and formulas in the composition of "new" incantations of the genre (for studies of the imagery of birth incantations, see e.g. Bergmann 2008; Couto-Ferreira 2014; Steinert 2017a).

The deities that play a role in the incantations of the Birth Compendium also reflect some interesting patterns (see also Stol 2000a, 63–72 for discussion). The healing goddess Gula is remarkably absent. The moon god (Nanna(r)/Sîn) is encountered in three incantations: in the first spell (lines 22–36), he intercedes with Enlil on behalf of the woman in labour; in "A Cow of Sîn" (lines 135–160) and a second spell (lines 163–172) the moon god is the main divine agent sending two protective spirits (*lamassu*) or deities who act as intermediaries. The moon god's links to birth are underlined in many other texts (outside the birth incantations) and can be traced back at least to Old Babylonian times (for the roots of this tradition in the ideology of the Ur III kingdom, see Stol 2000a, 68). The sun god Šamaš, acting as a divine birth helper (beside the moon god) already in Old Babylonian texts, makes an appearance in one incantation in the Compendium (lines 48–52), where he commands the mother goddess Bēlet-ilī to deliver the baby.

The god of magic *par excellence* Marduk/Asalluḫi is clearly the most important deity in the spells of the Compendium, while the mother goddess and other birth goddesses (more prominent in earlier texts) play a subordinate limited role. Marduk/Asalluḫi clearly seems to have absorbed traditional roles of the mother/birth goddesses, since he is called or calls himself "(male) midwife" (ŠÀ.ZU, *šabsû*) in at least two incantations (lines 194–195, 198–199). The lengthy Akkadian incantation in lines 56–130 of the Compendium is further witness to this shift. Thus, in the first preserved part of the text, the mother goddess Mami is asked to intercede on behalf of the woman in travail. But her role seems to be only subordinate, since further on in the spell, she appears to inform Marduk of the woman's suffering, beseeching him to have compassion and take action to bring forth the baby. The final lines of the composition again underline the primary authority of Marduk/Asalluḫi and Ea, since the spell is attributed to them, while Mami only "requested" the spell to be performed.

Further noteworthy is the invocation of Elamite deities (Kiririša, Napiriša, Naḫḫunte, Narunde) acting as intermediaries or messengers (of Sîn or Marduk) in two incantations of the Compendium (lines 40–47, 163–172), which seems to be a reflex of an old tradition of birth incantations in the Elamite language (attested on Old Babylonian tablets) which feature the same deities (e.g. YOS 11, 18 // OECT 11, 5; van Dijk 1982, 100; Krebernik 2018, 31). Naḫḫunte and Narunde are also encountered in an incantation in the first millennium BCE exorcistic series Ḫulbazizi (Finkel 1976, 53, 58–59, 108, 187–188 on line 179).

The importance of the Neo-Assyrian Birth Compendium within the medical literature of the first millennium BCE and its role in scholarly learning is also reflected in two Neo-/Late Babylonian manuscripts of commentaries on the Compendium that stem from Nippur and Ur (α: 11N-T3 and β: U. 30654 (= UET 6/3, 897), edited in section G of the volume). Besides giving revealing insights into textual hermeneutics, these commentaries are crucial for improving our reconstruction and knowledge of some damaged or lost passages in mss. A and B_{1-5}. Several passages from the commentaries are also discussed in the notes below, whenever they quote preserved passages from the base text or give information on lost sections of the Birth Compendium.

List of Manuscripts

Siglum	Museum Number	Copy	Collation	Format; Ductus	Provenience
A	VAT 8869	KAR 196 BAM 248	Coll.	Two-column tablet; Neo-Assyrian script; 8th/7th cent. BCE	Assur; library N4[336]
B_1 + B_4 + B_5 (+)	K. 2413 + K. 18482 + K. 16363	AMT 67/1 (only K. 2413)	Coll.	Fragments of a two-column tablet; Neo-Assyrian script; 7th cent. BCE	Nineveh; Ashurbanipal's library
B_3 (+)	K. 3485 + K. 10443 (+)	Geers, Folio J93 Pl. 36	Coll.	Fragment of a two-column tablet; Neo-Assyrian script; 7th cent. BCE	Nineveh; Ashurbanipal's library
B_2 (+)	K. 8210	Pl. 37	Coll.	Fragment of a two-column tablet; Neo-Assyrian script; 7th cent. BCE	Nineveh; Ashurbanipal's library
C	Rm. 376	*AS* 16, 287–288	Coll.	Fragment of a two-column tablet; Middle Assyrian script; ca. 11th cent. BCE	Nimrud

336 Pedersén 1986, 63 No. 146.

(continued)

Siglum	Museum Number	Copy	Collation	Format; Ductus	Provenience
D	–	*Iraq* 31, pl. V–VI	Photo Coll.	single-column tablet; Middle Assyrian script; ca. 12th/11th cent. BCE	Assur(?)
E	VAT 8943	KAR 205 BAM 183	–	single-column tablet, Neo-Assyrian script; 7th cent. BCE	Assur; library N4
F	K. 3628 + K. 4009 + Sm. 1315 + K. 19939	Finkel 1976, pl. 26	–	single-column tablet; Neo-Assyrian script; 7th cent. BCE	Nineveh; Ashurbanipal's library
G	K. 11956 + K. 14200	Pl. 38	Coll.	Fragment of a single-column tablet (excerpt); Neo-Assyrian script; 7th cent. BCE	Nineveh; Ashurbanipal's library
H	VAT 13972	BAM 249	Coll.	Fragment of a two-column tablet; Neo-Assyrian script; 8th/7th cent. BCE	Assur
I	K. 10507	AMT 66/4	Coll.	Fragment of a two- or multi-column tablet; Neo-Assyrian script; 7th cent. BCE	Nineveh
a	BM 36339 (80-6-17, 65)	Pl. 35	Coll.	Fragment of a single-column tablet; Neo-Babylonian script	Babylon
b	Bo 4822	KUB 4, 13	Photo Coll.	Fragment of a single-column tablet; non-Hittite script; ca. 13th cent. BCE	Hattuša
c	RS 25.436	*AuOr Suppl.* 23, pl. 11 (no. 20)	–	Fragment of a single-column tablet; Middle Babylonian script; ca. 13th cent. BCE	Ugarit
d	BM 38624 (80-11-12, 508) + BM 38828 (80-11-12, 713) + BM 45414 (81-7-1, 3175)	Pl. 12–13	Coll.	Fragments of a two-column tablet; Late Babylonian script; ca. 6th/5th cent. BCE	probably Babylon
e	N. 1568	*NABU* 2019, 141	–	Fragment of a tablet; Neo-Babylonian script	Nippur

The Main Sources of the Compendium
Ms. A (BAM 248):
Photo: CDLI P285333

Ms. B_1: K. 2413 + (AMT 67/1):
Photo: CDLI P394413

Ms. B_2: (K. 8210 (+)):
Photo: CDLI P397536

Ms. B_3: (K. 3485 + K. 10443):
Photo: CDLI P395046 (without photo)

Ms. B_4: K. 18482 +
Photo: CDLI P403690

Ms. B_5: K. 16363 +
Photo: CDLI P404833

Mss. $B_{1–5}$: It is not entirely certain whether all five fragments $B_{1–5}$ belong to the same tablet. In 2018, E. Jiménez (*Electronic Babylonian Library* (eBL) *Project*) identified K. 16363 (B_5) as a new fragment that can be joined directly with both K. 2413 (B_1) and K. 18482 (B_5). Inspection of the fragments showed that ms. B_3 (K. 3485 + 10443) does not belong to the same tablet as B_1+B_5+B_4, since the overlapping sections on the top of the reverse do not fit together. Therefore, it is possible that B_2 (K. 8210) as well as B_3 (K. 3485 + 10443) are fragments of at least another two-column tablet duplicating K. 2413(+). Ms. A differs slightly from ms. B_1 in its text alignment (B_2 rev. iii 1 = A rev. iii 7). The textual overlaps of the Nineveh fragments B_1–B_5 with ms. A can briefly be summarized as follows:

- **B_1 + B_4 + B_5** preserve a larger portion of the upper half of the reverse (col. iii and iv), the obverse is completely lost.[337] **B_1 +B_4 + B_5** rev. iii 1–33 // A rev. iii 7–39, **B_1** rev. iv 1–32 // A rev. iv 8–39
- **B_5** allows to join **B_1** and **B_4** directly. B_4 + B_5 preserve part of the first lines of col. iii on the reverse.[338] B_4 + B_5 rev. iii 5 overlaps with the first line preserved on B_1; B_4 + B_5 rev. iii 1–5 // A rev. iii 7–11
- **B_2** is a small fragment of the middle portion of the obverse of a two-column tablet.[339] **B_2** obv. i 1'–14' // A obv. i 28–41; **B_2** obv. ii 1'–13' // A obv. ii 31–43
- **B_3** consists of two joined fragments of the bottom right-hand portion of a two-column tablet; they preserve 14 lines of text of the bottom of col. ii and the ends of the first four lines of col. iii.[340] **B_3** obv. ii 1'–22' // A obv. ii 54–rev. iii 6; **B_3** rev. iii 1–4 // A rev. iii 7–10

Previous Edition and Discussion

Meloni 1911–1912, *Rivista degli Studi Orientali* 4, 560–571 (edition of ms. B_1)
Ebeling 1923, *AGM* 14, 65–78 (edition of ms. A)
Röllig 1985, *OrNS* 54, 260–273 (synoptic edition of mss. A rev. iii 10–35, B_1(+) rev. iii 5–29; C obv. 19–36; D 51–62; b 1'–12')
Farber 1987a, *TUAT* II/2, 274–277 (translation of A rev. iii 10–iv 5)
Veldhuis 1989, *ASJ* 11, 239–260 (partial edition of mss. A and B_1, with addition of commentary passages of 11N-T3 and older sources (mostly Old Babylonian texts); pp. 255–257 (edition of mss. B_2–B_4))
Veldhuis 1991, *A Cow of Sîn*, 8–15, 61–65 (edition of A iii 10–35, iii 36–iv 1, B_1(+) rev. iii 4–29, C obv. 19–36, D 51–62, b 1'–13')
Foster 2005, *Before the Muses*, 1007–1009 IV.53b-d (ms. A rev. iii 10–35 ("Cow of Sîn"); rev. iv 2–3; obv. ii 49–59)
Scurlock 2014a, *Sourcebook*, 594–604 (edition of A obv. i–rev. iv 38); 626–627 (A rev. iv 39–45)
Scurlock 2014b, 128–130, 131–133 (translation of ms. A obv. i 37–rev. iii 9, rev. iii 10–iv 5)
Couto-Ferreira 2014, *Dynamis* 34/2, 289–315 (overview, discussion)
Steinert 2017a, 331–336 with n. 135 (ms. A obv. i 52–53, ii 44, 47–54)
Steinert 2021a, *Byzantinische Forschungen* 33, 44 (ms. A obv. i 52–53, i 68–69, rev. iii 46–53), 49 (ms. A rev. iv 13–20), 50 (ms. A rev. iv 25, 27)
Electronic Babylonian Library (eBL) (edition of ms. B_1 (+) B_4 (+) B_5; https://www.ebl.lmu.de/library/K.2413)

Parallels and Additional Sources

Ms. C: Rm. 376
Copy: Lambert 1965, *AS* 16, 287–288
Photo: CDLI P282433
Edition: Lambert 1965, *AS* 16, 283–288; Röllig 1985, *OrNS* 54, 260–273; Veldhuis 1991, 10–11, 63; SEAL No. 7228; Collins 1999, 255–256 (obv. ii 1–11); Böck 2007, *Muššu'u*, 263, 290–293 Tablet VIII/1 (ms. U, obv. 1ff.)
Discussion: Albertz 1978, 51–55; Nowicki 2013 (*NABU* 2013/61); Marquéz Rowe 2015, *AuOr* 33, 51–62; Zomer 2018, 28, 29, 89 n. 389, 117, 233, 235, 341, 346, 363, 383

This fragment of a Middle Assyrian two-column tablet (ca. 1100 BCE) was registered in the Nineveh Collection of the British Museum. However, the tablet was excavated in the area of the Kidmuru temple at Nimrud (Kalhu) dedicated to Ištar of Kidmuru (for the rediscovery of the findspot information, see Reade 1986, 218). The preserved text is a collection of incantations for different purposes, e.g. against Lamaštu and *maškadu*-disease (obv. ii 1–11 and 12–18, see Zomer 2018, 270–272, 326–330, 341–342). The last section on the obverse (ii 19–36) contains a close variant of the birth incantation "A Cow of Sîn".

337 Measurements: ca. 10.5 x 11 x 0.5 cm (B_4).
338 Measurements: ca. 2 x 2 x 0.8 cm.
339 Measurements: ca. 4.5 x 4.3 x 0.3 cm.
340 Measurements: ca. 7.6 x 6.5 x 1.8 cm.

Arbøll (2018, 270–272; 2023, 273) has argued that the incantations of this collective tablet may have been intended for use in connection with matters having to do with pregnancy and difficult childbirth. The findspot of the text therefore confirms a connection of Ištar of Kidmuru with female fertility and childbirth.

Ms. D: *Iraq* 31, pl. V–VI
Copy: Lambert 1969, pl. V–VI
Photo: Fales 1989, 195
Edition: Lambert 1969, *Iraq* 31, 28–39; Röllig 1985, *OrNS* 54, 263–270 (lines 51–62); Fales 1989, 195–196; Veldhuis 1991, 12–13 (lines 51–62), 64; Scurlock 2014a, 605–608; Zomer 2018, 254–256 (lines 33–50); SEAL No. 7231, 7232; *infra* text II.1.4
Discussion: Foster 2005, 1006 (lines 33–50); Nowicki 2013, *NABU* 2013/4, No. 61; Zomer 2018, 30, 34, 76, 89, 118, 200 n. 765, 233, 234 n. 991; CDLI P282478

This Middle Assyrian tablet in the Signor Ligabue collection at Venice may originate from Assur, from the palace of Tiglath-pileser I). It contains prescriptions for postpartum conditions followed by two birth incantations, one of which (lines 51–62) presents a varying version of the spell "A Cow of Sîn". A second incantation in ms. D (lines 33–50) shares close resemblances to several passages in a much longer birth incantation in ms. A (see especially ms. A obv. ii 2–29, 44–45, 54–56). The prescriptions and the incantations in ms. D were assembled from two different sources (see the annotation in line 32).

Ms. E: VAT 8943 = BAM 183 (KAR 205)
Photo: CDLI P285275
Edition: Farber 1989a, *Schlaf, Kindchen*, 124–125 § 44, 126–127 § 45 *passim* (ms. t); Scurlock 2014a, 626–627; Farber 2014, *Lamaštu*, 49, 137 (ms. Rc); *BabMed Corpora Online*

This Neo-Assyrian excerpt tablet from Assur (from the N4 library; Pedersén 1986: 59 No. 7) contains prescriptions for infants, against Lamaštu, TU.RA.KÌLIB.BA ("all illnesses"). Two passages duplicate the prescriptions for the baby protecting it from the "Hand of the god" and the *lilû*-demon, appended at the end of BAM 248 col. iv (E obv. 8–9, 10–13 // A rev. iv 39–40, 41, 43).

Ms. F: K. 3628 + K. 4009 + Sm. 1315 + K. 19939
Photo: CDLI P395132
Copy: Finkel 1976, *Hulbazizi*, pl. 25–26
Edition: Finkel 1976, *Hulbazizi*, 266–278 (ms. P); Farber 1989a, *Schlaf, Kindchen*, 126–127 § 45 (ms. u); Scurlock 2014a, 621–626
Discussion: Schmidtchen 2019, *JMC* 33, 32–33 (new joined fragment K. 19939, colophon)

This Neo-Assyrian single-column tablet from Nineveh is designated as an excerpt (*nisḫu*) in the tablet colophon. The text contains prescriptions and diagnostic passages concerning infants suffering from epileptic seizures (AN.TA.ŠUB.BA, "Lord of the roof") or attacked by the "Hand of the god", the "Hand of the goddess", *lilû* and *alû*-demon. Lines 19'–22' of the text duplicate the final prescription in BAM 248 rev. iv 41–43, to protect the baby from the "Hand of the *lilû*-demon".

Ms. G: K. 11956 + K. 14200
Photo: CDLI P399540 (K. 11956); CDLI P400683 (K. 14200)
Copy: Pl. 38
Edition: *Electronic Babylonian Library* (eBL) (transliteration; https://www.ebl.lmu.de/library/K.11956); *infra* text D.1.2

The two fragments of this Neo-Assyrian excerpt tablet from Nineveh joined by the author preserve treatments for easing difficult delivery. One prescription (obv. 3–5) duplicates ms. A obv. i 52–53.

Ms. H: BAM 249 (VAT 13972)
Photo: CDLI P285334
Edition: *BabMed Corpora* (https://www.geschkult.fu-berlin.de/e/babmed/Corpora/BAM-3/BAM-3_-249; transliteration); *infra* text D.1.3

This fragment of a two-column tablet from Assur (N4 library) preserves recipes for speeding up a protracted and difficult delivery (column i'). Part of these prescriptions are duplicated in treatments in the Birth Compendium (mss. A and B). In column ii', ms. H contained other textual material that is unrelated to the Birth Compendium; for example, a section with prescriptions to ward off frightening nightmares (see *infra* for discussion).

Ms. I: AMT 66/4 (K. 10507)
Photo: CDLI P398722
Edition: Thompson 1934a, *Babyloniaca* 14, 83 and 133ff.
BabMed Corpora (https://www.geschkult.fu-berlin.de/e/babmed/Corpora/AMT-2/AMT66-4/index.html) (transliteration)
Electronic Babylonian Library (eBL) (transliteration; https://www.ebl.lmu.de/library/K.10507)
Infra text D.1.4
Discussion: Parpola 1983b, *JNES* 42, 21 (note on 1.1: 2'); Schuster-Brandis 2008, 60–61, 192–197; Böck 2014b, *OLZ* 109, 173–178

This fragment of a two- or multicolumn tablet from Nineveh preserves a mixture of materials related to women's healthcare, including amulet necklaces (e.g. for protecting pregnant women) and remedies for difficult delivery. It includes an incantation (lines 6' and 7', zalaḫ zalaḫ) for a woman in difficult labour duplicated in manuscripts of the Neo-Assyrian Birth Compendium. Some lines in ms. I refer to connections to the compendium *kunuk ḫalti*, a series collecting prescriptions for amulet necklaces destined for different purposes (see *infra* for discussion).

Ms. a: BM 36339 (80-6-17, 65)
Copy: Pl. 35
Photo: *Electronic Babylonian Library* (eBL) (https://www.ebl.lmu.de/library/BM.36339)
Edition: *Electronic Babylonian Library* (eBL) (transliteration)

This Neo-Babylonian fragment of a single-column tablet (presumably from Babylon)[341] preserves five sections with incantations and remedies for easing difficult delivery duplicating five passages in the Neo-Assyrian Birth Compendium that are found in column i of ms. A. Ms. a appears to present an extract or a varying collection of therapies in comparison with the Compendium represented by mss. A and B.

Ms. b: KUB 4, 13 (CTH 810; Bo 4822)
Photo: hethiter.net:/ fotarch N05373, fotarch BoFN00106a
Copy: Weidner 1922, KUB 4, No. 13
Edition: Röllig 1985, *OrNS* 54, 260–273 (lines 7'–14'); Veldhuis 1991, 12–13, 65; Zomer 2013, *NABU* 2013, 45–46 no. 27 (lines 15'–23'); SEAL Nos. 7233, 7234; *Thesaurus Linguarum Hethaeorum digitalis* (TLHdig; https://www.hethport.uni-wuerzburg.de/TLHdig/tlh_xtx.php?d=KUB%204.13)
Discussion: Schwemer 1998, 6 n. 26, 125; Stol 2000a, 64 fn. 101; Schwemer 2013, 156; Marquéz Rowe 2015, *AuOr* 33, 51–62; Zomer 2018, 35, 30, 31, 89 fn. 389, 119, 233, 234, 235, 341, 346, 363, 382, 383

The fragment found at the Hittite capital Hattuša is written in a 'Non-Hittite' script. It preserves remnants of two Akkadian birth incantations, the first of which parallels a couple of lines in "A Cow of Sîn", while the second is closely related to another spell in the Birth Compendium (BAM 248 obv. i 36–50 //) focusing on the cow in travail beloved by the moon god that also has precursors in Old Babylonian birth incantations.

Ms. c: RS 25.436 (Damascus DO 6726)
Copy: Arnaud 2007, AuOr Suppl. 23, pl. 11 (no. 20)
Photo: Del Olmo Lete 2014, *SANER* 4, pl. XXII
Edition: Arnaud 2007, AuOr Suppl. 23, 75–77 No. 20; SEAL No. 7229; Marquéz Rowe 2014, *SANER* 4, 77–78

341 Leichty, Finkel and Walker 2019, *CBT* IV–V, 316, 319; Reade 1986, in *CBT* VI, xxx. Measurements: ca. 5.5 x 5.0 x 2.3 cm.

Discussion: Caquot, Sznycer and Herdner 1974, 386 n. 1; Zomer 2018, 12, 18, 57, 89 fn. 389, 107, 165, 233, 235, 341, 345–346, 363, 383; Marquéz Rowe 2015, *AuOr* 33, 51–62

This tiny fragment from Ugarit found in the so-called "House of the Lamaštu tablets" preserves part of a Middle Babylonian precursor of the incantation "A Cow of Sîn".

Ms. d: BM 38624+
Photo: *Electronic Babylonian Library* (eBL) (https://www.ebl.lmu.de/library/BM.38624)
Copy: Pl. 12–13
Edition: *infra* text A.2.1

The fragmentary two-column tablet in Late Babylonian script may perhaps be best described as a therapeutic compendium or handbook on women's health that covers all the major relevant topics. Two prescriptions to speed up difficult delivery in the Neo-Assyrian Birth Compendium (mss. A and B) are duplicated in ms. d.

Ms. e: N. 1568
Photo: CDLI P276694
Copy: Jiménez 2019, *NABU* 2019/3, 141
Edition: Jiménez 2019, *NABU* 2019/3, 140–141 (No. 77); *Electronic Library Project* (eBL) (https://www.ebl.lmu.de/library/N.1568)

This fragment was recognized by E. Jiménez as the first Neo-Babylonian fragment stemming from Nippur that preserves a few damaged lines of the first birth incantation included in the Neo-Assyrian Birth Compendium (BAM 248 obv. i 1–35 = ms. A lines 1–21), a Sumerian spell going back to Old Babylonian precursors, with an interlinear Akkadian translation. Because the text of ms. A is so badly preserved, the exact placement of ms. e in relation to ms. A is currently uncertain. Therefore, the text of ms. e is briefly presented and discussed in the notes to ms. A below (lines 6–11).

Several birth incantations of older date in Sumerian or Akkadian offer parallels in wording or specific motifs to incantations found in the Birth Compendium, which are listed here for convenience (parallel passages from these texts are discussed in the notes below):

VAT 12597 = Deimel, SF 54 vi 1–viii 4 // Jestin **TSŠ 170** iv 6–vii 3 (Sumerian, Pre-Sargonic; Fara/Šuruppak; Krebernik 1984, 36–37 no. 6A-B; Cunningham 1997, Text 13a–b; Rudik 2011, 321–326 FSB 57)

UM 29-15-367 (Sumerian, Ur III period; van Dijk 1975, 53–57, Römer 1987; Cunningham 1997, 69–75 Text 62)
AUAM 73.1425 iii 3–iv 14 (Sumerian, Ur III period; Sigrist 1980, 153–167; Cunningham 1997, Text 70; Rudik 2011, 327–331 FSB 58)
VAT 8381 (= VS 17, 33; Sumerian, Old Babylonian period; van Dijk 1975, 62–63; parallels UM 29-15-367)
MLC 1207 (= YOS 11, 85; Sumerian, Old Babylonian period; van Dijk 1975, 66–67)
John Rylands Library Box 24 E6 (24) (Sumerian, Old Babylonian period; Wilcke 1973, 13–14; van Dijk 1975, 69)
E 47.190 (Sumerian; Old-Babylonian period; G. Farber 1984, *JNES* 43, 311–316)
BM 97093 (Sumerian; Old Babylonian period; *see infra* text II.1.1)

AUAM 73.3094 (bilingual, Old Babylonian period; Cohen 1976, *RA* 70, 135–139; Bergmann 2008, 28–29; Wasserman and Zomer 2022, No. 10)

***BiOr* 75, 19–20** (Akkadian, Old Babylonian period; Wasserman 2018, 18–20; Wasserman and Zomer 2022, No. 3)
BM 113625 (= CCT 5, 50e) (Akkadian, Old Assyrian period; Kouwenberg and Fincke 2012–2013; Barjamovic 2015, 75; Wasserman and Zomer 2022, No. 5)
Kt 90/k 178: 1–23 (Akkadian, Old Assyrian period; Michel 2004, *FS Larsen*, 395–420; Barjamovic 2015, 74; Wasserman and Zomer 2022, No. 9)
Kt 94/k 429 (Akkadian, Old Assyrian period; Barjamovic 2015, 75–77; Wasserman and Zomer 2022, No. 11)

CUSAS 32, No. 29b (Akkadian, Old Babylonian period; George 2016, 47–48; Pl. LXXVIII; Wasserman and Zomer 2022, No. 8)
VAT 8539 (= VS 17, 34) (Akkadian, Old Babylonian period; van Dijk 1972, 343–344; Bergmann 2008, 22; Wasserman and Zomer 2022, No. 12)

Overview

i	Fragmentary Sumerian incantation with partial interlinear Akkadian translation (boat motif): [munus ù-tu-ud-da-a-ni] A obv. i 1–35 // B_2 obv. i 1'–8'; cf. e 1'–9'	1–21
ii	Akkadian incantation: [. . .] *šupšuqat alāda* A obv. i 36–50 // B_2 obv. i 9'-14'; cf. b 15'-21'	22–36
iii	Rubric: KA.INIM.MA ^{munus}LA.RA.AḪ.A.KÁM A obv. i 51 // a obv. 1' // G obv. 2 (cf. b 22')	37
iv	Procedure (DÙ.DÙ.BI): oil/dust filled into a hollow reed applied to the woman's belly A obv. i 52–53 // G obv. 3–5 // a obv. 2'–4'	38–39
v	Akkadian incantation: šišik e laraḫ A obv. i 54–61 // a obv. 5'–rev. 1	40–47
vi	Akkadian incantation (boat motif): *ina kār mūti k*[*alât*] *eleppu* A obv. i 62–66 // a rev. 2–5	48–52
vii	Rubric: KA.INIM.MA ^{munus}LA.RA.AḪ.A.KÁM A obv. i 67	53
viii	Procedure (DÙ.DÙ.BI): massage the woman's belly in downward movement with oil that has been stirred with an arrow A obv. i 68–69 // a rev. 6–8	54–55
ix	Akkadian incantation A obv. ii 1–rev. iii 5 // B_2 obv. ii 1'–13'; B_3 obv. ii 1'–21'; cf. D 33–50	56–130
x	Rubric: KA.INIM.MA ^{munus}LA.RA.AḪ.A.KÁM A rev. iii 6 // B_3 obv. ii 22'	131
xi	Procedure (DÙ.DÙ.BI): massage the woman's belly in downward movement with different types of dust in oil A rev. iii 7–9 // B_1 + B_4 + B_5 rev. iii 1–3 // B_3 rev. iii 1–3	132–134
xii	Akkadian incantation ("A Cow of Sîn"): *iltēt littu ša Sîn Geme-Sîn šumša* A rev. iii 10–35 // B_1 + B_4 + B_5 rev. iii 4–28 // B_3 rev. iii 4 cf. C obv. 19–36; D 51–62; b 1'–12'; c 1'–10'	135–160
xiii	Rubric and fragmentary prescription b 13'–14'	161–162
xiv	Akkadian incantation (motif of the cow): *Narunde Naḫḫunte u Nanamgišir* A rev. iii 36–45 // B_1 + B_4 + B_5 rev. iii 29–33	163–172
xv	Procedure (DÙ.DÙ.BI): massage the woman's belly in downward movement with different types of dust mixed with oil and filled into a hollow reed A rev. iii 46–53	173–180
xvi	Akkadian incantation (motif of the cow, speaking in the first person): *litti Sîn ša Sîn anāku* A rev. iii 54–iv 1 // a rev. 9–11	181–193
xvii	Akkadian incantation (addressing the baby): *lusma kīma ṣabīti* A rev. iv 2–3	194–195
xviii	Procedure (DÙ.DÙ.BI): moving a staff or *e'ru*-wood crosswise over the woman's belly A rev. iv 4–5	196–197
xix	Akkadian incantation: *šupšuqta rēmi Marduk* A rev. iv 6–7	198–199

xx	Procedure: moving a staff or *e'ru*-wood over the woman's belly A rev. iv 8–9 // // $B_1 + B_4 + B_5$ rev. iv 1–2	200–201
xxi	(Pseudo-)Sumerian incantation: zalaḫ (iz)zalaḫ A rev. iv 10 // B_1 rev. iv 3 // I rev. i' 7'	202
xxii	Rubric: KA.INIM.MA munusLA.RA.AH.A.KÁM A rev. iv 11 // $B_1 + B_4 + B_5$ rev. iv 4	203
xxiii	Prescription: potion of *maštakal*-plant (and) roasted barley A rev. iv 12 // $B_1 + B_4 + B_5$ rev. iv 5	204
xxiv	Remedy for a woman who has difficulty in labour (*šumma sinništu ina alādi uštapšiq*): Potion of fox grape, 'dog's tongue'-plant, *tuḫlu*-plant A rev. iv 13–15 // $B_1 + B_4 + B_5$ rev. iv 6–8 // H i' 8'–10'	205–207
xxv	Prescription: Potion of excrement of a wall lizard (*zê ṣurāri*) A rev. iv 16 // // $B_1 + B_4 + B_5$ rev. iv 9	208
xxvi	Prescription: salve with dust dug out by a dog mixed in oil A rev. iv 17 // $B_1 + B_4 + B_5$ rev. iv 10	209
xxvii	Prescription: Salve with 'nest of a *šinūnūtu*-swallow' mixed in oil A rev. iv 18 // $B_1 + B_4 + B_5$ rev. iv 11	210
xxviii	Prescription: salve with male *pillû*-plant in oil A rev. iv 19–20 // $B_1 + B_4 + B_5$ rev. iv 12–13	211–212
xxix	Prescription: potion with fox grape or 'dog's tongue'-plant A rev. iv 21 // $B_1 + B_4 + B_5$ rev. iv 14	213
xxx	Prescription: potion of 'dog's tongue'-plant and *nīnû*-plant A rev. iv 22 // $B_1 + B_4 + B_5$ rev. iv 15	214
xxxi	Prescription: potion of 'spur of a bat' A rev. iv 23 // $B_1 + B_4 + B_5$ rev. iv 16 // d obv. ii 26'	215
xxxii	Prescription: potion of 'dog's tongue' plant and *maštakal*-soapwort[342] A rev. iv 24 // $B_1 + B_4 + B_5$ rev. iv 17	216
xxxiii	Dietetic recommendation: eat meat of a turtle A rev. iv 25 // $B_1 + B_4 + B_5$ rev. iv 18	217
xxxiv	Dietetic recommendation: eat meat of a white pig A rev. iv 26 // // $B_1 + B_4 + B_5$ rev. iv 19	218
xxxv	Dietetic recommendation: eat meat of a female fox A rev. iv 27 // $B_1 + B_4 + B_5$ rev. iv 20	219
xxxvi	Prescription: potion with *atā'išu*-plant A rev. iv 28 // // $B_1 + B_4 + B_5$ rev. iv 21	220
xxxvii	Prescription: potion with *kalgukku*-mineral A rev. iv 29 // $B_1 + B_4 + B_5$ rev. iv 22 // d obv. ii 25'	221
xxxviii	Dietetic recommendation: chew Kaniš-acorn (hazelnuts) A rev. iv 30 // $B_1 + B_4 + B_5$ rev. iv 23	222
xxxix	Prescription (amulet): shoot of a plant tied to a band is bound to the woman's thigh A rev. iv 31–38 // // $B_1 + B_4 + B_5$ rev. iv 24–31	223–230
lx	Prescription: amulet for the baby to protect from the Hand of the god[343] A rev. iv 39–40 // $B_1 + B_4 + B_5$ rev. iv 32 // E obv. 8–9	231–232
lxi	Prescription: fumigation for the baby to protect from Hand of the *lilû*-demon A rev. iv 41 // E obv. 10–11; F obv. 22'	233
lxii	Prescription: Salve for the baby to protect from Hand of the *lilû*-demon A rev. iv 42 // F obv. 20'	234

342 Note that the prescriptions in A rev. iv 24–38 // B_1 rev. iv 17–31 (lines 216–230) form one ruled-off section.

343 The prescriptions in A rev. iv 39–43 (lines 231–235) form one ruled-off section.

lxiii	Prescription: Salve for the baby to protect from Hand of the *lilû*-demon A rev. iv 43 // E obv. 12–13; F obv. 21'	235
lxiv	Catchline A rev. iv 44	236
lxv	Colophon A rev. iv 45	237

Transliteration

1	A obv. i 1	[ÉN munus ù-tu-ud-da-a-ni ....]
	A obv. i 2	[.......................................]
2	A obv. i 3–4	*completely lost*
3	A obv. i 5	[$^{\text{(ĝiš)}}$m]á ^{ĝiš}ere[n ....]
	A obv. i 6	[x]x *ri-qí* [*e-re-ni*] *ri-qí e-re-*⸢*ni*⸣ *ma*-[*lat*$^{?}$]
4	A obv. i 7	[^{ĝiš}má$^{?}$ $^{\text{na4}}$za]-gìn$^{?}$ s[a$_5$$^{?}$ x x x x] s[a$_5$$^{?}$ x x (x)]
	A obv. i 8	⸢x x⸣ [*uq*]-*na*$^{?}$-[*a* x x x x] ⸢$^{\text{giš!}}$MÁ$^{?}$⸣ *šá* MIN$^{?}$ [x x x]
5	A obv. i 9	[gug nu-zu] ù ZA.GUL$^{!}$ n[u-zu]
	A obv. i 10	[*lu-ʾ-at-ma a-na ni*]-*qí*$^{!}$-*i ul* [*na-ṭa-at*]
6	A obv. i 11	[...........] bi nu [...............]
	A obv. i 12	[...................................]
7–10	A obv. 13–20	*completely lost* *for ms. e (N. 1568) see the notes below*
11	A obv. i 21	[..............] x ĝiš$^{?}$ [..................]
	A obv. i 22	[.........] ⸢SAḪAR$^{?}$⸣ x [............]
12	A obv. i 23	[........ munus ḫé]-a ^{ĝiš}bala [^{ĝiš}kirid$^{?}$ ......]
	A obv. i 24	[............ *pi*]-*laq-qí* [............]
13	A obv. i 25	[x x]-⸢bi$^{?}$⸣ ⸢a-ri-a⸣ lag$^{?}$ ki ĝar [...........]
14	A obv. i 26	[..............] ⸢x bi GAR-*an* x *šá si*-x[...........]
15	A obv. i 27	[..............] ⸢GAR-*nu*$^{?}$⸣ *ana* ŠÀ$^{?}$ [.............]
16	A obv. i 28	[................]x ⸢nu-nu⸣ ⸢šika$^{?}$⸣ x [...................]
	B$_2$ obv. i 1'	[..] x
17	A obv. i 29	[.................] ⸢qar ma$^{?}$⸣ [x] an [................]
	B$_2$ obv. i 2'	[...]-[í]b-šú-šú
	A obv. i 30	[..............] ⸢ud$^{?}$⸣ *ana*$^{?}$ *ú-ri*-[..................]
	B$_2$ obv. i 3'	[..-*t*]*ab*$^{?}$-*ka*
18	A obv. i 31	[...................] an ul ma$^{?}$ [x] ⸢x x x⸣
	B$_2$ obv. i 4'	[....................................]-⸢x⸣-è
	A obv. i 32	[.................]x ^{d}UTU *li*-⸢x⸣-[x]-*ma*
	B$_2$ obv. i 5'	[............................ *li-ṣ*]*a-am-ma*
19	A obv. i 33	[.................. p]a ḫé$^{!}$-è$^{!}$-a-⸢ke$_4$⸣
	B$_2$ obv. i 6'	[inim ^{d}en-ki-ke$_4$ pa ḫé]-è-a-ke$_4$

20	A obv. i 34	[........................] ⌜ḫé⌝-en-⌜si-sá⌝-⌜e$^{!}$⌝
	B_2 obv. i 7'	[^{d}dam-gal-nun-na s]i ḫé-en-si-sá-e
21	A obv. i 35	[..]
	B_2 obv. i 8'	[^{d}asar-alim-nun-na dumu saĝ ab]zu-ke$_4$ sa$_6$-ga zíl-zíl-le-bi za-a-kám
A, B, b		
22	A obv. i 36	[ÉN ....]x *šup-šu-[qat a-la-da]*
	B_2 obv. i 9'	[............................] *šup-šu-qat a-la-da*
	b 15'	ÉN É.NU.RU *ar-ḫi-mi i-da-*[...................]
23	A obv. i 37	[ÁB GAL ^{d}NANNA A.RI.A *i-l]e$^{?}$-qé-ma ep-ri* DÙ-*uš ma-*[................]
	B_2 obv. i 10'	[..]x *ma-la-at* GIN$_7$ *na-a-di*
	b 16'	*sú-ú-pu$^{!}$*(MU)*-ur* ^{d}ŠÁKKAN *ar-ḫi-m[i* ....]
24	A obv. i 38	[*ina qar-ni-šú qaq*]*-qa-ru* [*ṭe-ra-at ina* KUN-*šá$^{?}$*]
	B_2 obv. i 11'	[........................]*-ra ṭe-ra-at*
	b 17'	*i-na* ⌜KUN⌝*-ša ú-še-iš-še-r[a* ....]
25	A obv. i 39	[*ú-šeš-še-ra tur-bu-'i$^{?}$*] ^{d}NANNA [*iṣ-bat ḫar-ra-na ina* IG]I$^{?}$ $^{d+}$EN.LÍL
	B_2 obv. i 12'–13'	[............................ *iṣ-ba]t$^{?}$ ḫar-ra-na* / [...........]
26	A obv. i 40	[(*i-bak-ki*) *il-la-ka di-ma-šú am-mi-ni-mi$^{?}$*] ^{d}[NANNA *i-bak*]*-ki*
	B_2 obv. i 13'$^{cont.}$	[..] *i-bak-ki*
	b 18'	*i-il-la-a-me-e il-la-k[a* ....]
27	A obv. i 41	[(*am-mi-ni-mi šá*) *el-la-me-e$^{?}$*] *il$^{!}$-la-*[*k*]*a$^{!}$* ⌜*di$^{!}$*⌝*-ma$^{?}$-šu$^{!}$*
	B_2 obv. i 14'	[......................................] *di-ma-šú*
	b 19'	*i-il-la-a-*⌜*me*⌝*-e il-l[a-ka* ....]
28	A obv. i 42	[..]-kal/dir
	B_2 obv. i 15'	*Illegible traces*
29	A obv. i 43	[*aš-šum ú-ni-qí-ia la pe-ti-tim aš-šum* ÁB*-ia*] ⌜*la$^{!}$*⌝ ⌜*a-lit*⌝*-ti*
	b 20'	*aš-šúm ú-ni-*⌜*í*⌝*-[qí* ....]
30	A obv. i 44	[*ina* KAR] *pu-uš-qí* [*k*]*a-lat* ^{giš}MÁ
31	A obv. i 45	[*ina* KAR] *dan-na-te ka-lat* ^{giš}MÁ.GUR$_8$
32	A obv. i 46	[*man-na(m) lu-uš*]*-pur a-na re-*[*me*]*-ni-*[*i*] ^{d}AMAR.UTU
33	A obv. i 47	[*ina* KAR] *pu-uš-qí lip-ru-ru* ^{giš}MÁ
34	A obv. i 48	[*ina* KAR] *dan-na-te li-maš-ši-ra* ^{giš}MÁ.GUR$_8$
35	A obv. i 49	[*ṣa-a* G]IN$_7$ MUŠ *né-šel-pa-a ki-ma ni-ra-ḫi*
36	A obv. i 50	[^{munus}LA.R]A.AḪ ⌜SILIM$^{?}$⌝*-ma šèr-ru lim-qu-ut-ma* ZÁLAG IGI
	b 21'	*li-i-šèr ár-d[a-tu$_4$* ....]
A		
37	A obv. i 51	[KA.INIM.MA] ^{munus}LA.RA.AḪ.A.KÁM
	G obv. 2	[KA.INIM.MA$^{?}$] ^{munus}L[A.RA.AḪ.A.KAM$^{?}$]
	a obv. 1'	[KA.INIM.MA ^{munus}LA.RA.AḪ.A.KA]M$^{?}$
	b 22'	TU$_6$ ÉN É.NU.[RU ....]
A, a, b, G		

38	A obv. i 52	[DÙ.DÙ.BI *ana* ŠÀ ^{gi}]⸢SAG⸣.KUD GI DU$_{10}$.GA Ì.GIŠ *ta-tab-bak*
	G obv. 3	[DÙ.DÙ.BI *ana* Š]À$^{?}$ ^{gi}SAG.KUD G[I DU$_{10}$.GA . . . .]
	a obv. 2'–3'	[. . . . . G]I ⸢DÙ$_{10}$⸣.GA SAḪAR ⸢SILA⸣.LÍM.MA / [DUB-*ak*$^{?}$]
39	A obv. i 53	[ÉN 7-*šú u* 7-*šú*$^{?}$ *ana* ŠÀ Š]ID$^{?}$-*nu ina* UGU ŠÀ-*šá* GAZ-[*ma*$^{?}$] *šèr-ru uš*-[*te-še*]-*ra*
	G obv. 4–5	[ÉN 7-*šú u* 7]-*šú ana* ŠÀ ŠID-*n*[*u* . . . .] / [*ár-ḫiš ul-lad-ma*$^{?}$] *šer-ru u*[*š-te-šir*]
	a obv. 3'–4'	[ÉN 7-*š*]*ú*$^{?}$ *u* 7-*šú ana* ŠÀ ŠID-*nu ana* UGU *lìb-bi-šú* / [x x *šè*]*r-ri uš-te-še*-<<*eš*>>-*ri*
A, a, G		
40	A obv. i 54	ÉN ši-[ši]-i[k$^{?}$] e la-ra-aḫ
	a obv. 5'	[ÉN š]i-ši-ik la-ra-aḫ
41	A obv. i 55	⸢nam⸣-maḫ [ši-ši-i]k la-ra-aḫ
	a obv. 5'$^{cont.}$	⸢nam$^{?}$⸣-maḫ ši-ši-ik la-ra-aḫ
42	A obv. i 56–57	[*ki*]-*ri-ri*-[*šá* x]-*ṭa-ab-ba nap-ri-šá* / [*k*]*i*$^{?}$-*ri ri*-[*šá*]
	a obv. 6'	[*ki-ri-r*]*i-šú uṭ*$^{?}$-*ṭa-ab-ba nap-ri-šú ki-ri-ri-šú*
43	A obv. i 57	[LÚ.TU]R$^{?}$ [*a*]-⸢*a*⸣ ⸢*ip*$^{!}$-*par*$^{!}$-*rik*⸣ *li-ṣa-a*
	a obv. 7'	[LÚ.TUR] *a-a ip-par-rik li-ṣa-a*
44	A obv. i 58	x x x [*na-ḫ*]*u-un-di e na-ru-un-di*
	a obv. 8'	[*na-ḫ*]*u-un-du na-ḫu-un-du e na-ru-un-du*
45	A obv. i 59	[*na-a*]*m*-[*l*]*i*-[*su*] *ki-ma ṣa-bi-ti*
	a obv. 9'	[*na-a*]*p*$^{?}$-*li-sa ki-ma* MAŠ.DÀ
46	A obv. i 60	⸢*ni*⸣-⸢*šal*$^{?}$⸣-[*l*]*i-l*[*a*] *ki-ma ni-ra-ḫi*
	a obv. 9'$^{cont.}$	*na-áš-li*-⸢*la*⸣ ⸢*ki*⸣-[*ma*] ⸢MUŠ.TUR⸣
47	A obv. i 61	*ana-ku* ^{d}⸢*asal-lú*⸣-*ḫi* DUMU [x x x x]-⸢*ku*$^{?}$⸣ *a-maḫ*$^{!}$-*ḫar-ka*$^{!}$ ÉN
	a rev. 1	[x x] ^{d}*asal-lú-ḫi* DUMU ^{d}IDIM ⸢*šab-sa-ku*⸣ *a*-⸢*maḫ*⸣-[*ḫar-ka* É]N
A		
48	A obv. i 62	ÉN *ina* KAR *mu-ti k*[*a-lat*] ^{giš}MÁ
	a rev. 2	[ÉN *ina*] KAR *mu-tu*$_{4}$ *ka-lat* ^{giš}⸢MÁ⸣
49	A obv. i 63	*ina* KAR *dan-na-ti* [*k*]*a*-[*lat*] ^{giš}MÁ.GUR$_{8}$
	a rev. 3	[*ina*] KAR *dan-na-tu*$_{4}$ *ka-lat* ^{giš}MÁ.GUR$_{8}$
50	A obv. i 64	*ul-la*$^{!}$(tu) ^{d}[UT]U E[N$^{?}$ *di-i*]-*ni*
	a rev. 4	[x x] ⸢^{d}⸣UTU EN *di-i-ni*
51	A obv. i 65	*ana* ^{d}*be-let-ì-lí* [*be-let*] *re-e-me qí-bi-ma*
	a rev. 4	*ana* ^{d}*be-let-ì-lí be-let* ⸢ARḪUŠ⸣ ⸢*qí*⸣-*bi-ma*
52	A obv. i 66	*ur-ḫu li-ši-ir šá* ŠÀ [*ek*]-⸢*le*⸣-*ti li-ṣa-a* <*ana*> ZÁ[LAG$^{?}$] ^{d}UTU-*ši*
	a rev. 5	[*ur-ḫ*]*u li-šir šá* ŠÀ *e*[*k*]-⸢*le*⸣-*tú* ⸢*li*⸣-*ṣa-a ana* ZÁLAG ^{d}UTU-*ši*
A, a		
53	A obv. i 67	KA.INIM.MA ^{munus}LA.RA.AḪ.A.KÁM
54	A obv. i 68	DÙ.DÙ.BI ⸢Ì.GIŠ⸣ ⸢BUR⸣ [*ina*] ⸢^{giš}⸣[GAG].⸢U$_{4}$⸣.[TAG.GA] *ana* ŠÀ x[x x]-*u*
	a rev. 6–7	[DÙ.DÙ.B]I Ì.GIŠ BUR *ina* ^{giš}GAG.U$_{4}$.TAG.GA *šá ina pi-i* ⸢^{giš}⸣PAN$^{?}$ / [*ú*]-*ṣu-ú*
55	A obv. i 69	*ta-maḫ-ḫa-aṣ* [TA *e-la-an ana*] *šap-la-an* [*tu-maš-šá-a'-ma*$^{?}$] SI.SÁ
	a rev. 7$^{cont.}$–8	*ta-maḫ-ḫaṣ*$^{?}$ ÉN 3-*šú ana* ŠÀ ŠID-*nu* / [TA] ⸢*e*⸣-*la-nu ana šap-la-nu tu-maš-šá-a'-ma šèr-r*[*i* SI.S]Á$^{?}$

a

56–68	A obv. ii 1–13	*almost entirely lost*
69	A obv. ii 14	[.......................................]-*ti*
70	A obv. ii 15	[.......................... *ša*]*p*$^{?}$-*la-an* x
71	A obv. ii 16	[......................... *sa-ni-iq*$^{?}$] KÁ
72	A obv. ii 17	[.......................................]x-*ti*
73	A obv. ii 18	[.......................................]x-*ši*
74	A obv. ii 19	[.......................................]-*e-šú*
75	A obv. ii 20	[.......................................]x-*su* šul *šá* ⸢x⸣
76	A obv. ii 21	[.......................................]-tu_4
77	A obv. ii 22	[.. *mu-ú*]-*ti*
	D 37	*ba-ni-tu u-bu-ḫa-at* SAḪAR$^{!}$(BA).MEŠ *mu-ú-te*
78	A obv. ii 23	[*ki-i*] ^{giš}APIN$^{!}$ *ub-b*[*u-ḫa-at* SAḪAR.MEŠ *ki*]-*di*$^{?}$
	D 39	*ki-i* ^{giš}APIN *u-bu-ḫa-at* SAḪAR$^{!}$(BA).MEŠ GIŠ.ÙR$^{!}$(TIR).MEŠ
79	A obv. ii 24	[*ki-i*] ⸢^{giš}GIGIR$^{?}$⸣ [*ub*]-*bu*-[*ḫa-at* SAḪAR.MEŠ *ta-ḫa-z*]*i*$^{?!}$
	D 38	*ki-i* ^{giš}GIGIR *u-bu-ḫa-at* SAḪAR$^{!}$(BA).MEŠ *ta-ḫa-zi*
80	A obv. ii 25	[*ki-i*] ⸢UR.SAG$^{!}$⸣ *mut*$^{!}$-*taḫ-i*[*ṣ*$^{?}$............. *ṣa*]-⸢*lat*$^{?}$⸣
	D 40	*ki-i* UR.SAG *mu-ut-taḫ-iṣ ina* MÚD.MEŠ-*šá ṣa-la-at*
81	A obv. ii 26	[x x] x [x IGI].MIN-*šá*................. *šap-ta-š*]*ú*$^{?}$
	D 41	*ú-ṭa-a* IGI.MEŠ-*šá ul ta-da-gal ka-at-ma šap-ta-šá*
82	A obv. ii 27	[x] x x [..................... *ul š*]*e*-⸢*ma-a*$^{!}$⸣ GEŠTU.[MIN$^{?}$]-*šú*
	D 43–44	*ú-ia* KA-*ša ik-ta-na-at-tam ul* ŠE.GA-*a* / GEŠTU.MEŠ-*šá*
83	A obv. ii 28	[*u*]*l* ⸢*sa*⸣-*an-q*[*a-at*... *s*]*a-pu*-[*ḫu*] ⸢*ku*⸣-*lu-lu*-[*šú*]
	D 44$^{cont.}$	*ul sa-qa-at* ^{uzu}GABA-*sa sà-pu-ḫu ku-lu-lu-ša*
84	A obv. ii 29	⸢*pu*⸣$^{!}$-*su-um-m*[*i*] ⸢*ul*⸣ ⸢*pu-su-na*⸣-[*at bul-t*]*a ul i*-[*ši*]
	D 45	*pu-ṣu-ni ul pa-ṣu-na-at bul-ta ul ti-šu*
85	A obv. ii 30	*uš*$^{!}$-*šu-rat ḫur-da-as-sa a*$^{?}$-[x x]x *sin-niš*-⸢*ti*$^{?}$⸣
86	A obv. ii 31	⸢*ki*$^{?}$-*ma*$^{?}$⸣ *mu-ti ù* ši ki$^{?}$ a$^{?}$ [........................]
	B_2 obv. ii 1'	x [...]
87	A obv. ii 32	*u*[*l-la*$^{?}$] ^{d}*a-ru-ru dan-na-tu* [.....................]
	B_2 obv. ii 2'	x [...]
88	A obv. ii 33	⸢^{giš}MÁ⸣.GUR_8 ^{d}*ma*-⸢*mi*⸣ qa$^{?}$ u$^{?}$ x[...............]
	B_2 obv. ii 3'	^{giš}M[Á.$GUR_8$$^{?}$.....................................]
89	A obv. ii 34	x x[............] *al*$^{?}$-x-*šá* x[........................]
	B_2 obv. ii 4'	*lem-n*[*u*...]
90	A obv. ii 35	[............]x-x-⸢*rat*/*ḫu*$^{?}$⸣ [........................]
	B_2 obv. ii 5'	*ina* KAR x[...]
91	A obv. ii 36	⸢*e-li*$^{?}$⸣ ⸢^{giš}MÁ⸣ ⸢^{d}*ma-mi*$^{?}$⸣ *me-ḫu*$^{?}$-⸢*ú*$^{?}$⸣ [............]
	B_2 obv. ii 6'	*e-l*[*i*$^{?}$...]

92	A obv. ii 37	[...............]-*ta li-ṣa-a*[*m*$^{?}$-*ma* ....]
	B_2 obv. ii 7'	*el*-x x[...]
93	A obv. ii 38	*ana* [..................] ⸢*la*$^{?}$⸣-*ke-e* x[..............]
	B_2 obv. ii 8'	*ana ṣe-ri* [..]
94	A obv. ii 39	*i*-[............................-*n*]*i*$^{?}$ *ki-ma* [*š*]*i*$^{?}$-x[x x]
	B_2 obv. ii 9'	*i-da-a*[*l*$^{?}$(-)..]
95	A obv. ii 40	*i-šá-pi* [.............]-⸢*qu*/*ti*$^{?}$⸣ *qa*-⸢*né*⸣-*e šá* [x x x]
	B_2 obv. ii 10'	*i-šá-pi ki*-[*ma* ....]
96	A obv. ii 41	*i-d*[*a-al* x x x *u*]*š*$^{?}$-*šu-rat pe-re-es-s*[*u*$^{?}$]
	B_2 obv. ii 11'	*i-da-al* x[..................................]
97	A obv. ii 42	GAL$_4$.LA$^{!?}$-[*šá* ....] ^{d}*ma*-⸢*mi*$^{?}$⸣
	B_2 obv. ii 12'	*ina ú-ri-š*[*á* ....]
98	A obv. ii 43	*aš*-⸢*šum*$^{?}$⸣ [^{giš}MÁ *šá*$^{?}$ ...... *u*]*d-dan-ni-na*$^{?!}$ *mar*$^{?}$-⸢*kas*⸣-[*s*]*a*$^{?}$
	B_2 obv. ii 13'	⸢*aš-šum*⸣ x x [......................................]
99	A obv. ii 44	*i*-⸢*na*⸣ ⸢*kit-tab-ri-šú*⸣ ⸢GUB⸣-*za*$^{?!}$ ^{d}AMAR.UTU
	D 46	GUB-*za*-<<*ma*>>-*am-ma* DUG$_4$.GA.MEŠ-*si re-ma-nu-ú* ^{d}AMAR.UTU
100	A obv. ii 45	*qí-i*[*p*$^{?}$ *nap-šá*]-*ti n*[*a*$^{?}$-*din*] *ši-pat* TI.LA
101	A obv. ii 46	*an-nu-ú me-ḫu-ú* ⸢*la-ma*⸣-*ku kul-dan-ni*
	D 47	*an-nu-ú te-šu-ú la-a-ma-ku-ma ku-ul-da-a-ni*
102	A obv. ii 47	*i-na* ⸢*ip-šu*$^{!}$⸣ *pi*-[*i-k*]*a liš-li-ma* ^{giš}MÁ
103	A obv. ii 48	*i-na* ⸢*ip-šu*⸣ ⸢*pi*$^{!}$-*i*$^{!}$⸣-[*k*]*a liš-te-še-ra* ^{giš}MÁ.GUR$_8$
104	A obv. ii 49	*dan-nu lip-pa-ṭir mar-kas-sa*
105	A obv. ii 50	*ù ed-lu lip-pe-ti* KÁ-*šá*
106	A obv. ii 51	*ṭur-da*$^{sic!}$ ^{giš}MÁ *a-na kar šul-me*
107	A obv. ii 52	*ṭur-da*$^{sic!}$ ^{giš}MÁ.GUR$_8$ *a-na kar* TI.LA
108	A obv. ii 53	*meš-re-e-tu lip-te-ṭi-ra li-ir-mu-ú* SA.MEŠ
109	A obv. ii 54	*ka-an-ga-tu*$_4$ *lip-taš-ši-ra li-ṣa-a nab-ni-tu*
	B_3 obv. ii 1'	[........................ *l*]*i-ṣa-a n*[*ab*-......]
	D 48	*še-li kak-ka ša-ti bu-nu-ut* DINGIR.MEŠ
110	A obv. ii 55	GÌR.PAD.DU *a-ḫi-tu*$_4$ *bi-nu-ut a-me*-⸢*lu*⸣-*ti*
	B_3 obv. ii 2'	[...........................] ⸢*a*⸣-*me*-[*lu-ti*]
	D 49	*bu-nu-ut* LÚ.U$_{18}$.LU *lu-ú-ṣa-ma*
111	A obv. ii 56	*ár-ḫiš li-ta-ṣa-am-ma li-ta-mar* ZÁLAG ^{d}UTU-*ši*
	B_3 obv. ii 3'	[.................... *l*]*i-ta-mar* ⸢ZÁLAG⸣ [^{d}UTU-*ši*]
	D 49$^{cont.}$	*li-mur* IZI.GAR
112	A obv. ii 57	*ki-ma ti-ik* AN-*e a-a i-tur a-na* EGIR-*šú*
	B_3 obv. ii 4'	[......... A]N-*e a-a i*-⸢*tur*⸣ [.........]
113	A obv. ii 58	*ki-ma ma-qit* BÀD *a-a i-né-e'* GABA-*su*
	B_3 obv. ii 5'	[........-*qi*]*t* BÀD *a-a i-né-e'* [........]

114	A obv. ii 59	*ki-ma pi-sa-an-ni šur-di-i a-a i-se-tu mu-ú-šá*
	B_3 obv. ii 6'	[. . . . *p*]*i-sa-an-ni šur-di-i a-a i-se-t*[*u* . . . .]
115	A obv. ii 60	*an-ni-ta* ^{d}*asal-lú-ḫi ina še-mé-e-šu*
	B_3 obv. ii 7'	[*a*]*n*-[*n*]*i-ta* ^{d}*asal-lú-ḫi ina še-mé*-[x]
116	A obv. ii 61	*ik-kud it-ta-id ba-laṭ-sa*
	B_3 obv. ii 8'	*ik-kud it-ta-id ba*-[. . . .]
117	A obv. ii 62	*ina*! *zik-ri ša* ^{d}*é-a ú-šar-bi šum-šu*
	B_3 obv. ii 9'	*ina zik-ri šá* ^{d}*é-a ú-šar-bi* [. . . . . .]
118	A obv. ii 63	*id-di* ÉN *ša* TI.LA *tu-ú ša šul*-[*me*]
	B_3 obv. ii 10'	*id-di* ÉN *šá* TI.LA *tu-ú šá šul-m*[*e*]
119	A obv. ii 64	*ú-ram-mi* DUR *ip-ta-ṭar ki-ṣ*[*ir-šá*]
	B_3 obv. ii 11'	⸢*ú*⸣-*ram-mi rik-sa ip*-[. . . . .]
120	A obv. ii 65	*ed-le-e-ti ba-ba-a-ti up*-[*te-et-te*]
	B_3 obv. ii 12'	[. . .-*l*]*e-e-ti ba-ba-a-t*[*i* . . . .]
121	A obv. ii 66	*up-te-eṭ-ṭi-ra meš-r*[*e-e-tu*]
	B_3 obv. ii 13'	[*up-te-e*]*ṭ-ṭi-ra* [. . . . .]
122	A obv. ii 67	*kan-ga-tu*$_4$ *up-taš-ši-ra ú*-[*ṣa-a nab-ni-tú*]
	B_3 obv. ii 14'	[. . . .]-⸢*a*⸣-*ti up*-[. . . . .]
123	A obv. ii 68	GÌR.PAD.DU *a-ḫi*-[*t*]*u bi-nu-ut* [*a-me-lu-ti*]
	B_3 obv. ii 15'	[. . . . . *a-ḫ*]*i-tu*$_4$ [. . . . .]
124	A obv. ii 69	*ár-ḫiš* [*i*]*t-ta-ṣa-am-ma i-ta-mar* [ZÁLAG ^{d}UTU-*ši*]
	B_3 obv. ii 16'	[. . . . .]
125	A obv. ii 70	*ki-ma ti-ik* AN-*e ul i-tur* [*ana* EGIR-*šú*]
	B_3 obv. ii 17'	⸢*ki-ma*⸣ ⸢*ti*⸣-*ik* ⸢AN-*e*⸣ *u*[*l* . . . .]
126	A rev. iii 1	*ki-ma ma-qit* BÀD *ul i-né-e*ʾ [GABA-*su*]
	B_3 obv. ii	*Omits*
127	A rev. iii 2	*ki-ma* ^{giš}PÍSAN *šur-di-i ul i-se-tu* [*mu-ú-šá*]
	B_3 obv. ii 18'	[*k*]*i-ma* ^{giš}PÍSAN *šur-di-i* ⸢*ul*⸣ ⸢*i-se-tu*⸣ [. . . .]
128	A rev. iii 3	ÉN *šá* ^{d}*asal-lú-ḫi ni-ṣir-tu šá e*[*ri-du*$_{10}$^{ki}]
	B_3 obv. ii 19'	[ÉN] *šá* ^{d}*asal-lú-ḫi ni-ṣir-tu šá eri*-[*du*$_{10}$^{ki}]
129	A rev. iii 4	*an-nu ki-nu šá* ^{d}*é-a i*$^{?}$-*di*$^{?}$-*tu*$_4$ ÉN *ša* ^{d}*ma-mi* ⸢*i-ri-šú*⸣ [. . . . .]
	B_3 obv. ii 20'	[*an-nu k*]*i-nu šá* ^{d}*é-a i-di-tu*$_4$ ÉN *šá* ^{d}*ma-mi i-ri-šú ana* $^{(m)}$*bu-luṭ-sa*$^{?}$-GA[L]$^{?}$
130	A rev. iii 5	^{d}40-LUGAL *id-di-nu ana šu-te-šur* ŠÀ.T[ÙR]
	B_3 obv. ii 21'	[. . . LU]GAL *id-di-nu ana šu-te-šur* ŠÀ.TÙR
A		
131	A rev. iii 6	KA.INIM.MA ^{munus}LA.RA.AḪ.A.K[ÁM]
	B_3 obv. ii 22'	[KA.]INIM.MA ^{munus}LA.RA.AḪ.A.KÁM[344]
A, B		

344 Bottom of B_3 obv. ii.

132	A rev. iii 7	DÙ.DÙ.BI NA$_4$ *ti-ik* AN-*e* SAḪAR *sa-mit* BÀD ŠUB-*t*[*i*]
	B$_1$ + B$_4$ + B$_5$ rev. iii 1	⸢DÙ.DÙ.BI⸣ [. . . . .] ⸢SAḪAR⸣ [. . . . .]-*ti*
	B$_3$ rev. iii 1	[. . . . .]-*ti*
133	A rev. iii 8	SAḪAR ^{giš}PÍSAN *šur-di-i ina* Ì BUR ḪI.ḪI TA *e-la-niš*
	B$_1$ + B$_4$ + B$_5$ rev. iii 2	⸢SAḪAR⸣ ^{giš}PÍSA[N] *šur*-[. . . . .]
	B$_3$ rev. iii 2	[. . . . .]-*niš*
134	A rev. iii 9	*ana šap-la-niš tu-maš-šá-a'-ma* MUNUS BI SI.SÁ
	B$_1$ + B$_4$ + B$_5$ rev. iii 3	*ana šap-l*[*a-n*]*iš tu*-⸢*maš-šá-a'*⸣-[. . . . .]
	B$_3$ rev. iii 3	[. . . . . SI.]SÁ

A, B

135	A rev. iii 10	ÉN 1-*et* ÁB *šá* ^{d}30 GÉME-^{d}EN.ZU.NA *šum-šá*
	B$_1$ + B$_4$ + B$_5$ rev. iii 4	ÉN 1-*et* ÁB [*š*]*á* ^{d}30 GÉME-[. . . . .]
	B$_3$ rev. iii 4	[. . . . .]-⸢*šá*⸣
	C obv. ii 19–20	ÉN É.NU.RÙ / GU$_4$.ÁB *šá* ^{d}30 GÉME-^{d}30
136	A rev. iii 11	*ti-iq-na-a-te tuq-qù-na-at*
	B$_1$+ B$_4$ + B$_5$ rev. iii 5	⸢*ti*⸣-*iq-na-a*-[*t*]*i* [. . . . .]
	C obv. ii 20$^{cont.}$	*ši-ik-na-te mu-tu-rat*
137	A rev. iii 12	*bi-nu-tam kaz-bat i-mur-ši-ma* ^{d}30 *i-ra-am-ši*
	B$_1$ (+) B$_4$ rev. iii 6	*bi-nu-tam k*[*az-ba*]*t* [. . . . .]
	C obv. ii 20$^{cont.}$–21	*mi-nu-ta ka-az*-[*bat*] / *e-mur-ši-ma* ^{d}30 *i-ra-am-ši*
	D 53–54	IGI.DU$_8$-*ši-ma* ^{d}30 / *i-ra-'-ši*
138	A rev. iii 13	*nam-ru šá* ^{d}30 *šu-ba-ḫi iš-ta-kan-ši*
	B$_1$ rev. iii 7	*nam-ru šá* ^{d}30 [. . . . .]
	C obv. ii 21$^{cont.}$	*mi-ḫi-ir* ^{d}30 *nam-ru te mu* [. . . . .]
139	A rev. iii 14	*uš-te-eṣ-bi-is-si-ma pa-an su-kul-lim*
	B$_1$ rev. iii 8	*uš-te-eṣ-bi-is-si*-[*ma* . . . .]
	C obv. ii 22	*ul-ta-aṣ-bi-si pa-nu su-ku-li-ša*
140	A rev. iii 15	*re-é-ú-tu il-la-ka* EGIR-*šá*
	B$_1$ rev. iii 9	*re-é-a-ú-tu i*[*l-la-ka* . . . .]
	C obv. ii 22$^{cont.}$	*la-tu i-la-ka-a i-n*[*a ar-ki-šá*]
141	A rev. iii 16	*ina nu-ru-ub šam-me i-re-'i šam-me*
	B$_1$ rev. iii 10	*ina nu-ru-ub šam-mi i*-[. . . . .]
	C obv. ii 23	*i-na nu-ru-ub* Ú.MEŠ *i-ra-'i-ši*
	D 54$^{cont.}$	*ana nu-ru-ub* Ú.MEŠ *ir-ta-na-'i*
142	A rev. iii 17	*ina šub-bé-e maš-qé-e i-šaq-qu-ši me-e*
	B$_1$ rev. iii 11	*ina šub-bé-e maš-qí-i* [. . . . .]
	C obv. ii 23$^{cont.}$	*i-na šub-be ša maš-qé*-⸢*e*⸣ [*i-šaq-qí-ši*]
	D 54$^{cont.}$–55	*ina sa-ḫi m*[*aš-q*]*í*$^{?}$ / NAG.MEŠ-[*ši* A].MEŠ
143	A rev. iii 18	*ina pu-zur ka-par-ri la a-mar re-'-i*
	B$_1$ rev. iii 12	*ina pu-zur ka-par-ri la a*-[. . .]
	C obv. ii 24	*i-na pu-zu*$^{!}$(KA)-*ur* ^{lú}SIPA *la la-mad ka-pár-ri*
144	A rev. iii 19	*ana* UGU ÁB *iš-ta-ḫi-iṭ mi-ru ek-du* $^{ḫe-pí}$<*zib*>-*ba-tuš-šá* ÍL-*ši*
	B$_1$ rev. iii 13	*ana* UGU ÁB *iš-ta-ḫi-iṭ mi*-[. . . . .]
	C obv. ii 24$^{cont.}$–25	GU$_4$.ÁB *il*-[*ta-ḫi-iṭ*] / AMAR *ek-du*
	D 55$^{cont.}$–56	*ana* UGU GU$_4$.ÁB *il-ti-ki-iṭ bu-ru* / *ek-du*

145	A rev. iii 20	U$_4$.MEŠ-*šá ina qu-ut-ti-i ár-ḫi-šá ina ga-ma-ri*
	B$_1$ rev. iii 14	U$_4$.MEŠ-*šá i-na qu-ut-ti-*⸢*i*⸣ [. . . . .]
	C obv. ii 25$^{cont.}$	*ar-ḫi-ša i-na ga-ma-ri* U$_4$.MEŠ-*ša i-n*[*a qut-ti-i*]
	D 56	U$_4$.MEŠ-*ša ana mu-le-e* ITI.MEŠ-*ša ana* [*ga-ma-ri*]
146	A rev. iii 21	ÁB *ig-ta-lit ú-ga-al-lit*
	B$_1$ rev. iii 15	ÁB *ig-da-lit i-ga-*[*al-lit*]
	C obv. ii 26	GU$_4$.ÁB *ik-ta-mi-ṣi i-ḫa-al ar-ḫu*
	D 57	*ta-aḫ-ti-me-iš ta-ha-al bu-ur-tu*
147	A rev. iii 22	*re-é-a-šá ap-pa-šu qá-di-is-su ka-par-ru ka-li-šú-nu sap-*⸢*du*⸣*-šú*
	B$_1$ rev. iii 15	*re-é-a-šá ap-pa-šu qá-di-*[. . . . .]
	C obv. ii 26$^{cont.}$–28	^{lú}SIPA x[x x x x] / *u ka-pár-ru*^{meš} DÙ.A.BI-*šu-nu sa-ap-du-ši sa-ap-*[*du* x x x] / [^{lú}S]IPA *na-ši* ŠU *ù ka-pár-ru ú-ka-na-šá*
	D	*Omits*
148	A rev. iii 23	*ana ik-kil-li-šá ana ri-gim ḫa-li-šá ne-pal-suḫ*$_4$(SAḪ)
	B$_1$ rev. iii 16	*ana ik-kil-li-šá ana ri-gim ḫa-*[*li-šá* . . . .]
	C obv. ii 28$^{cont.}$–29	*a-na* [*ik-kil-li-šá*] / [*a-na ri-g*]*i-im ḫi-li-šá*
	D 57$^{cont.}$–58	*ina i*[*k-ki-li-ša*$^?$] / *ina* GÙ.MEŠ *ḫi-li-ša*
149	A rev. iii 23$^{cont.}$–24	^{d}NANNA-*ru* / ^{d}30 *ina* AN-*e iš-tam-me ri-gim-šá iš-ši qa-as-su šá-ma-me*
	B$_1$ rev. iii 17	^{d}30 *ina* AN-*e iš-tam-me ri-*[. . . . .]
	C obv. ii 29$^{cont.}$–30	<^{d}30 *i*>-*na* AN *iš-ta-ma-a ri-gi-i*[*m-šá* x x x] / [x x (x)]
	D 58$^{cont.}$	^{d}30 *na-an-na-ar* AN-*e* [x x x x (x)]
	b 4'[345]	[*iš-š*]*i q*[*à-as-su* . . . .]
	c 1'–2'	^{d}NANNA-*ru* [. . . . .] / *iš-ši* ŠU-*su a-n*[*a* . . . .]
150	A rev. iii 25	2 ^{d}LAMMA.MEŠ AN-*e ú-ri-da-ním-ma* 1-*et* Ì.GIŠ BUR *na-šá-at*
	B$_1$ rev. iii 18	2 ^{d}LAMMA.MEŠ AN-*e ú-ri-*[*da-nim-ma* . . . .]
	C obv. ii 30$^{cont.}$–31	2-*ta* ^{d}ALAD AN-*e ú-ri-da-ni il-t*[*i-it* x x x] / [x x x]x
	D 59	2 *ši-na* DUMU.MUNUS ^{d}*a-nim* TA AN-*e ú-ri-da-a-ni* 1-*te na-ša-at* A.MEŠ [*ḫ*]*i-i-li*
	b 4'$^{cont.}$–5'	[. . . . .] / [1-*e*]*t*$^?$ x[. . . . .]
	c 3'–4'	2 *la-mas-sa-at* [. . . . .] / 1-*et* Ì BUR *na-*[*šá-at*]
151	A rev. iii 26	*šá-ni-tu*$_4$ *ú-šap-pa-la me-e ḫa-li il-pu-ut* Ì.GIŠ BUR *pu-us-sa*
	B$_1$ rev. iii 19	*šá-ni-tu*$_4$ *ú-šap-pa-la me-*[*e* . . . .]
	C obv. ii 31$^{cont.}$	KAŠ ⸢KÙ⸣.GA$^!$ *na-šá-*⸢*at*⸣ A.MEŠ *šul-me* x[x x x]
	D 59$^{cont.}$–60	*ša-ni-tu* / *na-ša-at* Ì *pu-ú-ri* A.MEŠ *ḫi-li* <<*li*>> *il-pu-ut* SAG.KI.MEŠ-*sa*
	b 5'$^{cont.}$–6'	[. . . . .] / *il-pu-u*[*t*. . . . .]
	c 4'$^{(cont.)}$–5'	[. . . . .] / *il-pu-ut* Ì [BUR . . . .]
152	A rev. iii 27	*me-e ḫa-li ú-šap-pi-ḫa ka-la zu-um-ri-šá*
	B$_1$ rev. iii 20	*me-e ḫa-li ú-šap-pi-*[*ḫa* . . . .]
	C obv. ii 32	[x x x x]x-*ip-ḫu p*[*u*$^?$-*t*]*am*$^{?!}$ *šá* GU$_4$.ÁB *š*[*a*$^?$-x x x]
	D 60$^{cont.}$–61	Ì *pu-ú-ri* <<x>> *ú*-<*šap*>-*pi*-<*ḫa*> / DÙ$^!$.A.BI SU.MEŠ-*ša*
	c 6'	*me-e ḫal-li u*[*š-tap-pi-ḫa* . . . .]
153	A rev. iii 28	*šá-na-a il-pu-ut* Ì.GIŠ BUR *pu-us-sa*
	B$_1$ rev. iii 21	*šá-na-a il-pu-ut* Ì+GIŠ$^!$(MA) BUR *p*[*u-us-sa*]

345 The traces in b 1'–3' cannot be read with certainty; cf. Marquéz Rowe 2015, *AuOr* 33, 54 who restores [. . . ^{ding}]^{ir}N[ANNA$^?$-*ru*$^?$ . . .] in ms. b 3' and in b 2': [*a*$^?$-*n*]*a*$^?$ *i*[*k*$^?$-*ki-li-ša/šu*$^?$ . . .] (ibid., 60), corresponding to the beginning of lines 148 and 149. These readings are not followed by SEAL and TLHdig.

	C and D	*Omit*
	b 7'	*i-na ša-⸢ni-i⸣ il-p[u-ut . . . .]*
	c 7'	*iš-ni-m[a . . . .]*
154	A rev. iii 29	*me-e ḫa-li ú-šap-pi-ḫa ka-la zu-um-ri-šá*
	B_1 rev. iii 22	*me-e ḫa-li ú-šap-pi-ḫa [. . . . .]*
	C and D	*Omit*
	b 8'	[. . . . .] *pa-na* SU-*šu*
	c 8'	*me ḫal-li [. . . . .]*
155	A rev. iii 30	*šal-šu*$^{!}$(la)-*ti-iš-šu ina la-pa-ti*
	B_1 rev. iii 23	*šal-šu*$^{!}$(la)-*ti-iš-šu ina la-[. . . . .]*
	C and D	*Omit*
	b 8'$^{\text{cont.}}$	*i-na ša-a[l-ši . . . .]*
	c 9'	*ina šal-ši [. . . . .]*
156	A rev. iii 31	*bu-ru* GIN$_7$ *ú-za-li im-ta-qut qaq-qar-šú*
	B_1 rev. iii 24	*bu-ru* GIN$_7$ *ú-za-li im-t[a-. . . . .]*
	C obv. ii 33	[x x x x-*l*]*i*$^{?}$ *im-qu-ta qaq*$^{!}$(a)-*qar-šu*
	D	*Omits*
	b 8'$^{\text{cont.}}$–9'	[. . . . .] / *im-qú-ut qa-aq-qár-šu*
	c 9'–10'	[. . . . .] / *a-na qa-[aq-qa-ri]*
157	A rev. iii 32	AMAR GA *iš-ta-kan šu-um bu-ú-ri*
	B_1 rev. iii 25	AMAR GA *iš-ta-kan šu-um bu-⸢ú⸣-[ri]*
	C obv. ii 33$^{\text{cont.}}$–34	*a-na mur*(-)[x x x] / [x x x x] x
	D	*Omits*
	b 9'$^{\text{cont.}}$–10'	x[. . . . .] / *il-ta-kan šu-ú-um* [. . . . . . .]
158	A rev. iii 33	*ki-ma* GÉME-^{d}EN.ZU.NA *i-šá-riš i-li-da*
	B_1 rev. iii 26	*ki-ma* GÉME-^{d}EN.ZU.NA *i-šá-r[iš . . . .]*
	C obv. ii 34$^{\text{cont.}}$	*ki-ma* GÉME-^{d}30 ⸢*li*⸣-*še*-⸢*ra*⸣ [x x x x x]
	D 61$^{\text{cont.}}$	GIN$_7$-*ma gi-i*-^{d}30 GÉME *ša* ^{d}30 *e-eš-ri-ši* Ù.TU-*du*
159	A rev. iii 34	*li-li-id ar-da-tu*$_4$ *mu-šap-šiq-tu*$_4$
	B_1 rev. iii 27	*li-li-id ar-da-tu*$_4$ *mu-[. . . . .]*
	C obv. ii 35	[x x x x]x-*du* x x x [x x] x x [x x x x x x]
	D 61$^{\text{cont.}}$-62	*lu*-Ù.TU-*id* / *ar-da-a-tu* ^{munus}LA.RA.AḪ.MEŠ
	b 11'	*li-il-dá ar-dá-t[u . . . .]*
160	A rev. iii 35	*šab-šu-tu*$_4$ *a-a ik-ka-li e-ri-tu li-ši-ir*
	B_1 rev. iii 28	*šab-su-tu*$_4$ *a-a ik-ka-l[i . . . .]*
	C obv. ii 36	------------------------ [*e-ri-tu l*]*i-še-er* [TU$_6$ ÉN É.NU.RU$^{?}$]
	D 62$^{\text{cont.}}$	-- ÉN$^{!}$(IGI) É.NU.RU
	b 12'	------------------------ PEŠ$_4$-*tu*$_4$ *li-še-e*[*r*] x[. . . . .]

A, B_1, C, b____

161	b 13'	KA.INIM.MA ÉN *mu-šap-ši-i[q-ti . . . .]*
162	b 14'	*iš-tu re-e-eš lìb-bi-šu a-[na . . . .]*

b____

163	A rev. iii 36	ÉN *na-ru-un-di na-ḫu-un-di u na-nam-gi-ši-ir*
	B_1 rev. iii 29	ÉN *na-ru-un-di na-ḫu-un-di n[a-. . . . .]*

164	A rev. iii 37	1-*et* ÁB *šá* ^{d}30 GÉME-^{d}30 *šum-šá*
	B$_1$ rev. iii 30	1-*et* ÁB *šá* ^{d}30 GÉME-^{d}30 [.........]
165	A rev. iii 38	*ana ik-kil-li-šá ana ri-gim ḫa-li-šá*
	B$_1$ rev. iii 31	*ana ik-kil-li-šá ana ri-gim ḫa-*[....]
166	A rev. iii 39	^{d}NANNA-*ru* ^{d}30 *iš-te-mi ri-gim-šá*
	B$_1$ rev. iii 32	^{d}NANNA-*ru* ^{d}30 *iš-t*[*e-*..........]
167	A rev. iii 40	*man-nu-um-ma na-ru-un-di man-nu-um-ma na-ḫu-un-di*
	B$_1$ rev. iii 33	⸢*man-nu*⸣-[.......................................]
168	A rev. iii 41	ÁB-*mi* EN *šup-šu-qat a-la-da*
	B$_1$ rev. iii	*Breaks*
169	A rev. iii 42	EN *me-e* BA.AN.DU$_8$.DU$_8$-*ka ana muḫ-ḫi-šá i-di-ma*
170	A rev. iii 43	*šá* ÁB *e-gi-*^{d}EN.ZU.NA *lip-pe-tu-ú pa-nu-šá*
171	A rev. iii 44	*li-ṣa-a* GIN$_7$ MUŠ *ki-ma* MUŠ.TUR *liš-šá-li-la*
172	A rev. iii 45	*ki-ma ma-qit* BÀD *le-es-su a-na ku-tal-li-šú a-a id-di* TU$_6$ ÉN

173	A rev. iii 46	DÙ.DÙ.BI SAḪAR SILA.LÍM.MA SAḪAR KUN$_4$ *maḫ-ri-tu*$_4$
174	A rev. iii 47	SAḪAR *pi-sa-an-ni e-li-i ù ši-ip-li-i*
175	A rev. iii 48	SAḪAR *pi-sa-an-ni* ^{giš}IG GI NÍG.GAL.GAL.LA
176	A rev. iii 49	*ap-pa ù il-da ta-sar-ri-im*
177	A rev. iii 50	SAḪAR.ḪI.A *šu-nu-ti a-na* ŠÀ Ì.GIŠ ŠUB-*di*
178	A rev. iii 51	ÉN *an-ni-tú* 7-*šú ana* ŠÀ ŠID-*nu*
179	A rev. iii 52	GI NÍG.GAL.GAL.LA DIRI-*ma ina* UGU ŠÀ-*šá zaq*$^{!}$(*qu*)-*pi*
180	A rev. iii 53	TA *e-le-nu ana šap-la-nu tu-maš-šá-a'*

181	A rev. iii 54	ÉN ÁB.GAL ^{d}30 *šá* ^{d}30 *ana-ku*
	a rev. 9	[ÉN x x] ⸢*e*⸣-*gi-zi-ni-tu*$_4$ *šá* ^{d}30 *r*[*a*$^{?}$-x-x x x]
182	A rev. iii 55	*e-ru-ú e-ra-ku-ma nu-uk-ku-pu ú-nak-kap*
	a rev. 10	[x x x x x x x *nu*]-*uk-ku-pu ú-*[*nak-kap*]
183	A rev. iii 56	*ina* SI-*ia*$_5$ *qaq-qa-ru ṭe-ra-ku*
	a rev. 10$^{cont.}$	[........................]
184	A rev. iii 57	*ina* KUN-*ia*$_5$ *uš-te-eš-še-ra tur-bu-'-i*
	a rev. 11	[...................... *tur-b*]*u*-⸢'⸣$^{?}$-[*i*]
185	A rev. iii 58	*ina* KAR *mu-ti ka-lat* ^{giš}MÁ
	a rev. 11$^{cont.}$	[........................]
186	A rev. iii 59	*ina* KAR *dan-na-ti ka-lat* ^{giš}MÁ.GUR$_8$
187	A rev. iii 60	[*man-na lu-uš-pu*]*r*$^{?}$ *ana*$^{?}$ ^{d}40 EN ÉN
188	A rev. iii 61	[*ina* KAR *mu*]-*ti lip-ṭu-ru* ^{giš}MÁ
189	A rev. iii 62	[*ina* KAR *dan-na-ti li*]-*ram-ma-a* ^{giš}MÁ.GUR$_8$

190	A rev. iii 63	[*ki-ma* GÉME-^{d}EN.ZU.NA *i-šá-riš*$^{?}$ *u*]*l-du-u l*[*i*$^{?!}$*-li-id*]
191	A rev. iii 64	[*ar-da-tu*$_4$ *mu-šap-šiq-tu*$_4$$^{?}$] ⸢*li*$^{?}$⸣*-ši-*[*ir šá* ŠÀ*-šá*$^{?}$]
192	A rev. iii 65	[. . . . .]
193	A rev. iv 1	*ár-ḫiš lit-ta-ṣa-am-ma li-mu-ra* ZALAG ^{d}UTU*-ši* TU$_6$ ÉN
194	A rev. iv 2	ÉN *lu-us-ma ki-ma* MAŠ.DÀ *né-er-ru-ba* GIN$_7$ MUŠ.TUR
195	A rev. iv 3	*ana-ku* ^{d}*asal-lú-ḫi šab-sa-ku a-maḫ-ḫar-ka* TU$_6$ ÉN
196	A rev. iv 4	DÙ.DÙ.BI ^{giš}GIDRU ^{giš}MA.NU *šá* ŠU *re-'-i ta-maḫ-ḫar*
197	A rev. iv 5	ÉN 7*-šú ana* UGU ŠID *ina* UGU ŠÀ*-šá ta-par-rik-ma ár-ḫiš* Ù.TU
198	A rev. iv 6	ÉN *šup-šuq-ta re-mi* ^{d}AMAR.UTU
199	A rev. iv 7	^{d}⸢ŠÀ$^{!}$.ZU$^{!}$⸣ *šab-su-ta-šá-ma at-ta šum-li-is-si* TU$_6$ EN
200	A rev. iv 8	DÙ.DÙ.BI ^{giš}GIDRU ^{giš}MA.NU *šá* ŠU *re-'-i*
	B$_1$ rev. iv 1	[DÙ.DÙ].BI ^{giš}GIDRU ^{giš}MA.NU *šá* [Š]U *re-'-*⸢*i*⸣
201	A rev. iv 9	ÉN 7*-šú* ŠID*-nu-ma* TA SAG ŠÀ*-šá ana šap-la-an* ŠÀ*-šá tuš-ga-ra-ár*
	B$_1$ rev. iv 2	[ÉN 7]*-šú* ŠID*-nu-ma* TA SAG ŠÀ*-šá ana šap-la-an* ŠÀ*-šá* ⸢*tuš*⸣*-g*[*a*-x-x]
A, B$_1$, I		
202	A rev. iv 10	ÉN za-la-aḫ iz-za-la-aḫ za-la-aḫ al-ti-la TU$_6$ ÉN
	B$_1$ rev. iv 3	[ÉN] ⸢za⸣-la-aḫ iz-za-la-aḫ za-la-aḫ al-ti-la ⸢TU$_6$⸣ É[N]
	I rev. i' 7'	ÉN za-la-aḫ za-la-[aḫ . . . . TU$_6$ ÉN]
A, B$_1$, I		
203	A rev. iv 11	KA.INIM.MA ^{munus}LA.RA.AḪ.A.KÁM
	B$_1$ rev. iv 4	⸢KA.INIM⸣.MA ^{munus}LA.RA.AḪ.A.KÁM
A, B$_1$		
204	A rev. iv 12	^{ú}I[N.NU.U]Š ZÌ ŠE.SA.A *ina* Ì.GIŠ *u* KAŠ NAG*-ši-ma uš-te-šer*
	B$_1$ rev. iv 5	^{ú}IN.NU.UŠ ZÌ ŠE.SA.A *ina* Ì.GIŠ *u* KAŠ NAG-⸢*ši-ma*⸣ *uš-te-šer*
A, B$_1$, H		
205	A rev. iv 13	DIŠ MUNUS *ina* Ù.TU *uš-tap-šiq* ^{giš}GEŠTIN.KA$_5$.A ⸢^{ú}EME⸣-UR.GI$_7$
	B$_1$ rev. iv 6	DIŠ MUNUS *ina* Ù.TU *uš-tap-šiq* ^{giš}GEŠTIN.KA$_5$.A ⸢^{ú}EME⸣-UR.GI$_7$
	H i' 8'	[DIŠ MUNUS *ina*$^{?}$] ⸢Ù.TU$^{?}$⸣ *uš*$^{!}$*-tap-šiq*$^{!}$*-šú* ^{ú}GEŠTIN.KA$_5$.A ^{ú}EME-UR.GI$_7$
206	A rev. iv 14	^{ú}*tuḫ-lam* SÚD ^{dug}LA.ḪA.AN KAŠ ^{lú}KÚRUN.NA DIRI*-ma*
	B$_1$ rev. iv 7	^{ú}*tuḫ-lam* SÚD ^{dug}LA.ḪA.AN KAŠ ^{lú}KÚRUN.NA DIRI*-ma*
	H i' 9'	[^{ú}*tuḫ-lam* ^{ú}IN].NU.UŠ DIŠ*-niš* SÚD ^{dug}LA.ḪA.AN KAŠ ^{lú}KÚRUN DIRI
207	A rev. iv 15	Ú.ḪI.A *an-nu-ti ana* ŠÀ SÌG*-aṣ la pa-tan* NAG*-ma ár-ḫiš* Ù.TU
	B$_1$ rev. iv 8	Ú.ḪI.A *an-nu-ti ana* ŠÀ SÌG*-aṣ la pa-tan* NAG*-ma ár-ḫiš* Ù.TU
	H i' 10'	[(. . .) Ú].ḪI.A ŠEŠ *ana* ŠÀ SÌG*-aṣ* NU *pa-tan* NAG*-ši-ma ár-ḫiš ul-lad*
A, B$_1$, H		

208	A rev. iv 16	DIŠ KI.MIN ŠE$_{10}$ EME.DIR *šá* IZ.ZI SÚD *ina* KAŠ *la pa-tan* NAG-*ma* KI.MIN
	B$_1$ rev. iv 9	DIŠ KI.MIN ŠE$_{10}$ EME.ŠID *šá* IZ.ZI ⸢SÚD⸣ *ina* KAŠ *la pa-tan* NAG-*ma* KI.MIN
	H i' 11'–12'	[DIŠ ^{munus}PE]Š$_4$$^?$ *ina* Ù.TU *uš-tap-šiq* ŠE$_{10}$ EME.DIR IZ.ZI SÚD / [*ina* KAŠ NU *p*]*a-tan* NAG-*ma ár-ḫiš ul-lad*
A, B$_1$, H		
209	A rev. iv 17	DIŠ KI.MIN SAḪAR *ni-pil-ti* UR.GI$_7$ SÚD *ina* Ì.GIŠ SÌG-*aṣ* ŠÀ-*šá* ŠÉŠ KI.MIN
	B$_1$ rev. iv 10	DIŠ KI.MIN SAḪAR *ni-pil-ti* UR.GI$_7$ SÚD *ina* Ì.GIŠ SÌG-*aṣ* ŠÀ-*šá* ŠÉŠ KI.MIN
A, B$_1$		
210	A rev. iv 18	DIŠ KI.MIN *qin-ni* SIM.MAḪ^{mušen} SÚD *ina* Ì.GIŠ ḪI.ḪI ŠÉŠ KI.MIN
	B$_1$ rev. iv 11	DIŠ KI.MIN *qin-ni* SIM.MAḪ^{mušen} SÚD *ina* Ì.GIŠ ḪI.ḪI ŠÉŠ KI.MIN
A, B$_1$		
211	A rev. iv 19	DIŠ KI.MIN SUḪUŠ ^{giš}NAM.TAR NITA *šá* $^{\text{tu15}}$SI.SÁ SÚD *ina* Ì.GIŠ ḪI.ḪI
	B$_1$ rev. iv 12	DIŠ KI.MIN SUḪUŠ NAM.TAR NITA *šá* $^{\text{tu15}}$SI.SÁ SÚD *ina* Ì.GIŠ ḪI.ḪI
212	A rev. iv 20	7-*šú ana* ⸢*muq-qal*⸣-*pi-ti pa-pan* ŠÀ-*šá* ŠÉŠ-*ma* KI.MIN
	B$_1$ rev. iv 13	7-*šú ana muq-qal-pi-ti pa-pan* ŠÀ-*šá* ŠÉŠ-*ma* KI.MIN
A, B$_1$		
213	A rev. iv 21	DIŠ KI.MIN ^{giš}GEŠTIN.KA$_5$.A SÚD [*ina*] KAŠ *la pa-tan* NAG-*ma* : ^{ú}EME-UR.GI$_7$ KI.MIN
	B$_1$ rev. iv 14	DIŠ KI.MIN ^{giš}GEŠTIN.KA$_5$.A SÚD [*ina*] KAŠ NU *pa-tan* NAG-*ma* : $^{\text{ú!}}$EME-UR.GI$_7$ KI.MIN
A, B$_1$		
214	A rev. iv 22	DIŠ KI.MIN ^{ú}EME-UR.GI$_7$ ^{ú}KUR.RA^{sar} SÚD *ina* KAŠ NU *pa-tan* NAG-*ma* KI.MIN
	B$_1$ rev. iv 15	DIŠ KI.MIN ^{ú}EME-UR.GI$_7$ ^{ú}KUR.RA^{sar} SÚD *ina* KAŠ NU *pa-tan* NAG-*ma* KI.MIN
A, B$_1$		
215	A rev. iv 23	DIŠ KI.MIN U$_5$ ARKAB^{mušen} SÚD KI.MIN
	B$_1$ rev. iv 16	DIŠ KI.MIN U$_5$ ARKAB^{mušen} SÚD KI.MIN
	d obv. ii 26'	DIŠ KI.MIN U$_5$ ARKAB^{mušen} S[ÚD . . . .]
A, B$_1$, d		
216	A rev. iv 24	DIŠ KI.MIN ^{ú}EME-UR.GI$_7$ ^{ú}IN.NU.UŠ SÚD KI.MIN
	B$_1$ rev. iv 17	DIŠ KI.MIN ^{ú}EME$^{!}$(NAG)-UR.GI$_7$ ^{ú}IN.NU.UŠ SÚD KI.MIN
217	A rev. iv 25	DIŠ KI.MIN ⸢UZU⸣ NÍG.BÚN.NA$^{\text{ku6}}$ GU$_7$-*ma* KI.MIN
	B$_1$ rev. iv 18	DIŠ KI.MIN ⸢UZU⸣ NÍG.BÚN.NA$^{\text{ku6}}$ GU$_7$-*ma* KI.MIN
218	A rev. iv 26	DIŠ KI.MIN UZU ŠAḪ BABBAR GU$_7$-*ma* KI.MIN
	B$_1$ rev. iv 19	DIŠ KI.MIN UZU ŠAḪ BABBAR GU$_7$-*ma* KI.MIN
219	A rev. iv 27	DIŠ KI.MIN UZU MUNUS.KA$_5$.A GU$_7$-*ma* KI.MIN
	B$_1$ rev. iv 20	DIŠ KI.MIN UZU MUNUS.KA$_5$.A GU$_7$-*ma* KI.MIN
220	A rev. iv 28	DIŠ KI.MIN ^{ú}KUR.KUR SÚD *ina* KAŠ NAG-*ma* KI.MIN
	B$_1$ rev. iv 21	DIŠ KI.MIN ^{ú}KUR.KUR SÚD *ina* KAŠ NAG-*ma* KI.MIN
221	A rev. iv 29	DIŠ KI.MIN ^{im}KAL.GUG SÚD *ina* KAŠ NAG-*ma* KI.MIN
	B$_1$ rev. iv 22	DIŠ KI.MIN ^{im}KAL.GUG SÚD *ina* KAŠ NAG-*ma* KI.MIN
	d obv. ii 25'	DIŠ MUNUS *a-lad uš-tap-šiq* ^{im}KAL.GU[G SÚD *ina* KAŠ NAG]

222	A rev. iv 30	DIŠ KI.MIN *al-la-an-ka-niš ina* KA-*šá i-mar-raq-ma* KI.MIN
	B$_1$ rev. iv 23	DIŠ KI.MIN *al-la-an-ka-niš ina* KA-*šá ú-mar-raq-ma* KI.MIN
223	A rev. iv 31	DIŠ KI.MIN ⸢ḪÉNBUR⸣ *ta-šab-bu-uš ina* KI.TA KIŠI$_{16}$
	B$_1$ rev. iv 24	DIŠ KI.MIN ⸢ḪÉNBUR⸣ *ta-šab-bu-uš ina* KI.TA ^{giš}KIŠI$_{16}$
224	A rev. iv 32	*šá* UGU *pi-ti-iq-ti a-ṣu-ú ta-tab-bak*
	B$_1$ rev. iv 25	*šá* UGU *pi-ti-iq-ti* È *ta-tab-bak*
225	A rev. iv 33	*ki-a-am* DU$_{11}$.GA-*ma um-ma at-ta-ma*
	B$_1$ rev. iv 26	*ki-a-am* DU$_{11}$.GA-*ma um-ma at-ta-ma*
226	A rev. iv 34	NÍG.BA-*ka maḫ-ra-ta* Ú *šá* TI *id-nam-ma*
	B$_1$ rev. iv 27	NÍG.BA-*ka maḫ-ra-ta* Ú *šá* TI *id-nam-ma*
227	A rev. iv 35	*šá* ^{munus}NENNI DUMU.MUNUS NENNI *šá* ŠÀ-*šá liš-te-šir*
	B$_1$ rev. iv 28	*šá* ^{munus}NENNI DUMU.MUNUS NENNI *šá* ŠÀ-*šá liš-te-šir*
228	A rev. iv 36	*an-nam* DU$_{11}$.GA-*ma* SUḪUŠ-*su u* SUḪUR-*su* ZI-*ma*
	B$_1$ rev. iv 29	*an-nam* DU$_{11}$.GA-*ma* SUḪUŠ-*su u* SUḪUR-*su* ZI-*ma*
229	A rev. iv 37	*ana* EGIR-*ka* NU IGI.BAR KI LÚ.NA.ME NU DU$_{11}$.DU$_{11}$-*ub*
	B$_1$ rev. iv 30	*ana* EGIR-*ka* NU IGI.BAR KI LÚ.NA.ME NU DU$_{11}$.DU$_{11}$-*ub*
230	A rev. iv 38	DUR NU.NU-*ú tara-kás ina* ^{uzu}ÚR 150-*šá* KÉŠ-*ma* TI
	B$_1$ rev. iv 31	⸢DUR⸣ NU.NU-*ú tara-kás ina* ^{uzu}ÚR GÙB-*šá* KÉŠ-*ma ina-eš*

A, B$_1$____

231	A rev. iv 39	DIŠ *a-na* LÚ.TUR ŠU.DINGIR.RA NU TE-*e* ŠE$_{10}$ ŠAḪ ŠE$_{10}$ UR.GI$_7$ GI$_6$
	B$_1$ rev. iv 32	[. . . . .] ⸢LÚ.TUR⸣ ⸢ŠU.DINGIR.RA⸣ [. . . . .]
	E obv. 8	--- ŠE$_{10}$ ŠAḪ ŠE$_{10}$ UR.GI$_7$ GI$_6$
232	A rev. iv 40	*il-la-at* ANŠE ḪI.ḪI *ina* ^{síg}ÀKA NIGIN-*mi ina* GÚ-*šú* GAR-*ma* TI-*uṭ*
	E obv. 8$^{\text{cont.}}$–9	ÚḪ ANŠE / *ina* Ì ḪI.ḪI *ina* ^{síg}ÀKA NIGIN *ina* GÚ-*šú* GAR-*an*[346]
233	A rev. iv 41	DIŠ *a-na* LÚ.TUR LÚ.LÍL.LÁ NU TE-*e* SÍG UR.GU.LA SÍG ÙZ *ina* DÈ SAR-*šú*
	E obv. 10–11	-- SÍG UR.GU.LA SÍG ÙZ / *ina* DÈ IGI.MEŠ-*šú* SAR-*šú*[347]
	F obv. 22'	DIŠ KI.MIN SÍG ⸢UR⸣.GU.L[A] : ⸢UR⸣.GI$_7$ SÍG ⸢ÙZ⸣ ⸢*ina*⸣ ⸢DÈ⸣ SAR-*šú*[348]
234	A rev. iv 42	DIŠ KI.MIN GÌR.PAD.DU LÚ.U$_{18}$.LU *ina* Ì.GIŠ *ka-a-a-na* ŠÉŠ.ME-*su*
	F obv. 20'	--------------- GÌR.PAD.DU LÚ.U$_{18}$.LU *ina* Ì *ka-a-a-na* ŠÉŠ.MEŠ-*su*[349]
235	A rev. iv 43	DIŠ KI.MIN $^{\text{na4}}$*mu-ṣu* ^{ú}*ṣa-ṣu-tú* GÌR.PAD.DU ŠAḪ *ina* Ì ŠÉŠ.ME-*su*
	E obv. 12–13	-------------- *mu-ṣa* ^{ú}*ṣa-ṣu-um-tú* GÌR.PAD LÚ.MEŠ / *ina* Ì EŠ-*su*
	F obv. 21'	DIŠ KI.MIN $^{\text{na4}}$*mu-ṣa* ^{ú}[*ṣ*]*a-ṣu-un-tú* GÌR.PAD.DU ŠAḪ SÚD *ina* Ì ŠÉŠ.MEŠ-*su*

A, E, F____

Catchline / Colophon:

236	A rev. iv 44	ÉN a idim-ta ba-ta-ĝen-na-ta mu-un-da-ús-sa
237	A rev. iv 45	LIBIR.RA.BI.GIN$_7$ AB.SAR-*ma* BA.AN.È

346 Ms. E inserts a ruling here.
347 Ms. E inserts a ruling here.
348 Ms. F inserts a ruling here.
349 Ms. F inserts a ruling here.

Bound Transcription and Translation

1 [ÉN munus ù-tu-ud-da-a-ni . . .]	1 [Incantation: "The woman giving birth . . .]
2 *completely lost*	2 *completely lost*
3 [$^{\text{(ĝiš)}}$m]á ^{ĝiš}ere[n . . . . . .]	3 [(*like*) a b]oat (loaded) with ced[ar . . .],
3 [x x]x *riqqī* [*erēni*] *riqqī erēni ma*[*liat*]	3 Akk. [(*like*) *a boat* (*loaded*)] with aromatics (and) [cedar], [*she is loa*]*ded* with aromatics (and) cedar.
4 [^{ĝiš}má$^?$ $^{\text{na4}}$za]-gìn$^?$ s[a$_5$$^?$ x x x x] s[a$_5$$^?$ x x (x)]	4 [(like) a boat] loa[ded(?) with lapis] lazuli, [she is load]ed with [*lapis lazuli*].
4 ⌜x x⌝ [*uq*]*nâ*$^?$ [x x x x] ⌜$^{\text{giš!}}$MÁ$^?$⌝ *šá* MIN$^?$ [x x x]	4 Akk. . . . [. . .] with lapis [lazuli(?)], a boat that [is loaded(?)] with ditto(?).
5 [gug nu-zu] ù ZA.GUL$^!$ n[u-zu]	5 [She does not know (whether) it is carnelian], and she does not [know] (whether) it is . . . .
5 [*lu''ât-ma ana ni*]*qî ul* [*naṭât*]	5 Akk. [She is defiled and] not [suited for (making) an off]ering.
6 *too fragmentary for transcription*	6 *too fragmentary for translation*
7–10 *completely lost*	7–10 *completely lost*
11 *too fragmentary for transcription*	11 *too fragmentary for translation*
12 [. . . . . . munus ḫé]-a ^{ĝiš}bala [^{ĝiš}kirid$^?$ . . . . . .]	12 [. . . . . . If] it is [a girl, a spindle (and) [a pin(?) . . . . . .]
12 [. . . . . . *pi*]*laqqi* [. . . . . .]	12 Akk. [. . . . . . a spi]ndle [. . . . . .]
13–17 *too fragmentary for transcription*	13–17 *too fragmentary for translation*
18 [. . .] . . . [. . .]-è	18 [. . . . . . . may it] come out.
18 [. . . . . .]x *Šamaš līṣâm-ma*	18 Akk. [. . . . . . .] may it come out [*to (see) the light*] of the sun!
19 [inim ^{d}en-ki-ke$_4$ pa ḫé]-è-a-ke$_4$	19 May [the word of Enki] become apparent,
20 [^{d}dam-gal-nun-na s]i ḫé-en-si-sá-e	20 [may Damgalnunna (= Damkina)] put things right,
21 [^{d}asar-alim-nun-na dumu saĝ ab]zu-ke$_4$ sa$_6$-ga zíl-zíl-le-bi za-a-kám	21 [O Asar-alim-nunna (= Marduk), foremost son of the Ap]sû, it is up to you to grant favour and kindness!"

---

22 [ÉN . . . . . .] *šupšuqat alāda* (var. ÉN É.NU.RU *arḫī-mi* [. . .])	22 [Incantation: "*The cow*(?) . . .], she has difficulty in her labour, (ms. b: Enuru-incantation: "O my cow . . .[. . .]")
23 [*littu rabītu ša Nanna riḫûta*(?) *il*]*eqqē-ma epri ippuš malât kīma nādi* (var. *supūr Šakkan arḫī-mi* [. . .])	23 [The big cow of Nanna(?)] took in [the semen] and she created 'dust'(?). She is full like a waterskin. (ms. b: The sheepfold of Šakkan, o my cow [. . .])
24 [*ina qarnīša*] *qaqqara ṭerât* [*ina zibbatīša*] (var. *ina zibbatīša ušeššera* [. . .])	24 She roots up the ground [with her horns] (ms. b: with her tail she sweeps [. . .]), [with her tail(?)]
25 [*ušeššera turbu'ī*] *Nanna* [*iṣba*]*t ḫarrāna* [*ina maḫ*]*ar Enlil*	25 [she whirls up dust clouds]. Nanna [too]k to the road, [bef]ore Enlil
26 [(*ibakki*) *illakā dīmāšu ammīni-mi Nanna*(?)] *ibakki* (var. *Ella-mê illakā* [. . . . . .])	26 [(he was crying), his tears were flowing down. 'Why is it that Nanna is] crying, (ms. b: Ella-mê's [tears] are flowing [. . .].)
27 [(*ammīni-mi ša*) *Ella-mê*] *illakā dīmāšu* (var. *Ella-mê illakā* [. . . . . .])	27 [(why) are Ella-mê's] tears flowing down?' (ms. b: Ella-mê's [tears] are flowing . . .)
28 [. . . . . .] . . .	28 [. . . . . .] . . .
29 [*aššum unīqīya lā petītti aššum littīya*] *lā ālitti*	29 '[Because of my kid (who is) unmated, (because) my cow] (who has) never given birth.'
30 [*ina kār*] *pušqi kalât eleppu*	30 [At the quay] of difficulty the boat is held back,

31 *[ina kār] dannate kalât makurru*
32 *[manna luš]pur ana rē[mē]nî Marduk*
33 *[ina kār] pušqi lipruru eleppu*
34 *[ina kār] dannate limaššera makurru*
35 *[ṣâ k]īma ṣerri nešelpâ kīma nirāḫi*
36 *[mušapši]qtu lišlim-ma šerru limqut-ma nūra līmur* (var. *līšer ard[atu . . . . . .]*)

31 [At the quay] of hardship the barge is held back.
32 [Whom should I se]nd to merciful Marduk,
33 (so that) the boat may break free [from the quay] of difficulty!
34 May he release the barge [from the quay] of hardship!
35 [Come out li]ke a snake, glide out like a *nirāḫu*-snake!
36 [May the woman in difficult] labour give birth safely, so that the baby may fall out and see the (sun)light!" (Ms. b: May the young woman give birth easily, [. . .]!)

---

37 [KA.INIM.MA] ^{munus}LA.RA.AḪ.A.KÁM (var. *tê* ÉN É.NU.RU [. . .])

37 [It is the wording (of an incantation)] for a woman who has difficulty in delivery (var.: Wording of an Enuru-incantation [. . . . . .]).

---

38 [DÙ.DÙ.BI *ana lib*]*bi takkussi qanî ṭābi šamna* (var. *eper sūq erbetti*) *tatabbak* 39 *[šipta sebîš]u u sebîšu ana libbi tamannu ina muḫḫi libbīša teḫeppī-ma* (var. adds: *[arḫiš ullad-ma*$^{?}$*] šerru uštešŝer*)

38 [The procedure for it:] You pour oil (var.: dust from a crossroads) [into] a hollow [reed] stem (taken from the) 'sweet reed'. 39 You recite [the incantation seven] and seven times into (the reed). (Then) you break (it) above her belly and (var. adds: she [will deliver quickly and(?)]) the child will be delivered easily.

---

40 ÉN ši-ši-ik e la-ra-aḫ
41 nam-maḫ ši-ši-ik la-ra-aḫ
42 *Kiririša uṭṭabba Napiriša Kiririša*
43 *[ṣeḫ]ru ay ipparrik liṣâ*
44 *Naḫḫunte Naḫḫunte e Narunde*
45 *[na]plisa* (var. *namlisu*) *kīma ṣabīti*
46 *našallila kīma nirāḫi*
47 *anāku Asalluḫi mār Ea šabsāku amaḫḫarka* ÉN

40 Incantation: "Šišik e laraḫ,
41 nammaḫ šišik laraḫ.
42 O Kiririša, *it shall be cleared up*(?)! O Napiriša (and) Kiririša –
43 [the ch]ild shall not lie athwart, may it come out!
44 [O Naḫḫunte], Naḫḫunte, hey Narunde!
45 *Look* (at me) (ms. A: Be plucked) like a gazelle,
46 glide out like a *nirāḫu*-snake!
47 I, Asalluḫi, son of Ea, I am the midwife! I will receive you." Incantation.

---

48 ÉN *ina kār mūti kalât eleppu*
49 *ina kār dannati kalât makurru*
50 *ulla Šamaš bēl dīni*
51 *ana Bēlet-ilī bēlet rēmi qibī-ma*
52 *urḫu līšer ša libbi eklēti liṣâ ana nūr šamši*

48 Incantation: "The boat is held back at the quay of death,
49 the barge is held back at the quay of hardship.
50 Now, Šamaš, lord of justice,
51 command Bēlet-ilī, the mistress of the womb,
52 that the road be straight, (and that) the one inside the darkness may come out into the sunlight!"

---

53 KA.INIM.MA ^{munus}LA.RA.AḪ.A.KÁM

53 It is the wording (of an incantation) for a woman who has difficulty in her delivery.

---

54 DÙ.DÙ.BI *šaman pūri ina šiltāḫi ana libbi* [. . .] (var. *ša ina pī qašti*(?) *[ū]ṣû*) 55 *tamaḫḫaṣ* (var. adds: *šīpta šalāšīšu ana libbi tamannu*) *[ultu] elānu ana šaplānu [tumašša'-ma]* (var. adds: *šerr[u]*) *uš(t)eššer*

54 The procedure for it: 55 You stir 54 oil-from-the-jar with an arrow into . . . (ms. a: with an arrow that *has [gone] out from the mouth of a bow*(?)). 55 (var. adds: You recite the incantation three times over (the oil)), you [massage (her) from] the top (of her belly) downwards, and she will deliver with ease (var. the child will come out straight away).

56–68 *Almost entirely lost*
69–70 *Too fragmentary for transcription*
71 *[. . . . . . san]iq bābu*
72–76 *Too fragmentary for transcription*
77 *[bānītu ubbuḫat eper mū]ti*
78 *kī epinni ubbuḫat [eper kī]di(?)* (var. *šukkuki(?)*)
79 *kī narkabti ubbuḫat [eper tāḫ]āzi*
80 *kī qurādi muttaḫḫiṣi [ina dāmīša ṣal]'at*
81 *[uṭṭâ] īnāša [ul tadaggal katmā šaptāš]a*
82 *[ūya pīša iktanattam] ul šemâ [uz]nāša*
83 *ul sanqat irassa sappuḫū kulūlūša*
84 *pusummī ul pussunat [būlta] ul īši* (var. *tīšu*)
85 *uššurat ḫurdassa . . .[. . .] sinništi*
86 *kīma mūti(?) . . .[. . .]*
87 *u[lla(?)] Aruru dannatu [. . . . . .]*
88 *makurru Mami . . .[. . . . . .]*
89 *lemnu [. . .]. . .[. . .]*
90 *ina kār [. . . . . .]*
91 *eli(?) eleppi Mami meḫû [. . . . . .]*
92 *. . .[. . . . . .]. . . līṣâ[m-ma(?) . . .]*
93 *ana ṣēri [. . .] lakê(?) [. . .]*
94 *idâl(?) [. . . . . .] kīma . . .[. . .]*
95 *išappi kī[ma(?) . . .]. . . qanê ša [. . . . . .]*
96 *idâl(?) . . .[. . .] uššurat pēressu*
97 *ina ūrīša [. . . . . .] Mami(?)*
98 *aššu [eleppi ša(?) . . .u]ddannina(?) markassa*
99 *ina kittabrīšu iziza Marduk* (var. *izizam-ma ištanassi(?) rēmānû Marduk*)
100 *qī[p napšā]ti n[ādin] šipat balāṭi*
101 *annû meḫû* (var. *tēšû*) *lamâku kuldanni*
102 *ina ipiš pîka lišlima eleppu*
103 *ina ipiš pîka lištēšera makurru*
104 *dannu lippaṭer markassa*
105 *u edlu lippeti bābša*
106 *ṭurda eleppa ana kār šulmi*
107 *ṭurda makurra ana kār balāṭi*
108 *mešrêtu lipteṭṭirā lirmû šer'ānū*
109 *kangātu liptašširā līṣâ nabnītu* (var. *šēli kakka šâti bunût ilāni*)
110 *eṣemtu aḫītu binût amēlūti* (var. *bunût a'īli lūṣâ-ma*)

56–68 *Almost entirely lost*
69–70 *Too fragmentary for translation*
71 [. . . .] the door [is made] fast(?),
72–76 *Too fragmentary for translation*
77 [The mother is covered with the dust of de]ath.
78 [Like] a plough, she is cov[ered with the dust of the open] land (ms. D: with the dust of harrowing(?)),
79 Like a chariot, she is covered with the dust of battle,
80 like a fighting warrior, she is cast down in her blood.
81 Her eyes [are dimmed, she cannot see]. Her [lips are closed (lit. covered)].
82 [The woe of her mouth keeps covering (her)], her ears do [not] hear.
83 Her chest is not restrained, her headdress is loosened (lit. scattered).
84 She is not veiled with a veil, (yet) she feels no [shame] (anymore).
85 Her vulva is set straight (to deliver the baby), [. . .] the woman's [. . .].
86 *Like death* . . . [. . .],
87 N[ow(?)], O mighty Aruru, [. . . .]!
88 The barge, O Mami, . . .[. . .],
89 The evil [. . . .] her, [. . .].
90 At the quay(?) of [. . .],
91 Against the boat, O Mami, a storm [*has risen*(?) . . .],
92 . . . [. . . . . .], let it *escape* [. . . .]!
93 Against [. . .] the suckling(?) [. . .].
94 She *wanders around in despair*(?) [. . .], like . . .[. . .],
95 she bellows(?) li[ke(?) a . . .], . . . (like) reeds that [. . .].
96 She *wanders around in despair*(?) . . .[. . .], her hair is loose,
97 (on) her vulva [. . . . . .], O Mami(?)!
98 Because of [the boat . . .]. . . whose rope *is made fast*(?) –
99 Stand by her side, O Marduk (ms. D: Stand by while *she keeps calling out*, O merciful Marduk!),
100 (you who) is entrusted with (giving) [lif]e, [(who) provides] the incantation of life –
101 'This is a storm (var. chaos) (that) I am surrounded (with) – reach for me!' –
102 At your command may the ship be safe,
103 At your command may the barge be steered right.
104 May her strong mooring rope be slackened,
105 May her closed gate be opened!
106 Send forth the boat to the quay of well-being!
107 Send forth the barge to the quay of life!
108 May the limbs relax, may the muscles loosen!
109 May the sealed (limbs) become relaxed, may the creature come forth! (ms. D: Bring forth that sealed one, a creation of the gods,)
110 a body (lit. bone) of its own, a human creature (ms. D: a creation of man! Let it come out)!

111 *arḫiš lītaṣâm-ma lītamar nūr šamši* (var. *līmur nūra*)	111 Let it come out quickly and from now on see the sunlight (ms. D: let it see the light)!
112 *kīma tīk šamê ay itūr ana arkīšu*	112 Like a (rain) shower from heaven, may it (the foetus) not turn back!
113 *kīma maqit dūri ay inē' irassu*	113 Like (someone who) has fallen from a wall, may it not turn (its breast) back!
114 *kīma pisanni šurdî ay isētū mûša*	114 Like a streaming drainpipe, may her waters not stay behind!
115 *annīta Asalluḫi ina šemêšu*	115 When Asalluhi heard this,
116 *ikkud itta'id balāssa*	116 he became anxious, he worried for her life.
117 *ina zikri ša Ea ušarbi šumšu*	117 At the command of Ea, he praised his name.
118 *iddi šiptu ša balāṭi tû ša šulmi*	118 He cast the incantation of life, the formula of well-being.
119 *urammi riksa iptaṭar kiṣi[rša]*	119 He loosened the bond, he untied [her] kn[ot].
120 *edlēti bābāti up[tette]*	120 He o[pened] the closed doors,
121 *upteṭṭirā meš[rētu]*	121 the li[mbs] became relaxed.
122 *kangātu uptašširā ū[ṣâ nabnītu]*	122 The sealed (limbs) became relaxed, [the creature] ca[me forth].
123 *eṣemtu aḫītu binût [amēlūti]*	123 A body (lit. bone) of its own, the [human] creature,
124 *arḫiš ittaṣâm-ma ītamar [nūr šamši]*	124 it came forth quickly and saw [the sunlight].
125 *kīma tīk šamê ul itūr [ana arkīšu]*	125 Like a rain shower from heaven, it did not turn back.
126 *kīma maqit dūri ul inē' [irassu]*	126 Like (someone who) has fallen from the wall, it did not turn back.
127 *kīma pisanni šurdî ul isētū [mûša]*	127 Like a streaming gutter, [her waters] did not stay behind.
128 *šiptu ša Asalluḫi niṣirtu ša Eri[du]*	128 (It is) the incantation of Asalluḫi, a secret of Eridu,
129 *annû kīnu ša Ea ēdītu šiptu ša Mami īrišu ana Buluṭ-sa-r[abi?]*	129 the reliable approval of Ea, the renowned incantation which Mami requested, (and which)
130 *Ea-šarru iddinu ana šutēšur šassūri*	130 (the god) Ea-šarru gave 129 to (the exorcist) Bullussa-ra[bi(?)], 130 to let the womb give birth easily."

---

131 KA.INIM.MA ^{munus}LA.RA.AḪ.A.KÁM	131 It is the wording (of an incantation) for a woman who has difficulty in delivery.

---

132 DÙ.DÙ.BI *aban tīk šamê eper samīt dūri maqti* 133 *eper pisanni šurdî ina šaman pūri tuballal ultu elāniš* 134 *ana šaplāniš tumašša'-ma sinništu šī uš(t)eššer*	132 The procedure for it: 'stone dripping from heaven' (hailstone), dust from the parapet of a dilapidated city wall (and) 133 dust from a streaming drainpipe you mix with oil-from-the-jar. From the top 134 downwards you massage (her with it). Then that woman will deliver easily.

---

135 ÉN (É.NU.RU) *iltēt littu ša Sîn Geme-Sîn šumša* (var. *littu ša Sîn Geme-Sîn*)	135 (Enuru)-Incantation: "There was a cow of Sîn, Geme-Sîn was her name (ms. C: A cow of Sîn was Geme-Sîn).
136 *tiqnāte tuqqunat* (var. *šiknāte mutturat*)	136 She was adorned with ornaments (ms. C: she was of imposing figure),
137 *binûta* (var. *minûta*) *kazbat īmuršī-ma Sîn irāmši* (var. *irā'ši*)	137 she was of alluring shape. Sîn saw her and fell in love with her.
138 *namru ša Sîn šubāḫi ištakanši* (var. *miḫir Sîn namru* . . .[. . .])	138 The brilliant (glow) of Sîn . . . he placed upon her (ms. C: the brilliant *gift*(?) of Sîn, [. . .]).
139 *ušteṣbissī-ma pān sukulli* (var. *pānu sukullīša*)	139 He let her take the lead of the herd,
140 *rē'ûtu illaka arkīša* (var. *lātu illakā ina [arkīša]*)	140 the shepherd(s) (ms. C: the cows) followed her.

141 *ina nurub šammē ire''i šammē* (var. *ira''īši*; *irtana''i*)

141 She(?) grazed on the lushest of grasses (ms. C: [he pastured her]; ms. D: she always grazed on).

142 *ina šubbê (ša) mašqê* (var. *ina saḫḫi m[ašq]î*) *išaqqûši mê* (var. [*išaqqīši*]; *iltanaqqī*[*ši*] *mê*)

142 They (the shepherds) gave her water to drink at the most satisfying of watering places (ms. D: he always gave her water to drink at a meadow with a wa[tering place]).

143 *ina puzur kaparrī lā amār rē'î* (var. *ina puzur rē'î lā lamād kaparrī*)

143 Hidden from the shepherd boys (ms. C: shepherd), unseen (ms. C: unnoticed) by the shepherd (ms. C: shepherd boys)

144 *ana muḫḫi litti ištaḫiṭ* (var. *iltaḫiṭ*; *iltikiṭ*) *mīru* (var. *būru*) *ekdu* (*ḫepi*) *zibbatušša išši*

144 the rampant bull (mss. C, D: calf) mounted the cow; he reared up at her (*broken*) tail.

145 *ūmēša ina quttî arḫīša ina gamāri* (var. *ūmēša ina gamāri arḫīša ina* [*quttî*]; *ūmēša ana mullê arḫēša ana* [*gamāri*])

145 When her days (of pregnancy) came to an end, when her months were finished (var. ms. C: when her days were finished, when her months [came to an end] / ms. D: when her days were up (fulfilled), her months [were finished]),

146 *littu igdalit igallit* (vars. *ugallit*; *littu iktamiṣi iḫâl arḫu*; *taḫtimiš taḫâl būrtu*)

146 the cow started to tremble severely. (var. ms. A: she frightened

147 her herdsman. / var. ms. C: the cow crouched, the cow went into labour. / var. ms. D: the cow bent down (and) was taken with labour pains).

147 *rē'âša appāšu qadissu kaparrū kalîšunu sapdūšu* (var. *rē'û* [. . .] *u kaparrū kalâšunu sapdūši sap*[*dū* . . .] *rē'û naši qāta u kaparru ukannaša*)

147 His head (lit. nose) was bowed, all the shepherd boys lamented (with) him. (var. ms. C: The herdsman [. . .]; and all the shepherd boys mourned for her, they mou[rned . . . .]. [One h]erdsman was lifting (his) hand (in prayer), and a shepherd boy (tried to) take good care of her.)

148 *ana ikkillīša ana rigim ḫâlīša* (var. *ḫīlīša*) *nepalsuḫ* (var. *ina rigmī ḫīlīša*)

148 At her crying, at her screaming in labour, he (the herdsman) was downcast.

149 *Nannāru Sîn ina šamê* (var.: *Sîn nannār šamê*) *ištamme* (var. *ištammâ*) *rigimša išši qāssu šamāmē* (var. *ana šamê*)

149 Nannaru-Sîn in heaven (var. ms. D: Sîn, the luminary of heaven) heard her screaming again and again, he raised his hand towards heaven.

150 *šittā lamassāt šamê ūridānim-ma* (var. *šittā šina mārāt Anim ultu šamê ūridāni*) *iltēt šaman pūri našât* (var. *ištēte našât mê ḫīlī*)

150 Two protective spirits descended from heaven, one carried oil-from-the-jar (var. ms. D: Two are they, the daughters of Anu, they descended from heaven. One carried 'water of labour'),

151 *šanītu ušappala mê ḫalli* (var. *šanītu našât šaman pūri*; [. . .] *šikara*? *ella*! *našât mê šulme* [. . .]) *ilput šaman pūri pūssa* (var. *mê ḫīlī ilput pūssa*)

151 the other brought down water-from-the-bowl (vars. ms. D: the other carried oil-from-the-jar / ms. C: *o*[*ne carried*(?) . . .] *pure beer*(?), one carried "water of well-being", [. . .]). She smeared her forehead with the oil-from-the-jar (var. ms. D: she smeared her forehead with 'water of labour'),

152 *mê ḫalli ušappiḫa kala zumrīša* (var. *šaman pūri ušappiḫa kala zumrīša*)

152 she sprinkled her whole body with water-from-the-bowl (var. ms. D: she sprinkled her whole body with oil-from-the-jar).

153 *šanâ* (var. *ina šanî*; *išnī-ma*) *ilput šaman pūri pūssa*

153 A second time she touched her forehead with oil-from-the-jar,

154 *mê ḫalli ušappiḫa kala* (var. *pān(a)*) *zumrīša*

154 she sprinkled her whole body (var. the front of her body) with water-from-the-bowl.

155 *šalšūtīšu* (var. *ina šalši*) *ina lapāti*

155 When she touched (her) for the third time,

156 *būru kīma uzāli imtaqut qaqqaršu* (var. *ana qaqqari*)

156 the calf fell on the ground like a gazelle's (young).

157 *būr šizbi ištakan šum būri*

157 She named the calf "Milk calf".

158 *kīma Geme-Sîn išariš ūlida(!)* (var. *kīma Gī-Sîn amtu ša Sîn eš(e)riš tūlidu; kīma Geme-Sîn līšera* [. . .])	158 Just as Geme-Sîn (var. ms. D: just as Gī-Sîn, the maidservant of Sîn) gave birth normally,
159 *līlid* (var. *lūlid, lilda*) *ardatu mūsapšiqtu*	159 may also the young woman who has difficulty in labour give birth!
160 *šabsūtu ay ikkali erītu līšer* (var. adds (TU_6) ÉN É.NU.RU)	160 May the midwife not be kept (waiting), may the pregnant woman be alright!" (var. ms. D adds: (Wording of an) Enu-ru-incantation.)

---

161 KA.INIM.MA *šipat mušapši[qti . . .]* 162 *ištu rēš libbīšu a[na . . . . . .]*	161 Wording of an incantation for a woman who has difficulty in (her) labour. [. . . . . .] 162 from the top of her belly towards [*her lower belly* . . . . . .].

---

163 ÉN *Narunde Naḫḫunte (u) Nanamgišir*	163 Incantation: "O Narunde, Naḫḫunte (and) Nanamgišir!
164 *ištēt littu ša Sîn Geme-Sîn šumša*	164 There was a cow of Sîn, Geme-Sîn was her name.
165 *ana ikkillīša ana rigim ḫâlīša*	165 At her crying, at her screaming in labour
166 *Nannāru-Sîn išteme rigimša*	166 Nannaru-Sîn heard her screaming, (saying)
167 *mannum-ma Narunde mannum-ma Naḫḫunte*	167 'Who is it, Narunde, who is it, Naḫḫunte?' –
168 *arḫum-mi bēl šupšuqat alāda*	168 'A cow, O lord, she has trouble in delivery!
169 *bēl mê banduddîka ana muḫḫīša idī-ma*	169 O lord, sprinkle water from your *banduddû*-bucket over her!
170 *ša litti Egi-Suena lippetû pānūša*	170 Let the 'face' of the cow Egi-Suena be opened,
171 *liṣâ kīma ṣerri kīma nirāḫi liššalila*	171 May it (the calf) come out like a snake! May it glide out like a *nirāḫu*-snake!
172 *kīma maqit dūri lēssu ana kutallīšu ay iddi tê šipti*	172 May it not turn back, like someone fallen down from a wall!'" Incantation formula.

---

173 DÙ.DÙ.BI *eper sūq erbetti eper askupp(at)i maḫrīti* 174 *eper pisanni elî u šaplî* 175 *eper pisanni dalti qanâ kabbara* 176 *appa u ilda tasarrim* 177 *eprī šunūti ana libbi šamni tanaddi* 178 *šipta annīta sebîšu ana libbi tamannu* 179 *qanâ kabbara tumalla-ma ina muḫḫi libbīša zaqpi* 180 *ultu elēnu ana šaplānu tumašša'*	173 The procedure for it: (You take) dust from a crossroads, dust from the front (door) threshold, 174 dust from the upper and lower drainpipe, 175 dust from the door socket; you cut off a very thick reed 176 (at) top and bottom. 177 You pour (all the mentioned types) of dust into oil, 178 you recite this incantation over it seven times, 179 you fill the thick (stem of) reed and 180 rub it 179 over her bulging belly 180 from top to bottom.

---

181 ÉN *litti(?) Sîn ša Sîn anāku* (var. [. . .] *Egizinītu ša Sîn* . . .[. . .])	181 Incantation: "I am the (big) cow of Sîn, belonging to Sîn (var.: "[. . .] Egizinītu belonging to Sîn [. . .]).
182 *erû erâku-ma nukkupu unakkap*	182 I am highly pregnant, and I am ready to gore.
183 *ina qarnīya qaqqara ṭerâku*	183 With my horns I root up the soil,
184 *ina zibbatīya ušteššera turbu'ī*	184 with my tail I sweep up dust clouds.
185 *ina kār mūti kalât eleppu*	185 At the quay of death the ship is held back,
186 *ina kār dannati kalât makurru*	186 at the quay of distress the ship is held back.
187 [*manna lušpu*]*r*(?) *ana Ea bēl šipti*	187 [Whom should I sen]d(?) to Ea, lord of the incantation?
188 [*ina kār mū*]*ti lipṭurū eleppa*	188 [At the quay of dea]th let them loosen the ship,
189 [*ina kār dannati li*]*rammâ makurra*	189 [At the quay of distress] let them (fem.) untie the cargo boat!
190 [*kīma Geme-Sîn*(?) *išariš ū*]*l*(*i*)*du l*[*īlid*]	190 [Just as Geme-Sîn(?)] gave birth [normally], may

191 [*ardatu mušapšiqtu*(?)] *līšer* [*ša libbīša*(?)] 192 [. . . . . .] 193 *arḫiš littaṣâm-ma līmura nūr šamši tê šipti*	191 [the young woman in difficult labour] 190 give [birth]! 191 May [her foetus(?)] come straight forth! 192 [. . . . . .] 193 May (it) come out quickly and see the sunlight!" Incantation formula.
194 ÉN *lusma kīma ṣabīti nerruba kīma nirāḫi* 195 *anāku Asalluḫi šabsāku amaḫḫarka tê šipti*	194 Incantation: "Run hither to me like a gazelle, slip out to me like a *nirāḫu*-snake! 195 I, Asalluḫi, am the midwife! I will receive you!" Incantation formula.
196 DÙ.DÙ.BI *ḫaṭṭi e'ri ša qāt rē'î tamaḫḫar* 197 *šipta sebîšu ana muḫḫi tamannu ina muḫḫi libbīša taparrik-ma arḫiš ullad*	196 The procedure for it: You take a staff of *e'ru*-wood from the hand of a shepherd, 197 you recite the incantation over it seven times, you place (it) across her belly. Then she will give birth quickly.
198 ÉN *šuqšuqta rēmi Marduk* 199 *Šazu šabsūtaša-ma attā šumlissi tê šipti*	198 Incantation: "Have pity on the woman in difficult labour, O Marduk! 199 You, Šazu, are her midwife, help her to give birth!" Incantation formula.
200 DÙ.DÙ.BI *ḫaṭṭi e'ri ša qāt rē'î* 201 *šipta sebîšu tamannū-ma ultu rēš libbīša ana šaplān libbīša tušgarrar*	200 The procedure for it: (You take) a staff of *e'ru*-wood from the hand of a shepherd. 201 You recite the incantation seven times, you roll (the staff) over her belly, from top to bottom.
202 ÉN za-la-aḫ iz-za-la-aḫ za-la-aḫ al-ti-la *tê šipti*	202 Spell: "*Slip out! It has slipped out. Slip out*, (so that) she will stay alive!" Incantation formula.
203 KA.INIM.MA ^{munus}LA.RA.AḪ.A.KÁM	203 Wording of a spell for a woman in difficult labour.
204 *maštakal labta ina šamni u šikari tašaqqīši-ma uštešser*	204 You give her *maštakal*-soapwort (and) roasted barley flour to drink in oil and beer, and she will deliver with ease.
205 *šumma sinništu ina alādi uštapšiq(šu) karān šēlebi lišān kalbi* 206 *tuḫlam* (var. adds *maštakal*) *tasâk laḫanna šikar sābî tumallā-ma* 207 *šammī annûti ana libbi tamaḫḫaṣ lā patān išattī-ma* (var. *tašaqqīši-ma*) *arḫiš ullad*	205 If a woman suffers severely during delivery, you pound fox grape, 'dog's tongue'-plant, 206 *tuḫlu*-plant (var. adds: *maštakal*-plant). You fill a bottle with beer from an innkeeper, and 207 you stir these plants into it. She shall drink (it) (var. you have her drink it) on an empty stomach, then she will give birth quickly.
208 DIŠ KI.MIN (var. [*šumma erī*]*tu ina alādi uštapšiq*) *zê ṣurāri ša igāri tasâk ina šikari lā patān išattī-ma* KI.MIN (var. *arḫiš ullad*)	208 Alternatively, (var. [If a pregnant wom]an has difficulty in delivery), you pound 'excrement of wall lizard' she shall drink (it) in beer on an empty stomach, and ditto (var. she will give birth quickly).

[209] DIŠ KI.MIN *eper nipilti kalbi tasâk ina šamni tamaḫḫaṣ libbaša tapaššaš* KI.MIN

[209] Alternatively, you pound the dust dug up by a dog, stir (it) in oil, rub her belly (with it), ditto (i.e. she will give birth quickly).

---

[210] DIŠ KI.MIN *qinni šinūnūti tasâk ina šamni tuballal tapaššaš* KI.MIN

[210] Alternatively, you pound 'nest of *šinūnūtu*-swallow', mix it with oil, rub (her), ditto.

---

[211] DIŠ KI.MIN *šuruš pillê zikari ša ištāni tasâk ina šamni tuballal* [212] *sebîšu ana muqqalpīti papān libbīša tapaššaš-ma* KI.MIN

[211] Alternatively, you pound the root of the male *pillû*-plant which (has grown on) the north side, mix it with oil, [212] you rub the area of her belly seven times (with it) 'going downstream', and ditto.

---

[213] DIŠ KI.MIN *karān šēlebi tasâk* [*ina*] *šikari lā patān išattī-ma* (var.) *lišān kalbi* KI.MIN

[213] Alternatively, you pound 'fox grape'-plant, she drinks (it) [in] beer on an empty stomach; (alternatively) 'dog's tongue'-plant, ditto.

---

[214] DIŠ KI.MIN *lišān kalbi nīnû tasâk ina šikari lā patān išattī-ma* KI.MIN

[214] Alternatively, you pound 'dog's tongue'-plant (and) *nīnû*-plant, she drinks (it) in beer on an empty stomach, and ditto.

---

[215] DIŠ KI.MIN *rikibti arkabi tasâk* KI.MIN

[215] Alternatively, you pound '*spur*(?) of a bat', ditto.

---

[216] DIŠ KI.MIN *lišān kalbi maštakal tasâk* KI.MIN

[216] Alternatively, you pound 'dog's tongue'-plant (and) *maštakal*-soapwort, ditto (i.e. she shall drink it in beer, and she will give birth quickly).

[217] DIŠ KI.MIN *šīr šeleppî ikkal-ma* KI.MIN

[217] Alternatively, she shall eat the meat of a turtle, and ditto.

[218] DIŠ KI.MIN *šīr šaḫî peṣî ikkal-ma* KI.MIN

[218] Alternatively, she shall eat the meat of a white pig, and ditto.

[219] DIŠ KI.MIN *šīr šēlebūti ikkal-ma* KI.MIN

[219] Alternatively, she shall eat the meat of a vixen, and ditto.

[220] DIŠ KI.MIN *atā'iša tasâk ina šikari išattī-ma* KI.MIN

[220] Alternatively, you pound *atā'išu*-plant, she shall drink (it) in beer, and ditto.

[221] DIŠ KI.MIN (var. *šumma sinništu alād(a) uštapšiq*) *kalgukka tasâk ina šikari tašattī-ma* KI.MIN

[221] Alternatively (var. if a woman has severe difficulty giving birth), you pound (red) *kalgukku*-ochre, give (it to her) to drink in beer, and ditto.

[222] DIŠ KI.MIN *allān-kaniš ina pîšu imarraq-ma* (var. *umarraq-ma*) KI.MIN

[222] Alternatively, she should chew Kaniš-acorn (hazelnuts) in her mouth, and ditto.

[223] DIŠ KI.MIN *ḫabbūra tašabbuš ina šapal ašāgi* [224] *ša eli pitiqti aṣû tatabbak* [225] *kīam taqabbī-ma umma attā-ma* [226] *qīštaka maḫrāta šamma ša balāṭi idnam-ma* [227] *ša annannīti mārat annanna ša libbīša lištēšer* [228] *annâ taqabbī-ma šurussu u qimmassu tanassaḫ-ma* [229] *ana arkīka lā tappallas itti mamma lā tadabbub* [230] *ṭurra taṭmû tarakkas ina pēmi šumēlīšu tarakkas-ma iballuṭ* (var. *ina"eš*)

[223] Alternatively, you collect a shoot, you spread it underneath an *ašāgu*-plant [224] that grows on a mudbrick wall. [225] Then you say as follows: [226] "You have received your gift (from me). Give me the Plant-of-Life, [227] so that Mrs. NN, daughter of NN, may easily deliver her baby (lit. that of her belly)!" [228] You shall say this, and then you tear off its root and its top, but [229] you shall not look behind you, nor shall you talk to anybody. [230] You shall tie (the plant) into a band that you have spun, you bind it to her left thigh, and she will get well.

[231] DIŠ *ana ṣeḫri šudingirakku lā ṭeḫê zê šaḫî zê kalbi ṣalmi* [232] *illāt imēri* (var. adds *ina šamni*) *tuballal ina itqi talammi ina kišādīšu tašakkan-ma iballuṭ* [233] DIŠ *ana ṣeḫri lilû lā ṭeḫê šārat urgulê* (var. adds (*šārat*) *kalbi*) *šārat enzi ina pēmti* (var. adds *pānīšu*) *tuqattaršu* [234] DIŠ KI.MIN *eṣemti amēli ina šamni kayyāna taptanaššassu* [235] DIŠ KI.MIN *mūṣa ṣaṣuntu eṣemti šaḫî* (var. *eṣemti amēli*) *ina šamni taptanaššassu*

[231] In order that the 'Hand of the god' does not approach a baby: [232] You mix [231] pig excrement, excrement of a black dog, [232] (and) donkey spittle (ms. E adds: with oil), you wrap it in a wad of wool, you put it around his neck. Then he will be well. [233] In order that the *lilû*-demon does not approach a baby: you fumigate him (var. his face) with lion hair (var.: (or) dog (hair)) and goat hair on (glowing) charcoal. [234] Alternatively, you regularly rub him with 'human bone' in oil. [235] Alternatively, you crush *mūṣu*-mineral, *ṣaṣumtu*-plant, (and) pig bone (var. 'human bone'), you repeatedly rub him (with these drugs) in oil.

Catchline:

[236] ÉN a idim-ta ba-ta-ĝen-na-ta mu-un-da-ús-sa

[236] Incantation: "The waters flowing from the source are flowing copiously."

Colophon:

[237] *kīma labirīšu šaṭer-ma bari*

[237] Written according to its original and checked.

Notes

Line 1: The restored incipit of ms. A, the introductory Sumerian phrase of a bilingual birth incantation, is quoted in the commentary from Nippur, 11N-T3 (both in line 1 and in line 53 in the colophon, see text G.1): ÉN munus ù-tu-ud-da-a-ni "Incantation: The woman giving birth." The incipit quoted here may be compared with the introduction of several Sumerian and bilingual birth incantations from the Old Babylonian period, in which the woman giving birth is compared with a boat (e.g. YOS 11, No. 85 obv. 4'–5' (van Dijk 1975, 66). A few parallel Sumerian texts present a textual variant – du-da-a-ni instead of ù-tu-ud-a-ni "giving birth" – which is interpreted in the interlinear Akkadian translation attested in one Old Babylonian manuscript as *ina atallukīša* "when she is walking about", a Gtn-stem form of *alāku* "to walk":

AUAM 73.3094 (Cohen 1976, *RA* 70, 135–139; Wasserman and Zomer 2022, No. 10):
[8] [. . . munus du-d]a-a-ni ma-gi$_4$ a mi-ni-ri / [9] [. . .] *i-na a-ta-al-lu-ki-ša ki-ma e-le-pi i-te-i-il*
[10] [x an-ú]r du-da-a-ni ma-gi$_4$ a mi-ni-ri / [11] [*i-ši*]*-id ša-me-e u er-ṣe-tim i-na a-ta-al-lu-ki-ša ki-ma e-le-pi i-te-i-il*
[8–9] "[The woman], *when she was walking about, wobbled* like a boat (Akk.),
[10–11] (From) the horizon, *when she was walking about*, she *wobbled* like a boat (Akk.)."

Other Old Babylonian manuscripts with a Sumerian version of the birth incantation show slightly varying spellings of the same passage, in which the phrase du-da-a(n)-ni presumably stands for (ù)-tud-a-ni), see notes on text II.1.1 (lines 1–4). For the notion of "steering" and for the boat as a metaphor for pregnant woman's body, see Steinert 2017, 323–324.

Line 3: This line can be reconstructed with the help of Sumerian (BM 97093 obv. 6–7 (see text II.1.1); YOS 11, No. 85 obv. 6'–7' (van Dijk 1975, 66ff.); EA 47.190: 4–6 (Farber 1984, 313ff.)) and bilingual birth incantations from the Old Babylonian period:

AUAM 73.3094: 12–17 (Cohen 1976, *RA* 70, 135–139; Wasserman and Zomer 2022, No. 10):
[12–13] ⌜ma še⌝-ma-ta še-em im-mi-in-si / *ki-ma e-le-ep ri-qí ri-qí ma-li-a-at*
[14–15] ma e-re-na-ta e-re-en im-mi-in-[si] / *ki-ma e-le-ep e-re-ni e-re-na-am ma-li-*[*a-at*]
[16–17] ma še-em e-re-na-ta še-em e-re-na im-mi-[in-si] / *ki-ma e-le-ep ri-qí e-re-ni ri-qí e-re-n*[*a-am ma-li-a-at*]
[12–13] "Like a boat (carrying) aromatics she is filled with aromatics (Akk.),
[14–15] Like a boat (carrying) cedar she is filled with cedar (Akk.),
[16–17] Like a boat (carrying) aromatics (and) cedar she is filled with aromatics (and) cedar (Akk.)."

Line 4: The Sumerian text in A obv. i 7 can be compared with older incantations, many of which mention that the boat is loaded with lapis lazuli (and carnelian), which refers to the gender of the baby to be born (cf. Bergmann 2008, 43–44 for discussion). See AUAM.73.3094 obv. 18–19 (Cohen 1976, *RA* 70, 135–139; Wasserman and Zomer 2022, No. 10); UM 29-15-367: 14 (van Dijk 1975, 53ff.); VS 17, No. 33: 13 (van Dijk 1975, 62–63); YOS 11, No. 85: obv. 6'–7', l. e. (van Dijk 1975, 66); E47.190: 6 (Farber 1984, 313ff.); BM 97093 obv. 8 (text II.1.1 with discussion). See further John Rylands Library Box 24 E 6 (24):

3 (Wilcke 1973, 13–14; van Dijk 1975, 69); AUAM 73.1425 iii 8 (Sigrist 1980, 154ff.). If deciphered correctly, ms. A reads sa_5 (for *malû* "to be full") instead of si in the older Sumerian texts (Veldhuis 1989, 241, 244).

The Akkadian translation in A obv. i 8 remains obscure for the moment (perhaps "her boat [is loaded] with ditto (i.e. lapis lazuli)" in the second half of the line. Commentary α (11N-T3: 1) quotes and comments on a passage from the Akkadian version of line 4, which cannot be completely reconciled with the traces in the first half of A obv. i 8 (see also text G.1): *e-lep-pi šá uq-na-a ṣa-na-at* "a boat that is loaded with lapis lazuli".

Line 5: The Sumerian text in ms. A obv. i 9 was transmitted in a corrupted form in comparison with the older precursors of birth incantations, which describe the woman's uncertainty about the sex of her foetus in terms of a ship that is loaded either with carnelian or with lapis lazuli (see Veldhuis 1989, 241, 245; Gabbay 2016, 175–177, 195–196):

YOS 11, No. 85 obv. 9' (van Dijk 1975, 66):
^{na4}[gug nu-zu] ^{na4}za-gìn nu-zu
"[She does not know (whether) it is carnelian]; she does not know (whether) it is lapis lazuli."

AUAM 73.3094 obv. 20–21 (Cohen 1976, *RA* 70, 135–139; Wasserman and Zomer 2022, No. 10):
ù gu-ug nu-zu ù za-gi-i[n nu-zu] / *ù sa-am-tum ú-ul i-di ù uq-nu-ú-um ú-u[l i-di]*
"Is it carnelian? She does not know; is it lapis lazuli? She does not know."

BM 97093 obv. 9 (*infra* text II.1.1):
[(x) ^{n}]$^{a4?}$ku-ug$^{?}$ nu-uz-zu za-gi-in nu-uz-zu
"She does not know (whether) it is carnelian; she does not know whether it is lapis lazuli."

Both the Sumerian line and its Akkadian translation in ms. A obv. i 9–10 are quoted in commentary α (11N-T3), which allow to restore the text in ms. A. But while the Sumerian line refers to the uncertainty of the gender of the baby to be born, the Akkadian translation in A obv. i 10 quoted in the commentary forms a reinterpretation of the corrupt Sumerian text. Commentary α quotes the passage from line 5, first the Sumerian followed by the corresponding Akkadian translation (see text G.1 for discussion):

α 2) **gug nu-zu ù ZA.GUL nu-zu : *lu-'-at-ma***
α 3) ***a-na ni-qí-i ul na-ṭa-at***
"(Sumerian:) 'She does not know (whether) it is carnelian, and she does not know (whether) it is . . . .' (Akkadian:) 'She is defiled and not fit for (making) an offering.'

The Sumerian text line quoted in the commentary shows in comparison with the older sources that during the transmission of the text the word za-gìn "lapis lazuli" was corrupted to gug (ZA.GUL) "carnelian", identical with the first word of the line. The Akkadian translation that was added in the first millennium BCE does not correspond to the meaning of the Sumerian text, perhaps due to the textual difficulties presented by the line. The commentary notes this divergence and explains how the Akkadian version related to the (corrupted) Sumerian text (see text G.1 for discussion). The Akkadian text refers to the notion of defilement or ritual impurity that affected women after a delivery and rendered them unfit for presenting offerings (or addressing the deity). For the ritual impurity of the parturient woman, more usually the postpartum woman (*mussukatu, ḫarištu*) in the period shortly after delivery, cf. the discussion in van der Toorn 1985, 31–32; 1994, 91–92; Böck 2013, 40; Stol 2016, 439–440; Feder 2016, 103–108, 112–116; Steinert 2023, 261–277).

Lines 6–11: These lines are completely lost but they appear to be commented on in both Babylonian commentaries on the Birth Compendium. The quotations from the base text together with parallels from the older incantations help to give a few glimpses of the lost text. The first relevant passage quoted in the commentary from Nippur is in Akkadian and concerned with the mother-goddess Bēlet-ilī being summoned by a herald, presumably to assist in delivery (see text G.1: 6–7).

The next passage in the Nippur commentary is on a quotation in Sumerian, from the dialogue between Enki and Asalluḫi, in which the former instructs the latter to use a reed from the marsh, dust from the street/crossroads and fat for treating the woman (see text G.1: 8–12). Several Old Babylonian incantations offer parallel passages (YOS 11, No. 85: 22'–23' (van Dijk 1975, 67); AUAM 73.3094 rev. 42–46 (Cohen 1976, *RA* 70, 135–139; Wasserman and Zomer 2022, No. 10); BM 97093 obv. 19–20 (see text II.1.1 with discussion).

E. Jiménez (2019, *NABU* 2019/3, 140–141 No. 77) has identified the Neo-Babylonian fragment N. 1568 (ms. e) from Nippur as a fragment preserving a passage of the present bilingual birth incantation in ms. A. Since N. 1568 cannot be placed in relation to ms. A with certainty, I offer here a transliteration and translation of the former fragment. Its fragmentary lines contain the Marduk-Ea-dialogue in an abbreviated form, with a partial Akkadian interlinear translation:

Beginning lost

1'	N. 1568: 1'	[. . . . .] x x [(x) (x)]
2'	N. 1568: 2'	[. . . . . . .] x-⸢bi⸣ ⸢bar⸣-šè in-kud [(x)]
	N. 1568: 3'	[. . . . . . .] x-⸢*šú*⸣ *a-ḫe-e up-tar-ri-*⸢?⸣[350]

3'	N. 1568: 4'	[^{d}asal-lú-ḫ]i igi : níĝ ĝá-e : ĝen-na dumu-ĝu$_{10}$ ⸢^{d}asal⸣-l[ú-ḫi]
4'	N. 1568: 5'	[gi èn-bar$^{?}$] bàn-da šu u-me-[ti]
	N. 1568: 6'	[x x *tak-k*]*u-si qa-né-e le-qé-e-ma* [(x)][351]
5'	N. 1568: 7'	[saḫar sila-lam$_{4}$-m]a ì kù šà-bi-šè u-me-ni-[dub]
	N. 1568': 8'	[*eper s*]*u-qí er-bet-ti šá-man el-lu ana lìb-b*[*i šupuk*]
6'	N. 1568: 9'	[. . . . .] x u-m[e-x-x]

Ms. e breaks; remainder lost

[1'] "[. . . . . .] . . . [. . .] [2'] [. . .] he/she has severed/cut off the *alien*(?) . . .[. . .].

[3'] [Asalluḫ]i saw it. <. . . Enki answered his son: . . . 'Whatever I <know, you know too.> Go, my son Asallu[ḫi]! Take a small [reed from the marsh] (Sum.) / Take a [hol]low reed tube [. . .] (Akk.), [pour dust from a cross]roads and pure oil into it, [. . .] . . .[. . .]."

The continuation of the Nippur commentary 11N-T3: 12 quotes from the lost base text, which gives an order about the crucial ritual action to be performed with the prepared reed, namely breaking the reed tube above the woman's belly: *e-li* LI.DUR-*šú ḫe-pi-ma* "Break (the reed) above her navel!" (see text G.1 for discussion). The quoted expression parallels a fragmentary passage in an Old Babylonian bilingual incantation (AUAM 73.3094 rev. 53; Cohen 1976, *RA* 70, 135–139; Wasserman and Zomer 2022, No. 10). The action described here recurs as a ritual instruction within the Birth Compendium in A obv. i 52–53 // (see the note on lines 38–39 below). A similar instruction using a reed filled with dust and oil is used to massage the woman giving birth in A rev. iii 46–53 (lines 173–180). For reed as the cutter of the umbilical cord, see also see also Stol 2000a, 142; Mayer 2016, *OrNS* 85, 182; BM 34208: 34' (text D.1.9).

Line 12: The traces in this line can be compared with passages in older birth incantations that speak of gender-specific objects given to or associated with the newborn. In texts from the third and second millennium BCE, spindle and (dress or hair) pin represent the female gender of the newborn baby, contrasting with male gendered objects (weapon or mace) representing a son (e.g., Rudik 2011). The pin (kirid/*kirissu*) is mentioned beside the spindle (balak, *pilakku*) in the birth incantations UM 29-15-367: 46–47 // VS 17, 33 rev. 7–10 (van Dijk 1975, 56–57, 63; Cunningham 1997, 70–71), YOS 11, 85:

---

350 The meaning of this line remains uncertain. For *parā'u* "to cut through, severe; to slit" (here presumably a D-stem perfect form is used, in the same meaning as the G-stem), see CAD P, 181–182. The word *aḫû* "strange, alien; hostile" occurs in another birth incantation as an attribute to *eṣemtu* "bone", referring to the baby. See below BAM 248 obv. ii 55 and dupl. (= line 110).

351 The restoration of line 4' is based on the Old Babylonian parallels quoted above. Note that the remedy used together with the present incantation in ms. A (lines 38–39) uses a *takkussi qanî ṭābi* "a hollow tube of the sweet reed", see below BAM 248 obv. i 52–53 and dupl. For *takkussu* "hollow(?) reed; tube", see CAD T, 78–79. The Sumerian equivalent (and logogram) of *takkussu* is usually ^{giš}saĝ-kud; thus, the restoration of the Sumerian text in this line (which is based on the Old Babylonian precursor texts) is not entirely certain.

27'–28' (van Dijk 1975, 67),[352] while AUAM 73.3094 rev. 54–57 (Cohen 1976, *RA* 70, 135–139; Wasserman and Zomer 2022, No. 10) speaks of "weapon" and "beer mash (container)".[353] See also *infra* text II.1.1 lines 22–24 for discussion.

Line 13: Here and in the following lines, it cannot be decided whether the interlinear sequences of Sumerian / Akkadian is continued. If that is the case, ms. A obv. i 25 should contain Sumerian text. The reading *pí*[!]*-laq-qí-šá* proposed by Veldhuis (1989, 245) in A obv. i 25 therefore remains uncertain.

Line 17: Veldhuis (1989, 255) reads KIN? at the end of ms. B_2, obv. i 2' but the spacing of the script could also suggest a reading -[í]b-šú-šú, as a Sumerian verbal form of the verb šuš "to cover, to spread over; to overwhelm; to slip through" (Attinger 2021, 1019). The next line may present the Akkadian translation, and the sign traces at the end of ms. B_2 obv. i 3' [. . .-*t*]*ab*[?]*-ka* may perhaps belong to a form of the verb *tabāku* "to pour out; to lay (down)", but this remains uncertain.

Line 18: Similar phrases as in the fragmentary Akkadian line of ms. A obv. i 32 // B_2 obv. i 5' are found in other Akkadian birth incantations of the compendium (see A obv. i 66, A obv. ii 56 and rev. iv 1 below).

Lines 19–21: As was seen by Veldhuis (1989, 242, 245–246), the Sumerian text of these lines can be reconstructed from identical formulaic expressions at the end of other bilingual incantations, see e.g. Udug-ḫul Tablet 4: 63–65 and Tablet 13–15: 118–120 (Geller 2016, 145, 468); see also Abusch and Schwemer 2016, CMAwR 2, text 7.11 sub 1, lines 12–13 (bilingual incantation against witchcraft).

Line 22: The ruling after A obv. i 35 is clearly visible on the museum photo Ass. S 4004, whereas the ruling drawn in Köcher's copy following line A obv. i 36 is doubtful (not clearly visible on the tablet/photograph); there is neither a ruling following ms. B_2 obv. i 9'. Line 22 is therefore regarded as the first line of an incantation (see also Veldhuis 1989, 246), not as a rubric for the preceding incantation (the latter is proposed by Scurlock (2014a, 595) who restores [KA.INIM.MA MUNUS] *šup-šu-*[(*qat a-la-da*)]. Line 22 may be commented on in commentary α (11N-T3):

α 14) ***šup-šuq-tùm-ma*** : *šup-šu-qa*
α 15) *ka-a-šú šá-niš dan-na-ti*
"(The word) *supšuqtum-ma* ('woman in difficult labour') stems from *šupšuqu* ('difficult, distressed') (which means) 'to be delayed' (i.e. in delivery), secondly (it means) 'woman in distress'."

The word *šupšuqtu* "woman in difficult labour" (the feminine adjective of the Š-stem of *pašāqu* "to be in dire straits") is used in other incantations in the Birth Compendium, see A rev. iii 41: ÁB-*mi* EN *šup-šu-qat a-la-da* "a cow, O lord, has difficulty in delivery"; A rev. iv 6: ÉN *šup-šuq-ta re-mi* [d]AMAR.UTU "Spell: Have pity, O Marduk, with the woman in hard labour" (see also the note on line 37 below). The wording of the quotation in commentary α (*supšuqtum-ma*) diverges slightly from *šupšuqat* mss. A and B. Note also the similar formulae in the Middle Assyrian birth incantation *Iraq* 31, 31: 33, which begins: [munus]LA.<RA>.AḪ-*tu šap-šu-qa-at* Ù.TU.MEŠ-*da* "the woman in difficult labour has great difficulty in delivery"; also ibid. 51: *gi-se-en* <<[d]30>> GÉME *šá* [d]30 *a-la-da šap-šu-qa-at* "Gī-Sîn, the maidservant of Sîn, has trouble in delivery".

Lines 22–36: Ms. b (from Hattuša) is included here as an older parallel, although that fragmentary spell is not an exact duplicate of mss. A and B. The earlier text is much shorter and leaves out several lines found in mss. A and B. For the text of ms. b, see also Zomer 2013, *NABU* 2013/2, 45–46 No. 27; Veldhuis 1989, 12–13, 65; SEAL no. 7233 and 7234. For similar older birth incantations with the motif of the cow, see e.g. *BiOr* 75, 19–20 (Old Babylonian; Wasserman 2018, 18–20; Wasserman and Zomer 2022, No. 3); VS 17, 34: 1–20 (Old Babylonian; Wasserman and Zomer 2022, No. 12), kt 90/k 178: 1–23 (Old Assyrian; Michel 2004, *FS Larsen*, 397, 399; Wasserman and Zomer 2022, No. 9); CCT 5, 50e: 1'–14' (Old Assyrian; Kouwenberg

352 Both items are also given in the Sumerian incantation AUAM 73.1425 iv 7–12 (Rudik 2011, 327–331, Ur III period). The keyword "pin; hair needle" (kirid; *kirissu*) is not preserved in ms. A, but commented on in commentary α (11N-T3: 14; text G.1).

353 See also Wasserman and Zomer 2022, 84 for discussion, who understand "weapon" (tukul, *kakku*) and "crucible" (ga-ri-im, for *agarin* = *agarinnu* "matrix, crucible, container for beer mash/sourdough") as euphemisms for the male and female sexual organs (cf. Steinert 2017a, 300–301). For the formula "if it is a boy . . . if it is a girl . . .", see further Michel and Wasserman 1997, *NABU* 1997/2, no. 64; VS 17, 34: 16–18 (Wasserman and Zomer 2022, No. 12). For spindle and pin ([giš]balak / *pilakk/qqu*; [giš]kirid / *kirissu*) as objects representing femininity, see further PSD B, 64 s.v. bala B; Attinger 2021, 630; CAD K 407 s.v. *kirissu*; CAD P 371–373 s.v. *pilakku*; Green 1998–2001, "Nadel", *RlA* 9, 70–71 § 3.2.1; Waetzoldt 2011–2013a, "Spinnen. A. Philologisch", *RlA* 13, 2 § 2.

and Fincke 2012–2013, *JEOL* 44, 141–146; Wasserman and Zomer 2022, No. 5); kt 94/k 429: 1–24 (Barjamovic 2015, *SANER* 9, 75–77 (Old Assyrian; Wasserman and Zomer 2022, No. 11). See also the compositions in lines 135–160 ("A Cow of Sîn", A rev. iii 10–35 //), lines 163–172 (A rev. iii 36–45 //) and lines 181–193 (A rev. iii 54–iv 1 //) in the Birth Compendium.

Line 23: The restoration of ms. A follows suggestions made by M. Stol (personal communication) and Scurlock 2014a, 618 note 41. Following Stol, I read *ep-ri* as *eperu* "dust", which may stand for a stage in the formation of the foetus from semen (and thus allude to the creation of humankind from clay in anthropogonic myths; cf. the creation of Adam from dust in Genesis 2). Scurlock (2014a, 595, 6) reads *ib-ri* instead and translates the line "([the cow of Sîn] took in [the semen] and so made clouds", presumably connecting the word *ib-ri* with *imbaru/ibbaru* "fog, cloud". Scurlock connects the reference to clouds with the following comparison of the woman as a full waterskin, which she interprets as a reference to the cow's udders filling with milk. However, the simile of the waterskin could also refer to the woman's/cow's womb/belly containing a full-term baby. This is reminiscent of similar imagery referring to the pregnant woman as a loaded boat (*eleppu malītu*, see KAR 223 and dupl., *infra* text D.3.1). For the image of the waterskin, see also K. 263 + 10934: line 43 (Steinert 2012b, 68, 70–71; *infra* text C.1.5).

For the particle *–mi* (in Ms. b 15': *ar-ḫi-mi*) is common in Old Assyrian and Old Babylonian incantations, see Farber 1996, *NABU* 1996/3, 71, no. 80; Wasserman 2012, 189, the latter of whom interprets it as indicating an address to the cow (*-mi* is also attested in Old Babylonian letters to introduce direct speech). See also line 168 (A rev. iii 71) below (ÁB-*mi*).

Lines 24–25: Ms. A is restored after ms. b and a similar passage in ms. A rev. iii 56–57 (see lines 182–184 below), in which the cow speaks: *ina* SI-*ia*$_5$ *qaq-qa-ru ṭe-ra-ku* / *ina* KUN-*ia*$_5$ *uš-te-eš-še-ra tur-bu-'-i* "With my horn(s) I root up the ground, with my tail I whirl up dust clouds". Ms. b uses a Š-stem form, ms. A rev. iii 57 the Št-form (durative) of *ešēru* in the meaning "to sweep; whirl up"; it is possible to restore either form here (*ušeššera* or *ušteššera*).

In addition to ms. b from Hattuša, two Old Assyrian birth incantations offer direct parallels, especially kt 90/k 178: 5–8 (Wasserman and Zomer 2022, No. 9): *i-na* / *a-pí-ša qá-qá-ra-am* | *té-sú-uq* / *i-zi-bi-tí-ša* | *ta-ša-bi-iṭ* / *bé-tám* "With her nose she *brushes* the ground; with her tail she sweeps the house."[354] The phrase "she roots up the ground with her horns" (*ina qar-ni-šú qaq-qar ṭe-ra-at*) in line 24 is also quoted and commented on in the commentaries α lines 15–17 and β obv. 1', which allows us to restore the original text (see texts G.1–G.2 for discussion). In ms. A obv. i 38, there is space for *ina* KUN-*šá* at the end of line 24, whereas ms. B$_2$ obv. i 11' ends with *ṭe-ra-at*. Thus, the text is spread out differently over lines 24 and 25 in mss. A and B$_2$ (the text distribution in line 25 also differs in both mss.). For the verb *ṭerû*, used in a transitive stative form with the meaning "to pierce, to penetrate", cf. CAD Ṭ, 104 s.v. *ṭerû* C sub b (differentiating this usage from *ṭerû* A "to squeeze out / rub" and *ṭerû* "to beat"), while AHw 1388–1389 and SAD 2, 116 assume one polysemous verb (cf. further Farber 1976, *BiOr* 33, 331–332 for discussion). Beside the passages from the Birth Compendium, the verb is also used with reference to the moon's "horns" piercing the sky.

Lines 26–27 and 29: Ms. A obv. i 41 (line 27) has been emended against Ebeling's copy and the parallel manuscripts. Most of the signs are not clearly visible on the photo. The present passage resembles the Old Babylonian birth incantation VS 17, 34 obv. 7–10:

> *am-mi-nim-mi* ^{d}UTU *i-bak-ki* / [*e*]*l-lam-me-e i-il-la-ka di-ma-šu* / [*a-n*]*a ar-ḫi-ia-mi la-a pe-ti-i-tim* / [*ú*]*-ni-qí-ia la wa-li-it-*⌈*tim*⌉
> "Why is Šamaš crying, (why) are Ella-mê's tears flowing down?" – "Over my cow, (who has) not yet mated, (over) my kid, (who has) never given birth!" (van Dijk 1972, 343–344; Stol 2000a, 64; Veldhuis 1989, 243; Wasserman and Zomer 2022, No. 12)

The moon god's name Ella-mê (lit. "the one pure of rites") restored in lines 26 and 27 of the Compendium is analysed in both commentaries (α 17–20 and β obv. 2'–5'). Commentary β obv. 2' (UET 6/3, 897) quotes a complete phrase from the base text: [*šá*? el-l]*am-me-e* DU.⌈MEŠ?⌉*-ak d*[*i*]-⌈*ma*⌉-[*a-šú* x x] "Ella(m)-mê's are tears flowing [. . .]".

The end of line 29 in ms. A can be restored from the commentaries which both quote and analyse the passage (see chapter G for discussion):

> α 21) ***aš-šum* ÁB*-ia la a-lit-ti*** *áš-šú* ^{d}30 EN *la-a-tu*$_4$ *el-le-e-ti*
> β obv. 6') ***áš-šú* ÁB*-ia*$_5$ *la a-lit-ti*** : ⌈*áš-šú*⌉ [^{d}30 EN *la*]-⌈*a-tim*⌉ KÙ.MEŠ
> "'Because of my cow (who has) never given birth': (this is said) because of Sîn, the lord of the pure cows."

354 This text shares similarities with CCT 5, 50e obv. 1'–5', likewise from Kaneš (Wasserman and Zomer 2022, No. 5).

On the sound play in the phrase (*aššum*) *littīya lā ālitti* "my cow (who has) never given birth", see Veldhuis 1989, 257 note 4; Veldhuis 1991, 20.

Line 32: For the *manna(m) lušpur*-formula, see Farber 1990. In the birth compendium, it is the healing gods Marduk/Asalluḫi and Ea who are "sent for" to intervene, see the parallel line A rev. iii 60 (with note below).

Lines 33–34: The "quay of difficulty/distress", where the woman (pictured as a boat) is held back, is found several times in the incantations of the Birth Compendium. The use of the verb *parāru* "to become detached; to be dissolved" (in the G-stem) in line 33 is unusual (cf. CAD P, 161–164), and the boat should probably be understood here as the subject of *liprur(u)*. AHw 830a s.v. *parāru* sub 3 regards the form as a possible mistake for *lipṭurū*, as in the parallel couplet in ms. A rev. iii 61–62: [*ina* KAR *mu*]-*ti lip-ṭu-ru* ^{giš}MÁ / [*ina* KAR *dan-na-ti li*]-*ram-ma-a* ^{giš}MÁ.GUR$_8$ "[At the quay of dea]th let them (masc.) loosen the ship, [at the quay of distress] let them (fem.) untie the cargo boat!"). A obv. i 47–48 and rev. iii 61–62 are parallel in structure, but the verbs differ in both passages (A obv. i 47–48: *parāru* / (*w*)*uššuru* vs. A rev. iii 61–62: *paṭāru* / *rummû*). CAD U/W, s.v. *uššuru* sub 1d translates the verb *limaššera* in line 34 "let him set free the barge", assuming a singular form with a ventive and the god Marduk as the subject rather than assuming a feminine plural form, which is followed here.

Line 35: The reconstruction follows A rev. iii 44, replacing verbal forms in the precative with imperative forms: *li-ṣa-a* GIN$_7$ MUŠ *ki-ma* MUŠ.TUR *liš-šá-li-la* "May it (the calf) come out like a snake! May it glide out like a *nirāḫu*-snake!" Both commentaries on the birth compendium comment on the words *nešelpû* (*nešalpû*) "to glide, slither" (the imperative form used in the base text is quoted first) and *nirāḫu* (a kind of snake, logographically written MUŠ.TUR, lit. "little snake") used in line 35 (see ms. α 23–26 and β obv. 7'; texts G.1–G.2). A Late Babylonian commentary on *Šumma ālu* Tablet 21 (SpTU 5, No. 259 obv. 12') explains *nirāḫu* as "a thin snake that is very long" (MUŠ *qát-nu šá ma-gal ár-ki*).

Line 36: For the reading ⸢SILIM⸣-*ma*, see Scurlock 2014a, 595. Perhaps, the text should be emended to ⸢*liš*$^!$-*lim*$^!$⸣-*ma*.

Line 37: For the rubric KA.INIM.MA ^{munus}LA.RA.AḪ.A.KÁM, which is also listed as an incantation genre in the so-called Exorcist's Manual (KAR 44: 15 and dupl.), see Stol 2000a, 129–130; Geller 2000a, *FS Lambert*, 253 ad line 15; Geller 2018a, 298; Heeßel 2023, 294. This rubric replaces the rubric KA.INIM.MA MUNUS.Ù.TU.(DA.KAM) "wording (of an incantation) for a woman in labour" common in Old Babylonian birth incantations (see Wasserman and Zomer 2022, No. 6 (CUSAS 32, 26a): 13', No. 8 (CUSAS 32, 29b): 30, No. 10 (RA 70, 137): 61, No. 12 (VS 17, 34): 20, No. 13 (YOS 11, 17): 6, No. 14 (YOS 11, 86a): 28.[355]

The incantation rubric KA.INIM.MA ^{munus}LA.RA.AḪ.A.KÁM is commented on in both commentaries (α 26–27 and β obv. 7'–8'); see chapter G for discussion), focusing on the term laraḫ, which is equated with Akkadian words that occur several times in the incantations within the birth compendium (*pušqu* "narrowness, straits", *dannatu* "difficulty, hardship").

For *muštapšiqtu* or *mušapšiqtu* as readings of ^{munus}LA.RA.AḪ, see CAD M/2, 259–260, 285. Note especially the Middle Assyrian birth incantation *Iraq* 31, 31: 33–50 having the rubric *šiptu ša multapšiqte*, as well as KUB 4, 13: 13' KA.INIM.(-)MA ÉN *mušapš*[*iqti*] (see line 161 ms. b). The equation is also found in the line *Iraq* 31, 31: 62 *lūlid ardatu* ^{munus}LA.RA.AḪ.(-)MEŠ (ms. D), which is parallel to A rev. iii 34 *līlid ardatu mušapšiqtu* "may the young woman who has difficulty in delivery give birth" (see line 159 below). Lexical texts furthermore equate ^{munus}LA.RA.AḪ with the feminine adjective *šupšuqtu* "(woman) having difficulty in delivery" (see CAD Š/3, 327). Stol (2000a, 123 n. 83) connects laraḫ with Akkadian *lā aruḫtu* "one who is not hastened" (i.e. a woman who is delayed in her delivery). Note in this connection that the term *aruḫtu* lit. "hastened woman" (i.e. woman in travail) is attested in the rubric *šipat aruḫtim* "incantation for a woman in labour" in the Old Babylonian birth incantation BM 115745 (Steinert 2017b, *FS Wiggermann*, 224–225; Wasserman and Zomer 2022, No. 4 line 15; *infra* text II.1.2).

Lines 38–39: In ms. a, the spelling *uš-te-še-<<eš>>-ri* is apparently an erroneous form of *uštešš*er (Št^2-stem durative of *ešēru*).

Scurlock (2014a, 596) emends the end of line 39 in A obv. i 53 to *ina* UGU ŠÀ-*šá* ḪÁŠ$^!$-[*šá* EŠ] "you [rub it gently] over her abdomen (and) [her] hypogastric region (*emšu*)". However, the parallel ritual found in the Old Babylonian birth incantation AUAM 73.3094 (Cohen 1976, *RA* 70, 135–139; Wasserman and Zomer 2022, No. 10 lines 42–53) and the Babylonian commentaries on the birth compendium commenting on the same ritual speak against the emendation. See the notes on lines 6–11 above.

355 For the varying sign forms of É in ÉN.É.NU.RU (in Ms. b lines 15' and 22'), see Zomer 2013, *NABU* 2013/2, no. 27.

The text of lines 38–39 suggests that the same ritual using a hollow reed filled with oil or dust from a crossroads that is described within the Old Babylonian birth incantation AUAM 73.3094 (Wasserman and Zomer 2022, No. 10) has become independent (in the form of a ritual instruction) and is utilized for performance together with another birth incantation (here lines 22–36). The ritual action of breaking (*ḫepû*) the reed filled with oil or dust from a crossroads above the woman's belly would release the materials contained in the reed onto the woman's abdomen; it probably symbolized a quick process of delivery. The commentaries on the Birth Compendium (text G.1–G.2) provide us with the explanation of the underlying symbolism or logic: The reed represents the woman's body or birth canal (equating the word gi "reed" with *sinništu* "woman"); the materials filled into the reed (dust and fat/oil) allude to semen and the baby/foetus, although in the present context oil could also represent the amniotic fluid. The ingredient "dust" may also be a pun for clay as the "fertile stuff or creation". For discussion of the interrelated text passages, see also Steinert 2017a, 335–340.

For a similar ritual in which dust and oil are filled into a reed, with which the woman is massaged, see A rev. iii 46–53 (with note below).

Lines 40–47: This incantation, only fragmentarily preserved in ms. A, can be restored with the help of the new duplicate ms. a. The divine names in this spell are of Elamite origin, and therefore perhaps all of lines 40–41 are to be interpreted as Elamite, if not mumbo-jumbo-like words (note however the word laraḫ "dire straits" at the end of lines 40 and 41). For a differing reading of lines 40–41, see *Electronic Babylonian Library* (eBL), sub BM.36339.

The deities Nap(i)riša (lit. "great god") and his consort Kiririša ("great lady") in line 42 (consisting of the Elamite words nap "god", kiri "goddess" and rišu/riša "great") form a divine triad of senior rank together with the god Inšušinak. Kiririša was a sky goddess and is called "mother of the gods"; she seems to have been responsible for battle and combat. Napiriša (often written DINGIR.GAL), was the lord of the earth. In a commentary on the incantation series *Šurpu* II 163 (where he occurs as [*Nap*]-*ru-šu* among other Elamite deities), he is equated with Ea (he is called "Ea of Elam" there; Reiner 1958, 17, 50 commentary B line 3). See further H. Koch 1998–2001a, "Napiriša", *RlA* 9, 163–164; Koch 2011, 55–56, 61–62, 127; Jahangirfar 2018, 108, 110–112.

The names of the Elamite deities Naḫ(ḫ)unte (Naḫunde) and Narunde (also Narudu/a/i) in line 44 are commented on in both commentaries (β obv. 9' and α 27). Both deities are addressed in another Akkadian incantation in the Birth Compendium (A rev. iii 40 = line 167, see below). Naḫ(ḫ)unte as the Elamite sun god belongs to the so-called "divine Seven of Elam"; the goddess Narunde is regarded as his sister (for Naḫ(ḫ)unte and Narunde as siblings, see also An = *Anum* VI 181 and 184). Commentaries α and β mistakenly equate Narunde with Šamaš and Naḫ(ḫ)unte with Sîn (see texts G.1–G.2).[356]

Both Narunde and Naḫḫunte are already attested in Old Elamite texts (from ca. 2300 BCE onwards). The occurrence of deities such as Kiririša, Napiriša and Narunde in birth incantations in Elamite on tablets from the Old Babylonian period (e.g. YOS 11, 18 // OECT 11, 5; van Dijk 1982, 100; Krebernik 2018, 31 Nos. 13–14) suggests a longstanding connection of the deities to childbirth and the protection of women and children. Moreover, Narunde and Naḫḫunte occur repeatedly in other Elamite incantations (for different purposes) on Old Babylonian tablets (Krebernik 2018, 23 Nos. 4–5 (LB 1003 // 1004, copied in Wasserman 2020, *BiOr* 77, 458), 25, 48 (HS 2338), 38 No. 45 (YOS 11, 5)). The preservation of these connections in first millennium BCE texts also implies that Elamite magical lore enjoyed continued popularity in the Mesopotamian healing traditions.[357]

Line 42: If the word *uṭ*$^?$-*ṭa-ab-ba* fully preserved in ms. a is to be understood as Akkadian, this could be interpreted as a Dt-stem present tense form of *ṭebû* "to sink, submerge", which in the D-stem can have the meaning "to settle, clear up" (a matter), especially in Old Assyrian texts (CAD Ṭ 70 sub mng. 4, SAD Vol. 2, 115). The Dt-stem of *ṭebû* could present a passive nuance here and refer to the elimination of the birthing difficulty/obstruction in delivery.

Line 45: This line is quoted and commented on in commentary α lines 28–30. The variant quoted is from ms. A: *na-am-li-su ki-ma ṣa-bi-tu*$_4$ "Be *plucked* like a gazelle" (from *malāsu* "to pluck"). Ms. a however, seems to preserve [*na-a*]*p*$^?$-*li-sa ki-ma*

356 For discussion, see also Civil 1974, *JNES* 33, 332: 27; van Dijk 1975, 53, 79; Vallat 1983, 95 note 4; Finkel 1997, *NABU* 1997/1, 22 with n. 3; Stolper 1998–2001, "Naḫḫunte", *RlA* 9, 82–84, esp. § 3; Koch 1998–2001b, "Narunde", *RlA* 9, 180; Koch 2011, 50–51, 63–64.

357 For discussion of incantations in Elamite and other alien languages including the question of abracadabra-spells, see also van Dijk 1982, 99–100, 104–105; Lambert 1983; van Dijk, Goetze and Hussey 1985, *YOS* 11, 3–4; Cunningham 1997, 156–157; Veldhuis 1999, 46–48; Prechel and Richter 2001, in: *FS Haas*, 334; George 2016, *CUSAS* 32, 90, 142–143 (No. 21b), 161–162; Finkel 2014, 62–63; Krebernik 2018; Baragli 2019, *KASKAL* 16, 293–321.

MAŠ.DÀ "[lo]ok (at me) like a gazelle" (N-stem of *palāsu*). The Nippur commentary offers explanations for the occurrence of both textual variants:

> α 28) ***na-am-li-su ki-ma ṣa-bi-tu***$_4$: zé : *ma-la-su* : zé : *ba-qa-mu*
> α 29) *šá-niš na-am-li-su lìb-bu-u nap-lu-su* : *a-ma-ra*
> "(In) '*Be plucked* like a gazelle', (Sumerian) zé (means) 'to pluck' (*malāsu*), (which is the same as) zé (which also means) *baqāmu* 'to pluck (hair or wool)'. Alternatively: *namlisu* (is the same) as in *naplusu* ("to look at"), (which is the same as) 'to see' (*amāru*)."

The commentary posits that *na-am-li-su* can also be interpreted as derived from the verb *naplusu* "to look", possibly because different variants of the source text were in fact known to the commentator(?).

Perhaps because of the similar line in BAM 248 rev. iv 2, *lusma kīma ṣabīti* "run hither to me (*lasāmu*) like a gazelle", CAD M/1, 161 (s.v. *malāšu*) suggests a translation "run(?)" for *namlisu* in BAM 248 iv 59. But taking seriously the meaning of *malāsu* pointed out in the commentary, the N-stem form should rather be translated as "Be plucked out like a gazelle!", unless *namlisu* is considered as a phonetic variant of *naplis(u)* "look" in ms. a. The word "to pluck" is used in a poetic way here as a metaphor for the desired easy delivery of child. The birth of gazelles and other wild animals (especially snakes) repeatedly appears as an image of ideal birth in the birth incantations (see e.g., Bergmann 2008, 45–46; Steinert 2017a, 328–329).

Line 47: The reading of ms. A follows ms. a and Ebeling's copy, which can be read [. . . *šab*]-*šá*-⌜*ku*$^{?}$⌝ *a*-⌜*maḫ*$^{!}$-*ḫar*⌝-[*k*]*a* ÉN; Köcher's copy differs and reads ([. . .]-⌜*ku*$^{?}$⌝ *a-maḫ*$^{!}$-*ḫar-šu* "I will receive him". See also the almost identical line in ms. A rev. iv 3 (line 195): *ana-ku* ^{d}*asal-lú-ḫi šab-sa-ku a-maḫ-ḫar-ka* "I, Asalluḫi, am the midwife! I will receive you". The specific nuance of the verb *maḫāru* "to receive, to confront" here may be "be ready for; to welcome" (see CAD M/1, 63–64 sub mng. 4a-1').

Lines 48–49: See also ms. A rev. iii 58–59 (lines 185–186) for the same couplet in another incantation of the Birth Compendium.

Line 50: The emendation of ms. A follows commentary β obv. 10' which quotes the exclamation *ulla Šamaš* "now, O Šamaš", while commentary α 30–31 provides explanations on the rare interjection *ulla* "well, now" (cf. CAD U/W, 74b):

> β obv. 10') ***ul-la*** ^{d}**UTU**: *ul-la* : *an*-[*na* x$^{?}$]
> α 30–31) . . . ***ul-la*** : *an-na* / *an-na* : *qí-bi-ti šá-niš ul-la* : *ul-la* Ì$^{i-'-u}$: *šá-am-nu*
> "(In) 'Well now (*ulla*), Šamaš', *ulla* (means) 'yes' (Akk. *anna*); *anna* (also means) 'divine pronouncement, command' (*qibītu*); alternatively, *ulla* means 'oil' (i.e. *ulû*), (because the sign) Ì (pronounced) *i'u* (means) 'oil' (*šamnu*)."

Line 52: A different reading of line 52 was proposed by Stol 2000a, 67 n. 117, but the line can now be restored completely with the help of ms. a. For lines 47–52, see also Reiner 1978, 192.

Lines 54–55: The prescription appears to differ slightly in mss. A and a. The end of line 54 in ms. A may contain a reference to a container(?) unless the signs read *ana* ŠÀ [. . .] should be emended to *šá*$^{!}$ ŠÀ [. . .] (i.e. an arrow *from the inside of* . . .). Ms. a gives a unique instruction: to use an arrow *šá ina pi-i* ⌜^{giš}⌝BAN$^{?}$ / [*ú*]-*ṣu-ú* "that has gone out from the *mouth of a bow*(?)". (The reading of the passage follows the *Electronic Babylonian Library Project* (eBL, BM.36339 rev. 6–7), improving the reading in Steinert 2021a, *Byzantinische Forschungen* 33, 44 n. 23, "(an arrow) that has been removed from a wound(?), *šá ina pi-i-tu*$_4^{?}$ / [*ú-š*]*e*$^{?}$-*ṣu-ú*). The unusual expression presumably refers to an arrow that has been shot from a bow before. The idiom "mouth of a bow" is otherwise unattested. The bow and arrow may be a metaphor for the penis and the male semen – a comparison that is found, for example, in the Talmud (M. J. Geller, personal communication). Within the cuneiform textual sources, bows, arrows, and bowstrings are intimately associated with the (erect) penis and male sexuality/potency in the ŠÀ.ZI.GA-rituals to promote sexual desire (Zisa 2021, 120, 105–200, 205 *passim*).

In line 55 in ms. A, there does not seem to be enough space for reconstructing *tu-maš-šá-a'-ma šèr-ri* SI.SÁ (as found in ms. a), and the word *šaplān* may have been followed by a genitive noun (e.g. *ana šaplān libbīša* ŠÉŠ-*ma* SI.SÁ "you rub (her from the top) toward the bottom of her belly and she will give birth easily"). For a similar instruction, see also A rev. iii 53 (line 180): TA *e-le-nu ana šap-la-nu tu-maš-šá-a'* "you rub it (over her bulging belly) from top to bottom" (ms. a has the variant *e-la-nu* found in some Standard/Late Babylonian texts, cf. AHw 198).

The ingredients of the prescription in lines 54–55 (*šaman pūri* (Ì.GIŠ BUR) "oil-from-the-jar" and the arrow (*šiltāḫu*, ^{giš}GAG.U$_4$.TAG.GA, with which the oil is stirred) are commented on in the commentaries on the birth compendium (11N-T3: 31–37; UET 6/3, 897 obv. 11'–13'; see texts G.1–G.2 for discussion).

Lines 56–130: It is not entirely certain whether ms. A obv. ii 1–rev. iii 5 contains the text of only one lengthy incantation (the longest of the whole compendium), since the first thirteen lines of column ii are completely lost. The commentaries on the birth compendium do not provide clarity on this point. In any case, the quoted text passages in commentaries α 37–40 (11N-T3) and β rev. 1'–4' (UET 6/3, 897) that cannot be assigned to another incantation in the compendium, appear to be concerned with the lost twenty-odd lines in ms. A col. ii (see below).

It is notable that several lines of the spell in ms. A obv. ii–rev. iii 5 share such close similarities with the text of a Middle Assyrian birth incantation (ms. D lines 33–49) that the latter text may be regarded as a shorter precursor or older model for the more elaborate and lengthy composition in ms. A obv. ii 1–rev. iii 5. The better-preserved parts of the spell in ms. A drawing on ms. D describe the suffering of the woman in difficult childbirth in vivid imagery (lines 77–86). In the following lines, the mother goddess (Mami, Aruru) is addressed in her capacity as a birth helper (lines 87–97). Then in lines 98–114, Marduk/Asalluḫi is called upon to take pity on the woman in travail and to bring forth the baby, perhaps by the mother goddess herself. This seems to be implied by the final lines of the spell (lines 128–130), which attribute the incantation to Ea and Asalluḫi saying it was created upon Mami's request. For the images encountered in this and other birth incantations (the woman as a warrior, doors and knots, the boat), see e.g. Bergmann 2008, 50–56; Couto-Ferraira 2014, 292, 310–311; Steinert 2017a, 323–335. For a complete edition of ms. D, see *infra* text II.1.4; Scurlock 2014a, 605–608; Zomer 2018, 254–256 (edition of lines 33–50).

Lines 56–68: The commentaries α 37–40 and β rev. 1'–4' appear to provide comments on the lost incantation passage in the upper section of ms. A obv. ii. The first respective entry in commentary α 37 quotes two name(s) of the cow in the famous incantation "A Cow of Sîn", Egizinītu and Geme-Sîn, and equates them with each other (see text G.1). However, these two names of the cow also appear in other incantations in the compendium. The incipit of the incantation "I am the (big) cow of Sîn, belonging to Sîn" (*litti Sîn ša Sîn anāku*) in ms. A rev. iii 54 has a variant in ms. a (BM 36339 rev. 9) that renders the name of the cow *E-gi-zi-ni-tu*$_4$, the form quoted in commentary α 37 (*e-gi-zi-ni-ti*). Egizinītu is the Akkadian rendering of the Sumerian names Egi-Suena, Gī-Sîn and Geme-Sîn. The latter names are found in the well-known incantation "A Cow of Sîn" (*iltēt littu ša Sîn Geme-Sîn šumša*, lines 135–160, ms. A rev. iii 10–35, especially line 135 and 158) and in a related spell (*Narunde Naḫḫunte u Nanamgišir*, lines 163–172, A rev. iii 36–45, especially lines 164 and 170). The form Egi-Suena is found in BAM 248 rev. iii 43 (line 170): *šá* ÁB *e-gi-*^{d}EN.ZU.NA *lip-pe-tu-ú pa-nu-šá* "let the 'face' of the cow Egi-Suena be opened". Note also ms. D (*Iraq* 31, 31: 51: *gi-se-en* <<^{d}30>> GÉME *šá* ^{d}30 *a-la-da šap-šu-qa-at* "Gī-Sîn, the maidservant of Sîn, has trouble in childbirth"; and ibid. 61: *gi-i-*^{d}30 GÉME *ša* ^{d}30.

The next passage in commentary α that most likely can be assigned to the lost beginning of A obv. ii concerns an unknown quotation from the base text, in which someone speaks in the first person:

α 37) ***ina* SAG.DU-*ia*$_5$ *na-ma-ra***
α 38) *na-ma-ra* : KASKAL.MIN *šá* ^{giš}GI *u* ^{giš}TIR
β rev. 1') ***na-ma-ri*** ⸢:⸣ ⸢KASKAL$^{?}$⸣ [. . . . . .]
"(In) 'The clearing in front of me' (lit. at my head) 'clearing' (*namāru*) (means) a path (in) a reed thicket or a forest."

The first-person perspective can be compared with a similar passage inserted in line 101 (A obv. ii 46) later in the text of the spell, the latter of which can be interpreted as the voice of the woman in dire straits, or as the voice of the baby to be born and trapped inside its mother (cf. note below). The image of a "clearing" or path that is opened for the baby out of the womb is found in other birth incantations, see Couto-Ferreira 2014, 310; Wasserman and Zomer 2022, No. 14 lines 12–17 and line 52 of the Birth Compendium.

The following commentary passages in α (11N-T3: 38–40) and β (UET 6/3, 897 rev. 2'–4') turn to yet another motif: the woman as a loaded boat travelling on a stream or sea, and the baby as the creature inside a shell – the latter is explained as another metaphor for the pregnant woman (for these images, see e.g. Bergmann 2008, 52–54; Couto-Ferreira 2014, 310; Steinert 2017a, 323–326, 332–335 and lines 1, 3–5, 30–34, 48–49, 91, 102–107 in the birth compendium). Both commentaries quote a complete sentence from the base text, unfortunately not preserved.[358] In this quotation, the agent who is to "show the one inside the shell the (day)light" (*ša libbi išqillati likallim nūru*) is the sun god Šamaš (for this motif, see also lines 36, 52, 111, 124 and 193 of the Birth Compendium).

Line 71: For the end of the line in ms. A compare a similar passage in ms. D (*Iraq* 31, 31: 36): *sa-ni-iq* KÁ-*bu ana ti-nu-qí ka*!(la)-*lu-ú pi-it* ARḪUŠ-*mu* "the door is *closed* (lit. fastened) against the suckling infant, the opening of the womb is blocked". See also *Iraq* 31, 31: 53: *sa-ni-iq* KÁ-*bu ana ti*!(nu)-*nu*!(ti)-*qí la-ku*!(lu) -*ú* "the door is *closed* for the suckling infant". See *infra* text II.1.4.

Lines 77–84: This passage is parallel to the text of the Middle Assyrian birth incantation of ms. D 37–45 (see text II.1.4 for this composition).

Line 78: The restoration proposed by Civil (1974, 335) and Veldhuis (1989, 244), [*iš-q*]*il*?-*la*-[*tu*$_4$ . . .] UB [. . . . . .] DI, is possible against the photograph of ms. A, but the end of the line does not fit the citation in commentaries α 38–39 and β rev. 3'–4' (*šá* ŠÀ *iš-qil-la-tu*$_4$ *li-kal-lim nu-ú-rum* "let him (Šamaš) expose the one inside the shell to the light"). The emendation gišAPIN! follows the parallel in ms. D. For reading *kīdu* at the end of line in ms. A, compare the equation *ra-aḫ ki-di* "inseminator of the open land" for *epinnu* "plough" (An IX 108, see CT 18, 6 rev. 48; *malku* = *šarru* III 63, see Hrůša 2010, 68–69, 230–231). For the emendation in ms. D 39, see Foster 2019, *NABU* 2019/2, no. 47 and *infra*.

Line 83: For the meaning of the stative of the verb *sanāqu* "to approach; to supervise, control" in *ul sanqat irassu* "her breast is not restrained", compare also the expression *saniq bābu* "the door is fastened" in *Iraq* 31, 31: 36 and 53 (ms. D, see note on line 71 above); CAD S, 140 s.v. *sanāqu* A sub 5b ("to be fastened"). Ms. D has *sa-qa-at* instead of *sa-an-q*[*a-at*] in ms. A; the former has been interpreted as an Assyrian feminine stative form of *sâqu* "to be(come) narrow, tight" (CAD S 169, translating this "her breast (or pectoral) is not restrained", see also Zomer 2028, 255). Commentary β which quotes the passage, also has *sanqat*, which raises the possibility of a defective writing in *sa-qa-at* of ms. D.

The form *sà-pu-ḫu* is interpreted as an Assyrian D-stem stative form (3rd masc. plural, instead of *suppuḫū*) of *sapāḫu* "to scatter, disperse" (CAD S, 154a sub 5a; CAD S, 169b translates "her headbands (*kulūlūša*) are flying"; cf. Zomer 2022, 255).

Commentary β rev. 5'–6' quotes line 83, but it presents a variation from the wording of the base text (see text G.2 for discussion).

Line 84: Note the variant *pu-ṣu-ni ul pa-ṣu-na-at bul-ta ul ti-šu* in ms. D against ⸢*pu*⸣!-*su-um-m*[*i*] ⸢*ul pu-su-na*⸣-[*at bul-t*]*a ul i*-[*ši*] in ms. A (cf. CAD P, 537 s.v. *pussunu*; CAD P, 537 s.v. *pusummu*). The word *pusummu/puṣunnu* "veil" appears to stand in the plural in both texts, as the ending in -*i* suggests.

Line 85: The traces at the end of the line in ms. A obv. ii 30 were not copied by F. Köcher in BAM 248. On line 85, see the commentaries α 40–44 and β rev. 7'–8' (texts G.1 and G.2) for discussion. The former quotes a phrase from this line: *uš-šu-rat ḫur-da-at-su* "her vulva is set straight".

Line 87: The word *dannatu* is ambiguous here due to the gaps. It can either be understood as the feminine form of the verbal adjective *dannu* "strong" and thus as an attribute of the mother goddess Aruru, or as the noun *dannatu*, which repeatedly occurs in the birth incantations in the meaning "difficulty, hardship".

Line 96: For the phrase *uššurat pēressa*, compare the Lamaštu incantation AO 6473 rev. 15 and dupl., describing the demoness: *uššurat pēressa buttuqā dīdāša* "her (Lamaštu's) hair is hanging loose, her loincloths are torn off" (CAD P, s.v. *pirtu* sub b; Farber 2014, 268, 298 and *infra* text D.3.9 line 43).

Line 97: At the beginning of A obv. ii 42, both Ebeling's and Köcher's copies read *mim-ma*, but this conflicts with ms. B$_2$ obv. ii 12', which reads *ina ú-ri-š*[*á*] "on her vulva"; hence the suggested emendation GAL$_4$.LA!?-[*šá*] in ms. A. In any case, the exact wording of this line appears to have differed in mss. A and B$_2$.

358 Both Civil (1974, 335) and Veldhuis (1989, 244) restore the line cited in the commentary in BAM 248 obv. ii 23 (against Ebeling's copy of KAR 196), reading [*iš-q*]*il*?-*la*-[*tu*$_4$ . . .] UB [. . .] DI. However, the remaining traces at the end of that line do not fit the citation given in both commentaries. BAM 248 obv. ii 23 can now be restored differently, see below line 78.

Line 98: The sign copied by Köcher after *dan-ni* looks like QA. The emendation [*u*]*d-dan-ni-na*$^{!}$ *mar*$^{?}$-⸢*kas*⸣-[*s*]*a*$^{?}$ is inspired by line 104 below: *dan-nu lip-pa-ṭir mar-kas-sa* "May her strong mooring rope be slackened". The verb *uddannina* can be interpreted as a Dt-stem form of *danānu*, which can have a passive nuance "to be reinforced", meaning that the rope of the boat is made fast.

Line 99: The rare body part term *kittabru* in the phrase *ina kittabrīšu* "at her side" is quoted and commented on in both commentaries on the Birth Compendium (α 43–44; β rev. 8'–9'), both of which consider it as a synonym to *idu* "arm, side" (see *infra*). Ms. D uses a different wording instead of *ina kittabrīšu iziza* "stand at her side".

The variant phrase GUB-*za*-<<*ma*>>-*am-ma* DUG$_4$.GA.MEŠ-*si* in ms. D could be read as two consecutive imperatives (i.e. "stand by and keep calling out (*šitassi*) (O Marduk)". Although the logogram DUG$_4$.GA usually stands for *qabû* "to speak", the phonetic complement -*si* suggests rather the verb *šasû* (Scurlock 2014a, 608 translates "stand by and say something to her", but in this case we would expect the pronominal suffix -*ši* not -*si*). Zomer (2018, 254–256) emends to DUG$_4$.GA.MEŠ-*ia*$^{!?}$(SI) and translates "*listen to my utterance* (*qabû*)", in which case the expected verb *šimi* "listen" would be completely missing. Given the first-person passage in line 101, a different interpretation may be proposed, in which DUG$_4$.GA.MEŠ-*si* refers to the woman in labour crying out in pain, assuming a durative form of the Gtn-stem of *šasû* (*ištanassi* "while she keeps crying out"). See also the note on line 101.

Line 100: The phrase *qīp napšāti* serving as a laudatory epithet of Marduk is quoted in commentary α lines 44–45: *qí-ip nap-šá-a-tu*$_4$: *qa-a-pa* : *na-da-nu* / túg $^{\text{tu-un}}$tun$_x$(DÚB) : *ka-ma-du* "(In) he who is entrusted with (their) lives", "to entrust" (means) "to grant"; (the expression) túg tun$_x$ (means) "to beat cloth". Curiously, the commentator does not comment on the noun *napšātu* "lives", derived from *napāšu* A "to breathe", but instead gives synonyms for the homonym *napāšu* B "to comb/clean wool". The verb *kamādu* means "to beat cloth" and is linked in the commentary with Sumerian túg tun$_x$(DÚB) (cf. Civil 1974, 335); it refers to a finishing procedure performed on woven fabrics, namely "beating the textile in order to thicken the cloth and to strengthen the weave of the fibres" (Wasserman 2013, *Iraq* 75, 264–265).

Line 101: Mss. A and D present a slightly differing wording (*meḫû* "storm" is replaced by *tēšû* "confusion, chaos" in ms. D). This line which suddenly switches to a first-person perspective has been understood as a cry of the baby trapped in the womb (e.g., Lambert 1969, *Iraq* 31, 36; Finkel 1980, 45; Zomer 2018, 256). However, the cry for help seems even more suited if coming from the woman's mouth, which is assumed here. Note, however, the Old Babylonian birth incantation CUSAS 32, No. 29b (Wasserman and Zomer 2022, No. 8), which preserves an even older parallel for the present passage, and in which indeed the baby may be speaking these words:

> ^{25} [*an-nu-ú*$^{?}$] *me-ḫu-ú e-li-a* ^{26} [*il*$^{?}$]-⸢*ka*$^{?}$⸣-*am* (or: [*i-zi-z*]*a-am*) ^{d}UTU *ku-uš-da-an-ni* . . . ^{28} [x x x *l*]*a*$^{?}$-*ma-ku-mi* ^{25} "[This(?)] is a storm upon me! ^{26} [*Co*]*me to me* (or: stand by me), o Šamaš, reach for me! . . . ^{28} [. . .] I am surrounded!"

However, the woman in labour appears to be speaking in other lines of this incantation. In line 20, she speaks of "my boat" (*eleppī*) detained in the quay of hardship, and in line 24, she may be introducing the baby's speech ([. . . *i*$^{?}$-*ša*$^{?}$]-⸢*a*$^{?}$⸣-*as-su-ú li-ib-bu-ú-a* "[*the one*] *that cries out* in my belly"; cf. Wasserman and Zomer 2022, 77–78). The imagery related to the boat held back or caught in a storm in the birth incantations is therefore often ambiguous, having potential relations to both the woman in delivery and her baby (both are threatened by death in the situation). For discussion, see also Kilmer 2007.

Lines 104–127: Lines 104–105 and 108–114 are composed as parallel to lines 119–127.

Lines 106–107: Previous editors have read DUR *ša* (^{giš}MÁ.(GUR$_8$) at the beginning of A obv. ii 51 and 52, which leads to an awkward sentence without a verb, translated as "(may) the mooring rope (*riksu*) of the boat (be moored) to the quay of well-being/life" (e.g., Ebeling 1923, 68–69; Stol 2000a, 65; Scurlock 2014a, 596, 601). This reading is inspired by line 119, which speaks of the woman's bond (DUR, *riksu*), which is loosened by Asalluḫi and is reminiscent of the boat's mooring rope. Accordingly, F. Köcher's copy renders the first two signs in lines 106–107 as DUR *ša* "the rope of (the boat)" in ms. A. However, Ebeling's copy in KAR 196 can in fact be read *ṭur-da*$^{!}$ "send away" (a G-stem imperative form of *ṭarādu* with a ventive). Commentary β (UET 6/3, 897) rev. 9'–10' now proves this reading as correct (for discussion of the commentary passage, see *infra* text G.2; Steinert 2017a, 323–324, 332–334). It quotes the beginning of line 106 and explains it as follows:

DUR$^{⌜\textit{ṭu}⌝\textit{-ur}}$***-da*** ^{giš}**MÁ** : *ṭú-ur-da* : ^{giš}MÁ / ^{giš}MÁ : ^{munus}PEŠ$_4$: *um-ma* ^{munus}PEŠ$_4$ *ṭú-ri-di*
"(For) DUR-*da* ^{giš}MÁ (read) *ṭu-ur-da* ^{giš}MÁ. (It means) 'send forth the boat'! Boat (means) 'pregnant woman'. Thus (the sentence means) 'Send away (*ṭurridī*?) the pregnant woman!'"

The metaphor of the pregnant woman or the woman in labour as a boat is attested already in Old Babylonian birth incantations discussed earlier (see notes on lines 1, 3–5). It is also found in the *Elegy on the Death of a Woman in Childbirth* (George 2010a) and in omen apodoses (e.g. Jeyes 1989, *Old Babylonian Extispicy*, 97 No. 1: 6), where the woman who died in delivery is equalled with a sunken or wrecked boat. In the ritual KAR 223 rev. 2' and dupl., the pregnant woman who has entered the month of her expected delivery refers to herself as a "full boat" (*eleppu malītu anāku*); see Hätinen 2017, *KASKAL* 14, 169–186 and *infra* text D.3.1.

Line 110: In ms. D, *kak-ka* stands for *kanka* "the sealed one", referring to the baby in the womb (CAD K, s.v. *kanku* adj. sub d). For the meaning *eṣemtu aḫītu*, lit. "strange bone", I follow AHw 251b sub mng. 4, translating "eine Gestalt für sich" (a body of its own). I.e. *eṣemtu* stands here *pars pro toto* for "body, figure", and *aḫû* "strange, extraneous" indicates the baby's existence as an independent organism or human being, to be separated from his mother's body (cf. Stol 2016–2018b, "Knochen (Material). A. Philologisch", *RlA* 15, 412a.

Lines 112–114 and 125–127: For the images, see also the note on lines 132–134 below. In lines 112, 113 and 126, the text requests that the foetus come out from the womb rather than turn backwards, through compelling similes. In line 112, the foetus should not turn back (*ay ītur ana arkīšu*), like a rain shower (does not return to heaven). In lines 113 and 126, the foetus should not turn back (*ay/ul inē' irassu*) like someone or something who has fallen from a wall (*kīma maqit dūri*). A similar expression is found in line 172 (A rev. iii 45): *lēssu ana kutallīšu ay iddi* "may it (the foetus) not throw its cheek toward its back (like someone who has fallen down from a wall)". This negative comparison with a person who has fallen from a wall (and died, unable ever to move again) has been interpreted as a reference to a breech position of the foetus (cf. CAD M/1, s.v. *maqtu* sub 1; CAD N/2, s.v. *nê'u* sub 1b-2'; Farber 1987a, *TUAT* II/1, 276 n. 45; Bergmann 2008, 45–46; Scurlock 2014a, 603, 618 n. 49). Cf. Deller and Mayer 1984, *OrNS* 53, 112 s.v. *maqtu*, who propose that the simile around *maqit dūri* refers to a piece of material that has fallen from a wall: the baby should not turn back into the womb just as a fallen-down piece from a wall does not return to its original place). See also Mayer 2019, *OrNS* 88, 299 *maqtum/maqittum* (resultative meaning).

Line 114: CAD Š/2, s.v. *šêtu* (*sêtu*) sub 1a translate this line: "may her waters (amniotic fluid), like (water in) a leaking vessel, not stay behind" (similarly in CAD Š/3, s.v. *šurdû* sub b: "just like (water from) an overflowing basket". However, the term *pisannu* does not only designate containers (basket, box), but also a "drainage passage, drainpipe" (s. CAD P, s.v. *pisannu* A sub 3). A comparison between the woman's amniotic fluid and water flowing unhindered through a drainpipe seems a more fitting image here (see also Steinert 2017a, 299 for similar imagery).

Line 116: Part of this line is quoted in commentary α 45–46: *ik-kud it-ta-'-id* "he became anxious (*ikkud*), he worried (for her life)" (see text G.1).

Line 129: The word *ēdītu* (spelled *i-di-tu*$_4$ in mss. A and B$_3$) is understood as a feminine form of the adjective (*w*)*ēdû* "prominent, high-placed" (following AHw 1495; cf. CAD E, 34–35 s.v. *edû* "well-known, renowned"). The word is picked up in commentary β (UET 6/3, 897) rev. 11': *e-di-ti* : *mi-di-ti* : *e-du-ú* : *mi-du-ú*. Although etymologically unrelated (according to AHw 1495), *ēdītu* is apparently explained in the commentary as a feminine form of the adjective *medû* "known" (presumably because of phonetic similarity). The second word pair stipulated by the commentator suggests that the verb *medû* (*madû*) is equated with *i/edû* "to know". CAD M/2, 3 regards *medû* as a secondary derivation from *i/edû* "to know" (cf. also AHw 640a s.v. *medû* "to become visible", with a meaning "is known" in the G-stem stative; Krebernik 2016, 207–208).

The word *i-ri-šú* in line 129 is ambiguous. Traces of this word are visible on the old museum photograph of BAM 248 following ^{d}*ma-mi*, although they were not copied by Köcher in BAM 248. Stol (2000a, 65), translates it as "the wise one". However, if the word was an attribute of the goddess Mami, one would rather expect the feminine form of *eršu* "wise" (*erištu*). Veldhuis (1989, 244, 247–248) interprets the word as an irregular spelling of *erešu* "queen", a loanword from Sumerian ereš (cf. CAD E, 281; AHw, 238). In both cases, the spelling of the word is irregular (i.e. one would expect *er-šu/e-riš-tu*$_4$ and *e-re-šú* respectively). A more convincing interpretation is to regard it as the regular preterite form of the verb *erēšu* "to ask for, to request" (with subjunctive ending; suggestion by E. Jiménez). Deities are often said to communicate requests (e.g. to build a temple, requests for offerings and gifts). In the context of the present incantation, the mother goddess requests a spell for easing delivery (from Ea), which befits her divine role linked to giving birth. Mami also plays a role earlier in the incantation.

The reading of the end of line 129 in ms. B$_3$ is difficult. Veldhuis (1989, 244, 247) reads: DIŠ-*niš* ⌜*ta*$^?$-*aq*$^?$-*ni*$^?$⌝ "(the incantation of Mami, the queen), is also well". Stol (2000a, 65 with n. 108, collation by M. J. Geller) instead proposed to read *ana bu-luṭ* Ú(?) "as medication . . .". After the suggested Ú, traces of another sign are visible in Ms. B$_3$, and the slightly damaged Ú could also be interpreted as SA. The reading *Bu-luṭ*-⌜*sa*⌝-G[AL] as the personal name *Bullussa-rabi* (missing the classifier for personal names) was proposed to me by I. Finkel (personal communication). However, the suggestion remains tentative for the time being (see also the next note). For discussion of Bullussa-rabi's role in this remarkable passage, see the *Introduction* section 2.2.

Line 130: The sign traces on BAM 248 at the beginning of the line, like those copied by F. Köcher, look like ^{d}40-LUGAL, see also Scurlock 2014a, 597, 602 who assumes LUGAL is an epithet of the god Ea here. Note however, that there is also a god Ea-šarru (lit. "Ea the king"), who presumably was originally a hypostasis of Enki/Ea (cf. Galter 1983, 14–16). The existence of temples for Ea-šarru (e.g. at Assur, Kalḫu) and the occurrence of Ea-šarru as theophoric element in personal names suggests that this was an independent deity in his own right (see Frankena 1954, *Tākultu*, 86 No. 46; CAD Š/2, 103b sub 2'). Ea-šarru is known from the Kassite to the Neo-Assyrian period. His first occurrence in Kassite times may fit well with the name Bullussa-rabi reconstructed in the preceding line. Nonetheless, the mentioning of the deity Ea-šarru together with the exorcist Bullussa-rabi is difficult to explain. Stol (2000a, 65 with n. 108) suggests a different divine name at the beginning of this line, Nisaba, ^{d}NIDABA(= ŠE-NAGA), but the sign traces on BAM 248 do not confirm this reading; ms. B$_3$ seems to confirm the sign [LU]GAL.

Lines 132–134: Ms. B$_3$ preserves no trace of a ruling between lines 134 and 135 (rev. iii 3 and 4), while it is visible on ms. B$_4$. For the ritual instruction, see Stol 2000a, 65–66, who wonders how the healers procured the ingredients for this prescription (especially *aban tīk šamê* "stone dripping from heaven", i.e. hailstone) and asks whether the prescription is realistic at all. In any case, the ingredients used in the prescription correspond directly with the images in the associated incantation (lines 112–114, 125–127), although there is a bit of divergence. The "rain shower" (*tīk šamê*) in the spell (lines 112 and 125) becomes "hailstone" (*aban tīk šamê*); someone/something "fallen from the city wall" (*maqit dūri*) is transposed to "dust from the parapets of a dilapidated city wall" (*eper samīt dūri maqti*); similarly, the "water running through a streaming drainpipe" becomes dust from a streaming drainpipe (*eper pisanni šurdî*). The images of the incantation are all linked to the concept of irreversibility, serving as compelling objects to evoke an unhindered and quick birth. For comments on the images, see Deller and Mayer 1984, *OrNS* 53, 112. For the image of the baby "falling" (to the ground) in birth incantations, see e.g. line 36 (A obv. i 50); Bergmann 2008, 45–46; Couto-Feirrera 2014, 298, 311. Note that the phrase *sa-mit* BÀD ŠUB-*t*[*i*] is ambiguous: it can be read *samīt dūri maqitti* "(dust) from the fallen parapet of a city wall" or *samīt dūri maqti* "(dust) from the parapet of a dilapidated city wall" (cf. CAD S, 117 s.v. *samītu* sub a).

For the commentary passages on lines 132–134, see commentary α 46–51and β rev. 12' (texts G.1 and G.2).

Lines 135–160: For the "Cow of Sîn" incantation, see especially Röllig 1985; Farber 1987, 275–276; Veldhuis 1991; Stol 2000a, 66–68; Foster 2005, 1007–1008; Bergmann 2008, 17–23, 25–26; Scurlock 2014a, 597–598, 602; Marquéz Rowe 2014, 77–78; 2015. Stol (2000a, 68) observed that the name of the cow in this incantation, Geme-Sîn, is identical with the name of a wife of the Ur III king Šulgi, Amat-Sîn. He concluded that the central role of the moon god in the incantation is perfectly in line with the Ur III ideology and proposed that the "Cow of Sîn" incantation was originally composed for the queen when she gave birth and had a difficult delivery. Nowicki (2013, *NABU* 2013/4, no. 61) proposed that the text may have been composed in the reign of Šulgi's son and successor Amar-Sîn and that it may originally have served an ideological purpose (thus, the name Amar-Sîn corresponds to the calf's name Amar-ga in the incantation). Note however that not Amat-Sîn, but Šulgi's first wife Tarām-Uram is now believed to have been Amar-Sîn's mother (Weiershäuser 2008, *Die königlichen Frauen der III. Dynastie von Ur*, 29, with Boese and Sallaberger 1996, *AoF* 23, 33–34). A similar ideologically charged composition from the Ur III period linked to royal birth is *A balbale to Bau for Šu-Suen*, in which king Šu-Sîn's mother (Abi-simtī, the wife of Amar-Sîn) assists in the delivery of Šu-Sîn's wife Kubātum, see Nowicki 2013; Widell 2011, *JNES* 70, 297–298.

Line 135: The text of "A Cow of Sîn" in ms. D 51–53 begins differently, introducing the cow as "Gī-Sîn, the maidservant of Sîn": *gi-se-en* <<^{d}30>> GÉME *šá* ^{d}30 *a-la-da šap-šu-qa-at še-er-ra / ku-na-at še-er-ra ku-na-at ana qa-tu-ú* ZI-*te* ŠU.RA *ši-ku-rum*

/ *sa-ni-iq* KÁ-*bu ana ti*$^{!}$(NU)-*nu*$^{!}$(TI)-*qí la-lu-ú* "Gī-Sîn, the maidservant of Sîn, has trouble in childbirth. The child is stuck, the child is stuck, to bring life to an end. The bolt is in place, the door is closed for the suckling babe." After this introduction, the text of D runs parallel to mss. A–C, telling the story of the cow loved by Sîn. Apparently, the introduction of the spell was modified, after the beginning of the preceding incantation in ms. D (lines 33–36), which, however, describes the suffering of a woman in labour, while mss. A–C describe the beauty of the cow Geme-Sîn (see the note on line 22 and the edition of ms. D *infra*). In ms. D 51, Veldhuis (1991, 64) regards the elided ^{d}30 in *gi-se-en* <<^{d}30>> in D 53 as a gloss, compare the spelling *gi-i-*^{d}30 GÉME *ša* ^{d}30 in D 61 (= line 158).

Line 164 (A rev. iii 37 //) is virtually identical to the incipit of "A Cow of Sîn" in mss. A (see the note below).

Line 136: The text of ms. A *tiqnāte tuqqunat* "she was adorned with ornaments" replaces the expression *šiknāte mutturat* "she was imposing of figure" in ms. C, which forms a closer parallel to *binûta kazbat* "she was alluring of shape" in line 137 (cf. Röllig 1985, 264; CAD Š/2, 430 s.v. *šikittu* A sub mng. 1b; CAD T, 199 s.v. *taqānu* D sub 3 ("to adorn"); CAD T, 422 s.v. *tiqnu* sub 1a).

Commentary β rev. 13' appears to comment on lines 136–137, but is unfortunately fragmentary: [*ti*]-⸢*iq*$^{?}$⸣-x x x-*ti kaz-bat* : *ba-na-at* ". . . she was alluring (of shape?)" (means) "she was beautiful". The reading [*b*]*i*$^{?}$-⸢*nu*$^{?}$⸣-*ti* (with Frahm 2011, 241) is difficult to reconcile with the sign traces (see also text G.2).

Line 137: The form *minûtu* in ms. C is regarded as a variant of *binûtu* "shape" in mss. A and B, as was suggested by Röllig 1985, 264 (*pace* AHw 657a and CAD M/2 99b sub 4). The form *i-ra-'-ši* in ms. D 54 is regarded here as a variant of *irāmši* "he loved her" in mss. A, B and C (*irā'ši*, with interchange of *m* > aleph; see thus Lambert 1969, *Iraq* 31, 32: 54; CAD R, 137b, 142b s.v. *râmu* A sub 1d-1'). Interchange between aleph and *m* is frequently attested in Middle Assyrian and later texts, e.g. in *amīlu/a'īlu* "(hu)man" or *zumru/zu'ru* "body" (GAG § 31d; CAD Z, 157a).

Line 138: The term *šubāḫu* in ms. A is a *hapax* (CAD Š/3, 168b s.v. *šubāḫu*); perhaps the term stands for some kind of ornament. It is not excluded that ms. A is corrupt since the wording of ms. C differs (the end of the line in C is not preserved). The syntax of the sentence in A is ambiguous. It is unclear whether *šu-ba-ḫi* stands in the singular or plural (CAD translates "he adorned(?) her with brilliant *š*.-s"), and in which syntactic relation it stands to the preceding *namru ša Sîn* "the brilliant (glow) of Sîn". Scurlock (2014a, 602) regards *namru* as an attribute to *šubaḫu* and translates "he put the shining *šubaḫu* of Sîn upon her".

Commentary β rev. 14' appears to equate the expression *namru ša Sîn* in the base text with *nūr Sîn* "the light of Sîn" (i.e. the moonlight), but the text is unfortunately fragmentary (see text G.2).

The variant *miḫir Sîn namru* in ms. C replacing *namru ša Sîn* is interpreted as "das glänzende Ebenbild des Sîn" ("the brilliant counterpart of Sîn") by Röllig (1985, 264 note A 13, 269). The noun *mi/eḫru* means "counterpart; equivalent", but occasionally it can refer to an offering (AHw 641b sub 8; cf. CAD M/2, 59 s.v. *miḫru* A sub 5, booking the passage under a meaning "front", however (ibid. sub 3). Close to the meaning "offering", I assume a word sense close to "gift" here, indicating an object that is perhaps the material carrier of Sîn's brilliant sheen (an ornament, pectoral?).

Line 140: For reading the spelling *é-a* in *re-é-a-ú-tu* (found in ms. B_1 rev. iii 9) as *e'u*, cf. Borger 2004, MZL, 344. Scurlock (2014a, 602) translates: "He had her take the lead of the herd, going as herdsman after her". The text literally means "the herdsmanship (*rē'ûtu*) went after her".

Line 141: Commentary β rev. 14' contains the corresponding phrase . . . *nu-ru-ub šam-*[*me* (x)] "the lushest grass" (see text G.2). Manuscripts A, C and D offer different forms or *re'û* (*ra'û*) "to pasture, to (let) graze" in the present line (cf. CAD R, 301 sub 1b). Ms. C uses an Assyrian G-stem form *i-ra-'i-ši* "her pastured her", while ms. D offers a Gtn-stem form *ir-ta-na-'i* without the feminine pronominal suffix *-ši*, which suggests that the cow is the subject here ("she always used to graze"; for the intransitive usage or *re'û* see CAD R, 301–302 sub mng. 2; for discussion see also de Ridder 2018, 412). For ms. A, CAD R, 301a sub 1b emends the spelling *i-re-'i* to *i-re-'u-*<*ši*>(!), in line with ms. C. The emendation is not followed here, but the form is translated as intransitive, in line with ms. D.

Line 142: The word *šub-bé-*(*e*) in mss. A, B and C has been interpreted as a textual corruption based on the misreading of *sa-ḫi* (*saḫḫu*) "meadow" in ms. D (thus Röllig 1985, 262, 265 who emends to *saḫ*$^{!}$-*ḫ*[*i*$^{!}$] in C). CAD Š/2, 26 s.v. *šaqû* sub 1b reads the word *ru-bi-e* instead, but translates it with "meadow", relying on the variant in ms. C. Veldhuis (1991, 9, 11) translates *ina šubbê* (*ša*) *mašqê* as "at the abundant well" and "at the abundance (of the) well". My translation follows Scurlock (2014a, 602), taking *šubbû* as a nominalised D-stem infinitive of *šebû* with the meaning "to sate, to satisfy, to quench (hunger or thirst)" (cf. CAD Š/2, 254 sub mng. 2a). The restoration *i-na sa-ḫi m*[*aš-qí*] in ms. D follows Röllig 1985, 262; the translation is inspired by Foster 2005, 1007 ("he would let her drink at a meadow wherein was a watering place").

Line 144: For the interchange of *ḫ/k* in *šaḫāṭu/šakāṭu*, see Lambert 1969, *Iraq* 31, 38; GAG § 25a. The reading of the second half of the line follows Farber 1987, 275 with n. 19a; Veldhuis 1991, 61, 62 n. 19; Scurlock 2014a, 598, 602. For the translation "he reared up (*iššî*) at her tail (*zibbatušša*)" (with a locative *-um*), compare the use of the verb *našû* "to rise up" in connection with sexual desire (Zisa 2021). For a different interpretation of ms. A, reading *ḫi-bi-ba-tuš-šá* ÍL-*ši* "(the bull) took her virginity", see CAD Ḫ 179a s.v. *ḫibibātu*; Röllig 1985, 265, 270.

Line 146: For comparison of the different manuscripts, cf. Röllig 1985, 265–266 who reads *ú-ga-al* ÁB instead of *ú-ga-al-lit* in mss. A and B, but interprets it as a mistake for *iḫâl* "(the cow) went into labour" (since no D-stem of *ḫâlu* is attested) found in mss. C and D. For the variants *igallit* vs. *ugallit* in mss. A and B, see the analysis of Veldhuis 1991, 36–37. In ms. B, the sequence *igdalit igal*[*lit*] (perfect and durative of *galātu* in the G-stem) may be seen as expressing an emphasis. The D-stem of *galātu* "to quiver, to become frightened" is only attested in the transitive meaning "to frighten" (CAD G, 13 sub 2; AHw 274). Therefore, I prefer to follow Veldhuis (1991, 10–11, 36) and Scurlock (2014a, 602), regarding *re'âša* "her herdsman" at the beginning of line 147 in ms. A as the direct object of *ugallit* (i.e. "it/she frightened her herdsman").

For the puns and word play involved in this line see Veldhuis 1991, note e.g. the homonymous verbs *ḫâlu* "to tremble" and *ḫâlu* "to be in labour". For *ḫamāšu* in ms. D, cf. AHw 315–316; Röllig 1985, 266 "die Beine einknicken".

Line 147: The reading *naši* ŠU "(the shepherd) lifted (his) hand (in prayer)" in ms. C obv. ii 28 follows Röllig 1985, 262, 266.

Line 148: For the reading *ne-pal-suḫ*$_4$(SAḪ), as a rendering of the stative of *napalsuḫu* "to (let oneself) fall to the ground (in despair)", cf. AHw 733b; CAD N/1, 271–272; GAG § 101d (for *napalsu/iḫ*).

Line 149: The text ms. C obv. ii 29 is apparently corrupt and different emendations have been proposed: most editors and commentors propose to restore either <^{d}30 *i*>*-na* AN *iš-ta-ma-a* "Sîn in heaven kept hearing" or <^{d}30 *na*>*-na-*<*ar*> AN-<*e*> "Sîn, the luminary of heaven (kept hearing)" (Lambert 1965, 284; Röllig 1985, 263, 267; Marquéz Rowe 2015, *AuOr* 33, 54). Arnaud (2007, 76 note on line 1') suggests reading *Na-an-*<. . .>. Veldhuis (1991, 11, 63) understood the verbal form *iš-ta-ma-a* in C obv. 29 as a feminine plural with the protective spirits (here: "two daughters of Anu" instead of "two *lamassu*-spirits") as the subject of the sentence. However, following Rowe (2015, 56–57), the verb can be regarded as an Assyrian (Gtn preterite) singular form with a ventive (*ištammâ*) "he (the moon god) heard again and again" (mss. A and B write *ištamme*).

In line with the older parallels, the subject of the verb *nepalsaḫ* in ms. A rev. iii 23 (line 148) should be the herdsman, not the moon god. Following other interpreters, ^{d}NANNA at the end of A rev. iii 23 is therefore taken as an apposition of ^{d}Sîn and therefore part of the clause in the following line 149 (since in some of the older manuscripts *Nannāru Sîn* stand in apposition in this line), see Marquéz Rowe 2015, 56; Röllig 1985, 267; Scurlock 2014a, 602; Farber 1987, 275.

Line 150: Ms. c apparently has a bound form *lamassāt* [*šamê*] "(two) protective spirit from heaven" indicating a genitive construction (and the origin of the protective spirits). The text of Middle Assyrian ms. D line 59 diverges, reading 2 *ši-na* DUMU.MUNUS ^{d}*a-nim* "two are they, the daughters of Anu, (they descended from heaven)". For a parallel passage, see e.g. *Maqlû* III 31–33 (Abusch 2016, 306): *šittā šina mārāt Ani ša šamê . . . ultu šamê urradāni* "Two are they, the heavenly Daughters of Anu, . . ., they descend to me from heaven".

Lines 150–152: The different manuscripts present several textual variations for the lines describing the actions of the divine helpers assisting the cow. In line 151, instead of emending the text of ms. D 60 to *ilput* "she touched" following the other manuscripts, Veldhuis (1991, 12–13) accepted *lilput* as a variant and translates "he must touch (her forehead)".

In ms. c 4'–6', Rowe (2014, 77) restores the text is as follows: 1-*et* Ì BUR *na-*[*ša-at šanītu ušappala mê ḫalli*] / *il-pu-ut* Ì [BUR *pūssa*] / *me-e ḫal-li u*[*š-tap-pi-ḫa kala zumriša*] "one ca[rried oil-from-the jar, [the other brought down water-from-the-bowl]; she (i.e. the former) smeared [her forehead] with oil-[from-the-jar]; she (i.e. the latter) sp[rinkled] [her whole body] with water from-the-bowl". Ms. D 59–60 reverses the order of the objects brought down by the two protective spirits. In most manuscripts, the first divine helper brings *šaman pūri* "oil-from-the-jar", but the second item is spelled differently in mss. A, B, D and c. Ms. c 6' and 8' from Ugarit has twice *me-e ḫal-li*, while mss. A and B_1 read *me-e ḫa-li*. The Middle Assyrian ms. D 59 and 60 spells A.MEŠ *ḫi-i-li* instead (compare the similar expression *ri-gim ḫi/ḫa-li-šá* "her screaming in labour" in lines 148 and 165). The expression *me-e ḫa-li/ḫi-i-li* in mss. A, B and D was usually understood as "water of labour", deriving the variant spellings from *ḫâlu* (*ḫiālu*) "to be in labour" and *ḫīlū* "birth pangs" respectively. This magic "water of (easy) labour" should not be confused with the amniotic fluid (cf. Stol 2000a, 125; notably, Michel (1997, 63–64) and CAD P, 544 sub 1b suggested that the amniotic fluid is rather called *mê bišri* or *mê pušqi* in Akkadian Lamaštu incantations, in addition to plain *mû* "water". However, the terms *me-e ḫa-li/ḫi-i-li* in mss. A, B and D may be re-interpretations of an older expression *mê ḫalli* "water-from-the-bowl" attested in ms. c from Ugarit, as was proposed by Marquéz Rowe 2015, *AuOr* 33, 58–59. The word *ḫallu* denotes a small earthen container for liquids (AHw 312; CAD Ḫ, 45; Sallaberger 1996, 111; Ḫh. X 223–237 (MSL 7, 88)), and the expression *mê ḫalli* would provide a closer parallelism to *šaman pūri* "oil-from-the-jar", which is also in line with the focus on the topos of pure waters in special containers that the spirits are said to bring down from heaven in other healings incantations (with the *mannam lušpur*-formula, see Farber 1990). The spelling *ḫa-li* in mss. A and B is ambiguous (it could be read either *ḫâli* or *ḫalli*); but it seems clear that the term *ḫallu* forms a pun on *ḫâlu* "to be in labour", just as *littu* "cow" alludes to *ālittu* "childbearing woman" in "A Cow of Sîn" and other birth incantations.

The text of ms. C ii 31–32 presents difficulties and seems to be corrupt. The proposed restoration [. . .] KAŠ ⸢KÙ⸣.GA$^{!}$ *na-šá-at* A.MEŠ *šul-me* [. . .] "[the other(?)] carried pure *beer*(?), [*she carried*(?)] water of well-being" in line 31 is a guess from context; we expect "pure oil" instead of beer, as in the other versions of the incantation. The very damaged line C obv. ii 32 does not align well with the text of line 152 found in the other manuscripts; only the sequence ⸢*pu*$^{?}$-*tam*$^{?}$⸣ *šá* GU$_4$.ÁB "the cow's forehead" bears some resemblance to the wording of the other manuscripts in line 151, which describes the smearing of the cow's forehead. Ms. C apparently differed to a considerable extent from the better-preserved manuscripts.

For reading *šapāḫu* (D-stem) "to sprinkle" in lines 152 and 154 instead of *sapāḫu* "to scatter" (as proposed in CAD S, 153–154 sub 5a; AHw 1024b D sub 3), see Marquéz Rowe 2015, *AuOr* 33, 58 following ms. c 6' (restored as *ušt*[*appiḫa*]); cf. CAD Š/1, 3, normalizing the verb as *šabāḫu* A "to sprinkle"; AHw 1167b "breit hinstreuen". The emendation in ms. D 60 *ú*-<*šap*>-*pi*-<*ḫa*> follows Rowe op. cit., 54.

In ms. b 8' (line 154), *pa-na* SU-*šu* "the front of her body" is apparently a variant for *ka-la zumrīša* "her whole body".

Line 152: At the end of ms. D line 60, Arnaud (2007, 76 note on line 8') proposed emending the text, reading *uk*$^{!}$-*tana-par*$_5$ (from *kapāru* Dtn-stem "to wipe (clean)").

Line 155: For *šal-la-ti-iš-šu* as a mistake for *šal-šu-ti-iš-šu* "for the third time", see Röllig 1985, 268, 271; CAD Š/1, 269.

Line 156: Instead of emending ms. C 32 to *qaq*$^{!}$-*qar-šu*, it would also be possible (although less likely) to read A.GÀR-*šu* "onto the meadow" (*ugāršu*) (thus Veldhuis 1991, 63). For discussion, see also Marquéz Rowe 2015, 59. In ms. c, the text breaks off at this point. On the left edge are traces of the signs [. . .] EGIR *šá*-[*tir* ...] "[...] is written after it(?)", possibly a colophon?

Line 157: Arnaud (2007, 77 note on line 10') restores in ms. C obv. 33 *a-na mur* [GU$_4$.ÁB/-*šá*] "for/to [the cow's / her] calf", presumably presenting a variant sentence referring to the naming of the calf (here the term *mūru* "young animal" instead of *būru* "calf" in the other manuscripts would be used). In line 156, the calf is compared with a gazelle's young (*uzālu*). For this comparison (wild animal birth as an ideal model of birth), see Steinert 2017a, 329; 2017b, *FS Wiggermann*, 227.

Line 158: The word *eš*(*e*)*riš* in ms. D 61 is the Assyrian form of *išariš* "normally".

Line 159: Röllig (1985, 270) regards the spelling *ar-da-a-tu* ^{munus}LA.RA.AḪ.MEŠ in ms. D line 62 as a plural; however, the verb (*lūlid*) is in the singular. Both mss. C and D omit text in line 160 and are presumably both marked with the phrase "Wording of an Enuru-incantation".

Lines 163–172: For different syllabic spellings of the cow's name (Geme-Sîn, Egi/Gī-Sîn, Egizinītu), compare BAM 248 rev. iii 43 (= line 170); see below BAM 248 rev. iii 54 (= line 181), with the variant in BM 36339 rev. 9 (ms. a). Compare the earlier version in *Iraq* 31, 31: 51: *gi-se-en* <<^{d}30>> GÉME *šá* ^{d}30 "Gī-Sîn, the maidservant of Sîn". For discussion, see note on lines 56–68 above and *infra* text II.1.4.

The Elamite deities Narunde and Naḫḫunte in lines 163 and 167 were already invoked in the incantation in ms. A obv. i 54–61 // (especially i 57 // = line 44) above, together with Napiriša and Kiririša (see the notes on lines 40–47 above). Nanamgišir in line 163 is understood here as a third obscure divine entity who is to intercede on the patient's behalf (see also Finkel 1997, *NABU* 1997/1, 22 n. 3, who found a similar triad of supernatural helpers in later Aramaic, Greek, Coptic, Syriac and Arabic texts; cf. Veldhuis 1991, 15; Stol 2000a, 69).

Line 168: For reading ÁB-*mi* as *arḫu-mi* or *arḫī-mi*, compare ms. b (KUB 4, 13: 15' and 16'), written in a syllabic spelling (*ar-ḫi-mi* "o my cow"), discussed above as an older parallel to the incantation in BAM 248 obv. i 36–50 (= lines 22–36). See also Veldhuis 1991, 65; Zomer 2013, *NABU* 2013/2, 45–46 No. 27. For the particle *-mi* (found already in Old Babylonian and Old Assyrian incantations, see Farber 1996, *NABU* 1996/3, 71–72 No. 80; Wasserman 2012, 189. However, ÁB-*mi* could also be read as *littī-mi* or *littu-mi* "o (my) cow", see the Old Babylonian birth incantation *BiOr* 75, 19–20 (Wasserman 2018, 18–20; Wasserman and Zomer 2022, 66–67; SEAL no. 7063), which begins with [*l*]*i-ti-mi* (line 1). Wasserman (ibid.) suggests the particle *-mi* denotes a direct address to a person present in the situation; but in the present context it may rather express an emphasized word within a direct speech (see GAG §123c).

Line 171: For *našallulu* "to slither, glide (said of snakes)" in a parallel phrase, see also A obv. i 59 // (= line 46) above.

Line 172: The expression *lēssu ana kutallīšu ay iddi* "may it not turn back (lit. may it not turn its cheek toward its back)" refers to an irreversible change. Someone who has fallen from a wall (and died as consequence) is not able to turn his neck anymore (see also CAD M/1, 255a; Veldhuis 1991, 14; Stol 2000a, 68; Scurlock 2014a, 603); the baby is to come out from the womb and not turn backwards. For different interpretations, see Farber 1987, *TUAT* II/2, 276 with n. 45; Scurlock 2014a, 618 n. 49, suggesting connotations with a breech position of the baby.

Line 174: The spelling *ši-ip-li-i* should perhaps be emended to *šap*$^{!}$*-li-i*, although the dictionaries have accepted the present attestation in BAM 248 iii 47 as a variant *šiplû* for *šaplû* (cf. CAD Š/1, 473a; AHw 1174 s.v. *šaplû* sub 2).

Line 175: For the equation of Sumerian gi-níĝ-gal-gal-(la) with Akkadian *qanû kabbaru*, see Ḫḫ. VIII 82 (MSL 7, 13; cf. ibid., VIII 91).

Line 179: For the emendation *zaq*$^{!}$*(qu)-pi*, see Stol 2000a, 69 note 129; Scurlock 2014a, 598. Translators agree that the word means "bulging" or "protruding". Farber (1987, 276 n. 52a) reads *quppi* and translates "gewölbt". The adjective *quppu* (derived from *qâpu* (D-stem) means "buckled; collapsed" (said of walls); Farber (ibid.) suggests the use of the term *quppu* in reference to the woman's belly (*libbu*) is a word play with line 172 above, which mentions a person who has fallen from a wall as a comparison with the baby. For semantic reasons, I prefer an emendation to *zaqpi* "erect" (following Stol op. cit).

Line 181: The Akkadian reading of ÁB.GAL is not entirely certain. Veldhuis (1991, 14) and Scurlock (2014a, 603) translate it with "big cow" in the present text line. Borger 2004, MZL, 397 No. 672 reads ÁB.GAL as *littu*, but notes following CAD B, 334 s.v. *burtu* (discussion) that in the present line (BAM 248 rev. iii 54) it may have to be read *burtu*.[359] Note the 1st millennium BCE commentary Rm. 307: 7–8 (quoted in CAD A/2, 263 lex. section and MSL 8/1, 63), which gives the following explanation: [ÁB].AL^{maḫ} : *bur-tú ar-ḫu rabītu*(GAL) *šá tu-lid-du* "[ÁB].AL (pronounced ÁB.MAḪ) means cow (*burtu*), being a full-grown (mature) cow that has (already) given birth (to a calf)". The term ÁB.MAḪ tends to be replaced by ÁB.GAL in Middle Babylonian texts. Cf. further the bilingual text BM 34208 obv. 11'–12' and 17'-18', for áb = *littu* (*infra* text D.1.9).

Ms. a rev. 9 presents a diverging formulation at the beginning of the incantation, replacing the expression "cow of Sîn" in ms. A with an Akkadian rendering of the cow's name bearing a feminine ending (which is elsewhere known as Geme-Sîn or Gī-Sîn), Egizinītu (⸢*e*⸣*-gi-zi-ni-tu*$_4$ *šá* ^{d}30 *r*[*a*$^{?}$-x-x x x]). In the gap before ⸢*e*⸣*-gi-zi-ni-tu*$_4$, there is room for two signs (e.g. ÁB.GAL). It is tempting to restore the line as [ÁB.(GAL)] ⸢*e*⸣*-gi-zi-ni-tu*$_4$ *šá* ^{d}30 *r*[*a*$^{?}$*-bi-tu*$_4$ *ana-ku*$^{?}$] "[I am the] b[ig cow] Egizinītu, belonging to Sîn".

Lines 182–184: The behaviour of the pregnant cow in labour (goring, rooting up the ground with her horns, whirling up dust with her tail or similar actions) is described in similar terms in other birth incantations, see lines 24–25 in the present text and the Old Assyrian incantations CCT 5, 50e obv. 1'–4' (BM 113625; Kouwenberg and Fincke 2012–2013, 141–146; Wasserman and Zomer 2022, No. 5); kt 90/k 178: 5–8 (Michel 2004, 397ff.; Wasserman and Zomer 2022, No. 9). See the note on lines 24–25 above. The paranomastic infinitive constructions in line 182 serve to emphasize the actions described by the finite verbs (GAG §150a), see also Veldhuis 1991, 14 ("I am pregnant and I am butting all the time") and Farber 1987, 276 ("Hochträchtig bin ich, und (daher) besonders stößig").

359 The same interpretation (reading *b/purti Sîn*) was proposed by Landsberger 1960, MSL 8/1, 66. The logogram ÁB is commonly read *littu* (cf. CAD L, 217 s.v. *littu* A sub a-2'; Veldhuis 1989, 8, 10 reading all instances of ÁB in the present incantation as *littu*). For 1st millennium BCE uses in literary texts of *arḫu* "cow" as correspondence to Sumerian áb (preserving an older tradition), see CAD A/2, 263 s.v. *arḫu* B sub b.

Lines 190–192: The restoration partially follows the similar wording in ms. A rev. iii 33–35 (= lines 158–160). The verb *līšer* may refer either to the woman (as in line 159 above) or to her foetus. Scurlock (2014a, 599) proposes a slightly different restoration of lines 190–192 following more closely the wording of lines 158–160. Since the preserved text of line 193 refers to the foetus, a restoration *līš[er ša libbīša]* "may her foetus be alright/come straight out" is proposed here already for the end of line 191. However, the foetus may have been mentioned only in the lost line 192, and we may have to restore *līš[er erītu]* "may the pregnant woman be alright/give birth easily" in line 191.

Lines 194–195: In line 194, the verb *nērubu* used in parallelism to *lasāmu* "to run" literally means "to flee, run away, escape" (CAD N/2, 182). For the spell, see also CAD Š/1, 16 s.v. *šabsû* "male midwife, accoucheur". Kouwenberg (2010, *The Akkadian Verb*, 292) regards the spelling *né-er-ru-ba* as a feminine plural imperative form (*nerrubā* instead of expected *nenrubā*). In the present edition, the ending *-a* (also present in *lusma*) is interpreted as a ventive instead (rendered as "to me").

Lines 196–197: The staff of *e'ru*-wood (possibly a type of cornel tree) is also used by the exorcist in Udug-ḫul as a powerful instrument, especially to drive off disease demons and foster healing by placing it close to the patient (Geller 2016, 22–23, 25–26; Tablet 3: 66; Tablet 7: 47, 92; Tablet 12: 83; Tablets 13–15: 74, 94, 134, 159). See also Wiggermann 1992, 65–66, 79ff. In the Birth Compendium, this staff specifically needs to be taken "from the hand (i.e. possession) of a shepherd" (*ša qāt rē'î*) (see also Stol 2000a, 69–70; CAD E, 320 s.v. *e'ru* b-3'a; CAD P, 154 sub 1a). See also lines 200–201 for a similar prescription and Veldhuis 1989, 252. Böck (2013, 48 n. 77) offers a differing interpretation of the passage, translating "take shepherd's staff and *e'ru*-wood from the hand of a shepherd, put them crosswise on top of her belly". For Böck, the crosswise placement (*parāku* "to lay across/crosswise") symbolizes the "barred exit" of the baby.

Lines 198–199: The reading *šup-šuq-ta re-mi* ᵈAMAR.UTU "have pity, o Marduk, on the woman who has trouble in delivery" in line 198 follows collation and CAD Š/3, 327 s.v. *šupšuqtu*, with CAD R, 263b s.v. *rēmu* (discussion section), assuming that *rēmi* is an irregular singular masculine imperative of *rêmu* "to be merciful, have compassion with". See also CAD Š/1, s.v. *šabsūtu* sub b. Alternative readings of line 198 proposed in Stol 2000a, 70 ("she with the sealed womb", reading *re-mi k[a-ni-i]k-tam*) and in Scurlock 2014a, 599, 603 (*re-mi* ⸢*ka*⸣*-[an-g]a-tú*) are based on Köcher's erroneous copy of ms. A in BAM III. For ᵈŠÀ.ZU (lit. "who know the inside (of the body)" as a name of Marduk associated with the womb, see CT 24, 42: 101 (god list): ᵈŠÀ.ZU = *Marduk ša rēmi*. For discussion of male deities assuming the role of the divine midwife in the Neo-Assyrian Birth Compendium, see also Stol 2000a, 71. Sumerian šà-zu also means "midwife". For the reading of line 199, see CAD A/1, 293 s.v. *alādu* sub 4a; Stol 2000a, 70 (translation).

Lines 200–201: In line 201, the text instructs to roll the staff of *e'ru*-wood over the woman's belly, in a downward movement (cf. AHw 1259–1260 s.v. *šugarruru* "abrollen; durch Rollen massieren"; CAD G, 48 s.v. *garāru* sub 2 ("to roll"). See also lines 196–197 for a parallel instruction and lines 211–212 for massaging the woman's belly in a downward movement.

Line 202: For this spell, cf. Veldhuis 1989, 257–258 note 9. The same incantation is to be recited in another compendium for women found at Nineveh, in AMT 66/4 rev. i' 6'–7' (here ms. I), where it is also applied to speed up difficult childbirth (for the context of this manuscript, see text D.1.4).

Although this short recitation (for which several variant examples are known) has been classified as pseudo-Sumerian or mumbo-jumbo words (Bácskay and Niederreiter 2023, 22–23 with n. 104), Veldhuis (1999, 47–48) has shown that such garbled words or phrases are not used in a random manner but often allude to real Sumerian terms that relate to the condition treated by the spell in question. Thus, in Sumerian bilingual texts, the verb za-la-aḫ is equated with Akkadian *zâqu* "to blow" (said of demons and other harmful agents), but its meaning is rather "to slip through an opening", in accordance with lexical passages equating it with *etēqu* "to pass through/by" (see CT 12, pl. 49 Sm. 1600 rev. i' 3'; CT 19, pl. 46 K. 4597 obv. i 1, quoted in ePSD2). Civil (2007, *FS Biggs*, 23 No. 82) regards za-la-aḫ as a Semitic loanword in Sumerian (with a cognate term in Arabic *zala'a* "to slide along, to slip"; compare perhaps also Assyrian *ṣalā'u* "to throw; to abort/miscarry a foetus"). The variant phrase iz-za-la-aḫ in mss. A and B (not in ms. I) perhaps just stands for ì-za-la-aḫ "it has slipped out". Veldhuis (1989, 257–258 n. 9) proposed a word play between za-la-aḫ with SAL(MUNUS).LA.RA.AḪ. There is possibly a double entendre in al-ti-la: Sumerian ti(l) may correspond to Akkadian *balāṭu* "to live" or *qatû* "to come to an end" (Veldhuis proposed the latter of these meanings in our passage).

Finkel (1976, 230–231 note on line 322) recognized a further variant of this formula in a spell from the series Ḫulbazizi. See also Bácskay and Niederreiter 2023, *JMC* 40, 22–23 n. 104 K. 3628 + 4009 + Sm. 1315 obv. 28: [ì-bi-za-<la>-a]ḫ ì-bi-za-<la>-aḫ.

Lines 205–215: This passage marks a sequence of prescriptions for speeding up difficult delivery (introduced in line 205 by the phrase *šumma sinništu ina alādi uštapšiq(šu)* "if a woman suffers severely in (her) delivery"), all separated by a ruling, which must have been taken as one block from an earlier source, when the compendium was assembled. Most of the remedies prescribe only a simple ingredient, either of herbal or animal origin, which is administered in a potion (on an empty stomach) or as an ointment. For discussion of the remedies, see also Stol 2000a, 70–71; Couto-Ferreira 2014, 298–303.

Some of the plant ingredients prescribed here and in the following section of remedies (lines 216–230) are also prescribed for difficult labour in pharmaceutical handbooks, such as *lišān kalbi* "dog's tongue plant", *karān šēlebi* "fox grape" and *atā'išu*-plant, see BAM 381 iii 25–26, 27–29, 31–32; BAM 380 rev. 31–32, 33–35, 36–37; BAM 379 iii 9 (Stol 2000a, 53–54).

Line 208: "Excrement of wall lizard" (ŠE$_{10}$ EME.DIR IZ.ZI) occurs in another context within the women's healthcare texts, namely in prescriptions to induce an abortion in BAM 246: 2 and 8 (see text B.1.6); in the latter text, one of the prescriptions specifies "multicoloured" (GÙN.A, *barmu*) wall lizard (*ṣurār igāri*), which may be a mere variant in wording. Both BAM 246 and 248 stem from the same archive (the library N4 at Assur). The uses of this ingredient, whether an alias name for a plant or not, indicate that this *materia medica* had expellant properties (and caused contractions of the uterus); cf. Böck 2013, 37–39 who suggests (multicoloured) wall lizard is a coded name, perhaps for the *adamantu*-plant.

Animal dung is also recommended as an abortifacient in Dioscorides *Materia Medica* (Book 2, 98), while Pliny the Elder (*Natural History* 28.29) asserts that chameleon (an animal belonging to the order of lizards) would be helpful to facilitate parturition. The multicoloured (wall) lizard is also attested in remedies to promote sexual desire (Zisa 2021, 408–409 Text K Prescription 31: 135–140 = Text N Prescription 8 (ii 3–8)); the excrement is likewise employed in prescriptions against discharge (*mūṣû*), see Geller 2005a, Text No. 8: 13).

Line 209: CAD N/2, 167b sub d lists the phrase *nipilti kalbi* under the lemma *nēpeštu* "work, handling", but acknowledged that *nipiltu* is preferably understood as a derivation from *napālu* "to dig up" (i.e. "soil pawed up by a dog"), see also Stol 2000a, 70 n. 134. Stol (ibid.) notes that this *materia medica* is so far unique in the Babylonian medical literature, but mentions a similar, though enigmatic expression *siḫipti litti* (see Stol *apud* Borger 1991, *BiOr* 48, 157 *ad* S.299), attested in BAM 476: 8 (cited in CAD S, 235a sub b): *eper bīt sinništi ša alāda parsat itti si-ḫi-ip-ti* ÁB *pa-gar-ti tuballal* (ḪI.ḪI) "you mix dust from the house of a woman who has stopped giving birth with the *siḫiptu* of a . . . cow". The meaning of the terms *siḫiptu* and *pak/gartu* are unclear in this context (cf. CAD P, 35 s.v. *pakartu*). The verb *saḫāpu* means "to envelop; overwhelm", and the derivation *siḫiptu* occurs as a disease designation together with divine names. A similar expression further occurs in BAM 469 rev. 13: "you mix together tamarisk seed with the afterbirth (ARḪUŠ/ÙŠ) of a woman who is *pakartu*" (MUNUS *pa-kar-ti*). The verb *pakāru* means "to tie up, tether", but this meaning seems unlikely here.

Line 210: The *šinūnūtu*-bird (also *šinuntu*, SIM.MAḪ^{mušen}) is probably closely related to *sinuntu* (SIM^{mušen}), the swallow (cf. CAD S, 295–296; CAD Š/3, 55–56). For a parallel remedy with *qinnu ša sinunti* "swallow's nest" in an orally consumed remedy against witchcraft, see Abusch and Schwemer 2011, CMAwR 1, text 10.3: 64''. In both instances, the ingredient presumably refers to an herbal ingredient (i.e. it is an alias name).

Line 211: For the root of the male *pillû*-plant growing on the north side of the tree, which is said to bear no fruit, see also BAM 578+ rev. iii 9 (Cadelli 2000, 201, 218; Johnson and Simkó 2024, 190 against *amurriqānu*-jaundice). Stol (2000a, 70) notes the contrast in line 211 between giving birth (bearing fruit) and the fruitless male *pillû* as the motivation for choosing it here as a remedy.

Line 212: The body part term *papān libbi* is translated as "(area of the) belly" or "diaphragm" (CAD P, 105–106 with medical references sub b; AHw 823 "Bauchwölbung"); Scurlock (2014a, 114 *passim*) and Schmidtchen (2021a, 663) translate the expression as "umbilical area" ("Bauchnabelregion"), following Adamson 1990, *RA* 84, 27–28. The expression is also attested in BAM 249 rev. i' 3' (text D.1.3), a fragmentary prescription to speed up difficult labour, where the woman's belly (*papān libbi*) is likewise rubbed. Note that like BAM 248, BAM 249 is a fragment of a collection of remedies from the library N4 at Assur, which contains a longer section of treatments for difficult delivery partly duplicating BAM 248 iv 13–16 (= see lines 205–208, ms. H). Interestingly, a similar, but simpler prescription applying an ointment to the *papān libbi* is already attested in an Old Babylonian tablet, following an Elamite incantation for a woman in labour:

CUSAS 32, No. 21b: 28'–29' (George 2016, 143; Krebernik 2018, 38):
ana Ì.GIŠ *ta-na-ad-di-ma* 7-*šu mi-š[a-r]a-am pa-ap-pa-al-li-ib-bi-šu ta-pa-aš-ša-aš*
"You cast (the spell) on oil and massage her(!) belly (with it) seven times straight down, (and massage her(!) shoulders seven times straight down)."

For *papān libbi*, see further *Diagnostic Handbook* Tablet 13: 136', 14: 136 (Schmidtchen 2021a, 527, 536, 552 (note on line 94), 572, 604). In a listing of body parts in a physiognomic omen text (Böck 2000, 208–209 CT 28, 25–27 rev. 1ff.), the term *papān libbi* is followed by LI.DUR (*abunnatu*) "area of the navel" and ÚR (*sūnu*) "genital area".

Anointing the woman's belly in a downward direction (*ana muqqalpīti* "going downstream") is reminiscent of the image of the woman in childbirth or the baby as a boat floating down a river.

Line 215: Within the women's healthcare texts, the ingredient *rikibti arkabi* is rare; see also BM 38624+ obv. ii 26' (text A.2.1: 59''') for its use to promote labour; cf. SpTU 1, No. 59: 4'-6' (text C.2.1) for *rikbti arkabi* in a fragmentary prescription to induce(?) the menses. See also the *Introduction* for discussion. Notably, *urânu*-plant (fennel or anise), for which *rikibti arkabi* may be an alias name, is encountered in the same context, see BM 47578 obv. 7 (text C.2.2).

Lines 216–230: This ruled-off text section presents a group of prescriptions and a peculiar ritual for making a band of plant fibres that is tied to the woman's body. The fact that the individual remedies in these lines are not ruled off from each other suggests that this group as a whole was extracted from a common textual source when the Compendium was assembled. See also Couto-Ferreira 2014, 298–306 for discussion.

Lines 217–219, 222: For the dietetic recommendations in these lines, see Couto-Ferreira 2014, 303–304. The exact logic behind recommendation to use specifically the meat of turtle, white pig and vixen for easy birth remains unknown. Although it is possible that these ingredients (especially vixen meat) might be alias names for plants, this latter possibility seems less likely, because concrete instructions for preparation are not given in the three lines. A similar instruction is given in line 222, recommending the consumption of hazelnuts (*allān-Kaniš*, lit. "Kaneš-acorns", a name that points to the northern areas of Mesopotamia and Anatolia as the place of origin; cf. Sturm 2008, *AoF* 35, 296–311), an ingredient that was also prescribed against conditions involving "constriction" (*ḫiniqtu*).

Lines 223–230: For a translation and discussion of these lines (ms. A rev. iv 31–38), see also Veldhuis 1989, 253 with notes; Stol 2000a, 71; Scurlock 2014a, 600; cf. Reiner 1995, 37–38; Couto-Ferreira 2014, 304–306; Steinert 2017a, 330. The passage presents a curious ritual on how to procure plant fibres from an *ašāgu*-plant (acacia shrub; camelthorn) which are spun into a band that is tied to the woman's left thigh. The *ašāgu*-plant is addressed and given a present (*qīštu*) of collected plant shoots, which the ritual expert presents as compensation for robbing it of part of its top and root to procure the needed fibres (cf. CAD Q, 253b s.v. *qimmatu* sub 2b: "you pull out (something from) the root and the top (of the acacia)"). Direct address (invocation, prayer) and offerings to plants and other healing entities are recurringly found in Mesopotamian (as well as Classical Greek and Latin) sources (Reiner 1995, 37–38 with examples). See also *infra*, text C.3.10; Maul 2019, Text 10, 33, 44, 62; Perdibon 2019, 61–63, 124–126, 134–169.

Lines 223–224: In line 223, ḪÉNBUR (ŠE-GAG) corresponds to Akkadian *ḫabbūru* "(green) shoot" or *ziqpu* "shoot, sapling", cf. CAD Ḫ, 15a; CAD Z, 127b sub 1b (with other attested lexical equations); correct CAD Š/1, 6b s.v. *šabāšu* sub 1b reading *ziq-pa ta-šab-bu-uš* "you collect a shoot (from a plant)"; CAD Š/1, 470a s.v. *šaplu* sub 3a-3': "you pour it under an acacia that grows on a garden wall". The *ašāgu*-plant is a type of acacia ("camelthorn, acacia shrub" (*Prosopis farcta*), see Stol 2000a, 71 n. 138; Civil 1987, *FS* Reiner, 47–48. In other healing texts, specifically an *ašāgu* that grows on a mudbrick wall is sought out, see CAD P, 437 s.v. *pitiqtu* sub b (BAM 494 i 43); cf. Reiner 1995, 39 (for *ašāgu* growing on a grave). For the motif see also Farber 1977, *Ištar and Dumuzi*, 61: 67. Couto-Ferreira (2014, 305) points out a parallel from Pliny's *Natural History* (23.71), in which a healing plant is picked, and care is taken that it does not touch the ground for special efficacy (or purity?) – a detail resembling the choice of the *ašāgu*-plant.

Lines 231–235: In ms. A (rev. iv 39–43), these lines form a kind of appendix of prescriptions (for an amulet, and ointment and a fumigation) not concerned with birth, but with protecting the newborn baby from malign divine and demonic influences (here especially from the "Hand of the god" and from the *lilû*-wind demon) that are associated with epilepsy or epilepsy-like afflictions (for discussion see also Volk 1999, 4, 17–18; Stol 1993, 33–38, 46–49, 131–132). The recipes were thus drawn from a different medical context and integrated into the Birth Compendium. This is clear from the duplicate ms. F from Nineveh (K. 3628+), which forms the second tablet of an excerpt series (*nisḫu*) that specifically focuses on children but deals with more conditions and superhuman agents responsible for them, see Scurlock 2014a, 621–626 text 2.13.1 for an edition of ms. F. For discussion of the colophon (on the joined fragment K. 19939) and context of ms. F, see Schmidtchen 2019, *JMC* 33, 32–34.

Lines 231–232: For these lines see also Farber 1989a, 124–125 § 44 with notes; Abusch and Schwemer 2011, CMAwR 1, 39. Ms. A has a syllabic spelling *il-la-at* instead of ÚḪ in ms. E, which may indicate that the logogram ÚḪ was read *illātu* instead of the more common *ru'tu* "spittle, saliva" here.

In lines 231 and 233, ms. E (BAM 183) omits the introductory clauses to the prescriptions found in mss. A. Ms. F obv. 22' has DIŠ KI.MIN, which resumes the introductory clause identical with ms. A rev. iv 41 (DIŠ *a-na* [L]Ú.TUR LÍL.LÁ.EN.NA NU TE-*e*), albeit in a preceding remedy (F obv. 19').

Lines 233–235: For these lines, see also Farber 1989a, 126–127 §45. The same recipe as in ms. F (K. 3628+) obv. 20' (= line 234) used here against the *lilû*-wind demon was applied to combat "Hand of the goddess" in ms. F obv. 13'; similarly, the recipe in F obv. 21' (against *lilû*, line 235) is also applied in F obv. 14' (Hand of the goddess), see Scurlock 2014a, 622 with diverging line count (translating *qāt ištari* as "Hand of Ištar" instead of "Hand of the goddess").

The Akkadian reading of SÍG(.)ÙZ "goat hair" in line 233 may be either *šārtu* or *šārat enzi*, cf. CAD Š/2, 129–130 sub mng. 3, with the present passage quoted sub 2b; CAD U/W, 216 s.v. *urgulû* sub 1a. For *urgulû* "lion", see also Wiggermann 1992, *Protective Spirits*, 90.

The ingredient *eṣemti amēli/amēlūti* "human bone" is an alias name for the "shepherd staff-plant" (ᵘGIDRU (SIPA), *ḫaṭṭi rē'î*), Rumor 2017, *JMC* 29, 9, 27 Uruanna III 36 (34); cf. Böck 2014a, 141, 147–148, 157–158 for other alias names of "shepherd staff-plant".

Lines 236–237: For the colophon see also Hunger 1968, 88 No. 281. The catchline cited in line 236 is the incipit of an unknown Sumerian incantation that was presumably recited against gynaecological haemorrhage, see Finkel 1980, *AfO* 27, 43b; Civil 1974, *JNES* 33, 331; Stol 2000a, 71 with n. 141; cf. van Dijk (et al.) 1985, YOS 11, 32. Finkel (ibid.) links the keyword idim in the catchline to *nagbu* "spring" and the waters of the Apsû; the waters of the spring/source flowing copiously are an image for the flow of blood or other fluids (e.g. amniotic fluid). The phrase a-idim "water of the source" also occurs in Old Babylonian Sumerian incantations against haemorrhage discussed by Finkel 1980, see especially 42–43 line 4, where the speaker of the spell says he is going a-idim BAD-e-dè "to shut off the spring water".

The citation of a catchline in BAM 248 (ms. A) implies that the text itself belonged to a longer medical compendium. However, the colophon does not identify the tablet as belonging to a specific series (*iškāru*) or compendium in a technical sense. Therefore, a straightforward connection of this Assur text and its closest Nineveh duplicate(s) (ms. B) with the medical compendium outlined in the Assur Medical Catalogue, especially with the treatise BIRTH remains to be proven by future evidence. However, the materials of the "Neo-Assyrian Birth Compendium" have close affinities to texts indicated by the incipits quoted in the AMC section BIRTH (see Steinert et al. 2018, 218, 272–276 lines 115–119 for discussion). The association of the catchline of BAM 248 with gynaecological bleeding matches with the inclusion of a tablet concerned with haemorrhage/menstrual bleeding (*sagû*) in the AMC treatise BIRTH (AMC line 118).

D.1.2 K. 11956 + 14200: An Excerpt with Treatments for Difficult Delivery

The fragments K. 11956 + 14200 belong to a small tablet in landscape format written in Neo-Assyrian script, of which the right portion is still missing. The tablet contains one line of symptom description introducing the topic (difficult birth), an incantation rubric (without the text of the incantation written out) and two rituals to go with it. The first of these procedures is duplicated in the Neo-Assyrian Birth Compendium (BAM 248 and duplicates) and may have been excerpted from the Nineveh copy of the compendium (K. 2413(+) = AMT 67/1), which like K. 11956+ belonged to Ashurbanipal's library. The second procedure, written down as an alternative treatment (DÙ.DÙ.BI 2-*ú*, *nēpešu šanû* "second/alternative procedure"), is hitherto unknown from other sources. The tablet ends with a colophon, marking the tablet as the property of Ashurbanipal's palace library. One could wonder whether the text was excerpted to serve for the performance of birth rituals when women in the palace gave birth.

List of Manuscripts

Siglum	Museum Number	Copy	Collation	Format; Ductus	Provenience
A	K. 11956 + K. 14200	Geers, Folio A135 (K. 11956) Pl. 38	Coll.	Fragments of a single-column tablet in landscape format; Neo-Assyrian script; 7th cent. BCE	Nineveh, Ashurbanipal's library[360]
B	VAT 8869	KAR 196 BAM 248	Coll.	Two-column tablet; Neo-Assyrian script; 8th/7th cent. BCE	Assur, N4 library
c	BM 36339 (80-6-17, 65)	Pl. 35	Coll.	Fragment of a single-column tablet; Neo-Babylonian script	Babylon

Overview

i	Fragmentary A obv. 1	1
ii	Incantation rubric A obv. 2 // B obv. i 51 / c obv. 1'	2
iii	Ritual procedure to speed up a difficult delivery A obv. 3–5 // B obv. i 52–53 // c obv. 2'–4' (variant)	3–5
iv	Alternative procedure to speed up a difficult delivery A obv. 6–rev. 2	6–14
v	Fragmentary colophon A rev. 3–5	15–17

Previous Edition and Discussion

Lambert, Folio 09741 (transliteration of K. 11956)
CDLI P399540 (photo of K.11956), P400683 (photo of K. 14200)
Electronic Babylonian Library Project (eBL) (transliteration of ms. A; https://www.ebl.lmu.de/library/K.11956) (photo and transliteration of ms. c, https://www.ebl.lmu.de/library/BM.36339)
Infra, text D.1.1 (edition mss. B and c)

Transliteration

1	A obv. 1	[DIŠ ^{munus}PEŠ$_4$$^?$ Ù.T]U-*ma šup-š*[*u-qat* . . . . . .]

2	A obv. 2	[KA.INIM.MA$^?$] ^{munus}L[A.RA.AḪ.A.KAM$^?$]
	B obv. i 51	[KA.INIM.MA] ^{munus}LA.RA.AḪ.A.KÁM
	c obv. 1'	[KA.INIM.MA ^{munus}LA.RA.AḪ.A.KA]M$^?$

3	A obv. 3	[DÙ.DÙ.BI *ana* Š]À$^?$ ^{giš}SAG.KUD G[I DU$_{10}$.GA . . . .]
	B obv. i 52	[DÙ.DÙ.BI *ana* ŠÀ ^{gi}]⸢SAG⸣.KUD GI DU$_{10}$.GA Ì.GIŠ *ta-tab-bak*
	c obv. 2'–3'	[. . . . . G]I ⸢DU$_{10}$⸣.GA SAḪAR ⸢SILA⸣.LÍM.MA / [. . . . . . .]

---

360 Measurements: ca. 5 x 4.3 x 2 cm.

4	A obv. 4	[ÉN . . .]-*šú ana* ŠÀ ŠID-*n*[*u* . . . .]
	B obv. i 53	[. . . . . Š]ID$^{?}$-*nu ina* UGU ŠÀ-*šá* GAZ-[*ma*$^{?}$]
	c obv. 3'$^{cont.}$–4'	[ÉN] 7$^{?}$ *u* 7-*šú ana* ŠÀ ŠID-*nu ana* UGU *lìb-bi-šú* / [GAZ-*ma*]
5	A obv. 5	[*ár-ḫiš ul-lad-ma*$^{?}$] *šer-ru u*[*š-te-še-ra*$^{?}$]
	B obv. i 53$^{cont.}$	*šèr-ru uš*-[*te-še*]-*ra*
	c obv. 4'$^{cont.}$	[*šè*]*r-ri uš-te-še*-<<*eš*>>-*ri*

6	A obv. 6	[DÙ.DÙ.B]I ⸢2⸣-*ú* 14 DUG KAŠ [. . . . .]
7	A obv. 7	[7 A]L.ŠEG$_{6}$.GÁ 7 NU AL.Š[EG$_{6}$.GÁ . . . .]
8	A obv. 8	[*n*]*a*$^{?}$-*aḫ-la* x[. . . . .]
9	A obv. 9	^{giš}SAG.KUD GI DU$_{10}$.GA [TI-*qí*$^{?}$]
10	A obv. 10	Ì.GIŠ *ḫal-ṣu a-n*[*a* ŠÀ *ta-tab-bak*$^{?}$]
11	A obv. 11	ÉN ŠID-*nu-ma* [*ina* UGU ŠÀ-*šá*$^{?}$]
12	A obv. 12	*tu-šag-r*[*a-ar*$^{?}$ (. . .)]
13	A rev. 1	*ina* UGU ŠÀ.TÙR-*šá* [GAZ-*ma*$^{?}$]
14	A rev. 2	*šer-ru uš-te*-[*še-ra*$^{?}$ (. . .)]

Colophon:

15	A rev. 3	[*ki-m*]*a la-bi-ri-šú šà*-[*ṭir-ma*$^{?}$ . . .]
16	A rev. 4	[É.GA]L ^{m}*Aš-šur*-DÙ-A LUGAL ŠÚ-*t*[*i*$^{?}$ LUGAL KUR *Aš-šur*^{ki}]
17	A rev. 5	[*šá a-na*] ⸢AN.ŠAR⸣ *u* ^{d}⸢*iš*$_{8}$-*tár*⸣ ⸢*tak*$^{?}$⸣-*lu*$^{?}$-[*ma* . . .]

Ms. A rev. breaks; remainder lost

Bound Transcription and Translation

[1] [*šumma erītu ulla*]*d-ma šupšu*[*qat* . . .]	[1] [If a pregnant woman] suffers severely during her delivery [. . .].
[2] [KA.INIM.MA$^{?}$] ^{munus}L[A.RA.AḪ.A.KAM$^{?}$]	[2] [Spell] for a woman who has difficulties in [delivery].
[3] [DÙ.DÙ.BI *ana lib*]*bi takkussi qanî ṭābi šamna* (var. *eper sūq erbetti*) *tatabbak* [4] [*šipta sebe u sebîšu*] *ana libbi tamannū-ma ana muḫḫi libbīšu teḫeppī*-[*ma*] [5] [*arḫiš ullad-ma*(?)] *šerru uš*[*teššera*]	[3] [The procedure for it:] you pour oil (var. dust from a crossroads)] [int]o a straw of 'sweet reed'. [4] You recite [the incantation seven and seven] times into it (the reed), [you break it above her belly. Then] [5] [she will deliver quickly and(?)] the child will [come out straight away].

6 [DÙ.DÙ.B]I *šanû* 14 *karpāt šikari* [. . .] 7 [7] *ṣarpūti* 7 *lā ṣarpūti* [. . .] 8 [*n*]*aḫla* [. . . . . .] 9 *takkussi qanî ṭābi* [*teleq-qe*(?)] 10 *šamna ḫalṣa ana li*[*bbi tatabbak*(?)] 11 *šipta tamannū-ma* [*ina muḫḫi libbīša*(?)] 12 *tušagr*[*ar* (. . .)] 13 *ina muḫḫi šassūrīša te*[*ḫeppī-ma*(?)] 14 *šerru ušte*[*ššera*]

6 Alternative [proce]dure: [You . . .] fourteen vessels of beer [. . .], 7 [seven] fired and seven unfired (vessels) [. . .]. 8 [You . . . si]fted(?) [flour(?) . . .]. 9 [You take(?)] a stem of the 'sweet reed', 10 [you pour(?)] pressed oil in[to it(?)]. 11 You recite the incantation. Then 12 you roll (it) 11[over her belly(?) (. . .)], 13 [you break it(?)] above(?) her womb (i.e. belly/vagina). [Then] 14 the baby will [come out straight away].

Colophon:

15 [*kīm*]*a labirīšu ša*[*ṭer* . . .] 16 [*ēkal*] *Aššur-bāni-apli šar kiš*[*šati šar māt Aššur*] 17 [*ša ana*] *Aššur u Ištar taklū-*[*ma* . . .]

15 Written according to its original [. . .]. 16 [Palace] of Ashurbanipal, king of the universe, [king of Assyria], 17 [who tr]usts in Aššur and ⌜Ištar⌝, [. . .]

Ms. A rev. breaks; remainder lost

Notes

Lines 1–2: The restoration of line 1 [DIŠ ^{munus}PEŠ$_4$ Ù.T]U-*ma šup-š*[*u-qat* . . .] is tentative and follows the incipit of Tablet 1 of the medical treatise BIRTH in the Assur Medical Catalogue (Steinert et al. 2018, 218, 272–273, line 115), reading: DIŠ ^{munus}PEŠ$_4$ *ina a-la-d*[*i-šá šu-up-šu-qat a-n*]*a šu-up-šu-ḫ*[*i*] "If a pregnant woman [suffers severely] during [her] delivery, [in] order to calm (her) down". A similar entry is found in AMT 66/4 (rev. i' 3'), beginning DIŠ ^{munus}PEŠ$_4$ *i-na a-l*[*a-di-šá šup-šu-qat*]. Passages with comparable, but not identical phrasing as in K. 11956: 1 occur also in incantations, e.g. in BAM 248 obv. i 36 (incipit), cf. rev. iii 41 // ([(ÉN) . . .]) *šup-šu-qat a-la-da* "([(Incantation): . . .], she has trouble in (her) delivery"). It is thus not excluded that K. 11956: 1 actually gives the incipit of an incantation for a woman in labour, which in fact could be the spell in BAM 248 obv. i 36–50, which is likewise followed by the rubric [KA.INIM.MA] ^{munus}LA.RA.AḪ.A.KÁM in BAM 248 obv. i 51, as in K. 11956: 2. This is rendered even the more likely, since K. 11956: 3–5 consists of a passage that duplicates BAM 248 i 52–53. In this light, we may suggest restoring K. 11956: 1 in a different way, as an incantation incipit: [ÉN MUNUS$^?$ . . .] x-*ma šup-š*[*u-qat a-la-da*] "[Spell. *The woman* . . .], and she has diffi[culty in (her) delivery]". This problem cannot be solved without additional textual evidence.

Lines 3–5: The restoration follows BAM 248 obv. i 52–53 (ms. B). Ms. c offers a textual variant, by using dust instead of oil to fill a hollow reed straw (*takkussu*). Lines 4–5 of ms. A could be restored in the light of mss. B or c. Reed straws (often from the "sweet/aromatic reed") were used, for instance, in rituals to whisper an incantation into the ritual subject's ear. In medical texts, they are often employed to suck *materia medica* or to blow them into a body opening, see CAD T 79, sub 2 for references.

Lines 6–14: The "alternative procedure" described in these lines seems to be more complex than that in lines 3–5, probably consisting of several actions. Lines 6–8 probably belong together and most likely describe an offering, as is indicated by the mention of 14 vessels of beer (seven fired and seven unfired ones) in lines 6–7, which may have been used for a libation. Another offering matter, presumably sifted (*naḫlu*) flour, may be mentioned in line 8. The following lines seem to describe two therapeutic actions, again involving a hollow reed. What is preserved of the text looks like a variant of the procedure in lines 3–5, i.e. a hollow reed straw of the "sweet reed" is filled with oil and applied in two different ways on the patient.

Line 12: The keyword here seems to be the verbal form *tu-šag-r*[*a-ar*$^?$] "you roll" (with an irregular durative form of *šugarruru*). A similar procedure using a staff or *e'ru*-wood is found in BAM 248 rev. iv 9 //: ÉN 7-*šú* ŠID-*nu-ma* TA SAG ŠÀ-*šá ana šap-la-an* ŠÀ-*šá tuš-ga-ra-ár* "you recite the incantation seven times, you roll (a shepherd's staff of *e'ru*-wood) over her belly, from top to bottom" (see text D.1.1).

Line 13: The action performed with the reed tube could be parallel to breaking (*teḫeppi*) it in the first procedure (the parallels BAM 248 // have *ina muḫḫi libbīša* "above her belly", but in the present case, the locus of the action is not the women's belly but her "womb"). The phrase *ina muḫḫi šassūrīša* "(you . . . it) above/over her womb" could either refer to the belly (i.e. the area where the womb is located seen from the outside) or to the vagina/vulva.

Lines 15–17: The colophon is similar to Hunger 1968, No. 319–320 ("Typ c-e and f"), with the difference that instead of the divine couple usually listed first in Ashurbanipal's colophons, Aššur and Ninlil, K. 11956 seems to read AN.ŠÁR *u* ^{d}U.DAR.

D.1.3 BAM 249: A Fragment of a Compendium with Prescriptions for Delivery

This quite damaged fragment of a two-column tablet from Assur (ms. A) in the collection of the Vorderasiatisches Museum, Berlin preserves in its column i' recipes for speeding up a protracted and difficult delivery. Part of these prescriptions are duplicated in treatments known from the so-called Neo-Assyrian Birth Compendium, whose main manuscript (ms. B) stems from the same library as ms. A (N4 library, the so-called "House of the incantation priest", Pedersén 1986, 75). A third fragment (ms. C_1) from Ashurbanipal's library at Nineveh presents a second manuscript of the Birth Compendium duplicating the same prescriptions. However, ms. A is only a partial duplicate to the Birth Compendium, since it also contained unrelated textual material that diverges from mss. B and C. Furthermore, two prescriptions of the section on delivery in ms. A are duplicated in a women's healthcare text from Sultantepe (STT 98, see text A.1.1 for an edition).

Due to the damaged state of ms. A, it is difficult to identify the purpose of the fragmentary lines at the beginning of column ii'. Remarkably, in col. ii' 11', shortly before the text breaks off, the text features a section with prescriptions to ward off frightening nightmares, which are very likely related to the apotropaic dream rituals and the series *Ziqīqu* (see Butler 1998 and below). Ms. A thus appears to have been a collection of diverse prescriptions for multiple problems which were not restricted to subjects concerned with women's health or delivery. This mixture of heterogeneous topics is unusual, since in the majority of Mesopotamian medical texts known to date, treatments concerned with women's health were usually not compiled together with remedies that are concerned with completely unrelated topics. Furthermore, ms. A includes instructions for protecting the newborn from "anything evil" (*mimma lemnu*), epilepsy (*bennu*) and "all troubles" (see col. i' 5'), which resembles the inclusion of similar protective treatments in the Neo-Assyrian Birth Compendium (see text D.1.1).

There is slight curving of the surface of the side of ms. A preserving text (see CDLI for a photograph of the fragment). It is therefore possible that col. i' and ii' actually have to be identified as the reverse rather than the obverse of the tablet (and would then need to be renumbered as col. iv and iii, respectively).

List of Manuscripts

Siglum	Museum Number	Copy	Collation	Format; Ductus	Provenience
A	VAT 13972	BAM 249	Coll.	Fragment of a two-column tablet; Neo-Assyrian script; ca. 8th/7th cent. BCE	Assur; N4 library
B	VAT 8869	KAR 196 BAM 248	Coll.	Two-column tablet; Neo-Assyrian script; 8th/7th cent. BCE	Assur; N4 library
C_1 + C_4 + C_5	K. 2413 + K. 18482 + K. 16363	AMT 67/1 (K. 2413 only)	Coll.	Fragments of a two-column tablet; Neo-Assyrian script; 7th cent. BCE	Nineveh; Ashurbanipal's library
D	SU 52/83 (+) 52/83A (+) 52/111 (+) 52/130 (+) 52/130A	STT 98	Coll.	Fragments of a single-column tablet; Neo-Assyrian script; 7th cent. BCE	Sultantepe

Overview

i'	Fragmentary prescription to speed up a difficult delivery A obv.? i' 1'–2' // D rev. 1'–3'	. . .]1'–2'
ii'	Fragmentary prescription to speed up a difficult delivery A obv.? i' 3'–5' // D rev. 4'–6'	3'–5'
iii'	Prescription to protect the newborn (ointment) A obv.? i' 6'–7'	6'–7'
iv'	Prescription to speed up a difficult delivery (potion) A obv.? i' 8'–10' // B rev. iv 13–15 // C rev. iv 6–8	8'–10'
v'	Prescription to speed up a difficult delivery (potion) A obv.? i' 11'–12' // B rev. iv 16 // C rev. iv 9	11'–12'
vi'	Fragmentary prescription to speed up a difficult delivery(?) A obv.? i' 13'	13'
vii'	Fragmentary prescription to speed up a difficult delivery(?) A obv.? i' 14'	14'
viii'	Fragmentary prescription to speed up a difficult delivery(?) A obv.? i' 15'	15'
ix'	Fragmentary prescription to speed up a difficult delivery(?) A obv.? i' 16'	16'
x'	Fragmentary prescription to speed up a difficult delivery (ointment) A obv.? i' 17'	17'
xi'	Fragmentary prescription to speed up a difficult delivery A obv.? i' 18'	18'
xii'	Fragmentary prescription to speed up a difficult delivery A obv.? i' 19'	19'
xiii'	Fragmentary prescription to speed up a difficult delivery A obv.? i' 20'	20'
xiv'	Fragmentary prescription to speed up a difficult delivery A obv.? i' 21'	21'[. . .
xv''	Fragmentary prescription A obv.? ii' 1'	. . .]22''
xvi''	Fragmentary prescription A obv.? ii' 2'–3'	23''–24''
xvii''	Fragmentary prescription A obv.? ii' 4'–5'	25''–26''
xviii''	Fragmentary prescription A obv.? ii' 6'	27''
xix''	Fragmentary prescription A obv.? ii' 7'-8'	28''–29''
xx''	Fragmentary prescription A obv.? ii' 9'	30''

xxii''	Fragmentary prescription to ward off frightening dreams(?) A obv.$^{?}$ ii' 10'–14'	31''–35''
xxiii''	Fragmentary prescription to ward off frightening dreams(?) A obv.$^{?}$ ii' 15'	36''[. . .

Previous Edition and Discussion

CDLI P285334 (transliteration; photo)

BabMed Corpora (https://www.geschkult.fu-berlin.de/e/babmed/Corpora/BAM-3/BAM-3_-249; transliteration)

Electronic Babylonian Library Project (eBL) (https://www.ebl.lmu.de/library/VAT.13972)

Infra text D.1.1 (edition of mss. B and C), text A.1.1 (edition of ms. D)

Transliteration

Beginning of ms. A obv.$^{?}$ i' lost

1'	A obv.$^{?}$ i' 1'	[. . . . .] an [x x] ⸢x x x⸣ [x x x x]
	D rev. 1'–2'	DIŠ ^{munus}PEŠ$_4$ ⸢*ina*⸣ [Ù.TU *uš-tap-šiq* . . .] / ^{giš}GEŠTIN.KA$_5$.A [. . . . .]
2'	A obv.$^{?}$ i' 2'	[. . . . .]x ⸢*ul*⸣ ⸢*uš*$^{?}$-*tap*$^{!}$⸣-*áš-šaq ár-ḫiš* <<*ḫiš*>> *ul-lad*
	D rev. 2'$^{\text{cont.}}$–3'	[. . . . .] / *ul uš-tap-pa-*⸢*áš*⸣-*ša*[*q* . . . .]
A, D		
3'	A obv.$^{?}$ i' 3'	[^{giš}GEŠTIN.K]A$_5$.A Ḫ[ÁD].⸢A⸣ ⸢SÚD$^{?}$⸣ ⸢*ina*⸣ ⸢Ì$^{?}$⸣ *pa-pa-an* ŠÀ-*šá*
	D rev. 4'	^{giš}⸢GEŠTIN.KA$_5$⸣.A ḪÁD.DA S[ÚD . . . .]
4'	A obv.$^{?}$ i' 4'	[x x] x [ŠÉŠ$^{?}$-*m*]*a*$^{?}$ *ár-ḫiš ul-lad šá*$^{?!}$ ŠÀ-*šá* ⸢SILIM$^{?!}$(BA)⸣
	D rev. 4'$^{\text{cont.}}$–5	[. . . . .] / *ár-ḫiš ul-lad šá* Š[À-*šá*$^{?}$ . . . .]
5'	A obv.$^{?}$ i' 5'	[*bul-ṭu*$^{?}$ *lat*]-⸢*ku*$^{?}$⸣ ⸢*mim*$^{?}$-*ma*$^{?}$⸣ *lem*$^{?}$-⸢*nim*⸣ *be-en-nu u* DÙ GIG-*te*
	D rev. 5'$^{\text{cont.}}$–6'	[. . . . .] / *be-en-nu* [. . . . .]
A, D		
6'	A obv.$^{?}$ i' 6'	[x x] ⸢x x⸣-*a-tú* ⸢ŠID$^{?}$⸣ x x ⸢du$^{?}$⸣ *la-am* UBUR$^{!?}$
7'	A obv.$^{?}$ i' 7'	[*ana* KA$^{?}$]-*šú* GAR-*ni ina* Ì ŠÉŠ-*ma* EN TI *mim-ma lem*$^{!}$-*nu* ⸢NU$^{!}$⸣ ⸢TE⸣
8'	A obv.$^{?}$ i' 8'	[DIŠ MUNUS$^{?}$ (*ina*)] ⸢Ù.TU$^{?}$⸣ *uš*$^{!}$-*tap-šiq*$^{!}$-*šú* ^{ú}GEŠTIN.KA$_5$.A ^{ú}EME-UR.GI$_7$
	B rev. iv 13	DIŠ MUNUS *ina* Ù.TU *uš-tap-šiq* ^{giš}GEŠTIN.KA$_5$.A ⸢^{ú}EME⸣-UR.GI$_7$
	C$_1$ rev. iv 6	DIŠ MUNUS *ina* Ù.TU *uš-tap-šiq* ^{giš}GEŠTIN.KA$_5$.A ⸢^{ú}EME⸣-UR.GI$_7$
9'	A obv.$^{?}$ i' 9'	[^{ú}*tuḫ-lam*$^{?}$ ^{ú}IN].NU.UŠ DIŠ-*niš* SÚD ^{dug}LA.ḪA.AN KAŠ ^{lú}KÚRUN DIRI
	B rev. iv 14	^{ú}*tuḫ-lam* SÚD ^{dug}LA.ḪA.AN KAŠ ^{lú}KÚRUN.NA DIRI-*ma*
	C$_1$ rev. iv 7	^{ú}*tuḫ-lam* SÚD ^{dug}LA.ḪA.AN KAŠ ^{lú}KÚRUN.NA DIRI-*ma*
10'	A obv.$^{?}$ i' 10'	[(x x x) Ú].ḪI.A ŠEŠ *ana* ŠÀ SÌG-*aṣ* NU *pa-tan* NAG-*ši-ma ár-ḫiš ul-lad*
	B rev. iv 15	Ú.ḪI.A *an-nu-ti ana* ŠÀ SÌG-*aṣ la pa-tan* NAG-*ma ár-ḫiš* Ù.TU
	C$_1$ rev. iv 8	Ú.ḪI.A *an-nu-ti ana* ŠÀ SÌG-*aṣ la pa-tan* NAG-*ma ár-ḫiš* Ù.TU
A, B, C		

11'	A obv.$^{?}$ i' 11'	[DIŠ ^{munus}PE]Š$_{4}$$^{?}$ *ina* Ù.TU *uš-tap-šiq* ŠE$_{10}$ EME.DIR IZ.ZI SÚD
	B rev. iv 16	DIŠ KI.MIN ŠE$_{10}$ EME.DIR *šá* IZ.ZI SÚD
	C$_{1}$ rev. iv 9	DIŠ KI.MIN ŠE$_{10}$ EME.ŠID *šá* IZ.ZI ⸢SÚD⸣
12'	A obv.$^{?}$ i' 12'	[*ina* KAŠ NU *p*]*a-tan* NAG-*ma ár-ḫiš ul-lad*
	B rev. iv 16$^{cont.}$	*ina* KAŠ *la pa-tan* NAG-*ma* KI.MIN
	C$_{1}$ rev. iv 9$^{cont.}$	*ina* KAŠ *la pa-tan* NAG-*ma* KI.MIN

B, C____

13'	A obv.$^{?}$ i' 13'	[DIŠ KI.MIN$^{?}$ . . . .-*m*]*a* MIN
14'	A obv.$^{?}$ i' 14'	[. . . . .-*m*]*a* MIN
15'	A obv.$^{?}$ i' 15'	[. . . . .-*m*]*a* MIN
16'	A obv.$^{?}$ i' 16'	[. . . . .-*m*]*a* MIN
17'	A obv.$^{?}$ i' 17'	[. . . . .] ŠÉŠ-*ma* MIN
18'	A obv.$^{?}$ i' 18'	[. . . . .] MIN
19'	A obv.$^{?}$ i' 19'	[. . . . . *ina* Ì.N]UN$^{?}$ MIN
20'	A obv.$^{?}$ i' 20'	[. . . . .] MIN
21'	A obv.$^{?}$ i' 21'	[. . . . .] MIN

Ms. A obv.$^{?}$ i' breaks; gap of unknown length

22''	A obv.$^{?}$ ii' 1'	*ina* Ì PÉŠ.ÙR.R[A . . . .]
23''	A obv.$^{?}$ ii' 2'	DIŠ KI.MIN PIŠ$_{10}$.^{d}ÍD ⸢^{ú}⸣[. . . . .]
24''	A obv.$^{?}$ ii' 3'	KA *tam-tim* ^{giš}x[. . . . .]
25''	A obv.$^{?}$ ii' 4'	DIŠ KI.MIN Ú.KU$_{6}$ ^{ú}KUR.KUR [. . . . .]
26''	A obv.$^{?}$ ii' 5'	ŠE$_{10}$ ARKAB<^{mušen}> šu [. . . . .]
27''	A obv.$^{?}$ ii' 6'	DIŠ KI.MIN ^{ú}*tar-muš*$_{8}$ ^{ú}IGI-*lim* [. . . . .]
28''	A obv.$^{?}$ ii' 7'	DIŠ KI.MIN *gul-gul* LÚ.[U$_{18}$.LU . . . .]
29''	A obv.$^{?}$ ii' 8'	NÍTA *u* MUNUS ^{na4}*mu-ṣa* [. . . . .]
30''	A obv.$^{?}$ ii' 9'	DIŠ KI.MIN ^{ú}x[. . . . .]

31''	A obv.$^{?}$ ii' 10'	kur ⸢x x⸣ [. . . . .]
32''	A obv.$^{?}$ ii' 11'	DIŠ NA MÁŠ.G[I$_{6}$.MEŠ *pár-da-ti iṭ-ṭul* MÁŠ.GI$_{6}$.MEŠ-*šú*]
33''	A obv.$^{?}$ ii' 12'	*ana* ḪUL-*tú* GAR-*š*[*ú*$^{?}$ . . . .]
34''	A obv.$^{?}$ ii' 13'	ḪUL-*ši*$^{!}$-*na* <*ana*> B[ÚR$^{?}$ *u ana* NA NU TE-*e*$^{?}$ . . .]
35''	A obv.$^{?}$ ii' 14'	^{ú}KUR.KUR ⸢MUN$^{?!}$⸣ [*eme-sal-lim* . . . *ina* KUŠ$^{?}$]
36''	A obv.$^{?}$ ii' 15'	DIŠ KI.MIN NUMUN ⸢$^{ú?}$⸣[. . . . .]

Ms. A obv.$^{?}$ ii' breaks; remainder lost

Bound Transcription and Translation

Beginning of ms. A obv.? i' lost

1' *šumma erītu ina [alādīša uštapšiq . . .] . . . karān šēlebi* [. . .] 2' [. . .] *ul uštapaššaq arḫiš ullad*

1' If a pregnant woman [suffers severely] during [delivery . . .], . . . 'fox grape'-plant [. . .] 2' [. . .]. She will not have an agonizing labour, (but) she will deliver quickly.

3' *karān šēlebi tubbal tasâk ina šamni*(?) *papān libbīša* 4' [. . .]. . . [*tapaššaš-m*]*a*(?) *arḫiš ullad ša libbīša išallim*(?) 5' [*bulṭu lat*]*ku*(?) *mimma lemni bennu u kal marušte*

3' You dry (and) crush 'fox grape'-plant, (mix it?) with oil(?), 4' [you rub(?)] 3' the area of her belly [. . .]. 4' Then she will deliver quickly, (and) her baby(?) will be healthy(?). 5' [*A pro*]*ven* [*remedy against*(?)] anything evil, *bennu*-epilepsy and all trouble.

6' [. . .] . . . [. . .]. . . *lām tulâ* 7' [*ana pī*]*šu*(?) *šakāni ina šamni tapaššaš-ma adi balṭu mimma lemnu ul iṭeḫḫe*

6' [. . .] . . . [. . .]. Before 7' putting 6' (his mother's) breast 7' [into] his (the baby's) [mouth], you should rub (the baby) with oil, and as long as he lives, anything evil will not approach (him).

8' [*šumma sinništu*] *alādu uštapšiqšu* (var. *ina alādi uštapšiq*) *karān šēlebi lišān kalbi* 9' *tuḫla maštakal ištēniš tasâk laḫanna šikar sābî tumallā-ma* 10' [(. . .)] *šammī annûti ana libbi tamaḫḫaṣ lā patān tašaqqīši-ma arḫiš ullad*

8' [If a woman] has an agonizing delivery, you pound 'fox grape'-plant, 'dog's tongue'-plant, 9' *tuḫlu*-plant (and) *maštakal*-plant together. You fill a bottle with beer from an innkeeper, 10' [(. . .)] you stir these [drug]s into it. You give (it) to her to drink on an empty stomach. Then she will deliver quickly.

11' [*šumma erītu*(?)] (var. DIŠ KI.MIN) *ina alādi uštapšiq zê ṣurār igāri tasâk* 12' [*ina šikari lā pa*]*tān išattī-ma arḫiš ullad* (var. KI.MIN)

11' [If a pregnant woman(?)] has an agonizing delivery (var. Alternatively), you pound 'excrement of wall lizard'. 12' She shall drink (it) [in beer on an empty] stomach. Then she will deliver quickly (var. ditto).

13' [DIŠ KI.MIN . . . . . .]-*ma* MIN

14' [. . . . . .]-*ma* MIN

15' [. . . . . .]-*ma* MIN

16' [. . . . . .]-*ma* MIN

17' [. . . . . .] *tapaššaš-ma* MIN

18' [. . . . . .] MIN

19' [. . . . . . *ina ḫim*]*ēti*(?) MIN

20' [. . . . . .] MIN

21' [. . . . . .] MIN

13' [Alternatively(?), ...], and ditto (i.e., she will deliver quickly).

14' [. . . . . .], and ditto (i.e., she will deliver quickly).

15' [. . . . . .], and ditto (i.e., she will deliver quickly).

16' [. . . . . .], and ditto (i.e., she will deliver quickly).

17' [. . . . . .] you rub, and ditto (i.e., she will deliver quickly).

18' [. . . . . .], ditto (i.e., you rub and she will deliver quickly).

19' [. . . . . . *with gh*]*ee*(?) ditto (i.e., you rub and she will deliver quickly).

20' [. . . . . .], ditto.

21' [. . . . . .], ditto.

Ms. A obv.? i' breaks; gap of unknown length

Beginning of ms. A obv.? ii' lost

22'' *ina šaman arra[bi . . . . . .]*

22'' with fat of an *arrabu*-dormou[se, ...].

23'' DIŠ KI.MIN *kibrītu . . .[. . . . . .]* 24'' *imbû tâmti . . .[. . . . . .]*

23'' Alternatively, [you . . .] *kibrītu*-sulphur, [. . .]-plant, [. . . . . .] 24'' *imbû-tâmti*-mineral, [. . .]-tree, [. . . . . .].

25'' DIŠ KI.MIN Ú.KU$_6$ *atā'išu* [. . . . . .] 26'' *zê arkabi . . .[. . . . . .]*

25'' Alternatively, [you . . .] Ú.KU$_6$-plant, *atā'išu*-plant, [. . . . . .], 26'' excrement of a bat, . . . [. . . . . .].

27'' DIŠ KI.MIN *tarmuš imḫur-līm* [. . . . . .]

27'' Alternatively, [you . . .] *tarmuš*-plant, 'heals thousand'-plant, [. . . . . .].

28'' DIŠ KI.MIN *gulgul amē[li . . . . . .]* 29'' *zikar u sinniš mūṣa* [. . . . . .]

28'' Alternatively, [you . . .] hu[man] skull, [. . . . . .], 29'' male and female 28''[. . .-stone/plant], 29'' *mūṣu*-stone, [. . . . . .].

30'' DIŠ KI.MIN . . .[. . . . . .]

30'' Alternatively, [. . .]-plant, [. . . . . .].

31'' *traces*

31'' *too fragmentary for translation*

32'' *šumma amēlu šunā[ti pardāti iṭṭul šunātūša(?)]* 33'' *ana lemutti šaknā-š[u . . . . . .]* 34'' *lumunšina* <*ana*> *pa[šāri u ana amēli lā teḫê? . . .]* 35'' *atā'išu ṭābat(?) [emesalli . . . ina maški(?)]* 36'' DIŠ KI.MIN *zēr . . .[. . . . . .]*

32'' If a man [sees frightening] dream[s, (and) his dreams], 33'' inflict misfortune on h[im . . . . . .] 34'' <in order to> dis[solve] their evil [so that it will not come close to (that) man: . . .], 35'' *atā'išu*-plant, [fine] salt(?), [. . . (wrapped up) in a piece of leather(?)]. 36'' Alternatively, [you . . .] seed of [. . .]-plant, [. . . . . .].

Ms. A obv.? ii' breaks; remainder lost

Notes

Lines 1'–2': The restoration of the passage could be confirmed by the duplicating prescription in STT 98 rev. 1'–3' (ms. D), which is, however, likewise fragmentary. The form *⸢ul⸣ ⸢uš?-tap!⸣-áš-šaq* "she will [not] have an agonizing delivery" in line 2' is a Št-stem verbal form of *pašāqu* "to be narrow, difficult" (the spelling *ul uš-tap-pa-⸢áš⸣-ša[q]* in ms. D rev. 3' is defective). The corresponding preterite *uštapšiq* also occurs in the introductory passages in lines 8' and 11', within the phrase *šumma sinništu/erītu ina alādi uštapšiq(šu)* "if a (pregnant) woman suffers severely during delivery", which is also attested several times in parallel passages in the Neo-Assyrian Birth Compendium (BAM 248 etc.). Similar phrases using a Š-stem stative form of *pašāqu* (with the same meaning) are found in other sources (see *infra*, K. 11956 + 14200 obv. 1 (text D.1.2); Assur Medical Catalogue lines 115 and 117 (Steinert et al. 2018, 218, 272–274 with discussion). For the context of childbirth, note also CT 39, 44: 5: *sinništu šī uštapaššaq* "that woman will suffer severely during delivery" (*Šumma Ālu* Tablet 104).

Lines 3'–5': The expression *papān libbīša* "the area of her belly" in line 3' occurs also in one prescription of the Neo-Assyrian Birth Compendium (BAM 248 rev. iv 19–20 and dupl., see text D.1.1 lines 211–212), in which the woman's belly is massaged downwards to promote delivery. Lines 3'–4' of BAM 249 very likely contained a similar, but shorter prescription (i.e., an ointment). The use of 'fox grape'-plant to speed up labour recurs in the following prescription (line 8'); see also AMT 66/4 rev. i' 5' (text D.1.4).

Interestingly, line 5' looks like a comment that the remedy in lines 3'–4' is a proven remedy(?) (*bulṭu latku*) against "anything evil (*mimma lemnu*), *bennu*-epilepsy and all hardship/trouble" (*kal maruštе*). Instead of DÙ GIG-*te*, interpreted here as *kal marušte* "all trouble", one would have expected the more common *kal murṣī* "(for) all illnesses". Should the text perhaps be emended to DÙ GIG <NU> TE "(a remedy that) anything evil, *bennu* and all illnesses <not> come near"? This would be in accordance with line 7', which clearly refers to keeping off anything evil from approaching the baby (see the next note). Line 5' thus appears to be a comment that explains alternative uses of a remedy described earlier. If this interpretation is correct, lines 3'–4' may have contained an ointment that could be used as a panacea (or prophylactic remedy) against any illness or trouble (perhaps to protect the newborn in particular). For discussion of epilepsy-related conditions and infants, see also Volk 1999, *OrNS* 68, 4, 17–18; Stol 1993, 34–35, 131–132; for plants/drugs against *bennu*-epilepsy, cf. Stol 1993, 103–104. For similar remedies to protect the newborn included in women's healthcare texts related to delivery, see also BAM 248 rev. iv 39–43 and duplicates (text D.1.1).

Lines 6'–7': The restoration of these lines is based on a parallel passage found in several texts concerned with protecting babies, edited by Farber 1989a, 65–67 §§ 15–15A lines 216–218. The sources presented by Farber attest to several varying versions of an ointment to protect a baby from illness. The main text preserving the ointment in question (K. 6901+ iii 62'–64' // LKU 32 l. e.) reads as follows:

> [*an*]*a* TU.RA *ana* LÚ.T[UR] N[U TE]-*e* ⸢^{giš}MA.NU⸣ [^{giš}ŠINIG BABBAR.ḪI^{sar}] / ^{túg}NÍG.DÁRA.ŠU.LÁL *tur-ár* SÚD *ina* ÌxG[IŠ ḪI.ḪI] / *la-am* UBUR *ana* KA-*šú* GAR-*nu* ŠÉŠ-*su-ma* TIN-*uṭ*
> "For illness not to come near/approach an infant: you roast and crush *e'ru*-wood, [tamarisk, *papparḫû*-plant], 'soiled rag'. [You mix] (it) with oil. You rub him (with it) before putting the breast into his mouth. Then (the baby) will be healthy."

A similar remedy is encountered in K. 3628 + 4009 + Sm. 1315 rev. 13–15 (Farber 1989a, 67; Scurlock 2014a, 623):

> *ana mim-ma lem-nu ana* LÚ.TUR NU TE-*e* NUMUN ^{giš}MA.NU NUMUN ^{ú}ŠAKIRA / NUMUN ^{ú}KU$_6$ TÚG.NÍG.DÁRA.ŠU.LÁL *ina* Ì.GIŠ ḪI.ḪI / [*l*]*a*-[*a*]*m* UBUR *ana* KA-*šú* GAR-*nu* ŠÉŠ-*su-ma* TI-*uṭ*
> "So that 'anything evil' not approach an infant: you mix seeds of *e'ru*-tree, seeds of *šakirû*-plant, seeds of *šimru*-plant and 'soiled rag' with oil. You rub him (with it) before putting the breast into his mouth. Then he will be healthy."

Based on these parallels, ms. A lines 6'–7' may have been concerned with a similar ointment. However, it is likely that lines 6'–7' expanded on the use of a salve described in the preceding lines of the text, since the space of the gap in line 6' seems rather limited to have contained a complete prescription. Judging from the context of ms. A, the treatment referred to here was very likely performed immediately after the baby had been born (to protect him from all evil for the rest of his life), before he was given the breast for the first time.

The sign form of UBUR in ms. A line 6' is written with the first element DÀG (NA$_4$) instead of DAG (i.e., DÀG-KISIM$_5$xGA), a variation attested for other compound signs with the element DAG-KISIM$_5$. For this variation and interchanges between DAG and DÀG, see Borger 2004, MZL, 124–126 Nos. 438, 440, 452, 455, 460. For further discussion of the sign forms and Sumerian/Akkadian terms for the female breasts, see Rodin 2019, in: *FS Pedersén*, 162–183; Güterbock 1973, in: *FS Otten*, 81–82 (the sign UBUR in the texts from Ḫattuša).

Lines 8'–10': The beginning of line 8' in ms. A has been restored and emended following the duplicates mss. B and C$_1$. However, while mss. B and C$_1$ have *šumma sinništu ina alādi uštapšiq* "if a woman suffers severely during delivery", the verbal form in ms. A *uš*$^{!}$-*tap-šiq*$^{!}$-*šú* with the pronominal suffix referring to the patient implies that *alādu* (Ù.TU) here functions as the subject of the verb *uštapšiq*, i.e. "delivery is extremely difficult for her". On the other hand, one could regard the suffix -*šú* here as an error and emend the text to [DIŠ MUNUS *ina*] ⸢Ù.TU⸣ *uš*$^{!}$-*tap-šiq*$^{!}$-<<*šú*>>.

Other texts feature further variants of this expression. A text from Nineveh in Neo-Babylonian script, K. 1930 + 11752 obv. 12' (text D.1.7) features an entry that probably has to be restored *šumma*(DIŠ) *sinništu*(MUNUS) *ūlid*(Ù.TU)-*ma u*[*š-tap-šiq*] "If a woman has difficulty while giving birth", presenting another variant formulation of the expression encountered in mss. A, B and C$_1$. This text preserves therapies for women, but also includes remedies for the baby, similar to texts such as BAM 248 and 249. Moreover, the Babylonian compendium with various prescription for women BM 38624+ (obv. ii 25) likewise contains a section with remedies DIŠ MUNUS *a-lad uš-tap-šiq* "for the case that a woman has difficulty giving birth" (see text A.2.1).

There are also attestations for expressions using the fem. stative form of *pašāqu* (Š) *šupšuqat*, as in K. 11956 + 14200, a small tablet with two rituals for delivery (duplicated in the Neo-Assyrian Birth Compendium BAM 248), whose incipit can be restored: [DIŠ MUNUS Ù.T]U-*ma šup-š*[*u-qat*] "[If a woman gives] birth, but suffers severely [from hard labour]" (see text D.1.2 for an edition).

The phrase *šumma sinništu ina alādi uštapšiq* is also listed as the incipit or title of a tablet belonging to the section BIRTH in the Assur Medical Catalogue (Steinert et al. 2018, 218, 274 line 117). So far, we are lacking actual witnesses for a therapeutic tablet bearing such an incipit, although the formulation is attested several times as introduction to prescriptions within women's healthcare texts concerned with delivery such as BAM 248 and the therapeutic collection encountered in BAM 249.

At the beginning of line 10' in ms. A, possibly no text is missing in the gap before [Ú].ḪI.A, judging from the duplicates mss. B and C$_1$.

Lines 11'–12': The text of mss. B and C_1 seem to differ slightly in comparison with ms. A. Thus, in mss. B and C_1 the text is slightly abbreviated through the use of ditto-signs at beginning and end of the prescription. While the former manuscripts begin with DIŠ KI.MIN, the traces in ms. A suggest a slightly different restoration [DIŠ ^{munus}PE]Š$_4$$^{?}$ *ina* Ù.TU *uš-tap-šiq* "[if a pregn]ant woman has an agonizing delivery". A parallel for such a variant formulation with *erītu*(^{munus}PEŠ$_4$) instead of mere *sinništu*(MUNUS) is found in the Nineveh text AMT 66/4, a fragment of a two- or multi-column tablet preserving among other topics, treatments and amulet charms for women to ease delivery (see text D.1.4 for an edition). One section in AMT 66/4 rev. i' 3ff. begins with DIS ^{munus}PEŠ$_4$ *i-na a-l*[*a-di-*(*šá*) *uš-tap-šiq/šup-šu-qat* . . .]. Which form of *pašāqu* was used here remains an open issue.

Another attestation for a parallel introductory phrase with *erītu* is presented by the first tablet incipit of the section BIRTH listed in the Assur Medical Catalogue (line 115), which may be restored as DIŠ ^{munus}PEŠ$_4$ *ina a-la-d*[*i-*(*šá*) *šu-up-šu-qat/uš-tap-šiq a-n*]*a šup-šu-ḫ*[*i*] "If a pregnant woman suffers severely during [(her) deliv]ery, in [order to] calm (her) down" (Steinert et al. 2018, 218, 272–273).

Lines 13'–21': It is unfortunate that this section of short prescriptions is so badly damaged. It is possible that these lines of ms. A actually contained remedies that have parallels in mss. B and C_1 (cf. the passages of short prescriptions in mss. B rev. iv 17–18, 21–30 // C_1 rev. iv 10–11, 14–23, *infra*).

Lines 31''–36'': There are no visible traces of a ruling following line 31''. Since line 32'' starts with a new prescription (beginning with DIŠ NA . . .), one wonders whether line 31'' contained some kind of introduction to lines 32''ff. or whether it stood on its own.

Although several differing restorations are possible in lines 32''–35'', the tentative reconstruction proposed here is inspired by a very similar prescription in the so-called *Assur Dream Ritual Compendium*, which belonged to the series *Zaqīqu* (Butler 1998, 281, 300 iii 61–63). The latter prescription, which offers a parallel phraseology and a common ingredient (*atā'išu*-plant) with ms. A lines 32''–35'' presents the first in a group of prescriptions for leather bags filled with various ingredients and worn around the patient's neck. These protective amulets aimed at dissolving the pending misfortune signalled by frightening dreams. The passage reads as follows:

> *šumma*(DIŠ) *amēlu*(NA) *šunāti*(MÁŠ.GI$_6$.MEŠ) *pardāte iṭṭul šunātu*(MÁŠ.GI$_6$.MEŠ)*-šu ana lemutti*(ḪUL) *šaknā*(GAR)*-šú* / *lumun*(ḪUL)*-šina* <*ana*> *pašāri*(BÚR) *u ana amēli*(NA) *lā*(NU) *ṭeḫê*(TE-*e*) *zēr*(NUMUN) *būšāni*(^{ú}ḪAB) *atā'iši*(^{ú}KUR.KUR) / *šamma peṣâ*(Ú BABBAR) *ṭābat*(MUN) *emesalli ina maški*(KUŠ)
> "If a man sees frightening dreams, (and) his dreams inflict misfortune upon him, <in order> to dissolve their evil, (so that) it will not come close to the man: (you place) seeds of *būšānu*-plant, *atā'išu*-plant, 'white drug' (and grains of) *emesallu*-salt in a leather (bag around his neck)."

For other possible restorations and introductory phrases encountered in dream omens and dreams rituals, see further Butler 1998, 241–410; Zgoll 2006. Protection from bad dreams and any form of evil and negative omens was also sought through Namburbi rituals and through protective amulets inscribed with prayers or apotropaic incantations (Maul 1994, 13, 181, 185; Panayotov 2020, 140–145).

D.1.4 K. 10507 (= AMT 66/4): Prescriptions and Amulets for Pregnant Women and for Delivery

This small fragment in Neo-Assyrian script belonged to a two- or multi-column tablet (preserving part of the middle section of the tablet). It shows traces of having been exposed to fire. The surface of the fragment is very flat. Whether it presents part of the reverse of a tablet, as suggested by Simo Parpola (1983b, 21 note to 1ine 1), remains uncertain.

The preserved text presents a mixture of contents. The fragmentary lines in the left-hand column i' consists of a prescription for an amulet (lines 1'–2') for a pregnant woman, which is also known from texts related to the compendium *kunuk ḫalti* (see below) specialized on amulet necklace prescriptions. The next sections (lines 3'–10') are concerned with difficult delivery and include an incantation (lines 6' and 7', zalaḫ zalaḫ) for a woman in difficult labour duplicated in manuscripts of the Neo-Assyrian Birth Compendium BAM 248 // (mss. B and C_1).

The first fragmentary four lines on the right-hand column ii' refer to amulets designated as the "sixth" and "seventh *ṭurru*" (string), providing an interesting link to the genres of amulet texts. In some witnesses of this genre, several amulets are grouped together in sections designated and numbered as "strings". The following two sections in ms. A appear to contain information resembling a colophon, referring to a "copy (of a tablet) from Assyria" (line 16''), which was presumably a source for the preceding text on the tablet. Remarkably, the following line 17'' appears to refer to the series *kunuk ḫalti* "Seal (or cylindrical bead) of *ḫaltu*-stone", a serialized compendium of amulet prescriptions. However, the scribe of ms. A appears to remark on a part of it that was "not written out" (NU SAR), i.e. left out in the copy of ms. A. Since the following line 18'' speaks of excerpted text, it is possible that the scribe noted that he had copied or extracted only a few passages from the series *kunuk ḫalti* to include them in the present tablet.

In his article on the so-called library records documenting incoming tablets that were integrated into Ashurbanipal's palace library at Nineveh, Parpola (1983b) discussed two attestations of the series title *kunuk ḫalti* in one of these inventory lists. According to this inventory, two copies of the series were included in the library, one on two clay tablets and one on a wooden writing board (polyptych wax tablets) consisting of five parts.[361] Thus, the series must have been quite extensive. A. Schuster-Brandis (2008, 192–197) has collected source materials (from Assyria and Babylonia) belonging or related to the series, of which, however, only two texts (K. 2542+ from Nineveh in Babylonian ductus and K. 9288+ from Babylon from the time of Nebukadnezzar II) preserve colophons mentioning the series title (K. 2542+ represents the "first extract (*pirsu*)", K. 9288+ presumably contains the first tablet (*tuppu*) of the series). Among the sources included by Schuster-Brandis, we find texts that contain sections involving the use of *ḫaltu*-stone (and other stones) in amulets for the protection of women. Some of the source texts exclusively deal with amulets for women, possibly forming excerpts or shorter collections. But there are also tablets with treatments for women that include or focus on amulets necklaces among other prescriptions, especially in the context of bleeding and pregnancy. This material may present overlaps to amulet prescriptions that were integrated into the series *kunuk ḫalti*, see e.g. BAM 237 (remedies against *naḫšātu*-haemorrhage, e.g. obv. i 6 and obv. ii 39 for the use of *ḫaltu*-stone; *infra* text C.1.4), AO 6473 (TCL 6, 49; amulets for pregnant women, *infra* text C.3.9). For tablets exclusively devoted to amulets, which may have belonged to *kunuk ḫalti*, see e.g. K. 4727 // (see *infra* text F.1).

List of Manuscripts

Siglum	Museum Number	Copy	Collation	Format; Ductus	Provenience
A	K. 10507	AMT 66/4[362]	Coll.	Fragment of a two- or multi-column tablet; Neo-Assyrian script; 7th cent. BCE	Nineveh; Ashurbanipal's library
B	VAT 8869	BAM 248	Coll.	Two-column tablet; Neo-Assyrian script; 8th/7th cent. BCE	Assur; N4 library
C_1 + C_4 + C_5	K. 2413 + K. 18482 + K. 16363	AMT 67/1	Coll.	Fragments of a two-column tablet; Neo-Assyrian script; 7th cent. BCE	Nineveh; Ashurbanipal's library

Overview

i'	Fragmentary prescription (amulet necklace?) A rev.? i' 1'–2'	1'–2'
ii'	Fragmentary prescription to ease difficult delivery A rev.? i' 3'–6'	3'–6'
iii'	(Pseudo-)Sumerian incantation (zalaḫ (iz)zalaḫ) A rev.? i' 7' // B rev. iv 10 // C_1 rev. iv 3	7'
iv'	Fragmentary prescription A rev.? i' 8'–10'	8'–10'[. . .
v''	Fragmentary instruction A rev.? ii' 1'–2'	. . .]11''–12''

361 See Parpola 1983b, 12 No. 1 obv. i 2' and rev. iv 5', now SAA 7, No. 49.
362 Measurements: 5.7 x 3.5 x 0.6 cm.

vi''	Fragmentary instruction A rev.$^{?}$ ii' 3'–4'	13''–14''
vii''	Fragmentary (rubric resembling colophon) A rev.$^{?}$ ii' 5'–6'	15''–16''
viii''	Fragmentary (rubric resembling colophon) A rev.$^{?}$ ii' 7'–8'	17''–18''
ix''	Fragmentary A rev.$^{?}$ ii' 9'–10'	19''–20''[. . .

Previous Edition and Discussion

Thompson 1934a, *Babyloniaca* 14, 83 and 133ff. (edition)
Finkel 1976, 230–231 (discussion of lines 6'–7')
BabMed Corpora (https://www.geschkult.fu-berlin.de/e/babmed/Corpora/AMT-2/AMT66-4/index.html) (transliteration)
CDLI P398722 (photo)
Parpola 1983b, *JNES* 42, 21 (note on 1.1: 2')
Schuster-Brandis 2008, 60–61, 192–197 (discussion)
Böck 2014b, *OLZ* 109, 176 (discussion of ms. A rev. ii' 3'–4')
Infra text D.1.1 (mss. B and C$_1$)

Transliteration

Beginning of ms. A rev.(?) i' lost

1'	A rev.$^{?}$ i' 1'	⸢^{na4}ÁŠ.GÌ.GÌ⸣ ⸢ZA.GÌN⸣ ⸢GUG⸣ ^{n}[$^{a4?}$. . . . .]
2'	A rev.$^{?}$ i' 2'	*šu-u* NITA *u* MUNUS 7 NA$_4$.[MEŠ . . . .]

3'	A rev.$^{?}$ i' 3'	DIŠ ^{munus}PEŠ$_4$ *ina a-l[a-di-(šá) šup-šu-qat/uš-tap-šiq* . . .]
4'	A rev.$^{?}$ i' 4'	U$_4$-*ma* ITI *šá* ⸢Ù$^{?}$⸣.[TU-*šá* . . . .]
5'	A rev.$^{?}$ i' 5'	^{giš}GEŠTIN.KA$_5$.A [. . . . .]
6'	A rev.$^{?}$ i' 6'	ÉN za-la-aḫ MIN *ana* Š[À . . . ŠID-*nu* . . . .]

A, B, C

7'	A rev.$^{?}$ i' 7'	ÉN za-la-aḫ za-la-[aḫ . . . .]
	B rev. iv 10	ÉN za-la-aḫ iz-za-la-aḫ za-la-aḫ al-ti-la TU$_6$ ÉN
	C$_1$ rev. iv 3	[ÉN] ⸢za⸣-la-aḫ iz-za-la-aḫ za-la-aḫ al-ti-la ⸢TU$_6$⸣ É[N]

A, B, C

8'	A rev.$^{?}$ i' 8'	DÙ.DÙ.BI ^{ú}[. . . . .]
9'	A rev.$^{?}$ i' 9'	*ina* Ì.GIŠ x[. . . . .]
10'	A rev.$^{?}$ i' 10'	⸢PA$^{?}$⸣ ⸢$^{giš?}$⸣[. . . . .]

Ms. A rev.(?) i' breaks; gap of unknown length

11''	A rev.$^{?}$ ii' 1'	[. . . . .]x ⸢*ina*⸣ ⸢GU⸣ È
12''	A rev.$^{?}$ ii' 2'	[. . . . .] 6-*šú* DUR

13''	A rev.$^{?}$ ii' 3'	[. . . . . S]UM^{sar} ^{ú}IGI-*lim* ^{ú}A.ZAL.LÁ
14''	A rev.$^{?}$ ii' 4'	[. . . . .] 7-*ú ṭú-ur-ru*

15''	A rev.$^{?}$ ii' 5'	[. . . . . š]ú$^{?}$ GÚ DAB-*bat u* Ú.MEŠ
16''	A rev.$^{?}$ ii' 6'	[. . . . . GAB]A.RI KUR AN.ŠÁR^{ki}

17''	A rev.$^{?}$ ii' 7'	[. . . . .]x ^{na4}KIŠIB *ḫal-ti* NU SAR
18''	A rev.$^{?}$ ii' 8'	[. . . . .] ZI.MEŠ-*ḫa*

19''	A rev.$^{?}$ ii' 9'	[. . . . . Š]À$^{?}$.ḪÚL.LA
20''	A rev.$^{?}$ ii' 10'	[. . . . .] TI

Ms. A rev.(?) ii' breaks; remainder lost

Bound Transcription and Translation

Beginning of ms. A rev.(?) i' lost

1' *ašgikû uqnû sāmtu* [. . . . . .] 2' *šû zikar u sinniš sebet abnī* [. . . . . .]	1' *Ašgikû*-stone (turquoise), lapis lazuli, carnelian, [. . . . . .], 2' 'male' and 'female' *šû*-stone, (these) seven stones [you thread on(?) . . . . . .].
3' *šumma erītu ina alād*[*i*(*ša*) *uštapšiq*/*šupšuqat* . . . . . .] 4' *enūma arḫu ša alādī*[*ša*(?) . . . . . .] 5' *karān šēlebi* [. . . . . .] 6' *šiptu* zalaḫ MIN *ana libbi* [*tamannu* . . . . . .]	3' If a woman [suffers severely] in [her deliv]ery [. . . . . .], 4' when the month of [her] de[livery(?) . . . . . .], 5' fox grape, [. . . . . .], 6' you recite the incantation "zalaḫ ditto" *over* it [. . . . . .].
7' ÉN za-la-aḫ (iz)-za-la-[aḫ za-la-aḫ al-ti-la *tê šipti*]	7' Incantation: "*Slip out, slip out*! [*Slip out*, (so that) she will stay alive." Incantation formula].
8' DÙ.DÙ.BI . . .[. . . . . .] 9' *ina šamni* . . .[. . . . . .] 10' *arat* . . .[. . . . . .]	8' The procedure for it: . . .-plant, [. . . . . .], 9' [. . .] with oil [. . . . . .], 10' twigs of [. . .]-tree(?), [. . . . . .].

Ms. A rev.(?) i' breaks; gap or unknown length

11'' [. . . . . .] *ina qê tašakkak* 12'' [. . . . . .] *šeššu ṭurru*	11'' [. . .] you thread on a string. 12'' [. . .]. The sixth string.
13'' [. . . . . . *šū*]*mū imḫur-līm azallû* [. . . . . .] 14'' [. . . . . .] *sebû ṭurru*	13'' [. . . . . . a gar]lic (bulb?), 'heals-thousand'-plant, *azallû*-plant, 14'' [. . . . . .]. The seventh string.

15'' [. . . . . .]. . . *kišāda tuṣabbat u šammī* 16'' [. . . . . .] *gabari māt Aššur*	15'' [. . . . . .] you attach [*the stones*(?)] to a neck(lace(?)) and the drugs/plants 16'' [*you* . . . . . .]. A copy (of a tablet) from Assyria.
17'' [. . . . . .] *kunuk ḫalti lā šaṭer* 18'' [. . . . . .] *nussuḫa*(?)	17'' [. . . . . .] (*other sections from the series*?) 'cylindrical (bead of) *ḫaltu*-stone' are not written down (i.e. included on the tablet). 18'' [. . . . . .] excerpted/copied.
19'' [. . . . . .] *ḫūd libbi*(?) 20'' *too fragmentary for transcription*	19'' [. . . . . .] joy(?) 20'' *too fragmentary for translation*

Ms. A rev.(?) ii' breaks; remainder lost

Notes

Lines 1'–2': These two fragmentary lines seem to run parallel to a prescription belonging to a group of amulets for protecting pregnant women, found in several tablets related to the series *kunuk ḫalti*. The group of amulets is ordered "from head to feet", listing instructions according to the different body parts around which the amulets were worn. The present one was tied around the woman's thigh.

The sources containing the parallel are: BAM 346 rev. 11'–14' // STT 278 rev. 2–3 // K. 4727+ obv. 22'–25' // K. 9071 obv. 13'–16' // BM 47904 + 47770 obv. 9' // KAL 2, 41 obv.$^{!}$ i' 6'–9' // DT 28 ii 1'–7' (see *infra* text F.1 for an edition of these sources and the textual variants). Guessing from the available space, it seems that ms. A may have contained a somewhat abbreviated instruction in comparison with the other sources.

Lines 3'–6': For line 3', compare the parallel passages in BAM 248 iv 13 // BAM 249 i' 8'–10' //, beginning: DIŠ MUNUS *ina* Ù.TU *uš-tap-šiq*, with a remedy likewise containing "fox grape-plant" (see text D.1.1). Nonetheless, the present recipe differs.

For line 4', compare, for example, SpTU 4, No. 153: 21 (text D.1.11): [DIŠ MUNUS] ITI *šá* Ù.TU-*šú iq-ri-ba-am-ma la u-*[*lid-ma* ^{lú}*lil-lid-su la ú*]-*ṣi-ma a-na* [*šu-ṣi-i*/ Ù.TU-*šú*$^{?}$] "[If a wom]an's month when the birth is due has approached, but she has not [(yet) given birth and her baby has not (yet)] emerged, t[o make it come out/to enable her to give birth] . . .". An alternative reading of the line could be proposed as well: U_4-*ma* ITI *šá-lim* "when the month is favourable".

"Fox grape-plant" (line 5') is repeatedly found in prescriptions to promote delivery, see BAM 248 rev. iv 13, 23 // (text D.1.1, lines 205, 213); BAM 249 i' 1', 3', 8' (text D.1.3); STT 98 rev. 2', 4' (text A.1.1); SpTU 4, No. 153 obv. 23, 26 (text D.1.11 lines 5, 8) with discussion.

Line 7': The parallels from the Neo-Assyrian Birth Compendium present a slight variant of this incantation for a woman in difficult labour (see text D.1.1 note on line 202 for discussion). In both mss. B and C_1, the spell is classified with the rubric ⸢KA.INIM⸣.MA ^{munus}LA.RA.AḪ.A.KÁM.

Lines 8'–10': I have not been able to identify a duplicating passage for this prescription, but compare BAM 248 rev. iv 12 // (Text D.1.1 line 204), for a potion of *maštakal*-soapwort (and) flour of roasted grain (*labtu*) in oil and beer to promote easy delivery.

Lines 11''–12'': Cf. CAD Š/2 338 for 6-*šú* (for *šeššu* "sixth"). For *ṭurru* "yarn, string; necklace" in amulet texts, see Schuster-Brandis 2008, 60–61 and *passim*; CAD Ṭ, 165a sub d. There are several amulet texts, in which groups of amulet necklaces for related purposes are subsumed and numbered as "first, second etc. string" (DUR/*ṭurru*), designating a section or division of the text, as encountered, for example in BAM 376 i 14', 27', ii 6', 18', iii 1, 12, 24, iv 4, 21 // (cf. Yalvaç 1968, 332–336):

PAB 39 NA_4.MEŠ 4 ŠU.MIN.MEŠ 6-*šú* DUR
"A total of 39 stones for four amulets (lit. parts, *qātātu*/ŠU.MIN.MEŠ), the sixth section ('string')." (BAM 376 ii 18')
PAB 44 NA_4.MEŠ 7 ŠU.MIN.MEŠ 7-*ú* DUR
"A total of 44 stones for seven amulets (lit. parts, *qātātu*/ŠU.MIN.MEŠ), the seventh section ('string')." (BAM 376 iii 1)

In parallel texts, the individual amulets ("portions; parts") are not given, but only the total of stones within the whole section (e.g. BAM 375). Incidentally, the amulets in BAM 376 belonging to the sixth and seventh "string" are not concerned with women, but with ailments such as epilepsy and other related and psychological conditions. It is difficult to say, however, what exactly the "sixth" and "seventh string" in lines 12'' and 14'' of our Nineveh text refer to, i.e. whether this referred to a collection of numbered amulets for women, or to actual sections in the series *kunuk ḫalti*. It also remains uncertain, whether the "sixth" and "seventh string" was part of the text on ms. A.

Lines 13''–14'': B. Böck in her review of Schuster-Brandis 2008, 60–61 (Böck 2014b, *OLZ* 109, 176), emends line 14'' to 7 Ú <*mû*> *tu-ur-ru*, i.e. seven plants for "zurückgehaltenes amniotisches Wasser" and refers e.g. to BAM 240 rev. 67. However, this reading seems unlikely given the parallel line 12'': 6-*šú* DUR (= *ṭurru*). I have thus refrained from adopting Böck's emendation but retain Schuster-Brandis' reading. Nonetheless, I agree with Böck that the enumeration of plants ([gar]lic$^{?}$, *imhur-līm*-plant, *azallû*-plant) in line 13'' is unusual in the context of amulets, unless the amulets in question were leather bags (*mêlu*), into which the plants were wrapped (see e.g. BAM 311: 13). However, occasionally, plants such as *imḫur-līm* occur as part of amulet necklaces, wound into a thread (see e.g., CT 23, 8: 40–43, combined with a leather bag).

Lines 15''–16'': The text in line 15'' may refer to earlier text sections on the tablet. Thus, it could give instructions that some ingredients (e.g. stones) would need to be attached to the body as a necklace, while others (e.g. plants) were to be worn wrapped in a leather bag (*mêlu*), but this remains uncertain. The word *kišādu* (GÚ) can mean both "neck" or "necklace" (Schuster-Brandis 2008, 61–62) and the word DAB-*bat* (*tuṣabbat* or *tušaṣbat*) occurs in the meaning "you attach" in amulet texts, see K. 4727+ obv. 16' (text F.1) and AO 6473 rev. 10, 12 (text C.3.9 lines 38 and 40) with discussion.

Line 16'' appears to have provide colophon-like information on the provenience of the original, from which the preceding text had been copied. It refers to a *Vorlage* from Assyria, but the line is fragmentary.

Lines 17''–18'': In line 17'', Parpola (1983b, 21 note on 1.1: 2') restores [*pir-su reš-tu*]-⌈*ú*⌉ $^{\text{na4}}$KIŠIB *hal-ti* "[first section (*pirsu*)] of (the series) *kunuk ḫalti*". But this restoration seems unlikely in my view, because of the following NU SAR (*lā šaṭer*) "is not written down" (on the tablet). Thus, one rather expects here information on a part(?) of the composition *kunuk ḫalti* that was not copied or included by the scribe of the tablet.

The logogram ZI.MEŠ-*ḫa* "excerpted" in line 18'' should probably be understood as a D-stem stative form of *nasāḫu* (*nussuḫa*), parallel to the more usual ZI-*ḫa* (*nasḫa*) in the G-stem (cf. CAD N/2, 13 sub 10e for other references). The reference to the text being an excerpt of selected passages rather than a complete copy of a *Vorlage* underscores the interpretation of line 17'' suggested here.

D.1.5 K. 11530: Childbirth Incantations and Instructions for the Midwife

K. 11530 is the fragment of a single-column tablet in Neo-Assyrian script. Livingstone (1989, xxi) assigned the text to the group of literary tablets from Nineveh written in the Neo-Assyrian dialect. The fragment preserves the lower part of a smaller tablet preserving fourteen fragmentary lines of text on the obverse and ten more lines around the lower edge and on the reverse. Judging from the curving of the tablet it appears that only a couple of lines are missing from the top of the tablet. The preserved text on the obverse appears to be part of an incantation, although no rubric is appended.[363] In the preserved lines, the main actor is a goddess who is described as kneeling before the weather god Adad, who is called her brother. This affiliation may speak for the mother goddess who is occasionally called Adad's sister (Krebernik 1993–1997, 507 sub 4.1; Schwemer 2001, 420–421; 2007c, *JANER* 7, 150–151). Interestingly, in the incantation, she asks the weather god to bestow on her the "inexhaustible art of medicine" (*asûtu*), which is an unusual feature reminding us of the *Gula Hymn of Bullussa-rabi*, in which Gula receives the art of medicine from Ea's hands (Lambert 1967; Foster 2005, 583–591 lines 144–146). It is thus possible that the goddess in the present incantation is also Gula or a goddess syncretised with her.

363 CDLI regards the fragment Rm. 908 (published by Livingstone 1989, 119–120 as No. 49; with Pl. XV) as part of K. 11530. However, as far as can be judged from the few fragmentary lines of Rm. 908, this text is unrelated to K. 11530; it mentions Gilgamesh and the "series of Gilgamesh", but also the city of Arbela, the Emašmaš (the temple of Ištar at Nineveh), and the goddess Bēlet-šamê (Ištar) who is described as a divine scribe holding writing tablets and stylus as insignia. Livingstone (1989, xxxi) suggested Rm. 908 could have been part of a composition with the god Nabû as the main character, but this remains uncertain.

The incantation on the obverse closes with a short performative utterance wishing that "the *phlegm* shall keep falling to the ground like a *meteor/flash* from heaven." In the text that follows, after a ruling on the lower edge of K. 11530, this topic features again in a three-line instruction, formulated, however, not in the second person, but in the third person feminine, implying a female subject. Stol (2000a, 177) wondered whether the mother or the midwife was the agent of these lines; however, the content of the instructions can be regarded as typical actions performed by the midwife having to do with cleaning the newborn. The present text states that she should rub (*muššu'u*) "his chest" with oil, put her fingers into "his mouth", so that *mucus* (*nīṣu*) is discharged (for unhindered breathing). A few other texts such as a Sumerian hymn to the goddess of medicine Ninisina (*Ninisina* A), describes her role performance as a divine midwife (nu-gig).[364] This comprises manipulations to assist delivery (directing the foetus downward, opening the mouth of the uterus), cutting the umbilical cord, but also turning the baby upside down, with its belly(?) pointing downwards to the ground, to make it cry loudly, and cleaning the breathing passage (IM-di luḫ). Comparable to rubbing (*muššu'u*) in K. 11530, "wiping off" (or cleaning, *kuppuru*) the newborn is mentioned as another typical action of the midwife, in an Old Babylonian Lamaštu incantation (Farber 2014, 260, 282–283 OB_3 obv. 3).

The reverse of K. 11530 continues with another incantation, of which only the first lines are preserved, and which speaks of the mother goddess' (Bēlet-ilī) temple and cattle pen, where pregnant ones give birth, thus further alluding to the birth context, and to the cow as a well-known comparison for the woman in delivery.

List of Manuscripts

Siglum	Museum Number	Copy	Collation	Format; Ductus	Provenience
A	K. 11530	ABRT 2, 19	Coll.	Single-column tablet; Neo-Assyrian script; 7th cent. BCE	Nineveh, Library of Ashurbanipal

Overview

i'	Fragmentary birth-related incantation A obv. 1'–14'	. . .]1'–14'
ii'	Instructions addressed at the midwife for cleaning the newborn A lo. e. 1–3	15'–17'
iii'	Fragmentary birth incantation: *ina bītīša ša Bēlet-ilī* A rev. 1–7	18'–24'[. . .

Previous Edition and Discussion

Livingstone 1989, SAA 3, 118 No. 48, pl. xvi (edition; photo)
Volk 2004, 87 n. 104 (lines 15'–17')
CDLI P334932 (photo)
Electronic Babylonian Library Project (eBL) (https://www.ebl.lmu.de/library/K.11530)
Oracc (http://oracc.museum.upenn.edu/saao/saa03/P334932; edition)

Transliteration

Beginning of ms. A obv. lost

1'	A obv. 1'	[x *ta-n*]*a*?-⸢*ad*?-*ki*?⸣ MU[NUS . . . .]
2'	A obv. 2'	[x x]-⸢*ni*?⸣ *šá* [x x] *ta-nak*-x [. . . . .]

364 See ŠRT 6 iii 4–5, Römer 2001, 113 lines 74–81, with discussions in Böck 2014a, 30–32; Steinkeller 2022, 26–27 and the *Introduction* sub 5 for discussion.

3'	A obv. 3'	*š[a i-la-u-ni i*$^{?}$*]-ba-ki la* ⸢*i*⸣-[*la-ʾi qa-la-tú*$^{?}$]
4'	A obv. 4'	[x x x x x *i*]-*ba-áš-ši a*-⸢*na*⸣ [x x x x]
5'	A obv. 5'	[x x x x x]x MUNUS x[x x x x]
6'	A obv. 6'	[x x x x x]x *ka-an-ṣa ki-i*[*n*$^{!}$*-ṣa-šá*]
7'	A obv. 7'	⸢*pa*⸣-[*ta-ni up-na*]-*šá ina pu-ut* ^{d}IŠKUR ŠE[Š-*šá*]
8'	A obv. 8'	*mi*-⸢*nu*⸣ ⸢*te-riš*⸣-[*i*]*n-ni* NIN *mi-nu li-di-n*[*u-ni-ki*]
9'	A obv. 9'	*li-di-nu-ni-ki* GU$_4$.MEŠ NIGA.MEŠ UDU.MEŠ *ma-ru-u-t*[*e*]
10'	A obv. 10'	*ul* GU$_7$ GU$_4$.MEŠ NIGA.MEŠ UDU.MEŠ *ma-ru-u-te*
11'	A obv. 11'	*li-din-u-ni a-a-ši zi-mu ša* KI.SIKIL.MEŠ *ba-nu-tú ša* GURUŠ.MEŠ
12'	A obv. 12'	^{lú}A.ZU-*u-tú ša la i-ga-ma-ru ina* ŠU.MIN-*ia šu-kun*
13'	A obv. 13'	*ni-ṣu ki-ma nab-li* TA *pu-ut* AN-*e*
14'	A obv. 14'	*li-ta-na-qu-ta ina qaq-qa-ri*

15'	A lo. e. 1	$^{[u]zu}$GABA-*su ina* Ì.MEŠ *tu-ma-áš-šá-aʾ*
16'	A lo. e. 2	$^{[u]zu}$ŠU.SI-*šá ina pi-i-šú tu-še-rab*
17'	A lo. e. 3	*ni-ṣu i-kar-ra-ár*

18'	A rev. 1	[É]N$^{!}$ *ina* É-*šá ša* ^{d}*be-let*-DINGIR.MEŠ *ina* TÙR-*šá ša* ^{d}NIN.É.GAL$^{!}$
19'	A rev. 2	[*e-ri*]-*a a-ri-a-te i-ḫi-la ḫa-a-a-la-te*
20'	A rev. 3	[*ša i-l*]*a-u-ni i-ba-ki la i-la-ʾi qa-la-tú*
21'	A rev. 4	[x *a*]-⸢*ši*$^{!}$-*pu*$^{!}$-*su*$^{?}$⸣ *man-nu* [x x] ⸢^{uzu}⸣GÌR.PAD.DU
22'	A rev. 5	[x x x x x x x x x x]-*ba-a-te*
23'	A rev. 6	[x x x x x x x x x-*g*]*a-a-te*
24'	A rev. 7	[x x x x x x x x x x] x [x]-*niš*

Ms. A rev. breaks; remainder lost

Bound Transcription and Translation

Beginning of ms. A obv. lost

$^{1'}$ [. . . *tanâ*]*dki sinniš*[*tu* . . .]	$^{1'}$ "[. . . *she prai*]*ses* you (fem.), the wom[an . . .],
$^{2'}$ [. . .]. . . *ša* . . . [. . .]	$^{2'}$ [. . .] who . . . does [. . .],
$^{3'}$ *š*[*a ilaʾʾûni i*]*bakki lā* [*ilaʾʾi qalātu*]	$^{3'}$ [whoever can cr]ies, un[able to *cease*(?)],
$^{4'}$ [. . . *i*]*bašši* . . .[. . .]	$^{4'}$ [. . . . .] there is . . .[. . .],
$^{5'}$ [. . .] *sinništu* [. . . .]	$^{5'}$ [. . . . .] *the woman* [. . . . . .],
$^{6'}$ [. . .]. . . *kanṣā ki*[*nṣāša*]	$^{6'}$ [. . . . . .] she knelt.
$^{7'}$ *pa*[*tâni upnā*]*ša ina pūt Adad aḫ*[*īša*]	$^{7'}$ Her [hands were ope]ned (in prayer) before Adad, [her] brot[her].
$^{8'}$ *mīnu terrišinni aḫātī mīnu liddin*[*ūnikki*]	$^{8'}$ 'What do you wish from me, (my) sister, what should they give [you]?
$^{9'}$ *liddinūnikki alpī marûti immerī marûti*	$^{9'}$ Should they give you fattened oxen, fattened sheep?'
$^{10'}$ *ul akkal alpī marûti immerī marûti*	$^{10'}$ 'I don't eat fattened oxen, fattened sheep.
$^{11'}$ *liddinūni yâši zīmū ša ardāti banûtu ša eṭlī*	$^{11'}$ Let them give me the attractiveness of maidens, the handsomeness of young men!
$^{12'}$ *asûtu ša lā igammaru ina qātīya šukun*	$^{12'}$ Place in my hand the inexhaustible craft of medicine (*asûtu*)!
$^{13'}$ *nīṣu kīma nabli issu pūt šamê*	$^{14'}$ May $^{13'}$ the *phlegm* $^{14'}$ keep falling on the ground $^{13'}$ like a fire flame from heaven!'"
$^{14'}$ *littan(a)quta ina qaqqari*	

15' *irassu ina šamnī tumašša'* 16' *qātīša ina pîšu tušerrab* 17' *nīṣu ikarrar*

15' She massages his (the baby's) chest with oil. 16' She inserts her finger into his mouth, 17' (and) he will discharge the *phlegm*.

18' [É]N! *ina bītīša ša Bēlet-ilī ina tarbāṣīša ša Bēlet-ēkalli*

18' [Incan]tation. "In Bēlet-ilī's own temple, in Bēlet-ēkalli's own cow pen

19' *[erī]ā ariāte iḫīlā ḫayyalāte*

19' pregnant ones are [pregnant], those in labour are in labour.

20' *[ša il]a''ûni ibakki lā ila''i qalātu*

20' [Whoever c]an cries, unable to *cease*(?).

21' *[. . . ā]šipūssu*(?) *mannu [. . .] eṣemtu*

21' His [exo]rcism(?) [is . . .], who [. . .] the bone?

22'–24' *too fragmentary for bound transcription*

22'–24' *too fragmentary for translation*

Ms. A rev. breaks; remainder lost

Notes

Line 1': The restoration of this and the following lines is tentative. Possibly restore *tanâdki* "she praises you (fem.)". It remains unclear who the addressed female is. The agent here may be a woman asking a female deity for assistance in a difficult(?) delivery. From the dialogue between Adad and the anonymous goddess later on one could surmise that the beseeched goddess went to ask her brother for special medical expertise to help the woman.

Line 3': For the restoration, see line 20' below.

Line 6': For kneeling (sitting or resting on the shins) as a prayer gesture (usually *ina kim/nṣī kamās/ṣu*), see CAD K, 375 sub 1b-1'c'. Oppenheim (1936, *Anthropos* 31, 475) noted that this is the typical posture of the supplicant in penitential *šigû*-prayers (cf. van der Toorn 1985, 117–121). Parallel to the construction with the stative in line 6' is a line in a Neo-Assyrian prophecy coming from Ištar of Arbela, addressed at king Esarhaddon's mother (Parpola 1997, SAA 9, No. 5: 2): *kin-ṣa-a-a kan-ṣa a-n[a pān* d(?). . .] "my knees are bent be[fore . . .]". What is interesting in the present context is further that *kamāsu* is also found as the posture of women giving birth, especially in birth incantations (e.g., "Cow of Sîn", see *infra*, *Iraq* 31, Pl. V–VI (ms. D) rev. 57; text II.1.4).

Line 7': A similar phrase occurs in the *Elegy on the Death of a Woman in Childbirth* (Livingstone 1989, No. 15 K. 890 obv. 9; Foster 2005, 949; George 2010a, *FS Foster*, 209, 213), in which the woman speaks about beseeching the mother goddess to help her in her difficult labour: *pa-ta-ni up-na-ia-a a-na* d*be-let*-DINGIR *ú-ṣal-la* "my hands were opened (in supplication), as I prayed to Bēlet-ilī". However, in K. 11530, we seem to have a dialogue between two divine siblings, with the unnamed female deity (probably the mother goddess) kneeling before her brother Adad, asking him for the gift of the medical arts. This request is unusual, because the storm god Adad is not known as a patron of medicine. However, it is interesting that among oracular questions addressed at Adad (and Šamaš) as patron(s) of divination found in Ashurbanipal's library, there are requests concerning women and concerning matters of pregnancy and successful delivery (will the wife get pregnant; will a sick pregnant wife survive; will she finally give birth to a boy after so many girls have been born; see Stol 2000a, 36, 131, 207; Lambert 2007, No. 12a–c col. i 11–ii 3, ii 4–15, rev. iii 1–17; No. 13). For the weather god as a deity addressed by women and praised for providing offspring, see also Schwemer 2001, 79ff. *passim*; Steinert 2017b, *FS Wiggermann*, 215.

Line 12': Compare the *Gula Hymn of Bullussa-rabi*, in which Gula praises herself (Lambert 1967, lines 124 lines 144, 146; Foster 2005, 589): *Ea ina apsî nēmeqšu igmura . . . asûtu pirišti ilāni ana qātēya umanni* "Ea in the Apsû gave me in full of his wisdom, . . ., the physician's craft, the secret of the gods, he entrusted to my hands."

Line 13': For *nīṣu*, which Livingstone provisionally translates as "phlegm", cf. CAD N/2, 279 s.v. *nīṣu*. AHw 782 includes the reference to our text under the lemma *nēṣ/su* "strong(?)", which is attested in synonym lists as a synonym for *gašru* "mighty". However, CAD N/2, 190 keeps both terms separate, as the meanings appear to be unrelated. The word *nīṣu* is a hapax in K. 11530 so far. That the word refers to a body substance that needs to be removed from the mouth of the newborn, becomes clear from lines 16'–17': *qātīša ina pîšu tušerrab / nīṣu ikarrar* "She inserts her finger into his mouth (and) he will discharge the *phlegm*." M. J. Geller (personal communication) suggests *nīṣu* may be related to *nezû* "to void" (urine, excrement). Scurlock (1991, 175 n. 133) reads Ì.ZUM instead of *ni-ṣu*, which she links with *ḫâlu* "to be in labour, to exude liquid" (written logographically with ZUM) and therefore translates the term as "amniotic fluid".

The incantation expresses the excretion of *nīṣu* with the verb "to fall" (*maqātu*) which is used in other birth incantations with reference to the baby, urging it to come out from the womb and to fall to the ground (e.g. BAM 248 i 50 and dupl. (text D.1.1): *šerru limqutma* "may the baby fall and (see the light)"; VS 17, 34: 18: *limqutam qaqqaršum* "let it fall down to the ground"). See also Stol 2000a, 127 for discussion. An incantation in the Neo-Assyrian Birth Compendium uses a similar meteorological simile for the baby as K. 11530, line 13': "like rainfall from heaven, may it not turn backwards" (*kīma tīk šamê ay itūr ana arkišu*, BAM 248 ii 57, 70).

The specific simile in K. 11530, *kīma nabli issu pūt šamê* "(may the *nīṣu* keep falling on the ground) like a flash/fireball/meteor(?) from heaven", can further be compared with a passage in an incantation recited "to remove chaff, a splinter or anything from the eyes", known from the series EYES (IGI) Tablet I (Geller and Panayotov 2020, 104–105 lines 189'–190'), which addresses the patient's eyes: *zunnāni kīma kakkabi mitaqqutāni kīma nabli* "Rain down like (a shooting) star, drop down like a meteor (oh eyes)!", alluding to the production of tears that will help remove the foreign body from the eyes.

Lines 15'–17': The verb *karāru* "to lay, to put in place; to throw, drop" is predominantly found in Middle and Neo-Assyrian texts; its meanings correspond to Babylonian *nadû*. A few times *karāru* is encountered in Neo-Assyrian letters sent by the exorcists Adad-šumu-uṣur and Marduk-šākin-šumi, and by the physician Urad-Nanaya to Esarhaddon, with reference to the discharge of sweat (*zu'tu*), described there as a symptom and as an effect of medical treatments (SAA 10, No. 241 obv. 11–12, SAA 10, No. 315 rev. 15, SAA 10, No. 217 rev. 7).

Lines 18'–19': For Ninegal(la) = *Bēlet-ēkalli* "Lady of the Palace", a minor deity possibly acting as the divine patron of the royal palace, sometimes serving as an epithet of Inanna/Ištar or other goddesses, see Behrens and Klein 1998–2001, "Ninegalla", *RlA* 9, 342–347; Meinhold 2009, 116–137. The reference to the cow pen of Ninegal(la)/Bēlet-ēkalli, parallel to the house/temple of the mother goddess, reminds one of the prominent association of women in labour with cows and of the association of the mother goddess(es) with a cow's uterus (manifested in the so-called "omega symbol", cf. Steinert 2017b). In other birth incantations, we find the image of the deity's sleeping chamber (in the temple) as a place of birth/or as a metaphor of the womb, cf. Steinert 2017a; Couto-Ferreira 2018c for discussion.

Line 19': For *ḫâlu/ḫiālu* "to be in labour" and *ḫayyaltu* "woman in labour", see Stol 2000a, 122–123 with n. 79, 126 fn. 104 *passim*; Couto-Ferreira 2014, *Dynamis* 34, 294. A similar phrasing as found in K. 11530 rev. 2, occurs, for example, in Westenholz 1997, 64–65: 20–21. For the comparison of women in labour with warriors, see also *infra* text II.1.4 (*Iraq* 31, 31: 40). For *ḫâlu/ḫiālu* in the gynaecological corpus, see also SpTU 4, No. 153 obv. 9 (text D.1.11).

Line 20': Crying is a few times found in connection with women in labour, cf. Stol 2000a, 123 fn. 79, especially in incantations about the Cow of Sîn (see text D.1.1, BAM 248 iii 23 and dupl.).

The meaning of the term *qa-la-tú* is uncertain, as it appears to be a hapax. The form is most likely an infinitive.

Line 21': If *āšipūssu* "his exorcism" is the correct reading of the first signs in this line, one might expect a male divine name in the gap at the beginning of the line. The word "bone" may refer here to the baby to be born, as in BAM 248 obv. ii 55 "(May the creature come forth), a body (lit. bone) of its own, the human creature" (*eṣemtu aḫītu binût amēlūti*)"; see also Lambert 2007, No. 12b col. ii 12: *eṣentu aḫītu ana libbiša* [. . .] "the *foetus* (body of its own) in her belly [. . .]". Thus, a statement such as that a certain god's exorcism (Ea's or Marduk's?) is capable to deliver the baby, may be expected in the present line of K. 11530.

D.1.6 Sm. 157 + 1134: Instructions for Difficult Delivery

The fragments Sm. 157 + 1134 form the top left-hand corner of a single-column tablet and preserve the beginning of fourteen lines on the obverse. The reverse preserves traces of a colophon written in a larger script, marking it as a tablet that belonged to king Ashurbanipal's personal tablet collection. This unusual Neo-Assyrian text contains a narrative passage describing interventions in connection with complications in the context of pregnancy and childbirth (Stol 2000a, 131 with n. 129). The main healthcare professional acting in this text is not the male healer, but the midwife, designated in this text with the exceptional term *lamittu* "knowledgeable/skilled/experienced one" (lines 9–10).

The text was previously edited by Kinnier Wilson (1969) who interpreted it as a fragment of the Etana legend, because a passage features the uncertain expression *sangû ša alādi*, which Kinnier Wilson interpreted as *"plants/drugs* (= *šammū*) of (giving) birth". A "plant of birth/childbearing" plays a crucial role in the Etana story (where Etana tries to procure it for his barren wife). However, as Stol (2000a, 131) has pointed out, Sm. 157 + 1134 is not part of the Etana legend, and the nature of the text seems to be rather technical and instructive than literary. Judging from what is preserved, Sm. 157 + 1134 may have contained recommendations and advice to male healers on how to recognise and manage complications arising around delivery (possibly connected with the premature death of the foetus in utero), although the instructions appear to be addressed at the midwife, who in this text is portrayed as the main agent intervening manually in the delivery process.

List of Manuscripts

Siglum	Museum Number	Copy	Collation	Format; Ductus	Provenience
A	Sm. 157 + Sm. 1134	Thompson 1930, pl. 54 (Sm. 157) *Iraq* 31, pl. III (Sm. 157 + 1134)	Coll.	Fragments of a single-col. tablet; Neo-Assyrian script, 7th cent. BCE	Nineveh, Ashurbanipal's library[365]

Overview

i Instructions for complications during a woman's delivery 1–14[. . .
A obv. 1–14
ii' Fragmentary colophon . . .]15'–16'
A rev. 1'–2'

Previous Edition and Discussion

Thompson 1930, *The Epic of Gilgamish*, pl. 54 (copy of Sm. 157)
Kinnier Wilson 1969, *Iraq* 31, 15–16 (edition)
Stol 2000a, 131 with n. 129; 171 (discussion)
Electronic Babylonian Library Project (eBL) (transliteration, https://www.ebl.lmu.de/library/Sm.157)
CDLI P426420

Transliteration

1 A obv. 1 [(x)]x *mim-ma šèr-t*[*i ina na-ma-ri*$^{?}$. . . . .]
2 A obv. 2 ⸢*la*⸣*-am a-dan-ni-šá* ⸢GENNA⸣ ⸢*šá*⸣ ⸢ŠÀ⸣-[*šá*$^{?}$. . . . .]
3 A obv. 3 *la ú-na-šá* [. . . . .]
4 A obv. 4 *ù sa-an-gu-u* *šá a-l*[*a-di* . . . .]
5 A obv. 5 *la e-mar-ma ki sa-an-gi šá* <*a*>*-la-d*[*u*$^{?}$ . . .]
6 A obv. 6 *ù ḫi-lu it-tab-tu-ši ina ḫa-li-*⸢*e*⸣*-*[*šá* . . . .]
7 A obv. 7 ⸢GENNA⸣ *šá* ŠÀ-*šá la i-pár-ri-ku i*[*na*$^{?}$ ŠÀ.TÙR-*šá*$^{?}$ . . . . . .]
8 A obv. 8 *ù-lu* GIN$_7$ *it-taḫ-ri-šú um-ma* [. . . . .]
9 A obv. 9 *la-mit-tu*$_4$ NÍ *šá* ŠÀ-*šá la* KUR-*ad-m*[*a* . . . .]
10 A obv. 10 *la-mit-tu*$_4$ *ana ri-du-ut da-*[. . . . .]
11 A obv. 11 *la ú-tar-ra-ši-ma la-mit-*[*tu*$_4$ . . . .]
12 A obv. 12 ⸢*ù*⸣*-lu šá* ŠÀ-*šá la-mit-t*[*u*$_4$ . . . .]
13 A obv. 13 [*ù*]*-lu šá* ŠÀ-*šá* TÉŠ.B[I$^{?}$ . . . .]
14 A obv. 14 [x x] AD *šá* MUNUS ⸢x⸣ [. . . . .]

365 Measurements: 4.8 × 6.2 × 1.7 cm.

Ms. A obv. breaks; remainder lost
Beginning of ms. A rev. lost

Colophon:

15' A rev. 1' [x x]x SUMUN$^{?}$ [......................]
16' A rev. 2' ⌜KUR⌝ ^{m}AN.ŠÁR-[DÙ-IBILA......]

Remainder of the reverse left blank

Bound Transcription and Translation

^{1} [...]... *mimma šērti* [*ina namārī*$^{?}$...] ^{2} *lām adannīša šerru ša libbī*[*ša*......] ^{3} *lā unâša* [......] ^{4} *u sangû ša al*[*ādi*......] ^{5} *lā emmar-ma kī sangû ša alād*[*i*......] ^{6} *u ḫīlū ittabtūši ina ḫâlē*[*ša*......] ^{7} *šerru ša libbīša lā iparriku i*[*na šassūrīša*(?)......] ^{8} *ūlu kīma ittaḫrišu umma* [...] ^{9} *lamittu zumra*(?) *ša libbīša lā ikaššad-m*[*a* ...] ^{10} *lamittu ana ridût* ...[...] ^{11} *lā utarrašī-ma lamit*[*tu* ...] ^{12} *ūlu ša libbīša lamit*[*tu* ...] ^{13} *ūlu ša libbīša ištēn*[*iš*......] ^{14} [...] *rigmu*(?) *ša sinništi*(?) ...[...]

^{1} [...]... at the first sign of dawn [...], ^{2} (if it happens) that before her appointed time (due date) the child of her womb [*dies in his mother's womb*(?)], ^{3} (the baby?) does not move (anymore in her womb?) [...], ^{4} and the *discharges* of labour [*flow*(?)... but] ^{5} she does not *experience colic*, (or) when the *discharges* of labour [*flow and she gets labour pains*(?)...], ^{6} but then the birth pangs *leave* her during [her] labour, [...], ^{7} (so that) the child of her womb will not get stuck (lit. lie crosswise) *i*[*n her womb*(?)...], ^{8} or when she *is in childbed*, [(and) *she gets*(?)] a fever(?) [...], ^{9} (or if) the midwife (lit. the experienced one) does not reach the *body*(?) of her foetus and [...], ^{10} the midwife [...] *in pursuit of*(?) [...], ^{11} the midwife shall not *retreat from her* [...], ^{12} or the midwife [...] her baby [...], ^{13} or her baby instantly/altogether(?) [...], ^{14} [...] the crying(?) of the woman [(in labour)...]...

Ms. A obv. breaks; remainder lost

Beginning of ms. A rev. lost

$^{15'}$ *only traces preserved*

$^{15'}$ *too fragmentary for translation*

Colophon:

$^{16'}$ *ēkal Aššur-*[*bāni-apli*......]

$^{16'}$ Palace of Ashur[banipal,......].

Rest of rev. uninscribed

Notes

Line 1: The reading of the opening line follows eBL; for similar phrases in ritual and medical texts, see CAD Š/2, 323 s.v. *šērtu* sub 1a-4'. It improves the reading proposed by Kinnier Wilson 1969, 15. The beginning of line 1 remains uncertain, as does the connection of line 1 to the rest of the text. At the beginning, perhaps restore [*u*$_{4}$-*m*]*u* "when" as a temporal expression (CAD U/W, 146–147 sub 1b-8'a)?

Line 2: My tentative interpretation of the fragmentary text is that it describes what to do in case of a serious complication during pregnancy, namely that the foetus dies in utero before the calculated due date (here designated with the term *adannu* referring to "a moment in time at the end of a specified period" or "a period of time of predetermined length", see CAD A/1, 97). Line 3 may refer to a crucial sign that the foetus is dead, namely that the woman does not feel it move anymore in her belly (which would mean that the woman was already in the third trimester of pregnancy). The death of the foetus would explain the urgency of the following actions and interventions described in the text, since that situation would have made it urgent to remove the foetus, i.e. to induce labour and cause the woman to expel the foetus. This intended procedure may be described in lines 4–6.

Line 3: *nâšu* in the D-stem can mean "to move, dislodge, shake" (often said of limbs or parts of the body), see CAD N/2, 115 sub 5b.

Lines 4–6: CAD S, 146b s.v. *sangu*, interprets the word *sa-an-gu-u/sa-an-gi* in Sm. 157 + 1134 as a variant or corrupted spelling for *šammu* "plant; drug". Alternatively, it may be connected with the word *sangû*, the meaning of which, however, is likewise uncertain. It designates an object that is enumerated beside charcoal, copper and lead in an Old Babylonian love incantation (VAS 17, 23: 6–7, see Wasserman, 2016, 249–250). For *šammu ša alādi*, see also Stol 2000a, 53, 55. In the Etana legend, the "plant of childbearing" is a remedy for infertility, enabling conception. In Sm. 157+1134, it could be possible that *sangû ša alādi* refers to drugs that were meant to bring on or intensify the uterine contractions (designated as labour pains, *ḫīlū*). In drug compendia, plants for conception/fertility and difficult labour are usually designated with other terms, viz. *šammi lā ālitti* "plant for a barren woman" and *šammi mušapšiqti* "plant for a woman in difficult labour" (see Stol 2000a, 52–54). The present passage could perhaps describe the failure in the progress of delivery despite administering abortive drugs (line 6 may describe a weakening of labour pains interfering with a prompt delivery).

A third possibility for interpreting *sangû* in the present text may be as a variant spelling for *sagû* "(flow of) blood, (menstrual) discharge" (suggestion by M. Stol, personal communication). For instances of a similar interchange between /ng/ and /gg/, cf. Soden GAG, § 32b. However, the specific phrase *sagû ša alādi* "the *blood* of childbirth" is not attested elsewhere in women's healthcare texts yet. Note the mention of *mû* "(amniotic) fluid" (describing the breaking of waters during labour) in SpTU 4, No. 153 obv. 26 (text D.1.11 line 8), and the reference to "fluids" (*mû*) and "blood" (*dāmu*) in BAM 240: 67', to refer to the postpartum discharges. For *sagû* "(menstrual) discharge", see especially *infra* sections C.1 and C.2.

The Assyrian form *e-mar* (for preterite *ēmar* or durative *emmar*) could be linked with *emēru*, which is equated with *napāḫu* "to be swollen, distended" in a medical commentary from Nippur (Civil 1973, 337–338 line 26). Scurlock and Andersen (2005, 286–287) translate *emēru* as "to have colic" and link the term with pain associated with distension (following CAD E, 148 s.v. *emēru* A), in contrast to *ebēṭu* "to cramp", which they link with cramping pain produced by contraction of the intestines (see further Johnson and Simkó 2024, 18, 64 *passim*). Pain in the abdomen also fits the context of delivery in Sm. 157 + 1134. It is possible that *emēru* refers to the woman's abdomen feeling hard to the touch (as well as painful) as a sign for the progress of labour. Note that the dictionaries only list stative forms for *emēru* in the G-stem so far; the present context requires a feminine subject (the patient).

Line 6: The passage is quoted in CAD Ḫ 189, s.v. *ḫīlū* "labour pains", translating the line "and the pangs of labor left her when (she) gave birth . . .". The form *ittabtūši*, can be analysed as perfect N-stem of *abātu* "to destroy"; the N-stem means "to collapse; to fall down; to become annihilated, ruined" (see CAD A/1 44 sub 4; AHw 5). A word with a similar meaning may be seen in *šalputtu*, literally "defeated; destroyed; annihilated" (from *lapātu* "to touch"; Š-stem "to defeat, to destroy"), which refers to a woman affected by a complication during birth (and is perhaps connected to foetal death due to prolonged labour and malpresentation), see Stol 2000a, 53–55 for discussion; *infra* text B.1.6 (BAM 246) note on lines 1–5. The term *šalputtu* may further be connected to the expression "to be touched by a touch" (TAG TAG.TAG, *lipta lupputu*(?)), which occurs in a similar context of expelling a dead foetus. Thus, KADP 22 ii 2 (discussed by Stol 2000a, 54) contains the following passage: DIŠ MUNUS TAG TAG.TAG-*át* : GENNA *ina lìb-bi-*[*šá* UG$_7^?$] "If a woman is 'touched by a touch': this means that the child in [her] womb [*is dead*(?)]". Another passage with this expression is found in K. 4206+ rev. 28 (Mirelman 2015, *JCS* 67, 177–178, 181), where a woman 'touched by a touch' is recommended to drink a potion containing *ḫulmittu*-snake so that she will expel (her foetus) (BAD-*ma* MUNUS TAG TAG.TAG-*at* NAG-*ma* ŠUB-*a*).

The case of a woman with a dead foetus in her belly appears to be presented in an Old Babylonian letter (ABIM 15: 8–9), in which she writes: ITI.7.KAM *annûm šerrum ina libbīya ištu* ITI.1.KAM *šerrum ina libbīya mīt-ma* "for seven months that (unborn) child has been in my belly, but for a month the child in my belly has been dead (now)" (quoted in CAD Š/2, 318 sub a-2'). In the letter the woman requests that someone may help her in her dangerous situation.

Line 7: CAD P, 155 s.v. *parāku* sub 2a quotes our passage, translating "may they not block (the birth of) the offspring of her womb", analysing the verb as a plural form. The basic meaning of the verb *parāku* is "to lay/lie across, crosswise" (CAD P, 153–155 mng. 1), which would fit the context if referring to the baby being stuck because it is in a transversal angle in the womb; if the baby is the subject, the form *iparriku* has a subjunctive ending.

Line 8: Kinnier Wilson (1969, 16) interpreted the form as the Gt infinitive of *naḫāru* "to become withered", referring to the plant of birth ("as it became withered"). However, the passage is listed in the dictionaries (with incorrect restoration) under the verb *ḫarāšu* "to be in childbed, confinement" (AHw 324b *ḫarāšu* I; CAD Ḫ, 96 s.v. *ḫarāšu* A sub mng. 3a; see also

Stol 2000, 123 n. 82). The form *it-taḫ-ri-šú* would be a rare attestation of an N-stem (perfect) form. This interpretation is tentatively followed here.

After the verb, Kinnier Wilson (1969, 16) restores *um-ma-*[*nu* . . .]. The word *ummânu* "scholar" is a possibility (if this refers to a male birth helper here), but perhaps *umma* "fever" is a better guess in the context, which would yield a reference to childbed fever.

Lines 9–10: For the exceptional term *lamittu* "knowledgeable, experienced, skilled" (also in lines 10–12), which is presumably an honorific designation for the midwife, cf. Kinnier Wilson 1969, 15; Stol 2000a, 172 (rendering the form as "she who learns"; CAD L, 67b s.v. *lamdu* "experienced", fem. *lamittu*). *Lamittu* is derived from *lamādu* "to learn; to become knowledgeable (in a craft)"; it can be interpreted as the feminine form of the verbal adjective *lamdu*.

Line 9: The sign NÍ is usually read *ramānu* "self" in Akkadian, and one may restore NÍ-*šá* "(the midwife by) herself". A second option is to read NÍ as Akkadian *zumra* "body (of her baby)". The latter equation is attested in lexical texts, see the CAD Z, 157a lex. section.

Line 10: The signs *ana ri-du-ut* could also be read *ana ri-du-tú* (for *ana ridûti*). The noun *ridûtu* means "succession, inheritance" and "following", none of which particularly suits the context, cf. CAD R, 325–326. Perhaps a different meaning derived from the verb *redû* (also "to control, to pursue") may be suggested for *ridûtu* here (cf. CAD R, 226ff.). An alternative restoration could be *ana ri-du-ut da-*[*mi* . . .] "in order to [. . .] the flow of blo[od?]" (cf. *ridût irrī* "(over)flowing of the bowels; diarrhoea").

Line 11: Most likely, *ú-tar-ra-ši-ma* is a present tense form of *târu* in the D-stem, which can mean "to make someone retract; to turn back, retreat" (CAD T, 273–274 s.v. *târu* sub mng. 11).

D.1.7 K. 1930 + 11752: A Fragment of Treatments for Delivery

The fragment K. 1930, now joined to K. 11752, was already published as hand copy in AMT 65/2 and again in CT 28, 40. The fragments stem from the lower left-hand corner of a single-column tablet written in Neo-Babylonian script. Previously, the fragment K. 1930 has been erroneously classified as "birth omens",[366] but in fact they contain recipes and incantations for women and for the baby. Line 12' on the obverse speaks of a woman giving birth and having a difficult delivery. The two fragments thus presumably belonged to a collection of remedies for women in labour, which included prescriptions for the newborn (see also Farber 1989a, 28 ms. v, who likewise identified the obverse as concerned with women's diseases and one salve recipe on the reverse (lines 1'–2') as used for a baby). A similar combination of materials is attested in other texts such BAM 248 and dupl. (text D.1.1), the Neo-Assyrian Birth Compendium, which similarly appends a short section for the baby at the end, although the rest of the text is concerned with treatments in case of a difficult delivery.

List of Manuscripts

Siglum	Museum Number	Copy	Collation	Format; Ductus	Provenience
a	K. 1930 + K. 11752	AMT 65/2 CT 28, No. 40 (K. 1930 only) Pl. 39	Coll.	Fragment of a single-column tablet; Neo-Babylonian script; 7th cent. BCE	Nineveh; Ashurbanipal's library

366 See Dennefeld 1914, *Geburts-Omina*, 193 (for K. 1930); J. Fincke, Nineveh Tablet Collection Database (http://www.fincke-cuneiform.com/nineveh/babylonian/index.htm); followed by CDLI P238115 and the British Museum Online Database (https://www.britishmuseum.org/collection/object/W_K-1930).

Overview

i'	Fragmentary prescription (potion) a obv. 1'–3'	. . .]1'–3'
ii'	Fragmentary prescription a obv. 4'–6'	4'–6'
iii'	Fragmentary prescription (bandage) a obv. 7'–11'	7'–11'
iv'	Fragmentary prescription for difficult delivery a obv. 12'–rev. 2	12'–20'
v'	Sumerian incantation a rev. 3–10(?)	21'–27'(?)
vi'	Fragmentary prescription for the newborn (ointment) a rev. 11(?)–13	28'(?)–30'
vii'	Fragmentary incantation a rev. 14–15	31'–32'[. . .

Previous Edition and Discussion

Farber 1989a, *Schlaf, Kindchen, Schlaf,* 130 ms. v (K. 11752 rev. 1'–4')
BabMed Corpora (https://www.geschkult.fu-berlin.de/e/babmed/Corpora/AMT-2/AMT65-2/index.html) (transliteration of K. 1930)
CDLI P238115 (K. 1930)
Electronic Babylonian Library Project (eBL) (photos; https://www.ebl.lmu.de/library/K.1930)
Fincke 2003–2004, 143

Transliteration

Beginning of ms. a obv. lost

1'	a obv. 1'	x x x[. . . . .]
2'	a obv. 2'	NU *pa-tan* NA[G$^?$ . . . .]
3'	a obv. 3'	NAG-*ši-ma* [. . . . .]

4'	a obv. 4'	DIŠ KI.MIN DÈ NÍG.NA [. . . . .]
5'	a obv. 5'	*ta-za-ru ana* KA$^?$ [. . . . .]
6'	a obv. 6'	*tu-ba-aḫ-ḫar* [. . . . .]

7'	a obv. 7'	ZÌ GÚ$^?$.G[AL$^?$ . . . .]
8'	a obv. 8'	ŠE$_{10}$ TU^{muš}[^{en} . . . .]
9'	a obv. 9'	[DIŠ]-*niš* ḪI.ḪI *ina* D[È$^?$ . . . .]
10'	a obv. 10'	⸢*ina*⸣ IZI ŠEG$_6$-[*šal*$^?$ . . . .]
11'	a obv. 11'	SÍG BABBAR LÁ *šum*$_4$-*ma* ⸢É⸣.[MEŠ$^?$ . . . .]

12'	a obv. 12'	DIŠ MUNUS Ù.TU-*ma u*[*š-tap-šiq*$^?$ . . . .]
13'	a obv. 13'	^{šim}LI ^{šim}G[ÚR.GÚR$^?$ . . . .]
14'	a obv. 14'	ILLU LI.TAR x[. . . . .]
15'	a obv. 15'	Ì *ḫal-ṣa* [. . . . .]
16'	a lo. e. 1'	GÌR.PAD.D[U . . . .]

17'	a lo. e. 2'	*ina* IZI ŠE[G$_6$-*šal* . . . .]
18'	a lo. e. 3'	*ta-šá-ḫal* [. . . . .]
19'	a rev. 1	*ina* KA$^?$ x[. . . . .]
20'	a rev. 2	*ana* ŠÀ-*šá* GAR-*ma* [. . . . .]

21'	a rev. 3	ÉN É.NU.RU x[. . . . .]
22'	a rev. 4	ki tur-ra bí-x[. . . . .]
23'	a rev. 5	ù ⸢ku$^?$⸣ bí-íb-[. . . . .]
24'	a rev. 6	šu-za-a bí-in-ĝar [. . . . .]
25'	a rev. 7	[x]x bí-ḫa-za [. . . . .]
26'	a rev. 8	[x x]x-ke$_4$ b[í$^?$-. . . . .]

Lines 27'-28' broken

29'	a rev. 11	[*ina*] Ì ḪI.ḪI 3-*šú*$^?$ [ÉN *an-ni-tú* ŠID-*nu*$^?$ (. . .)]
30'	a rev. 12	LÚ$^?$.TUR ŠÉŠ-*m*[*a*$^?$. . . . .]

31'	a rev. 13	ÉN É.NU.RU x[. . . . .]
32'	a rev. 14	si x x[. . . . .]

Ms. a rev. breaks; remainder lost

Bound Transcription and Translation

Beginning of ms. a obv. lost

1' *traces* 2' *lā patān išatti* [. . . . . .] 3' *tašaqqīši-ma* [. . . . . .]

1' . . .[. . . . . .], 2' she shall drink (it) on an empty stomach [. . . . . .]. 3' You give (it) to her to drink and [. . . . . .].

4' DIŠ KI.MIN *dikmēn nignakki*(?) [. . . . . .] 5' *tazarru ana pî*(?) [. . . . . .] 6' *tubaḫḫar* [. . . . . .]

4' Alternatively, ashes from a censer(?) [. . . . . .] 5' you sprinkle. Into *the opening of* [. . . . . .]. 6' you heat (it) [. . . . . .].

7' *qēm ḫallūri* [. . . . . .] 8' *zê summati* [. . . . . .] 9' *ištēniš tuballal ina diqmēni*(?) [. . . . . .] 10' *ina išāti tušabšal* [. . . . . .] 11' *ina šīpāti peṣâti taṣammid šumma um*[*mātu*(?) . . . . . .]

7' Flour of *ḫallūru*-peas(?), [. . . . . .], 8' 'dove excrement', [. . . . . .] 9' you mix toge[ther]. With ashes(?) [. . . . . .]. 10' You boil (it) over a fire, [. . . . . .]. 11' You make a bandage with white wool. If it is (in the) summertime(?), [. . . . . .].

12' *šumma sinništu ūlid-ma uš*[*tapšiq* . . . . . .] 13' *burāšu kuk*[*ru* . . . . . .] 14' *ḫīl abukkati* [. . . . . .] 15' *šamna ḫalṣa* [. . . . . .] 16' *eṣemti* [. . . . . .] 17' *ina išāti tušabšal* [. . . . . .] 18' *tašaḫḫal* [. . . . . .] 19' *ina* . . .[. . . . . .] 20' *ana libbīša tašakkan-ma* [. . . . . .]

12' If a woman suf[fers severely] during delivery, [. . . . . .], 13' juniper, *kuk*[*ru*-plant, ...], 14' resin of *abukkatu*-aromatic, [. . . . . .], 15' pressed oil [. . . . . .], 16' bone of [. . . . . .]. 17' You boil (it) over a fire [. . . . . .], 18' you filter (it) [. . . . . .], 19' *with* . . .[. . . . . .]. 20' You place (it) on her belly(?) [. . . . . .].

21' ÉN É.NU.RU . . .[. . .] 22' ki tur-ra bí-x[. . . . . .] 23' ù ⸢ku$^?$⸣ bí-íb-[. . . . . .] 24' šu-za-a bí-in-ĝar [. . . . . .] 25' [x]x bí-ḫa-za [. . . . . .] 26' *too fragmentary for transcription*

21' Enuru-incantation. "[. . . . . .], 22' where the little one . . .[. . . . . .], 23' sleep(?) . . . [. . . . . .], 24' . . . he/she placed in your hand [. . .]. 25' [. . .] . . . he/she held [. . .]. 26' *too fragmentary for translation*

Gap of two lines

29' *ina šamni tuballal šalāšīšu* [*šipta annītu tamannu* (. . .)] 30' *ṣeḫra tapaššaš-m*[*a* . . . . . .]	29' (. . .) you mix [with] oil, [you recite the incantation] three times [(. . .)], 30' you rub the baby (with it) [. . .].
31' ÉN É.NU.RU . . .[. . . . . .] 32' *traces*	31' Enuru-incantation. "[. . . . . .] 32' *too fragmentary for translation*

Ms. a rev. breaks; remainder lost

Notes

Lines 12'–20': The purpose of this as well as the preceding remedies remains unclear. In line 20', one expects *ana* ŠÀ.TÙR-*šá* GAR-*ma* "you insert (it) into her womb (i.e., vagina)" instead of *ana* ŠÀ-*šá* GAR-*ma* "you put it on her belly". Since there are no parallels to assist in the restoration of the prescription, I refrain from emending the text.

Lines 21'–30': Due to the fragmentary state of the text it remains uncertain whether the Sumerian spell in lines 21'–27'(?) was recited with the preceding remedy to assist delivery or whether it was used for the following prescription, an ointment for the baby, in lines 28'(?)–30'. Line 22' perhaps referred to the emergence of the baby from the womb.

Lines 27'–28' are unfortunately lost completely, and therefore the end of the incantation and beginning of the following prescription cannot be determined with certainty. However, line 29' does not appear to represent the beginning of the prescription, which must have started at least one line earlier.

D.1.8 A Bilingual Incantation for a Woman in Childbirth Afflicted by Witchcraft

The bilingual incantation is known from two tablets written in Neo-Babylonian script, both of which were found in the collection of Ashurbanipal's library. The incantation addresses the sun god Utu/Šamaš, beseeching him to help a woman in difficult childbirth and to save her life and that of the baby.[367] The difficult labour is attributed to witchcraft in the incantation, in particular to sorcerous knots that are obstructing the emergence of the baby. Neither of the tablets does contains ritual or therapeutic instructions, and the text of the incantation does not provide any information on the actions that would be performed with the recitation.

List of Manuscripts

Siglum	Museum Number	Copy	Collation	Format; Ductus	Provenience
a	K. 3025 + K. 5982 + K. 8917	Meek, *BA* 10/1, 66–69 Schollmeyer, HGŠ, 138–139 (K. 3025) Gray, ŠRT pl. VIII (K. 5982) Macmillan, BA 5/V, 695, no. XLVIII (K. 8917) Abusch et al., CMAwR 3, pl. 6–7	Coll.	Single-column tablet; Neo-Babylonian script; 7th cent. BCE	Nineveh, Ashurbanipal's library
b	K. 879 + K. 2769 + K. 10527	Meek, BA 10/I, 65 (K. 897), 70–71 (K. 2769) Macmillan, BA 5/V, 711–712, no. XLVI (K. 2769) Gray, ŠRT pl. VIII (K. 10527) Abusch et al., CMAwR 3, pl. 8	Coll.	Single-column tablet; Neo-Babylonian script; 7th cent. BCE	Nineveh, Ashurbanipal's library

367 Cf. also Geller 1995, *ASJ* 17, 110: 112 for another incantation to Utu mentioning either the mother in childbirth or the newborn child.

Overview

i	Incantation addressed to Utu-Šamaš a obv. 1–rev. 11 // b obv. 1–rev. 10	1–26

Previous Edition and Discussion

Schollmeyer 1912, HGŠ, 66–68, No. 10 (K. 2769, K. 3025); 69–70, no. 11 (K. 8917); 108–109, no. 23 (K. 5892 + 10527)
Meek 1913, BA 10/I, 1–5 (ms. a, K. 879 and K. 2769)
Falkenstein 1953, SAHG, 221–222, No. 43 (translation)
Seux 1976, *Hymnes et prières*, 216–217 (translation; notes)
Borger 1985, *OrNS* 54, 14–26, esp. 14–18 (edition)
Scurlock 1991, *Incognita* 2, 143 (translation of lines 14–20)
Stol 2000a, 134 (translation of lines 14–26)
Polonsky 2002, 608–622, esp. 610–614 (edition; discussion)
Polonsky 2006, *Studies Leichty*, 297–300 (edition; discussion)
Abusch et al. 2020, CMAwR 3, 77–81 text 5.6 with pls. 6–8
CDLI P237921 (photo of K. 879+); CDLI P238249 (photo of K. 3025+)
Electronic Babylonian Library Project (eBL) (https://www.ebl.lmu.de/library/K.879; https://www.ebl.lmu.de/library/K.3025)

Transliteration

1	a obv. 1	⸢ÉN⸣ ^{d}utu dumu an-n[a-ke$_4$ . . . . . .][368]
	b obv. 1	[É]N ^{d}utu dumu an-na-k[e$_4$ . . .]
	a obv. 1	^{d}UTU DUMU ^{d}*a-nim e-⸢tel⸣*(-)[. . .]
	b obv. 1	^{d}UTU DUMU ^{d}*a-nim ⸢e⸣-[tel*(-) . . .]
2	a obv. 2	^{d}utu ibila zálag an-ki-b[i-da-ke$_4$]
	b obv. 2	⸢^{d}⸣utu ibila zálag an-ki-bi-[da-ke$_4$]
	a obv. 2	^{d}UTU *ap-lu muš-na-mir* [AN-*e u* KI-*tim*]
	b obv. 2	^{d}UTU *ap-lu muš-na-m*[*ir* AN-*e u* KI-*tim*$^{?}$]
3	a obv. 3	⸢peš⸣-tur-zi $^{d+}$suen-na ^{d}ni[n-gal-la-ke$_4$]
	b obv. 3	[peš]-tur-zi $^{d+}$suen-na ^{d}ni[n-gal-la-ke$_4$]
	a obv. 3	*lìb-bìb-bi* ^{d}30 *u* ^{d}NI[N.GAL]
	b obv. 3	*lìb-bìb-bi* ^{d}30 [*u* ^{d}NIN.GAL]
4	a obv. 4	en zimbir^{ki} an-dùl ⸢é⸣-[babbar-ra-ke$_4$]
	b obv. 4	[en zim]bir^{ki} an-⸢dùl⸣ <<en>> é-bab[bar-ra-ke$_4$]
	a obv. 4	EN *sip-par ṣu-lul é-babbar-r*[*a*]
	b obv. 4	[x x x] *ṣu-lu-lu é-babbar-r*[*a*]
5	a obv. 5	ki-áĝ ^{d}a-a é-gi$_4$-a ki-tuš an ⸢kù⸣-g[a]
	b obv. 5	[x x ^{d}]⸢a⸣-a é-gi$_4$-a ki-tuš an kù-g[a]
	a obv. 5	*na-ram* ^{d}MIN *kal-lat a-šib-bat* AN-*e* KÙ.MEŠ
	b obv. 5	[x x] ^{d}*a-a kal-lat a-ši-bat* AN-*e* KÙ.MEŠ
6	a obv. 6	^{d}utu an-šà kù-ga-ta e-ti-a-zu-ne
	b obv. 6	[x x an-š]à kù-ga-ta e-ti-zu-ne
	a obv. 6	^{d}UTU *ul-tu* AN-*e* KÙ.MEŠ *ina a-ṣe-k*[*a*]
	b obv. 6	[x x *u*]*l-tu* AN-*e* KÙ.MEŠ *ina a-ṣe-ka*
7	a obv. 7	kur ḫa-šur-ra-ta ⸢bal⸣-$_{\text{<<zu>>}}$dè-zu-ne
	b obv. 7	[kur ḫa-šur-r]a-ta bal-dè-zu-ne

368 The line numbering of mss. a and b follows Abusch et al. 2020, CRMAwR 3, pl. 6–8.

	a obv. 7	*šá-du-u ḫa-⸢šur⸣ ina na-bal-kut-ti-ka*
	b obv. 7	*[šá-d]u-u ḫa-šur ina na-bal-kut-ti-ka*
8	a obv. 8	[^{d}]⸢pap-nun⸣-[na sukkal š]à-ḫúl-la-zu-šè <<ne>>$^{over\ erasure}$ du$_{11}$-g[a-ab]
	b obv. 8	[^{d}pap-nu]n-na sukkal šà-ḫúl-la-zu-šè du$_{11}$-ga-ab
	a obv. 8	[x x x x *su*]*k-kal-⸢lum⸣ ḫu-ud lìb-bi-ka* [x x]
	b obv. 8	[^{d}*b*]*u-ne-ne suk-kal-li ḫu-⸢ud⸣ lìb-bi-ka liq-bi*
9	a obv. 9	[^{d}n]í[ĝ-zi-da á z]i-⸢da⸣-zu$^{!}$(ĝu$_{10}$) al-gub-b[a]
	b obv. 9	[^{d}níĝ-z]i-da á zi-da-zu al-gub-bu
	a obv. 9	*kit-tú l[i-iz-ziz] ina im-ni-ka*
	b obv. 9	*[ki]t-ti li-iz-ziz ina im-ni-ka*
10	a obv. 10	^{d}níĝ-si-sá ⸢á⸣ ⸢gùb⸣-bu-zu al-gub-b[a]
	b obv. 10	[^{d}níĝ-si]-sá á gùb-bu-zu al-gub-ba
	a obv. 10	*mi-šá-ri li-iz-ziz ina šu-me-li-ka*
	b obv. 10	*[mi]-šá-ri li-iz-ziz ina šu-me-li-ka*
11	a obv. 11	máš-saĝ kur-kur-ra-me-en
	b obv. 11	[máš-sa]ĝ kur-kur-ra-me-en
	a obv. 11	*a-šá-red ma-ta-ta at-ta*
	b obv. 11	*[a-š]á-red ma-ta-ta at-ta*
12	a obv. 12	⸢di-ku$_{5}$⸣ maḫ kur igi-nim kur igi-sig ḫé-em-ma-an-si-sá-e-dè
	b obv. 12	[di-ku$_{5}$ maḫ] kur igi-nim kur igi-⸢sig⸣ ḫé-em-ma-rab-si-sá-e-dè
	a obv. 12	*da-a-a-nu ṣi-rim šá ma-a-tú e-lit u šap-lit uš-te-ši-ri*
	b obv. 12	*[da-a-a-n]u ṣi-⸢rim⸣* [. . . . . *š*]*ap-lit at-ta*
13	a obv. 13	^{d}utu di-ku$_{5}$ maḫ [a]-⸢a⸣ saĝ-gi$_{6}$-ga
	b	*Omits*
	a obv. 13	^{d}UTU *da-a-a-nu ṣ[i-r]im a-bi ṣal-mat qaq-qa-du*
	b	*Omits*
14	a obv. 14	munus-⸢bi⸣ ⸢pa$_{4}$-ḫal⸣-l[a dumu-munus diĝir]-ra-na
	b obv. 13	[. . . . . diĝir-ra-n]a
	a obv. 14	*⸢sin-niš⸣-[tu$_{4}$ ši-i mut-tal-lik-tu$_{4}$] mar-ti* DINGIR-*šú*
	b obv. 13	*⸢sin-niš⸣-tu$_{4}$ š[i-i* . . . . DINGIR-*š*]*ú*
15	a obv. 15	[. . . . . du$_{8}$-ù]-da
	b obv. 14	⸢zú⸣-kéš-bi igi diĝir-⸢zu⸣ ⸢du$_{8}$-ù⸣-[d]a
	a obv. 15	[. . . . . *lip-pa-ṭi*]*r*$^{?}$
	b obv. 14	*[ki-ṣ]ir-ú-šá ina ma-ḫar* DINGIR-*ú-ti-ka lip-pa-ṭír*
16	a rev. 1	munus-bi$^{!}$ silim-ma ù-[t]u-ud-da
	b obv. 15	[x x sili]m-ma ù-tu-ud-da
	a rev. 1	*sin-niš-tú ši-i šal-míš [l]i-lid*
	b obv. 15	[x x x] *⸢ši-i⸣ šal-míš li-lid*
17	a rev. 2	ù-tu-ud-da ti-la šà-bi silim-ma
	b rev. 1	[ù-t]u-ud-da ti-la šà-bi silim-ma
	a rev. 2	*li-lid-ma lib-luṭ šá lìb-bi-šú li-šèr*
	b rev. 1	*⸢li⸣-lid-ma lib-luṭ šá lìb-bi-šú li-šèr*
18	a rev. 3	igi diĝir-zu silim-ma ḫé-en-du-du$^{!}$
	b rev. 2	igi diĝir-zu silim-ma ḫé-en-du-du
	a rev. 3	*ina ma-⸢ḫar⸣* DINGIR-*ti-ka šal-míš lit-tal-lak*
	b rev. 2	*ina ma-ḫar* DINGIR-*ú-⸢ti⸣-ka šal-míš lit-tal-lak*
19	a rev. 4	silim-ma ù-tu-ud-da ka-tar-zu ḫé-en-si-il-lá
	b rev. 3	silim-ma ⸢ù⸣-[tu-ud-da ka]-⸢tar⸣-zu ḫé-si-il
	a rev. 4	*šal-míš li-lid-ma dà-lí-lí-ka lid-lul*
	b rev. 3	*⸢šal⸣-[míš* x x x *dà-lí-lí*]*-ka lid-lul*

20	a rev. 5	⸢uš$_{11}$⸣-z[u] níĝ-ḫul-dím-ma igi diĝir$^{!}$-zu ḫé-en-búr-re
	b rev. 4	u[š$_{11}$-zu . . . . ḫé-e]n-búr-ra
	a rev. 5	⸢*kiš*⸣-*p*[*u*] *up-šá-su*$^{!}$-*u ina ma-ḫar* DINGIR-*ti-ka lip-pa-áš-ru*
	b rev. 4	[. . . . . *lip-pa-š*]*ar*
21	a rev. 6	šu-sa[r]-gin$_{7}$ ḫé-en-búr-re : (empty)
	b rev. 5	[. . . . . : *kīma pitilti lippašir*]
22	a rev. 7	šúm$^{⸢sar⸣}$-gin$_{7}$ ḫé-en-bar-ra : (empty)
	b rev. 6	[. . . . . : *kīma šūmī liq-q*]*a*-⸢*lip*⸣
23	a rev. 8	⸢munus⸣-[bi] ḫé$^{!}$-en$^{!}$-ti-la : *MUNUS* *ši*-i lib-luṭ
	b rev. 7	[. . . . . ḫé-en-ti-l]a : MUNUS *ši-i lib-luṭ*
24	a rev. 9	en-⸢e⸣ u$_{4}$-da al-ti-la nam-maḫ-zu ḫ[é-é]b-bé
	b rev. 8	[. . . . . al-ti-l]a nam-maḫ-zu ḫé-éb-bé
	a rev. 9	*a-di* ⸢*u*$_{4}$-*mu*⸣ *bal-ṭa-tu nar-bi-ka* [*liq-b*]*i* (*unclear traces on the edge*)
	b rev. 8	[. . . . . *bal-ṭ*]*a-tu nar-bi-ka liq-bi*
25	a rev. 10	nam-maḫ ⸢$^{d+}$en⸣-ki ^{d}asal-lú-ḫi ùĝ-bi ḫé-[en-zu-zu]
	b rev. 9	[. . . . . ^{d}asal-lú-ḫ]i ùĝ-bi ḫé-[e]n-zu-zu
	a rev. 10	*erasure* *nar-bi* ⸢^{d}*é*⸣-*a u* ^{d}AMAR.UTU UN.MEŠ [x x x]
	b rev. 9	[. . . . . ^{d}]AMAR.UTU UN.MEŠ *lil-tan-du*
26	a rev. 11	u ĝá lú-⸢mu$_{7}$-mu$_{7}$⸣ uru$^{?rù}$-du-zu \ k[a-tar-zu x x x]
	b rev. 10	[. urd]u-zu ka-tar-zu ḫé-si-il
	a rev. 11	*u ana-ku a*-⸢*ši*⸣-*pi* ⸢ÌR⸣-*k*[*a* . . . .]
	b rev. 10	[. . . . . ÌR-*k*]*a dà-lí-lí-ka lud-lul*

Bound Transcription and Translation

1 ÉN ^{d}utu dumu an-na-k[e$_{4}$ . . .]	1 Incantation: "Utu, son of An, [. . .],
1 *Šamaš mār Ani et*[*el* . . .]	1 "Šamaš, descendant of Anu, pr[ince . . .],
2 ^{d}utu ibila zálag an-ki-bi-[da-ke$_{4}$]	2 Utu, first-born son, illuminator of heaven [and] earth,
2 *Šamaš aplu mušnammir* [*šamê u erṣeti*]	2 Šamaš, first-born son, illuminator of [heaven and earth],
3 peš-tur-zi $^{d+}$suen-na ^{d}ni[n-gal-la-ke$_{4}$]	3 offspring of Sîn and Ni[ngal],
3 *liblibbi ša Sîn u Ni*[*kkal*]	3 offspring of Sîn and Ni[kkal],
4 en zimbir^{ki} an-dùl é-bab[bar-ra-ke$_{4}$]	4 lord of Zimbir, protection of Eba[bbar],
4 *bēl Sippar ṣulūl Ebabba*[*r*]	4 lord of Sippar, protection of Ebabbar,
5 ki-áĝ ^{d}a-a é-gi$_{4}$-a ki-tuš an-kù-ga	5 beloved of Aya, the bride who dwells in the pure heavens!
5 *narām Aya kallāt āšibat šamê ellūti*	5 beloved of Aya, the bride who dwells in the pure heavens!
6 ^{d}utu an-šà kù-ga-ta e-ti-((a))-zu-ne	6 Utu, as you rise from the interior of the pure heavens,
6 *Šamaš ultu šamê ellūti ina aṣêka*	6 Šamaš, as you rise from the pure heavens,
7 kur ḫa-šur-ra-ta bal-dè-zu-ne	7 as you cross mount Ḫašur,
7 *šadû Ḫašur ina nabaluttīka*	7 as you cross mount Ḫašur,
8 ^{d}pap-nun-na sukkal šà-ḫúl-la-zu-šè du$_{11}$-ga-ab	8 let the vizier Papnuna proclaim your happiness!
8 [*B*]*unene sukkallu ḫūd libbīka liqbi*	8 let the vizier Bunene proclaim your happiness!
9 [^{d}níĝ-z]i-da á zi-da-zu al-gub-bu	9 Truth stands at your right side,
9 *kittu lizziz ina imnīka*	9 May Truth stand at your right side,
10 ^{d}níĝ-si-sá á gùb-bu-zu al-gub-ba	10 Justice stands at your left side.
10 *mīšari lizziz ina šumēlīka*	10 may Justice stand at your left side!
11 máš-saĝ kur-kur-ra-me-en	11 You are the foremost of (all) the lands,
11 *ašarēd mātāta attā*	11 You are the foremost of (all) the lands,

12 di-ku$_5$-maḫ kur igi-nim kur igi-sig ḫé-em-ma-an-si-sá-e-dè	12 may you, the exalted judge, set the upper and lower lands in order!
12 *dayyānu ṣīri ša mātu elīt u šaplīt uštešširi* (var. *attā*)	12 the exalted judge, who sets the upper and lower lands in order (var. you are the exalted judge of the upper and lower lands).
13 ^{d}utu di-ku$_5$ maḫ [a]-a saĝ-gi$_6$-ga	13 Utu, exalted judge, father of the black-headed people,
13 *Šamaš dayyānu [ṣīr]i abi ṣalmāt qaqqadu*	13 Šamaš, [exalt]ed judge, father of the black-headed people,
14 munus-bi pa$_4$-ḫal-l[a dumu-munus diĝir]-ra-na	14 This troubled woman, [daughter] of her [god],
14 *sinništu š[ī muttalliktu] mārti ilīšu*	14 Th[is troubled] woman, daughter of her god,
15 zú-kéš-bi igi diĝir-zu du$_8$-ù-[d]a	15 her knot(s) having been loosened before your divinity,
15 *[kiṣ](i)rūša ina maḫar ilūtīka lippaṭir(ū)*	15 may her [kno]ts be loosened before your divinity,
16 munus-bi silim-ma ù-tu-ud-da	16 when this woman has safely given birth,
16 *sinništu šī šalmiš līlid*	16 may this woman give birth safely,
17 ù-tu-ud-da ti-la šà-bi silim-ma	17 having given birth, being alive (and) her baby being well,
17 *līlid-ma libluṭ ša libbīšu līšer*	17 may she give birth and live, may her baby be well,
18 igi-diĝir-zu silim-ma ḫé-en-du-du	18 may she live well before your divinity!
18 *ina maḫar ilūtīka šalmiš littallak*	18 may she live well before your divinity!
19 silim-ma ù-tu-ud-da ka-tar-zu ḫé-((en))-si-il-((lá))	19 Having given birth safely, may she praise your glory!
19 *šalmiš līlid-ma dalīlīka lidlul*	19 Let her give birth safely, so that she may praise your glory!
20 uš$_{11}$-z[u] níĝ-ḫul-dím-ma igi-diĝir-zu ḫé-en-búr-re	20 May witchcr[aft] [and] evil machinations be undone before your divinity,
20 *kišp[ū] upšašû ina maḫar ilūtīka lippašrū*	20 May witchcr[aft] (and] evil) machinations be undone before your divinity,
21 šu-sa[r]-gin$_7$ ḫé-en-búr-re	21 may they be unravelled like a palm-fibre cord,
21 *[kīma pitilti lippašir]*	21 [may they be unravelled like a palm-fibre cord],
22 šúm^{sar}-gin$_7$ ḫé-en-bar-ra	22 may they be peeled away like garlic!
22 *[kīma šūmī liqq]alip*	22 [may they be peeled away like garlic]!
23 munus-[b]i ḫé-en-ti-la	23 May [th]is woman live!
23 *sinništu šī libluṭ*	23 May this woman live!
24 en-e u$_4$-da al-ti-la nam-maḫ-zu ḫé-éb-bé	24 As long as she lives, may she proclaim your greatness!
24 *adi ūmi balṭatu narbīka liqbi*	24 As long as she lives, may she proclaim your greatness!
25 nam-maḫ $^{d+}$en-ki ^{d}asal-lú-ḫi ùĝ-bi ḫé-en-zu-zu	25 May these people know the greatness of Enki and Asalluḫi!
25 *narbî Ea u Marduk nišū liltandū*	25 May the people learn the greatness of Ea and Marduk!
26 u ĝá lú-mu$_7$-mu$_7$ urdu-zu ka-tar-zu ḫé-si-il	26 And I, the exorcist, your servant, will praise your glory!"
26 *u anāku āšipi aradka dalīlīka ludlul*	26 And I, the exorcist, your servant, will praise your glory!"

Notes

Line 7: As pointed out by Abusch et al. 2020, CMAwR 3, 81 (note on line 7), the scribe of ms. a added a small ZU under the signs BAL and NE. According to Abusch et al., this mistaken addition was triggered by the sequence -zu-ne at the end of both lines 6 and 7.

Mount Ḫašur is a mythical cedar mountain in the east (George 2003, *Gilgamesh Epic*, 864–865).

Line 8: Against earlier readings of silim$^?$ after šà-ḫúl-la-zu-šè$^?$ (Borger and Polonsky), that sign DI (or NE) has been erased by the scribe, as Abusch et al. observed.

Line 15: CAD K, 437a reads *ki-ṣir* ŠÀ-*šá*, a reading that was accepted by earlier editors. Borger emends the text, reading a singular *ki-ṣir-šá*. Abusch et al. note, however, that the tablet has *[ki-ṣ]ir-ú-šá* and accept this as a first-millennium spelling (for the plural *kiṣrūša*). They also regard *lip-pa-ṭir* as a representation of *lippaṭrū* and refer to similar spellings (where a CVC sign is employed to represent CCV and CV_1CV_2), see Schwemer 2017, 79–80.

Lines 21–22: PSD B, 195a s.v. búr E, bilingual meaning 3) reads line 21 as ma-m[ú]-gin$_7$ ḫé-en-búr-re "may they be resolved like a dream". Line 22 is read in PSD B, 113a s.v. bar E, meaning 9) as zú-lu[m-m]a-gin$_7$ ḫé-en-bar-ra (both readings followed by Polonsky 2006, 299 n. 13). However, these readings were corrected by Borger (1985, 17), noting the parallel in *Šurpu* V–VI 52–53, and 56–57 (Reiner 1958, 31). See now also Abusch et al. 2020, with new copies of both manuscripts on pls. 7–8.

Line 26: Abusch et al. (2020, 80–81) elucidated the syllabic spelling uru$^{?rù}$-du "servant" (with gloss) in ms. a against [urd]u in ms. b.

D.1.9 BM 34208: A Bilingual Birth Incantation Featuring the Cow in Dire Straits

This remarkable Sumerian birth incantation with partial interlinear Akkadian translation is preserved on a fragmentary tablet in an elegant Neo-Babylonian script (BM 34208; ms. a). The interlinear Akkadian text provides glosses rather than a true translation.[369] Each text line (or each double-line with Sumerian-Akkadian text respectively) is separated by a horizontal ruling. The upper part of the tablet is missing.

The small fragment BM 37476 (ms. b) appears to be a duplicate or close parallel of BM 34208. It preserves the end of several lines on its damaged obverse and reverse, which run parallel to lines 1'–12' and 25'–32' on the obverse of ms. a (= lines 1'–9' and 17'–20').[370] This could suggest that the format of mss. a and b differed from each other. It is also possible that the text of the incantation in ms. b diverged at points from ms. a, or that the text was arranged differently on both tablets.

The incantation itself is related to older Sumerian incantations on the cow of the moon god Sîn serving as a model for women having a difficult delivery – a tradition reaching back to texts from the Ur III and the Old Babylonian period (such as UM 29-15-367 and VS 17, 33; van Dijk 1975; Cunningham 1997, Text 62). The fragmentary beginning of mss. a and b speaks about giving birth and mentions the cow who in the present incantation belongs to the god Dumuzi, "the great/true herdsman of heaven" (udul gal/sipa zi an-na-ke$_4$). Lines 9'–14' describe how the cow is impregnated by the bull, in similar phrases as found in the older Sumerian incantations on the cow; in lines 15'–19' the cow is in dire straits, having a difficult delivery. Her cries are heard by the god Asalluḫi (line 20'), followed by the well-known but abbreviated Marduk-Ea formula in which Asalluḫi promptly receives instructions from his father Enki how to help the cow. Similar to other birth incantations about the cow, she is rubbed and a spell is recited to facilitate birth (lines 21'–27').

The last twenty lines preserved in ms. a turn to a different scene and setting: the temple of the birth goddess Nintur at Keš (line 28'), where the child (or calf) is born, assisted by the healing goddess Ninisina/Nintinuga, who acts as midwife (line 29'). The following lines describe the goddess performing the proper rites and purifications, how she then cuts the umbilical cord of the newborn, cleans the baby, anoints him and gives him his name. Lines 38'–49' are very fragmentary but once again resume the setting of delivery taking place in the temple of Nintur at Keš, with actions performed by the divine midwife. Line 34' and 46' mention the determination of destiny (for the newborn), which is usually associated with cutting the umbilical cord.

List of Manuscripts

Siglum	Museum Number	Copy	Collation	Format; Ductus	Provenience
a	BM 34208 (Sp. 314 + 412 + Sp-2, 365 + Sp-2, 599 + Sp-2, 695 + Sp-2, 701 + 4 unnumbered fragments)	Pl. 40–41	Coll.	Fragment of a single-col. tablet; Neo-Babylonian script	Babylonia[371]
b	BM 37476 (80-6-17, 1233)	Pl. 42	Coll.	Fragment of a single-col.(?) tablet; Neo-Babylonian script	Babylon

369 See also Leichty, Finkel and Walker 2019, *CBT* Vol. IV-V, 239. The fragments of BM 34208 were identified and joined by I. L. Finkel in 1981. Measurements: ca. 10 x 12 x 2.6 cm.

370 I owe this insight to Zsombor Földi and Henry Stadhouders (from the *Electronic Babylonian Library* Project) who identified the duplicate and shared a transliteration of ms. b with me. Cf. Leichty, Finkel and Walker 2019, *CBT* Vol. IV–V, 361, who classify the fragment as lexical.

371 The Sp and Sp-2 collections of the British Museum were purchased from Messrs. Spartali & Co., London, in 1879. The register gives the proveniences Babylon or Babylonia for the different fragments, see Leichty, Finkel and Walker 2019, CBT IV–V.

Overview

i	Bilingual birth incantation a obv. 1'–rev. 44 // b obv. 1'–rev. 6'	. . .]1'–49'[. . .

Previous Edition and Discussion

Electronic Babylonian Literature Project (eBL) (https://www.ebl.lmu.de/library/BM.34208, transliteration of ms. a; https://www.ebl.lmu.de/library/BM.37476, transliteration of ms. b)

Transliteration

Beginning of mss. a obv. and b obv. lost

1'	a obv. 1'	[. . . . .] ⸢du⸣
	b obv. 1'	[. . . . .] du
2'	a obv. 2'	[. . . . .]-a
	b obv. 2'	[. . . . .] a ri-a
3'	a obv. 3'	[. . . . . ù-tu-ud]-da
	b obv. 3'	[. . . . .] ⸢ù⸣-tu-ud-da
4'	a obv. 4'	[. . . . .] ⸢ù⸣-[tu]-ud-da
	b obv. 4'	[. . . . .] ⸢ù⸣-tu-ud-da
5'	a obv. 5'	[. . . . .]x-⸢ke$_4$$^?$⸣ áb maḫ-e ù-⸢tu⸣-[ud]-da
	b obv. 5'	[. . . . .] ⸢ù⸣-tu-ud-⸢da⸣
6'	a obv. 6'	[. . . . .] ^{kuš}ùsan [nu t]ag$^?$-ga
	b obv. 6'	[. . . . .] x ti ⸢^{kuš}ùsan⸣ <nu> ⸢tag$^?$⸣-ga
	a obv. 7'	[. . . . .] *šá ina qin-na-zu l[a$^?$ lap-t]a$^?$-tu$_4$*
7'	a obv. 8'	[áb diĝir bara-ga-ni] ú-dúl gal a[n-na-ke$_4$]
	b obv. 7'	[. . . . . ú-dúl ga]l$^?$ ⸢an⸣-na-ke$_4$
8'	a obv. 9'	^{d}d[umu-zi$^?$] sipa zi a[n-na-ke$_4$]
	b obv. 8'	[. . . . . sipa-zi an]-⸢na⸣-ke$_4$
	a obv. 10'	[. . . . .] *ki-num šá* ⸢AN⸣-[*e*]
	b obv. 9'	[. . . . .] ⸢x x-*ni*$^?$⸣
9'	a obv. 11'	[x] kù tùr a[maš kù-ga]-ta gu$_4$ gal áb maḫ-e [ba-u$_5$]
	b obv. 10'	[. . . . .] x
	a obv. 12'	*lit-tu$_4$ ṣir-tu$_4$* [*ir-kab*]
	b obv. 11'	[. . . . .] x
10'	a obv. 13'	[gu$_4$] gal a du$_{10}$-ga [. . .]x šà-bé ba-ni-[in-ri$^?$]
	a obv. 14'	*ri-ḫu-t*[*ú$^?$ ṭa-ab-t*]*u$_4$* *ina lìb-bi-šú* [*ir-ḫi*]
11'	a obv. 15'	ú ki-áĝ-ĝá-[né x x]-da$^?$ mú ḫé-en-⸢x-x-x⸣ [. . . . .]
	a obv. 16'	*ú-kul-li* x[x x x *šam-m*]*i$^?$ na-ra-mi-*[*šá$^?$* . . . .]
12'	a obv. 17'	áb šà-ḫú[l . . . .]
	a obv. 18'	*lit-tu$_4$ ḫu-*[*ud lìb*]*-bi* [. . . . .]
13'	a obv. 19'	áb diĝir ⸢bara⸣-ga-ni ú-dúl gal [an-na-kam$^?$]
14'	a obv. 20'	⸢áb⸣ ^{d}dumu-zi-da sipa zi an-na-kam
15'	a obv. 21'	áb u$_4$-da-a-ni iti$^!$(ITI-gunû)-da ì-ak-a
	a obv. 22'	*ar-ḫi-šá* <*ina*> ⸢*qut*$^?$⸣*-ti-šá*
16'	a obv. 23'	áb kù-ga gú$^!$(GÀR) ki-šè ba-ni-in-ĝar gù mu-un-na-an-dé-dé-e
	a obv. 24'	*qa-da-da-niš* *iš-ta-na-as-si*
17'	a obv. 25'	gù-bi an-e ba-te gù ki-⸢šè⸣ ba-te
	b rev. 1'	[. . . . .] ⸢ba⸣-t[e]
	a obv. 26'	*ri-gim-šá* x-[x]

18'	a obv. 27'	gù-bi an-úr-ra túg-⌜gin$_7$⌝ mi-ni-in-dul gada-gin$_7$ [ki$^?$] ⌜mi-ni-in-bàra⌝	
	b rev. 2'	[............ mi-ni]-⌜in⌝-bàra	
	a obv. 28'	*ri-gim-šá i-šid* AN-*e ki-ma ṣu-ba-tú ik-tùm ki-ma k[i-ti-e er-ṣ]e-tú* ⌜*uš*⌝-*p[ar-ri-ir$^?$]*	
	b rev. 3'	[............ *ki*]-⌜*ma*⌝ GADA ⌜*uš*⌝-*par-r[i-ir]*	
19'	a obv. 29'	[gab]a$^?$ kur-ra-ke$_4$ gú$^!$(GÀR) ki-šè [b]a-ni-in-ĝar gù m[u-u]n-na-an-dé-[dé-e]	
	b rev. 4'	[............ gù mu-un-na-an]-⌜dé-dé⌝-[e]	
	a obv. 30'	*i-rat* KI-*tim qa-d[a-da-ni]š*	*iš-t[a-n]a-as-si*
	b rev. 5'	[............] x x [x x (x)]	
20'	a obv. 31'	[^{d}as]al-⌜lú-ḫi⌝ ⌜igi⌝ [im-ma$^?$]-⌜an$^?$⌝-sig$_{10}$-g[e]	
	b rev. 6'	[............ i]m$^?$-⌜ma$^?$⌝-a[n$^?$- sig$_{10}$-ge]	
21'	a obv. 32'	[............ šu] ù-me-ti	
22'	a obv. 33'	[............ š]à-bé u-me-ni-lù	
	a obv. 34'	[............ *ina*] *lìb-bi bu-lul-ma*	
23'	a obv. 35'	[............ u]-me-ni-šéš	
	a obv. 36'	[............] *ta-pa-áš-ša-aš*	
24'	a rev. 1	[............ u]-me-ni-šid	
25'	a rev. 2	[............ ḫ]é-em-ma-an-ĝen	
	a rev. 3	[............] *lil-li-ka*	
26'	a rev. 4	a ⌜bísaĝ⌝ ⌜ùr-ra-gin$_7$⌝	ḫé-em-ma-ni-in-ĝar
	a rev. 5	*ki-ma me-e pi-sa-an-ni*	*a-a is-sa-ḫer*
27'	a rev. 6	igi ^{d}utu-šè	ḫé-em-ma-ra-è
	a rev. 7	*ma-ḫar* ^{d}UTU	*li-ṣa-a*
28'	a rev. 8	é kèš^{ki}-ke$_4$ é ^{d}nin-tu-ra-ke$_4$	ḫé-ù-tu-du
	a rev. 9	*ina* *ina* É ^{d}MIN	*lu i'-a-lid*
29'	a rev. 10	^{d}nin-tin-ug$_5$-ga	mí zi-dè-eš du$_{11}$-ga
	a rev. 11		*ki-niš u-kan-ni-šú*
30'	a rev. 12	⌜^{d}⌝nin-ì-si-in-na	ama kalam-ma-ke$_4$
31'	a rev. 13	nin ⌜en$^?$⌝-e ù-tu-ud	ama é-[ku]r-ra-ke$_4$
	a rev. 14	*be-l[e-et ú-al$^?$]-lá-ád e-n[i-im$^?$]*	*um-mu*
32'	a rev. 15	šu-luḫ-[ḫa kù-ga$^?$ ....]	si-sá-e
	a rev. 16	*šu-luḫ-[ḫi el-lu]-ti*	*uš-te-šer-šu*
33'	a rev. 17	me-bi $^{\text{par-ṣ[i-š]u}}$	šu $^{\text{⌜ú⌝-šak-lil}}$du$_7$
34'	a rev. 18	⌜^{gi}⌝z[ú$^{!?}$ èn-d]ur ku$_5$-da	nam ⌜tar⌝-tar-re
	a rev. 19	*[le-ṭu-ú$^?$] ba-ti-iq a-bu-un-na-tú šim-tú* ⌜*i*⌝-*šim-šú*	
35'	a rev. 20	[x x u$_4$-d]a-a-ni mu-ni bi-[in-s]a$_4$-a	
	a rev. 21	[..............] *šum-šú* [*i*]*b-bi*	
36'	a rev. 22	[^{d}kù-sù sáĝa]-maḫ ^{d}en-líl-lá-ke$_4$ lú-ba a-gúb-ba níĝ-na gi-izi-lá šu-n[é$^?$ kù-g]a ⌜dadag-ge⌝	
	a rev. 23	[............]	*ina* ŠU.MIN-*šú e[l-l]e$^?$-tu$_4$ [ub-bi-ib-šú$^?$]*
37'	a rev. 24	[x x x ì b]ur	šéš-š[éš]
	a rev. 25	[...........]	*ip-šu-us-su-ma* [(x)]
38'	a rev. 26	[é kèš^{ki}-k]e$_4$ é ^{d}nin-tu-ra-ke$_4$ ḫé-ù-tu-ud-d[a]	
	a rev. 27	[...........] *ina*	*lu i'-a-lid*
39'	a rev. 28	[.............-r]a-ke$_4$	mu-ni-in-gub
	a rev. 29	[..........]	*uš-zi-is-su*
40'	a rev. 30	[..............]x	mu-ni-in-ḫa-la[m]
	a rev. 31	[..........-š]*ú*	*ú-ḫal-liq*
41'	a rev. 32	[................ mu$^?$] sa$_4$-a	bí-in-s[a$_4$]
	a rev. 33	[.............]	*ib-bi*

42'	a rev. 34	[. . . . .]	mi-ni-in-[mu$_4$$^?$] *ú-lab-b[i-iš?]*[372]
43'	a rev. 35	[. . . . .]	saĝ-ĝá-na [mu-ni]-i[n-ĝar$^?$]
	a rev. 36	[. . . . .]	*ina qa-qa-di-šú* [*iš-k*]*un* x[. . . .]
44'	a rev. 37	[. . . . .]	mu-ni-in-[ĝar]
	a rev. 38	[. . . . .]	*iš-kun*
45'	a rev. 39	[. . . . .]	⌜diĝir⌝-ra-⌜na⌝ x ḫé-en-ši-in-x[-x]
46'	a rev. 40	[. . . . .]	[. . . . . . . nam$^?$. . . m]i-ni-in-[tar$^?$]
	a rev. 41	[. . . . .]	[. . . . . . . *šim-tú i-š*]*im-šú*
47'	a rev. 42	[. . . . .] an-n[a-x]	
48'	a rev. 43	[. . . . .] ⌜an-na⌝-[x]	
49'	a rev. 44	[. . . . . an]-n[a$^?$-x]	

Ms. a rev. breaks; remainder lost

Bound Transcription and Translation

Beginning lost

1' *only traces preserved*	1' *only traces preserved*
2' [. . . . . .] a ri-a	2' "[. . . . . .] impregnated,
3' [. . .] ù-tu-ud-da	3' [. . .] giving birth,
4' [. . .] ù-tu-ud-da	4' [. . .] giving birth,
5' [. . .]x-ke$_4$$^?$ áb maḫ-e ù-tu-[ud]-da	5' [. . .]. . . the mature cow giving birth,
6' [. . .] x ti ^{kuš}ùsan [nu-t]ag$^?$-ga	6' [. . .]. . ., who was [never] beaten with a whip,
6' [. . .] *šá ina qinnāzi l[ā lapt]atu*	6' [. . .] who was ne[ver bea]ten (lit. touched) with a whip,
7' [áb diĝir bara-ga-ni] ú-dúl gal [an-na-ke$_4$]	7' [the cow whose divine lord is] the great herdsman [of heaven],
8' ^{d}d[umu-zi] sipa zi an-na-ke$_4$	8' D[umuzi], the true shepherd of heaven.
8' [. . .] *kīnu ša šamê*	8' [. . .] the true [. . .] of heaven.
9' [x] kù tùr a[maš kù-ga]-ta gu$_4$ gal áb maḫ-e [ba-u$_5$]	9' [In the] pure [. . .], the pen, the [pure] fold, the mighty bull [mounted] the mature cow,
9' [. . .] *littu ṣīrtu* [*irkab*(?)]	9' [. . . mounted] the exalted cow,
10' [gu$_4$] gal a du$_{10}$-ga [. . .]. . . šà-bi ba-ni-[in-ri]	10' the mighty [bull pour]ed the good semen [. . .] into her belly.
10' *riḫût[u ṭābt]u ina libbīšu* [*irḫi*]	10' [he poured goo]d semen into her belly.
11' ú ki-áĝ-ĝá-[né x x]-da mú ḫé-en-⌜x-x-x⌝ [. . . . .]	11' [Her] beloved herbs, growing in [. . .], she certainly [*fed on* . . .],
11' *ukullî* . . .[. . . *šamm*]*i narāmī*[*ša* . . . . . .]	11' The food . . .[. . ., her] beloved [her]b(s) [. . .],
12' áb šà-ḫú[l . . .]	12' the cow (was the) joy of the heart [. . .].
12' *ḫūd* [*lib*]*bi* [. . .]	12' joy of the heart [. . .].
13' áb diĝir ⌜bara⌝-ga-ni ú-dúl gal [an-na-kam$^?$]	13' The cow whose divine lord [is$^?$] the great herdsman [of heaven$^?$],
14' ⌜áb⌝ ^{d}dumu-zi-da sipa zi an-na-kam	14' she is (truly) the cow of Dumuzi, the shepherd of heaven.
15' áb u$_4$-da-a-ni iti-da ì-ak-a	15' The cow – when she had completed her days and months(?),
15' *arḫīša* <*ina*> *quttîša*	15' When she had completed her months,
16' áb kù-ga gú! ki-šè ba-ni-in-ĝar gù mu-un-na-an-dé-dé-e	16' the pure cow bent down to the ground and kept crying out.
16' *qadadāniš ištanassi*	16' bowed down (to the ground), she kept crying out.
17' gù-bi an-e ba-te gù ki-šè ba-te	17' Her cries reached the heavens, her cries reached the netherworld,
17' *rigimša* [. . .]	17' Her cries [. . .],

372 Or *ú-lab-b[i-is-su]* "she clothed [him/her]".

18' gù-bi an-úr-ra túg-gin$_7$ mi-ni-in-dul gada-gin$_7$ [ki] ⌜mi-ni-in-bàra⌝	18' her cries covered the horizon like a garment, they spread over [the earth] like (a) linen (garment).
18' *rigimša išid šamê kīma ṣubāti iktum kīma kitê [erṣ]eta ušp[arrir]*	18' her cries covered the horizon like a garment, sp[read] over the [ea]rth like linen (garment).
19' [gab]a$^?$ kur-ra-ke$_4$ gú$^!$ ki-šè [b]a-ni-in-gar gù m[u-u]n-na-an-dé-dé-[e]	19' She bent down to the bosom of the netherworld (and) kept crying out.
19' *irat erṣeti qad[adāni]š išt[an]assi*	19' Bent down to the bosom of the earth she kept crying out.
20' [^{d}as]al-lú-ḫi igi [i]m$^?$-ma$^?$-an$^?$-sig$_{10}$-g[e]	20' Asalluḫi saw her (there).
21' [. . . šu] ù-me-ti	21' 'Take [. . .],
22' [. . . š]à-bi u-me-ni-lù	22' mix [. . .] with it,
22' [. . . *ina*] *libbi bulul-ma*	22' mix [. . .] with it. Then
23' [. . . u]-me-ni-šéš	23' [. . .] rub (her).
23' [. . .] *tapaššaš*	23' [. . .] you shall rub (her).
24' [. . . u]-me-ni-šid	24' After you have recited [*the incantation* . . .],
25' [. . . ḫ]é-em-ma-an-ĝen	25' may it come forth [*like* . . .],
25' [. . .] *lillika*	25' may it come forth [. . .],
26' a ⌜bísaĝ⌝ ⌜ùr-ra-gin$_7$⌝ ḫé-em-ma-ni-in-ĝar	26' may it be set (on its course) like drainpipe water from a roof,
26' *kīma mê pisanni ay issaḫḫer*	26' like drainpipe water may it not turn back,
27' igi ^{d}utu-šè ḫé-em-ma-ra-è	27' may it come out to (see) the face of the sun (god Utu)!
27' *maḫar Šamaš līṣâ*	27' may it come out into the presence of Šamaš!
28' é kèš^{ki}-ke$_4$ é ^{d}nin-tu-ra-ke$_4$ ḫé-ù-tu-ud	28' In the temple of Keš, the temple of Nintur, it (the calf/child) was indeed born.
28' *ina* < > *ina bīt Nintur lū i'alid*	28' In < >, in the temple of Nintur, he/it was indeed born.
29' ^{d}nin-tin-ug$_5$-ga mí zi-dè-eš du$_{11}$-ga	29' Nintinuga, who treats with tender care,
29' < > *kīniš ukannīšu*	29' < > she treated him kindly,
30' ^{d}nin-ì-si-in-na ama-kalam-ma-ke$_4$	30' Ninisina, the mother of the land,
31' nin en$^?$-e ù-tu-ud ama é-[ku]r-ra-ke$_4$	31' the lady who gives birth to the lord(?), the mother of the Ekur,
31' *bēl[et u'al]lad ēn[i(?)] ummu*	31' the la[dy (who) gives] birth to the lord(?), the mother,
32' šu-luḫ-[ḫa kù-ga] si-sá-e	32' properly performed the [sacred] purification rites,
32' *šuluḫ[ḫī ellū]ti uštēšeršu*	32' properly carried out the [sac]red purification rites for him,
33' me-bi šu du$_7$	33' she performed her cultic rites perfectly.
33' *parṣ[īš]u ušaklil*	33' she performed her cultic rites perfectly.
34' ^{gi}z[ú$^{!?}$ èn-d]ur ku$_5$-da nam tar-tar-re	34' While cutting [the umbilical] cord with a sh[arp(?)] reed, she determined the fate (for the baby).
34' [*leṭû*(?)] *bātiq abunnati šīmta išīmšu*	34' [The (reed) sliver(?)] that cuts the umbilical cord determined the fate for him.
35' [x x u$_4$-d]a-a-ni mu-ni bi-[in-s]a$_4$-a	35' [. . .on] that [day] wh]en she called his name,
35' [. . .] *šumšu* [*i*]*bbi*	35' [. . .] she called his name,
36' [^{d}kù-sù sáĝa]-maḫ ^{d}en-líl-lá-ke$_4$ lú-ba a-gúb-ba níĝ-na gi-izi-lá šu-n[é kù-g]a ⌜dadag-ge⌝	36' [Kusu], the (divine) high [priest(ess)] of Enlil, cleansed that person with holy water vessel, censer (and) torch in his/her [pu]re hand(s).
36' [. . .] *ina qātīšu e*[*ll*]*ētu* [*ubbibšu*]	36' [. . . he/she cleansed him] with his/her p[ur]e hands.
37' [x x x ì b]ur šéš-š[éš]	37' [. . .] rubbed with p[ot oil].
37' [. . .] *ipšussu-ma*	37' [. . .] rubbed him, so that

38' [é kèš^{ki}-k]e$_4$ é ^{d}nin-tu-ra-ke$_4$ ḫé-ù-tu-ud-d[a]

38' [. . .] *ina <. . .> lū i'alid*
39' [. . .-r]a-ke$_4$ mu-ni-in-gub
39' [. . .] *ušzissu*
40' [. . .] mu-ni-in-ḫa-la[m]
40' [. . .-š]*u uḫalliq*
41' [. . . mu$^?$] sa$_4$-a bí-in-s[a$_4$]
41' [. . .] *ibbi*
42' [. . .] mi-ni-in-[mu$_4$]
42' [. . .] *ulabb*[*iš*$^?$]
43' [. . .] saĝ-ĝá-na [mu-ni]-i[n-ĝar$^?$]
43' [. . .] *ina qa-qa-di-šú* [*iš-k*]*un* x[. . .]
44' [. . .] mu-ni-in-[ĝar]
44' [. . .] *iš-kun*
45' [. . .] ⸢diĝir$^?$⸣-ra-⸢na x⸣ ḫé-en-ši-in-x[-x]
46' [. . . nam$^?$ . . . -m]i-ni-in-[tar$^?$]
46' [. . . *šīmtu iš*]*īmšu*
47' [. . .] an-n[a-x]
48' [. . .] ⸢an-na⸣-[x]
49' [. . . an]-n[a$^?$-x]

Ms. a rev. breaks; remainder lost

38' [In the temple of Keš], the temple of Nintur, where it/he (the calf/child) was indeed born,
38' it/he was indeed born [. . .] in <. . .>.
39' She placed him in the [. . .] of [. . .],
39' [. . .] she made him/it be present,
40' she removed [. . .],
40' [. . .] she removed [hi]s/its [. . .].
41' [. . .] she called him by (his) given [name],
41' [. . .] she named,
42' [with . . .] she [clothed] him,
42' [. . .] she cloth[ed],
43' [. . .] she p[ut] on his(?) head,
43' [. . . she p]ut on her/his head, [. . .]
44' [. . .] she p[ut/placed],
44' [. . .] she put/placed,
45' [. . .] she certainly . . .[. . .-ed] for his god(?),
46' [. . .] she [determined the destiny] for him,
46' [. . .] she determined [the destiny] for him,
47'–49' *too fragmentary for translation*

Notes

Lines 3'–5': For similar repetitive opening lines in Old Babylonian birth incantations, see e.g., BM 97093 obv. 1–4 (*infra* text II.1.1); AUAM 73.3094 obv. 1ff. (Cohen 1976, *RA* 70, 136–139; SEAL No. 5.1.3.4; Wasserman and Zomer 2022, 81–84 No. 10), E.47190 obv. 1–3 (G. Farber 1984, *JNES* 43, 313–316), although these compositions focus on a differing motif (the woman as a cargo boat), not on the woman giving birth as a cow.

Line 6': In ms. b, eBL reads ⸢^{kuš}ùsan⸣ nu-tag-ga "not beaten with a whip" instead, but there does not seem enough space for the nu. However, the line is heavily worn off and difficult to decipher. In ms. a, exactly this passage in line 6' is also damaged, but there is enough space in the gap to restore a negation both in the Sumerian and Akkadian. Since the cow in dire straits is usually described as beloved to her divine shepherd, it seems reasonable to assume that she is described here as an exceptional animal that was never beaten with a whip. Note that in contrast to ms. a, ms. b does not include a line of Akkadian translation for this Sumerian text line. The compound sign ÙSAN in ms. a is written in an irregular manner; the first element looks like GÁN rather than NUNUZ.

Line 8': In ms. b 9', perhaps read ⸢^{d}*A-ni*⸣ "of the god Anu", as the Akkadian translation of the Sumerian [sipa-zi an]-⸢na⸣-ke$_4$. In ms. a, the end of the line is not preserved, but provisionally restored as [. . .] *ki-num šá* ⸢AN⸣-[*e*] "true [shepherd] of heaven". A restoration *šá* ^{d}[*a-nim*] is likewise possible.

Line 9': For restoration, compare the similar sentence in UM 29-15-367: 2 (Ur III period) // VS 17, 33: 1 (Old Babylonian period): [munus-e$^?$] é-tùr amaš-kug-ga [ní]nda-zi ba-u$_5$ "The fecund (breeding) bull has mounted the [*woman*(?)] in the pen, the pure fold" (with parallel VS 17, 33: 1; see van Dijk, 1975, *OrNS* 44, 53ff., 62ff.; Cunningham 1997, 70–71 Text 62). Cf. CAD R, 87 s.v. *rakābu* sub 3. In the present text, instead of [ní]nda-zi we have gu$_4$-gal "mighty bull", the woman(?) is replaced by the cow (áb, *littu*). For áb-maḫ (rendered as *littu ṣīrtu* "splendid cow" in the Akkadian translation), compare the commentary Rm. 307: 7–8 (MSL 8/1, 63), where áb-maḫ is explained as a full-grown cow that has delivered a calf (*būrtu arḫu* GAL *ša tu-lid-du*), see CAD A/2, 263a lex. For discussion, see further BAM 248 and dupl. (text D.1.1 note on line 181).

In ms. b obv. 11', perhaps rather read [*ir-ḫ*]*i* "he inseminated", which is restored at the end of line 14' in ms. a.

Line 10': Compare UM 29-15-367: 3 // VS 17, 33: 3: [numun z]i nam-lú-ùlu šà-ga ba-ni-in-ri "he has poured the fecund seed of mankind into the belly"; see van Dijk, 1975, *OrNS* 44, 53ff., 62ff.; Cunningham 1997, 70–71 Text 62. Cf. CAD R 252–253 s.v. *reḫû* for ri = *reḫû* "to inseminate, impregnate".

Line 11': For the cow / pregnant woman eating the food "beloved to her" and thereby getting "a big belly", see also UM 29-15-367: 7–8 (// VS 17, 33: 6; van Dijk 1975, *OrNS* 44, 52, 62, 64; Cunningham 1997, 70–71 Text 62): ú-làl ninda ki-áĝ-ĝá-ni [z]ú bí-in-gub šà gal b[a-n]i-i[n-ĝa]r "she put her teeth in the 'Honey Plant', her beloved food, (and) became full on it" (lit. she got a big belly from it). See also Jacobsen 1973, *OrNS* 42, 279–280; Stol 2000a, 60–61; CAD U/W, s.v. *ukullû*.

Line 13': bar(a)-ga is understood as a phonetic spelling for bara(g) "dais", which can also mean "king, ruler" (Akk. *šarru*), see PSD B, 140–141, 143 s.v. bara$_2$ A sub 2 and lex.; Attinger 2021, 837 s.v. para$_{10}$-k "souverain".

Line 15': For completing the days/months (of pregnancy), cf. also VS 17, 33: 7: munus-e u$_4$-da-ni iti-da-ni n[a]-nam "this woman, her day, her month was there" (van Dijk 1975, *OrNS* 44, 62, 64). For a parallel phrase see also BAM 248 rev. iii 20 (and dupl.): U$_4$.MEŠ-*šá ina qu-ut-ti-i ár-ḫi-šá ina ga-ma-ri* "When her days came to an end, her months were finished, . . ." (see text D.1.1 line 145). In the present text, iti-da // *arḫīša* may have to be understood in the sense of "month by month" (i.e. Akkadian *arḫiša(m)* "monthly") rather than "her months" (suggestion by H. Stadhouders, personal communication).

Lines 16' and 19': The sign gàr in both lines appears to be an error for gú "neck". Sumerian gàr can be read as Akkadian *abbuttu* "forelock", but the sign more likely presents a corruption.

Lines 17'-18': Very close to UM 29-15-367: 10–11 (// VS 17, 33: 9–10; van Dijk 1975, *OrNS* 44, 54–55, 62; Cunningham 1997, 70–71 Text 62): gù an-⸢e⸣ ⸢bí⸣-te gù ki-šè ba-te / gù šu-nígin-na an-úr-ra túg-gin$_7$ im-mi-in-dul "(her) cries reached heaven, (her) cries reached the earth; all (her) cries covered the base of heaven (= horizon) like a garment".

For the formulation of line 19', compare also Borger 1967, *JCS* 21, 8: 63 (from the Third House of *Bīt rimki*): ázag nu[mun-b]i túg-gin$_7$ ba-an-dul gada-gin$_7$ ba-an-bàra: *a-s[a]k-ku lil-lid-su ki-ma ṣu-ba-ti ik-tùm ki-ma ki-te-e uš-pa-ri-ir* "the *asakku*-demon has covered its offspring as with a garment, he has spread (it) out like linen". Cf. CAD Š/3, 117 s.v. *šuparruru* lex. section.

Lines 26'–27': For the drainpipe with water gushing forth as an image of unimpeded birth (and the breaking of amniotic water), see also Couto-Ferreira 2014, e.g. UM 29-15-367 iii 7 and dupl. (van Dijk 1975, *OrNS* 44, 56–57: 43; Cunningham 1997, 71–72 Text 62): a-pìsan-ùr-bàd-da-k[a-gin$_7$] nam-ma-ra-DU-DU "(may it be released like rain from heaven), may it (i.e. the baby) come running like drainpipe water from a high roof". See also BAM 248 obv. ii 57, 59, 70 (and dupl., *infra* text D.1.1 lines 112, 114, 125).

The motif of the baby coming out to see the light of the sun (god) is attested in numerous birth incantations, see e.g. AUAM 73.3094 (Cohen 1976, *RA* 70, 136–139; SEAL No. 5.1.3.4; Wasserman and Zomer 2022, 81–84 No. 10 lines 59–60); BAM 248 i 66, ii 56, iv 1 (and dupl., *infra* text D.1.1); Stol 2000a: 69; Polonsky 2006, 302. Cf. also BM 115745 rev. 13 (Wasserman and Zomer 2022, 68–69 No. 4; *infra* text II.1.2) for Šamaš as a birth helper.

Line 28' and 38': Keš, the city of the mother/birth goddess Nintur (often equated with the goddesses Ninḫursaĝa and Aruru), was also called "Keš, the brick of giving birth" (sig$_4$ tud-tud, Biggs 1971, *ZA* 61, 195–196; Jacobsen 1973, *OrNS* 42, 288). In her temple at Keš, Nintur/Aruru established giving birth (*tigi-song to Nintur*, ETCSL c.4.26.1 lines 14, 18; for a first millennium BCE version of this text, see Hallo 1989, *Studies Sjöberg*, 240–246).

The temple of Nintur/Ninḫursaĝa at Keš is celebrated in the Sumerian temple hymns, see ETCSL c.4.80.1, edited in Sjöberg and Bergmann 1969, 22 TH No. 7, especially lines 87–100, the section on the "house of Ninḫursaĝa in Keš"). In the Keš Temple Hymn, the sanctuary is also associated with birth (see ETCSL c.4.80.2; edited by G. B. Gragg in Sjöberg and Bergmann 1969, 155–188; see also Edzard 1974, *OrNS* 43, 103–113; Moran 1976, *Kramer Anniversary Volume*, 335–342). It is called "house which gives birth to kings, which determines the destinies of the land" (line 58: é lugal ù-tu nam kalam-ma tar-re); there "Ninḫursaĝa sits within (the temple) like a serpent. Nintur the great mother assists at births there" (lines 78–79: ^{d}nin-ḫur-saĝ-ĝá ušumgal-àm šà im-mi-in-tuš / ^{d}nin-tur$_5$ ama gal-la tud-tud mu-un-ĝá-ĝá). For Nintur at Keš, see also Jacobsen 1973, *OrNS* 42, 274–298; Krebernik 1993–1997, "Muttergöttin A.I.," *RlA* 8, 511, 514. Another text on Keš was edited by Kramer 1971, *Gratz College Anniversary Volume*, 165–175 (edition of CT 36, 47–50).

The verbal forms in lines 28' and 38' with the modal proclitic ḫé- and the corresponding Akkadian particle *lū* are understood here as expressing an assertion (or epistemic certainty), translated with "indeed, truly, certainly", see Jagersma 2010, 562–563, Huehnergard 2005, 326.

Lines 29'–30': After introducing the birth goddess Nintur, two healing goddesses, Ninisina and Nintinuga, are invoked in their capacity as a divine midwife assisting in birth. Both goddesses tend to be equated with the goddess Gula by the first millennium BCE or appear to be at times interchangeable, but they sometimes still appear as individual deities (cf. Böck 2014a, 9–14; Sibbing-Plantholt 2022, 52–56, 87, 137, 150–153, 156–161). In the present text, they seem to be conceptualized as two manifestations of a single deity.

Line 31': Akkadian *ēnu* (from Sumerian en), is a title for the ruler or king, but it also refers to the high priest of certain deities. Both meanings of en/*ēnu* are possible in the present context. The title "mother of the Ekur" given to Ninisina refers to Enlil's sanctuary at Nippur. Both Ninisina, the main goddess of Isin, and Nintinuga were venerated at Nippur (Nintinuga being a goddess from the Nippur tradition belonging to Enlil's circle), especially within the temples of Ninlil and Ninurta. As healing deities, both goddesses became closely associated with each other already in the Old Babylonian period (Edzard 1998–2001b, "Nin-tin-uga, Nin-tila-uga", *RlA* 9, 506; Richter 1999, AOAT 257, 110–113; Sibbing Plantholt 2022, 125–126, 146–148, 150–152). For Ninisina and Nintinuga as midwives, see also Sibbing Plantholt 2022, 130 (on the epithets šà-zu an ki "midwife of heaven and earth" and ama kalam-ma "mother of the land"); Steinkeller 2022, 26–29 (on Ninisina's role as "nu-gig (midwife) of the gods").

Because of their role as a midwife, the healing goddesses are also linked to the circle of the mother/birth goddesses. As is Ninisina in the present incantation, the birth goddess Nintur or her temple at Keš are praised in hymns for "giving birth" to the (offices of the) en- and lagar-priest, as well as to kings. A tigi-song to Nintur (*Nintur* A; ETCSL t.4.26.1, edited by Wilcke 1976, 237 lines 1–18) states: "Lady Aruru of the house Keš (nin ^{d}a-ru-ru é kèš^{ki}-a), . . . mother Nintur (ama ^{d}nin-tur$_{5}$), . . . supreme mother of all lands (ama maḫ kur-kur-ra-[ka], . . ., she has given birth to the en-priest, has given birth to the lagar-priest. On the holy throne dais, Nintur has given birth to the king (lugal barag kug-ga ^{d}nin-tur$_{5}$ bí-in-ù-tu)." Our present text thus draws on old literary motifs dating back more than a millennium, based on the idea that birth goddesses – with various names – have given birth (metaphorically) to the elite of the land.

Lines 32'–37': For the activities of the (divine) midwife, see Jacobsen 1973, *OrNS* 42, 289–293; Stol 2000a, 74–80, 112–117, 141–145, 177; Böck 2014, 30–32. The moment when the umbilical cord is cut is usually when the fate of the child is determined, see Stol 2000a, 143. The birth incantation UM 29-15-367 iii 13–14 (lines 49–50), dupl. VS 17, 33: 25–26 (van Dijk 1975, *OrNS* 44, 56–57, 63; Cunningham 1997, 71–72 Text 62) explicitly mentions the healing goddess Gula in this capacity: ^{d}gu-la agrig-zi [šu]-dim$_{4}$-ma-ke$_{4}$ ^{gi}dur kud-rá-a-ni nam ḫé-em-mi-íb-tar-re "Gula, the just administrator with capable hands, while cutting the (umbilical) cord, indeed determines the destiny."

The reading at the beginning of line 34' is not entirely certain. In the Sumerian version, eBL suggests reading gi nu-x[. . .] "reed, (which is) not(?) [. . .]", while Mayer (2016, *OrNS* 85, 182) restores merely [^{uzu}èn]-dur ku$_{5}$-da, without reading the traces at the very beginning of the line. The reading suggested here, Sumerian ^{gi}z[ú$^{!?}$], may relate to ĝíri-(gi)-zú$^{(zabar)}$ (Akkadian *leṭû/luṭû*), referring to a dagger or knife, in our case made from a sharp reed. For the proposed restoration of the Akkadian equivalent in line 34', note the *Atramḫasīs* myth, which mentions the reed for severing the umbilical cord, together with the birth brick among the utensils of the divine midwife Mami/Bēlet-ilī (Lambert and Millard 1969, 60, 154 K. 3399 + 3943 iii 7 (Neo-Assyrian version): *[le-ṭ]a-a ap-pa-ri ba-ti$^{!}$-iq a-bu-un-na-te* "the reed (sliver) of the canebrake, the cutter of the umbilical cord"). A diverging restoration for line 34' is proposed by Mayer (2016, *OrNS* 85, 182): *[ib]-ba-ti-iq a-bu-na-tú šim-tú i[š-šim]* "die Nabelschnur ist abgeschnitten worden, das Schicksal bestimmt". See further Stol 2000a, 113–114 with n. 24; 141–142. Interestingly, such a tool to cut the umbilical cord, here made of silver, is mentioned in a document from the Ur III-period listing objects belonging to the temple of the mother goddess Ninḫursaĝa (Hilgert 1998, OIP 115, 19: 5: 1 ^{gi}dur-ku$_{5}$ kù-babbar). A knife representing the tool to cut the umbilical cord is also depicted together with the so-called omega symbol representing the mother goddess Ninḫursaĝa, on the *kudurru* stones (see e.g. the *kudurru* of Meli-Šipak; Steinert 2017b, *FS Wiggermann*, 208–209 Fig. 5; Jacobsen 1973, 280; Seidl 1989, 132).

For the mother goddess cutting the umbilical cord, note further the hymn *Nungal* A 72 (ETCSL t.4.28.1), where the goddess says of herself that she assists Nintur in delivery, that she knows how to cut the umbilical cord (^{gi}dur ku$_{5}$-da) and favourable words when determining destiny (nam tar-re-da). See also the hymn *Ninisina* A 75 (ETCSL t.4.22.1; Böck 2014a,

30 ŠRT 6 iii 2 //: ^{gi}dur ku$_5$-dè nam tar-re-dè); OB Gilgameš (George 2003, 178 OB II line 163). For ^{gi}dur "umbilical cord", see Attinger 2021, *Glossaire*, 313; ePSD2.[373]

Lines 36'–37' refer to cleansing (with holy water, censer and torch) and anointing (the baby). In the Neo-Assyrian text K. 11530: 13–17 (SAA 3, No. 48; *infra* text D.1.5), the midwife similarly massages the baby with oil and puts her finger in the baby's mouth to remove matter (*nīṣu*) that may obstruct free breathing. "Wiping off" (or cleaning, *kuppuru*) the newborn is mentioned as another typical action of the midwife, in an Old Babylonian Lamaštu incantation (Farber 2014, 260, 282–283 OB$_3$ obv. 3; see also Stol 2000a, 177).

Lines 35' and 41' mention name-giving (mu sa$_4$) in association with the very first actions when the baby is born, which is rarely mentioned in other birth incantations (see, however, BAM 248 rev. iii 32 and dupl. (the "Cow of Sîn" incantation, text D.1.1 line 157), in which the born calf receives its name directly after birth). In the *Gilgamesh Epic* (I 47; George 2003, 540), we read that "Gilgamesh was his name from the day he was born" (*ultu ūm i'aldu nabû šumšu*); see also *Enūma eliš* VI 123 (Lambert 2013, 116–117), where the god Marduk receives fifty names, and Marduk appears as the first of these names, since this was "as he was named by his 'father' Anu from his birth" (*ša ultu ṣītīšu imbûšu abūšu Anu*).

Line 33': Here and in line 42', the scribe inserted in smaller characters Akkadian glosses in-between the Sumerian terms instead of placing them underneath the Sumerian text.

Line 36': Kusu is a deity of purification and a personification of the censer (*nignakku*), see Livingstone 1986, 172: 8; Michalowski 1993, *FS Hallo*, 158–159. For recent discussion on the gender of this deity, see Simons 2018, *RA* 112, 123–148. The epithet "high priest(ess) (*šangamaḫḫu*) of Enlil" is found in An = Anum I 308 (CT 24, 10: 12) and in incantations, see CAD Š/1, 376 lex. section; Conti 1997, *MARI* 8, 256–257; Sallaberger and Huber Vulliet 2003–2005, *RlA* 10, 631 § 5.4.2; Jursa 2006–2008, *RlA* 11, 228 §4; Geller 2016, 304 Udug-ḫul Tablet 9: 8' (with note 8'); Simons 2018, 123, 131, 134,137 for further references.

Lines 38'–46': Presumably, the divine midwife continues to be the agent in these lines, given the parallelism of line 38' with line 28'. But it is not always clear in these fragmentary lines whether the pronominal suffixes of the third person sg. always refer to the newborn baby. Certainly, however, name-giving and determining the destiny in lines 41' and 46' are done for the baby. Putting on clothing and a headdress may refer to the midwife or the baby (cf. Lambert and Millard 1969, 62 *Atramḫasīs* I 284–286, where Nintur performing as midwife puts on a headcover and girds her hips; cf. Stol 2000a, 177 for the practice of swaddling in the (ancient) Near East). In line 44', something is put/placed in someone's hand; this may perhaps allude to the practice of bringing gender-specific objects into contact with the newborn (especially weapons for boys and a spindle for girls).

D.1.10 BM 54846: A Birth Ritual for Banītu'a

This fragment stems from excavations by Hormuzd Rassam in Babylonia and may originate from Babylon or Sippar (CBT VI/1, xxxii–xxxiii, 158). It preserves a portion from the bottom of a single-column tablet. The fragment can be dated to the Achaemenid period, thanks to a fragmentary colophon preserved on the reverse dated to the 28th of Simanu (III) in the 31st year of Artaxerxes, which may be Artaxerxes I (465–424 BCE) or Artaxerxes II (404–359 BCE) (i.e. 434 BCE or 374 BCE).

The fragmentary lines on the obverse belong to the final sentences of an Akkadian incantation that seems to have been recited in a ritual for a specific female patient whose name and affiliation is inserted in the text. The name of the woman is perhaps to be restored as Banītu'a, daughter of Ea-[. . .]. The preserved text of the incantation seems to indicate the context of a birth ritual (mentioning *lillidu* "child, baby"). Notably a goddess (possibly the mother goddess Aruru) is

373 In *Enki and the World Order* (lines 393–400), the goddess Aruru receives these paraphernalia: "Aruru, the sister of Enlil, the lady of birth, has received the pure brick of birth, the sign of her office as en-priestess, she took with her the reed that cuts off the (umbilical) cord, the stone imman, her leeks (. . .). She is certainly the midwife of the land" (ETCSL c.1.1.3; Stol 2000a, 111–112). Scurlock (1991, 149) identifies the imman(akku)-stone with sand and interprets its use together with the leeks as substances that were applied to the navel of the newborn, to soothe the wound from severing the umbilical cord. In a Sumerian incantation to Utu (Alster 1991, *ASJ* 13, 47, 73, line 57) it is said: "Utu, without you Ninmaḫ, the lady who creates everything, who cuts the umbilical cord, could not decide the fate for humankind."

addressed (line 4'), and the epithet *bēlet balāṭi* "lady of life" is mentioned at least twice in the text. This is a title of Gula. So possibly, the help of the healing goddess as a divine midwife was invoked in this incantation.

List of Manuscripts

Siglum	Museum Number	Copy	Collation	Format; Ductus	Provenience
a	BM 54846 (82-5-22, 1175)	Pl. 47	Coll.	Fragment of a single-col. tablet; Late Babylonian script; 5th/4th cent. BCE	Babylon or Sippar[374]

Overview

i'	Fragmentary Akkadian incantation a obv. 1'–9'	. . .]1'–9'
ii'	Colophon a rev. 1'–4'	10'–13'

Previous Edition and Discussion

Electronic Babylonian Library Project (eBL) (https://www.ebl.lmu.de/library/BM.54846; without edition)

Transliteration

Beginning of ms. a obv. lost

1' a obv. 1' [. . . . .] x [x x x]
2' a obv. 2' [. . . . . *i*]*š-ku-na*$^{?}$ *ni-il-š*[*u*$^{?}$ *ina qer-bi-*(*ti*)$^{?}$]
3' a obv. 3' [. . . . .] ⸢*i*⸣*-la-nu be-le-*[*et ba-la-ṭu*]
4' a obv. 4' [. . . . . ^{d}*a-r*]*u*$^{?}$*-ru* NU *ṣal-tu*$_{4}$ NUMUN$^{?}$ [x x x]
5' a obv. 5' [. . . . . *ru-u*]*m-*⸢*mu*⸣*-'u sik-kur-ru meš-*[*re-e-tu*$_{4}$$^{?}$]
6' a obv. 6' [. . . . . *l*]*u*$^{?}$*-ṣa-a lil-li-d*[*u* x x]
7' a obv. 7' [. . . . . ^{munus}*ba-ni-t*]*u*$^{?}$*-ú-a* DUMU.MUNUS *šá* ^{md}IDIM-[x-x]
8' a obv. 8' [. . . . . *ina qí-bit*(?) . . . IGI.GÁ]L$^{?}$*-lu*$_{4}$ *i-la-nu be-let ba-la-ṭ*[*u*] ⸢x (x)⸣
9' a obv. 9' [. . . . . GAŠAN$^{?}$ *re-me*$^{?}$]*-ni-tu*$_{4}$ ⸢*mu*⸣*-bal*$_{x}$(BUL)*-liṭ-ṭu*$_{4}$ *te* ÉN

Remainder of the obv. left blank

Colophon:

10' a rev. 1' [DUB(?) ^{m}. . . . .]x ⸢^{d}INNIN⸣*-a-a* DUMU BA$^{?}$ rin x[x]x
11' a rev. 2' [*pāliḫ* ^{d}. . .] ⸢*i*⸣*-na sar-tu*$_{4}$ NU TÙM$^{?}$ [(x)]
12' a rev. 3' [. . . . . ^{it}]^{i}SIG$_{4}$ U$_{4}$ 28 MU 31[(+x).KAM]
13' a rev. 4' [. . . . . . ^{m}*ar-taḫ*]*-šá-as-su* LUGAL KUR.[KUR]

Remainder of the rev. left blank

374 Measurements: ca. 4 x 4.3 x 2.3 cm.

Bound Transcription and Translation

Beginning of ms. a obv. lost

1' *only traces preserved*
2' [. . . . . .] *iškuna nīlš[u ina qerbīti(?)]*
3' [. . . . . .] *ilāni bēle[t balāṭi]*
4' [. . . . . . *Ar]uru(?) lā ṣāltu zēri(?)* [. . .]
5' [. . . . . . *ru]mmû sikkūrū meš[rêtu(?)]*
6' [. . . . . .] *lūṣâ lillidu* [. . .]
7' [. . . . . . *Banīt]u'a(?) mārtu ša Ea-*[. . .]
8' [. . . *ina qibīt(?) . . . igigal]li(?) ilāni bēlet balāṭi . . .*
9' [. . . . . . *bēltu rēmē]nītu muballiṭṭu tê šipti*

1' *only traces preserved*
2' "[. . .], he deposited h[is] semen [in the womb(?)],
3' [. . . . the . . .] of the gods, the lad[y of life],
4' [. . . Ar]uru(?), (who) does not 'drop' (i.e. abort) the child (lit. "seed") [. . .],
5' [. . .], the bolts are removed, the li[mbs(?)]
6' [*may become relaxed* . . .] 'I(?), the child, want to come out!' [. . .].
7' [. . . Banī]tu'a(?), the daughter of Ea-[. . .],
8' [. . . *by the command of* . . . *the wise*(?)] one of the gods, the lady of life, . . .,
9' [. . . the mer]ciful [lady] who keeps alive." Incantation formula.

Remainder of the obv. left blank

Colophon:
10' [*tuppi(?)* . . .] *Ištarāya mār* . . .[. . .] 11' [*pāliḫ* . . .] *ina sarti lā itabbal* 12' [. . .] *simānu ūmu 28 šattu 31.*[(+x).KAM] 13' [(. . .) *Artaḫ]šassu šar māt[āti]*

10' [Tablet(?) of . . .] Ištarāya, son of . . .[. . .]. 11' [Who respects . . .], will not take it away by theft. 12' [. . .] 28th day of Simānu (III), 31st(?) year (of) 13' [(. . .) Arta]xerxes, king of the land[s].

Remainder of the rev. left blank

Notes

Line 2': Perhaps this passage describes the conception of the baby. For the depositing of semen (*nīlu*) in the womb in similar expressions, see e.g. Römer 1966, *JAOS* 86, 138 ii 1–2: *i-na e-er-ši id-di-i-ni-lu* / ^{d}*en-líl i-zi-ib ri-ḫi-is-sú ik-ka-ar-ši* "On the bed they were lying again and again. Enlil left his semen in (Ninlil's) belly (womb)." The Sumerian correspondence is found in the expression a šà-gá ĝar "to deposit semen in the womb/inside" (e.g. Sjöberg 1972, *JCS* 24, 109; UM 29-15-367 i 3–4, ii 1–2 (van Dijk 1975, *OrNS* 44, 53ff., 62ff.; Cunningham 1997, 69ff.)), beside the synonymous a ri(-a), the latter of which is equated with Akkadian *reḫû* "to inseminate; to impregnate". See e.g., *Enki and Ninḫursaĝa* 73–74: ^{d}nin-ḫur-saĝ-ĝá-ke$_{4}$ a šà-ga ba-ni-in-ri / a šà-ga šu ba-ni-in-ti a ^{d}en-ki-ga-ka "He (Enki) poured semen into Ninḫursaĝa's womb and she conceived the semen in the womb, the semen of Enki" (Attinger 1984, 14–15 lines 75–76; ETCSL text 1.1.1). Note further, the bilingual incantation BM 34208 line 10' (see *infra* text D.1.9): [gu$_{4}$]-gal a du$_{10}$-ga [. . .]x šà-bi ba-ni-[in-ri$^{?}$] : *ri-ḫu-t[ú$^{?}$ ṭa-ab-t]u$_{4}$ ina lìb-bi-šú [ir-ḫi]* "the great bull [pour]ed the good semen into her (the cow's) belly". See also Couto-Ferreira 2015–2016, *Korot* 23, 55–57 for discussion.

Line 3': The restoration follows line 8'. See note on lines 8'–9' below.

Line 4': The restoration Aruru is tentative, although it fits the context of the incantation. The mother goddess Aruru is addressed in other birth incantations, e.g. AUAM 73.1425 iii 5 (Ur III period, beside Nintur; Sigrist 1980, 157–158; Rudik 2011, 327–331).

If interpreted correctly, the form *ṣāltu* may be linked to the verb *ṣalā'u* "to drop, to cast, set down; to abort/miscarry (a foetus)" (cf. CAD Ṣ, 41 sub 1d; AHw 1076–1077); it can be analysed as a feminine participle or verbal adjective. A noun *ṣāltu* is not attested in the dictionaries.

Line 5': Undoing the door bolts probably serves as an image for easy delivery, standing for the birth canal that is open for the baby to pass through (e.g., BAM 248 ii 65 //: *ed-le-e-ti ba-ba-a-ti up-*[*te-et-te*] "he o[pened] the closed doors" (text D.1.1). Similarly in Old Babylonian birth incantations, e.g. YOS 11, No. 86: 23–24: *p*[*a-a*]*ṭ-ru sí-ik-ku-ru-*[(*ka*?)] / [*ru-u*]*m-ma-a da-la-t*[*u*]-[*ka*?] "[your(?)] bolts are unbarred, / [your(?)] doors are ⌜unfastened⌝" (Wasserman and Zomer 2022, No. 14). As a contrast, closed doors stand for obstructed labour in birth incantations, see e.g. *Iraq* 31, 31 lines 33–36 and 51–53 (see *infra* text II.1.4).

Lines 8'–9': For ***bēlet balāṭi*** as an epithet of Gula in healing incantations, see e.g. BAM 549 rev. iv 9'; BAM 543 rev. iii 51', also BAM 105: 10. The goddess Gula (or one of her other divine manifestations such as Ninisina) act as midwife in other birth incantations, see e.g. UM 29-15-367 iii 13–14 // VAS 17, No. 33 rev. 11–13 (from the Ur III/Old Babylonian period; van Dijk, *Or NS* 44, 1975, 53ff., 62ff.; Cunningham 1997, 69ff.), where Gula cuts the umbilical cord. Noteworthy is further the bilingual birth incantation BM 34208 lines 29ff., where Ninisina/Nintinugga occurs in the same role (see text D.1.9). See further the *Gula Hymn of Bullussa-rabi* (Lambert 1967, *OrNS* 36, 128 line 182 ***bēltu ša balāṭi anāku-ma***); Böck 2014a, 30–34 for further sources (e.g. the Sumerian hymn *Ninisina* A which describes the actions the goddess performs in her role as a midwife).

For *muballiṭṭu* in line 9', compare the equation of the name ^{d}Nin-tin-ug$_{5}$-ga with ***bēltu muballiṭat mīti*** "lady who revives the dead" (*Šurpu* VII 73–74; Reiner 1958, 38). In line 9', possible restorations are ***bēltu/iltu rēmēnītu*** "merciful lady/goddess".

D.1.11 SpTU 4, No. 153 (Part 2): Prescriptions for Difficult Delivery from Uruk

This Late Babylonian text in the collection of the Iraq Museum Baghdad preserves a part of a longer collection of remedies for women inscribed on a single-column tablet. The fragment preserves the upper part of the tablet's obverse and contains two thematic sections. The obverse begins with remedies to stop gynaecological haemorrhage (lines 1–18) and is followed by a section on procedures to speed up a contracted delivery (lines 19–31). The latter part of the tablet is edited here; the first section on bleeding is treated in chapter C of this volume (text C.1.10).

The tablet belonged to the collection of the descendants of Ekur-zakir, a family of *āšipu*s, whose members lived in the 4th–3rd cent. BCE (cf. Clancier 2009a, 53, 59–61, 396). It was found in association with SpTU 2, No. 5, a tablet owned by the renowned scholar and exorcist Iqīšâ, son of Ištar-šumu-ēreš, a descendant of Ekur-zakir (active in the late 4th cent. BCE). Collations from photos kindly provided by Anmar Fadhil revealed that the preserved upper edge of the tablet contained one additional line of text and a fragmentary colophon which was not previously copied by E. von Weiher in his *editio princeps* (cf. von Weiher 1993, 181). Unfortunately, the name of the tablet owner/scribe cannot be read with certainty. As previously noted, SpTU 4, No. 153 may belong to the same tablet as SpTU 5, No. 253, a badly preserved fragment that stems from the same library, also dealing with treatments for conditions specific to women (see text E.2.6).

The present text has several highly remarkable and unusual features often found in Late Babylonian medical manuscripts. It has been discussed as a parallel (in its approaches to a similar medical condition) to a text passage in the Hippocratic treatise *Diseases of Women* I, a roughly contemporary text from Greece, describing procedures to expel a dead foetus stuck in the mother's womb or birth canal (Geller 2021, 346–347; cf. Potter 2018, 149–151). The parallel passage in SpTU 4, No. 153 is remarkable, because it explicitly refers to procedures for the case that the foetus has died during delivery and is still stuck inside the woman, which is rare in Babylonian texts on difficult labour.

The Greek parallel from *Diseases of Women* I shows that Babylonian and Greek healers had to cope with similar life-threatening cases of difficult deliveries. But at the same time, the prescriptions and interventions found in the Babylonian text also differ in many regards and details from their Greek counterparts. For example, *Diseases of Women* I recommends shaking the woman lying in her bed, to induce downward movement of the foetus through the commotion. The passages in SpTU 4, No. 153 feature similar methods, when repeatedly recommending that the woman should get up, walk around and finally, take a bumpy ride in a cart – methods not described in any other Mesopotamian text on difficult labour so far. The only means of speeding up labour beyond the administration of drugs mentioned in other texts is the application of massage to the woman's belly.

The remedies in SpTU 4, No. 153 however recommend a selection of drugs that are well known from similar prescriptions found in earlier first millennium BCE gynaecological texts from Babylonia and Assyria. On the other hand, the style and format of the prescriptions in SpTU 4, No. 153 is much less formalistic compared with other Mesopotamian texts. While the descriptions of remedy preparation are at times less detailed than in many other medical texts, the recipes include additional explanations and recommendations, for example on the effect of specific drugs, which are reminiscent of the genre of medical commentaries.

The section dealing with protracted, delayed labour treated here consists of two sections, including a longer continuous section of text that likewise adds unusual contextual information mostly missing from other prescriptions. For example, the text explains that the vaginal suppositories prescribed in one passage had the desired effect of dilating the birth canal. It is possible that due to potential negative impact of applying these suppositories, which are explicitly mentioned, healers usually refrained from using this method (and preferred to administer potions), so as not to interfere with the process of delivery (cf. Steinert 2021a, 48–49 for discussion). As another remarkable feature, the text mentions the presence, utterings and interventions of the midwife, apparently interacting with the male healer.

List of Manuscripts

Siglum	Museum Number	Copy	Collation	Format; Ductus	Provenience
a	W. 22649 IM 76998	SpTU 4, No. 153 Pl. 26	Photo coll.	Fragment of a single-column tablet; Late Babylonian script; 4th/3rd cent. BCE	Uruk; library of the descendants of Ekur-zakir

Overview

i	Prescription for a woman in difficult labour a obv. 19–20	1–2
ii	Prescriptions for a woman in difficult labour a obv. 21–31	3–13[. . .
iii	Prescription for a woman suffering from bile(?) a u. e. 1	. . .]14'
iv	Colophon a u. e. 2–3	15'–16'

Previous Edition and Discussion

Von Weiher 1993, *SpTU* 4, 89–91 (edition)
Geller 1995–1996, *AfO* 42–43, 246–247 (transliteration and translation of obv. 21–31; discussion)
Volk 2004, 82–83 n. 73 (obv. 21–25)
Böck 2010a, *TUAT NF* 5, 113 (translation of obv. 21–31)
Steinert 2021a, 49–50 (obv. 21–26)
Geller 2021, *AfO* 54, 346–347 (obv. 21–31)
CDLI P348746

Transliteration

For edition of ms. a obv. 1–18 see infra text C.1.10

1	a obv. 19	⸢DIŠ$^{?}$⸣ ⸢MUNUS$^{?}$⸣ ⸢*šá*⸣ ⸢x x-*šú*$^{?}$⸣ *i-ku-la* : MUNUS *šá* 1 *u*$_4$*-mu* 2 *u*$_4$*-mu i-ḫi-lu* [x x x x x x] ZÌ ŠE.SA.A [(. . .)]
2	a obv. 20	x ⸢*ina*⸣ ⸢A⸣ SÚD-*ma* NAG$^{!}$-*šú* ZÌ ŠE.SA.A *a-na* IGI *pa-t*[*an*$^{?}$] D[UB$^{?}$ GU$_7$-*šú-ma*$^{?}$ *ár-ḫiš*$^{?}$] *ul-lad šá* [ŠÀ-*šá* SI.SÁ$^{?}$]

3	a obv. 21	[DIŠ MUNU]S ITI *šá* Ù.TU-*šú iq-ri-ba-am-ma la ú-*[*lid-ma* ^{lú}*lil-lid-su la*] ⸢*ú*⸣-*ṣi-ma a-*[*na šu-ṣi-i*/Ù.TU-*šú*$^{?}$]
4	a obv. 22	ŠE$_{10}$ BURU$_5$^{ur5}.ḪABRUD.DA^{mušen} *u* ^{ú}*ka-mun* <*ina*> ⸢*me-e*$^{?}$⸣ [GAZI$^{sar?}$] ⸢*tu*⸣-[*šab*]-*šal-m*[*a* SU]M-*su a-di maš-qa-a-*[*ti šá*]
5	a obv. 23	^{ú}GEŠTIN.KA$_5$.A ^{ú}IN$_6$.ÚŠ NAG-*šú tu-šá-*⸢*as-ge-eš*⸣ ^{lú}*lil-lid-su i-qar-ri-ba-am-m*[*a ki-i*$^{?}$]

6	a obv. 24	^{munus}ŠÀ.ZU *tam-mar-ú-ma i-qab-bak-ka um-ma* Ù.TU.DA *qé-ru-ub* EGIR *maš-šit šá* ŠE$_{10}$ BU[RU$_5^{ur5}$.(-) ḪABRUD.DA^{mušen} *u*]
7	a obv. 25	^{ú}*ka-mun* SUM-*su* ŠE$_{10}$ BURU$_5^{ur5}$.ḪABRUD.DA^{mušen} *u* ^{ú}*ka-mun ma-'-diš i-pét-ti ki-i kab-*[*ta-at*]
8	a obv. 26	SUM-*ši* A.MEŠ-*šá ú-šá-ra-qam-m*[*a*] ^{lú}*lil-lid-su i-ma-at* ^{ú}GEŠTIN.KA$_5$.A ^{ú}IN$_6$.ÚŠ *u* EME-UR.[GI$_7$]
9	a obv. 27	1.TA.ÀM NINDA.ḪI.A *ina* KAŠ ŠE.BAR *eš-šú* SÚD-*ma ta-šá-ḫal-ma ina* MUL$_4$ *tuš-bat ina še-rim* A.MEŠ *šú-nu* ḪÁD.A$^{!}$ *id-d*[*a-at* A.MEŠ$^?$]
10	a obv. 28	*ta-dal-ú-ma* NAG-*šú u tu-šá-as-ge-eš mim-ma šá i-ka-lu lu-ú* KU$_6$ *lu-ú* SUM^{sar} [*ina* UGU]
11	a obv. 29	DUB-*šú ina* 2-*i u*$_4$-*mu* 1 NINDA ZÌ ŠE.SA.A 1 NINDA Ì *ḫal-ṣa la* ŠEG$_6$ KI 1 SÌLA GAZ-*lu* ZÚ.LUM.MA [*ina*]
12	a obv. 30	*me*$^{!}$-*e*$^{!}$(NÍG LA) GAZI^{sar} *šá* KA ^{dug}NÍG.DÚR.BÙR <*ta*>-*pa-aṣ-ma* NAG-*šú u tu-šá-as-ge-eš lu-ú li-i-li-*[*a-tam*]
13	a obv. 31	[*lu*]-*ú um ma*[*š*]-*lu u-ka-*⌜*ba*⌝$^{!}$-*as li-še-et-ba lit-tal-lak-*[*m*]*a a-na* ^{giš}*sa-par-ri* ⌜U$_5$⌝-*ma* [(...)]

Ms. a obv. breaks; remainder of obv. and reverse not preserved

14'	a u. e. 1	[DIŠ$^?$] *ki-i šu-ru-ú šá* MUNUS ZÉ$^?$ *šu-a-tú* PA.MEŠ *šá* E-*ú* ⌜SAG$^?$⌝ ⌜*šá*⌝ GEŠTIN$^?$ $^{giš?}$ḪAŠḪUR ^{giš}[........]
Colophon:		
15'	a u. e. 2	⌜IM⌝ ⌜^{m}⌝^{d}60-x-x MU$^?$ x x ^{d}[................][375]
16'	a u. e. 3	*up-puš*$_4$ *u ba-rù*

Bound Transcription and Translation

[1] (*šumma*) *sinništu ša . . .-ša īkulā : sinništu ša ištēn ūmu šina ūmī iḫīlu* [......] *qēm labti* [(...)] [2] ... *ina mê tasâk-ma tašaqqīšu qēm labti ana pān pat*[*āni*] *tas*[*arraq*(?) *tušak-kalšī-ma*(?) *arḫiš*] *ullad ša* [*libbīša iššer*]

[1] (If) a woman's ... hurt: (this means) a woman who has birth pangs for one or two days, [(*but cannot give birth*). . . .] flour of roasted barley [. . .], [2] [. . .] you pound in water and give it to her to drink. You [sprinkle(?)] the flour of roasted barley onto (her) me[als(?)], you have [her eat it(?), then] she will deliver [quickly]; her [foetus will be well].

---

[3] [*šumma sinni*]*štu arḫu ša alādīšu iqribam-ma lā ū*[*lid-ma lillidsu lā ū*]*ṣī-ma a*[*na šūṣî/šūludīšu*(?)] [4] *zê iṣṣūr ḫurri u kamūna* <*ina*> *mê* [*kasî*(?)] *tu*[*šab*]*šal-m*[*a tanad*]*dissu adi mašqâ*[*ti ša*] [5] *karān šēlebi maštakal tašaqqīšu tušasgēšu lillidsu iqarribam-m*[*a kī*(?)] [6] *šabsūtu tammarū-ma iqab-bâkka umma alādu qerub arki maššītu ša zê iṣṣ*[*ūr ḫurri*] [7] *kamūni tanaddissu zê iṣṣūr ḫurri u kamūnu mādiš ipetti kī kab*[*tat*] [8] *tanaddinši mêša uš(a)râq-ma lillidsu imât karān šēlebi maštakal u lišān kal*[*bi*] [9] *ištēnâ akal ina šikar uṭṭati ešši tasâk-ma tašaḫḫal-ma ina kakkabi tušbât ina šēri mê šunu tubbal idd*[*āt*(?) *mê*] [10] *tadallū-ma tašaqqīšu tušas-gēšu ša ikkalu lū nūnu lū šūmū* [*ina muḫḫi*] [11] *tasarraqšu ina šanî ūmi ištēn akal labta ištēn akal šamna ḫalṣa lā bašāl itti ištēn qa ḫašlū*<*tī*> *suluppī* [*ina*] [12] *mê*(!) *kasî ša pī namzīti* <*ta*>*pâṣ-ma tašaqqīšu-ma tušasgēšu lū līlia*[*ttam*] [13] *lū ūmu mašlu ukabbas lišetbâ littallak-ma ana saparri lirkab-ma* [(...)] ...

[3] [If a wom]an's month when the birth is due has approached, but she has not [yet given birth and her baby has not yet] emerged, t[o make *it come out/enable her give birth*(?)]: [4] You boil *ḫurru*-bird excrement and cumin <in> juice of [*kasû*-plant(?)] a[nd admin]ister it to her, together with potio[ns of] [5] 'fox grape'-plant (and) *maštakal*-soapwort (which) you have her drink. You let her walk around. Her baby will start to approach (come out) and [when(?)] [6] the mid-wife examines (the woman), she will tell you thus: "Birth is near!" Afterwards [7] you administer to her [6] (another?) suppository of *ḫur*[*ru*-bird] excrement [7] (and) cumin. The *ḫurru*-bird excrement and cumin should dilate (lit. "open") (her) considerably. You (also) administer (it) to her when [she has] a lot of pain(?) (lit. "is in difficulty"). [8] Should she let her (amniotic) fluid flow out completely, her baby will die. (In this case) you should pound 'fox grape', *maštakal* and 'dog's tongue-(plant)', [9] (taking) one tenth of a litre(?) of each (ingredient), in new barley beer. You filter and leave (the liquid mixture) outside overnight. In the morning you dry that liquid. There[after], [10] you draw [9] [water (from a

375 This line seems to have been partially erased.

well)] [10] and you have her drink (it). Then you make her walk around. [11] You sprinkle (the mixture) [on] anything [10] she eats, be it fish or garlic. [11] On the second day [12] <you> pound one tenth of a litre of roasted barley flour, one tenth of a litre of pressed, non-boiled oil with one litre of crushed dates [in] [12] juice(!) of *kasû*-plant (and beer poured?) from the mouth of a brewing vessel and you have her drink (it). Then you make her walk around. Be it in the evening [13] or during midday, she shall walk about. Let her get up, let her walk around and let her ride in a cart. Then [(. . .)] . . .

Ms. a obv. breaks; remainder of obv. and rev. lost

[14'] [*šumma*] *kī šūrû*(?) *ša sinništi marta šuātu arātu ša iqbû rēšu*(?) *ša karāni ḫašḫūri* . . .[. . . . . .]

[14'] [For the case that], when causing that bile of a woman to be vomited(?): the leaves which are prescribed, (should be taken from?) the top (part) of grapevine, apple tree (or) [. . .]-tree [. . . . . .].

Colophon:
[15'] *tuppi Anu-*. . . . . .[. . . . . .] [16'] *uppuš u bari*

[15'] Tablet of Anu-. . ., . . .[. . . . . .]. [16'] (Properly) executed and collated.

Notes

Lines 1–2: The form *īkulā* suggests that the verb is a feminine plural form of *akālu* "to eat; to hurt", presumably with a body part in the dual as a subject. One may ask whether the usual meaning "to hurt" forms the best interpretation in the present context, since usually a pronominal suffix referring to the patient would be attached to the verb. The appended explanation "a woman who has birth pangs for one, two days" points to a protracted labour and complicated delivery process. The following prescription aims at speeding up delivery, which may hint at a decrease in uterine contractions or pain as the described problem treated here.

For flour of roasted barley in a remedy for difficult delivery (also in line 11), see also BAM 248 iv 12 // (potion) (text D.1.1): ^{ú}IN.NU.UŠ ZÌ ŠE.SA.A *ina* Ì.GIŠ *u* KAŠ NAG-⸢*ši-ma*⸣ *uš-te-šer* "You give her *maštakal*-soapwort (and) roasted barley flour to drink in oil and beer, and she will deliver with ease." *Maštakal* is among the drugs prescribed for delivering a dead foetus in line 8, see the note below. For the phrase *arḫiš ullad* "she will give birth quickly" describing the effect of another potion for delivery, see also BAM 248 iv 15 //.

The restoration of line 2, *ana* IGI *pa-ta*[*n*] D[UB] "you spr[inkle] (the roasted barley flour) onto (her) meal(s)" is tentative. It assumes an infinitive *patānu* "to eat a meal" in a nominal use ("what she eats").

Lines 3–13: For this text passage, significant improvements were made by Geller 1995–1996, *AfO* 42–43, 246–247; Finkel 1994, *NABU* 1994/3, No. 69; Stol 2000a, 130–131. Interestingly, the use of *kamūnu* (cumin) and "*ḫurru*-bird excrement" to speed up delivery is only attested in the present text so far. I assume that the instruction SUM-*su* found here and in other prescriptions in SpTU 4, No. 153 refers to the application of suppositories. The insertion of suppositories to "dilate" the woman in labour is not recommended elsewhere in other Mesopotamian remedies for difficult birth. The logogram KU in KU BURU$_5^{\text{ur5}}$.ḪABRUD.DA^{mušen} is understood here as ŠE$_{10}$ = *zû* "excrement" instead of *sīktu* "powder" usually found with plant materials. The name raises the possibility of the drug "*ḫurru*-bird excrement" being an alias name for an herbal drug ingredient, similar to *zê summati* "dove excrement" (= seed of *ašāgu*-thorn, false carob), see CAD Z, 151 with Uruanna I 189; CAD S, 380 sub mng. 3.

Line 3: At the end of line 3, restore possibly *a*[*na šūṣî*] "to let it (the baby) come out" or an infinitive form of (*w*)*alādu* in the Š-stem (*ana šūludīša* "to enable her to give birth"). Geller (2021, 346) restores *a*-[*di* . . .] "until [. . .]" instead.

Line 4: Geller (1995–1996, 246) interpreted the verb SUM-*su* not as a form of *nadānu* "to give", because the pronominal suffix -*su* instead of -*šu*/-*ši* (which mostly likely refers to the patient) usually points to a verb with a dental as the final root consonant. He suggested that the verb *paqādu* "to take care of (a person)" may stand behind the logogram SUM here, which seems unlikely, since *paqādu* is not attested elsewhere in a similar context in medical texts. The spelling SUM-*su* (obv. 2–3, 6–9, 12–13, 25) interchanges with SUM-*šú/ši* in the present text (-*šú* in line 12, -*ši* in lines 2, 26). The suffix -*su* in SUM-*su* most likely points to an assimilated form of *nadānu* "to give, to administer", i.e. *tanaddissu* (> *tanaddin+-šu*); see GAG § 102l for irregular assimilated forms of *nadānu* + pronominal suffixes of the 3rd person in Late Babylonian texts.

After the word ^{ú}*ka-mun*, Geller (2021, 346) restores [*mál-ma-liš*]. However, the sign traces following ^{ú}*ka-mun*, which look like NÍG or ME (or LÁL), do not support the reading *m*[*al/mál-ma-liš*]. In the gap, one expects the designation of a liquid or vessel, in which the substances are boiled or heated up. The traces on photos of SpTU 4, 153 perhaps suggest a reading *me-*⸢*e*?⸣ [GAZI^{sar}] before *tu-šab-šal-ma*, which is syntactically difficult. Cf. also line 12.

Lines 5–6: The verb *tu-šá-as-ge-eš* in line 5 can be understood as a Š-stem form of *segû* "to move about" with abbreviated pronominal suffix -*ši*, cf. CAD S, 206–207 sub 2a. The verb is a loan from Aramaic *sgy* "to go" (AHw 1034a; Geller 2021, 346; Finkel 2000, 170 note on Text 16 rev. 4). It occurs again in lines 10 and 12, but interchanges with *littallak* "let her walk around" in line 13. The commentary SpTU 1, No. 49: 38 (Hunger 1976, 59) equates the participle *sēgû* with *murtappidu* "roaming". Finkel (2000, 176 Text 21 Source B: 12) tentatively read the phrase MUNUS *tu-šá-as-ge-eš* in another Late Babylonian medical prescription; however, due to the badly damaged text, this reading is uncertain.

The meaning of *amāru* "to see" in ^{munus}ŠÀ.ZU *tam-mar-ú-ma* at the beginning of line 6 has been interpreted in differing ways as a 2nd person masc. sg. or 3rd person fem. sg. form, cf. Finkel 1994, *NABU* 1994/3, No. 69; Geller 1995–1996, 246; 2021, 347; Böck 2010a, 113. Since the ending -*ú* seems to indicate a subjunctive form, I propose to restore the subordinating conjunction [*kī*] "when" at the end of line 5. I understand the midwife as the subject of the clause, and the verb *amāru* in the sense of "to examine", i.e. the midwife oversees the progress of labour and reports on it to the healer. This would mean that the text uses both the prefixes *i*- and *ta*- interchangeably for the 3rd person fem. sg. verbal forms (the form *i-qab-ba-ka* follows immediately after *tam-mar-ú-ma*). For *amāru* in the context of a medical examination performed by a physician (*asû*), compare e.g. CAD A/2, 14b sub 2h (*amāru*) and 344b (s.v. *asû*); de Boer 2021, 93 No. 23: 9–10 (Old Babylonian letter), in which the letter writer sends for a physician (A.ZU) that he may "examine a wound" (*simmam līmur-ma*); Heeßel 2000, 356, 369 *Diagnostic Handbook* Tablet 33 lines 53–54 (recommending inspection of a skin disease, *asû*(A.ZU) *līmur*(IGI)); SAA 8, No. 463 rev. 5–6 (A.ZU . . . *līmuršu*).

Line 8: Note that the plants prescribed here, "dog's tongue-plant", "fox grape" and soapwort (*maštakal*) are frequently used for difficult delivery, often in combination, in other texts, see e.g. BAM 248 iv 13–15 and duplicates (especially ms. H (= BAM 249) i' 8'–10'), iv 21, iv 22, iv 24 (see texts D.1.1, D.1.3). Note the first enumerated parallel as preserved in BAM 249 i' 8'–10' mentioning beer from an innkeeper. Compare with the mention of beer from an innkeeper, the occurrence of a brewing vessel in line 12 of the present text (cf. the note below).

Following Geller (1995–1996, 246; 2021, 347), the verb *ú-šá-ra-qam-m*[*a*] in line 8 is assumed to be a variant form of *râqu/riāqu* (Š-stem) "to empty out"; the regular durative form would be *ušrâqam-ma* (cf. AHw 979; CAD R, 178 sub 7–9 with similar forms in first millennium BCE texts). The text anticipates the death of the baby (in the birth canal?) if the amniotic fluid is "emptied out" (discharged too quickly?). For the breaking of the waters in the context of delivery, see e.g. Old Assyrian birth incantations such as Kt 90/k 178 (Michel 2004, 397, 399; Wasserman and Zomer 2022, 79–80 No. 9: 4–5 with commentary) and *SANER* 9, 77 (Barjamovic 2015, 75–77; Wasserman and Zomer 2022, 85–86 No. 11: 4–5). Several lines in *Šumma izbu* Tablet 4 concern the discharge of amniotic fluid (discussed beside labour pains and giving birth at locations such the river and the street), see Schmidtchen, *NABU* 2023/18, 35 lines 72–77. Cf. also the incipit of Tablet 38 of the *Diagnostic Handbook* (If a woman's (amniotic) fluid flows for three days", see Schmidtchen 2018, 316; Schmidtchen 2021a, 48–50 and LKU 126 (*infra* text I.1.6) for discussion.

Lines 9–10: The reading *id-d*[*a-at*] for *iddāt* "thereafter" at the end of line 9 and the restoration [*ina* UGU] at the end of line 10 follows Geller 2021, 347. In addition, I assume that the logogram A.MEŠ or *me-e* followed *iddāt* in the gap, because of *tadallū-ma* "you draw (water) from a well" (from *dalû*) at the beginning of line 10. See also Böck 2010a, 113. The procedure for the potion described here may be reconstructed as follows: Herbal drugs were crushed in beer, filtered and left to stand outside overnight. The instruction "to dry" (ḪÁD.A, *tubbal*) this liquid mixture (reading A.MEŠ *šunu* "the aforementioned liquid" rather than A.MEŠ-*šunu* "their liquid") the next morning may mean that the liquid had to be thickened in consistency. The instructions in lines 10–11 presumably say that the drug mixture could be administered as a potion, diluted with fresh water from a well, or added to (sprinkled on) the patient's food.

The sequence 1.TA.ÀM NINDA.ḪI.A at the beginning of line 9 has not previously been understood as a measurement ("one tenth of a litre (of) each (ingredient listed before)". However, in my view, this interpretation provides the best sense in the context. Previous editors have translated 1.TA.ÀM (*ištēnâ*) as "consecutively" (Geller 2021, 347), "one at a time" (Geller 1995–1996, 246) or "einzeln" (von Weiher 1993, 91). The following NINDA.ḪI.A is usually interpretated as "(with?) bread", but all editors recognized the syntactical difficulty, because NINDA.ḪI.A is left unconnected to the rest of the sentence (we would expect *itti* "with" preceding NINDA.ḪI.A). Interestingly, however, the following prescription requests that exactly one NINDA of each ingredient should be used, which can be seen as corresponding to 1.TA.ÀM NINDA.ḪI.A in line 9. For the counted item after the distributive number 1.TA.ÀM occasionally standing in the plural rather than singular in Late Babylonian texts, see Streck 1995, *Zahl und Zeit*, 71 § 65. For the measurement NINDA written with the plural marker ḪI.A with numbers higher than one, see e.g. VS 5, No. 4: 13 (San Nicolò and Ungnad 1935, 71–74 with note 5): *ki-i pi* 6.ÀM NINDA.ḪI.A ("according to (the price of) six NINDA for each (shekel)"; here, NINDA refers to an area of land).

For using water drawn fresh from the well, see also Ebeling 1950, *Parfümrezepte*, 26 ii 14, 26 "(water) from the mouth of the bucket" (*ša pī dāli*); CAD P, 469 s.v. *pû* sub 9b.

Line 11: For Ì *ḫal-ṣa la* ŠEG$_6$ as "pressed, non-boiled/unheated oil", compare also SpTU 5, No. 253: 27' (text E.2.6), using KAŠ$^?$.(-)SAG$^?$ *la ba-šal* "non-boiled beer(?)". Usually, liquids in medical prescriptions are used in the "boiled" state (AL.ŠEG$_6$.GA), cf. also AHw 111–112 s.v. *bašālu* and *bašlu* sub 1c; CAD B, 140 s.v. *bašlu* sub 2. This procedure would have killed off bacteria or other germs. Thus, "non-boiled" or "unheated" oil in the present example presumably does not refer to a specific form of oil production (like pressing, extracting), but to its preparation for the remedy.

Line 12: The emendation *me*$^!$-*e*$^!$ (text: NÍG LA) GAZI^{sar} "juice/infusion of *kasû*-plant" at the beginning of line 12 follows Geller 2021, 347. The restoration [*ina*] at the end of line 11 is necessitated by the syntax. The following genitive *šá* KA ^{dug}NÍG.DÚR.BÙR "from the mouth/opening of *namzītu*-brewing vessel" appears at first sight to be incomplete; one expects a reference to an alcoholic substance in the vessel. For this reason, one could assume that the text passage is missing the term for the fluid carrier substance for the potion, which has accidentally been omitted after GAZI^{sar}, presumably beer drawn or poured directly from the brewing vessel. However, it is known that *kasû*-plant was also used as a condiment and ingredient in making date beer and *billatu*-beer (cf. Stol 1994, 175–179, identifying *kasû* with *Cuscuta*, dodder); Eypper 2019, *JMC* 33, 44–45, suggesting an identification with tamarind). The *kasû*-plant had a red colour, so the fluid extracted from the plant would look similar to the blood and fluids of childbirth. Moreover, the fact that an ingredient needed to be taken from the "opening of a brewing vessel" may also be influenced by associations between the brewing vessel and the female reproductive organs/womb and the gestation of the foetus (cf. Steinert 2013; 2017a).

The *namzītu*-vessel occurs in other prescriptions for women, as do other containers (for beer). For example, a "lubricating" substance "from the opening of a vat" is taken in a recipe for a suppository to enhance fertility, cf. BM 42313+ rev. 35 // BM 42333+ obv. 9: (you mix ingredients) *ina ḫu-li-bi šá* KÁ *dan-nu* "with the fatty material from the opening of a *dannu*-vat" (see text A.2.2). However, in BM 38624+ obv. i 14'–15' (text A.2.1), an unidentified substance from the mouth of a *namzītu*-vessel is prescribed in a potion to expel the retained placenta. The brewing vessel had two openings, a larger one at the top, and a hole in its narrow bottom (see Stol 1994, 170–171; Gaspa 2014, *Contenitori*, 135–138 s.v. *nazzītu*). One may thus think of an association of the opening(s) of the *namzītu*-vessel with the birth canal (cervix and vagina), see Steinert 2013, *JMC* 22, 10–14 with n. 34, as well as text C.1.4 (BAM 237 ii 1'ff. // SpTU 4, No. 129 i 21') for discussion. The substances taken "from the mouth" of the brewing vessel may sometimes be particles of residues sticking to the inside of the vessel (similar to the foetus and placenta stuck in the womb/birth canal). For the broader symbolic significance of the *namzītu*-brewing vessel, see also Maul 1994, 101–105.

The emendation *<ta>-pa-aṣ* in line 12 follows Geller 1995–1996, 246; 2021, 347, although it is likewise possible to restore *<tu>-pa-aṣ* or to assume an imperative form *pāṣ* (although instructions given as imperatives are rare in first millennium BCE medical texts).

Line 13: The reading [*lu*]-⸢*ú*⸣ *um ma*[*š*]-*lu* follows Geller 1995–1996, 246; 2021, 347. However, collation of the tablet photo throws doubt reading of the following signs as *ul ta*$^?$-*pa-aṣ* "you shall not pound" (proposed by Geller 1995–1996, 246; 2021, 347). One rather expects a continuation of the instructions starting with *tušasgêš* "you make her move about" in line 12. The tentative reading *u*-[*k*]*a-ba*$^!$-*as* (D-stem of *kabāsu* "to step, to tread") "(be it evening or midday,) she shall walk around" proposed here is that the text emphasises that the woman should constantly move about. The following precatives *li-še-*

et-ba-a lit-tal-lak-[*m*]*a* instead of 3rd person singular durative forms are noteworthy, but occasionally occur in other Late Babylonian texts from Uruk (e.g., SpTU 5, No. 248 line 70, see text C.3.10).

Line 14': The reading of this line is tentative due to lacking context. At the beginning of the line, one or perhaps two signs are missing. The topic appears to concern a woman suffering from bile (*martu*), which would be a unique gender-specific condition not yet attested in the women's healthcare texts. The following comment appears to specify that the leaves or twigs of the drug recommended for that condition should be taken from specific plants or trees such as grapevine and apple tree. A similar specification using the expression *ša iqbû* "as is said" occurs in line 13 of the same text, where the powder of an old log among the ingredients of the preceding prescription should be of poplar and not of date palm wood (see *infra* text C.1.10).

The specified drugs in line 14', if understood correctly, were meant to cause the patient to vomit up (*arû* Š-stem) the bile. Inducing vomiting by way of potions is a common therapeutic strategy to treat conditions caused by bile and associated with intestinal disorders (e.g. *pāšittu, tugānu*). Several prescriptions in the treatise STOMACH Tablet 3 concerned with bile-disease(s) recommend such a treatment to rid the body of the pathological substance, see Cadelli 2000, 187ff.; Johnson and Simkó 2024, 163–188; BAM 578 (and duplicates) i 14, 50–64, ii 20–22, ii 67–iii 3; cf. also Stadhouders and Johnson 2018, *FS Geller*, 568–571 BM 78963 §§ 1–2 (treatments for intestinal fever, *ṣētu*), with the verbs *arû* or *parû*. Note also SAA 10, No. 217, a letter by the healer Adad-šumu-uṣur to Esarhaddon, in which the king is diagnosed as suffering from bile, and in which "purging upward and downward" (*ana eliš u šapliš šūšuru*) (i.e. through the mouth and anus) is seen as a suitable intervention to restore health.

D.2 Texts Treating Postpartum Conditions

D.2.1 BAM 240: Treatments for Pregnant Women and Postpartum Conditions

The Neo-Assyrian single-column tablet BAM 240 (ms. A) found at Assur (N4 library) presents a collection of recipes for complications during pregnancy and after delivery, which is almost completely preserved. Remarkably, the text does not mention or include any incantations and consists solely of prescriptions. The ailments treated in the text concern intestinal complaints during pregnancy or after birth (bloating, being full of wind) and more serious conditions after delivery, including diarrhoea, abdominal pain, fever, infection, pus, retention of the lochia and skin problems. A second Neo-Assyrian fragment on women's health, presumably likewise from Assur (A. 3461 = ms. B, text A.1.2), duplicates two prescriptions in ms. A (lines 20'–24').

The last preserved lines on the reverse turn to the topic of conception and relate to treatments for women that are unable to conceive. Two lines of the text (69'–70') present diagnostic entries without a prescription, which suggests these may have been extracted and integrated here from a diagnostic text, because of similar subject matter.

On the obverse (lines 10' and 16'), the scribe specifically noted that two sections of the text stemmed from two different sources. One of these sections with numerous peculiar linguistic features may point to orally transmitted traditions with a more popular origin (cf. Stol 2007b and the discussion below).

List of Manuscripts

Siglum	Museum Number	Copy	Collation	Format; Ductus	Provenience
A	VAT 8881	KAR 195 BAM 240	Coll.	Single-column tablet in portrait format; Neo-Assyrian script; 8th/7th cent. BCE	Assur; N4 library[376]
B	A. 3461	Pl. 9	Coll.	Fragment of a single-column(?) tablet; Neo-Assyrian script; 8th/7th cent. BCE	Assur

376 Pedersén 1986, 61 (94).

Overview

i'	Fragmentary prescription A obv. 1'	. . .]1'
ii'	Fragmentary prescription A obv. 2'–3'	2'–3'
iii'	Fragmentary prescription (for a problem during pregnancy) A obv. 4'–5'	4'–5'
iv'	Prescription (ointment and suppository) A obv. 6'–9'	6'–9'
v'	Scribal note A obv. 10'	10'
vi'	Prescriptions (bandages?) A obv. 11'–15'	11'–15'
vii'	Scribal note A obv. 16'	16'
viii'	Prescription for NI.RA-disease (postpartum pain) A obv. 17'–19'	17'–19'
ix'	Prescription against bloating due to wind (suppository) A obv. 20'–22' // B obv. 8'–11'	20'–22'
x'	Prescription against bloating due to wind (enema) A obv. 23'–24' // B obv. 12'–13'	23'–24'
xi'	Prescription against bloating due to wind (after delivery; bandage) A obv. 25'	25'
xii'	Prescription against bloating due to wind (after delivery) A obv. 26'	26'
xiii'	Prescription against bloating due to wind (after delivery; potion) A obv. 27'	27'
xiv'	Prescription against bloating due to wind (during pregnancy) A obv. 28'	28'
xv'	Prescription for postpartum problem (*birdu*-spots; prolapse of the anus) (potion) A obv. 29'	29'
xvi'	Prescription for postpartum problem (loose navel) (powder) A obv. 30'	30'
xvii'	Prescription for postpartum problem (loose navel) (bandage) A obv. 31'–32'	31'–32'
xviii'	Prescription for postpartum problem (diarrhoea) (ingesting) A obv. 33'	33'
xix'	Prescription for postpartum problem (diarrhoea) (ingesting) A obv. 34'–35'	34'–35'
xx'	Prescription for postpartum problem (diarrhoea) (potion) A obv. 36'–38'	36'–38'
xxi'	Prescription for postpartum problem (fever; retention of the lochia) A rev. 1–4	39'–42'
xxii'	Prescription for postpartum problem (fever; retention of the lochia) (tampon) A rev. 5–8	43'–46'
xxiii'	Prescription for postpartum problem (fever; retention of the lochia) (tampon) A rev. 9–11	47'–49'

xxiv'	Prescription for postpartum problem (fever; retention of the lochia) (bandage) A rev. 12–13	50'–51'
xxv'	Prescription for postpartum problem (fever; retention of the lochia) (tampon) A rev. 14–15	52'–53'
xxvi'	Prescription for postpartum problem (fever; retention of the lochia) (tampon) A rev. 16	54'
xxvii'	Prescription for postpartum problem (fever; retention of the lochia) (potion) A rev. 17	55'
xxviii'	Prescription for postpartum problem (fever; retention of the lochia) (massage and suppository) A rev. 18–19	56'–57'
xxix'	Prescription for postpartum problem (fever; retention of the lochia) (wash) A rev. 20	58'
xxx'	Prescription for postpartum problem (fever; skin disease) (wash) A rev. 21–22	59'–60'
xxxi'	Prescriptions for postpartum problem (fever; skin disease) (wash, enema, bandage) A rev. 23–25	61'–63'
xxxii'	Prescription for postpartum problem (fever; skin disease) (ointment, suppository) A rev. 26	64'
xxxiii'	Prescription for postpartum problem (pain, pus) (suppository; potion) A rev. 27–28	65'–66'
xxxiv'	Prescription for postpartum problem (pain; "blocked fluids") (suppository) A rev. 29–30	67'–68'
xxxv'	Diagnostic-prognostic entry (concerning conception) A rev. 31	69'
xxxvi'	Diagnostic-prognostic entry (concerning conception) A rev. 32	70'
xxxvii'	Prescription for a woman who cannot retain the male semen A rev. 33–36	71'–74'
xxxviii'	Fragmentary prescription A rev. 37–38	75'–76'[. . .

Previous Edition and Discussion

Scurlock 1991, *Incognita* 2, 149–151 and 176–177 notes 139–149 (discussion of selected lines)
Scurlock 2014a, *Sourcebook*, 608–616
Böck 2010a, *TUAT NF* 5, 109 (lines 70'–74'), 112 (translation of lines 17'–22'), 113–114 (lines 26'–29', 39'–42', 50'–58')
Böck 2013, 30–31 (lines 70', 71'–74'), 47 (lines 33', 34'–35')
Bácskay 2018a, 108–112 No. 42 (lines 39'–68')
CDLI P285326 (photo; transliteration)
BabMed Corpora (https://www.geschkult.fu-berlin.de/e/babmed/Corpora/BAM-3/BAM-3_-240) (transliteration)
Steinert 2017a, 305–306 (lines 69'–71')
Steinert 2020, *JMC* 36, 60–61 (lines 59'–63'), 63–64 (lines 71'–74')
Steinert 2021a, *Byzantinische Forschungen* 33, 48 (lines 47'–48'), 50 (line 33'), 51 (line 26'), 52 (lines 39', 58', 59'–61', 62'–63'), 67 (lines 6'–9', 20', 23'-24', 26'), 68 (lines 36'–38')
Infra text A.1.2 (edition of ms. B)

Transliteration

Beginning of ms. A obv. lost

1'	A obv. 1'	[x x] ^{ú}x[. . . . .]
2'	A obv. 2'	[DIŠ K]I.MIN ⸢SI⸣ DÀ[RA!.MAŠ . . . .]
3'	A obv. 3'	DIŠ-*niš ta-sàk* [. . . . .]
4'	A obv. 4'	DIŠ MUNUS PEŠ$_4$-*ma* Š[À].M[EŠ-*šá*? . . . .]
5'	A obv. 5'	ZÀ.ḪI.LI *ta-ma-*⸢*raq*⸣ x[. . . . .]
6'	A obv. 6'	GEŠTIN SUR.RA KAŠ KALA.GA NA[G x x x x x x x x x x]
7'	A obv. 7'	*it-ti qí-lip* ZÚ.LUM.MA *ina* Ì.UDU ⸢*ta*⸣-x-[x x x x x x x x x]
8'	A obv. 8'	*za-mar* ⸢x x⸣ *ši-i* SA$_5$ *i-tab-ba-ka* A GAZI^{sar} ⸢KÁ⸣ ⸢ŠÀ.TÙR-*šá*⸣ [ŠÉŠ-*aš*]
9'	A obv. 9'	*saḫ-le-e ina* Ì.UDU ḪI.ḪI *ana* ŠÀ.TÙR-*šá* GAR-*ma kal u$_4$-me ú-k*[*al*?]
10'	A obv. 10'	*a-nu-ú šá pi-i tup-p*[*i*]
11'	A obv. 11'	*ta-ḫap-šá la-bi-ra it-ti gu-un-ni li-taḫ-ḫi-ḫu-ma pur-qa liš-ši*
12'	A obv. 12'	*mu-un-da šá* GÚ.TUR ^{šim}ḪAB *ina* GA *li-taḫ-ḫi-ḫu-ma pur-qa liš-ši*
13'	A obv. 13'	*mu-ṣip-ti la-bir-ta ina* GA *li-taḫ-ḫi-ḫu-ma pur-qa liš-ši*
14'	A obv. 14'	*gul-gul* NAM.LÚ.U$_{18}$.LU *ina* IZI *li-ir-ri-*<*ru*>*-ma ina* ^{síg}*pu-šik-ki liš-ši*
15'	A obv. 15'	EN *ina ṭé-mi-šá* ⸢*iṭ-ṭi-ra*⸣ ⸢*di*?*-ú*?⸣ [*di-li*]*p-*⸢*tu$_4$*?⸣ *ana muḫ-ḫi la i-qar-ru-ub*
16'	A obv. 16'	*a-gan-nu-ú šá šum-'u-ut-tu*
17'	A obv. 17'	DIŠ MUNUS Ù.TU-*ma e-la-an u-ri-šá ú-sa-ḫal-ši em-ša-ša* TAG.MEŠ-*ši*
18'	A obv. 18'	MUNUS BI NI.RA DAB-*si e-ra-a šá* DIDA *baḫ-ru-su* LÁ-*si* EME-UR.GI$_7$
19'	A obv. 19'	GEŠTIN.KA$_5$.A SÚD *ina* KAŠ ŠEG$_6$-*šal ta-šá-ḫal ana* GAL$_4$.LA-*šá ta-ak*(*a*)*-ra* ^{ú}IGI-*lim ina* GEŠTIN NAG-*ši*
A, B		
20'	A obv. 20'	DIŠ MUNUS TU$_{15}$ *iš-biṭ-ma ma-lit ù* SU-*šá* KÚR.KÚR *ana* TI-*šá* ^{giš}GÚR.GÚR GAZI^{sar} ^{ú}KUR.RA
	B obv. 8'–9'	[DIŠ MUNUS T]U$_{15}$ *iš-biṭ-ma ma-lit ù* [. . . . .] / [^{giš}GÚR.G]ÚR GAZI^{sar} ^{ú}KUR.RA
21'	A obv. 21'	^{šim}LI ^{ú}ḪAR.ḪAR ^{ú}NU.LUḪ.ḪA *saḫ-lé-e* NUMUN GADA Ú *a-ši-e* ^{šim}ḪAB
	B obv. 9'$^{cont.}$–10'	^{š}[^{im}LI . . . .] / [*saḫ-l*]*é-e* NUMUN GADA Ú ⸢*a*⸣*-ši-*⸢*i*⸣ [. . . . . .]
22'	A obv. 22'	Ú BABBAR 11 Ú.ḪI.A ŠEŠ *ina* KAŠ.SAG *u* Ì ŠEG$_6$-*šal* ÍL-*ma ina-eš*
	B obv. 11'	[x Ú].ḪI.A ŠEŠ *ina* KAŠ.SAG *u* Ì [. . . . .]
A, B		
23'	A obv. 23'	DIŠ KI.MIN ^{giš}*ḫa-šu-u* ^{ú}NU.LUḪ.ḪA ^{giš}ŠE.NÁ.A ZÚ.LUM.MA ^{ú}*a-ṣú-ṣi-im-tú*
	B obv. 12'	DIŠ KI.MIN ^{giš}*ḫa-šu-u* ^{ú}NU.LUḪ.ḪA [. . . . .]
24'	A obv. 24'	5 Ú *an-nu-ti ina* KAŠ.SAG ŠEG$_6$-*šal ana* ŠÀ.TÙR-*šá* DUB
	B obv. 13'	⸢Ú⸣ BABBAR 6 Ú.ḪI.A ŠEŠ *ina* KA[Š.SAG . . . .]
A, B		

25'	A obv. 25'	DIŠ MUNUS Ù.TU-*ma* TU$_{15}$ *ud-du-pat* ^{ú}GÚR.GÚR ^{giš}LI SÚD *ina* DIDA SIG ḪI.ḪI *e-ma* GAL$_{4}$.LA-*šá* LÁ-*ma ina-eš*
26'	A obv. 26'	DIŠ MUNUS Ù.TU-*ma ṣe-em-rat u* TU$_{15}$ *ud-du-pat* SAḪAR ^{urudu}NÍG.KALA.GA *tu-še-ṣe-en-ši-ma ina-eš*
27'	A obv. 27'	DIŠ KI.MIN ^{šim}LI SÚD *ina* KAŠ.SAG NAG-*ši-ma ina-eš*
28'	A obv. 28'	DIŠ MUNUS *'e-re-et-ma u* TU$_{15}$ *ud-du-pat* DIM$_{10}$.ME DAB SAḪAR ^{urudu}NÍG.KALA.GA-*e tu-še-ṣe-en-ši*
29'	A obv. 29'	DIŠ MUNUS Ù.TU-*ma* SU-*šá bir-di* DIRI DÚR-*šá ma-qit* PA ^{giš}ḪA.LU.ÚB *ina* Ì EŠ *ina* KAŠ NAG
30'	A obv. 30'	DIŠ MUNUS MIN-*ma* LI.DUR-*sa* DU$_{8}$-*at* IR *a-la-ka la i-kal-la* $^{\text{na4}}$IŠKILA *tur-ár* SÚD *ana* IGI ŠUB
31'	A obv. 31'	DIŠ KI.MIN ^{ú}KIŠI$_{16}$.ḪAB ^{ú}ŠAKIRA ^{ú}EME-UR.GI$_{7}$ ^{ú}ḪAB ^{ú}SIKIL ḪÁD.A *mál-ma-liš* SÚD
32'	A obv. 32'	$^{\text{na4}}$IŠKILA ḪI.ḪI-*ma* Ì.GIŠ ŠÉŠ *ana* IGI LI.DUR-*šá ta-sár-raq* LÁ-*id*
33'	A obv. 33'	DIŠ MUNUS MIN-*ma ir-ru-šá* SI.SÁ ^{giš}GÚR.GÚR SÚD NINDA.Ì.DÉ.A ZÌ.KUM Ì.NUN GU$_{7}$ *ir-ru-šá ik-*[*ka*$^{?}$*-ṣ*]*a-ru*
34'	A obv. 34'	DIŠ MUNUS MIN-*ma ri-du-ut ir-ri* TUKU ZÌ.KUM ZÌ ZÍZ.ÀM Ì.UDU ÉLLAG UDU Ì.UDU GU$_{4}$ PIŠ$_{10}$.(-)⌜^{d}?⌝[ÍD]
35'	A obv. 35'	ŠE.LÚ^{sar} SÚD KI Ì.UDU *tu-sa-maḫ ina* DUḪ.LÀL ŠUB-*ma* ŠEG$_{6}$-*šal* GU$_{7}$-*ši-ma* [*ina-eš*$^{?}$]
36'	A obv. 36'	⌜DIŠ⌝ ⌜^{munus}⌝*ḫa-riš-tú* ŠÀ SI.SÁ DAB-*si* NÍG.ÀR.RA ZÍZ.ÀM ZÚ.LUM.MA x[x x]
37'	A obv. 37'	[*ina* ^{d}]^{ug}NÍG.DÚR.BÙR *tàra-sà-an ina ši-mi-tan tu-*[x x x]
38'	A obv. 38'	NAG-*ši-ma* [*ina-eš*$^{?}$]

(*Bottom of ms. A obv.*)

39'	A rev. 1	DIŠ MUNUS Ù.TU-*ma* KÚM *ir-ri* TUKU.[TUKU]-*ši i-ár-ru* ŠÀ *ši-*[x x x x x x x x x]
40'	A rev. 2	MÚD *ḫa-riš-ti šá ina* ŠÀ-*šá it-te-*[*es*]*-ki-ru* MUNUS BI *ina* Ù.TU-*š*[*á* x x x x x x]
41'	A rev. 3	ZÌ ŠE.GIG KU GAZI^{sar} BÍ[L].MEŠ KU ^{giš}ŠE.NU ^{šim}GÚR.GÚR ^{giš}L[I x x x x x]
42'	A rev. 4	DUḪ.ŠE.GIŠ.Ì ŠE$_{10}$ TU^{mušen}.MEŠ [*ina*] $^{\text{na4}}$NA.ZÀ.ḪI.LI SÚD *ina* DID[A ḪI.ḪI x x x x x]
43'	A rev. 5	DIŠ MIN DIDA SIG ^{giš}GÚR.GÚR ^{giš}LI ^{šim}BULUḪ GAZI^{sar} BÍL.MEŠ ^{ú}NU.LAḪ.Ḫ[A x x x SÚD$^{?}$]
44'	A rev. 6	*saḫ-lé-e* BÍL.MEŠ *bu-ṭu-tú ina* ŠÀ DUB-*ak ina* Ì ḪI.ḪI *ina* TÚG$^{?}$ *šú-nu-ti tála-pap ana* Š[À.TÙR-*šá* GAR]
45'	A rev. 7	ÍL-*ma ú-kal* GIN$_{7}$ *ši-i i-te-mu pa-gar-šá it-tan-pa-ḫu ú-na-kar-ma* LÀ[L x x x]
46'	A rev. 8	DIŠ-*niš tuš-tab-bal ina* MUD A.BÁR *ana pag-ri-šá i-nap-paḫ-ma ina-*[*eš*]
47'	A rev. 9	DIŠ MIN ^{giš}GÚR.GÚR ^{giš}LI GAZI^{sar} ^{giš}EREN.BAD ^{šim}MUG ^{ú}NU.LAḪ.ḪA ^{giš}MAN.DU ^{giš}*ti-ía-tú*
48'	A rev. 10	^{šim}ḪAB ILLU ^{šim}BULUḪ ^{ú}AN.DAḪ.ŠUM ^{ú}*šu-un-ḫu* ^{ú}MAŠ.TAB.BA DIDA SIG
49'	A rev. 11	DIŠ-*niš te-ṭe*$_{4}$*-en ina* Ì ^{šim}GÍR *u* KAŠ ŠEG$_{6}$-*šal líp-pa tála-pap* Ì SUD *ana* ŠÀ.TÙR-*šá* GAR-*an*

50'	A rev. 12	DIŠ MIN ZÌ ŠE.GIG KU GAZI^{sar} BÍL.MEŠ KU ^{giš}ŠE.NÁ.A ^{giš}LI ^{šim}BULUḪ ZÌ ŠE.MUŠ$_5$ ZÌ GÚ.GAL
51'	A rev. 13	DABIN GÚ.TUR DUḪ.ŠE.GIŠ.Ì ŠE$_{10}$ TU^{mušen} NUMUN GADA KU ^{giš}*ḫa-ru-bi* DIDA SIG *mál-ma-liš* ⸢SÚD⸣ ḪI.ḪI LÁ
52'	A rev. 14	DIŠ MIN ^{ú}ḪAR.ḪAR ^{ú}NU.LUḪ.ḪA Ú *a-ši-e* ^{giš}GÚR.GÚR ^{giš}LI GAZI^{sar} Ú BABBAR NUMUN GADA
53'	A rev. 15	DIŠ-*niš* BÍL-*lu*$_4$ SÚD KI DIDA ILLU LI.DUR *ina* Ì ŠEG$_6$-*šal ana* ŠÀ.TÙR-*šá* DUB *ina* ^{síg}ÀKA NIGIN *ina* ŠÀ.TÙR GAR-*an*
54'	A rev. 16	DIŠ MIN ^{ú}*a-zu-ki-ra-ni* SÚD *ina* Ì *u* KAŠ *ina* ŠÀ.TÙR$^{!}$-*šá* GAR-*an* ^{giš}MAN.DU ^{šim}BULUḪ ^{giš}LI KI DIDA ḪI.ḪI MIN
55'	A rev. 17	DIŠ MIN ^{giš}GÚR.GÚR Ú *a-ši-e saḫ-lé-e* MUN ^{šim}ḪAB ŠIM.ḪI.A DÙ.A.BI *ina* KAŠ ḪI.ḪI ⸢NAG⸣-*ma ina-eš*
56'	A rev. 18	DIŠ MIN ^{giš}GÚR.GÚR ^{giš}LI GAZI^{sar} Ú *a-ši-e* ^{šim}HAB ^{giš}MAN.DU *sik-ka-tú* DIDA SIG DIŠ-*niš* ḪI.ḪI
57'	A rev. 19	⸢MUNUS⸣ ⸢ÍL⸣ KAŠ AL.ŠEG$_6$.GÁ *sú-un-šá ú-maš-šá-a'* ÍL-*ma ina-eš*
58'	A rev. 20	^{giš}*šu-šum* ^{giš}ŠE.NÁ.A ^{ú}*ak-tam* GAZI^{sar} GI DU$_{10}$ ^{giš}LUM.ḪA ^{giš}*ár-gá-nu ina* A ŠUB ŠEG$_6$ *ina* ŠÀ RA.MEŠ-*si*
59'	A rev. 21	DIŠ MUNUS MIN-*ma* KÚM *li-'-ba u ter-ku ina* UZU.MEŠ-*šá u* SA.MEŠ-*šá* ⸢TUKU$^{!}$.MEŠ⸣ *qer-bé-nu*
60'	A rev. 22	LUGUD *ú-kal ana šup-šú-ḫi ina*$^{!}$ A GAZI^{sar} *ina* A ^{giš}*bu-uṭ-na-nu* RA.MEŠ
61'	A rev. 23	A.GAR.GAR *ša* IGI MU.AN.NA *ina* NINDU ÚŠ-*ir* RA-*si* Ì *u* KAŠ *ana* ŠÀ.TÙR-*šá* DUB-*ak*
62'	A rev. 24	1 SÌLA KU ^{giš}*šu-še* 1 SÌLA KU DUḪ.ŠE.GIŠ.Ì 1 SÌLA ZÌ MUNU$_6$ 1 SÌLA KU ^{giš}GÚR.GÚR 1 SÌLA ^{šim}LI
63'	A rev. 25	*ina* A GAZI^{sar} SILA$_{11}$-*aš ina* TÚG SUR-*ri tu-kàṣ-ṣa ina ruq-qí* LÁ-*id*
64'	A rev. 26	DIŠ KI.MIN $^{\text{ú!(GA)}}$GA.RAŠ^{sar} *tu-kàṣ-ṣa-ma* EŠ-*aš ana* ŠÀ.TÙR-*šá* GAR-*an*
65'	A rev. 27	DIŠ MUNUS MIN-*ma* ⸢*qer-bi-sà*⸣ SÌG.SÌG-*si qer-bé-nu* LUGUD TUKU GAZI^{sar} ^{giš}GÚR.GÚR BÍL ZÀ.ḪI.LA SÚD ḪI.ḪI ALLA DÙ *ana* ŠÀ.TÙR-*šá* GAR-*an*
66'	A rev. 28	^{ú}ḪAR.ḪAR ⸢ú⸣[x.x] ⸢Ì⸣.UDU ÚKUŠ.LAGAB ḪÁD.DU SÚD *ina* Ì *u* KAŠ NAG-*ši*
67'	A rev. 29	DIŠ MUNUS MIN-*ma qer-bi-s*[*a* SÌG.SÌG-*si*$^{?}$ *nap*$^{?}$]-⸢*šá*⸣-*tu-šá ik-te-ner-ra-a* MUNUS BI A *tur-re-ti* GAR
68'	A rev. 30	^{ú}GUR$_5$.UŠ SIG$_7$-[*su*] ⸢SÚD⸣ *ina* ⸢^{síg}ÀKA⸣ ⸢NIGIN-*mi*⸣ *ana* ŠÀ.TÙR-*šá* GAR-*an*
69'	A rev. 31	DIŠ MUNUS *qer-bi-sa ri-ḫu-tú im-ḫur-ma* IBILA ⸢*mu-tir*$^{?}$⸣ *gi-mil-li* T[UKU$^{?}$]
70'	A rev. 32	DIŠ MUNUS *qer-bi-sa ri-ḫu-tú im-ḫur-ma* NU Ù.TU *šib-sat* DINGIR NU DU$_{10}$-*ub* [ŠÀ-*bi*]
71'	A rev. 33	DIŠ MUNUS ⸢*ina*⸣ ⸢ŠÀ⸣ TUKU-*at ka-la-a la i-le-'e-e ana* MUNUS *nu-uḫ-ḫi* GÌR.PAD.DA.GÍ[D.DA]
72'	A rev. 34	^{munus}ÁŠ.GÀR GÌŠ.NU.ZU *ki-la-la-*⸢*an*⸣ [*te-ṭe*$_4$-*en*$^{?}$] ⸢NÍG$^{?}$⸣.ÀR.RA *ina* A *ta-maḫ-ḫa-a*[*ṣ*]
73'	A rev. 35	GÌR.PAD.DU.GÍD.DA *šú-nu-ti ina lìb-b*[*i* ŠUB$^{?}$. . . . .] ⸢x x⸣ [x x]
74'	A rev. 36	*ina* GAL$_4$.LA-*šá* GAR-*an tu-u*[*l*$^{?}$-. . . . .]

75'	A rev. 37	^{ú}*ku-li-*⌜*li*$^{?}$⌝*-*[*tú*$^{?}$ ....]
76'	A rev. 38	^{ú}[..]

Ms. A rev. breaks; remainder lost

Bound Transcription and Translation

Beginning of ms. A obv. lost

1' *only traces preserved*	1' *too fragmentary for translation*
2' [DIŠ K]I.MIN *qaran ayyali* [......] 3' *ištēniš tasâk* [......]	2' [Alter]natively, 3' you pound 2' stag horn, [......] 3' together, [......].
4' *šumma sinništu erât-ma qer*[*būša*(?) ......] 5' *saḫlê tamarraq* ...[......]	4' If a woman is pregnant and [her] intest[ines *are* ......], 5' you pulverise *saḫlû*-cress, [......].
6' *karāna ṣaḫta šikara danna iša*[*tti* ......] 7' *itti qilip suluppī ina lipî ta-*[......] 8' *zamar* ... *šī sāma itabbaka mê kasî bāb šassūrīša* [*tapaššaš*] 9' *saḫlê ina lipî tuballal ana šassūrīša tašakkan-ma kal ūme uk*[*âl*]	6' She shall drin[k] grape juice (and) strong beer. [......], 7' you [...] with date skin in fat [......]. 8' (If) suddenly ... (and) she(?) pours out red (fluid?), you [rub] the opening of her womb with juice of *kasû*-plant. 9' You mix *saḫlû*-cress with tallow, insert (it) into her womb (viz. vagina), and she [shall keep it (there)] all day long.
10' *annû ša pī tuppi*	10' This is (copied) according to the wording of a tablet.
11' *taḫapša labira itti gunni littaḫḫiḫū-ma purqa lišši*	11' Let them moisten an old (piece of) felt <with> medium quality (oil), let her wear (it) in a *purqa*-manner.
12' *munda ša kakkî ṭūra ina šizbi littaḫḫiḫū-ma purqa lišši*	12' Let them moisten groats made from *kakkû*-lentils (and) *ṭūru*-aromatic with milk and let her wear (it) in a *purqa*-manner.
13' *muṣipti labirta ina šizbi littaḫḫiḫū-ma purqa lišši*	13' Let them moisten an old cloth with milk and let her wear (it) in a *purqa*-manner.
14' *gulgul amēlūti ina pēmti lirri*<*rū*>*-ma ina pušikki lišši* 15' *adi ina ṭēmīša iṭṭira di'u*(?) [*dilip*]*tu*(?) *ana muḫḫi lā iqarrub*	14' Let <them> roast 'human skull' on charcoals and let her wear (it) in combed wool, 15' until it is removed from her mind(?). (If she does this), *di'u*-disease(?) and [sleepless]ness will not approach (her).
16' *agannû ša šum'uttu*	16' This is according to oral tradition.
17' *šumma sinništu ūlid-ma elān ūriša usaḫḫalši emšaša iltanappataši* 18' *sinništu šī* NI.RA *iṣbassi erâ ša billati baḫrūssu taṣammissi lišān kalbi* 19' *karān šēlebi tasâk ina šikari tušabšal tašaḫḫal ana ūriša tak(â)ra imḫur-līm ina karāni tašaqqīši*	17' If a woman gives birth and subsequently feels a piercing pain (in) her pubic region (and) her lower abdomen continually hurts her, 18' that woman is afflicted by NI.RA-disease. You bandage her with (a poultice soaked in) warm dregs of beer-wort. You pound 'dog's tongue'-(plant) (and) 19' 'fox grape', you boil (them) in beer, drain (it). You apply (*it by insertion*) into her vagina. You have her drink 'heals thousand'-plant in wine.

[20'] *šumma sinništu šāru išbiṭ-ma malît u zumurša ittanakker ana bulluṭīša kukru kasû nīnû* [21'] *burāšu ḫašû nuḫurtu saḫlê zēr kitê sammi ašî ṭūru* [22'] *šammu peṣû* 11 *šammī annûti ina šikari u šamni tušabšal inaššī-ma ina''eš*

[20'] If 'wind' has 'blown' (into) a woman so that she is filled up (with it), but (the look of) her body keeps changing (for the worse), to cure her: *kukru*-plant, *kasû*-plant, *nīnû*-plant, [21'] *burāšu*-juniper, *ḫašû*-plant, *nuḫurtu*-plant, *saḫlû*-plant, linseed, *ašû*-disease plant, *ṭūru*-aromatic, [22'] (and) 'white drug' – these eleven plants you boil in beer and oil. She shall apply (it). Then she will get well.

[23'] DIŠ KI.MIN *ḫašû nuḫurtu šunû suluppū aṣuṣimtu* [24'] (var. *šammu peṣû*) *ḫamšat* (var. *šeššet*) *šammī annûti ina šikari tušabšal ana šassūriša tatabbak*(?)

[23'] Alternatively: *ḫašû*-plant, *nuḫurtu*-plant, chaste tree, date(s) (and) *aṣuṣimtu*-plant, [24'] (var. adds: 'white drug') – these five (var. six) plants you boil in beer, you pour (it) into her womb (viz. vagina).

[25'] *šumma sinništu ūlid-ma šāra uddupat kukra burāša tasâk ina billat našpi tuballal ēma ūraša taṣammid-ma ina''eš*

[25'] If a woman gives birth and subsequently is bloated with wind: you pound *kukru*-plant (and) *burāšu*-juniper, you mix (it) with *billatu*-substance (used for making) *našpu*-beer. Whenever you bandage her vulva (with it), she will get well.

[26'] *šummu sinništu ūlid-ma ṣemrat u šāra uddupat eper nigkalagî tušeṣṣenšī-ma ina''eš*

[26'] If a woman gives birth and subsequently is distended and bloated with wind, you have her sniff (lit. smell) the dust from a copper bell(?). Then she will get well.

[27'] DIŠ KI.MIN *burāša tasâk ina šikari tašaqqīši-ma ina''eš*

[27'] Alternatively, you pound *burāšu*-juniper, you give (it) to her to drink in beer, and she will get well.

[28'] *šumma sinništu 'erêt-ma u šāra uddupat Lamaštu iṣbat eper nigkalagê tušeṣṣenši*

[28'] If a woman is *pregnant* and bloated with wind, Lamaštu has seized (her). You have her sniff (lit. smell) the dust from a copper bell.

[29'] *šumma sinništu ūlid-ma zumurša birdī mali šuburraša maqit arat ḫaluppi ina šamni tapaššaš ina šikari išatti*

[29'] If a woman gives birth and subsequently her body is full of *birdu*-spots(?), (and) she has a prolapse of the rectum (lit. her anus has fallen), you rub (her) with leaves of *ḫaluppu*-tree (mixed) with oil, (and) she shall drink (it) in beer.

[30'] *šumma sinništu* MIN-*ma abunnassa paṭrat zu'ta alāka lā ikalla išqillata turrar tasâk ana pāni tanaddi*

[30'] If a woman ditto (i.e. gives birth) and subsequently her umbilical area (lit. navel) (feels) supple (lit. loose), (and) she cannot stop the sweat from flowing, you roast and pound a shell (and) sprinkle it onto (the navel).

[31'] DIŠ KI.MIN *dadāna šakirâ lišān kalbi būšāna sikilla tubbal malmališ tasâk* [32'] *išqillata tuballal-ma ina šamni tapaššaš ana pān abunnatīša tasarraq taṣammid*

[31'] Alternatively, you dry and pound *dadānu*-carob, *šakirû*-plant, 'dog's tongue'-plant, *būšānu*-plant, (and) *sikillu*-plant in equal quantities. [32'] You mix (the ingredients) with *išqillatu*-shell and smear (them) with oil, you scatter (the mixture) over her navel (and) cover (it) with a bandage.

33' *šumma sinništu* MIN-*ma irrūša iššerū*(?) *kukra tasâk miris isqūqi ḫimēti ikkal irrūša ik*[*kaṣ*]*ṣarū*

33' If a woman ditto (i.e. gives birth) and subsequently she has diarrhoea (lit. her intestines are straight): you pound *kukru*-plant, she shall eat (it with) *mersu*-confection made of *isqūqu*-flour (and) ghee. (Then) her bowels will [*become bound*] *up* (again).

34' *šumma sinništu* MIN-*ma ridût irrī irašši isqūqa qēm kunāši lipî kalīt immeri šaman alpi kibrīta* 35' *kisibirra tasâk itti šamni tusammaḫ ina iškūri tanaddī-ma tušabšal tušakkalšī-ma* [*ina''eš*(?)]

34' If a woman ditto (i.e. gives birth) and subsequently gets diarrhoea (lit. flowing of the intestines): you pound *isqūqu*-flower, emmer flour, fat from the kidney of a sheep, ox fat, sulp[hur], 35' (and) coriander. You mix (it) with tallow, you pour (the mixture) into wax and boil it. You have her eat (it). Then [she will get well(?)].

36' *šumma ḫarištu libbu išaru iṣbassi munda kunāši suluppī* . . .[. . .] 37' [*ina*] *namzīti tarassan ina šimētān tu*-[. . . . . .] 38' *tašaqqīši-ma* [*ina''eš*(?)]

36' If a woman in confinement is afflicted with diarrhoea (lit. 'straight inside'), you soak emmer groats, dates (and) . . .[. . .] 37' [in] a fermenting vessel. In the evening you [. . . (it and)] 38' have her drink (it). Then [she will get well(?)].

39' *šumma sinništu ūlid-ma ummi irrī irtanašši i'arru libbi* . . .[. . . . .] 40' *dām ḫarišti ša ina libbīša itteskiru sinništu šī ina alādīša* [. . . . . .] 41' *qēm kibti sīkti*(?) *kasî qalûti sīkti*(?) *šunî kukra burāša* [. . . . . .] 42' *kupsa zê summati* [*ina*] *urṣi tasâk ina billat*[*i tuballal*(?) . . . . . .]

39' If a woman gives birth, and subsequently she constantly has intestinal fever, (and) vomits, the inside of [. . . . . .], 40' (it is) the blood of the woman in childbed (the lochia) which has been locked in her womb. This woman [. . .] during her labour [. . . . . .]. 41' You pound wheat flour, powder of roasted *kasû*-plant, powder of chaste tree(?) (*šunû*), *kukru*-plant, *burāšu*-juniper, [. . .], 42' sesame bran (and) seed of false carob (lit. 'dove excrement') [in] a stone pestle, [mix (it)] with *billatu*-substance, [. . . . . .].

43' DIŠ KI.MIN *billat našpi kukra burāša buluḫḫa kasî qalûti nuḫurta* [. . . *tasâk*] 44' *saḫlê qalûti buṭuttu ina libbi tašappak*(?) *ina šamni tuballal ina lubāri šunūti talappap ana ša*[*ssūrīša tašakkan*] 45' *inaššī-ma ukâl kīma šī ītem*(*i*)*mu pagarša ittanpaḫu unakkar-ma diš*[*pa* . . .] 46' *ištēniš tuštabbal ina uppi abāri ana pagrīša inappaḫ-ma ina''*[*eš*]

43' Alternatively, [you pound] *billatu*-substance (for making) *našpu*-beer, *kukru*-plant, *burāšu*-juniper, *baluḫḫu*-aromatic, roasted *kasû*-plant, *nuḫurtu*-plant, (and) [. . .]. 44' You pour roasted *saḫlû*-plant (and) terebinth into it, you mix (it) with oil, you wrap the aforementioned (drugs) in a cloth. [You insert (it)] into [her womb]. 45' She wears it and keeps (it there). When *she becomes hot*(*ter than before*?) and her body becomes increasingly bloated, she should remove (the tampon). Then 46' you mix 45' syr[up (and) . . .] 46' together. (Someone) should blow (the medication) into her body with a lead tube. Then she will get [well].

47' DIŠ KI.MIN *kukra burāša kasî šupuḫra ballukka nuḫurta suāda tīyata* 48' *ṭūra ḫīl baluḫḫi andaḫšu šunḫu māštu billat našpi* 49' *ištēniš teṭên ina šaman asi u šikari tušabšal lippa talappap šamna tasallaḫ ana šassūrīša tašakkan*

47' Alternatively, 49' you grind up together 47' *kukru*-plant, *burāšu*-juniper, *kasû*-plant, *šupuḫru*-cedar, *ballukku*-aromatic, *nuḫurtu*-plant, *suādu*-plant, *tīyatu*-plant, 48' *ṭūru*-aromatic, resin of *baluḫḫu*-aromatic, *andaḫšu*-vegetable, *šunḫu*-plant, *māštu*-plant (and) *billatu*-substance (used for making) *našpu*-beer. 49' You boil down (these ingredients) in myrtle oil and beer. You wrap (the mixture) into a wad (of wool), sprinkle it with oil, (and) insert (it) into her womb (viz. vagina).

50' DIŠ KI.MIN *qēm kibti sīkti(?) kasî qalûti sīkti(?) šunî burāša baluḫḫa qēm šegušši qēm ḫallūri* 51' *tappinna kakkâ kupsa zê summati zēr kitê sīkti(?) ḫarūbi billat našpi malmališ tasâk tuballal taṣammid*	50' Alternatively, 51' you crush and mix in equal quantities 50' wheat flour, powder of roasted *kasû*-plant, powder of *šunû*-tree, *burāšu*-juniper, *baluḫḫu*-aromatic, *šeguššu*-flour, pea flour, 51' coarse flour, lentil(s), sesame bran, seed of false carob (lit. 'dove excrement'), linseed, powder of carob-tree (and) *billatu*-substance (for making) *našpu*-beer, you bandage (her with the mixture).
52' DIŠ KI.MIN *ḫašâ nuḫurta šammi ašê kukra burāša kasî šamma peṣâ zēr kitê* 53' *ištēniš taqallu tasâk itti billati ḫil abukkati ina šamni tušabšal ana šassūrīša tatabbak*(?) *ina itqi talammi ina šassūri(ša) tašakkan*	52' Alternatively, you roast and crush together *ḫašû*-plant, *nuḫurtu*-plant, *ašû*-disease plant, *kukru*-plant, *burāšu*-juniper, *kasû*-plant, 'white drug' (and) linseed. 53' You boil (the mixture) together with *billatu*-substance (and) *abukkatu*-resin in oil, you *pour*(?) (this) into her womb (viz. vagina). (Or) you wrap (the ingredients) in a wad of wool, (and) insert (it) into (her) womb (viz. vagina).
54' DIŠ KI.MIN *azukirāni tasâk ina šamni u šikari ina šassūrīša tašakkan suāda baluḫḫa burāša itti billati tuballal* MIN	54' Alternatively, you pound *azukirānu*-plant in oil and beer, you insert (it) into her womb (viz. vagina). You mix *suādu*-plant, *baluḫḫu*-aromatic (and) *burāšu*-juniper with *billatu*-substance, ditto (i.e. you insert it into her womb).
55' DIŠ KI.MIN *kukru šammi ašê saḫlê ṭābtu ṭūru riqqē kalāma ina šikari tuballal išattī-ma ina''eš*	55' Alternatively, *kukru*-plant, *ašû*-disease plant, *saḫlû*-plant, salt, *ṭūru*-aromatic – all these aromatics you mix together with beer. She shall drink (it). Then she will get well.
56' DIŠ KI.MIN *kukra burāša kasî šammi ašê ṭūra suāda sikkatu billat našpi ištēniš tuballal* 57' *sinništu inašši šikara bašla sūnša umašša' inaššī-ma ina''eš*	56' Alternatively, you mix together *kukru*-plant, *burāšu*-juniper, *kasû*-plant, *ašû*-disease plant, *ṭūru*-aromatic, *suādu*-plant, *sikkatu*-beer ingredient and *billatu*-substance (for making) *našpu*-beer, 57' the woman shall apply it (as a suppository). She shall (also) rub her genitals with boiled beer. She applies (the suppository again). Then she will get well.
58' *šūšu šunâ aktam kasî qanâ ṭāba barīrāta argānu ina mê tanaddi tušabšal ina libbi tartanaḫḫassi*	58' You pour *šūšu*-plant, *šunû*-chaste tree, *aktam*-plant, *kasû*-plant, 'sweet reed', *barīrātu*-plant, *argānu*-conifer into water (and) boil (it). You wash her repeatedly with (the liquid).
59' *šumma sinništu* MIN-*ma ummu li'ba terku ina šīrīša u šer'ānīša irtanašši(?) qerbēnu* 60' *šarka ukâl ana šupšuḫi ina mê kasî ina mê buṭnāni tartanaḫḫas*	59' If a woman ditto (i.e. gives birth) and subsequently she keeps getting(?) fever, *li'bu*-disease and dark spots on her flesh and her muscles, 60' she has pus 59' internally. 60' To calm (down the fever?): you wash (her) repeatedly with *kasû*-juice (and) *buṭnānu* (lit. 'terebinth-like plant') infusion.

61' *piqanna ša pān šatti ina tinūri tesekker taraḫḫassi šamna u šikara ana šassūrīša tatabbak(?)* 62' *ištēn qa sīkti(?) šūše ištēn qa sīkti(?) kupsi ištēn qa qēm(?) buqli ištēn qa kukri ištēn qa burāši* 63' *ina mê kasî talâš ina lubāri teṭerri tukasṣṣa ina ruqqi taṣammid*

61' You heat dung pellets from the springtime in an oven, you wash her (with it). You pour(?) oil and beer into her womb (viz. vagina). 63' You knead 62' one litre of powder of *šūšu*-plant, one litre of powder of sesame draff, one litre of malt flour(?), one litre of powder of *kukru*-aromatic, one litre of *burāšu*-juniper 63' with *kasû*-juice. You *smear* (the mixture) on (a piece of) cloth, you let it cool down (and) make a bandage with a thin (cloth?).

64' DIŠ KI.MIN *karaša tukaṣṣā-ma tapaššaš ana šassūrīša tašakkan*

64' Alternatively, you cool down leek, and you rub (her with it?). (Or) you insert (it) into her womb (viz. vagina).

65' *šumma sinništu* MIN-*ma qerbīssa umaḫḫassi qerbēna šarka iraššī kasî kukra qalâ saḫlê tasâk tuballal allāna teppuš ana šassūriša tašakkan* 66' *ḫašâ* [. . .] *lipî irrê tubbal tasâk ina šamni u šikari tašaqqīši*

65' If a woman ditto (i.e. gives birth) and subsequently her womb gives her a sharp pain, she has pus internally. You pound (and) mix *kasû*-plant, roasted *kukru*-plant (and) *saḫlû*-cress. You form an acorn-shaped suppository (of the mixture), you insert (it) into her womb (viz. vagina). 66' You dry (and) pound *ḫašû*-plant, [. . .]-plant, fat (pith of) *irrû*-colocynth. You have her drink (the mixture) with oil and beer.

67' *šumma sinništu* MIN-*ma qerbī*[*ssa umaḫḫassi nap*]*šātuša*(?) *iktenerrâ sinništu šī mê turrūti*(?!) *šaknat*(?) 68' *šarmada arqūs*[*su*] ⸢*tasâk*⸣ *ina* ⸢*itqi talammi*⸣ *ana šassūrīša tašakkan*

67' If a woman ditto (i.e. gives birth) and subsequently her womb [gives her a sharp pain (and) her brea]thing(?) becomes increasingly short, this woman is afflicted by *blocked* fluids(?). 68' ⸢You pound⸣ fresh *šarmadu*-plant, ⸢wrap⸣ it in a ⸢wad of wool⸣, you insert it into her womb (viz. vagina).

69' *šumma sinništu qerbīssa riḫûtu imḫur-ma apla muter gimilli i*[*rašši*(?)]

69' If a woman's womb receives the semen, she will g[et(?)] a male child, an avenger.

70' *šumma sinništu qerbīssa riḫûtu imḫur-ma lā ittalad šibsāt ili lā ṭūb* [*libbi*]

70' If a woman's womb receives the semen, but she does not bear: anger of the god, unhappi[ness].

71' *šumma sinništu ina libbi rašât kalâ lā ile"e ana sinništi nuḫḫi sāq*[*ī*] 72' *unīqi lā petīti kilallān* [*teṭên*(?)] *munda ina mê tamaḫḫaṣ* 73' *sāqī šunūti ina libb*[*i tanaddi* . . . . . .] . . .[. . .] 74' *ina ūrīša tašakkan tu*[*l*-. . . . . .]

71' If a woman has acquired (the semen) in (her) belly, (but) cannot retain it (inside), to calm the woman: [you grind(?)] both thigh bones 72' of a virgin she-goat, you sti[r] *mundu*-flour into water. 73' [You *add*(?)] these thigh bones to (it), [. . . . . .]. 74' You insert (it) into her vagina, you [. . . . . .].

75' *kulīl*[*ītu*(?) . . . . . .] 76' *traces*

75'–76' *too fragmentary for translation*

Ms. A rev. breaks; remainder lost

Notes

Line 1': The small top piece with sign traces of line 1', rendered in Köcher's copy, is not preserved anymore on the tablet today.

Lines 4'–5': The identification of *saḫlû* (ZÀ.ḪI.LI$^{(sar)}$) with "garden cress" is contested, cf. CAD S, 62ff. with discussion; Stol 1983–1984, *JEOL* 28, 24–32; Powell 2003–2005, *RlA* 10, 14; Köcher 1995, *AUWE* 10, 212 note 19'. Edzard (1985, *ZA* 75, 125) suggests "Salat".

Lines 6'-9': For *karānu ṣaḫtu* "grape-juice" (pressed grapes)", cf. Stol 2016–2018a, *RlA* 15, 38b §3. The text at the beginning of line 8', *za-mar* ⸢x x⸣ *ši-i* SA$_5$ *i-tab-ba-ka*, is difficult to read with certainty. Scurlock (2014a, 613) translates "(If) suddenly that [. . .] pours out red (liquid)". It is possible that *šī* refers to the patient discharging a reddish fluid or blood (thus Scurlock and Andersen 2005, 12.46). The following treatment, in which *kasû*-juice (which is likewise of a red colour) was applied to the opening of the patient's vulva followed by the application of a suppository introduced into the vagina, likewise seems to indicate this interpretation.

Lines 11'–16': The numerous unusual features of lines 11'–16' have been discussed by Stol 2007b, *JMC* 10, 1–3. For example, the word *purqa* or *burqa*, occurring in lines 11'–14' with the form and function of an adverb, is a hapax (CAD P, 521 s.v. *purqa*). The word may be related to the adverb *purqidam* "on one's back, supine" (CAD P, 521, also attested in Aramaic *prqdn*, from PRQD "to fall on the back"; see Comprehensive Aramaic Lexicon; https://cal.huc.edu). The references to textiles and to the patient "wearing" or applying a blanket or a piece of cloth specially prepared (moistened) suggests that the medications in lines 11'–13' were applied as some sort of bandage.

Line 11': The word *taḫapšu* (probably of Hurrian origin) was first defined as a kind of woollen blanket but has been shown to designate felt (cf. CAD T, 40–41, with our passage quoted sub sub d; SAD, Vol. 2, 51b; Cancik-Kirschbaum 1999, *FS Renger*, 85–87; Postgate 2000, *FS Saporetti*, 213–217; Gaspa 2018, *Textiles*, 91, 279). For another medical passage, in which this word occurs, see AMT 61/2 ii 3'ff. // BAM 559: 3'–5': *ta-ḫap-ša ina libbi taṣappu* "you soak a felt-rug with it". In this remarkable, but unfortunately damaged passage treating an affliction of the pelvis and lower back, it appears a baked brick was heated and then wrapped into the *taḫapšu*, which was previously soaked in a liquid, to be applied to the patient's hips (a sort of heating treatment).

The term *gunnu/gurnu* in line 11' means "of average quality" and qualifies products such as dates, wool, beer, but also oil (AHw 299a, s.v. *gurnu, gunnu*; CAD G, 139b sub d). That it may refer to oil in the present line, may be suggested from the verb *taḫāḫu* "to sprinkle with a liquid; to moisten(?)" (D-stem), which is equated with Sumerian sud in lexical lists (CAD T, 39b). The Akkadian verb occurs only rarely in the texts. AHw 299a, s.v. *gurnu* sub 5 proposes to emend the passage to <*ina*> *itti gunni* "<with> medium-quality bitumen".

Line 13': The word *muṣīptu* (or *muṣiptu*) refers to a (standard-size) piece of cloth (CAD M/2, 242–243; Gaspa 2018, *Textiles*, 159, 266). The term occurs also in BM 57853: 7' (CT 55, 377 = text E.2.5).

Line 14': Lambert and Millard (1969, 156) regard *li-er-ri-ma* in line 14' as a reference for a verb *urrû* "to parch, to dry" (and render it *li'erri*), which they see as the same verb as the form *li-e-er-ri* "let him parch (the ground)" in *Atramḫasīs* II 15. However, CAD A/2, 317 s.v. *arû* D emends our passage to *li-ir-ri-*<*ir*> (following Köcher 1965, *FS Landsberger*, 323–325) and connects the verb with *urruru* "to dry; to char". Because of the other precative plural verbal forms in lines 11'–13', Stol 2007b, *JMC* 10, 1 prefers the emendation *li-ir-ri-*<*ru*>*-ma*, which is followed here. For the use of charred (and pulverized) human skull, cf. also AMT 103 ii 18 (ointment); AMT 15/3 rev. iv 10'; BAM 104: 32 (bandage; Geller 2005a, No. 28). The instruction to wear the skull in combed wool in line 14' may refer to a kind of amulet; certainly, only a piece or sherd of a skull must have been used.

Line 15': The reading of this line tentatively follows Scurlock 2014a, 609. The text is highly unusual and may imply that the prescription had an apotropaic function. CAD I/J, 232a sub 3' proposed a different reading; cf. CAD Q, 234 sub 3c.

Line 16': The word *šum'uttu* in line 16' is a hapax. CAD Š/III, 300 (also CAD A/1, 143b; CAD M/1, 24a) derives it from the verb *mâdu* (*ma'ādu*) "to become numerous" (Š-stem) and renders it as "additional(?)"; similarly, AHw 1276a "(Text)-Zusatz(?)"; Scurlock (2014a, 613) "supplemental". However, Stol (2007b, *JMC* 10, 1) interprets the word as *šum'ūtu* "hear-say" (derived from *šemû*, i.e. "oral tradition", related to Aramaic *šm*^{c}*th* or *šm*^{c}*tt'* "tradition"). Stol draws on the unusual and difficult textual features of the recipes in the preceding lines, which perhaps point to folklore and popular medicine as a source.

In contrast to this section marked by the scribe as special, the beginning of the tablet reflects a more scholarly medical language. These lines are commented on in line 10 as having been copied "according to the wording of a tablet".

Lines 17'–19': For the symptom description in lines 17'–18', compare BM 38624+ i 24'–25' (text A.2.1), where similar symptoms receive a different diagnosis ("blocked fluids"). For this condition, see the notes below on lines 67'–68' and the *Introduction* in this volume.

The symptom "her pubic region gives her a piercing pain" (*elān ūrīša usaḫḫalši*) in line 17' of ms. A also occurs as an explanation for a different disease name in KADP 22 ii 5: DIŠ MUNUS ^gišGIDRU DAB-*si*^!? : *e-la-an* GAL_4.LA-*šá ú-saḫ-ḫal-*⸢*ši*^?⸣ "If a woman is seized by the 'staff/sceptre' (*ḫaṭṭu*): (it means) her pubic region gives ⸢her⸣ a piercing pain".

The reference to a "staff" is interesting in comparison with the disease name NI.RA encountered in line 18'. Scurlock interprets it as a Sumerogram Ì.RA "striking" (or "it strikes", see Scurlock 1991, 173 n. 133; Scurlock and Andersen 2005, 12.120; Scurlock 2014b, 111). The Akkadian equivalent to Sumerian ra is indeed *maḫāṣu* "to beat" (see also CAD M/2, 61 s.v. *miḫṣu* sub 3–4 "wound, blow (by a weapon); attack (of a demon or disease)"). Elsewhere, "being hit (by the weapon)" is a euphemistic expression for gynaecological haemorrhage (see BAM 235: 4 (*infra* text C.1.1): if a woman ^gišTUKUL *maḫṣat* "is hit by the weapon"). There is a second disease name in women's healthcare texts with the likely element Ì (NI.NE) (see BAM 237 rev. iv 9–14, *infra* text C.1.4 with discussion), which may be interpreted in the same way as Ì.KÚM/BIL ("it has burned"), to denote a burning pain (cf. KÚM = *ummu* "fever"). The disease name NI/Ì.RA would thus allude to the leading symptom (pain) described in lines 17'–18'.

Line 18': For *iri'u* / *erû* "(beer) dregs", see CAD I/J, 177b, AHw 386a. However, CAD B, 227a, lists the present attestation of *e-ra-a* as an erroneous spelling for *bit-ra-a* under the term *bitru* (see CAD B, 279a, correcting CAD I/J, 177b; CAD B, 227a). The expression *bit-ra ša* DIDA SIG "dregs of *billatu*-substance (for making) *našpu*-beer" is attested in BAM 558 rev. iv 9. Scurlock (2014a, 481, 486 n. 21) reads the word there as *é-ra* for "dregs". Stol (personal communication) suggests that the word for dregs might actually be *piṭru* and not *erû* or *bitru* (cf. CAD P, 449–450; AHw 870b listed under *pitru*). The term *piṭru* means "fissure, separation", which would allude to the dregs as a product of separation from a liquid.

Line 19': The verb *kâru* "to rub, apply medication" in line 19' is usually spelled *ta-kar* in medical texts (CAD K, 239–240), whereas ms. A reads *ta-ak-ra* (for *takâra* with a ventive?). The verb usually refers to an external application of medicine to the body by rubbing.

Lines 20'–22': The feminine stative form of *malû* in line 20' should have read *malât* (*maliat*) rather than *malît*. The aetiological condition of being "blasted by wind" (*šāru išbissu*(*ma*) (referencing a male patient) or "wind blasting" (*šibiṭ šāri*) elsewhere in cuneiform medical texts can be linked with either internal conditions (bloating, fever) or with external symptoms (e.g., skin rashes, affected eyes, penis), see Steinert et al. 2018, 211, 231 ad line 31; Schmidtchen 2021a, 41 with further references. Since the following sections in BAM 240 continue with problems of internal bloating with wind (*šāra uddupat*) after delivery and during pregnancy (see lines 25–28 below), it seems likely that in line 20' also an intestinal problem rather than a skin condition is meant. The additional symptom "her body (or skin?) keeps changing" refers to a worsening of the patient's state. For KÚR.KÚR (Gtn-stem of *nakāru*), "to keep changing (for the worse)" in line 20', cf. Scurlock and Andersen 2005, 92 4.15; CAD N/1, 164a sub 2g.

The treatment instruction *inaššī-ma* "she shall wear/apply (it)" in line 22' is ambiguous. In instructions given in women's healthcare texts, the verb *našû* "to wear; to apply" can indicate the recommended insertion of a suppository or tampon into the vagina (see explicitly below, lines 44'–45'; cf. CAD N/2, 100a; Reiner 1982, *ZA* 72, 131 n. 24 with parallels from ancient Greek texts). Scurlock (2014a, 111) simply translates "she takes (it)", leaving open the form of application. For discussion of the prescriptions in lines 20'–24', see also Steinert 2021a, *Byzantinische Forschungen* 33, 62, 67–68.

A partial parallel to this prescription is found in BAM 408 obv.^? i' 5'–8' (text A.2.7).

Line 25': Because the logographic writings for *našpu* interchange between SIG and SIG_5, Böck (2010a, 113 line 51') translates DIDA SIG as "gutes *billatu*-beer". Dictionary references suggest reading either *billat našpi* or *billatu našiptu* (CAD B, 228; CAD N/2, 78). For *billatu*-substance, a dry and crumbly substance used in beermaking and for producing a kind of instant beer, see Stol 1971, *BiOr* 28, 161b; 1994, 165; Maul 1994, 51. For *billat našpi*, see also Abusch and Schwemer 2011, CMAwR 1, 55 text 1.6 note on lines 9'–10'. For *našpu* as a kind of light-coloured beer, see Powell 1994, 105–106.

The word *ēma* in *ēma ūraša taṣammid-ma* "whenever you bandage her vulva (with it)" seems to be used here as instead of *šumma* "if", cf. AHw 210b, CAD E, 136.

Lines 26'–28': This section of BAM 240 is concerned with the key symptom bloating by wind (*šāra uddupat*), both found in lines 26' and 28'. I interpret both entries offering variant cases of a postpartum vs. a pregnant woman bloated by wind. Line 28' offers the additional phrase *ṣemrat* "she is distended/swollen". With Landsberger (MSL 9, 86–87 as well as AHw 72b sub *arû, erû*; von Soden 1995, GAG § 106k), I consider *'e-re-et* in line 28' as an irregular stative form instead of *erât* "she is pregnant", and not as a form of the verb *emēru* "to be swollen" used as a synonym or variant of *ṣemrat* in line 26' (cf. Scurlock and Andersen 2005, 19.226 and Scurlock 2014a, 614). Landsberger (op. cit.) discusses semantic differences between *ṣemēru* and *emēru*, which despite their semantic similarities (distention), seem to exclude that both verbs are just variant forms.

Lines 26' and 28' employ the same treatment, which consists in the patient sniffing (lit. smelling) dust (SAḪAR) taken from the musical instrument called ^{urudu}NÍG.KALA.GA.[377] The aim of this treatment based on the principle of analogy was to induce sneezing and thus expel the wind from the patient's body, in a sonorous manner resembling the sound of the ^{urudu}NÍG.KALA.GA. The musical instrument ^{urudu}NÍG.KALA.GA "hardened/powerful copper-thing" has been understood variously as cymbals, a drum or a bell, cf. AHw 787b (kettledrum); CAD N/2, s.v. **nigkalagû*; Livingstone 1986, 179; Panayotov 2013, *NABU* 2013/3, 80–85. Reiner (1969, *RA* 63, 170–171) suggested ^{urudu}NÍG.KALA.GA should be read in Akkadian as *tigû* (a drum or string instrument), not as *nigkalagû*. See further Geller 2016, 24–26 *passim*; Rendu-Loisel 2015; 2016, 181–199 for the use of the ^{urudu}NÍG.KALA.GA in Udug-ḫul rituals, where its loud sound is employed by the healer to drive away disease demons.

BAM 575 ii 54–55, a passage from the treatise STOMACH (Tablet 2), uses a similar therapy for a male patient bloated by wind:

> [DIŠ NA ŠÀ-*šú*] TU$_{15}$ *ṣe-en* ^{urudu}ŠUM$^{!}$(DÌM).GAM.ME ZABAR *lu* GÍR ZABAR *i-lek-ma* TI
> [SAḪAR ^{urudu}NÍG].KALA.GA *tu-uš-ṣe-en-šú i-še$_{20}$-ḫe-eq-ma* TI
> "[If a man's belly] is bloated with 'wind', he shall lick a bronze saw or a bronze dagger and he will recover.
> [(Alternatively)] you have him sniff the [dust from a copper] bell(?), he will sneeze and get well." (see Cadelli 2000, 133, 157; Johnson and Simkó 2024, 127–128 lines 124–125)

The irregular spelling *tu-uš-ṣe-en-šú* in this passage (against *tu-še-ṣe-en-ši-ma* in BAM 240: 26' and 28') was apparent influenced by *ṣe-en* "he is bloated" in the preceding line (for the verb *ṣânu/ṣênu* "to fill up, to bloat", see AHw 1081–1082 "auffüllen, aufschwemmen").[378] The verbal form *i-ši-ḫi-iq* (a hapax) was first proposed in AHw 1209a to represent a verb *šeḫēqu* with the meaning "to sneeze" (related to West Semitic *ś/ṣḥq* "to laugh"; see also Stol 1991–1992, *JEOL* 32, 60; CAD Š/2, 263b).

Both the similarities as well as the differences between BAM 240: 26', 28' and BAM 575 ii 54–55 are interesting. On the one hand, there are variations in the terms describing the symptom of distention and bloating (*ṣênu, ṣemēru, edēpu* (D-stem); on the other, BAM 575 ii 54 features a curious therapy (licking a bronze or iron dagger), which is not recommended in BAM 240 for a female patient (perhaps because weapons are associated with men).

Line 29': The skin condition designated as *birdu* has been interpreted as striae (stretch marks), cf. Labat 1951, TDP 1, 76 n. 138. However, *birdu* is not a gender-specific condition restricted to postpartum women but mostly attested outside the women's healthcare texts. For *birdu* as a type of skin lesion, see Adamson 1969, *JRAS* 101, 12 with n. 7; Scurlock and Andersen 2005, 95, 221–222).

For *ḫaluppu*-tree (perhaps willow?) in the prescriptions for women, see Steinert 2021a, *Byzantinische Forschungen* 33, 58 and BAM 380 rev. 29 // BAM 381 iii 22 (further discussed in text A.2.7 note on lines 26'–34').

377 Instead of SAḪAR "dust", it is not excluded that the scribe meant to write SAḪAR.URUDU <^{urudu}>NÍG.KALAG.GA "patina from a copper bell" (cf. Scurlock 2014b, 111).

378 The verb *eṣēnu* "to smell, to sniff" in the Š-stem further occurs in a prescription in BM 78963: 53 (Stadhouders and Johnson 2018, *FS Geller*, 578–579, 600–601 §13, likewise misspelled: *tu-še-en-ṣe-šu-ma* "you have him sniff it (i.e. black pulverized cumin against cough)".

Line 30': For a different reading of this prescription and its purpose (which is not followed here), see Kinnier Wilson 2011, *JMC* 17, 12–13. The same postpartum problem appears to be described and treated in the Babylonian compendium BM 38624 + i 34'–35' (see *infra* text A.2.1).

The exact meaning of *paṭāru* "to be loose, supple" in line 30' describing the woman's navel (*abunnatu*) is difficult to specify exactly, but suppleness may be most likely. The suggested translations in CAD P, 289b sub 2' for *paṭāru* in connection with body parts alternate between "split" (open) and "loose" (CAD A/1, 89 s.v. *abunnatu* sub 1 translates with "broken"). Compare, for example, *Diagnostic Handbook* Tablet 40 (lines 44 and 45): *šumma lā'û šibīt qaqqadišu paṭrat* "if the suture of an infant's skull is open (and subsequently his skull widens)" (Scurlock 2014a, 260, 265). *Diagnostic Handbook* Tablet 36 (line 27) describes the tip of the pregnant woman's breast as "open" (*paṭir*) and an "unravelled (*pašir*) navel" (line 85, probably referring to a protruding navel). Both these features are regarded as positive (i.e. normal) phenomena (see *infra* text I.1.1), in contrast to the problem treated in BAM 240: 30', which also includes heavy sweating (probably due to puerperal fever; see Scurlock and Andersen 2005, 282 12.123).

For the reading ^{na4}IŠKILA(ŠÀxA), corresponding to Akkadian *išqillatu*, see Borger, MZL, 385 no. 608. However, the word refers to a shell rather than to a "pebble" (thus CAD I/J, s.v. *išqillatu*) or "Kies" (gravel; thus Borger 2004, MZL, 385). The shell carries strong associations with pregnant women and female genitals, see Steinert 2017a, 334–335; UET 6/3, 897 rev. 3'–4' and 11N-T3: 38–40 (texts G.1–G.2), commenting on a passage of a lost birth incantation that was probably included in the birth compendium BAM 248 // (text D.1.1). The Sumerogram literally means "stone of pregnancy", see Stol 2000a, 51–52.

Lines 31'–32': Some of the ingredients used in this prescription resemble the fragmentary treatment in BM 38624+ i 34'–37' (text A.2.1), applied for the same problem, but because the latter text is so damaged, it remains unclear whether both passages are proper duplicates.

Line 33': Contrary to Böck (2013, 47), lines 33'–35' treat diarrhoea in women after delivery, not during pregnancy (prescriptions from line 29' onward resume the introductory DIŠ MUNUS Ù.TU-*ma* "if a woman gives birth and then . . ." with MIN-*ma* "ditto"). The verbal form behind SI.SÁ may be the stative *išarū* (see CAD I/J, 226 sub *išaru* 4), although a G-stem or Š-stem form of *ešēru* is also possible (see also Schmidtchen 2021a, 562 note on *Diagnostic Handbook* Tablet 13, lines 159'–160').

At the end of line 33', the verb *kaṣāru* "to be knotted, bound, constricted" (N-stem) is suggested in contrast to the treated problem of diarrhoea, which is described as 'straightness' (*ešēru*) of the intestines. Thus, it seems that diarrhoea is conceptualised here in terms of the bowels assuming a straight instead of the natural coiled position in the body. For a similar context, see Geller 2005a, *BAM* 7, No. 37 i 17: *qerbū*(ŠÀ.MEŠ)-*šú ik-ka-ṣa-ru* "his intestines will become bound up (again)". This prognosis similarly concludes the treatment instruction for some kind of discharge or perhaps diarrhoea. See further Steinert 2021a, *Byzantinische Forschungen* 33, 50–51.

Lines 34'–35': The reading PEŠ$_{10}$.$^{⌈d?⌉}$[ÍD] at the end of line 34' follows Köcher's copy. However, the traces of the damaged sign after PEŠ$_{10}$ do not look like DINGIR, but like a double vertical wedge. Perhaps, the traces should be read PEŠ$_{10}$.Í[D$^{!}$].

Lines 36'–38': At the end of line 37', perhaps restore *tu-*[*sà-a-ak*] "you strain (the liquid)" (*sâku* D-stem).

Lines 39'–42': This passage shows that Mesopotamian healers recognized the retention of the lochia as cause of the patient's symptoms. A parallel recipe with many identical ingredients can be found in BM 38624+ obv. i 24'–29' (text A.2.1). The latter prescription is used against "blocked fluids" (MUNUS BI A.MEŠ *tur-rat*).[379]

As indicated by the form BÍL.MEŠ = *qalûti* "roasted" specifying GAZI^{sar} in line 41' and 43', the word *kasû* is a plurale tantum like *saḫlû* "cress"; other drugs are sometimes constructed as plural words in medical recipes to indicate a plurality of pieces (e.g. seeds, leaves) used, e.g. *ḫašû, atā'išu, nīnû*, see Abusch and Schwemer 2011, 36 note to text 1.1 lines 22'–24'.

Line 42': For *zê summati* "dove excrement" as an alternative name for "seed of *ašāgu*-thorn" (a type of acacia), see Uruanna I 189, cited in CAD S, 380; CAD Z, 151a; cf. also BRM 4, 32: 11 describing the appearance of the *ēdu*-plant (^{ú}DILI) as *kīma ḫallā summati* "like the thigh(s) of a dove".

379 For the condition of "blocked fluids", see the *Introduction* of this volume, with BM 38624+ (text A.2.1), *Iraq* 31, 29: 1ff. (text II.1.4), K. 8678+ rev. 3' (text A.1.4) edited in this volume. See also line 67' below.

In line 42', perhaps restore *ina* DID[A ḪI.ḪI NAG-*ši-ma ina-eš*(?)] "[mix (it)] with *billatu*-beer, [*you give it to her to drink and she will get well*(?)]". It is also possible that dry *billatu*-substance was used and that the resulting pharmakon was a solid substance eaten (*akālu*) by the patient.

Lines 43'–46': In line 43', ᵘNU.LAḪ.ḪA is apparently a variant writing or error for ᵘNU.LUḪ.ḪA. The orthography is also used in line 47' below.

In line 44', Scurlock (2014a, 112) translates *ina ṣubāti šunūti talappap*: "(you) wind them into burls with a cloth". The expression *lippa talappap* "you wrap into a wad/burl (of wool)" is encountered in line 49'; both prescriptions refer to tampons introduced into the vagina. The expression *lippī talappap* is, however, more often encountered in amulet prescriptions (see Chapter F for discussion).

There have been different interpretations of the verbal form *i-te-mu* in line 45'. CAD E, 414b sub 1d interprets *i-te-mu* as a form of *ewû* with the meaning "to change; to turn into", translating: "when it (the mixture) had 'turned' (*kīma šī ītemu*)". Similarly, Scurlock 2014b, 112 "to change (colour)"; Bácskay 2018a, No. 42: 7. In this case, the pronoun *šī* would need to refer to a feminine noun (presumably to TÚG "cloth", which then would need to be read as Akkadian *lubuštu*). In contrast to this, CAD N/1, 270a (s.v. *napāḫu* sub 12, Ntn-stem) normalises the verb as *ītemmu*, analysing it as a form of *emēmu* "to become hot" and regards *šī* as referring to the patient: "as soon as she (the patient) has become hot, and her body has swelled (she? changes the compress)". The use of the pronoun *šī* in reference to the female patient is attested in other texts. AHw 213b also lists this passage for *emēmu* "to become hot" (G perfect form). In this case, the form is irregular (for correct *ītemimu*). We follow the latter interpretation because of the context. The text may perhaps acknowledge here that the treatment (tampon) described in lines 43'–45' could sometimes lead to an aggravation of the initial symptoms (fever, inflammation). For *napāḫu* "to be bloated" as a term for abdominal distention (perhaps caused by gas in the abdominal cavity), see Johnson and Simkó 2024, 12, 62 with n. 138 *passim*.

Line 46': One wonders whether the last part of the treatment may have been intended to alleviate the adverse effects of the suppository described in line 45'. For the instruction *ina uppi abāri ana pagriša inappaḫ* "one shall blow (the medicine) into her body (i.e. via the vagina) with a lead tube in line 46', compare BAM 241 ii 10'; var. BM 42313+ rev. 4 (text A.2.2): "one (var. you?) pour(s) (the medicine) into her womb (var. urethra) with a (bronze) tube" (*ina up-pí* (var. MUD ZABAR) *ina šà-su-ri-šá* (*múš-tin-ni-šú*) *i-ta-b*[*a-ak*]/DUB-[*ak*]). In other contexts, a tube is used to blow or pour medicine into the patient's urethra, see also Geller 2005a, *BAM* 7, No. 1 i 28', ii 10', ii 17', iv 10; No. 2 i 19, 22, 23 *passim* (usually a bronze tube is used here); Geller 2000b, *From Athens to Jerusalem*, 23 n. 72; CAD N/1, 204b; Goltz 1974, 82–83. The abrupt change from a 2nd to a 3rd person verbal form in line 46' is presumably an error for *tanappaḫ* "you blow".

Lines 47' and 54': Note that the *suādu*-plant (ᵍⁱˢMAN.DU), which is used in compound prescriptions in lines 47' and 54', was known to be effective against febrile conditions. See, e.g., Uruanna II 98–99, 101 (cf. CAD S, 338b; CAD U/W, 131b), which characterizes the *suādu*-plant as Ú KÚM ŠÀ.SUR "a plant for the fever/heat of the *womb*(?)" (cf. CAD Š/2, 145–146, with ŠÀ.SUR perhaps being an error or variant for ŠÀ.TÙR, *šassūru*) and KÚM ŠÀ-*bi* ZI-*ḫi* "(plant) to remove the fever/heat of the inside/belly".

Line 48': The drug name ᵘMAŠ.TAB.BA or Ú.MAŠ.TAB.BA in line 48' literally means "twin (disease)-plant". In Uruanna II 168 (cited in CAD M/1, 395b s.v. *māštu* lex. sect.), the drug name Ú *maš-tú/-te* is equated with "seed of the *ašû*-disease plant" (NUMUN *šammi ašî*), which could suggest that Ú.MAŠ.TAB.BA could be read *māštu* or *šammi māšti*. The drug *šammi ašî* (written syllabically) is also part of a compound remedy in lines 21', 52', 55 and 56' of ms. A. For discussion, see BM 42587+ (text B.2.4) line 11'.

Line 54': The term *azukirānu* is a variant spelling of the *azupīrānu*-plant, probably indicating a plant similar to the *azupīru*-plant (a spice and medicinal plant perhaps to be identified with saffron), cf. CAD A/2, 530–531.

Lines 56'–57': For *sikkatu* as a beer ingredient (perhaps yeast), see CAD S, 254b s.v. *sikkatu* C; AHw 1042a s.v. *sikkatu* III; Landsberger 1962, MSL 8/2, 108; Stol 1971, *BiOr* 28, 168.

Line 58': See CAD R, 73b s.v. *raḫāṣu* sub 1a. For a longer variant of this prescription using most of the ingredients listed in line 58' (with additional ingredients), see the Middle Assyrian text *Iraq* 31, 31 lines 19–26 (*infra* text II.1.4).

Lines 59'–60': For *li'bu* as a disease associated with fever, see Stol 2007a, 11–15; Scurlock and Andersen 2005, 29–32; Bácskay 2018a, 5–6 and *passim*. The term *li'bu* as a disease is sometimes associated with other symptoms (skin disease or odious discharges). It is not clear which symptoms of *li'bu* are indicated in the enumeration in line 59' together with fever and dark spots on the patient's body. The symptoms overall may point to puerperal fever and infection (cf. Scurlock 1991, 150 with n. 143; Scurlock and Andersen 2005, 10.61, 12.125 for discussion and below lines 65' and 67' for related symptoms).

CAD Š/2, 64 s.v. *šarku* sub a-4' reads the verb in line 59' as GÁL.MEŠ. Scurlock (2014a, 612) reads KAB.ME(Š) and translates "(dark spots) accumulate(?) (on her flesh and veins)", possibly thinking of the Akkadian verb *kamāru* "to heap up", "to accumulate" (Gt-stem). The sign in question indeed looks like KAB rather than GÁL. However, to my knowledge, this verb is not attested in this context in medical texts. Bácskay (2018a, 110) emends to ⸢TUKU⸣!-*ši*. The logogram GÁL!.MEŠ may be a mistake for the more common TUKU.MEŠ or TUKU-*ši*, "to develop symptoms of a disease" (Gtn-stem of *rašû*, cf. CAD R, 201 sub 5). However, it is also possible to read GÁL.MEŠ as a plural *ibaššû* "(fever, *li'bu* and *terku*-spots) are present (in her flesh and muscles)". Compare, for example, BAM 584 ii 27', 31': *bubu'tu peṣītu/sāmtu ina zumur amēli ibašši*(GÁL-*ši*) "(if) a white pustule appears on a man's body"; for other examples, see CAD U/W, 131–132 s.v. *ummu* sub 1.

Lines 61'–63': For the reading RA-*si* = *taraḫḫassi* "you wash/bathe her" in line 61', see CAD R, 182a s.v. *rasīnu*.

It is not certain whether the signs ZÌ/ŠE$_{10}$ MUNU$_6$ in line 62' should be read as Akkadian *qēm/zê buqli* "malt flour" / "refuse of malt", or as ZÌ.MUNU$_6$ = *isimmānu*. The latter two terms denote a leftover product of malt in beer production, see Borger, MZL no. 808 and 810; CAD I/J, s.v. *isimmānu* disc. and CAD Z, s.v. *zû* sub 2c (*zê buqli*). See also Borger, *BiOr* 55, 821–822. For sesame draff/bran (*kupsu*), see Stol 1985a, *BSA* 2, 122.

The meaning of the word *ruqqu* in line 63' is likewise unclear (cf. CAD R, 419b sub 4). AHw 995a differentiates two homonymous words: *ruqqu* I designates a vessel ("kettle, cauldron" or "Schale", written ^{urudu}ŠEN), and *ruqqu* II is rendered as "dünne, schmale Stelle" (from *raqāqu* "to be thin", logographically written as SAL.LA), which is used to describe a feature of body parts (cf. also CAD R, 418–419 sub 3, regarding *ruqqu* as one lexeme with different meanings). Perhaps the word is used here to refer to a thin piece of textile used as a bandage.

In line 63', see, for similar instructions, the Middle Assyrian text *Iraq* 31, 30: 30 (*ina lubāri*(TÚG) *te-ṭe$_4$-ri*), where a mixture is likewise used as a bandage for a woman suffering from a postpartum condition. Because of the instruction *tukaṣṣa* "you let (it) cool down" following *teṭerri* in line 63', one would expect the phrase "you heat (it) in an oven, you take it out" earlier in the instruction, as in *Iraq* 31, 30: 29, where the mixture is enclosed in an oven before application. The recipe in lines 61'–63' thus seems to have been transmitted in an abbreviated form. For the possible meanings of *ina lubāri ṭerû* "to press through a cloth" or "to smear on a cloth", see also CAD Ṭ, 103 s.v. *ṭerû* A sub 1b; Farber 1976, *BiOr* 33, 331–332; Goltz 1974, 54–55; see also the discussion of BAM 408 line 16'' (text A.2.9).

Line 64': For the instruction, cf. CAD P, 246b s.v. *pašāšu* sub 1a–2'a-2''. The emendation $^{ú!}$GA.RAŠ^{sar} follows Bácskay (2018a, 110). Since the signs Ú and GA look very similar, a scribal error is likely. However, it is not excluded that the sign GA should be read as another ingredient (*šizbu* "milk"; see Scurlock (2014a, 616), translating "you cool *karašu*-leek with milk"). The instructions of line 64' seem to be abbreviated, as one would expect an instruction to previous processing and heating/boiling of the leek, before letting it cool down. The instruction to rub the patient is likewise elusive, since there is no mention of oil. Would the patient first be rubbed with oil, before a suppository of leek was applied? Or does the recipe recommend two alternative or supplementary forms of applying the leek, i.e. externally and internally?

Lines 65'–66': Scurlock (2014a, 611) and Bácskay (2018a, 110) read ⸢ŠÀ-*bi-šá*⸣ "her insides" instead of ⸢*qer-bi-sà*⸣ SÌG.SÌG-*si* "her womb (*qerbītu*) gives her a sharp pain". However, the sign traces and the following lines 65'–70', all of which feature *qer-bi-sa* instead of ŠÀ or ŠÀ.TÙR, speak for the latter reading. For *maḫāṣu* "to beat" in the D-stem (often written SÌG.SÌG) taking on the meaning "to hurt", when the verb is used with body parts as subject, see CAD M/1, 82–83 sub 7a.

In line 65', ZÀ.ḪI.LA presents another variant spelling of a drug name; usually the logogram for *saḫlû* is ZÀ.ḪI.LI$^{(sar)}$.

Lines 67'–68': For different restorations of line 67', compare Steinert 2013, *JMC* 22, n. 19; Scurlock 2014a, 612, 616 n. 79; Bácskay 2018a, 110. The expression *napištašu/napšātušu iktenerru/iktanerrâ* (ZI.(MEŠ)-*šú* LÚGUD.MEŠ) is attested in medical texts in the meaning "to (constantly) be short of breath, to gasp for breath", see CAD K, 230a s.v. *karû* for references.

The condition of "blocked fluids" is attested in a few other women's healthcare texts and appears to refer to the retention of the lochia, the discharges of a postpartum woman, which normally occur in the first weeks after delivery. The premature stopping of the lochia is associated with other symptoms (e.g., pain in the abdomen) pointing to puerperal infection (see the *Introduction* for discussion). See also BM 38624+ obv. i 24'–25', 30'–31', ii 19'ff.; K.8678+ rev. 3', written A.MEŠ GUR-*át* or *tur-rat* (texts A.2.1 and A.1.4). For the meaning of the verb *târu* "to return" in the D-stem (stative) in the sense of "to (be) locked, closed (from the inside)" in connection with doors or gates, see CAD T, 237b sub 11d; CAD S, 143 sub 11. In the Middle Assyrian text *Iraq* 31, 29: 1–3 (text II.1.4), the form GUR.MEŠ-*ru* should probably be read as a stative plural form *turrū* "(her fluids and blood) are blocked". In BAM 240: 67' another variant expression is used instead, which one may perhaps interpret as *sinništu šī mê*(A) *tur-re-ti šaknat*(GAR) "that woman is afflicted with blocked fluids" (or perhaps as "(concerning) that woman, *blocked* fluids are present (*šaknū*)"). The form *tur-re-ti* is problematic but might be the verbal adjective of the D-stem *turru* "turned", with an irregular plural ending *-ēti* instead of *-ūti*. Alternatively, *tur-re-ti* may perhaps be related to the noun *tūrtu* "return", presenting a similar variation as found in *ṣertu/ṣerretu* "breast" (cf. also the nouns *tūrtu* and *turrūtu* "turning", listed in CAD T, 489, 491; AHw 1373). The passage in BAM 240: 67' remains difficult and is probably corrupt, but a connection with the condition of "blocked fluid" in the textual parallels nonetheless appears to be likely.

Line 69': For the idea of the womb "accepting" or "receiving" (*maḫāru*) the male semen, as a precondition for conception, see, e.g., Stol 2000a, 5–6; Steinert 2017a, 305–306. Previous readings in the second half of this line diverge from the one suggested here. Scurlock (2014a, 613, 616) suggests restoring DUMU.NITA [Ù.TU] *gi-mil-li* [DINGIR] "(If a woman's womb receives the semen and) [she gives birth] to a son, (it means) [divine] favor" (similarly Stol 2000a, 5). This reading is based on the parallel entry in line 70', which features a contrasting diagnostic statement for the contrasting case that a woman receives the male semen but does not get pregnant, namely *šibsāt ili lā ṭūb* [*libbi*] "(it means) wrath of the god (and) unhappiness". However, the traces on the tablet (and copied by Köcher in BAM III) better fit the reading proposed here. For the expression *muter gimilli*, which means "one who returns a favour/kindness" (mostly attested in personal names) and "avenger" (in literary texts), usually as an epithet of deities or kings, see CAD M/2, 299 s.v. *mutīr gimilli*; CAD G, 73–75 s.v. *gimillu*. The expression seems to be idiomatic in the present passage.

Interestingly, lines 69'–70' consist only in diagnostic entries, without any treatment instructions, and seem to be insertions that look as if they were quoted perhaps from a passage in the *Diagnostic Handbook*, since they attribute the woman's inability to conceive to divine wrath rather than to other causes (see also Stol 2000a, 5 suggesting that such a view may have had "a widespread, popular origin"). For the different causes of infertility in medical texts and a discussion of this passage, see also Steinert 2017a, 305–306.

Line 70': See also CAD R, 343 s.v. *riḫûtu* sub 1e. There may not be enough space for restoring NU DU$_{10}$-*ub* [ŠÀ TUKU-*ši*] "[she will suffer] from misery" at the end of line 70', as was suggested by Böck 2013, 31 n. 12. Cf. also Stol 2000a, 5; CAD Ṭ, 119b, 120b.

Lines 71'–74': For this passage, cf. Stol 2000a, 28; Böck 2010a, *TUAT* NF 5, 109 ("to prevent the untimely loss of the male semen"); Böck 2013, 30 n. 10; Scurlock 2014a, 616; Steinert 2020, 63–64. The first signs in lines 71'–74' copied by Köcher are unfortunately not preserved anymore on the tablet but have been worn off. The reading of the beginning of line 71' DIŠ MUNUS ⌜*ina* ŠÀ⌝ TUKU-*at* suggested by Köcher's copy was confirmed through the collation of an older museum photograph (Ph. Ass. S 3968). Böck (2013, 30 n. 10) reads DIŠ MUNUS ⌜NUMUN ŠÀ⌝ TUKU-*at* with same meaning. In my view, there is unlikely enough space at the end of line 71' for the restoration [UDU NÍTA *u*] "(the thigh bones) of [a ram and] (an unmated she-goat)" suggested by Böck 2013, 30 n. 10. For GÌR.PAD.DU.GÍD.DA, Akkadian *sāqu* "thigh bone, femur", lit. "long bone" (cf. AHw 1028a "Oberschenkel"), see Stol 2016–2018b, *RlA* 15, 411b § 2.1; Pongratz-Leisten 1994, *WO* 25, 68: 3' UZU MIN (= GÌR.PAD.DU) GÍD.DA = *sa-a-qu* (Ḫh. XV 193); Civil 2010, *CUSAS* 12, 157 col. 10: 21': gìr-gíd-da-ĝu$_{10}$: *sa-qí* (Ugu-mu). The term *sāqu* also refers to the thigh as a cut of meat. For the use of the bone in medical prescriptions, see also BAM 152 i 6' // BAM 155 iii 10 (thigh bone of a ram (GÌR.PAD.DU UDU.NÍTA) is roasted and crushed and applied externally, against lesions on the head); BAM 480 i 43 (GÌR.PAD.DU UDU.NÍTA is crushed with tallow and daubed on against feverish head and throbbing of the temples; Worthington 2005, *JMC* 5, 8).

In line 74', Scurlock (2014a, 616), without restoring *tu-u*[*l-lad . . .*], translates "⌜she should be able to give birth⌝". However, the use of the verbal prefix *tu-* (or *ta-*) for a 3rd person sg. feminine subject is not attested anywhere else in the present text.

The present passage in BAM 240, in which the patient has "received" or "acquired" (*rašû*) something in her belly, but cannot "retain" it (*kalû*), i.e. discharges it. Although the word *riḫûtu* is missing in line 71', the preceding lines speaking of the woman's ability or inability to "receive" (*maḫāru*) the semen suggest that a similar situation is meant here. Stol (2000a, 28) compared the passage with the concept of a "flow" (*rhúsis, ékrhusis*) in Greek texts, designating a discharge in the first seven days of pregnancy, which is not regarded as a miscarriage yet (only after the seventh day). The passage in BAM 240 may also be compared to similar notions encountered in the Hippocratic treatise *Diseases of Women* I (Chapters 10–13; see Potter 2018, 42–55), where a woman's inability to conceive is connected to the observation that the patient discharges the semen within the first seven days after intercourse: "Women who cohabit but are still unable to become pregnant you must question . . . whether the seed is immediately discharged (sc. after intercourse), or on the next day, or on the third, sixth or seventh day. Now if she says the seed is discharged immediately after intercourse, the mouth (sc. of the uterus) is not straight, but folded over and it fails to take up the seed. If she says this happens on the second or third day, then her uterus is full of moisture and the seed gets washed away. If it is on the sixth or seventh day, the seed is decomposing and being discharged in that state" (Potter 2018, 43). A detailed description of different treatment regimes to straighten the mouth of the uterus or to dry the woman's overly moist uterus or body follows. The treatment performed in BAM 240, a suppository prepared with animal bones, may have been intended as a barrier that would prevent the loss of the semen; the choice of bones as *materia medica* suggests an association with both semen and the foetus that would eventually be formed from it (cf. Steinert 2020, 63–64).

D.3 Rituals Dealing with Inauspicious Birth

D.3.1 Two Rituals to Delay the Delivery of a Child in the Month Nisannu

The present text of two rituals for a pregnant woman is known from six witnesses. The main witness (ms. A) written in Neo-Assyrian script was found at Assur in the library of the "House of the incantation priest" and bears a colophon of Kiṣir-Nabû, son of Šamaš-ibni and nephew Kiṣir-Aššur, all of whom belonged to an Assur-based family of ritual specialists who also served as exorcists (*mašmaššu*) of the Aššur temple. The colophon states that the text was copied "for performance".[380] It has been known since Erich Ebeling published the copy in 1920 and edited the tablet in 1931 as KAR 223. Four other witnesses are written in Neo-Babylonian script, and three of them (mss. b, c, e) stem from Ashurbanipal's library. Ms. b is an almost complete tablet running parallel to ms. A, but contains several textual variations,[381] while mss. c and e are fragments duplicating part of the text. Ms. d (BM 68458 + K. 11550) was first edited by Stadhouders and Steinert (2018) together with the other manuscripts as two separate tablet fragments (designated there as mss. D and F), but A. Hätinen (2019) recognized that the two fragments in fact join and published a copy of the pieces. The provenience of ms. d remains uncertain: while one of the fragments (BM 68458 = 82-9-18, 8456) was registered in the Sippar collection of the British Museum (Leichty 1987, CBT VII, 234), the other (K. 11550) was registered as a fragment from Nineveh (Bezold 1889–1899, Vol. III, 1176). Since the majority of tablets in the 82-9-18 collection stems from excavations of Hormuzd Rassam in Sippar (Leichty 1986, CBT VI, xxxiii), this provenience seems most likely, and the assignment of K. 11550 to texts from Kuyunjik was probably due to an error during the processing of the incoming tablets in the museum (Leichty 1986, in CBT VI, xxvi–xxvii; Lambert 1992, ix–x; see also Hätinen 2019 for discussion). The sixth manuscript BM 47459 (ms. f) is a tablet written by Iprā'ya, a member of the Ēṭiru family and known from colophons of scholarly texts (especially commentaries and texts of medical, astrological and divinatory content). According to the information gleaned from other colophons of tablets owned by Iprā'ya, he may have lived in the fifth or fourth century BCE during the Achaemenid period. BM 47459 was recently recognised by E. Jiménez and the *Electronic Babylonian Library* Project; another text copied by Iprā'ya related to the women's healthcare text is BM 47491 (see text A.2.6).

The two rituals preserved on mss. A–f were performed to avert the birth of a child in the month of Nisannu and sought to bring about a postponement of the delivery through divine intervention ("to let the month of her delivery pass by"). The first of the two procedures addresses the moon god Sîn, the other the sun god Šamaš. Both gods are well-known as deities taking care of matters linked to fertility, pregnancy and birth (e.g. Stol 2000a, 61–72; Polonsky 2006; Hätinen 2021, 229–249). In the present context, the role of moon god and sun god as regulators of the calendar and guardians of the correct order of things also comes to the fore. The view that the birth of a child in the month Nisannu is a bad omen is known from the hemerological/menological tradition. Thus, a passage in the series *Iqqur īpuš* predicts that a child born in this month

380 For the find spot, see Pedersén 1986, 61 (98).

381 The tablet was first mentioned by Reiner and Civil 1967, *JNES* 26, 191 n. 15 and identified as a duplicate of KAR 223 (ms. A) by M. Stol (2000a, 93).

will cause disaster for his family (Labat 1965, 132ff. §64 line 1; Stol 2000a, 93ff.; Stadhouders and Steinert 2018, 58, 63–64). In the case that the birth of the child could not be postponed successfully to the next month Ayyaru, a Namburbi ("release") ritual could nonetheless be performed to save the parents from the evil portended by the event (Reiner and Civil 1967, 191; Maul 1994, 400–408).[382] In fact, the catchline of ms. b (line 33) is identical with the opening line of the Namburbi ritual in question (Maul 1994, 401–402 line 1). The complete prediction, also found in *Iqqur īpuš*, reads as follows: "If a child is born in the month Nisannu, from the first to the thirtieth day, by his feet (i.e. through the child's actions) his father's house will be disrupted; either the hand of his god or the hand of the king will reach his father and his mother. As to that baby: it will fare well in future days. Release-ritual so that the evil of that child does not reach his father and his mother, in order to make that disaster go by, that this evil goes away and does not come near to his father and his mother . . ." (Stol 2000a, 95; Maul 1994, 401–402: 1–7).

The first of the two rituals (Ritual 1) to postpone delivery begins with instructions for an amulet that was to be worn by the pregnant woman during the critical month Nisannu. In the manuscript from Assur (ms. A), the amulet was more elaborate and consisted of multiple strings or cords on which various materials were strung, while in the Babylonian manuscripts, the prescription is reduced to the first string described in ms. A. This consisted of a cord of multicoloured wool onto which sixty spindle whorls of two types of wood (thirty each of tamarisk and sissoo-wood) were threaded and sixty knots tied into the cord. Ms. A specifies a second cord of red wool on which thirty kernels (or seeds) of sissoo-wood should be strung, again tying a corresponding number of thirty knots. A third cord of red wool was threaded with fifteen pieces of cornel wood (*e'ru*) and the same number of knots. To this ensemble stone beads were added which are specified as "stones worn around the hips by a woman who has difficulty bringing her pregnancies to term" (for these stones see sections C.3 and F), i.e. materials that were believed to save pregnant women from miscarriage or premature delivery. The amulet was then worn by the woman who had to cut off a varying number of spindle whorls every day and throw them away on the staircase of her house. In all manuscripts except ms. A, the woman removed two spindle whorls each day, and all sixty spindle whorls would have been cut off on the last day of month Nisannu, signalling that the favourable time for her delivery had now arrived. In ms. A, however, the ritual is scheduled to last sixty days (through Nisannu and the following month Ayyaru), and the woman had to discard only one spindle whorl per day.

In addition to the preparation of the amulet, a ritual was performed (presumably on the first day of Nisannu), during which an offering was set up for Sîn on the roof of the woman's house. The patient uttered a prayer to the moon god asking him to let her carry her unborn child through the critical period and to let her give birth safely after that period was over. The ritual ends with instructions for supportive treatments (an ointment and a fumigation) to be performed for the patient during the critical period.

Ritual 2 presumably took place in the morning of the first day of Nisannu with an offering to Šamaš, during which the patient recited a prayer to the sun god whilst standing or stepping on an architectural feature or elevated object usually translated as "ramp" (*šukbusu*), perhaps referring to a staircase situated at the exterior of the house, or to a movable object such as a foot step, but apparently having the same significance marking a liminal space, parallel to the staircase (*bīt simmilti*) in Ritual 1. In her prayer, the woman calls herself a "fully laden boat" (*eleppu malītu*), asking the sun god to let her pass the critical month safely and thereby to cancel the evil omen threatening her family. The ritual concludes with further precautionary actions: the woman's ears are filled up with red wool, she was (regularly?) rubbed with a salve, and she had to put on a special garment (^{túg}MA.AN.DUL) which also plays a role in Ritual 1 (see below for discussion). Moreover, the text warns that the woman should not exhaust herself physically during her waiting period, in order to avoid an untimely delivery.

382 Compare also TCL 6, 14 obv. 22 (Sachs 1952, *JCS* 6, 66), in a section making predictions on personal fate related to the twelve zodiac signs – probably connected to the date of birth. Here, the zodiac sign Aries (replacing the month Nisannu) similarly portends "death of his (the child's) family" (ÚŠ IM.RI.A-*šú*).

List of Manuscripts

Siglum	Museum Number	Copy	Collation	Format; Ductus	Provenience
A	VAT 8004	KAR 223 Hätinen 2021, pl. 11–12	Coll.	Single-column tablet in landscape format; Neo-Assyrian script; 7th cent. BCE	Assur; N4 library
b	K. 8666	Hätinen 2021, pl. 13–14 Pl. 44–45	Coll.	Single-column tablet in portrait format; Neo-Babylonian script; 7th cent. BCE	Nineveh; Ashurbanipal's library
c	79-7-8, 95	Pl. 46	Coll.	Fragment of a single-column tablet in landscape format; Neo-Babylonian script; 7th cent. BCE	Nineveh; Ashurbanipal's library
d	BM 68458 (82-9-18, 8456) + K. 11550	*NABU* 2019/3, 139 Figs. 1–2	Coll.	Fragments of a single-column tablet in portrait format; Neo- or Late Babylonian script; ca. 6th–4th cent. BCE(?)	provenience uncertain; perhaps Sippar
e	K. 13315	Geers, Folio M117 Pl. 47	Coll.	Fragment of a tablet; Neo-Babylonian script; 7th cent. BCE	Nineveh; Ashurbanipal's library
f	BM 47459 (81-11-3, 164	-	Coll.	Single-column tablet in landscape format; Late Babylonian script; 5th or 4th cent. BCE[383]	Babylon or Borsippa

Overview

i Ritual 1 to postpone the birth of child scheduled for month Nisannu: 1–15
- Introductory statement (line 1)
- Prescriptions for an amulet tied around the pregnant woman's hips; ritual instructions for handling the amulet (lines 2–7)
- Offering to Sîn and further ritual actions (lines 8–10)
- Prayer *Sîn nannār šamê u erṣeti* "Sîn, light of heaven and earth" spoken by the woman (lines 11–13)
- Prescription for a salve and fumigation (lines 14–15)

A obv. 1–15 // b obv. 1–18 // c obv. 1'–13' // d obv. 1'–11' // e obv. 1'–5' // f obv. 1–16

ii Ritual 2 to postpone the birth of child scheduled for month Nisannu: 16–32
- Offering to Šamaš (lines 16–17)
- Incantation *Šamaš bēlu šurbû* "Šamaš, exalted lord" recited by the pregnant woman (lines 18–27)
- Further ritual actions (lines 28–32)

A obv. 16–rev. 12 // b obv. 19–rev. 12' // c rev. 1–12 // d rev. 1'–9' // e rev. 1'–5' // f rev. 1–13

iii Rubric(?) 33

f rev. 14

iv Alternative procedure(?) 34–36

f rev. 15–17

iv Catchline / colophons 37–39

A rev. 13–15; b rev. 13'–15'; f u. e. 1–2

Previous Edition and Discussion

Ebeling 1931, 3–8 (edition of ms. A)
Stol 2000a, 93–95 (translation of lines 2–15; discussion)
Hätinen 2017, *KASKAL* 14, 169–186 (discussion)
Stadhouders and Steinert 2018, *JMC* 32, 56–76 (edition)
Hätinen 2019, *NABU* 2019, 138–139 No. 76 (transliteration of ms. d)
Hätinen 2021, 508–519 (edition)

---

383 Measurements ca. 10.5 × 7.3 × 2.9 cm.

CDLI P369187 (ms. A, copy); P238752 (ms. b, photo); P236879 (ms. c, photo); P239012 (ms d K. 11550, photo); P239201 (ms. e, photo)
Geers, Folio Ab 54 (ms. c, copy); Geers, Folio N95 (ms. d K. 11550, copy) Geers, Folio M117 (ms. e, copy)
Electronic Babylonian Library Project (eBL) (transliteration of ms. f, https://www.ebl.lmu.de/library/BM.47459), (transliteration of ms. d, https://www.ebl.lmu.de/library/K.11550)

Transliteration

1	A obv. 1	{*e*$^{?}$-*nu*$^{!}$-*ma*$^{!}$ MUN}US ⸢ITI⸣ *šá* Ù.TU-*šá* KU$_4$-*ma* ⸢ITI$^{?}$⸣ [B]I$^{?}$ ^{iti}BÁRA <*ana*> *šu*-[x-x]
	b obv. 1	⸢*e*⸣-*nu-ma* MUNUS ITI *šá* Ù.TU-*šá* *i-ru-ba-am-ma* ^{iti}BÁRA <*ana*> *šu*-⸢*tu*⸣-*qí*
	c obv. 0'	[..]
	f obv. 1	⸢*ana*⸣ ⸢^{munus}⸣P[EŠ$_4$] ^{iti}BÁRA ITI-*šá* *šu-t*[*u-q*]*í-ma la a-la-di*
b, c, f		____
2	A obv. 2	{DÙ.DÙ.B}I 1 *šu-ši* SAG.DU ^{giš}BAL 30 *ša* ^{giš}ŠINIG 30 *šá* ^{giš}MES.MÁ.GAN.[NA x x]
	b obv. 2–3	DÙ.DÙ.BI 60+*šu* SAG.DU ^{giš}BAL 30 SAG.DU ^{giš}BAL ŠINIG / 30 SAG.DU ^{giš}⸢BAL⸣ ⸢^{giš}MES⸣.MÁ.GAN.NA DÙ-*uš*
	c obv. 1'	[.. ^{giš}M]ES.MÁ.⸢GAN.(-) NA⸣ ⸢DÙ⸣-[*uš*]
	f obv. 1$^{cont.}$–2	⸢DÙ$^{?}$⸣.[DÙ.BI$^{?}$] / ⸢60(DIŠ)⸣+*šu* SAG.⸢DU⸣ ^{giš}BAL 30 *šá* ^{giš}ŠINIG 30 *šá* ^{giš}MES.⸢MÁ⸣.GAN.NA DÙ-*u*[*š*]
3	A obv. 3	{*ina* $^{síg!(éš)}$*ba*}-*ru-un-di* È-*ak* 1 *šu-ši* KA.KÉŠ KÉŠ 30 ŠE ^{giš}MES.MÁ.GAN.NA *ina* SÍG SA$_5$.A [È-*ak*]
	b obv. 3$^{cont.}$–4	*ina* ^{síg}*ba-ru-un-du* È-*ak* / ⸢60+*šu*⸣ ⸢KA.KÉŠ⸣ KÉŠ --
	c obv. 2'	[...] ----------------------------------
	f obv. 3	*i-na* ⸢^{síg}*ba*⸣-*ru-un-du* È-⸢*ak*⸣ 60(UŠ)+⸢*šu*⸣ KA.KÉŠ KÉŠ-*ár ina* GÚ-*šú* GAR-*an*
4	A obv. 4	{30 KA.K}ÉŠ KÉŠ 15$^{!}$ GIG ^{giš}MA.NU *ina* SÍG SA$_5$.A È-*a*[*k*]
	b	*Omits*
	c	*Omits*
	f	*Omits*
5	A obv. 5	[15 KA.KÉŠ K]ÉŠ NA$_4$.MEŠ MURUB$_4$.MEŠ *šá* MUNUS NU SI.SÁ *it-ti-šú-nu ta-ṣa-m*[*id*]
	b	*Omits*
	c	*Omits*
	f	*Omits*
6	A obv. 6	[x x-*š*]*á* KÉŠ-*si ul-tú*$^{!}$(te) U$_4$.1.KÁM *šá* ^{iti}BÁRA EN U$_4$.30.KÁM *šá* ^{iti}GU$_4$ *u$_4$-mu* 1-*en* SAG.DU ^{giš}⸢BAL⸣
	b obv. 4$^{cont.}$–5	⸢*ina*⸣ ⸢MURUB$_4$.MEŠ-*šá*$^{?}$⸣ ⸢KÉŠ$^{?}$⸣ [T]A U$_4$.1.KAM *šá* ^{iti}⸢BÁRA⸣ EN U$_4$.⸢30.KAM⸣ / [*u$_4$-mu*] ⸢1-*en*⸣ SAG.DU ^{giš}BAL
	c obv. 2'–3'	[............................ TA U$_4$.1].KAM *šá* ^{iti}BÁRA EN U$_4$ 30.K[AM] / [........................]
	f obv. 4	------------------------------------ TA U$_4$.1.KAM *šá* ^{iti}BÁRA EN U$_4$.⸢30.KAM⸣ ⸢*u$_4$-mu*⸣ ⸢2$^{?}$⸣ SAG.DU ^{giš}BAL
6a	A	*Omits*
	b obv. 5$^{cont.}$–6	⸢^{giš}ŠINIG⸣ *ù* 1-*en* SAG.DU ^{giš}⸢BAL⸣ / [^{giš}]⸢MES⸣.MÁ.GAN.NA
	c	*Omits*
	f obv. 4–5	1+*et šá* ^{giš}⸢ŠINIG⸣ / 1+*et šá* ^{giš}MES.MÁ.GAN.NA
7	A obv. 7	[*ina* É *sim-mi*]*l-tu$_4$ i-bat-taq-ma i-na-suk*
	b obv. 6$^{cont.}$–7	*ina* ⸢É⸣ ⸢*sim-mil-ti*⸣ *i-bat-taq-ma* / [*i*]-⸢*na*⸣-[*as*]-*suk*
	c obv. 3'$^{cont.}$–4'	[........................ *i-ba*]*t-taq-m*[*a*] / [..............]
	e obv. 0–1'	[...] / ⸢*i*$^{?}$⸣-[.........]
	f obv. 5$^{cont.}$	*i-na* ⸢É⸣ ⸢*sim*⸣-*mil-ti i-bat-taq-ma* ⸢*i*⸣-*na*-⸢*suk*⸣
8	A obv. 8	[x x x-*m*]*a*$^{?}$ ⸢*ana*⸣ IGI ^{d}30 GI.DU$_8$ *tara-kás* NÍG.NA ^{š}{^{im}L}I GAR-*an* KAŠ BAL-*qí-ma*
	b obv. 7$^{cont.}$–8	*a-na ú-ri il-li-ma ana* IGI ^{d}30 ⸢GI.DU$_8$⸣ KÉŠ-*as* / [...................... KAŠ.S]AG$^{?}$ BAL-*qí-ma*$^{!}$ *tuš*-^{ki}*ken*
	c obv. 4'$^{cont.}$–5'	[..................]x *ana* IGI ^{d}30 GI.DU$_8$ KÉŠ / [...................... BA]L-*qí-ma tuš-ken* ^{erasure}

	e obv. 1'$^{cont.}$–2'	[. . . . .] / NÍG.NA [. . . . .]
	f obv. 6–7	*a-na* ÙR $_{(gloss)}$: É : E$_{11}$-*ma a-na* IGI ^{d}30 GI.DU$_{8}$ KÉŠ-*as* NÍG.NA ^{šim}LI GAR-⸢*an*⸣ / KAŠ.SAG BAL-*qí-ma tuš-*⸢*ken-ma*$^{?}$⸣
9	A obv. 9	[^{túg}MA.AN.DU]L *ul-tú* KI ÍL-*ma i-šad-da-ad-ma* ⸢TA⸣ É *sim-mil-tu*$_{4}$ ------------------------ *ana* ÙR E$_{11}$-*ma*
	b obv. 8–10	⸢$_{túg}$MA.AN.DUL⸣ / ⸢*ul-tu*⸣ [*qaq-qa-r*]*i*$^{?}$ ÍL-*ma* ⸢*i-šad-da*⸣-*ad-ma ul-tu* É ------ / *a-di* ⸢ÙR⸣ [*ú*]-⸢*šel*⸣-*le* ⸢*a*⸣-*na* ⸢ÙR⸣ *il-li-ma*
	c obv. 5'$^{cont.}$–7'	MA.AN.DUL / [. . . . . *i*]-⸢*šad-da*⸣-*ad-ma* TA É *sim-mil-ti* / [x x] ⸢ÙR⸣ *ú-šel-le ana* ÙR E$_{11}$-*ma*
	e obv. 2'$^{cont.}$–4'	[. . . . .] / TA *qaq-*[*qa-ri* . . . .] / *a*$^{?}$-*di* ⸢*ú*⸣-[*ri* . . . . . .]
	f obv. 7$^{cont.}$–8	⸢^{túg}MA⸣.AN.DUL TA *qaq-qa-ru* ÍL-*ma i-šad-da-ad-m*[*a*] / *ul-tu* É *sim-mil-tú a-d*[*i*] ⸢ÙR⸣ ⸢*ú-šel-le*⸣-*ma a-na* ÙR E$_{11}$-*ma*
10a	A obv. 10	[x x x x] *i-ma-kà-a*{*k*$^{sic!}$-*m*}*a*
	b obv. 11	^{túg}MA.AN.DUL ⸢*i-ma-ak-ka*⸣-*a*[*k-ma*]
	c obv. 7'$^{cont.}$–8'	^{túg}MA.AN.DUL / *i-ma-ak-ka-ak-ma*
	e obv. 4'$^{cont.}$–5'	[. . . . .] / ⸢*i*⸣-*m*[*a-* . . . .]
	f obv. 8$^{cont.}$–9	⸢^{túg}MA⸣.AN.DUL / *i-ma-ak-ka-ak-ma*
10b	A	*Omits*
	b obv. 11$^{cont.}$–12	[*ina mu*]*ḫ*-⸢*ḫi*⸣ *i-ke-ri* / *i-teb-bi-ma iz-za-*⸢*az*⸣-*ma*
	c obv. 8'$^{cont.}$–9'	*ina muḫ-ḫi i-ke-er-ri* / *i-teb-bé-e-ma* GUB-*az-ma*
	d obv. 0–1'	[. . . . .] / ⸢GUB-*zu-ma*⸣
	f obv. 9$^{cont.}$	*ina m*[*uḫ*]-⸢*ḫi*⸣ *i-*⸢*ke*⸣-*er-ri i-teb-bi-ma* GUB-*az-ma*
10c	A obv. 10$^{cont.}$	⸢*ina*⸣ ⸢IGI⸣ ^{d}30 ŠU.MIN-*šá* LUḪ-*s*{*i*} *ana* ^{d}30 *kam* DU$_{11}$.GA
	b obv. 12$^{cont.}$–13	*ana* I[GI ^{d}30] ŠU.MIN-*šú* LUḪ-*si* / ⸢*ana*⸣ ^{d}30 *ki-a-am i-qab-bi*
	c obv. 9'$^{cont.}$–10'	*ana* IGI ^{d}30 ŠU.MIN-*šá* LUḪ-*si* / *ana* IGI ^{d}30 UR$_{5}$.GIM DU$_{11}$.GA
	d obv. 1'$^{cont.}$–2'	[. . . . .] / *a-na* ^{d}30 UR$_{5}$.G[IM . . . .]
	f obv. 10	*ana* IGI ^{d}30 ŠU+⸢MIN⸣-*šá* LUḪ-*si* ⸢*a-na*⸣ IGI ^{d}30 *ki-a-am* DU$_{11}$.GA

d, f ____

11a	A	*Omits*
	b obv. 13$^{cont.}$	ÉN ⸢30⸣ [*na-a*]*n-na-ra* AN-[*e*] *u* KI-*tim*
	c	*Omits*
	d obv. 3'	ÉN 30 $^{d+}$EN$^{!}$.ZU.KI-*ra* A[N . . . .]
	f obv. 11	[É]N ^{d}30 ^{d}NANNA-*ra* AN-⸢*e*⸣ *u* KI-*tim*
11b	A obv. 11	[x x U$_{4}$].1.KÁM *šá* ^{iti}BÁRA EN U$_{4}$.30.KÁM *šá* ^{iti}GU$_{4}$
	b obv. 14	*ul-tu* U$_{4}$.1.KAM *šá* ^{iti}BÁRA *ana* U$_{4}$.1.⸢KAM *šá*⸣ ^{iti}GU$_{4}$
	c obv. 10'$^{cont.}$	TA U$_{4}$.1.KAM *šá* ^{iti}BÁRA EN U$_{4}$.1.KAM *šá* ^{iti}GU$_{4}$
	d obv. 4'	U$_{4}$.1.KAM *šá* ^{iti}BÁRA *a-na* U$_{4}$.1.KAM ⸢*šá* ^{iti}GU$_{4}$⸣
	f obv. 11$^{cont.}$–12	*ul-tu* U$_{4}$.1.KAM *šá* ^{iti}BÁRA *a-di* U$_{4}$.1.KAM / [*šá*] ⸢^{iti}⸣GU$_{4}$
12	A obv. 12	[x x x]x *lu-uš-te-šer* IGI-*ka*
	b obv. 14$^{cont.}$	*piq-dan-ni* -----------------
	c obv. 11'	*piq-dan-ni* -----------------
	d obv. 5'–6'	*piq-dan-ni-ma lu-uš-lim lu-ši-r*[*a*] / [IG]I-*ka*
	f obv. 12$^{cont.}$	*piq-dan-ni-ma* ⸢*lu*⸣-*u*[*š*]-*te-ši-ra* IGI-*ka*
13	A obv. 13	[x x *l*]*i-mur nu-u-ru* {*n*}*àr-bi-ka lu-*{*š*}*á-pí dà-lí-lí-ka lud-lul*
	b	*Omits*
	c	*Omits*
	d obv. 6'–7'	*šèr-ri li-mu-ra nu-ru* / [x]-*bi-ka lu-šá-pi dà-lí-lí-ka lid-lul*
	f obv. 12$^{cont.}$–13	*šèr-ra li-mu-ra nu-ru* / [*nàr-b*]*i-ka lu-šá-*⸢*pí*⸣ *d*[*à*]-*lí-lí-ka lud-lul*

d, f ____

14	A obv. 14	[*kam*$^{?}$ DU$_{11}$.G]A-*ma ina* ⸢*qaq*⸣-{*qa-ri ur*}-[*ra*]-*dam-ma* ^{ú}*ak-tam* ^{ú}IGI-*lim ina* Ì+GIŠ ŠÉŠ-*si*
	b obv. 15–16	3-*šú* ⸢*i*⸣-*qab-bi* ⸢*ana*⸣ ⸢*qaq*⸣-*qa-ra ur-ra-dam-ma* ^{ú}⸢*ak-tam*⸣ / x[x x *ina* Ì.G]IŠ *i-nam-di ip-pa-áš-ši*-⸢*iš*$^{?}$⸣
	c obv. 11'$^{cont.}$–12'	3-*šú* DU$_{11}$.GA-*ma a-na qaq-qa-ri ur-ra-dam-ma* / ^{ú}*ak-tam* ------- *ana* Ì.GIŠ ŠUB-*ma* ŠÉŠ
	d obv. 8'–10'	[x x] DU$_{11}$.GA-*ma ana qaq-qa-ru ur-ra-dam-ma* / [^{ú}*a*]*k-tam* ^{ú}IGI-*lim ana* Ì.GIŠ ŠUB-*di-ma* / [*ip-p*]*a-ši-iš*$^{!}$(ka)
	f obv. 14–15	[3-*šú*$^{?}$ *ana*] ⸢^{d}⸣30 D[U$_{11}$.G]A-*ma* ⸢*a-na*⸣ *qaq-qa-ri ur-ra-dam-ma* ^{ú}*ak-tam* ^{ú}IGI-*lim* / [*a-na* (*lìb-bi*)] ⸢Ì⸣.(-)GIŠ ⸢ŠUB-*di-ma*⸣ ⸢ŠÉŠ-*si*⸣
15	A obv. 15	[x x x *s*]*aḫ*-⸢*lé-e*⸣ *m*{*u-šá-ṭa* NUMUN GADA *a-d*}*i* Ù.TU *ina* DÈ SAR-*ši*
	b obv. 17–18	[x x x]x^{sar} ZÀ.ḪI.LI^{sar} *mu-šá-ṭi* ⸢NUMUN⸣ [GADA] / [*a-di ul-l*]*a-du ina* DÈ ⸢SAR⸣-[*ši*]
	c obv. 12'$^{cont.}$–13'	^{šim}GÚR.GÚR GAZI^{sar} / *saḫ-lé-e mu-šá-ṭi* NUMUN GADA *a-di* Ù.TU *ina* DÈ SAR-*š*[*i*]
	d obv. 10'$^{cont.}$–11'	ILLU$^{?!}$(kal) GÚR.GÚR GAZI^{sar} ZÀ.ḪI.LI / [. . . . . *a-d*]*i*$^{?}$ [*u*]*l-la-d*[*u* . . . .]
	f obv. 15$^{cont.}$–16	^{šim}GÚR.GÚR GAZI^{sar} ZÀ.ḪI.LI^{sar} / [*mu-šá-ṭi* NUMUN GA]DA *a-di ul-la-di i-na* DÈ SAR-*šú*

A, c, f____

(*Ms. d obv. breaks*)

16	A obv. 16	[x x x] {^{d}UTU GI.DU$_{8}$ KÉŠ-⸢*as*⸣ NÍG.N}A ^{šim}LI GAR-*an* KAŠ.SAG BAL-*qí*
	b obv. 19–20	[. . . . . . .] ^{d}UTU GI.DU$_{8}$ ⸢KÉŠ-*as*⸣ ⸢NÍG⸣.NA ^{š}[^{im}LI] / [. . . . . BAL-*qí* MUN]US$^{?}$ ⸢BI⸣
	c rev. 1	DIŠ KI.MIN *ina še-rim ana* IGI <^{d}UTU> GI.DU$_{8}$ KÉŠ-⸢*as*⸣ NÍG.NA ^{šim}LI GAR KAŠ BAL-*qí* [x x]
	f rev. 1–2	[x x x x x x x x x x x] x [x x] ⸢^{šim}LI⸣ ⸢GAR⸣-*an* ⸢KAŠ.SAG⸣ BAL-*qí* / [MUNUS BI]
17	A obv. 17	[x x x] {*šuk-bu-si* GUB-*ma* ÉN ^{d}UTU EN} *šur-bu-u* 3-*šú* ŠID-*nu*
	b obv. 20$^{cont.}$–21	⸢*ina*⸣ UGU ⸢*šuk-bu-si*⸣ ⸢GUB⸣-[*ma*] / [. . . . .] x [. . . . .]
	c rev. 2	*ina* UGU *šuk-bu-si* GUB-*az-ma* ÉN ^{d}UTU EN *šur-bu-ú* 3-*šú* [ŠID-*nu*]
	f rev. 2$^{cont.}$	[*i-na* UG]U ⸢*šuk*⸣-[*bu-si* GUB-*az*]-*ma* ÉN ^{d}UTU E[N *šu*]*r*-⸢*bu-ú*⸣ 3-*šú* ŠID-⸢*nu*⸣

A, c, f____

(*Ms. b obv. breaks*)

18	A obv. 18	[x x x] {*šur-bu-u* ZÁLAG AN.TA}.[MEŠ] *u* KI.TA.[MEŠ]
	c rev. 3	[ÉN] ⸢^{d}UTU⸣ ⸢EN⸣ *šur-bu-ú* ZÁLAG AN.TA.MEŠ *u* KI.TA.MEŠ
	e rev. 1'	ÉN ⸢^{d}⸣[UTU . . . .]
	f rev. 3	[ÉN ^{d}UTU EN] ⸢*šur-bu-ú*⸣ ZÁLAG AN.TA.M[EŠ *u* KI.T]A.M[EŠ]
19	A obv. 19	[x x] {*í-gì-gì* ^{d}*a-nun-na-ki* NUN$^{!}$(sag) *pa*$^{!}$-*ri*$^{!}$}-*i*[*s*$^{!}$ x x] x x [x x x]
	c rev. 3$^{cont.}$	DI.KUD ^{d}*í-gì-gì* NUN *pa-ri-is* ⸢EŠ.BAR⸣ [x x (x)]
	d rev. 1'	[. . . . .] *p*[*a-r*]*i-is* EŠ.BA[R] x [x x x]
	f rev. 3$^{cont.}$–4	[D]I.⸢KUD⸣s ^{d}*í-gì-gì pa*-⸢*ri*⸣-*is* EŠ.⸢BAR⸣ / [AN-*e u*] KI-*tim*
20	A obv. 20	{[*mu-ši*]*m*$^{?}$ NAM.MEŠ} [. . . . .] *ka-su-u i-še-su*-{*ka*} *k*[*a-a-šá*]
	c rev. 4	[x x NAM.M]EŠ *ṣab-ta šal-la ù ka-su-ú i-šá-as-si-ka ka*-<<*šá*>>-*a-šú*
	d rev. 2'–3'	[x x NA]M.⸢MEŠ⸣ *ṣab-tu šal-la u ka-s*[*u-ú*] / [*i-š*]*e-su-ka ka-a-šá*
	e rev. 2'	*mu-šim* N[A]M.[MEŠ . . . .]
	f rev. 4$^{cont.}$	*mu-šim* NAM.MEŠ *ṣ*[*ab-ta šal-la*] ⸢*ù*$^{?}$⸣ ⸢*ka-su-ú*$^{?}$⸣ [*i-šá*]-⸢*as-su*⸣-*ka ka-a-šu*
21	A rev. 1	[*šá-pal-k*]{*a ak-mis*} (. . .)] *ana-ku* ^{munus}N[ENNI-*tu*$_{4}$ x x x x]
	c rev. 4$^{cont.}$–5	*šá-pal-ka ak-mi*[*s*] / [x x x ^{munus}NE]NNI-*tu*$_{4}$ DUMU.MUNUS NENNI-*tu*$_{4}$
	d rev. 3'$^{cont.}$–4'	*šá-pal-ka ak-mis* / [*a*]-*n*[*a-k*]*u*$^{?}$ *al-si-ka* ^{munus}NENNI-*tú* DUMU.MUNUS NENNI-*tu*$_{4}$
	e rev. 2'$^{cont.}$–3'	[. . . . .] / *ana-ku al-si-ka* [. . . . .]
	f rev. 5	[*šá-pal-k*]*a ak-mis ana-ku al-s*[*i-ka* ^{munus}NENNI-*t*]*u*$_{4}$ ⸢DUMU.MUNUS⸣ ⸢NENNI⸣-[*tu*$_{4}$]

22	A rev. 2	[*šá* DINGIR-*šá* NEN]{NI$^{?!}$ ^{d}15-*šá*} ⸢NENNI⸣-*tu*$_{4}$ ⸢^{giš}MÁ⸣ *ma-li-tú ana-ku*
	b rev. 0–1'	[. . . . .] / [^{d}]⸢*iš*$_{8}$-*tár-šú*⸣ ⸢NENNI-*tu*$_{4}$⸣ ^{giš}M[Á] *m*[*a*-x x x x]
	c rev. 5$^{cont.}$–6	*šá* DINGIR-*šú* NENNI ^{d}15-*šú* NENNI-*t*[*u*$_{4}$] / [. . . . .]
	d rev. 5'	⸢*šá*⸣ DINGIR-*šú* NENNI ^{d}⸢15⸣-*šú* NENNI-*tu*$_{4}$ ^{giš}MÁ *ma-li-ti ana-ku*
	e rev. 3'$^{cont.}$–4'	[. . . . .] / ^{giš}MÁ *ma-lit ana-k*[*u*$^{!}$(ki)]
	f rev. 5$^{cont.}$–6	[*š*]*á* ⸢DINGIR⸣-*šú* NENNI / [^{d}15-*šú* NENNI]-*tu*$_{4}$ ^{giš}⸢MÁ⸣ [*ma-li-t*]*i a-na-ku*
23	A rev. 2$^{cont.}$–3	^{d}[UTU$^{?}$ x x x] / [x x x]-*ma mu-gur tés-li-ti* MU *šu-tu-qí* I[TI x x x x]
	b rev. 1'$^{cont.}$–3'	[x x x x x] / [*re*]-⸢*man-ni*$^{?}$⸣-*ma* ⸢*mu*$^{?}$⸣-*gur tés-li-t*[*u*$_{4}$ . . . .] / [(x) ITI]-⸢*ia*⸣ ⸢^{iti}BÁRA⸣
	c rev. 6$^{cont.}$–7	[^{d}U]TU *ši*-⸢*man-ni*⸣ *re-man-ni mu-gur tés-l*[*iti*] / [. . . . .]
	d rev. 6'–7'	^{d}UTU *ši-man-ni* [*r*]*e-man-né-e-ma mu-gur tés-li-tú* / *áš-šú šu-tu-qí* IT[I]-*ia* ^{iti}BÁRA
	e rev. 4'$^{cont.}$–5'	[. . . . .] / *áš*$^{!}$(pa)-*šú šu-tu-qí* ITI-[. . . . .]
	f rev. 6$^{cont.}$–7	^{d}⸢UTU⸣ [*ši*]-*man-ni* / [*re-man-ni*] ⸢*mu-gur*⸣ *tés*$^{?}$-[*li-ti áš*$^{?}$]-⸢*šú*$^{?}$⸣ ⸢*šu-tu-qu*⸣ ⸢Ù.TU-*ia*⸣ ⸢ITI⸣-*ia* ^{iti}BÁRA
24	A rev. 4	[x-x-*k*]*a a-š*[*e*]-{*e*}-*ka* ^{túg}SÍG-[*ka* x x]
	b rev. 3'	*as-ḫur-ka eš-e-ka* ⸢^{túg}SÍG⸣-⸢*ka*⸣ *a*[*ṣ-bat*$^{?}$]
	c rev. 7	[. . . . . .] *eš-e-ka* ^{túg}SÍG-*ka aṣ*-⸢*bat*⸣
	d rev. 7'$^{cont.}$–8'	*as-ḫur-ka eš-e*-⸢*ka*⸣ / ^{túg}SÍG-*ka aṣ-bat*
	e rev. 5'$^{cont.}$	[. . . . .]
	f rev. 8	[*as-ḫur-k*]*a* ⸢*eš*$^{?}$-*šim*$^{?}$-*ka*⸣ ⸢^{túg}⸣[SÍG-*ka aṣ-bat*]
25	A rev. 5	[x x] ⸢ḪUL⸣-*tì šu-tu-qu* {*ki*}-*ṣir lum-ni pa-ṭa-r*[*i* x x x (x)]
	b rev. 4'–5'	⸢GISKIM⸣ ⸢ḪUL⸣-*tì šu-tu-qu ki-ṣir lum-ni pa-ṭ*[*a-ri*] / KI-[*ka ba-š*]*u-ú*
	c rev. 8	[. . . . .]x *lum-ni* DU$_{8}^{!}$ KI-*ka ba-šú*-⸢*ú*⸣
	d rev. 8'–9'	*áš*-⸢*šú*⸣ GISKIM ḪUL-*tì šu-t*[*u-qu*] / *ki-ṣir lum-nu pa-ṭ*[*a-r*]*i* KI-*ka ba-šu*-[x]
	e rev. 6'	GISKIM ḪUL-*tì* [. . . . .]
	f rev. 8$^{cont.}$–9	[*áš-šú* GISKIM] ⸢ḪUL⸣ ⸢*šu-tu*⸣-[*q*]*u* ⸢*ki-ṣir*⸣ ⸢ḪUL⸣ / ⸢*pa-ṭa*⸣-[*ru* K]I-*ka ba*-[*šu-ú*]
26	A rev. 6	[x x Ù].TU-*ia*$_{5}$ *an-né*-[*e*] *šu-ti-q*[*a-an-ni-ma*]
	b rev. 5'	ITI Ù.TU-*ia an-ni-i šu-ti-qa-an*-⸢*ni*⸣-*ma*
	c rev. 9	[. . . . .-*m*]*a*
	e rev. 7'	ITI Ù.T[U-*ia* . . . .]
	f rev. 9$^{cont.}$	[ITI] ⸢Ù.TU-*ia*⸣ ⸢*an-ni-i*⸣ ⸢*šu*⸣-*ti-qa-an*-[*ni*]-*ma*
27	A rev. 7	[x x]-*ka lu-šá-pi dà-l*{*í-lí-k*}*a lud-lul* T[U$_{6}$ ÉN]
	b rev. 6'	⸢*nar*⸣-*bi-ka lu-šá-pi dà-lí-lí*-⸢*ka*⸣ ⸢*lud*⸣-*lul* T[U$_{6}$ ÉN]
	c rev. 9$^{cont.}$	[*n*]*a*[*r-b*]*i-ka lu-šá-pi dà-lí-lí-ka lud*-⸢*lul*⸣
	e rev. 7'$^{cont.}$	[. . . . .]
	f rev. 10	[*nar-bi-k*]*a lu-šá*-[*pi dà-lí-lí-ka lud-l*]*ul*$^{?}$ [TU$_{6}$ É]N

A, c, e, f

28	A rev. 8	[ÉN *an*]-*ni-tú* 3-*šú t*{*u-ša*}*d-bab-šú* MUNUS BI *tuš-ken-ma tu-še-eš-šeb-š*[*i*]
	b rev. 7'–8'	⸢ÉN⸣ *an-ni-ti* 3-*šú tu-šad-bab-šú* MUNUS BI *tuš-ken-m*[*a*] / ⸢*tu-še*⸣-*šeb-ši-ma*
	c rev. 10–11	[. . . . .] ⸢*tuš*⸣-*ken-ma* / [. . . . .]
	e rev. 8'–9'	ÉN *an-ni-t*[*ú* . . . .] / [TU]Š-⸢*ši*⸣-*m*[*a*]
	f rev. 11	⸢ÉN⸣ ⸢*an*⸣-*ni-ti* 3-*šú t*[*u-ša*]*d*-⸢*bab*⸣-[*šú* MUNUS] ⸢BI⸣ ⸢*tuš*⸣-[*ken-ma tu-še-šeb-ši-ma*]
29	A rev. 9	[^{síg}ḪÉ.ME].DA GEŠTU.MIN.MEŠ-*šá* DIRI-*ma*
	b rev. 8'$^{cont.}$	^{síg}ḪÉ.ME.DA GEŠTU.MIN-*šú* DIRI-[*ma*]
	c rev. 11$^{cont.}$	[. . . . .]
	f rev. 11$^{cont.}$–12	[^{síg}]⸢ḪÉ⸣.M[E.DA GEŠTU.MIN-*šá*] / ⸢DIRI⸣-*ma*
30	A rev. 10	[x x x x] {M}U$_{4}$. {M}U$_{4}$-*si* Ì.GIŠ *sír-di* ^{ú}*tar-muš*$_{8}$ NUMUN ^{giš}ŠINIG
	b rev. 9'–10'	[⸢]^{úg}MA.AN.DUL MU$_{4}$.MU$_{4}$-*si* Ì.GIŠ *sír-di* / ⸢^{ú}*tar*⸣-*muš* NUMUN ŠINIG

c rev. 11$^{\text{cont.}}$–12 [. . . . . MU$_4$.MU$_4$-*s*]*i* Ì.GIŠ *sír-*[*d*]*i* ^{ú}*tar-*⸢*muš*⸣ / [. . . . .]
f rev. 12$^{\text{cont.}}$ ^{túg}MA.⸢AN.DUL⸣ ⸢MU$_4$.MU$_4$-*su*⸣ ⸢Ì.GIŠ⸣ ⸢*sír*⸣*-d*[*i* ^{ú}*tar-muš*$_8$ NUMUN ^{giš}ŠINIG]

31 A rev. 11 [x x ŠÉ]Š-*si a-di* ITI *šá* Ù.TU *ú-še-et-te-qu-ma*
b rev. 10'–11' *ina* Ì.GIŠ BUR ŠÉŠ-*su* / ⸢EN⸣ ITI *šá* Ù.TU-*šá ú-še-ti-iq*
c rev. 12$^{\text{cont.}}$ [. . . . .-*q*]*u*
f rev. 12$^{\text{cont.}}$–13 [*i-na* Ì.GIŠ BUR / Š]ÉŠ-*su* ⸢EN⸣ [IT]I-*šá* ⸢*ú-še*⸣*-et-*[*ti-qu*]

32 A rev. 12 [x x]-*šá la i-da-'i-ip* ^{iti}BÁRA *ú-qa-ta-ma* Ù.TU
b rev. 12' *ra-man-šá la ú-da-'a-ap*
c rev. 12$^{\text{cont.}}$ [*r*]*a-*⸢*man*⸣*-šá la ú-d*[*a*]-⸢*'a-ap*⸣
f rev. 13$^{\text{cont.}}$ [*ra*]-⸢*man*⸣*-š*[*ú la ú-da-'a-ap*]

A, b, f____

(*Ms. c breaks*)

33 f rev. 14 ⸢*šá*$^?$*-niš*$^?$⸣ x [x] x x x x [. . . . .]

f____

34 f rev. 15 ⸢30⸣ ⸢ŠE⸣ [^{giš}ME]S.MÁ.GAN.NA *ina* ^{síg}⸢*ba*⸣*-r*[*u-un-di* È*-ak* . . . .]
35 f rev. 16 1[5$^?$ GI]G$^?$ x x x x [. . . . .]
36 f rev. 17 [x K]A.⸢KÉŠ⸣ KÉ[Š$^?$] x x x x [. . . . .]

f____

(*Ms. f: bottom of the reverse*)

Ms. b: Catchline and colophon

37 b rev. 13' <DIŠ> ⸢*i-na*⸣ ^{iti}BÁRA <TA> U$_4$.1.KAM EN U$_4$.30.KAM ⸢LÚ⸣.TUR Ù.TU
38 b rev. 14' ⸢*ki*⸣*-ma la-bi-ri-šú* <*šá*>*-ṭir-ma*
39 b rev. 15' IGI.⸢KÁR⸣ IM.GÍD.DA *up-x x x x-*DINGIR

Ms. A: Colophon

37 A rev. 13 *ina* ZAG *la-bi-ri-šú* SAR*-ma* IGI.KÁR
38 A rev. 14 {*a-na*} *ṣa-bat* DÙ-*ši* ^{m}*ki-ṣir-*^{d}AG *šá* ^{d}AG NIR-*su*
39 A rev. 15 {A ^{m}}⸢^{d}⸣UTU-*ib-ni* ^{lú}MAŠ.MAŠ É AN.ŠÁR

Ms. f: Colophon

37 f u. e. 1 [GIN$_7$ K]A ^{giš}*le-u*$_5$ *ša* ⸢GIN$_7$⸣ SUMUN-*š*[*ú*] ⸢SAR-*ma*⸣ U$_6$ IM.GÍD.DA ⸢^{m}ŠE⸣.B[A$^?$-*'a-a* DUMU]
38 f u. e. 2 ^{md}*za-ba*$_4$*-ba*$_4$-NUNUZ-Ù[R]U DUMU ^{m}*e-ṭi-ru* ^{iti}BÁRA ⸢U$_4$⸣.[x.KAM]

Bound Transcription and Translation

[1] *enūma sinništu arḫu ša alādīša īrubam-ma arḫu? šū? nisannu* <*ana*> *šūtuqi* (var. ms. f: *ana erītu nisannu araḫša šūt[uq]ī-ma lā alādi*) [2] DÙ.DÙ.BI *šūši qaqqad pilaqqi šalāšā* (ms. b adds: *qaqqad pilaqqi*) *ša bīni šalāšā* (ms. b adds: *qaqqad pilaqqi*) *ša musukkanni teppuš* [3] *ina barundi tašakkak šūši kiṣrī takaṣṣar* (var. ms. f adds: *ina kišādīšu tašakkan*) *šalāšā uṭṭāt musukkanni ina šīpāti sāmāti* [*tašakkak*] [4] *šalāšā kiṣrī takaṣṣar ḫamiššer ḫerṣī e'ri ina šīpāti sāmāti tašakkak* [5] [*ḫamiššer kiṣrī takaṣ*]*ṣar abnē qablē sinništi lā muštēšerti ittīšunu taṣammid* [6] *ina qablēšu tarakkas*(*sî*) *ultu* (*ūmi*) *maḫrî ša Nisanni adi* (*ūmi*) *šalāšî* (ms. A adds: *ša Ayyāri*) *ūmu ištēn qaqqad pilaqqi* [6a] *bīni u ištēn qaqqad pilaqqi musukkanni* (var. ms. f: *šitta qaqqad pilaqqi ištēt ša bīni ištēt ša musukkanni*) [7] *ina bīt simmilti ibattaq-ma inassuk* [8] *ana ūri* (var. ms. f adds gloss: *bīti*) *illī-ma ana pān Sîn paṭīra tarakkas nignak burāši tašakkan šikara tanaqqī-ma tuškên* [9] túgMA.AN.DUL *ultu qaqqari inaššī-ma išaddad-ma ultu bīt simmilti adi* (var. *ana*) *ūri ušelle ana ūri illī-ma* [10a] túgMA.AN.DUL *imakkak-ma* [10b] *ina muḫḫi ikerri itebbē-ma izzaz-ma* [10c] *ana pān Sîn qātēša imessi ana Sîn kīam iqabbi*

[1] When the month in which a woman is due to give birth has arrived and that month is Nisannu – (to) make it pass by (var. "to make a pregnant woman pass by Nisannu, her month (of delivery) and (to) avoid that she gives birth) – [2] (this is) the procedure for it: [3] You make [2] sixty spindle whorls (lit. "heads") – thirty (spindle whorls) of tamarisk wood (and) thirty (spindle whorls) of sissoo-wood. [3] You thread (them) on multi-coloured wool. You tie sixty knots (between them). (Var. adds: you put it around her neck.) [You thread] thirty 'grains' of sissoo-wood on (a thread of) red wool, [4] you knot thirty knots (between them). You string fifteen(!) cut-off pieces of *e'ru*-wood on (a thread of) red wool, [5] you ti[e fifteen knots (between them)]. Together with these (strings) you fasten stone beads (worn around) the hips by a woman who has difficulty bringing pregnancies to term (and) [6] you fasten (the strings) around her hips. From the first day of Nisannu until the thirtieth day (ms. A adds: of Ayyāru) [7] the [wo-m]an shall cut off [6] one spindle whorl [6a] (var.) of tamarisk wood and one spindle whorl of *musukkannu*-wood [6] every day (var. ms. f: two spindle whorls, one of tamarisk wood and one of *musukkannu*-wood), [7] (whilst standing) on the staircase (in the house where she lives), and she shall throw (them) away. [8] She goes up to the roof (var. adds gloss: (of the) house) and you set up an offering table in front of Sîn. You prepare a censer (burning) juniper (wood), you libate beer. Then you shall bow down. [9] She lifts up a MA.AN.DUL-garment from the ground and brings (it) up from the staircase onto the roof, dragging it (along). When she arrives on the roof, [10a] she spreads out the MA.AN.DUL-garment [10b] and she bows down on it. (Then) she rises and standing upright [10c] she washes her hands in front of Sîn. (Then) she speaks to Sîn as follows:

[11a] ÉN *Sîn nannār šamê u erṣeti*
[11b] [*ultu* (*ūmi*)] *maḫrî ša nisanni adi* (*ūmi*) *maḫrî ša Ayyāri* (ms. A: *adi* (*ūmi*) *šalāšî ša Ayyāri*)
[12] *piqdannī-ma luštēšir(a) maḫarka* (var. d: *lušlim lūšira maḫarka*)
[13] *šerrī* (var. *šerra*) *līmur nūru narbîka lušāpi dalīlīka ludlul*

[11a] Incantation: "Sîn, light of heaven and earth (mss. b and d)!
[11b] [From the] first [day] of Nisannu until the first day of Ayyāru (ms. A: until the thirtieth of Ayyāru)
[12] take care of me and let me bring my pregnancy to term before you! (var. ms. d: let me be well, let me be alright, let me prosper before you!)
[13] May my child see the light, (then) I shall glorify your greatness (and) praise you."

---

[14] *šalāšīšu* (var. adds: *ana Sîn*) *iqabbī-ma ana qaqqari urradam-ma aktam imḫur-līm ana* [*(libbi)*] *šamni tanaddī-ma ippaššiš* (var. ms. f: *tapaššassi*) [15] *kukra* (var. *ḫīl*(?) *kukri*) *kasê saḫlê mušāṭi zēr kitê adi ulladu ina pēmti tuqattarši*

[14] She says thus three times (var. adds: to Sîn). Then she goes downstairs. Then you put *aktam*-plant and 'heals thousand'-plant into oil and she shall rub herself (with it) (var.: you rub her). [15] You fumigate her (regularly) with *kukru*-aromatic (var. resin(?) of *kukru*), *kasû*-plant, cress, combed-out hair, linseed (thrown) on charcoals, until she gives birth.

---

[16] DIŠ KI.MIN *ina šēri ana pān Šamaš paṭīra tarakkas nignak burāši tašakkan šikara tanaqqi* [*sin*]*ništu šī* [17] *ina muḫḫi šukbusi izzaz-ma šipta Šamaš bēlu šurbû šalāšīšu tamannu*

[16] Alternatively (ms. c): in the morning you set up an offering table before Šamaš, you prepare a censer (burning) juniper, you libate beer. While that woman [17] is standing on a *stair*, you shall recite the incantation "Šamaš, exalted lord" three times.

---

[18] ÉN [*Šamaš bēlu*] *šurbû nūr elâti u šaplâti*

[19] *dayyān Igigi u Anunnakī rubû pāris purussê* [*šamê u*] *erṣeti*

[20] *mušīm šīmāti ṣabta šalla kasû išessûka kâša*

[21] *šapalka akmis anāku alsīka* (*anāku*) *annannītu mārat annannītu*

[22] [*ša ilšu annanna*] *ištaršu annannītu eleppu malītu anāku*

[23] *Šamaš šimânni rēmanni-ma mugur teslītī aššu šūtuqi* (var. ms. f adds: *alādīya*) *arḫīya nisannu*

[24] *asḫurka eš'eka sissiktaka aṣbat*

[25] *aššu itti lemutti šūtuqu kiṣir lumni paṭāri ittīka bašû*

[26] *araḫ alādīya annê šūtiqanni-ma*

[27] *narbîka lušāpi dalīlīka ludlul tê šipti*

[18] Incantation: "[Šamaš], exalted [lord], light of the upper and lower regions,

[19] judge of the Igigi and the Anunnaki, prince who makes decisions [for heaven and] earth,

[20] who determines fates! It is you whom the captive, deportee and prisoner invoke.

[21] I kneel in supplication at your feet, I have called out to you, (I), Mrs. So-and-so, daughter of Mrs. So-and-so,

[22] [whose god is So-and-so], whose goddess is So-and-so. I am a full boat.

[23] Šamaš (ms. d), listen to me, have mercy upon me and accept my prayer: concerning letting pass by (var. adds: my delivery,) Nisannu, the month of my (due delivery),

[24] I have turned to you, sought you out, grasped the hem of your garment.

[25] Since it is in your power to let the evil-boding sign pass by, to loosen the knot of evil,

[26] make this month of my (due) delivery pass by for me, then

[27] I shall glorify your [greatness] (and) praise you." Incantation formula.

---

[28] *šipta annītu šalāšīšu tušadbabšu sinništu šī tuškên-ma tušeššebšī-ma* [29] *tabarra uznēša tumallā-ma* [túg]MA.AN.DUL *tulabbassi šaman serdi tarmuš zēr bīni* [31] *ina šaman pūri tapaššassi adi arḫa ša alādīša ušettequ* [32] *ramānša lā uda''ap nisanna uqatta-ma ullad*

[28] You have her say this incantation three times. That woman prostrates herself. Then you have her sit down, and [29] you fill her ears with red wool, [30] and clothe her up with a MA.AN.(-)DUL-garment. [31] You rub her [30] with olive oil, *tarmuš*-plant, tamarisk seed, [31] (mixed) with oil-from-the-jar. Until she has passed the month of her delivery by, [32] she *must avoid bumping* (lit. "must not push") her[self]. (Ms. A adds:) She will complete the month Nisannu and then give birth.

---

[33] *šanîš*(?) . . .[. . . . . .]

[33] Alternatively(?), . . .[. . . . . .].

---

34 *šalāšā uṭṭāt* [*mus*]*ukkanni ina bar*[*undi tašakkak* . . . . . .] 35 *ḫami*[*ššer ḫer*]*ṣī*(?) . . . [. . . . . .] 36 [. . . *ki*]*ṣrī takaṣṣar*(?) . . . [. . . . . .]

34 [You thread] thirty 'grains' of [sis]soo-wood on (a thread of) multi[coloured] wool, [. . . . . .] 35 fif[teen cut-off] pieces(?) . . . [. . . . . .], 36 [. . .] . . . you tie(?) [kn]ots . . . [. . .].

Ms. b Catchline and colophon

37 *<šumma> ina nisanni <ultu> (ūmi) maḫrê adi (ūmi) šalāšī šerru i'allad* 38 *kīma labirīšu šaṭer-ma* 39 *bari imgiddû* . . .

39 "(If) a baby is born in the month Nisannu, (from) the first until the thirtieth day". 38 Copied according to its original and 39 collated. Oblong tablet of . . . .

Ms. A: Colophon

37 [(. . .)] *ina pūt labirīšu šaṭer-ma bari* 38 *ana ṣabāt epēši Kiṣir-Nabû ša tuklassu Nabû* 39 [(. . .)] *mār Šamaš-ibni mašmašši bīt Aššur*

37 [. . .] copied according to its original and collated 38 for the execution of a ritual performance by Kiṣir-Nabû, whose trust is Nabû, 39 [. . .], son of Šamaš-ibni, conjurer of the Aššur temple.

Ms. f: Colophon

37 [*kīma p*]*ī lē'i ša* ⸢*kīma*⸣ *labirīšu šaṭer-ma bari imgiddû Iprā*[*'ya*] [*mār*] 38 *Zababa-pir'u-uṣur mār Ēṭiru Nisannu* ⸢U$_4$⸣. [x.KAM]

37 [According to the word]ing of a wooden writing-board, which was written ⸢according⸣ to its original and collated. Oblong tablet of Iprā['ya], [son] of 38 Zababa-pir'u-uṣur, a descendant of (the) Ēṭiru (family), (written on) the [x-th] ⸢day⸣ of Nisannu.

Notes

General note: Passages that have deteriorated on the tablet of ms. A since Ebeling's copy and are now lost are indicated by curly brackets.

Line 1: For the reading of the line beginning, see the copy of ms. b (pl. 44). For understanding *arḫu* "month" as the subject of the first sentence rather than the woman, see Stadhouders and Steinert 2018, 71; cf. CAD A/1, 289a; Stol 2000a, 93 with n. 21. See similarly, SpTU 4, No. 153: 21: [DIŠ] ITI *šá* Ù.TU-*šú iq-ri-ba-am-ma* "if the month when she is due to give birth has arrived" (*infra* text D.1.11). For *erēbu* "to enter" in the sense of "to be coming" (said of spans of time), see AHw 236 s.v. *erēbu* G sub 9. The restoration follows ms. b, although it is possible that ms. A ended in ^{iti}BÁRA *šu-*[*u ana šu-ti-qí*] "(and) it is the month Nisannu, [in order to let it pass by]". The reading *šu-tu-qí* at the end of line 1 in ms. b was proposed by Reiner and Civil 1967, 191 n. 15 and has been confirmed by collation. The recently discovered ms. f presents a slightly varying formulation: ⸢*ana*⸣ ⸢^{munus}⸣P[EŠ$_4$] ^{iti}BÁRA ITI-*šá šu-t*[*u-q*]*í-ma la a-la-di* "to make a pregnant woman pass by Nisannu, her month (of delivery) and (to) avoid that she gives birth".

Lines 2–6a: As pointed out above, the instructions for the amulet in ms. A are considerably longer and more complex than in mss. b, c and f (the latter omit lines 3b–5). Ms. f presents a variant instruction to put the amulet around the patient's neck (rather than the hips specified in ms. A line 6). Note that ms. f contains a passage appended to the text as lines 34–36, which resembles lines 3b–5 in ms. A (cf. the note on line 34–36 below). The text passage of line 6a is only found in mss. b and f, with a slightly different wording.

For the symbolism and significance of the "spindle whorls" (*qaqqad pilaqqi*) of tamarisk and *musukkannu*-wood, see Stadhouders and Steinert 2018, 59. The "grains" (ŠE = *uṭṭatu*) of *musukkannu*-wood (perhaps small kernels of wood rather than seeds) and the fifteen(!) pieces (*ḫerṣu*) of *e'ru*-wood (perhaps cornel), which are used for an additional component of the amulet in ms. A, may have presented a similar colour contrast as the spindle whorls of tamarisk and *musukkannu*-wood (cf. CAD U/W, s.v. *uṭṭatu* sub mng. 2).

Line 4: Against Ebeling's and Hätinen's copy of line 4, collation of ms. A confirmed that the scribe actually wrote the number 15 (and not 14), which yields a much better correlation with the numbers thirty and sixty found in the preceding lines.

Line 5: For stones worn around the hips by a woman who has difficulties bringing to term (*sinništu lā muštēšertu*), which are not further specified in the present text, see sections C.3 and F in the present volume. Explicit reference to these stones is made in STT 241: 7 (text C.3.1). See also Schuster-Brandis 2008, 149–150.

Line 6: In ms. b, only faint traces are visible in the passage referring to attaching the amulet; the restoration here follows Ms. A. It is possible that one should read GAR-*an* "you put (it around her hips)" instead of KÉŠ "you tie (it around her hips)".

The addition of "(until the thirtieth day) of Ayyāru" in ms. A diverges from the other manuscripts; however, the variant instructions reveal that the ritual was staged to last 60 days rather than 30 days (from the first to the thirtieth day of Nisannu in the other manuscripts); i.e. instead of two spindle whorls the woman discarded only one spindle whorl per day. See also the text of the prayer in line 11, which requests divine protection during the month of Nisannu, and which contains the same variant in ms. A (speaking of the thirtieth instead of the first day of Ayyāru).

Line 8: The scribe of ms. f inserted the curious gloss É "house" underneath the phrase *ana ūri illī-ma* "she goes up to the roof", serving either as an explanation or as the notation of a textual variant.

At the end of the line, Stadhouders and Steinert (2018, *JMC* 32, 65) propose to read *la tuš-ken* "you shall not prostrate yourself" in ms. b, against positive *tuš-ken* in ms. c (see also Hätinen 2021, 509). Ms. b seems to be corrupt in that passage; I read the passage in question as *tuš-*^{ki}*ken*, interpreting the sign KI as a gloss. It is possible that *tuškên* should be translated as "she shall prostrate herself" here (see also line 28 below). However, it seems more likely that in line 8 *tuškên* references an action of the healer which concludes the presentation of the offering to Sîn.

Line 9: Hätinen (2021, 513, 515–516) improved Stadhouder's and Steinert's (2018, 60 note 28) reading ^{túg}BA.AN.DUL and its interpretation as "reed mat" in lines 9, 10 and 30 of the present text. Hätinen proposes to read ^{túg}MA.AN.DUL instead, which is attested in Middle Babylonian texts and designates a type of garment given to women as part of their dowry (she refers to Aro 1970, 16 HS 157: 89–90, spelled ^{túg}MAN.DUL). The Akkadian reading of the logogram and the exact nature of the garment remains unknown; the patient is clothed with it in line 30; here it is spread out on the ground.

This line varies slightly in mss. A, b, c and f; only the Babylonian texts explicitly state that the woman should bring up the MA.AN.DUL-garment from the ground floor to the roof.

The scribe of ms. c appears to have misunderstood his *Vorlage* in obv. 5', i.e. that the determinative ^{túg} is part of ^{túg}MA.AN.DUL, since he erased a sign following *tuš-ken*, which looks a bit like a damaged TÚG. After that, he left a space to spread out the signs MA.AN.DUL towards the right edge of the tablet. In contrast to this, the scribe clearly copied ^{túg}MA.AN.DUL at the end of ms. c obv. 7'.

Line 10a–b: Line 10b is omitted in ms. A, but found in all the Babylonian manuscripts. The verb *i-ke-er-ri* in line 10b has posed difficulties for previous interpreters. Stadhouders and Steinert (2018, 60–61, 69, 71–72) proposed a derivation from *karû* "to be(come) short" and suggested a derived meaning "to crouch down" from the context. Hätinen (2021, 513, 517) prefers a derivation from *qerû* "to invite" and translates "she extends an invitation (while being) on it" (i.e. on the MA.AN.(-)DUL-garment). However, SAD Vol. 3, 59, following the lead of AHw 1566, offers a better alternative in the verb *karā'u* "to bow down" (a loan from Aramaic *kr'*), which is attested in a late Babylonian text from Uruk (SpTU 2, No. 24: 8, with p. 128) in the strong form *ak-ta-ra-'* "I bowed down". The form *i-ke-er-ri* would indicate a weak variant *ka/erû* of this verb. For the tendency of some ultimae aleph verbs to be inflected as ultimae weak verbs (with an "Umlaut" *e*), cf. GAG § 99a, § 105c–d.

Lines 11–13: For the prayer to Sîn, cf. Mayer 1976, 295, 409 "Sîn 12". The manuscripts vary in the wording of the woman's address. Line 11a is only found in mss. b, d and f, while mss. A and c omit the opening. Furthermore, mss. b and c omit most of lines 12 and 13, and the address is shortened down to only one sentence.

Line 11a: For $^{d+}$EN$^{!}$.ZU.KI-*ra*, which seems to be an otherwise unattested spelling for ^{d}ŠEŠ.KI-*ra* = *Nannar*, see Stadhouders and Steinert 2018, 72.

Line 14: Ms. f presents a variant instruction ŠÉŠ-*si* "you rub her" (for *tapaššassi*) in this line in contrast to the other manuscripts. Ms. c is emended to *ippaššiš*, understood as N-stem durative form meaning "she rubs herself". See also Stadhouders and Steinert 2018, 72).

Line 17: For the difficulty of understanding the precise meaning of *šukbusu* "step, ramp" in the present text, see the comments in Stadhouders and Steinert 2018, 61–62; Hätinen 2021, 517; CAD Š/3, 214; AHw 1263). Hätinen suggests *šukbusu* may stand for the lowest step of the staircase in this text rather than a separate location. It is not excluded that the word referred to a movable household object here (e.g. a stool, step or the like).

Lines 18–27: For this prayer, see also Mayer 1976, 417 "Šamaš 55".

Line 19: Ms. f now allows us to restore the phrase *pāris purussê šamê u erṣeti* "who makes decisions for heaven and earth" (lost in all other manuscripts), following the suggestion of Hätinen 2019, 165.

Line 21: In ms. d, Hätinen (2021, 511) reads *[a]-n[a-k]u al-si-ka* at the beginning of line 4'. This restoration is followed here. Ms. A may have presented a reversed word order, since *anāku* is found preceding the formula introducing the patient.

Line 22: For the metaphor of the pregnant woman as a laden (cargo-)boat (*eleppu malītu*), see e.g. Steinert 2017a, 325–326, 332–334; Hätinen 2017, 169–186; 2021, 518. See also the edition of BAM 248 ii 47–54 *passim* (text D.1.1) and the commentary UET 6/3, 897 rev. 9'–10' in this volume (text G.2).

Line 28: Context requires to understand the form *tuš-ken-ma* following MUNUS BI "that woman" in this line as a 3rd person feminine verbal form, in contrast to *tuškên* in line 11 above. Forms with *ta-/tu*-prefixes standing for a 3rd person fem. sg. referent in Late Babylonian texts presumably reflect Aramaic influence, cf. Stadhouders and Steinert 2018, 73 with GAG § 75h. Hätinen 2021, 512, 516 suggests the reading *uš*$_{4}$*-ken* here.

Line 31: For *šaman pūri* "oil-from-the-jar", an ingredient often encountered in texts related to birth and delivery, see e.g. BAM 248 and dupl. (*infra* text D.1.1).

Line 32: The unusual expression *ramānša lā uda''ap* "she should not push herself", from the verb *da'āpu* clearly refers to refraining from a certain behaviour to avoid the onset of an early labour. Hätinen (2021, 518–519) draws attention to the usage of the verb *da'āpu* in astrological-astronomical contexts, where it can indicate the "act of movement [of a planet] after a stationary phase". Whether the expression in the present text recommended that the woman should avoid trauma, movement or overly exhaustion remains a matter of interpretation. See also Stadhouders and Steinert 2018, 69, 73.

Lines 33: The reading of this largely damaged line in ms. f, which is ruled off from the preceding ritual and the following concluding lines 34–36, is difficult. The eBL project's transliteration suggests to read ⸢1-*niš*⸣ K[A.KÉ]Š$^{?}$, which is difficult to translate without more context. The reading *šanîš* (*šá-niš*) "alternative(ly)" proposed here draws its inspiration from a ritual text (Gurney 1960, *Iraq* 22, 224: 21), which introduces a varying ritual stemming from a different source with the words *šanîš ša pī tuppi šanê* "Alternatively, according to another tablet" (with the text of the ritual following). Perhaps line 33 in ms. f presented a similar scribal note, which introduced the following lines 34–36, which may present the text of a shorter, varying ritual performed for the same purpose.

Lines 34–36: Unfortunately, these lines in ms. f are too damaged to allow an exact interpretation. However, certain deciphered keywords make it clear that these lines contained a set of ritual instructions for an amulet which share certain similarities with lines 3–5 of ms. A, which were omitted in the other (Babylonian) manuscripts: notably the thirty 'grains' of *musukkannu*-wood and fifteen knots(?) (cf. fifteen pieces of *e'ru*-wood in ms. A).

Colophons and catchline: For the colophon of ms. A, see also Hunger 1968, No. 208; Arbøll 2021, 117 n. 55.

The catchline in ms. b refers to the Namburbi ritual performed to ward off the consequences of an ill-boding birth in Nisannu (see Maul 1994, 400–408). For the parallels in *Iqqur īpuš*, see Labat 1965, 132ff. § 64, with discussion in Stadhouders and Steinert 2018, 63–64; Hätinen 2021, 519. The last signs of the colophon in ms. b were erased by the scribe and are only barely visible. Possibly, restore *up-pu-uš* "(properly) executed", followed by the scribe's personal name. Cf. Hunger 1968, 161.

For the colophon of ms. f, compare also the colophon of BM 47491 edited in this volume (text A.2.6), likewise written by Iprā'ya, son of Zababa-pir'u-uṣur, a descendant of (the) Ēṭiru (family).

Chapter E
Women's Healthcare Texts for Other or Uncertain Purposes

This chapter discusses eleven fragments and tablets of medical texts related to the corpus of women's healthcare texts that could not be clearly assigned to a specific thematic group as defined in Chapters A–D and F. These texts consist of three Neo-Assyrian fragments from Assur and Nineveh, and eight Late Babylonian fragments and small tablets from Sippar, Babylon and Uruk, including tablets from the Bēl-rēmanni archive, the Ebabbar temple (Sippar) and from the library of the descendants of Ekur-zakir (Uruk).

Among the fragments in Chapter E are pieces that belonged to two-column tablets that contained longer collections of remedies (E.1.2–E.1.3, E.2.4). Text E.2.8 may have contained therapies for diverse topics including women's health and non-gender-specific problems. Among the more unusual texts of Chapter E is the fragment of a ritual for a woman that resembles the Namburbi rituals and was concerned with removing the impact of an ominous negative sign (text E.2.3). Furthermore, the remedies on the Uruk fragment SpTU 5, No. 253 (text E.2.6) deal with treatments for a serious condition of the uterus not known so far from other women's healthcare texts. The sources from the Bēl-rēmanni archive included in Chapter E (texts E.2.1–E.2.2) are small students' tablets that contain only one or a few remedies; one of these texts (E.2.1) is preserved in three copies reflecting the teaching activities linked with the family of Bēl-rēmanni.

E.1 Texts from Assyria

E.1.1 BAM 251: A Fragment from Assur with Prescriptions for Women

This small fragment from the top of a tablet preserves ten damaged lines of text with recipes for a fumigation, an ointment and an amulet. The fragment can be assigned to the therapeutic texts for women's health due to the occurrence of the feminine pronominal suffix. The exact purpose of the prescriptions remains unclear, but the instructions for the amulet in the present fragment share similarities with prescriptions for amulets to stop bleeding (during pregnancy; see sections C.1., C.3. and F in this volume).

List of Manuscripts

Siglum	Museum Number	Copy	Collation	Format; Ductus	Provenience
A	VAT 13897	BAM 251	Coll.	Fragment of a tablet; Neo-Assyrian script; ca. 8th/7th cent. BCE	Assur; N4 library

Overview

i Fragmentary prescription 1–6
A obv.? 1–6

ii Fragmentary prescription 7–10 [. . .
A obv.? 7–10

Previous Edition and Discussion

Köcher 1964, BAM Vol. 3, xix and pl. 57 (copy; discussion)
Böck 2013, *JA* 103, 36 fn. 32 (transliteration)
CDLI P285336 (photo; transliteration)
BabMed Corpora (https://www.geschkult.fu-berlin.de/e/babmed/Corpora/BAM-3/BAM-3_-251) (transliteration)

https://doi.org/10.1515/9781501506475-008

Transliteration

1 A obv.$^{?}$ 1 [...... *k*]*ib-rit* ^{ú}KUR.KUR NUMUN [.........]

2 A obv.$^{?}$ 2 [.......]^{sar} ḪAMANZER(SÍK.ŠAB) *ina* DÈ [SAR$^{?}$ ....]

3 A obv.$^{?}$ 3 [........... Ú.ḪI].⸢A⸣ *an-nu-ti ina* DÈ *tur-á*[*r* ....]

4 A obv.$^{?}$ 4 [.......... ŠÉ]Š-*si* ^{ú}*ak-tam* [.................]

5 A obv.$^{?}$ 5 [.......... $^{\text{na4}}$GIŠ.NU$_{11}$.G]AL$^{?}$ $^{\text{na4}}$ÁŠ.GÌ.GÌ $^{\text{na4}}$[............]

6 A obv.$^{?}$ 6 [.......... KA A.A]B.BA $^{\text{na4}}$KUR-*nu* [DAB ....]

---

7 A obv.$^{?}$ 7 [................] NA$_{4}$.MEŠ *an-nu-t*[*i ina* DUR ... È ....]

8 A obv.$^{?}$ 8 [...... KA.KÉŠ KÉŠ]-*ma*$^{?!}$ *e-ma* KÉŠ [..........]

9 A obv.$^{?}$ 9 [................] ⸢Ú⸣.MEŠ *an-nu-t*[*i* ....]

10 A obv.$^{?}$ 10 [...............]x ^{síg}Ḫ[É.ME.DA ....]

Ms. A obv.$^{?}$ breaks; remainder lost

Bound Transcription and Translation

[1] [. . . . . .] *kibrītu atā'išu zēr* [. . . . . .] [2] [. . . . . .] ... *mušāṭa ina pēnti* [*tuqattar*(?) . . . . . .] [3] [. . . . . . *šam*]*mī annûti ina pēnti turrar* [. . . . . .] [4] [. . . . . . *tapa*]*ššassi aktam* [. . . . . .] [5] [. . . . . . *ašnuga*]*llu ašgikû* [. . . . . .] [6] [. . . . . . *imbu' tâ*]*mti šadânu* [*ṣābitu* . . . . . .]

[1] [. . . . . .] sulphur, *atā'išu*-plant, seed of [. . . . . .], [2] [you fumigate (her?) with . . . . . .]-plant (and) combed hair over charcoal [. . . . . .]. [3] [. . . . . .] you roast these [drug]s(?) over charcoal, [. . . . . .] [4] [. . . . . . you r]ub her (with it). [*You* ...] *aktam*-plant, [. . . . . .], [5] [. . . . . . alabas]ter, turquoise, ...-stone, [. . . . . .] [6] [. . . . . . *imbu' tâ*]*mti*-mineral, magnet[ite, ...].

---

[7] [. . . . . .] *abnī annûti* [*ina ṭurri . . . tašakkak*(?) . . . . . .] [8] [. . . . . . *kiṣra takaṣṣar*]-*ma*(?) *ēma taktaṣru* [. . . . . .] [9] [. . . . . .] *šammī annûti* [. . . . . .] [10] [. . . . . .]. . . *ta*[*barru*(?) . . . . . .]

[7] [. . . . . . *you thread*] these stones [*on a string of* ..., ...] [8] [. . . . . . *so and so many times* you knot a knot (into it)]. Wherever you have made a knot, [. . . . . .]. [9] [. . . . . .] these drugs [. . . . . .] [10] [. . . . . . red] wool(?) [. . . . . .] ...

Ms. A breaks; remainder lost

Notes

Lines 1–6: This section presents several amalgamated prescriptions. Lines 1–2 may have to be understood as remnants of a prescription for a fumigation, followed by an alternative remedy for an ointment (lines 2–4). The list of ingredients in lines 4–6 may belong to the instructions for making an amulet necklace in lines 7–10, since it includes mostly stones/minerals.

Lines 7–10: For similar instructions, see e.g. BAM 235 obv. 15–16 // BAM 236 rev. 7'–9' (text C.1.1 lines 15–16; C.1.2 lines 27'–28'); KAR 247 l. col. 4'–7' (text C.3.6 lines 52''''–55'''').

E.1.2 K. 14028: A Fragment from Nineveh with Treatments for Women

This small Neo-Assyrian medical fragment from Nineveh must have formed part of a large two-column tablet. Although only offering a few damaged lines, the tablet in question may have contained a collection of treatments for women's health matters, since one line in the fragment features an instruction pointing to a female patient (line 8'). Similar Nineveh fragments in Neo-Assyrian script of two-column tablets belonging to the corpus of women's healthcare texts are K. 11647 (AMT 66/3) and K. 17499 (see texts C.3.2 and E.1.3 in this volume).

List of Manuscripts

Siglum	Museum Number	Copy	Collation	Format; Ductus	Provenience
A	K. 14028	Geers, Folio A164 Pl. 37	Coll.	Fragment of a two(?)-column tablet; Neo-Assyrian script; 7th cent. BCE[384]	Nineveh; Ashurbanipal's library

Overview

i'	Fragmentary instruction A obv.$^{?}$ 1'–6'	...]1'–6'
ii'	Fragmentary prescription A obv.$^{?}$ 7'–9'	7'–9'
iii'	Fragmentary instruction A obv.$^{?}$ 10'	10'
iv'	Fragmentary instruction A obv.$^{?}$ 11'–12'	11'–12'[...

Previous Edition and Discussion
CDLI P400591 (photo)
Electronic Babylonian Library Project (eBL) (https://www.ebl.lmu.de/library/K.14028) (transliteration; photo)

Transliteration

Beginning of ms. A obv.(?) lost

1' A obv.$^{?}$ 1' [......] x [......]

2' A obv.$^{?}$ 2' [......] x x [......]

3' A obv.$^{?}$ 3' [......] x ši [......]

4' A obv.$^{?}$ 4' [......] ⸢*i*$^{?}$⸣-*tab-bal* [......]

5' A obv.$^{?}$ 5' [...... ^{d}UTU *ina*$^{?}$] È-*šú* [......]

6' A obv.$^{?}$ 6' [. . . . . .] *e-ru*$^{?}$-⸢*u*$^{?}$⸣ x x KAŠ *ana* GÙB ŠUB BAD U$_{4}^{?}$.[MEŠ-*šá*$^{?}$ . . . . . .]

---

384 Measurements: ca. 3.4 x 4.7 x 1.5 cm.

7' A obv.$^{?}$ 7' [DIŠ MUNUS$^{?}$ ... -*š*]*á* IGI-*mar* [...]

8' A obv.$^{?}$ 8' [... ŠE]G$_{6}$$^{?}$-*šal ba-lu pa-tan* GU$_{7}$-*ši-ma* ⸢*i*$^{?}$⸣-[...]

9' A obv.$^{?}$ 9' [... *ana*$^{?}$] ⸢U$_{4}$$^{?}$⸣.MEŠ TAG$_{4}$.MEŠ [...]

10' A obv.$^{?}$ 10' [DIŠ MUNUS$^{?}$ ... GI]G$^{?}$ DUGUD *i-mar-ra-a*[*ṣ*$^{?}$ ...]

11' A obv.$^{?}$ 11' [DIŠ MUNUS$^{?}$ ...] *u* ⸢ḪUL⸣ ⸢IGI$^{?}$⸣-*m*[*ar*$^{?}$ ...]

12' A obv.$^{?}$ 12' [...] x[...]

Ms. A obv.(?) breaks; remainder lost

Bound Transcription and Translation

Beginning of ms. A obv.(?) lost

$^{1'-3'}$ *too fragmentary for transcription and translation*

$^{4'}$ [. . . . . .] *itabbal*(?) [. . . . . .] $^{5'}$ *Šamaš ina*(?)] *aṣîšu* [. . . . . .] $^{6'}$ [. . . . . .] *erû*(?) . . . *ana šumēli tanaddi šumma ūm*[*īša*(?) . . . . . .]	$^{4'}$ [...] she takes away(?) [...], $^{5'}$ [... at sun]rise(?) [...], $^{6'}$ [...] dregs(?) (of) ...-beer(?) you pour out toward the left. If(?) [her?] day[s(?) . . . . . .].
$^{7'}$ [*šumma sinništu*(?) ...-*š*]*a immar* [. . . . . .] $^{8'}$ [. . . . . . *tušab*]-*šal*(?) *balu patān tušakkalšī-ma i-*[. . . . . .] $^{9'}$ [. . . . . . *ana*] *ūmī*(?) *rēḫūti*(?) [. . . . . .]	$^{7'}$ [If a woman(?) ...] sees her(?) [...], [. . . . . .] $^{8'}$ [...] you boil(?), you have her eat on an empty stomach, and she will [...]. $^{9'}$ [...] (for all) *remaining days*(?) [. . . . . .].
$^{10'}$ [*šumma sinništu*(?) ... *mur*]*ṣa kabta imarra*[*ṣ* . . . . . .]	$^{10'}$ [If a woman(?) ...], she will get sick with a serious [dis-e]ase, [. . . . . .].
$^{11'}$ [*šumma sinništu*(?) ...] *u lumna imm*[*ar*(?) . . . . . .] $^{12'}$ [...]... [...]	$^{11'}$ [If a woman(?) . . .] and experiences misfortune, [...], $^{12'}$ [...] ... [...]

Ms. A obv.(?) breaks; remainder lost

Notes

Lines 1'–6': The restorations are tentative. In line 6', eBL reads *e-reb* ... instead of *e-ru-u* "dregs". For the use of beer dregs, see also BAM 240: 18' (text D.2.1): *e-ra-a šá* DIDA *baḫ-ru-su* "hot (= steaming) dregs of *billatu*-substance". The context of the present instruction is different, however.

Lines 7'–9': Within the women's healthcare texts, the verb *amāru* "to see" sometimes occurs in a euphemistic phrase in the contexts of a missed menstrual period, in which the woman is described as "not seeing her *trouble*" (*maruštu*), see SpTU 1, No. 59: 12' (text C.2.1). Compare also below line 11', for a similar entry mentioning the experience of misfortune/calamity. The reading and meaning of line 9' are not certain.

Line 10': Following eBL, I restore GI]G$^{!?}$ DUGUD "a serious [dise]ase".

Line 11': The reference to experiencing misfortune (lit. "seeing evil") recalls sorcerous practises described in the anti-witchcraft texts, where the victim of evil magic receives frightening messages or signs. In the context of women's healthcare texts concerned with protecting pregnant women from sorcery causing miscarriage, a similar phrase is attested referring to the woman as "having been shown something" (*kullumu*). The Assur Medical Catalogue (Steinert et al. 2018, 218, 271–272, lines 113–114) cites three entries from therapeutic texts that refer to this bewitchment: DIŠ ^{munus}PEŠ$_4$ *kul-lu-mat* "If a pregnant woman has been 'shown' (something)", DIŠ MUNUS Ù.TU-*ma kul-l*[*u-mat*$^?$] "If a woman gives birth and is 'shown' (something)", and [(*ana*) *ḫ*]*a-riš-te ša kul-lu-ma-tú* BÚR "(treatments for) a woman in confinement who has been 'shown' (something)". The Assur text LKA 9 rev. iii 2'–3' (text C.3.5) contains a remedy for "a leather bag to release a pregnant woman or a woman in confinement to whom (something evil) has been shown" (*me-e-lu šá* ^{munus}PEŠ$_4$ *u* ^{munus}*ḫa-riš-t*[*i*] *šá kul-lu-ma-tu*$_4$ *pa-šá-ri*). It is possible that the present treatment had a similar purpose.

E.1.3 K. 17499: A Fragment Related to Women's Health?

This tiny Neo-Assyrian fragment from Nineveh has been included here, as it may have belonged to a medical tablet with treatments for women. This interpretation is based on the reading of two partially restored phrases that appear to indicate a female patient. The attribution to the gynaecological corpus remains tentative for the time being.

List of Manuscripts

Siglum	Museum Number	Copy	Collation	Format; Ductus	Provenience
A	K. 17499	Pl. 53	Coll.	Fragment of a two(?)-column tablet; Neo-Assyrian script; 7th cent. BCE[385]	Nineveh; Ashurbanipal's library

Overview

i' Fragmentary instruction ...]1'–11'[...
A obv.$^?$ 1'–11'

Previous Edition and Discussion

Lambert, Folio 11281 (transliteration)
CDLI P 420836 (photo)
Electronic Babylonian Library Project (eBL) (https://www.ebl.lmu.de/library/K.17499) (transliteration; photo)

Transliteration

Beginning lost

1' A obv.$^?$ 1' [...]-*na*$^?$ ⸢*lem*$^?$-*ni*⸣ ⸢*e*$^?$⸣-⸢*lu*$^?$⸣ [...]

2' A obv.$^?$ 2' [...]x NITA KI x[...]

3' A obv.$^?$ 3' [... *šá*(?) U]ZU-*šá ik-ka-l*[*u-ši* ...]

4' A obv.$^?$ 4' [... *ina*$^?$ ... *š*]*á* A.ZU *kat-me* [...]

385 Measurements: 2.4 x 4.1 x 0.8 cm.

5' A obv.$^?$ 5' [...*ina*$^?$] U$_4$ *a-a-i* GIG-*ṣa-a*[*t*$^?$ ...]

6' A obv.$^?$ 6' [...] *ú-sa-*⸢*niq*$^?$⸣ [...]

7' A obv.$^?$ 7' [...] [...]

8' A obv.$^?$ 8' [...]x ti x[...]

9' A obv.$^?$ 9' [...] x[...]

10' A obv.$^?$ 10' [...] N[AG$^?$ ...]

11' A obv.$^?$ 11' [...] r[i ...]

Text breaks; remainder lost

Bound Transcription and Translation

1'–2' *too fragmentary for transcription and translation*

3' [. . . . . . *ša*(?) *š*]*ērša ikkal*[*uši* ...] 4' [... *ina* ... *š*]*a asî katme* [. . . . . .] 5' [. . . . . . *ina*] *ūmi*(?) *ayyi marṣa*[*t* . . . . . .] 6' [. . . . . .] *usanniq* [. . . . . .]

3' [. . . . . . (a woman) who]se(?) flesh hur[ts her . . . . . .], 4' [. . . . . . *in a*] covered(?) [...] of a physician ... [...], 5' [. . . . . . on(?)] whatever day(?) she is sick(?) [...], 6' [. . . . . .] he/she has checked [. . . . . .],

7'–11' *for transcription and translation*

Text breaks; remainder lost

Notes

Line 3': The verbal form *ikkal*[*uši*] can be read as a singular form with a subjunctive or to a masc. pl. form (with a preceding enumeration of body parts).

Line 4': Medical texts often mention specific utensils or treatments of the *asû*, see e.g. BAM 244 obv. 28 (text B.1.1): "[you boil(?) (the ingredients)] in a small *tangussu*-vessel like (one) from the hand of an *asû*$^?$" (*ina* ŠEN.TUR GIN$_7$ ŠU A.Z[U ŠEG$_6$-*šal*$^?$]). See further BAM 229 obv. 16': *an-nu-ú* ŠU.MIN A.ZU "this (lotion) is from the hands of a physician". Cf. CAD A/2, 345 sub a).

Line 5': The reading of the traces as [*ina*] *ūmi ayyi* "on whatever day" is tentative, cf. CAD A/1 234–236. eBL restores [... -*n*]*a*$^?$-*a-a-i* GIG-*za* [...].

Line 6': The D-stem form of *sanāqu* could also be a perfect form (*ussanniq*); the verb also means "to harass, to plague; to interrogate" (cf. CAD S, 141–144 s.v. *sanāqu* sub 10–13).

E.2 Texts from Babylonia

E.2.1 A Recipe for a Woman in Three Late Babylonian Sources

Among the school tablets with medical content associated with the archive of the family of Bēl-rēmanni (stemming from Sippar and dating to the 6th/5th cent. BCE), I. L. Finkel (2000, 157–159) edited three small tablets bearing the same prescription (for the archive, see Jursa 1999). That the tablets come from the same find spot is also suggested by the similar staining (black dots) of the surfaces of mss. a and c.

The exact purpose of the prescription is contested because the purpose statement presents several difficulties. According to the interpretation offered here, the prescription concerned the treatment of pain via an enema into the anus.

According to a different reading of the text (Scurlock and Andersen 2005, 270 12.62), the remedy aimed at inducing delayed labour pains and at speeding up delivery.

List of Manuscripts

Siglum	Museum Number	Copy	Collation	Format; Ductus	Provenience
a	BM 42507 (81-7-1, 267)	Finkel, *FS Lambert*, Fig. 9	Coll.	Single-column tablet in landscape format; Late Babylonian script; 6th/5th cent. BCE	Sippar
b_1 (+) b_2	F 238 (81-7-1 unnumbered) (+) BM 43268 (81-7-1, 1032)	Finkel, *FS Lambert*, Fig. 10	Coll.	Fragments of a single-column tablet; Late Babylonian script; 6th/5th cent. BCE	Sippar
c	BM 43229 (81-7-1, 993)	Finkel, *FS Lambert*, Fig. 11	Coll.	Single-column tablet in portrait format; Late Babylonian script; 6th/5th cent. BCE	Sippar

Overview

i Prescription for treating pain (enema into the anus?) 1–17
a obv. 1–rev. 7 // b_1 (+) b_2 obv. 1–rev. 2' // c obv. 1–rev. 6'

Previous Edition and Discussion

Finkel 2000, *FS Lambert*, 157–159 Text 5
Scurlock and Andersen 2005, 270 12.62 with note 53 (alternative readings for BM 43229 rev. 3'–6')
Electronic Babylonian Library Project (eBL) (https://www.ebl.lmu.de/library/BM.42507; https://www.ebl.lmu.de/library/BM.43268; https://www.ebl.lmu.de/library/BM.43229)

Transliteration

1	a obv. 1	1 GÍN *nu-ḫur-tu*$_4$ [(x x x)]
	b_1 obv. 1	1 GÍN *nu-*[*ḫur-tu*$_4$ (...)]
	c obv. 1	1 GÍN *nu-ḫur-tu*$_4$
2	a obv. 2	1 GÍN ^{ú}*ka-m*[*u-nu*]
	b_1 obv. 2	1 GÍN [...........]
	c obv. 2	1 GÍN *ka-mu-nu*
3	a obv. 3	1 GÍN *ak-tam* 1 [GÍN *qa-nu-ú*]
	b_1 obv. 3	⸢1⸣ [GÍN ....]
	c obv. 3$^{cont.}$–4	1 GÍN ⸢*ak*⸣-*tam* / 1 GÍN *qa-nu-ú*

4	a obv. 4	1 GÍN $^{\text{[ši]m}}$⸢MUG⸣ [*sa-pan*]
	b$_2$ obv. 1'	⸢1⸣ [x x x x]
	c obv. 5	2 GÍN ^{šim}MUG *sa-pan*
5	a obv. 5	⸢1⸣ NINDA *si-*[*i*]*n-du* ⸢$^{\text{ú?}}$⸣[*ba-r*]*a*$^{?}$-[*ra*$^{?}$-*tu*$_4$]
	b$_2$ obv. 2'–3'	1 NINDA *si-in-d*[*u* (…)] / 1 NINDA ^{ú}*ba-r*[*a*$^{?}$-*ra-tu*$_4$$^{?}$]
	c obv. 6–7	1 NINDA *si-in-du* G[IG] / 1 [NINDA *si-in-d*]*u* M[UNU$_4$]
6	a obv. 6	[*ina*] 5 SÌLA [KA]Š ⸢ŠE⸣.BAR ⸢SUMUN$^{?}$⸣ [2 SÌLA *m*]*e*-⸢*e*⸣
	b$_2$ obv. 4'	*ina* 2 SÌLA *me-e*
	c obv. 8	[............] ⸢x x⸣ [x]
7	a obv. 7	[*t*]*a-ḫa-qu* ⸢*tu-šab*⸣-*šal a-d*[*i*]
	b$_2$ obv. 4'$^{\text{cont.}}$–5'	*t*[*a-ḫa-qu*] / *tu-šab*$^{!}$(ib)-*šal a-*[*di*]
8	a obv. 8	⸢2⸣ SÌLA GUR *su-u*[*m-m*]*u-nu šam*$^{!}$-*ni*
	b$_2$ obv. 5'$^{\text{cont.}}$–6'	[.............] / *su-um-mu-*[*nu* ....]
9	a obv. 9	1/2 NINDA LÀL 1/2 GÍN *i*[*n*]-*za-ru-ú*$^{!}$
	b$_2$ lo. e. 1	1/2 NINDA LÀL [.......]
10	a lo. e. 1	⸢*a*⸣-*na* 3-*ta zi-*⸢*it*⸣-*tu*$_4$ ŠUB
	b$_2$ rev. 1	*a-na* 3-*t*[*a* ....]
11	a rev. 1	*a-na ṭúr-*⸢*ru*⸣-*šú ta-šap-pak*
	b$_2$ rev. 2	*a-na ṭúr-ri-šú* [........]
12	a rev. 2	*a-na zi-*⸢*it*⸣-*tu*$_4$ *ku-tal-la-tu*$_4$
	b$_2$ rev. 3	*a-na zi-it-tu*$_4$ *k*[*u-*..........]
13	a rev. 3	^{ú}*ni-na-a-tu*$_4$ ⸢*lu*⸣ ⸢^{ú}⸣*a-tar-*[*tu*$_4$]
	b$_2$ rev. 4	^{ú}*ni-na-a-tu*$_4$ *l*[*u* ....]
	c rev. 1'	⸢*lu*⸣ ⸢^{ú}⸣x[x x x x]
14	a rev. 4	*me-e* Ú.ZAL.L[A *tu-š*]*e-ep-*[x]
	b$_2$ rev. 5	[*me*]-⸢*e*⸣ ⸢Ú.ZAL⸣.L[A ....]
	c rev. 2'	Ú.ZAL.LA *tu-še-ep-su*
15	a rev. 5	*a-na* MUNUS *šá tu-*[x x] ⸢x⸣ [x]
	c rev. 3'	*a-na* MUNUS *šá tu-lu-ša*$^{!?}$(di)
16	a rev. 6	[*t*]*a-kul-la* GA[L$_4$.LA$^{?}$-*ša*]
	b$_1$ rev. 1'	*ta-kul-*⸢*lu-ú*$^{?}$⸣
	c rev. 4'	*ta-kul-lu-ú*

17	a rev. 7	⌜*ik*⌝*-kal-lu-šú* S[IG$_5$ (...)]
	b$_1$ rev. 1'$^{\text{cont.}}$–2'	[.........] / SIG$_5$
	c rev. 5'–6'	*ik-kal-lu-ši* / SIG$_5$

Bound Transcription and Translation

[1] *šina šiqil nuḫurtu* [(...)] [2] *šina šiqil kamūnu* [3] *ištēn šiqil aktam ištēn šiqil qanû* [4] *ištēn* (var. *šina*) *šiqil ballukku sapān* [5] *ištēn akal(?) sindu* (var. adds: *kibti*) *ištēn akal bar*[*īrātu*] (var. *ištēn* [*akal sind*]*u buqli*) [6] *ina ḫamšat qa šikar uṭṭati labiri šina qa mê* [7] *taḫâq tušabšal adi* [8] (*ana*) *šina qa iturru summunu šamni* [9] *mišil akal dišpu ištēn šiqil inzarû* [10] *ana šalašta(?) zittu tanaddi* [11] *ana ṭurrīšu tašappak* [12] *ana zittu kutallatu* [13] *nīnâtu lū atar*[*tu*] [14] *mê azallê tušep<pes>su* [15] *ana sinništi ša tulûša(?)* [16] *takullâ* (ms. a adds *ū*[*rīša(?)*]) [17] *ikkalūši damiq*

[7] You mix [1] two shekels of *nuḫurtu*-(plant), [(...)], [2] two shekels of *kamūnu*-plant, [3] one shekel of *aktam*-plant, one shekel of reed, [4] one (var. two) shekel(s) of *ballukku*-soap, [5] a tenth of a litre of milled *simdu*-cereal (var. (prepared from) wheat), (and) a tenth of a litre of *bar*[*īrātu*-plant] (var. a [tenth of a litre of *simd*]*u*-cereal (prepared from) malt). [7] You boil (the mixture) [6] in five litres of old barley beer (and) [two litres of] water (var. in two litres of water), [7] until [8] it is reduced to two litres. [10] You add [8] an eighth of a litre of oil, [9] half a tenth litre of (date) syrup (and) one shekel of *inzarû*-aromatic, [10] (dividing it) into three *portions* (lit. parts). [11] You pour it into her anus. [12] As an *after-treatment*(?) [13] you *make use of*(?) *nīnû*-plants(?) or *atartu*-plant [14] (with) an infusion of *azallû*-plant. [15] It is good for a woman whose breasts(?) [17] are affected [16] by pain (*takullû*) (var. adds (of the) genitals?).

Notes

Line 4: For the word *sapān* (Aramaic loan) indicating a soapwort or alkaline plant and often occurring as an attribute of *ballukku*-aromatic, see the discussion of BM 42450+ obv. 5' (text B.2.3), with Finkel 2000, Text 16; eSAD S, s.v. *sapān(u)*.

Line 5: Ms. c (obv. 6–7) does not seem to use *simdu* and *barīrātu*-plant, but instead two different types *simdu* (also *sindu*), a milled cereal product or type of flour (cf. AHw 1045; CAD S, 272a for specifications of *simdu*). Based on the traces at the end of line 6 in Ms. c, I suggest reading "*sindu*-cereal (prepared from) wheat (GIG)", parallel to "*sindu*-cereal (prepared from) malt" in line 7. Note also BAM 52 rev. 1 (cf. Bácskay 2018, 208): LAGAB MUNU$_4$ *si-in-du šá ser-*[*qi*(?) . . .] "lumps of malt, milled *simdu*-cereal for a *ser*[*qu*-offering of strewn flour(?)]".

Line 7: For *ḫiāqu/ḫâqu* "to mix (mostly liquids)", cf. CAD Ḫ, 86–87; AHw 342b; SAA 10, No. 321: 14 (restored following SAA 10, No. 336 rev. 3; see Parpola 1983, *LAS* II, 247 (No. 251). For other attestations, see eBL (Dictionary; https://www.ebl.lmu.de/dictionary/hiāqu%20I). For Late Babylonian *mediae infirmae* verbal forms with an "overhanging" vowel, see e.g. von Soden 1995, GAG § 104g.

Line 8: Ms. b$_2$ obv. 4' uses only two litres of water and therefore would have to stipulate a lower capacity than two litres after boiling down the liquid in obv. 5'.

Both Finkel (2000, note on Text 22: 15–16) and CAD S, 381 regard the word *summunu* as a foodstuff. However, the context requires a quantity or measurement here. For *summunu* as "one eighth (of a litre)", see AHw 1058b sub *summunu*; Streck 1995, 66 § 57c with n. 151. See also Stadhouders and Johnson 2018, *FS Geller*, 575, 595 BM 78963 §7 (line 37), with a reference to a similar medical passage using *su-um-*<*mu*>*-nu* Ì *ḫal-ṣa* "one eighth litre of pressed oil".

Lines 10–14: These lines contain textual difficulties, but also close parallels to other Late Babylonian medical texts, which help to elucidate the procedure described here. A remarkably similar instruction is found in BAM 391: 10–26 // BM 42404 rev. 1'–6' (Finkel 2000, 155–156 Text 4), a prescription for a lotion (*marḫaṣu*) to treat the skin condition *rašûtu* (*rišûtu*).

Similar to the remedy for a woman described in mss. a–c, different ingredients are first boiled down in a liquid, after which further ingredients (in this case oil and *kamūnu*) are added (*ana libbi* ŠUB). Then the text continues:

> *a-na* 2-*ta* [21] ḪA.LA ŠUB-*šú a-na* [22] *ṭù-ur-ri* (var. *ṭù-ur-ru*)-*šú* ŠUB [23]A.MEŠ Ì.GIŠ *ina pa-ni* (var. IGI) [24] *tu-še-ep*-SU$^{?!}$ (var. *tu-še-ep*-<SU>)
> "You apply(?) it in two portions, by pouring it into his anus. Before (that treatment?) you *make use of*(?) water and oil."

The first parallel to mss. a–c, is the expression *a-na* 2-*ta* [21] ḪA.LA ŠUB-*šú*, which corresponds to *ana* 3-*ta zittu* ŠUB in line 10. Finkel (2000, 157) translated the latter passage as "three times for each half(?) (you add)", which makes little sense. Moreover, he suggested a very different interpretation of *a-na* 2-*ta* [21] ḪA.LA ŠUB-*šú* in BAM 391, translating "Twice you apply(?)" (ibid., 155 Text 4). However, both formulations are so parallel that they should have the same basic meaning. There are divergent analyses of numerals with the form 2-*ta*, 3-*ta* etc. Streck (1995, 21–25) showed that the TA should be understood as a phonetic complement reflecting a feminine form of the numeral and collected evidence for the rise of gender congruence between numeral and counted item (and for the decline of gender polarity between numeral and counted item) in the Late Babylonian texts. Numerals of this form stand for cardinal numbers (i.e., the TA does not have a distributive function). The word *zittu* (ḪA.LA) means "share, portion" (e.g., of an inheritance, property, payment), and is used in Late Babylonian texts in reference to the twelve sections of the zodiac signs (CAD Z, 139–148, esp. sub 5d). Although the dictionaries do not give references from medical texts, it seems likely that the expression *ana* 2/3-*ta zittu nadû*(ŠUB) means that the prepared medication was divided into two or three portions (*zittu*), applied one after another.

The expression *ana ṭú-ur-ri-šú tanaddi*(ŠUB) in BAM 391: 22 // is apparently parallel to *ana ṭúr-ri/ru-šu ta-šap-pak* in line 11 of the present text represented in mss. a and b. Although it is possible to read the latter phrase partially logographically *ana* DÚR-*ri-šú* "into her anus (*šuburru*)", SAD Vol. 2, 120a and CAD Ṭ, 166b *ṭurru* D (citing our passage sub a) convincingly argue for a loanword *ṭurru* II (also *durru*) "anus, rectum" (from Sumerian dúr) in both prescriptions (see also Streck 2009, *ZA* 99, 136–140). Thus, both prescriptions apply an enema injected into the anus (designated in BAM 391 // as *marḫāṣu* "lotion, rinse"). Cf. CAD Š/1, s.v. *šapāku* sub 2b.

In line 12, Finkel (2000, 156 (note to text 4 lines A 20–21), as well as 157, 159) erroneously reads *ana zittu kutallatu* ŠUB, translating this as "you apply it(?) to the dividing line of her back(?)". However, there is no sign ŠUB at the end of line 12 in ms. a (see Finkel's correct copy of BM 42507 on p. 157); the sentence beginning in line 12 continues up to the verb *tu-še-ep*-SU in line 14. The word *kutallatu* in the expression *ana zittu kutallatu* in line 12 should probably be understood as an attribute to *zittu*, "part, portion" (cf. the commentary in Finkel 2000, 156 for differing considerations). The form may be related to *kutallu* "back (of the neck); rear part; later time", for which a feminine plural form *kutallātu* is attested. But the dictionaries do not list an adjective or a feminine noun derived from *kutallu*. It may be a parallel formation as in (*w*)*arkatu* "rear, backside; buttocks", which is linked to "(*w*)*arki* "after, behind" and the adjective (*w*)*arkû* "rare, later". Thus, *zittu kutallatu* may be understood as the final part of the treatment or perhaps as an "after-treatment", administered after the three previous portions. Lines 13–14 apparently add a short instruction for this "after-treatment".

In mss. a–c, a combination of two plants (*nīnâtu* and *atartu*) and an infusion of *azallû*-plant are prescribed for the "after-treatment". The latter ingredient is spelled Ú.ZAL.LA in all manuscripts instead of ^{ú}A.ZAL.LÁ, which Finkel (2000, 156) regards as an indicator that the scribes of mss. a–c wrote the text from oral dictation). The term *nīnâtu* is tentatively interpreted as a fem. pl. of the medicinal plant *nīnû*, following the spelling ^{ú}*ni-na-a-tu*^{meš} in Prechel and Freydank 2014, No. 21: 1; SAD Vol. 4, 143. The *azallû*-plant was used by Mesopotamian healers as a plant to drive away sorrow/depression. The proposed identification with *Cannabis sativa* (Thompson 1949, 220–222) should be rejected. Cf. Böck 2022, 123–124, 130, 132 who describes the plant as a sedative or stimulant drug.

The analysis of the verb *tu-še-ep*-SU in line 14 is difficult. But it occurs several times in the Late Babylonian medical texts from Sippar discussed by Finkel (2000) in a comparable context:

> BAM 391 // BM 42404 rev. 4'–5': [23]A.MEŠ Ì.GIŠ *ina pa-ni* (var. IGI) [24] *tu-še-ep*-SU$^{?!}$ (var. *tu-še-ep*-<SU>)
> Finkel 2000, 164 Text 10 (*marḫāṣu* against "stricture" (*ḫiniqtu*)) line 45: A.MEŠ Ì.GIŠ *ina* IGI DÙ-*uš*
> "Before (the treatment(?), you *make use of*(?) water and oil."
>
> BM 79308: lines 8, 11 and 13: (*ana* 4 ḪA.LA ...) *tu-še-ép-pi-is-su* "you *use it*(?) (the medication) ... (in four portions)"

Notably, Finkel (2000, 156) read [*tu-š*]*e-ep-p*[*i*$^{?}$-x] in ms. a rev. 4, but the traces at the end of the line are not conclusive. He (ibid. 156 note to text 4 A 23–24) suggests that the form *tu-še-ep*-SU (or *tušeppessu*) should be connected with *epēšu* ("to make, to perform, to act") Š-stem ("to let someone make something"; occasionally also "to use", see CAD E, s.v. *epēšu* mng.

5b–3', also mng. 2f–6'). One would need to assume that the sign SU has a value /piš/ or /peš/ here (unattested so far). Alternatively, the interplay with the spelling *tu-še-ép-pi-is-su* may suggest that *tu-še-ep*-SU is a defective or abbreviated spelling omitting a syllable. Significant for the understanding of the whole sentence may also be the adverbial *ina pāni* "before" in two of the texts quoted above, which appears to contrast with *zittu kutallatu* in line 12 of our text under discussion (see above). Do the texts speak here of an "introductory" and a "concluding" part of the treatment?

It is not excluded that a more specific meaning stands behind *tu-še-ep-(pi)*-SU in the present context. Cf. possibly the Aramaic verbal roots šp' "to flow/pour out abundantly" and šwp "to pour out" (Sokoloff 2001, *A Dictionary of Jewish Babylonian Aramaic*, 1122b; cf. Geller (2024, 206) giving the meanings "to strain" and "to rub" respectively for attestations in the *Syriac Book of Medicines*).

Lines 15–17: The purpose statement formulated in these three lines also presents difficulties. Scurlock and Andersen (2005, 270 12.62, with n. 53) translate "(it is good for a woman) for whom giving birth and birth pangs are delayed". Apparently, they understand the word *tu-lu-di* as a noun for "birthgiving" (related to *(w)alādu*) but leave the word and its form unexplained (there is no attestation of such a word elsewhere). In this light, SAD Vol. 2, 58b suggests emending the text to *ana* MUNUS *ša tulûša*(?!) *takullû* (var. *takullâ*) *ikkaluši* "for a woman whose breasts(?) are affected by pain". See similarly, Reiner 2007, *JNES* 66, 49–50 ("for woman who is plagued by an itch"), sub *takullû* (also *tākulû*) "pain, itch".

Scurlock and Andersen (2005, 270 with n. 53) argue against interpreting the verb *ik-kal-lu-ši* in line 17 as a form of *akālu* "to eat" (in the sense of "to hurt") and assume an N-stem form of *kalû* "to hold back" (meaning "to be delayed"). Although the verb form *ik-kal-lu* would be the correct present tense form of *kalû* "to hold back" (N-stem), similar spellings of forms of *akālu* "to eat" with a geminated final consonant, are attested in first millennium BCE texts, often in Neo-Assyrian and Neo-Babylonian letters (Luukko 2004, 32). See, e.g., TCL 9, 101: 9–10 (Ebeling 1930–1934, *Neubabylonische Briefe aus Uruk*, 260–261 No. 326): *ḫa-bu-ru ik-kal-lu-ú* "(the sheep) eat the green grass"; YOS 3, 76: 33 (Ebeling 1930–1934, 64–65 No. 76): *li-kul-lu*$_4$ "let (the donkeys) eat (green grass)".

Mss. a–c appear to present slight variations in their formulation of the purpose statement. Thus, in ms. a rev. 6, the word [*t*]*a-kul-la* is followed by another word not found in mss. b and c, which I provisionally read as a second body part, namely GA[L$_4$.LA$^?$-*ša*] "her vulva/genitals". The word order suggests that GA[L$_4$.LA$^?$-*ša*] is a genitive attribute to *takullû* (i.e. "her breasts hurt her (stemming) from pain of her ge[nitals]"). Notably, if read correctly, the present prescription would be the first attestation of a treatment for women's breasts within Mesopotamian gynaecological materials.

E.2.2 BM 43110+: A School Tablet with Prescriptions for Women

The fragments of a small school tablet identified as one of the medical texts from Sippar which belonged to the archives of the Bēl-rēmanni-family (Jursa 1999; Finkel 2000) preserve a handful of prescriptions for women, two of them for suppositories.[386] One of the remedies is perhaps concerned with the promotion of fertility, while another one may have formed a treatment preparing the pregnant woman for delivery (perhaps to induce labour). Since no duplicates are known for the fragmentary remedies, these conclusions remain provisional.

List of Manuscripts

Siglum	Museum Number	Copy	Collation	Format; Ductus	Provenience
a	BM 43110 + BM 43291 + BM 43470 (81-7-1, 874 + 1055 + 1234)	Finkel, *FS Lambert*, Fig. 25	Coll.	Fragments of a single-column tablet in landscape format(?); Late Babylonian script; 6th/5th cent. BCE	Sippar

386 Cf. Leichty, Finkel and Walker 2019, *CBT* IV–V, 535.

Overview

i'	Prescription for a pregnant woman(?) (suppository) a obv. 1'–3'	1'–3'
ii'	Fragmentary prescription (suppository) a obv. 4'–5'	4'–5'
iii'	Fragmentary (rubric?) a obv. 6'	6'
iv'	Fragmentary prescription to promote conception / fertility a obv. 7'–9'	7'–10'[...
v''	Fragmentary prescription a rev. 1'–2'	...]11''–12''

Previous Edition and Discussion

Finkel 2000, *FS Lambert*, 173–174 Text 18 (copy; transliteration)
Electronic Babylonian Library Project (eBL) (https://www.ebl.lmu.de/library/BM.43110)

Transliteration

Beginning of ms. a obv. lost

1' a obv. 1' [DIŠ MUNUS *šà* ŠÀ-Š]À-*šú šá-pil-ma* MUNUS [BI x x x]

2' a obv. 2' [x x x x] ⌜x⌝ ÚḪ-*tú* PIŠ$_{10}$$^{!}$(KI).Í[D x x x x]

3' a obv. 3' [x x x x] ⌜ÚKUŠ⌝.LAGAB *ina* Ì ḪI.Ḫ[I-*ma ana* Š]À.T[ÙR-*šú* GAR-*an*]

4' a obv. 4' [DIŠ KI.MIN$^{?}$ x x] x x x ri [x x] GÁN.GÁN

5' a obv. 5' [x x x x x *ina* Ì.GIŠ$^{?}$ ^{šim}G]IG SUMUN Ì.UDU ḪI.ḪI

6' a obv. 6' [.......................................].GA

7' a obv. 7' [^{munus}NU.PEŠ$_{4}$ *ana šu-r*]*e*$^{?}$-*e* Ù.⌜TU$^{?}$⌝

8' a obv. 8' [..........................] x 1/2$^{?}$ ⌜GAM⌝.M[A$^{?}$ x x]

9' a obv. 9' [..........................] x [x x x]

10' a obv. 10' [..........................] x [x x x]

Ms. a obv. breaks

11'' a rev. 1' [............. B]URU$_{5}$.ḪABRUD.D[A^{mušen} (x)]

12'' a rev. 2' [............. *ina me*]-⌜*e*$^{?}$⌝ NU *pa-tan* NA[G]

remainder of ms. a rev. left blank (except for erased signs)

Bound Transcription and Translation

Beginning lost

1' [*šumma sinništu ša liblibb*]*īšu*(?) *šapil-ma sinništu* [*šī*(?) . . . . . .] 2' [...]... *ru'tīta kibrīta* [. . . . . .] 3' [. . . . . .] *errâ ina šamni tubal*[*lal-ma ana*] *šassūr*[*īšu tašakkan*]

1' [If a woman's foe]tus(?) is low and [that] woman [. . . . . .] 2' [. . . . . .]... *ru'tītu*-sulphur, *kibrītu*-sulphur, [. . . . . .] 3' [. . . . . .] (and) colocynth you mix with oil. [Then you insert (it) into her womb (viz. vagina).

4' [DIŠ KI.MIN$^?$ ...] ... [. . . . . .] ... 5' [. . . . . . *ina šaman*] *kanakti labiri lipî tuballal*

4' [Alternatively(?), ...] ... [...]... 5' [. . . . . .], you mix (it) [with] old [oil of] *kanaktu*-aromatic (and) tallow.

6' [. . . . . .] ...

6' *too fragmentary for translation*

7' [*lā erītu ana šūr*]*ê šūludi*(?) 8' [. . . . . .] . . . *mišil ṣum*[*lalû*(?) . . .] 9'–10' *traces*

7' [To enable a woman who is not pregnant to get] pregnant (and) to bear (children): 8' [. . . . . .]... half (a shekel?) of *ṣum*[*lalû*-aromatic$^?$, . . .] 9'–10' *too fragmentary for translation*

Ms. a obv. breaks; gap of unknown length

11'' [. . . . . .] *iṣṣūr ḫurri* 12'' [. . . . . . *ina m*]*ê lā patān iš*[*atti*]

11'' [. . . . . . of a] partridge 12'' [. . . . . .] she dr[inks] (it) [in] [wa]ter on an empty stomach.

Remainder of rev. left blank (except for erased signs)

Notes

Lines 1'–3': The restoration [*šà* ŠÀ-Š]À-*šú* instead of [*šà* Š]À-*šú* in line 1' assumes a superfluous pronominal suffix -*šú*, which was added because the usual expression *ša libbīša* "her foetus" (sometimes written *šà* ŠÀ-*šà*, as a variant to *šá* ŠÀ-*šá*) had become a frozen logogram (thus also Finkel 2000, 174). Compare the spelling in BM 42313+ rev. 11 (text A.2.2). However, if we take the spelling *šà* ŠÀ-ŠÀ-*šú* seriously, it might have to be read as a variant expression *ša liblibbīša*, with the same meaning as *ša libbīša* "her foetus". The duplicated form *liblibbu* for "foetus" was probably influenced by the parallel expression *līp*(*i*) *līpi* (also *lib*(*bi*)*libbi*), "descendent", from *līpu* "son" (cf. AHw 555a; CAD L, 179–181; written with a different logogram ŠÀ.BAL.BAL, however).

The interpretation of line 1' follows Finkel (2000, 173–174), who suggests the prescription was concerned with inducing labour in a woman in an advanced stage of pregnancy (shortly before delivery, when the foetus shifts its position downward towards the birth canal). An alternative restoration at the beginning of line 1' could be [DIŠ MUNUS Š]À-*šú šá-pil-ma* "if a woman's heart is low", standing for a depressed mood, cf. CAD Š/1, 424 s.v. *šapālu* sub 1f, with examples from medical texts. So far, no other text concerned with depression in a female patient is known.

The logogram for *ru'tītu*-sulphur in line 2' is written in an unusual form (ÚḪ-*tú* instead of ÚḪ-^{d}ÍD), similar to the following ingredient *kibrītu*-sulphur, which is rendered as KI.Í[D] instead of PIŠ$_{10}$-^{d}ÍD.

Lines 4'–5': Perhaps the first fragmentary signs in line 4' should be read ⸢3 1/2 NINDA⸣ "three and a half NINDA" (= 350 ml). For oil perfumed with *kanaktu*-aromatic in line 5', often mentioned beside other types of oil or fat, see CAD K, 135–136. The present prescription appears to have been for a suppository.

Line 6': Perhaps, this single line contained a Sumerian rubric.

Lines 7'–8': For similar purpose statements, see e.g., BM 42313+ rev. 33 // BM 42333 obv. 5: DIŠ MUNUS NU PEŠ$_4$ *a-na šu-ri-i* "If a woman does not get pregnant, to enable (her) to get pregnant"; BM 424313+ rev. 37 // BM 42333 obv. 1: ^{munus}*la a-lit-ti* [*ana*] *šu-ri-*⸢*i* "to enable a barren woman to get pregnant" (text A.2.2); STT 98: 2', 4' (text A.1.1): [DIŠ$^{?}$] ⸢MUNUS⸣ NU PEŠ$_4$ *ana* ⸢PEŠ$_4$⸣ "[If] a woman does not get pregnant, to let her get pregnant"; BAM 244: 8 (text B.1.1): [^{munus}]*la a-lit-ta* <*ana*> *šu-*[*ri*]*-im-m*[*a* ...] "<to> enable an infertile [woman to get] pregnant"; BAM 243: 1': DIŠ MUNUS NU Ù.TU ⸢*ana*⸣ *š*[*u-ri-i*] "If a woman does not bear, to en[able her to get pregnant]". Note also BAM 241 iii 7': [MUNUS N]U *a-li-da-at ana ur-re-*⸢*e*⸣ [...] "to impregnate a barren woman [...]" (see also N. 4001: 11' (text B.2.1) for another example of the D-stem of *erû*).

For *ṣumlalû*-aromatic (^{šim}GAM.MA), see also BAM 244 obv. 27 (text B.1.1, there used in the form of a powder, as an ingredient for a poultice to make an infertile woman conceive). For this plant, see Stol 1979, *On Trees*, 18–19; cf. Köcher 1995, AUWE 10, 211b.

E.2.3 BM 47801: A Fragment of a Ritual for a Woman Related to an Eclipse

This fragment of a tablet completely ruled with lines is written in a Late Babylonian script; it was excavated by Hormuzd Rassam and may perhaps stem from Babylon.[387] On the reverse of ms. a (lines 28''–31''), there is a fragmentary colophon preceded by a partially preserved catchline (line 28''), reading [*e-nu-ma*] ⸢MUNUS⸣ ⸢ITI⸣ Ù.TU-*šú* KU$_4$-*am-ma* [^{iti}BÁRA (*ana šūtuqi*)] "[When] the month of a woman's delivery has arrived and [it is the month Nisannu – (in order to let it pass by)]". This is the incipit of a ritual (known from KAR 223 and duplicates), recently presented in a new edition (Stadhouders and Steinert 2018; Hätinen 2019) and included again in this volume (text D.3.1). The latter ritual was concerned with delaying the inauspicious birth of a child scheduled to take place in the month Nisannu. The ritual in BM 47801 has a different objective, but it seems to have belonged to a thematically related group of texts concerned with removing an evil omen.

The obverse of BM 47801 contains a purificatory ritual for a woman, featuring offerings to Ea, Šamaš and Asalluḫi and the fabrication of a substitute figurine, followed by a prayer to the sun god, who is also addressed in KAR 223 // as a deity responsible for pregnant women and women in childbirth (see text D.3.1). Significantly, the addressed deities and the ritual procedure making use of a substitute figurine connect BM 47801 with the Namburbi rituals to remove evil signaled by a negative ominous sign (Maul 1994). The reverse of BM 47801 confirms this conclusion, mentioning an eclipse (*anta(l)lû*/AN.TA.LÙ, line 27'') as the source of the woman's impurity. It is possible that BM 47801 contained a Namburbi-like ritual dealing with evil signs affecting women. Similar to the apotropaic rituals in KAR 223 //, the present ritual may have averted negative signs that occurred during pregnancy or delivery.

List of Manuscripts

Siglum	Museum Number	Copy	Collation	Format; Ductus	Provenience
a	BM 47801 (81-11-3, 508)	Pl. 48	Coll.	Fragment of a single-column tablet; Late Babylonian script; ca. 5th–3rd cent. BCE[388]	uncertain; perhaps Babylon

387 Leichty, Finkel and Walker 2019, *CBT* IV–V, 656, 672.

388 Measurements: ca. 3.5 x 5.8 x 2.5 cm.

Overview

i'	Ritual for purifying a woman from evil signaled by an omen (eclipse)	...]1'–27''
	– Fragmentary ritual instructions: preparation of two substitutes for the patient (a obv. 1'–9')	...]1'–9'
	– Fragmentary prayer to the sun god Šamaš: [*Šamaš šar ša*]*mê u erṣeti bēl kitti* [*u mīšari muštēšer el*]*âti u šaplâti* (a obv. 10'–16')	10'–16'[...
	– Further ritual instructions and recitation (*ašḫuṭ ašḫuṭ*): washing over the substitute and disposal (a rev. 1'–11')	...]17''–27''
ii'	Catchline and colophon (a rev. 12'–15')	28''–31''[...

Previous Edition and Discussion

Electronic Babylonian Library Project (eBL) (https://www.ebl.lmu.de/library/BM.47801; photo, transliteration)

Transliteration

About one or two lines lost from the beginning of ms. a obv.

1' a obv. 1' [x x x x] ⸢x x x x x x⸣ [.............]

2' a obv. 2' [*ina še-rim ina* ^{d}U]TU.È ÙR SAR A KÙ.[(GA) SUD ......]

3' a obv. 3' [KEŠDA.MEŠ *ana* ^{d}]⸢*é*⸣-*a* ^{d}UTU *u* ^{d}*asal-lú-ḫi tara-kás* UDU KÙ [BAL-*qí* ......]

4' a obv. 4' [x x x MUNUS *šu*]-⸢*a*⸣-*tu*$_{4}$ NÍG.NA GI.IZI.LÁ [*tuš-ba-a'-šú* ....]

5' a obv. 5' [NU *di-na-ni-šá šá*$^{?}$] ⸢ZÌ⸣.DA *ina* KI *te-ṣir* [................]

6' a obv. 6' [x x x]-*ma ina* UGU NU$^{!}$(PAP) *di-na-ni-šá šá* ZÌ.D[A ...]

7' a obv. 7' [NU *di-na-ni-š*]*á*$^{?}$ NITA *u* MUNUS *šá* [IM DÙ-*uš*$^{?}$ (. . .)]

8' a obv. 8' [x x x MUNUS$^{?}$ *ina*] ŠU.MIN-*šú* ÍL-*ma at-ta k*[*i-am* DU$_{11}$.GA$^{?}$ . . . .]

9' a obv. 9' [GIN$_{7}$ *an-nam* DU$_{11}$.GA$^{?}$]-*ú* MUNUS BI *ana* ^{d}UTU U[R$_{5}$.GIM DU$_{11}$.GA (...)]

10' a obv. 10' [ÉN ^{d}UTU LUGAL A]N-*e u* KI-*tim* EN *kit-ti* [*u mi-šá-ri*]

11' a obv. 11' [*muš-te-šir* A]N.TA.MEŠ *u* KI.TA.MEŠ [(...) ^{lú}TI.LA *u* ^{lú}ÚŠ]

12' a obv. 12' [x x x *b*]*a*$^{?}$-*ar kal mim-ma šum-šú* [............]

13' a obv. 13' [x x x x] *at-ta-ma* DU$_{8}$ *ka-si*-⸢*i*⸣ [...............]

14' a obv. 14' [x x x m]an$^{?}$ *mu-kal-lim*$^{!}$ ZALAG$^{!}$ GAR$^{?!}$ *kit*-[*ti*$^{?}$.......]

15' a obv. 15' [x x x] ⸢MAḪ$^{?}$⸣-*ti* ^{d}UTU ḪUL *š*[*u*$^{?}$-*ú* ....]

16' a obv. 16' *only traces preserved*

Ms. a obv. breaks; gap of unknown length

Beginning of ms. a rev. lost

17'' a rev. 1' [x x x x] ⸢x x x x⸣ [...............]

18" a rev. 2' [GIN$_7$ *tu-u*]*š*$^?$*-ta-ad-bi-bu* $^{\textit{he-pí}}$ $^{\ulcorner \textit{eš-šú} \urcorner}$ [......]

19" a rev. 3' [x x x x]x *ana* ^{d}UTU.ŠÚ.A [......]

20" a rev. 4' [*ana* UGU NU *di-na-n*]*i-šá* A TU$_5$*-šú* UR$_5$.GIM [DU$_{11}$.GA (...)]

21" a rev. 5' [(NU *at-ta*) *ana pu-ḫi*$^?$]*-ia ad-din-ka ana di-*⌜*na-ni*⌝*-í*[*a*$^?$ *ad-din-ka*$^?$]

22" a rev. 6' [*aš-ḫu-uṭ mim*]*-ma lem-nu šá* SU*-ia*$_5$ [*ana* UGU*-ka*]

23" a rev. 7' [*aš-ḫu-uṭ mim*]*-ma lem-nu šá* UZU*-ia*$_5$ [*ana* UGU*-ka*]

24" a rev. 8' [*aš-ḫu-uṭ mim*]*-ma lem-nu šá* SA*-ia*$_5$ [*ana* UGU*-ka*]

25" a rev. 9' [x x x x]x ⌜x*-ma*⌝ *le-qé* [......]

26" a rev. 10' [x x x x]*-di*$^?$*-šú* KEŠDA DU$_8$*-ma* [......]

27" a rev. 11' [x x *ina* ḪUL *šá*$^?$ A]N.TA.LÙ *el-let ip-qid* x[......]

Catchline:

28" a rev. 12' [*e-nu-ma*] ⌜MUNUS⌝ ⌜ITI⌝ ⌜*šá*⌝ Ù.TU*-šú* KU$_4$*-am-ma* [^{iti}BÁRA (*ana šu-tu-qí*)$^?$]

Colophon:

29" a rev. 13' [x x x x] *blank* [...............][389]

30" a rev. 14' [x x x DU]B$^?$ ⌜$^{md+}$AG$^?$⌝*-i-din-*⌜*nam*⌝ ⌜^{d}AMAR.UTU⌝-[............]

31" a rev. 15' [x x x x x] ⌜x x x⌝ [....................]

Ms. a rev. breaks; one to two lines lost

Bound Transcription and Translation

About one or two lines lost from the beginning of the obv.

1' [...] . . . . . .[...] 2' [*ina šēri ina*] *ṣīt* [*š*]*amši ūra tašabbiṭ mê ell*[*ūti tasallaḫ* . . .] 3' [*riksī ina maḫar*] *Ea Šamaš u Asalluḫi tarakkas immera ella* [*tanaqqi* . . .] 4' [. . . *sinništu šu*]*ātu nig-nakka gizillâ* [*tušbaʾšu* . . .] 5' [*ṣalam dinānīša ša*] *qēmi ina qaqqari teṣṣer* [. . . . . .] 6' [. . .]*-ma ina muḫḫi ṣalam dinānīša ša qēmi* [*izzaz*(?) . . .] 7' [*ṣalam dinānīš*]*a zikar u sinniš ša*(?) [*ṭīdi teppuš*(?) ...] 8' [... *sinništu ina*] *qātīšu inaššī-ma attā k*[*īam taqabbi*(?) ...] 9' [*kīma annâ taqtab*]*û sinništu šī ana Šamaš k*[*īam iqabbi* (. . .)]

1' [. . . . . .] ... [. . . . . .]. 2' [In the morning, at s]unrise you sweep the roof, [you sprinkle] pure water, [...] 3' [... in front] of Ea, Šamaš and Asalluḫi you set up [offering arrangements]. [You sacrifice] a pure sheep [...], 4' [...] you move] censer and torch [past th]at [woman ...]. 5' You draw [an image of her substitute] with flour on the ground [...], 6' [....] and [she steps(?)] on the substitute image of flour [...]. 7' [You make a] male or(?) female [clay figurine (serving) as a substitute for h]er [...]. 8' [..., the woman] shall lift (it) up in her hands. Then you [speak] as foll[ows: "...]." 9' [When you have said this], that woman [speaks] to Šamaš as fo[llows: (...)]

---

389 Presumably, this line was left blank.

10' [ÉN *Šamaš šar ša*]*mê u erṣeti bēl kitti* [*u mīšari* (. . .)]

11' [*muštēšer el*]*âti u šaplâti* [(. . .) *balṭi u mīti*]

12' [...] *bār*(*i*) *kal mimma šumšu* [. . . . . .]
13' [. . .] *attā-ma pāṭir kasî* [. . . . . .]
14' [. . .]. . . *mukallim nūri šākin*(?) *kit*[*ti*(?) . . .]
15' [. . .] *ṣīrti Šamaš lumnu š*[*ū*(?) . . . . . .]
16' *only traces preserved*

10' [Incantation: "Šamaš, king of hea]ven and earth, lord of truth [and justice, (...)],
11' [who guides right] the upper world and lower world, [(...) the living and the dead(?)],
12' [...] who oversees everything that exists, [...],
13' you are [...], one who releases the bound one, [...],
14' [...] ..., who brings light, who establishes(?) just[ice(?), ...],
15' [...] foremost [...], Šamaš – th[at(?)] evil [. . . . . .]
16' *only traces preserved*

Ms. a obv. breaks; gap of unknown length

Beginning of ms. a rev. lost

17'' [...] ... [. . . . . .] 18'' [*kīma tu*]*štadbibu*(*šu*?) *ḫepi eššu* [. . . . . .] 19'' [...]... *ana ereb šamši* [...] 20'' [*ana muḫḫi ṣalam dinān*]*īša mê turammukšu kīam* [*iqabbi*(?) (. . .)] 21'' [*ana pūhī*]*ya addinka ana dinānīy*[*a addinka*] 22'' [*ašḫuṭ mim*]*ma lemnu ša zumrīya* [*ana muḫḫīka*] 23'' [*ašḫuṭ mim*]*ma lemnu ša šīrīya* [*ana muḫḫīka*] 24'' [*ašḫuṭ mim*]*ma lemnu ša šer'ānīya* [*ana muḫḫīka*] 25'' [. . .] . . .-*ma leqe* [. . .] 26'' [. . .]. . . *riksa tapaṭṭar-ma* [. . .] 27'' [. . . *ina lumni ša a*]*ttallî ellet ipqid* . . .[. . .]

17'' [...] ... [. . . . . .], 18'' [*When you*] have let (her) recite (the prayer?); *new break* (in the original) [...]. 19'' [...] towards sunset [...]. 20'' You wash her with water [over] her [substitute figurine]. (Then) [she says(?)] as follows: [(...)] 21'' "I have given you as my [substitute], [I have given you] as m[y] replacement. 22'' [I have cast off any]thing bad from my body [onto you], 23'' [I have cast off any]thing evil from my flesh [onto you], 24'' [I have cast off any]thing evil of my sinews [onto you]! 25'' [...] and take (it away) [...]!" 26'' [...] ..., you remove the ritual arrangement. Then [...] 27'' [... *from the evil*(?) of the ec]lipse she is cleaned, she(?) has been entrusted [*to* ...].

Catchline:
28'' [*enūma*] *sinništu arḫu ša alādīšu īrubam-ma* [*nissanu* (*ana šūtuqi*)]

28'' [When] the month in which a woman (is due to) deliver has arrived, and [(it is) the month Nisannu, (to make it pass by).]

Colophon:
29'' [(...)] *blank* [(...)]
30'' [... *tup*]*pi*(?) *Nabû-iddina*(?) *Marduk*-[. . . . . .]
31' *only traces preserved*

29'' [...] (*one line left blank*?) [...]
30'' [... tabl]et(?) of Nabû-iddina(?), Marduk-[. . .],
31'' [...] ... [...]

Ms. a rev. breaks; one to two lines lost

Notes

Lines 1'–4': These ritual instructions share many similarities with the Namburbi rituals. The latter rituals usually began in the morning, with setting up offerings to the gods Ea, Šamaš and Asalluḫi (Maul 1994, 48ff.), before the sun god could be asked to undo the evil omen that threatened the patient. Often, portable offering tables (*paṭīru*, GI.DU$_8$) were set up for that purpose, but in ms. a line 3', the formulation seems to be *riksī rakāsu* "to arrange offerings", suggested by the verb *tarakkas*. The offering materials in the Namburbi rituals usually consist of bread, *mersu*-confection, drinks such as beer, water or milk, and fragrant incense burned on a censer. In some cases, also an animal had to be sacrificed. In ms. a line 3', a "pure sheep" (*immeru ellu/ebbu*, UDU KÙ) is sacrificed (for similar instructions in Namburbi rituals, see Maul 1994, 54 *passim*).

Lines 5'–6': The reading and restoration of lines 5'–6' is inspired by the Namburbi rituals. At first sight, a restoration [ZÌ.(-)SUR.RA] "(magic) flour circle" at the beginning of line 5' seems most likely, since in magic rituals the site of an offering is often separated and protected by surrounding it with a circle of flour. The usual expression in this context is *zisurrâ lamû* "to surround with a flour circle". In ms. a, however, the practitioner has to "draw" (*eṣēru*) something on the ground with flour. In Namburbi rituals, the expression *šiddī ša qēmi*(ZÌ.DA) *šadādu* "to draw lines of flour" is attested in this context (Maul 1994, 56, 59), and the missing word at the beginning of line 5' might be *šid-di*. Yet, the following line 6', explicitly speaks of a "substitute figurine of flour" representing the patient, which rather suggests the restoration [NU *di-na-ni-šá šá*?] ⌜ZÌ⌝.DA *ina* KI *te-ṣir* at the beginning of line 5'. This means an image of the patient was drawn on the ground with flour used for a first rite of transfer and purification.

In order to undo the impact of the omen affecting the patient, Namburbi rituals instruct the healer to make a figurine representing the omen carrier (often an animal), which was later removed and destroyed, and which took the evil away from the patient (Maul 1994, 72ff., 85ff., 250: 10–11, 265: 9', 278: 1'). However, Namburbi rituals also mention "substitute figurines/images" (*ṣalam andunāni/dināni*) representing the patient that were used for similar rites of transfer and purification (Maul 1994, 74–75). In ms. a line 6' flour is mentioned as the substance of the substitute image before the line breaks. Possible restorations in the break may be *izzaz* (GUB-*az*) "she (the patient) should stand (on the substitute figure)", *ikabbas* "she should tread on" or (*qātīša*) *mê irammuk* "she washes (her hands) with water" (over the substitute figure). Similar actions are performed in a Namburbi ritual against "a fall of fire", a fire that was caused in a man's house by lightning (Maul 1994, 138: 118–121).

For washing oneself over the substitute figurine, see also Borger 1967, 6 line 47; Maul 1994, 68–69, with 138: 121ff.; 72ff. and further references. Later in line 20'' of ms. a, the patient also washes herself over a second substitute (figurine), see the notes below.

Lines 7'–9': It is not entirely clear whether the line separating lines 6' and 7' is a ruling indicating a new section. However, the ritual seems to continue in line 7' with the preparation of a second substitute. In contrast to the flour drawing in lines 5'–6', that substitute was probably a figurine made of clay, since the patient appears to lift up the substitute figurine in her hands in line 8', presenting it to Šamaš, before she utters the prayer to the sun god written out in lines 10'ff. It remains uncertain whether a pair of figurines (a male and female one) had to be made here, or only one figurine which could be male or female. At least in the recitation in line 21'', the substitute figurine is addressed in the singular.

The reading MUNUS BI "that woman" in line 9' is crucial for identifying the gender of the patient, also indicated by feminine pronominal suffixes that occur several times in the text (lines 6', 7', 20''). A different reading of line 9' is proposed by eBL. See also the comment on the catchline (line 28'').

Lines 10'–16': The beginning of the prayer (lines 10'–11') appears to be identical with the opening of the prayer "Šamaš 45": *Šamaš šar šamê erṣeti bēl kitti u mīšari muštēšer elâti u šaplâti* "Šamaš, king of heaven and earth, lord of truth and justice, who guides right the upper and the lower world", which was recited in the sixth house of the *Bīt rimki* ritual (cf. Mayer 1976, *Gebetsbeschwörungen*, 416; that prayer may be identical to "Šamaš 86" or "Šamaš 91"; Mayer 1976, 420–421; cf. Abusch and Schwemer 2016, CMAwR 2, text 9.5). However, the remainder of the prayer in ms. a does not duplicate that text.

Alternatively, it is possible to restore the beginning of the prayer in ms. a following the prayer "Šamaš 8", *Šamaš dayyān elâti u šaplâti* (*bēl kitti u mīšari muštēšer elâti u šaplâti*) "Šamaš, judge of the upper and lower world", which was used in a Namburbi ritual to ward off the evil signaled by a monstrous birth (*izbu*) of a domestic animal in a man's household (Mayer 1976, 411; Maul 1994, *Zukunftsbewältigung*, 336ff. LKA 114 obv. 15–22 //). However, also "Šamaš 8" differs from the text in lines 12'ff.

In the gap at following *muštēšer elâti u šaplâti* in line 11', eBL suggests restoring ^{lú}ÚŠ TI-*ṭu* "(you guide right) the dead (and) the living (person)", see similarly BMS 6: 99 and dupl. (Ebeling 1953a, *Handerhebung*, 48; Mayer 1976, 504 "Šamaš 1"): ^{d}UTU *muš-te-šir mīti*(^{lú}ÚŠ) (*u*) *balṭi*($^{(lú)}$TI.(LA)).

Line 12': For the phrase *bār(i) kal mimma šumšu*, see also the prayer "Šamaš 1" (BMS 6: 99 and dupl.; Ebeling 1953a, 48; Mayer 1976, 504).

Line 14': Some of the preserved signs in this line seem to be corrupt; the text should list two further laudatory epithets of Šamaš. For *mukallim nūri*, see also "Šamaš 1" (BMS 6: 98 and dupl.; Ebeling 1953a, 48; Mayer 1976, 504). The signs following ZALAG are read as *ía*? *kal*? [...] in eBL; the reading GAR!? *kit*-[*ti*] proposed here is tentative; the usual epithet is *bēl kitti u mīšari* "lord of truth and justice".

Line 15': At the beginning of the line, perhaps restore *ina ilūtika/qibītika/uznīka ṣirti* "through your excellent divinity/command/wisdom".

Line 18'': Another possible restoration here is [*u*]*š-ta-ad-bi-bu* "(when) she has been made to recite".

Line 19'': The phrase "towards the west / sunset" could be restored to *pānīšu ana ereb šamši tašakkan* "you direct its (the figurine's) face toward sunset", reminiscent of similar passages found elsewhere in rituals disposing of magical substitutes / figurines, cf. Abusch and Schwemer 2011, CMAwR 1, 186 text 7.8, line 36' (addressing the witch in an incantation: *ana ḫurri ša ereb šamši pānīki aš[kun]* "I have dir[ected] your face to a hole toward sunset". In that anti-witchcraft ritual, a representation of witchcraft in the form of a tongue is buried in a hole.

Line 20'': Very likely there is nothing missing after the restored [DU_{11}.GA] (similar to line 9'); either a second or a third person subject is possible here (*iqabbi* or *taqabbi*, or possibly also *tušadbabšu* "you make her say (the following) words"), but most likely the patient was reciting the following prayer formula, since it is phrased in the first person.

Lines 21''–24'': The restoration of lines 21''–24'' follows similar incantation formulas known by the title *ašḫuṭ ašḫuṭ* which are recited in Namburbi and other rituals in connection with rites of transfer, see e.g. Maul 1994, 72ff., with 139: 137–139 (Namburbi against "fall of fire"); 306: 10'–11' (Eidechsen-Namburbi); 317–318: 36–40 (Hunde-Namburbi); 487: 38–41 (Universalnamburbi 2); Lambert 1957–1958, 297–298; Borger 1967, 10. The verb *šaḫāṭu* in this context refers to rinsing off the impurity or evil from the patient's body onto the substitute, see e.g. Maul 1994, 139: 137. Fittingly, ms. a line 20'' requests that the patient washes herself (*ramāku*) over the substitute figurine.

Line 25'': This line still seems to belong to the recitation spoken by the woman, addressing the substitute figurine. A possible restoration could be [*lumnī ta-ba*]*l-ma le-qé* [*ana* . . .] "[Take away the evil affecting me] and take it (with you) [to ... (perhaps to the netherworld or Apsû?)]!"

Line 26'': A plausible restoration from the context at the beginning of the line may be [*ana* ÍD ŠUB]-*di*?-*šú* "you throw it (*tanaddīšu*) into the river", signaling the disposal of the substitute figurine. See similarly in Namburbi rituals, e.g. Maul 1994, 85ff., 140: 140, 307: 24', 319: 57, 488: 60 for the disposal of substitutes in the river. Alternatively, the pronominal suffix -*šú* may refer to the patient.

Line 27'': It is uncertain whether the present ritual was concerned with a lunar or a solar eclipse, and why this sign was particularly problematic for a woman (eclipses are usually seen as omens affecting the king in particular). A possible background for the ritual in ms. a may have been the occurrence of an eclipse during a woman's delivery, but there is no further confirmative textual evidence. However, Late Babylonian horoscopes and nativity omens sometimes refer to the case of a baby born during the time of an eclipse. Rochberg (1998, *Babylonian Horoscopes*, 40–42, 44–45) notes that the eclipses mentioned in horoscopes do not coincide with the day of birth but often took place weeks or months earlier or later. One example of a Late Babylonian text with nativity omens (BM 32488) concerns predictions for a child born during a lunar or solar eclipse. Several of the predictions are negative for the child (e.g. predicting early death or poverty). Perhaps significantly for the ritual edited here, in some cases the dispersal of "the house of his father" is predicted (col. i 10', 17').[390] Another Late Babylonian text with nativity omens deals with the case that during the day of conception of a child an eclipse took place under the influence of different signs of the zodiac (VAT 7851 rev. circular diagram; Weidner 1967, 12–15; Monroe 2016, *Advice from the Stars*, 129–135). The predictions resemble each other in that they signal that the child will be attacked by different agents of disease from its birth (lit. "from (the moment it leaves) the womb of its mother").

For a Namburbi ritual against the effects of a lunar eclipse, cf. Maul 1994, 458ff., and 51 n. 56 for a Namburbi ritual against a solar eclipse. There is also an earlier tradition of birth omens found in the hemerological series *Iqqur īpuš*, which contains a passage making predictions for the birth of a child in the months of the year (Labat 1965, 132–135 §64). Here, specifically birth in the month Nisannu predicts disaster for the household of that child, for which case we have prophylactic rituals to postpone the birth to the next month to avoid the envisaged misfortune (see *infra* text D.3.1).

Interestingly, in line 27'' of ms. a, the patient is said to be "pure" (*ellet*), presumably referring to the removal of the malignant influence of the omen. The end of line 27'' remains unclear to me; the verb *ipqid* "he/she entrusted" usually occurs with reference to deities who are supposed to entrust the patient to his or her personal gods or protective spirits. In comparable contexts when the patient is the subject of *paqādu*, the stative form is normally used instead of a preterite.

Line 30'': The name Nabû-iddin(a) tentatively restored as the name of the scribe is attested for numerous individuals in Neo-/Late Babylonian times (see https://prosobab.leidenuniv.nl/). The following divine name Marduk may belong to a second personal name; however, it is lacking a personal name classifier.

390 I am grateful to Marvin Schreiber, who is preparing an edition of this text and shared his transliteration and translation with me.

E.2.4 BM 48710: A Fragment of a Remedy Collection for Women

This fragment of a two-column tablet comes from the excavations of Hormuzd Rassam in Babylonia and is listed in the register of the British Museum's Babylonian Collection as originating from Babylon.[391] The fragment presumably belonged to a larger collection of remedies for women, since the remnants of a few lines of text in columns i' and ii' written in a small script indicate that the prescriptions in question were employed for female patients (see line 8'). The fragment may have represented a similar compendium of material as found in texts such as BM 38624+ or BM 40152, likewise from Babylon (see texts A.2.2, C.1.8).

List of Manuscripts

Siglum	Museum Number	Copy	Collation	Format; Ductus	Provenience
a	BM 48710 (81-11-3, 1421)	–	Coll.	Fragment of a two-column tablet; Late Babylonian script; ca. 6th/5th cent. BCE(?)[392]	Babylon

Overview

i' Fragmentary prescription (suppository) ...]1'–9' [...
a obv.$^?$ i' 1'–9'
ii'' Fragmentary 10''
a obv.$^?$ ii' 1'
iii'' Fragmentary prescription 11''–13'' [...
a obv.$^?$ ii' 2'–4'

Previous Edition and Discussion

Electronic Babylonian Library Project (eBL) (https://www.ebl.lmu.de/library/BM.48710) (transliteration; photos)

Transliteration

Beginning of ms. a obv.$^?$ i' lost

1' a obv.$^?$ i' 1' [...............] ^{ú}KUR.⌈RA$^?$⌉

2' a obv.$^?$ i' 2' [...............]x 1 GÍN ^{šim}LI

3' a obv.$^?$ i' 3' [......... x GÍN ^{ú}AN.D]AḪ.ŠUM 1 GÍN Ú BABBAR

4' a obv.$^?$ i' 4' [......... x GÍN *zi*]-*bu-u* 2 GÍN ^{ú}*nam-ruq-qa*

5' a obv.$^?$ i' 5' [......... URUDU SUMUN *šá*$^?$] ⌈*šá*$^?$⌉-*ḫi-tú* ŠUB

6' a obv.$^?$ i' 6' [. .. .. x G]ÍN$^?$ ILLU 1 GÍN MÚD ^{giš}EREN

7' a obv.$^?$ i' 7' [. .. ..] GAR *ana* DIDA SIG$_5$-*tú*

8' a obv.$^?$ i' 8' [. .. ..] *ana* ŠÀ.TÙR-*šá* GAR

9' a obv.$^?$ i' 9' [. .. ..]x [(x)]

Ms. a obv.$^?$ i' breaks; gap of unknown length

391 Leichty, Finkel and Walker 2019, CBT IV–V, 695.
392 Measurements: 3.1 cm x 3.6 cm x 1.5 cm.

Beginning of ms. a obv.? ii' lost

10''	a obv.? ii' 1'	i[m . . . .]

11''	a obv.? ii' 2'	DIŠ MUNUS *š*[*à* ŠÀ-*šà*? ŠUB? . . . .]
12''	a obv.? ii' 3'	ú x[. . . . .]
13''	a obv.? ii' 4'	K[A? . . . .]

Ms. a obv.(?) ii' breaks; remainder lost; reverse not preserved

Bound Transcription and Translation

Beginning of ms. a obv.? i' lost

1' [. . . . . .] *nīnû* 2' [. . . . . .] *ištēn šiqil burāšu* 3' [. . . . . . *šiqil and*]*aḫšu ištēn šiqil šammu peṣû* 4' [. . . . . . *šiqil z*]*ibû šina šiqil namruqqa* 5' [. . . *erû labiru ša*(?)] *šaḫittu*(?) *nadû*(?) 6' [. . . . . . *šiq*]*il ḫīlu ištēn šiqil dām erēni* 7' [. . . . . .] *tašakkan*(?) *ana billati našipti* 8' [. . . . . .] *ana šassūrīša tašakkan* 9' [. . . . . .] . . . [. . . . . .]

1' [. . . . . .], *nīnû*-plant, 2' [. . . . . .] a shekel of *burāšu*-juniper, 3' [. . . . . ., shekel(s) of *and*]*aḫšu*-plant, a shekel of 'white drug', 4' [. . . . . . shekel(s) of bl]ack cumin, two shekels of *namruqqu*-plant, 5' [... old copper which(?)] has produced *patina*(?), 6' [. . . . . . she]kel(s) of resin, a shekel of cedar 'blood', 7' [. . . . . .] you put(?), into *billatu*-substance for *našpu*-beer 8' [you . . . . . .], you insert (it) into her womb (viz. vagina), 9' *too fragmentary for translation*

Ms. a obv.(?) i' breaks; gap of unknown length

Beginning of ms. a obv.(?) ii' lost

10' *only traces preserved*

10' *too fragmentary for translation*

11'' *šumma sinništu š*[*a libbīša*(?) *inaddi*(?) . . . . . .] 12'' ...[. . . . . .] 13'' *only traces preserved*

11'' If a woman [*aborts her*] *foe*[*tus*(?) . . . . . .] 12'' [...]-plant, [. . . . . .], 13'' *too fragmentary for translation*

Ms. a obv.(?) ii' breaks; remainder lost; reverse not preserved

Notes

Lines 1'–9': A similar prescription sharing some of the ingredients is found in BAM 240: 47'–49' (see text D.2.1), but also in BM 42587+ obv. 11'–18' (text B.2.4). The latter remedy may be a variant of the present prescription: both ms. a and BM 42587+ mention *nīnû*-plant, *burāšu*-juniper, black cumin, cedar 'blood' and possibly old copper as ingredients (see also the next note). The purpose of the prescription is lost in both texts, but the remedy is inserted into the vagina as a tampon or suppository in both cases.

Line 5': The passage is restored after the parallel in BM 42587+ obv. 15' (text B.2.4), which mentions URUDU SUMUN *ša-ḫi-it-tu*$_4$ "old copper with a *patina*". According to CAD Š/2, 415, *šiḫittu* (also *šahittu*) may be a feminine adjective that qualifies plants (especially *šambaliltu* "fenugreek"), which is attested mostly in lexical lists and in Uruanna. AHw 1232a, however, lists *šiḫittu* II as the name of a garden plant. The term qualifies copper (*erû*) in BM 42587+, which is a masculine noun. Therefore, it was suggested in the analysis of BM 42587+ that *šaḫittu* in the present context could be related to *šuḫtu* (SAḪAR.(-)URUDU) "verdigris, patina (lit. "copper dust)" (see *infra* text B.2.4). The restoration [URUDU SUMUN *šá*?] ⌜*šá*?⌝-*ḫi-tú* ŠUB "[old copper], which has produced *patina*" in ms. a seems highly plausible and confirmative in this regard. The sign ŠUB following *šá-ḫi-tú* in ms. a line 5' is interpreted as *nadû* "to put, to throw", here in the sense of "to excrete (a substance), to produce (a feature)" (CAD N/1, 89–90 sub 3). Notably the verb *nadû* is used with *šuḫtu* "verdigris" in this sense in the *Erra*

Epic I 91 (Cagni 1969, 66–67): *patarn[i] ina lā*[!] *ṭabāḫi itt[ad]i šuḫtu* "our dagger is corroded (has produced verdigris) for want of slaughter".

Line 6': The ingredient ILLU "resin" may be an abbreviation for ILLU [šim]BULUḪ (*ḫīl baluḫḫi*) "resin of *baluḫḫu*-aromatic".

Line 7': The Akkadian reading of DIDA SIG_5 is not certain, but the references in CAD N/2, 78 s.v. *našpu* suggest either *billat našpi* or *billatu našiptu.* The spelling DIDA SIG_5-*tú* in line 7' indicates that the second word should be read as a feminine attribute (*našiptu*). For discussion of *billat našpi*, see also Abusch and Schwemer 2011, CMAwR 1, 55 text 1.6 note on lines 9'–10' with further references; Stol 1971, *BiOr* 28, 161; Maul 1994, 51.

Line 11'': An alternative interpretation for the line beginning could be *ana* [munus]P[$EŠ_4$ *šà* ŠÀ-*šà*[?] ŠUB[?]] "so that a pr[egnant] woman [aborts her foetus]"; cf. K. 8678+ line 34'' (text A.1.4).

E.2.5 BM 57853: A Fragment with Prescriptions for Women from Sippar

This fragment of a tablet from the temple archive of the Ebabbar temple in Sippar preserves the beginnings of ten lines of text, which have been identified as medical prescriptions, although the exact purpose of the recipes remains unclear. That the text was concerned with treatments for women's health, is suggested by line 2' mentioning the interior or a woman's womb (ŠÀ ŠÀ.TÙR).

List of Manuscripts

Siglum	Museum Number	Copy	Collation	Format; Ductus	Provenience
a	BM 57853 (82-7-14, 261)	CT 55, No. 377	Coll.	Fragment of a single-column(?) tablet; Neo-/Late Babylonian script; ca. $6^{th}/5^{th}$ cent. BCE[393]	Sippar; Ebabbar temple

Overview

i'	Fragmentary prescription a obv.[?] 1'–7'	...]1'–7'
ii'	Fragmentary prescription a obv.[?] 8'-9'	8'–9'
iii'	Fragmentary prescription(?) a obv.[?] 10'	10'[...?

Previous Edition and Discussion

Electronic Babylonian Library Project (eBL) (https://www.ebl.lmu.de/library/BM.57853)
CDLI P314769 (copy)
Achemenet (www.achement.com) (transliteration)
Reiner 1995, *Astral Magic*, 35 n. 145 (line 4')
Stol 2007, *JMC* 10, 2 (line 7')
Jursa 2009, 161 n. 68 (line 4')

Transliteration

Beginning of ms. a obv.(?) lost

393 Leichty 1986, *CBT* VI, 244. Measurements: ca. 4.4 x 4.7 x 1.5 cm.

1'	a obv.? 1'	*tu*-⌜x⌝-[.....................................]	
2'	a obv.? 2'	ŠÀ ŠÀ.TÙR-*šú* x[................]	
3'	a obv.? 3'	*tál-tál* GIŠIMMAR u_4-*ḫi-nu* SIG_7 x[..........]	
4'	a obv.? 4'	šimGIG *qu-un-nab áp-ru*-[*šú* ....]	
5'	a obv.? 5'	*ba*!(MA)-*al-ta-ma ina* GEŠTIN 3 u_4-*mu* [................]	
6'	a obv.? 6'	KÚM-*am* na4*gab-u nam-ruq* ú[.................................]	
7'	a obv.? 7'	*ana* IGI ŠUB *ina* UD.DA GAR-*an mu-ṣip-t*[u_4 ....]	
8'	a obv.? 8'	šimŠEŠ *ka-mu-nu nam-ruq* x[...............................]	
9'	a obv.? 9'	úKUR.KUR GÚR.GÚR *ta*-ŠUB *ina* LÀL [................]	
10'	a obv.? 10'	A? GI_6 *šup-li šá* ŠEN *šá*? [................]	

After one or two uninscribed(?) lines, ms. a obv.? breaks; remainder lost

Bound Transcription and Translation

Beginning of ms. a obv.(?) lost

1' *tu*-[. . . . .] 2' *qereb*(?) *šassūrīšu* ...[. . . . . .] 3' *taltal*(?) *gišimmari uḫinnu arqu* ...[. . . . . .] 4' *kanaktu qunnab apru*[*šu* . . . . . .] 5' *baltāma*(?) *ina karani šalāšat umī* [. . . . . .] 6' *emma*(?) *gabû namruq*(*qu*) . . .[. . . . . .] 7' *ana pāni tanaddi ina ṣēti tašakkan muṣiptu* [. . . . . .]	1' you ...[. . . . . .] 2' the inside of her womb [. . . . . .], 3' pollen(?) of the date palm, green fresh dates, [. . . . . .], 4' *kanaktu*-aromatic, *qunnabu*-aromatic, *apru*[*šu*-plant, ...], 5' *balsam*(?) [*you* ...] in wine (for) three days. [. . . . . .] 6' (still) hot(?), alum, *namruqqu*-plant, [...]-plant, [. . . . . .] 7' you pour over (it). You set (it) out in the bright daylight/open air, [*you* ... (it) *with*(?)] a *muṣiptu*-garment [. . . . . .].
8' *murra kamūnu namruq*(*qa*) ...[. . . . . .] 9' *atā'iša kukra tanaddi*(?) *ina dišpi* [. . . . . .]	8' [You ...] *murru*-aromatic, *kamūnu*-aromatic, *namruqqu*-plant, [. . . . . .]; 9' you *add atā'išu*-plant (and) *kukru*-aromatic. [You ...(it)] in syrup [. . . . . .].
10' *mû ṣalmūtu*(?) *šupli*(?) *ša ruqqi* ... [. . . . . .]	10' Dark water(?) from the bottom(?) of a kettle, ...[...]

After one or two lines without preserved text, ms. a obv.(?) breaks; remainder lost

Notes

Line 2': The phrase ŠÀ ŠÀ.TÙR-*šá/šú* "the inside/interior of her womb" is not attested elsewhere in the women's healthcare texts. Most likely, ŠÀ stands for *qerbu* "interior, middle" rather than *libbu* "inside, belly" here.

Line 3': Our passage is cited in CAD U/W, 46 s.v. *uḫinnu* sub 2, with a different interpretation, emending to PI $^{\text{giš!}}$GIŠIMMAR, but without offering a translation. More likely in my view, the signs TÁL.TÁL at the beginning of line 3' may be read as the logogram for the plant *urânu* (written without the plant determinative, as are other ingredients in this text). However, *tál-tál* could also be interpreted as the word *taltallu*, the pollen of the date palm, see CAD T, 104 with references from medical texts.

Line 4': Our passage is quoted in CAD Q, 306 s.v. *qunnabu* sub a. Reiner (1995, 35 n. 145) and Jursa (2009, 161 n. 68) regard *qunnabu* here as a gloss, as an equation for the preceding ^{šim}GIG (= *kanaktu*-aromatic). However, there is no *Glossenkeil* between these two plant names. For *qunnabu* as *Cannabis sativa*, the word being a loan (and wide-spread *Kulturwort*) from Persian *qu/innab* (the latter referring both to the plant and to ropes made from hemp fibres), see recently Böck 2022, 130; Jursa 2009, 163; Stein 2009, 585–596, 601. It is interesting that the drug name is written as *qu-un-nab*, without a case ending, perhaps underlining its nature as a loanword. So far *qunnabu* has been attested only in first millennium BCE sources, mostly in lists of aromatic substances and in the context of religious ceremonies. Its occurrence in a medical prescription for a woman is therefore remarkable. The equation of *qunnabu* with "the aromatic plant of the goddess Išḫara" (ŠIM ^{d}*Išḫara*) has been interpreted as an indication that *qunnabu* was used as an aphrodisiac (Prechel 1996, 153–154; Reiner 1995, 35; Fales 1983, *ZA* 73, 245).

The term *aprušu* is a medicinal and aromatic plant recommended in pharmaceutical texts for the treatment of fevers, see CAD A/2, 192 s.v. *aprušu* for references.

Line 5': The word *ma-al-ta-ma* at the beginning of the line may stand for the word *martû* (*mertû*, also *maštû, maltû*), which means "stick" but also occurs as the name of a tree (cf. CAD M/1, 200 s.v. *martû*, 395 s.v. *maštû*). The sign MA following *ma-al-ta* could also be read separately from the preceding signs, as a logogram for *tittu* "fig", written without a determinative (and not as the particle *-ma*). However, in light of the Late Babylonian attestations of the West Semitic loanword *baltām(mu)* "balsam" (*Commiphora opobalsamum*) identified by Jursa (2009, 156–157; see also SAD Vol. 1, 8), which is found in lists of aromatic substances from the Ebabbar archive, I propose to emend the first sign in line 5' to *ba*$^{!}$*-al-ta-ma*.

Line 6': The sequence KÚM/NE-*am* at the beginning of the line may be a mistake for KÚM-*em* = *ēm* ("it is hot"), or it could indicate an accusative (or adverbial) form (such as *baḫra* "(boiling) hot" or *emma* "hot".

The plant *namruqqu* encountered here and in the following prescription was used, for example, in complications during delivery, with the aim of expelling the foetus (see Stol 2000a, 53–55, with BAM 380 rev. 40 // BAM 381 iii 35), as a plant to expel the afterbirth (BAM 422 rev. iii' 5, see CAD S, 264b s.v. *silītu*), to induce abortion (see BAM 246: 1, text B.1.6) and as a plant promoting fertility (see BAM 244: 31, 33, text B.1.1). It also occurs in SpTU 5, No. 253: 4 (text E.2.6).

Line 7': The rulings after lines 7' and 9' were omitted in Pinches' copy. The word *muṣiptu*, referring to a standard sized piece of cloth, is also attested in BAM 240 obv. 13' (see text D.2.1), where such a garment is applied to the patient's body (probably in the form of a bandage), see Stol 2007, *JMC* 10, 2; CAD M/2, 243. In the present passage, the cloth may also have been used to cover the mixture of drugs while it was left in the open air.

For leaving medical substances in the open air or bright daylight (*ina ṣēti*), see CAD Ṣ, 152–153 sub f.

Line 9': Instead of reading *ta*-ŠUB (for *tanaddi* "you pour, steep, set up"), one may also emend to *ta-<za>-ru* "you sprinkle". The website of the *Achemenet* Project emends to *<qu>-ta-ru* "fumigant".

Line 10': The reading of the sign traces in line 10' is very ambiguous due to the broken context. At the beginning of the line, an interpretation of the signs a mi ru as the word *āmiru* "ill-wisher" does not seem likely. Therefore, I prefer a logographic rendering A GI$_{6}$ "black/dark water/fluid". The expression *mû ṣalmūtu* (A.MEŠ GI$_{6}$.MEŠ) is attested in omens in *Šumma ālu*, describing the appearance of water in a river or well (see CAD Ṣ, 78 sub 2c). I have tentatively rendered the following signs as *šup-li šá* ŠEN "from the bottom(?) (lit. depth) of a kettle/cauldron". A kettle (*ruqqu*) is occasionally used in medical procedures to heat or boil ingredients (e.g. BAM 393 rev. 20). However, in BAM 417: 20, a remedy for bandage against a skin disease mentions an unidentified substance taken from a kettle among other, similar ingredients (such as plaster from an oven; quoted in CAD R, 416–417 sub 1a; for *ruqqu*, see also Gaspa 2014, *Contenitori*, 90–92, 524 Fig. 11). The term *šuplu* "depth" may be a mistake for *šaplu* "bottom" (cf. CAD Š/3, 324–325). Note that *šupul mê* "depth of the waters" also refers to the groundwater table (CAD Š/3, 324 sub 1a).

The remainder of the tablet following line 10' may have been left blank.

E.2.6 SpTU 5, No. 253: Treatments for "Spots" on the Uterus

This poorly preserved fragment from Late Babylonian Uruk may belong to the same single-column tablet as SpTU 4, No. 153 (texts C.1.10 and D.1.11), as was proposed by Oelsner (2001, *OLZ* 96, 481). Both fragments were unearthed in the scholarly library of the descendants of Ekur-zakir. SpTU 5, No. 253 was found in association with SpTU 3, No. 65, a tablet with an extract from the bilingual incantation series SAG.GIG.GA.MEŠ, bearing a colophon of the well-known scholar and exorcist Iqīšâ, son of Ištar-šumu-ereš, descendant of Ekur-zakir (who was active in the late 4th century BCE).

The present fragment preserves the lower portion of the obverse and the upper portion of the reverse, about 45 lines of text altogether.[394] The subject on the first thirty lines on the tablet's obverse preserved in SpTU 4, No. 153 are abnormal haemorrhage and difficult birth. It is uncertain whether the text first sections on the obverse of SpTU 5, No. 253 were concerned with the same subject.

The topic of the final sections on the obverse and the sections on the reverse are treatments for a visible pathological symptom of the womb called *tikpū* "spots, dots" (rev. 1: *tikpī ina rēmīša ittakkip*). It is difficult to say exactly what *tikpu* refers to (e.g., cysts, ulcers), but it is clear that the "spots" were regarded as a serious condition that could cause painful sensations. Comparisons of this Late Babylonian text with the topics dealt with in the Hippocratic treatise *Diseases of Women* I and II show a similar scope and order of topics. These Greek treatises, roughly contemporary with the Late Babylonian medical texts, deal with menstrual disorders, conception and disorders of pregnant women, postpartum disorders, complications during delivery (e.g. retention of a dead foetus) and disorders of the uterus. Among the latter conditions, *Diseases of Women* I and II include treatments for ulceration (*hélkos* "ulcer") of the uterus – a condition that, according to the Hippocratic authors, tends to occur as a complication following a difficult delivery or an abortion (see Potter 2018, *Diseases of Women* I, chapters 36, 38, 49, 63–67, 78).

The laconic reference to the *tikpu*-spots on the womb in SpTU 5, No. 253 has been read as an indication that Mesopotamian healers undertook examinations of female patients' vagina and cervix with the help of an instrument to spread open the vagina (Scurlock and Andersen 2005, 259). Such instruments are attested from Roman medical practice (the so-called *speculum*), but no comparable instruments have been identified in the archaeological record from ancient Mesopotamia.

Due to its badly preserved state, the decipherment of several passages in the present fragment remains difficult. These issues notwithstanding, the fragment exhibits a high number of unusual features that diverge from standard characteristics of Mesopotamian medical prescriptions, such as the vocabulary used as well as the structure and format of the text. For example, several verbal forms giving instructions for processing medical ingredients are of uncertain meaning and otherwise unattested, which may point to Aramaic influence. The preserved prescriptions make only rare use of KI.MIN "ditto; alternatively" at the beginning of the recipes; instructions how to apply the remedies are at times sparse or ambiguous. The format of the prescriptions resembles other Late Babylonian medical texts, for example in the high frequency of measurements specifying the exact amount of the ingredients used. Several of the prescriptions in SpTU 5, No. 253 end with a short statement specifying the condition for which the remedy is applied, another feature resembling Late Babylonian women's healthcare texts edited in this volume (see e.g. section A).

List of Manuscripts

Siglum	Museum Number	Copy	Collation	Format; Ductus	Provenience
a	W. 22668/0 IM 77020	SpTU 5, No. 253	Photo coll.	Fragment of a single-col. tablet; Late Babylonian script; 4th/3rd century BCE	Uruk; library of the descendants of Ekur-zakir

394 It is unnecessary to switch obverse and reverse of SpTU 5, No. 253 (*pace* Biggs 2001, *JNES* 60, 291).

Overview

i'	Fragmentary prescription a obv. 1'–3'	...]1'–3'
ii'	Prescription (unknown purpose) a obv. 4'–12'	4'–12'
iii'	Prescription (unknown purpose) a obv. 13'–18'	13'–18'
iv'	Prescription against spots on a woman's womb a obv. 19'–22'	19'–22'
v'	Prescription against spots on a woman's womb a obv. 23'–24'	23'–24'
vi'	Prescription against spots on a woman's womb a rev. 1–2	25'–26'
vii'	Prescription against spots on a woman's womb a rev. 3–5	27'–29'
viii'	Prescription against spots on a woman's womb a rev. 6–8	30'–32'
ix'	Prescription against spots on a woman's womb a rev. 9–12	33'–36'
x'	Prescription a rev. 13–14	37'–38'
xi'	Prescription a rev. 15	39'
xii'	Prescription a rev. 16–17	40'–41'
xiii'	Fragmentary prescription a rev. 18–21	42'–45'[...

Previous Edition and Discussion

Von Weiher 1998, SpTU 5, 67–70 (edition) and 168 (copy)
Scurlock and Andersen 2005, 219 (10.62), 259 (12.1) (rev. 1)

Transliteration

Beginning lost

1' a obv. 1' [x x x t]a x x x 2 NINDA ZÌ x[. . . . .]

2' a obv. 2' [x x GAZ]I^{sar} BIL.ME *ina* ŠÀ ŠEG$_6$-*šal-ma* A *šá* ^{du}[^{g}. . . . .]

3' a obv. 3' [x]x-*niš* *ša*$^{?!}$ KA IGI [x] x [.]

4' a obv. 4' [x]x ŠE.GIŠ.Ì *ta-ḫap-pap ina* KEŠDA *tara-kás* 3 NINDA *nam-ruq ina* x[x x x x x x]

5' a obv. 5' [*a-n*]*a ú-de-e šá* KÀŠ *taq-né-e-ti ke*$^{?!}$-*ṣe-e-tú ta*-[*šak-kan*$^{?}$ x x (x)]

6' a obv. 6' [*a-n*]*a ú-de-e* 2-*i šá* KÀŠ *ta-na-dín ki-i lu* $^{\text{ḫe-pí}}$ *ut*$^{?}$-x[x x x x x]

7' a obv. 7' [*šá-maš*$^{?}$]-*šá*$^{?}$-*mi* ḪÁD.DU ŠE.GIŠ.Ì *ta-kap-par lu-pár* DUḪ GEŠ.TIN ri da$^{?}$ [x x x x]

8' a obv. 8' [1.TA.À]M$^{?}$ SÚD *si-ik-ta-šú-nu ina* ŠÀ *a-ḫa-a-meš* ḪI.ḪI *ta-ṣa-ḫat* ḫ[u$^{?}$ x x x x]

9' a obv. 9' [x x *a*]-*ḫa-meš* ḪI.ḪI-*ma* 2 GÍN KU ^{ú}KUR.RA 2 GÍN KU ^{ú}*ak-tam* 1 G[ÍN x x x x x]

10' a obv. 10' [1 GÍN KU *u*]*r-nu-ú* 1 GÍN KU ^{šim}GÚR.GÚR 1 GÍN KU *šu*$^{!}$-*nu-ú* 1 GÍN KU I[N.NU.UŠ DIŠ-*niš* SÚD$^{?}$]

11' a obv. 11' [*si-ik*$^{?}$]-*ta*$^{?}$-*šú* GA ÈME *ana* ŠÀ ŠUB-*di ina ú-de-e šá* Ì.GIŠ x x [x x x x x]

12' a obv. 12' [*ina* K]I$^{?}$ *te-qeb-ber-šú* E$_{11}$$^{!}$-*ma ki-i pat-ra-at ina*$^{?}$ KU$^{?}$.MEŠ *an-na-a-tú* x[x x x x x] | *ina* GA x[x x x x x]

13' a obv. 13' [L]ÀL$^{?}$ Ì.NUN ILLU MÚD EREN ^{šim}ḪAB DIŠ-*niš* ḪI.ḪI-*ma ina ú-de-e* GAR-*an ina* MÚD$^{?}$ [x x x x]

14' a obv. 14' [*t*]*u-rab-bak* ÍL-*ma ina* Ì.GIŠ *šá tu-šaḫ-ḫi-ru u* Ì.ŠAḪ *tu-ša-a*[*k-kal-ši*$^{?}$]

15' a obv. 15' [EN$^{?}$] *šá ka*$_{4}$-*an-ni-šú tam-ma-ru ina 4-i u*$_{4}$-*mu šá ina* IGI-*šú i-kam-mi-su* [x x x *kīma*$^{?}$]

16' a obv. 16' [*m*]*aḫ-ri-i* SUM-*su ina* 5 *u*$_{4}$-*mu* TA ŠÀ *ri-bi-ku šá i*$^{!}$-*na*$^{!}$(GIM) *qaq-qar* [*taq-bi-ru*$^{?}$]

17' a obv. 17' x x-*né-e* SUM-*nu-šú ma-la maš-ši-ti* TA ŠÀ ÍL-*ma* 4 *u*$_{4}$-[*mu ú-kal*$^{?}$]

18' a obv. 18' [x x]-*ú-tú-šá* BABBAR$^{?}$ $^{\text{na4}}$*gab-u ana* ŠÀ ḪI.ḪI *pat*$^{?}$-[x x]

19' a obv. 19' [DIŠ MUNUS$^{?}$ *ṣer*$^{?}$]-*ḫi* LÍL-*ma ti-ik-pi ina* ARḪUŠ-*šá i-tak-kip* NINDA$^{?}$ 4 SÌLA *šal-šá-a*-[*tú šá*]

20' a obv. 20' [KAŠ ŠE] SUMUN 15 GÍN GÚ.GAL *sa-an-du-tú* 2/3 MA.NA UZU EGIR AM$^{?!}$ Ú$^{?}$ BABBAR x[x]

21' a obv. 21' [DIŠ-*niš*$^{?}$ *t*]*a-sal-laq* EN *a-na* 2 SÌLA GUR 4 NINDA Ì.ŠAḪ 1 NINDA Ì *gu-un-nu ana* UGU GAR *šá tak-ṣa*-⸢*a*⸣-[*tú*]

22' a obv. 22' ŠUB-*ma* DÙ-*su šá ti-ik-pi*

23' a obv. 23' 3 SÌLA *šal-šá-a-tú šá* KAŠ ŠE SUMUN 1 GÍN *saḫ-lé-e ana* ŠÀ ŠUB ⸢*ta*$^{?}$-*sal*$^{?}$⸣-*laq* 2 GÍN NÍG.⸢GU$_{7}$$^{?}$⸣ 1/2 SÌLA$^{!}$ ZÌ$^{?}$ [x]

24' a obv. 24' 2 GÍN ^{šim}ḪAB *ana* ŠÀ *ta-se-ḫi* 3 NINDA Ì.NUN 3 NINDA Ì *gu-un-nu ana* IGI ŠUB 5-*šú* 6-*šú* DÙ-*s*[*u*$^{?!}$] | *šá* DÙ [x] ⸢x⸣ *is-li-it*

25' a rev. 1 DIŠ MUNUS *ti-ik-pi ina* ARḪUŠ-*šá i-tak-kip* 4$^{?!}$ GÍN$^{?!}$ x x RU 1/2$^{?}$ GÍN ⸢ŠE.GIŠ.Ì⸣ [x GÍN]

26' a rev. 2 ^{šim}ḪAB 1/2 GÍN MÚD ^{giš}EREN *ina* Ì KU$_{6}$ *u* Ì.ŠAḪ$^{!}$(KU$_{6}$) *te-se-eḫ-ḫi* Ì.ŠAḪ *šá tu-šab*$^{!}$-*š*[*i*$^{?}$-*lu*$^{?}$ x x] \ *tu-ṭa-pí* Ì.ŠAḪ SUD [DÙ-*su*(?)]

27' a rev. 3 DIŠ KI.MIN *ḫu-um-mu-ṭu pe-ṣu-ú* 1 *ú-de-e* ⸢KAŠ$^{?}$.SAG$^{?}$⸣ *la ba-šal te-pe*$^{?}$-*ḫ*[*i*$^{?}$ x x (x)]

28' a rev. 4 ḪÁD.DU *ina* ⸢NINDU$^{!}$⸣ *tuš-bat* E$_{11}$$^{!?}$-*ma ina ur-ṣa* SÚD *gi-na-a* DU$_{10}$ *la ba-šal ina* ŠÀ *tu-sak* [x x]

29' a rev. 5 *ana* IGI *ur*$_{5}$-*ri la* ÍL-*šú šá* TU$_{15}$ *u ti-ik-pi* SIG$_{5}$

30' a rev. 6 DIŠ KI.MIN 5 GÍN GÚ.GAL *sa-an-du-tu* 2 GÍN ^{ú}NU.LUḪ.ḪA 2 GÍN ^{šim}MUG *sa-pan*

31' a rev. 7 *ina* 3 SÌLA *šal-šá-a-tú šá* KAŠ ŠE SUMUN [ŠE]G$_6$-*šal* EN *a-na* 1/2 SÌLA GUR 2 GÍN ^{šim}ḪAB *ana* ŠÀ *ta-ḫap-pu*

32' a rev. 8 4 NINDA Ì.ŠAḪ 2 NINDA Ì *gu-un-nu ana* ŠÀ ŠUB-*di* DÙ-*su*

33' a rev. 9 DIŠ KI.MIN 5 GÍN GÚ.GAL *sa-an-du-tu* 5 GÍN *sim-di* KUR DU 1/2 SÌLA KÀŠ SUMUN

34' a rev. 10 1 SÌLA *šal-*[*šá-a-tú*] *šá* KAŠ ŠE SUMUN ŠEG$_6$-*šal a-di a-na* 7 NINDA GUR$^{!}$ 3 NINDA Ì *gu-un-nu* 3 NINDA Ì.ŠAḪ

35' a rev. 11 1 GÍN ^{šim}ḪAB *ina* ŠÀ *ta-se-ḫi ana* IGI ŠUB 4 NINDA GA UDU$^{?}$ KU$_7^{?}$ *ana*$^{!}$ UGU *maš-šit*$^{?!}$ ŠUB-*ma*$^{!}$(BA) *šum*$_4$-*ma* ÚTU(U+GA)

36' a rev. 12 *ana*$^{?}$ [UG]U$^{?}$ *ku*$^{?}$-*uṣ-ṣu* ŠUB 3 NINDA GA UDU$^{?}$ KU$_7^{?}$ 2 NINDA *ku-ru-nu šá* KAŠ ŠE SUMUN *ana* UGU ŠUB-*ma* DÙ-*su*

37' a rev. 13 5 GÍN GÚR.GÚR 3 GÍN MUG 3 GÍN NU.LUḪ.ḪA *ina* 3 SÌLA *šal-šá-a-tú šá* KAŠ ŠE SUMUN ŠEG$_6$-*šal* EN

38' a rev. 14 *a-na* 1 SÌLA GUR 2 GÍN *ka-mun ina mar-ḫaṣ šá tu-šab-ši-lu* DIŠ-[*niš* ḪI.ḪI$^{?}$]

39' a rev. 15 *ana* ŠÀ *ta-kar*$_5^{?}$-*aš* 2 <NINDA$^{?}$> ⸢GA⸣ ⸢UDU⸣ ⸢KU$_7^{?}$⸣ 3 GÍN ^{šim}ḪAB 5 NINDA Ì ŠE.BAR-*tú* 5 GÍN Ì.Š[AḪ x x]

40' a rev. 16 KU$^{?!}$ ⸢ÚKUŠ$^{?}$⸣ ŠIM.⸢ḪI.A⸣ ŠEŠ.ME *ina* 5 SÌLA *šal-šá-a-tú šá* KAŠ ŠE SUMUN ŠEG$_6$-*šal* EN [*ana* x SÌLA]

41' a rev. 17 GUR Ì.GIŠ *ana* IGI ŠUB *ku-um* A.MEŠ Ì [x x (x)]

42' a rev. 18 x ⸢GÍN$^{?}$⸣ Ì *reš-ti*$^{!}$ *ana* 3 SÌLA ⸢*šur*$^{?}$-*šum*$^{?}$⸣-*mi* KAŠ ŠE SUMUN ŠUB ŠEG$_6$-*šal* EN *a-n*[*a* x SÌLA GUR]

43' a rev. 19 [x x KU ^{ši}]^{m}ḪAB KU GAM$^{!}$.<MA> GÚR.GÚR x KU MUG *sa-pan* KU KUR.KUR KU *ak-tam* KU x[x x x]

44' a rev. 20 [x x x KU] NU.LUḪ.ḪA *qa-li-tu*$_4$ KU [*gu-š*]*u*$^{!}$-*ri* SUMUN *ana* ŠÀ ŠUB [x x x x]

45' a rev. 21 [. . . . .] ⸢x x x⸣ [. . . . .]

Ms. a rev. breaks; remainder lost

Bound Transcription and Translation

Beginning of ms. a obv. lost

1' [...]... *šina akal qēm* ...[. . . . . .] 2' [... *kas*]*ê qalûti ina libbi tušabšal-ma mê ša* [. . . . . .] 3' [...]... *ša pî* ...[...]

1' [...] ... two tenths of a litre flour of [. . . . . .], 2' [...] roasted *kasû* you boil with it, [you ...] water from a [...]-vessel [...]. 3' [...] from the mouth of ...[. . . . . .].

4' [...]... *šamaššammī taḫappap ina riksi tarakkas šalāšat akal namruq(qu) ina* ...[. . . . . .] 5' [*an*]*a udê ša šīnāti taqnēti keṣêtu*(?) *ta*[*šakkan*(?)] . . . . . .] 6' [*an*]*a udê šanî ša šīnāti tanaddin*(?) *kī* ... ḫepi ...[...] 7' [*šamaš*]*šammī*(?) *tubbal šamaššammī takappar lupāra tuḫḫī karāni* ...[...] 8' [*ištē*]*nâ tasâk sīktašunu ina libbi aḫāmeš tuballal taṣaḫḫat* ...[. . . . . .] 9' [... *a*]*ḫāmeš tuballal-ma šina šiqil sīkti*(?) *nīnê šina šiqil sīkti*(?) *aktam ištēn ši*[*qil* . . . . . .] 10' [*ištēn šiqil sīkti*(?) *u*]*rnû ištēn šiqil sīkti*(?) *kukri ištēn šiqil sīkti*(?) *šunû ištēn šiqil sīkti*(?) *m*[*aštakal ištēniš tasâk*(?)] 11' [*sīk*]*tašu šizib atāni ana libbi tanaddi ina udê ša šamni* ...[. . . . . .] 12' [*ina qaqq*]*ari*(?) *teqebberšu tušellâ-ma kī paṭrat ina sikāti*(?) *annâtu* ...[. . . . . .] *ina šizib* [. . . . . .]

4' [...]... you pound(?) sesame, you tie it into a bandage(?). [You ...] three tenths of a litre of *namruqqu*-plant in [. . . . . .]. 5' You [put (it)] into a container with normal, cold(?) urine, [. . . ...] 6' you *transfer*(?) (it) [t]o a second container of urine. When . . . broken ...[...], 7' you dry [the ses]ame(?), you *wipe* the sesame *clean*(?). *Lupāru*-tree(?), bran, wine, . . .[. . . . . .] 8' you pound [separ]ately, you mix their powders together with it (the sesame?). (Then) you press (it) out, ...[. . . . . .] 9' [. . .] you mix (it) together. Then [you crush together(?)] two shekels powder of *nīnû*-plant, two shekels powder of *aktam*-plant, one she[kel . . . . . .] 10' [one shekel powder of *u*]*rnû*-plant, one shekel powder of *kukru*-plant, one shekel powder of *šunû*-tree, one shekel powder of *ma*[*štakal*-soapwort] 11' [. . . . . .], you add *that* [pow]der(?) (and) donkey's milk to it. In a vessel with oil . . .[... . . .]. 12' You bury it (the vessel) [in the grou]nd(?). You take it out (again), and when it *is dissolved*(?), [you ...] with/in these *powders*(?) [. . . . . .], with milk (of) ... [. . . . . .].

13' [*diš*]*pa ḫimēṭa ḫīl dām erēni ṭūra ištēniš tuballal-ma ina udê tašakkan ina dāmi*(?) [. . . . . .] 14' [*t*]*urabbak inaššī-ma ina šamni ša tušaḫḫiru*(?) *u nāḫi tuša*[*kkalši*(?)] 15' [*adi*] *ša kannīšu tammaru ina rebî ūmu ša ina maḫrīšu ikammisu* [... *kīma*] 16' [*m*]*aḫrî tanaddissu ina ḫamši ūmu ultu libbi ribīku ša ina*(?) *qaqqari* [*taqbiru*(?)] 17' ... *tattadnušu*(?) *mala maššīti ultu libbi inaššī-ma erbet ū*[*mū ukâl*(?)] 18' [...]...-*ša peṣû*(?) *gabû ana libbi tuballal* ...[...]

13' You mix [syr]up(?), ghee, cedar 'blood' (and) *ṭūru*-aromatic together, you put it into a vessel, with blood(?) of [. . . . . .], 14' you make a paste (from it), she applies it (as a suppository). And you (also) have [her eat(?) (it)] with oil which you have *heated*(?), and (with) lard, 15' [until (the day?)] that she sees/you see (a discharge on) her menstrual bandage. On the fourth day that *she submits*(?) *to it* (the menses?) [. . . . . .] 16' you give (it) to her [as be]fore(?). On the fifth day: from the paste that [you have buried(?)] in(!) the ground 17' (and which) . . . you have administered to her(?), she applies from it as much as (is appropriate in) a suppository. And for four days [she shall keep it (there?)]. 18' [*If*] her(?) [...] are white(?), you mix alum with it, ...[. . .].

19' [*šumma sinništu ṣer*]*ḫi*(?) *isalla'-ma tikpī ina rēmīša ittakkip akalu*(?) *erbet qa šalšā*[*tu ša*] 20' [*šikar uṭṭati*] *labiri* 15 *šiqil ḫallūru sandūtu* 2/3 *mana šīr arkat rīmi*(?) *šammu peṣû* ...[...] 21' [*ištēniš ta*]*sallaq adi ana šina qa iturru erbet akal nāḫu ištēn akal šamnu gunnu ana muḫḫi tašakkan ša takṣâ*[*tu*] 22' *tanaddī-ma teppussu ša tikpī*

19' [If a woman(?)] is ill [with feverish] heat(?), and she is covered with spots on her womb: 21' you boil [together(?)] 19' bread(?), four litres of old third-class 20' [barley beer], fifteen shekels of ground peas (and) two thirds of a mina of meat from the rear of a wild bull(?), 'white drug', [...] 21' until (the liquid) is reduced to two litres. You add four tenths of a litre of lard (and) one tenth of a litre of average-quality oil to it. For cooling(?) 22' you set (it) out. Then you can *treat her* (with it?). (A treatment) for spots.

23' *šalāšat qa šalšātu ša šikar uṭṭati labiri ištēn šiqil saḫlê ana libbi tanaddi tasallaq šina šiqil ukultu*(?) *mišil qa qēm*(?) [...] 24' *šina šiqil ṭūru ana libbi taseḫḫi*(?) *šalāšat qa ḫimētu šalāšat qa šamnu gunnu ana pāni tanaddi ḫamšīšu šeššīšu teppuss*[*u*(?)] *ša epēš* [...]... *islit*(?)

23' (Alternatively,) you add to it three litres of old third-class barley beer, one shekel of *saḫlû*-plant (and) boil it. Two shekels of ..., half a litre of [. . .]-flour(?), 24' two shekels of *ṭūru*-plant you *mix* with it. You add three tenths of a litre of ghee (and) three tenths of a litre of standard-quality oil to it. You *apply the treatment* for h[er] five or six times. (It is also good?) for *treating* [. . . (which)] *has been lacerated*(?).

25' *šumma sinništu tikpī ina rēmīša ittakkip erbet*(?) *šiqil* ... *zūz* (*šiqil*) *šamaššammū* [... *šiqil*] 26' *ṭūru zūz* (*šiqil*) *dām erēni ina šaman nūni u nāḫi*(!) *teseḫḫi nāḫu ša tušabš*[*ilu*(?) ...] *tuṭappi nāḫa tasallaḫ* [*teppussu*(?)]

25' If a woman is covered with 'spots' on her womb: You *mix*(?) four shekels(?) of ..., half a shekel of sesame, [. . . shekel(s)] 26' *ṭūru*-plant (and) half a shekel of cedar 'blood' with fish oil and lard(!). The lard, which you have boil[ed, . . .] you (can) apply (as a compress). You sprinkle (it) with the lard, [*you treat her* (with it?)].

27' DIŠ KI.MIN *ḫummuṭū peṣû ištēn udê šikari*(?) *lā bašal tepeḫ*[*ḫi*(?) ...] 28' *tubbal ina tinūri*(?) *tušbât tušellâ-ma*(?) *ina urṣi tasâk ginâ ṭāba lā bašal ina libbi tusâk* [...] 29' *ana pān urrî*(?) *lā tušaššāšu ša šāri u tikpī damiq*

27' Alternatively, (if) they (the spots) are burning hot (and) white: you se[al(?)] a vessel with non-boiled beer(?). [. . .] 28' you dry(?), you let (it) spend the night in an oven(?). (In the morning), you take it out(?) and pound (it) in a mortar. You pulverize good *ginû*-flour(?) with it without boiling, [...]. 29' You should not let her apply (it) before *sexual intercourse* (lit. "impregnation"?). It is good for "wind" and spots.

30' DIŠ KI.MIN *ḫamšat šiqil ḫallūru sandūtu šina šiqil nuḫurta šina šiqil ballukku-sapān* 31' *ina šalāšat qa šalšātu ša šikar uṭṭati labiri* [*tuša*]*bšal adi ana mišil qa iturru šina šiqil ṭūru ana libbi taḫappu* 32' *erbet akal nāḫu šina akal šamnu gunnu ana libbi tanaddi teppussu*(?)

30' Alternatively, you boil five shekels ground peas, two shekels *nuḫurtu*-plant (and) two shekels *ballukku*-soap 31' in three litres of old third-class barley beer, until it is reduced to half a litre. You *pour*(?) two shekels of *ṭūru*-aromatic into it, 32' you add four tenths of a litre of lard (and) two tenths of a litre of standard-quality oil to it. You *treat her* (with it).

33' DIŠ KI.MIN *ḫamšat šiqil ḫallūru sandūtu ḫamšat šiqil simdi* ... *mišil qa šīnātu labirātu* 34' *ištēn qa šal*[*šātu*] *ša šikar uṭṭati labiri tušabšal adi ana sebet qa iturru šalāšat qa šamnu gunnu šalāšat qa nāḫu* 35' *ištēn šiqil ṭūru ina libbi taseḫḫi*(?) *ana pāni tanaddi erbet akal šizib immeri matqu*(?) *ana muḫḫi maššīt*(?) *tanaddī-ma*(!) *šumma diktu* 36' *ana* [*muḫ*]*ḫi*(?) *kuṣṣu tanaddi šalāšat akal šizib immeri matqu*(?) *šina akal kurunnu*(?) *ša šikar uṭṭati labiri ana muḫḫi tanaddī-ma teppussu*(?)

33' Alternatively, you boil five shekels ground peas, five shekels of . . . *simdu*-cereal, half a litre of old urine (and) 34' one litre of old third-quality barley beer, until it is reduced to seven tenths of a litre. You *mix*(?) with it three tenths of a litre of standard-quality oil, three tenths of a litre of lard (and) 35' one shekel of *ṭūru*-plant. You add to *the mixture* four tenths of a litre of *sweet sheep milk*(?). And(!) if (you're using) *diktu*-flour, 36' you add (it) *to* (the mixture when it is) *cooled*. You (then) add to it three tenths of a litre of *sweet sheep milk*(?) and two tenths of a litre of *kurunnu*(?) made from old barley beer, and you *treat her* (with it?).

37' *ḫamšat šiqil kukru šalāšat šiqil ballukku šalāšat šiqil nuḫurtu ina šalāšat qa šalšātu ša šikar uṭṭati labiri tušabšal adi* 38' *ana ištēn qa iturru šina šiqil kamūnu ina marḫaṣi ša tušabšilu ištē*[*niš tuballal*(?)]

37' You boil five shekels of *kukru*-aromatic, two shekels of *ballukku*-aromatic, three shekels of *nuḫurtu*-plant in three litres old third-quality barley beer, until 38' it is reduced to half a litre. [You mix] toge[ther(?)] two shekels of *kamūnu*-plant with the lotion that you have boiled.

39' *ana libbi takâraš*(*i*) *šina* <*akal*> *šizib immeri matqu*(?) *šalāšat šiqil ṭūru ḫamšat akal šamnu uṭṭatu ḫamšat šiqil nā*[*ḫu* ...]

39' You rub(?) her with(?) it. Two <tenths of a litre?> *sweet sheep milk*(?), three shekels of *ṭūru*-plant, five tenths of a litre of oil, barley (and) five shekels of la[rd, . . .].

40' *sīkti*(?) *qiššê*(?) *riqqī annûti ina ḫamšat qa šalšātu ša šikar uṭṭati labiri tušabšal adi* [*ana* ... *qa*] 41' *iturru šamna ana pāni tanaddi kūm mê šamnu* [...]

40' You (can also) boil powder of cucumber(?) (and?) these (i.e., the aforementioned) aromatics in five litres of old third-class barley beer, until it is reduced [to ... litres]. 41' You add oil to it. Instead of water, [. . .] oil.

42' ... *šiqil šamnu rēštî ana šalāšat qa šuršummi šikar uṭṭati labiri tanaddi tubšabšal adi an*[*a* ... *qa iturru*] 43' [... *sīkti*] *ṭūri sīkti ṣumlalî kukru* ... *sīkti ballukku-sapān sīkti atā'iši sīkti aktam sīkti* ...[...] 44' [... *sīkti*] *nuḫurtu qalītu sīkti* [*gu-š*]*ūri labiri ana libbi tanaddi* [. . . . . .] 45' [. . . . . .] ... [. . . . . .]

42' You pour ... shekels(?) of premium oil into three litres of dregs of old barley beer. You boil it, until it [is reduced] t[o . . . litres]. 43' You add [. . ., powder] of *ṭūru*-plant, powder of *ṣumlalû*-plant, *kukru*-aromatic, . . . powder of *ballukku*-soap, powder of *atā'išu*-plant, powder of *aktam*-plant, powder of [. . . . . .], 44' [. . . . . .], roasted *nuḫurtu*-[powder], powder of an old [b]eam(?), [. . . . . .] 45' [. . . . . .] ... [. . . . . .]

Ms. a rev. breaks; remainder lost

Notes

Line 3': The sign traces in this line are inscribed with blank spaces in between, but unfortunately barely readable anymore on the photos. Von Weiher copied the signs TA KA, which can be read *ultu pî* "from the mouth". This phrase could be part of an editorial note referring to the source of the recipe or of a group of recipes on the tablet. However, the usual phrase referring to authorship, oral lore or dictation is *ša pî* or *šūt pî*, not *ultu pî* (cf. CAD P, 466 sub 6a). The following traces could be read (*ša* KA) IGI.[GÁ]L "(from the mouth) of a sage" (*igigallu*), as a variation of the more common phrase *ša pī ummâni* "from the mouth of a scholar". For similar editorial notes referring to authorship or oral lore in other women's healthcare texts, see BM 50700: 11'; BM 38624+: 86'''''' (texts A.2.1, A.2.3). See further Frahm 2011, 44–45, 51–52 *passim*; Gabbay 2016, 51–52.

Line 4': At the beginning of the line, von Weiher, SpTU 5, 67–68 reads [*ana ti-k*]*lip* "[für den Tup]fer(?)" (i.e. "for the swab"), but there is hardly room for more than one short sign before the assumed [K]IB to the left margin. Von Weiher's restoration is based on an interpretation of the term *tikpu* in lines 19' and 25', where it occurs in the introduction to the prescription: (DIŠ MUNUS) *ti-ik-pi ina* ARḪUŠ-*šá i-tak-kip* "if a woman is covered with spots on her womb". Based on a suggestion by I.L. Finkel, von Weiher assumes a meaning "swab" for *tikpu* (cf. the notes below). This interpretation is not followed here. The damaged beginning of line 4' could start with (DIŠ) KI.MIN or with a term for an ingredient. If one takes the sign [KI]B for granted, one could also restore [^{giš}ŠEN]NUR = *šallūru* "plum". The copied sign traces may perhaps be emended to [LÀ]L$^{!}$ "syrup", but do not support the reading [DU]Ḫ (for DUḪ.ŠE.GIŠ.Ì = *kupsu* "sesame pomace").

Von Weiher, SpTU 5, 68 translates *ta-ḫap-pap* in line 4' as "du zerkleinerst", from *ḫapāpu* I "to pound; to smash" (AHw 321b). This verb also occurs in BM 50700: 8' (text A.2.3). However, a derivation of *ta-ḫap-pap* in line 4' from *ḫapāpu* II "to wash, clean" is not excluded (an Aramaic loanword well attested in Babylonian Aramaic and Syriac; cf. CAD Ḫ, 84 s.v. *ḫapāpu*). For another occurrence of the latter verb in a Neo-Assyrian medical text from Assur, see e.g. Geller 2007, *JMC* 10,

9–10 AO 11447: 28, 38; see also Fincke 2011, in: *The Empirical Dimension*, 190 BM 41282+ obv. ii 4', 11' (G-stem). The following *ina* KEŠDA *tara-kás* "you tie into a band (of cloth)" in line 4' is unexpected. The word *riksu*(KEŠDA) can designate a "band, strap" or a "package, bundle". Perhaps the operation served to drain the washed(?) sesame before further processing.

The *namruqqu*-plant (also *nabruqqu*) is used several times in recipes in abortive remedies, see e.g., BAM 246: 4 (text B.1.6); K. 8678+ line 37'' (text A.1.4). Cf. also Stol 2000a, 53–55 for its use in the context of promoting delivery. The *nabruqqu*-plant is also used in prescriptions to promote conception (BAM 244: 31, 33; text B.1.1).

Lines 5'–6': A similar procedure of putting drugs into urine is found in K. 8678+ lines 39''–40'' (in a prescription for a tampon to induce an abortion, see text A.1.4). In SpTU 5, No. 253: 5'–6', drugs appear to be soaked or steeped in two different vessels (*udû* "container, jar") with urine. The word *udû* occurs several times in the present fragment (see also line 13': *ina ú-de-e* GAR-*an*).

The term *taq-né-e-ti* in line 5' appears to be an attribute qualifying *šīnātu* "urine". There is a noun *taknītu/teknītu* "care, solicitude" (CAD T, 84; AHw 1344b), but it is not clear what this term would mean in the present context. We therefore assume a feminine plural form of the adjective *taqnu* "in order; good; secure" here (cf. CAD T 199; AHw 1324a). The following sign before *ṣe-e-tú* is not entirely clear from the copy (it may be GIM), but the context suggests a second attribute to *šīnātu* with a feminine plural ending. The word *ṣētu* means "sunlight, heat; open air", but reading this as *kīma*(GIN$_7$) *ṣēti* does not make good sense here. If one emends the text to *ki*$^{!}$-*ṣe-e-tú*, this could be understood as a variant spelling of *kaṣâtu*, the feminine plural of the adjective *kaṣû* "cold", or as the adverb *kaṣâtam* "in the early morning" (to *kaṣâtu* "early morning"). Cf. also *kīṣu* "cool (of the day)".

Line 6': Von Weiher's copy reads *ta-na*-DIR, which, however, does not yield a verb with a suitable meaning. The faint traces of the assumed sign DIR could also be read KAL (compare thus also the sign KAL in ILLU(A.KAL) in line 13'). The present reading *ta-na-dín* "you *transfer*" (from *nadānu* "to give") is provisional for lack of a better solution. For the value *dín* of the sign KAL, see von Soden and Röllig 1991, *Akkadisches Syllabar*, 173.

Line 7': The signs LU BAR could be read *lubāru* "cloth", but the occurrence within a list of medical ingredients does not make this reading very likely. Therefore, a tentative reading *lu-pár* for the *lupāru*-tree is proposed here. The verb *kapāru* "to wipe clean; to smear" is not found elsewhere in connection with the processing of medical ingredients nor with sesame, in particular.

Although rarely written syllabically, the restoration [*šá-maš*]-*šá-mi* for *šamaššammū* "sesame" is proposed here, since the word (written logographically, however) recurs in the same line.

Lines 8'–11': The occurrence of the syllabically written term *sīktu* "powder" in lines 8' and 11' in connection with powdered ingredients written with the logogram KU suggests that the sign KU has to be read as Akkadian *sīktu* rather than ZÌ = *qēmu* "flour" in the present text (the verb *sâku* "to pound" also precedes the first mention of *sīktu* in line 8'). Note that in line 12' of our text, several powdered ingredients used in the prescription are referred to with the plural *sīkātu* (see next note).

Similar prescriptions using powdered ingredients are found e.g., in BAM 240: 41', 50'–61', 61'–63' (text D.2.1); BM 38624+ lines 24'–29' (text A.2.1), often in recipes for bandages.

Line 12': Elsewhere in medical texts, drugs are buried for a couple of days in the ground, see e.g. CAD Q 202–203 s.v. *qebēru* sub 2b; CAD T 336–337 s.v. *temēru* sub 1d; Geller and Panayotov 2020, 121, 123, 132 (IGI 2 lines 28, 59', 103' under a threshold). The phrase [*ina* K]I may be read in Akkadian as *ina erṣeti* "in the earth" or *ina qaqqari* "in the ground".

The meaning of the feminine stative *paṭrat* in this specific context is not clear; its referent – are presumably the "powder(s)" (*sīktu*) referred to earlier in lines 8' and 11' that have been buried in the ground in a vessel with oil. Possible meanings here are "to be loosened, detached, dissolved" (cf. CAD P, s.v. *paṭāru*).

Von Weiher, SpTU 5, 70 reads the signs following *ki-i paṭ-ra-at* as *ina* SI$^{?}$.MEŠ *an-na-a-tú* and interprets SI.MEŠ as *qarnāte* "horn-shaped vessels, rhytons" (cf. AHw 904 s.v. *qarnu* sub 3; CAD Q 138–139 sub 4). In medical recipes or rituals, substances are sometimes filled into an ox horn (*qaran alpi*), see e.g. Scurlock 2006, 48, No. 5: 4, No. 7; No. 8: 3, 12; AMT 89/3 iii 2(!) (in prescriptions and rituals against a ghost-induced ailment). However, in the present context, the use of such a vessel seems unexpected. The sign read as SI is also not entirely beyond doubt. Instead of SI.MEŠ, a reading KU$^{!}$.MEŠ is thus proposed here, standing for *sīkātu* (*annâtu*) "(these) powders". This would refer again to the mixed powders of several plants enumerated in lines 9'–11'. The word *sīktu* in the singular occurs two more times in this prescription (in lines 8' and 11', written syllabically), which further supports the new reading.

Line 13': Von Weiher, SpTU 5, p. 67 suggests to restore [*ana ti-k*]*ip*? "[Für den Tup]fer(?)" (*tikpu*), but there is no room for two more signs before the sign read as [K]IB. The copied sign traces look a bit like DU rather than KIB. The reading [L]ÀL (for *dišpu* "syrup") proposed here is a mere guess from the context.

Line 14': In women's healthcare texts, the verb *našû* (written ÍL) usually refers to inserting suppositories (*maššītu*) into the vagina, see also line 17' below; BAM 240: 44'–45' (text D.2.1); UET 7, No. 123 obv. 8 and rev. 11 (text B.2.2) and *passim*.

For *turabbak* "you make a compound/paste" (from *rabāku* "to concoct", D-stem), note also the derived noun *ribīku* in line 16'. The latter is a variant spelling for *rabīku* or *ribku* often encountered in Late Babylonian texts (see also BM 50700 (text A.2.3) lines 3', 4', 6' with comments). The dictionaries render the word as "decoction" or "mash" (CAD R, 20 and 321; AHw 935a "ein Absud" and AHw 980b "ein (Drogen-) Absud"); for the more appropriate meaning "to make a paste", see Cadelli 2000, 111 fn. 25; Attia 2021, *JMC* 38, 77–78. The spelling *ri-bi-ku* possibly points to Aramaic influence. The cognate Aramaic term *rbyk*, *rbykh*, which means "flour paste" (Comprehensive Aramaic Lexicon, https://cal.huc.edu), denotes "a pulp of flour mixed with hot water or oil" (Jastrow, *A Dictionary of the Targumim*, 1442b).

The signs *tu*-ŠAḪ-*ḫi-ru* in line 14' may be read *tu-šaḫ/sáḫ/ṣeḫ-ḫi-ru*. Neither the D-stem of *ṣeḫēru* ("to make small, to reduce, to deduct, to break up into small pieces") nor the D-stem of *saḫāru* ("to turn around") offer meanings that seem appropriate in the present context. An unclear verb *šaḫāru* is only attested lexically, listed beside *ḫamāṭu* ("to burn; to heat up(?)") and *u''ulu* ("to bind, coagulate") as Akkadian renderings of Sumerian šu-úr-ĝar, see CAD Š/1, 81 quoting Nabnitu J 196 (MSL 16, 160–161). Therefore, I tentatively translate *ša tušaḫḫiru* as "(oil) which you have *heated*". See in these terms also the similar passage Ì.ŠAḪ *šá tu-šab*!-*š*[*i*?-*lu*] "lard which you have boi[led]" in lines 26' and 38' below.

Line 15': For *kannu* "menstrual bandage", see also AO 6473 line 40 (text C.3.9). The *ta-* infix in the form *tammaru* may refer to the third person fem. sg. or to a second person sg., cf. also SpTU 4, No. 153 obv. 24 (text D.1.11).

The expression *šá ina* IGI-*šú i-kam-mi-su* is unclear and probably idiomatic. The verb *kamāsu* I means "to gather; to finish up (doing something)" and *kamāsu* II "to squat, to kneel, to crouch". Since the latter verb is attested with *ina maḫar* "before someone" (= to kneel in submission; cf. CAD K, 118–119 sub 1b), the expression *ina* IGI-*šú i-kam-mi-su* is presumably used here in a similar meaning.

Lines 17'–18': This passage is still difficult to understand, but there are some similarities with texts such as UET 7, No. 123 (text B.2.2). In line 17' of the present text, the patient applies (ÍL) a suppository (*maššītu*), presumably to the vagina. For the uses of suppositories in women's healthcare texts, see also SpTU 4, No. 153: 2; FLP 1306 rev. 20 (for stopping haemorrhage); BM 42313+ obv. 8–9, rev. 22 (for promoting conception/pregnancy); BM 50700: 11', 12', 28''' (for treating 'wind'); BM 38624+: 1'–5', 10', 52'''; UET 7, No. 123 lines 6, 23'–29' (see *infra* text A.2.1, A.2.2, A.2.3, B.2.2, C.1.9, C.1.10 with notes).

The restoration at the end of line 17' follows UET 7, No. 123, e.g. lines 8, 10, where it is stated that the patient should wear (*našû*) a tampon (*itqu*) filled with medical ingredients for three days and then remove it. This is found in prescriptions for fertility/pregnancy tests. If understood correctly, the fragmentary text in line 18' of SpTU 5, No. 253 could be reminiscent of UET 7, No. 123. Thus, it appears that the beginning of line 18' describes the appearance of something related to the patient's body as "white/shiny" (BABBAR?), which could be the womb or a vaginal discharge (cf. UET 7, No. 123 lines 3, 12). But the traces at the beginning of line 18' still defy a restoration (von Weiher's copy does not support reading [ŠÀ.(-) T]ÙR-*šá* or [ARḪ]UŠ-*šá*). Perhaps restore [DIŠ *ru*]-*ú-tú-šá* BABBAR "if her *mucus* (*ru'tu*) is white", denoting some kind of discharge (the usual meaning of *ru'tu* is "saliva, phlegm, mucus" coming out of the mouth)?

Line 19': The phrase (DIŠ MUNUS) *ti-ik-pi ina* ARḪUŠ-*šá i-tak-kip* "(if a woman) is covered with spots on her womb" occurs here and in line 25'. The key term *tikpū* "spots" is only attested in this medical text as a symptom or condition, and it is also without parallel in the corpus of women's healthcare texts. Against the interpretation of von Weiher (in SpTU 5) as a swab ("Tupfer"), *tikpu* clearly refers to a symptom here, since the *tikpu*-spots are described as "white" (*peṣû*) and "burning hot" (*ḫummuṭu*) in line 27'. Furthermore, two remedies are summarized as "(good) for spots" (*ša tikpī* (*damiq*) in lines 22' and 29'). Beyond the medical texts, the word *tikpu* (often together with the verb *takāpu*) is found in descriptions of stones having spots or dots. It also refers to the imprints of the stylus made in the clay in the expression *tikip santakki* ("cuneiform"). See SAD Vol. 2, 91; cf. CAD T, 403–404; and the notes on lines 22', 25', 29' below.

The form *i-tak-kip* used here and in line 25' has been recognized as an N-stem form of *takāpu* ("to pierce, to puncture; to speckle, dapple; to cover with dots, spots") in SAD Vol. 2, 54, cf. CAD T, 68–69; Mayer 2009, *OrNS* 78, 424.

The proposed restoration [DIŠ MUNUS? *ṣer*?]-*ḫi* LÍL-*ma* at the beginning of line 19' is tentative. The logogram LÍL is to be read as the verb *salā'u* "to be ill", which is used as a synonym of GIG = *marāṣu*. In a similar manner, the noun *silīʾtu* often simply means "disease" (as does *murṣu*). In some contexts, *salāʾu* and *silīʾtu* refer to a serious and protracted illnesses (for discussion see Stol 2009a; CAD S, 96 translates *salāʾu* as "to be seriously ill; to enter a critical stage of illness"). The verb *salāʾu* is mostly attested in the N-stem in medical texts, when written syllabically. Stol (ibid., 33–34) discusses references to women (mostly from letters) being "ill" (*salāḫu/salāʾu*), but these are usually unspecific about the nature of the illness. Interestingly, the verb is also found in an oracle question for a woman in confinement (*tāmīt ḫarišti*), (Lambert 2007, *Babylonian Oracles Questions*, 90 no. 12c: 11–13): "Every day she is overwhelmed (*ik-kàt-ta-mu*), she is chronically ill (*is-sa-la-'u*), bread and beer are displeasing to her, her appetite is diminished, her illness [...]". Since *salāʾu* is so far only attested in SpTU 5, 253 and not in other therapeutic women's healthcare texts, the verb may have a more specific meaning here (e.g. to suffer seriously/chronically from a condition).

The restoration [DIŠ MUNUS? *ṣer*?]-*ḫi* LÍL-*ma* "[if y woman is ill with [burning] heat / inflammation(?)" (*ṣerḫu*) at the beginning of line 19' is a guess from the context. However, *silīʾtu* and *salāʾu* are found several times in the context of fever (e.g. *ṣētu, liʾbu*), see Stol 2009. For *ṣerḫu* "fever(ish) heat, burning, inflammation", related to *ṣarāḫu* "to become hot (with fever)", see AHw 1092 s.v. *ṣerḫu* III, Bácskay 2018, 6, e.g. in BAM 174 rev. 31 (Bácskay 2018, no. 39: 3); BAM 124 iii 15 (*naṣmatti ṣerḫi* "a bandage for *inflammation*", Scurlock 2014a, 454, 458). The association of "spots" on the womb with fever or inflammation may be compared with passages dealing with ulcers of the uterus in the Hippocratic treatise *Diseases of Women* I (chapters 36, 38, 49, 63–67, 78), stating that ulceration often develops as a result of physical injuries from a delivery or from the abortion of a foetus or as a result of undischarged lochia putrefying in the womb, and that ulcers are usually accompanied by inflammation or fever as well as pain, purulent discharges and swelling (i.e. severe symptoms that are often lethal in the end), see Potter 2018, *Diseases of Women* I, chapters 36, 38, 49, 63–67, with treatments in chapter 78 (53)–(60). For inflammation of the uterus, see also *Diseases of Women* I, chapters 50, 53–54. The Hippocratic doctors often treated these conditions with injections (enemas) of *materia medica* into the vagina or with ointments or suppositories applied to the ulcers. These informative passages may perhaps serve as points of comparison for a better understanding of the remedies in SpTU 5, 253.

For *šalšātu* (fem. plural of *šaluštu* "third"), understood as "third-class" (beer), which repeatedly occurs with KAŠ ŠE SUMUN "old barley beer" in the present text (lines 19', 23', 31', 34', 37', 40'), cf. CAD Š/1, 285–288 esp. sub 1c; AHw 1150b s.v. *šalšu* sub 2b. Note that the specific expression *šikaru šaluštu* refers to beer that is diluted to/by a third.

Line 20': The emended sign AM in 2/3 MA.NA UZU EGIR AM?! "two-thirds of a mina (= ca. 300 g) of meat from the rear of a wild bull(?)" looks more like the signs MA and ḪI in von Weiher's copy, but the two signs in question are written very close together by the scribe, as revealed by photos of the tablet. For *arkatu* "rear, back" as a cut of meat, cf. CAD A/2, 276 sub 1c-2b'. The use of meat in the present prescription finds a fascinating parallel in remedies with beef found in catalogues of prescriptions for uterine ulcers or genital blisters/aphthae in *Diseases of Women* I, chapter 90 and in *Diseases of Women* II, chapter 64. One of these remedies consists in a suppository of beef covered with a mixture of fat, anise and saffron that is inserted into the vagina (Potter 2018, *Diseases of Women* I, chapter 90 (2). In a similar prescription a piece of beef is applied to genitalia affected by aphthae (ibid., *Diseases of Women* I, chapter 90 (5)).

Lines 21' and 23': For *salāqu* "to boil", see CAD S, 92–93; AHw 1014.

Line 21'-22': The expression *ša takṣâtu tanaddi* "you set it out for cooling" is interpreted here as one phrase. For *takṣâtu*, compare SpTU 4, No. 153 obv. 7, where *maštakal*-soapwort and *simbirru*-plant(?) are used for "cooling a pregnant woman" (*ana takṣâtu ša erīti*). The cooling through remedies is associated with stopping bleeding in SpTU 4, No. 153 obv. 9: *ina libbi šīrīšu ikaṣṣû u dāmū ikkallû* "her body will cool down through it and the blood will be held back" (see text C.1.10). Here in line 21', it seems more likely, however, that the remedy which has been boiled is cooled before application. See also SAD Vol. 2, 57; Steinert 2020, *JMC* 36, 59.

DÙ-*su* is understood here as *teppussu* "you treat her (with it)", analogous to SUM-*su* "you administer (it) to her". Von Weiher, SpTU 5, 67, 69, 70 reads the DÙ-*su šá ti-ik-pi* differently as *epēssu* (infinitive of *epēšu* + pronominal suffix) and translates "(das) ist die Herstellung des Tupfers". This interpretation is followed by SAD Vol. 2, 91 s.v. *tikpu* with the translation "its (the medicine's) preparation for spots". Although Late Babylonian medical prescriptions often feature such concluding rubrics stating the form and purpose of treatment, these formulations usually use a more specific term (e.g. "suppository (*maššītu*) for (*ša*) ..."). Moreover, the pronominal suffix -*su* before *ša tikpi* would be very unusual, if the whole phrase DÙ-*su šá ti-ik-pi* was to be understood as a genitive construction. Moreover, it is not unusual to find a short purpose statement with *ša* + disease term appended at the end of prescriptions from the Late Babylonian period, see e.g.

BM 50700 obv. 12' (text A.2.3). The occurrence of *epēšu* "to do; to make; to carry out, perform" instead of more specific verbs informing the reader how a medical treatment was to be administered is nonetheless highly unorthodox; compare however text E.2.1 above for a similar use of *epēšu* (Š-stem).

Line 23': NÍG.GU$_7$ = Akk. *ukultu* usually means "food, fodder", but can also refer to a kind of sauce or soup (see CAD U/W, 65 s.v. *ukultu* sub 3; the references for the latter meaning listed there are from the Neo-Assyrian period). The reading of the end of line 23' is uncertain.

Line 24': The phrase *ana pāni tanaddi* replaces *ina muḫḫi tašakkan* in line 21'. Ingredients and procedure of the two prescriptions in lines 19'–22' and 23'–24' are so similar that they appear to be variant prescriptions.

The last sign copied by von Weiher at the end of line 24' looks like EŠ. However, as in line 22', the traces should probably be read DÙ-*s*[*u*!]. The indented text written on the ruling is presumably to be interpreted as a purpose statement introduced by *ša* "(this is) for ...". The following DÙ can either be read as the infinitive *epēšu* or as DÙ-[*ti*] = *nēpešti* "(for) the treatment of ...". After a short gap, the term *is-li-it*, if read correctly, is part of the purpose statement specifying the condition for which the remedy was used. The form may reflect the verb *salātu* "to split off, to cut off, to notch", but due to the preceding gap and uncertain sign traces, the reading of this passage remains provisional. The verb may describe some condition of the uterus, e.g. some form of injury stemming from a difficult delivery and linked to the condition of *tikpu*-spots.

Lines 24' and 26': As seen already by von Weiher, SpTU 5, 70, the verb forms *ta-se-ḫi* (also in line 35') and *te-se-eḫ-ḫi* are very likely variant forms of the same unknown verb. The context suggests a probable meaning "to mix". The forms could be related to the verb *esēḫu* "to allocate, to assign" (with overhanging vowel) or to *seḫû* "to rise up, revolt", but neither verb offers a fitting sense here. The verb is presumably an Aramaic loan (cf. *sḫy* "to wash; to bathe", Jastrow 1903, 971; Sokoloff 2002, 797; Geller 2024, 206).

Line 26': The sign traces after Ì.ŠAḪ differ from the parallel phrase *šá tu*-ŠAḪ-*ḫi-ru* in line 14' (see the note above). For another occurrence of *šá tu-šab-ši-lu*, see line 38' below (there referring to a lotion, *marḫaṣu*).

At the beginning of the indented passage in rev. 2, von Weiher (SpTU 5, 67) reads *tu-ṭa-bi* "du tauchst ein", from *ṭebû* "to submerge" (D-stem "to immerse"), but the verb *ṭepû* "to apply medication" (said of poultices, compresses (*ṭīpu*) applied to affected body parts) seems more suitable here (see CAD Ṭ, 101 sub 2b, cf. 1c; Mayer 2022, *OrNS* 91, 349 "hinbreiten; auftragen"; Stol 2018, in: *FS Geller*, 761 with fn. 46 (for a Dt-stem form). If understood correctly, the remedy in lines 25'–26' could be used as a compress, or as a suppository.

Line 27': The word *ḫummuṭu* (D-stem of *ḫamāṭu* "to burn, to be inflamed, to be feverish") can mean "to burn; to cause a burning pain" or "to make feverish" (CAD Ḫ, 65 s.v. *ḫamāṭu* B sub 2). In reference to the "spots" (*tikpū*) the patient is suffering from, the term may describe a burning painful sensation the spots cause in the patient (cf. Scurlock and Andersen 2005, 288). In addition, the spots are described here as "white" (*peṣû*).

The reading *te-pe-ḫ*[*i*] "you seal off" (the container) in this line is not certain; however, *peḫû* is found in connection with enclosing ingredients in a sealed container or oven, see CAD P 317 sub d ("to lute").

Line 28': Von Weiher's copy shows a sign that looks like GIŠxA, but the traces on the tablet photos look very much like NINDU (LAGABxNINDA). Therefore, a reading *ina tinūri*(NINDU!) *tuš-bat* is proposed here. The signs copied by von Weiher after *tuš-bat* "you leave overnight" are SIG DU-*ma*, which is presumably a mistake for E$_{11}$-*ma* "you take out".

The word *gi-na-a* in line 28' should refer to a (solid) substance here because of the following instruction "you pulverise with it" (*ina* ŠÀ *tu-sak*) rather than the adverb *ginâ* "constantly, normally". The noun *ginû* usually refers to regular offerings but can also designate a quality of flour (cf. CAD G 82 s.v. *ginû* A sub c-3'; AHw 290a sub 3c). Von Weiher elides the following ḪI, but perhaps this is simply to be read DU$_{10}$ = *ṭābu* "good".

Line 29': The phrase *ana pān*(IGI) *ur$_5$-ri la tušašša*(ÍL)-*šú* is provisionally rendered here as "you should not let her apply it before *intercourse*(?)". Von Weiher reads *ḫur-ri* "hole" ("vor ein Loch(?) darfst du es nicht nehmen(?)"), but this makes little sense. The word *ur$_5$-ri* could be understood as *urru* "early morning" (i.e. "do not let her apply it before the early morning"). Alternatively, a reading *mur-ri* or *ur$_5$-ri* could be interpreted as the infinitive *urrû* (also *ḫurrû, murrû*) "to severe, separate; to cut off" (cf. CAD U/W, 245–246 s.v. *urrû* A; AHw 1433 s.v. *urrû* III, 1497 s.v. *wurrû*; Stol 2000a, 116 n. 35). This verb is used in reference to women giving birth and is either understood in terms of the parturient separating herself from the baby or in terms of her separation/isolation after delivery. Furthermore, the word ur_5-*ri* may be understood as the D-stem infinitive of *erû* "to be(come) pregnant" (lit. "impregnating"), which could refer to having sexual intercourse here. For the D-stem of *erû*, see also N. 4001 line 13: KA.INIM.MA munusNU.Ù.TU *a-na ur-*⌜*ri*⌝*-i* "recitation to make a barren woman get pregnant" (text B.2.1); BAM 241 rev. iii 7': [MUNUS N]U *a-li-da-at ana ur-re-*⌜*e*⌝ [...] "to make an infertile woman get pregnant" (text II.1.3). In other words, the present passage would state that the woman should not insert the remedy (suppository) before intercourse. Compare for example, statements in other texts recommending that the woman's husband "should not approach her" (sexually) during certain treatments (to promote fertility), see e.g. UET 7, No. 123 rev. 5' (text B.2.2).

I understand the phrase *šá* TU_{15} *u ti-ik-pi* SIG_5 as a purpose statement, with SIG_5 standing for *damiq* "it is good for (treating) wind and spots", with *šá* as a variation for the usual *ana* ... SIG_5. For the treatment of "wind" in women's healthcare texts, see e.g. BAM 240: 20'–28' (text D.2.1), BM 50700: 28''' (text A.2.3). Incidentally, the Hippocratic treatises *Diseases of Women* I and II speak of a similar condition, in which the patient's uterus becomes inflated with wind (*anemos*) or air (*phusa*), causing pain and other symptoms, which may perhaps serve as a point of comparison to the present Babylonian text. See Potter 2018, 83 *Diseases of Women* I chapter 34, 367 *Diseases of Women* II chapter 45, 399 *Diseases of Women* II chapter 68, 429 *Diseases of Women* II chapter 93 (recipe), 451 *Diseases of Women* II chapter 102 (recipe).

Line 30': For the word *sapān* (an Aramaic loan) here and in line 43', which is a soapwort or alkaline plant often occurring as an attribute of *ballukku*-aromatic, see the discussion to BM 42450+ obv. 5' (text B.2.3), with Finkel 2000, Text 16. See also BM 42507 obv. 4 (text E.2.1), with a similar procedure. In the latter text, the remedy is applied as an enema.

Lines 31'–32': For similar procedures, in which mixtures or ingredients are boiled down in a liquid until reduced to a certain amount (with the verb *târu*(GUR) "to turn (into)"), see e.g. CAD T, 260 sub 4b; Köcher 1978, 21–22; Finkel 2000, *FS Lambert*, 159 text 6: 9, 164 text 10: 37, 164 text 11 obv. 4', 165 text 12: 17, 175 text 19 rev. 4', 181 text 23: 14, 15; SpTU 1, No. 63: 1–8; SpTU 1, No. 63: 8–12; BM 42507 // lines 7–8 (*infra* text E.2.1). See also the following prescriptions in SpTU 5, No. 253 (lines 33'–43').

Line 31': The verbal form *ta-ḫap-pu* (or *ta-ḫab-bu*) is unclear. Cf. *ḫabû* "to draw water", AHw 306; CAD Ḫ 19, but this verb is not really fitting in the present context; *ḫâb/pu* "to purify, wash" (cf. Aramaic *ḥpp* / *ḥwp* "to wash (hair); rub together"), CAD Ḫ, 20–21 s.v. *ḫâbu* A; AHw 306a, 1557b. None of these verbs fit the present context well. The adverb *ana libbi* preceding the verb suggests a meaning such as "to pour" (into it) or "to add" (to it). However, note the Aramaic verb *ḥph* / *ḥpy* "to cover; to strew/spread over" (Jastrow 1903, 491; Sokoloff 2002, 477), the latter sense of which may provide a better fit.

Line 33': For the use of milled *simdu*-cereal in a similar context, see also BM 42507 and dupl. line 5 (text E.2.1). The attribute or qualification KUR DU following *sim-du* in the present text is not yet understood; cf. CAD S, 272a for other specifications of *simdu*.

Line 35': The second half of line 35' has been heavily emended here and the new proposed readings are tentative; the signs are not clearly visible on the tablet photos. Von Weiher copied the signs ÍL.DU here as well as in lines 36' and 40', each time following a measurement, which signals the name of an ingredient; however, a logogram ÍL.DU is not otherwise attested. The emendation GA UDU KU_7 "sweet sheep milk" is a guess from the context resembling the signs rendered in von Weiher's copy.

For the reading *maš-šit*! "suppository", see also line 17' above.

For ÚTU = *diktu/tiktu*, a type of flour (not a dairy product, as stated in CAD D s.v. *dīktu*), see AHw 1357a; CAD T, 404 disc. s.v. *tīktu*.

Line 36': The reading of the beginning of the line is not certain; the passage is damaged. If understood correctly, the final ingredients are added after the boiled mixture has cooled down (*kuṣṣu*, D-stem stative of *kaṣû*). Note the parallel expression *šá tak-ṣa-*⌜*a*⌝*-*[*tú*] ŠUB-*ma* "you set (the mixture) down for cooling" (before administering the remedy to the patient) in lines 21'–22' above.

Although von Weiher, SpTU 5, 70 doubts the reading *kurunnu* for *ku-ru-nu* in line 36', I do not see a better solution. Presumably, *kurunnu* from old barley beer designates a better quality of beer than the type called *šalšātu* (*šá* KAŠ ŠE SUMUN) found several times in this text (lines 19', 23', 31', 34', 37', 40'; cf. CAD K, 579 "a choice kind of beer or wine"; eSAD K, s.v. *kurunnu* "fine beer"; AHw 513b "ein Feinbier").

Line 37': The scribe omits the usual classifiers preceding names of plants/aromatics in the substances enumerated in this line.

Line 38': For *marḫaṣu* "ablution", usually constructed with *raḫāṣu*(RA) "to wash", see e.g. BAM 240: 58 (text D.2.1): *ina libbi* RA.MEŠ-*si*; *Iraq* 31, 29: 25 *ina libbi* RA-*si* "you wash her with it" (text II.1.4); BAM 244: 19–20, 72 (text B.1.1).

Line 39': If the text is deciphered correctly, the final instruction for the preceding remedy in lines 37'–38' is written at the beginning of line 39', which is highly unusual, since there is a ruling between lines 38'–39'. The same phenomenon may be seen between lines 39' and 40' (likewise separated by a ruling). The reading of the beginning of the line as *ana* ŠÀ *ta-ka-r*$_5^?$*-aš* "you rub her with(?) it" (with a durative form of *kâru* "to rub (in medication)", followed by the abbreviated suffixed pronoun) is proposed here in lack of a better solution.

After the sign MIN, von Weiher (SpTU 5, 68) adds the measurement NINDA, but this sign is neither preserved on the copy nor on the photo.

The reading ŠE.BAR-*tú* (for *uṭṭatu* "barley"), directly following Ì "oil", without a specified measurement, is unusual. One would rather expect the specification of a type of oil.

Line 40': The "aromatics" (ŠIM.ḪI.A ŠEŠ.ME) referred to here should sum up several ingredients listed before and are therefore presumably the plants enumerated in the first half of line 37', since there is only room for one ingredient name at the very beginning of line 40' (cf. KU$^!$.MEŠ *annâtu* in line 12'). The reading of the first two signs (KU$^{?!}$ (text: ŠU) ÚKUŠ$^?$) in line 40' is uncertain. These unusual features suggest that lines 39' as well as 40'–41' describe variant(s) of the earlier prescription.

Line 44': Powder of an old wooden beam (KU ^{giš}ÙR/ŠU.ÙR SUMUN) is also an ingredient in prescriptions to stop bleeding, see e.g. SpTU 4, No. 153 obv. 12–13; FLP 1306 obv. 13 and parallels (texts C.1.9–C.1.10).

E.2.7 BM 48997: A Late Babylonian Fragment of Prescriptions for Women

This small fragment has been identified by H. Stadhouders of the *Electronic Babylonian Library Project* (eBL) as a piece of a tablet containing remedies for women. It belongs to tablets excavated by Hormuzd Rassam in Babylonia and listed in the British Museum registers with the provenience Babylon.[395] The external features and the handwriting of BM 48997 and BM 49133 (text E.2.8) resemble each other to a high degree, and both fragments likely belong to the same tablet, although they do not join (see below). BM 48997 preserves the ends of several lines with prescriptions (potions, tampons/suppositories, amulets), and a short incantation. The combination of therapies in these lines may be indicative of their purpose as treatments to stop bleeding, but this remains uncertain for the time being. The fragment is included here for convenience of the reader.

List of Manuscripts

Siglum	Museum Number	Copy	Collation	Format; Ductus	Provenience
a	BM 48997 (81-11-3, 1708)	–	Coll.	Fragment of a tablet in Late Babylonian script; ca. 6th–3rd cent. BCE	Babylon

Overview

i'	Fragmentary prescription a obv.$^?$ 1'	...] 1'
ii'	Fragmentary prescription (potion) a obv.$^?$ 2'	2'
iii'	Fragmentary prescription (potion, tampon) a obv.$^?$ 3'–5'	3'–5'

395 See Leichty, Finkel and Walker 2019, *CBT* IV–V, 702 and the dossier on BM 48997 in the online collection of the British Museum (https://www.britishmuseum.org/collection/object/W_1881-1103-1708).

iv'	Fragmentary prescription a obv.? 6'–9'	6'–9' [...
v''	Fragmentary prescription (suppository?) a rev.? 1'-3'	...]10''–12''
vi''	Fragmentary incantation a rev.? 4'–5'	13''–14''
vii''	Rubric a rev.? 6'	15''
viii''	Fragmentary prescription (amulet?) a rev.? 7'–8'	16''–17'
ix''	Fragmentary prescription a rev.? 9'–10'	18''–19''
x''	Fragmentary prescription (tampon?) a rev.? 11'	20''
xi''	Fragmentary a rev.? 12'	21''[...

Previous Edition and Discussion

Electronic Babylonian Library Project (eBL) (https://www.ebl.lmu.de/library/BM.48997; photo; transliteration)

Transliteration

Beginning of ms. a obv. lost

1' a obv.? 1' [................................] ⸢*ina-eš*⸣

2' a obv.? 2' [................................] x NAG

3' a obv.? 3' [.......................... *ina* MUL] ⸢*tuš*⸣*-bat* NAG

4' a obv.? 4' [................................] x *an-nu-ḫa-ra*

5' a obv.? 5' [..................... *ana* ŠÀ.T]ÙR-*šá* GAR-*an*

6' a obv.? 6' [................................] x NIGIN-*mi*

7' a obv.? 7' [.......................... Ì.G]IŠ ⸢DU?!10.GA?⸣

8' a obv.? 8' [................................ S]AR?

9' a obv.? 9' [................................] x

Ms. a obv. breaks; gap of unknown length

Beginning of ms. a rev. lost

10'' a rev.? 1' [................................] x

11'' a rev.? 2' [................................] ⸢ALLA?⸣

12'' a rev.? 3' [................................] MIN

13'' a rev.? 4' [................................]-*ma/la*?

14" a rev.? 5' [................................] x ÉN?

15" a rev.? 6' [KA.INIM.MA MUNUS *šá* ...... GIG]-*at*

16" a rev.? 7' [................................] KÉŠ

17" a rev.? 8' [................................] *ina-eš*

18" a rev.? 9' [.............................. DIŠ-*n*]*iš* ḪI.ḪI

19" a rev.? 10' [................................ *i*]*na-eš*

20" a rev.? 11' [..................... *ana* ŠÀ.TÙR-*šá*? GAR]-*an*

21" a rev.? 12' [................................]x MIN

Ms. a rev. breaks; remainder lost

Bound Transcription and Translation

Beginning of ms. a obv. lost

1' [. . . . . .] *ina"eš(?)*	1' [. . . . . .] she will get well.
2' [. . . . . .] *išatti*	2' [. . . . . .] she shall drink (it).
3' [. . . . . . *ina kakkabi*] *tušbât išatti* 4' [. . . . . .] ... *annuḫara* 5' [. . . . . . *ana šas*]*sūrīša tašakkan*	3' [. . . . . .] you let (it) stand outside overnight [under the star(s)]. (Then) she shall drink it. 4' [. . . . . .] (white) *annuḫaru*-pigment 5' [. . . . . .] you insert (it) [into] her [wo]mb (viz. vagina).
6' [. . . . . .]... *talammi* 7' [. . . . . . *šam*]*nu ṭābu(?)* 8' [. . . . . .] ... 9' [. . . . . .] ...	6' [. . . . . .] ... you wrap, 7' [. . . . . .] fragrant (sweet-smelling) oil(?), 8' [. . . . . .] ... 9' [. . . . . .] ...

Ms. a obv. breaks; gap of unknown length

Beginning of ms. a rev. lost

10'' [. . . . . .] ... 11'' [. . . . . .] *allānu(?)* 12'' [. . . . . .] MIN	10'' [. . . . . .] ... 11'' [. . . . . .] an acorn-shaped suppository(?) 12'' [. . . . . .] ditto.
13'' [. . . . . .]... 14'' [. . . . . .] ÉN	13'' "[. . . . . .]... 14'' [. . . . . .]." Incantation (formula).

15'' [KA.INIM.MA *šinništi ša ... marṣ*]*at*	15'' [Wording (of an incantation) for woman who] is [sick with ...].
16'' [. . . . . .] *takaṣṣar*(?) 17'' [. . . . . .] *ina"eš*	16'' [. . . . . .] you tie (knots), 17'' [. . . . . .] she will get well.
18'' [. . . . . .] *ištēniš taballal* 19'' [. . . . . .] *ina"eš*	18'' [. . . . . .] you mix together, 19'' [. . . . . .] she will get well.
20'' [. . . . . . *ana šassūrīša tašak*]*kan*	20'' [. . . . . . you ins]ert (it) [into her womb (viz. vagina)].
21'' *fragmentary*	21'' *too fragmentary for translation*

Notes

Lines 3'–5': For similar instructions to leave a remedy outside overnight before administering it to the patient, specifically in texts concerned with gynaecological haemorrhage, see e.g. BM 40152 rev. iv 13' (text C.1.8, line 58''); BAM 237 obv. i 29' (text C.1.4).

Line 10'': Acorn-shaped suppositories (ALLA, *allānu*) are prescribed in other women's healthcare texts, see e.g. K. 8893 obv.(?) 5', 9' (text C.1.6); BAM 240: 65' (text C.2.1).

Line 15'': Note a comparable rubric in the Neo-Assyrian text BAM 237, KA.INIM.MA MUNUS *ša naḫšāti marṣat* "wording (of an incantation) for a woman who suffers from *naḫšātu*" (bleeding during pregnancy). This condition is not attested in women's healthcare texts from Babylonia, however. Other disease terms are also possible in the gap.

E.2.8 BM 49133: A Fragment Related to Women's Health?

This Late Babylonian fragment, like the fragment BM 48997 (text E.2.7 above), stems from excavations of Hormuzd Rassam in Babylon.[396] It was brought to my attention by H. Stadhouders and the *Electronic Babylonian Library* Project (eBL). The external features and the handwriting of BM 48997 and BM 49133 resemble each other to a high degree, so both fragments may belong to the same tablet, although they do not join (BM 49133 preserves the beginning of a couple of lines of the obverse and reverse of the tablet including the left edge; BM 48997 preserves several line endings of the obverse and reverse and the right edge). One section on the obverse of BM 49133 begins with DIŠ MUNUS "if a woman" followed by a reference to the month of delivery or to a month of pregnancy, which suggests that the fragment is a tablet dealing with medical treatments for women. However, the first line on the reverse starts with DIŠ NA "if a man", after a double ruling. This may indicate that the fragment belonged to a collective tablet that dealt with a mixture of different topics, including remedies for women (gynaecological material) and remedies for other non-gender-specific conditions. Such a mixture of topics is unusual but occasionally attested among the first millennium BCE cuneiform medical texts (see BM 61975 (text C.2.4), K. 8678+ (text A.1.4), BAM 249 (text D.1.3).

List of Manuscripts

Siglum	Museum Number	Copy	Collation	Format; Ductus	Provenience
a	BM 49133 (81-11-3, 1844)	–	Coll.	Fragment of a tablet; Late Babylonian script; ca. 6th–3rd cent. BCE	Babylon

396 Leichty, Finkel and Walker 2019, 705. Geller and Panayotov (2020, 10) list BM 49133 as a Late Babylonian text on eye diseases, but that tablet number is presumably a typo.

Overview

i'	Fragmentary prescription a obv. 1'–2'	1'–2'
ii'	Fragmentary prescription (to induce labour?) a obv. 3'–7'	3'–7'[...
iii''	Fragmentary instructions a rev. 1'–6'	...]8''–13''

Previous Edition and Discussion

Electronic Babylonian Library Project (eBL) (https://www.ebl.lmu.de/library/BM.49133; photo; transliteration)

Transliteration

Beginning of ms. a obv. lost; gap of unknown length

1' a obv. 1' ⌜ILLU⌝ L[I.DUR ....]

2' a obv. 2' Ì.UDU *m*[*al*?-*ma-liš* ḪI.ḪI? ....]

3' a obv. 1' DIŠ MUNUS *šá* ITI [Ù.TU-*šá* KU_4-*ma* NU Ù.TU?]

4' a obv. 2' *ša* ŠÀ-*šá ana š*[*u-ṣi-i*? ....]

5' a obv. 3' *lu-ú ina* gìš[GEŠTIN? ....]

6' a obv. 4' *ra-man-šú i*-[...]

7' a obv. 5' EGIR-*šú* x [..]

Ms. a obv. breaks; gap of unknown length

Beginning of ms. a rev. lost

8'' a rev. 1' DIŠ NA [...................................]

9'' a rev. 2' ZÚ.L[UM.MA ....]

10'' a rev. 3' *ina* ILLU [.................................]

11'' a rev. 4' *ana lìb-bi* [................................]

12'' a rev. 5' *ana* SU/KUŠ? [.............................]

13'' a rev. 6' x [..]

Ms. a rev. breaks; remainder lost

Bound Transcription and Translation

Beginning of ms. a obv. lost; gap of unknown length

1' *ḫīl abu*[*kkati* . . . . . .] 2' *lipâ m*[*almališ tuballal*(?) . . . . . .]	1' resin of *abu*[*kkatu*, ...] 2' (and) tallow [you mix] e[qually(?) . . . . . .].

3' *šumma sinništu ša arḫu [ša alādīša īrubam-ma lā ūlid(?)]* 4' *ša libbīša ana š[ūṣî(?)* ......] 5' *lū ina [karāni(?)* ......] 6' *ramānšu i-[*......] 7' *arkīšu* ...[......]

3" If the month in which a woman [is due to give birth has arrived, but she doesn't give birth(?)], 4" to make her foetus [come out(?) ......] 5' or in [wine(?) ......] 6' she herself(?) will [......] 7' afterwards [......]

Ms. a obv. breaks; gap of unknown length

Beginning of ms. a rev. lost

8" *šumma amīlu* [......] 9" *sul[uppū* ......] 10" *ina ḫīl* [......] 11" *ana libbi* [......] 12" *ana* ...[......] 13" *traces*

8" If a man [......] 9" da[tes ......] 10" with resin of [......] 11" into [......] 12" onto [......] 13" *too fragmentary for translation*

Ms. a rev. breaks; remainder lost

Notes

Lines 3'–4': Parallels from other women's healthcare texts offer several possible restorations for the fragmentary purpose statement in lines 3'–4'. The word ITI (*arḫu*) "month" may either refer to a month of pregnancy or to the month of birth, in which a woman was supposed to deliver. A few prescriptions to protect a woman from miscarriage mention bleeding or miscarriage in the first trimester of pregnancy, e.g. BM 42313+ rev. 9 and dupl. (text A.2.2 line 50): DIŠ MUNUS *lu* (*šá*) ITI *lu* (*šá*) 2 ITI *lu* (*šá*) 3 ITI *šá* ŠÀ-ŠÀ-*šà* ŠUB.ŠUB-*a* "If a woman, (being) either one month or two months or three months (pregnant) keeps having a miscarriage (lit. keeps aborting her foetus) ...". See also BM 42313+ rev. 12 (text A.2.2 line 53). The second option for restoring lines 3'–4' (followed here) are parallel introductions in prescriptions to induce labour and promote delivery, such as found in SpTU 4, No. 153: 21 (text D.1.11 line 3): [DIŠ MUNU]S ITI *šá* Ù.TU-*šú iq-ri-ba-am-ma la ú-[lid-ma* [lú]*lil-lid-su la]* ⌜*ú*⌝*-ṣi-ma a-[na šu-ṣi-i*/Ù.TU-*šú*?] "[If a wom]an's month when the birth is due has approached, but she has not [yet given birth and her baby has not yet] emerged, t[o make *it come out/enable her give birth*(?)]". The context and following prescription in BM 49133 lines 5'ff. is too fragmentary to reach any certainty which of these readings and restorations is more likely.

Chapter F
Texts on Amulet Charms for (Pregnant) Women

In Mesopotamian healing traditions, amulet charms played an eminent role. They came in the form of strings of (mostly) beads – made from stones, metals, shells as well as other materials – beside phylacteries in the form of leather bags filled with various materials. They were used for apotropaic, protective and curative purposes. The beads and other components of an amulet were usually strung on threads of wool of different colour (sometimes strings of other materials such as linen or tendons were used as well). In many prescriptions, a specific number of knots had then to be tied into the strings. In addition, spells were recited over the prepared amulet strings before they were attached to the patient's body (for an overview see Schuster-Brandis 2008, 51–69).

The "magic binding" of pregnant women with amulets and the use of specific stones to protect them from miscarriage is a common practice in many cultures, past and present; and certain aspects of this magic lore were transmitted from ancient times to later centuries (e.g. Hanson 1995; Stol 2000a, 49–50 (on the "eagle stone"); Michel 1995; 2004, 178–202; Obermeyer 2000). Mesopotamian healing texts on women's health matters from the first millennium BCE can serve as early examples for such practices (Stol 2000a, 49–52). Amulet charms for women are incorporated in several texts devoted to pregnancy. They were prescribed especially for protection from miscarriage and against bleeding (during pregnancy) and other discharges; they were also applied for fertility (see texts B.1.4, C.1.1–C.1.4, C.1.8, C.3.1, C.3.3–C.3.7, C.3.9). The use of amulets to protect from miscarriage and stop haemorrhage goes back to a much older tradition (Finkel 1980; Scurlock 1991). The texts edited in this chapter (F.1–F.2) illustrate the integration of amulet charms for pregnant women into multi-purpose compilations (serialized compendia) of amulet charms and their use in practice, which signals the popularity of such charms in first millennium BCE healing traditions.

F.1 A Group of Amulet Charms for Women Incorporated into the Series *kunuk ḫalti*

When Mesopotamian scholars in the first millennium BCE assembled compilations of amulet charm prescriptions for different purposes extracted from various healing texts, they also included amulets for women in such compilations. The group of amulet necklaces for the protection of pregnant women discussed here was incorporated as a thematic section into compendia of amulet prescriptions. The amulets were meant to be used as a whole ensemble of necklaces for different body parts, arranged from head to feet. Five of the texts grouped together in this chapter have been discussed by Schuster-Brandis (2008, 192–197) among the sources for the series *kunuk*(^{na4}KIŠIB) *ḫalti* "cylindrical *ḫaltu*-stone" (with a preliminary reconstruction of the series). This series is a specialized compendium of amulet prescriptions used for various apotropaic, protective and curative purposes. The name of the series *kunuk ḫalti* is attested in a library inventory from Nineveh (SAA 7, No. 49 i 2', iv 5'), but so far only two tablet fragments can be attributed to the series through a colophon referring to the series title.

Since most of the manuscripts containing the amulets for pregnant women are fragments, they cannot be identified with certainty as witnesses of a specific edition of the series *kunuk ḫalti* yet. The single-column tablet Ms. A_1 (K. 4727+) (+) A_2 (K. 6688) could represent an extract or excerpt from the series *kunuk ḫalti*.[397] It begins with the amulets for women and later turns to amulets for SAG.KI.DAB.BA (migraine) and other (unidentified) problems. Mss. B (K. 9071) and g (BM 47770+) are too fragmentary to be certain, but the former, with its overlaps to the sequence of the sections in ms. A_1 (+) A_2, could present a similar compilation of amulets. Two of the source texts contain only the amulets for pregnant women, likely forming excerpts or shorter extracts from the series (mss. D (= BAM 346), F (= STT 278)). Mss. c (DT 28) and E (KAL 2, No. 41) are fragments of two- or three-column tablets that seem to assemble treatments for women, although these may focus on amulets; ms. E seems to be a collection of procedures (mostly amulets) for protecting pregnant women (including recited incantations).

Schuster-Brandis (2008, 194 n. 485) observes that the place of the section with amulets for women in the series *kunuk ḫalti* is not completely certain yet. According to the reconstruction by Schuster-Brandis, amulets for stopping nosebleed may have formed the beginning of the series, preceding the amulets for pregnant women. This sequence has a thematic

397 K. 4727+ and K. 6688 have not been identified as fragments of the same tablet. Although the pieces barely touch each other, the textual overlap as well as shape of the fragments and script suggests that they actually form part of one tablet.

https://doi.org/10.1515/9781501506475-009

link, since the source texts for the ten amulets for pregnant women include one amulet between the amulet for the waist and the thigh, which was used to stop bleeding during pregnancy. This amulet was added to and worn together with the amulet for the woman's waist. Mss. A obv. 21' and E obv.! i 5' sum up the two amulets (attached to the waist) as "a string (of amulet stones) for a pregnant woman" (*takṣīru ša erīti*).

The inventory or memorandum BAM 363, which was found (like mss. D and E) in the N4 (exorcist's) library at Assur (edited as text F.2) attests to the application of the group of amulets for pregnant women from the series *kunuk ḫalti* in practice. It lists sums of stone beads and other ingredients, many of which have correspondences in the actual amulet prescriptions, which are referred to in a total of items (similar to mss. A and B) as "knotted (strings) for a pregnant woman" (*kuṣarū ša erīti*).

As a related piece of evidence, a similar group of amulets from head to feet for a pregnant woman who cannot bring to term, comparable to the ensemble discussed here (however, diverging in the ingredients), is found on a Neo-Assyrian tablet from Sultantepe (STT 241; text C.3.1), together with the text of an incantation recited over the amulet strings (see the table below). Another text with a longer collection of amulets and incantations for protecting pregnant women from miscarriage that contains ensembles of amulets attached to different body parts is AO 6473 from Hellenistic Uruk (text C.3.9).

A new text fragment for the amulet prescriptions for women edited in this chapter is DT 28 (ms. c). This Neo-Babylonian fragment found at Nineveh belonged to a two- or three-column tablet. The few preserved lines of its first column contain ritual instructions mentioning a "woman for whom childbearing has stopped", and an incantation with the incipit *māḫiṣ muḫḫi* "(You) who hits (my) skull" that was to be recited over amulet stones (for transliteration of the passage, see below). An incantation with this incipit (*māḫiṣ muḫḫi mubbil liq pīya* "The one who hits (my) skull, who dries my palate") is recited over amulets for a pregnant woman in STT 241 (see text C.3.1 and below). It is not entirely certain whether the "woman for whom childbearing has stopped" in DT 28 refers to the patient/treated problem, or whether it refers to a post-menopausal woman as a ritual agent who has to perform a specific action (e.g. spin a thread), as is sometimes required in ritual texts. In the second column of DT 28, the partial instructions for an amulet for the thigh is preserved, which is a duplicate to that respective amulet for pregnant women in the sources relating to the series *kunuk ḫalti*.

Another fragment of a large library tablet from Nineveh (AMT 66/4) with treatments for women preserves a fragmentary passage related to the amulets discussed here: thus, one of the amulets edited here (the amulet for the thigh) is followed there by other treatments for women (including amulets). The fragment also contains a colophon-like note referring to the series *kunuk ḫalti*. The note seems to be a scribal remark that only a selection of contents (i.e. amulets for pregnant women?) was extracted from the series and included on the tablet (see text D.1.4 for discussion).

The ensemble of amulets for pregnant women consisted of ten parts, each attached to a different body part, from the head down to the feet (see the table below; see also Schuster-Brandis 2008, 146–150 for discussion). The manuscripts differ slightly in their attribution of the amulets to specific body parts, but usually the forehead/temples, neck, both hands and feet as well as the waist/hips including the navel are specified. A similar, but less complex ensemble of amulets in STT 241 specifies seven bodily locations for the amulets. As mentioned above, one of the ten amulets was intended specifically to stop bleeding. This amulet can be seen as an additional element added to the amulet for the waist, since it had to be fastened together with the latter (see lines 28–32 in the edition below).

Overview of the amulets for pregnant women according to body parts.

BAM 346 (D)	**STT 278 (F)**	**K. 4727 (+) K. 6688 (A1 (+) A2) BM 47770 (g)**	**STT 241 (text C.3.1)**
Forehead (SAG.KI; "Kette 154"; 2 stones)	[Right and(?)] left [temple](?)	[. . .]	Temples (SAG.KI.MEŠ)
Forelock (*abūsātu*; "Kette 155"; 6 stones)	[. . .]	Left [. . .]	–
Neck (GÚ; "Kette 156"; 4 stones)	Neck	Neck	–
Right hand (ŠU 15 "Kette 157"; 4 stones)	Right hand	Right hand	Right hand
Left hand (ŠU 150; "Kette 158"; 5 stones)	Left hand	[. . .]	Left hand
Waist (MURUB$_4$; "Kette 159"; 14 stones)	Waist	Waist	Hips (MURUB$_4$.MEŠ)
Amulet to stop bleeding during pregnancy (45 stones tied to the waist)	[. . .]	(Bleeding)	Navel

(continued)

BAM 346 (D)	STT 278 (F)	K. 4727 (+) K. 6688 (A1 (+) A2) BM 47770 (g)	STT 241 (text C.3.1)
[Thigh][398] (ÚR; "Kette 160"; 8 (var. 7) stones)	[. . .]	Thigh	–
Right [foot(?)] ("Kette 161"; 6 stones)	Right [. . .]	Right foot	Right foot
Left foot ("Kette 162"; 8 stones)[399]	[. . .]	Left [foot?]	Left foot

Taken together, the ten amulets for pregnant women are quite complex and costly in their composition. Beside 102 different stones and plant materials serving as main components (in the form of perforated beads), various strings as well as wads (or burls) made of wool of various colours are indicated as central material elements of the amulets. In comparison, the inventory BAM 363 (text F.2) lists even a higher total of 130 components ("stones") that were used for a similar ensemble of amulets.

The textual structure of the amulet sections can be summarized as follows:

- Name of body part
- List of main components (stone beads, shells, plant materials etc.) with total
- Indication of string(s) of wool, on which components are threaded
- Indication of different wads or burls of wool (*lippu*, *ḫuppu*, *ubānu*) attached to the amulet string
- Knots tied into the string (only in the amulet for the waist/hips)
- Indications for application

The variations in this structure are discussed in the notes to the text below.

List of Manuscripts

Siglum	Museum Number	Copy	Collation	Format; Ductus	Provenience
A_1 (+)	K. 4727 + K. 9426 + 81-2-4, 386 (+)	Geers, Folio D93 (K. 4727 + K. 9426 + 81-2-4, 386) Pl. 49–50	Coll.	single-column tablet, portrait format;[400] Neo-Assyrian script; 7th cent. BCE	Nineveh
A_2	K. 6688	Geers, Folio G16 (K. 6688) Pl. 49–50	Coll.	Fragment of a single-column tablet, portrait format;[401] Neo-Assyrian script; 7th cent. BCE	Nineveh
B	K. 9071	Geers, Folio D95 Pl. 51	Coll.	Fragment of a single-column(?) tablet;[402] Neo-Assyrian script; 7th cent. BCE	Nineveh
c	DT 28	Geers, Folio G18 Pl. 53	Coll.	Fragment of a two(?)-column tablet;[403] Neo-Babylonian script; 7th cent. BCE	Nineveh
D	A 624	BAM 346	Coll.	Single-column tablet, portrait format; Neo-Assyrian script; ca. 8th/7th cent. BCE	Assur; N4 library

398 KAL 2, No. 41 (ms. E) uses this amulet for the "right thigh" (ÚR 15).
399 KAL 2, No. 41 (ms. E) uses this amulet for the "left thigh" (ÚR 150) instead.
400 Measurements: ca. 7 x 13.5 x 1.9 cm.
401 Measurements: ca. 5 x 4.8 x 2 cm.
402 Measurements: ca. 4 x 6.3 x 1.8 cm.
403 Measurements: ca. 6.5 x 2.5 x 2.9 cm.

(continued)

Siglum	Museum Number	Copy	Collation	Format; Ductus	Provenience
E	VAT 13629 + 13866	KAL 2, No. 41 (p. 193)	-	Two- or three-column tablet; Neo-Assyrian script; ca. 8th/7th cent. BCE	Assur; N4 library
F	SU 52/146 + 173 + 338	STT 278	Coll.	Single-column tablet; landscape format;[404] Neo-Assyrian script; ca. 911–612 BCE	Huzirina (Sultantepe)
g	BM 47770 + BM 47904 (81-11-3, 475 + 81-11-3, 611)	Pl. 52	Coll.	fragment of a single(?)-column tablet; Neo-/Late Babylonian script; ca. 6th cent. BCE(?)	probably Babylon

Overview

i	Amulet string for protecting a pregnant woman (for the forehead, var. right and left temple(?)) A_2 obv. 1–3 // D obv. 1–3 // F obv. 1–2	1–3
ii	Amulet string for protecting a pregnant woman (for the forelock, var. left . . .) A_2 obv. 4–9 // D obv. 4–8 // F obv. 3–5	4–8
iii	Amulet string for protecting a pregnant woman (for the neck) A_2 obv. 10–12 // D obv. 9–11 // F obv. 6–7	9–11
iv	Amulet string for protecting a pregnant woman (for the right hand) A_2 obv. 13–A_1 obv. 3' (+) A_2 obv. 15 // D obv. 12–14 // F obv. 8–9	12–14
v	Amulet string for protecting a pregnant woman (for the left hand) A_1 obv. 4'–6' // D obv. 15–17 // F. obv. 10–11	15–17
vi	Amulet string for protecting a pregnant woman (for the waist) A_1 obv. 7'–16' // B obv. 1'–7' // D obv. 18–22 // F obv. 12–17 // g obv. 1'–4'	18–27
vii	Amulet string for protecting a pregnant woman (against bleeding) A_1 obv. 17'–21' // B obv. 8'–12' // D rev. 7'–10' // E obv.! i' 1'–5' // F obv. 18–rev. 1 // g obv. 4'–7'	28–32
viii	Amulet string for protecting a pregnant woman (for the thigh, var. right thigh) A_1 obv. 22'–25' // B obv. 13'–16' // c ii 1'–6' // D rev. 11'–14' // E obv.! i' 6'–11' // F rev. 2–3 // g obv. 8'–9'	33–35
ix	Amulet string for protecting a pregnant woman (for the right foot) A_1 obv. 26'–28' // B obv. 17' // D rev. 15'–17' // E obv.! i' 17' // F rev. 4 // g obv. 10'–11'	36–38
x	Amulet string for protecting a pregnant woman (for the left foot, var. left thigh) A_1 obv. 29'–31' // D rev. 18'–19' // E obv.! i' 12'–16' // g obv. 12'	39–41

Previous Edition and Discussion

K. 4727+ (Ms. A_1):

Photo: CDLI P395702

Edition: *Electronic Babylonian Library* (eBL) (transliteration) https://www.ebl.lmu.de/library/K.4727; Schuster-Brandis 2008, Kette 255 (K. 4727+ rev. 26"–28")

Discussion: Köcher, BAM IV, p. XIII (sub BAM 346); Schwemer 2007, *KAL* 2, p. 100; Schuster-Brandis 2008, 148 (Kette 154–162), 193 text “G”

K. 6688 (Ms. A_2):

Although the fragments barely touch each other, K. 6688 most likely should be identified as part of K. 4727+, preserving the upper right corner of the obverse and bottom right corner of the reverse.

Photo: CDLI P396732

404 Measurements: ca. 10 x 7 x 2 cm.

Edition: *Electronic Babylonian Library* (eBL) (https://www.ebl.lmu.de/library/K.6688; transliteration)

K. 9071 (Ms. B):
Photo: CDLI P397891
Edition: *Electronic Babylonian Library* (eBL) (https://www.ebl.lmu.de/library/K.9071; transliteration)
Discussion: Köcher, BAM IV, p. XIII (sub BAM 346); Schwemer 2007, *KAL* 2, p. 100; Schuster-Brandis 2008, 148 (Kette 154–162), 193 text "H"

DT 28 (Ms. c):
Photo: CDLI P237716
Edition: *Electronic Babylonian Library* (eBL) (https://www.ebl.lmu.de/library/DT.28; transliteration)
Discussion: Fincke 2003–2004, *AfO* 50, 143

BAM 346 (A 624; Ms. D):
Photo: –
Edition: *BabMed Corpora*; CDLI P285418 (transliteration)
Discussion: Schuster-Brandis 2008, 193 text "E"; Limet 1984, 332–333 (transliteration and translation of lines 1–14)

VAT 13629 + 13866 (KAL 2, No. 41; Ms. E):
Photo: –
Edition and Discussion: Schwemer 2007, *KAL* 2, 100–102 No. 41 obv.$^{!}$ i' 1'–17';[405] Abusch et al. 2020, CMAwR 3, text 5.2 (summary notes); CDLI P480934

STT 278 (Ms. F):
Photo: –
Edition: –
Discussion: Schwemer 2007, *KAL* 2, p. 100; Schuster-Brandis 2008, 148 (Kette 154–162), 193 (ms. "F"); CDLI P338596

BM 47770 + 47904 (Ms. g)
Edition: –
Discussion: Schwemer 2007, KAL 2, p. 100; Schuster-Brandis 2008, 148 (Kette 154–162), 193 (ms. "I"); Leichty, Finkel and Walker 2019, *CBT* IV–V, part 5, 671; *electronic Babylonian Library* (eBL) (https://www.ebl.lmu.de/library/BM.47770)

Transliteration

1	A$_2$ obv. 1–2	[x x]x x ⸢2$^{?}$⸣ ^{na4}ZÚ ZALAG$^{?}$.⸢MEŠ$^{?}$⸣ / [. . . . . . .]
	D obv. 1	SAG.KI 2 ^{na4}⸢ZÚ⸣ ⸢ZALAG$^{?}$⸣ ⸢*ina*⸣ ⸢DUR$^{?}$⸣ ⸢SÍG$^{?}$⸣ x [È]
	F obv. 1	[. . . . .]
2	A$_2$ obv. 2$^{cont.}$–3	[^{síg}GA.RÍG.A]K.A 4 ⸢ŠU.SI$^{?}$⸣ / [. . . . .]
	D obv. 2	^{síg}GA.RÍG.AK.A ⸢4$^{?}$⸣ ŠU.SI *ina bi-ri-šú-n*[*u*]
	F obv. 1$^{cont.}$	[. . . . .] *bi-r*[*i*]-*š*[*u-nu*]
3	A$_2$ obv. 3$^{cont.}$	[*t*]*ála-pap ina* ⸢PIŠ$_{10}$.^{d}ÍD$^{?}$⸣ x x x ⸢*tara*⸣-*k*[*ás*$^{?}$]
	D obv. 3	*ina* PIŠ$_{10}$.^{d}ÍD *tála-pap ina* SAG.KI-*šá tara-kás*
	F obv. 2	[. . . . . *ina* SAG.KI-*šá šá* 15$^{?}$] *u* ⸢150$^{!?}$⸣ ⸢*tara-kás*⸣

A, D, F ______________________________

405 As observed by Abusch et al. 2020, text 5.3 (notes), the assignment of the fragment's obverse and reverse in KAL 2, No. 41, needs to be reversed. Abusch et al. 2020, 54 (summary) believe that obv.$^{!}$ i' is in fact column ii of the tablet, but nothing is preserved of the assumed column i to know with certainty.

4	A$_2$ obv. 4	[x x x x ^{na4}]PA *šá* 7 ⸢GÙN⸣.MEŠ-⸢*šá*⸣
	D obv. 4	*a-bu-us-sa-tú* ^{na4}PA *kús-bir-rat-*⸢*tú*⸣
	F obv. 3	[. . . . .]
5	A$_2$ obv. 5	[. . . . . ^{n}]^{a4}*àba-aš-mu* ^{na4}G[UG$^{?}$]
	D obv. 5	^{na4}*àba-aš-mu* ^{na4}NÍR ^{na4}*aš-pu-u* ^{na4}G[UG$^{?}$]
	F obv. 3$^{cont.}$	[. . . . .] ⸢x x x x⸣ ⸢^{na4}GUG$^{?}$⸣
6	A$_2$ obv. 6–7	[. . . . .] PAP 6 NA$_4$.MEŠ / [. . . . . . .]
	D obv. 6	PAP 6 NA$_4$.MEŠ *ina* SÍG GÙN.A È
	F obv. 4	[. . . . .] ⸢x x x⸣
7	A$_2$ obv. 7$^{cont.}$–8	[*líp-p*]*i ḫúp-pi tála-pap* / [. . . . . . ^{síg}ḪÉ.ME.D]A$^{?}$ *tála-pap*
	D obv. 6$^{cont.}$–7	⸢*líp-pi*$^{?}$⸣ ⸢*ḫúp*⸣-[*pi*] / 3 *líp-pi šá* ^{síg}ḪÉ.ME.DA *tála-*[*pap*]
	F obv. 4$^{cont.}$–5	[x x x x] 3 *lí*[*p-pi šá* ^{síg}ḪÉ.M]E$^{!}$.⸢DA$^{?!}$⸣ / [. . . . . .]
8	A$_2$ obv. 9	[. . . . .] ⸢GÙB⸣ *tara-kás*
	D obv. 8	*ina el-li-ti-šá šá* 150 ⸢*tara*⸣-[*kás*]
	F obv. 5$^{cont.}$	[. . . . . *tara*]-*kás*$^{!}$
A, D, F		
9	A$_2$ obv. 10–11	[. . . . .]x ^{na4}ZA.GÌN / [. . . . . .]
	D obv. 9	GÚ ^{na4}KIŠIB *ḫal-ti* ^{na4}PA ^{na4}ZA.GÌN ^{na4}⸢MUŠ⸣.[GÍR]
	F obv. 6	[. . . . . G]ÍR$^{?}$
10	A$_2$ obv. 11$^{cont.}$–12	[. . . . .] ⸢NA$_4$⸣.MEŠ *ina* SÍG GÙN / [. . .]
	D obv. 10	^{na4}ZÚ PAP 4 NA$_4$.MEŠ *ina* SÍG GÙN.A È-⸢*ak*$^{?}$⸣
	F obv. 6$^{cont.}$	⸢x x⸣ *ina* x[. . . . .]
11	A$_2$ obv. 12$^{cont.}$	[. . . . . ^{síg}]ḪÉ.ME.DA *tála-pap ina* ⸢GÚ-*šú*⸣ GAR-*an*
	D obv. 11	3 *líp-pi ša* ^{síg}ḪÉ.MID *tála-pap ina* GÚ-*šá tara-*⸢*kás*⸣
	F obv. 6$^{cont.}$–7	3 *líp-p*[*a*] / [. . . . .] *ina* GÚ-*šú* ⸢GAR⸣-*an*
D, F		
12	A$_1$ obv. 1'(+)A$_2$ obv. 13	[x x x x] ⸢^{na4}⸣[x x ^{n}]^{a4}*šu-u* NÍTA ^{na4}ZÚ
	D obv. 12	ŠU 15 ^{na4}GUG ^{na4}ZA.GÌN ^{na4}*šu-u* NÍTA ⸢$^{na4!}$ZÚ$^{!}$⸣ ⸢SIG$_7$$^{?}$⸣
	F obv. 8	⸢ŠU$^{?}$⸣ [. . . . . . ^{n}]^{a4}ZA.⸢GÌN⸣ ^{na4}⸢*šu-u*⸣ ⸢NÍTA$^{?!}$⸣ ⸢^{na4}ZÚ$^{?}$⸣ 4 ⸢NA$_4$.MEŠ$^{?}$⸣
13	A$_1$ obv. 2'(+)A$_2$ obv. 14	[x x *ina* SÍ]G GÙN.A ^{sí}[^{g}ZA].GÌN.NA ^{síg}GA.RÍG.AK.A
	D obv. 13	*ina* SÍG GÙN.A ^{síg}ZA.GÌN.NA ^{síg}GA.RÍG.A[K].A ⸢È⸣
	F obv. 8$^{cont.}$–9	⸢*ina*⸣ ⸢SÍG⸣ x *ina* ⸢^{síg}⸣[Z]A.GÌN.⸢NA⸣ / ⸢^{síg}⸣[. . . . .]
14	A$_1$ obv. 3'(+)A$_2$ obv. 15	[x *líp*]-*pi šá* ^{síg}ḪÉ.M[E.D]A ⸢*tála-pap*⸣ ⸢*ina*⸣ ⸢ŠU⸣ [15]-⸢*šá*⸣ GAR-⸢*an*⸣
	D obv. 14	3 *líp-pi ša* ^{síg}ḪÉ.MID *tála-pap ina* ŠU 15-⸢*šá*⸣ ⸢*tara-kás*⸣
	F obv. 9$^{cont.}$	[x *lí*]*p-pa šá* ⸢^{síg}ḪÉ.ME.DA⸣ *tála-pap* <<pap>> ⸢*ina*⸣ ⸢ŠU⸣ ⸢ZAG$^{?}$⸣-[*šá*] ⸢GAR⸣-*a*[*n*$^{?}$]
A, D, F		
15	A$_1$ obv. 4'	[x x] ^{na4}ÁŠ.GÌ.GÌ ^{na4}BA[BBAR.DILI$^{?}$ . . . .]
	D obv. 15–16	ŠU 150 ^{na4}AŠ.GÌ.GÌ ^{na4}BABBAR.DILI ^{na4}*šu-*[*u* x x x x] / ^{na4}ZÚ ZALAG
	F obv. 10	⸢ŠU⸣ 150 ^{n}[^{a4}x x x ^{n}]^{a4}BABBAR.DILI ^{na4}*šu-u* ⸢MUNUS$^{?!}$⸣ ⸢^{na4}⸣ZA.GÌN ⸢^{na4}ZÚ⸣
16	A$_1$ obv. 5'	[x N]A$_4$.MEŠ *ina ba-ru-un-*[*di* . . . .]
	D obv. 16$^{cont.}$–17	PAP 5 NA$_4$.MEŠ *ina ba-r*[*u-un-di*$^{?}$] / ^{síg}ZA.GÌN.NA
	F obv. 10$^{cont.}$–11	5$^{!}$(4) ⸢NA$_4$$^{!?}$(LAGAB)⸣.MEŠ *ina b*[*a*$^{?}$-. . . . .] / ⸢^{síg}ZA.GÌN⸣

17	A$_1$ obv. 6'	[^{síg}]GA.RÍG.AK.A È [..........................]
	D obv. 17$^{cont.}$	^{síg}GA.RÍG.AK.A [È (. . .) *ina* ŠU 150-*šá tara-kás*$^?$]
	F obv. 11$^{cont.}$	^{síg}GA$^{?!}$.[RÍG.A]K$^?$.⸢A⸣ 3 *líp-pa šá* ^{síg}ḪÉ.ME.D[A] *tála-pap* <<pap>> *ina* ŠU ⸢150⸣-[*šá*$^?$] ⸢GAR⸣-*a*[*n*] ⸢x$^?$⸣
	g obv. 1'	⸢x x x x⸣ [...]
A, D, F, g		________________
18	A$_1$ obv. 7'	[MURU]B$_4$ ^{na4}KIŠIB ŠUBA ^{n}[^{a4} ....]
	D obv. 18	MURUB$_4$ ^{na4}KIŠIB ŠUBA ^{na4}ŠU[BA$^?$ x x x x]
	F obv. 12	⸢MURUB$_4$⸣ ^{na4}KIŠIB ŠUBA ^{na4}ŠU[BA$^?$] ^{na4}⸢KIŠIB⸣ KUR-*nu*
	g obv. 2'	[x] ^{na4}KIŠIB ŠU[BA] ^{na4}ŠUBA ^{na4}KIŠIB ⸢KUR-*nu*⸣
19	A$_1$ obv. 8'	[^{n}]^{a4}KIŠIB *ḫal-tu*$_4$ 3 ^{na4}x[.........................]
	D obv. 19	^{na4}KIŠIB *ḫal-ti* 3 ^{na4}ZÁ[LAG$^?$ ....]
	F obv. 12$^{cont.}$	^{na4}⸢KIŠIB⸣ *ḫal-tú* ⸢x x⸣ [x]-*nu* ^{na4}G[UG$^?$]
	g obv. 2'	⸢^{na4}KIŠIB⸣ ⸢*ḫal-tu*$_4$$^?$⸣ 3 [x x] x ⸢^{na4}GUG⸣ ⸢^{na4}⸣[...........]
20	A$_1$ obv. 9'	[KA].⸢KÉŠ⸣ ^{giš}ḪAB ŠIKA ⸢E⸣.[SÍR ....]
	D obv. 20	[x x ^{g}]^{iš}⸢ḪAB⸣ ⸢ŠIKA$^?$⸣ ⸢E.SÍR⸣.⸢KA⸣.[LÍM.MA$^?$ ......]
	F obv. 13	[K]A.⸢KÉŠ⸣ ^{giš}ḪAB ŠIKA ⸢E⸣.[SÍR].⸢KA.LÍMMU-*te*$^?$⸣
	g obv. 2'$^{cont.}$–3'	[....................] / [ŠIKA SI]LA.LÍM.MA
21	A$_1$ obv. 10'	[K]A A.AB.BA ^{na4}*z*[*i*-É ....]
	B obv. 1'	[(x)] x x [..................................]
	D obv. 21	[........... ^{na4}*zi*]-⸢É$^!$⸣ ⸢^{na4}⸣[..................]
	F obv. 13$^{cont.}$	KA *tam-tim* [^{na4}]*zi*-É ^{na4}*šu-u* NÍTA ^{n}[^{a4}x x]
	g obv. 3'	KA ⸢*tam*⸣-*tim* ^{na4}*zi*-É ^{na4} *šu-u* NÍTA ^{na4}⸢*sa*$^?$⸣-[*a*]-⸢*bu*$^?$⸣
22	A$_1$ obv. 11'	[x x x x *ina*] S[ÍG ....]
	B obv. 2'	14 NA$_4$.MEŠ *ina* S[ÍG$^?$ ....]
	F obv. 14	[x x x]x *ina* ⸢SÍG$^{?!}$⸣.MEŠ ⸢GÙN$^{!?}$⸣.A ⸢x⸣ ⸢*líp-pa*⸣ ⸢^{síg}ḪÉ⸣.[ME.DA]
	g obv. 3'$^{cont.}$	PAP 14 NA$_4$.MEŠ *ina* SÍG ⸢GÙN.A⸣ [È ....]
23	A$_1$ obv. 12'	[.................................]
	B obv. 3'	[*tál*]*a-pap* 4 KA.KÉŠ [KÉŠ$^?$ ....]
	F obv. 14$^{cont.}$	[*tála-p*]*ap* 4 K[A.KÉŠ KÉŠ (x x)]
F		________________
24	A$_1$ obv. 13'	[...]
	B obv. 4'	DUR SÍG BABBAR È [..........................]
	F obv. 15	[x x x x] ⸢DUR⸣ ⸢SÍG⸣ BABBAR È [x x] ⸢KA.KÉŠ⸣ x x[..............]
25	A$_1$ obv. 14'	[x x x x x KI N]A$_4$.MEŠ MURUB$_4$ D[AB-*bat*$^?$ x x x x]
	B obv. 4'$^{cont.}$–5'	[.......] / KI NA$_4$.MEŠ MURUB$_4$ DAB$^?$-*b*[*at*$^?$ ....]
	F obv. 16	[..]
26	A$_1$ obv. 15'	[x x x x x x] SA$_5$ DUR ^{síg}⸢ZA⸣.[GÌN.NA ....]
	B obv. 6'	DUR SÍG SA$_5$-*tim*$^{?!}$ DU[R ....]
	F obv. 16$^{cont.}$	[........] S[A$_5$ DU]R$^?$ SÍG ⸢GI$_6$$^{?!}$⸣ *ina*$^?$ x[.............]
27	A$_1$ obv. 16'	[x x] ⸢7$^?$⸣ ⸢KA.KÉŠ⸣ KÉŠ KI NA$_4$.MEŠ MURUB$_4$ DAB-*bat ina* MURUB$_4$-⸢*šá*⸣ [*tara-kás*$^?$]
	B obv. 7'	KA.KÉŠ KÉŠ KI NA$_4$.M[EŠ ....]
	F obv. 17	[......... K]A.KÉŠ [(x) KÉ]Š$^?$.KÉŠ ⸢KI⸣ NA$_4$.M[EŠ ....]
	g obv. 4'	[x *lí*]*p*-⸢*pi*⸣ *šá* ^{síg}⸢ḪÉ.ME.DA⸣ *tála-pap* 7 KA.KÉŠ KÉŠ-*ár ina* MURUB$_4$-*šú tara-kás*
D		________________

28	A_1 obv. 17'	⸢*šum*⸣-[*ma*] MUNUS MÚD.MEŠ-*šá* DU-*ku-ši*$^?$ 14 ^{na4}GUG *kup-pu-ut-*⸢*tu*⸣
	B obv. 8'	*šum-ma* MUNUS MÚD.MEŠ-*šá* DU-*k*[*u* . . . .]
	D rev. 7'	*šum*$_4$-[*ma* x x].⸢MEŠ$^?$⸣ x x x[. . . . .]
	F obv. 18	[. . . . . D]U-*ku* [NU KU]D$^?$ 14$^?$ ^{na4}GUG$^!$ *k*[*u*$^!$*-up-pu-ut-tu*]
	g obv. 4'$^{cont.}$	--- 14 ^{na4}⸢GUG *kup-*⸢*pu*⸣*-u*[*t-tu*]
29	A_1 obv. 18'	14 ⸢KA.KÉŠ⸣ ^{giš}ḪAB *ina* SÍG GÙN.A È 14 ^{na4}*šu-u* NÍTA.MEŠ
	B obv. 9'	14 KA.KÉŠ ^{giš}ḪAB *ina* SÍG G[ÙN.A . . . .]
	D rev. 8'	x x x x x x [. . . . .]
	F obv. 19	[. . . . . G]ÙN$^?$.A [. . . . . . .] ^{na4}*šu-u* NÍTA
	g obv. 5'	[x K]A.KÉŠ ^{giš}ḪAB *ina* SÍG SA$_5$ È 14 ^{na4}*šu-u* NÍTA.MEŠ
30	A_1 obv. 19'	*ina* SÍ[G] ⸢BABBAR⸣ SÍG SA$_5$ È KI NA$_4$.MEŠ *šá* MURUB$_4$ *tu-kàṣ-ṣar* ŠIKA SI[LA].⸢LÍM⸣.MA
	B obv. 10'–11'	*ina* SÍG BABBAR$^{?!}$ SÍG SA$_5$ È [. . . . .] / ŠIKA SILA.LÍM.MA
	D rev. 8'$^{cont.}$–9'	[*ina* SÍG] / ⸢SA$_5$$^?$⸣ SÍG⸣ ⸢BABBAR⸣ ⸢SÍG⸣ ⸢GÙN⸣.A$^?$ ⸢È⸣ [. . . . .]
	E obv.$^!$ i' 1'–2'	⸢KI⸣ N[A$_4$].⸢MEŠ⸣ ⸢x x⸣ [x x x] / ŠIKA ⸢SILA.LÍM.MA⸣
	F obv. 19–20	*ina* ⸢DUR⸣ [. . . . .] / [. . . . .]-*ru* ŠI[KA SILA$^?$.LÍMMU]-*te*$^?$
	g obv. 5'$^{cont.}$–7'	*ina* SÍG GÙN.A È 3 ^{na4}ZÚ ZALAG.MEŠ [*ina* SÍG x È$^?$] / ⸢*ina*⸣ DUR SÍG BABBAR *ina* DUR SÍG GI$_6$ *ina* DUR SÍG SA$_5$ *ina* D[UR ^{síg}]ZA.GÌN.NA <<*ina*>> 7.TA.ÀM KA.K[ÉŠ KÉŠ-*ár*] / [x x x MUR]UB$_4$ DAB-*bat* ⸢ŠIKA⸣ SILA.LÍM.MA
31	A_1 obv. 20'	⸢*a*⸣-*n*[*a*] ⸢*pi-in*⸣-*gi ina* LI.DUR-⸢*šá*⸣ GAR-*an* PAP 59 NA$_4$.MEŠ *šá* MU[RUB$_4$ EN 14 KA.KÉ]Š$^?$
	B obv. 11'–12'	*ana pi-i*[*n-gi* . . . .] / *šá* MURUB$_4$ EN 14 KA.K[ÉŠ . . . .]
	D rev. 10'	PAP x ⸢NA$_4$⸣.M[EŠ$^?$]
	E obv.$^!$ i' 2'–4'	*ana pi-*[*i*]*n-g*[*i*] / *ina* LI.DUR-⸢*šá*⸣ GAR-*an* / PAP 59 NA$_4$.MEŠ *šá* MURUB$_4$.MEŠ / EN 14 KA.KÉŠ ^{giš}ḪAB
	F obv. 20$^{cont.}$–rev. 1	*ina pi*$^!$-⸢*in-gi*⸣ *ina* L[I.DUR-*šá*$^?$ x x] / [. . . . . 10]+⸢4⸣ ⸢KA.KÉŠ⸣ ^{giš}Ḫ[AB$^?$ . . . . . .]
	g obv. 7'$^{obv.}$	*a-na pi-in-*⸢*gi*⸣ ⸢*i*⸣*-na* LI.DUR-*šú* [x x x x]
32	A obv. 21'	*tak-ṣi-ru šá* ^{munus}⸢PEŠ$_4$⸣
	D rev. 10'$^{cont.}$	[x x x M]ÚD ⸢MUNUS⸣ ⸢KUD$^?$⸣ x
	E obv.$^!$ i' 5'	*tak-ṣi-ri šá* ^{munus}PEŠ$_4$

A, B, d, E, F, g

33	A_1 obv. 22'	ÚR ^{na4}ÁŠ.GÌ.GÌ ^{na4}GUG ^{na4}ZA.GÌN ^{na4}PA ^{na4}*ka-pa-*⸢*ṣu*⸣
	B obv. 13'	ÚR ^{na4}ÁŠ.GÌ.GÌ ^{na4}G[UG . . . .]
	c ii 1'–3'	⸢ÚR⸣ ⸢^{na4}⸣ÁŠ.GÌ.GÌ $^{n[a4}$ . . . . .] / ^{na4}ZA.GÌN ^{na4}PA $^{n[a4}$ . . . .] / ^{na4}*zi-É*
	D rev. 11'	⸢x x x⸣ $^{n[a4]}$x x x x x x x
	E obv.$^!$ i' 6'–7'	ÚR 15 ^{na4}ÁŠ.GÌ.GÌ ^{na4}GUG ^{na4}ZA.GÌN / ^{na4}PA ^{na4}*ka-pa-*⸢*ṣu*⸣ ⸢^{na4}⸣*zi-É*
	F rev. 2	[. . . ^{na4}ÁŠ].GÌ.GÌ ⸢^{na4}GUG$^?$⸣ ⸢^{na4}ZA.GÌN$^?$⸣ [. . . . .]
	g obv. 8'	[x ^{n}]^{a4}AŠ.GÌ.GÌ ^{na4}GUG ^{na4}ZA.G[ÌN] ^{na4}PA ^{na4}*ka-pa-*⸢*ṣa*⸣ ⸢^{na4}⸣*zi-É*
34	A_1 obv. 23'	^{na4}*šu-u* NÍTA *u* MUNUS PAP 7 NA$_4$.MEŠ *ina* SÍG GÙN.A È x[(x)]
	B obv. 14'	^{na4}*šu-u* NÍTA *u* MUNUS x[. . . . .]
	c ii 3'$^{cont.}$–4'	$^{n[a4}$. . . . .] / PAP 8 NA$_4$.MEŠ *ina* [. . . . .]
	D rev. 13'–14'	⸢^{na4}*šu-u*⸣ ⸢NÍTA$^?$⸣ ⸢^{na4}ZÚ$^?$⸣ PAP ⸢8$^?$⸣ ⸢NA$_4$⸣.[MEŠ] / ⸢*ina*$^?$⸣ ⸢^{síg}⸣ZA.GÌN.NA È
	E obv.$^!$ i' 8'–9'	[^{n}]^{a4}*šu-u* NÍTA *u* MUNUS PAP ⸢8⸣ ⸢NA$_4$⸣.[M]EŠ *ina* SÍ[G] GÙN$^!$.A / ⸢È-*ak*$^?$⸣
	F rev. 3	[. . . . . SÍ]G GÙN.A$^!$ ⸢È$^!$⸣
	g obv. 8'$^{cont.}$–9'	^{na4}*šu-u* NÍTA *u* MUNUS ⸢PAP⸣ [. . . . .] / ⸢È⸣*-ak*

35	A_1 obv. 24'–25'	[*líp*]-*pi ḫúp-pa tála-pap* 3 *líp-pi šá* ^{síg}ḪÉ.ME.D[A] / [*tála-p*]*ap ina* ÚR-*šá* *tara-k*[*ás*]
	B obv. 14'$^{\text{cont.}}$–16'	[*líp-pi*] / *ḫúp-pa tála-pap* [. . . . .] / *ina* ÚR-*š*[*á* . . . .]
	c col. ii 5'–6'	*líp-pi ḫúp-*[*pi* . . . .] / ⸢x x⸣ [. . . . .][406]
	D rev. 14'$^{\text{cont.}}$	3 *líp-*⸢*pi*⸣ ⸢*tála-pap*$^{?}$⸣ x x x x [x]
	E obv.$^{!}$ i' 9'$^{\text{cont.}}$–11'	[x x x x x *l*]*íp-pi* / [. . . . .] / [. . . . .]
	F rev. 3$^{\text{cont.}}$	⸢*líp-pa*$^{?}$⸣ *ḫ*[*úp-pa* . . . .]
	g obv. 9'$^{\text{cont.}}$	*líp-pi ḫúp-pi šá* ^{síg}ḪÉ.ME.D[A] / [*t*]*ála-pap i-na* ÚR-[. . . . .]

A, B, D, F, g____

36	A_1 obv. 26'	[GÌR 15 ^{n}]$^{\text{a4}}$BABBAR.DILI $^{\text{na4}}$PA $^{\text{na4}}$*zi*-É $^{\text{na4}}$GUG $^{\text{na4}}$*šu-u*
	B obv. 17'	[GÌR] 15 [. . . . .][407]
	D rev. 15'–16'	[GÌR$^{?}$] 15 $^{\text{na4}}$BABBAR.DILI $^{\text{na4}}$PA $^{\text{na4}}$*z*[*i*]-⸢É⸣ ⸢$^{\text{na4}}$⸣[x] / ⸢$^{\text{na4}}$*šu*⸣-*u*
	E obv.$^{!}$ i' 17'	[GÌR 15$^{?}$ $^{\text{na4}}$BABBAR.DILI ^{n}]$^{\text{a4}}$PA ^{n}[$^{\text{a4}}$*zi*-É][408]
	F rev. 4	[x] ⸢15⸣ ⸢$^{\text{na4}}$BABBAR.DILI$^{?}$⸣ ⸢$^{\text{na4}}$PA$^{?!}$⸣ ⸢$^{\text{na4}}$*zi*-É$^{?}$⸣ [. . . . .]
	g obv. 10'	[x 1]5$^{?}$ $^{\text{na4}}$BABBAR.DILI $^{\text{na4}}$PA $^{\text{na4}}$*zi*-É $^{\text{na4}}$⸢GUG⸣ ⸢$^{\text{na4}}$*šu*⸣-*u*
37	A_1 obv. 27'	[NÍTA *u* MUNUS] PAP 6 NA$_4$.MEŠ *ina ba-ru-un-di* SÍG BABBAR ^{síg}ZA.[GÌN.NA]
	D rev. 16'$^{\text{cont.}}$–17'	NÍTA $^{\text{na4}}$ZÚ [(ZALAG?)] PAP 6 ⸢NA$_4$.MEŠ$^{?}$⸣ ⸢*ina*⸣ [x x x] / ⸢SÍG BABBAR⸣ ^{síg}ZA.GÌN.NA
	F rev. 4$^{\text{cont.}}$	[. . . . .]
	g obv. 10'$^{\text{cont.}}$–11'	NÍTA *u* MUNUS $^{\text{na4}}$ZÚ ZAL[AG . . . .] / ⸢^{síg}⸣ZA.GÌN.NA
38	A_1 obv. 28'	[È-*ak*] ⸢3$^{?}$⸣ *líp-pi šá* ^{síg}ḪÉ.ME.DA *tála-pap ina* GÌR 15-*šá ta*[*ra-kás*]
	D rev. 17'$^{\text{cont.}}$	È 3 ⸢*líp-pa*⸣ ⸢*tála-pap*$^{?}$⸣ [x x x x]
	F rev. 4$^{\text{cont.}}$	[. . . . .]
	g obv. 11'	È-*ak* 3 ⸢*líp*⸣-*pi šá* ^{síg}ḪÉ.ME.DA *tála-pap* [. . . . .]

A, D, g____

39	A_1 obv. 29'	[GÌR 150 x x ^{n}]$^{\text{a4}}$*zi*-É $^{\text{na4}}$BABBAR.DILI ^{n}[$^{\text{a4}}$x x x x]
	D rev. 18'	⸢GÌR$^{?}$⸣ 150 $^{\text{na4}}$PA $^{\text{na4}}$⸢*zi*-É⸣ ⸢$^{\text{na4}}$BABBAR.DILI⸣ [x x x]
	E obv.$^{!}$ i' 12'–13'	[ÚR 150 $^{\text{na4}}$]⸢PA⸣ ⸢$^{\text{na4}}$*zi*-É⸣ ⸢$^{\text{na4}}$⸣BABBAR.DILI / [$^{\text{na4}}$x]x
	g obv. 12'	[. . . . . ^{n}]$^{\text{a4}}$*zi*-É $^{\text{na4}}$BABBAR.DILI ^{n}[$^{\text{a4}}$M]UŠ.GÍR
40	A_1 obv. 30'	[. . . . .] ⸢$^{\text{na4?}}$⸣[. . . . .]
	D rev. 19'	⸢$^{\text{na4}}$⸣[. . . . .]
	E obv.$^{!}$ i' 13'$^{\text{cont.}}$–14'	$^{\text{na4}}$*šu-u* MUNUS $^{\text{na4}}$NÍ[R] / [$^{\text{na4}}$x x ^{n}]$^{\text{a4}}$⸢x⸣ [PAP] ⸢8⸣ ⸢NA$_4$⸣.ME[Š]
	g obv. 12'$^{\text{cont.}}$	$^{\text{na4}}$*šu-u* MUNUS $^{\text{na4}}$NÍR $^{\text{na4}}$[. . . . .]
41	A_1 obv. 31'	[. . . . .]
	E obv.$^{!}$ i' 15'–16'	[*ina ba-ru-un-d*]*i* SÍG BABBAR ^{síg}ZA.G[ÌN.NA] / [È-*ak* 3$^{?}$ *líp-pi tála*]-*pap ina* ÚR ⸢150⸣-[*šá tara-kás*]
	g obv. 12'$^{\text{cont.}}$	[. . . . .]

A, E, g____

For convenience, the preserved lines of ms. c (DT 28) column i' are added here:
Beginning of ms. c col. i' lost; gap of unknown length

---

406 Ms. c breaks off here.
407 Ms. B obv. breaks off here.
408 With this line, the bottom of the tablet in ms. E is reached. The continuation of the amulet prescription which must have been inscribed in the first lines of obv.$^{!}$ ii' is not preserved.

c i' 1' [. . . . . ÉN *ma-ḫi-iṣ* UG[U]-⌈*ḫi*⌉[409]
c i' 2' [. . . ÉN . . . *lu-u*] ⌈*ta-ma-ta*⌉ *ana* UGU NA_4.MEŠ
c i' 3' [. . .] ⌈7⌉.TA.ÀM ŠID-*ma*
c i' 4' [x x x] ⌈*ana*⌉ ⌈MUNUS⌉ ⌈*šá*⌉ Ù.TU KUD-*at*
c i' 5' [. . . . .]x-*ka-tu*
c i' 6' [. . . . .]x

Ms. c col. i' breaks; remainder lost
Bound Transcription and Translation

1' [. . . . . .] ÉN *māḫiṣ muḫḫi* 2' [. . . ÉN . . . *lū*] *tamâta ana muḫḫi abnī* 3' [. . .] 7.TA.ÀM *tamannu* 4' [. . .] *ana sinništi ša alāda parsat* 5' [. . . . . .]. . . 6' [. . . . . .]

1' "[. . . . . .] the incantation 'The one who hits (my) skull, 2' [. . .' (and) the incantation '. . . be] conjured' 3' you recite seven times each 2' over the stones, 4' [. . .] for a woman for whom childbearing has stopped. 5' [. . . . . .] . . ., 6' [. . . . . .]"

For the sections of ms. E not edited here, see infra text C.3.7

Summary of the sections of ms. A_1 (+) A_2 not edited here

A_1 obv. 32'–35':	List of eight stones against abnormal flow of semen (*riḫûtu*) // Sm. 1071 obv. ii 1
A_1 obv. 36'–37':	List of ten stones against throbbing of the head // Sm. 1071 obv. ii 2–6 // BAM 480+ iv 10–11 (= CRANIUM 1 lines 211–212)[410]
A_1 obv. 38'–rev. 5	List of 21(?) stones against SAG.KI.DAB.BA (with total and instruction) ("Kette 119") // AMT 102/1 i 20–23 (= CRANIUM 3)[411]
A_1 rev. 6–16	List of 25 (/24) stones against SAG.KI.DAB.BA (with total) ("Kette 120") // K. 9288+ ii 1–4 // K. 9071 rev. 1'–2' // K. 3304+ ii 6'–11' // AMT 102/1 i 30–34, 37 (= CRANIUM 3)
A_1 rev. 17–19	List of eight stones against SAG.KI.DAB.BA ("Kette 121") // K. 9288+ ii 8–12 // K. 9071 rev. 3'–4'
A_1 rev. 20–22	List of 11 stones for [. . .] ("Kette 122") // K. 9288+ ii 17–20 // K. 9071 rev. 5'–7'
A_1 rev. 23–24	List of three stones against [seeing ghosts?] (cf. "Kette 140")[412] // K. 9071 rev. 8'–9'
A_1 rev. 25–27	List of nine stones for [. . .] // K. 9071 rev. 10'–11'
A_1 rev. 28	Fragmentary list of stones // K. 9071 rev. 12'–13'
A_1 rev. 29–31	Fragmentary list of stones (with total)
A_1 rev. 32–34	Fragmentary list of stones (with total)
A_1 rev. 25–A_2 rev. 5'	Fragmentary

The last two fragmentarily preserved lines on the obverse of ms. g (BM 47770+) contain a new section of uncertain context. The traces can be read as follows:

409 Note that an incantation with the incipit *māḫiṣ muḫḫi mubbil liq pīya* is recited over an amulet with stones for a woman who does not bring her pregnancies to term in STT 241: 8–28 (there written out in full, see *infra* text C.3.1); the incipit is also mentioned in AO 6473 obv. 26 (text C.3.9). Presumably, the same spell is quoted here in ms. c i' 1'.
410 See Worthington 2005; Geller and Panayotov 2020, 206–220.
411 For CRANIUM 3, see *NinMed (The Nineveh Medical Project).*
412 Scurlock 2006, No. 20.

g obv. 13' [..............]x *ina*$^{?}$ PIŠ$_{10}$.^{d}ÍD ÚḪ.^{d}ÍD ^{na4}x[................]
g obv. 14' [........]x NÍTA$^{?}$ ⌜SA⌝ MAŠ.DÀ$^{?}$ [x] ⌜KUR$^{?}$⌝ ⌜ŠURUN$^{?}$⌝ [GU$_4$$^{?}$......]

The reverse is almost completely worn off, except for a few signs, insufficient for transliteration.

Bound Transcription and Translation

1 *pūtu šina ṣurrū namrūtu* ⌜*ina*⌝ ⌜*ṭurri*$^{?}$⌝ ⌜*šīpāti*⌝ ... [*tašakkak*] 2 *pušikku erbe ubānātu ina birīšunu* 3 *ina kibrīti talappap ina pūtīša* (var. [*ina nakkaptīša ša imitti*(?)] *u šumēli*) *tarakkas*	1 (For) the forehead: [*you thread*] two light-coloured *ṣurru*-stones ⌜on a string of⌝ [. . .] ⌜wool⌝. 2 You wind four finger-(shaped wads) of combed wool (filled?) with sulphur between them. 3 You tie (it) around her forehead (var. [on her right(?)] and left [temple?]).
4 *abūsātu ayyartu* (var. adds: *ša sebe tikpūša*) *kusibirrātu* 5 *abašmû ḫulālu ašpû sāmtu* 6 *napḫar šeššet abnī ina šīpāti barmāti* 7 *lippī ḫuppi talappap šalāšat lippī ša tabarri talappap* 8 *ina elītīša ša šumēli tarakkas*	4 (For) the forelock: *ayyartu*-shell (var. an *ayyartu*-shell with seven dots), a coriander (fruit-shaped bead), 5 *abašmû*-stone, *ḫulālu*-stone, *ašpû*-stone, carne[lian] – 6 a total of six stones. You thread (them) on multi-coloured wool, 7 you wind *ḫuppu*-wads (and) three wads of red-dyed wool (between them). 8 You bind (it) on her . . . of the left side.
9 *kišādu kunuk ḫalti ayyartu uqnû muššaru* 10 *ṣurru napḫar erbet abnī ina šīpāti barmāti tašakkak* 11 *šalāšat lippī ša tabarri talappap ina kišādīša tarakkas* (var. *tašakkan*)	9 (For) the neck: a cylindrical *ḫaltu*-stone, *ayyartu*-shell, lapis lazuli, *muššaru*-stone 10 (and) *ṣurru*-stone – a total of four stones. You thread (them) on multi-coloured wool. 11 You wind three wads of red wool (between them). You tie (var. put) (it) around her neck.
12 *qāt imitti sāmtu uqnû šû zikaru ṣurru* (var. adds: *arqu*(?); var. adds: *erbet abnī*) 13 *ina šīpāti barmāti uqnâti pušikki tašakkak* 14 *šalāšat lippī ša tabarri talappap ina qāt imittīša tarakkas* (var. *tašakkan*)	12 (For) the right hand: carnelian, lapis lazuli, 'male' *šû*-'stone', (var. adds: yellow-green(?)) *ṣurru*-stone – (var. adds: (these) four stones) 13 you thread on multi-coloured wool, blue-dyed (and) combed wool. 14 You wind three wads of red wool (between them). You tie (var. put) (it) around her right hand.
15 *qāt šumēli ašgikû pappardilû šû sinnišu uqnû ṣurru* (var. *ṣurru namru*) 16 *napḫar ḫamšat abnī ina barun*[*di*] *uqnâti* 17 *pušikki tašakkak* (var. adds: *šalāšat lippī ša tabarri talappap*) *ina qāt šumēlī*(*ša*) [*tarakkas*] (var. *tašakkan*)	15 (For) the left hand: *ašgikû*-stone (turquoise), *pappardilû*-stone, 'female(?)' *šû*-'stone', lapis lazuli, 16 (var. light-coloured) *ṣurru*-stone – a total of five stones. You thread (them) on multi-colo[ured wool], blue-dyed wool (and) 17 combed wool (var. adds: you wind three wads of red wool). [You tie] (var. put) (it) around (her) left hand.

[18] *qablu kunuk šubî šubû kunuk šadâni* [19] *kunuk ḫalti šalāšat zalāqū sāmtu* [. . .] [20] *kiṣir ḫûrati ḫaṣab sūq erbetti* [21] *imbu' tâmti zibītu šû zikaru sābu*(?) [22] *napḫar* 14 *abnī ina šīpāti barmāti* [*tašakkak*] . . . *lippī tab*[*arri*] [23] *talappap erbet kiṣrī* [*takaṣṣar* (. . .)]

[18] (For) the waist: a cylindrical (bead of) *šubû*-'stone', a *šubû*-'stone', a cylindrical (bead of) *šadânu*-stone (haematite), [19] a cylindrical (bead of) *ḫaltu*-stone, three *zal*[*āqu*-stones(?)], carnelian, [. . .]-stone, [20] a 'knot' of *ḫûratu*-plant, a potsherd from a crossroads, [21] *imbu' tâmti*-mineral, *zibītu*-'stone', 'male' *šû*-'stone', *sābu*-stone(?) – [22] a total of fourteen 'stones'. [You thread] (them) on multi-coloured wool. You wind [. . .] wads of red-[dyed] wool (between them). [23] [You tie] four knots (into the cord) [(. . .)].

---

[24] *ṭurri šīpāti peṣâti tašakkak* [. . .] *kiṣrī* . . .[. . .] [25] [. . .] *itti abnī ša qabli tuṣabb*[*at*(?). . .] [26] [. . .] *ṭurri šīpāti sāmāti ṭurri uqnâti* (var. *šīpāti ṣalmāti*?) [. . .] [27] [. . .] (var. adds: *lippī ša tabarri talappap*) *sebet kiṣrī takaṣṣar itti abnī qabli tuṣabbat*(?) *ina qablīša tarakkas*

[24] You thread a string of white wool, [. . .] knots [*you tie* (into it?)]. [25] You fas[ten (it)] to the stones for the waist, [. . .]. [26] [*You twine together*(?)] a string of red wool, a string of blue (var. black?) wool, [. . .]. [27] (var. adds: You wind [. . .] wads of red wool). You tie seven knots (into the string). You fasten (it) to the stones for the waist, (then) you bind (it) around her waist.

---

[28] *šumma sinništu dāmūša illakū* [*lā iparr*]*asū* 14 *sāmtu kupputtu* [29] 14 *kiṣrī ḫûrati ina šīpāti barmāti* (var. *šīpāti sāmāti*) *tašakkak* 14 *šû zikaru* [30] *ina* (var. adds: *ṭurri*) *šīpāti peṣâti šīpāti sāmāti* (var. adds: *šīpāti barmāti*) *tašakkak* (var. adds: *šalāšat zalāqū* [*ina šīpāti* . . . *tašakkak*(?)] / *ina ṭurri šīpāti peṣâti ina ṭurri šīpāti ṣalmāti ina ṭurri šīpāti sāmāti ina ṭurri uqnâti* 7.TA.ÀM *kiṣ*[*rī takaṣṣar*]) *itti abnī ša qabli tukaṣṣar* (var. *tuṣabbat*) *ḫaṣab sūq erbetti* [31] *ana pingi ina abunnatīša tašakkan napḫar* 59 *abnī ša qabli* (var. *qablāti*) *adi* 14 *kiṣrī ḫûrati* [32] *takṣīru ša erīti* (var. [. . .] *dām sinništi parāsi*(?))

[28] If a woman's blood flows (and) [does not sto]p, you thread fourteen block-shaped beads of carnelian (and) [29] fourteen 'knots' of *ḫûratu*-plant on multi-coloured (var. red) wool. You thread fourteen 'male' *šû*-'stones' [30] on (var. adds: a thread of) white, red (var. (adds): (and) multi-coloured) wool. (ms. g adds: [*you thread*] three *zalāqu*-stones [*on* . . . *wool*(?)]. [You tie] seven kn[ots] each into a string of white wool, into a string of black wool, into a thread of red wool, into a thr[ead] of blue [wool]). You tie (var. fasten) (all this together) to the stones for the waist. You put (var. b[ind]) a potsherd from a crossroads [31] as a final on her navel. A total of fifty-nine 'stones' for the waist (var. hips) including fourteen 'knots' of *ḫûratu*-plant. [32] A string of amulet stones for a pregnant woman (var. ms. D: [. . . *to*] stop(?) a woman's blood).

---

[33] *pēmu* (var. *pēm imitti*) *ašgikû sāmtu uqnû ayyartu kapāṣu* (var. adds: *zibītu*) [34] *šû zikaru u sinnišu* (var. *šû zikaru ṣurru*) *napḫar sebet* (var. *samānat*) *abnī ina šīpāti barmāti* (var. *uqnâti*?) *tašakkak* [35] *lippī ḫuppī* (var. adds: *ša tabarri*) *talappap šalāšat lippī ša tabarri* [*talapp*]*ap ina pēmīša tarakkas*

[33] (For) the (var. right) thigh: *ašgikû*-stone, carnelian, lapis lazuli, *ayyartu*-shell, *kapāṣu*-shell (var. adds *zibītu*-'stone'), [34] 'male' and 'female' *šû*-'stone' (var. male *šû*-'stone', *ṣurru*-stone) – a total of seven (var. eight) stones. You thread (them) on multi-coloured wool (var. on blue(?) wool). [35] You wind *ḫuppu*-wads (var. adds: of red-dyed wool) (and) three wads of red-dyed wool (between them). You tie (it) around her thigh.

---

[36] *šēp imitti pappardilû ayyartu zibītu sāmtu šû* [37] *zikaru u sinnišu* (var. *zikaru*; var. adds: *ṣurru namru*) *napḫar šeššet abnī ina barundi šīpāti peṣâti uqnâti* [38] *tašakkak šalāšat lippī ša tabarri talappap ina šēp imittīša ta*[*rakkas*]

[36] (For) the right foot: *pappardilû*-stone, *ayyartu*-shell, *zibītu*-'stone', carnelian, [37] 'male' and 'female' (var. 'male') [36] *šû*-'stone', (var. adds: light-coloured *ṣurru*-stone) – [37] a total of six stones. [38] You thread (them) [37] on multi-coloured wool, white wool (and) blue wool, [38] you wind three wads of red-dyed wool (var. ms. D: you wind three wads). You t[ie] (it) around her right foot.

---

[39] *šēp* (var. [*pēm*]) *šumēli ayyartu zibītu pappardilû papparminu* [40] *šû sinnišu ḫulālu* [. . . . . .] *napḫar* 8 *abnī* [41] [*ina barund*]*i šīpāti peṣâti uqnâti* [*tašakkak šalāšat*(?) *lippī tala*]*p-pap ina* [*šēp*] (var. *pēm*) *šumēlī*[*ša tarakkas*]

[39] (For) the left foot (var. [thigh]): *ayyartu*-shell, *zibītu*-stone, *pappardilû*-stone, *papparminu*-stone, [40] 'female' *šû*-'stone', *ḫulālu*-stone, [. . .-stone], [. . .]-st[one] – a total of eight stones. [41] You thread (them) [on multi-coloure]d wool, white wool (and) bl[ue] wool. You [wi]nd [three(?) wads (between them)]. [You tie (it) around her] left [foot] (var. left thigh).

Notes

Lines 1–3: Ms. D presumably prescribes this amulet for the forehead (SAG.KI, *pūtu*), while ms. F appears to present a variant. Unfortunately, the corresponding text line in ms. F does not preserve the body part term, but only a fragmentary 150 "left (side)". Presumably, the amulet was tied around the right and left temple (*nakkaptu*). Compare also STT 241: 1 (text C.3.1), where the first amulet in a similar group of amulets for different body part is destined for the temples (SAG.KI.MEŠ), but with different beads. The use of two "light-coloured *ṣurru*-stones" as main components of the amulet in ms. A and D may correspond with the idea of the two temples.

For the reading of ^{na4}ZÚ ZALAG as *ṣurru namru* "light-coloured *ṣurru*-stone" (not (^{na4}ZÚ) BABBAR = *peṣû* "white"), see the syllabic spelling in Maul 1994, 341: 49. The mineral *ṣurru* without colour indication is usually regarded as obsidian or flint, see Schuster-Brandis 2008, 457–458 (including black, yellow-green and light-coloured varieties). The amulets for women in texts F.1 and F.2 mention the light-coloured and yellow-green varieties as well as *ṣurru* without colour indication, see below lines 10, 12, 15, 34, 37 and text F.2: 1 and 11.

Line 2: The interpretation of *ubānu* (ŠU.SI) as "finger-shaped wads or burls of wool" proposed here and in AO 6473 obv. 2 differs from the interpretation of the dictionaries, as a unit of length (CAD U/W, 7 s.v. *ubānu* sub 3a; CAD P, 542 s.v. *pušikku*; AHw 1399 sub 2). "Fingers" (ŠU.SI) of combed wool (*pušikku*) are also a component of one of the amulets in AO 6473 obv. 2 (text C.3.10), which seems to offer a variant to the present amulet for the forehead in lines 1–3. In the AO 6473, five "fingers" of combed wool are tied (*rakāsu*) on the cord "between" several light-coloured *ṣurru*-stones. In the present instruction, four "fingers" are placed "between" two light-coloured *ṣurru*-stones, but here they appear to be filled with sulphur (*kibrītu*). As with the woolen *lippu*-wads that form an element of the other amulets for pregnant women, the "fingers" are attached by "winding/wrapping" (*lapāpu*) them around the cord in the present text (cf. discussion of *lippu ḫuppu* below). Unfortunately, all manuscripts preserving the instruction are fragmentary; the text of ms. A_2 and D seems to display slight variation in the wording and syntax (in line 3). Note that elsewhere in medical texts, the term *ubānu* refers to suppositories introduced into the anus or other body openings, see CAD U/W, 6 sub 1c-2'; Goltz 1974, 75 (written ŠU.SI or U).

Lines 4–8: Only ms. D preserves the beginning and final instruction of the amulet indicating the body part to which it had to be tied. In contrast to the other amulet sections, ms. D presents a discrepancy in the body part designations at the beginning of line 4 and at the end of line 8. Line 4 refers to *abūsātu*, the "forelock", usually denoting to a lock of hair covering the forehead (CAD A/1, 92 sub *abusātu*; AHw 9, s.v. *abūsu, abussu* sub 3). Line 8, however, instructs to attach the amulet *ina el-li-ti-šá šá* 150 "on the left . . .". Ms. A_2 preserves the sign GÙB "left", but the body part term is broken. The spelling *el-li-ti* in ms. D presumably stands for *elītu* "that which lies above; upper" (note a similar spelling of *a-bu-us-sa-tú* with a double consonant in line 4). This word can refer to the upper or outer part of body parts (in such cases, *elītu* is followed by a body part term in the genitive), but it can also denote an "upper or outer garment" (CAD E, s.v. *elītu* sub 4 and 7c, 7f; AHw 202 sub mng. 4 and 6). Perhaps, the patient had to attach the amulet to her headdress, because it would have been difficult to tie it to her actual hair.

Line 4: For beads in the shape of a coriander fruit pod (designated as *kisibirrum/kusibirru* or the variant terms *kisibirrītu/ kusibirrītu* and *kusibirrātu*), see also Arkhipov 2018, 50, 52, 62; Schuster-Brandis 2008, 148 "Kette" 155 with notes 384 and 386, and 426–427; CAD K, 420–421; SAD Vol. 3, 86.[413] Examples of *kusibirrīt ḫurāṣi* "coriander-(shaped beads) of gold" mentioning the material show that "coriander" refers to a specific shape (round beads with striations) rather than the actual coriander fruit. The parallel inventory of amulet ingredients BAM 363: 3 (text F.2) lists 1 *kús-bir-r*[*at-tú*] "one coriander-(shaped bead)" as corresponding entry to the amulet described here in detail.

Line 6: For multicoloured wool ((*šīpātu*) *barmātu*), see CAD B, 112–113. The synonymous term *burrumu* (adjective of the D-stem) is attested in reference to garments, linen or leather objects, but not in reference to wool, see CAD B, 332 sub b.

Lines 7 and 35: In lines 7 and 35, we find the item *lippu ḫuppu*, which probably indicates a type of wad or burl, in addition to the more common term *lippu* "wad, wrapping", which occurs as a component in all except one of the ten amulet prescriptions for pregnant women discussed here (see lines 7, 11, 14, 17, 22, 27, 35, 38, 41). In all completely preserved instances, the prescriptions require that three *lippu*-wads of red-coloured wool (*tabarru*) had to be "wrapped" (*lapāpu*) around the cord. Two amulets of the amulet prescriptions additionally require *lippu ḫuppu*, mentioned alongside the wads of red wool. The term *lippu* in amulet texts is usually rendered as "wrappings", "wads" or "burls" ("Umschlag, Wickel", cf. CAD L, 200; AHw 554b; Schuster-Brandis 2008, 62, 66–67). Similar to *mêlu* "leather pouches", *lippu*-wads could be filled with different materials, before being attached as components to amulet strings, but the present text does not indicate this practice. Elsewhere in medical texts, *lippu* is a term for a tampon into which medical ingredients are wrapped and inserted into body openings (Goltz 1974, 72; SAA 10, No. 321).

The reading and meaning of *lippu ḫuppu* (the spellings *líp-pi/pa ḫúp-pi/pa* could indicate a variation between an accusative plural/singular case ending) are not entirely certain. The present author interprets *lippu ḫuppu* as a type of wad or burl made of wool (see also Steinert 2016, *ZA* 106, 250; cf. CAD L, 200 s.v. *lippu*; Landsberger 1967, *JCS* 21, 147 n. 39). Schwemer (2007b, KAL 2, 101–102 No. 41 rev. iv/vi 9' = ms. E) reads *kappu* "feather" rather than *ḫuppu*, inspired by rare references from ritual texts in which bird feathers are wrapped into leather and put around a patient's neck (see BAM 311: 59, 63, written logographically PA); Schwemer (2007b, 101) translates our passage "eine Feder wickelst du ein, indem du drei Wickel aus roter Wolle wickelst". CAD K, 176 books the references in question under *kapāpu* "to roll", translating *lippī kappu* (or *ḫuppu*) as "wads wrapped(?) with", assuming a verbal adjective. However, as Farber (2014, 254) pointed out, in this case one would expect a plural adjective ending. Moreover, ms. g speaks of *ḫuppu*-burls of red wool, which supports our reading of *ḫuppu* as an apposition to *lippu*. See also AO 6473: 11, mentioning *líp-pi ḫúp-pi šá* ^{síg}ZA.GÌN.NA "*ḫuppu*-wads of blue wool" (text C.3.10). Abusch et al. (2020, CMAwR 3, text 5.1: note on line 4) now accept the reading *ḫuppu* but leave the word *ḫuppu* untranslated.

A similar occurrence of *lippu ḫuppu* is attested in the amulet prescriptions in the Lamaštu series Tablet III 36: 7 *líp-pi ḫúp-pu šá* 7 *ṣir-pa-a-ni tala-pap* "you roll seven *ḫuppu*-burls from seven (strands of) dyed wool" (see Farber 2014, 132, 188, 254, see also Tablet III 48). The meaning of *ḫuppu* in the present context is uncertain. Since in the Lamaštu example, these burls are used to wrap up other materials (plants, dust) that had previously been rolled up into bands/coils, the term *ḫuppu* may be related to *ḫuppu* "basket", less likely to *ḫuppu* "hole" (CAD Ḫ, 238–239 s.v. *ḫuppu* A and B; Gaspa 2014, *Contenitori*, 249–250).[414] The verb *ḫapû* "to wrap up" may likewise be related (AHw 332a "verpacken"; CAD Ḫ, 85–86). Note perhaps a cognate noun *ḥwpy, ḥwpy'* in Aramaic, designating a material made from palm leaves (Jastrow 1903, 437b; Sokoloff 2002, 442a; Comprehensive Aramaic Lexicon, https://cal.huc.edu).

Line 9: For *kunukku* "cylinder seal" as a term for a necklace bead in the shape of a cylinder, see Arkhipov 2018, 52, 62–63. Cylindrical *ḫaltu*-stone beads (*kunuk ḫalti*) are encountered repeatedly as an element in amulet prescriptions for pregnant women (see also line 19 in the present text; BAM 237 obv. i 4 (text C.1.4); AOAT 6473: 2 (text C.3.10); the inventory BAM 363: 8 (text F.2) also mentions two *kunuk ḫalti*-beads). As observed by Stol (2000a, 49–50), the popularity of the *ḫaltu*-stone in

413 AHw 1562a, Köcher (1971, BAM 4, p. XVIII) and Limet (1984, 332–333 n. 15) prefer to read the word in question in the present text as *ḫum-bir-rat-t*[*ú*] instead, but since there are no attestations for the assumed lexeme from other texts, this reading is unlikely to be correct.

414 Other, though less likely candidates are *ḫūpu/ḫuppu* designating a metal ring (AHw 357b s.v. *ḫūpu* I "Ring, Reifen"; CAD Ḫ, 239a s.v. *ḫuppu* D) and *kappu* designating a kind of bead made from different kinds of stone, which may be derived from *kapāpu* "to curve" (rather than *kappu* "wing"), see Arkhipov 2012, *ARM* 32, 47.

this context may have to do with the sound of the word *ḫaltu*, which resembles *ḫâlu* "to be in labour" (or *ḫayyaltu* "woman in labour"). Other cylindrical beads are prescribed for the amulet in lines 18–19 (of *šadânu* (haematite) and *šubû*-'stone').

Line 12: Collation of ms. D obv. 12 suggests a reading ^{na4}ŠU.U NITA ^{na4}ZÚ SIG$_7$ "male *šû*-'stone', yellow-green *ṣurru*-stone" against Köcher's copy which suggests ^{na4}ŠU.U NITA *u* MUNUS "male and female *šû*-'stone'".[415] The present reading is confirmed by the duplicating manuscripts A and F (which, however, have ^{na4}ZÚ without a colour indication. Yellow-green *ṣurru*-stone is also mentioned in BAM 363 obv. 11 (text F.2).

Lines 18–23: Cylindrical beads of *ḫaltu*-stone, *šubû*-'stone' and 'male' *šû*-'stone' are also used together in an amulet for the pregnant woman's neck in AO 6473: 2 (there 'male' and 'female' *šû*-'stones' are required); see also BAM 237 obv. i 4'–8' (*ḫaltu*-stone, *šubû*-'stone', 'male' and 'female' *šû*-'stone' (and several other shells), blood-red carnelian). Several of the ingredients used here carry symbolic connotations, especially related to their colour. Thus, the red colour of some the stones (haematite, carnelian, *sābu*-stone) and of the *ḫûratu*-plant (madder, the source of a red dye) alludes to blood and is reminiscent of the use of these stones in amulets and other prescriptions to stop gynaecological bleeding, e.g. during pregnancy (see e.g. Scurlock 1991, 138–141; Steinert 2012b, *Sudhoffs* Archiv 96, 70–71, 76–77 for discussion; for the *sābu*-stone, see Schuster-Brandis 2008, 439–440). *Šubû* and the male/female varieties of *šû*-'stone' (like *zibītu*, *ayyartu* and *kapāṣu* repeatedly found as components of the amulets discussed here) may refer to shells or cowrie snails ('stones of the sea', see Oppenheim 1963, *OrNS* 32, 411; Schuster-Brandis 2008, 446, 449). Shells are associated with the female sexual organs and with the embryo, so they likewise feature prominently in the amulets for women (e.g. Stol 2000a, 51–52; Scurlock 1991; Steinert 2012b, 82; Steinert 2017a). A diverging interpretation of the *šubû*-stone as a kind of agate is given in CAD Š/3, 185b s.v. *šubû* A). Cf. also Civil (2011, 182) who regards the šuba-jewels worn by goddesses associated with birth (e.g. Ninisina in the hymn *Ninisina* A) as tokens of fertility and fecundation symbolizing male semen rather than shells.

Lines 20–21: The ingredient "potsherd from a crossroads" is again encountered in lines 30–31, where it is used as a final piece (*pingu*) for an amulet string and tied on the woman's navel (see note below). The ingredients "knot of *ḫûratu*-plant" (madder), "potsherd from a crossroads" and *imbu' tâmti*-mineral found together in lines 20–21 also occur side by side in the inventory BAM 363 rev. 9'–11' (text F.2). The amulet prescription in lines 28–32 (to stop bleeding) further required 14 "knots of *ḫûratu*-plant" (see below). However, the inventory BAM 363 gives a total of only 13 knots of *ḫûratu*-plant. For the symbolism of obstruction and blockage (preventing miscarriage) linked to the use of a potsherd in rituals to stop bleeding during pregnancy, see e.g. BAM 237 obv. i 9'–16' (text C.1.4); Scurlock 1991, 138–140.

Line 20: For *kiṣru* "knot" as a joint or node of a plant (such as of reed or wood), see CAD K, 440–441 sub 7. The *ḫûratu*-plant is identified as madder (*Rubia tinctorum*), the root of which contains a red dye used for dying wool and other fabrics, see Stol 1980–1983, "Leder(industrie)", *RlA* 6, 532, 534–535; Thavapalan 2020, 296–298, 331–338. My guess is that pieces of the plant's root were used as amulet components here and may have been indicated by the term *kiṣru*. The root of madder is of a red colour, very long and thick, developing side roots from which new plant shoots grow (Böck 2022, 134 n. 16) – characteristics providing symbolisms that fit well with the present use context. A differing interpretation of *kiṣir ḫûrati* as the fruit of tanner's sumac (*Rhus coriaria*) is proposed in Schwemer 2007, KAL 2, 102 (note on IV 5'). For "knots" of *ḫûratu*-plant in a treatment to stop bleeding, see also BAM 235 obv. 15 // BAM 236 rev. 8' (text C.1.1–C.1.2).

Line 21: The sign traces copied by Köcher in ms. D (BAM 346) obv. 21 are not preserved anymore. The last lines inscribed on the bottom of the tablet are missing, but it can be estimated that no more than two or three lines of text are lost in the lacuna. The first six fragmentary lines of the reverse of BAM 346 are not legible. The reading of the very slight traces from ms. D rev. 7 onwards is very tentative and based on the duplicates.

Lines 24–27: These lines are only ruled off from the preceding and following sections (lines 18–23 and 28–32) in mss. F and D, respectively. Thus, the passage still forms part of the instructions for the amulet for the waist. As the most complex of all the amulets in the group, additional strings of wool (of different colour) had to be twined together, wrapped with *lippu*-wads, after which knots were tied into them. These strings were then fastened to the string with the stones for the waist (see next note).

415 For the varieties of 'male' and 'female' stones/minerals (attested e.g. with *šû*-'stone' and *šubû*-'stone'), which may refer to 'darker' and 'lighter' coloured varieties of a particular stone, see CAD Š/3, 161–162 sub c-1', 186 sub c-3'; Schuster-Brandis 2008, 449 *passim*; Thavapalan 2020, 158.

Lines 27 and 30: In ms. F obv. 15, the reading [. . . KÉ]Š.KÉŠ is not entirely certain, but it may indicate an exceptional D-stem of *kaṣāru* ("to tie multiple knots"?) instead of the usual G-stem. The decipherment of the fragmentary signs in ms. F obv. 16 is also tentative (especially the sign read GI$_6$ in SÍG ⸢GI$_6^{!}$⸣ "black wool", which would be a variant for "lapis lazuli wool" in the other manuscripts).

An abbreviated parallel to the instruction in lines 27 and 30 is encountered in the Lamaštu series Tablet III 35–43, especially line 43: seven 'eye stones', seven 'mule-stones' and burls of wool KI NA$_4$.MEŠ GÚ DAB-*bat* "you fasten with the stones for/of the neck" (cf. Farber 2014, 132, 188 and 254). Our present text confirms that the collocation NA$_4$.MEŠ + body part (DAB-*bat*) can be regarded as a genitive construction, since an instruction to attach the amulet to the body follows: KI NA$_4$.MEŠ MURUB$_4$ DAB-*bat ina* MURUB$_4$-⸢*šá*⸣ [*tara-kás*$^?$] "you fasten (this) with the stones for the waist (and) [tie (it)] around her waist".[416] Farber (2014, 188–189, 254 note on III 43) interprets the verb DAB-*bat* as a Š-stem form of *ṣabātu* (*tušaṣbat*) with a causative meaning. For reading DAB-*bat* as a D-stem (*tuṣabbat*), with the specific meaning "to fasten; to tie; to link", see also AO 6473: 38 and 40 (text C.3.10) for a comparable context.

Lines 28–29: The three-fold number of 14 ingredients in this amulet (14 block-shaped beads of carnelian, 14 'knots' of *ḫûratu*-plant, 14 'male' *šû*-'stones') is significant. The inventory BAM 363 rev. 9' directly related to the present amulets for women lists 13 *kiṣir ḫûrati*(^{giš}ḪAB) "13 'knots' of *ḫûratu*-plant" as amulet items instead of 14 found in mss. A and B. For 'knots' of *ḫûratu*-plant, see also lines 20–21 above.

Line 28: In ms. A$_1$, the verbal form DU-*ku-ši* instead of DU-*ku* (with the 3rd person feminine pronominal suffix) is otherwise unattested. Therefore, the sign ŠI is perhaps a scribal mistake. An option may be to read DU-*ku* IGI "(her blood) is seen flowing"?

For the adjective *kupputu* "lump-shaped" or "in a block", often said of carnelian (*sāmtu*), see CAD K, 552b. See also AO 6473: 9: 2 ^{na4}KUR-*nu* DAB *kup-pu-tú* "two magnetite stones in nugget form" (text C.3.10).

Lines 31–32: There is a ruling following the last line of the obverse of F (obv. 20), but the first line of the reverse (also followed by a ruling) appears to form the text of the summarizing rubric written out over lines 31b–32 in the other manuscripts. The remainder of the text on the reverse of ms. F has two more ruled sections (2+1 lines = 33–35 and 36–38). The rest of the tablet's reverse was left blank. If the reconstruction presented here is correct, the final amulet for the left foot (lines 39–41) was omitted from ms. F.

Line 31: The term *pingu* (*pinku*) "knob, cap, final (of a necklace)", related to the verb *panāgu* (*panāku*) "to mount; to cap", is frequently attested in texts referring to the production of necklaces (GÚ, *kišādu*) or other types of jewellery and decorative objects (see CAD P, 78; CAD P, 383a sub c; AHw 818a, 864; Hirsch 1987, *AfO* 34, 50–51 with note 9).[417] The *pingu*-caps serving as final pieces of necklaces (holding the components together in place) can be of different form (e.g. in the shape of "coriander-fruit/pod", "seed of *šakirû*-plant", or "date-shaped") and are mostly made of precious stone or gold.[418]

In the present amulet prescription, a potsherd served as the final (or central?) element, which had to be placed on the woman's navel. A parallel passage is found in the similar group of amulets for a pregnant woman in STT 241: 6: ^{na4}ŠIKA SILA.LÍMMU-*ti ina* LI$^!$.DUR-*šá* "a potsherd from a crossroads on her navel" (text C.3.1). As one further parallel, the inventory BAM 363 rev. 11' lists a potsherd from a crossroads as an item for amulet strings (*kuṣāru*) for a pregnant woman (see text F.2 and the next note on line 32).

The total of 59 "stones" given here was not understood literally, since the scribe explicitly points out that this number includes 14 "knots" of *ḫûratu*-plant (madder). Incidentally, the total of 59 refers to the number of the main components (beads) for the two amulets for the waist (14 ingredients) and against bleeding (45 ingredients) that are fastened together to the patient's waist (lines 18–27 and 28–32).

---

416 A different interpretation was proposed by Farber (ibid.), regarding GÚ as a direct object of *ṣabātu* in the accusative (*itti abnī kišāda tušaṣbat* "you *attach* . . . together with the stones, *to the* neck").

417 For *pingu/pinku* as a body part associated with the genitals/anus (perhaps the clitoris) and as an archaic title of a priestess (only attested in the LÚ-lists, cf. Stol 2020a, *BiOr* 77, 109; Lecompte 2016, 37, 38, 42).

418 See Durand 1983, ARM 21, 237–238; Limet 1985, *MARI* 4, 520–521 sub 3.5 and 3.6; Limet 1986, *ARM* 25, no. 55: 4; Talon 1985, ARM 24, 84–85 no. 149: 8, 4', 10'; Arkhipov 2012, ARM 32, 88–89; Sassmannshausen 2001, 428: 31–33; Arkhipov 2018, 54; Joannès 1992, *RA* 86, 180 no. 93 (CT 55, 320: 15').

Line 32: For the term *takṣīru* lit. "knotting; attachment" (derived from *kaṣāru* D-stem "to tie a knot") as a word for a string of amulet stones, see CAD T, 87 s.v. *takṣīru*; Schuster-Brandis 2008, 59–60; Kraus 1970, *RA* 64, 59–61 ("Gebinde", "Geknotetes"). The term relates to the central, magically significant practice of tying knots into amulet strings. The same expression *takṣīru ša erīti* "string (of amulet stones) for a pregnant woman (to protect her from miscarriage)" is also used as a classifying rubric in AO 6473 obv. 7, rev. 10, 12 (text C.3.10). Note also the fragment K. 4782: 12' related to the corpus of amulet texts: PAB-*ma* 13 *tak-ṣi-ru ša* SAG.[KI$^?$. . .] "a total of 13 strings (of amulet stones) for the fore[head(?) . . .]" (used against nosebleed, see *Electronic Babylonian Library* (eBL).

The inventory BAM 363 rev. 13' features the synonymous expression *kuṣarū ša erīti* "knottings for a pregnant woman" in a passage giving a total of amulet ingredients (such as beads of stones, shells, plants) closely resembling those used in the group of amulets discussed here (see text F.2, line 34').

Lines 33–35: For the variant attribution of this amulet in ms. E, see the note to lines 39–41 below.

Line 34: Ms. A_1 lists and sums up seven stones instead of eight in mss. c, D and E (omitting *zibītu*-stone).

Lines 39–41: Collation revealed that at least two more lines of text are inscribed on the upper edge of ms. D (BAM 346) following rev. 19', but they are now illegible. These lines supposedly contained the end of the amulet prescription for the left foot. Thus, BAM 346 presumably follows the same order of body parts as ms. A.

In contrast to the other manuscripts, ms. E prescribes this amulet for the left thigh, not for the left foot. All manuscript except ms. E prescribe only one amulet for the thigh, without a "left/right" distinction. Thus, ms. E (KAL 2, No. 41) presents a varying attribution of the amulets: the amulet for the thigh (= lines 33–35) in the other sources is specified for the "right thigh" in ms. E obv.$^!$ i' 6'–11'; the amulet for the "left thigh" in ms. E obv.$^!$ i' 12'–16' is prescribed for the "left foot" in the other manuscripts (= lines 39–41).

F.2 BAM 363: A Memorandum of Items for Amulet Charms to Protect Pregnant Women

This almost completely preserved tablet from Assur contains a list (inventory) of materials and items used for making amulets, designated as *kuṣarū* "knottings" for the protection of a pregnant woman. The list of stones (including minerals, metals, shells and plant ingredients) is followed by two shorter sections inventorising other ingredients. One lists wool of different colours and strings (items that are typically used as components of amulets, e.g. for cords on which the amulet stones are strung), the other lists fatty substances and honey destined for an ointment.

As is typical for memoranda such as BAM 363, each listed item is preceded by a number; and a total (here of 130 "stones") is given at the end of the list. There are numerous close correspondences between the items in BAM 363 and the ingredients of a group of amulets for pregnant women attached to different body parts, which were incorporated into the series *kunuk ḫalti* and are attested in several sources discussed in the preceding chapter F.1 (K. 4727+ //). Two of the source texts for this group of amulets (BAM 346 and KAL 2, No. 41) come from the same archive as BAM 363 (the exorcists' library N4). Thus, BAM 363 could reflect the practical application of a very similar group of amulets for a female patient on a particular occasion (for similarities and differences to the text sources of K. 4727+ // see the notes below). In this light, the BAM 363 could represent a memorandum of the materials needed for the amulets and additional utensils for the performance of an associated ritual and for an ointment (see also Maul 1994, 32 for an interpretation of the text as an order list). Similar inventories of items, including stones for amulets or necklaces used in a ritual or cultic context, have been identified among the texts from the N4 collection as well as from other places and can serve as points of comparison (Schuster-Brandis 2008, 189–191). Like in BAM 363, the inventories list items supplied with a number/total and rarely bear a colophon:

VAT 13605 (from Assur), an inventory list of materials, especially clay figurines, needed for a ritual against Lamaštu (Farber 2014, 278–279, 310–313, 337–338, 457 pl. 76), with similar terminology (see below);

BAM 355 (from Assur, N4 library; Pedersén 1986, 60 no. 58), a tiny inventory of stones;

BAM 356 (from Assur), combines a stone list for six amulets (obv.) and an inventory of the amulet items with totals (rev.) (Schuster-Brandis 2008, 199–203 Text 1);

BAM 364 (from Assur), combines a stone list for different amulet necklaces (col. i–ii) and an inventory of the amulet items with totals (col. iii–vi) (Schuster-Brandis 2008, 204–207, Text 2);

BAM 366 (from the N4 library, Assur; Pedersén 1986, 67 no. 307), an inventory of stones for necklace(s) (*kišādu*) of Marduk, with fragmentary colophon of Kiṣir-[Aššur?] (Schuster-Brandis 2008, 61–62, 190; Arbøll 2021, 165, 166–168, interpreted as a stock-taking list of items needed for a specific purpose and available to the practitioner);

BAM 420 (Neo-Babylonian), an inventory of stones with occasional numbers (Schuster-Brandis 2008, 190–191);

SpTU 4, No. 219 (from Uruk; Late Babylonian), an inventory of stones with numbers/totals (von Weiher 1993, 132);

STT 401 (from Sultantepe, Neo-Assyrian), inventory of stones with numbers/totals (*Geography of Knowledge Corpus* (CAMS/GKAB; http://oracc.museum.upenn.edu/cams/gkab/corpus/)

List of Manuscripts

Siglum	Museum Number	Copy	Collation	Format; Ductus	Provenience
A	A 265[419]	BAM 363	Coll.	Single-column tablet; Neo-Assyrian script, ca. 8th/7th cent. BCE	Assur; N4 library[420]

Overview

i	List of 130 items for amulet strings (*kuṣarū*) for a pregnant woman A obv. 1–rev. 13'	1–34'
ii	List of items for a ritual (?) A rev. 13'–19'	35'–40'
iii	List of items for an ointment A rev. 20'–u. e. 1	41'–43'

Previous Edition and Discussion

CDLI P285434

BabMed Corpora (https://www.geschkult.fu-berlin.de/e/babmed/Corpora/BAM-4/BAM-4_-363/index.html)

Limet 1984, 333 notes 15, 17, 336–337 nn. 26, 31

Schuster-Brandis 2008, 148–149 Kette 154–162 (discussion of parallels)

Stol 2000a, 49

Transliteration and Translation

1	A obv. 1	10 ^{na4}Z[Ú ZALAG]	Ten [light-coloured] *ṣurru*-stones,
2	A obv. 2	7 ^{na4}P[A]	seven *ayyartu*-stones (shells),
3	A obv. 3	1 *kús-bir-r*[*at-tú*]	one coriander (shaped bead),
4	A obv. 4	1 ^{na4}*àba-*[*aš-mu*]	one *abašmû*-stone,
5	A obv. 5	3 ^{na4}N[ÍR]	three *ḫul*[*ālu*]-stones,

419 Measurements: 3.5 x 10 x 1.5 cm.

420 Pedersén 1986, 60 (64).

6	A obv. 6	1 $^{\text{na4}}$*aš-pu-u*	one *ašpû*-stone,
7	A obv. 7	4 $^{\text{na4}}$GUG	four carnelian (beads),
8	A obv. 8	2 $^{\text{na4}}$KIŠIB *ḫal-ti*	two cylindrical *ḫaltu*-stones,
9	A obv. 9	4 $^{\text{na4}}$ZA.GÌN	four lapis lazuli (beads),
10	A obv. 10	⸢3?⸣ $^{\text{na4}}$MUŠ.GÍR	⸢three(?)⸣ *muššaru*-stones,
11	A obv. 11	2 $^{\text{na4}}$ZÚ SIG$_7$	two green *ṣurru*-stones,
12	A obv. 12	18 $^{\text{na4}}$*šu-u* NITA	eighteen 'male' *šû*-'stones',
13	A obv. 13	3 $^{\text{na4}}$AŠ.GÌ.GÌ	three *ašgikû*-stones (turquoise),
14	A obv. 14	⸢1?⸣ $^{\text{na4}}$BABBAR.DILI	⸢one(?)⸣ *pappardilû*-stone,
15	A obv. 15	5 $^{\text{na4}}$*šu-u* MUNUS	five 'female' *šubû*-'stones',
16	A obv. 16	1 $^{\text{na4}}$KIŠIB ŠUBA	one cylindrical *šubû*-'stone',
17	A obv. 17	2 $^{\text{na4}}$ŠUBA	two *šubû*-'stones',
18	A obv. 18	2 $^{\text{na4}}$KIŠIB KUR-*ni*	two cylindrical *šadânu*-stones (haematite),
19	A obv. 19	⸢4?⸣ $^{\text{na4}}$KUR-*ni*	⸢four(?)⸣ *šadânu*-stones,
20	A obv. 20	2 $^{\text{n}[\text{a4}}$x]	two [. . .]-stones,
21	A obv. 21	⸢x⸣ [$^{\text{na4}}$x]	. . . [. . .-stones],
Ms. A obv. breaks; gap of a few lines			
22'	A rev. 1'	[x] $^{\text{n}[\text{a4}}$x]	[. . . . . .]-stone(s),
23'	A rev. 2'	14 $^{\text{na4}}$x[x]	fourteen [. . .]-stones,
24'	A rev. 3'	1 $^{\text{na4}}$*ka-pa-ṣu*	one *kapāṣu*-shell,
25'	A rev. 4'	1 $^{\text{na4}}$GIŠ.NU$_{11}$.GAL	one *gišnugallû*-stone,
26'	A rev. 5'	1 $^{\text{na4}}$URUDU NÍTA	one 'male' copper (bead),
27'	A rev. 6'	1 $^{\text{na4}}$ḪI.LIB	one *ḫilibû*-stone,
28'	A rev. 7'	1 $^{\text{na4}}$KÙ.SI$_{22}$	one gold (bead),
29'	A rev. 8'	1 MUN *eme-sal-lim*	one (lump of) *emesallu*-salt,
30'	A rev. 9'	13 *ki-ṣir* ^{giš}ḪAB	thirteen 'knots' of *ḫûratu*-plant,
31'	A rev. 10'	1 ŠIKA SILA.LÍMMU.BA	one potsherd from a crossroads,
32'	A rev. 11'	1 KA A.AB.BA	one *imbu' tâmti*-mineral.
33'	A rev. 12'	PAP-*ma* 1 *me* 30 NA$_4$.MEŠ	A total of 130 stones
34'	A rev. 13'	*ku-ṣa-ri šá* ^{munus}PEŠ$_4$	(for) amulets ('knottings') for a pregnant woman.
35'	A rev. 14'	SÍG BABBAR SÍG GI$_6$ SÍG SA$_5$	White wool, black-(dyed) wool, red wool,
36'	A rev. 15'	^{síg}ZA.GÌN.NA *tab-ri-mu*	blue-(dyed) wool (and) red-dyed wool
37'	A rev. 16'	*tab-ri-bu*	(also called) *tabribu*,
38'	A rev. 17'	⸢*ni*⸣-*ri šá* GU	braided strings (made) of thread(s),

39'	A rev. 18'	*ša* 1 GI.DU$_8$ *e-si-iḫ-*⸢*tu*?⸣	(This is) for one portable altar (*paṭīru*),
40'	A rev. 19'	*gab-bu* [(x)]	40' everything 39' that was assigned.
41'	A rev. 20'	⸢Ì⸣ DU$_{10}$.GA Ì ^{giš}ER[EN]	Fragrant oil, ce[dar] oil,
42'	A rev. 21'	⸢LÀL⸣ Ì.NUN.NA	syrup, ghee.
43'	A u.e. 1	AŠ-*ma nap-šal-*[*tu*?]	(This is for) one(?) ointment.

Notes

Line 1: Light-coloured *ṣurru*-stones (^{na4}ZÚ ZALAG, *ṣurru namru*) are used in three of ten amulets for a pregnant woman in K. 4727+ and dupl., lines 1, 15, 36 (see text F.1 with notes for discussion). The number of 10 stones given in line 1 is higher than the number in the source texts. However, not in all cases where *ṣurru*-stone is mentioned in the respective amulet prescriptions, a colour indication is given. Line 11 of our inventory additionally lists "green *ṣurru*-stones", see also K. 4727+ // line 12 (ms. D).

Line 2: *Ayyartu*-shell is used as a component in several of the amulet strings for pregnant women in K. 4727+ // (lines 4, 9, 33, 36, 39).

Line 3: The same spelling *kús-bir-rat-tú* is also attested in BAM 346: 4, see text F.1 (ms. D) for discussion.

Lines 4–7: The stones listed in these four lines (*abašmû, ḫulālu, ašpû*, carnelian) are used together in one of the amulets for pregnant women in K. 4727+ // (line 5). Carnelian (*sāmtu*) is a component of four more of the amulets; in one case a set of "fourteen carnelians in nugget form" (*sāmtu kupputtu*) was used (K. 4727+ // lines 12, 19, 28, 33).

Line 8: For *kunukku* "cylinder seal" as a cylindrical stone bead, see Arkhipov 2018, 62–63. For *kunuk ḫalti* "cylindrical bead of *ḫaltu*-stone" as a recurring element in the amulets for women, see Stol 2000a, 49–50. This component is found in two of the amulets for women in K. 4727+ // (lines 9 and 19).

Lines 9 and 10: Lapis lazuli and *muššaru*-stone are likewise attested in the amulets for women, see K. 4727+ // (lines 9, 12, 15, 33 lapis lazuli; line 9 *muššaru*).

Line 12: 'Male' *šû*-'stone' is a component in four of the amulets for pregnant women in K. 4727+ // (lines 12, 21, 29 and 34). The 'female' variety is perhaps attested in one of the amulets (K. 4727+ // (line 15, only in ms. F). All taken together correspond exactly with the number 18 given BAM 363: 12. Note also 'male' and 'female' *šû*-'stone' in AO 6473: 2 (text C.3.10). Male *šû*-'stone' is attested in other amulet prescriptions to protect women from miscarriage, see e.g. LKA 9 rev. r. col. 14'; SpTU 3, No. 84 rev. 6 (and dupl., see *infra* texts C.3.5 and C.3.6).

Line 13: A bead of *ašgikû*-stone (a green stone, perhaps turquoise) is part of two amulets in K. 4727+ // (lines 15 and 33). See Schuster-Brandis 2008, 400–401.

Line 14: Possibly read the number as ⸢4⸣ instead of 1 ^{na4}BABBAR.DILI. The *pappardilû*-stone (banded agate) is utilized in three amulets in K. 4727+ // (lines 15, 36, 39).

Lines 15–18: The three entries in lines 15–17 are concerned with different beads of *šubû*-'stone', which may have to be interpreted as a type of shell or cowrie snail rather than a stone, see Schuster-Brandis 2008, 446; Arkhipov 2018, 50. Two of the items, *šubû* and a cylindrical bead of *šubû*, are used together in one of the amulets in K. 4727+ // (line 18, for the waist). The 'female' *šubû*-'stone' is not attested in K. 4727+ //. For other instances of 'male' and 'female' *šūbû*-stone, see CAD Š/3, 186 sub c-3'. The item "cylindrical haematite" (*kunuk šadâni*) in line 18 is likewise part of the amulet for the waist in K. 4727+ // (line 18).

Line 24': *Kapāṣu*-shell is part of one amulet (for the thigh) in K. 4727+ // (line 33).

Lines 25'–29': The items listed in these lines (*gišnugallu*, copper, gold, *ḫilibû*-stone and *emesallu*-salt) are not mentioned in the amulets for pregnant women in K. 4727+ //. The mention of *emesallu*-salt is unusual; perhaps this ingredient was intended for filling it into a leather bag.

Line 27': The *ḫilibû*-stone (a mineral of reddish, translucent colour) is equated with *yānibu*-'stone' (a shell) in Ḫg. B IV 111 and E 17; cf. Schuster-Brandis 2008, 416–417. Neither of these minerals is mentioned in the amulet prescriptions in K. 4727+ //.

Lines 30'–32': The three ingredients listed here, "knot of *ḫûratu*-plant" (madder), "potsherd from a crossroads" and *imbu' tâmti* (a mineral from the seashore, perhaps coral?) are also used together in one of the amulets (for the waist) in K. 4727+ // lines 20–21. In addition, a second amulet in the group (K. 4727+ // lines 28, 31, to stop bleeding) required 14 "knots of *ḫûratu*-plant". In BAM 363 rev. 9', only 13 knots are listed.

Line 34': For *kuṣāru/ū ša erīti* "knot(tings) for a pregnant woman", see also Stol 2000a, 49. The noun *kuṣāru* is so exceptional (a hapax?) that it is not listed in the Akkadian dictionaries yet. The synonymous term *takṣīru* lit. "knotting; attachment" (like *kuṣāru* derived from *kaṣāru* "to tie a knot") is used to refer to strings of amulet stones for a pregnant woman in K. 4727+ and duplicates (see text F.1, line 32 for discussion).

Lines 35'–37': The types of different coloured wool enumerated here (together with "braided strings") are commonly found in the amulet prescriptions, in the form of strings. The items white wool (SÍG BABBAR), black/dark wool (SÍG GI_6), red wool (SÍG SA_5) indicate naturally coloured/pigmented fleece, while the other two terms "blue (lapis lazuli-coloured) wool" (^{síg}ZA.GÌN.NA) and red-dyed wool (*tabribu*) refer to wool dyed with woad and madder (Thavapalan 2020, 138, 149, 176–177, 295–308, 314–322).

Lines 36'–37': CAD T, 30–31 regards *tabribu* as a variant spelling of *tabrimu* and as a term for red-dyed wool, while AHw 1299 s.v. *tabrīmu* and *tabrīmu* differentiates two lemmas (this view is revised in von Soden 1957, *ZA* 52, 233). The term is considered as a loanword from Hurrian *tawarriwa* (with intervocalic *w* rendered as *b* in Assyrian and *m* in Babylonian, respectively), as is the more common term *tabarru* "red wool"; cf. CAD T, 21–24; Thavapalan 2020, 298–304. Gaspa (2018, 64–65) understands *tabribu* as "red wool", but *tabrimu* as a variety of polychrome wool. While the word *tabarru* comes into use in the second millennium BCE, attestations of the word *tabribu* (spelled syllabically) are only found in Neo-Assyrian texts. Here and in the inventory of ritual items BAM 304: 19', the ingredient name *tabribu* seems to be a gloss on the word *tabrimu* preceding it (Köcher BAM 3, p. XXIII on BAM 304; *BabMed Corpora*), which points to their understanding as synonyms. See also Meinhold 2017, *KAL* 7, 16 no. 1–2 (Neo-Assyrian ritual text), where ^{síg}*tab-ri-bu* (a+6) interchanges with ^{síg}*tab-ri-mu* (a+11).

Line 38': For *nīru* "braided string", see CAD N/2, 265 s.v. *nīru* B; Schuster-Brandis 2008, 64–65.

Lines 39'–40': The expression *isiḫtu gabbu* "everything that was assigned" (cf. CAD I/J, 191–192 s.v. *isiḫtu* "allocation; assigned working material (of craftsmen, for performing a specific task)") also occurs in the Assur inventory VAT 13605 (Farber 2014, 278–279, 310–313, 457 pl. 76). In the latter text, it introduces a list of ritual items (mostly clay figurines) for rituals involving Lamaštu; the same phrase may also have been inscribed on the left edge of the tablet. The first line also mentions a portable altar: *ša* 1-*en* GI.DU_8 / *a-nu-ut* BÁḪAR / *i-si-iḫ-tú gab-bu* "For one portable altar; potter's utensils; everything that was assigned". This parallel helps to confirm the reading of lines 39'–40' in our present text, especially the phrase *ša* 1(DIŠ) GI.DU_8 (instead of *ša ana* GI.DU_8), cf. Maul 1994, 50 fn. 31.

The mention of a portable altar (GI.DU_8; *paṭīru*), often used for presenting food offerings, is somewhat unexpected in the present text. Maul (1994, 32) suggests part of the items listed in BAM 363 were used for ritual actions associated with the consecration of the amulets, but we have no textual evidence for such actions fitting the mentioned items. Wool and strings of different colour mentioned in lines 35'–38' are also common components of the amulet strings.

Line 41'–43': The first two signs of the rubric in line 43', AŠ-*ma*, are presumably to be analysed as a variant spelling for *ištēn*(DIŠ)-*ma* "it is (for) one (ointment)". The particle -*ma* marks a nominal clause. The enumeration of different oils, ghee and honey in the preceding lines suggests the restoration *nap-šal-*[*tu*] "ointment" following AŠ-*ma*.

Chapter G
Two First Millennium BCE Commentaries on the Neo-Assyrian Birth Compendium

The two commentaries edited here provide ancient scholarly discussions on the same text, the so-called Neo-Assyrian Birth Compendium (text D.1.1), a compendium of incantations, rituals and prescriptions to promote easy delivery and deal with difficult labour (Frahm 2011, 231, 241, 302, 312). That fact that among the small group of commentaries on medical therapeutic texts from first millennium BCE Babylonia two manuscripts preserve a commentary on the Neo-Assyrian Birth Compendium underlines the importance of this text within the medical literature of the first millennium BCE and its role in scholarly learning. The two manuscripts (11N-T3 and UET 6/3, 897) stem from different sites in Babylonia (Nippur and Ur) and probably date roughly to the same era (the Achaemenid period). While they comment on largely overlapping text sections of the Birth Compendium and present many similarities and parallel passages (in the text passages selected from the base text as well as in the comments and explanations), the two commentaries are clearly no duplicates. Thus, the two texts present many differences in detail.

11N-T3 (text G.1) from Nippur is often more extensive in its explanations, which may be linked to its role in a teaching setting alluded to in its colophon (which defines the text as "oral explanations, and (materials for) a 'questioning', following the sayings of a (master)-scholar", see below). Both commentaries contain many lexical explanations of terms and expressions in the base text, but they also engage in textual hermeneutics, seeking to show the intimate relations between certain words in the incantations, the *materia medica* in the prescriptions of the Birth Compendium and the central aim of the prescribed medical and ritual interventions, namely successful delivery. Moreover, the relevance of medical commentaries such as 11N-T3 and UET 6/3, 897 is that they are precious sources that aid in the reconstruction and interpretation of the fragmentary base text.

G.1 The Commentary 11N-T3 from Nippur

The tablet 11N-T3 (kept in the National Museum of Iraq, Baghdad) can be regarded as the best-preserved medical commentary known to date. It was excavated in Nippur, in a trash pit dating to the Achaemenid period (5th/4th cent. BCE) and may be approximately contemporary with the other commentary on the Neo-Assyrian Birth Compendium from Ur (see G.2 below). It has been translated and discussed several times in the secondary literature. The edition included here has profited much from the study of the text by Jiménez (2014).

The colophon of the tablet identifies it as an IM.GÍD.DA ("oblong tablet") belonging to Enlil-kāṣir, a lamentation-priest (*kalû*) of Enlil, son of Enlil-šumu-imbi, and descendant of Lú-dumu-nun-na, "the Sumerian" (i.e. Nippurean).[421] In its rubric, the commentary is referred to as a *ṣâtu*-commentary containing *šūt pî u maš'altu ša pī ummâni ša libbi* én munus ù-tu-du-da-a-ni "oral explanations, and (materials for) a 'questioning', following the sayings of a (master)-scholar, (relating to lemmas/passages) from (the text entitled) 'Incantation: The woman giving birth'" (cf. Frahm 2011, 54, 231).

11N-T3 contains lexical explanations of difficult terms in the base text. But at the same time, the intention of the commentary can be described as "speculative philology", the main purpose of which was to show that words drawn from the incantations and *materia medica* of the base text have hidden connections with the aim of the base text, i.e. successful delivery (Frahm 2011, 231; Jiménez 2014). Thus, the commentator applies various hermeneutical techniques (such as *notarikon*, false etymologies) with ingenuity, reflecting his detailed knowledge and creative handling of lexical traditions and literary texts.

421 On the owner of the tablet, see Gordin 2016, *WdO* 18, 184; on the family name Lú-dumu-nun-na, see George 2009, *Babylonian Literary Texts in the Schøyen Collection*, 124–128, 130, 145 No.17; Wunsch 2014a, 289–290; Jiménez 2017, *The Babylonian Disputation Poems*, 46–47.

https://doi.org/10.1515/9781501506475-010

List of Manuscripts

Siglum	Museum Number	Copy	Collation	Format; Ductus	Provenience
α	11N-T3	–	–	Single-column tablet; Late Babylonian script; 5th/4th cent. BCE	Nippur

Previous Edition and Discussion

Civil 1974, *JNES 33*, 331–337 (edition)
Frahm 2010b, *TUAT NF* 5, 175–176 (partial translation)
Jiménez 2014, CCP, no. 4.2.A.a (edition)
Civil 1975, "Appendix A: Cuneiform Texts", in *OIC* 22, 131–132 No. 20 (discussion)
Cavigneaux 1976, *Die sumerisch-akkadischen Zeichenlisten. Überlieferungsprobleme* (Diss. München), 152–154 (discussion of lines 2–6, 43–44)
Cavigneaux 1987, *AuOr* 5, 252–255 (discussion)
Frahm 2011, 38–39, 54, 65–67, 69, 71, 73–74, 92, 99, 104, 231, 237, 241, 302, 312, 389 (discussion of lines 8–9, 10, 13, 18–23, 28, 38–39, 40–41, 42–43)
Veldhuis 1989, *Acta Sumerologica* 11, 239–260 ("ms. c"; discussion of selected lines)
Steinert 2017a, 331–340 (discussion of lines 8–9, 11–12, 39–40)
Jiménez 2019, *NABU* 2019, 140–141 No. 77 (lines 8–12)

Transliteration

1 **ÉN munus ù-tu-ud-da-a-ni** : ***e-lep-pi šá uq-na-a ṣa-na-at***[422]

2 *ṣa-na* : *ma-lu-ú* : **gug nu-zu ù ZA.GUL nu-zu** : ***lu-ʾ-at-ma***

3 ***a-na ni-qí-i ul na-ṭa-at*** : *pu-uḫ-*tu_4 *ši-i* : gug : *el-lum*

4 nu : *la-ʾ* : zu : *na-ṭu-u* : *a-ma-ra* : *a-na ni-qí-i ul na-ṭa-at*

5 *šá* E-*u* : siskur : *ni-qu-ú* : siskur : *ṣu-le-e um-ma lu-ʾ-at-ma*

6 *a-na ṣu-le-e ul am-ra-at* : ***na-gi-ri um-ma*** **^{d}GAŠAN-DINGIR**

7 ***iš-ta-na-as-si*** : ${}^{na\text{-}gi\text{-}ri}$nigru(KAxAD.KÙ) *šá ka-ga-ak-ku* AD.KÙ *i-gub* : *a-ši-pu*

8 **gi èn-barbàn-da šu u-me-ti** : gi : *sin-niš-tì* : bar : *a-ṣu-u* : bàn-da

9 *še-er-ri* : *ṣa-aḫ-ri* : **saḫar sila^{la}** : saḫar : *e-pe-ri* : sa-ḫar *u ṣa-ḫar iš-ten-ma*

10 **sila-**$\mathbf{lam_4}$**-ma** : si : *e-še-ri šá a-la-ku* : la : *la-a* : *ṣa-ḫar* : *am-ma* : *ze-ri*

11 ***šá-am-nu*** : ${}^{ni\text{-}ig}$níĝ : *sin-niš-tì* : *am* : *ze-ri* : nu : *ba-nu-u šá-niš* $^{!}$ì(NI)

12 *šá-am-nu* : i : *a-ṣu-u šá* NUMUN : ***e-li* LI.DUR-*šú ḫe-pi-ma*** *aš-šum* GI

13 *na-ki-is ab-bu-un-na-ti* : *ab-bu-un-na-tú ri-ik-si šá* LÚ *ši-i*

14 ^{giš}[${}^{ki\text{-}ri\text{-}is}$]**kirid** : *ki-ri-is-su* : É *ú-ba-nu* : ***šup-šuq-tùm-ma*** : *šup-šu-qa*

15 *ka-a-šú šá-niš dan-na-ti* : ***ina qar-ni-šú qaq-qar ṭe-ra-at*** : *ṭa-ru-u* SAG.ÚS

16 *šá-niš ṭe-ra-at* : *ḫe-eṣ-ne-et* : *ṭa-ru-u* : *ha-ṣa-nu lìb-bu-u* gú-da ri

17 *na-an-du-ra* : gú$^{!}$(e)-lá : *e-de-ri* : ***el-la-me-e*** : AGA *taš-ri-iḫ-ti*

422 Text in bold characters marks quotations of words or phrases from the base text or from other identified texts.

18 *lìb-bu-u* é-lam$_4$-ma : É *er-bé šá-niš* si é-gar$_8$-bi til-la : *el-lam-mu-u*

19 *šá nu-ú-ru la-ni-šu ú-qat-ta-a* : si : *nu-ú-rù* : é-gar$_8$: *la-a-nu*

20 bi : *šu-u* : til : *qa-tu-u áš-šú* ^{d}30 *šá* AN.TA.LÙ *gam-mar-ti i-šak-kan*

21 ***aš-šum* ÁB-*ia la a-lit-ti*** *áš-šú* ^{d}30 EN *la-a-tu*$_4$ *el-le-e-ti*

22 **zi ^{d}nin-dar-a sipa udul$_{10}$(ÁB-LU)-lu-ú-a ḫé-pàd : *niš* ^{d}MIN SIPA**

23 ***ú-tul-la-a-tú lu-ú ta-ma-at*** : ^{d}nin-dar-a : ^{d}30 : ***né-šel-pa-a***

24 *né-šal-pú-u* : *e-te-qu* : *né-šal-pú-u* : *a-la-ka* : gir$_5$-gir$_5$: *na-ḫal-ṣu-u*

25 gir$_5$-gir$_5$: *na-šal-pú-u* : $^{ni-ra-aḫ}$ ^{d}GU$_4$: ***ni-ra-ḫu*** : an : *ze-ri*

26 gud : *šá-ḫa-ṭu* : **KA.INIM.MA** <<:>> ^{munus}**LA.RA.AḪ.A.KÁM** : la-ra-aḫ : *pu-uš-qa*

27 *dan-na-ti* : ***na-ḫu-un-di*** : ^{d}30 : ***na-ru-un-di*** : ^{d}UTU

28 ***na-am-li-su ki-ma ṣa-bi-tu*$_4$** : zí : *ma-la-su* : zí : *ba-qa-mu*

29 *šá-niš na-am-li-su lìb-bu-u nap-lu-su* : *a-ma-ra* : ***ki-ma* MAŠ.DÀ**

30 bar$^{ba-ár}$: *a-ṣu-u šá* NUMUN : $^{du-u}$dù : *lil-li-du* : ***ul-la*** : *an-na*

31 *an-na* : *qí-bi-ti šá-niš ul-la* : *ul-la* ì$^{i-'u-u}$: *šá-am-nu* : **Ì BUR**

32 Ì *kan-nu šá* ^{lú}Ì.SUR *šá-niš* bur : *bi-'-il-ti* : ^{urudu}**GAG.U$_4$.TAG.E**

33 mul-mul : *mul-mul* : *šil-ta-ḫu* : mul-mul : *ze-ri*

34 ^{gi}mul-mul : *ze-ri šá-niš* gi : *sin-niš-ti* : urudu : *e-ru-u*

35 *a-na a-re-e* : $^{du-u}$dù : *lil-li-du* : $^{za-al}$zalag(UD) : *nu-úr* : tag-ga

36 *e-ze-bi šá-niš* $^{du-u}$dù : *lil-li-du* : si : *e-še-ri šá a-la-ku aš-šum*

37 ^{mul}KAK.SI.SÁ : ***e-gi-zi-ni-ti*** : GÉME-^{d}30 : ***ina* SAG.DU-*ia*$_5$ *na-ma-ra***

38 *na-ma-ra* : KASKAL.MIN *šá* GIŠ.GI *u* ^{giš}TIR : ***šá* ŠÀ *iš-qil-la-tu*$_4$ *li-kal-lim nu-ú-rù***

39 *ana* ^{munus}PEŠ$_4$ *iq-ta-bi* : ^{na4}iškila(ŠÀxA) : *ṣi-il-la-tu*$_4$: ia$_4$(NA$_4$) : *a-ṣu-u šá ze-rù*

40 a : *ma-ra* : šà : *lìb-bi* : ***uš-šu-rat ḫur-da-at-su*** : *hur-da-tú* : *ú-ru-u*

41 *šá sin-niš-ti lìb-bu-u* ***qa-at-ka šu-ta-am-ṣa-am-ma lu-pu-ut ḫur-da-at-na***

42 *šá-niš ḫur-da-ti* : *qim-ma-ti* : *šal-šiš ḫur-da-ti* : *ḫur-ri da-di*

43 *da-du* : *ma-ra* : ***ina kit-tab-ri-šú*** : *ina i-di-šú* : *kit-tab-ri* : *i-di* : še : *i-di*

44 še : *kit-tab-ra* : ***qí-ip nap-šá-a-tu*$_4$** : *qa-a-pa* : *na-da-nu*

45 túg $^{tu-un}$dun$_x$(DÚB) : *ka-ma-du* : ***ik-kud it-ta-'i-id*** : *ta-an-ki-tu*$_4$

46 *ḫi-is-sa-tu*$_4$: *it-mu-du* : *še-mu-ú* : ***ab-nu ti-ik-ku* AN-*e*** : *ab-nu*

47 ab : *ba-nu-u šá a-la-du* : nu : *ze-rù* : u-gu$_4$: *ti-ik-ku* : u : *ba-nu-u*

48 gu : *a-la-du* : an : AN-*e* : an : *ze-ri* : **SAḪAR BÀD ŠUB-*tú***

49 bàd : *du-ú-ru* : kéš : *ri-ik-si* : bad : *pe-tu-u*

50 ŠUB-*tú šá* E-*u áš-šú* dirig(SI.A) : *qa-a-pa šá* É.GAR$_8$: si : *e-še-ri šá a-lak*

51 a : *ṣa-ḫar* : **SAḪAR PISAN *šur-di-i*** : $^{ma-a}$ĝá : *pi-sa-an-nu* : ĝá : *a-la-ku*

Colophon:

52 *ṣa-a-ti šu-ut* KA *u maš-'a-al-ti šá* KA *um-ma-nu šá* ŠÀ

53 ÉN munus ù-tu-ud-da-a-ni IM.GÍD.DA ^{d}50-KÁD

54 ^{lú}GALA ^{d}*en-líl* A *šá* ^{md}*en-líl*-MU-*im-bi* ŠÀ.BAL.BAL

55 ^{m}LÚ-DUMU-NUN.NA *šu-me-ru-u*

Bound Transcription and Translation

1 **én munus ù-tu-ud-da-a-ni** : ***eleppi ša uqnâ ṣânat***	1 "Incantation: The woman giving birth". (In) "a ship which is loaded with lapis lazuli"
2 *ṣâna* : *malû* : **gug nu-zu ù ZA.GUL nu-zu** : ***lu''ât-ma***	2 "to be loaded" (*ṣânu*) (means) "to be full". (Sumerian:) gug nu-zu ù ZA.GUL nu-zu "She does not know (whether) it is carnelian, and she does not know (whether) it is … ." (Akkadian:) "She is impure and
3 ***a-na niqî ul naṭât*** : *pūḫtu šī* : gug : *ellu*	3 not fit for (making) an offering." – This is a (word) replacement. (The Sumerian word) gug (means) "pure" (Akk. *ellu*),
4 nu : *lā'* : zu : *naṭû* : *amāra* : ***ana niqî ul naṭât***	4 nu (means) "not" (Akk. *lā*), zu (means) "to be appropriate", (which is synonymous to) *amāru* ("to see"). (In) "she is not fit for (making) an offering",
5 *ša iqbû* : siskur : *niqû* : siskur : *ṣulê umma lu''ât-ma*	5 which it (= the base text) said: (Sumerian) siskur (means) "offering" (*niqû*) (and) siskur (also means) "prayer", thus: "she is impure and
6 *ana ṣulê ul amrat* : ***nāgiri umma Bēlet-ilī***	6 (should) not to be seen (*amrat*) for prayer." (In) "the herald (*nāgiru*) 7 summons 6 the goddess Bēlet-ilī as follows",
7 ***ištanassi*** : $^{na\text{-}gi\text{-}ri}$nigru(KAxAD.KÙ) *ša kagakku* AD.KÙ *igub* : *āšipu*	7 (the word) "herald" (means) "exorcist" (nigru), (because the sign) KA with (the signs) AD.KÙ put inside it, (means) "exorcist".
8 **gi èn-bar bàn-da šu u-me-ti** : gi : *sinništi* : bar : *aṣû* : bàn-da	8 (In the Sumerian phrase) gi èn-bar bàn-da šu u-me-ti ("Take a small reed from the marsh"), gi ("reed") means "woman"; bar (the second element of the word èn-bar "marsh") means "to go out", bàn-da ("small")
9 *šerri* : *ṣaḫri* : **saḫar sila^{la}** : saḫar : *eperi* : saḫar *u ṣaḫar ištēn-ma*	9 means "baby" (or) "small (child)". (In) "dust (saḫar) from the street (sila)", saḫar means "dust". "Dust" (saḫar) and "baby" (*ṣaḫar*) are one and the same (phonetically).
10 **sila-lam$_4$-ma** : si : *ešēri ša alāku* : la : *la'û* : *ṣaḫar* : *amma* : *zēri*	10 (In) "crossroads" (sila-lam$_4$-ma), si means 'to go straight", said of "going"; la means "child" (*la'û*, which means) "little one"; and "people" (*ammu*) means "seed".
11 ***šamnu*** : $^{ni\text{-}ig}$níĝ : *sinništi* : *am* : *zēri* : nu : *banû šanîš* ^{i}ì(NI)	11 (In) "oil" (*šamnu*), the sign NÍG (= *šá* in *šá-am-nu*), read níĝ, means "woman"; *am*(*mu* "people") means "seed"; nu (means) "to create". Secondly, the sign NI, pronounced i,
12 *šamnu* : i : *aṣû ša zēri* : ***eli abunnatīšu ḫepī-ma*** *aššum qanû*	12 (means) "oil"; i (also means) "to go out" (i.e. sprout), said of seed. (In) "Break it (i.e. the reed) over her navel", (it is said) because reed
13 *nākis abunnati* : *abunnatu riksi ša amēli šī*	13 is the cutter of the umbilical cord; the umbilical cord is the bond of human(kind).

14 ^{giš}[$^{\text{ki-ri-is}}$]**kirid** : *kirissu* : *bīt ubāni* : ***šupšuqtum-ma*** : *šupšuqa*

14 (Sum.) kirid (means) "pin, needle" (Akk. *kirissu*), (which also means) "thimble" (lit. "house for the finger"). (The word) *supšuqtum-ma* ("woman in difficult labour") stems from *šupšuqu* ("to be in difficult labour"),

15 *kâšu šanîš dannati* : ***ina qarnīšu qaqqar(a) ṭerât*** : *ṭarû kayyānu*

15 (which means) "to be delayed"; alternatively (it means) "woman in distress". (In) "she roots up the earth with her horns", (the word *ṭerât* "she roots up" stems from) *ṭarû* "to root up" – (this is the) usual meaning.

16 *šanîš ṭerât* : *heṣnet* : *ṭarû* : *ḫaṣānu libbū* gú-da ri

16 Alternatively, *ṭerât* ("she strikes") (is equivalent to) *ḫeṣnet* "she hugs", (because) *ṭarû* (is equivalent to) *ḫaṣānu* ("to hug"), as in (Sumerian) gú-da ri (which equates with)

17 *nandura* : gú$^{?!}$-lá : *edēri* : ***ella(m)mê*** : *agû tašriḫti*

17 *nanduru* "to embrace one another", (and because Sumerian) gú$^{?!}$-lá (is) *edēru* ("to embrace"). (The name) Ella(m)mê (means) "Crown of Splendour" (i.e. an epithet of the moon god, referring to the full moon).

18 *libbū* é-lam$_4$-ma : ***bīt erbe*** *šanîš* si é-gar$_8$-bi til-la : *el-lam-mû*

18 (The pronunciation is the same) as in é-lam$_4$-ma (which means) "house (of) four". Secondly, si é-gar$_8$-bi til-la (refers to) Ellam-mû.

19 *ša nūr lānīšu uqattâ* : si : *nūru* : é-gar$_8$: *lānu*

19 (It means) "he who brings the light *of* his figure to an end", (since) si (means) "light", é-gar$_8$ (is synonymous to) "figure" (*lānu*),

20 bi : *šu* : til : *qatû aššu Sîn ša attalû gamarti išakkan*

20 bi (means) "his", til (means) "to finish"; (this is said) concerning the moon god when he sets a total eclipse.

21 ***aššum littīya lā ālitti*** *aššu Sîn bēl lâti ellēti*

21 "Because of my cow who has not given birth": (this is said) because Sîn (is) the lord of the pure cows.

22 **zi ^{d}nin-dar-a sipa udul$_{10}$(ÁB-LU)-lu-ú-a hé-pàd** : ***nīš*** **^{d}MIN** ***rē'î***

22 (As in the Sumerian phrase) "Be conjured by Nindara, the shepherd of the herdsmen", (Akk.) "by the life of ditto (Nindara), the shepherd

23 ***utullāti lū tamât*** : ^{d}nin-dar-a : *Sîn* : ***nešelpâ***

23 over the herdsmen, you are conjured". (The god) Nindara (is) Sîn. (The word) *nešelpâ* ("glide out!" stems from)

24 *nešalpû* : *etēqu* : *nešalpû* : *alāka* : gir$_5$-gir$_5$: *naḫalṣû*

24 *nešalpû* (which means) "to pass" (Akk. *etēqu*); *nešalpû* (also means) "to go" (*alāku*). (Since Sumerian) gir$_5$-gir$_5$ (means) *neḫelṣû* ("to slip; to slide; to glide"),

25 gir$_5$-gir$_5$: *našalpû* : ^{niraḫ} ^{d}GU$_4$: ***nirāḫu*** : an : *zēri*

25 gir$_5$-gir$_5$ (can also be equated with) *nešelpû*. Niraḫ (is the pronunciation of the logogram) ^{d}GU$_4$ (which is the same as) *nirāḫu* ("little snake"). (The sign) an (same as the divine classifier) (also means) "semen, seed"

26 GUD : *šaḫāṭu* : **KA.INIM.MA** <<:>> **^{munus}LA.RA.AḪ.A.KÁM** : la-ra-aḫ : *pušqa*

26 (and) GUD (means) *šaḫāṭu* "to jump; to leap". (In) "it is the wording (of an incantation)] for a woman who has difficulty during delivery", laraḫ (means) "(dire) straits" (Akk. *pušqu*),

27 *dannati* : ***naḫundi*** : *Sîn* : ***narundi*** : *Šamaš*

27 (which is the same as) "hardship, distress" (*dannatu*). Naḫḫunte (is) Sîn, Narunde (is) Šamaš.

28 ***namlisu kīma ṣabītu*** : zí : *malāsu* : zí : *baqāmu*

28 (In) "*Be plucked* like a gazelle", zí (means) "to pluck" (*malāsu*) (which is the same as) zí (which also means) *baqāmu* "to pluck (hair or wool)".

29 *šanîš namlisu libbū naplusu* : *amāra* : ***kīma*** **MAŠ.DÀ**

29 Alternatively, *namlisu* (is the same) as in *naplusu* ("to look at"), (which is synonymous to) *amāru* "to see". (In) "like a gazelle" (MAŠ.DÀ),

30 bar$^{\text{ba-ár}}$: *aṣû ša zēri* : $^{\text{du-u}}$dù : *lillidu* : ***ulla*** : *anna*	30 (the sign) MAŠ (pronounced) bar means "to come out", referring to "seed". The sign KAK (= DÀ) (pronounced) dù (means) *lillidu* "child." (In) "Well now (*ulla*)", (*ulla* means) "yes" (Akk. *anna*);
31 *anna* : *qibīti šanîš ulla* : *ulla* ì$^{\text{i-'u-u}}$: *šamnu* : **Ì BUR**	31 *anna* (also means) "divine pronouncement; command" (*qibītu*). Alternatively, *ulla* means "oil" (i.e. *ūlu*), (because the sign) Ì (pronounced as) *i'u* (means) "oil" (Akk. *šamnu*). "Oil-from-the-jar" (Ì BUR) is
32 *šaman kanni ša ṣāḫiti šanîš* bur : *bi'ilti* : ^{urudu}**GAG.(-) U$_4$.TAG.E**	32 "oil from the oil-presser's vessel". Alternatively, bur ("pot") means "container" (*bi'iltu*). "Arrow" (the logogram ^{urudu}GAG.(-) U$_4$.TAG.E)
33 mul-mul : *mulmul* : *šiltāḫu* : mul-mul : *zēri*	33 (is the same as Sumerian) mul-mul (which is) *mulmul(lu)* (or) *šiltāhu* "arrow" (in Akkadian). (Sumerian) mul-mul (also means) "seed" (*zēru*);
34 ^{gi}mul-mul : *zerri šanîš* gi : *sinništi* : urudu : *erû*	34 (furthermore) ^{gi}mul-mul (also means) "reed fence" (Akk. *zerru*). Alternatively, gi means "woman". Urudu (means) "copper" (Akkadian *erû*, which is phonetically the same as)
35 *ana arê* : $^{\text{du-u}}$dù(KAK) : *lillidu* : $^{\text{za-al}}$zalag(UD) : *nūr* : tag-ga	35 "to be pregnant" (Akk. *arû*). The sign KAK (pronounced as) dù means "baby". The sign UD (pronounced) zal(ag) means "light". (Sumerian) tag-ga (i.e. tag$_4$) means
36 *ezēbi šanîš* $^{\text{du-u}}$dù(KAK) : *lillidu* : si : *ešēri ša alāku aššum*	36 "to leave (behind)". Alternatively, the sign KAK (pronounced) dù means "baby", (and Sumerian) si means "to go straight", said of "going". (This is relevant) because of
37 ^{mul}KAK.SI.SÁ : ***egizinīti*** : *Geme-Sîn* : ***ina qaqqadīya namāra***	37 the constellation "Arrow" (^{mul}KAK.SI.SÁ, Sirius). Egizinīti (is the same as) Geme-Sîn ("the slave-girl of Sîn"). (In) "The clearing in front of me" (lit. at my head)
38 *namāra* : *ḫarrānu ša api u qišti* : ***ša libbi išqillati likallim nūru***	38 "clearing" (*namāru*) (means) a path (in) the reed thicket or a forest. (In) "let him (Šamaš) show the light to the one inside the shell" –
39 *ana erīti iqtabi* : $^{\text{na4}}$iškila(ŠÀxA) : *ṣillatu* : na$_4$: *aṣû ša zēri*	39 it (the base text) said it in reference to the pregnant woman. $^{\text{na4}}$iškila (lit. "pregnancy stone") means "shell"; na$_4$ (means) "to come out", said of seed/offspring;
40 a : *māra* : šà : *libbi* : ***uššurat ḫurdatsu*** : *ḫurdatu* : *urû*	40 (in the sign iškila(ŠÀxA)) a (means) "son"; šà (means) "inside, belly". (In) "her vulva is set straight" – the vulva (is) the pubic triangle
41 *ša sinništi libbū* ***qātka šūtamṣâm-ma luput ḫurdatna***	41 of a woman; as in: "Let your hand be stretched out and stroke our vulva!"
42 *šanîš ḫurdati* : *qimmati* : *šalšiš ḫurdati* : *ḫurri dādi*	42 Alternatively, "vulva" (means) "(pubic?) hair"; thirdly: "vulva" (is) "the hole of the darling";
43 *dādu* : *māra* : ***ina kittabrīšu*** : *ina idīšu* : *kittabri* : *idi* : še : *idi*	43 "darling" (means) "child". "At her side" (*ina kittabrīšu*) (is the same as) "at her side" (*ina idīšu*), (because) "side, arm" (*kittabru*) (is the same as) "side, arm" (*idu*). (Moreover) še means "arm" (*idu*),
44 še: *kittabra* : ***qīp napšāti*** : *qa-a-pa* : *nadānu*	44 (and) še (also means) "side" (*kittabru*). (In) "he who is entrusted with (their) lives", "to entrust" (means) "to grant".
45 túg $^{\text{tu-un}}$tun$_x$(DÚB) : *kamādu* : ***ikkud itta'id*** : *tankittu*	45 túg tun$_x$ (means) "to beat cloth". (In) "he was anxious (*ikkud*) and concerned", "anxiety" (*takkittu*)
46 *ḫissatu* : *itmudu* : *šemû* : ***abnu tikku šamê*** : *abnu*	46 means "understanding" and "to be concerned" means "to listen". (In) "hailstone from heaven" (*abnu tīk šamê*), "stone" (*abnu*) (can be explained as)

47 ab : *banû ša alādu* : nu : *zēru* : u-gu$_4$: *tikku* : u : *banû*

47 ab (which means) “to create”, said of giving birth; nu (which means) “seed”. (Furthermore) ugu (corresponds to) “neck” (*tikku*), where u (stands for) “to create” (*banû*)

48 gu : *alādu* : an : *šamê* : an : *zēri* : *eper dūri maqti* (**SAḪAR BÀD ŠUB-*tú***)

48 (and) gu (stands for) “to give birth” (*alādu*); an (stands for) “heaven” (*šamû*), (and for) “seed” (*zēru*). (In) “dust from a dilapidated city wall” (SAḪAR BÀD ŠUB-*tú*),

49 bàd : *dūru* : kéš : *riksi* : bad : *petû*

49 BÀD (= KÉŠxBAD) means “wall” (*dūru*); (its component) KÉŠ (means) “bond” (*riksu*) (and) BAD (means) “to open” (*petû*).

50 *maqtu ša iqbû aššu* diri(SI.A) : *qâpa ša dūri* : si : *ešēri ša alāk(u)*

50 (The wall is) “fallen”, which it said, (this is) because diri(-SI.A) (means) “to collapse”, said of a wall; si (means) “to go straight”, said of walking (and)

51 a : *ṣaḫar* : *eper pisanni šurdî* (**SAḪAR PISAN *šur-di-i***) : ma-a ĝá : *pisannu* : ĝá : *alāku*

51 a (means) “little one” (*ṣaḫar*). (In) “dust from a streaming drainpipe”, (the sign) GÁ (= PISAN), when pronounced /ma/ means “drainpipe” (*pisannu*); ĝá (can also mean) “to walk” (*alāku*).

Colophon:

52 *ṣâtī šūt pî u mašʾalti ša pî ummâni ša libbi*

52 Lemmata, oral explanations, and (materials for) a “questioning” *by* a master-scholar, related to (the text with the incipit)

53 ÉN munus ù-tu-ud-da-a-ni *imgiddû Enlil-kāṣir*

53 “Incantation: The woman giving birth”. Oblong tablet of Enlil-kāṣir,

54 *kalû Enlil māru ša Enlil-šuma-imbi liblibbi*

54 lamentation-priest of Enlil, son of Enlil-šuma-imbi, descendent of

55 *Lu-dumununna šumerû*

55 Ludumununna, the Sumerian (i.e. Nippurean).

Notes

Line 1: The quotation én munus ù-tu-ud-da-a-ni in line 1 is the incipit or title of the base text commented on (again referred to in line 53 of the colophon). It can thus be surmised that it also formed the incipit of BAM 248 etc., i.e. that this tablet started with an incantation beginning “the woman giving birth ...”. The following lines in 11N-T3 comment on the first text section of BAM 248 (obv. i 1–35), which is unfortunately almost completely lost. However, it is clear from the remaining traces that this first section of BAM 248 must have contained a Sumerian incantation with interlinear Akkadian translation, and that this composition has precursors in Sumerian birth incantations from the Old Babylonian period (see text D.1.1 in the present volume).

The Akkadian phrase *e-lep-pi šá uq-na-a ṣa-na-at* must be a quotation from BAM 248 obv. i 8, which appears to refer to the boat loaded with lapis lazuli but is very fragmentary. Several Old Babylonian precursors to the incantation offer parallel lines (cf. discussion of BAM 248, text D.1.1). On the image of the woman as a boat loaded with lapis lazuli and other precious materials, see also Woods 2009, *JANER* 9, 222 fn. 162; Hätinen 2017, *KASKAL* 14, 174–175. For the verb *ṣênu/ṣânu* “to load”, see AHw 1091; CAD Ṣ, 131–132.

Lines 2–6: The Sumerian phrase gug nu-zu ù ZA.GUL nu-zu forms a citation from the base text BAM 248 obv. i 9, and the following *lu-ʾ-at-ma a-na ni-qí-i ul na-ṭa-at* “she is defiled and unfit for (making a) sacrifice” appears to quote the interlinear Akkadian translation in BAM 248 obv. i 10, which can be restored with the help of the commentary (following Veldhuis 1989, 241, 245). As elucidated by Gabbay (2016, 175–177), the Sumerian line presents a textual corruption, in which the sign gug (ZA.GUL) is a corruption of za-gìn “lapis lazuli”, the latter of which is found in the Old Babylonian parallels to BAM 248 obv. i 9 (in Sumerian birth incantations, see the discussion of BAM 248 in this volume (text D.1.1)). The Akkadian rendering presents a complete divergence from the meaning of the Sumerian text, which explains the commentary’s need for exegesis.

The word *pūḫtu* “substitute, replacement, exchange” has been understood by Cavigneaux (1987, 152–153) to signify a substitution of one word by another. For an overview of different interpretations of the word *pūḫtu* (lit. “replacement”), see Frahm 2011, 69; Seminara 2001, 531–533; AHw 877 (“Austauschwort, Synonym”); Civil 1974, *JNES* 33, 333 (in the sense of metonym or antonym). According to Gabbay (2016, 169–170, 175–177) the term *pūḫtu* "(word) replacement" in the commentary flags a deviation from the regular word order, implied by the Akkadian rendering and interpretation of the corrupt Sumerian text. However, the word *pūḫtu* could also simply denote the divergence in meaning between the Sumerian and Akkadian version of the base text and refer to the word replacements that the commentary then posits to establish a coherence between the Sumerian and Akkadian versions. In particular, the commentator explains that Sumerian gug (which usually means "carnelian") also means *ellu* "pure" and nu means *lā* "not", which in the Akkadian base text corresponds to *lu"âtma* "she is defiled". Thus, the Akkadian text refers to the notion of defilement or ritual impurity that affected women after a delivery and rendered them unfit for presenting offerings (or addressing the deity).

The second half of the quoted Akkadian line of the base text is explained on the basis of other word replacements: the Sumerian word zu in the base text (which usually means "to know") is equated with *naṭû* "to be fitting, appropriate, suitable" which is further equated with *amāru* "to see"; and the term gug ("carnelian", which can also stand for Akkadian *niqû* "sacrifice" and *guqqû* "(monthly) offering") is (implicitly) replaced by siskur "offering", which corresponds to Akkadian *niqû* (in the base text) and is further equated with *ṣulû* "prayer" (for analysis, see Cavigneaux 1976, 153–154; 1982, *JCS* 34, 236 n. 22). For the association of *naṭû* "to be suitable, proper" and *amāru* "to see, observe; to look favourably upon someone", see also the *Šurpu* Commentary B (Reiner 1958, 50 line 8), equating *la na-ṭa-a-tum* with *la a-ma-ra-a-tú*.

For the expression *ša iqbû* "which it (= the base text) said", in line 5, see Gabbay 2016, 203, noting that this phrase refers to a preceding quoted lemma or passage from the base text that is about to be commented on. In other words, *ša iqbû* marks the end of a cited text passage before introducing a commentary on it.

Lines 6–7: I understand the phrase *na-gi-ri um-ma* ᵈGAŠAN-DINGIR *iš-ta-na-as-si* "the herald summons Bēlet-ilī as follows" as a citation from the Akkadian base text, which must have belonged to the lost lines in BAM 248 obv. i 12–20. The word *um-ma* is ambiguous, as it may be "mother" or "as follows", introducing a direct speech. The following commentary, in my view, dwells on a phonetic link between of Akkadian *nāgiru* "herald" and a similar pronunciation of the Sumerian word nigru(KAxAD+KÙ), which is equated with *āšipu* "conjurer" in the lexical tradition (Ea Tablet 3 (MSL 14, 308: 122); Lú = *ša* (MSL 12, 133: 153)). On this commentary passage, cf. also Sassmannshausen 1995, *BaM* 26, 183–184; Wee 2017, *ZA* 107, 240–241 with fn. 41. For the commentary's description of the composite nature of the sign nigru (the incorporation of a cuneiform sign into another sign) with the phrase ša ...ak+u ...a i-gub "... written inside of ...", cf. Gong 2000, *Die Namen der Keilschriftzeichen*, 27–30.

Lines 8–13: The quotations from the base text commented on in these lines are not preserved in the base text BAM 248 (see text D.1.1 line 11 with discussion), but Old Babylonian birth incantations offer precursors; moreover, the Neo-Babylonian fragment N. 1568 from Nippur (published by Jiménez 2019) preserves a fragmentary passage of a couple of lines belonging to the bilingual incantation of the base text (see notes on BAM 248 obv. i 1–36 (text D.1.1) in this volume). The quoted passages in lines 8–13 refer to ritual actions to promote delivery: taking a reed from the marsh (gi èn-bar bàn-da), filling it with dust (from a street or crossroads) and oil and breaking it above the woman's umbilical area / navel). The commentary explains certain keywords from the quotes by pointing out meanings inherent in the component signs that relate to the birth situation and the aim of the ritual.

For the reed from the marsh in lines 8–9, see Cavigneaux 1987, *AuOr* 5, 253; Maul 1997, *FS Röllig*, 264–265; Frahm 2011, 231; Steinert 2017a, 337–338; Jiménez 2019, 140: 5'–6' (read *[tak-k]u-si qa-né-e* "a hollow reed stem" in line 6', see *infra* text D.1.1 notes on lines 6–11). For the quoted keywords saḫar sila[la] "dust from a street" and sila-lam$_4$-ma "crossroad" in lines 9–10, see Steinert 2017, 338–339; N. 1568: 7'–8' (Jiménez 2019, 140; *infra* text D.1.1). Dust from a crossroads is a popular ingredient of ointments used to massage the woman giving birth in other sections of BAM 248 (see obv. i 52–53, with the variant in ms. a (BM 36339 obv. 2'–3'), BAM 248 rev. iii 46). For *ištēn-ma* "(it) is one (and the same)" in line 9, see Gabbay 2016, 92–93, who notes that the term does not mean simple lexical equations, but that the explanation "dust (saḫar) and child (*ṣaḫar*) are one (*ištēn-ma*)", employs an etymology (based on homophony of saḫar and *ṣaḫar*). See also Frahm 2011, 73.

In the equation si = *ešēru* found in line 10 (as well as in lines 36 and 51), si is understood here as an abbreviation for si-sá.

For the commented keyword *šamnu* "oil, fat" (lines 11–12), see also the duplicating passage in commentary UET 6/3, 897 l. e. 1–2 (edited below as text G.2). The commentator's exegesis of these key words and phrases revolves around stating connections between the component signs and syllables in the cited words and Sumerian and Akkadian words that mean "woman", "baby", "to come out (easily)". In this way, the exegete points out a deeper connection of the incantation text with the birth situation, during which it was recited, and implicitly provides a rationale for the assumed effectivity of the incantation.

On lines 8–12 of the commentary, see also CAD S, 287a; CAD Š/1, 322a (lex. section); Frahm 2010a, 96; Frahm 2014, 324; Maul 1999, 12; Reiner and Civil 1990, 109–110; Scurlock 1991, *Incognita* 2, 143–144, 173 n. 129; Wee 2017, *ZA* 107, 240; Steinert 2017a, 339.

Lines 12–13: For the instruction *e-li abunnati*(LI.DUR)*-šú ḫe-pi-ma* "break it above her navel" quoted in line 12, see AUAM 73.3094 rev. 53; Cohen 1976, *RA* 70, 133ff.; Wasserman and Zomer 2022, No. 10, with a similar instruction in BAM 248 obv. i 52–53 (*infra* text D.1.1); Steinert 2017a, 336, 339. For reed as the cutter of the umbilical cord, see also Stol 2000, 142; Mayer 2016, *OrNS* 85, 182; BM 34208: 34' (*infra* text D.1.9). The commentary draws a link between the treatment performed in the ritual of the base text (breaking a reed above the woman's navel) and the positive outcome of the delivery completed by severing the baby's umbilical cord (both navel and umbilical cord are referred to with the Akkadian term *abunnatu*), see Gabbay 2016, 164. Furthermore, the element DUR in LI.DUR (= *abunnatu*) corresponds to *riksu* "bond" in Akkadian, providing the link to the explanation "the umbilical cord is the bond of human(kind)" in line 13; cf. Frahm 2011, 65–66.

Line 14: The Sumerian word kirid "pin" commented upon here is not preserved but may be restored in the fragmentary line BAM 248 obv. i 23 (text D.1.1). In older birth incantations from the third and second millennium BCE, spindle (^{giš}bala-k / *pilak-k/qqu*) and (dress or hair) pin / needle (kirid/*kirissu*) are gender-specific objects representing the female gender of the newborn baby, which are contrasted with male gendered objects (weapon or mace) representing a son (e.g., Rudik 2011, 323–325, 328, 330–331). For discussion see text D.1.1 line 12; BM 42327+ (text C.3.3) line 34' and SpTU 3, No. 84 (text C.3.4) note on line 56. The commentary adds the complementary term "thimble" (*bīt ubāni*, lit. "house of the finger") to match the term *kirissu*.

Lines 14–15: The commentary here begins to comment on the second incantation preserved in the Neo-Assyrian Birth Compendium (BAM 248 obv. i 36–50 //; cf. text D.1.1). The first cited keyword is *šup-šuq-tùm-ma*, "woman having difficulty in labour" (the feminine form of the verbal adjective *šupšuqu*, from the Š-stem of *pašāqu*, see CAD Š/3, 327). This term has been previously restored in the fragmentary line BAM 248 obv. i 36 and interpreted as a rubric: [KA.INIM.MA *ša*] *šup-šu-[uq-ti]* (CAD Š/3 327, s.v. *šupšuqtu*). However, since the ruling following BAM 248 obv. i 36 is doubtful, it is also possible to restore the fem. stative form *šupšu[qat (alāda)]* "she has difficulty (giving birth)" in BAM 248 obv. i 36 (ms. A) and ms. B_2 obv. i 9', and to understand it as the first line of the incantation.

The commentary explains the term *šupšuqtu* with the verb *kâšu* "to be late" (CAD K, 294–295), the latter of which is attested in the gynaecological texts in other contexts (in the connection with the placenta delayed in being expelled after delivery; see BM 38624+, text A.2.1). The second explanation given for *šupšuqtu* in the commentary is the term *dannatu*. Jiménez (2014, CCP) understands this as the feminine form of the adjective *dannu* "difficult; distressed" (i.e. "distressed woman"), rather than as the noun *dannatu* "hardship, distress", the latter of which occurs several times in the incantations in BAM 248 etc. (text D.1.1).

Lines 15–17: The phrase cited in line 15 is also commented on in the commentary UET 6/3, 897 obv. 1' (see below text G.2), but the exegesis (lost in the lacuna) is much more concise in the latter text. The quoted incantation passage describing the cow in birth pangs who roots up the earth with her horns can be reconstructed with the help of the commentaries in the base text BAM 248 (ms. A) obv. i 38: [*ina qar-ni-šú qaq*]*-qa-ru* [*ṭe-ra-at ina* KUN*-šá*?], duplicated in ms. B_2 obv. i 11': [...]-*ra ṭe-ra-at*. See also BAM 248 rev. iii 56 (*infra* text D.1.1).

For SAG.ÚS = *kayyān(u)* "permanent; regular; normal; actual" in commentaries, as a technical expression referring to the "literal" or "usual meaning" (of a word) in the quoted base text, see Frahm 2011, 38; Gabbay 2016: 182–194.

For different interpretations of the present commentary passage, see Cavigneaux 1987, 253–254; George 1991, *RA* 85, 155; Rochberg 2016, 268–269. The word *ṭarû* in lines 15–16 appears to be a phonetic variant of *ṭerû* "to beat; to pierce" (AHw 1388–1389 "tief eindringen"; differently read as *dārû* "permanent" by CAD Ṭ, 104 s.v. *ṭerû* B sub b, followed by Rochberg 2016, 268, understanding the following *kayyānu* as a synonym). The equation gú-da ri = *nanduru* "to meet; embrace each other" (N-stem of *edēru*) is a quotation from the lexical literature (Ḫḫ. II 287; MSL 5, 72), introduced by *libbū* "as in" in the commentary. According to George (1991, 155), the commentator draws a connection between the cow's horns rooting up the ground in the incantation and astronomical observations describing the moon crescent's "horns" "piercing" (*ṭerû*, or "sticking into") the sky. He assumes that the commentator then points out semantic connections between *ṭerû*, and the words *ḫaṣānu* "to shelter", *nanduru* (N-stem of *edēru*) "to embrace each other" and *nanduru* (*na'duru*, N-stem of *adāru*) "to become darkened, obscured, eclipsed" (said of heavenly bodies). The commentator elucidates different semantic associations evoked by the keyword *ṭerû* by drawing on phonological similarities to other Akkadian terms.

Marten Stol (1992, 257–258) further suggested that the word *nanduru* in the commentary was to be interpreted as "darkened" and referred to the moon god's sadness and weeping about the cow's trouble, manifesting in an eclipse. He suggested that in the following equation of e-lá = *edēru* "to embrace", the former may have to be linked with *elallu*, a poetic word for one who carries water, used in reference to clouds (and connected to Sumerian e_4 "water" and lal/lá "to carry"). This expression may be "a reference to the appearance of the moon in eclipse as covered by a cloud, hence carrying the water that was the source of his tears" (see Rochberg 2018, 293). Stol further surmised that *edēru* "to embrace" may allude to the sexual union between the moon god and the cow Geme-Sîn. Since in Old Babylonian texts, gú-lá means "to embrace", Gabbay (2016, 189–190) suggests e-lá is in fact a mistake for gú-lá. Gabbay interprets the second explanation given in the commentary passage (i.e. the word *ṭarû* meaning "to give shelter, to protect") as a reference to the positive outcome of the delivery, namely that the woman/cow will protect her young, which the commentator associates with the gesture of "embracing". The commentary here also draws on (approximate) homophony between the associated verbs (*ṭerû, edēru, nanduru*, gú-da ri). For *libbū* "as in" before homophones, see also Gabbay 2016, 129 and lines 17–18 and 28–29 below.

Lines 17–20: Instead of only citing the name *Ella(m)-mê* ("pure of rites", a title of the moon god, see CAD E 100–101), the commentary passage in UET 6/3, 897 obv. 2' cites the complete line of the base text (BAM 248 obv. i 41 //), from which it is drawn, which refers to the moon god crying because of his cow's birthing difficulties (see text D.1.1 and below G.2). According to Stol (1992, 257–258), the commentator may have understood the title *Ella-mê* to mean "pure of water", linking it to the metaphor of the moon god's tears and weeping during a lunar eclipse (see also Rochberg 2016, 118–119).

The exegesis in 11N-T3: 17–20 and UET 6/3, 897 obv. 2'–5' runs almost entirely parallel. 11N-T3 offers two additional explanations or comparisons. One of these associates the title of the moon god *Ella-mê* with Sumerian é-lam$_4$-ma "house of four" (rendered as Akkadian *bīt erbe*), which may allude to the four quadrants (or houses) of the moon that could be obscured during an eclipse (see Wee 2017, *ZA* 107, 241, with Stol 1992, 258, 271 n. 116). Gabbay (2016, 129 n. 6) notes that the word *libbū* "as in" introducing é-lam$_4$-ma may indicate a homonymous expression rather than a quotation from an unknown textual source. An equation not found in UET 6/3, 897 is the connection of *Ella-mê* with *agû tašriḫti* "crown of splendour" (line 17), a designation for the full moon (Stol 1992, 250). For discussion of this passage, see also Cavigneaux 2000, *BaM* 31, 225 (on line 18); Rochberg 2016, 118–119; 2018, 292–294.

For the second explanation of *Ella-mê* in lines 18–20, see the discussion in Gabbay 2016, 157–158. The commentary equates *Ella-mê* with Sumerian si é-gar$_8$-bi til-la "he who brings the light *of* his figure to an end" and explains this by analysing the meanings of the different components of the Sumerian phrase and by relating that expression to the moon god making a complete eclipse (the latter explanation is introduced by *aššu* "because of").

Lines 21–23: The phrase of the base text (BAM 248 obv. i 43) cited here describes how the moon god cries over his cow that is unable to deliver. The same phrase is also commented upon in UET 6/3, 897 obv. 6'–7' (see below). The first explanation provided by both commentaries is identical (*áš-šú* ÁB-*ia*$_5$ *la a-lit-ti* : ⌜*áš-šú*⌝ [^{d}30 EN *la*]-⌜*a-tim*⌝ KÙ.MEŠ "(the phrase) 'because of my cow who has not given birth' – (this is said) because Sîn is the lord of the pure cows"). The explanation *bēl lâti ellēti* "the lord of the pure cows" creates a "homophonic paraphrase of the description of the cow in the base text" (*littīya lā ālitti*), see Gabbay 2016, 161–162 for discussion.

To further support the first explanation, the commentator then cites a bilingual incantation passage from Udug-ḫul Tablet 5: 59 (Geller 2016, 188), in which the god Nindara is said to be the shepherd of the herdsmen (udul$_{10}$(ÁB-LU)-lu-ú-a : *utullātu*), i.e. is likewise associated with cattle. For contamination with *utul lâti* "herdsman of cows", cf. OB Diri Oxford 283 (MSL 15, 43; cf. CAD U/W 342 lex. section). For the equation of Nindara (originally a god of Lagaš/Girsu and husband of Nanše) with Sîn, see also An = Anum III 65; Litke 1998, 124; Lambert and Winters 2023, 20, 140 (= III 59); Edzard 1998–2001a, "Nindar(a)", *RlA* 9, 338.

Lines 23–26: Cf. UET 6/3, 897 obv. 7' (see below). The words *nešelpû* and *nirāḫu* commented upon are quoted from a birth incantation (BAM 248 obv. i 49: [*ṣa-a* G]IN$_7$ MUŠ *né-šel-pa-a ki-ma ni-ra-ḫi* "[come out li]ke a snake, glide out like a little snake!"). The word *nirāḫu* "little snake" is written syllabically in the commentary (instead of logographic MUŠ.TUR in BAM 248). In lines 25–26, the commentary connects the word *nirāḫu* with the chthonic god Niraḫ, usually written with the logogram ^{d}MUŠ. However, in BAM 499 iii 3', GU$_4$/GUD is glossed with MUŠ, see also Wiggermann 1998–2001, "Niraḫ, Irḫan", *RlA* 9, 570; Peterson 2009, 68.

The image of the baby slipping out from the womb like a snake triggered the associations and lexical equations given by the commentator in lines 23–25 (focusing on the verbs *nešalpû* "to glide" and its synonyms *naḫalṣû* "to slide", *etēqu* "to pass" and *alāku* "to go"). The equation of an = *zēru* "semen; seed" in line 25 is not attested lexically, but an may be a phonetic variant for a "water; semen" (for discussion of the passage, see Cavigneaux 1987, 254); GUD is known as a variant logogram for *šaḫāṭu* "to jump" (usually spelled GU_4.UD).

Lines 26–27: Cf. also the commentary UET 6/3, 897 obv. 7'–8' (below text G.2). 11N-T3 cites the incantation rubric encountered in BAM 248 obv. i 51 (and *passim*) attached to the incantations in the Birth Compendium. For ^{munus}LA.RA.AḪ (*mušapšiqtu, šupšuqtu*) "woman having difficulty in childbirth" and the rubric KA.INIM.MA ^{munus}LA.RA.AḪ.KAM, see also Stol 2000, 123, n. 83, 129, 132; the Exorcist's Manual (KAR 44: 15 and dupl.; Geller 2018a, 298; Heeßel 2023, 294); Stadhouders 2011, *JMC* 18, 7 fn. 18 (for a possible occurrence of a "plant for dystocia" (*šammi pušqi*, Ú LA.RA.AḪ in *šammu šikinšu*) and *infra* text D.1.1.

The Elamite deities Naḫunde (Naḫ(ḫ)unte) and Narunde, which are here (mistakenly) equated with the Babylonian moon god and sun god, are addressed in two incantations in the Birth Compendium, in BAM 248 obv. i 58 and in BAM 248 rev. iii 36, 40. For comments, see notes on BAM 248 obv. i 40–47 (*infra* text D.1.1).

Lines 28–30: The quoted text passage *na-am-li-su ki-ma ṣa-bi-tu*$_4$ is from BAM 248 obv. i 59 (ms. A) // BM 36339 obv. 9' (ms. a) (text D.1.1 line 45). Interestingly, BM 36339 has a textual variant, which is also discussed in the commentary:

A obv. i 59 [*na-a*]*m-*[*l*]*i-*[*su*] *ki-ma ṣa-bi-ti*
a obv. 9' [*na-a*]*p*$^?$*-li-sa ki-ma* MAŠ.DÀ
"Be plucked out (var. ms. a: Look (at me)) like a gazelle!"

In line 29, the commentary posits that *na-am-li-su* can also be interpreted as the verb *naplusu* "to look" (synonymous to *amāru* "to see"), introduced by *libbū* "as in", which is used to introduce homonymic or homophonic explanations (Gabbay 2016, 129 with n. 6). Possibly, the attested variants of the base text were known to the commentator. For parallels to the lexical equations in this commentary passage, see also CAD M/1 161 s.v. *malāšu*; CAD B 97 s.v. *baqāmu*. The verbs *malāsu* and *baqāmu* refer to plucking or tearing out of hair / wool of animals or plants. For discussion of the equations in line 30, see also Civil 1974, 330. The equation of the sign KAK, pronounced as dù with Akkadian *lillidu* "baby", may be due to homonymy with dú (TU) = *alādu* "to give birth" or with dù-a "young (animal); child" (cf. Attinger 2021, *Glossaire*, 594 n. 594; see also lines 35 and 36 for the same equation).

Lines 30–31: The commentary cites the word *ulla* from the incantation in BAM 248 obv. i 64 // BM 36339 rev. 4 (see text D.1.1 line 50). The duplicating commentary UET 6/3, 897 obv. 10' cites the full phrase *ulla Šamaš* "well now, Šamaš" from the base text (cf. below). Gabbay (2015, CCP 4.2.A.b with note 4) understands *ulla* and *anna* in UET 6/3, 897 obv. 10' as deictic or adverbial particles (status absolutus of *ullû* and *annû*, meaning "that, this" (or, alternatively "here, there"). The parallel, but better-preserved passage in 11N-T3: 30–31 appears to comment on several homonymous Akkadian words. Thus, it is also possible that the commentator equated the interjection *ulla* "well, now" (used in the base text) with *anna* "yes" (or *annu* "yes-word; consent") or with the interjection *anna* "well" (cf. CAD A/2, 125, 134–136; CAD U/W, 74–75), which may be implied by the following equation of *anna* with *qibītu* "command" in line 31. Interesting is further the (implicit) association of *ulla* with the homonymous *ūlu* "oil", implied by the equation with ì = *šamnu* "oil" in line 31. This explanation also builds a bridge to the following section commenting on *šaman pūri* "oil-from-the-jar" (the latter is used as *materia medica* in the base text). For *ulû*/*ūlu* "finest oil", see also CAD U/W, 88 s.v. *ulû*; cf. the discussion in Civil 1974, 334–335 note on lines 30ff.; Veldhuis 1989, 246–247.

Lines 31–37: This commentary passage is similar to UET 6/3, 897 obv. 11'–13'. However, 11N-T3 extracts isolated words and phrases, while UET 6/3, 897 quotes a longer passage from the base text: Ì.GIŠ BUR *šá ina* ^{giš}GAG.U_4.TAG.GA *in-d*[*aḫ-ṣu*$^?$] "oil-from-the-jar (*šaman pūri*) which has been st[irred] with an arrow". The expression occurs similarly in the prescription in BAM 248 obv. i 68–69 // BM 36339 rev. 6–7 (cf. text D.1.1 lines 54–55). In line 32, the commentator lists synonyms or explanations for *šaman pūri* "oil-from-the-jar" (Ì BUR) and *pūru* (BUR) "jar; bowl": the former is explained as *šaman kanni ša ṣāḫiti* "oil from the oil-presser's vessel" (see CAD K, s.v. *kannu* A lex. and sub 3), and *pūru* is associated with the *bi'iltu*-vessel (alabastron(?), see CAD B, s.v. *bi'iltu* lex. section). The medical commentary BRM 4, 32: 17 (Scurlock 2014a, 342, 345) also associates *pūru*-oil with pressed oil and with the *bi'iltu*-vessel. See further Guichard 2005, ARM 31, 183–185 on the variant spelling *baḫiltum* "phial, ampulla" in Old Babylonian texts from Mari.

The next keyword analysed in lines 32–37 is “arrow” (here written ^{urudu}GAG.U_4.TAG.E, while the manuscripts BAM 248 and BM 36339 of the base text use the logogram ^{giš}GAG.U_4.TAG.GA). The first explanations in lines 33–34 giving synonymous and homonymous (Sumerian and Akkadian) terms for “arrow” are parallel to UET 6/3, 897 obv. 12'–13' (although the latter commentary is slightly shorter). For these lexical equations, see CAD M/2, 190–191 s.v. *mulmullu*; CAD Š/2 s.v. *šiltāḫu*; CAD Z s.v. *zirru* “reed fence” (the reference to the equation mul-mul = *zerru* “reed fence” is based on homophony with *zēru*). See also Gabbay 2016, 158–159 for discussion.

In lines 34–37, the commentator turns to analysing the meanings of the component signs of $^{gi/urudu}$GAG.U_4.TAG.GA “arrow”, in order to point out relations between the ritual use of the arrow and the situation of the woman giving birth and her baby. The comment gi = *sinništu* “woman” may have been introduced in line 34 due to the variant $^{gi/urudu}$GAG.U_4.TAG.GA. For this unusual equation, compare gi (Emesal) = *ardatu* “young woman”, which also occurs in the commentary SpTU 1, No. 39: 6'–7' (see Wee 2017, 240; *infra*, Chapter I.1.2). The commentator proceeds to give Akkadian equations for the component signs in ^{urudu}GAG.U_4.TAG.GA. The equation urudu = *erû* “copper” is further associated with the homonym *erû/arû* “to be pregnant”; TAG.GA (for Sumerian taka) is equated with *ezēbu* “to leave (behind), to let go” (see Gabbay 2016, 136–137; Cavigneaux 1987, 254 for discussion). In lines 36–37, the commentator further brings in the term ^{mul}KAK.SI.SÁ “Arrow-star” (Akkadian *Šukūdu*, Sirius), whose component signs KAK (GAG) and SI he analyses by providing lexical equations that are directly related to the aim of the commented ritual (the unhindered birth of the baby).

Lines 37–38: These lines in the commentary presumably provide comments on the lost passage in the first half of BAM 248 obv. ii. The name of the cow of Sîn cited here as *e-gi-zi-ni-ti* (an Akkadian rendering of the cow’s name Geme-Sîn or Gī-Sîn) is also attested in the incantation in BM 36339 rev. 9–11, which begins with the name of the cow, *e-gi-zi-ni-*tu_4 *šá* ^{d}30 “(I am) Egizinītu, belonging to Sîn” (cf. text D.1.1 line 181, variant of BAM 248 rev. iii 54).

The next quoted passage *ina* SAG.DU-ia_5 *na-ma-ra* “the path in front of me” in line 37 cannot be identified yet in BAM 248, but probably stemmed from the incantation in the first lost lines of obv. ii. Notably, the word *namāru* “path, clearing” is also commented on in UET 6/3, 897 rev. 1' (see below). For *namāru*, which is derived from *naw/māru* “to be light, to shine” and related to *taw/mirtu* “watered field, cultivated land”, see also Stol 1988, *BSA* 4, 180.

Lines 38–40: For discussion, see also CAD N/2, 349b; Frahm 2011, 67, 241; Gabbay 2016, 234; Steinert 2017a, 334–335. The commentary draws on the recurring image in birth incantations of the baby as the creature inside a shell, in which the shell is a euphemism for the pregnant woman’s body or genital organs. For the motif of the baby coming out to see the daylight and the sun god, see also Polonsky 2006, 302 with fn. 24.

Both Civil (1974, 335) and Veldhuis (1989, 244) restore the line cited in the commentary in BAM 248 obv. ii 23 (against Ebeling’s copy of KAR 196), reading [*iš-q*]*il*$^{?}$-*la*-[tu_4 ...] UB [...] DI. However, the remaining traces at the end of that line do not fit the citation given in both commentaries as *šá* ŠÀ *iš-qil-la-*tu_4 *li-kal-lim nu-ú-rum*. For a different restoration of BAM 248 obv. ii 23, see *infra* text D.1.1 (line 78). The quoted line is probably to be found before BAM 248 obv. ii 23, in the lost beginning of col. ii, which contained the beginning of the birth incantation commented on in 11N-T3 lines 37ff. The commentary UET 6/3, 897 rev. 3'–4' cites the same line from the base text. Interestingly, the first part of the exegesis in 11N-T3 and UET 6/3, 897 is the same (explaining that the word *išqillatu* “shell” refers to the pregnant woman; see Gabbay 2016, 234 for the phrase *ana ... iqtabi*, used for contextualising or spelling out the intention of the base text). But the former commentary then continues to provide word equations for the constituent signs in ^{na4}IŠKILA($PEŠ_4$): the sign na_4 (the classifier for “stone”, but here presumably to be pronounced /i/ or /ia/) is equated with *aṣû* “to come out” (here linked with *zēru* “seed, offspring”; cf. CAD A/2, 356b sub lex. section; Borger 2004, MZL, No. 385; Cavigneaux 1987, 254–255; Attinger 2021, *Glossaire*, 542, 755 for ia_4(NA_4) = è “to go out”). The sign IŠKILA (which can also be read $peš_4$ “(to be) pregnant”) consists of the signs ŠÀ and A, and thus the commentator explains relevant meanings of the latter signs (šà = *libbu* “inside, womb” and a = *māru* “son”). UET 6/3, 897 rev. 4' instead points out alternative readings or metaphorical meanings of the word IŠKILA($PEŠ_4$) “shell” (the equation *ummu* “mother” for Sumerian $peš_4$ is not attested lexically). See also below text G.2.

Lines 40–43: For comments, see Frahm 2011, 104; Gabbay 2016, 132. The citation from the base text in line 40 is found in BAM 248 obv. ii 30 (see text D.1.1 line 85): *uš*$^{!}$*-šu-rat ḫur-da-as-sa* “her vulva is set straight” (to deliver the baby). The commentary dwells on the rare literary word *ḫurdatu* “vulva”, which it explains as *urû* (*ūru*) *ša sinništi* “female pudenda”. In support of this explanation, line 41 then offers a quotation from the *Gilgamesh Epic* VI 69 featuring the word *ḫurdatu* (see George 2003, 622–623, 837). The commentary UET 6/3, 897 rev. 7'–8' runs parallel to 11N-T3: 40–41 (with minor variants, cf. below), but only quotes the central keyword *ḫurdatsu* “her vulva”. The folk-etymological explanation of *ḫurdati* “vulva” as *ḫurri dādi* “hole of the darling” in line 42 makes it the hole where the child emerges (Cavigneaux 1987, 255 “cavité du chéri”; Frahm 2011, 71; Gabbay 2016, 77; differently CDA^2 121b, translating the expression as “hole of love”). For discussion, cf. also Civil 1974, 335; Taylor 2005, *RA* 99, 23 (on ḪAR-ra-tu-da). For *dādu* “darling” (and the homonym *dādu* referring to an aquatic animal with a shell), see also Wasserman and Zomer 2022, 51, 92; Wasserman 2016, 52.

Lines 43–44: The quotation *ina kittabrīšu* in line 43 stems from BAM 248 obv. ii 44 (text D.1.1 line 99), which can be restored as: *i-⸢na⸣ ⸢kit-tab-ri-šú⸣* ⸢GUB⸣-*za*$^{?!}$ ^{d}AMAR.UTU “⸢Stand by her side⸣, O Marduk”. The quotation and exegesis are very similar to UET 6/3, 897, but more detailed. The terms *kittabru* and *idu* are known as synonyms in the lexical tradition, as is the equation še = *kittabru* (see CAD K, 468b sub lex. section; Cavigneaux 1976, 152–153).

Lines 44–45: Line 44 introduces the phrase *qīp napšāti* “the one entrusted with the lives” (of mother and baby) quoted from the base text (BAM 248 obv. ii 45, D.1.1 line 100), which is used as a laudatory epithet of Marduk. The first explanation dwells on the verb *qâpu* (*qiāpu*) “to (en)trust”, from which the adjective *qīpu* “entrusted” is derived. In the following, the commentator, somewhat curiously, does not comment on the noun *napšātu* “lives”, derived from *napāšu* A “to breathe”, but instead gives synonyms for the homonym *napāšu* B “to comb/clean wool”. The verb *kamādu* means “to beat cloth”, which the commentary links with Sumerian túg tun$_x$(DÚB) (cf. Civil 1974, 335; on the related profession of the ^{lú}túg-du$_8$, see Waetzoldt 2011–2013b, *RlA* 13, 620a § 4.7); it refers to a finishing procedure performed on woven fabrics, namely “beating the textile in order to thicken the cloth and to strengthen the weave of the fibres” (Wasserman 2013, *Iraq* 75, 264–265). For *kamādu*, see also Schmidtchen 2020, *NABU* 2020/2, 174 No. 81 (ad Schmidtchen 2018c, *FS Geller*, 499: 7, for a D-stem form *kummudā* “interwoven (lines of the hand?)”).

Lines 45–46: The complete line from the base text (BAM 248 obv. ii 61) quoted in line 45 reads *ik-kud it-ta-id ba-laṭ-sa* “he (= Marduk) became anxious (*nakādu*), he worried (*na’ādu*) for her (the woman’s) life”. The commentary expands on the keywords *nakādu* “to worry, to be anxious” and *na’ādu* “to be attentive, concerned, anxious” by noting words derived from both terms and giving partial synonyms. The noun *tankittu* “worry, anxiety(?)” derived from *nakādu* is not attested elsewhere (CAD T, 175; Civil 1974, 335–336); it is explained with *ḫissatu* “understanding, wisdom”. The form *itmudu* is a variant of *it’udu* “to watch carefully” (infinitive Gt-stem of *na’ādu*) is associated by the commentator with *šemû* “to hear; listen; understand”. The terms *ḫissatu* and *šemû* focus more on perceptive and mental faculties than on emotive aspects (of worrying and caring) that are linked to the verbs *nakādu* and *na’ādu* (cf. CAD N/1, 1 and 153 sub lex. section).

Lines 46–51: The last lines of the commentary focus on magical substances that are applied in the base text BAM 248 (and dupl.) to speed up a difficult delivery. These substances (which are mixed with oil and used to massage the woman’s belly) also have a symbolic or metaphorical significance that is made explicit via corresponding images in the incantations that are recited with the remedies in question (see text D.1.1 for discussion). The substances represent objects that become symbols for an easy and normal birth. These links are also drawn on in the explanations of the commentary. The objects and *materia magica* commented on are found in the prescription BAM 248 rev. iii 7–8 // (text D.1.1 lines 132–133) and in the preceding incantation BAM 248 obv. ii 57–59 and obv. ii 70–rev. iii 2 (text D.1.1 lines 112–114 and 125–127).

Lines 46–48: The first substance commented on is *aban tīk šamê* “hailstone” (lit. ‘stone dripping from heaven’) quoted from BAM 248 rev. iii 7 // (text D.1.1 line 132). See CAD T, 404b sub a-3’. The commentator points out connections between this *materia magica* and the purpose of the treatment by analysing the component signs and their different readings. Thus, the syllables ab and nu in *ab-nu* “stone” are explained as Sumerograms that mean *banû* “to create” (i.e. to bear offspring, probably stemming from the correspondence of ab(-ba) with *bānû* “father; creator”) and *zēru* “seed, offspring”. In a similar manner, the commentary explains the sign AN in AN-*e* (“heaven”) as a logogram for *zēru* “seed”. For *tikku* (*tīku*) “shower”, the commentator first points out a corresponding Sumerogram u-gu$_4$ (which, however, stems from the equation of gú with the homonym *tikku* “nape of the neck”) and then analyses the component syllables as u = *banû* “to create” (for this equation see also CAD B, 81) and gu = *alādu* “to give birth” (cf. also Ea I 137). For the lexical equations in these lines, see also Cavigneaux 1987, 255. The commentary UET 6/3, 897 rev. 12' (text G.2) comments only on *aban tīk šamê*, but not on the other two substances (see below).

Lines 48–51: For the commentary passage, see also Gabbay 2016, 209, 223. As pointed out by Civil (1974, 336), the commentary quotes an abbreviated phrase from the base text dropping the word *samītu* “parapet” (i.e. SAḪAR BÀD ŠUB-*tú* “dust from a dilapidated city wall” instead of SAḪAR *sa-mit* BÀD ŠUB-*tú*), see BAM 248 rev. iii 7 // (text D.1.1 line 132). The commentator first dwells on the sign BÀD, which corresponds to Akkadian *dūru* “city wall”; then he splits up the sign BÀD (consisting of the signs EZENxBAD) into its components and lists other values of these signs in Sumerian with their Akkadian renderings. Thus, the sign EZEN can also be read kéš in Sumerian which corresponds to Akkadian *riksu* "bond", a word appearing several times in incantations within the base text in reference to severing the bond that keeps the baby from coming out of his mother's womb. Furthermore, the Sumerian word bad corresponds to *petû* "to open", which likewise features in the spells in BAM 248 and dupl. in connection with the baby's blocked exit out of the womb (text D.1.1 lines 105, 170). The commentary then turns to the word *maqtu* "fallen; dilapidated" (written ŠUB-*tú*) from the base text. Thus, the commentator links this term with synonymous word dirig (written with the signs SI.A), which corresponds to Akkadian *qâpu* "to buckle, collapse" (said of walls). He then points out links to the ritual context of the base text by providing meaningful equations for the Sumerian words si and a, namely si = *ešēru* "to be straight", which is used in the meaning "to be born / delivered easily" in the birth contexts, and a = *ṣeḫru* (*ṣaḫar*) "little one; baby".

Line 51: "Dust from a streaming drainpipe" (*eper pisanni šurdî*, written SAḪAR gišPÍSAN *šur-di-i*) is the symbolic ingredient of a remedy for difficult birth in BAM 248 (A) rev. iii 8 // (text D.1.1 line 133). The substance relates directly to the simile of the waters flowing through a "streaming drainpipe" in the incantation recited with the remedy (A obv. ii 59 and rev. iii 2 // text D.1.1 lines 114 and 127). The commentary quotes this phrase in a slightly varying spelling compared with the base text (SAḪAR PISAN *šur-di-i*). The commentator dwells only on the word *pisannu* "box, container; drainpipe", which is written with the sign GÁ but usually pronounced pisan in Sumerian (see CAD P, 421 lex. section). However, the commentator gives ma-a as the pronunciation gloss (for Sumerian ĝá). This is presumably because of the following equation gá = *alāku* "to go" (which is known from lexical sources, see CAD A/1, 300b lex. section, e.g. Ea IV 229; Idu II 157).

Lines 52–55: For the subscript and colophon see Frahm 2011, 54, 231. For introducing the title of the commented base text with *ša libbi* (followed by an incantation incipit), see also the medical commentary BAM 401: 35 (Frahm 2011, 236–237).

G.2 The Commentary UET 6/3, 897

UET 6/3, 897 (U. 30654) is a fragmentary tablet possibly dating to the Achaemenid period. It is one of only two commentaries currently known from the city of Ur (Gabbay 2015). The text was first identified by Marten Stol as a partial duplicate of the commentary on the Neo-Assyrian Birth Compendium, 11N-T3 from Nippur (Römer 2007, 182). In comparison with the latter, UET 6/3, 897 cites more passages from other texts to expand on the base text. Among these, citations from the *Gilgamesh Epic* (rev. 7'), the exorcistic incantation series Udug-ḫul (rev. 6') and from a compendium of incantations (obv. 8') have been identified. In comparison with the commentary from Nippur, UET 6/3, 897 draws on more passages from the base text; thus, the last fragmentary lines on the reverse comment on the incantation known as "A Cow of Sîn" (BAM 248 rev. iii 10–35 and duplicates, see text D.1.1).

List of Manuscripts

Siglum	Museum Number	Copy	Collation	Format; Ductus	Provenience
β	U. 30654	UET 6/3, 897	Coll.	Fragment of a single-column tablet in landscape format; Neo-/ Late Babylonian script; ca. 6th–4th cent. BCE	Ur

Previous Edition and Discussion

Gabbay 2015, CCP 4.2.A.b (edition; photos)
CDLI P346934 (photo)
Römer 2007, *BiOr* 64, 182 (review of A. Shaffer, UET 6/3)
Frahm 2011, 67, 104, 231, 241, 312 (discussion of rev. 3'–4', 7'–8', 13'–15')
Gabbay 2016, *The Exegetical Terminology of Akkadian Commentaries*, 77, 131, 132, 157–158, 161–162, 196, 234 (discussion of obv. 3'–5', 6', 8', 12'–13', rev. 3'–5', 6', 7'–8')
Hätinen 2017, *KASKAL* 14, 179 (discussion of rev. 9'–10')
Steinert 2017a, 331–335 (discussion of rev. 3'–4', 9'–10')

Transliteration

Beginning of ms. β obv. lost

1'	β obv. 1'	**[*ina qar-ni*]-*šá qaq-qar ṭe-r*[*a-at* ...]**[423]
2'	β obv. 2'	**[*ša*$^?$ *el-l*]*am-me-e* DU.⸢MEŠ⸣-*ak d*[*i*]-⸢*ma*⸣-[*a-šú*** x x]
3'	β obv. 3'	[*šá-niš*] si é-gar$_8$-bi til-la : *el-lam-mu-ú* [: ^{d}30$^?$]
4'	β obv. 4'	⸢*šá*⸣ *nu-ru la-ni-šú ú-qé-et-ta-a* [: si : *nu-ú-r*]*u*$^?$: ⸢é⸣-gar$_8$: ⸢*la*$^?$-*nu*$^?$⸣
5'	β obv. 5'	bi : *šu-ú* : til : *qa-tu-ú* : *šá* A[N.TA.LÙ TI]L-*tim* GAR-*nu*
6'	β obv. 6'	***áš-šú* ÁB-*ia*$_5$ *la a-lit-ti*** : ⸢*áš-šú*⸣ ⸢^{d}⸣[30 EN *la*]-⸢*a-tim*⸣ KÙ.MEŠ
7'	β obv. 7'	***né-šal-pa-a*** : *e-té-qa* : **la-[ra-aḫ** : ... ...]x
8'	β obv. 8'	*lìb-bu-ú* **la-ra-aḫ gig-⸢ga⸣ ⸢su-ni-ta$^?$⸣ ⸢kéš-da⸣**
9'	β obv. 9'	***na-ḫu-un-di*** : ^{d}30 : ***na-ru-un-du*** : ^{d}U[TU]
10'	β obv. 10'	***ul-la* ^{d}UTU**: *ul-la* : *an-*[*na* (x)]
11'	β obv. 11'	**Ì.GIŠ BUR *šá ina* ^{gi}GAG.U$_4$.TAG.GA *in-d*[*aḫ-ṣu*$^?$]**
12'	β obv. 12'	⸢^{gi}⸣GAG.U$_4$.TAG.GA : *šil-ta-ḫu* : ⸢^{gi}GAG.U$_4$.TAG⸣.GA : [mul-mul$^?$]
13'	β obv. 13'	[*mul-m*]*ul* : *šil-ta-ḫu* : ⸢mul⸣-m[ul : *ze-ri*$^?$]

Ms. β obv. breaks; ca. three lines missing to the bottom of the tablet
Beginning of ms. β rev. lost

14"	β rev. 1'	***na-ma-ri*** ⸢:⸣ ⸢KASKAL$^?$⸣ [......................]
15"	β rev. 2'	**^{giš}MÁ** : *tam-tim šá*$^?$-*niš*$^?$ x[...........] ⸢x *ḫu* x⸣
16"	β rev. 3'	***šá* ŠÀ ^{na4}*iš-qil-lat* ⸢*li-kal-lim*⸣ ⸢*nu-ru*$^?$⸣** *a-na* ^{munus}PEŠ$_4$ *iq-ta-bi*
17"	β rev. 4'	^{na4}IŠKILA(PEŠ$_4$) *ṣil-lat šá-niš um-mi šal-šiš* ^{munus}PEŠ$_4$
18"	β rev. 5'	**[*u*]*l sa-an-qa-at* GABA-*sa*** ⸢:⸣ *šá ku-lu-lu-ša la kut-tu-mu*
19"	β rev. 6'	⸢*lìb*⸣-*bu-ú* ***ir-tu*$_4$ ár-da-at pa-su-um-tu$_4$ ⸢*iš-ḫu*⸣-*ṭu***
20"	β rev. 7'	***ḫur-da-at-su*** : *su-un* MUNUS$^?$: *lìb-bu-ú* **ŠU.MIN-*ka šu-ta-am-ṣa-am-ma***
21"	β rev. 8'	***lu-pu-ut ḫur-da-at-ni* : *ina kit-tab-ri-šú*** : *ina i-di-šú*
22"	β rev. 9'	*kit-tam-ri* : *i-di* : **DUR$^{⸢ṭu⸣-ur}$-*da* ^{giš}MÁ** : *ṭú-ur-da* : ^{giš}MÁ
23"	β rev. 10'	^{giš}MÁ : ^{munus}PEŠ$_4$: *um-ma* ^{munus}PEŠ$_4$ ⸢*ṭú*⸣-*ri-di*
24"	β rev. 11'	***e-di-ti*** : *mi-di-ti* ⸢:⸣[424] *e-du-ú* : *mi-du-ú*
25"	β rev. 12'	**NA$_4$ *ti-ki* AN-*e*** ⸢MIN$^?$⸣ ⸢*aq*$^?$⸣-*qul* DU$_{11}$.DU$_{11}$-*ub*
26"	β rev. 13'	**[*ti*]-⸢*iq*$^?$⸣-x x x-*ti kaz-bat*** : *ba-na-at*

423 In the transliteration, citations from the base text and other identified texts are rendered in bold.
424 Disjunction sign written over erasure?

27''	β rev. 14'	[***nam-ru šá*** ^{d}**30**$^{?}$:] *nu-úr*$^{?}$ *šá* ^{d}30 : ***nu-ru-ub šam-[me]***
28''	β rev. 15'	[.....................] ⸢x x⸣ : ni x[............]

Ms. β rev. breaks

29'''	β l. e. 1	[............]x x-*ú* : *i* : Ì : Ì.GI[Š$^{?}$ ....]
30'''	β l. e. 2	[............ : *a-ṣu-ú*] *šá ze-er*[425]

Bound Transcription and Translation

Beginning of ms. β obv. lost

1' [***ina qarnī*]*ša qaqqara ṭer*[*ât*** ...]	1' "[With her horns] she roo[ts up] the ground" [...].
2' [***ša***$^{?}$ ***ell*]*am-mê illakā dimā*[*šu*** x x]	2' "Ella(m)-mê's tears were flowing", [...];
3' [*šanîš*] si é-gar$_8$-bi til-la : *ellam-mû* [: *Sîn*$^{?}$]	3' [Alternatively,] si é-gar$_8$-bi til-la (refers to) "Ella(m)-mû" [(which) means Sîn(?)];
4' ⸢*ša*⸣ *nūr lānīšu uqettâ* [: si : *nūr*]*u* : ⸢é⸣.gar$_8$$^{?}$: *lānu*$^{?}$	4' (it means) "he who brings the light *of* his figure to an end", [(since Sumerian) si means "li]ght"; é-gar$_8$ means "figure",
5' bi : *šū* : til : *qatû* : *ša at*[*talî gamar*]*ti išakkanu*	5' bi means "that", til means "to come to an end". (This is said) on account of (the moon) making a complete eclipse.
6' ***aššu littīya lā ālitti*** : *aššu Sîn bēl lâti ellēti*	6' "Because of my cow who has not yet given birth"; (this is said) because Sîn (is) the lord of the pure cows.
7' ***nešalpû*** : *etēqu* : **la-[ra-aḫ** : ... ...]x	7' "To glide out" means "to pass". "(Dire) stra[its" means ...],
8' *libbū* **la-ra-aḫ gig-⸢ga⸣ ⸢su-ni-⸢ta$^{?}$⸣ ⸢kéš-da⸣**	8' as in (the Sumerian sentence) "dire straits are bound to his body".
9' ***Naḫundi*** : *Sîn* : ***Narundu*** : *Ša*[*maš*]	9' Naḫḫunte means Sîn. Narunde means Šamaš.
10' ***ulla Šamaš*** : *ulla* : *an*[*na* (x)]	10' (In) "Well now (*ulla*), Šamaš", *ulla* (means) "yes/well" (*anna*).
11' ***šaman pūri ša ina*** ^{gi}**GAG.U$_4$.TAG.GA** ***ind*[*aḫṣu*]**	11' (In) "oil-from-the-jar that has been st[irred] with an arrow",
12' ⸢^{gi}⸣GAG.U$_4$.TAG.GA : *šiltāḫu* : ⸢^{gi}GAG.U$_4$.TAG⸣.GA : [mul-mul$^{?}$]	12' (the logogram) ^{gi}GAG.U$_4$.TAG.GA means "arrow", (and) ^{gi}GAG.U$_4$.TAG.GA (is the same as Sumerian) [mul-mul]
13' [*mulm*]*ul* : *šiltāḫu* : mul-m[ul : *zēru*$^{?}$]	13' (which is) *mulmul(lu)* (or) *šiltāhu* "arrow" (in Akkadian). (Sumerian) mul-mul (also means) ["seed" (*zēru*)].

Ms. β obv. breaks; ca. three lines missing to the bottom of the tablet
Beginning of ms. β rev. lost

14'' ***namāru*** ⸢:⸣ ⸢*ḫarrānu*$^{?}$⸣ [... ...]	14'' "Clearing" means "path" [... ...].
15'' ***eleppu*** : *tâmti šanîš*$^{?}$ ...[... ...] ...	15'' "Boat" means "(that of the?) sea", alternatively(?) [... ...].
16'' ***ša libbi išqillati likallim nūru***$^{?}$ *ana erīti iqtabi*	16'' "Let him show the light to the one inside the shell!" – it (the base text) said it with regard to the pregnant woman, (because)
17'' ^{na4}IŠKILA(PEŠ$_4$) *ṣillatu šanîš ummu šalšiš* ^{munus}PEŠ$_4$	17'' ^{na4}IŠKILA(PEŠ$_4$) (lit. pregnant stone) (means) "shell". Alternatively, (it means) "mother", (and) thirdly (it can mean) "pregnant woman".

425 The remainder of the line is left blank, so presumably the commentary finished here.

18'' **[u]l sanqat irassa** ⸢:⸣ *ša kululūša lā kuttumu*

18'' "Her chest is not *'restrained'*" (means) "one whose head-dress is uncovered";

19'' *libbū* **irti ardati pasumti išḫuṭū**

19'' as in: "they stripped the veil from the woman's chest".

20'' **ḫurdatsu** : *sūn sinništi* : *libbū* **qātīka šutamṣâm-ma**

20'' "Her vulva" means "female lap", as in: "Stretch out your hand(s) and

21'' **luput ḫurdatni** : **ina kittabrīšu** : *ina idīšu*

21'' stroke our vulva!" "At her side" (*ina kittabrīšu*) (is the same as) "at her side" (*ina idīšu*),

22'' *kittamri* : *idi* : **DUR**$^{\text{⸢tu⸣-ur}}$**-da** ^{giš}**MÁ** : *ṭurda* : ^{giš}MÁ

22'' (because) "side, arm" (*kittamru*) (is the same as) "side" (*idu*). For DUR-*da* ^{giš}MÁ (read) *ṭurda* ^{giš}MÁ. (It means) "send forth (namely) the boat!"

23'' ^{giš}MÁ : ^{munus}PEŠ$_4$: *umma* ^{munus}PEŠ$_4$ *ṭurridī*

23'' "Boat" means "pregnant woman". Thus (the sentence means) "Send away(?) the pregnant woman!"

24'' **ēdīti** : *medīti* : *edû* : *medû*

24'' "Renowned" (*ēdītu*) (is the same as) "known" (*medīti*); (just as) "to know" (*edû*) (is the same as) "to know" (*medû*).

25'' **aban tīk šamê** MIN? *aqqul(li) idabbub*

25'' "Stone dripping from heaven" – one also says this with regard to(?) the *aqqullu-phenomenon.*

26'' **[ti]-⸢iq?⸣-x x x-ti kazbat** : *banât*

26'' "... she was alluring" (of shape) means "she was beautiful".

27'' **[namru ša Sîn?** :] *nūr? ša Sîn* : **nurub šam[mē]**

27'' "[The brilliant (glow) of Sîn(?)" means] "the light of Sîn". "The lushest grass" (means)

28'' [... ... ...] x x : ni x[... ...]

28'' [...] ... [...]

Ms. β rev. breaks

29''' [... ...] ... : *i* : Ì : *šam[nu?* ....]

29''' [...]... *i* is (the pronunciation of the sign) Ì (which means) "oil" (Ì.GIŠ?) [....].

30''' [... ... : *aṣû*] *ša zēri*

30''' [... ... means "to come out"], said of seed.

Notes

Line 2': Cf. the parallel commentary passage in 11N-T3: 17–20 commenting on the word *Ella(m)-mê*, a title of the moon god (see above text G.1). However, UET 6/3, 897 quotes the complete line from the base text BAM 248 obv. i 41 and duplicates (see text D.1.1 line 27). The line is completely preserved in the Old Babylonian birth incantation VS 17, 34: 8: *el-la-me-e i-il-la-ka di-ma-ša* (Wasserman and Zomer 2022, No. 12).

Lines 3'–5': This passage runs parallel to 11N-T3: 18–20 (see Gabbay 2016, 157–158 and above for discussion). The phrase ⸢*šá*⸣ *nu-ru la-ni-šú ú-qé-et-ta-a* is the Akkadian rendering of the Sumerian phrase si é-gar$_8$-bi til-la in line 3'. At the end of line 4', Gabbay (2015, CCP 4.2.A.b) reads *la?-ni?* instead of *la?-nu?*. In this passage, the tears (weeping, sadness) of the moon god are associated with an eclipse (because his tears/sadness metaphorically darken his shape/body). For the moon god crying and eclipses of the moon, see also Stol 1992, 257–258.

Line 6': For the citation and parallel commentary passage, see also the discussion on 11N-T3: 21 above and the base text BAM 248 obv. i 43 // (text D.1.1 line 29). The explanation *bēl lâti ellēti* "(because Sîn is) the lord of the pure cows" relies on homophony with the base text's *aššu littīya lā ālitti* "because of my cow who has not (yet) given birth" (see Gabbay 2016, 161–162 for discussion). The exegesis of 11N-T3 is longer than that in UET 6/3, 897, by introducing a second passage from a different source text in support of the explanation (the moon god's connection with herding and cattle/cows).

Line 7': For the parallel, but much longer commentary passage on the word *nešalpû* "to glide" in 11N-T3: 23–25 see above. The keyword relates to the base text BAM 248 obv. i 49 (text D.1.1 line 35).

Line 8': Also the Nippur commentary 11N-T3: 26–27 comments on the term laraḫ "(dire) straits; difficulty", drawing on the rubric KA.INIM.MA ^{munus}LA.RA.AḪ.A.KÁM "wording of (an incantation) for a woman who has difficulty during delivery" found several times in the base text (see BAM 248 obv. i 51 *passim*; text D.1.1 line 37). The Sumerian quotation in line 8' (not found in 11N-T3) was identified by E. Jiménez as a passage from the Incantation Compendium 3: 39 (Schramm 2008, 36): la-ra-aḫ gig-ga su-a-n[i-t]a kéš-⸢da⸣ "dire straits are bound to his body". For laraḫ "dire straits", see also Maul and Strauß 2011, *KAL* 4, 80; Frayne 1990, *RIME* 4, 302: 6.

Line 9': See the parallel commentary passage in 11N-T3: 27 (text G.1) and the base text BAM 248 obv. i 58 (text D.1.1 line 44).

Line 10': See also 11N-T3: 30–31 and the base text BAM 248 obv. i 64 // (text D.1.1 line 50). Gabbay (2015, CCP 4.2.A.b) understands *ulla* and *anna* in the explanation as deictic or adverbial particles (status absolutus of *ullû* and *annû*, meaning "that, this" (or, alternatively "here, there"). The parallel, more extended passage in 11N-T3 appears to comment on several homonymous Akkadian words of different meaning. Thus, it is also possible that the commentator equated the interjection *ulla* "well, now" (used in the base text) with *anna* "yes" or with the interjection *anna* "well" (cf. discussion of 11N-T3: 30–31 above; CAD A/2, 125; CAD U/W, 74–75). Note further that Sumerian ul-la is equated with *annu* "consent, approval" in bilingual and lexical texts, see CAD A/II, s.v. *annu* lex.

Lines 11'–13': Gabbay (2015, CCP 4.2.A.b) restores *in-⸢di⸣* at the end of line 11', understanding it as *emdu* (from *emēdu* "to come into contact"; "to place"; "to lean"). However, since the base text preserving this passage (BAM 248 obv. i 68–69 and BM 36339 rev. 6–7) speaks of stirring (*maḫāṣu*) the oil with an arrow, an alternative restoration is suggested here. The phrase encountered in UET 6/3, 897 is not an exact quotation from the base text, but more a paraphrase (cf. text D.1.1 lines 54–55). The parallel commentary passage in 11N-T3: 32–37 comments both on the terms "oil-from-the-jar" and "arrow" from the base text; UET 6/3, 897 instead focuses on the latter. The restoration of line 12' follows the verbatim parallel in 11N-T3: 33.

Line 14'': Compare 11N-T3: 37–38 above. The passage commented on here is not preserved in the base text, but it probably belonged to the beginning of a long Akkadian incantation which takes up BAM 248 obv. ii (the first twenty lines of col. ii are almost completely lost).

Line 15'': This fragmentary line does not have a correspondence in 11N-T3. It is possible that UET 6/3, 897 commented on the very fragmentarily preserved lines in BAM 248 obv. ii 33ff. // (text D.1.1 lines 88ff.). On the image of the woman in labour as a boat see also line 22''–23'' below.

Lines 16''–17'': For discussion of this passage, see the parallel quotation and exegesis in commentary 11N-T3: 38–40 above; Frahm 2011, 241; Gabbay 2016, 234–235; Steinert 2017a, 334–335. The commentary on this passage in 11N-T3: 38–40 presents some variants in comparison with UET 6/3, 897.

Line 18'': This line is best preserved in the Middle Assyrian ms. D (*Iraq* 31, 31: 44; *infra* text II.1.4): *ul sa-qa-at* ^{uzu}GABA-*sa sà-pu-ḫu ku-lu-lu-šá* "her chest is not 'fastened', her headdress is loosened (lit. scattered)". See also BAM 248 obv. ii 28 (text D.1.1 line 83), which runs parallel to ms. D. For *sanāqu* "to fasten", cf. CAD S, s.v. *sanāqu* A sub 5b; Durand 2012, *FS Fales*, 260–261; Mayer 2022b, *OrNS* 91, 346 sub *tēniqu*. It is not entirely certain whether the second phrase in line 18'' is part of the commentary or a citation from the base text differing from the preserved sources.

Line 19'': Gabbay (2015, CCP 4.2.A.b) reads *ar-da-at* instead of *ár-da-at*. The text quoted here has been identified by E. Jiménez as a line from Udug-ḫul Tablet 13–15: 32, which presents a slight variant: [ga]ba ⸢šú-ki-(a)⸣ ⸢dam-ra$^{?}$⸣ ba-an-[sìg-ga-eš] : ⸢*ir-ti áš-ša-ti*⸣ *pa-su-un-tu iš-ḫu-ṭu* "they stripped the breast of a veiled wife" (cf. Geller 2016, 443 with n. 32). *Pa(s)-sum/ntu* may be connected either to the word *pu(s)sumtu* "veil", or to the feminine adjective form *pussum/ntu* "veiled" (cf. CAD P, 537–538). The commentary picks up the word *kulūlu* "headdress" from the base text to comment on the parallel expression "her chest is not restrained" (*ul sanqat irassu*). The commentator appears to understand the word *passumtu* in the quote from Udug-ḫul as synonymous to *kulūlu*, a term for a headdress made from a woven fabric (often of rulers and deities); in the present context, "headband" and "veil" have been suggested as senses of *kulūlu* (the plural is used in BAM 248 obv. ii 28 = text D.1.1 line 83). Therefore, the commentator may have had the word *pussumtu* "veil" in mind in the Udug-ḫul passage rather than the feminine adjective *pussumtu* "veiled" (cf. CAD P 537 s.v. *pussunu*; CAD P 538 s.v. *pusumtu*). This may have been triggered by the occurrence of the word *pussumu* "veil" in the next line of the base text (line 84: *pusummī ul pussunat* "she is not veiled with a veil").

A similar line (though not cited in the commentary) is found in BAM 248 obv. ii 29: ⸢*pu*⸣$^{!}$-*su-um-m*[*i*] ⸢*ul pu-su-na*⸣-[*at bul-t*]*a ul i-*[*ši*], parallel to the Middle Assyrian ms. D (*Iraq* 31, 31: 45): *pu-ṣu-ni ul pa-ṣu-na-at bul-ta ul ti-šu* "she is not veiled with a veil, she does not feel [shame] (anymore)" (see text D.1.1 line 84).

Lines 20''–22'': For lines 20''–21'' see also 11N-T3: 40–43, which runs partially parallel to the Ur commentary, but equates *ḫurdatu* "vulva" with *ūru ša sinništi* "the genitals of a woman" instead of the synonymous *sūn sinništi*(MUNUS?) "female lap". The following citation is from *Gilgamesh Epic* Tablet VI 69 (cf. George 2003, 622–623, 883). The complete phrase found in the base text (BAM 248 obv. ii 30 = text D.1.1 line 85) is *uš*!-*šu-rat ḫur-da-as-sa* "her vulva is set straight" (to deliver), quoted in full in 11N-T3. Compared with UET 6/3, 897, the exegesis of 11N-T3 on the word *ḫurdatu* is more extensive (see above for discussion; Gabbay 2016, 77, 132).

The next quotation in line 21'' stems from BAM 248 obv. ii 44; the complete text line reads: *i-*⌜*na*⌝ ⌜*kit-tab-ri-šú* GUB⌝-*za*?! dAMAR.UTU "⌜Stand by her side⌝, Marduk". The text of the Middle Assyrian parallel ms. D (*Iraq* 31, 31 rev. 46) differs (text D.1.1 line 99). The parallel passage in the Nippur commentary 11N-T3: 43–44 is more detailed than in UET 6/3, 897; the latter introduces a lexical variant *kittamru* for *kittabru* "side" in line 22'' not found in 11N-T3 (see above text G.1 for discussion).

Line 22'': For a slightly differing translation, cf. Gabbay 2015 (CCP). The cited base text in BAM 248 obv. ii 51, after collation, reads *ṭur-da*sic! gišMÁ *a-na kar šul-me* "Send forth the boat to the quay of wellbeing!" (see text D.1.1 line 106 and Steinert 2017: 332–334 for discussion). The commentary quotes the ambiguous spelling *ṭur*(DUR)-*da* from the base text and inserts a pronunciation gloss and clarifying rendering of the verb (*ṭu/ṭú-ur-da*). For the boat as an image for the pregnant woman, see also Hätinen 2017, esp. 179.

Line 23'': The reconstructed form *ṭú-ri-di* would be a fem. sg. imperative form of the D-stem of *ṭarādu* "to send" (cf. CAD Ṭ, 59–60 s.v. *ṭarādu* A; usually the D-stem has the meanings "to harass; to drive away"). As discussed by Gabbay (2016, 195–197), the word *umma* "thus" is used in some commentaries as a technical term introducing a paraphrase of the base text in light of the preceding explanation.

Line 24'': The base text BAM 248 rev. iii 4 // ms. B_3 obv. 20 has the following passage: *an-nu ki-nu šá* d*é-a i*?-*di*?-*tu*$_4$ ÉN *šá* d*ma-mi i-ri-šu* "(it is) the reliable approval of Ea, the renowned spell which Mami requested" (text D.1.1 line 129). The word *ēdītu* (spelled *i-di-tu*$_4$ in BAM 248 and dupl.) commented on in line 24'' is understood as a feminine form of the adjective (*w*)*ēdû* "prominent, high-placed" (following AHw 1495; cf. CAD E, 34–35 s.v. *edû* "well-known, renowned"). Although etymologically unrelated (according to AHw 1495), *ēdītu* is apparently explained in the commentary as a feminine form of the adjective *medû* "known" (presumably because of phonetic similarity). The second word pair stipulated by the commentator suggests that the verb *medû* (*madû*) is equated with *i/edû* "to know". CAD M/2, 3 regards *medû* as a secondary derivation from *i/edû* "to know" (cf. also AHw 640a s.v. *medû* "to become visible", with a meaning "is known" in the G-stem stative; Krebernik 2016, 207–208).

Line 25'': Compare the much more extensive commentary passage in 11N-T3: 46ff. and the corresponding ritual instruction in BAM 248 rev. iii 7: NA$_4$ *ti-ik* AN-*e* SAḪAR *sa-mit* BÀD ŠUB-*t*[*i*] "stone dripping from heaven (hailstone), dust from the parapets of a dilapidated city wall" (cf. also BAM 248 obv. ii 56 and 70, where *tīk šamê* "rain shower" is mentioned within the incantation, see text D.1.1 lines 112–114, 125–127 and 132–133). Gabbay 2015 (CCP 4.2.A.b) suggests that the latter half of the line likewise represents a citation from a ritual instruction in the base text, which is not preserved or written out in BAM 248. He translates DUG$_4$.DUG$_4$-*ub* as "you recite" (cf. CAD D, 7-8 sub 4). My tentative suggestion is that DUG$_4$.DUG$_4$-*ub* "one speaks/says" is part of an explanation concerning *aban tīk šamê* "hailstone", identifying it with a similar phenomenon. For *anqullu* (*aqqullu*) as an atmoshperic phenomenon, perhaps a dust cloud, see Scarpelli 2024, 262–264. The use of *dabābu* instead of the expected verb *qabû* "to say" is irregular, however (cf. Gabbay 2016, 231–259 for explanations in commentaries introduced with *qabû*). Alternatively, read ⌜*a*?-*na*?⌝ NUMUN DUG$_4$.DUG$_4$-*ub* "one *says* (this) to/for(?) the offspring (seed)".

Line 26'': The corresponding passage in the source text BAM 248 rev. iii 11–12, from the beginning of the Cow of Sîn incantation, reads: *ti-iq-na-a-te tuq-qù-na-at / bi-nu-tam kaz-bat* "she was adorned with ornaments, she was alluring of shape" (text D.1.1 lines 136–137). Thus, the beginning of line 26'' in the commentary may be the word *tiqnu* "ornament" (or *tiqnāti*) drawn from the base text. Frahm (2011, 241) tentatively suggests reading the following signs as ⌜*bi-nu*⌝-*ti kaz-bat*, although ⌜*bi-nu*⌝-*ti* cannot be entirely reconciled with the traces on the tablet.

Line 27'': The complete passage in BAM 248 rev. iii 13 // reads (text D.1.1 line 138): *nam-ru šá* d30 *šu-ba-ḫi iš-ta-kan-ši* "the brilliant (glow) of Sîn ... he laid upon her". The second citation in line 27'' is from BAM 248 rev. iii 16 // (text D.1.1 line 141): *ina nu-ru-ub šam-me i-re-'i šam-me* "she grazed on the lushest of grasses".

Lines 29'''–30''': The two fragmentary lines visible on the left edge of the tablet were not copied by A. Shaffer and are not transliterated by U. Gabbay in CCP 4.2.A.b. The first fragmentary line may be compared with 11N-T3: 31–32, which comments on the phrase *šaman pūri* (Ì.(GIŠ) BUR) "oil-from-the-jar" in the base text (BAM 248 obv. i 68; cf. above). The fragmentary phrase in line 30''' is presumably parallel to 11N-T3: 30, commenting on MAŠ.DÀ "gazelle" in BAM 248 obv. i 59 (see discussion above). The phrase *aṣû ša zēri* is found a second time in the commentary passage 11N-T3: 11–12.

Chapter H
Appendix – Treatments for Women's Hair

Treatments for women's hair in first millennium BCE Mesopotamian medical texts present an interesting case, where prescriptions for women are included in a "non-gynaecological" section or treatise of the therapeutic corpus, among remedies formulated for a (generalized) male patient. Since prescriptions for women's hair are otherwise not attested within the women's healthcare texts, but nonetheless present related material, these prescriptions have been included here due to the interest for the subject of women's healthcare in ancient Mesopotamia. The exclusion of these treatments from the immediate corpus of gynaecological material provides a clue to Mesopotamian healing specialists' classification of medical topics, suggesting that the focus of the women's healthcare texts was on conditions of the female sexual organs and on topics having to do with reproduction. However, it is worth mentioning that cosmetic prescriptions are occasionally found in Late Babylonian medical collections for women's health issues (see text A.2.2).

The main text presented in Chapter H are Neo-Assyrian fragments of a two-column tablet from Nineveh, (BAM 498–500+) preserving remedies for specific conditions of the head (e.g. the *ašû*-disease) as well as recipes to counter hair loss, which also include a few prescriptions specifically for women's hair. The tablet belongs to the first section of the *Nineveh Medical Compendium* (the therapeutic series with "remedies from head to toes"), which is known in Assyriology as UGU (or CRANIUM).[426] Recently identified new fragments and joins make it worthwhile to present here the sections for women in this text together with a few parallel or duplicating passages in other first millennium medical texts. If one compares the preserved recipes for women's and men's hair in the treatise CRANIUM, it is conspicuous that all the preserved treatments for women (whose hair becomes thin or falls out) are amulets attached to the head, while the treatments for men (e.g. against grey hair) involve topical applications of oils and different substances by anointing, bandaging or washing, but this choice may correlate with the purpose rather than the sex of the patient.

H.1 Treatments for Female Hair Loss in a Chapter of the Treatise CRANIUM (BAM 498–500+)

The present text (ms. A) can currently be assembled from fragments published by F. Köcher as BAM 498, BAM 499 and BAM 500, with the addition of several other fragments identified by the *Nineveh Medical Project* and the *electronic Babylonian Library* Project.[427] The first column on the obverse is still lost. The treatments in obv. ii deal with hair loss, grey hair and dull hair in male patients, while rev. iii preserves treatments for hair loss in women, the latter of which are edited here. The preserved passages in A rev. iv deal with *ašû*-disease, also referred to as *māštu*-disease in this text. These sections duplicate a longer passage in BAM 494 (= K. 6224+) ii 16–58. The latter tablet may represent Tablet 4 or 5 of the Nineveh treatise CRANIUM. However, in contrast to BAM 498–500+, BAM 494 is mainly concerned with skin conditions befalling the head, including *ašû* (ii 3–58), *guraštu* (iii 1–6) and *kurāru* (iii 21'–iv 7), while the two last preserved remedies in col. iv 8–10 interestingly deal with hair loss (the hair falling out in tufts).[428] Thus, while sharing overlapping topics and text sections, BAM 498–500+ and BAM 494 do not represent manuscripts of the same chapter of CRANIUM.

Two prescriptions for women countering hair loss in ms. A also occur, with minor differences, in two other texts related to the treatise on diseases of the head (CRANIUM), where they are recommended for a male patient. The amulet making use of the patient's combed out hair to produce an amulet in ms. A 23'–25' is also included in BAM 3 (ms. B), an Assur extract tablet collecting material from the treatise *šumma amēlu muḫḫašu umma ukâl* (CRANIUM). The compound amulet and ointment prescribed in ms. A lines 34'–35' resembles a prescription in BAM 497 (ms. C), another Nineveh fragment dealing with ailments of the head (hair loss, *ašû*-disease).

426 See Steinert et al. 2018, 207, 209, 220–222 *passim* for discussion, where the title CRANIUM is introduced for this treatise, matching the title UGU.

427 K. Simkó suggests further indirect joins for BAM 498–500 with the following Nineveh fragments containing remedies for the hair (not exclusively recommended for women): K. 2532 (AMT 5/1), K. 3719 (AMT 76/6) (+) K. 10549 (AMT 3/6), and Sm. 712 (AMT 3/1). The former fragments offer treatments to blacken white hair.

428 For discussion and edition of BAM 494, see Bácskay and Simkó 2017, *JMC* 30, 1–71. For the treatise CRANIUM in the Assur Medical Catalogue and in the textual record, see also Steinert et al. 2018, 209, 220ff.

https://doi.org/10.1515/9781501506475-011

Ms. A (lines 7–8) features a short alliterative spell, of which varying longer versions or variations are encountered in ms. A lines 26'–30' (an incantation likewise used for women's hair), in BAM 526 (K. 13366): 7'–10' (used against nosebleed), in STT 277 iv 1–4 (unclear context) and in A. 3461 rev. 4'–7' (see *infra*, text A.1.2). The latter fragment focuses on women's diseases, but its exact purpose or context of use remains unclear.

List of Manuscripts

Siglum	Museum Number	Copy	Collation	Format; Ductus	Provenience
A	K. 2416 + K. 9224 + K. 10624 + K. 11172 + K. 16402 + DT 215 + Rm. 254 (+) K. 2424 + 7016 (+?) K. 6206 + K. 16449 (+) K. 20128 (+?) K. 18178	BAM 498 BAM 499 BAM 500 AMT 3/2 AMT 4/1 AMT 26/4 AMT 16/4 AMT 25/8 AMT 46/3	Coll.	Fragments of a two-column tablet; Neo-Assyrian script; 7th cent. BCE	Nineveh; Ashurbanipal's library
B	VAT 9029	KAR 202 BAM 3	Coll.	Two-column tablet; Neo-Assyrian script; 7th cent. BCE	Assur; N4 library
C	K. 54	BAM 497	Coll.	Fragment of a two-column tablet; Neo-Assyrian script; 7th cent. BCE	Nineveh; Ashurbanipal's library

Overview

i	Incantation rubric (referring to women's hair) A rev. iii 1	1
ii	Prescription (KÌD.KÌD.BI) (amulet and ointment?) A rev. iii 2–6	2–6
iii	(Pseudo-)Sumerian incantation (tuḫul tuḫul) A rev. iii 7–8	7–8
iv	Incantation rubric referring to women's hair A rev. iii 9	9
v	Fragmentary prescription A rev. iii 10	10
vi'	Fragmentary prescription A rev. iii 11'–13'	11'–13'
vii'	Fragmentary A rev. iii 14'	14'
viii'	Fragmentary rubric(?) A rev. iii 15'	15'
xi'	Procedure (KÌD.KÌD.BI) for a woman's hair (amulet) using hair combings (*mušāṭu*) A rev. iii 16'–18'	16'–18'
x'	Pseudo-Sumerian incantation A rev. iii 19'–21'	19'–21'
xi'	Incantation rubric (to prevent a woman's hair from falling out) A rev. iii 22'	22'
xii'	Prescription (amulet) making use of hair combings A rev. iii 23'–25' /// B obv. ii 24–26	23'–25'
xiii'	(Pseudo)-Sumerian incantation A rev. iii 26'–30'	26'–30'

xiv'	Incantation rubric (to prevent a woman's hair from falling out) A rev. iii 36'	31'
xv'	Prescription (ointment) A rev. iii 32'–35'; variant ms. C obv. ii 1'–3'	32'–35'
xvi'	Fragmentary Akkadian incantation A rev. iii 36'–39'	36'–39'

Previous Edition and Discussion

Thompson 1924, *PRSM* 17, 10–12
Thompson 1929, *RA* 26, 68 (only AMT 26/4)
Köcher 1980a, BAM V, xxxi-xxxii and pl. 103–106
Scurlock and Andersen 2005, 10.99 (A rev. iv 2), 10.193 (A rev. iii 1)
BabMed Corpora (transliterations of BAM 498–500)
CDLI P424664 (transliteration, photo of BAM 498), P394416 (transliteration, photo of BAM 499), P398787 (transliteration, photo of BAM 500)
Nineveh Medical Project (https://oracc.museum.upenn.edu/asbp/ninmed/)
Electronic Babylonian Library (eBL) (https://www.ebl.lmu.de/library/K.2416)
Thomsen 1987, *Zauberdiagnose*, 82 n. 113 (lines 23'–24')
Scurlock and Andersen 2005, 10.192 (lines 31', 35'), 10.193 (line 22')
Worthington 2006, *JMC* 7, 21–22, 26 (lines 23'–25')
Steinert 2020, *JMC* 36, 65–66 (discussion of lines 22'–25')

Sections of BAM 498–500+ (ms. A) not edited here

Obv. i 1'	Fragmentary
Obv. ii 1'-6'	Prescription (ointment to blacken grey hair, SÍG BABBAR GI_6)[429]
Obv. ii 7'–13'	Prescriptions (ointments, bandages) to blacken prematurely grey hair (*šībtu*) (line 7' // AMT 5/1: 5')[430]
Obv. ii 14'–18'	Prescription to blacken grey hair (SÍG BABBAR)
Obv. ii 19'–21'	Incantation
Obv. ii 22'	Incantation rubric for dull (unpleasant) hair (*šārat qaqqadi lā ṭābi*)
Obv. ii 23'–25'	Prescription (ointment) against grey hair
Obv. ii 26'–29'	Fragmentary prescription
Rev. iv 1	Prescription
Rev. iv 2–6	Prescription for "fleeting *ašû*" (*ašû muttaprišu*) // BAM 494 ii 16–18[431]
Rev. iv 7	Prescription (purpose unknown) // BAM 494 ii 19
Rev. iv 8–11	Prescription (purpose unknown) // BAM 494 ii 20–22
Rev. iv 12	Beginning of a prescription (purpose unknown)
Rev. iv 13'–15'	Fragmentary prescriptions for *ašû*-disease // BAM 494 ii 28–29 etc.
Rev. iv. 16'–17'	Prescription for *ašû*-disease // BAM 494 ii 30 etc.
Rev. iv 18'–22'	Incantation // BAM 494 ii 31–34
Rev. iv 23'–24'	Incantation rubric and prescription (referring to *māštu*-disease) // BAM 494 ii 35–36
Rev. iv 25'-27'	Fragmentary incantation // BAM 494 ii 37–38 etc.
Rev. iv 28'–29'	Incantation rubric and prescription (referring to *māštu*-disease) // BAM 494 ii 39–40 etc.
Rev. iv 30'–31'	Prescription for *ašû*-disease // BAM 494 ii 41–43

429 See Scurlock and Andersen 2005, 10.203. For other prescriptions for this purpose, see also AMT 76/6: 9', 11', 13'; AMT 3/6 ii 7' (Scurlock and Andersen 2005, 10.202). For discussion, see also Kwasman 1999, NABU 1999/3, No. 60.

430 See Scurlock and Andersen 2005, 245 10.201 with n. 211; CAD Š/2, 387a s.v. *šībtu*.

431 For edition of BAM 494 and duplicates, see Bácskay and Simkó 2017, *JMC* 30, 10–11. For *ašû muttaprišu* "fleeting *ašû*", see also BAM 1 i 67 (Scurlock 2014a, 277); *Diagnostic Handbook* Tablet 33: 6 (Scurlock 2014a, 231); BAM 543 iv 25' and 36' (written RI.RI, within incantation).

Rev. iv 32'–33'	Prescription for *ašû*-disease // BAM 494 ii 43–44
Rev. iv 34'–35'	Incantation // BAM 494 ii 47–48
Rev. iv 36'–40'	Incantation rubric and prescription for *ašû*-disease // BAM 494 ii 49–51
Rev. iv 41'–42'	Prescription for *ašû*-disease // BAM 494 ii 52
Rev. iv 43'–44'	Fragmentary incantation // BAM 494 ii 53 etc.
Rev. iv 45'–46'	Fragmentary prescription for *māštu*-disease // BAM 494 ii 54–55 etc.
Rev. iv 47'–48'	Incantation // BAM 494 ii 56 etc.
Rev. iv 49'–50'	Fragmentary prescription // BAM 494 ii 57–58 etc.

Transliteration

1	A rev. iii 1	KA.INIM.MA SÍG SAG.DU MUNUS [*i-šaḫ-ḫu-uḫ*]
2	A rev. iii 2	KÌD.KÌD.BI SÍG SA$_5$ SÍG ⸢BABBAR⸣ ^{síg}ZA.GÌN.NA ^{ú}NINNI$_5$ NITA DIŠ-*niš* [NU.NU (x)]
3	A rev. iii 3	^{na4}GUG ^{na4}PA *šá* 7 GÙN.MEŠ-*šá* È 7 KA.KÉŠ ⸢KÉŠ⸣ *e-m*[*a* KÉŠ ÉN ŠID-*nu*]
4	A rev. iii 4	*ina* SAG.KI-*šá* KÉŠ *mu-šá-*⸢*ṭí-šá*⸣ NU.NU 7 KA.⸢KÉŠ⸣ KÉŠ [x x x]
5	A rev. iii 5	⸢*mu*⸣-*šá-ṭí-šá tur-ár* ⸢SÚD⸣ ^{ú}SI.⸢SÁ⸣ [x x x x]
6	A rev. iii 6	^{ú}*ak-tam šá* KUR Ú.⸢ḪI⸣.A *an-nu-t*[*i* x] x [x x x x]
7	A rev. iii 7	ÉN tu-ḫu-ul tu-ḫu-ul [x x x x x x x]
8	A rev. iii 8	ma-da ḫul ma-da ḫul-ḫul [x x x x x (TU$_6$ ÉN)]
9	A rev. iii 9	[K]A.INIM.MA ⸢SÍG⸣ SA[G.DU MUNUS$^?$ x x x x]
10	A rev. iii 10	[x x x $^{n]a4}$GUG ^{na4}Z[A.GÌN$^?$ ....]

Break of unknown length

11'	A rev. iii 11'	⸢kin⸣ [...]
12'	A rev. iii 12'	kin-k[in$^?$ ....]
13'	A rev. iii 13'	an-k[i ....]
14'	A rev. iii 14'	*ḫa-a*[*ṣ*-...]
15'	A rev. iii 15'	K[A.INIM.MA$^?$ ....]
16'	A rev. iii 16'	[KÌD.KÌ]D.BI *mu-šá-ṭi-šá ina* ⸢ŠÀ⸣ [......................]
17'	A rev. iii 17'	⸢*mu*⸣-*šá-ṭi-šá ta-qal-lu ana* ŠÀ [KÉ]Š$^?$-⸢*ru*⸣ ÉN 7-*šú* ŠID-*nu*
18'	A rev. iii 18'	ÍB.TAG$_4$ *mu-šá-ṭi ši-*[*i*$^?$ T]I-*qé* DUR NU.NU 7 *u* 7 KA.KÉ[Š KÉŠ] ⸢ÉN⸣ [ŠID$^?$]
19'	A rev. iii 19'	ÉN ki ḫuš x[x]-⸢u-uš$^?$⸣ ḫé-em-⸢il$^?$⸣
20'	A rev. iii 20'	èš-sa$^!$-du [x x] gu dím-ma ti-la-šè ki-bé-eš
21'	A rev. iii 21'	ki-⸢ri⸣-ri-šá nap-ri-šá ki-ri-ri-šá : ki-ri-ri ki-lu-ur-šá ⸢TU$_6$⸣ ÉN

22'	A obv. iii 22'	KA.INIM.MA SÍG SAG.DU MUNUS *i-šaḫ-ḫu-uḫ*
23'	A obv. iii 23'	KÌD.KÌD.BI *mu-šá-ṭi-šá* TI-*qé ku-niš-tú ta-ṣa-pir ur-ṭe-e* TÚG ^{giš}GIŠIMMAR *šá* ^{tu15}SI.SÁ
	B obv. ii 24–25	DIŠ KI.MIN *mu-šá-ṭi-šú* TI-*qé ku-niš-tú ta-ṣap-pir ur-ṭe-e* / ^{giš}GIŠIMMAR *šá* IGI ^{tu15}SI.SÁ
24'	A obv. iii 24'	NU.NU *zap-pi* ANŠE.KUR.RA BABBAR 7 *u* 7 KA.KÉŠ KÉŠ *ina* SÍG-*šá* KÉŠ ÉN 7-*šú* ŠID-*nu*
	B obv. 25–26	*zap-pi* ANŠE.KUR.RA *pu-ḫa-li* BABBAR 7 *u* 7 / KA.KÉŠ KÉŠ *ina* SÍG-*šú* KÉŠ-*as* ⸢ÉN⸣ ⸢7-*šú*⸣ ŠID-*nu*
25'	A obv. iii 25'	⸢x x x⸣ U$_{4}$.3.KÁM *ti-ik-ka-šá* GU$_{7}$-*ši a-di* SÍG-*šá* GUB-*zu* NU DU$_{8}$
	B	*Omits*
26'	A rev. iii 26'	[ÉN SÍG$^{?}$ *k*]*a-le-e* ḫul-a tu-ḫu-ul ḫu-ul
27'	A rev. iii 27'	[ma-da ḫ]u-ul ḫu-ul ḫu-ul ma-da ma-da
28'	A rev. iii 28'	[x ki-l]i ki-li : šà ke-še-da-ni ke-še-da-nu
29'	A rev. iii 29'	[x x x] imin a-rá ka-kéš-da-šè hé-en-zálag-ga
30'	A rev. iii 30'	[ḫé-en-sikil ḫé]-en-dadag eme ḫul-ĝál bar-šè ḫé-em-ta-gub
31'	A rev. iii 31'	[KA.INIM.MA SÍ]G MUNUS *ka-le-e*
32'	A rev. iii 32'	[KÌD.KÌD.BI x x x]x NU.NU ^{na4}PA *šá* 7 GÙN.MEŠ-*šá* ^{na4}*ia-ni-ba*
33'	A rev. iii 33'	[^{na4}x x x ^{n}]^{a4}*zíb-tú gu-ti-tú* URUDU ZABAR
	C obv. ii 1'	[...............] ⸢^{na4}GUG⸣ ^{na4}ZA.GÌN *šá-da-a*
34'	A rev. iii 34'	[x x x x È] 7 *u* 7 KA.KÉŠ KÉŠ *e-ma* KÉŠ ÉN ŠID-*nu*
	C obv. ii 2'	[.................. KA.KÉ]Š KÉŠ *e-ma* KÉŠ ÉN ŠID-*nu*
35'	A rev. iii 35'	[*ina* SAG.KI-*ša* KÉŠ Ì.GIŠ ŠÉŠ$^{?}$-*m*]*a* SÍG *a-lik-tu$_{4}$ ik-kal-la*
	C obv. ii 3'	[........................]x *ta-pa-šá-áš-ma* SÍG *a-lik-tú ik-kal-la*
36'	A rev. iii 36'	[ÉN x x x x x x *gul-g*]*ul*$^{?}$-*la* SAG.DU *up-te-ti bi-la-am*
37'	A rev. iii 37'	[x x x x x x x x] ur *li-ḫi-ia-aq*
38'	A rev. iii 38'	[x x x x x x x]x AN.TA *ku-ku ki-šá-*⸢*'a*$^{?}$⸣
39'	A rev. iii 39'	[x x x x x x x x x x]-⸢*ta*⸣ ⸢*ṣe-en*⸣ ÉN

For the continuation of ms. A see above

Bound Transcription and Translation

1 KA.INIM.MA SÍG SAG.DU MUNUS [*išaḫḫuḫ*]	1 Wording (of an incantation for the case that) the hair of a woman's head [falls out].

2 KÌD.KÌD.BI *šipāti sāmāti šipāti peṣêti uqnâti ašla zikar ištēniš [taṭammi (...)]* 3 *sāmta ayyarta ša sebet tikpūša tašakkak sebet kiṣrī takaṣṣar ēma [taktaṣru šipta tamannu]* 4 *ina pūtī/nakkaptīša tarakkas mušāṭīša taṭammi sebet kiṣrī takaṣṣar [... ...]* 5 *mušāṭīša turrar tasâk šurdunû [... ...]* 6 *aktam ša šadê šammī annûti [... ...]*

2 The procedure for it: [You twine] red wool, white wool, blue-coloured wool and male *ašlu*-rush together. [(...)], 3 you thread carnelian and an *ayyartu*-shell with seven dots (on it). You knot seven knots (into the thread). Whenever [you have tied a knot, you recite the incantation.] 4 You tie it around her forehead/temples. You twine together her combed out hair, you tie seven knots. [...]. 5 You desiccate her combed out hair, crush (it), (you take) *šurdunû*-plant, [...], 6 (and) *aktam*-plant of the mountains – (all) these plants [*you* ... ...].

---

7 ÉN tu-ḫu-ul tu-ḫu-ul [... ...]
8 ma-da ḫul ma-da ḫul ḫul [... (*tê šipti*)]

7 Incantation. Tuḫul tuḫul [... ...]
8 mada ḫul mada ḫul ḫul [... (Incantation formula)].

---

9 [K]A.INIM.MA *šārat qaq[qad sinništi*(?) ...]

9 Wording (of an incantation) [to ... a woman's(?)] hair.

---

10 [...] *sāmtu* ...[... ...]

10 [...] carnelian, [lapis lazu]li, [... ...]

Break of unknown length

11'–13' *fragmentary*

11'–13' *too fragmentary for translation*

14' *fragmentary*

14' *too fragmentary for translation*

15' K[A.INIM.MA(?) ... ...]

15' In[cantation(?) for ...].

16' [KÌD.KÌ]D.BI *mušāṭīša ina libbi [... ...]* 17' *mušāṭīša taqallu ana libbi takaṣṣar*(?) *šipta sebîšu tamannu* 18' *rīḫti mušāṭi š[ī i]leqqe*(?) *ṭurra iṭammi sebet u sebet kiṣ[rī takaṣṣar] šipta*(?) *[tamannu*(?)*]*

16' The [proced]ure for it: [You put(?) ...] her hair combings into(?) [... ...], 17' you roast her hair combings, you tie (them) together with it(?). You recite the incantation seven times. 18' She (i.e. the patient) takes(?) the rest of the hair, she twines a string (with it). [You(?) knot] seven and seven knots (into it). [You recite(?)] the incantation(?).

19' ÉN ki ḫuš x[x]-˹u-uš?˺ hé-em-˹íl?˺
20' èš-sa!-du [...] gu dím-ma ti-la-šè ki-bé-eš
21' ki-˹ri˺-ri-šá nap-ri-šá ki-ri-ri-šá ki-ri-ri ki-lu-ur-šá *tê šipti*

19' Incantation: *Pseudo-Sumerian spell*
21' Kiririša Napiriša Kiririša kiriri kilurša. Incantation formula.

22' KA.INIM.MA *šārat qaqqad sinništi išaḫḫuḫ*

22' Wording (of an incantation for the case that) the hair of a woman's head falls out.

23' KÌD.KÌD.BI (var. DIŠ KI.MIN) *mušāṭīša teleqqe kuništa taṣappir urṭê ṣubāti gišimmari ša pān ištāni taṭammi* 24' *zappi puḫāli peṣî sebet u sebet kiṣrī takaṣṣar ina šārtīša tarakkas šipta sebîšu tamannu* 25' ... U$_4$.3.KAM *tikkaša ikkal adi šārtīša izzazu lā tapaṭṭar*

23' The procedure for it (var. Alternatively): You take combings from her, you strand it into a strand of hair, you twine (it with) fibres from the texture surrounding the date palm (from the side) facing north (and with) 24' bristles from a white stallion. You knot seven and seven knots, you bind (this) into her hair, you recite the incantation seven times. 25' ... for three days her neck will hurt (her), (but) you shall not remove it until her hair stops (falling out).

26' [ÉN *šārta k*]*alê*(?) ḫul-a tu-ḫu-ul ḫu-ul	26' [Incantation for] *holding back*(?) [the hair (from falling out)]: "Ḫula tuḫul ḫul
27' [ma-da ḫ]u-ul ḫu-ul ḫu-ul ma-da ma-da	27' [mada ḫ]ul ḫul ḫul mada mada
28' [x ki-l]i ki-li : šà ke-še-da-ni ke-še-da-nu	28' [... kil]i kili ša kešedani kešedanu
29' [...] imin a-rá zú-kéš-da-šè hé-en-zálag-ga	29' [...] seven times over. Due to the knotting may she become radiant,
30' [ḫé-en-sikil ḫé]-en-dadag eme-ḫul-gál bar-šè ḫé-em-ta-gub	30' [May she become pure, may] she become bright! May the evil tongue step aside!"
31' KA.INIM.MA *šārat qaqqad sinništi kalê*	31' [Wording (of an incantation)] to hold back the hair of a woman's head (from falling out).
32' [KÌD.KÌD.BI ...]... *taṭammi ayyartu ša sebet tikpūša yāniba* 33' [...] *zibtu gutītu erû siparru* (var. *sāmtu uqnû šadâ*) 34' [... ...] *sebet u sebet kiṣrī takaṣṣar ēma taktaṣru šipta tamannu* 35' [*ina pūtīša/nakkaptīša tarakkas šamna tapaššaš*]-*ma šārtu āliktu ikkalla*	32' [The procedure for it: you twine [*a thread of* ...], 34' [you thread (on it)] 32' an *ayyartu*-shell with seven dots, *yānibu*-'stone', 33' [...]-stone, Gutian *zibtu*-stone, copper, bronze (var. [...], carnelian, lapis lazuli of the *mountains*), 34' [...], you make seven and seven knots. Wherever you have made a knot, you recite the incantation. 35' [you tie it around her forehead/temples. You rub (her) with oil(?)]. Then the 'going' hair will be retained.
36' [ÉN ... *gul*]*gulla*(?) *qaqqada uptetti bila*	36' [Incantation. "...]... I have bared(?) the skull, the head. Bring it to me!
37' [... ...] ... *liḫiaq*(?)	37' [... ...] let him mix(?) ....
38' [.. ...] *eliš ku-ku ki-šá-*˹'*a*?˺	38' [... ...] above ... ...,
39' [... ...]-˹*ta*˺ *ṣe-en-šú*? ÉN	39' [... ...] ...!" Incantation (formula).

Notes

Line 1: The reconstruction of the rubric is based on BAM 499 ii 7' (see below and Scurlock and Andersen 2005, 10.193).

Lines 2–6: These lines offer at least two prescriptions: a recipe for an amulet to be worn around the forehead (lines 2–4), and a second prescription (lines 4–6), using combed out hair of the patient, which is spun as well as desiccated and crushed and then combined with plant materials. Perhaps the latter remedy was applied as a second amulet. For the *šurdunû*-plant (reading the logogram as ᵘSI.SÁ rather than ᵘ*si-di*), cf. CAD Š/3, 343–344; perhaps to be identified with rocket.

Lines 7–8: For other spells containing the formula tuḫul tuḫul, see *infra* text A.1.2). The incantation can be classified as an example of a string of "poetic Mumbo-Jumbo Sumerian" often encountered in incantations in Mesopotamian medical texts (see e.g. Veldhuis 1999, 47–48; Baragli 2019; Geller and Panayotov 2020, 87, 90, 91–93 IGI I 110'–111', 119'–120', 125', 132'–133'; Bácskay and Niederreiter 2024, 22–23 for examples). As Veldhuis (op. cit.) has shown, the elements in such formulae which are used in a repetitive, rhythmic fashion, can sometimes be recognized as meaningful words (in our case tuḫul "thigh, hip(bone), mada "(low) land; plain" (= Akk. *mātu*) and ḫul "bad").

Lines 16'–18': If the restoration ÍB.TAG$_4$ *mu-šá-ṭi ši-*[*i*? T]I-*qé* in line 18' is correct, the fem. sg. pronoun *šī* "she" probably refers to the female patient as subject of the sentence, and not to the feminine noun *rīḫtu* "rest".

Lines 19'–21': Line 21' presents a mixture of Elamite divine names and *abracadabra*-phrases, perhaps reminiscent of Sumerian words. The theonyms Kiririša "great lady" and Nap(i)riša "great god" also occur in a few birth incantations from the second and first millennium BCE (see BAM 248 obv. i 56–57 (text D.1.1) for discussion).

Line 22': The verb *šaḫāḫu* "to fall out" (CAD Š/1, 75–76 sub 1c) contrasts with *kalû* "to retain, to hold back" (the hair) in line 31' and 35'. A similar contrast is found in *šārtu āliktu* "hair falling out ('going')" and *izuzzu* "to stop moving, to stand still" in line 35' (CAD A/1, 347b sub c; CAD U/W, 375–376 sub 2c).

Lines 23'–25': Mss. A and B slightly vary in a few details. Ms. B omits the complete line 10' found in ms. A. In line 8', ms. A reads *ur-ṭe-e* TÚG ^{giš}GIŠIMMAR "fibres from the texture (*ṣubātu*) of the date palm", whereas ms. B only has *ur-ṭe-e* ^{giš}GIŠIMMAR. Both expressions refer to the fibres resembling horse's hair (together resembling a kind of garment), which surround the bases of the flower and leaf stalks and sometimes cover the fruit. From these fibres ropes of great stability can be made.[432]

In line 23', the form of the verb *ṣapāru/ṣepēru* "to strand (hair)" can be read *ta-ṣa-par* or *ta-ṣa-pir*, since according to AHw 1082a, this verb can have an *a/u* or *i/i* vocalization (cf. CAD Ṣ, 132–133). For *kuništu* "strand, twist (made of hair)", related to *kunšu* "ball/braid of hair", see Köcher 1980a, BAM V, xxxv *ad* BAM 503: 12; CAD K, 540a, 542–543 (both terms are rarely attested).

Lines 32'–35': Ms. C appears to use different amulet ingredients than ms. A with the same instruction and for the same purpose. Among the amulet ingredients are shells, which likewise form popular materials in amulets for other female health issues (e.g. haemorrhage). For *ayyartu*-shell with seven dots, see also BAM 237 obv. i 47'–48', rev. iii 2, 28 (text C.1.4), KAL 7, No. 16 line 2' (text C.1.3) and line 3 above.

The *zibtu*-stone (^{na4}*zíb-tú/tu*$_4$) in line 33' is also attested in BAM 237 obv. i 47'–48' in an amulet prescription to stop haemorrhage (*infra* text C.1.4). Instead of ^{na4}*zíb-tu*$_4$, Stol (2000a, 49 n. 7) proposes to read ^{na4}*ḫáš-tum* (a stone attested in the Old Babylonian version of Lugale 603–611, which Stol regards as a variant for the *ḫaltu*-stone, cf. Schuster-Brandis 2008, 416; Joannès 1989, *RA* 83, 122–123). The *zibtu*-stone may refer to a shell, as it is elsewhere mentioned among "stones of the sea".[433] In the present text of ms. A, a "Gutean" variety (*zibtu gutītu*) is prescribed, not attested elsewhere to my knowledge (cf. CAD Q, 328; AHw 931a s.v. *qutû*).[434]

The variant in ms. C ii 1' preserves different minerals than ms. A, namely carnelian and ^{na4}ZA.GÌN *šá-da-a*, which I interpret as "lapis lazuli of the mountain(s)" (i.e. genuine stone, usually written *uqnû šadî*, ^{na4}ZA.GÌN KUR.RA).[435] However, the glass texts also attest to a colourant *šadû* (spelled *ša-da-a*) that was an ingredient for making blue (lapis lazuli-coloured glass), perhaps yielding a source of cobalt or iron oxide, see CAD Š/1, 61 s.v. *šadû* C; Thavapalan 2021, *JCS* 73, 147, 149 n. 34. Therefore, it is not entirely certain whether *šá-da-a* in ms. C is identical with this colourant.

Line 36': For the D-stem of *petû* "to open" in the sense of "to bare (the head), to unveil", see CAD P, 355 sub 6j (see also sub 3b).

Line 38': *ki-šá-'a* is perhaps best be understood as an imperative (fem. plural?) of *kašû* (also *kašā'u*) "to increase (strongly)". At least in the D-stem (stative), the verb can also mean "to be plentifully endowed (with hair)" (CAD K, 297; AHw, 463), which would also suit the present context (perhaps the verb references a feminine plural *šārātu* "hair").

Lines 39': The sign copied by Köcher before ÉN looks a bit like GÙB, but a reading *ṣe-en*$^{!?}$ seems more plausible. If correct, this may be an imperative (with pron. suffix) of *ṣênu* "to load; to heap up" (cf. AHw, 1091 s.v. *ṣênu* I; CAD Ṣ, 131–132).

H.2 A Treatment for Hair Loss Applicable for Men and Women in BAM 480

The Nineveh text BAM 480 (K. 2354+) presents the first tablet of the treatise CRANIUM (UGU) dealing with diseases of the head. It focuses on the topic fever/heat (or inflammation) of the head.[436] Other sections of the tablet deal with ointments, amulets and incantations to treat hair loss. The problem is described as occurring as a side-effect of fever/inflammation

432 See Landsberger 1967, *Date Palm*, 19–20 for discussion and references; see also CAD U/W, 256 s.v. *urṭû*; CAD Ṣ, 221, 225 lex. section and sub 2 (translating "bark of the palm"); Streck 2004, *ZA* 94, 268–270; correct the reading ÉŠ (for *ašlu* "rope") instead of TÚG in Steinert 2020, *JMC* 36, 65; 2021a, *Byzantinische Forschungen* 33, 69

433 Cf. Oppenheim 1963, *OrNS* 32, 411; Schuster-Brandis 2008, 456; Arkhipov 2012, 39, 58; 2018, 50.

434 The geographical designation Gutium (*G/Qutû*) in second and first millennium BCE texts is applied to regions of the Zagros highlands north-east of the lower Tigris and in geographical and astronomical texts may replace or join Subartu (Assyria), standing for a general eastern direction (Horowitz 1998, 82–84, 91–92, 323–324 *passim*). The geographical associations of Gutium appear to contradict an association of *zibtu* with sea shells in the present context and rather point to a stone.

435 CAD Š/1, 54 sub 1d; CAD U/W, 196–197 sub 1a-1'; Oppenheim et al. 1970, *Glass*, 9–10, 12; Thavapalan 2020, 312.

436 For further discussion, see also Heeßel 2010e, 158; Steinert et al. 2018, 209, 220.

('heat') of the head (col. iii 22–56). This section of the text begins with the words: "If a man's head is hot, and the hair of his head falls out, to [remove$^{?}$] the inflammation (heat) of [his] head and to bring hair loss (lit. 'going' hair) to a standstill" (DIŠ NA SAG.DU-*su* KÚM-*ma* S[ÍG S]AG.DU-*su i-šaḫ-ḫu-uḫ ana* KÚM SAG.DU-[*šú* ZI-*ḫi*] / *u* SÍG DU-*tú* GUB-*zi*; Worthington 2005, 12 rev. iii 22–23; Scurlock 2014a, 314, 315; Wee 2010a, 301, 443 §P). Since BAM 480 rev. iii 48–56 deals with hair on a man's cheek that is falling out, the preceding prescriptions may also have been used for treating hair loss independent of additional symptoms affecting the head. The section, as a whole (which prescribes mostly ointments, in addition to a bandage and an amulet), does not contain prescriptions reserved specifically for women. But one of the treatments explicitly states that it could be used both "for a man or [a woman]" (iii 38–39 *lū ša zikari lū* [*ša sinništi*]). This passage of interest consists of a prescription for an ointment applied to the head and a Sumerian incantation recited over the remedy. The remedy promises that "the hair that is 'going' (i.e. falling out) will be prevented (from falling out)" (SÍG DU-*tú ik-kal-la*).

List of Manuscripts

Siglum	Museum Number	Copy	Collation	Format; Ductus	Provenience
A	K. 2354 + K. 2412 + K. 2453 + K. 2491 + K. 3237 + K. 6774 + K. 7086 + K. 8356 + K. 8800 + K. 8842 + K. 9828 + K. 10428 + K. 11868 + K. 13398 + K. 13399 + K. 16541 +$^{?}$ K. 17155 +$^{?}$ K. 17315 +$^{?}$ K. 17359 +$^{?}$ K. 20138 + Sm. 637 + Sm. 1156 (+$^{?}$) K. 13417	CT 23, 23–38 AMT 92/3 BAM 480	Photo Coll.	Two-column tablet; Neo-Assyrian script; 7th cent. BCE	Nineveh; Library of Ashurbanipal

Previous Edition and Discussion

Worthington 2005 (edition)
Worthington 2006
Worthington 2007
Heeßel 2010d, *TUAT NF* 5, 48–50 (partial translation)
Scurlock 2014a, 306–328 (edition)
Panayotov 2016a
Panayotov 2016b
Bácskay 2018a, 47–66 (partial edition)
Wee 2019a, 300–301, 443
Geller and Panayotov 2020, 206–220, 303–305, pl. 36–39 (edition; photos)
CDLI P365742
Electronic Babylonian Library (eBL) (https://www.ebl.lmu.de/library/K.2354)
The Nineveh Medical Project (NinMed) (https://oracc.museum.upenn.edu/asbp/ninmed/)

Transliteration

1 A rev. iii 36 ÉN i-bi gi ⸢i-bi⸣ ⸢gi⸣ ḫé-en-z[álag-g]e saĝ-ki zí saĝ-ki zí ḫé-en-zálag-ge saĝ-ki iz saĝ-ki iz

2 A rev. iii 37 ḫé-en-zálag-g[e] še-er zi ⸢ḫé⸣-e[n-zálag-g]e ma-al-lal *i-di* mu-ra-an-gub ḫul-bi ḫul-ḫul <TU$_{6}$> ÉN

---

3 A rev. iii 38 KÌD.KÌD.[BI SA]G.⸢DU⸣ ⸢BURU$_{5}$⸣ K[UR.RA S]AG.DU ÍGIRA^{mušen} SAG.DU BURU$_{5}$.ḪABRUD.DA NÍTA ^{giš}U$_{4}$.(-)ḪI.IN ^{giš}GIŠIMMAR [(x)]

4 A rev. iii 39 x x [........ É]N 3-*šú ana* ŠÀ ŠID-*nu* EŠ.MEŠ-*su-ma* SÍG DU-*tú ik-kal-la lu šá* NITA *lu* [*šá* MUNUS]

Bound Transcription and Translation

1 ÉN i-bi gi ⸢i-bi⸣ ⸢gi⸣ ḫé-en-z[álag-g]e saĝ-ki zí saĝ-ki zí ḫé-en-zálag-ge saĝ-ki iz saĝ-ki iz	1 Incantation: "Turn the eyes away, turn the eyes away, so that it may become bright for him! Rise from the forehead, rise from the forehead, so that it may become bright for him! It has risen from the forehead! It has risen from the forehead!
2 ḫé-en-zálag-g[e] še-er zi ⸢ḫé⸣-e[n-zálag-g]e ma-al-lal *idi* mu-ra-an-gub ḫul-bi ḫul-ḫul <TU$_6$> ÉN	2 May it become bright for him! Remove the *sheen*, so that it may become [bright for] him! It (the illness) will diminish for me, it will stand *aside* for me. Destroy its (the disease's) evil!" Incantation <formula>.
3 KÌD.KÌD.[BI] *qaqqad āribi šadî qaqqad igirê qaqqad iṣṣūr ḫurri zikari uḫinnī gišimmari* 4 … [… …] *šipta šalāšīšu ana libbi tamannu taptanaššassū-ma šārtu āliktu ikkalla lū ša zikari lū [ša sinništi]*	3 The procedure [for it: 4 You […] 3 the head of a mountain raven, the head of a heron, the head of a male partridge (*iṣṣur ḫurri*), fresh dates from a date palm, 4 […]. You recite the spell three times over it. You repeatedly rub him (with it), and the falling hair will be held back, be it that of a man or that [of a woman].

Notes

Line 1: The phrase i-bi gi could be understood as i-bí-gin$_7$ "like smoke" (Akk. *qutru*). However, Emesal i-bí can also stand for igi "eye; face" (Attinger 2021, *Glossaire*, 555). The sign GIŠ could be understood as "to be straight, alright, well" (= Akkadian *ešēru*); see Worthington 2005, 20. Scurlock (2014b, 315) interprets zí and iz as Akkadian imperatives *iṣ(i)*, and *ṣī* (from *aṣû* "to depart"); I prefer to render zí and iz as phonetic, variant spellings of Sumerian verb forms of zi(g) "to rise; to remove" (with iz perhaps standing for i-zi).

Line 2: Scurlock (2014a, 315) interprets the word še-er(-zi) "radiance, sheen" as an allusion to a shiny bald spot. The interpretation of i-di preceding mu-ra-an-gub is uncertain. Scurlock (2014a, 335 n. 112) regards i-di as a pseudo-Sumerogram, from Akkadian *idu* "arm, side". The expected Sumerian expression would be bar-šè "aside, to the side". Worthington (2005, 20) suggests i-di could stand for idim "furious, raging" (Akk. *ekdu*). Alternatively, i-di may be interpreted as i$_7$-d (íd) "river, canal" or as idim "source, spring". The verb gub "to stand (up, firm)" in the passage is reminiscent of *izuzzu* "to stand still; to stop moving" (i.e. stop the hair from falling out) used elsewhere in BAM 480 (e.g. iii 22–23) in contrast to 'going' hair (cf. CAD U/W, 375–376 s.v. *uzuzzu* sub 2c; CAD A/1, 347b sub b). Thus, the "falling hair" (illness) may have been compared with a flowing river or water source, which should come to a halt.

References

Abusch, Tzvi. 2008. "Witchcraft, Omens, and Voodoo-death in Ancient Mesopotamia," in: R. J. van der Spek (ed.), *Studies in Ancient Near Eastern World View and Society: Presented to Marten Stol on the Occasion of His 65th Birthday, 10 November 2005 and His Retirement from the Vrije Universiteit Amsterdam.* Bethesda, 53–68.

Abusch, Tzvi. 2016. *The Magical Ceremony Maqlû: A Critical Edition.* Ancient Magic and Divination 10. Leiden/Boston.

Abusch, Tzvi and Daniel Schwemer. 2011. *Corpus of Mesopotamian Anti-Witchcraft Rituals, Volume 1.* Ancient Magic and Divination 8/1. Leiden/Boston.

Abusch, Tzvi and Daniel Schwemer, with Mikko Luukko and Greta van Buylaere. 2016. *Corpus of Mesopotamian Anti-Witchcraft Rituals, Volume 2.* Ancient Magic and Divination 8/2. Leiden/Boston.

Abusch, Tzvi Schwemer, Daniel, Luukko, Mikko and Greta van Buylaere. 2020. *Corpus of Mesopotamian Anti-Witchcraft Rituals, Volume 3.* Ancient Magic and Divination 8/3. Leiden/Boston.

Adamson, P. B. 1969. "*Bubu'tu* and *Birdu* Lesions in Akkadian Texts," *Journal of the Royal Asiatic Society* 101, 10–12.

Adamson, P. B. 1990. "Some Anatomical and Pathological Terms in Akkadian," *Revue d'Assyriologie* 84, 27–32.

Albertz, Rainer. 1978. *Persönliche Frömmigkeit und offizielle Religion: Religionsinterner Pluralismus in Israel und Babylon*, Stuttgart.

Alster, Bendt. 1972. *Dumuzi's Dream: Aspects of Oral Poetry in a Sumerian Myth.* Copenhagen.

Alster, Bendt. 1991. "Incantation to Utu," *Acta Sumerologica* 13, 27–96.

Arbøll, Troels P. 2018. "Tracing Mesopotamian Medical Knowledge: A Study of *maškadu* and Related Illnesses," in: G. van Buylaere, M. Luukko, D. Schwemer and A. Mertens-Wagschal (eds.), *Sources of Evil: Studies in Mesopotamian Exorcistic Lore.* Ancient Magic and Divination 15. Leiden/Boston, 261–284.

Arbøll, Troels P. 2019. "A Newly Discovered Drawing of a Neo-Assyrian Demon in BAM 202 Connected to Psychological and Neurological Disorders," *Le Journal des Médecines Cunéiformes* 33, 1–31.

Arbøll, Troels P. 2021. *Medicine in Ancient Assur: A Microhistorical Study of the Neo-Assyrian Healer Kiṣir-Aššur.* Ancient Magic and Divination 18. Leiden/Boston.

Arbøll, Troels P. 2023. "Venomous Scorpions and Venerable Women: The Relationship between Scorpions, the Goddess Išḫara, and Queens in the Neo-Assyrian Period," in: N. Brisch and F. Karahashi (eds.), *Women and Religion in the Ancient Near East and Asia.* Berlin/Boston, 263–287.

Arkhipov, Ilya. 2012. *Le vocabulaire de la métallurgie et la nomenclature des objets en métal dans les textes de Mari.* Archives Royales de Mari 32. Paris.

Arkhipov, Ilya. 2018. "Les perles de pierre et de métal dans les textes sumériens et akkadiens," in: S. Léon (aves une contribution d'I. Arkhipov), *Chaga Bazar (Syrie) VI. Les tombes ordinaires de l'âge du Bronze ancien et moyen des chantiers D-F-H-I (1999–2011). Les objets.* Louvain, 43–70.

Arnaud, Daniel. 1985. *Emar. Recherches du pays d'Aštata: Textes sumériens and accadiens. Planches.* Emar 6/1–2. Paris.

Arnaud, Daniel. 1987. *Emar. Recherches du pays d'Aštata: Textes sumériens and accadiens. Textes de la bibliothèque – transcriptions et traduction.* Emar 6/4. Paris.

Arnaud, Daniel. 1992. "Tablettes de genres divers du Moyen-Euphrate," *Studi Micenei ed Egeo-Anatolici* 30, 195–245.

Arnaud, Daniel. 2007. *Corpus des textes de bibliothèque de Ras Shamra-Ougarit (1936–2000) en sumérien, babylonien et assyrien.* Aula Orientalis Supplementa 23. Sabadell/Barcelona.

Aro, Jussi. 1955. *Studien zur mittelbabylonischen Grammatik.* Helsinki.

Aro, Jussi. 1970. *Mittelbabylonische Kleidertexte der Hilprecht-Sammlung Jena, mit einem Anhang: Fünf alt-, mittel- und neubabylonische Texte aus der gleichen Sammlung.* Berlin.

Asher-Greve, Julia and Joan Goodnick Westenholz 2013. *Goddesses in Context. On Divine Powers, Roles, Relationships and Gender in Mesopotamian Textual and Visual Sources.* Orbis Biblicus et Orientalis 259. Fribourg/Göttingen.

Attia, Annie. 2018. "The *libbu* our Second Brain? (part 1)," *Le Journal des Médecines Cunéiformes* 31, 67–88.

Attia, Annie. 2021. "Cabinet de lecture: *Corpus of Mesopotamian Anti-Witchcraft Rituals,* AMT 8/3 et 8/4," *Le Journal des Médecines Cunéiformes* 38, 76–84.

Attia, Annie and Gilles Buisson. 2003. "Edition de texte: Si le crâne d'un homme contient de la chaleur, deuxième tablette," *Le Journal des Médecines Cunéiformes* 1, 1–24.

Attia, Annie and Gilles Buisson. 2012. "BAM 1 et consorts en transcription," *Le Journal des Médecines Cunéiformes* 19, 22–50.

Attinger, Pascal. 1984. "Enki et Ninḫursaĝa," *Zeitschrift für Assyriologie und Vorderasiatische Archäologie* 74, 1–52.

Attinger, Pascal. 2007 [2015]. "La malédiction d'Agade (2.1.5)." http://www.iaw.unibe.ch/ueber_uns/amm_amp_va_personen/prof_dr_attinger_pascal#pane122850.

Attinger, Pascal. 2008. "La médecine mésopotamienne," *Le Journal des Médecines Cunéiformes* 11–12, 1–96.

Attinger, Pascal. 2021. *Glossaire sumérien-français principalement des textes littéraires paléobabyloniens.* Wiesbaden.

Bácskay, András. 2018a. *Therapeutic Prescriptions against Fever in Ancient Mesopotamia.* Alter Orient und Altes Testament 447. Münster.

Bácskay, András. 2018b. "'Seize a frog!' The use of the frog in medical and magical texts," *Le Journal des Médecines Cunéiformes* 32, 1–23.

Bácskay, András. 2018c. "The 34th Extract of the UGU Series from Babylon: An Edition of the Tablet BM 35512," in: S. V. Panayotov and L. Vacín (eds.), *Mesopotamian Medicine and Magic: Studies in Honor of Markham J. Geller.* Ancient Magic and Divination 14. Leiden/Boston 93–115.

Bácskay, András. 2019. "Two Sumerian Incantations against Migraine (SAG-KI-DAB-BA) on Amulets and Cuneiform Tablets," *Revue d'Assyriologie* 113, 175–188.

Bácskay, András. 2021a. "Medical Treatments against Respiratory Diseases, Ear Complaints and Migraine: An Edition of a Late Babylonian Medical Compendium Tablet BM 32277+," *Revue d'Assyriologie* 115, 159–174.

Bácskay, András. 2021b. *Glosses and Embedded Variants in Mesopotamian Therapeutic Texts.* Münster.

https://doi.org/10.1515/9781501506475-012

Bácskay, András. 2023. "Therapeutic Prescriptions and Magical-Medical Rituals against Fever: An Edition of a Late Babylonian Tablet BM 55516 + 55577 + 1882,0704.188," *Journal of Cuneiform Studies* 75, 155–169.
Bácskay, András and Zoltán Niederreiter. 2023. "Clay cylindrical amulets inscribed with incantations, tools for medical-magical rituals," *Le Journal des Médecines Cunéiformes* 40, 1–41.
Bácskay, András and Krisztián Simkó. 2012. "*Leitfaden der Beschwörungskunst*, some remarks on a well-known text," *NABU* 2012/3, 67–70, no. 52.
Bácskay, András and Krisztián Simkó. 2017. "Edition of BAM 494. The fifth tablet of UGU or a compilation of recipes against the skin diseases of the head," *Le Journal des Médecines Cunéiformes* 30, 1–71.
Bácskay, András and Krisztián Simkó. 2021. "Medical Tablets from the Archive of the Egibi Family? An Edition of BM 30918 and BM 31071," *Iraq* 83, 183–203.
Baker, Heather D. 2002. "Sīn-iddina," in: H. D. Baker et al. (ed.), *The Prosopography of the Neo-Assyrian Empire*, Vol. 3/1. Helsinki, 1134–1135.
Baragli, Beatrice. 2019. "Abracadabra Incantations: Nonsense or Healing Therapies?", *KASKAL – Rivista di storia, ambienti e culture del Vicino Oriente Antico* 16, 293–321.
Barjamovic, Gojko. 2015. "Contexualizing Tradition: Magic, Literacy and Domestic Life in Old Assyrian Kanesh," in: P. Delnero (ed.), *Texts and Contexts: The Circulation and Transmission of Cuneiform Texts in Social Space*. Studies in Ancient Near Eastern Records 9. Berlin, 48–86.
Bartelmus, Alexa. 2018. "Formale Besonderheiten mittelbabylonischer Schülertafeln," in: E. Cancik-Kirschbaum and B. Schnitzlein (eds.), *Keilschriftartefakte: Untersuchungen zur Materialität von Keilschriftdokumenten*. Gladbeck, 63–94.
Battini, Laura. 2006. "Les images de la naissance en Mésopotamie," in: L. Battini and P. Villard (eds.), *Médecine et médecins au Proche-Orient ancien. Actes du Colloque International organisé à Lyon les 8 et 9 novembre 2002, Maison de L'Orient et de la Méditerranée*. Oxford, 1–37.
Beaulieu, Paul-Alain. 1999. "Un inventaire de joaillerie sacrée de l'Eanna d'Uruk," *Revue d'Assyriologie* 93, 141–155.
Beaulieu Paul-Alain. 2003. *The Pantheon of Uruk during the Neo-Babylonian Period*. Cuneiform Monographs 23. Leiden.
Beck, Susanne. 2015. "Sāmānu as a Human Disease," *Le Journal des Médecines Cunéiformes* 26, 33–46.
Beckman, Gary. 1993. "From Cradle to Grave: Women's Role in Hittite Medicine and Magic," *Journal of Ancient Civilization* 8: 25–39.
Beckman, Gary. 2003–2005. "Pantheon A.II. Bei den Hethitern", in: D. O. Edzard, M. P. Streck et al. (eds.), *Reallexikon der Assyriologie und Vorderasiatischen Archäologie* 10. Berlin/New York, 308–316.
Behrens, Hermann and Jacob Klein. 1998–2001. "Ninegalla," in: D. O. Edzard et al. (ed.), *Reallexikon der Assyriologie und Vorderasiatischen Archäologie* 9. Berlin/New York, 342–347.
Bergmann, Claudia D. 2008. *Childbirth as a Metaphor for Crisis: Evidence from the Ancient Near East, the Hebrew Bible, and 1QH XI, 1–18*. Berlin/New York.
Bezold, C. 1889–1899. *Catalogue of the Cuneiform Tablets in the Kouyunjik Collection of the British Museum*. 5 Vol. London.
Biggs, Robert D. 1967. *ŠÀ.ZI.GA: Ancient Mesopotamian Potency Incantations*. Locust Valley.
Biggs, Robert D. 1971. "An Archaic Sumerian Version of the Kesh Temple Hymn from Tell Abū Ṣalābīkh," *Zeitschrift für Assyriologie und Vorderasiatische Archäologie* 61, 193–207.
Biggs, Robert D. 2000. "Conception, Contraception, and Abortion in Ancient Mesopotamia," in: A. R. George and I. L. Finkel (eds.), *Wisdom, Gods and Literature: Studies in Assyriology in Honour of W. G. Lambert*. Winona Lake, 1–13.
Biggs, Robert D. 2002. "The Babylonian Sexual Potency Texts," in: S. Parpola and R. M. Whiting (eds.), *Sex and Gender in the Ancient Near East: Proceedings of the 47th Rencontre Assyriologique Internationale, Helsinki, July 2–6, 2001. Volume* 1, Helsinki, 71–78.
Biggs, Robert D. 2001. Review of W. von Weiher, Uruk: Spätbabylonische Texte aus dem Planquadrat U 18. Teil 5, *Journal of Near Eastern Studies* 60, 290–291.
Biggs, Robert D. 2006. "The Human Body and Sexuality in the Babylonian Medical Texts," in: L. Battini and P. Villard (eds.), *Médecine et médecins au Proche-Orient ancien. Actes du Colloque International organisé à Lyon les 8 et 9 novembre 2002, Maison de L'Orient et de la Méditerranée*. Oxford, 39–52.
Bird, Phyllis A. 2019. *Harlot or Holy Woman? A Study of Hebrew Qedešah*. University Park.
Black, Jeremy A. 1987. "Sumerian balag Compositions," *Bibliotheca Orientalis* 44, 36–79.
Böck, Barbara. 2000. *Die babylonisch-assyrische Morphoskopie*. Archiv für Orientforschung, Beiheft 27. Wien.
Böck, Barbara. 2003. "Hauterscheinungen in altorientalischer Divination und Medizin, Teil 1: Das *kurāru*-Mal," *Aula Orientalis* 21, 161–184.
Böck, Barbara. 2007. *Das Handbuch Muššu'u "Einreibung": Eine Serie sumerischer und akkadischer Beschwörungen aus dem 1. Jt. v. Chr.* Madrid.
Böck, Barbara. 2009. "On Medical Technology in Ancient Mesopotamia," in: A. Attia and G. Buisson (eds.), *Advances in Mesopotamian Medicine from Hammurabi to Hippocrates. Proceedings of the International Conference "Oeil Malade et Mauvais Oeil", Collège de France, Paris, 23rd June 2006*. Cuneiform Monographs 37. Leiden/Boston, 105–128.
Böck, Barbara. 2010a. "Konzeption, Kontrazeption, Geburt, Frauenkrankheiten," in: B. Janowski and D. Schwemer (eds.), *Texte zur Heilkunde. Texte aus der Umwelt des Alten Testaments. Neue Folge* 5, Gütersloh, 107–114.
Böck, Barbara. 2010b. "Pharmakologische Texte," in: B. Janowski and D. Schwemer (eds.), *Texte zur Heilkunde. Texte aus der Umwelt des Alten Testaments, Neue Folge Band* 5. Gütersloh, 163–168.
Böck, Barbara. 2011. "Sourcing, organising and administering medical ingredients," in: K. Radner and E. Robson (eds.), *The Oxford Handbook of Cuneiform Cultures*. Oxford, 690–705.
Böck, Barbara. 2013. "Medicinal Plants and Medicaments Used for Conception, Abortion, and Fertility Control in Ancient Babylonia," *Journal Asiatique* 301, 27–52.
Böck, Barbara. 2014a. *The Healing Goddess Gula: Towards an Understanding of Ancient Babylonian Medicine*. Leiden.
Böck, Barbara. 2014b. "Bemerkungen zur Literatur über Amulettsteine," *Orientalistische Literaturzeitung* 109, 173–178.
Böck, Barbara. 2014–2016. "Vulva. A. Philologisch," in: M.-P. Streck et al. (ed.), *Reallexikon der Assyriologie und Vorderasiatischen Archäologie* 14. Berlin/Boston, 598–600.

Böck, Barbara. 2015. "Shaping texts and text genres: On the drug lore of Babylonian practitioners of medicine," *Aula Orientalis* 33, 21–37.
Böck, Barbara. 2016. "On the Ancient Mesopotamian Concept of 'Taboo'": Transgression and Delimitation," in: A. Weissenrieder (ed.), *Borders: Terminologies, Ideologies, and Performances.* Tübingen, 305–321.
Böck, Barbara. 2021. "Ancient Mesopotamian Physic Gardens: On Medicinal Plants, Vegetables and Spices," in: H. Perdicoyianni-Paléologou (ed.), *Health, Disease and Healing from Antiquity to Byzantium: Medicinal Foods, Plants and Spices. Byzantinische Forschungen* 33, Amsterdam, 1–19.
Böck, Barbara. 2022. "Mind-altering Plants in Babylonian Medical Sources," in: D. L. Stein, S. K. Costello and K. Polinger Foster (eds.), *The Routledge Companion to Ecstatic Experience in the Ancient World.* London, 121–137.
Böck, Barbara. 2023. "Zur medizinischen Verwendung von Zedernteer, Rote Zaunrübe und Gemeine Schmerzwurz im alten Mesopotamien, " in: C. Ambos, N. P. Heeßel and W. Meinhold (eds.), *kullat ṭupšarrūti. Festschrift für Stefan M. Maul.* Wiesbaden: Harrassowitz, 121–136.
Böck, Barbara, Shanina A. Ghazanfar and Mark Nesbitt. 2023. *An Ancient Mesopotamian Herbal.* Kew: Royal Botanic Gardens.
Boese, Johannes and Walter Sallaberger. 1996. "Apil-kīn von Mari und die Könige der III. Dynastie von Ur," *Altorientalische Forschungen* 23, 24–39.
Boiy, Tom. 2004. *Late Achaemenid and Hellenistic Babylon.* Orientalia Lovaniensia Analecta 135. Leuven.
Bonechi, Marco. 2003. "The Second Prescription in the Pharmaceutical Text TM.75.G.1623 (III Millennium Ebla)," *NABU* 2003/1, 19–20 No. 24.
Borelli, Noemi. 2021. "An Ur III Account of Fish from Umma," *NABU* 2021/1, 13–14 no. 7.
Borger, Rykle. 1954. "Ein Omentext aus der Sammlung Liagre Böhl," *Bibliotheca Orientalis* 11, 88–89.
Borger, Rykle. 1957–1958. Review of A. L. Oppenheim, The Interpretation of Dreams in the Ancient Near East. With a Translation of the Assyrian Dream Book, *Archiv für Orientforschung* 18, 415–418.
Borger, Rykle. 1967. "Das dritte 'Haus' der Serie *bīt rimki* (VR 50–51, Schollmeyer HGŠ Nr. 1)," *Journal of Cuneiform Studies* 21, 1–17.
Borger, Rykle. 1969. "Die erste Tafel der zi-pà-Beschwörungen (ASKT 11)," in: W. Röllig and M. Dietrich (eds.), *Lišān mitḫurti: Festschrift Wolfram Freiherr von Soden zum 19. VI. 1968 gewidmet von Schülern und Mitarbeitern.* Alter Orient und Altes Testament 1. Kevelaer/Neukirchen-Vluyn, 1–22.
Borger, Rykle. 1971. "Weiteres Materials zu VR 50–51 (JCS 21, 1–17)," *Zeitschrift für Assyriologie und Vorderasiatische Archäologie* 61, 84–88.
Borger, Rykle. 1985. "Einige Texte religiösen Inhalts," *Orientalia Nova Series* 54, 14–26.
Borger, Rykle. 1991. Review of CAD S, *Bibliotheca Orientalis* 48, 154–157.
Borger, Rykle. 2000. "*Šurpu* II, III, IV und VIII in 'Partitur'," in: A. R. George and I. L. Finkel (eds.), *Wisdom, Gods and Literature: Studies in Assyriology in Honour of W. G. Lambert.* Winona Lake, 15–90.
Borger, Rykle. 2001. "Johannisbrot in der Bibel und im Midrasch: Über Fortschritt, Rückschritt und Stillstand in der biblischen Philologie," *Zeitschrift für Althebraistik* 14, 1–19.
Borger, Rykle. 2004. *Mesopotamische Zeichenlexikon.* Alter Orient und Altes Testament 305. Münster.
Bosworth, David A. 2016. *Infant Weeping in Akkadian, Hebrew, and Greek Literature.* Winona Lake.
Bottéro, Jean. 1949. "Les inventaires de Qatna" and "Les inventaires de Qatna (Suite)", *Revue d'Assyriologie* 43, 1–40 and 137–215.
Boyarin, Daniel. 1993. *Carnal Israel: Reading Sex in Talmudic Culture.* Berkeley.
Brinkman, John A. 2007. "Notes on AO 4422 (TCL 12 1)," *NABU* 2007/1, 10 No. 10.
Butler, Sally A. L. 1998. *Mesopotamian Conceptions of Dreams and Dream Rituals.* Alter Orient und Altes Testament 258. Münster.
Butz, Kilian. 1977. "Bemerkungen zu den Jagdtieren in Mesopotamien," *Bibliotheca Orientalis* 34, 282–290.
Butz, Kilian. 1982. "Altbabylonische Beschwörungen um den 'Blasensprung' bei Graviden herbeizuführen, " *Oriens Antiquus* 21, 221–226.
Caballero-Navas, Carmen. 2004. *The Book of Women's Love and Jewish Medieval Medical Literature on Women. Sefer Ahavat Nashim.* London/New York.
Cadelli, Danielle S. 2000. *Recherche sur la médecine mésopotamienne: La serie šumma amêlu suâlam maruṣ.* PhD Dissertation Université de Paris I, Panthéon-Sorbonne. Paris.
Cadelli, Danielle S. 2019. "Symptomatologie dans Suâlam (première partie)," *Le Journal des Médecines Cunéiformes* 34, 4–68.
Cagni, Luigi. 1969. *L'epopea di Erra.* Roma.
Cancik-Kirschbaum, Eva. 1999. "[lú]*sāpi'u/sēpû.* Eine akkadische Berufsbezeichnung aus dem Bereich der Textilherstellung," in: B. Böck, E. Cancik-Kirschbaum and T. Richter (eds.), *Munuscula Mesopotamica: Festschrift für Johannes Renger.* Alter Orient und Altes Testament 267. Münster, 79–93.
Caquot, André, Sznycer, Maurice, Herdner, Andrée (eds.). 1974. *Textes ougaritiques, I. Mythes et legends.* Littératures anciennes de Proche-Orient 7. Paris.
Cavigneaux, Antoine. 1976. *Die sumerisch-akkadischen Zeichenlisten. Überlieferungsprobleme.* PhD Dissertation. München.
Cavigneaux, Antoine. 1982. Remarques sur les commentaires à Labat TDP 1," *Journal of Cuneiform Studies* 34, 231–241.
Cavigneaux, Antoine. 1987. "Aux Sources du Midrash: l'herméneutique babylonienne," *Aula Orientalis* 5, 243–255.
Cavigneaux, Antoine. 1994. "Magica Mariana," *Revue d'Assyriologie* 88, 155–161.
Cavigneaux, Antoine. 1995a. "Textes magiques de Tell Haddad (Textes de Tell Haddad II). Deuxième partie," *Zeitschrift für Assyriologie und Vorderasiatische Archäologie* 85, 19–46.
Cavigneaux, Antoine. 1995b. "Textes magiques de Tell Haddad (Textes de Tell Haddad II). Troisième partie," *Zeitschrift für Assyriologie und Vorderasiatische Archäologie* 85, 169–220.
Cavigneaux, Antoine. 1996. *Uruk: Altbabylonische Texte aus dem Planquadrat Pe XVI-4/5.* Ausgrabungen in Uruk-Warka Endberichte 23. Mainz.
Cavigneaux, Antoine. 1999. "A Scholar's Library in Meturan?", in: T. Abusch and K. van der Toorn (eds.), *Mesopotamian Magic: Textual, Historical, and Interpretative Perspectives.* Ancient Magic and Divination 1. Groningen, 253–273.
Cavigneaux, Antoine. 2000. "Neue Texte historischen Inhalts aus den irakischen Grabungen von Babylon, *Baghdader Mitteilungen* 31, 213–244.
Cavigneaux, Antoine and Farouk al-Rawi. 1993. "Textes magiques de Tell Haddad (Textes de Tell Haddad II)," *Zeitschrift für Assyriologie und Vorderasiatische Archäologie* 83, 170–205.
Cavigneaux, Antoine and Farouk al-Rawi. 2002. "Liturgies exorcistiques agraires (Textes de Tell Haddad IX)," *Zeitschrift für Assyriologie und Vorderasiatische Archäologie* 92, 1–59.
Chalendar, Verène. 2016. "What reality for animals in Mesopotamian medical texts? Plant vs. animal," *Anthropozoologica* 51, 97–103.

Chalendar, Verène. 2017. *Quand l'animal soigne … Les utilisations thérapeutiques de l'animal dans le corpus médical cunéiforme assyro-babylonien.* PhD dissertation. École Pratique des Hautes Études, Paris.

Chalendar, Verène. 2018. "Éléments de pharmacopée mésopotamienne: retour sur l'ingrédient *rikibtu*," *Le Journal des Médecines Cunéiformes* 32, 24–55.

Chalendar, Verène. 2020. "Le dosage des ingrédients dans les prescriptions thérapeutiques mésopotamiennes: Quelques observations à partir du texte BAM 579," *Histoire et mésure* 35, 55–76.

Charpin, Dominique. 1984. "Une pratique administrative méconnue," *MARI* 3, 258–259.

Charpin, Dominique. 2017. "Chroniques bibliographiques 20. Pour une diplomatique des documents paléo-babyloniens," *Revue d'Assyriologie* 111, 155–178.

Charpin, Dominique. 2018. "Chroniques bibliographiques 21. À l'occasion des dix ans du projet Archibab," *Revue d'Assyriologie* 112, 177–208.

Civil, Miguel. 1960. "Prescriptions médicales sumériennes," *Revue d'Assyriologie* 54, 57–72.

Civil, Miguel. 1961. "Une nouvelle prescription médicale sumérienne," *Revue d'Assyriologie* 55, 91–94.

Civil, Miguel. 1974. "Medical Commentaries from Nippur," *Journal of Near Eastern Studies* 33, 329–338.

Civil, Miguel. 1975. "Appendix A: Cuneiform Texts", in: M. Gibson (ed.), *Excavations at Nippur Eleventh Season.* Oriental Institute Communications 22. Chicago, 125–142.

Civil, Miguel (with the collaboration of Margaret W. Green and Wilfred G. Lambert). 1979. Ea A = *nâqu*, Aa A = *nâqu, with Their Forerunners and Related Texts.* Materialien zum Sumerischen Lexikon 14. Rome.

Civil, Miguel. 1983. "Enlil and Ninlil: The Marriage of Sud," *Journal of the American Oriental Society* 103, 43–66.

Civil, Miguel. 1987. "Feeding Dumuzi's Sheep: The Lexicon as a Source of Literary Inspiration," in: F. Rochberg-Halton (ed.), *Language, Literature, and History: Philological and Historical Studies Presented to Erica Reiner.* New Haven, 37–55.

Civil, Miguel. 2005. "Texts from the Series Urra = *ḫubullu*," in: I. Spar and W. G. Lambert (eds.), *Literary and Scholarly Texts of the First Millennium B.C.* Cuneiform Texts in the Metropolitan Museum of Art, Vol. 2. New York, 230–244.

Civil, Miguel. 2007. "Early Semitic Loanwords in Sumerian," in: M. T. Roth, W. Farber, M. W. Stolper and P. von Bechtolsheim (eds.), *Studies Presented to Robert D. Biggs June 4th, 2004.* Chicago, 11–33.

Civil, Miguel. 2008. *The Early Dynastic Practical Vocabulary A (Archaic ḪAR-ra A)*. Archivi reali di Ebla Studi 4. Roma.

Civil, Miguel. 2010. *The Lexical Texts in the Schøyen Collection.* Cornell University Studies in Assyriology and Sumerology 12. Bethesda.

Civil, Miguel. 2011. "The Law of Collection of Ur-Namma," in: A. R. George (ed.), *Cuneiform Royal Inscriptions and Related Texts in the Schøyen Collection.* Cornell University Studies in Assyriology and Sumerology 17. Bethesda, 221–286.

Clancier, Philippe. 2009a. *Les bibliothèques en Babylonie dans le deuxieme moitié du 1er millénaire av. J.-C.* Alter Orient und Altes Testament 363. Münster.

Clancier, Philippe. 2009b. "SpTU 1, 040 [Sakikku 39 commentary]." *The Geography of Knowledge in Assyria and Babylonia: A Diachronic Analysis of Four Scholarly Libraries.* http://oracc.org/cams/gkab/P348461.

Clancier, Philippe. 2009c. "SpTU 1, 039 [Sakikku 36 commentary]." *The Geography of Knowledge in Assyria and Babylonia: A Diachronic Analysis of Four Scholarly Libraries.* http://oracc.org/cams/gkab/P348460.

Clanicer, Philippe. 2014. "Teaching and Learning Medicine and Exorcism at Uruk during the Hellenistic Period," in: A. Bernard and C. Proust (eds.), *Scientific Sources and Teaching Contexts Throughout History: Problems and Perspectives.* Dordrecht, 41–66.

Clemens, David M. 2001. *Sources for Ugaritic Ritual and Sacrifice. Vol.* I. *Ugaritic and Ugarit Akkadian Texts.* Alter Orient und Altes Testament 284/1. Münster.

Cohen, Mark E. 1976. "Literary Texts from the Andrew University Museum", *Revue d'Assyriologie* 70, 129–144.

Cole, Steven W. 1996. *Nippur IV. The Early Neo-Babylonian Governor's Archive from Nippur.* Oriental Institute Publications 114. Chicago.

Collins, Timothy J. 1999. *Natural Illness in Babylonian Medical Incantations.* PhD Dissertation, University of Chicago.

Conti, Giovanni. 1997. "Incantation de l'eau bénite et de l'encensoir et textes connexes," *MARI* 8, 253–272.

Cooper, Jerrold S. 1972. "Bilinguals from Boghazköi II," *Zeitschrift für Assyriologie und Vorderasiatische Archäologie* 62, 62–81.

Cooper, Jerold S. 1983. *The Curse of Agade.* Baltimore.

Cooper, Jerrold S. 1988. "Warrior, Devastating Deluge, Destroyer of Hostile Lands: A Sumerian Šuila to Marduk," in: E. Leichty, M. de Jong Ellis and P. Gerardi (eds.), *A Scientific Humanist: Studies in Memory of Abraham Sachs*. Philadelphia, 83–93.

Cooper, Jerrold S. 1996. "Magic and M(is)use," in: M. E. Vogelzang and H. L. J. Vanstiphout (eds.), *Mesopotamian Poetic Language: Sumerian and Akkadian.* Cuneiform Monographs 6. Groningen, 47–55.

Coreil, Jeannine, Barnes-Josiah, Debora, Augustin, Antoine and Michel Cayemittes. 1996. "Arrested Pregnancy Syndrome in Haiti: Findings from a National Survey," *Medical Anthropology Quarterly* 10/3, 424–436.

Couto-Ferreira, M. Erica. 2008. "Si una mujer tiene la cabeza grande: Fisionomía y carácter femenino en un texto assirobabylónico," *Asclepio* 60, 19–36.

Couto-Ferreira, M. Erica. 2010. "It Is the Same for a Man and a Woman: Melancholy and Lovesickness in Ancient Mesopotamia," *Quaderni di Studi Irano-Mediterranei* 3, 21–39.

Couto-Ferreira, M. Erica. 2013. "The River, the Oven, the Garden: The Female Body and Fertility in a Late Babylonian Ritual Text," in: C. Ambos and L. Verderame (eds.), *Approaching Rituals in Ancient Cultures. Proceedings of the Conference, November 28–30, 2011, Roma.* Supplemento No. 2 Alla Rivista Degli Studi Orientali Nuova Serie, Vol. 86. Pisa/Roma, 97–116.

Couto-Ferreira, M. Erica. 2014. "She will give birth easily: therapeutic approaches to childbirth in 1st millennium BCE cuneiform sources," *Dynamis* 34, 289–315.

Couto-Ferreira, M. Erica. 2015. "Agency, Performance and Recitation as Textual Tradition in Ancient Mesopotamia", in: M. de Haro Sanchez (ed.), *Écrire la magie dans l'antiquité. Actes du colloque international (Liège, 13–15 octobre, 2011)*. Liège, 187–200.

Couto-Ferreira, M. Erica. 2015–2016. "In the Womb: Embryological Ideas in Mesopotamian Cuneiform Texts," *Korot* 23, 47–71.

Couto-Ferreira, M. Erica. 2017. "'Let Me Be Your Canal': Some Thoughts on Agricultural Landscape and Female Bodies in Sumero-Akkadian Sources," in: L. Feliu, F. Karahashi and G. Rubio (eds.), *The First Ninety Years: A Sumerian Celebration in Honor of Miguel Civil.* Berlin, 54–69.

Couto-Ferreira, M. Erica. 2018a. "Politics of the Body Productive: Agriculture, Royal Power and the Female Body in Sumerian Sources," in: S. L. Budin, M. Cifarelli, A. Garcia-Ventura and A. Millet Alba (eds.), *Gender and Methodology in the Ancient Near East: Approaches from Assyriology and Beyond.* Barcelona, 3–9.

Couto-Ferreira, M. Erica. 2018b. "Putting Theory into Practice: Kiṣir-Aššur's Expertise between Textual Knowledge and Practical Experimentation," in: S. V. Panayotov and L. Vacín (eds.), *Mesopotamian Medicine and Magic: Studies in Honor of Markham J. Geller.* Ancient Magic and Divination 14. Leiden/Boston, 149–166.

Couto-Ferreira, M. Erica. 2018c. "Uterine Architecture: Womb and Space in Sumero-Akkadian Sources," in: M. E. Couto-Ferreira and L. Verderame (eds.), *Cultural Constructions of the Uterus in Pre-modern Societies, Past and Present.* Newcastle, 34–54.

Couto-Ferreira, M. Erica. 2018d. "When Women Get Ill: Gendered Constructions of Health and Disease in Cuneiform Texts on Healing," in: S. Svärd and A. Garcia-Ventura (eds.), *Studying Gender in the Ancient Near East.* University Park, 109–131.

Couto-Ferreira M. Erica and Lorenzo Verderame (eds.). 2018. *Cultural Constructions of the Uterus in Pre-modern Societies, Past and Present.* Newcastle.

Cunningham, Graham. 1997. *Deliver Me from Evil. Mesopotamian Incantations 2500–1500 BC.* Rome.

De Boer, Rients. 2021. *The Ikūn-Pîša Letter Archive from Tell ed-Dēr.* PIHANS 131. Leiden/Leuven.

De Ridder, Jacob J. 2018. *Descriptive Grammar of Middle Assyrian.* Wiesbaden.

De Zorzi, Nicla. 2014. *La serie teratomantica Šumma izbu: Testo, tradizione, orizzonti culturali.* 2 Vol. History of the Ancient Near East / Monographs, 15. Padova.

Deimel, Anton. 1969. *Die Inschriften von Fara Vol. 2, Schultexte aus Fara.* Wissenschaftliche Veröffenlichungen der Deutschen Orient-Gesellschaft 43. Osnabrück.

Deller, Karlheinz and Werner R. Mayer. 1984. "Akkadische Lexikographie: CAD M," *Orientalia Nova Series* 53, 72–124.

Deller, Karlheinz, Werner R. Mayer and Walter Sommerfeld. 1987. "Akkadische Lexikographie: CAD N," *Orientalia Nova Series* 56, 176–218.

Del Monte, Giuseppe F. 1997. *Testi dalla Babilonia ellenistica. Vol. 1: Testi cronografici.* Roma.

Delnero, Paul. 2011–2013. "Šulpa'e," in: M. P. Streck et al. (ed.), *Reallexikon der Assyriologie und Vorderasiatischen Archäologie* 13. Berlin/New York, 284–286.

Del Olmo Lete, Gregorio. 2014. *Incantations and Anti-Witchcraft Texts from Ugarit. With a Contribution by Ignacio Márquez Rowe.* Studies in Ancient Near Eastern Records 4. Boston/Berlin.

Dennefeld, Ludwig. 1914. *Babylonisch-assyrische Geburts-Omina, zugleich ein Beitrag zur Geschichte der Medizin.* Leipzig.

Dietrich, Manfried. 1969. "Untersuchungen zur Grammatik des Neubabylonischen I. Die neubabylonischen Subjunktionen, " in: W. Röllig and M. Dietrich (eds.), *Lišān mitḫurti: Festschrift Wolfram Freiherr von Soden zum 19. VI. 1968 gewidmet von Schülern und Mitarbeitern.* Alter Orient und Altes Testament 1. Kevelaer/Neukirchen-Vluyn, 65–100.

Dioscorides. *De Materia Medica. Being an Herbal with Many Other Medical Materials Written in Greek in the First Century of the Common Era. A New Indexed Version in Modern English by T. A. Osbaldeston and R. P. A. Wood.* Johannesburg [Published in 2000].

Dittrich, Carolin and Eva Götting-Martin. 2021. "'Green Frog in the Water': A Herpetological Approach to the Magico-medical Use of Frogs and Frog-Amulets in Mesopotamia," in: C. W Hess and F. Manuelli (eds.), *Bridging the Gap: Disciplines, Times, and Spaces in Dialogue, Vol. 1. Sessions 1, 2, and 5 from the Conference Broadening Horizons 6 Held at Freie Universität Berlin, 24–28 June 2019.* Oxford, 99–115.

Dornauer, Aron. 2018. *Proso, Sorghum, Tiger Nut: Some Minor Crops in the Cuneiform Sources.* Gladbeck.

Duke, James A. (with Peggy-Anne K. Duke and Judith L. duCellier). 2008. *Duke's Handbook of Medicinal Plants of the Bible.* Boca Raton.

Durand, Jean-Marie. 1983. *Textes administratifs des salle 134 et 160 du Palais de Mari.* Archives royales de Mari 21. Paris.

Durand, Jean-Marie (avec une contribution épigraphique de Michaël Guichard). 2012. "La guerre ou la paix? Réflexions sur les implications politiques d'une prophétie," in: G. B. Lanfranchi, D. M. Bonacossi, C. Pappi, and S. Ponchia (eds.), *Leggo! Studies Presented to Frederick Mario Fales on the Occasion of His 65th Birthday.* Wiesbaden, 251–272.

Ebeling, Erich. 1923. "Keilschrifttexte medizinischen Inhalts", *Archiv für Geschichte der Medizin* 14, 65–78.

Ebeling, Erich. 1930–1934. *Neubabylonische Briefe aus Uruk.* Berlin.

Ebeling, Erich. 1931. *Aus dem Tagewerk eines assyrischen Zauberpriesters.* Mitteilungen der Altorientalischen Gesellschaft V/3. Leipzig.

Ebeling, Erich. 1949. "Beschwörungen gegen den Feind und den bösen Blick aus dem alten Zweistromlande," *Archiv Orientální* 17, 172–211.

Ebeling, Erich. 1950. *Parfümrezepte und kultische Texte aus Assur.* Roma.

Ebeling, Erich. 1951. *Bruchstücke einer mittelassyrischen Vorschriftensammlung für die Akklimatisierung und Trainierung von Wagenpferden.* Berlin.

Ebeling, Erich. 1953a. *Die akkadische Gebetsserie "Handerhebung".* Berlin.

Ebeling, Erich. 1953b. "Sammlungen von Beschwörungsformeln teils in sumerisch-akkadischer, teils in sumerischer oder akkadischer Sprache," *Archiv Orientální* 21, 357–423.

Edzard, Dietz O. 1974. "Zur sumerischen Hymne auf das Heiligtum Keš," *Orientalia Nova Series* 43, 103–113.

Edzard, Dietz O. 1985. Review of CAD S, *Zeitschrift für Assyriologie und Vorderasiatische Archäologie* 75, 124–128.

Edzard, Dietz O. 1998–2001a. "Nindar(a)", in: D. O. Edzard et al. (ed.), *Reallexikon der Assyriologie und Vorderasiatischen Archäologie* 9. Berlin/Boston, 338.

Edzard, D. O. 1998–2001b. "Nin-tin-uga, Nin-tila-uga," D. O. Edzard et al. (ed.), *Reallexikon der Assyriologie und Vorderasiatischen Archäologie* 9. Berlin/Boston, 506.

Eidem, Jesper. 1991. "An Old Assyrian Treaty from Tell Leilan," in: D. Charpin (ed.), *Marchands, diplomates et entrepreneurs: Études sur la civilization mésopotamienne offerts à Paul Garelli.* Paris, 185–208.

Englund, Robert. 1990. *Organisation und Verwaltung der Ur-III-Fischerei.* Berliner Beiträge zum Vorderen Orient 10. Berlin.

Eypper, Sona C. 2016. "Diseases of the Feet in Babylonian-Assyrian Medicine: A Study of Text K.67+," *Le Journal des Médecines Cunéiformes* 27, 1–58.

Fales, Mario F. 1983. "Studies on Neo-Assyrian Texts II: 'Deeds and Documents' from the British Museum", *Zeitschrift für Assyriologie und Vorderasiatische Archäologie* 73, 232–254.

Fales, Mario F. 1989. *Prima dell'alfabeto: la storia della scrittura attraverso testi cuneiformi inedita.* Venezia.

Fales, Mario F. 2016. "Anatomy and surgery in Ancient Mesopotamia: A bird's-eye view," in: H. Perdicoyianni-Paléologou (ed.), *Anatomy and Surgery from Antiquity to the Renaissance*, Amsterdam, 3–71.

Fales, Mario F. (with Francesca Minen). 2018. *La medicina assiro-babilonese.* Roma.

Falkenstein, Adam. 1931a. *Literarische Keilschrifttexte aus Uruk.* Berlin.

Falkenstein, Adam. 1931b. *Die Haupttypen der sumerischen Beschwörung.* Leipzig.

Falkenstein, Adam. 1953. *Sumerische und akkadische Hymnen und Gebete.* Zürich.

Farber, Gertrud. 1984. "Another Old Babylonian Childbirth Incantation," *Journal of Near Eastern Studies* 43, 311–316.

Farber, Walter. 1973. "*ina* KUŠ DÙ.DÙ(.BI) = *ina maški tašappi*," *Zeitschrift für Assyriologie und Vorderasiatische Archäologie* 63, 59–68.

Farber, Walter. 1976. Review of D. Goltz, *Studien zur altorientalischen und griechischen Heilkunde*, *Bibliotheca Orientalis* 33, 329–333.

Farber, Walter. 1977. *Beschwörungsrituale an Ištar und Dumuzi: Attī Ištar ša Ḫarmaša Dumuzi.* Wiesbaden.

Farber, Walter. 1985. "Akkadisch 'blind'," *Zeitschrift für Assyriologie und Vorderasiatische Archäologie* 75, 210–233.

Farber, Walter. 1987a. "'Die Kuh des Sin': Ritual für schwierige Geburt," in: W. Farber, H. M. Kümmel and W. H. Ph. Römer, *Texte aus der Umwelt des Alten Testaments* II/2, *Rituale und Beschwörungen* I, Gütersloh, 274–277.

Farber, Walter. 1987b. "Zur 'Bibliothek des Iqīša'," *Die Welt des Orients* 18, 26–42.

Farber, Walter. 1987c. "Tamarisken – Fibeln – Skolopender: Zur philologischen Deutung der 'Reiseszene' auf neuassyrischen Lamaštu-Amuletten," in: F. Rochberg-Halton (ed.), *Language, Literature, and History: Philological and Historical Studies Presented to Erica Reiner.* New Haven, 85–105.

Farber, Walter. 1989a. *Schlaf, Kindchen, schlaf! Mesopotamische Baby-Beschwörungen und -Rituale.* Mesopotamian Civilizations 2. Winona Lake.

Farber, Walter. 1989b. "Lamaštu, Enlil, Anu-ikṣur: Streiflichter aus Uruks Gelehrtenstuben," *Zeitschrift für Assyriologie und Vorderasiatische Archäologie* 79, 223–241.

Farber, Walter. 1990. "*Mannam lušpur ana Enkidu*: Some New Thoughts about an Old Motif," *Journal of Near Eastern Studies* 49, 299–321.

Farber, Walter. 1993–1997. "Myrrhe B. Philologisch", in: D. O. Edzard et al. (eds.), *Reallexikon der Assyriologie und Vorderasiatischen Archäologie* 8. Berlin/New York, 536–537.

Farber, Walter. 1996. "*qanu'ummi qanu'um*," *NABU* 1996/3, 71–72 No. 80.

Farber, Walter. 2010. "Ištar und die Ehekrise: Bemerkungen zu STT 257, RA 18, 21ff. ("Tisserant 17"), und STT 249," in: D. Shehata, F. Weiershäuser and K. V. Zand (eds.), *Von Göttern und Menschen: Beiträge zur Literatur und Geschichte des Alten Orients. Festschrift für Brigitte Groneberg.* Cuneiform Monographs 41. Leiden, 73–85.

Farber, Walter. 2014. *Lamaštu: An Edition of the Canonical Series of Lamaštu Incantations and Rituals and Related Texts from the Second and First Millennia B.C.* Winona Lake.

Feder, Yitzhaq. 2010. "The Mechanics of Retribution in Hittite, Mesopotamian and Ancient Israelite Sources," *Journal of Ancient Near Eastern Religions* 10, 119–157.

Feder, Yitzhaq. 2016. "Defilement, Disgust, and Disease: The Experiential Basis of Hittite and Akkadian Terms for Impurity," *Journal of the American Oriental Society* 136, 99–116.

Feldman, David M. 1975. *Marital Relations, Birth Control, and Abortion in Jewish Law.* 2nd printing. New York.

Figulla, Hugo H. 1951. "Law Suit concerning a Sacrilegious Theft at Erech," *Iraq* 13, 95–101.

Fincke, Jeanette C. 2000. *Augenleiden nach keilschriftlichen Quellen. Untersuchungen zur altorientalischen Medizin.* Würzburg.

Fincke, Jeanette C. 2003–2004. "The Babylonian Texts of Nineveh: Report on the British Museum's *Ashurbanipal Library Project*," *Archiv für Orientforschung* 50, 111–149.

Fincke, Jeanette C. 2006–. *Nineveh Tablet Collection.* http://www.fincke-cuneiform.com/nineveh/index.htm, last accessed 23 June, 2024.

Fincke, Jeanette C. 2011. "Spezialisierung und Differenzierung im Bereich der altorientalischen Medizin: Die Dermatologie am Beispiel der Symptome *simmū matqūtu*, *kalmātu* (*matuqtu*), *kibšu*, *kiṣṣatu* und *gurištu*," in: G. J. Selz and K. Wagensonner (eds.), *The Empirical Dimension of Ancient Near Eastern Studies.* Wiener Offene Orientalistik 6. Wien, 159–208.

Fincke, Jeanette C. 2017a. "Assyrian Scholarship and Scribal Culture in Kalḫu and Niniveh," in: E. Frahm (ed.), *A Companion to Assyria.* Hoboken/Chichester, 378–397.

Fincke, Jeanette C. 2017b. "The Library of Ashurbanipal," in: L. P. Petit and D. Morandi Bonacossi (eds.), *The Great City: Symbol of Beauty and Power.* Leiden, 208–211.

Fincke, Jeanette C. 2018. "Of *tirku*, Moles and Other Spots on the Skin according to the Physiognomic Omens," in: S. V. Panayotov and L. Vacín (eds.), *Mesopotamian Medicine and Magic: Studies in Honor of Markham J. Geller.* Ancient Magic and Divination 14. Leiden/Boston, 203–231.

Fincke, Jeanette C. 2021. *An Ancient Mesopotamian Herbal Handbook: The Series URU.AN.NA and MÚD-UR.MAḪ. Volume 1: The Tablets.* Leuven.

Finkel, Irving L. 1976. *ḪUL.BA.ZI.ZI: Ancient Mesopotamian Exorcistic Incantations.* PhD Dissertation University of Birmingham. Birmingham.

Finkel, Irving L. 1980. "The Crescent Fertile," *Archiv für Orientforschung* 27, 37–52.

Finkel, Irving L. 1988. "Adad-apla-iddina, Esagil-kīn-apli, and the Series SA.GIG," in: E. Leichty, M. de Jong Ellis and P. Gerardi (eds.), *A Scientific Humanist: Studies in Memory of Abraham Sachs.* Philadelphia, 143–155.

Finkel, Irving L. 1994. "A Late Babylonian *lillidu*," *NABU* 1994/3, 60 No. 69.

Finkel, Irving L. 1997. "Babylonian Elements in Aramaic Childbirth Magic?", *NABU* 1997/1, 21–22 No. 22.

Finkel, Irving L. 1998. "A Study in Scarlet: Incantations against Samana," in: S. M. Maul (ed.), *Festschrift für Rykle Borger zu seinem 65. Geburtstag am 24. Mai 1995, tikip santakki mala bašmu ... .* Groningen, 71–97.

Finkel, Irving L. 2000. “On Late Babylonian Medical Training,” in: A. R. George and I. L. Finkel (eds.), *Wisdom, Gods and Literature: Studies in Assyriology in Honour of W. G. Lambert*. Winona Lake, 123–223.

Finkel, Irving L. 2008a. “The Babylonian Inheritance,” in: I. L. Finkel and M. J. Seymour (eds.), *Babylon: Myth and Reality*. London, 190–202.

Finkel, Irving L. 2008b. “On the Rules for the Royal Game of Ur,” in I. L. Finkel (ed.), *Ancient Board Games in Perspective: Papers from the 1990 British Museum Colloquium with Additional Contributions*. London, 16–32.

Finkel, Irving L. 2014. *The Ark Before Noah. Decoding the Story of the Flood*. London.

Finkel, Irving L. 2018. “Amulets against Fever,” in: S. V. Panayotov and L. Vacín (eds.), *Mesopotamian Medicine and Magic: Studies in Honor of Markham J. Geller*. Ancient Magic and Divination 14. Leiden/Boston, 232–271.

Fitzmeyer, Joseph A. 1995. *The Aramaic Inscriptions of Sefire*. Second revised edition. Roma.

Flemming, Rebecca. 2000. *Medicine and the Making of Roman Women: Gender, Nature, and Authority from Celsus to Galen*. Oxford.

Flemming, Rebecca. 2002. “The Pathology of Pregnancy in Galen’s Commentaries on the ‘Epidemics’, *Bulletin of the Institute of Classical Studies, Supplement* 77 (*The Unknown Galen*), 101–112.

Flemming, Rebecca. 2007. “Women, writing, and medicine in the classical world,” *Classical Quarterly* 57, 257–279.

Flemming, Rebecca. 2021. “Fertility Control in Ancient Rome,” *Women’s History Review* 30/6, 896–914.

Foster, Benjamin R. 1996. *Before the Muses: An Anthology of Akkadian Literature*. 2nd edition. Potomac.

Foster, Benjamin R. 2005. *Before the Muses: An Anthology of Akkadian Literature*. 3rd edition. Bethesda.

Foster, Benjamin R. 2019. “A Harrowing Birth,” *NABU* 2019/2, 79 no. 47.

Frahm, Eckart. 2010a. “Reading, the Tablet, the Exta, and the Body: The Hermeneutics of Cuneiform Signs in Babylonian and Assyrian Text Commentaries and Divinatory Text,” in: A. Annus (ed.), *Divination and Interpretation of Signs in the Ancient World*. Chicago, 91–141.

Frahm, Eckart. 2010b. „Kommentare zu medizinischen Texten“, in: B. Janowski and D. Schwemer (eds.), *Texte zur Heilkunde. Texte aus der Umwelt des Alten Testaments. Neue Folge* 5, Gütersloh, 171–176.

Frahm, Eckart. 2011. *Babylonian and Assyrian Text Commentaries: Origins of Interpretation*. Guides to the Mesopotamian Textual Record 5. Münster.

Frahm, Eckart. 2014. “Traditionalism and Intellectual Innovation in a Cosmopolitan World: Reflections on Babylonian Text Commentaries from the Achaemenid Period,” in: U. Gabbay and S. Secunda (eds.), *Encounters by the Rivers of Babylon*. Tübingen, 317–333.

Frahm, Eckart. 2018. “The Exorcist’s Manual: Structure, Language, *Sitz im Leben*,” in: G. van Buylaere, M. Luukko, D. Schwemer and A. Mertens-Wagschal (eds.), *Sources of Evil: Studies in Mesopotamian Exorcistic Lore*. Ancient Magic and Divination 15. Leiden/Boston, 9–47.

Frahm, Eckart, Mary Frazer and Enrique Jiménez. 2013a. “Commentary on Sagig 36 (CCP 4.1.36),” *Cuneiform Commentaries Project* (E. Frahm, M. Frazer, and K. Wagensonner), 2013–2024, accessed 17 June, 2024 at https://ccp.yale.edu/P348460. DOI: 10079/f1vhj0d.

Frahm, Eckart, Mary Frazer and Enrique Jiménez. 2013b. “Commentary on Sagig 39 (CCP 4.1.39),” *Cuneiform Commentaries Project* (E. Frahm, M. Frazer, and K. Wagensonner), 2013–2024, accessed 17 June, 2024 at https://ccp.yale.edu/P348461. DOI: 10079/98sf7zx.

Frahm, Eckart, Mary Frazer and Enrique Jiménez. 2013c. “Commentary on Therapeutic (*šumma amēlu qerbūšu ittanappaḫū), bulṭu bīt Dābibi* 22 (*CCP* 4.2.P),” *Cuneiform Commentaries Project* (E. Frahm, E. Jiménez, M. Frazer, and K. Wagensonner), 2013–2024; accessed July 20, 2024, at https://ccp.yale.edu/P285472. DOI: 10079/6djhb7w.

Frame, Grant. 2014–2016. “Ulai, Ulaja,” in: M. P. Streck et al. (ed.), *Reallexikon der Assyriologie und Vorderasiatischen Archäologie* 14. Berlin/New York, 302–303.

Frame, Grant and Andrew R. George. 2005. “The Royal Libraries of Nineveh: New Evidence of King Ashurbanipal’s Tablet Collecting,” *Iraq* 67, 265–284.

Frankena, Rintje. 1954. *Tākultu: De sacrale maaltijd in het assyrische ritueel. Met een overzicht over de in Assur vereerde goden*. Leiden.

Frayne, Douglas R. 1990. *Old Babylonian Period (2003–1595 B.C.). The Royal Inscriptions of Mesopotamia, Early Periods Volume* 4. Toronto.

Frazer, Mary. 2015. “Commentary on Therapeutic (*šumma amēlu qablāšu ikkalāšu, bulṭu bīt Dābibi* 24) (*CCP* 4.2.B),” *Cuneiform Commentaries Project* (E. Frahm, E. Jiménez, M. Frazer, and K. Wagensonner), 2013–2024; accessed July 20, 2024, at https://ccp.yale.edu/P459065. DOI: 10079/8cz8wpc.

Frazer, Mary. 2017. “Commentary on Therapeutic *(šumma amēlu qāt eṭemmi iṣbassū-ma), bulṭu bīt Dābibi* (*CCP* 4.2.Q),” *Cuneiform Commentaries Project* (E. Frahm, E. Jiménez, M. Frazer, and K. Wagensonner), 2013–2024; accessed June 23, 2024, at https://ccp.yale.edu/P461270. DOI: 10079/2ngf27c.

Freedman, Sally M. 2006. *If a City Is Set on a Height: The Akkadian Omen Series Šumma Ālu ina Mēlê Šakin. Volume 2: Tablets 22–40*. Philadelphia.

Friberg, Jöran. 2007. *A Remarkable Collection of Babylonian Mathematical Texts*. New York.

Friberg, Jöran, Hermann Hunger and Farouk N. H. al-Rawi. 1990. “Seed and Reeds, a Metro-mathematical Topic Text from Late Babylonian Uruk,” *Baghdader Mitteilungen* 21, 483–557, pl. 46–48.

Fritzsche, Elifta. 2011. “GA.KIN.AG *EMṢU* im Hethitischen,” *Altorientalische Forschungen* 38, 15–62.

Fronzaroli, Pelio. 1998. “A Pharmaceutical Text at Ebla (TM.75.G.1623),” *Zeitschrift für Assyriologie und Vorderasiatische Archäologie* 88, 225–239.

Gabbay, Uri. 2015. “Commentary on Therapeutic (én munus ù-tu-ud-da-a-ni) (*CCP* 4.2.A.b),” *Cuneiform Commentaries Project* (E. Frahm, E. Jiménez, M. Frazer, and K. Wagensonner), 2013–2024; accessed June 19, 2024, at https://ccp.yale.edu/P346934. DOI: 10079/d2547s7.

Gabbay, Uri. 2016. *The Exegetical Terminology of Akkadian Commentaries*. Leiden/Boston.

Galter, Hannes D. 1983. *Der Gott Ea/Enki in der akkadischen Überlieferung. Eine Bestandsaufnahme des vorhandenen Materials*. Graz.

Garroway, Kristine Henriksen. 2023. “Abortion in the Ancient Near East and Greco-Roman World.” https://thetorah.com/article/abortion-in-the-ancient-near-east-and-greco-roman-world.

Gaspa, Salvatore. 2014. *Contenitori neoassiri: Studi per un repertorio lessicale*. Wiesbaden.

Gaspa, Salvatore. 2018. *Textiles in the Neo-Assyrian Empire: A Study of Terminology*. Boston/Berlin.

Geller, Markham J. 1990. “Taboo in Mesopotamia: A Review Article,” *Journal of Cuneiform Studies* 42, 105–117.

Geller, Markham J. 1995. “Very Different Utu Incantations,” *Acta Sumerologica* 17, 101–126.

Geller, Markham J. 1995–1996. Review of E. von Weiher, *Uruk. Spätbabylonische Texte aus dem Planquadrat U 18. Teil IV*, *Archiv für Orientforschung* 42–43, 245–248.

Geller, Markham J. 2000a. "Incipits and Rubrics," in: A. R. George and I. L. Finkel (eds.), *Wisdom, Gods and Literature: Studies in Assyriology in Honour of W. G. Lambert*. Winona Lake, 225–258.

Geller, Markham J. 2000b. "An Akkadian Vademecum in the Babylonian Talmud," in: S. Kottek and M. Horstmanshoff (eds.), *From Athens to Jerusalem: Medicine in Hellenized Jewish Lore and in Early Christian Literature*. Rotterdam, 13–32.

Geller, Markham J. 2002. "Mesopotamian Love Magic: Discourse of Intercourse?", in: S. Parpola and R. M. Whiting (eds.), *Sex and Gender in the Ancient Near East: Proceedings of the 47th Rencontre Assyriologique Internationale, Helsinki, July 2–6, 2001. Volume* 1, Helsinki, 129–139.

Geller, Markham J. 2004. *Akkadian Healing Therapies in the Babylonian Talmud*. Berlin.

Geller, Markham. J. 2005a. *Renal and Rectal Disease Texts*. Die babylonische-assyrische Medizin in Texten und Untersuchungen 7. Berlin/New York.

Geller, Markham J. 2005b. "Discourse or intercourse revisited," *NABU* 2005/4, 4–5 No. 81.

Geller, Markham J. 2006. "Les maladies et leurs causes, selon un texte médical paléo-babylonien," *Le Journal des Médecines Cunéiformes* 8, 7–12.

Geller, Markham J. 2007a. "Textes médicaux du Louvre, nouvelle édition: AO 11447, AO 7760 et AO 66774. Première partie," *Le Journal des Médecines Cunéiformes* 10, 4–18.

Geller, Markham J. 2007b. "Médecine et magie: l'*asû*, l'*âšipu* et le *mašmâšu*," *Le Journal des Médecines Cunéiformes* 9, 1–8.

Geller, Markham J. 2010. *Ancient Babylonian Medicine: Theory and Practice*. Chichester.

Geller, Markham J. 2014. *Melothesia in Babylonia: Medicine, Magic and Astrology in the Ancient Near East*. Berlin/Boston.

Geller, Markham J. 2015. "Encyclopaedias and Commentaries," in: J. C. Johnson (ed.), *In the Wake of the Compendia: Infrastructural Contexts and the Licensing of Empiricism in Ancient and Medieval Mesopotamia*. Berlin/Boston, 31–45.

Geller, Markham J. 2016. *Healing Magic and Evil Demons: Canonical Udug-hul Incantations*. With the Assistance of Luděk Vacín. Die babylonisch-assyrische Medizin in Texten und Untersuchungen 8. Berlin/Boston.

Geller, Markham J. 2018a. "The Exorcist's Manual," in: U. Steinert (ed.), *Assyrian and Babylonian Scholarly Text Catalogues: Medicine, Magic and Divination*. Die babylonisch-assyrische Medizin in Texten und Untersuchungen (BAM) 9. Berlin/Boston, 292–312.

Geller, Markham J. 2018b. "Babylonian Medicine as a Discipline," in: A. Jones and L. Taub (eds.), *The Cambridge History of Science, Volume 1. Ancient Science*. Cambridge, 29–57.

Geller, Markham J. 2020. "An Apothecary's Handbook," *Le Journal des Médecines Cunéiformes* 35, 1–33.

Geller, Markham J. 2021. "Babylonian Gynaecology in Greek (or vice versa)," *Archiv für Orientforschung* 54, 343–347.

Geller, Markham J. 2023. "Male Doctors and Female Patients," *Le Journal des Médecines Cunéiformes* 41, 1–15.

Geller, Markham J. 2024. *The Syriac Book of Medicines – Section Three – The Local Recipes*. In cooperation with Stephanie Rudolf. Preprint No. 517. Max Planck Institute for the History of Science. Berlin.

Geller, Markham J. and Strahil V. Panayotov. 2020. *Mesopotamian Eye Disease Texts: The Niniveh Treatise*. Die babylonisch-assyrische Medizin in Texten und Untersuchungen 10. Berlin/Boston.

Genty, Thomas. 2010. "Les commentaires à TDP 3–40, première partie," *Le Journal des Médecines Cunéiformes* 16, 1–38.

George, Andrew R. 1991. "Babylonian Texts from the Folios of Sidney Smith, Part Two: Prognostic and Diagnostic Omens, Tablet 1," *Revue d'Assyriologie* 85, 137–163.

George, Andrew R. 1992. *Babylonian Topographical Texts*. Leuven.

George, Andrew R. 2003. *The Babylonian Gilgamesh Epic: Introduction, Critical Edition and Cuneiform Texts*. 2. Vol. Oxford.

George, Andrew R. 2009. *Babylonian Literary Texts in the Schøyen Collection*. Cornell University Studies in Assyriology and Sumerology 10. Bethesda.

George, Andrew R. 2010a. "The Assyrian Elegy: Form and Meaning," in: S. C. Melville and A. L. Slotsky (eds.), *Opening the Tablet Box: Near Eastern Studies in Honor of Benjamin R. Foster*. Leiden/Boston, 203–216.

George, Andrew R. 2010b. "Babylonian Literary Texts in the Schøyen Collection, Nos. 18 and 19," *NABU* 2010/1, 5–6 No. 5.

George, Andrew R. 2013. *Babylonian Divinatory Texts Chiefly in the Schøyen Collection*. Cornell University Studies in Assyriology and Sumerology 18. Bethesda.

George, Andrew R. 2015. "On Babylonian Lavatories and Sewers," *Iraq* 77, 75–106.

George, Andrew R. 2016. *Mesopotamian Incantations and Related Texts in the Schøyen Collection*. Cornell University Studies in Assyriology and Sumerology 32. Bethesda.

George, Andrew R. 2018. "Kamadme, the Sumerian Counterpart of the Demon Lamaštu," in: G. van Buylaere, M. Luukko, D. Schwemer and A. Mertens-Wagschal (eds.), *Sources of Evil: Studies in Mesopotamian Exorcistic Lore*. Ancient Magic and Divination 15. Leiden/Boston, 150–157.

George, Andrew R. and Manfred Krebernik. 2022. "Two Remarkable Vocabularies: Amorite-Akkadian Bilinguals!", *Revue d'Assyriologie* 116, 113–166.

George, Andrew R. and Junko Taniguchi (with a contribution by Markham J. Geller). 2010. "The Dogs of Ninkilim, Part Two: Babylonian Rituals to Counter Field Pests," *Iraq* 72, 79–148.

Gesenius, William. 1930 [1906]. *Hebrew and English Lexicon of the Old Testament*. Oxford.

Goltz, Dietlinde. 1974. *Studien zur altorientalischen und griechischen Heilkunde. Therapie – Arzneibereitung – Rezeptstruktur*. Wiesbaden.

Gong, Yushu. 2000, *Die Namen der Keilschriftzeichen*. Alter Orient und Altes Testament 268. Münster.

Gordin, Shai. 2016. "The Cult and Clergy of Ea in Babylon," *Die Welt des Orients* 18, 177–201.

Gourevitch, Danielle. 1996. "La gynécologie et l'obstétrique à l'époque impériale," in: W. Haase (ed.), *Aufstieg und Niedergang der Römischen Welt*. Berlin, 2083–2146.

Gray, Clifton D. 1901. *The Šamaš Religious Texts*. PhD Dissertation. Chicago.

Green, Anthony. 1998–2001. "Nadel", in: D. O. Edzard et al. (ed.), *Reallexikon der Assyriologie und Vorderasiatischen Archäologie* 9. Berlin/Boston, 68–73.

Groneberg, Brigitte. 1997. *Lob der Ištar: Gebet und Ritual an die altbabylonische Venusgöttin. Tanatti Ištar*. Cuneiform Monographs 8. Groningen.

Güterbock, Hans G. 1973. "Einige seltene oder schwierige Ideogramme in der Keilschrift von Boğazköy", in: E. Neu and C. Rüster (eds.), *Festschrift Heinrich Otten, 27. Dezember 1973*. Wiesbaden, 71–88.

Guichard, Michaël. 2005. *La vaisselle de luxe des roi de Mari. Matériaux pour le dictionnaire de babylonien de Paris tome II* (Archives Royales de Mari 31). Paris.

Guichard, Michaël. 2014. *L'Épopée de Zimrī-Lîm.* Florilegium marianum 14. Paris.

Guinan, Ann. 1996. "Left/Right Symbolism in Mesopotamian Divination," *State Archives of Assyria Bulletin* 10, 5–10.

Gurney, Oliver. 1960. "A Tablet of Incantations against Slander," *Iraq* 22, 221–227.

Hämeen-Anttila, Jaakko. 2000. *A Sketch of Neo-Assyrian Grammar.* State Archives of Assyria Studies 13. Helsinki.

Hätinen, Aino. 2017. "'I Am a Fully Laden Boat!' A Mesopotamian Metaphor Revisited," *KASKAL – Rivista di storia, ambienti e culture del Vicino Oriente Antico* 14, 169–186.

Hätinen, Aino. 2019. "Sippar meets Kuyunjik: Join of BM 68458 and K. 11550," *NABU* 2019/3, 138–139 No. 76.

Hätinen, Aino. 2021. *The Moon God Sîn in the Neo-Assyrian and Neo-Babylonian Times.* Münster.

Hallo, William W. 1985. "Biblical Abominations and Sumerian Taboos," *The Jewish Quarterly Review* 76, 21–40.

Hallo, William W. 1989. "Nippur Originals," in: H. Behrens, D. Loding and M. T. Roth (eds.), *Dumu-e$_2$-dub-ba-a: Studies in Honor of Åke W. Sjöberg.* Philadelphia, 237–248.

Hallo, William W. and Jan J. A. van Dijk. 1968. *The Exaltation of Inanna.* New Haven, Conn.

Hanson, Ann Ellis. 1995. "Uterine Amulets and Greek Uterine Medicine", *Medicina nei Secoli: Journal of the History of Medicine* 7, 281–299.

Haussperger, Marta. 1997. "Ein kleines medizinisches Kompendium aus altbabylonischer Zeit," *Würzburger medizinhistorische Mitteilungen* 16, 131–149.

He, Wei, Huang, Xiaodong, Zhang, Jun, Zhu, Jue, Liu, Yajun, Lio, Bo, Wang, Qilong, Huang, Xiaonan and Da He. 2021. "$CaCo_3$ Chitosan Composites Granules for Instant Hemostasis and Wound Healing," *Materials* 14, article no. 3350. https://doi.org/10.3390/ma14123350.

Hecker, Karl. 2008. "Rituale und Beschwörungen," in: B. Janowski and D. Schwemer (eds.), *Omina, Orakel, Rituale und Beschwörungen. Texte aus der Umwelt des Alten Testaments Neue Folge* 4. Gütersloh, 63–127.

Heeßel, Nils P. 2000. *Babylonisch-assyrische Diagnostik.* Alter Orient und Altes Testament 43. Münster.

Heeßel, Nils P. 2001–2002. "'Wenn ein Mann zum Haus des Kranken geht ...': *Archiv für Orientforschung* 48–49, 29–49.

Heeßel, Nils P. 2002a. *Pazuzu: Archäologische und philologische Studien zu einem altorientalischen Dämon.* Ancient Magic and Divination 4. Leiden.

Heeßel, Nils P. 2002b. "Ein neubabylonisches Rezept zur Berauschung und Ausnüchterung," in: C. Wunsch (ed.), *Mining the Archives: Festschrift for Christopher Walker on the Occasion of His 60th Birthday 4 October 2002.* Dresden, 99–106.

Heeßel, Nils P. 2005. "Stein, Pflanze und Holz: Ein neuer Text zur 'medizinischen Astrologie'," *Orientalia Nova Series* 74, 1–22.

Heeßel, Nils P. 2006. "Der verschwiegene Unterschied: Die Geschlechterdifferenz in medizinischen Texten aus dem Alten Mesopotamien," in: B. Heininger and R. Lindner (eds.), Krankheit und Heilung. Gender – Religion – Medizin. Münster, 9–24.

Heeßel, Nils P. 2007. *Divinatorische Texte I. Terrestrische, teratologische, physiognomische und oneiromantische Omina.* Keilschrifttexte aus Assur literarischen Inhalts 1. Wiesbaden.

Heeßel, Nils P. 2008. "Astrological Medicine in Babylonia," in: A. Akasoy, C. Burnett and R. Yoeli-Tlalim (eds.), *Astro-Medicine: Astrology and Medicine, East and West.* Firenze, 1–16.

Heeßel, Nils P. 2009. "The Babylonian Physician Rabâ-ša-Marduk. Another Look at Physicians and Exorcists in the Ancient Near East," in: A. Attia and G. Buisson (eds.), *Advances in Mesopotamian Medicine from Hammurabi to Hippocrates. Proceedings of the International Conference "Oeil Malade et Mauvais Oeil", Collège de France, Paris, 23rd June 2006.* Cuneiform Monographs 37. Leiden/Boston, 13–28.

Heeßel, Nils P. 2010a. "Rechts oder links – wörtlich oder dem Sinn nach?", in: A. Imhausen and T. Pommerening (eds.), *Writings of Early Scholars in the Ancient Near East, Egypt, Rome, and Greece: Translating Scientific Texts.* Berlin/New York, 175–188.

Heeßel, Nils P. 2010b. "Diagnostische Texte," in: B. Janowski and D. Schwemer (eds.), *Texte zur Heilkunde. Texte aus der Umwelt des Alten Testaments. Neue Folge* 5. Gütersloh, 8–31.

Heeßel, Nils P. 2010c. "Einleitung zu Struktur und Entwicklung der therapeutischen Texte," in: B. Janowski and D. Schwemer (eds.), *Texte zur Heilkunde. Texte aus der Umwelt des Alten Testaments. Neue Folge* 5. Gütersloh, 31–35.

Heeßel, Nils P. 2010d. "Erkrankungen des Kopfes," in: B. Janowski and D. Schwemer (eds.), *Texte zur Heilkunde. Texte aus der Umwelt des Alten Testaments. Neue Folge* 5. Gütersloh, 45–52.

Heeßel, Nils P. 2010d. "Gebinde mit Amulettsteinen und anderen therapeutischen Substanzen," in: B. Janowski and D. Schwemer (eds.), *Texte zur Heilkunde. Texte aus der Umwelt des Alten Testaments. Neue Folge* 5. Gütersloh, 157–163.

Heeßel, Nils P. 2010e. "Neues von Esagil-kīn-apli: Die ältere Version der physiognomischen Omenserie *alamdimmû*," in: S. M. Maul and N. P. Heeßel (eds.), *Assur-Forschungen. Arbeiten aus der Forschungsstelle »Edition literarischer Keilschrifttexte aus Assur« der Heidelberger Akademie der Wissenschaften.* Wiesbaden, 139–187.

Heeßel, Nils P. 2012. *Divinatorische Texte II. Opferschau-Omina.* Keilschrifttexte aus Assur literarischen Inhalts 5. Wiesbaden.

Heeßel, Nils P. 2016. "Medizinische Texte aus dem Alten Mesopotamien," in: A. Imhausen and T. Pommerening (eds.), *Translating Writings of Early Scholars in the Ancient Near East, Egypt, Greece and Rome: Methodological Aspects with Examples.* Berlin/Boston, 17–73.

Heeßel, Nils P. 2017. "On the Fortune – or Misfortune – of Having Children," in: O. Drewnowska and M. Sandowicz (eds.), *Fortune and Misfortune in the Ancient Near East: Proceedings of the 60th Rencontre Assyriologique Internationale at Warsaw, 21–25 July 2014.* Winona Lake, 59–74.

Heeßel, Nils P. 2018. "A New Medical Therapeutic Text on Rectal Disease," in: S. V. Panayotov and L. Vacín (eds.), *Mesopotamian Medicine and Magic: Studies in Honor of Markham J. Geller.* Ancient Magic and Divination 14. Leiden/Boston, 310–342.

Heeßel, Nils P. 2019. "K. 11939: fragment d'un commentaire de SA.GIG 37 en provenance de Ninive," *Le Journal des Médecines Cunéiformes* 34, 1–3.

Heeßel, Nils P. 2023. "Der „Leitfaden der Beschwörungskunst" in Assur," in: C. Ambos, N.P. Heeßel and W. Meinhold (eds.), *kullat ṭupšarrūti. Festschrift für Stefan M. Maul.* Wiesbaden: Harrassowitz, 289–305.

Heimpel, Wolfgang. 1976–1980. "Insekten," in: D. O. Edzard et al. (ed.), *Reallexikon der Assyriologie und Vorderasiatischen Archäologie* 5. Berlin/New York, 105–109.

Heimpel, Wolfgang. 1996. "Moroccan Locusts in Qaṭṭunan," *Revue d'Assyriologie* 90, 101–120.
Herréro, Pablo. 1984. *La thérapeutique mésopotamienne.* Paris.
Hinz, Walther and Heidemarie Koch. 1987. *Elamisches Wörterbuch: in 2 Teilen.* Berlin.
Hilgert, Markus. 1998. *Drehem Administrative Documents from the Reign of Šulgi.* Oriental Institute Publications 115. Chicago.
Hirsch, Hans. 1966. *"Idi and idi," Orientalia Nova Series* 35, 413–416.
Hirsch, Hans. 1987. "Interpretationsversuche II," *Archiv für Orientforschung* 34, 45–53.
Hölscher, Monika. 1996. *Die Personennamen der kassitenzeitlichen Texte aus Nippur.* Münster.
Horstmanshoff, Manfred, Helen King and Claus Zittel (eds.) 2012. *Blood, Sweat and Tears: The Changing Concepts of Physiology from Antiquity into Early Modern Europe*. Leiden.
Hrůša, Ivan. 2010. *Die akkadische Synonymenliste malku = šarru. Eine Textedition mit Übersetzung und Kommentar.* Alter Orient und Altes Testament 50. Münster.
Hsu, Elisabeth. 2010. "Introduction. Plants in medical practice and common sense: On the interface of ethnobotany and medical anthropology," in: E. Hsu and S. Harris (eds.), *Plants, Health and Healing: On the Interface of Ethnobotany and Medical Anthropology*. Oxford, 1–48.
Huehnergard, John. 2005. *A Grammar of Akkadian. Second Edition.* Winona Lake.
Hunger, Hermann. 1968. *Babylonische und assyrische Kolophone.* Alter Orient und Altes Testament 2. Kevelaer/Neukirchen-Vluyn.
Hunger, Hermann. 1975. "Zur Ordnung der diagnostischen Omenserie," *Zeitschrift für Assyriologie und Vorderasiatische Archäologie* 65, 63–68.
Hunger, Hermann. 1976. *Spätbabylonische Texte aus Uruk. Teil* 1. Berlin.
Hunger, Hermann. 1992. *Astrological Reports to Assyrian Kings.* State Archives of Assyria 8. Helsinki.
Hunger, Hermann. 1994. "Wachstum eines Kindes vor der Geburt," *NABU* 1994/2, 32 No. 34.
Hunger, Hermann. 1996. "Noch einmal: Wachstum eines Kindes vor der Geburt," *NABU* 1996/2, 35 No. 39.
Hunger, Hermann. 2004. "Stars, Cities, and Predictions," in: C. Burnett, J. Hogendijk, K. Plofker and M. Yano (eds.), *Studies in the History of the Exact Sciences in Honour of David Pingree.* Leiden, 16–32.
Hunger, Hermann and David E. Pingree. 1989. *MUL.APIN: An Astronomical Compendium in Cuneiform*. Archiv für Orientforschung Beiheft 24. Horn.
Jacobsen, Thorkild. 1973. "Notes on Nintur," *Orientalia Nova Series* 42, 270–298.
Jagersma, Bram. 2010. *A Descriptive Grammar of Sumerian.* PhD Dissertation, Universiteit Leiden. Leiden.
Jahangirfar, Milad. 2018. "The Elamite Triads: Reflections on the Possible Continuities in Iranian Tradition," *Iranica Antiqua* 53, 105–124.
Jaques, Margaret. 2015. *Mon dieu qu'ai-je fait? Les diĝir-šà-dab$_{(5)}$-ba et le piété privée en Mésopotamie. Avec une contribution de Daniel Schwemer.* Orbis Biblicus et Orientalis 273. Fribourg/Göttingen.
Jastrow, Marcus. 1903. *A Dictionary of the Targumim, the Talmud Babli and Yerushalmi, and the Midrashic Literature.* London/New York.
Jean, Cynthia. 2006. *La magie néo-assyrienne en contexte. Recherches sur le métier d'exorciste et le concept d'āšipūtu.* State Archives of Assyria Studies 17. Helsinki.
Jeyes, Ulla. 1989. *Old Babylonian Extispicy: Omen Texts in the British Museum.* Istanbul.
Jestin, Raymond. 1937. *Tablettes sumériennes de Šuruppak conservé au Musée de Stamboul*, Paris.
Jiménez, Enrique. 2014. "Commentary on Therapeutic (én munus ù-tu-ud-da-a-ni) A," *Cuneiform Commentaries Project* (CCP), no. 4.2.A.a (E. Frahm, E. Jiménez, M. Frazer, and K. Wagensonner), 2013–2024; accessed June 18, 2024, at https://ccp.yale.edu/P459066. DOI: 10079/ht76hsq.
Jiménez, Enrique. 2015. "Commentary on Therapeutic (*bulṭu bīt Dābibi* 2) (*CCP* 4.2.G)," *Cuneiform Commentaries Project* (E. Frahm, E. Jiménez, M. Frazer, and K. Wagensonner), 2013–2024; accessed July 20, 2024, at https://ccp.yale.edu/P348472. DOI: 10079/mkkwhm0.
Jiménez, Enrique. 2016a. "Loose Threads of Tradition: Two Late Hemerological Compilations," *Journal of Cuneiform Studies* 68, 197–227.
Jiménez, Enrique. 2016b. "May the Reader Not Withhold the Tablet! On a Formulae in Late Babylonian Colophons," in: L. Kogan (ed.), *Babel und Bibel* 9, *Proceedings of the Sixth Biennial Meeting of the International Association for Comparative Semitics and Other Studies*. University Park, 227–239.
Jiménez, Enrique. 2017. *The Babylonian Disputation Poems. With Editions of the* Series of the Poplar, Palm and Vine, *the* Series of the Spider, *and the* Story of the Poor, Forlorn Wren. Culture and History of the Ancient Near East 87. Leiden/Boston.
Jiménez, Enrique. 2019. "Marginalia on the Cuneiform Commentaries Project. No. 2: An Incantation for Childbirth," *NABU* 2019/3, 140–141 No. 77.
Jiménez, Enrique. 2023. "Quotations from Lexical Lists and Other Texts in Later Mesopotamian Commentaries," in: T. Bernheimer and R. Vollandt (ed.), *Synopses and Lists: Textual Practices in the Pre-modern World.* Cambridge, 1–22.
Jiménez, Enrique, Aino Hätinen, Zsombor J. Földi, Adrian C. Heinrich and Tonio Mitto. 2019. "From the Electronic Babylonian Literature Lab 1–7," *KASKAL – Rivista di storia, ambienti e culture del Vicino Oriente Antico* 16, 75–94.
Joannès, Francis. 1984. "Textes N° 91 à 245," in: G. Bardet et al. (ed.), *Archives administratives de Mari 1.* Archives Royales de Mari 23. Paris, 83–226.
Joannès, Francis. 1989. "La culture matérielle à Mari: (IV): Les méthodes de pesée. À propos d'un ouvrage récent," *Revue d'Assyriologie* 83, 113–152.
Joannès, Francis. 1992. "Les temples de Sippar et leurs trésors à l'époque néo-babylonienne," *Revue d'Assyriologie* 86, 159–184.
Johnson, J. Cale and Krisztián Simkó. 2024. *Gastrointestinal Disease and Its Treatment in Ancient Mesopotamia: The Nineveh Treatise.* Babylonisch-assyrische Medizin in Texten und Untersuchungen 11. Boston/Berlin.
Jones, William H. S. 1931. *Hippocrates Vol. IV.* Loeb Classical Library 150. Cambridge, Mass.
Jursa, Michael. 1999. *Das Archiv des Bēl-rēmanni.* Leiden.
Jursa, Michael. 2006–2008. "Räucherung, Rauchopfer. A. In Mesopotamien," in: M. P. Streck et al. (eds.), *Reallexikon der Assyriologie und Vorderasiatischen Archäologie* 11. Berlin/New York, 225–229.
Jursa, Michael. 2009. "Die Kralle des Meeres und andere Aromata," in: A. Werner (ed.), *Philologisches und Historisches zwischen Anatolien und Sokotra: Analecta Semitica in Memoriam Alexander Sima.* Wiesbaden, 147–180.
Karahashi, Fumi. 2017. "Royal Nurses and Midwives in Presargonic Lagaš Texts," in: L. Feliu, F. Karahashi, and G. Rubio (eds.), *The First Ninety Years. A Sumerian Celebration in Honor of Miguel Civil.* Berlin, 159–171.

Katz, Dina. 2003. *The Image of the Netherworld in the Sumerian Sources.* Bethesda.

Kienast, Burkhart. 1978. *Die altbabylonischen Briefe und Urkunden aus Kisurra.* 2 Vol. Wiesbaden.

Kilmer, Anne D. 2007. "On Babies, Boats, and Arcs," in: M. T. Roth, W. Farber, M. W. Stolper and P. von Bechtolsheim (eds.), *Studies Presented to Robert D. Biggs June 4th, 2004.* Chicago, 159–166.

King, Helen. 1998. *Hippocrates' Woman: Reading the Female Body in Ancient Greece.* London.

Kinnier Wilson, James V. 1969. "Some Contributions to the Legend of Etana", *Iraq* 31, 8–17.

Kinnier Wilson, James V. 2005. "On the Cryptograms in the Lexical and Related Texts," *Le Journal des Médecines Cunéiformes* 6, 1–21.

Kinnier Wilson, James V. 2011. "A Journey through the Prescriptions," *Journal des Médecines Cunéiformes* 17, 1–24.

Kirsch, Elisabeth. 1996. *Die Behandlung von Frauenkrankheiten auf der Grundlage ausgewählter medizinischer Keilschrifttexte* aus dem ersten Jahrtausend v. Chr. Master Thesis, Freie Universität Berlin. Berlin.

Klan, Matthias. 2007. *Als das Wünschen noch geholfen hat oder: wie man in Mesopotamien Karriere machte. Eine Untersuchung zur ‚dunklen' Seite der akkadischen Beschwörungsliteratur des 1. Jt. v. Chr.* Hamburg.

Klein, Harald. 1983. "Tudittum," *Zeitschrift für Assyriologie und Vorderasiatische Archäologie* 73, 255–284.

Koch, Heidemarie. 1998–2001a. "Napiriša", in: D. O. Edzard et al. (ed.), *Reallexikon der Assyriologie und Vorderasiatischen Archäologie* 9. Berlin/Boston, 163–164.

Koch, Heidemarie. 1998–2001b. "Narunde," in: D. O. Edzard et al. (ed.), *Reallexikon der Assyriologie und Vorderasiatischen Archäologie* 9. Berlin/Boston, 180.

Koch, Heidemarie. 2011. "Die Religion der Elamer," in: V. Haas and H. Koch (ed.), *Religionen des Alten Orients 1. Hethiter und Iran.* Göttingen, 19–79.

Koch, Ulla S. 2000. *Babylonian Liver Omens: The Chapters Manzāzu, Padānu and Pān tākalti of the Babylonian Extispicy Series Mainly from Aššurbanipal's Library.* Copenhagen.

Koch, Ulla S. 2015. *Mesopotamian Divination Texts: Conversing with the Gods. Sources from the First Millennium BCE.* Guides to the Mesopotamian Textual Record 7. Münster.

Köcher, Franz. 1957–1958. "Ein Assur-Fragment der Series igi-duḫ.a = *tāmartu*," *Archiv für Orientforschung* 18, 86–88.

Köcher, Franz. 1964. *Keilschrifttexte aus Assur 3.* Die babylonisch-assyrische Medizin in Texten und Untersuchungen, Band 3. Berlin.

Köcher, Franz. 1965. "*Urruru*, '(am Feuer)' dörren," in: H. G. Güterbock and T. Jacobsen (eds.), *Studies in Honor of Benno Landsberger on his Seventy-Fifth Birthday April 21, 1965.* Assyriological Studies 16. Chicago, 323–325.

Köcher, Franz. 1966. "Die Ritualtafel der magisch-medizinischen Tafelserie 'Einreibung'," *Archiv für Orientforschung* 18, 13–20.

Köcher, Franz. 1971. *Keilschrifttexte aus Assur 4, Babylon, Nippur, Sippar, Uruk und unbekannter Herkunft.* Die babylonisch-assyrische Medizin in Texten und Untersuchungen, Band 4. Berlin.

Köcher, Franz. 1978. "Spätbabylonische medizinische Texte aus Uruk", in: C. Habrich, F. Marguth and J. H. Wolf (eds.), *Medizinische Diagnostik in Geschichte und Gegenwart. Festschrift für Heinz Goerke zum sechzigsten Geburtstag.* München, 17–39.

Köcher, Franz. 1980a. *Keilschrifttexte aus Ninive 1.* Die babylonisch-assyrische Medizin in Texten und Untersuchungen, Band 5. Berlin/New York.

Köcher, Franz. 1980b. *Keilschrifttexte aus Ninive 2.* Die babylonisch-assyrische Medizin in Texten und Untersuchungen, Band 6. Berlin/New York.

Köcher, Franz. 1995. "Ein Text medizinischen Inhalts aus dem neubabylonischen Grab 405", in: R. M. Boehmer, F. Pedde and B. Salje (eds.), *Die Gräber.* Ausgrabungen in Uruk-Warka Endberichte 10. Mainz, 203–217.

Köcher, Franz, A. Leo Oppenheim and Hans G. Güterbock. 1957–1958. "The Old-Babylonian Omen Text VAT 7525," *Archiv für Orientforschung* 18, 62–80.

Kouwenberg, Bert and Jeanette C. Fincke. 2012–2013. "A 'New' Old Assyrian Incantation," *Jaarbericht van het Vooraziatisch-Egyptisch Genootschap "Ex Oriente Lux"* 44, 141–146.

Kouwenberg, Norbertus J. C. 2010. *The Akkadian Verb and Its Semitic Background.* Winona Lake.

Kramer, Samuel N. 1971. "Keš and Its Fate: Laments, Blessings, Omens," in: I. D. Passow and S. T. Lachs (eds.), *Gratz College Anniversary Volume: On the Occasion of the Seventy-Fifth Anniversary of the Founding of the College, 1895–1970.* Philadelphia, 165–175.

Kraus, Fritz R. 1970. "Akkadische Wörter und Ausdrücke, I–III," *Revue d'Assyriologie* 64, 53–61.

Kraus, Fritz R. 1986. "Lexikalisches und Lexikographisches zu einem akkadischen Verbum," in: W. Meid and H. Trenkwalder (eds.), *Im Bannkreis des Alten Orients: Studien zur Sprach- und Kulturgeschichte des Alten Orients und seines Ausstrahlungsraumes. Karl Oberhuber zum 70. Geburtstag gewidmet.* Innsbruck, 125–141.

Krebernik, Manfred. 1984. *Die Beschwörungen aus Fara und Ebla.* Hildesheim.

Krebernik, Manfred. 1987–1990a. "Lil (Lil(lu))", in: D. O. Edzard et al. (ed.), *Reallexikon der Assyriologie und Vorderasiatischen Archäologie* 7. Berlin/New York, 19–20.

Krebernik, Manfred. 1987–1990b. "Lugal-AMAŠ-pa'e", in: D. O. Edzard et al. (ed.), *Reallexikon der Assyriologie und Vorderasiatischen Archäologie* 7. Berlin/New York, 111.

Krebernik, Manfred. 1993–1997. "Muttergöttin. A.I. In Mesopotamien", in: D. O. Edzard et al. (ed.), *Reallexikon der Assyriologie und Vorderasiatischen Archäologie* 8. Berlin/New York, 502–516.

Krebernik, Manfred. 2009–2011a. "Šarrat-Kidmuri", in: M. P. Streck et al. (ed.), *Reallexikon der Assyriologie und Vorderasiatischen Archäologie* 12. Berlin/New York, 75.

Krebernik, Manfred. 2009–2011b. "Šar-ur und Šar-gaz", in: M. P. Streck et al. (ed.), *Reallexikon der Assyriologie und Vorderasiatischen Archäologie* 12. Berlin/New York, 84–86.

Krebernik, Manfred. 2014–2016. "Ulai, Ulaja," in: M. P. Streck et al. (ed.), *Reallexikon der Assyriologie und Vorderasiatischen Archäologie* 14. Berlin/New York, 303.

Krebernik, Manfred. 2016. "'Wissen' im Akkadischen, Semitischen, Afroasiatischen", in: H. Rechenmacher (ed.), *In Memoriam Wolfgang Richter.* St. Ottilien, 205–238.

Krebernik, Manfred. 2018. "Eine neue elamische Beschwörung aus der Hilprecht-Sammlung (HS 2338) im Kontext alloglotter Texte der altbabylonischen Zeit", in: *Elamica* 8 (= B. Mofidi-Nasrabadi, D. Prechel and A. Pruß (eds.), *Elam and Its Neighbors: Recent Research and New Perspectives. Proceedings of the International Congress Held at Johannes Gutenberg University Mainz, September 21–23, 2016*). Hildesheim, 13–48.

Kuntner, Liselotte. 1994. *Die Gebärhaltung der Frau: Schwangerschaft und Geburt aus geschichtlicher, völkerkundlicher und medizinischer Perspektive*. 4. ergänzte Auflage. München.

Kwasman, Theodore. 1999. "*bunbullu*," *NABU* 1999/3, 59 No. 60.

Labat, René. 1939, *Hémérologies et Ménologies d'Assur.* Paris.

Labat, René. 1951. *Traité akkadien de diagnostics et prognostics médicaux* (TDP). 2 Vol. Leiden.

Labat, René. 1957–1971a. "Frauenkrankheiten," in: E. Weidner and W. von Soden (eds.), *Reallexikon der Assyriologie und Vorderasiatischen Archäologie* 3. Berlin/New York, 109.

Labat, René. 1957–1971b. "Geburt," in: E. Weidner and W. von Soden (eds.), *Reallexikon der Assyriologie und Vorderasiatischen Archäologie* 3. Berlin/New York, 178.

Labat, René. 1960. "Ordonnances médicales ou magiques," *Revue d'Assyriologie* 54, 169–176.

Labat, René. 1965. *Un calendrier babylonien des travaux des signes et des mois (séries iqqur îpuš)*. Paris.

Labat, René. 1974. *Textes littéraires de Suse.* Mémoires de la Délégation Archéologique en Iran 57. Paris.

Laessøe, Jørgen. 1955. *Studies on the Assyrian Ritual and Series bît rimki.* Copenhagen.

Lambert, Wilfred G. 1957–1958. "An Incantation of the *Maqlû* Type," *Archiv für Orientforschung* 18, 288–299.

Lambert, Wilfred G. 1960. *Babylonian Wisdom Literature.* Oxford.

Lambert, Wilfred G. 1962. "A Catalogue of Texts and Authors," *Journal of Cuneiform Studies* 16, 59–77.

Lambert, Wilfred G. 1965. "A Middle Assyrian Tablet of Incantations," in: H. G. Güterbock and T. Jacobsen (eds.), *Studies in Honor of Benno Landsberger on his Seventy-Fifth Birthday April 21, 1965.* Assyriological Studies 16. Chicago, 283–288.

Lambert, Wilfred G. 1967. "The Gula Hymn of Bulluṭsa-rabi (Tab. VIII–XXIII)," *Orientalia Nova Series* 36, 105–132.

Lambert, Wilfred G. 1969. "A Middle Assyrian Medical Text," *Iraq* 31, 28–39.

Lambert, Wilfred G. 1970. "Fire Incantations," *Archiv für Orientforschung* 23, 39–45.

Lambert, Wilfred G. 1972–1975. "Ḫuškia," in: D. O. Edzard et al. (ed.), *Reallexikon der Assyriologie und Vorderasiatischen Archäologie* 4, Berlin/Boston, 522–523.

Lambert, Wilfred G. 1974. "Dingir.šà.dib.ba Incantations," *Journal of Near Eastern Studies* 33, 267–270, 272–322.

Lambert, Wilfred G. 1975. "The Problem of the Love Lyrics," in: H. Goedicke and J. J. M. Roberts (eds.), *Unity and Diversity: Essays in the History, Literature, and Religion of the Ancient Near East.* Baltimore, 98–135.

Lambert, Wilfred G. 1976–1980. "Karašul," in: D. O. Edzard et al. (ed.), *Reallexikon der Assyriologie und Vorderasiatischen Archäologie* 5, Berlin/Boston, 408.

Lambert, Wilfred G. 1980. "The Twenty-One 'Poultices'," *Anatolian Studies* 30, 77–83.

Lambert, Wilfred G. 1982. "The Hymn to the Queen of Nippur," in: G. van Driel, Th. J. H. Krispijn, M. Stol and K. R. Veenhof (eds.), *Zikir Šumim: Assyriological Studies Presented to F. R. Kraus on the Occasion of His Seventieth Birthday.* Leiden, 173–218.

Lambert, Wilfred G. 1983. "Exorcistic mumbo jumbo," *Revue d'Assyriologie* 77, 94–95.

Lambert, Wilfred G. 1987–1990. "Lugal-me/Lugal-mea/Mea and Lugal-namENna," in: D. O. Edzard et al. (ed.), *Reallexikon der Assyriologie und Vorderasiatischen Archäologie* 7, Berlin/Boston, 149.

Lambert, Wilfred G. 1992. *Catalogue of the Cuneiform Tablets in the Kouyunjik Collection of the British Museum, Third Supplement.* London.

Lambert, Wilfred G. 1997. "Processions to the Akītu House," *Revue d'Assyriologie* 91, 49–80.

Lambert, Wilfred G. 2007. *Babylonian Oracles Questions.* Winona Lake.

Lambert, Wilfred G. 2013. *Babylonian Creation Myths.* Winona Lake.

Lambert, Wilfred G. and Millard, Alan R. 1969. *Atra-ḫasīs: The Babylonian Story of the Flood. With the Sumerian Flood Story by Miguel Civil.* Oxford.

Lambert, Wilfred G. and Ryan D. Winters. 2023. *An = Anum and Related Lists. God Lists of Ancient Mesopotamia, Volume I.* Edited by A. George and M. Krebernik. Tübingen.

Landsberger, Benno. 1934. *Die Fauna des alten Mesopotamien nach der 14. Tafel der Serie ḪAR-ra = ḫubullu.* Leipzig.

Landsberger, Benno. 1937. *Die Serie ana ittišu.* Materialien zum sumerischen Lexikon 1. Roma.

Landsberger, Benno (in cooperation with Anne Draffkorn Kilmer and Edmund I. Gordon). 1960. *The Fauna of Ancient Mesopotamia, First Part. Tablet XIII.* Materialien zum sumerischen Lexikon 8/1. Roma.

Landsberger, Benno. 1962. *The Fauna of Ancient Mesopotamia, Second Part. ḪAR-ra = ḫubullu XIV and XVIII.* Materialien zum sumerischen Lexikon 8/2. Roma.

Landsberger, Benno. 1967. *The Date-Palm and its By-products according to the Cuneiform Sources.* Archiv für Orientforschung, Beiheft 17. Graz.

Landsberger, Benno and Oliver R. Gurney. 1957–1958. "Practical Vocabulary of Assur," *Archiv für Orientforschung* 18, 328–341.

Lapinkivi, Pirjo. 2004. *The Sumerian Sacred Marriage in the Light of Comparative Evidence.* State Archives of Assyria Studies 15. Helsinki.

Lecompte, Camille. 2016. "Representation of Women in Mesopotamian Lexical Lists," in: B. Lion and C. Michel (eds.), *The Role of Women in Work and Society in the Ancient Near East.* Boston/Berlin, 29–56.

Lehmhaus, Lennart. 2023. "Re-reading Gynaecology in the Ancient World: A Transcultural and Interdisciplinary Survey," in: L. Lehmhaus (ed.), *Female Bodies and Female Practitioners: Gynaecology, Women's Bodies, and Expertise in the Ancient to Medieval Mediterranean and Middle East.* Tübingen, 3–83.

Leichty, Erle. 1970. *The Omen Series Šumma Izbu.* Texts from Cuneiform Sources 4. New York.

Leichty, Erle. 1973. "Two Late Commentaries," *Archiv für Orientforschung* 24, 78–86.

Leichty, Erle. 1986. *Catalogue of the Babylonian Tablets in the British Museum, Volume VI. Tablets from Sippar 1.* London.
Leichty, Erle. 1987. *Catalogue of the Babylonian Tablets in the British Museum, Volume VII. Tablets from Sippar 2.* London.
Leichty, Erle. 1988. "Guaranteed to Cure," in: E. Leichty, M. de Jong Ellis and P. Gerardi (eds.), *A Scientific Humanist: Studies in Memory of Abraham Sachs*. Philadelphia, 261–264.
Leichty, Erle, Finkel, Irving L. and Christopher B. F. Walker. 2019. *Catalogue of the Babylonian Tablets in the British Museum. Volumes IV–V.* Münster.
Leick, Gwendolyn. 1994. *Sex and Eroticism in Mesopotamian Literature.* London.
Lenzi, Alan. 2008a. *Secrecy and the Gods: Secret Knowledge in Ancient Mesopotamia and Biblical Israel.* State Archives of Assyria Studies 19. Helsinki.
Lenzi, Alan. 2008b. "The Uruk List of Kings and Sages and Late Mesopotamian Scholarship," *Journal of Ancient Near Eastern Religions* 8, 137–169.
Lenzi, Alan. 2015. "Mesopotamian Scholarship: Kassite to Late Babylonian Periods," *Journal of Ancient Near Eastern History* 2, 145–201.
Lieberman, S. J. 1990. "Canonical and Official Cuneiform Texts: Towards an Understanding of Ashurbanipal's Personal Tablet Collection," in: T. Abusch, J. Huehnergard and P. Steinkeller (eds.), *Lingering over Words: Studies in Ancient Near Eastern Literature in Honor of William L. Moran*. Atlanta, 305–336.
Limet, Henri. 1984. "Amulettes babyloniennes et lapidaire zoroastrien," in: *Orientalia J. Duchesne-Guillemin emerito oblata.* Acta Iranica 23. Leiden, 327–339.
Limet, Henri. 1985. "Bijouterie et orfèvrerie à Mari," *MARI* 4, 509–521.
Linton, Deirdre. 1970. *The Series SAG.GIG.GA.MEŠ and Related Incantations.* PhD Dissertation, University of Birmingham.
Limet, Henri. 1986. *Textes administratifs relatifs aux métaux.* Archives Royales de Mari 25. Paris.
Lion, Brigitte and Cécile Michel. 1997. "Criquets et autres insectes à Mari," *MARI. Annales de Recherches Interdisciplinaires* 8. Paris, 707–724.
Lion, Brigitte, Michel, Cécile and Pierre Noël. 2000. "Les crevettes dans la documentation du Proche-Orient ancien," *Journal of Cuneiform Studies* 52, 55–60.
Litke, Richard L. 1998. *A Reconstruction of the Assyro-Babylonian god-lists, AN: ^{d}A-nu-um and AN: Anu šá amēli.* New Haven.
Livingstone, Alasdair. 1986. *Mystical and Mythological Explanatory Works of Assyrian and Babylonian Scholars.* Oxford.
Livingstone, Alasdair. 1989. *Court Poetry and Literary Miscellanea.* State Archives of Assyria 3. Helsinki.
Livingstone, Alasdair. 2013. *Hemerologies of Assyrian and Babylonian Scholars.* Cornell University Studies in Assyriology and Sumerology 25. Bethesda.
Luukko, Mikko. 2004. *Grammatical Variation in Neo-Assyrian.* State Archives of Assyria Studies 16. Helsinki.
Luukko, Mikko and Greta van Buylaere. 2020. *Corpus of Mesopotamian Anti-Witchcraft Rituals: Glossaries and Indices.* Ancient Magic and Divination 8/4. Leiden/Boston.
Macgregor, Sherry Lou. 2012. *Beyond Hearth and Home: Women in the Public Sphere in Neo-Assyrian Society.* State Archives of Assyria Studies 21. Helsinki.
Macmillan, Kerr D. 1906. *Some Cuneiform Tablets Bearing on the Religion of Babylonia and Assyria.* Beiträge zur Assyriologie und semitischen Sprachwissenschaft 5/V. Leipzig.
Malbran-Labat, Florence. 1995. *Les inscriptions royales de Suse: briques de l'époque paléo-élamite à l'Empire néo-élamite.* Paris.
Marquéz Rowe, Ignacio. 2014. "The Babylonian Incantation Texts from Ugarit," in: Del Olmo Lete, Gregorio, *Incantations and Anti-Witchcraft Texts from Ugarit.* Studies in Ancient Near Eastern Records 4. Boston/Berlin, 36–80.
Marquéz Rowe, Ignacio. 2015. "Water of labour? A Note on the Story of Sin and the Cow", *Aula Orientalis* 33, 51–62.
Martin, Emily. 1987. *The Woman in the Body: A Cultural Analysis of Reproduction.* Boston.
Matsushima, Eiko. 2014. "Ištar and Other Goddesses of the So-Called 'Sacred Marriage' in Ancient Mesopotamia," in: D. T. Sugimoto (ed.), *Transformation of a Goddess: Ishtar – Astarte – Aphrodite.* Orbis Biblicus et Orientalis 263. Fribourg/Göttingen, 1–14.
Maul, Stefan M. 1994. *Zukunftsbewältigung: Eine Untersuchung altorientalischen Denkens anhand der babylonisch-assyrischen Löserituale (Namburbi).* Baghdader Forschungen 18. Mainz.
Maul, Stefan M. 1997. "Küchensumerisch oder hohe Kunst der Exegese? Überlegungen zur Bewertung akkadischer Interlinearübersetzungen von Emesal-Texten," in: B. Pongratz-Leisten, H. Kühne and P. Xella (eds.), *Ana šadî Labnāni lū allik. Beiträge zu altorientalischen und mittelmeerischen Kulturen. Festschrift für Wolfgang Röllig.* Alter Orient und Altes Testament 247. Kevelaer/Neukirchen-Vluyn, 253–267.
Maul, Stefan M. 1999. "Das Wort im Worte. Orthographie und Etymologie als hermeneutische Verfahren babylonischer Gelehrter," in: G. W. Most (ed.), *Commentaries – Kommentare.* Göttingen, 11–18.
Maul, Stefan M. 2010. "Die Tontafelbibliothek aus dem sogenannten »Haus des Beschwörungspriesters«," in: S. M. Maul and N. P. Heeßel (eds.), *Assur-Forschungen. Arbeiten aus der Forschungsstelle »Edition literarischer Keilschrifttexte aus Assur« der Heidelberger Akademie der Wissenschaften.* Wiesbaden, 189–228.
Maul, Stefan M. 2013. "Ein altorientalischer Pferdesegen – Seuchenprophylaxe in der assyrischen Armee," *Zeitschrift für Assyriologie und Vorderasiatische Archäologie* 103, 16–37.
Maul, Stefan M. 2019. *Bannlösung (nam-érim-búr-ru-da): Die Therapie eines auf eidliche Falschaussage zurückgeführten Leidens.* Keilschrifttexte aus Assur literarischen Inhalts 10. Wiesbaden.
Maul, Stefan M. and R. Strauß. 2011. *Ritualbeschreibungen und Gebete I. Mit Beiträgen von Daniel Schwemer.* Keilschrifttexte aus Assur literarischen Inhalts 4. Wiesbaden.
May, Natalie N. 2018a. "Exorcists and Physicians at Assur: More on Their Education and Interfamily and Court Connections," *Zeitschrift für Assyriologie und Vorderasiatische Archäologie* 108, 63–80.
May, Natalie N. 2018b. "Female Scholars in Mesopotamia?", in: S. L. Budin, M. Cifarelli, A. Garcia-Ventura and A. Millet Alba (eds.), *Gender, Methodology and the Ancient Near East: Proceedings of the Second Workshop Held in Barcelona, February 1–3, 2017.* Barcelona, 149–162.
May, Natalie M. 2022. "Women in Cult in First Millennium BCE Mesopotamia," in: K. de Graef, A. Garcia-Ventura, A. Goddeeris and B. Alpert Nakhai (eds.), *The Mummy Under the Bed: Essays on Gender and Methodology in the Ancient Near East.* Münster, 125–156.
Mayer, Werner R. 1976. *Untersuchungen zur Formensprache der babylonischen „Gebetsbeschwörungen“.* Rome.

Mayer, Werner R. 1987. "Ein Mythos von der Erschaffung des Menschen und des Königs," *Orientalia Nova Series* 56, 55–68.
Mayer, Werner R. 1992. "Ein Hymnus auf Ninurta als Helfer in der Not," *Orientalia Nova Series* 61, 17–57.
Mayer, Werner R. 2009. Review of CAD T and Ṭ, *Orientalia Nova Series* 78, 423–439.
Mayer, Werner R. 2010. "Die Tätigkeiten und Regungen, Haltungen und Zustände des Menschen im Spiegel der Sprache: zur akkadischen Idiomatik," *Orientalia Nova Series* 79, 304–341.
Mayer, Werner R. 2014. "Nachlese," *Orientalia Nova Series* 83, 380–406.
Mayer, Werner R. 2016. "Zum akkadischen Wörterbuch: A–L," *Orientalia Nova Series* 85, 181–235.
Mayer, Werner R. 2017. "Zum akkadischen Wörterbuch: M–S," *Orientalia Nova Series* 86, 1–41.
Mayer, Werner R. 2019. "Zum Verbaladjektiv im Akkadischen," *Orientalia Nova Series* 88, 293–305.
Mayer, Werner R. 2022a. "Neues zum akkadischen Wörterbuch I," *Orientalia Nova Series* 91, 265–294.
Mayer, Werner R. 2022b. "Neues zum akkadischen Wörterbuch II," *Orientalia Nova Series* 91, 334–350.
Meek, Theophile J. 1913. *Cuneiform Bilingual Hymns, Prayers and Penitential Psalms.* Beiträge zur Assyriologie und semitischen Sprachwissenschaft 10/I. Leipzig.
Meier, Gerhard. 1939. "Ein akkadisches Heilungsritual aus Boğazköy," *Zeitschrift für Assyriologie und Vorderasiatische Archäologie* 45, 195–215.
Meinhold, Wiebke. 2009. *Ištar in Assur. Untersuchung eines Lokalkultes von ca. 2500 bis 614 v. Chr.* Alter Orient und Altes Testament 367. Münster.
Meinhold, Wiebke. 2017. *Ritualbeschreibungen und Gebete II.* Keilschrifttexte aus Assur literarischen Inhalts 7. Wiesbaden.
Meissner, Bruno. 1932–1933. Review of A. Falkenstein, *Literarische Keilschrifttexte aus Uruk, Archiv für Orientforschung* 8, 57–62.
Meloni, Gerardo. 1911–1912. "Testi assiri del British Museum", *Rivista degli Studi Orientali* 4, 559–598.
Menzel, Brigitte. 1989. *Assyrische Tempel.* 2 Vol. Roma.
Michalowski, Piotr. 1978. Review of O. R. Gurney and S. N. Kramer, Sumerian Literary Texts in the Ashmolean Museum, *Journal of Near Eastern Studies* 37, 343–345.
Michalowski, Piotr. 1986. "An Early Old Babylonian Loan Document," *Journal of Cuneiform Studies* 38, 167–171.
Michalowski, Piotr. 1993. "The Torch and the Censer," in: M. E. Cohen, D. C. Snell and D. B. Weisberg (eds.), *The Tablet and the Scroll: Near Eastern Studies in Honor of William W. Hallo.* Bethesda, 152–162.
Michel, Cécile. 1992. "Les fractions dans les tablettes économiques du début de second millénaire en Assyrie et en Babylonie," in: P. Benoit, K. Chemla and J. Ritter (eds.), *Histoire de fractions, fractions d'histoire.* Boston/Berlin, 87–101.
Michel, Cécile. 1997. "Une incantation paléo-assyrienne contre Lamaštu," *Orientalia Nova Series* 66, 58–64.
Michel, Cécile. 2004. "Deux incantations paléo-assyriennes: une nouvelle incantation pour accompagner la naissance," in: J. G. Dercksen (ed.), *Assyria and Beyond: Studies Presented to Mogens Trolle Larsen.* Leiden, 395–420.
Michel, Cécile and Nathan Wasserman. 1997. "Du nouveau sur *šumma zikar a-li-da-ni šumma sinnišat na-ap-TA-ar-ta-ni*," *NABU* 1997/2, 62 No. 64.
Michel, Simone. 1995. "Medizinisch-magische Amulettgemmen. Schutz und Heilung durch Zauber und edle Steine der Antike", *Antike Welt* 26: 379–387.
Michel, Simone. 2004. *Die magischen Gemmen. Zu Bildern und Zauberformeln auf geschnittenen Steinen der Antike und Neuzeit.* Berlin.
Militarev, Alexander and Leonid Kogan. 2000. *Semitic Etymological Dictionary. Vol. I: Anatomy of Man and Animals.* Alter Orient und Altes Testament. Münster.
Militarev, Alexander and Leonid Kogan. 2005. *Semitic Etymological Dictionary. Vol. II: Animal Names.* Alter Orient und Altes Testament 278/2. Münster.
Millard, Alan. 1994. *The Eponyms of the Neo-Assyrian Empire (910–612 BC).* State Archives of Assyria Studies 2. Helsinki.
Minen, Francesca. 2018. "Discendenza, gravidanza e nascita in Mesopotamia antica: i testi ostetrico-ginecologici", in: F. M. Fales and F. Minen, *La medicina assiro-babilonese.* Roma, 167–204.
Minen, Francesca. 2020. Engendering Healthy, Royal Heirs: Some Notes on the Rationale behind the 'Female' Sub-series in *Alamdimmû* and *Sakikkû*," *Le Journal des Médecines Cunéiformes* 36, 10–22.
Mirelman, Sam. 2015. "Birds, Balaĝs, and Snakes (K.4206+)," *Journal of Cuneiform Studies* 67, 169–186.
Monroe, M. Willis. 2016. *Advice from the Stars: The Micro-zodiac in Seleucid Babylonia.* PhD Dissertation, Brown University.
Moore, Ellen W. 1935. *Neo-Babylonian Business and Administrative Documents.* Ann Arbor.
Moran, William L. 1976. "The Keš Temple Hymn and the Canonical Temple List," in: B. Eichler (ed.), *Kramer Anniversary Volume: Studies in Honor of Samuel Noah Kramer.* Alter Orient und Altes Testament 25. Kevelaer, 335–342.
Morgan, Kathryn R. and Seth Richardson. 2020. "Wine from Mamma: *Alluḫarum*-Pots in 17th-Century BC Trade Networks," *Iraq* 82, 179–205.
Müller, Hans-Peter. 1995. "Das Problem der Tierbezeichnungen in der althebräischen Lexikographie," *Studi Epigrafici e Linguistici sul Vicino Oriente antico* 12, 135–147.
Nerlich, Brigitte. 2011. "The Role of Metaphor Scenarios in Disease Management Discourses: Foot and Mouth Disease and Avian Influenza," in: S. Handl and H.-J. Schmid (eds.), *Windows to the Mind: Metaphor, Metonymy and Conceptual Blending.* Berlin, 115–142.
Neumann, Hans. 2008. "Sumerische und akkadische Texte des 3. Jt. v. Chr.," in: B. Janowski and G. Wilhelm (eds.), *Texte aus der Umwelt des Alten Testaments, Neue Folge Band* 4. *Omina, Orakel, Rituale und Beschwörungen.* Gütersloh, 1–15.
Neumann, Hans. 2010. "Texte des 3. Jt. v. Chr.," in: B. Janowski and D. Schwemer (eds.), *Texte aus der Umwelt des Alten Testaments, Neue Folge Band* 5, *Texte zur Heilkunde.* Gütersloh, 3–7.
Nougayrol, Jean. 1949. "Conjuration ancienne contre Samanu," *Archiv Orientální* 17/3–4, 213–226 and Pl. III–V.
Nougayrol, Jean. 1963. "Aleuromancie babylonienne," *Orientalia Nova Series* 32, 381–386.
Nougayrol, Jean. 1965. "Du bon usage des faux," *Syria* 42, 227–234.
Nougayrol, Jean. 1968. "Textes suméro-accadiens des archives et bibliothèques privées d'Ugarit," *Ugaritica* V, 1–367.
Nowicki, Stefan. 2013. "Some Notes about "The Cow of Sin": A Proposal for a New Interpretation", *NABU* 2013/4, 103–104 no. 61.

Obermeyer, Carla M. 2000. "Pluralism and Pragmatism: Knowledge and Practice of Birth in Morocco." *Medical Anthropology Quarterly* 14/2, 180–201.
Oelsner, Joachim. 1996. "Die Entwicklung der Kolophone im neu- und spätbabylonischen Uruk", in: J.-P. Weiss, M. Dubrocard and C. Kircher (eds.), *Hommage au Doyen Weiss.* Publications de la Faculté des Lettres, Art et Sciences Humaines de Nice. Nice, 429–444.
Oelsner, Joachim. 2000. "Von Iqīšâ und einigen anderen spätgeborenen Babyloniern", in: S. Graziani (ed.), *Studi Vicino Orienta Antico dedicati alla Memoria di Luigi Cagni.* Naples, 797–814.
Oelsner, Joachim. 2001. Review of W. von Weiher, Uruk: Spätbabylonische Texte aus dem Planquadrat U 18. Teil 5, *Orientalistische Literaturzeitung* 96, 478–488.
Oppenheim, A. Leo. 1936. "Die akkadischen Personennamen der 'Kassiten-Zeit'," *Anthropos* 31, 470–488.
Oppenheim, A. Leo. 1956. *The Interpretation of Dreams in the Ancient Near East. With a Translation of the Assyrian Dream Book.* Philadelphia.
Oppenheim, A. Leo. 1963. "Mesopotamian Conchology," *Orientalia Nova Series* 32, 407–412.
Oppenheim, A. Leo, R. H. Brill, B. Barag and A. von Saldern. 1970. *Glass and Glassmaking in Ancient Mesopotamia: An Edition of the Cuneiform Texts Which Contain Instructions for Glassmakers with a Catalogue of Surviving Objects.* New York.
Oshima, Takayoshi. 2011. *Babylonian Prayers to Marduk.* Tübingen.
Ossendrijver, Mathieu. 2019. "Babylonian Market Predictions," in: J. Haubold, J. Steele and K. Stevens (eds.), *Keeping Watch in Babylon. The Astronomical Diaries in Context.* Leiden: 53–78.
Otto, Adelheid. 2016. "Professional Women at Work in Mesopotamia and Syria (3rd and early 2nd millennia BC): The (rare) information from visual images," in: B. Lion, C. Michel (Hg.), *The Role of Women in Work and Society in the Ancient Near East.* Boston, 112–148.
Panayotov, Strahil V. 2013. "A Copper Bell to Expel Demons in Berlin," *NABU* 2013/3, 80–87 No. 50.
Panayotov, Strahil V. 2016a. "Fragments of the Nineveh Medical Composition IGI Join UGU," *Le Journal des Médecines Cunéiformes* 27, 59–67.
Panayotov, Strahil V. 2016b. "Addenda and Corrigenda to 'Fragments of the Nineveh Medical Composition IGI Join UGU'," *Le Journal des Médecines Cunéiformes* 28, 66–67.
Panayotov, Strahil V. 2017. "Eye Metaphors, Analogies and Similes within Mesopotamian Magico-Medical Texts," in: J. Z. Wee (ed.), *The Comparable Body: Analogy and Metaphor in Ancient Mesopotamian, Egyptian, and Greco-Roman Medicine*. Studies in Ancient Medicine 49, Leiden/Boston, 204–246.
Panayotov, Strahil V. 2018. "Notes on the Assur Medical Catalogue with Comparison to the Nineveh Medical Encyclopaedia," in: U. Steinert (ed.), *Assyrian and Babylonian Scholarly Text Catalogues: Medicine, Magic and Divination.* Die Babylonisch-assyrische Medizin in Texten und Untersuchungen 9. Berlin/Boston, 89–120.
Panayotov, Strahil V. 2020. "Healing in Images and Texts: The Sickbed Scene," in: J. C. Johnson (ed.), *Patients and Performative Identities: At the Intersection of the Mesopotamian Technical Disciplines and Their Clients.* University Park, 129–158.
Pangas, J. C. 1990. "Notas sobre el aborto en la antigua Mesopotamia," *Aula Orientalis* 8, 213–218.
Parpola, Simo. 1983a. *Letters from Assyrian Scholars to Esarhaddon and Ashurbanipal.* 2 Vol. Alter Orient und Altes Testament 5/1–2. Kevelaer.
Parpola, Simo. 1983b. "Assyrian Library Records", *Journal of Near Eastern Studies* 42, 1–29.
Parpola, Simo. 1997. *Assyrian Prophecies.* State Archives of Assyria 9. Helsinki.
Parpola, Simo and Kazuko Watanabe. 1988. *Neo-Assyrian Treaties and Loyalty Oaths.* State Archives of Assyria 2. Helsinki.
Parys, Magalie. 2014. "Édition d'un texte médical thérapeutique retrouvé à Assur (BAM 159)," *Le Journal des Médecines Cunéiformes* 23, 1–88.
Pedersén, Olof. 1984–1986. "The Reading of the Neo-Assyrian Logogram U.U," *Orientalia Suecana* 33–35, 313–315.
Pedersén, Olof. 1985. *Archives and Libraries in the the City of Assur: A Survey of the Material from the German Excavations. Part I.* Uppsala.
Pedersén, Olof. 1986. *Archives and Libraries in the the City of Assur: A Survey of the Material from the German Excavations. Part II.* Uppsala.
Pedersén, Olof. 1998. *Archives and Libraries of the Ancient Near East 1500–300 B.C.* Bethesda.
Peled, Ilan. 2020. *Law and Gender in the Ancient Near East and the Hebrew Bible.* London.
Perdibon, Anna. 2019. *Mountains and Trees, Rivers and Springs: Animistic Beliefs and Practices and Ancient Mesopotamian Religion.* Leipziger Altorientalische Studien 11. Wiesbaden.
Peterson, Jeremiah. 2009. *God Lists from Old Babylonian Nippur in the University Museum, Philadelphia.* Alter Orient und Altes Testament 362. Münster.
Petschow, Herbert P. H. 1976–1980. "Inzest," in: D. O. Edzard at al. (ed.), *Reallexikon der Assyriologie und Vorderasiatischen Archäologie* 5. Berlin/New York, 144–150.
Philip, Tanja. 2006. *Menstruation and Childbirth in the Bible: Fertility and Impurity.* New York.
Polonsky, Janice. 2002. *The Rise of the Sun God and the Determination of Destiny in Ancient Mesopotamia.* PhD Dissertation, University of Pennsylvania. Ann Arbor.
Polonsky, Janice. 2006. "The Mesopotamian Conceptualization of Birth and the Determination of Destiny at Sunrise," in: Ann K. Guinan et al. (eds.), *If a Man Builds a Joyful House: Assyriological Studies in Honor of Erle Verdun Leichty.* Leiden/Boston, 297–311.
Pommerening, Tanja. 2006. "Überlegungen zur Beurteilung der Wirksamkeit altägyptischer Arzneimittel aus heutiger Sicht," in: K. Zibelius-Chen and H.-W. Fischer-Elfert (eds.), *"Von reichlich ägyptischem Verstande" – Festschrift für Waltraud Guglielmi zum 65. Geburtstag.* Wiesbaden, 103–112.
Pommerening, Tanja. 2015. "Milch einer Frau, die einen Knaben geboren hat," in: P. Kousoulis and N. Lazaridis (eds.), *Proceedings of the Tenth International Congress of Egyptologists. University of the Aegean, Rhodes, 22–29 May, 2008. Vol.* 2. Leuven, 2083–2095.
Pommerening, Tanja. 2023. "The Female Body in Ancient Egypt: Sources, Terminology, and Concepts," in: L. Lehmhaus (ed.), *Female Bodies and Female Practitioners: Gynaecology, Women's Bodies, and Expertise in the Ancient to Medieval Mediterranean and Middle East.* Tübingen, 133–174.
Pommerening, Tanja and Ulrike Steinert. 2019. "Hilfreiche Rezepte überschreiten Grenzen: Zur Behandlung von Würmern mit der Granatapfelwurzel im alten Ägypten und Mesopotamien," in: A. Schubert, W. Leitmeyer and S. Zanke (eds.), *Medicus: Die Macht des Wissens.* Begleitkatalog zur Sonderausstellung, Speyer/Darmstadt, 54–55.
Pongratz-Leisten, Beate. 1994. "Ein neuassyrisches Duplikat zu ḪAR-ra : ḫubullu XV", *Welt des Orients* 25, 66–70.

Postgate, John N. 1994. "Rings, torcs and bracelets", in: P. Calmeyer (ed.), *Beiträge zur altorientalischen Archäologie und Altertumskunde: Festschrift für Barthel Hrouda zum 65. Geburtstag.* Wiesbaden, 235–246.

Postgate, John N. 2000. "Assyrian Felt," in: P. Negri Scafa and P. Gentili (eds.), *Donum natalicium: Studi presentati a Claudio Saporetti in occasione del suo 60. compleanno.* Rome, 213–217.

Postgate, John N. 2001. "Assyrian Uniforms," in: W. H. van Soldt, J. G. Dercksen, N. J. C. Kouwenberg and Th. J. H. Krispijn (eds.), *Veenhof Anniversary Volume: Studies Presented to Klaas R. Veenhof on the Occasion of His Sixty-Fifth Birthday.* Leiden, 373–388.

Potter, Paul. 1988. *Hippocrates. Volume* V. Loeb Classical Library 472. Cambridge, Mass.

Potter, Paul. 2018. *Hippocrates. Volume* XI. Loeb Classical Library 538. Cambridge, Mass.

Powell, Marvin A. 1973. Review of E. Sollberger, Cuneiform Texts from Babylonian Tablets in the British Museum, Part L, *Zeitschrift für Assyriologie und Vorderasiatische Archäologie* 63, 99–106.

Powell, Marvin A. 1987–1990. "Masse und Gewichte," in: D. O. Edzard et al. (ed.), *Reallexikon der Assyriologie und Vorderasiatischen Archäologie* 7. Berlin/New York, 457–517.

Powell, Marvin A. 1994. "Metron Ariston: Measure as a Tool for Studying Beer in Ancient Mesopotamia, in: Lucio Milano (ed.), *Drinking in Ancient Societies: History and Culture of Drinks in the Ancient Near East*, Padova, 91–119.

Powell, Marvin A. 2003–2005. "Obst und Gemüse (Fruits and Vegetables) A.1. Mesopotamien", in: D. O. Edzard, M. P. Streck et al. (eds.), *Reallexikon der Assyriologie und Vorderasiatischen Archäologie* 10. Berlin/New York, 13–22.

Prechel, Doris. 1996. *Die Göttin Išḫara: Ein Beitrag zur altorientalischen Religionsgeschichte.* Münster.

Prechel, Doris and Helmut Freydank. 2014. *Urkunden der königlichen Palastverwalter vom Ende des 2. Jt. v. Chr.: Das "Archiv" Assur 21101 (M7 F).* Studien zu den Assur-Texten 5. Wiesbaden.

Prechel, Doris and Thomas Richter. 2001. "Abrakadabra oder Althurritisch. Betrachtungen zu einigen altbabylonischen Beschwörungstexten," in: T. Richter (ed.), *Kulturgeschichten: Altorientalistische Studien für Volkert Haas zum 65. Geburtstag.* Saarbrücken, 333–371.

Pritzker, Sonya. 2003. "The Role of Metaphor in Culture, Consciousness, and Medicine: A Preliminary Inquiry into the Metaphors of Depression in Chinese and Western Medical and Common Languages," *Clinical Acupuncture and Oriental Medicine* 4, 11–28.

Ramez, Manon. 2019. " «Tu représenteras parfaitement la force de mon héroïsme!» La diorite come vecteur de l'idéologie royale au pays de Sumer et d'Akkad (IIIe et IIe millénaires av. J.-C.)," in: G. Chambon, M. Guichard and A.-I. Langlois (eds.), *De l'argile au numérique: Mélanges assyriologiques en l'honneur de Dominique Charpin.* Leuven, 841–878.

Reade, Julian E. 1986. "Archaeology and the Kuyunjik Archives", in: K. Veenhof, (ed.), *Cuneiform Archives and Libraries: Papers Read at the 30e Rencontre Assyriologique Internationale Leiden, 4–8 July1983.* Leiden, 213–222.

Reade, Julian E. 1998–2001. "Ninive (Nineveh)," in: D. O. Edzard et al. (ed.), *Reallexikon der Assyriologie und Vorderasiatischen Archäologie* 9. Berlin/Boston, 388–433.

Reiner, Erica. 1956. "Lipšur Litanies," *Journal of Near Eastern Studies* 15, 129–149.

Reiner, Erica. 1958. *Šurpu: A Collection of Sumerian and Akkadian Incantations.* Archiv für Orientforschung Beiheft 11. Osnabrück (Reprint 1970).

Reiner, Erica. 1959–1960. "ME.UGU = *mēlu*," *Archiv für Orientforschung* 19, 150–151.

Reiner, Erica. 1961. "The Etiological Myth of the 'Seven Sages'," *Orientalia Nova Series* 30, 1–11.

Reiner, Erica. 1966. "La magie babylonienne," in: *Le monde du sorcier: Egypte, Babylone, Hittites, Israël, Islam, Asie centrale, Inde, Népal, Cambodge, Vietnam, Japon.* Paris, 67–98.

Reiner, Erica. 1969. "Deux cryptogrammes akkadiens," *Revue d'Assyriologie* 63, 170–171.

Reiner, Erica. 1971. "Notes Brèves," *Revue d'Assyriologie* 65, 180–181.

Reiner, Erica. 1973. "Inscription from a Royal Elamite Tomb," *Archiv für Orientforschung* 24, 87–102.

Reiner, Erica. 1978. "Die akkadische Literatur," in: W. Röllig (ed.), *Altorientalische Literatur. Neues Handbuch der Literaturwissenschaft Band* 1. Wiesbaden, 151–210.

Reiner, Erica. 1982a. "Babylonian Birth Prognoses," *Zeitschrift für Assyriologie und Vorderasiatische Archäologie* 72, 124–138.

Reiner, Erica. 1982b. "A Manner of Speaking," in: G. van Driel, Th. J. H. Krispijn, M. Stol and K. R. Veenhof (eds.), *Zikir Šumim: Assyriological Studies Presented to F. R. Kraus on the Occasion of His Seventieth Birthday.* Leiden, 282–289.

Reiner, Erica. 1990. "Nocturnal Talk," in: T. Abusch, J. Huehnergard and P. Steinkeller (eds.), *Lingering over Words: Studies in Ancient Near Eastern Literature in Honor of William L. Moran*. Atlanta, 421–424.

Reiner, Erica. 1995. *Astral Magic in Babylonia.* Transactions of the American Philosophical Society Vol. 85, Part 4. Philadelphia.

Reiner, Erica. 2007. "Supplement to *Chicago Akkadian Dictionary* T (Volume 18)," *Journal of Near Eastern Studies* 66, 47–61.

Reiner, Erica and Miguel Civil. 1967. "Another Volume of Sultantepe Tablets," *Journal of Near Eastern Studies* 26, 177–211.

Reiner, Erica and Miguel Civil. 1990. "La linguistica del Vicino e Medio Oriente," in: G. C. Lepschy (ed.), *Storia della Linguistica, Vol. I.* Bologna, 85–118.

Rendu-Loisel, Anne-Caroline. 2015. "The Voice of Mighty Copper in a Mesopotamian Exorcistic Ritual," in: B. Pongratz-Leisten and K. Sonik (eds.), *The Materiality of Divine Agency.* Boston/Berlin, 211–227.

Rendu-Loisel, Anne-Caroline. 2016. *Les chants du monde: Le paysage sonore de l'ancienne Mésopotamie.* Toulouse.

Renger, Johannes. 1973. "*mārat ilim*: Exogamie bei den semitischen Nomaden des 2. Jt. v. Chr.," Archiv *für Orientforschung* 24, 103–107.

Richter, Thomas. 1999. *Untersuchungen zu den lokalen Panthea Süd- und Mittelbabyloniens in altbabylonischer Zeit.* Alter Orient und Altes Testament 257. Münster.

Richter, Thomas. 2014–2016. "Tutu," in: M. P. Streck et al. (ed.), *Reallexikon der Assyriologie und Vorderasiatischen Archäologie* 14. Berlin/New York, 241–242.

Riddle, John M. 1992. *Contraception and Abortion from the Ancient World to the Renaissance.* Cambridge, Mass.

Ritter, Edith K. 1965. "Magical-Expert (= *Āšipu*) and Physician (= *Asû*): Notes on Two Complementary Professions in Babylonian Medicine," in: H. G. Güterbock and T. Jacobsen (eds.), *Studies in Honor of Benno Landsberger on His Seventy-Fifth Birthday, April 21, 1965.* Assyriological Studies 16. Chicago, 299–322.

Rittig, Dessa. 1977. *Assyrisch-babylonische Kleinplastik magischer Bedeutung vom 13.–6. Jh. v. Chr.* Munich.

Rochberg, Francesca. 1998. *Babylonian Horoscopes*. Transactions of the American Philosophical Society 88/1. Philadelphia.

Rochberg, Francesca. 2016. *Before Nature: Cuneiform Knowledge and the History of Science.* Chicago/London.

Rochberg, Francesca. 2018. *"Ina lumun attalî Sîn: On Evil and Lunar Eclipses,"* in: G. van Buylaere, M. Luukko, D. Schwemer and A. Mertens-Wagschal (eds.), *Sources of Evil: Studies in Mesopotamian Exorcistic Lore*. Ancient Magic and Divination 15. Leiden/Boston, 287–315.

Rochberg-Halton, Francesca. 1988. *Aspects of Babylonian Celestial Divination: The Lunar Eclipse Tablets of Enūma Anu Enlil.* Archiv für Orientforschung Beiheft 22. Horn.

Rodin, Therese. 2014. *The World of the Sumerian Mother Goddess: An Interpretation of Her Myths.* Uppsala. http://urn.kb.se/resolve?urn=urn:nbn:se:uu:diva-228932).

Rodin, Therese. 2019. "The Female Breasts in Sumerian Literature: the sign(s), the contexts and the Akkadian correspondences", in: Mattias Karlsson (ed.), *The Rod and Measuring Rope: Festschrift for Olof Pedersén.* Wiesbaden, 162–183.

Röllig, Wolfgang. 1985. "Der Mondgott und die Kuh: Ein Lehrstück zur Problematik der Textüberlieferung im Alten Orient", *Orientalia Nova Series* 54, 260–273.

Römer, Willem H. Ph. 1966. "Studien zu altbabylonischen hymnisch-epischen Texten (2). Ein Lied über die Jugendjahre der Götter Sîn und Išum (CT 15, 5–6)," *Journal of the American Oriental Society* 86, 138–147.

Römer, Willem H. Ph. 1987. "Rituale und Beschwörungen in sumerischer Sprache", in: *Texte aus der Umwelt des Alten Testaments* II/2. *Rituale und Beschwörungen* I. Gütersloh, 204–207.

Römer, Willem H. Ph. 2001. *Hymnen und Klagelieder in sumerischer Sprache.* Alter Orient und Altes Testament 276. Münster.

Römer, Willem H. Ph. 2007. Review of A. Shaffer, UET 6/3, *Bibliotheca Orientalis* 64, 180–182.

Root-Bernstein, Robert and Michèle Root-Bernstein. 1997. *Honey, Mud, Maggots, and Other Medical Marvels: The Science Behind Folk Remedies and Old Wives' Tales.* Boston/New York.

Roth, Marta. 1997. *Law Collections from Mesopotamia and Asia Minor.* Atlanta.

Rudik, Nadezda. 2011. *Die Entwicklung der keilschriftlichen Beschwörungsliteratur von den Anfängen bis zur Ur III-Zeit.* PhD Dissertation, University of Jena.

Rüster, Christel. 1989. *Hethitisches Zeichenlexikon: Inventar und Interpretation der Keilschriftzeichen aus den Boğazköy-Texten.* Wiesbaden.

Rumor, Maddalena. 2016. "Aluzinnu Versus Ἀλαζών: On the Use of Medical Terminology in the Babylonian and Greek Comic Traditions," in: E. Devecchi, P. Corò, M. Maiocchi and N. de Zorzi (eds.), *Libiamo ne' lieti calici: Ancient Near Eastern Studies Presented to Lucio Milano on the Occasion of his 65th Birthday by Pupils, Colleagues and Friends*. Alter Orient und Altes Testament 436. Münster, 587–603.

Rumor, Maddalena. 2017a. "The 'AŠ-section' of Uruanna III in *Partitur*," *Le Journal des Médecines Cunéiformes* 29, 1–34.

Rumor, Maddalena. 2017b. "There's No Fool like an Old Fool: The Mesopotamian *Aluzinnu* and Its Relationship to Greek *Alazôn*," *KASKAL – Rivista di storia, ambienti e culture del Vicino Oriente Antico* 14, 187–210.

Rumor, Maddalena. 2018. "At the Dawn of Plant Taxonomy: Shared Structural Design of Herbal Descriptions in *Šammu šikinšu* and Theophrastus' *Historia plantarum* IX," in: S. V. Panayotov and L. Vacín (eds.), *Mesopotamian Medicine and Magic: Studies in Honor of Markham J. Geller.* Ancient Magic and Divination 14. Leiden/Boston, 446–461.

Rumor, Maddalena. 2020. "*Dreck-*, *Deck-*, or what the heck?", *Le Journal des Médecines Cunéiformes* 36, 37–53.

Rumor, Maddalena. 2021. "Medicinal Plants, Foods, and Spices in Ancient Mesopotamia," in: H. Perdicoyianni-Paléologou (ed.), *Health, Disease and Healing from Antiquity to Byzantium: Medicinal Foods, Plants and Spices. Byzantinische Forschungen* 33, Amsterdam, 21–37.

Rumor, Maddalena. 2024. *Perplexing Remedies in Mesopotamian Medicine. Dreckapotheke in Mesopotamia and the Graeco-Roman World.* Berlin/Boston.

Rutz, Matthew T. 2011. "Threads for Esagil-kīn-apli: The Medical Diagnostic-Prognostic Series in Middle Babylonian Nippur," *Zeitschrift für Assyriologie und Vorderasiatische Archäologie* 101, 294–308.

Rutz, Matthew T. 2013. *Bodies of Knowledge in Ancient Mesopotamia: The Diviners of Late Bronze Age Emar and their Tablet Collection.* Ancient Magic and Divination 9. Leiden/Boston.

Rutz, Matthew T. 2016. "Anti-Witchcraft Prescriptions from Hattuša and Nippur," *Zeitschrift für Assyriologie und Vorderasiatische Archäologie* 106, 42–61.

Sachs, Abraham. 1952. "Babylonian Horoscopes," *Journal of Cuneiform Studies* 6, 49–75.

Sachs, Abraham J. and Hermann Hunger. 1996. *Astronomical Diaries and Related Texts from Babylonia, Vol. 3: Diaries from 164 B.C. to 61 B.C.* Wien.

Sallaberger, Walter. 1996. *Der babylonische Töpfer und seine Gefäße: Nach Urkunden altsumerischer bis altbabylonischer Zeit sowie lexikalischen und literarischen Zeugnissen.* Ghent.

Sallaberger, Walter and Fabienne Huber Vulliet. 2003–2005. "Priester. A. I. Mesopotamien," in: D. O. Edzard, M. P. Streck et al. (eds.), *Reallexikon der Assyriologie und Vorderasiatischen Archäologie* 10. Berlin/New York, 617–640.

Salonen, Armas. 1973. *Vögel und Vogelfang im Alten Mesopotamien.* Helsinki.

San Nicolò, Mariano and Arthur Ungnad. 1935. *Neubabylonische Rechts- und Verwaltungsurkunden. Band 1: Rechts- und Wirtschaftsurkunden der Berliner Museen aus vorhellenistischer Zeit.* Leipzig.

Sandowicz, Małgorzata. (forthcoming). *Their Mothers' Children: Neo- and Late Babylonian Matronyms.* [non videt]

Sassmannshausen, Leonard. 1995. "Funktion und Stellung der Herolde (NIGIR / *nāgiru*) im alten Orient," *Baghdader Mitteilungen* 26, 85–194.

Sassmannshausen, Leonard. 2001. *Beiträge zur Verwaltung und Gesellschaft Babyloniens in der Kassitenzeit.* Baghdader Forschungen 21. Mainz am Rhein.

Scarpelli, Tommaso. 2024. *Das Wetter in der mesopotamischen Kulturgeschichte des II. und I. Jahrtausends v. Chr.* Wiesbaden.

Schmidtchen, Eric. 2018a. "Esagil-kīn-apli's Catalogue of *Sakikkû* and *Alamdimmû*," in: U. Steinert (ed.), *Assyrian and Babylonian Scholarly Text Catalogues: Medicine, Magic and Divination.* Die Babylonisch-assyrische Medizin in Texten und Untersuchungen 9. Berlin/Boston, 137–157.

Schmidtchen, Eric. 2018b. "The Edition of Esagil-kīn-apli's Catalogue of the Series *Sakikkû* (SA.GIG) and *Alamdimmû*," in: U. Steinert (ed.), *Assyrian and Babylonian Scholarly Text Catalogues: Medicine, Magic and Divination.* Die Babylonisch-assyrische Medizin in Texten und Untersuchungen 9. Berlin/Boston, 313–333.

Schmidtchen, Eric. 2018c. "Simplicia and Unpublished Fragments of *Alamdimmû* from the British Museum," in: S. V. Panayotov and L. Vacín (eds.), *Mesopotamian Medicine and Magic: Studies in Honor of Markham J. Geller.* Ancient Magic and Divination 14. Leiden/Boston, 462–500.

Schmidtchen, Eric. 2019. "A Short Note on a New Join to K. 3628+ (Epileptic and Demonic Afflictions of Infants)," *Le Journal des Médecines Cunéiformes* 33, 32–34.

Schmidtchen, Eric. 2020. "Corrigenda to Schmidtchen, E., Simplicia and Unpublished Fragments of *Alamdimmû* from the British Museum," *NABU* 2020/2, 174 No. 81.

Schmidtchen, Eric. 2021a. *Mesopotamische Diagnostik: Untersuchungen zu Rekonstruktion, Terminologie und Systematik des babylonisch-assyrischen Diagnosehandbuchs und eine Neubearbeitung der Tafeln 3–14.* Babylonisch-assyrische Medizin in Texten und Untersuchungen 13. Berlin/Boston.

Schmidtchen, Eric. 2021b. "Demons, Deputies of the Gods, and How to Get Rid of Them: CTN 4, 72 and Some New Duplicates," *Le Journal des Médecines Cunéiformes* 37, 31–68.

Schmidtchen, Eric. 2023. "New Joins for the Reverse of *Šumma izbu* Tablet 4, Including a Reconstruction of *Iqqur īpuš* §64," *NABU* 2023/1, 33–40 No. 18.

Schnitzlein, Babette. 2023. *Untersuchungen zur Schreibkultur Mesopotamiens im 1. Jahrtausend v. Chr.* Boston/Berlin.

Schollmeyer, Anastasius. 1912. *Sumerisch-babylonische Hymnen und Gebete an Šamaš.* Paderborn.

Schramm, Wolfgang. 2008. *Ein Compendium sumerisch-akkadischer Beschwörungen.* Göttinger Beiträge zum Alten Orient 2. Göttingen.

Schreiber, Marvin. 2018a. "Spiegel des Himmels: Synchronisation von Himmel und Erde in der babylonischen Leberschau, Iatromathematik und dem 20-Felder-Spiel," in: S. V. Panayotov and L. Vacín (eds.), *Mesopotamian Medicine and Magic: Studies in Honor of Markham J. Geller.* Ancient Magic and Divination 14. Leiden/Boston, 501–527.

Schreiber, Marvin. 2018b. *Die astrologische Medizin der spätbabylonischen Zeit.* PhD Dissertation Humboldt-Universität Berlin.

Schretter, Manfred K. 1990. *Emesal-Studien: Sprach- und literaturgeschichtliche Untersuchungen zur sogenannten Frauensprache des Sumerischen.* Innsbruck.

Schuster-Brandis, Anais. 2008. *Steine als Schutz- und Heilmittel. Untersuchung zu ihrer Verwendung in der Beschwörungskunst Mesopotamiens im 1. Jt. v. Chr.* Alter Orient und Altes Testament 46. Münster.

Schwemer, Daniel. 1998. *Akkadische Rituale aus Hattuša: Die Sammeltafel KBo XXXVI 29 und verwandte Fragmente.* Heidelberg.

Schwemer, Daniel. 2001. *Die Wettergottgestalten Mesopotamiens und Nordsyriens im Zeitalter der Keilschriftkulturen: Materialien und Studien nach den schriftlichen Quellen.* Wiesbaden.

Schwemer, Daniel. 2007a. *Abwehrzauber und Behexung: Studien zum Schadenzauberglauben im alten Mesopotamien.* Wiesbaden.

Schwemer, Daniel. 2007b. *Rituale und Beschwörungen gegen Schadenzauber.* Keilschrifttexte aus Assur literarischen Inhalts 2. Wiesbaden.

Schwemer, Daniel. 2007c. "The Storm-Gods in the Ancient Near East: Summary, Synthesis, Recent Studies, Part I," *Journal of Ancient Near Eastern Religions* 7, 123–168.

Schwemer, Daniel. 2009. "Washing, Defiling and Burning: Two Bilingual Witchcraft Incantations," *Orientalia Nova Series* 78, 44–68.

Schwemer, Daniel. 2010a. "Fighting Witchcraft before the Moon and Sun: A Therapeutic Ritual from Neo-Babylonian Sippar," *Orientalia Nova Series* 79, 480–504.

Schwemer, Daniel. 2010b. "Altbabylonische therapeutische Texte," in: B. Janowski and D. Schwemer (eds.) *Texte zur Heilkunde. Texte aus der Umwelt des Alten Testaments, Neue Folge Band* 5. Gütersloh 2010, 35–38.

Schwemer, Daniel. 2010c. "Therapeutische Texte aus Hattuša und Emar," in: B. Janowski and D. Schwemer (eds.) *Texte zur Heilkunde. Texte aus der Umwelt des Alten Testaments, Neue Folge Band* 5. Gütersloh 2010, 38–45.

Schwemer, Daniel. 2011. "Magic rituals: Conceptualization and performance," in: K. Radner and E. Robson (eds.), *The Oxford Handbook of Cuneiform Culture.* Oxford, 419–441.

Schwemer, Daniel. 2013. "Gauging the Influence of the Babylonian Magic: The Reception of Mesopotamian Traditions in Hittite Ritual Practice," in: E. Cancik-Kirschbaum, J. Klinger and G. G. W. Müller (eds.), *Diversity and Standardization: Perspectives on Social and Political Norms in the Ancient Near East.* Berlin, 145–171.

Schwemer, Daniel. 2015. "Secret Knowledge of Lu-Nanna, the Sage of Ur," in: A. Müller-Karpe, E. Rieken and W. Sommerfeld (eds.), *Saeculum. Gedenkschrift für Heinrich Otten anlässlich seines 100. Geburtstags.* Wiesbaden, 211–228.

Schwemer, Daniel. 2017. *The Anti-Witchcraft Ritual Maqlû: The Cuneiform Sources of a Magic Ceremony form Ancient Mesopotamia.* Wiesbaden.

Schwemer, Daniel. 2021. "KU.KU = *supantu, supandu*," *NABU* 2021/2, 117 No. 48.

Scurlock, JoAnn. 1988. *Magical Means of Dealing with Ghosts in Ancient Mesopotamia.* PhD. Dissertation, University of Chicago.

Scurlock, JoAnn. 1991. "Baby-Snatching Demons, Restless Souls and the Dangers of Childbirth: Medico-Magical Means of Dealing with Some of the Perils of Motherhood in Ancient Mesopotamia," *Incognita* 2, 137–185.

Scurlock, JoAnn. 1999. "Physician, exorcist, conjurer, magician: A tale of two healing professionals," in: T. Abusch and K. van der Toorn (eds.), *Mesopotamian Magic: Textual, Historical, and Interpretative Perspectives.* Groningen, 69–79.

Scurlock, JoAnn. 2002. "Translating Transfers in Ancient Mesopotamia," in: P. Mirecki and M. Meyer (eds.), *Magic and Ritual in the Ancient World.* Leiden/Boston, 209–223.

Scurlock, JoAnn. 2003. "Collation of the 'Jastrow'," *Le Journal des Médecines Cunéiformes* 2, 16–17.

Scurlock, JoAnn. 2005. "Ancient Mesopotamian Medicine," in: D. C. Snell (ed.), *A Companion to the Ancient Near East.* Malden, 302–315.

Scurlock, JoAnn. 2006. *Magico-Medical Means of Treating Ghost-Induced Illness in Ancient Mesopotamia.* Ancient Magic and Divination 3. Leiden/Boston.

Scurlock, JoAnn. 2014a. *Sourcebook for Ancient Mesopotamian Medicine*, Atlanta.

Scurlock, JoAnn. 2014b. "Medicine and Healing Magic", in: M. W. Chavalas (ed.), *Women in the Ancient Near East: A Sourcebook.* London/New York, 101–143.

Scurlock, JoAnn. 2017. "Medical Texts," in: K. Lawson Younger (ed.), *The Context of Scripture. Volume 4: Supplements.* Leiden, 277–312.

Scurlock, JoAnn. 2020. "Blind mice and despairing rats: the uses of *kurkanû*-tumeric in ancient and modern medicine," *Le Journal des Médecines Cunéiformes* 35, 34–68.
Scurlock, JoAnn and Burton R. Andersen. 2005. *Diagnoses in Assyrian and Babylonian Medicine: Ancient Sources, Translations, and Modern Medical Analyses.* Urbana/Chicago.
Seidl, Ursula. 1989. *Die babylonischen Kudurru-Reliefs. Symbole mesopotamischer Gottheiten.* Orbis Biblicus et Orientalis 87. Fribourg/Göttingen.
Seminara, Stefano. 2001. *La versione accadica del Lugal-e: La tecnica babilonese della traduzione dal sumerico e le sue "regule".* Roma.
Seux, Marie-Joseph. 1976. *Hymnes et prières aux dieux de Babylonie et d'Assyrie.* Paris.
Sibbing-Plantholt, Irene. 2014. "A New Look at the Kassite Medical Letters, and an Edition of Šumu-libši Letter N 969," *Zeitschrift für Assyriologie und Vorderasiatische Archäologie* 104, 171–182.
Sibbing-Plantholt, Irene. 2021. "Visible Death and Audible Distress: The Personification of Death (*Mūtu*) and Associated Emotions as Inherent Conditions of Life in Akkadian Sources," in: S.-W. Hsu and J. Llop-Raduà (eds.), *The Expression of Emotions in Ancient Egypt and Mesopotamia.* Culture and History of the Ancient Near East 116. Leiden/Boston, 335–389.
Sibbing-Plantholt, Irene. 2022. *The Image of Mesopotamian Divine Healers: Healing Goddesses and the Legitimization of Professional asûs in the Mesopotamian Medical Marketplace.* Cuneiform Monographs 53. Leiden/Boston.
Sigrist, Marcel. 1980. "Une tablette d'incantation sumérienne", *ASJ* 2, 153–167.
Simkó, Krisztián. 2017. "Sm. 1402: a new manuscript of the 'Kette Hammurapis'?", *NABU* 2017/4, 185–188 No. 105.
Simkó, Krisztián. 2018. "*BAM* 7 44: Suppositories for Rectal and Gastro-Intestinal Diseases," in: S. V. Panayotov and L. Vacín (eds.), *Mesopotamian Medicine and Magic: Studies in Honor of Markham J. Geller.* Ancient Magic and Divination 14. Leiden/Boston, 537–555.
Simons, Frank. 2018. "The Goddess Kusu," *Revue d'Assyriologie* 112, 123–148.
Sjöberg, Åke W. 1972. "'He Is a Good Seed of a Dog' and 'Engardu, the Fool' *Journal of Cuneiform Studies* 24, 107–119.
Sjöberg, Åke W. 1973. "Der Vater und sein missratener Sohn," *Journal of Cuneiform Studies* 25, 105–169.
Sjöberg, Åke W. 1975. "in-nin šà-gur$_4$-ra: A Hymn to the Goddess Inanna by the en-Priestess Enḫeduanna," *Zeitschrift für Assyriologie und Vorderasiatische Archäologie* 65, 161–253.
Sjöberg, Åke W. and Eugen Bergmann. 1969. *The Collection of the Sumerian Temple Hymns (and The Keš Temple Hymn by Gene B. Gragg).* Texts from Cuneiform Sources 3. Locust Valley.
Sokoloff, Michael. 2002. *A Dictionary of Jewish Babylonian Aramaic of the Talmudic and Geonic Periods.* Ramat-Gan.
Spar, Ira and Eva van Dassow. 2000. *Private Archive Texts from the First Millennium B.C.* Cuneiform Texts in the Metropolitan Museum of Art 3. New York.
Stadhouders, Henry. 2011. "The Pharmacopoeial Handbook *Šammu šikinšu* – An Edition," *Le Journal des Médecines Cunéiformes* 18, 3–51.
Stadhouders, Henry. 2012. "The Pharmacopoeial Handbook *Šammu šikinšu* – A Translation," *Le Journal des Médecines Cunéiformes* 19, 1–21.
Stadhouders, Henry. 2018a. "The Unfortunate Frog: On Animal and Human Bondage in K. 2581 and Related Fragments with Excurses on BM 64526 and *YOS* XI, 3," *Revue d'Assyriologie* 112, 159–176.
Stadhouders, Henry. 2018b. "A posological curiosity: the date stone as a unit of measurement (being an edition of BM 59626, ft. BM 40051, 54914, 59623, 64526)," *NABU* 2018/3, 125–129 No. 81.
Stadhouders, Henry and J. Cale Johnson. 2018. "A Time to Extract and a Time to Compile: The Therapeutic Compendium Tablet BM 78963," in: S. V. Panayotov and L. Vacín (eds.), *Mesopotamian Medicine and Magic: Studies in Honor of Markham J. Geller.* Ancient Magic and Divination 14. Leiden/Boston, 556–622.
Stadhouders, Henry and Ulrike Steinert. 2018. "Two Rituals to Postpone an Ill-omened Childbirth: An Edition of KAR 223 and Duplicates," *Le Journal des Médecines Cunéiformes* 32, 56–78.
Stamm, Johann J. 1939. *Die akkadische Namengebung.* Leipzig.
Stein, Diana. 2009. "Winged Disks and Sacred Trees at Nuzi: An Altered Perspective on Two Imperial Motifs," *Studies on the Culture and Civilization of Nuzi and the Hurrians* 18, 573–603.
Steinert, Ulrike. 2012a. *Aspekte des Menschseins im Alten Mesopotamien: Eine Studie zu Person und Identität im 2. und 1. Jt. v. Chr.* Cuneiform Monographs 44. Leiden/Boston.
Steinert, Ulrike. 2012b. "K. 263+10934, A Tablet with Recipes Against the Abnormal Flow of a Woman's Blood", *Sudhoffs Archiv. Zeitschrift für Wissenschaftsgeschichte* 96/1, 64–94.
Steinert, Ulrike. 2013. "Fluids, Rivers, and Vessels: Metaphors and Body Concepts in Mesopotamian Gynaecological Texts," *Le Journal des Médecines Cunéiformes* 22, 1–23.
Steinert, Ulrike. 2014a. "I smell a rat! Fumigation in Mesopotamian and Hippocratic recipes for women's ailments – Part 1", The Recipes Project. Food, Magic, Art, Science and Medicine (posted 11 March, 2014). http://recipes.hypotheses.org/3278.
Steinert, Ulrike. 2014b. "I smell a rat! Fumigation in Mesopotamian and Hippocratic recipes for women's ailments – Part 2", The Recipes Project. Food, Magic, Art, Science and Medicine (posted 13 March, 2014). http://recipes.hypotheses.org/3284.
Steinert, Ulrike. 2015. "Tested Remedies in Mesopotamian Medical Texts: A Label for Efficacy Based on Empirical Observation?", in: J. C. Johnson (ed.), *In the Wake of the Compendia: Infrastructural Contexts and the Licensing of Empiricism in Ancient and Medieval Mesopotamia.* Boston/Berlin, 103–145.
Steinert, Ulrike. 2016. Review of Walter Farber, Lamaštu. An Edition of the Canonical Series of Lamaštu Incantations and Rituals and Related Texts from the Second and First Millennia B.C., *Zeitschrift für Assyriologie und Vorderasiatische Archäologie* 106, 240–251.
Steinert, Ulrike. 2017a. "Concepts of the Female Body in Mesopotamian Gynecological Texts", in: J. Z. Wee (ed.), *The Comparable Body: Analogy and Metaphor in Ancient Mesopotamian, Egyptian, and Greco-Roman Medicine.* Studies in Ancient Medicine 49. Leiden/Boston, 275–357.
Steinert, Ulrike. 2017b. "Cows, Women and Wombs: Interrelations between Texts and Images from the Ancient Near East," in: D. Kertai and O. Nieuwenhuyse (eds.), *From the Four Corners of the Earth: Studies in Iconography and Cultures of the Ancient Near East in Honour of F. A. M. Wiggermann.* Alter Orient und Altes Testament 441. Münster, 205–258.

Steinert, Ulrike. 2018. "Catalogues, Texts, and Specialists: Some Thoughts on the Assur Medical Catalogue and Mesopotamian Healing Professions," in: U. Steinert (ed.), *Assyrian and Babylonian Scholarly Text Catalogues: Medicine, Magic and Divination.* Die babylonisch-assyrische Medizin in Texten und Untersuchungen 9. Berlin/Boston, 158–200.

Steinert, Ulrike (ed.). 2018. *Assyrian and Babylonian Scholarly Text Catalogues: Medicine, Magic and Divination.* Die Babylonisch-assyrische Medizin in Texten und Untersuchungen 9. Berlin/Boston.

Steinert, Ulrike. 2020. "Healing Substances and Therapies in Mesopotamian Women's Health Care Texts: Properties, Effects and Cultural Meanings," *Le Journal des Médecines Cunéiformes* 36, 54–72.

Steinert, Ulrike. 2021a. "Medicinal Substances in Ancient Mesopotamian Women's Health Care Texts," in: H. Perdicoyianni-Paléologou (ed.), *Health, Disease and Healing from Antiquity to Byzantium: Medicinal Foods, Plants and Spices. Byzantinische Forschungen* 33, Amsterdam, 39–80.

Steinert, Ulrike. 2021b. "Disease Concepts and Classifications in Ancient Mesopotamian Medicine," in: U. Steinert (ed.), *Systems of Classification in Premodern Medical Cultures: Sickness, Health and Local Epistemologies.* London, 140–194.

Steinert, Ulrike. 2022. "Ecstatic Experience and Possession Disorders in Ancient Mesopotamia," in: D. Stein, S. K. Costello and K. Polinger Foster (eds.), *The Routledge Companion to Ecstatic Experience in the Ancient World.* London, 369–396.

Steinert, Ulrike. 2023. "Created to Bleed: Blood, Women's Bodies and Gender in Ancient Mesopotamian Medicine," in: L. Lehmhaus (ed.), *Female Bodies and Female Practitioners. Gynaecology, Female Bodies, and Expertise in the Ancient to Medieval Mediterranean and Middle East.* Tübingen, 233–305.

Steinert, Ulrike. 2024. "Mesopotamian Amulet Prescriptions for Preventing and Averting Fear," in: A. Berlejung and G. Bohak (eds.), *Amulets of Protection and Texts for Fears in Antiquity.* Tübingen, 117–146.

Steinert, Ulrike and Paola Paoletti. 2014–2016. "Uterus," in: M. P. Streck et al. (ed.), *Reallexikon der Assyriologie und Vorderasiatischen Archäologie* 14. Berlin/New York, 513–516.

Steinert, Ulrike and Luděk Vacín. 2018. "BM 92518 and Old Babylonian Incantations for the 'Belly'," in: S. V. Panayotov and L. Vacín (eds.), *Mesopotamian Medicine and Magic: Studies in Honor of Markham J. Geller.* Boston/Leiden, 694–740.

Steinkeller, Piotr. 2022. "On Prostitutes, Midwives and Tavern-Keepers in Third Millennium BC Babylonia," *KASKAL – Rivista di storia, ambienti e culture del Vicino Oriente Antico* 19, 1–38.

Stol, Marten. 1971. "Zur altmesopotamischen Bierbereitung," *Bibliotheca Orientalis* 28, 167–171.

Stol, Marten. 1979. *On Trees, Mountains, and Millstones in the Ancient Near East.* With a chapter by K. van Lerberghe. Leiden.

Stol, Marten. 1980–1983. "Leder(industrie)," in: D. O. Edzard et al. (ed.), *Reallexikon der Assyriologie und Vorderasiatischen Archäologie* 6. Berlin/New York, 527–543.

Stol, Marten. 1983–1984. "Cress and Its Mustard," *Jaarbericht van het Vooraziatisch-Egyptisch Genootschap "Ex Oriente Lux"* 28, 24–32.

Stol, Marten. 1984. "Beer in Neo-Babylonian Times," in: L. Milano (ed.), *Drinking in Ancient Societies: History and Culture of Drinks in the Ancient Near East. Papers of a Symposium Held in Rome, May 17–19, 1990.* Padova, 155–183.

Stol, Marten. 1985a. "Beans, Peas, Lentils and Vetches in Akkadian Texts," *Bulletin on Sumerian Agriculture* 2, 127–139.

Stol, Marten. 1985b. "Fragment of a Herding Contract," in: J.-M. Durand and J.-R. Kupper (eds.), *Miscellanea Babylonica: Mélanges offers à Maurice Birot.* Paris, 273–275.

Stol, Marten. 1987a. "Garlic, Onion, Leek," *Bulletin on Sumerian Agriculture* 3, 57–80.

Stol, Marten. 1987b. "The Cucurbitaceae in the Cuneiform Texts," *Bulletin on Sumerian Agriculture* 3, 81–92.

Stol, Marten. 1987–1990. "Malz," in: D. O. Edzard et al. (ed.), *Reallexikon der Assyriologie und Vorderasiatischen Archäologie* 7. Berlin/New York, 322–329.

Stol, Marten. 1988a. "Old Babylonian Fields," *Bulletin on Sumerian Agriculture* 4, 173–188.

Stol, Marten. 1991–1992. "Diagnosis and Therapy in Babylonian Medicine," *Jaarbericht van het Vooraziatisch-Egyptisch Genootschap "Ex Oriente Lux"* 32, 42–65.

Stol, Marten. 1992. "The Moon as Seen by the Babylonians", in: D. J. W. Meijer (ed.), *Natural Phenomena: Their Meaning, Depiction and Description in the Ancient Near East.* Amsterdam, 245–277.

Stol, Marten. 1993. *Epilepsy in Babylonia.* Cuneiform Monographs 2. Groningen.

Stol, Marten. 1993–1997a. "Mohrhirse," in: D. O. Edzard et al. (ed.), *Reallexikon der Assyriologie und Vorderasiatischen Archäologie* 8. Berlin/New York, 348–349.

Stol, Marten. 1993–1997b. "Milch(produkte). A. In Mesopotamien", in: D. O. Edzard et al. (ed.), *Reallexikon der Assyriologie und Vorderasiatischen Archäologie* 8. Berlin/New York, 189–201.

Stol, Marten. 1994. "Beer in Neo-Babylonian Times", in: Lucio Milano (ed.), *Drinking in Ancient Societies: History and Culture of Drinks in the Ancient Near East.* Padova, 155–183.

Stol, Marten. 1998. "Einige kurze Wortstudien," in: S. M. Maul (ed.), *Festschrift für Rykle Borger zu seinem 65. Geburtstag am 24. Mai 1994: Tikip santakki mala bašmu ... .* Groningen, 343–352.

Stol, Marten. 2000a. *Birth in Babylonia and the Bible. With a Chapter by F.A.M. Wiggermann.* Cuneiform Monographs 14. Groningen.

Stol, Marten. 2000b. Review of J. A. Black, A. R. George, N. Postgate (eds.), A Concise Dictionary of Akkadian. *Bibliotheca Orientalis* 57, 626–629.

Stol, Marten. 2002–2005a. "Pflanzenkunde. A. Nach schriftlichen Quellen," in: D. O. Edzard and M. P. Streck (eds.), *Reallexikon der Assyriologie und Vorderasiatischen Archäologie* 10. Berlin/New York, 503–506.

Stol, Marten. 2002–2005b. "Pharmakologie," in: D. O. Edzard and M. P. Streck (eds.), *Reallexikon der Assyriologie und Vorderasiatischen Archäologie* 10. Berlin/New York, 524–525.

Stol, Marten. 2006–2008. "Rasieren," in: M. P. Streck et al. (ed.), *Reallexikon der Assyriologie und Vorderasiatischen Archäologie* 11. Berlin/New York, 260–262.

Stol, Marten. 2007a. "Fevers in Babylonia," in: I. L. Finkel and M. J. Geller (eds.), *Disease in Babylonia.* Cuneiform Monographs 36. Leiden/Boston, 1–39.

Stol, Marten. 2007b. "An unusual prescription: oral tradition?", *Le Journal des Médecines Cunéiformes* 10, 1–3.

Stol, Marten. 2007c. Review of A. Militarev and L. Kogan, Semitic Etymological Dictionary. Vol. I: Anatomy of Man and Animals," *Bibliotheca Orientalis* 64, 332–335.

Stol, Marten. 2009a. "'To be ill' in Akkadian: The Verb *Salā'u* and the Substantive *Sili'tu*," in: A. Attia and G. Buisson (eds.), *Advances in Mesopotamian Medicine from Hammurabi to Hippocrates. Proceedings of the International Conference "Oeil Malade et Mauvais Oeil", Collège de France, Paris, 23rd June 2006.* Cuneiform Monographs 37. Leiden/Boston, 29–46.

Stol, Marten. 2009b. "Embryology in Babylonia and the Bible," in: J. M. Law and V. R. Sasson (eds.), *Imagining the Fetus: The Unborn in Myth, Religion, and Culture*. Oxford Scholarship Online, DOI: 10.1093/acprof:oso/9780195380040.001.0001.

Stol, Marten. 2008. Review of CAD P, *Orientalistische Literaturzeitung* 103, 348–355.

Stol, Marten. 2009–2011. "Schwefel," in: M. P. Streck et al. (ed.), *Reallexikon der Assyriologie und Vorderasiatischen Archäologie* 12. Berlin, 317–319.

Stol, Marten. 2011. "Pferde, Pferdekrankheiten und Pferdemedizin in altbabylonischer Zeit," in: O. Loretz, *Hippologica Ugaritica: Das Pferd in Kultur, Wirtschaft, Kriegführung und Hippiatrie Ugarits.* Alter Orient und Altes Testament 386. Münster, 363–402.

Stol, Marten. 2011–2013. "Thymian," in: M. P. Streck et al. (ed.), *Reallexikon der Assyriologie und Vorderasiatischen Archäologie* 13. Berlin/Boston, 641–642.

Stol, Marten. 2012. "Birth. Ancient Near East and Hebrew Bible/Old Testament," in: H.-J. Klauck et al. (ed.), *Encyclopedia of the Bible and Its Reception*, Vol. 4. Berlin/New York, 1–6.

Stol, Marten. 2013. Review of T. Abusch and D. Schwemer, Corpus of Mesopotamian Anti-Witchcraft Rituals, Volume 1, *Bibliotheca Orientalis* 70, 125–130.

Stol, Marten. 2016a. *Women in the Ancient Near East.* Berlin/Boston.

Stol, Marten. 2016b. Review of U. Steinert, Aspekte des Menschseins im Alten Mesopotamien, *Bibliotheca Orientalis* 73, 418–423.

Stol, Marten. 2016–2018a. "Wein. A. In Mesopotamien," in: M. P. Streck et al. (eds.), *Reallexikon der Assyriologie und Vorderasiatischen Archäologie* 15. Berlin/Boston, 37–42.

Stol, Marten. 2016–2018b. "Knochen (Material). A. Philologisch," in: M. P. Streck et al. (eds.), *Reallexikon der Assyriologie und Vorderasiatischen Archäologie* 15. Berlin/Boston, 411–413.

Stol, Marten. 2017. Review of T. Abusch and D. Schwemer, with M. Luukko and G. van Buylaere, Corpus of Mesopotamian Anti-Witchcraft Literature, Volume 2, *Bibliotheca Orientalis* 74, 371–379.

Stol, Marten. 2018. "Teeths and Toothache," in: S. V. Panayotov and L. Vacín (eds.), *Mesopotamian Medicine and Magic: Studies in Honor of Markham J. Geller.* Ancient Magic and Divination 14. Leiden/Boston, 745–770.

Stol, Marten. 2020a. Review of M. P. Streck, Supplement to the Akkadian Dictionaries, Vol. 1, *Bibliotheca Orientalis* 77, 101–110.

Stol, Marten. 2020b. Review of T. Abusch et al., Corpus of Mesopotamian Anti-Witchcraft Literature, Volume 3 and M. Luukko and G. van Buylaere, Corpus of Mesopotamian Anti-Witchcraft Literature, Volume 4, *Bibliotheca Orientalis* 77, 567–573.

Stol, Marten. 2021. Review of Michael P. Streck (ed.), Supplement to the Akkadian Dictionaries, Vol. 2 (D, T, Ṭ). *Bibliotheca Orientalis* 78, 431–458.

Stol, Marten. 2022. Review of D. L. Stein, S. K. Costello and K. Pollinger Foster (eds.), The Routledge Companion to Ecstatic Experience in the Ancient World, *Bibliotheca Orientalis* 79, 325–329.

Stol, Marten. Forthcoming. "The Asafoetida in Cuneiform Texts," in: *PIHANS* 136, 313–330.

Stolper, Matthew W. 1998–2001. "Nahhunte," in: D. O. Edzard et al. (ed.), *Reallexikon der Assyriologie und Vorderasiatischen Archäologie* 9. Berlin/Boston, 82–84.

Streck, Michael P. 1995. *Zahl und Zeit: Grammatik der Numeralia und des Verbalsystems im Spätbabylonischen.* Cuneiform Monographs 5. Groningen.

Streck, Michael P. 2004. "Dattelpalme und Tamariske in Mesopotamien nach dem akkadischen Streitgespräch," *Zeitschrift für Assyriologie und Vorderasiatische Archäologie* 94, 250–290.

Streck, Michael P. 2009. Review of CAD Ṭ, *Zeitschrift für Assyriologie und Vorderasiatische Archäologie* 99, 135–140.

Streck, Michael P. 2011–2013. "Tamariske (tamarisk)", in: M. P. Streck et al. (ed.), *Reallexikon der Assyriologie und Vorderasiatischen Archäologie* 13. Berlin/Boston, 428–431.

Streck, Michael P. 2021. "Old Babylonian," in: J.-P. Vita (ed.), *History of the Akkadian Language, Volume 1: Linguistic Background and Early Periods.* Handbook of Oriental Studies 152/2. Leiden, 993–1038.

Sturm, Thomas. 2008. "*Allānū* – Haselnüsse als Delikatesse im *kārum*-zeitlichen Handel von Anatolien nach Nordmesopotamien (ca. 1930–1730 v. Chr.)," *Altorientalische Forschungen* 35, 296–311.

Tallquist, Knut L. 1918. *Assyrian Personal Names*. Helsingfors.

Talon, Philippe. 1985. *Textes administratifs des salles «Y et Z» du Palais de Mari*. Archives royales de Mari 24. Paris.

Taylor, Jon. 1999. "The Sumerian Proverb Collections," *Revue d'Assyriologie* 99, 13–38.

Temkin, Oswei. 1991. *Soranus' Gynecology.* Baltimore (Paperbacks edition).

Thavapalan, Shiyanthi. 2020. *The Meaning of Color in Ancient Mesopotamia.* Culture and History of the Ancient Near East 104. Leiden/Boston.

Thavapalan, Shiyanthi. 2021. "Keeping Alive Dead Knowledge: Middle Assyrian Glass Recipes in the Yale Babylonian Collection," *Journal of Cuneiform Studies* 73, 125–176.

Thompson, R. Campbell. 1924. "Assyrian Medical Texts," *Proceedings of the Royal Society of Medicine* 17, 1–34.

Thompson, R. Campbell. 1929. "Assyrian Medical Prescriptions for Diseases of the Stomach," *Revue d'Assyriologie* 26, 47–92.

Thompson, R. Campbell. 1930. *The Epic of Gilgamish: Text, Transliteration and Notes.* Oxford.

Thompson, R. Campbell. 1934a. "Assyrian Prescriptions for Diseases of the Urinary Tract etc.," *Babyloniaca* 14, 57–151.

Thompson, R. Campbell. 1934b. "Assyrian Prescriptions for Diseases of the Chest and Lungs," *Revue d'Assyriologie* 31, 1–29.

Thompson, R. Campbell. 1949. *A Dictionary of Assyrian Botany.* London.

Thomsen, Marie-Louise. 1987. *Zauberdiagnose und schwarze Magie in Mesopotamien.* Copenhagen.

Thureau-Dangin, François. 1921. "Rituel et amulettes contre Labartu," *Revue d'Assyriologie* 18, 161–198.

Totelin, Laurence M. V. 2007. "Sex and vegetables in the Hippocratic Gynaecological Treatises," *Studies in History and Philosophy of Biological and Biomedical Sciences* 38, 531–540.
Totelin, Laurence M. V. 2009. *Hippocratic Recipes: Oral and Written Transmission of Pharmacological Knowledge in Fifth- and Fourth-century Greece.* Leiden.
Tsukimoto, Akio. 1999. "'By the Hand of Madi-Dagan, the Scribe and *Apkallu*-Priest' – A Medical Text from the Middle Euphrates Region," in: K. Watanabe (ed.), *Priests and Officials in the Ancient Near East. Papers of the Second Colloquium on the Ancient Near East – The City and its Life Held at the Middle Eastern Culture Center in Japan (Mitaka, Tokyo) March 22–24, 1996.* Heidelberg, 187–200.
Vallat, François. 1983. "Le dieu Enzak: Une divinité dilmunite venerée à Suse", in: D. T. Potts (ed.), *Dilmun: New Studies in the Archaeology and Early History of Bahrain.* Berlin, 93–100.
Van Buren, Elizabeth D. 1939. *The Fauna of Ancient Mesopotamia as Represented in Art.* Analecta Orientalia 18. Roma.
Van der Geest, Sjaak, Susan R. Whyte and Anita Hardon. 1996. "The anthropology of pharmaceuticals: A biographical approach," *Annual Review of Anthropology* 25, 153–178.
Van der Toorn, Karel. 1985. *Sin and Sanction in Israel and Mesopotamia: A Comparative Study.* Assen/Maastricht.
Van der Toorn, Karel. 1989. "La pureté rituelle au Proche-Orient ancien," *Revue de l'Histoire des Religions* 206, 339–356.
Van der Toorn, Karel. 1994. *From Her Cradle to Her Grave: The Role of Religion in the Life of the Israelite and the Babylonian Woman.* Sheffield.
Van Dijk, Jan J. A. 1972. "Une variante du thème de 'l'Esclave de la Lune'," *Orientalia Nova Series* 41, 339–348.
Van Dijk, Jan J. A. 1973. "Une incantation accompagnant la naissance de l'homme," *Orientalia Nova Series* 42, 502–507.
Van Dijk, Jan J. A. 1975. "Incantations accompagnant la naissance de l'homme," *Orientalia Nova Series* 44, 52–79.
Van Dijk, Jan J. A. 1982. "Fremdsprachige Beschwörungstexte in der südmesopotamischen literarischen Überlieferung", in: H. J. Nissen and J. Renger (eds.), *Mesopotamien und seine Nachbarn: Politische und kulturelle Wechselbeziehungen im alten Vorderasien vom 4.–1. Jahrtausend v. Chr.* Berliner Beiträge zum Vorderen Orient 1. Berlin, 97–110.
Van Dijk, Jan J. A. 1983. *Lugale ud me-lám-bi nir-ĝál: le récit épique et didactique des travaux de Ninurta, du déluge et de la nouvelle création.* 2 vol. Leiden.
Van Dijk, Jan J. A. 1989. "Ein spätaltbabylonischer Katalog einer Sammlung sumerischer Briefe," *Orientalia Nova Series* 58, 441–452.
Van Dijk, Jan A. A. and Markham J. Geller. 2003. *Ur III Incantations from the Frau Professor Hilprecht Collection, Jena.* Münster.
Van Dijk, Jan J. A., A. Goetze and M. I. Hussey. 1985. *Early Mesopotamian Incantations and Rituals.* Yale Oriental Series, Babylonian Texts 11. New Haven.
Van Rijn-van Tongeren, Geraldine W. 1997. *Metaphors in Medical Texts.* Amsterdam.
Van Soldt, Wilfred H. 1990. "Fabrics and Dyes at Ugarit," *Ugarit-Forschungen* 22, 321–357.
Van Soldt, Wilfred H. 1991. Review of A. J. Sachs and H. Hunger, Astronomical Diaries and Related Texts from Babylonia, Vol. I, Diaries from 652 B.C. to 262 B.C., *Zeitschrift für Assyriologie und Vorderasiatische Archäologie* 81, 153–155.
Van Soldt, Wilfred H. 2015. *Middle Babylonian Texts in the Cornell University Collections 1: The Later Kings.* Cornell University Studies in Assyriology and Sumerology 30. Bethesda.
Veldhuis, Niek. 1989. "The New Assyrian Compendium for a Woman in Childbirth", *ASJ* 11, 239–260.
Veldhuis, Niek. 1991. *A cow of Sîn.* Groningen.
Veldhuis, Niek. 1999. "The Poetry of Magic", in: T. Abusch and K. van der Toorn (eds.), *Mesopotamian Magic: Textual, Historical and Interpretative Perspectives.* Groningen, 35–48.
Veldhuis, Niek. 2000. "Kassite Exercises: Literary and Lexical Extracts," *Journal of Cuneiform Studies* 52, 67–94.
Verderame, Lorenzo. 2018. "Ninmaḫ and Her Imperfect Creatures: The Bed Wetting Man and Remedies to Cure Enuresis (*STT* 238)," in: S. V. Panayotov and L. Vacín (eds.), *Mesopotamian Medicine and Magic: Studies in Honor of Markham J. Geller.* Ancient Magic and Divination 14. Leiden/Boston, 779–800.
Viano, Maurizio. 2014. "Writing Sumerian in the West," in: A. Archi and A. Bramanti (eds.), *Tradition and Innovation in the Ancient Near East: Proceedings of the 57th Rencontre Assyriologique Internationale at Rome 4–11 July 2011.* Winona Lake, 381–392.
Viano, Maurizio. 2016. *The Reception of Sumerian Literature in the Western Periphery.* Venezia.
Volk, Konrad. 1999. "Kinderkrankheiten nach der Darstellung babylonisch-assyrischer Keilschrifttexte," *Orientalia Nova Series* 68, 1–30.
Volk, Konrad. 2004. "Vom Dunkel in die Helligkeit: Schwangerschaft, Geburt und frühe Kindheit in Babylonien und Assyrien," in: V. Dasen (ed.), *Naissance et petite enfance dans l'Antiquité: Actes du colloque de Fribourg, 28 novembre–1er décembre 2001.* Orbis Biblicus et Orientalis 2003. Fribourg/Göttingen, 71–92.
Von Soden, Wolfram. 1936. "Schwer zugängliche russische Veröffentlichungen altbabylonischer Texte. 1. Ein Opferschaugebet bei Nacht," *Zeitschrift für Assyriologie und Vorderasiatische Archäologie* 36, 305–308.
Von Soden, Wolfram. 1939. "Aus einem Ersatzopferritual für den assyrischen Hof," *Zeitschrift für Assyriologie und Vorderasiatische Archäologie* 45, 42–61.
Von Soden, Wolfram. 1952. "Zur Wiederherstellung der Geburtsomen-Serie *šumma izbu*," *Zeitschrift für Assyriologie und Vorderasiatische Archäologie* 50, 182–191.
Von Soden, Wolfram. 1957. "Ein neues Bruchstück des assyrischen Kommentars zum Marduk-Ordal," *Zeitschrift für Assyriologie und Vorderasiatische Archäologie* 52, 224–234.
Von Soden, Wolfram. 1957–1958. "Die Hebamme in Babylonien und Assyrien," *Archiv für Orientforschung* 18, 119–121.
Von Soden, Wolfram. 1968. "Aramäische Wörter in neuassyrischen und neu- und spätbabylonischen Texten: Ein Vorbericht. II (n-z und Nachträge)," *Orientalia Nova Series* 37, 261–271.
Von Soden, Wolfram. 1995. *Grundriß der akkadischen Grammatik.* Dritte, ergänzte Auflage. Roma.
Von Soden, Wolfram and Wolfgang Röllig. 1991. *Das akkadische Syllabar.* 4th rev. ed. Rom.
Von Weiher, Egbert. 1983. *Spätbabylonische Texte aus Uruk. Teil* 2. Berlin.
Von Weiher, Egbert. 1988. *Spätbabylonische Texte aus Uruk. Teil* 3. Berlin.
Von Weiher, Egbert. 1993. *Uruk: Spätbabylonische Texte aus dem Planquadrat U 18. Teil* 4. Mainz am Rhein.

Von Weiher, Egbert. 1998. *Uruk: Spätbabylonische Texte aus dem Planquadrat U 18. Teil* 5. Mainz am Rhein.

Waetzoldt, Hartmut. 2011. "Die Textilproduktion von Garšana," in: D. I. Owen (ed.), *Garšana Studies.* Cornell University Studies in Assyriology and Sumerology 6. Bethesda, 405–454.

Waetzoldt, Hartmut. 2011–2013a. "Spinnen. A. Philologisch," in: M. P. Streck et al. (ed.), *Reallexikon der Assyriologie und Vorderasiatischen Archäologie* 13, Berlin/Boston, 1–3.

Waetzoldt, Hartmut. 2011–2013b. "Textilien A. Philologisch," in: M. P. Streck et al. (ed.), *Reallexikon der Assyriologie und Vorderasiatischen Archäologie* 13, Berlin/Boston, 617–624.

Walker, Christopher B. F. 1988. "Introduction," in: E. Leichty, J. J. Finkelstein and C. B. F. Walker, *Catalogue of the Babylonian Tablets in in the British Museum, Volume 8: Tablets from Sippar* 3. London, xi–xxv.

Waschow, Heinz. 1936. *Babylonische Briefe aus der Kassitenzeit.* Mitteilungen der Altorientalischen Gesellschaft 10. Leipzig.

Wasserman, Nathan. 1996–1997. "An Old Babylonian Medical Text against the *kurārum*-Disease, *Revue d'Assyriologie* 90, 1–5 and *Revue d'Assyriologie* 91, 31–32.

Wasserman, Nathan. 2012. *Most Probably. Epistemic Modality in Old Babylonian.* Winona Lake.

Wasserman, Nathan. 2013. "Treating Garments in the Old Babylonian Period: 'At the Cleaners' in a Comparative View," *Iraq* 75, 255–277.

Wasserman, Nathan. 2016. *Akkadian Love Literature of the Third and Second Millennium BCE.* Leipziger Altorientalische Studien 4. Wiesbaden.

Wasserman, Nathan. 2018. "Labor Pains, Difficult Birth, Sick Child: Three Old Babylonian Incantations from a Private Collection," *Bibliotheca Orientalis* 75, 14–25.

Wasserman, Nathan. 2019. "Mesopotamian Underwear and Undergarments," in: G. Chambon, M. Guichard and A.-I. Langlois (eds.), *De l'argile au numérique: Mélanges assyriologiques en l'honneur de Dominique Charpin.* Leuven, 1125–1144.

Wasserman, Nathan. 2020. "A Hybrid Magical Text from the Böhl Collection," *Bibliotheca Orientalis* 77, 446–452.

Wasserman, Nathan and Elyze Zomer. 2020. *Akkadian Magic Literature. Old Babylonian and Old Assyrian Incantations: Corpus – Context – Praxis.* Leipziger Altorientalische Studien 12. Wiesbaden.

Watanabe, Kazuko. 1989. Review of S. Dalley and J. N. Postgate, The Tablets from Fort Shalmaneser, *Zeitschrift für Assyriologie und Vorderasiatische Archäologie* 79, 272–278.

Watson, Rita and Wayne Horowitz. 2011. *Writing Science before the Greeks: A Naturalistic Analysis of the Babylonian Astronomical Treatise MUL.APIN.* Leiden/Boston.

Wee, John Z. 2006. "Virtual Moons over Babylonia: The Calendar Text System, Its Micro-Zodiac of 13, and the Making of Medical Zoology," in: J. M. Steele (ed.), *The Circulation of Astronomical Knowledge in the Ancient World.* Leiden, 139–229.

Wee, John Z. 2016. "A Late Babylonian Astral Commentary on *Marduk's Address to the Demons,*" *Journal of Near Eastern Studies* 75, 127–167.

Wee, John Z. 2017a. "Pan-astronomical Hermeneutics and the Arts of the Lamentation Priest," *Zeitschrift für Assyriologie und Vorderasiatische Archäologie* 107, 236–260.

Wee, John Z. (ed.). 2017b. *The Comparable Body: Analogy and Metaphor in Ancient Mesopotamian, Egyptian, and Greco-Roman Medicine*. Studies in Ancient Medicine 49, Leiden/Boston.

Wee, John Z. 2018. "Five Birds, Twelve Rooms, and the Seleucid Game of Twenty Squares," in: S. V. Panayotov and L. Vacín (eds.), *Mesopotamian Medicine and Magic: Studies in Honor of Markham J. Geller.* Ancient Magic and Divination 14. Leiden/Boston, 833–876.

Wee, John Z. 2019a. *Knowledge and Rhetoric in Medical Commentary: Ancient Mesopotamian Commentaries on a Handbook of Medical Diagnosis (Sa-gig).* Cuneiform Monographs 49/1. Leiden/Boston.

Wee, John Z. 2019b. *Mesopotamian Commentaries on the Handbook Sa-gig: Edition and Notes on Medical Lexicography.* Cuneiform Monographs 49/2. Leiden/Boston.

Wee, John Z. 2021. "A Systematic Etiology of Sicknesses from Ancient Iraq: Organ Systems and the Functional Holism of the Babylonian Body," in: C. Thumiger (ed.), *Holism in Ancient Medicine and Its Reception.* Leiden/Boston, 318–326.

Weidner, Ernst. 1922. *Akkadische Keilschrifttexte.* Keilschrifturkunden aus Boghazköi 4. Berlin.

Weidner, Ernst. 1952–1953. "Die Bibliothek Tiglatpilesers I," *Archiv für Orientforschung* 16, 197–215.

Weidner, Ernst. 1967. *Gestirn-Darstellungen auf babylonischen Tontafeln.* Wien.

Weiershäuser, Frauke. 2008. *Die königlichen Frauen der III. Dynastie von Ur.* Göttinger Beiträge zum Alten Orient 1. Göttingen.

Westendorf, Wolfhart. 1999. *Handbuch der altägyptischen Medizin. 1. Band.* Leiden/Boston.

Westenholz, Joan Goodnick. 1989. "Tamar, *Qědēšā, Qadištu*, and Sacred Prostitution in Mesopotamia," *Harvard Theological Review* 82, 243–265.

Westenholz, Joan Goodnick. 1997. *Legends of the Kings of Akkade: The Texts.* Winona Lake.

Westenholz, Joan Goodnick. 2010. "Ninkarrak – An Akkadian Goddess in Sumerian Guise", in: D. Shehata, F. Weiershäuser and K. V. Zand (eds.), *Von Göttern und Menschen: Beiträge zur Literatur und Geschichte des Alten Orients. Festschrift für Brigitte Groneberg.* Cuneiform Monographs 41. Leiden, 377–405.

Westenholz, Joan Goodnick and Marcel Sigrist. 2006. "The Brain, the Marrow and the Seat of Cognition in Mesopotamian Tradition," *Le Journal des Médecines Cunéiformes* 7, 1–10.

Westenholz, Joan Goodnick and Marcel Sigrist. 2008. "The Measure of Man: The Lexical Series Ugu-mu," in: R. D. Biggs, J. Myers and M. T. Roth (eds.), *Proceedings of the 51st Rencontre Assyriologique Internationale Held at the Oriental Institute of the University of Chicago July 18–22, 2005.* Chicago, 221–230.

Widell, Magnus. 2011. "Who's Who in 'A balbale to Bau for Šu-Suen' (Šu-Suen A)," *Journal of Near Eastern Studies* 70, 289–302.

Wiggermann, Frans A. M. 1983. "Exit *Tlalim*! Studies in Babylonian Demonology I," *Jaarbericht van het Vooraziatisch-Egyptisch Genootschap "Ex Oriente Lux"* 27, 90–105.

Wiggermann, Frans A. M. 1992. *Mesopotamian Protective Spirits. The Ritual Texts.* Cuneiform Monographs 1. Groningen.

Wiggermann, Frans A. M. 1998–2001. "Niraḫ, Irḫan," in: D. O. Edzard et al. (ed.), *Reallexikon der Assyriologie und Vorderasiatischen Archäologie* 9. Berlin/Boston, 570–574.

Wiggermann, Frans A. M. 2003–2005. "Pāšittu," in: D. O. Edzard, M. P. Streck et al. (eds.), *Reallexikon der Assyriologie und Vorderasiatischen Archäologie* 10. Berlin/Boston, 363–364.

Wilcke, Claus. 1969. *Das Lugalbandaepos.* Wiesbaden.

Wilcke, Claus. 1973. "Sumerische literarische Texte in Manchester und Liverpool," *Archiv für Orientforschung* 24, 1–18.

Wilcke, Claus. 1976. "Formale Gesichtspunkte in der sumerischen Literatur," in: S. J. Lieberman (ed.), *Sumerological Studies in Honor of Thorkild Jacobsen on His Seventieth Birthday, June 7, 1974.* Assyriological Studies 20. Chicago/London, 205–316.

Wilhelm, Gernot. 1994. *Medizinische Omina aus Hattuša in akkadischer Sprache.* Studien zu den Boğazköy-Texten 36. Wiesbaden.

Wiseman, Donald J. 1953. *The Alalakh Tablets.* London.

Woods, Christopher. 2009. "At the Edge of the World: Cosmological Conceptions of the Eastern Horizon in Mesopotamia," *JANER* 9, 183–239.

Worthington, Martin. 2005. "Edition of UGU 1 (= BAM 480 etc.)," *Le Journal des Médecines Cunéiformes* 5, 6–43.

Worthington, Martin. 2006. "Edition of BAM 3," *Le Journal des Médecines Cunéiformes* 7, 18–48.

Worthington, Martin. 2007. "Addenda and Corrigenda to 'Edition of UGU 1 (= BAM 480 etc.)' and 'Edition of BAM 3'," *Le Journal des Médecines Cunéiformes* 9, 43–46.

Wunsch, Cornelia. 1993. *Die Urkunden des babylonischen Geschäftsmannes Iddin-Marduk: Zum Handel mit Naturalien im 6. Jh. v. Chr.* 2 Vol. Cuneiform Monographs 3. Groningen.

Wunsch, Cornelia. 2000. *Das Egibi-Archiv, Band I. Die Felder und Gärten.* Cuneiform Monographs 20A. Groningen.

Wunsch, Cornelia. 2003. *Urkunden zum Ehe-, Vermögens- und Erbrecht aus verschiedenen neubabylonischen Archiven.* Dresden.

Wunsch, Cornelia. 2014a. "Babylonische Familiennamen," in: M. Krebernik and H. Neumann (eds.), *Babylonien und seine Nachbarn in neu- und spätbabylonischer Zeit. Wissenschaftliches Kolloquium aus Anlaß des 75. Geburtstages von Prof. Dr. Joachim Oelsner, 2.–3. März 2007 in Jena.* Münster, 289–314.

Wunsch, Cornelia. 2014b. "Double Family Names in Neo-Babylonian Records: The Case of the Ēṭiru and Ṭābiḫu Families and Their Butcher's Prebends," in: Z. Csabai (ed.), *Studies in Economic and Social History of the Ancient Near East in Memory of Péter Vargyas.* Budapest, 751–787.

Yalvaç, Kadriye. 1968. "Eine Liste von Amulettsteinen im Istanbuler Museum," in: H. G. Güterbock and T. Jacobsen (eds.), *Studies in Honor of Benno Landsberger on his Seventy-Fifth Birthday April 21, 1965.* Assyriological Studies 16. Chicago, 329–336.

Yu, Ning. 2008. "The Relationship between Metaphor, Body and Culture," in: R. M. Frank, R. Dirven, T. Ziemke and E. Bernárdez (eds.), *Body, Language and Mind, Vol. 2: Sociocultural Situatedness.* Berlin/New York, 387–407.

Zgoll, Annette. 1997. "Inana als nu-gig," *Zeitschrift für Assyriologie und Vorderasiatische Archäologie* 87, 181–195.

Zgoll, Annette. 2003. *Die Kunst des Betens: Form und Funktion, Theologie und Psychagogik in babylonisch-assyrischen Handerhebungsgebeten zu Ištar.* Alter Orient und Altes Testament 308. Münster.

Zgoll, Annette. 2006. *Traum und Welterleben im antiken Mesopotamien: Traumtheorie und Traumpraxis im 3.-1. Jahrtausend v. Chr. als Horizont einer Kulturgeschichte des Träumens.* Alter Orient und Altes Testament 333. Münster.

Zisa, Gioele. 2021. *The Loss of Male Sexual Desire in Ancient Mesopotamia. Nīš Libbi Therapies.* Berlin/Boston.

Zomer, Elyze. 2013. "KUB 4, 13: 15'–23' revisited," *NABU* 2013/2, 45–45 No. 27.

Zomer, Elyze. 2018. *Corpus of Middle Babylonian and Middle Assyrian Incantations.* Leipziger Altorientalische Studien 9. Wiesbaden.

Glossaries

The glossary of Akkadian words contains all reconstructed words in the texts edited in this volume. The attestations of the forms and orthographies of a specific lemma are listed in alphabetical order, with completely preserved instances listed first, followed by increasingly damaged or questionable ones. Verbal adjectives and participles are listed separately from the verbs; statives are listed under the corresponding verb rather than the adjective. For each attested verbal form the stem is added in square brackets for convenience. Bipartite phrases with a specific meaning distinct from the components or forming fixed expressions are usually listed as a single unit alphabetised under the first term, with minor exceptions. Logograms for which the Akkadian reading is unclear or ambiguous are listed under the logographic form. Terms for cardinal numbers are listed under the masculine absolute form. Complex prepositions or adverbials are listed under the nominal component. Only one occurrence of a word is listed if the same word occurs more than once in a given line. Distinct orthographies of the same term preserved in multiple text manuscripts (or orthographies that are damaged to a differing extent) are listed separately.

The normalised forms of lemmas in the Sumerian glossary follow ePSD2.

Akkadian Words

abāku G “to send; to dispatch, to bring along”: ***ib-bak*** [G] A.2.4: 7'; C.3.10: 12

abālu I G “to dry (up)”; D “to dry (up, out)”: **ḪÁD.A** [D] A.2.2: 50, 79; D.2.1: 31'; **ḪÁD.A$^{!}$** [D] D.1.11: 9; **HÁD.⸢A⸣** [D] C.3.3: 2; **ḪÁD.⸢A$^{?}$⸣** [D] A.2.7: 26'; **[Ḫ́Á]D.A** [D] A.2.2: 16; **Ḫ[ÁD].⸢A⸣** [D] D.1.3: 3'; **⸢ḪÁD⸣.[A]** [D] A.2.2: 79; **ḪÁD.DA** [D] A.1.1: 47'''; A.2.2: 34; **ḪÁD.D[A$^{?}$]** [D] A.2.5: 22''; **ḪÁD.DU** [D] A.2.3: 13'; A.2.7: 2; C.1.2: 14; C.1.4: 92'', 125'', 158''', 159'''; C.3.5: 10'; D.2.1: 66'; E.2.6: 7', 28'; ***i-b[a-lu$^{?}$]*** [G] C.1.10: 4; ***mu-bíl*** [D] C.3.1: 8, 9; ***mu-ub$^{!}$-bil*** [D] C.3.9: 26; ***tu-bal*** [D] A.2.2: 34; ***[tu-b]al$^{?}$*** [D] A.2.2: 31; ***tu-ub-⸢bal⸣*** C.1.9: 4; ***ub-bal*** [D] C.1.2: 25'; C.1.10: 11; ***ub-[bal$^{?}$]*** [D] C.1.10: 14

abālu II G “to bring; to carry (off)”; Gtn iter. of G; Št “to stir”: ***bi-la*** [G] C.3.10: 71, 72; ***bi-la-⸢a⸣-ni*** [G] C.3.3: 22; ***bi-[la-a-ni]*** [G] C.3.4: 66; ***bi-la-am*** [G] H.1: 36'; ***bí-la-ni*** [G] C.3.9: 47; ***it-ta-nab-ba-lu*** C.3.4: 91; ***tuš-tab-bal*** [Št] D.2.1: 46'; ***ub-ba-lu*** [G] C.1.2: 22'

aban alādi “stone of giving birth”: **NA$_4$** ***a-la$^{?}$-<di>*** A.1.3: 8'

aban gabî “alum” see ***gabû***

abāru “lead”: **A.BÁR** D.2.1: 46'

abašmû (a stone): ^{na4}***àba-aš-mu*** F.1: 5; ^{na4}***àba-[aš-mu]*** F.2: 4

abātu G “to destroy; to ruin”; N “to collapse; to fall down; to become annihilated, ruined”: ***it-tab-tu-ši*** [N] D.1.6: 6

abnu “stone; bead; pit”: ***ab-nu*** G.1: 46; **NA$_4$** A.1.3: 8'; C.1.4: 25'; C.1.10: 18; C.3.4: 15; C.3.9: 4, 6, 9; D.1.1: 132; G.2: 25''; **NA$_4$.⸢ME$^{?}$⸣** C.3.9: 1; **NA$_4$.MEŠ** B.1.4: 14; C.1.4: 5', 8', 14'; C.3.1: 7, 30; C.3.6: 58''''; C.3.9: 5, 29, 37, 40; D.3.1: 5; E.1.1: 7; F.1: 6, 10, 16, 22, 25, 30, 31, 34, 37; F.2: 33'; **NA$_4$.[MEŠ]** D.1.4: 2'; **⸢NA$_4$.MEŠ$^{?}$⸣** F.1: 12; **⸢NA$_4$⸣.ME[Š]** F.1: 40

abru “brushwood”: ***ab-ra*** C.3.10: 68

absinnu “furrow”: **AB.SÍN** B.2.1: 9

abu “father”; *ab*(*i*) *abi* “grandfather”: ***a-bi*** C.3.4: 50; D.1.8: 13; I.1.1: 111; ***⸢a⸣-bi*** B.1.1: 53; C.3.10: 47; ***a-bi-ia*** C.3.4: 50; ***a-bi-ía*** C.3.4: 50; ***a-bi-ka*** C.3.5: 21'; **AB.BA** I.1.1: 89; **AD-*ka*** C.3.9: 57; **AD-*ki*** C.3.3: 36; C.3.4: 76; **[A]D-*šá*** C.3.3: 25; **AD-*šú*** B.1.1: 52; C.3.1: 25; C.3.4: 15; C.3.9: 49; I.1.3: 6, 21, 22

abukkatu (an aromatic plant and its resin): ***a-bu-ka-ta*** II.1.4: 5; ***a-bu-ka-tu$_4$*** C.1.4: 171'''; **LI.DUR** A.2.1: 6'; D.2.1: 53'; **L[I.DUR]** E.2.8: 1'; **LI.TAR** D.1.7: 14'; **LI.TA[R]** A.1.1: 22'; **[LI$^{?}$].⸢TAR⸣** A.2.3: 3'

abunnatu “navel; umbilical cord”: ***ab-bu-un-na-ti*** G.1: 13; ***a-bu-un-na-ti-šá*** I.1.1: 85; ***a-b[u-u]n-na-ti-šú*** A.2.1: 30'; ***a-bu-un-na-tú*** D.1.9: 34'; ***ab-bu-un-na-tú*** G.1: 13; **LI.DUR-*sa*** C.1.4: 3'; D.2.1: 30'; **LI.DUR-*šá*** D.2.1: 32'; **LI$^{!}$.DUR-*šá*** C.3.1: 6; **LI.DUR-⸢*šá*⸣** F.1: 31; **LI.DUR-*šú*** F.1: 31; G.1: 12

aburriṣānu, *burriṣānu* (an animal; rodent): ***bur-i-ṣa-n[u]*** B.1.1: 43

abūsātu “forelock”: ***a-bu-us-sa-tú*** F.1: 4

adannu “fixed date; time limit”: ***a-dan-ni-šá*** D.1.6: 2

adāru I (a tree, probably a type of poplar): **ÍLDAG** C.1.2: 24'

adāru II G “to be afraid of”; Št “to give a fright”: ***tul-te-e'-⸢di-ir⸣*** [Št] C.3.5: 20'; ***tu-uš-ta-dir*** [Št] C.3.5: 20'

adi (prep.) “until; together with; up to; just before; as”; (conj.) “as long as; until; when”: ***a-di*** B.2.1: 23; B.2.2: 20'; C.3.1: 21; C.3.5: 18'; C.3.6: 62''''; C.3.10: 5; D.1.8: 24; D.1.11: 4; D.3.1: 9, 31, 11b, 15; E.2.6: 34'; H.1: 25'; ***a-di$^{?}$*** A.2.5: 17''; ***a-d[i]*** E.2.1: 7; ***a-di-i*** A.2.4: 6'; **EN** A.2.2: 33; A.2.3: 22''; A.2.4: 46'''; B.1.1: 18; C.3.3: 13; C.3.9: 35, 40; C.3.10: 90; D.1.3: 7'; D.2.1: 15'; D.3.1: 6, 11b; E.2.6: 21', 31', 37', 40', 42'; **⸢EN⸣** C.3.6: 59''''; C.3.10: 88; D.3.1: 31

agammu “marsh(es)”: ***a-gam-ma*** C.3.10: 57; ***a-gam-me*** C.3.4: 61; ***a-gam-mi*** C.3.3: 12; ***a-gam-mu*** C.3.10: 15

agannû “these”: ***a-gan-nu-ú*** D.2.1: 16'

agargarītu “black sulphur”: **A.GAR.GAR-^{d}ÍD** C.1.4: 39'

agû “crown”: **AGA** G.1: 17

agubbû, *egubbû* “holy water vessel”: **A.GÚB.BA** C.3.4: 39

agusīgu a green stone (turquoise?): ^{na4}**U[GU.AŠ.GÌ.GÌ$^{?}$]** A.1.3: 8'

aḫāmiš “each other; one another”; *ana aḫāmiš* “together”: ***a-ḫa-meš*** A.2.5: 23''; C.2.3: 23'; E.2.6: 8'; ***[a]-ḫa-meš*** E.2.6: 9'

aḫātu “sister”: **NIN** D.1.5: 8'

aḫāzu G “to take; to marry; to learn”; D “to mount, plate, inlay (with metal, stone)”; N “to catch; to spread (fire)”: ***na-an-ḫu-za-at*** [N] C.3.10: 27; ***tu-uḫ-ḫa-za*** [D] C.3.9: 8

aḫu I “arm; side; bank; shore”: ***a-aḫ*** C.3.4: 47

https://doi.org/10.1515/9781501506475-013

aḫu II "brother": ŠE[Š-šá] D.1.5: 7'

aḫû "strange; foreign": a-ḫi-[t]u D.1.1: 123; a-ḫi-tu$_4$ D.1.1: 110; a-ḫu-ú C.3.4: 44; BAR-t[i] C.3.4: 23

akalu "bread; food"; (a unit of capacity): NINDA A.1.4: 31'', 32''; A.2.1: 11', 51''', 88'''''', 89''''''; A.2.2: 22; A.2.3: 2', 3'; A.2.4: 11'; B.2.2: 18'; B.2.4: 4', 6', 7'; B.2.6: 4; C.1.9: 17; C.2.3: 19'; C.3.10: 5, 77; D.1.11: 11; E.2.1: 5, 9; E.2.6: 1', 4', 21', 24', 32', 34', 35', 36', 39'; NINDA$^?$ E.2.6: 19'; ⸢NINDA$^?$⸣ A.2.4: 11'; NINDA.ḪI.A A.2.2: 74; C.3.10: 8; D.1.11: 9; NINDA.MEŠ C.3.10: 76, 79

akālu G "to eat; to devour; to hurt; to take"; Gtn iter. of G; Š "to feed; to have someone eat": GU$_7$ [G] D.1.5: 10'; D.2.1: 33'; GU$_7$-ma [G] D.1.1: 217, 218, 219; G[U$_7$.MEŠ-ši$^?$] [Gtn] A.2.4: 8'; GU$_7$.MEŠ-šú [Gtn] A.2.1: 25'; GU$_7$-ši [G] H.1: 25'; GU$_7$-ši-ma [Š] D.2.1: 35'; E.1.2: 8'; GU$_7$-šú-ma [G] A.2.2: 49; Ì.GU$_7$ [G] I.1.3: 25; i-ka-lu [G] D.1.11: 10; i-ku-la [G] D.1.11: 1; ik-ka-lu [G] C.3.4: 87, 88; ik-ka-l[u-ši] [G] E.1.3: 3'; ik-kal-lu-ši [G] E.2.1: 17; ⸢ik⸣-kal-lu-šú [G] E.2.1: 17; li-ku-lu [G] C.1.8: 36'; šu-ku-ul [Š] C.1.4: 174'''; tu-ša-a[k-kal-ši$^?$] [Š] E.2.6: 14'; ⸢tu-šá⸣-[kal-ši] [Š] A.2.8: 8; tu-šak-kal [Š] A.2.4: 5'; t[u-šak-kal-ši$^?$] [Š] B.2.1: 24; ú-šá-kal-ma [Š] C.3.10: 86

ākilu "one who eats; eater, devourer": [a]-kil C.3.1: 9

aktam (unidentified plant): ak-tam A.1.3: 1'; A.2.3: 3'; B.2.4: 20'; E.2.1: 3; E.2.6: 43'; ^{ú}ak-tam A.1.1: 16'; D.2.1: 58'; D.3.1: 14; E.1.1: 4; E.2.6: 10'; H.1: 6; ⸢^{ú}⸣ak-tam B.2.4: 14'

alādu G "to bear; to give birth"; Š caus. of G; N pass. of G: a-la-da [G] II.1.4: 51; B.1.2: 5'; D.1.1: 22, 168; a-la-di [G] D.3.1: 1; a-la$^?$-<di> [G] A.1.3: 8'; a-l[a-di] [G] D.1.4: 3'; D.1.6: 4; a-lad [G] A.2.1: 56''', 58''', 69'''', 91''''''; D.1.1: 221; a-la-du [G] G.1: 47, 48; a-⸢la⸣-⸢du$^?$⸣ A.2.6: 25; <a>-la-d[u$^?$] [G] D.1.6: 5; i'-a-lid [N] D.1.9: 28', 38'; i'-al-du [N] C.3.6: 63''''; i-li-da [G] D.1.1: 158; li-il-dá [G] D.1.1: 159; li-li-id [G] D.1.1: 159; li-l[i-id$^?$] [G] II.1.1: 34; l[i$^{?!}$-li-id] [G] D.1.1: 190; li-lid [G] D.1.8: 16; li-lid-ma [G] D.1.8: 17, 19; lu-Ù.TU-id [G] II.1.4: 61; MUD [G] C.2.3: 11'; šum-li-is-si [Š] D.1.1: 199; [ú-al$^?$]-lá-ád [D] D.1.9: 31'; ú-lid [G] C.3.4: 10; ⸢ú$^?$⸣-[li]d [G] A.2.2: 11; ú-lid-ma [G] A.2.8: 28'; ⸢ú⸣-lid-ma A.2.8: 15; ⸢ú-lid⸣-ma [G] C.3.8: 10; [ú]-⸢lid⸣-[ma] [G] A.2.8: 20'; ú-[lid-ma] [G] D.1.11: 3; [u]l-du-u [G] D.1.1: 190; ul-la-di [G] D.3.1: 15; ul-la-du [G] C.3.6: 62''''; ul-la-d[u] [G] C.3.10: 52; [u]l-la-d[u] [G] D.3.1: 15; ul-la-du-ma [G] C.3.10: 45; ul-lad [G] A.1.1: 48'''; D.1.3: 2', 4', 10', 12'; D.1.11: 2; ⸢TU$^?$⸣ [G] B.2.1: 36; Ù.TU [G] A.2.3: 5'; B.1.1: 1'; B.1.5: 2'; B.2.6: 1; C.3.9: 35; D.1.1: 197, 205, 207; D.1.3: 11'; D.2.1: 70'; D.3.1: 15, 31, 32; I.1.1: 61, 114, 115; I.1.3: 7; I.1.6: 23', 24', 25', 26', 27', 28', 29'; Ù.TU [Š] B.1.3: 1; Ù.TU [N] D.3.1: 37(b); ⸢Ù.TU⸣ [G] C.3.6: 59''''; ⸢Ù.TU$^?$⸣ [G] D.1.3: 8'; Ù.⸢TU$^?$⸣ [Š] E.2.2: 7' Ù.T[U] [G] I.1.6: 11', 12', 30'; Ù$^!$.T[U$^?$] [Š] C.3.10: 75; Ù.[TU] [G] I.1.6: 13', 14', 16', 17'; ⸢Ù⸣.[TU$^?$] [G] II.1.3: 41'''; I.1.6: 9', 10', 15'; Ù.TU.DA D.1.11: 6; Ù.⸢TU-di⸣ [G] C.3.10: 88; Ù.TU-du [G] II.1.4: 61; Ù.TU-ia [D] D.3.1: 26; ⸢Ù.TU-ia⸣ [G] D.3.1: 23; [Ù].TU-ia$_5$ [G] D.3.1: 26; Ù.TU-ma [G] II.1.4: 1; A.2.4: 40'''; A.2.9: 12''; C.1.10: 7; D.1.7: 12'; D.2.1: 17', 25', 26', 29', 31', 32', 33', 34'; I.1.6: 18', 19', 20', 21', 22'; Ù.TU-m[a] [G] I.1.6: 37'; Ù.T[U-ma] [G] I.1.6: 35'; Ù.[TU-ma] [G] I.1.6: 38'; ⸢Ù⸣.[TU-ma] [G] A.1.1: 36''; [Ù].TU-m[a] [G] B.1.3: 1; [Ù.T]U-ma A.2.7: 18; D.1.2: 1; Ù.TU.MEŠ [G] II.1.4: 34; Ù.TU.MEŠ-da [G] II.1.4: 33; Ù.TU-šá [G] D.3.1: 1, 31; Ù.TU-š[á] [G] D.2.1: 40'; ⸢Ù$^?$⸣.[TU-šá] [G] D.1.4: 4'; Ù.TU-šú [G] C.3.9: 14; D.1.11: 3; E.2.3: 28''

alaktu "course (of life); way": [a-l]ak-tu$_4$ C.1.5: 44

alāku G "to go; to flow; to walk about; to come (vent.)"; Gtn iter. of G; Gt "to go away": a-la-ka [G] A.2.1: 34'; D.2.1: 30'; G.1: 24; a-la-ku [G] G.1: 10, 36, 51; a-lak [G] G.1: 50; a-lik [G] B.1.1: 56; DU [G] I.1.1: 87, 88; DU-ak [G] A.2.2: 53; A.2.6: 2; A.2.7: 37'; I.1.1: 115; ⸢DU-ak$^!$⸣ [G] C.3.4: 23; DU.DU-ak [Gtn] C.1.4: 56''; [D]U.DU-ku [Gtn] C.1.4: 55''; DU-ki-ma [G] C.3.4: 16; DU-ku [G] II.1.3: 46'''; A.2.2: 57, 61; A.2.7: 35', 36'; C.1.1: 7; C.1.4: 26', 64'', 65''; C.1.9: 21; I.1.1: 82, 117; I.1.3: 24, 31', 33'; DU-⸢ku⸣ [G] A.1.2: 14'; DU-⸢ku$^?$⸣ [G] A.1.1: 5'; C.3.4: 19; DU-[ku] [G] C.1.4: 189'''; [D]U-ku F.1: 28; [DU$^?$]-⸢ku$^?$⸣ [G] C.1.2: 1; [DU-k]u$^?$ [G] C.1.5: 1; ⸢DU$^!$⸣-ku$^!$ [G] C.3.4: 23; DU-ku-ma [G] C.1.8: 21'; DU-ku-m[a$^?$] [G] C.1.4: 174'''; DU-ku-ši$^?$ [G] F.1: 28; DU-ma [G] C.3.4: 13; ⸢DU$^?$⸣-[ma] [G] I.1.3: 27; DU.ME [Gt] I.1.1: 42; DU.⸢MEŠ⸣-ak [Gtn] G.2: 2'; DU.MEŠ-ma [Gtn] C.1.10: 1; i-la-ka-a [G] D.1.1: 140; il-lak [G] C.3.4: 65; ⸢il⸣-[lak] C.3.3: 19; il$^!$-lak [G] C.3.9: 44; il-la-ka [G] D.1.1: 140; il-la-k[a] [G] D.1.1: 26; il$^!$-la-[k]a$^!$ [G] D.1.1: 27; il-la-ku [G] C.1.4: 51''; il-lak-ma [G] C.3.10: 7, 12, 26; it-<tal>-l[u-ku$^?$] [Gtn] C.1.4: 136''; lil-li-ka [G] D.1.9: 25'; lit-tal-lak [Gtn] D.1.8: 18; lit-tal-lak-[m]a [Gtn] D.1.11: 13

alālu G "to hang up": tal-lal-ma [G] C.3.10: 88

alamû (a medicinal plant): ^{ú}a-la-me-e C.1.4: 168'''

alap asurrî "ox of the sewer" (a name for the scorpion): a-la-ap a-su-ri B.1.1: 44

alapû, *elap(p)û* "seaweed; algae": a-lap B.2.2: 14; ⸢e⸣-lap-pu-ú A.2.6: 24

ālidu, fem. *ālittu* "one who begets": a-li-da-at II.1.3: 47'''; a-li-id C.3.4: 98; TU I.1.1: 1, 2, 9, 13, 15, 16, 24, 26, 49, 52, 56, 57, 59, 72, 73, 76, 77, 78, 79, 80, 81, 82, 83, 84, 85, 87, 89, 90, 92, 93, 94, 96, 99, 100, 101, 102, 107, 108, 109, 110, 111, 112, 113, 116; I.1.3: 32'; T[U] I.1.1: 105, 106; ⸢TU⸣ I.1.1: 18, 88, 103; TU.UD.DA C.3.4: 15

āliku "going (one); flowing; moving": a-lik C.3.5: 25'; a-lik-tú H.1: 35'; a-lik-tu$_4$ H.1: 35'; DU-tú H.2: 4

ālittu "one who gives birth; fertile (woman)"; *lā ālittu* "barren; infertile (woman)": la a-lit-ti G.1: 21; G.2: 6'; ⸢la$^!$⸣ ⸢a-lit⸣-ti D.1.1: 29; la a-⸢lit⸣-tu$_4$ B.2.1: 8; [^{munus}]la a-lit-ta B.1.1: 8; ^{munus}la a-lit-ti A.2.2: 78; ⸢^{munus}⸣la a-lit-tu$_4$ A.2.7: 8; MUNUS.MUD C.1.4: 7'; ^{munus}NU.Ù.TU B.2.1: 13; [^{mun}]^{us}NU.⸢Ù⸣.TU A.2.7: 10

allān Kaniš "hazelnut" (lit. Kaniš oak): al-la-an-ka-niš D.1.1: 222

allānu "acorn; acorn-shaped suppository": al-⸢la-na$^?$⸣ C.2.3: 5'; al-la-nu A.1.4: 4'; A.2.2: 27; al-⸢la-nu⸣ A.1.4: 7'; a[l-la]-nu A.1.4: 9'; ALLA A.1.4: 18'; D.2.1: 65'; ⸢ALLA$^?$⸣ E.2.7: 11''; alla-an A.2.2: 76; alla-nu A.2.4: 15'; C.1.6: 6', 9'; ^{giš}AL.LA.AN C.1.4: 163'''; ^{giš}al-la-nu C.3.6: 19'

alluḫara see ***annuḫaru***

alluttu "crab": [a]l-lu-tú C.1.4: 160'''

alpu "ox; bull": a-la-ap B.1.1: 44; al-pi C.3.5: 25'; GU$_4$ A.2.2: 23, 25; A.2.4: 12'; A.2.6: 3, 19; C.1.4: 170'''; C.3.3: 19; C.3.4: 65; C.3.9: 44; D.2.1: 34'; GU$_4$.MEŠ B.1.1: 7; D.1.5: 9', 10'

amāru G "to see; to look at; to experience"; Gtn iter. of G; Gt "to see from now on(?)"; N "to be seen; to appear; to be visible": a-ma-ra [G] G.1: 4, 29; a-mar [G] D.1.1: 143; a-mur [G] C.3.8: 10; a-tam-ma-ru [Gtn] C.3.10: 40; am-ra-at [G] G.1: 6; e-mur-ši-ma [G] B.1.1: 49; D.1.1: 137; IGI [G] II.1.4: 26; A.1.1: 18'; A.2.2: 18; C.2.2: 2; D.1.1: 36; [I]GI$^?$ [G] A.2.2: 14; IGI.DU$_8$.MEŠ-ma [N] B.2.6: 3; IGI.DU$_8$-ši-ma [G] II.1.4: 53; IGI.IGI [Gtn] B.2.2: 14; IGI.LÁ C.3.1: 24, 25; I[GI.LÁ$^?$] [G] A.2.6: 27; IGI-mar [G] II.1.4: 13; E.1.2: 7'; I.1.1: 114; ⸢IGI$^?$⸣-m[ar$^?$] [G] E.1.2: 11'; I[GI-mar] [G] C.3.4: 60; IGI-mar-ma [G] II.1.4: 18; IGI-mur [G] II.1.4: 19; IGI-šú [G] C.3.9: 14; ⸢IGI⸣-šú-ma$^?$ [G] A.2.1: 76''''; i-mur-ši-ma [G] D.1.1: 137; [i-mu]r-ši-na-ti-ma [G] C.1.4: 50''; i-mu-ur-šu-ma [G] II.1.2: 11; i-ta-mar [G] D.1.1: 124; i-ta-[nam-mar$^?$] [Gtn] A.2.5: 1'; i-ta-nam-ma-ru [Gtn] C.1.10: 8; I.1.2: 8'; ⸢i$^?$⸣-[ta-nam-ma-ru$^?$]

[Gtn] C.1.9: 1; ***im-mar*** [G] A.2.1: 63'''; C.2.1: 12'; ***im-ma-ru*** [G] A.2.1: 54'''; ***li-mi-ra*** [G] C.3.6: 26'; ***li-mu-ra*** [G] D.1.1: 193; D.3.1: 13; ***li-mur*** [G] II.1.4: 49; ***[l]i-mur*** [G] D.3.1: 13; ***li-ta-mar*** [Gt] D.1.1: 111; ***lu-m[u-u]r*** [G] C.3.10: 32; ***ta-mu-r[u]*** [G] C.3.5: 18'; ***tam-ma-ru*** [G] C.3.5: 18'; E.2.6: 15'; ***tam-mar-ú-ma*** [G] D.1.11: 6; ***ta-⸢ta-mar⸣*** [G] C.3.3: 11; ***ta-ta-nam-mar*** [Gtn] C.1.10: 10

amātu "word; command; matter": ***a-mat*** C.1.4: 136''; **INIM.MEŠ-*ki-na*** C.3.9: 20

amēlu, *amīlu*, *awīlum*, *a'īlu* "(hu)man": **LÚ** B.2.6: 4, 10; G.1: 13; **⸢LÚ⸣** C.3.4: 54; **LÚ.MEŠ** D.1.1: 235; **LÚ.U$_{18}$.LU** II.1.4: 49; **LÚ.[U$_{18}$.LU]** D.1.3: 28''; D.1.1: 234; **LÚ.⸢ÙLU⸣** C.3.4: 15; **NA** C.2.1: 15'; C.3.3: 41; C.3.4: 17; D.1.3: 32''; E.2.8: 8''; **⸢NA⸣** C.3.4: 18; **NA$^{?}$** C.3.4: 19

amēlūtu "humankind": ***a-me-lu-te$^{!}$*** C.3.6: 12'; ***a-me-lu-ti*** C.3.6: 11', 12'; ***a-me-⸢lu⸣-ti*** D.1.1: 110; ***a-me-lu-tu*** C.1.4: 48''; ***a-me-lu-tú*** C.3.4: 48; ***a-mi-lu-te*** C.3.6: 11'; ***a-mi-lu-[ti]*** C.3.5: 16'; ***a-wi-l[u-ti]*** C.3.5: 16'; **LÚ-*tú*** C.3.9: 49; **L[Ú-*t*]*u*$_4$** C.3.3: 26; **LÚ-*ut-tu*$_4$** C.3.4: 69; **NAM.LÚ.U$_{18}$.LU** A.2.2: 9; C.1.4: 60''; D.2.1: 14'; **NAM$^{!}$.LÚ.U$_{18}$.LU** C.1.4: 164'''; **NAM.LÚ.U$_{19}$.LU** C.1.4: 26'

amḫara (an unidentified medicinal plant): ***^{ú}am-ḫa-ra*** C.1.4: 154'''; ***[^{ú}am-ḫa-r]a*** II.1.3: 33'''

āmiru "one who sees": ***a-m[i]-⸢ri⸣*** C.3.3: 10; ***a-mi-ru*** C.3.4: 60

ammaki/u "instead of": ***am-ma-ki*** C.3.3: 27, 28; C.3.4: 69, 70; C.3.9: 49, 50, 51; ***am-ma-ku*** C.3.3: 25

ammatu "cubit; forearm": **KÙŠ** C.4.1: 13'

ammīni "why?": ***am-me-ni*** C.3.4: 8; ***am-mi-ni*** C.3.5: 17'

ammu, *ḫammu* "people": ***am*** G.1: 11; ***am-ma*** G.1: 10

amtu "maid": **GÉME** II.1.4: 51, 61; C.3.4: 37; C.3.10: 35

ana "to; into; for": ***a-na*** II.1.1: 29, 34; II.1.2: 13; A.2.2: 61, 74; A.2.5: 23''; A.2.8: 1, 10; B.2.1: 19, 20; B.2.2: 22'; B.2.3: 13'', 16''; C.1.5: 1; C.2.3: 3'; C.3.4: 9, 68; C.3.6: 11', 45'''; C.3.9: 48; C.3.10: 11, 12, 15, 19, 55, 59, 79, 86; D.1.1: 23, 106, 107, 112, 148, 156, 157, 172, 177, 231, 233; D.1.11: 2, 13; D.3.1: 8, 9, 14, 38(A); E.2.1: 15; E.2.6: 21', 31', 34', 38'; F.1: 31; G.1: 3, 4, 6, 35; G.2: 16''; I.1.1: 118; ***a-n[a]*** A.2.7: 37'; D.1.2: 10; E.2.6: 42'; ***a-⸢na⸣*** D.1.5: 4'; ***a-[na]*** D.1.1: 162; D.1.11: 3; ***⸢a⸣-na*** A.2.8: 18; D.3.1: 9; E.2.1: 10; ***⸢a-na⸣*** B.2.1: 28, 40; ***⸢a⸣-[na]*** A.2.7: 8, 10; B.2.1: 18; ***[a-n]a*** E.2.6: 5', 6'; ***[a$^{?}$]-⸢na⸣*** C.3.7: 12''; ***[a-n]a$^{?}$*** B.2.1: 29; ***ana*** II.1.3: 45''', 47; II.1.4: 3, 8, 12, 16, 17, 24, 25, 28, 35, 52, 53, 54, 55, 56; A.1.1: 2', 4'; A.1.2: 17''; A.1.3: 12'; A.2.1: 5', 17', 19', 54''', 61'''; A.2.2: 5, 8, 9, 10, 13, 17, 18, 28, 29, 31, 39, 42, 45, 47, 51, 53, 68, 70, 77, 78, 79, 80, 82; A.2.3: 28'''; A.2.4: 3', 15', 18', 43''', 46'''; A.2.5: 4', 5', 24''; A.2.6: 2, 27; A.2.7: 1, 3, 40'; A.2.10: 10''; B.1.1: 7, 15, 16, 17, 20, 52, 72; B.1.3: 10; B.1.4: 15; B.1.5: 2'; B.1.6: 1; B.2.1: 13, 37; B.2.2: 8, 10, 20'; B.2.5: 1; B.2.6: 5, 15, 19; C.1.1: 2, 9, 12; C.1.3: 12', 13'; C.1.4: 3', 8', 11', 15', 25', 26', 28', 33', 34', 35', 36', 39', 41', 43', 45', 61'', 75'', 81'', 87'', 108'', 110'', 138'', 147''', 152''', 155''', 156''', 160''', 161''', 173''', 175''', 177''', 178'''; C.1.5: 3, 9, 37, 38, 40; C.1.6: 9'; C.1.7: 5', 8'; C.1.8: 23', 27', 29', 32', 35', 38', 39', 43'; C.1.9: 9, 22, 25, 32; C.1.10: 1, 5, 7, 10, 17; C.2.1: 6', 11'; C.2.3: 6', 11', 22'; C.3.1: 32; C.3.2: 4''; C.3.3: 4, 8, 24; C.3.4: 1, 3, 11, 12, 13, 14, 16, 19, 23, 24, 25, 35, 36, 40, 41, 43, 46, 47, 55, 56, 57, 78, 86, 87, 90, 95; C.3.5: 7'; C.3.6: 6', 11', 15', 16', 17', 20', 50''''; C.3.8: 8; C.3.9: 10, 11, 12, 13, 15, 16, 19, 22, 24, 39; C.3.10: 13, 26, 62, 68, 70, 73, 74, 75, 83, 90, 91; D.1.1: 15, 39, 51, 52, 54, 55, 93, 129, 130, 134, 144, 148, 165, 169, 178, 180, 197, 201, 207, 212, 229; D.1.2: 4; D.1.3: 10', 33''; D.1.4: 6'; D.1.6: 10; D.1.7: 5', 20'; D.2.1: 9', 15', 19', 20', 24', 30', 32', 44', 46', 49', 53', 60', 61', 64', 65', 68', 71'; D.3.1: 8, 9, 10c, 11b, 14, 16; E.1.2: 6', 9', 19'', 21''; E.2.4: 7', 8'; E.2.5: 7'; E.2.6: 11', 18', 21', 23', 24', 29', 31', 39', 41', 42', 44'; E.2.8: 4', 11'', 12''; F.1: 31; G.1: 39; H.1: 17'; H.2: 4; I.1.1: 59, 60, 61, 62, 63, 64, 65, 73, 74, 115, 117; I.1.2: 15'; I.1.3: 9, 36'; I.1.7: 10; ***ana$^{?}$*** A.2.8: 28'; C.2.3: 7'; D.1.1: 17, 187; E.2.6: 36'; E.2.8: 4', 11', 12'; ***ana$^{!}$*** E.2.6: 35'; ***⸢ana⸣*** II.1.3: 46'''; 52'''; A.1.1: 8'; A.2.1: 20'; A.2.2: 51, 57; B.1.2: 1; B.2.1: 9; C.1.5: 32; C.2.3: 14'; C.3.10: 29, 33; I.1.3: 27, 33'; ***a[na$^{?}$]*** A.2.10: 5'; ***⸢ana$^{?}$⸣*** A.2.7: 39'; C.3.1: 33; ***[an]a$^{?}$*** C.3.2: 18'''

anāku "I": ***a-na-ku*** C.3.4: 46; C.3.5: 30'; C.3.10: 29, 34; D.3.1: 22; ***a-n[a-k]u*** B.2.6: 21; ***[a]-n[a-k]u$^{?}$*** D.3.1: 21; ***ana-ku*** C.3.4: 11, 44, 45, 46, 51a; C.3.8: 7; C.3.9: 20; C.3.10: 31; D.1.1: 47, 181, 195; D.1.8: 26; D.3.1: 21, 22

andaḫšu (an alliaceous or apiaceous plant): ***an-da$^{?}$-[aḫ]-šú$^{?}$*** A.2.8: 23'; ***an-daḫ-šú*** A.2.4: 13'; ***[an]-daḫ-šú*** A.2.4: 10'; **^{ú}AN.DAḪ.ŠUM** A.2.1: 60'''; D.2.1: 48'; **[^{ú}AN.D]AḪ.ŠUM** E.2.4: 3'

anduḫallatu (a kind of lizard): **EME.ŠID.Z[I.DA]** A.2.2: 16

anḫu "tired (one)": ***an-ḫu*** B.2.6: 21

anḫullû (a medicinal plant, especially against witchcraft): **^{ú}AN.ḪÚL** C.3.9: 21; **^{ú}AN.ḪÚL.LA** C.3.9: 21; **$^{⸢ú⸣}$AN.ḪÚL.LA** B.1.1: 63

ankibītu "of heaven and earth" (epithet of Ištar): ***an-ki-bi-i-tu$_4$*** C.1.4: 20'

ankinūtu (a medicinal plant): **[^{ú}A]N.KI.NU.DI** B.1.6: 3; ***^{ú}an-ki-nu-te*** A.2.6: 4; C.1.4: 181'''; ***^{ú}⸢an-ki⸣-[nu]-⸢te⸣*** A.2.7: 33'

anna "yes; certainly": ***an-na*** G.1: 30; ***an-[na]*** G.2: 10'

annaku "tin; tin stone": **^{na4}⸢AN.NA⸣** C.3.5: 1'

annanna, fem. *annannītu* "so-and-so": **^{munus}NENNI** C.3.4: 91, 94; D.1.1: 227; **^{munus}NENNI-*tú*** D.3.1: 21; **NENNI** C.3.4: 91, 94; C.3.6: 13', 14'; D.1.1: 227; D.3.1: 22; **⸢NENNI⸣** C.3.6: 16'; **⸢NENNI$^{?}$⸣** C.3.6: 15'; **NENNI-*tu*$_4$** C.3.4: 16; C.3.6: 13'; C.3.8: 7; D.3.1: 21, 22; **⸢NENNI⸣-*tu*$_4$** C.3.6: 14'

annu "approval; consent": ***an-na*** G.1: 31; ***an-nu*** D.1.1: 129

annû "this": ***a-nu-ú*** D.2.1: 10'; ***an-na-a*** II.1.4: 13; C.1.4: 12'; ***an-na-a-tú*** E.2.6: 12'; ***an-nam*** C.1.4: 13'; C.3.4: 43, 47, 49, 95; C.3.6: 44'''; C.3.10: 83; D.1.1: 228; ***an-né-[e]*** D.3.1: 26; ***an-ni-a-am*** B.2.6: 26; ***an-ni-i*** D.3.1: 26; ***an-ni-ta*** C.3.5: 15'; C.3.10: 77, 86; D.1.1: 115; ***an-<ni>-ta*** B.2.2: 25'; ***an-ni-ti*** C.3.4: 14; D.3.1: 28; ***an-n[i-t]i$^{?}$*** A.2.5: 12'; ***[an-ni]-ti*** C.3.4: 78; ***an-ni-tu*** B.1.1: 72, 73; ***an-ni-tú*** C.3.6: 9', 28'; C.3.7: 23''; C.3.10: 78, 81, 83; D.1.1: 178; ***an-ni-t[ú]*** D.3.1: 28; ***[a]n-ni-tú*** C.3.7: 16''; ***[an-n]i-tú*** C.3.6: 55''''; ***an-n[i-tu$_4$]*** C.3.3: 39; ***an-[ni-tu$_4$]*** C.3.1: 29; ***an-nit*** C.1.10: 6; ***an-n[it]*** C.1.10: 2; ***an-nu-ti*** II.1.4: 7, 23; A.1.2: 17''; A.2.7: 12; B.2.1: 16; C.1.4: 5', 183'''; C.3.4: 48; D.1.1: 207; D.2.1: 24'; E.1.1: 3; ***⸢an⸣-nu-ti*** C.1.4: 2'; ***[an-n]u-ti*** C.1.4: 176''; ***an-nu-t[i]*** E.1.1: 7, 9; H.1: 6; ***an-[nu-ti]*** II.1.3: 67'''; ***an-nu-tì*** C.3.4: 16; ***an-nu-tu*** C.1.10: 4; ***⸢an-nu⸣-tu*** A.2.6: 11; ***an-nu-tú*** C.3.9: 5; ***an-nu-ú*** II.1.4: 47; A.2.7: 39'; C.3.4: 91; D.1.1: 101; **ŠEŠ** A.1.2: 11', 13'; D.1.3: 10'; D.2.1: 22'; **Š[EŠ]** A.2.1: 42''; **ŠEŠ.ME** E.2.6: 40'; **ŠEŠ.MEŠ** A.2.1: 67''''; **⸢ŠEŠ⸣.MEŠ** II.1.4: 27; **ŠEŠ-*ti*** B.1.6: 5

annuḫaru, *alluḫara* (a type of alum): ***an-nu-ḫa-ra*** E.2.7: 4'; ***an-nu-ḫa-r[a]*** A.2.2: 51; **IM.SAḪAR.BABBAR.KUR** C.1.4: 36'; **IM.SAḪAR.BABBAR.KUR.RA** C.1.4: 33', 42', 112''; **[IM].SAḪAR.BABBAR.KUR.RA** C.1.8: 10'; **[IM.SAḪ]AR.BABBAR.KUR.RA** A.1.3: 7'; **IM.[SAḪAR].BABBAR.KUR.RA** C.1.2: 15; **[IM.SAḪAR.BABBAR.K]UR.RA** C.1.4: 162'''; ***[^{ú}a]n-nu-ḫa-ra*** A.1.1: 19'

antal(l)û, *attalû* "eclipse": **AN.TA.LÙ** G.1: 20; **[A]N.TA.LÙ** E.2.3: 27''

AN.ZA.GUL.MEŠ (a stone): **^{na4}AN.ZA.GUL.MEŠ** C.3.1: 1

anzaḫḫu (a frit-like glass): **AN.ZAḪ** C.1.4: 42'; **[AN].ZAḪ** C.1.1: 8; **[AN.Z]AḪ** C.1.4: 74''

anzanu(n)zû "subterranean waters": ***an-za-nu-zi*** II.1.2: 7

apālu I G "to answer": ***i-[ip-pal]*** [G] B.1.1: 55

apālu II G "to be (too) late"; Dt "to be delayed": ***ú-tap-pi-il*** [Dt] B.2.6: 1

apāniš "through the window": ***a-pa-niš*** C.3.3: 21; C.3.4: 66; C.3.9: 45

aplu "heir; son": ***ap-la*** B.2.6: 24; ⸢***ap-li***⸣***-ia*** B.2.6: 22; ***ap-lu*** D.1.8: 2; **IBILA** C.3.6: 15'; D.2.1: 69'

appu "nose": ***ap-pa*** D.1.1: 176; ***ap-pa-šu*** D.1.1: 147; ***ap-pi*** I.1.1: 26; ***ap-pi-šá*** I.1.1: 70; ***ap-pi-šú*** C.1.4: 54''; **KIR**$_4$ C.1.8: 32'; C.3.9: 8; **KIR**$_{14}$ I.1.1: 26, 36, 52; **KIR**$_4$**-*šá*** I.1.1: 87, 88; **K[IR**$_4$**]-*šá*** I.1.1: 15; **[K]IR**$_4$**-*šá*** I.1.1: 16, 18; **KIR**$_4$**-*šú*** C.1.4: 65''

aprušu (an unidentified plant): ***áp-ru-[šú]*** E.2.5: 4'

apsû "subterranean waters": ***ap-si-i*** C.3.10: 55

aptu "window": ***ap-ti*** C.3.10: 88; ⸢***ap***$^?$***-ti-šá***⸣ C.3.6: 60''''

apu "reed marsh; canebrake": ***a-pi*** C.3.4: 64; C.3.9: 43; **GIŠ.GI** G.1: 38; **GIŠ.**⸢**GI**$^?$⸣ A.2.6: 5; **GIŠ.[GI]** C.3.9: 43

apû G "to be(come) visible; to appear"; Š "to manifest; to glorify": ***lu-šá-pi*** [Š] D.3.1: 13, 27

aqqullu (an atmospheric phenomenon): ⸢***aq***$^?$⸣***-qul*** G.2: 25''

arādu G "to descend; to go down; to come down (vent.)"; Š "to make descend; to let down; to take down": ***it-tar-da-ni*** [G] C.3.9: 12, 16; ***it-tar-du-ni*** [G] C.3.9: 16; ***šu-ri-da*** [Š] C.1.4: 61''; ***tu-še-re-du-šum-ma*** [Š] C.3.9: 14; ***tu-še-ri-sa*** [Š] B.1.1: 18; ***ur-rad*** [G] C.3.10: 12; ***ur-ra-dam-ma*** [G] D.3.1: 14; ***ur-ra-da-ni*** [G] I.1.3: 10; ***ú-ri-da-a-ni*** [G] II.1.4: 59; ***ú-ri-da-ni*** [G] D.1.1: 150; ***ú-ri-da-ním-ma*** [G] D.1.1: 150; ***ur-rad-m[a]*** [G] C.3.10: 33

arāku G "to be long; to last long": **GÍD.DA** [G] C.1.4: 175'''; **GÍD-*ma*** [G] I.1.3: 23

arāqu G "to be yellow-green, pale": **SIG**$_7$ [G] A.2.2: 61; I.1.1: 1, 24, 32; I.1.3: 32'; **SIG**$_7$**-*at*** [G] B.2.2: 4; **SIG**$_7$**.M[EŠ]** [G] I.1.6: 20'

arari(y)ānu (a plant): **PA-<*àri*>-*a-n[u]*** C.1.4: 164'''

arāru G "to be convulsed; to tremble"; Gtn iter. of G: ***[i]-ta-nàr-ra-[ar***$^?$***]*** [Gtn] I.1.4: 10'

ardatu "young woman": ***ar-da-a-tu*** II.1.4: 62; ***ár-da-at*** G.2: 19''; ***ár-d[a-tu***$_4$***]*** D.1.1: 36; ***ar-da-tu***$_4$ D.1.1: 159; I.1.2: 7'; ***a[r-da]-tu***$_4$ I.1.2: 6'; ***ar-dá-t[u]*** D.1.1: 159; **KI.SIKIL** C.1.4: 54''; **KI.SIKIL.MEŠ** C.3.9: 19; D.1.5: 11'

ardu "servant; slave": **ÌR** C.3.4: 37; C.3.10: 35; **ÌR-*ka*** B.2.6: 21; ⸢**ÌR**⸣**-*k[a]*** D.1.8: 26

argānu, *argannu* (an aromatic plant/tree and its resin): ^{giš}***ar-ga-na*** II.1.4: 10; $^{\text{[gi]š}}$***ar-ga-nu*** B.1.1: 5; ^{giš}***ar-[ga-nu]*** B.1.1: 13; ^{giš}***ár-ga-n[u]*** C.1.4: 14'; ^{giš}***ár-gá-nu*** D.2.1: 58'; ^{ú}***ar-ga-na*** II.1.4: 22

arḫiš "quickly": ***ár-ḫiš*** A.1.1: 48'''; C.2.1: 10'; D.1.1: 111, 124, 193, 197, 207; D.1.3: 2', 4', 10', 12'

arḫu I "month": ***ar-ḫi-ša*** D.1.1: 145; ***ar-ḫi-šá*** D.1.9: 15'; ***ár-ḫi-šá*** D.1.1: 145; **ITI** A.2.2: 50, 53; B.2.5: 2; C.3.9: 14; C.4.1: 12'; D.1.4: 4'; D.1.11: 3; D.3.1: 1, 26, 31; E.2.8: 3'; I.1.1: 106, 107, 108, 109, 110, 111, 112, 113; I.1.2: 13'; I.1.3: 1, 2, 3, 4, 5, 6, 7; I.1.6: 23', 36'; ⸢**ITI**⸣ E.2.3: 28''; ⸢**ITI**⸣$^{!}$ B.2.1: 36; **IT[I]-*ia*** D.3.1: 23; **ITI.MEŠ** C.4.1: 13'; **ITI.MEŠ-*ša*** II.1.4: 56; **ITI.MEŠ-*šú*** C.1.10: 8; **ITI-*šá*** D.3.1: 1; **[IT]I-*šá*** D.3.1: 31; **ITI-*šú*** I.1.2: 15'

arḫu II, fem. ***aruḫtu*** "quick; fast": ***a-ru-uḫ-tim*** II.1.2: 15

arḫu III "cow": **ÁB-*mi*** D.1.1: 168; ***ar-ḫi-mi*** D.1.1: 22; ***ar-ḫi-m[i]*** D.1.1: 23; ***ar-ḫu*** D.1.1: 146

arḫussu "every month; monthly": **[IT]I-*us-su*** C.3.9: 14

āribu, *ēribu* or *arību*, *erēbu*, *ḫerēbu* "raven; crow": ***a-ri-bi***^{mušen} A.2.6: 12; ***a-ri-bi***$^{\text{mu[šen]}}$ A.2.6: 2; ⸢**BURU**$_5$⸣ H.2: 3; **UGA**^{mušen} C.1.4: 179'''

arītu, *erītu* "pregnant (woman)"; *lā erītu* "woman (who is) not pregnant": ***a-ri-a-te*** D.1.5: 19'; ⸢***a***$^?$***-ri***$^?$***-ti***⸣ C.3.10: 1; ***e-ri-tu*** D.1.1: 160; ***l[a***$^?$ ***e-ri-tu]*** B.1.1: 75; ^{munus}***e-ri-ti*** C.3.5: 7'; ^{munus}***la e-ri-tu***$_4$ A.2.8: 1; ^{munus}***la*** ⸢***e***$^?$⸣***-[ri-tu]*** B.1.1: 71; ^{munus}**NU.PEŠ**$_4$ A.2.1: 5'; ^{munus}**NU.PEŠ**$_4$ B.1.4: 15; B.2.5: 1; ^{munus}**NU.**⸢**PEŠ**$_4$$^?$⸣ A.2.2: 9'; ^{munus}**PEŠ**$_4$ A.1.1: 44'''; A.2.2: 57; C.1.10: 7, 8; C.3.2: 6''; C.3.3: 1, 40; C.3.4: 56, 88; C.3.5: 2'; C.3.9: 7, 40; C.3.10: 70, 88; D.1.4: 3'; F.1: 32; F.2: 34'; G.1: 39; G.2: 16'', 17'', 23''; I.1.1: 116; I.1.2: 13'; I.1.3: 1; ^{munus}⸢**PEŠ**$_4$⸣ A.2.2: 61; ^{munus}**PE[Š**$_4$**]** A.2.2: 10; ⸢^{munus}⸣**PEŠ**$_4$ A.2.7: 1; ⸢^{munus}**PEŠ**$_4$$^?$⸣ A.2.2: 59; C.1.9: 1; ⸢^{munus}⸣**P[EŠ**$_4$**]** D.3.1: 1; **[**^{munus}**P]EŠ**$_4$ B.1.6: 1; **[**^{munus}**PE]Š**$_4$ C.3.7: 11'', 17''; **[**^{munus}**PE]Š**$_4$$^?$ D.1.3: 11'; **[**^{munus}**]**⸢**PEŠ**$_4$$^?$⸣ A.1.4: 41''; ⸢^{munus}**PEŠ**$_4$$^?$⸣***-ti*** A.2.1: 70''''; ^{munus}**PEŠ**$_4$**-*tú*** C.3.9: 13, 38; ⸢**PEŠ**$_4$⸣ A.2.7: 35'; **PEŠ**$_4$ C.3.10: 69, 70, 85; **PEŠ**$_4$**-*tu***$_4$ D.1.1: 160

arka, *arki* (adv.) "afterwards": **EGIR** A.2.4: 44'''; C.1.10: 2, 6; C.2.3: 23'; **EGIR-*šú*** E.2.8: 7'

arkabu "bat": **[ARK]AB**^{mušen} C.2.1: 6'; **ARKAB**<^{mušen}> D.1.3: 26''

arkatu "rear; back": **EGIR** E.2.6: 20'

arki, *urki* (prep., conj.) "behind; after": **EGIR** C.1.4: 10'; C.1.10: 6, 10; D.1.11: 6; **EGIR-*ka*** D.1.1: 229; **EGIR-*šá*** B.2.2: 20'; C.1.4: 11'; D.1.1: 140; **EGIR-*šú*** B.2.3: 15''; C.3.4: 23, 55; D.1.1: 112; ***ur-ki*** C.3.5: 25'

armû "young gazelle": ***á[r]-m[e]-e*** C.3.3: 12; ***ár-***⸢***mé-e***⸣ C.3.4: 61

arnu "guilt; sin; punishment": ***an-ni-ia*** C.3.4: 8; ***ar-na*** I.1.1: 89; ***ár-ni*** C.3.4: 8; ***ár-nu*** C.3.10: 14, 34, 44, 55, 58; ***[á]r-nu*** B.1.1: 45; ***ár-nu-šú*** C.3.10: 43; ⸢***ár***⸣***-nu-šú*** C.3.10: 56

arqu I "garden green(s); greenery; vegetables": **SAR** II.1.3: 66'''

arqu II "yellow-green; pale": **SIG**$_7$ A.2.6: 15; B.2.2: 18', 24', 28'; E.2.5: 3'; F.2: 11; ⸢**SIG**$_7$$^?$⸣ F.1: 12; **SIG**$_7$**.MEŠ** I.1.1: 55

arqūtu "greenness; freshness": **SIG**$_7$**-*su*** A.2.2: 10; C.1.9: 27; **SIG**$_7$**-*[su]*** D.2.1: 68'

arrabu "dormouse": **PÉŠ.ÙR.R[A]** D.1.3: 22''; ⸢**PÉŠ.ÙR**⸣$^{!}$**.R[A**$^?$**]** A.2.7: 23'

artu "twig; branch; leaves": ⸢***a***⸣***-rat*** B.1.1: 10; **PA** D.2.1: 29'; ⸢**PA**$^?$⸣ D.1.4: 10'; **[P]A** B.1.3: 6; **PA.MEŠ** D.1.11: 14'

arû, *erû* I G "to be(come) pregnant; to conceive"; D "to make pregnant; to impregnate"; Š caus. of G: ***a-re-e*** [G] G.1: 35; ***e-ra-ku-ma*** [G] D.1.1: 182; ***e-ra-at*** [G] I.1.1: 99; ⸢***e***⸣***-ra-at*** [G] I.1.1: 26; ***[e-r]a-at*** I.1.1: 36; ***[e-ra-a]t*** [G] I.1.1: 52; ***'e-re-et-ma*** [G] D.2.1: 28'; ***e-ri*** [G] C.3.4: 10; ***[e-ri]-a*** [G] D.1.5: 19'; ***[e-r]i***$^?$***-i***$^?$ [G] A.2.2: 70; ***e-ru-ú*** [G] D.1.1: 182; ***er-re-e-ma*** [G] C.3.10: 29; ***i-***⸢***ri***⸣***-ka*** [G] C.3.10: 20; ***ir-ri*** [G] II.1.3: 30'''; A.2.2: 73, 77, 79; A.2.9: 3'; ⸢***ir-ri***⸣ [G] B.2.1: 33; ***[ir]-ri*** [G] II.1.3: 53'''; ***[ir-r]i*** [G] B.2.1: 32; A.2.8: 10; ***ir-ri-ma*** [G] I.1.5: 2'; **PEŠ**$_4$ [G] A.1.1: 2', 4', 9', 18', 21'; A.2.2: 8, 63, 74; A.2.7: 34'; B.2.1: 30; B.2.2: 4, 7, 9, 27'; B.2.4: 26'; **PEŠ**$_4$ [Š] B.1.4: 15; **P[EŠ**$_4$**]** [G] A.1.1: 5'; ⸢**PEŠ**$_4$$^?$⸣ [G] A.2.2: 72; **PEŠ-*at*** [G] I.1.1: 57, 58, 59, 60, 63, 64, 65, 66, 67, 68, 70, 71, 72, 73, 74, 75, 76; **PEŠ**$_4$**-*at*** [G] I.1.1: 28, 29, 30, 45, 49, 50, 51, 52, 53, 54, 90, 91, 92, 93, 94, 95; ⸢**PEŠ**$_4$⸣**-*at*** [G] I.1.1: 31; **PEŠ**$_4$**-*át*** [G] I.1.1: 33, 34, 35; **PEŠ**$_4$**-*ma*** [G] D.2.1: 4'; I.1.1: 1; **PEŠ**$_4$**-**⸢***ma***⸣ [G] I.1.1: 116; **[PEŠ**$_4$$^?$**-*m]a*** [G] B.1.1: 40; ***[šu-r]e***$^?$***-e*** [Š] E.2.2: 7'; ***šu-ri-'-***⸢***i***⸣ [Š] A.2.8: 10; ***šu-ri-'-[i]*** [Š] A.2.8: 1; ***šu-ri-i*** [Š] A.2.1: 5'; A.2.2: 8, 78; ***šu-ri-***⸢***i***⸣ [Š] A.2.2: 78; ***šu-r[i-i]*** [Š] A.2.2: 74; B.2.5: 1; ***š[u-ri-i]*** [Š] B.1.2: 1'; ***šu-[ri]-im-m[a]*** [Š] B.1.1: 8; ***ur-re-***⸢***e***⸣ [D] II.1.3: 47'''; ***ur-***⸢***ri***⸣***-i*** [D] B.2.1: 13; ***ur***$_5$***-ri*** [D] E.2.6: 29'

arû II G "to vomit"; Š "to make vomit": **BURU$_8$-*šú*** [Š] B.2.2: 7; ***i-ár-ru*** [G] D.2.1: 39'; ***šu-ru-ú*** [Š] D.1.11: 14'

arzallu (a multi-coloured stone): ^{na4}***ár-zal-la*** C.3.5: 5'

askuppu, *askuppatu* "threshold": **KUN$_4$** C.3.3: 5; C.3.4: 58; D.1.1: 173

asnû "(date) from Dilmun": ***as-⸢né-e⸣*** A.1.4: 2'; ***as-né-[e]*** A.1.4: 19'; ***is-sa-nu*** B.2.2: 17'

asu "myrtle": **AZ** A.2.7: 28'; ^{šim}**GÍR** B.1.1: 27; D.2.1: 49'; **GÍR** A.2.5: 21''

asurrû "sewer": ***a-su-ri*** B.1.1: 44

asû "physician": **A.ZU** E.1.3: 4'; **A.Z[U]** B.1.1: 28; ^{lú}**A.ZU** B.2.1: 40

asurrakku, *esurakku* "depths; subterranean waters": ***e-s[u-ur-ra-ak-ki-im]*** II.1.1: 32

asûtu "profession of physician; medical skill": ^{lú}**A.ZU-*u-tú*** D.1.5: 12'

aṣû G "to go out; to emerge; to escape; to come out (vent.)"; Gt "go away (for good)"; Š "to let/make go out; to take/bring out; to set free; to let go; to expel; to release; to make/let grow, sprout; to deliver; to disclose; reveal"; Štn iter. of Š: ***a-ṣe-ka*** [G] D.1.8: 6; ***a-ṣu-u*** [G] G.1: 8, 12, 30, 39; ***a-ṣu-ú*** [G] D.1.1: 224; **È** [G] C.3.4: 66, 70; D.1.1: 224; **È** [Š] C.3.9: 39; **⸢È$^?$⸣** [G] C.3.4: 19; **È-*am-ma*** [G] C.3.3: 11; C.3.4: 60; **È-*ma*** [G] C.3.1: 22; **È-*ma*** [Š] C.3.10: 74; **È-*šá*** [G] C.3.10: 74; **È-*šú*** [G] E.1.2: 5'; ***[i]t-ta-ṣa-am-ma*** [G] D.1.1: 124; ***li-ṣa-a*** [G] D.1.1: 43, 52, 109, 171; D.1.9: 27'; ***li-ṣa-a[m$^?$-ma]*** [G] D.1.1: 92; ***[li-ṣ]a-am-ma*** [G] D.1.1: 18; ***li-še-ṣa-a'*** [Š] C.3.10: 58; ***⸢li⸣-še-ṣa-a'*** [Š] C.3.10: 16; ***li-ta-ṣa-am-ma*** [Gt] D.1.1: 111; ***lit-ta-ṣa-am-ma*** [Gt] D.1.1: 193; ***[l]u$^?$-ṣa-a*** [G] D.1.10: 6'; ***lu-ú-ṣa-ma*** [G] II.1.4: 49; **NÍNDA** [Š$^?$] B.2.4: 8', 10'; ***š[u-ṣi-i$^?$]*** [Š] E.2.8: 4'; ***šu-ṣu-ú*** [Š] C.1.8: 29'; ***šu-ta-am-ṣa-am-ma*** [Štn] G.1: 41; G.2: 20''; ***tu-ṣa-am-ma*** [G] C.3.5: 18'; ***tu-ṣa-am-ma-a*** [G] C.3.5: 18'; ***tu-ṣi-i*** [G] C.3.3: 28; C.3.9: 51; ***u-ṣi*** [G] B.2.2: 5; ***ú-ṣa-a*** [G] I.1.7: 9; ***ú-[ṣa-a]*** [G] D.1.1: 122; ***⸢ú⸣-ṣi-ma*** [G] D.1.11: 3; ***[ú]-ṣu-ú*** [G] D.1.1: 54; ***ú-še-ṣi*** [Š] A.2.7: 8; B.2.1: 8; ***[u]ṣ-ṣa*** [G] C.3.3: 22; ***uṣ-ṣi*** [G] C.3.10: 73; ***uṣ-ṣu*** [G] C.3.9: 46

aṣuṣimtu (a medicinal plant): ^{ú}***a-ṣú-ṣi-im-tú*** D.2.1: 23'

AŠ *zikari* (reading uncertain; a 'male' stone): ^{na4}**AŠ *zi-ka-ri*** C.3.10: 3

ašābu G "to sit (down); to squat; to dwell"; Š "to have someone sit": ***áš-ba-ak*** C.3.10: 34; ***áš-ba-ku*** [G] C.3.6: 2', 4'; C.3.8: 9; ***áš$^!$-ba$^!$-ku*** [G] C.3.4: 11; ***áš-ba-t[u$_4$]*** [G] C.3.4: 16; ***áš-bak*** C.3.10: 32; ***tu-še-šab*** [Š] II.1.4: 9; ***[t]u-še-ša-ab*** [Š] II.1.4: 15; ***tu-še-eš-šeb-š[i]*** [Š] D.3.1: 28; **TUŠ-*⸢ab⸣*** [G] C.3.6: 51''''; **⸢TUŠ⸣-*[(šeb)-ši$^?$]*** [Š] A.1.4: 33''; **TUŠ-*šeb-ši-ma*** [Š] A.1.4: 28''; **TUŠ-*ši*** [Š] C.1.4: 26', 27'; **[TU]Š-*⸢ši⸣-m[a]*** [Š] D.3.1: 28

ašāgu (a thorny shrub): ^{giš}**KIŠI$_{16}$** II.1.4: 7; B.1.1: 12; C.1.4: 147''', 150'''; D.1.1: 223; **[^{giš}KI]ŠI$_{16}$$^?$** A.2.1: 18'; **[^{giš}KI]ŠI$_{16}$$^?$** A.2.1: 97'''''''; **KIŠI$_{16}$** D.1.1: 223

ašarēdu "foremost (one); leader": ***a-šá-red*** D.1.8: 11

ašāru D "to release; to set free": ***li-maš-ši-ra*** [D] D.1.1: 34; ***⸢tu$^?$-maš$^?$⸣-šar*** [D] B.2.6: 20; ***uš-šu-rat*** [D] C.3.3: 18; C.3.4: 64; ***uš-šu-rat*** [D] G.1: 40; ***uš$^!$-šu-rat*** [D] D.1.1: 85; ***[u]š$^?$-šu-rat*** [D] D.1.1: 96; ***uš-šú-rat*** [D] C.3.9: 43

ašāšu G "to be distressed, aggrieved"; Gtn/Ntn "to constantly become distressed": ***i-ta-na-aš-šá-šu*** [Gtn/Ntn] I.1.1: 105; **⸢ZI.IR.ME⸣** [Gtn] I.1.3: 23; **ZI.IR.MEŠ** [Gtn] I.1.3: 23

ašgigû, ***ašg/kikû*** (a stone, perhaps turquoise): ^{na4}**AŠ.GÌ.GÌ** C.3.1: 3; C.3.9: 4; E.1.1: 5; F.1: 15, 33; F.2: 13; **⸢^{na4}ÁŠ.GÌ.GÌ⸣** D.1.4: 1'

āšibu "sitting; dwelling; inhabitant": ***a-ši-bat*** D.1.8: 5; ***a-ši-ib*** C.3.5: 16'; ***a-šib*** C.3.3: 8, 10; C.3.4: 59, 60; C.3.5: 16'

āšipu "conjurer; incantation priest; healer": ***a-⸢ši⸣-pi*** D.1.8: 26; ***a-ši-pu*** G.1: 7; **KA.PIRIG** I.1.1: 117; I.1.3: 33'; **⸢KA⸣.PÌRIG** B.2.6: 4; **[^{lú}]MU$_7$$^!$.MU$_7$$^!$** C.3.4: 39

āšipūtu "profession of conjurer; exorcistic lore; exorcism": ***[a]- ⸢ši$^!$-pu$^!$-su$^?$⸣*** D.1.5: 21'

ašlu "rope, rush": **[^{ú}]*aš-la*** C.1.2: 25'; ^{ú}***aš-lam*** C.1.4: 7'; ***⸢$^{ú?}$áš$^?$⸣-lam*** A.1.3: 3'; ^{ú}**NINNI$_5$** H.1: 2

ašnugallu, *išnugallu*, *gišnugallu* "alabaster": ^{na4}**GIŠ.NU$_{11}$.GAL** F.2: 25'; **[^{na4}GIŠ.NU$_{11}$.G]AL$^?$** E.1.1: 5

ašpû (a chalcedony): ^{na4}***aš-pu-u*** F.1: 5; F.2: 6

ašqulālu (an aquatic, medicinal plant): **LAL** C.2.2: 3;**⸢^{ú}⸣LAL$^?$** A.2.7: 34'

ašru "place"; *ašar* "where": ***a-ša-ar*** II.1.2: 8; ***a-šar*** C.3.6: 19'; C.3.10: 7, 37; **KI** C.1.4: 10'; C.3.4: 40

aššum, *aššu* "because (of); as for; concerning": ***aš-šu*** C.3.5: 18'; ***áš-šú*** A.2.1: 55'''; D.3.1: 23; G.1: 20, 21, 50; G.2: 6'; ***áš-⸢šú⸣*** D.3.1: 25; ***aš-šum*** B.2.6: 22; G.1: 12, 21, 36; ***⸢aš-šum⸣*** D.1.1: 98; ***aš-šúm*** D.1.1: 29; **MU** D.3.1: 23; ***šum*** C.3.6: 14'

ašû (a disease): ***⸢a⸣-ši-⸢i⸣*** A.1.2: 10'

ašūhu "pine-tree": **[^{giš}]Ù.<SUḪ$_5$>$^?$** B.1.3: 8

atā'išu (an unidentified plant): **KUR.KUR** E.2.6: 43'; ^{ú}**KUR.KUR** II.1.4: 4, 6, 21; A.1.4: 14'; A.2.6: 3; C.1.4: 11'; C.1.9: 16; C.1.10: 5; C.2.1: 9'; C.3.6: 17'; D.1.1: 220; D.1.3: 25'', 35''; E.1.1: 1; E.2.5: 9'; **⸢^{ú}⸣KUR.KUR** B.2.4: 12'; **[^{ú}KU]R.KUR$^?$** A.2.6: 13; ^{ú}**KUR.KUR.R[A]** II.1.3: 61'''; **⸢^{ú}⸣KUR.KUR.RA** II.1.3: 66'''

atānu "she-ass; jenny": **ÈME** A.2.3: 29'''; A.2.5: 5'; C.3.10: 85, 86, 87; E.2.6: 11'

atappu "(small) canal": ***a-da-ap-a-ta*** C.3.10: 15; ***a-da-ap-⸢a⸣-[ta]*** C.3.10: 57; ***a-tap*** C.1.1: 10; ***a-⸢tap⸣*** C.1.2: 21'; **PA$_5$.MEŠ-*šú*** C.1.5: 42

atartu (a medicinal plant): ***⸢^{ú}⸣a-tar-[tu$_4$]*** E.2.1: 13

atāru G "to be excessive"; D "to enlarge; to increase; to make huge": ***at-ru-ma*** [G] A.2.5: 13'; **⸢DIRI$^?$⸣.MEŠ-*šú*** [G] C.2.3: 8'; ***mu-tu-rat*** [D] D.1.1: 136

atbaru (a stone; basalt): ^{na4}**AD.BAR** C.1.4: 23', 31', 39', 40', 94''; 107'', 108'', 110''

attā "you" (masc. sg.): ***at-ta*** B.2.6: 17; C.1.4: 60''; C.3.4: 8, 48; D.1.1: 199; D.1.8: 11, 12; E.2.3: 8'; ***at-ta-ma*** C.3.10: 41, 54; D.1.1: 225; E.2.3: 13'; ***⸢at⸣-ta-ma*** C.3.10: 48; ***[a]t-ta-ma*** C.3.10: 53

attī "you" (fem. sg.): ***at-ti-ma*** C.3.6: 10'

ay, *ē* I "not": ***a-a*** C.1.4: 136''; C.3.4: 94; D.1.1: 43, 112, 113, 114, 160, 172; D.1.9: 26'; ***e*** C.3.7: 10''

ay II "alas!": ***a-a*** C.3.10: 34

ay(y)aba "sea": ***a-a-ba*** II.1.2: 5; C.3.9: 18

ayyalu "stag": **DÀRA.MAŠ** C.1.4: 111'', 159'''; **DÀRA.<MAŠ>** C.2.2: 5; **DÀ[RA$^!$.MAŠ]** D.2.1: 2'

ayyartu (a shell): ^{na4}***ía-ár-tú*** C.1.4: 45', 46'; ^{na4}***ía-ár-[t]ú*** C.1.4: 133''; ^{na4}**PA** A.2.6: 15; C.3.1: 4; C.3.6: 56''''; F.1: 4, 9, 33, 36, 39; H.1: 3, 32'; **^{na4}⸢PA$^?$⸣** C.3.1: 3; **⸢^{na4}PA$^?$⸣** A.1.1: 32''; ^{na4}**P[A]** F.2: 2; **PA** C.1.3: 2'

ayyu, *ayyû* "which; what": ***a-a-i*** E.1.3: 5'

azallû (an unidentified plant): ^{ú}**A.ZAL.LÁ** A.1.1: 7'; D.1.4: 13''; ^{ú}**A.Z[AL.LÁ]** A.2.8: 13; **[^{ú}]⸢A.ZAL.LÁ$^?$⸣** C.2.3: 13'; ^{ú}***a-zal-le-e*** C.1.4: 146'''; **Ú.ZAL.L[A]** E.2.1: 14

azupīrānu, *azukirānu* (a medicinal plant): ^{ú}*a-zu-ki-ra-ni* D.2.1: 54'; ^{ú}*a-zu-pi-ra-nu* A.2.1: 57'''; ^{ú}*a-zu-pi-*⸢*ra*⸣*-nu* A.2.1: 55'''; [$^{(ú)}$*a-zu*]*-*⸢*pi*⸣*-ra-nu* A.2.4: 9'; ^{ú}*a-zu-pi*$_4$*-ra-nu* B.1.6: 3

azupīru (a medicinal plant; saffron(?)): ^{ú}**ḪUR.SAG** B.1.1: 25; C.1.4: 146'''; [^{ú}**Ḫ**]**UR.SAG** A.1.1: 6'; ^{ú}**ḪU[R].SAG** II.1.3: 61'''

bābu "gate; door(way); opening; entrance": *ba-ba-a-ti* D.1.1: 120; **KÁ** II.1.4: 36; A.2.2: 76; C.1.4: 3'; D.1.1: 71; ⸢**KÁ**⸣ D.2.1: 8'; **KÁ-*bu*** II.1.4: 53; **KÁ-*šá*** D.1.1: 105; ⸢**KÁ**⸣**-*šá*** A.2.10: 11''; ⸢**KÁ**⸣**-*šu*** C.3.4: 95; **KÁ-*šú*** C.1.4: 43, 44; **KÁ-[*šú*]** C.1.8: 18'; **[K]Á-<*šú*>** C.1.5: 45

baḫru "(steaming) hot": *ba-ḫír*$^?$ A.2.2: 21; *ba-*⸢*ḫír*$^?$⸣ A.2.8: 22'; **KÚM** II.1.3: 59'''; **KÚM**$^!$ B.2.2: 23'

baḫrūtu "boiling condition"; *baḫrūssu* "when (steaming) hot": *baḫ-ru-su* D.2.1: 18'

bakû G "to cry"; Š caus. of G: *i-ba-ki* [G] D.1.5: 20'; [*i*$^?$]*-ba-ki* [G] D.1.5: 3'; *i-bak-ki* [G] C.1.4: 50''; D.1.1: 26; *lu-ub-ki* [G] C.3.4: 46; *ta-tab-ki* [G] C.3.5: 17'; *tab-ki* [G] C.3.5: 17'; *tul-te-eb-ki* [Š] C.3.5: 19'; *tu-uš-tab-ki* [Š] C.3.5: 19'; *ú-šab-ku-ú* [Š] C.3.4: 92

balālu G "to mix"; D "to mix up": *ba-li-*[*i*]*l* [G] I.1.3: 8; *bu-lul-ma* [G] D.1.9: 22'; **ḪI.ḪI** [G/D] II.1.4: 12; 28; A.1.4: 23''; A.2.1: 52''', 62''', 90''''', 104''''''; A.2.2: 7, 30, 31, 32, 38, 63, 76, 79; A.2.3: 4', 12', 28''', 30'''; A.2.4: 14'; A.2.9: 11''; B.1.1: 28; B.1.3: 7; B.2.4: 8', 17', 31'; C.1.4: 126'', 157'''; C.1.5: 2; C.1.6: 4', 6'; C.1.8: 25'; C.1.9: 9, 32; D.1.1: 133, 210, 211, 232; D.1.7: 9', 29'; D.2.1: 9', 25', 44', 51', 54', 55', 56', 65'; E.2.2: 5'; E.2.6: 8', 18'; E.2.7: 18''; **ḪI.Ḫ[I]** A.2.2: 64; A.2.9: 14''; C.1.4: 3'; C.3.3: 3; **ḪI.**⸢**ḪI**⸣ C.1.4: 154'''; **ḪI.**⸢**ḪI**⸣$^?$ A.2.3: 28'''; **ḪI.[ḪI]** A.2.5: 23''; B.2.5: 8; C.1.5: 34; **ḪI**$^?$**.[ḪI]** A.2.2: 13; **[Ḫ]I.ḪI** A.1.4: 38''; A.2.3: 11'; A.2.9: 1'; **[ḪI].ḪI** B.1.1: 32; **[ḪI.Ḫ]I**$^?$ A.1.4: 40''; **ḪI.ḪI-*ma*** [G/D] B.1.1: 64; C.1.9: 19; C.3.4: 57; C.3.5: 11'; D.2.1: 32'; E.2.6: 9', 13'; **ḪI.Ḫ[I-*ma*]** E.2.2: 3'; *i-bal-lal-ma* [G] I.1.3: 8; *ta-bal-lal* [G] A.2.2: 51; A.2.8: 3, 32', 34'; *ta-b*[*al-la*]*l* [G] A.2.8: 24'; [*ta-b*]*al-lal* [G] A.2.10: 5'; *t*[*a-bal-lal*$^?$] [G] II.1.3: 35'''

balāṭu I "life; well-being": *ba-la-ṭ*[*u*] D.1.10: 8'; *ba-laṭ-sa* D.1.1: 116; **NAM.TI.[LA]** I.1.1: 106, 107, 110; **TI** D.1.1: 226; **TI.LA** B.1.1: 70; D.1.1: 100, 107, 118

balāṭu II G "to be(come) healthy; to live; to recover"; D "to heal; to restore health; to revive": **AL.TI** [G] I.1.3: 1, 5; I.1.3: 16; *bal-ṭa-tu* [G] D.1.8: 24; *bal-ṭa-tú* [G] B.2.2: 27'; [*i*$^?$]*-bal-lu-ṭu* [G] A.2.5: 17''; *lib-luṭ* [G] C.3.10: 87; D.1.8: 17, 23; **TI** [G] II.1.4: 18, 31; B.1.5: 5'; D.1.1: 230; D.1.3: 7'; D.1.4: 20''; I.1.1: 17; **TI.[LA-*ma*]** [G] I.1.6: 32'; **TI.MEŠ** [D] A.2.1: 31'; **TI-*šá*** [D] D.2.1: 20'; **TI-*uṭ*** [G] II.1.3: 64'''; I.1.1: 40, 41, 113; I.1.3: 6, 7; **T[I-*uṭ*$^?$]** A.2.2: 10; **TIN** [G] I.1.1: 20; I.1.1: 82, 86; I.1.3: 36'; **TIN-*šú*** [D] A.2.2: 61; **TIN-*uṭ*** [G] A.2.1: 29'; C.3.3: 4; D.1.1: 232

ballukku (an aromatic plant/shrub and its resin): **MUG** A.2.5: 21''; E.2.6: 37', 43'; ^{šim}**BAL** II.1.4: 4; ⸢^{šim}⸣**BAL** B.1.1: 27; ^{šim}**MUG** A.1.4: 16'; A.2.9: 15''; B.2.3: 5'; C.3.10: 80; D.2.1: 47'; E.2.1: 4; E.2.6: 30'; [^{ši}]^{m}**MUG** A.2.1: 27'; ^{š}[^{im}]⸢**MUG**⸣ A.2.3: 4'

baltām(mu) "balsam": *ba*$^!$*-al-ta-ma* E.2.5: 5'

baltu (a thorny shrub, perhaps camel-thorn): ^{giš}**DÌḪ** A.2.6: 6; B.1.1: 12; C.1.4: 150'''

balṭu "alive; fresh; living (person)": **TI.LA** A.2.1: 89'''''

balṭūtu "state of being alive/healthy": [*bal-ṭ*]*ú-ti-šá* I.1.3: 19

balu "without": *ba-lu* C.1.8: 26'; C.2.1: 2'; E.1.2: 8'; *ba-lu-uk-ki* C.3.6: 10'; **NU.ME** C.3.1: 19

baluḫḫu (an aromatic plant and its gummy resin; sagapenum?): **BULUḪ** A.2.3: 28''', 30'''; C.1.9: 9, 19, 32; **BULUḪ**$^?$ A.2.4: 12'; ^{šim}**BULUḪ** II.1.4: 6; A.1.1: 22'; A.1.4: 10', 20'; A.2.1: 4', 12', 68'''', 90'''''; A.2.9: 13''; C.2.1: 4'; D.2.1: 43', 48', 50', 54'; ⸢^{šim}⸣**BULUḪ** A.2.1: 62'''; A.2.2: 8; ^{ši}[^{m}**BULUḪ**$^?$] B.1.1: 32

banduddû "bucket": **BA.AN.DU$_8$.DU$_8$-*ka*** D.1.1: 169

bāntu "mother": *ba-an-ta* C.3.10: 47

banû I G "to create; to fashion; to form; to grow"; N "to be created; to be formed": *ba-nu-u* [G] G.1: 11, 47; **DÙ-*ú*** [G] C.1.4: 48''; **DÙ-*ú*** [G] C.4.1: 2'; *ab-ni* [G] C.3.4: 10; ⸢*ib*⸣*-ba-ni* [N] II.1.2: 2; *ib-nu* [G] II.1.2: 4; *ib-ni* [G] C.1.4: 49''; *li-ib-ni* [G] B.2.1: 10; *ta-ba-an-ni* [G] C.3.4: 8; *tab*$^?$*-ni*$^?$ [G] C.3.6: 23'; *tab-ni-i* [G] C.3.4: 48

banû II G "to be(come) good, beautiful"; D "to make good; to beautify; to execute well": *ba-na-at* [G] G.2: 26''; *tu-ban-ni* [D] A.2.5: 19''

bānû, fem. *bānītu* "creator; begetter": *ba-ni-ti* C.3.4: 11; *ba-ni-tu* II.1.4: 37; D.1.1: 77; *ba-nu-ú* C.3.9: 57; C.3.10: 53; [*ba-nu-ú*]*-ki* C.3.3: 38; ⸢*ba-nu-šú*⸣*-nu* C.3.10: 54; **DÙ-*ki*** C.3.4: 77

banûtu "beauty": *ba-nu-tú* D.1.5: 11'

baqāmu G "to pluck; to tear out"; D "to pluck out (hair)": *ba-qa-mu* [G] G.1: 28; *ú-baq-qam* [D] I.1.3: 21

barāmu I G "to be multicoloured, variegated"; Gt "to be(come) speckled, multicoloured": *ba-ru-um* [G] I.1.1: 5; *bar-mat* [G] I.1.1: 8; **GÙN.A** [G] I.1.1: 5, 20, 21; *ib-tar-rum* [Gt] B.2.2: 9

barāmu II G "to seal (up)": ⸢*ta*⸣*-bar-ram* [G] C.1.5: 45

barbartu "she-wolf": *bar-bar-rat* C.3.4: 62; C.3.9: 41; [*bar-ba*]*r-rat* C.3.3: 15

barbaru "wolf": **UR$^?$.BAR$^?$.RA** A.2.6: 7; **[UR.BA]R.RA$^?$** II.1.3: 27'''

barīrātu (an aromatic plant and its gummy resin): *ba-ri-ra-te* B.1.1: 24; ^{giš}*ba*$^!$*-ri-ra-*[*t*]*a* II.1.4: 27; ^{giš}**LUM.ḪA** D.2.1: 58'; ^{ú}*ba-ri-ra-ta* II.1.4: 10, 22; [^{ú}*b*]*a-ri-ra-t*[*u*] C.1.4: 14'; ^{ú}*ba-r*[*a*$^?$*-ra-tu*$_4$$^?$] E.2.1: 5

barmu "multicoloured": **GÙN** F.1: 10; **GÙN.A** B.1.6: 2; C.3.6: 57''''; F.1: 6, 10, 13, 29, 30, 34; ⸢**GÙN.A**⸣ F.1: 22

barû G "to collate; to watch over; to behold": *ba-a-ri* [G] B.2.1: 34; **BA.AN.È** [G] D.1.1: 237; [*b*]*a*$^?$*-ar* E.2.3: 12'; *ba-ri* [G] C.3.4: 99; *ba-rù* [G] D.1.11: 16'; *bir* [G] I.1.1: 118; *ib-ri*$_{12}$ [G] C.2.1: 17'; **IGI.KÁR** [G] B.2.1: 41; D.3.1: 37(A); **IGI.**⸢**KÁR**⸣ [G] D.3.1: 39(b); **U$_6$** [G] D.3.1: 37(f)

bâru G "to catch": ⸢*i*$^?$⸣*-bar-ru* [G] B.1.5: 4'

bārû "diviner": ^{lú}⸢**AZU**$^?$⸣ C.3.6: 37''

barumtu, *barundu* "coloured wool": *ba-ru-un-di* F.1: 37; *ba-ru-un-*[*di*] F.1: 16; [*ba-ru-un-d*]*i* F.1: 41; $^{síg!}$*ba-ru-un-di* D.3.1: 3; ^{síg}⸢*ba*⸣*-r*[*u-un-di*] D.3.1: 34; ^{síg}*ba-ru-un-du* C.3.9: 5; D.3.1: 3; ; ^{síg}*ba-ru-*<<*DA*>>*-un-du* C.3.9: 30

bašālu G "to boil"; Š "to boil; to cook": **ŠEG$_6$** [Š] A.2.2: 40; D.2.1: 58'; **ŠEG$_6$-*al*** [Š] B.2.1: 18; **ŠEG$_6$-**⸢***al***⸣ [Š] A.2.7: 19; **ŠEG$_6$-*šal*** [Š] A.2.2: 18; A.2.3: 12', 28'''; A.2.7: 27'; A.2.9: 16''; C.1.4: 125''; C.2.1: 5'; D.2.1: 19', 22', 24', 35', 53'; E.2.6: 34', 37', 40', 42', 49'; **ŠEG$_6$-*š*[*al*]** [Š] B.1.2: 4'; **ŠEG$_6$-[*šal*$^?$]** [Š] D.1.7: 10'; **ŠE[G$_6$-*šal*]** [Š] D.1.7: 17'; **ŠE[G$_6$$^?$-*šal*]** [Š] A.2.2: 9; **Š[EG$_6$-*šal*$^?$]** [Š] A.1.1: 1'; **[ŠE]G$_6$-*šal*** [Š] A.1.1: 3'; E.2.6: 31'; **[ŠE]G$_6$$^?$-*šal*** [Š] E.1.2: 8'; **[ŠEG$_6$-*š*]*al*$^?$** [Š] A.2.2: 17; **ŠEG$_6$-*šal-ma*** [Š] E.2.6: 2'; *tu-šab-šal* [Š] II.1.4: 14, 24; ⸢*tu-šab*⸣*-šal* [Š] E.2.1: 7; ⸢*tu*⸣*-*[*šab*]*-šal-m*[*a*] [Š] D.1.11: 4; *tu-šab-ši-lu* E.2.6: 38'; *tu-šab*$^!$*-š*[*i*$^?$*-lu*$^?$] [Š] E.2.6: 26'

bašlu "boiled": **AL.ŠEG$_6$.GÁ** D.2.1: 57'; *ba-šal* E.2.6: 27', 28'; **ŠEG$_6$** D.1.11: 11; **Š[EG$_6$]** A.1.2: 5'

bašû G "to be available; to exist; to occur"; Š "to bring into being; to create; to procreate"; N "to be available; to come into being; to occur; to happen; to befall": ***ba-šu-ú*** [G] C.3.10: 35; ***ba-šú-⸢ú⸣*** [G] D.3.1: 25; ***[ba-š]u-ú*** [G] D.3.1: 25; **GÁL** [G] I.1.4: 5'; **GÁL-*ši*** [G] B.2.1: 43; ***[i]-ba-áš-ši*** [G] D.1.5: 4'; ***ib-ba-šu***$^{?}$ [N] A.2.2: 65; ***lib-ba-ši*** [N] C.3.6: 25'; ***tu-šab-šú*** [Š] C.3.10: 37
batāqu G "to cut off; divide; tear off"; D "to cut off": ***i-bat-taq-ma*** [G] D.3.1: 7; ***bu-ut-tu-qa*** [D] C.3.4: 64; C.3.9: 43
bātiqu "one who cuts": ***ba-ti-iq*** D.1.9: 34'
bâtu G "to stand overnight"; Š "to let stand overnight": ***i-ba-a-tú*** [G] C.3.10: 6; ***tuš-bat*** [Š] A.1.1: 18'; A.2.1: 84'''''; A.2.2: 60; A.2.7: 30'; A.2.9: 4'; C.1.4: 28'; C.1.8: 58''; D.1.11: 9; E.2.6: 28'; ***tuš***$^{!}$***-bat*** B.2.1: 22; ***⸢tuš⸣-bat*** E.2.7: 3'; ***⸢tuš-bat⸣*** C.1.5: 10; ***t[uš-bat***$^{?}$***]*** [Š] II.1.3: 45'''; A.1.1: 8'; ***[tu]š-bat*** C.1.4: 75''; C.1.5: 29
batūltu "adolescent, nubile girl": **MUNUS.GURUŠ.TUR** C.3.1: 33
bâ'u G "to go along, across; to pass; to overtake"; Š "to move past": ***a***$^{?!}$***-i-ba-am*** [G] B.2.1: 37; ***tuš-ba-a'-šú*** [Š] C.3.4: 55
bēltu "mistress": ***be-le-[et]*** D.1.10: 3'; ***be-l[e-et]*** D.1.9: 31'; ***be-let*** C.3.10: 18; D.1.1: 51; D.1.10: 8'; **GAŠAN** B.1.1: 70; C.3.6: 10'; C.3.10: 64; **⸢GAŠAN⸣-*tu***$_4$ C.3.6: 12'
bēlu "lord": ***be-el*** C.3.4: 98; ***be-[el]*** C.3.1: 14; ***be-lu*** C.3.4: 98; **EN** C.3.1: 28; C.3.5: 29'; C.3.7: 4'; D.1.1: 50, 168, 169, 187; D.1.8: 4; D.3.1: 17; G.1: 21; I.1.3: 10; **⸢EN⸣** D.3.1: 18; E.2.3: 10'; **EN-*šú-nu*** C.3.10: 41; **UMUN-*šú*** I.1.2: 15'
bennu "epilepsy": ***be-en-nu*** A.1.1: 49'''; D.1.3: 5'; ***[be-e]n-nu*** A.1.3: 6'
berû G "to be hungry; to starve"; D "to starve; to let go hungry": ***ú-bar-re-e-ma*** [D] C.2.3: 17', 20'; ***[ú-b]ar-re-e-ma*** [D] C.2.3: 15'
bêru G "to choose; to select; to be thin (of hair)": ***bé-e-er*** I.1.3: 9; ***bé-e-[er]*** [G] I.1.5: 8'
bi'iltu "container (for oil, ghee)": ***bi-'-il-ti*** G.1: 32
billat našpi, see ***našpu***
billatu (a dry substance used in the preparation of beer; beerwort): ***bi-il-le-tu***$_4$ A.2.8: 23'; **DIDA** II.1.4: 11, 28; A.1.1: 22'; A.2.4: 13'; B.1.1: 6; B.2.4: 25'; D.2.1: 18', 25', 43', 48', 51', 53', 54', 56'; E.2.4: 7'; **DID[A]** D.2.1: 42'; **[DID]A** A.1.3: 10'; A.2.1: 98''''''
biltu "load; burden": ***bil-tu***$_4$ C.3.10: 45; ***bil-lat-su*** C.3.10: 57
binītu "creation; creature; shape; limbs": ***bi-ni-it*** II.1.1: 32
binna "give!": ***bi-in-nim-ma*** C.3.10: 30
bīnu "tamarisk": ⸢$^{giš?!}$***bi***$^{?}$***-ni***$^{?}$⸣ C.3.4: 49; ^{giš}**ŠINIG** C.1.4: 147''', 165'''; D.3.1: 1, 30; ^{giš}**⸢ŠINIG⸣** D.3.1: 6a; [^{gi}]^{š}**ŠINIG** B.1.1: 58; ^{giš}**ŠI[NIG]** C.3.6: 46'''; **ŠINIG** C.1.5: 18; C.1.10: 16; C.3.4: 44, 49, 54; D.3.1: 2, 30
binûtu "creation; creature; product; form": ***bi-nu-tam*** D.1.1: 137; ***bi-nu-ut*** C.3.5: 16'; D.1.1: 110, 123; ***bi-nu-⸢ut***$^{?}$⸣ B.1.1: 58; ***bu-nu-ut*** II.1.4: 48, 49
birdu nodule; skin spot: ***bi***$^{!}$***-ir***$^{!}$***-da***$^{?!}$ A.2.8: 15; ***bir-di*** D.2.1: 29'
biri- "among, between": ***bi-ri-šú-nu*** C.3.9: 2; ***bi-ri-šú-n[u]*** F.1: 2
birītu I "space between"; *ina birīt* "between; among": ***bi-ri-it*** B.2.6: 10; ***bi-ri***$^{?}$***-it***$^{!}$ B.2.6: 5; ***bi-rit*** C.1.4: 8'; C.3.4: 9; C.3.10: 76
birītu II "clasp": ***bir-rat*** C.3.9: 9
biṣṣūr atāni "donkey vulva" (name of a shell or cowrie snail): ^{na4}**PEŠ**$_4$**.ANŠE** C.1.4: 156'''; **PEŠ**$_4$**.ANŠE** C.1.5: 20
biššu a garden plant: ***bi-iš-<šú>*** A.2.6: 22
bītānû "inner": ***b[i-ta-ni-tú]*** C.3.4: 58; **É-*a-ni-tú*** C.3.3: 5
bītu "house; temple": ***bi-i-tú*** C.3.9: 45; **É** II.1.4: 25; A.2.2: 46; A.2.7: 40'; B.2.6: 4; C.1.4: 10'; C.3.3: 22, 28; C.3.4: 11, 16, 66, 70; C.3.6: 2', 4', 61''''; C.3.8: 9; C.3.9: 51; C.3.10: 32, 34; D.1.9: 28'; D.3.1: 9, 39(A); G.1: 14, 18; I.1.1: 115, 117; I.1.3: 21, 22, 33'; **⸢É⸣** D.3.1: 7; **⸢É**$^{?}$**⸣** C.2.1: 15'; **É-*sà*** I.1.3: 20; **É-*šá*** D.1.5: 18'; **É-*šú*** C.3.4: 23, 55; C.3.10: 91
buḫḫuru D "to heat": ***tu-ba-aḫ-ḫar*** [D] D.1.7: 6'
bukru "son": ***bu***$_{12}$***-kúr*** C.3.10: 92
bulṭu "prescription; remedy": ***bul-ṭu*** A.2.7: 41'; C.1.4: 17'; C.2.1: 15'; ***[b]u-ul-ṭú*** C.1.8: 29'
būlu "animals; livestock": ***[bu]-ul*** C.3.4: 45
buppānu a plant: ^{ú}***bu-up-pa-nu*** A.2.6: 5
buqlu "malt": **MUNU**$_4$ A.2.4: 18'; C.3.2: 5''; **MUNU**$_4^{?}$ A.2.8: 34'; **M[UNU**$_4$**]** E.2.1: 5; **MUNU**$_5^{?}$ A.2.5: 12'; **[MUN]U**$_5^{?}$ A.2.2: 18; **MU[NU**$_5^{?}$**]** A.2.2: 22; **MUNU**$_6$ B.1.1: 5; D.2.1: 62'; **⸢MUNU**$_6^{?}$**⸣** A.2.2: 65
buqlu qarnānû "sprouted malt": **MUNU**$_4^{?}$**.È.⸢A**$^{?}$**⸣** A.2.3: 13'
burāšu "juniper": ^{giš}**LI** A.2.1: 64'''; B.2.4: 19'; D.2.1: 25', 43', 47', 50', 52', 54', 56'; E.2.4: 2'; ^{giš}**L[I]** D.2.1: 41'; $^{giš.šim}$**LI** C.3.10: 69; **LI** B.2.2: 7; B.2.4: 13'; B.2.6: 7; **⸢LI**$^{?}$**⸣** B.2.2: 7; **[L]I** B.2.2: 15; ^{šim}**LI** II.1.4: 21; A.1.4: 5'; A.2.1: 60'''; A.2.2: 8, 74; A.2.6: 7, 12, 22; B.1.1: 59; C.1.4: 10', 149''', 181'''; C.3.4: 6, 42; C.3.10: 62; D.1.7: 13'; D.2.1: 21', 27', 62'; D.3.1: 8, 16; [^{ši}]^{m}**LI** A.2.2: 83; ⸢^{šim}**LI**⸣ II.1.4: 3; ⸢^{šim}⸣**[LI]** B.2.1: 19; ^{š}[^{im}**LI]** A.1.2: 9'; [^{šim}]**⸢LI**$^{?}$**⸣** A.2.1: 103'''''''; [^{šim}**L]I** A.2.3: 17'; C.2.1: 3'; C.3.6: 9'
burku "knee; lap": ***bur-ki-šá*** A.2.4: 8'
burrumu "multicoloured": ***⸢bur⸣-ru-mu*** A.2.6: 12
būrtu I "hole; pit; cistern": **PÚ** A.1.4: 30''; C.3.4: 81
būrtu II "cow": ***bu-ur-tu*** II.1.4: 57
būru I "(bull) calf": **AMAR** C.1.4: 3'; D.1.1: 144, 157; **AMAR**$^{!?}$ C.2.2: 6; ***bu-ru*** II.1.4: 55; D.1.1: 156; ***bu-ú-ri*** D.1.1: 157
būru II "well": ***bu-ú-ri*** C.3.5: 23'
burzigallu (a bowl): ^{dug}**BUR.ZI.GAL** B.2.1: 18; C.3.4: 3
burzisallû (a bowl): **BUR.ZI.SAL** C.3.6: 58''''
buṣinnu (a plant, perhaps mullein (*Verbascum*); wick (made from *Verbascum* leaves)): ^{ú}***bu-ṣi-ni*** B.1.6: 4
būšānu, *bu'šānu* (unidentified plant, lit. 'stinking plant'): ^{ú}**ḪAB** II.1.3: 37'''; A.2.1: 51''', 73''''; D.2.1: 31'; ^{ú}**ḪAB**$^{?}$ A.2.1: 102'''''''
būštu, *būltu* "shame; modesty; dignity": ***bul-ta*** II.1.4: 45; ***[bul-t]a*** D.1.1: 84
buṭnānu (a garden plant, lit. "terebinth-like"): ^{giš}***bu-uṭ-na-nu*** D.2.1: 60'

buṭumtu, *buṭuttu*, *buṭuntu* "terebinth": ***bu-ṭu-tú*** D.2.1: 44'

bu''û D "to look for": ***ub-be-ak-ka*** [D] C.3.10: 43, 54

bu''ušu "stinking": ***bu-'u-ú-šu-tú*** A.2.2: 75

da'āmu G "to be(come) dark (red)": **DARA$_{4}$$^{!}$-⸢*im*⸣** [G] I.1.1: 52

da'āpu G "to push away; to knock against (part of body)"; D "to injure": ***i-da-'i-ip*** [G] D.3.1: 32; ***ú-da-'a-ap*** [D] D.3.1: 32

dabābu G "to speak; to talk"; Š caus. "to let/make someone speak": **DU$_{11}$.DU$_{11}$** [G] A.2.7: 40'; **DU$_{11}$.DU$_{11}$-*ub*** [G] D.1.1: 229; G.2: 25''; **DU$_{11}$-*ma*** [G] C.3.4: 23; ***id-bu-bu*** [G] B.2.2: 25'; ***šu-ud-bu-bu*** [Š] A.2.6: 11, 14, 17; ***tu-šad-bab-šú*** [Š] D.3.1: 28; ***[tu-u]š$^{?}$-ta-ad-bi-bu*** [Š] E.2.3: 18''

dadānu (a thorny shrub, probably *Prosopis farcta*): **^{ú}KIŠI$_{16}$.ḪAB** D.2.1: 31'

dādu "darling": ***da-di*** G.1: 42; ***da-du*** G.1: 43

dagālu G "to see; to look at": ***i-da-ga-la*** [G] II.1.2: 10; ***ta-da-gal*** [G] II.1.4: 41

dâku G "to kill": **GAZ-*ma*** [G] C.3.10: 80

dalālu G "to praise": ***lid-lul*** [G] C.3.10: 61; D.1.8: 19; D.3.1: 13; ***lu-ud-lul*** [G] B.2.6: 25; ***lud-lul*** [G] C.3.10: 17, 40; D.1.8: 26; D.3.1: 13, 27

dalīlu "praise; glory": ***da-li-li-ka*** B.2.6: 25; C.3.10: 40, 61; ***dà-lí-lí-ka*** C.3.10: 17; D.1.8: 19, 26; D.3.1: 13, 27; ***[d]a$^{?}$-li-li-ki*** C.3.6: 27'

daltu "door": **^{giš}IG** C.1.4: 10', 15'; D.1.1: 175

dalû G "to draw water (with bucket)": ***ta-dal-ú-ma*** [G] D.1.11: 10

dâlu G "to walk/run/move around; to roam": ***i-da-al*** [G] D.1.1: 96; ***i-da-a[l$^{?}$]*** [G] D.1.1: 94

dām erēni "cedar blood" (cedar tar?): **MÚD EREN** E.2.6: 13'; **MÚD ^{giš}EREN** A.2.2: 26; 38; C.1.5: 2; C.1.9: 8; E.2.4: 6'; E.2.6: 26'

damāmu G "to wail; to moan"; Š caus. of G: ***ú-š[a]d-ma-mu*** [Š] C.3.4: 92

damāqu G "to be good; to prosper": **SIG$_{5}$** [G] B.2.3: 16''; E.2.1: 17; E.2.6: 29'; **[SI]G$_{5}$$^{?}$** [G] A.2.2: 18; **SIG$_{15}$** [G] A.2.5: 14'

dāmātu, *da'mātu* (a dark-yellow paste): **IM.SIG$_{7}$.SIG$_{7}$** C.1.4: 148'''

damiqtu "good fortune; favour; good will": ***da-mi-iq-ta-šá*** C.1.4: 64''

damqu "good; fine; favourable": ***dam-qa*** B.1.1: 50; ***[da]m-qa*** B.1.1: 42; **SIG.GI** A.2.7: 31'; **SIG$_{5}$** A.2.2: 39; B.1.1: 23; **[SI]G$_{5}$$^{?}$** A.2.4: 13'; **SIG$_{15}$** A.2.5: 11'

dāmu "blood": ***[da$^{?}$]-mi-šú*** A.2.8; ***da-mu*** I.1.2: 6', 8'; **MÚD** A.2.1: 13', 17', 20'; A.2.2: 28, 29, 31; A.2.6: 16; A.2.7: 2; A.2.10: 5'; B.2.2: 3; B.2.3: 19''; B.2.4: 4'; C.1.1: 4, 14, 19; C.1.2: 26'; C.1.4: 65'', 185'''; C.1.5: 25, 37; C.1.8: 32'; C.1.9: 1, 3, 6, 10, 15, 20, 25; C.1.10: 8, 9, 17; C.3.3: 3, 20; C.3.4: 57, 65, 70; C.3.5: 10'; C.3.9: 44, 50; D.2.1: 40'; I.1.1: 31, 93; I.1.6: 8', 9'; **⸢MÚD⸣** A.2.1: 21', 23'; A.2.2: 18, 23; **[M]ÚD** F.1: 32; **MÚD$^{?}$** E.2.6: 13'; **MÚD.ME-*šú*** A.2.5: 13'; C.1.8: 21; **[M]ÚD.ME-*šú*** C.1.9: 26; **MÚD.MEŠ** A.2.2: 61; C.1.3: 15''; C.1.4: 5'; **MÚD.MEŠ-*ša*** C.1.8: 11'; **MÚD.M[EŠ-*ša*]** II.1.4: 2; **MÚD.MEŠ-*šá*** II.1.4: 40; C.1.2: 17; C.1.8: 21'; F.1: 28; **MÚD.ME[Š-*šá*]** C.1.3: 14'; **MÚD.[MEŠ-*šá*]** C.1.3: 12'; **[M]ÚD$^{!}$.MEŠ-*šá*** C.1.1: 3; **⸢MÚD.MEŠ⸣-*šá*** C.1.8: 28'; **MÚD.MEŠ-*šú*** A.2.2: 42; C.1.4: 55''; C.1.10: 1, 7; **MÚD-*šá*** C.1.1: 10; C.1.5: 30; C.2.1: 14'; C.2.2: 2; **MÚD-⸢*ša*$^{?}$⸣** C.1.2: 21'; **MÚD-*ši-na*** C.1.4: 49''; **MÚD-*šú*** A.2.2: 53; C.1.5: 10, 36; **MÚD$^{?}$-*š[ú$^{?}$]*** A.2.2: 23; **MÚD$^{?}$-[*šú*]** A.2.2: 13

da'mu "dark (blood)": **MUD** I.1.1: 82, 87, 88

danānu G "to be(come) strong; to be heavy, difficult, severe"; D "to strengthen": ***dan-na-áš-šú*** [G] I.1.2: 5'; ***dan-na-a[t]*** [G] C.3.9: 27; ***dan-na-niš-šú*** [G] I.1.7: 10; ***⸢dun⸣-nu-nu*** [D] C.1.4: 59''; ***[u]d-dan-ni-na$^{?!}$*** [D] D.1.1: 98

dannatu "hardship; trouble; distress": ***dan-na-te*** D.1.1: 31, 34; ***dan-na-ti*** D.1.1: 49, 186; G.1: 27; ***dan-na-tu$_{4}$*** D.1.1: 49

dannu I "strong; powerful; mighty; severe; hard": ***dan-na-ti*** G.1: 15; ***dan-na-tu*** D.1.1: 87; ***dan-nu*** D.1.1: 104; ***dan-nu-ti*** A.1.4: 8'; **KALA** A.2.6: 15; C.3.7: 4'; **KALA.GA** C.1.8: 57''; D.2.1: 6'; **⸢KALA.GA$^{?}$⸣** A.2.2: 15

dannu II "(large) vat; barrel": ***dan-nu*** A.2.2: 76

dânu G "to judge; to administer justice": ***i-din-nu*** [G] B.2.6: 3

dapīnu "overbearing; savage": ***[da-p]i-ni*** C.3.3: 17; ***da-pi-nu*** C.3.4: 63; C.3.9: 42

daprānu "juniper": ***^{giš}dap-ra-nu*** B.1.2: 6'; ***^{šim}dáp-ra-na*** II.1.4: 20

dāt, *dāti*, *dātu* "behind; after; then"; *ina dāt*, *iddāt* (prep., conj.) "behind; after": ***id-d[a-at]*** D.1.11: 9

dayyānu "judge": ***da-a-a-nu*** D.1.8: 12, 13; **DI.KUD** D.3.1: 19

dekû, *dakû* G "to raise; to lift up": ***da-ke-e*** [G] I.1.7: 10; ***[da-k]e-e*** [G] I.1.2: 4'

dīdū (a women's undergarment): ***[di-d]a-a-šá*** C.3.3: 19; ***di-da-a-šú*** C.3.9: 43; ***d[i-da-a-šú]*** C.3.4: 64; ***di$^{!}$-da-šá*** C.3.9: 43; ***di-di*** A.2.2: 55

dikšu "bulge; pressing pain": ***⸢di$^{?}$⸣-ik-šú*** A.2.1: 24'

diktu, *tiktu* (a type of flour): **ÚTU** E.2.6: 35'

diliptu "sleeplessness": ***di-lip-tu$_{4}$*** C.3.10: 35; ***[di-li]p-⸢tu$_{4}$$^{?}$⸣*** D.2.1: 15'

dimtu "tear": ***d[i]-⸢ma⸣-[a-šú]*** G.2: 2'; ***di-ma-šá*** C.1.4: 51''; ***di-ma-šú*** C.1.4: 55''; D.1.1: 27; ***di-ma-ta*** C.3.5: 22'

dinānu "replacement; substitute": ***di-⸢na-ni⸣-i[a$^{?}$]*** E.2.3: 21''; ***di-na-ni-šá*** E.2.3: 6'; ***[di-na-n]i-šá*** E.2.3: 20''; ***[di-na-ni-š]á$^{?}$*** E.2.3: 7'

dīnu "(legal) case; legal decision": ***di-i-ni*** D.1.1: 50; ***di-in*** B.2.6: 3; ***di-in-šú*** C.3.10: 49; ***di-ni$_{7}$-šu-ma*** C.3.10: 56; ***di-ni$_{7}$-šú-n[u]*** C.3.10: 42

diqāru "pot": **$^{⸢dug⸣}$ÚTUL** C.1.10: 14

diqmēnu, *ṭikmēnu*, *dikmennu* "ashes": **DÈ** A.2.2: 43, 64; C.1.2: 13; C.1.4: 166''', 167''', 168'''; D.1.7: 4'; **DÈ.LÁ** C.1.4: 175'''; ***dì-iq-mé-[en]*** II.1.3: 31'''; ***dì-iq-m[é-en]*** II.1.3: 32'''; ***di-iq-me-en-na*** B.2.2: 22'; ***di-iq-me-en-na-šú-nu*** C.1.10: 15

dišpu "syrup; honey": **LÀL** A.2.2: 80; A.2.4: 11'; C.1.4: 3', 12'; C.3.6: 8'; E.2.1: 9; E.2.5: 9'; **LÀ[L]** D.2.1: 45'; **⸢LÀL⸣** A.2.2: 17; C.3.4: 41; F.2: 42'; **[L]ÀL** C.3.4: 90; **[L]ÀL$^{?}$** A.2.2: 24; E.2.6: 13'

di'u (a disease): ***di-'u*** C.3.10: 35; ***⸢di$^{?}$-ú$^{?}$⸣*** D.2.1: 15'

dudittu "dress-pin": ***du-di-it-ti*** C.3.4: 75; C.3.9: 56

DÙ.DÙ.BI (reading uncertain); "the procedure for it": **DÙ.DÙ.BI** A.1.1: 31''; C.1.4: 22'; C.3.6: 6'; C.3.10: 62; D.1.1: 54, 132, 173, 196, 200; D.1.4: 8'; D.3.1: 2; **DÙ.DÙ.[B]I** C.1.5: 42; **[DÙ].DÙ.BI** C.1.2: 27'; **[DÙ.D]Ù.BI** C.1.1: 15; **[DÙ.DÙ.B]I** D.1.2: 6

dullu "trouble; work; craft; ritual; treatment": ***dul-la-šá*** B.2.2: 5

dumqu "goodness; good (thing); good fortune": ***du-muq*** C.1.4: 63''
dūru "(city) wall": **BÀD** C.3.4: 96; D.1.1: 113, 126, 132, 172; G.1: 48; ***du-ú-ru*** G.1: 49
durugiqqu "rectal disease": **DÚR.GIG** A.1.4: 7', 9'; **⸢DÚR.GIG⸣** A.1.4: 4'
dušû "steatite; chlorite": ^{na4}**DUḪ.ŠI.A** A.2.7: 26'

ē (an interjection): ***e*** D.1.1: 44
ebēbu G "to be pure/clean/bright"; D "to purify": ***ub-ba-bu*** B.1.1: 59
ebēḫu G "to gird"; D "to be surrounded with": ***u-bu-ḫa-at*** [D] II.1.4: 37, 38, 39; ***ub-b[u-ḫa-at]*** D.1.1: 78; ***[ub]-bu-[ḫa-at]*** D.1.1: 79
ebertu "opposite bank; other side": ***e-ber-ti*** C.3.4: 14
ebēru G "to cross over"; Š "to make cross; bring across": ***tu-še-ber*** [Š] C.3.4: 14
ebēṭu G "to swell up; to be swollen": ***eb-ṭù*** [G] I.1.1: 66
ēdēnu, *ēdānu* "alone": ***⸢e$^{?}$-da$^{?}$-na$^{?}$⸣*** B.2.6: 18
ēdēnû, *ēdānû* "single; sole; alone": ***e-de-na-a*** C.1.8: 33'
edēpu G "to blow (away); to be inflated"; D "to be inflated": ***i-di-ip*** [G] I.1.7: 1; ***ud-du-pat*** [D] D.2.1: 25', 26', 28'
edēru G "to embrace"; N "to embrace one another": ***e-de-ri*** [G] G.1: 17; ***na-an-du-ra*** [N] G.1: 17
ēdiššī- "alone": ***e-diš-ši-šú*** C.3.4: 44
edlu "locked": ***ed-le-e-ti*** D.1.1: 120; ***ed-lu*** D.1.1: 105
edû I "flood, wave": ***e-de-e-em*** II.1.1: 32
edû II G "to know"; Š "to make known; to show": ***e-de-e*** [G] C.3.10: 39; ***e-du-ú*** [G] G.2: 24''; ***i-di*** [G] C.3.10: 40; ***⸢tu$^{?}$-še$^{?}$⸣-du-ši*** [Š] C.1.4: 78''; **ZU-*šá*** [G] I.1.5: 5'; **ZU-*ú*** [G] A.2.1: 55'''
ēdu I "single; sole; solitary": ***⸢e⸣-da*** B.1.1: 58
ēdu II, *šammu ēdu* (unidentified plant), lit. "solitary (plant)": ^{d}**DILI** A.2.1: 81'''''; B.1.6: 2; C.1.4: 7'; ^{d}**DILI$^{?}$** A.1.1: 7'
ēdû "prominent; renowned": ***e-di-ti*** G.2: 24''; ***i-di-tu$_{4}$*** D.1.1: 129
ēkallu "palace": **[É.GA]L** D.1.2: 16; **⸢KUR⸣** D.1.6: 16''
ekdu "wild; fierce": ***⸢ek$^{?}$⸣-[di$^{?}$]*** C.3.1: 10; ***ek-du*** II.1.4: 56; D.1.1: 144
ekkēmu "robber": ***ek-ke-mu*** C.3.4: 82
eklētu "darkness": ***ek-le-ti*** C.3.3: 8, 10; C.3.5: 16'; ***[ek]-⸢le⸣-ti*** D.1.1: 52; ***ek-le-tim*** C.3.5: 16'; ***e[k]-⸢le⸣-tú*** D.1.1: 52; ***ek-let*** C.3.4: 59, 60
elāniš "above": ***e-la-niš*** D.1.1: 133
elēnu, *elānu* "above (of)" (adv., prep.): ***e-la-an*** D.2.1: 17'; ***⸢e⸣-la-nu*** D.1.1: 55; ***e-le-nu*** D.1.1: 180
elēḫu G "to strew; to sprinkle"; D "to strew; to sprinkle": ***ul-lu-ḫa-tú*** [D] B.2.2: 3; ***[ul]-⸢lu⸣-ḫat*** [D] A.2.2: 73
elēlu G "to be pure"; D "to purify": ***el-let*** [G] C.3.10: 27; E.2.3: 27''; ***[tu-u]l-lal-ma*** [D] C.3.4: 36; ***[t]úl-lal-šú-ma*** [D] C.3.4: 36
elēnītu, *eliyanītu* (fem.) "the superior one": ***e-li-ia-na-ti*** C.3.9: 16
eleppu "boat": ***e-lep-pi*** G.1: 1; ^{giš}**MÁ** C.3.4: 14; D.1.1: 30, 33, 48, 102, 106, 185, 188; D.3.1: 22; G.2: 15'', 22'', 23''; [^{gi}]^{š}**MÁ$^{?}$** C.1.5: 25; ⸢^{giš}**MÁ**⸣ D.1.1: 91; ⸢$^{giš!}$**MÁ$^{?}$**⸣-***šá*** D.1.1: 4
eli (prep.) "on; upon; over; above": D.1.1: 224; ***e-li*** G.1: 12; ***⸢e-li$^{?}$⸣*** D.1.1: 91; ***e-li-ía*** C.3.4: 11: **UGU** C.1.4: 63''
eliš "above": **AN.TA** H.1: 38'; I.1.1: 64; ***e-liš*** C.3.10: 41
elītu "that which is above; upper world": **AN.TA.MEŠ** D.3.1: 18; **[A]N.TA.MEŠ** E.2.3: 11'; ***⸢e-la-a-te⸣*** C.3.4: 98; ***el-li-ti-šá*** F.1.: 8; ***e-lit*** D.1.8: 12
ellu "pure": ***el-le-e-ti*** G.1: 21; ***el-le-tu$_{4}$*** A.2.8: 37'; ***e[l-l]e$^{?}$-tu$_{4}$*** D.1.9: 36'; E.2.3: 3'; ***el-lim*** B.2.6: 23; ***[el-lu]-ti*** D.1.9: 32'; ***el-lum*** G.1: 3; **KÙ** C.3.4: 25, 40; **KÙ.GA** II.1.4: 11; B.1.1: 64, 65, 66; C.3.4: 40; **KÙ.[(GA)]** E.2.3: 2'; **⸢KÙ⸣.GA$^{!}$** D.1.1: 151; **KÙ.MEŠ** D.1.8: 5, 6; G.2: 6'
elû I "upper": ***e-li-i*** D.1.1: 174
elû II G "to go up; to come up; to rise"; Š "to take out; to remove": ***e-li-ma*** [G] C.1.4: 61''; **E$_{11}$**-***la-ma*** [Š] II.1.4: 14; **E$_{11}$**-***ma*** [Š] II.1.4: 25, 29; **E$_{11}$$^{!}$**-***ma*** [Š] E.2.6: 12'; **E$_{11}$**-***ma*** [G] D.3.1: 8, 9; **E$_{11}$$^{!?}$**-***ma*** [Š] E.2.6: 28'; **E$_{11}$**-***ši-ma*** [Š] B.1.1: 19; ***i-lam-ma*** [G] C.3.4: 64; C.3.9: 43; ***[i-l]am-ma*** [G] C.3.3: 18; ***il-la-a'*** [G] C.3.10: 31; ***il-lam-ma*** [G] C.3.10: 26; ***il-li-ma*** [G] D.3.1: 8, 9; ***še-li*** [Š] II.1.4: 48; ***tu-še-il-la-a*** [Š] B.1.1: 16; ***⸢ú$^{?}$⸣-še-[li$^{?}$]*** [Š] B.1.1: 42; ***ú-šel-le*** [Š] D.3.1: 9; ***⸢ú-šel-le⸣-ma*** [Š] D.3.1: 9; ***⸢uš$^{?}$⸣-[e]l$^{?}$-lam-ma*** [Š] A.2.2: 71
ēm, *ēma* "wherever; whenever": ***e-ma*** C.3.6: 53''''; C.3.10: 73; D.2.1: 25'; E.1.1: 8; H.1: 34'; ***e-m[a]*** H.1: 3; ***[e-m]a*** C.1.1: 16; ***⸢e⸣-[ma]*** C.1.4: 186'''; ***e-ma-a'*** C.3.10: 9
emēdu G "to lean on; to impose; to load"; Št "to mix": ***en-de-et*** [G] C.3.10: 44, 55; ***en-de-tu-nu*** [G] C.3.10: 25; ***i-mid-da*** [G] C.3.10: 59; ***tuš-te-mid*** [Št] C.1.4: 177'''
emēmu G "to be hot": ***i-te-mu*** [G] D.2.1: 45'; **KÚM** [G] I.1.3: 8; **KÚM$^{?}$** [G] A.2.4: 41'''
emēru G "to be swollen, bloated; to have a colic": ***e-mar-ma*** [G] D.1.6: 5; ***em-rat*** [G] II.1.4: 1
emesallu (a type of salt), see *ṭābat emesalli*
emmu "hot": **KÚM** A.2.2: 32; **KÚM**-***am*** E.2.5: 6'
emšu "abdomen": ***em-ša-ša*** D.2.1: 17'; ***em-ši-ša*** C.3.5: 12'; I.1.1: 59, 60, 61, 62, 63, 64, 65; ***em-ši-šá*** I.1.1: 74; ***[em]-ši-šú*** A.2.1: 24'; **ḪÁŠ**-***šá*** C.1.4: 23', 108''; **ḪÁŠ**-***[šá]*** C.1.4: 94''; ^{uzu}***em-ši-e-ša*** II.1.4: 30
ÉN É.NU.RU: "Enuru incantation": **ÉN É.NU.RU** C.1.4: 76'', 90'', 95'', 114'', 123'', 127'', 130'', 139'', 143''; D.1.1: 22, 135; D.1.7: 31', 21'; **ÉN$^{!}$ É.NU.RU** II.1.4: 50, 62; **[ÉN] É.NU.RU** B.1.1: 76; **[É]N É.NU.RU** C.1.4: 79''; **ÉN É.NU.R[U]** C.1.4: 88'', 136''; **ÉN É.NU.[RU]** C.1.4: 135''; C.3.5: 16'; D.1.1: 37
enēqu G "to suck"; Dt "to be suckled"; Š "to suckle; to give the breast": ***i-ni-iq-ma*** [G] A.2.4: 7'; ***lu-še-niq*** [Š] C.3.4: 67; C.3.9: 47; ***lu-še-ni-i[q]*** [Š] C.3.3: 23; ***ú-ta-naq*** [Dt] C.3.4: 86
engisû, *engišû* (a stone): [^{n}]^{a4}***en-gi$^{?}$-⸢su$^{?}$⸣*** C.3.6: 64''''
ennēnu, *inninnu* (a type of barley): ***in-ni-ni*** B.1.1: 23

enu "lord": ***e-n[i-im***$^{?}$**]** D.1.9: 31'

enzu "goat": **ÙZ** C.1.4: 38'; C.3.6: 51''''; D.1.1: 233; **Ù[Z**$^{?}$**]** A.2.1: 47''

eperu "earth; soil; dust": ***e-pe-ri*** G.1: 9; ***ep-ri*** D.1.1: 23; **SAḪAR** C.1.4: 28'; C.3.5: 9'; D.1.1: 38, 132, 133, 173, 174, 175, 209; D.2.1: 26', 28'; G.1: 48, 51; **⸢SAḪAR**$^{?}$**⸣** A.1.1: 19'; **SAḪAR.ḪI.A** D.1.1: 177; **SAḪAR**$^{!}$**.MEŠ** II.1.4: 37, 38, 39; **⸢SAḪAR⸣-*ru*** C.3.3: 2

epēšu G "to do; to perform; to commit"; Gtn iter. of G; D "to perform; to execute properly (tablet)"; Š caus. of G: **⸢AK**$^{?}$**⸣** [G] C.2.3: 11'; **DÙ** [G] D.2.1: 65'; E.2.6: 24'; **DÙ-*su*** [G] E.2.6: 22', 32', 36'; **DÙ-*s[u*** $^{?!}$**]** [G] E.2.6: 24'; **DÙ-*ši*** [G] D.3.1: 38(A); **DÙ-*šu*** [G] C.3.10: 22, 23, 24; **DÙ-*uš*** [G] A.2.1: 54'''; A.2.2: 76; A.2.4: 15'; B.2.2: 23'; C.1.6: 9'; C.1.10: 4; C.3.4: 39; C.3.9: 7; C.3.10: 89, 90; D.1.1: 23; D.3.1: 2; **DÙ-*u[š]*** [G] C.1.6: 6'; C.3.4: 2; **DÙ.DÙ-*šu*** [Gtn] C.1.4: 13'; **DÙ.DÙ-*uš-ma*** [Gtn] C.3.10: 83; **DÙ.MEŠ-*uš-ma*** [Gtn] II.1.4: 13; ***e-pu-uš*** [G] B.2.2: 5; C.3.10: 56; ***[e]-pu-uš*** [G] C.3.10: 49; ***ep-šu-ši-ma*** [G] C.3.7: 17''; ***te-ep-pu-ši-ma*** [G] C.3.10: 2; ***te-ep-pu-šu***$^{?!}$ [G] C.2.3: 12'; ***te-pu-u[š]*** [G] II.1.3: 50'''; ***tu-še-ep-su*** [Š] E.2.1: 14; ***up***$^{!}$***-pu-ša-ta*** [D] II.1.4: 32; ***up-puš***$_4$ [D] D.1.11: 16'

epinnu "(seed) plough": ^{giš}**APIN** II.1.4: 39; ^{giš}**APIN**$^{!}$ D.1.1: 78

ēpištu "sorceress": ***⸢e-piš-ti⸣*** C.3.6: 42'''; ***e-piš-tú*** C.3.10: 42, 44; ***e-piš-t[ú]*** C.3.10: 58; ***e-piš-tu***$_4$ C.3.10: 23, 24

ēpišu "sorcerer": ***e-piš*** C.3.10: 23, 24, 42, 44, 58

eqlu "field": **A.ŠÀ** B.2.1: 7

equ G "to daub; to apply": **MAR-*qú*** [G] A.2.5: 11'; ***te-qu*** [G] A.2.6: 17

erbe, fem. *erbet* "four": **4** A.1.4: 13', 14'; A.2.2: 74; A.2.4: 42'''; B.2.6: 7; C.1.4: 103''; C.1.10: 5, 8; C.4.1: 9', 10'; E.2.6: 17', 19', 21', 32', 35'; F.1: 2, 10, 12, 23; F.2: 7, 9; I.1.1: 37; I.1.3: 34'; **⸢4⸣** C.1.8: 38'; **4**$^{?!}$ E.2.6: 25'; **⸢4**$^{?}$**⸣** F.2: 19; ***er-bé*** G.1: 18

erbēšer "fourteen"; U$_4$.14.KAM "the fourteenth day": **14** II.1.3: 33'''; A.2.2: 54; C.1.1: 8; C.1.4: 22', 47', 109'', 155'''; C.1.4.1: 5'; D.1.2: 6; F.1: 22, 28, 29, 31; F.2: 23'; I.1.1: 44; **U**$_4$**.14.KAM** B.2.6: 2

erbêšu "four times": **4-*šú*** A.2.4: 38'''

erbu "locust": **BU[RU**$_5$$^{?}$**]** A.2.2: 19

ereb šamši "sunset; west": ^{d}**UTU.ŠÚ.A** C.1.8: 16', 34'; E.2.3: 19''; ^{d}**UTU.ŠÚ.⸢A⸣** A.2.7: 37'; **KU**$_4$ ***šam-ši*** C.3.4: 13

erēbu G "to enter"; Š "to bring in; to insert": ***e-ru-ub*** [G] II.1.4: 17; ***e-ru-um-ma*** [G] B.1.1: 52; ***i-ru-ba-am-ma*** [G] D.3.1: 1; ***i-ru-bu*** [G] C.3.9: 45; ***ir-ru-ub*** [G] C.3.9: 46; ***ir-r[u-ub]*** [G] C.3.3: 22; **KU**$_4$ [G] C.3.4: 55, 66; **KU**$_4$**-*am-ma*** [G] E.2.3: 28''; **KU**$_4$**-*bi*** [G] C.3.4: 70; **KU**$_4$**-*eb*** [Š] C.1.4.2: 7'; **⸢KU**$_4$$^{?}$**⸣-*⸢eb⸣*** [Š] C.1.4.2: 8'; **KU**$_4$**-*ma*** [G] D.3.1: 1; **KU**$_4$**-*ub*** [G] A.2.7: 40'; C.3.4: 66; C.3.10: 91; ***te-ru-⸢ba⸣*** [G] C.3.10: 90; ***⸢ter-ru-bi-ma⸣*** [G] C.3.4: 16; ***ter-[ru-bi]*** [G] C.3.3: 28; ***ter-ru-bu*** [G] C.3.9: 51; ***tu-še-rab*** [Š] D.1.5: 16'; ***tu-še-rab-ši*** [Š] II.1.4: 26

erēnu "cedar": ***e-re-⸢ni⸣*** D.1.1: 3; **EREN** B.2.3: 19''; **⸢EREN⸣** A.2.1: 8'; **[ER]EN**$^{?}$ A.2.1: 100''''''; ^{giš}***⸢e⸣-re-ni*** B.1.1: 26; ^{giš}**EREN** A.2.2: 26; A.2.9: 15''; B.1.3: 6; B.2.4: 16', 30'; C.1.4: 113'', 167'''; C.3.10: 80; ^{giš}**⸢EREN⸣ C.1.9: 31;** ^{giš}**ER[EN]** F.2: 41'; ^{g}**[**^{iš}**E]REN** C.1.9: 19; ^{šim}**EREN.NA** II.1.4: 20

erēšu I G "to sow; to cultivate; to plough": ***⸢i⸣-ri-iš*** [G] A.2.7: 8; ***i-⸢ri⸣-iš*** B.2.1: 7; ***⸢i-te-riš-ka-ma⸣*** C.3.10: 21

erēšu II G "to desire; to request": ***i-ri-šú*** [G] D.1.1: 129; ***⸢te-riš⸣-[i]n-ni*** [G] D.1.5: 8'

ergilu (a type of locust): **BURU**$_5$**.IR.GI.L[UM]** A.2.7: 24'

erib karāni "grapevine locust": **⸢BURU**$_5$$^{?}$**⸣.GEŠTIN.NA** A.2.7: 26'

erib tâmti "sea locust (shrimp?)": **BURU**$_5$ **A.AB.BA** A.2.4: 13'; ***e-ri-bi ti*-GÉME** B.2.3: 18''

erib turbu'ti "dust locust": **BU[RU**$_5$**].⸢SAḪAR.RA⸣** B.2.1: 16

erištu "wish; request; need": **⸢KAM-*ti***$^{?}$**⸣-*šú-nu*** A.2.2: 37; **URU**$_4$$^{!}$**-*tú*** B.2.2: 23'

erru, *irru* "intestine(s)": ***ir-ri*** D.2.1: 34', 39'; ***ir-ru-šá*** D.2.1: 33'

errû, *irrû* "colocynth; wild melon(?)": ***ir-re-e*** C.3.4: 46; ***ir-re-e***$^{!?}$ A.2.2: 30; **ÚKUŠ.LAGAB** A.2.2: 54; A.2.7: 35'; D.2.1: 66'; **ÚKUŠ.LAG[AB]** C.2.1: 9'; **⸢ÚKUŠ⸣.LAGAB** E.2.2: 2'

erṣetu "earth": ***[er-ṣ]e-tú*** D.1.9: 18'; **KI** C.3.4: 15; **KI-*tim*** D.1.9: 19'; D.3.1: 11a, 19; E.2.3: 10'

eršu "bed": ^{giš}**NÁ-*šú*** A.2.2: 48

erû "copper": ***e-ru-u*** G.1: 34; ^{na4}**URUDU** C.3.10: 3; F.2: 26'; **URUDU** B.1.4: 13; B.2.4: 15'; H.1: 33'; **[UR]UDU**$^{?}$ C.1.5: 46

ēru, *e'ru* (a tree and its wood, possibly cornel): ^{giš}**MA.NU** C.1.4: 103'', 153''', 185'''; D.1.1: 196, 200; D.3.1: 4; **[**^{giš}**]MA.NU** II.1.3: 67'''

esēlu G "to inflate; to be constipated": ***es-lu*** [G] II.1.4: 2

esēpu G "to gather together": ***te-si-ip*** [G] II.1.4: 8, 28; ***te-sip*** [G] B.1.1: 15

esēru G "to enclose"; D "to enclose, imprison; to wrap(?)": ***tu*-ŠIR-*ši*** [D] II.1.4: 9, 15

eṣēlu G "to paralyze"; N "to be become paralysed"; Ntn iter. of N: ***it-te-nen-ṣi-la*** [Ntn] I.1.1: 84; ***it-te-ne[n-ṣi-la]*** Ntn I.1.4: 4'

eṣemtu "bone": ***e-ṣe-em-tum*** II.1.2: 2; ***e-ṣe-et*** C.1.9: 11; **GÌR.PAD** D.1.1: 235; **GÌR.PAD.DU** C.1.4: 26', 175'''; C.1.10: 11; C.2.2: 6; D.1.1: 101, 123, 234, 235; **GÌR.PAD.D[U]** D.1.7: 16'; **⸢GÌR.PAD⸣.DU** A.2.2: 28; **[GÌR.PAD.D]U**$^{?}$ A.2.2: 67; **⸢**^{uzu}**⸣GÌR.PAD.DU** D.1.5: 21'

eṣēnu G "to smell"; Š caus. of G; "to let sniff": ***tu-še-ṣe-en-ši*** [Š] D.2.1: 28'; ***tu-še-ṣe-en-ši-ma*** [Š] D.2.1: 26'

eṣēru G "to draw": ***te-ṣir*** [G] E.2.3: 5'

ešer "ten": **10** A.1.4: 7'; A.2.2: 7; C.3.10: 76; C.4.1: 1'; F.2: 1; I.1.1: 43

ešēru G "to go well/straight; to be well/successful; to prosper"; Š "to put in order; to make successful; to cause to prosper; to have a bowel movement; to give birth easily/normally; to sweep (out)"; Št "to set aright; to deliver easily; to sweep (out)": ***e-še-ri*** [G] G.1: 10, 36, 50; ***eš-re-tú*** [G] C.3.10: 16; ***eš-re-tu***$_4$ [G] C.3.10: 13; ***i-še***$^{!?}$***-[er-ši***$^{?}$**]** [G] I.1.6: 18'; ***li-i-šèr*** [G] D.1.1: 36; ***[l]i-še-er*** [G] D.1.1: 160; ***⸢li⸣-še-⸢ra⸣*** [G] D.1.1: 158; ***li-šèr*** [G] D.1.8: 17; ***li-ši-ir*** [G] D.1.1: 52, 160; ***⸢li***$^{?}$***⸣-ši-[ir]*** [G] D.1.1: 191; ***liš-te-še-ra*** [Št] D.1.1: 103; ***liš-te-šir*** [Št] D.1.1: 227; ***lu-še-ši-ir*** [Š] C.3.4: 11; ***[lu-še***$^{?}$***-š]i-ir*** [Š] C.3.6: 4'; ***lu-ši-ir*** [G] C.3.4: 11; ***lu-ši-r[a]*** [G] D.3.1: 12; ***lu-uš-te-šer*** [Št] D.3.1: 12; ***⸢lu⸣-u[š]-te-ši-ra*** [Št] D.3.1: 12; **SI.SÁ** [G] C.3.4: 23; D.2.1: 33'; **SI.SÁ** [Š/Št] C.3.10: 62; D.1.1: 55, 134; I.1.1: 26, 27, 39, 55; ***šu-ši-ra-an-ni-ma*** [Š] C.3.10: 16; ***šu-šu-ri*** [Š] C.3.6: 6'; ***šu***$^{?}$***-šu-ri*** [Š] B.2.6: 19; ***šu-š[u-ri***$^{?}$**]** [Š] A.2.4: 3'; ***šu-šu-ru*** [Š] C.3.10: 13; 16; ***šú-šú-ru*** [Š] I.1.1: 49; ***šu-te-šur*** [Št] D.1.1: 130; ***uš-te-eš-še-ra*** [Št] D.1.1: 184; ***uš-[te-še]-ra*** [Št] D.1.1: 39; ***uš-te-[še-ra***$^{?}$**]** [Št] D.1.2: 14; ***u[š-te-še-ra***$^{?}$**]** [Št] D.1.2: 5; ***uš-te-še-<<eš>>-ri*** [Št] D.1.1: 39; ***uš-te-šer*** [Št] D.1.1: 204; ***uš-te-šer-šu*** [Št] D.1.9: 32'; ***uš-te-ši-ri*** [Št] D.1.8: 12; ***ú-še-iš-še-r[a]*** [Š] D.1.1: 24

ešrā "twenty": **20** B.2.4: 23'; C.1.4: 2'
ešrû "tenth; one-tenth"; *ina ešrî ūmi* "on the tenth day": **10** I.1.1: 113; ***10-i*** C.4.1: 11', 13'; **10.KAM** I.1.3: 7; **[U$_4$.10].KÁM** I.1.1: 113
eššu "new": ***eš-še-tu$_4$*** C.3.10: 3; ***eš-šú*** C.3.9: 28; D.1.11: 9; **GIBIL$_4$** C.1.10: 14
etellu "supreme; prince": ***e-⸢tel⸣*** D.1.8: 1; ***e-tel-lu*** C.3.4: 98; ***e-tel-lu$_4$*** C.3.4: 98
etēqu G "to cross over; to pass by; to go past"; Š "to make pass by": **BAL** [G] A.2.5: 25''; **DIB** [G] C.3.6: 5'; C.3.8: 13'; C.3.10: 82, 84; **DI[B]** [G] C.3.8: 13'; **[DI]B$^{?}$** [G] C.3.4: 55; ***DIB-iq-šú*** [G] C.3.9: 40; ***DIB-ma$^{!?}$*** [G] C.3.4: 55; ***e-té-qa*** [G] G.2: 7'; ***e-te-qu*** [G] G.1: 24; ***i-te-ti-iq-šú*** [G] C.3.4: 24; ***šu-ti-qa-an-⸢ni⸣-ma*** [Š] D.3.1: 26; ***šu-tu-qí*** [Š] D.3.1: 23; ***šu-⸢tu⸣-qí*** [Š] D.3.1: 1; ***šu-t[u-q]í-ma*** [Š] D.3.1: 1; ***šu-tu-qu*** [Š] C.2.3: 19'; D.3.1: 23, 25; ***ú-še-et-te-qu-ma*** [Š] D.3.1: 31; ***⸢ú-še⸣-et-[ti-qu]*** [Š] D.3.1: 31; ***ú-še-ti-iq*** [Š] D.3.1: 31
eṭēru G "to take away; to save"; N "to be taken away, saved": ***e-ṭe-ri*** [G] C.3.4: 80; ***in-né-ṭe-ru*** [N] C.3.4: 97; ***⸢iṭ-ṭi-ra⸣*** D.2.1: 15' [G] D.2.1: 15'; **KAR** [G] C.3.4: 1; **KAR.MEŠ** [Ntn] C.3.4: 1
eṭlu "young man": **GURUŠ** C.1.4: 54'', 62''; **GURUŠ.MEŠ** C.3.9: 19; D.1.5: 11'; **⸢GURUŠ$^{?}$⸣.MEŠ** C.3.10: 70
eṭṭeru "eager to save": ***eṭ-ṭe-ru*** C.3.4: 82
eṭû G "to be(come) dark, dim"; D "to darken": ***ú-ṭa-a*** [D] II.1.4: 41
ezēbu G "to leave"; Š "to rescue; to save": ***e-ze-bi*** [G] G.1: 36; ***šu-zu-bu*** [Š] C.3.10: 59; ***TAG$_4$-šú*** [G] C.3.10: 74; ***⸢ú$^{?}$⸣-še-zi-bu*** [Š] C.3.4: 83
ezēzu G "to be furious, raging, fierce": ***ez-ze-et*** [G] A.2.7: 3; C.3.3: 4; C.3.4: 62; C.3.9: 41; ***⸢ez-ze⸣-[et]*** [G] C.3.3: 14; ***ez-ze-ta*** [G] C.3.9: 27

gabarû "copy; opponent": **GABA.RI** B.2.2: 29'; C.2.1: 16'; C.3.4: 79, 97, 99; C.3.10: 91; I.1.1: 117; I.1.3: 35'; **[GAB]A.RI** C.1.8: 30'; D.1.4: 16''; ***gaba-rì*** C.3.9: 7, 39
gabbu "totality; all (of)": ***gab-bi*** A.2.5: 10'; B.2.2: 2; C.1.10: 13; ***gáb-bi*** B.2.2: 21'; ***gab-bu*** F.2: 40
gabû, *aban gabî* "alum": **IM.SAḪAR.NA$_4$.KUR.RA** C.1.4: 42', 112'', 148''', 162'''; C.2.2: 8; **⸢IM.SAḪAR⸣.[NA$_4$.KUR.RA]** C.1.4: 1'; **⸢IM⸣.SAḪ[AR.NA$_4$].KUR.RA** C.1.8: 9'; **[IM.SAḪAR.N]A$_4$.⸢KUR⸣.RA** A.1.4: 37''; **[IM.SAḪA]R.N[A$_4^{!}$].KUR.RA** C.1.2: 16; **NA$_4$** ***ga-bi-i*** A.1.1: 31''; C.1.5: 12; **[NA$_4$** ***g]a-bi-⸢i⸣*** A.1.1: 10'; **⸢NA$_4$⸣** ***g[a-bi-i]*** A.1.1: 20'; ^{na4}***E-ú*** B.2.4: 9'; ***ga-bi-[e]*** C.1.4: 169'''; ^{na4}***ga-bu-u*** A.1.4: 6'; A.2.1: 12'; ^{na4}***ga-bu-[u]*** C.1.6: 8', 10'; ^{na4}***gab-b[u-u]*** A.2.1: 2'; ^{na4}***ga-⸢bu⸣-[u]*** A.2.1: 86''''''; ⸢^{na4}***gab-bu-u⸣*** A.2.1: 8'; ^{na4}***gab-bu-ú*** A.2.2: 36, 70; C.1.9: 18, 22; ^{na4}***gab-u*** A.2.4: 9'; B.2.2: 1, 13; B.2.4: 14'; E.2.5: 6', 18'; ^{na4}***gab-ú*** C.1.10: 1, 3, 6, 16; ^{na4}***[ga]b-⸢ú⸣*** B.2.4: 29'; ^{n}[^{a4}***ga-bu-u$^{?}$]*** A.2.10: 7'; ***gab-⸢ú⸣*** C.1.10: 10
galātu G "to tremble; to be afraid"; Gtn iter. of G; D "to frighten": ***ḪULUḪ.ḪULUḪ-ut*** [Gtn] I.1.3: 14; ***i-ga-[al-lit]*** [G] D.1.1: 146; ***ig-da-lit*** [G] D.1.1: 146; ***ig-ta-lit*** [G] D.1.1: 146; ***ú-ga-al-lit*** [D] D.1.1: 146
gallābūtu "function of a barber; (to perform) shaving": ***gal-la-bu-us*** C.3.10: 2
gamāru G "to complete; bring to conclusion": ***ga-am-rat*** [G] II.1.4: 32; ***ga-ma-ri*** [G] D.1.1: 145; ***i-ga-ma-ru*** [G] D.1.5: 12'; ***ig-mu-ru$^{!?}$*** [G] C.3.4: 45
gamru, fem. *gammirtu* "complete; total": ***gam-mar-ti*** G.1: 20; **TIL** C.3.4: 18; ***TIL-šú*** C.1.10: 8; ***[TI]L-tim*** G.2: 5'
GAN.U$_5$ (reading uncertain; a medicinal plant): ^{giš}**GAN.U$_5$** C.3.6: 17'; C.3.9: 21
gaṣṣu "gypsum": **IM.BABBAR** C.3.4: 54
gašīrû (an unidentified plant): ⸢^{ú}⸣***ga-ši-ru-u*** A.2.1: 35'
gašru "powerful (one); very strong (one)": ***ga-aš-ru*** C.3.4: 98; ***ga-aš-rù*** C.3.4: 98
gešû G "to belch": ***i-geš-sú*** [G] I.1.7: 1
gillatu "misdeed; crime; error; sin": ***gíl-la-a-ti*** B.1.1: 45; ***gíl-lat*** C.3.10: 14, 34; ***⸢gíl-lat-su⸣*** C.3.10: 56
gilšu, *giššu* "hip-(bone)": ***giš-šú*** A.2.5: 9'
gimillu "favour; friendly deed; vengeance": ***gi-mil-li*** D.2.1: 69'
ginû "regular offerings"; a quality of flour: ***gi-na-a*** E.2.6: 28'
girû "1/24 shekel; carat": ***gi-re-e*** A.1.4: 13', 14', 15', 16'; ***gír-u$^{?}$*** A.2.5: 8'; ***gír-⸢e⸣*** A.2.8: 14
gišimmaru "date palm": ^{giš}**GIŠIMMAR** A.2.4: 4'; C.1.4: 147'''; C.1.10: 13, 33; H.1: 23'; H.2: 3; [^{gi}]^{š}**GIŠIMMAR** B.1.1: 60; **GIŠIMMAR** E.2.5: 3'; ***giš-ma-ru*** A.2.5: 8'
gišnugallu see *ašnugallu*
gizillû "torch": **GI.IZI.LÁ** C.3.4: 55; E.2.3: 4'
GI.ZÚ.LUM.MA (reading uncertain; unidentified medicinal plant, perhaps mullein; see the dictionaries under *buṣinnu*, *kūru*, *kurṣiptu*): **GI.ZÚ.LUM** C.1.4: 171'''; ^{giš}**GI.ZÚ.LUM.MA** C.1.4: 182'''; ^{giš}**GI.Z[Ú.LUM.MA]** A.2.1: 1'; $^{ú?}$**G[I.ZÚ.LUM.MA$^{?}$]** A.2.1: 65''', 103'''''''
gūdu (a plant/drug): ^{ú}***gu-ú-du*** A.2.2: 31, 35
guḫlu "antimony; black paint for the eyes; kohl": ***⸢gu⸣-uḫ-lu*** A.2.8: 14
gulgullu "skull": ***gul-gul*** D.1.3: 28''; D.2.1: 14'; ***[gul-g]ul$^{?}$*** A.2.7: 24'; ***[gul-g]ul$^{?}$-la*** H.1: 36'; ***gul-g[ul-li]*** A.2.5: 8'
gurnu, *gunnu* "of average quality": ***gu-un-ni*** D.2.1: 11'; ***gu-un-nu*** E.2.6: 21', 24', 32', 34'
gušūru "beam": ^{giš}**ÙR** C.1.10: 12, 13; C.2.2: 5; ^{giš}**Ù[R]** A.2.10: 3'; C.1.6: 2'; ***[gu-š]u$^{!}$-ri*** E.2.6: 44'; **[ŠU.Ù]R** C.1.7: 4'; **ŠU.ÙR** C.1.9: 13

ḫabātu G "to rob; to plunder"; Gtn iter. of G: ***iḫ-t[a-n]a-b-ba-tu*** [Gtn] C.3.4: 91
ḫabbātu "plunderer": ***ḫab-ba-ta*** C.3.4: 91; ***ḫab-ba-tu*** C.3.4: 83
ḫabbūru "sprout; shoot": **⸢ḪÉNBUR⸣** D.1.1: 223
ḫābilu, fem. *ḫābiltu* "evildoer; criminal": ***ḫe-bi-il$_5$*** C.3.10: 43; ***ḫe-bil-ti*** C.3.10: 43
ḫalāpu G "to slip into, through": ***i-ḫal-lu-um-ma*** [G] C.3.10: 85; ***i-ḫal-lu-up*** [G] C.3.4: 66; C.3.9: 45; ***i-ḫal-lu-up$^{!}$*** [G] C.3.10: 87; ***i-ḫal-lu-⸢up⸣*** [G] C.3.3: 21
ḫalāqu G "to be lost; to disappear; to perish"; D "to destroy; to annihilate": ***ú-ḫal-liq*** [D] D.1.9: 40'; **ZÁḪ** [G] C.3.1: 31; I.1.3: 21
ḫallu I "loins": ***ḫal-li*** C.1.4: 177'''; ***ḪAŠ$_4$-šà*** I.1.1: 60
ḫallu II (a clay vessel): ***ḫa-li*** [G] D.1.1: 151, 152, 154; ***ḫal-li*** D.1.1: 154
ḫallulāya "centipede(?)": **UB.PAD** B.1.5: 4'

ḫallūru "pea": **GÚ.GAL** B.1.1: 24; C.1.4: 126''; C.2.2: 12; D.2.1: 50'; E.2.6: 20', 30', 33'; **GÚ$^?$.G[AL$^?$]** D.1.7: 7'; **G[Ú.GA]L** A.2.1: 27'
ḫalṣu "pressed; filtered": ***ḫal-ṣa*** A.2.3: 12'; A.2.4: 11', 45'''; B.2.2: 19', 23'; D.1.7: 15'; D.1.11: 11; ***⌜ḫal-ṣa⌝*** A.2.3: 10'; ***[ḫ]al$^?$-<ṣa>*** A.1.4: 17'; ***ḫal-ṣu*** D.1.2: 10
ḫaltu (a stone): ***ḫal-ti*** D.1.4: 17''; F.1: 9, 19; F.2: 8; ***ḫal-tú*** C.3.9: 2; F.1: 19; ***ḫal-tu$_4$*** F.1: 19; $^{\text{na4}}$***ḫal-ta*** C.1.4: 4', 184'''; $^{\text{na4}}$***⌜ḫal-tu$^?$⌝*** C.3.1: 2
ḫaluppu (a tree): ^{giš}**ḪA.LU.ÚB** D.2.1: 29'
ḫamāṭu G "to inflame; to burn"; D "to burn (up); to incinerate": ***ḫu-um-mu-ṭu*** [D] E.2.6: 27'; ***tu-ḫa-[a]m-maṭ*** [D] A.2.4: 17'
ḫamedīrānu (a plant/drug?): ***ḫa-me-di-ra-an-ni*** A.2.8: 6
ḫamiš, fem. *ḫamšat* "five"; *ḫamšat ūmī* "five days": **5** A.2.5: 21''; C.3.9: 2; C.4.1: 11'; D.2.1: 24'; E.2.1: 6; E 2.6: 16', 30', 33', 37', 39', 40'; F.1: 16; F.2: 15; I.1.1: 38, 47, 48; **U$_4$.5.KAM$^!$** I.1.6: 32'
ḫamiššer "fifteen": **15** B.2.4: 22', 29'; E.2.6: 10'; I.1.1: 45; **15$^!$** D.3.1: 4; **1[5$^?$]** D.3.1: 35
ḫamiššerīšu "fifteen times": **15-*šu*** C.1.4: 177'''
ḫāmītu "sand-wasp": **NIM.UR$_4$.UR$_4$** C.1.4: 151'''
ḫamšīšu "five times": **5-*šú*** C.3.10: 9; E.2.6: 24'
ḫamšu "fifth; one-fifth"; *ina ḫamši ūmi* "on the fifth day": **5** I.1.1: 108; **5-*aš*** A.1.4: 15'; A.2.8: 30'; **5-*šú*** C.4.1: 6'; **5.KAM** I.1.3: 3; **⌜U$_4$⌝.5.KÁM** I.1.1: 108
ḫāmū "rubbish": ***ḫa-mu*** C.3.10: 39
ḫanāqu G "to press; to strangle, throttle": ***ta-ḫa-naq-ma*** [G] C.3.4: 4; C.3.9: 13
ḫanqu "strangled": ***ḫa-ni-⌜iq$^?$-ti⌝*** C.1.8: 13'
ḫapāpu G "to break up; to smash; to pound": ***ta-ḫap-pap*** [G] E.2.6: 4'; ***⌜ta$^?$⌝-ḫap-pap*** [G] A.2.3: 8'
ḫapû G (meaning uncertain): ***ta-ḫap-pu*** [G] E.2.6: 31'
ḫâqu G "to mix up": ***[t]a-ḫa-qu*** [G] E.2.1: 7; ***[ta-ḫa]-qú-ma*** [G] A.2.4: 12'
ḫarāšu G/N "to be in childbed, confinement": ***it-taḫ-ri-šú*** [N] D.1.6: 8
ḫarpu "early": ***ḫar-pu*** C.3.10: 37
ḫarištu "woman in childbed": ***ḫa-riš-ti*** A.2.3: 5'; D.2.1: 40'; ^{munus}***ḫa-riš-ti*** I.1.7: 1; ^{munus}***ḫa-riš-t[i]*** C.3.5: 2'; $^{⌜\text{munus}⌝}$***ḫa-riš-tú*** D.2.1: 36'
ḫarmunu (a medicinal plant): $^{⌜\text{ú}⌝}$**ḪAR.ḪUM.BA.ŠIR** B.1.1: 37
ḫarrānu "way; road; journey": ***⌜ḫa-ra⌝-na-am*** II.1.2: 10; ***ḫar-ra-na*** D.1.1: 25; **KASKAL** C.3.10: 90; **⌜KASKAL$^?$⌝** G.2: 14''; **[K]ASKAL.A$^?$** A.2.10: 10''; **KASKAL.MIN** C.3.10: 8; G.1: 38
ḫarūbu "carob": ^{giš}***ḫa-ru-bi*** D.2.1: 51'; ***ḫa-ru-bu*** A.2.1: 28'; A.2.2: 31
ḫaṣabtu "(pottery) sherd": **ŠIKA** C.1.4: 9', 99''; C.3.3: 5; C.3.4: 58; **ŠIKA-*tú*** A.2.1: 18'
ḫaṣānu G "to embrace; to take under one's protection": ***ha-ṣa-nu*** [G] G.1: 16; ***ḫe-eṣ-ne-et*** [G] G.1: 16; ***i-ḫaṣ-ṣí-in-ma*** [G] C.3.10: 26, 33
ḫaṣāṣu G "to snap off": ***ta-ḫa-aṣ-ṣa-aṣ-ma*** [G] II.1.1: 30
ḫaṣbu "(pottery) sherd": $^{\text{na4}}$**ŠIKA** C.3.1: 6; **ŠIKA** A.2.2: 28, 37, 40; A.2.5: 7', 8', 9'; C.1.4: 112'', 168''', 180'''; C.1.9: 12, 23; C.1.10: 11, 14; F.1: 20, 30; F.2: 31'; **ŠIKA$^?$** A.2.2: 30
ḫašālu G "to crush": **GAZ** [G] A.1.1: 6'; A.1.4: 39''; A.2.1: 75''''; A.2.2: 16; A.2.3: 7', 27'''; C.1.4: 87''; C.1.9: 5, 9; **⌜GAZ⌝** A.2.5: 11'; C.1.9: 31; C.2.2: 6; **⌜GAZ$^?$⌝** II.1.3: 56'''; **KUM** [G] A.2.1: 16'; A.2.6: 13; **⌜KUM⌝** A.2.1: 28'; ***ta-ḫaš-šal*** [G] II.1.3: 35'''; ***[t]a-ḫaš-šal*** II.1.3: 50'''
ḫašḫūru "apple (tree)": $^{\text{giš?}}$**ḪAŠḪUR** D.1.11: 14'
ḫašlu "crushed": **GAZ-*lu*** D.1.11: 11
ḫašû (a medicinal plant and spice, probably thyme): ^{giš}***ḫa-šu-u*** A.1.2: 12'; D.2.1: 23'; **ḪAR.ḪAR** B.2.2: 7; ^{ú}**ḪAR.ḪAR** C.1.4: 170''', 181'''; C.2.1: 3', 9'; C.3.6: 17'; D.2.1: 21', 52', 66'; I.1.5: 3'; ^{ú}**ḪAR.[ḪAR]** II.1.3.1: 5'
ḫaṭṭi rē'î "shepherd's staff-plant": ^{giš}**NÍG.GIDRU SIPA** C.1.8: 33'
ḫaṭṭu "staff": ^{giš}**GIDRU** D.1.1: 196, 200
ḫâṭu G "to examine; to seek out": **LÁ-*šú*** [G] B.2.2: 21'
ḫayyaltu "woman in labour": ***ḫa-a-a-la-te*** D.1.5: 19'
ḫepû G "to break; to smash": **GAZ-[*ma*$^?$]** [G] D.1.1: 39; ***ḫe-pí*** [G] A.2.7: 7; C.1.10: 18; C.3.9: 28; D.1.1: 144; I.1.1: 46; ***⌜ḫe⌝-pí*** [G] A.2.7: 38'; ***ḫe-pi-ma*** [G] G.1: 12; ***ḫé-pu-u*** [G] I.1.7: 5
ḫerṣu "fragment; cut (piece)": **GIG** C.1.4: 103''; D.3.1: 4; **[GI]G$^?$** D.3.1: 35; ***ḫe-re-eṣ*** C.1.4: 28'; ***ḫe-er-ṣi*** C.1.4: 185'''
ḫiālu, *ḫâlu* G "to be in labour; exude (fluid)": ***ḫa-li-⌜e⌝-[šá]*** [G] D.1.6: 6; ***ḫa-li-šá*** [G] D.1.1: 148, 165; ***i-ḫa-al*** [G] D.1.1: 146; ***i-ḫi-la*** [G] D.1.5: 19'; ***i-ḫi-lu*** [G] D.1.11: 1; ***ta-ḫa-al*** [G] II.1.4: 57
ḫiāqu, *ḫâqu* G "to mix": ***li-ḫi-ia-aq*** [G] H.1: 37'
ḫilibû (a dark red, translucent stone): $^{\text{na4}}$**ḪI.LIB** F.2: 27'
ḫīlu "resin, gum": ***ḫi-li*** A.1.4: 10', 32''; ***⌜ḫi-li⌝*** A.2.2: 17; ***ḫi-l[i$^?$]*** A.2.2: 24; **ILLU** II.1.4: 5, 6; A.2.1: 4', 6', 12', 64''', 68''''; A.2.3: 30'''; A.2.4: 19'; A.2.9: 13''; B.2.2: 7; B.2.4: 5', 7', 25'; C.1.4: 171'''; C.1.9: 9, 19, 32; C.1.10: 11; D.1.7: 14'; D.2.1: 48', 53'; E.2.4: 6', 13'; E.2.8: 10''; **ILL[U]** B.2.4: 23'; **IL[LU]** A.2.8: 33'; A.2.9: 13''; C.2.1: 4'; **[IL]LU** A.1.4: 20'; **[ILL]U** A.1.1: 22'; A.2.1: 90''''''; **⌜ILLU⌝** A.2.1: 62'''; A.2.3: 28'''; B.2.4: 3'; E.2.8: 1'; **ILLU$^{?!}$** D.3.1: 15
ḫīlū "labour pains": ***[ḫ]i-i-li*** II.1.4: 59; ***ḫi-li*** II.1.4: 60; ***ḫi-li-ša*** II.1.4: 58; ***ḫi-li-šá*** C.3.10: 89; D.1.1: 148; ***ḫi-lu*** D.1.6: 6
ḫimētu "ghee": **Ì.NUN** A.2.3: 4'; C.1.4: 3', 87''; C.3.4: 41; D.2.1: 33'; E.2.6: 13', 24'; **[Ì.N]UN$^?$** D.1.3: 19'; **Ì.NUN.NA** C.1.4: 12'; C.3.6: 8'; F.2: 42'; **⌜Ì.NUN.NA⌝** C.3.4: 90
ḫissatu "understanding; wisdom; intelligence": ***ḫi-is-sa-tu$_4$*** G.1: 46
ḫišiḫtu "requirement; needed thing": ***ḫi-ši-iḫ-tú*** C.3.4: 5
ḫiṭītu "crime; sin; defect": ***ḫi-ṭi-ti*** C.3.10: 34; ***ḫi-ṭi-tu$_4$*** C.3.10: 14
ḫīṭu "crime; sin; wrongdoing": ***ḫi-ṭu*** B.1.1: 45
ḫubur (a plant): ^{ú}***ḫu-bur*** C.3.9: 9
ḫubūtu "thicket": ***ḫu-bu-ta*** A.2.3: 20'

ḫūdu "joy; happiness; satisfaction"; *ḫūd libbi* "happiness; contentment": ***ḫu-ud*** D.1.8: 8; ***ḫu-[ud]*** D.1.9: 12' **ŠÀ.ḪÚL.LA** A.2.5: 18''; **[Š]À$^{?}$.ḪÚL.LA** D.1.4: 19''
ḫulālu (a stone with black and white stripes; banded agate): ^{na4}**NÍR** C.1.8: 24'; C.3.9: 4; F.1: 5, 40; ^{na4}**N[ÍR]** F.2: 5
ḫulibu (a fatty substance): ***ḫu-li-bi*** A.2.2: 76
ḫultuppû, *ḫaltappû* "rod (of the incantation priest)": ***ḫal-dap-pu-ú*** A.2.8: 39'
ḫulû "shrew": ***ḫu-la-a*** A.2.2: 50
ḫuluqqā'u, *ḫuluqqû*, *ḫulqû* "(financial) losses": ***ḫu-lu-uq-šú*** C.3.4: 38
ḫummušu "one-fifth of a shekel": **5-*šú*** A.2.8: 13
ḫumṣirtu, *ḫam(a)ṣirtu*, *ḫab(a)ṣirtu* "female mouse": ***ḫa-am-ṣi-ir-ta*** C.3.10: 80
ḫumṣiru "(large) mouse": **⸢PÉŠ SAR⸣.R[A$^{?}$]** A.2.7: 23'
ḫunṭu "ripeness; maturity": ***[ḫ]u-un-ṭu*** A.2.4: 17'
ḫuppu (meaning uncertain): ***ḫúp-pa*** F.1: 35; ***ḫúp-pi*** C.3.9: 11; F.1: 7, 35
ḫupû "disposable (lit. 'broken') pot; sherds": ***ḫu-pa-a*** C.3.4: 18
ḫurāṣu "gold": **KÙ.SI$_{22}$** A.2.7: 27'; C.1.4: 2'; C.3.4: 85; C.3.9: 8, 9; **K[Ù.S]I$_{22}$** B.1.4: 12; ^{na4}**KÙ.SI$_{22}$** F.2: 28'
ḫûratu "madder": ^{giš}**ḪAB** A.2.1: 51'''; A.2.5: 6'; C.1.2: 28'; C.2.2: 11; F.1: 20, 29, 31; F.2: 30'; [^{g}]^{iš}**ḪAB** B.2.4: 20'
ḫurbabillu "chameleon(?)": **BAR.GÙN.<GÙN>.NA** C.1.4: 180'''
ḫurdatu "(female) pudenda": ***ḫur-da-as-sa*** D.1.1: 85; ***ḫur-da-ti*** G.1: 42; ***hur-da-tú*** G.1: 40; ***ḫur-da-at-na*** G.1: 41; ***ḫur-da-at-ni*** G.2: 21''; ***ḫur-da-at-su*** G.1: 40; G.2: 20''
ḫurru "hole; garbage pit": **[ḪABR]UD$^{?}$** C.1.8: 16'; ***ḫur-ri*** G.1: 42; ***⸢ḫur⸣-ri*** C.1.5: 42
ḫuṣābu "twig; stick; splinter; chip": ***ḫu-ṣa-bu*** A.2.1: 64'''; ***ḫu-ṣab*** A.1.4: 32''; B.2.4: 5'
ḫuššû "red": ***ḫuš-sa-a*** C.1.4: 78''
ḫuzālu, *uzālu* "gazelle kid": ***ú-za-li*** D.1.1: 156

idu "arm; side; strength"; *ina idi* "at (someone's) side, beside"; *idi ana idi* "on each side": **Á** C.3.9: 10, 11, 12, 32; **⸢Á$^{?}$⸣** B.2.6: 9; **Á-*šá*** C.1.4: 11'; ***i-da-šu*** II.1.2: 9; ***i-di*** G.1: 43; G.2: 22''; ***i-[di-šá]*** C.1.4: 16'; ***i-di-šú*** G.1: 43; G.2: 21''
igāru "wall": **É.GAR$_{8}$** G.1: 50; ***i-gàr*** C.3.10: 25; ***i-ga-ri*** C.3.10: 7; **IZ.ZI** D.1.1: 208
igigallu "wise person; wisdom": **[IGI.GÁ]L$^{?}$-*lu*$_{4}$** D.1.10: 8'
igirû "heron": **ÍGIRA^{mušen}** H.2: 3
ikkibu "taboo": **NÍG.GIG-*šá*** I.1.3: 25
ikkillu "clamour": ***ik-kil-li-šá*** D.1.1: 148, 165; ***i[k-ki-li-ša$^{?}$]*** II.1.4: 57; ***ik-kil-lu$_{4}$*** C.3.4: 82
ikribu "prayer": **SISKUR$^{!}$** A.2.5: 7'
īku "dyke; ditch; small canal; bank of earth": ***i-k[u$^{?}$]-šá*** B.1.1: 53
illātu "saliva; spittle": ***il-la-at*** D.1.1: 232; **ÚḪ** D.1.1: 232
illūr pānī, *lurpânu* (a red cosmetic pigment): **IM.KÙ.SI$_{22}$** C.1.4: 148'''
illurê, *illuru* (an exclamation): ***il-lu-ra*** C.3.9: 17; ***il-lu$^{!}$-ru*** C.3.9: 17
illūru (a plant with a red flower): ^{ú}***el-lu-ra*** C.1.4: 28'; ^{ú}***el-⸢lu-ra⸣*** C.1.4: 30'; ^{ú}**NÍNDA** C.1.4: 156'''; **[^{ú}NÍN]DA$^{?}$** C.1.5: 26
iltu "goddess": **DINGIR-*at*** C.3.4: 62; ***i-lat*** C.3.3: 14; C.3.9: 41; ***i-la-ti*** C.3.8: 5, 6
ilu "god": **DINGIR** B.1.1: 46, 70; C.1.4: 60''; D.2.1: 70'; **DINGIR-*ía*** C.3.10: 39; **DINGIR.MEŠ** II.1.4: 48; C.1.4: 48'', 52''; C.3.4: 51a; **DINGIR-*šá*** A.2.5: 7', 14'; **[DINGI]R-*šá*** C.3.6: 13', 14'; **DINGIR-*šú*** C.3.6: 13'; D.1.8: 14; D.3.1: 22; I.1.3: 19, 20; ***i-la-nu*** D.1.10: 8'; ***⸢i⸣-la-nu*** D.1.10: 3'
ilūtu "deity; divinity": **DINGIR-*ti-ka*** C.3.6: 16'; D.1.8: 18, 20; **DINGIR-*ti-ki*** C.3.6: 20'; **DINGIR-*ú-ti-ka*** D.1.8: 15, 18
imbu'/imbû tâmti (a mineral): **KA A.AB.BA** A.2.2: 29; C.1.4: 160''', 181'''; F.2: 32'; **[K]A A.AB.BA** F.1: 21; **[KA A.A]B.BA** E.1.1. 6; **KA *tam-tim*** A.2.1: 18'; A.2.2: 47; A.2.5: 9'; C.1.9: 12; C.1.10: 12; D.1.3: 24''; F.1: 21
imēru "donkey": **ANŠE** C.1.9: 23; D.1.1: 232
imgiddû "(a type of) tablet; school exercise tablet": **IM.GÍD.DA** B.2.1: 37; D.3.1: 37(f), 39(b); G.1: 53; I.1.2: 14'
imḫur-ešrā "it heals (lit. opposes) twenty (diseases)-plant" (unidentified plant): ^{ú}**IGI-20** A.1.1: 19'; A.2.1: 45''; A.2.7: 11; B.1.1: 36; C.2.1: 12'; C.2.2: 10; C.3.9: 10, 22; ⸢^{ú}⸣**IGI-20** B.1.1: 34; ⸢^{ú}⸣**[IGI]-20** A.1.1: 6'; ^{ú}**IGI-⸢20$^{?}$⸣** B.1.1: 62; ⸢^{ú}**IGI-20**⸣ C.2.1: 9'; ^{ú}***im-ḫur-20*** B.2.1: 14; C.1.4: 37'; ⸢^{ú}⸣***[im-ḫur-20$^{?}$]*** C.1.4: 171'''; ^{ú}***im-ḫur-aš-ra*** II.1.3: 48'''; ^{ú}***⸢im-ḫur⸣-aš-⸢ra⸣*** C.3.9: 22
imḫur-līm "it heals (lit. opposes) thousand (diseases)-plant" (unidentified plant): ^{ú}**IGI-*lim*** A.1.1: 6', 17'; A.2.6: 26; C.1.4: 37', 181'''; C.1.5: 13; C.2.1: 7'; D.1.3: 27''; D.1.4: 13''; D.2.1: 19'; D.3.1: 14; ^{ú}**IGI-*lim*$^{?}$** C.2.2: 10; ⸢^{ú}⸣**IGI-*lim*** B.1.1: 62; C.1.2: 6; **[^{ú}]IGI-*lim*** A.2.7: 11; **[^{ú}IG]I-*lim*** B.1.1: 36; ⸢^{ú}⸣**[IGI-*li*]*m*$^{?}$** A.1.1: 19'; **[^{ú}]⸢IGI-*lim*⸣** C.2.1: 9'; ^{ú}***im-ḫur-lim*** A.2.7: 28', 35'; B.2.1: 14; C.1.4: 171'''; ^{ú}***im-⸢ḫur⸣-lim*** II.1.3: 62'''
imitta "on the right": **15** I.1.1: 18, 20, 22
imittu I "right (hand, side, foot)": **15** C.3.9: 36; F.1: 12, 33, 36; **15-*šá*** A.2.7: 4; C.3.3: 7; F.1: 38; **15-⸢*šá*⸣** F.1: 14; **15-*šú*** C.2.3: 3'; C.3.4: 59; C.3.9: 4, 34; C.3.10: 5; ***i-mi-⸢it$^{?}$⸣-t[i$^{?}$-šú$^{?}$]*** C.2.3: 5'; **ZAG** I.1.1: 71, 87, 90, 92, 94, 95, 96, 98; **ZAG-*šá*** C.3.1: 2, 3; **⸢ZAG$^{?}$⸣-[*šá*]** F.1: 14
imittu II "shoulder": **ZAG.LU** C.1.4: 180'''
immanakku (a type of stone or sand): $^{n[a4]}$***⸢im-ma-an⸣-na-ku*** A.2.6: 10
immertu "ewe": ***im-mer-tú*** C.3.10: 65, 71
immeru "(male) sheep": ***im-mé-er*** C.3.5: 24'; **UDU** A.2.5: 15''; C.1.10: 16; D.2.1: 34'; E.2.3: 3'; **UDU$^{?}$** E.2.6: 35', 36'; **⸢UDU⸣** E.2.6: 39'; **⸢UDU$^{?}$⸣** A.2.3: 28'''; **UDU.MEŠ** D.1.5: 9', 10'; **UDU.NITA** A.2.5: 9'; **UDU.NÍTA** A.2.2: 28; C.1.9: 11; C.1.10: 11, 15; C.3.3: 20; C.3.4: 65; C.3.9: 44; C.3.10: 5, 75; **UDU.⸢NÍTA⸣** A.2.2: 67; **[UDU$^{?}$].NÍTA** C.1.7: 3'; **⸢UDU.NÍTA⸣** C.3.10: 77
imna "on the right": **ZAG** I.1.1: 11, 16, 63
imnu "right (side/hand)": ***im-ni-ka*** D.1.8: 9

ina "in; on; by; with; from; through": ***ina*** II.1.3: 34''', 35''', 36''', 37''', 39''', 49''', 51'''; II.1.4: 9, 11, 12, 14, 15, 25, 29, 54, 57, 58; A.1.1: 7', 17', 18', 20', 21', 29'', 39'', 51'''; A.1.2: 6', 11', 13'; A.1.3: 2', 9'; A.1.4: 31'', 33'', 39''; A.2.1: 4', 9', 12', 14', 28', 29', 32', 40'', 41'', 56''', 57''', 62''', 75'''', 84''''', 91''''''; A.2.2: 5, 6, 7, 9, 16, 18, 20, 21, 25, 27, 28, 29, 31, 33, 34, 38, 40, 44, 45, 47, 48, 55, 56, 58, 60, 62, 63, 68, 71, 72, 79, 80; A.2.3: 6', 9', 10', 14', 17', 28''', 29'''; A.2.4: 16', 26'', 42'''; A.2.5: 7', 14', 20'', 25''; A.2.6: 3, 13, 16, 20, 22, 23, 26; A.2.7: 2, 4, 12, 13, 14, 19, 20, 25', 28', 30', 31', 33', 34', 35', 28', 38'; A.2.8: 9, 24', 27', 35'; A.2.9: 4', 11'', 16''; A.2.10: 11''; B.1.1: 28, 29, 32, 33, 34, 35, 36, 37, 28, 42, 50, 54, 65; B.1.2: 4'; B.1.3: 9; B.1.4: 16, 17; B.1.5: 3'; B.1.6: 6; B.2.1: 17; B.2.2: 8, 10, 11, 19', 22', 23', 26'; B.2.3: 4', 20''; B.2.4: 4', 7', 10', 17'; B.2.5: 2, 6, 8; B.2.6: 1, 4, 5, 10, 23; C.1.1: 2, 5, 16, 17; C.1.2: 12, 16, 18, 29'; C.1.3: 3', 6', 9'; C.1.4: 3', 6', 8', 10', 14', 23', 24', 26', 28', 29', 30', 31', 32', 37', 38', 40', 41', 47', 54'', 65'', 74'', 75'', 77'', 92'', 94'', 102'', 104'', 105'', 108'', 136'', 138'', 146''', 147''', 148''', 149''', 150''', 152''', 153''', 157''', 158''', 159''', 171''', 174''', 183''', 189'''; C.1.5: 2, 11, 27, 29, 31, 32, 35, 40, 41, 42; C.1.6: 4'; C.1.7: 3', 4'; C.1.8: 7', 10', 17', 23', 26', 37', 47'', 48'', 49'', 50'', 51'', 58''; C.1.9: 2, 5, 9, 11, 13, 14, 19, 24, 32; C.1.10: 8, 11, 15; C.2.1: 7', 8', 13'; C.2.2: 3, 4, 5,6 7, 8, 10, 11, 12; C.2.3: 7', 13', 22'; C.3.1: 2, 3, 4, 5, 6, 13, 17, 18, 19, 30; C.3.3: 3, 5, 7, 20, 27; C.3.4: 6, 11, 12, 21, 22, 39, 49, 57, 59, 65, 70, 79, 83, 85, 88, 93, 96, 97; C.3.5: 3', 6', 11', 14', 17'; C.3.6: 2', 4', 10', 16', 51'''', 55'''', 57'''', 61'''', 62''''; C.3.7: 13'', 20''; C.3.9: 1, 2, 3, 4, 5, 6, 10, 29, 30, 31, 33, 34, 35, 36, 37, 50; C.3.10: 2, 3, 4, 5, 6, 7, 8, 21, 27, 28, 30, 31, 32, 34, 35, 39, 60, 68, 73, 74, 80, 81, 85, 87, 88, 89, 90; C.4.1: 2', 6', 7', 12', 13'; D.1.1: 48, 49, 54, 90, 97, 115, 117, 133, 141, 142, 143, 145, 149, 155, 179, 183, 184, 185, 186, 197, 204, 205, 209, 210, 211, 214, 220, 221, 222, 223, 230, 232, 233, 234, 235; D.1.2: 13; D.1.3: 7', 11', 22''; D.1.4: 3', 9'; D.1.5: 7', 12', 14', 15', 16', 18'; D.1.6: 6, 7; D.1.7: 9', 17', 19'; D.1.8: 6, 9, 10, 15, 18, 20; D.1.9: 6', 10', 28', 36', 38', 43'; D.1.11: 9, 11; D.2.1: 7', 9', 13', 14', 15', 19', 22', 24', 25', 27', 29', 35', 37', 40', 42', 44', 49', 53', 54', 55', 58', 59', 60', 61', 63', 66', 68', 72', 73', 74'; D.3.1: 3, 4, 7, 10b, 14, 15, 16, 17, 31, 34, 38(A); E.1.1: 2, 3, 6; E.2.2: 3'; E.2.3: 5', 6'; E.2.5: 5', 7', 9'; E.2.6: 2', 4', 8', 11', 12', 13', 14', 15', 16', 19', 25', 26', 28', 31', 35', 37', 38', 40'; E.2.8: 5', 10''; F.1: 2, 3, 6, 8, 10, 11, 13, 14, 16, 17, 22, 27, 29, 30, 31, 34, 35, 37, 38, 41; G.1: 15, 37, 43; G.2: 11', 21''; H.1: 4, 16', 24'; I.1.1: 42, 56, 77, 78, 79, 82, 83, 87, 88, 94, 103, 104, 105, 118; I.1.2: 3', 8', 15'; I.1.3: 10, 11, 12, 13, 14, 15, 16, 17, 19; I.1.5: 5'; I.1.6: 15', 16', 17', 35'; ***ina***$^{?}$ A.1.4: 40'; E.2.6: 12'; F.1: 26; ⸢***ina***⸣ A.1.1: 44'''; A.1.4: 17'; A.2.2: 15, 23, 79; A.2.3: 30'''; A.2.4: 23''; A.2.7: 18; B.1.1: 15, 16; B.2.3: 12''; C.1.5: 43; C.1.8: 46''; C.2.1: 5'; C.3.5: 1'; C.3.7: 9''; C.3.8: 9; C.3.10: 76; D.1.3: 3'; D.1.4: 11''; D.1.7: 10'; D.1.11: 2; D.2.1: 71'; D.3.1: 6, 10c; F.1: 1; ⸢***ina***$^{?}$⸣ B.1.5: 1'; C.2.3: 5'; ***ina***$^{!}$ C.1.5: 45; C.3.4: 93; ***[i]na*** C.3.4: 82; ***[in]a*** II.1.3: 59'''; A.2.3: 20''; C.1.4: 134''; ***i[na]*** A.1.4: 27''; C.1.5: 26; ***i[na***$^{?}$***]*** C.1.4: 185'''; D.1.6: 7; ***i-na*** II.1.2: 5, 7; A.2.4: 10'; B.2.1: 17, 19; B.2.6: 2, 10; C.3.5: 10', 21'; C.3.9: 44; C.4.1: 3', 4', 5', 8', 9', 10', 11'; D.1.1: 24, 102, 103, 141, 142, 143, 145, 153, 155; D.3.1: 3, 7, 15; F.1: 35; ***i***$^{!}$***-na***$^{!}$ E.2.6: 16'; ⸢***i***⸣***-na*** F.1: 31; D.1.10: 11'; ***i-***⸢***na***⸣ D.1.1: 99; ***i-n[a]*** D.1.1: 140; ***[i-n]a*** A.2.3: 7'; ⸢***i-na***⸣ D.3.1: 37(b) ⸢***i***$^{?}$***-na***⸣ B.2.1: 21

inanna "now": ***i-***⸢***na***⸣***-an-na*** C.3.4: 92; ***i-na-an-ni*** C.3.4: 16

inbu "fruit": **GURUN** C.1.4: 176'''; ***in-bi*** C.3.10: 38

inṣabtu "earring": ***in-ṣab-ti*** C.3.4: 73; ***in-ṣa-ab-tú*** C.3.9: 54; ***in-ṣab-tu***$_4$ C.3.3: 32

īnu "eye; (water) source": ⸢**IGI**⸣ C.1.10: 15; **IGI.DIDLI-*šá*** I.1.1: 80; **IGI.MEŠ-*šá*** II.1.4: 41, 42; ⸢**IGI.MIN**⸣**-*šá*** I.1.1: 89; **[IGI].MIN-*šá*** D.1.1: 81; **IGI.MIN-*šú*** A.2.6: 16; I.1.7: 8; ***i-in*** C.3.5: 21'; ***i-na-šu*** II.1.2: 10; ***i-ni-šú*** I.1.7: 9

inūma, *enūma* "when": ***e-nu-ma*** A.2.5: 18''; A.2.7: 38'; C.3.4: 17; ⸢***e***⸣***-nu-ma*** C.3.4: 1; ***[e-nu]-ma*** A.2.5: 13'; ***e-nu-***⸢***ma***⸣ I.1.1: 117; I.1.3: 33'; ***e***$^{?}$***-nu***$^{!}$***-ma***$^{!}$ D.3.1: 1; **U$_4$*-ma*** D.1.4: 4'

inzarû (an aromatic plant): ***[i]n-za-ru-ú*** B.2.3: 9'; ***in-***⸢***za-ru***⸣***-[ú]*** B.2.3: 19''; ***i[n]-za-ru-ú***$^{!}$ E.2.1: 9

ipšu "sorcery; deed; act": ***ip-ši*** C.3.7: 17''; ⸢***ip-šu***⸣ D.1.1: 103; ⸢***ip-šu***$^{!}$⸣ D.1.1: 102

iri'u, *erû* "dregs; lees": ***e-ra-a*** D.2.1: 18'; ***e-ru***$^{?}$***-***⸢***u***$^{?}$⸣ E.1.2: 6'

irtu "breast; chest": **GABA** C.3.3: 6; **GABA-*sa*** G.2: 18''; **GABA-*su*** D.1.1: 113; ***i-rat*** D.1.9: 19'; ***ir-tu***$_4$ G.2: 19''; ^{uzu}**GABA-*sa*** II.1.4: 44; [^{u}]^{zu}**GABA-*su*** D.1.5: 15'

isiḫtu "allocation; assigned materials": ***e-si-iḫ-***⸢***tu***$^{?}$⸣ F.2: 39'

isqūqu (a flour): **ZÌ.KUM** D.2.1: 33', 34'

iṣ pišri "wood of release": **GIŠ BÚR** C.3.9: 21; **GIŠ BÚR**$^{!}$ C.3.9: 10; ***iṣ piš-ri*** A.2.6: 6

iṣṣūr ḫurri "*ḫurru*-bird" (partridge?): **BURU$_5$.ḪABRUD.DA** C.3.4: 57; H.2: 3; **BURU$_5$.ḪABRUD$^{!}$.DA** C.3.5: 10'; **BU[RU$_5$.Ḫ]ABRUD**$^{?mu[šen?]}$ II.1.3: 60'''; **BURU$_5$.Ḫ[ABRUD.DA^{mušen}]** A.2.7: 2; **[B]URU$_5$.ḪABRUD.D[A^{mušen}]** E.2.2: 11''; **BURU$_5$.[ḪABRUD.DA^{mušen}]** C.1.1: 4; **BURU$_5$^{ur5}.ḪABRUD.DA^{mušen}** D.1.11: 4, 7; **BU[RU$_5$^{ur5}.ḪABRUD.DA^{mušen}]** D.1.11: 6; **BURU$_5$.ḪABRUD^{ru}.DA^{mušen}** C.3.3: 3; **[BURU$_5$.ḪABRUD]^{u}.DA** C.1.5: 9

iṣṣūru "bird": **MUŠEN**$^{?}$ A.2.2: 26

iṣu "wood": **GIŠ** A.2.2: 84; ***i-ṣi*** A.2.5: 8'; C.1.10: 10; ***iṣ-ṣi*** C.3.10: 38

īṣu "small; little": ***i-ṣ[i]*** A.2.3: 11', 15'; ⸢***i-ṣi***⸣ A.2.8: 9

išāriš "correctly; normally": ***e-eš-ri-ši*** II.1.4: 61; ***i-šá-riš*** D.1.1: 158

išaru "straight; normal; fortunate; just": **SI.SÁ** D.2.1: 36'; I.1.1: 30, 33, 34, 54, 92, 102; **S[I].**⸢**SÁ**$^{?}$⸣ C.1.8: 15'

išātu "fire; fever": **IZI** A.2.2: 28, 31; A.2.6: 3, 13, 22; B.1.2: 4'; B.2.1: 17; C.1.4: 170'''; C.1.7: 3'; C.1.9: 11; C.1.10: 11, 15; D.1.7: 10', 17'; D.2.1: 14'; **IZI**$^{?}$ A.2.10: 4'; ⸢**IZI**⸣ C.3.10: 38

išdu "foundation; base; lower extremities": ***i-šid*** D.1.9: 18'; ***il-da*** D.1.1: 176; **SUḪUŠ** C.3.9: 8

išippu "purification priest": ***i-šip-pu*** C.3.2: 18'''

iškūru "wax": **DUḪ.LÀL** A.1.4: 9', 11'; A.2.1: 90''''''; A.2.4: 2', 12'; A.2.10: 9'; B.2.2: 19'; B.2.4: 26'; C.3.4: 39; D.2.1: 35'; **[D]UḪ.LÀL** A.2.3: 16'; **[D]UḪ.LÀL**$^{?}$ A.2.3: 12'; **[DU]Ḫ.LÀL** A.1.4: 3'; **DUḪ.LÀ[L]** A.1.4: 5', 19'

išqillatu, *ṣillatu*, *(is)sillatu* (a shell): ^{na4}**IŠKILA** D.2.1: 30', 32'; G.2: 17''; ^{na4}***iš-qil-lat*** G.2: 16''; ***iš-qil-la-tu***$_4$ G.1: 38; ***ṣi-il-la-tu***$_4$ G.1: 39; ***ṣil-lat*** G.2: 17''

ištānu "north (wind)": ^{tu15}**SI.SÁ** D.1.1: 211; H.1: 23'

ištarītu an epithet of Ištar: ^{d}***iš-ta-ri-tu***$_4$ C.1.4: 20'

ištaru "goddess": ^{d}**15-*ia*** C.3.10: 39; ^{d}**15-*šá*** C.3.6: 13', 14'; ^{d}**15-*šú*** D.3.1: 22; ^{d}***iš-tar*** B.1.1: 46; ^{d}***iš***$_8$***-tár-šú*** C.3.6: 13'; [^{d}]⸢***iš***$_8$***-tár-šú***⸣ D.3.1: 2

ištēn, fem. *ištēt* "one": **1** II.1.3: 31''', 32'''; II.1.3.1: 4'; A.1.4: 10', 19', 31''; A.2.1: 3', 16', 88''''''; A.2.2: 24, 25, 26, 27, 28, 63, 70; A.2.3: 2', 3'; A.2.4: 9', 35''', 45'''; A.2.5: 21''; A.2.7: 35'; A.2.8: 25', 33'; B.2.2: 18', 23'; B.2.3: 5'; B.2.4: 2', 4', 5', 11', 12', 13', 14', 16', 27', 32'; B.2.6: 8; C.1.4: 154'''; C.1.9: 7, 8, 16, 17; C.1.10: 18; C.3.9: 28, 33, 35, 40; C.4.1: 13'; D.1.11: 1, 11; D.2.1: 62'; D.3.1: 2, 6; E.2.1: 1, 2, 3, 4, 5; E.2.4: 2', 6'; E.2.6: 9', 10', 21', 23', 27', 34', 35', 38'; F.2: 3, 4, 6, 16, 24', 25', 26', 27', 28', 29', 31', 32', 33', 39'; I.1.1: 116; I.1.3: 34'; **1**$^{?}$ A.2.2: 21; ⸢**1**⸣ A.2.4: 9', 36'''; B.2.4: 1'; B.2.6: 7; ⸢**1**$^{?}$⸣ B.2.3: 7'; F.2: 14; **1-*en*** B.2.2: 29';

B.2.5: 2; C.3.9: 31; D.3.1: 6, 6a; **1-*e*[*n*$^?$]** A.2.2: 84; **1+*en*** C.3.9: 14; **1+*et*** B.2.3: 14''; C.1.10: 16; D.3.1: 6a; **1-*et*** D.1.1: 135, 150, 164; **1-*te*** II.1.4: 59; **AŠ-*ma*** F.2: 43'; ***iš-ten-ma*** G.1: 9; ***il-t*[*i-it*]** D.1.1: 150

ištēnâ, *ištēnû* "one each; one by one; single": **1-*en* TA.ÀM** C.2.3: 22'; **1.TA.ÀM** C.1.4: 155''', 178'''; C.1.10: 4, 12, 18; C.3.9: 11, 34, 36; D.1.11: 9; **[1].TA.ÀM** B.1.1: 28; **1.⸢TA⸣.ÀM** A.2.5: 10'; **[1.T]A.ÀM** C.1.1: 9; C.2.3: 23'; **[1.TA.À]M** II.1.3: 34'''; **[1.TA.À]M$^?$** E.2.6: 8'; **1-*ú*** A.2.4: 17'

ištēniš "together": **DIŠ-*niš*** A.1.1: 7'; A.2.4: 14'; A.2.9: 11''; B.1.1: 28, 35, 36; C.1.1: 5, 15, 34; C.1.2: 16, 27'; C.1.4: 3', 7', 171''', 177''', 183'''; C.1.5: 4; C.1.8: 10', 25'; C.2.1: 7', 8', 13', 46', 49'; C.3.4: 5; C.3.6: 52''''; D.1.3: 9'; D.2.1: 3', 53', 56'; E.2.6: 13'; H.1: 2; **DIŠ$^?$-*niš*$^?$** C.1.1: 20; **DIŠ-[*niš*]** E.2.6: 38'; **[DIŠ]-*niš*** B.1.1: 64; D.1.7: 9'; **[DIŠ-*n*]*iš*** B.2.4: 16'; E.2.7: 18''; **TÉŠ.BI** II.1.4: 7, 24; B.2.6: 3; C.1.4: 126''; C.3.6: 38''; **TÉŠ.B[I$^?$]** D.1.6: 13; **[TÉ]Š.BI** II.1.3: 64'

ištēnšeret, *išteššer* "eleven"; *išteššer ūmī* "eleven days": **11** II.1.4: 6, 23; D.2.1: 22'; I.1.6: 36'; **U$_4$.11.KAM** II.1.3: 29'''

****ištēnšerû*** "eleventh": **11.KÁM** I.1.1: 118

išti "with" ***iš-te*$^?$** A.2.8: 38'; **[T]A** A.2.7: 38'

ištiššu "once": **[1]-*en-šú*** A.2.5: 10'; **1-*šú*** B.2.2: 20'; C.1.9: 28; **[1]-*šú*** B.2.2: 7

ištu, *ultu*, *issu* "from; out of; since; after": ***iš-tu*** C.3.4: 64; C.3.9: 43; D.1.1: 162; **[*i*]*š-tu*** C.3.4: 16; ***i*[*š-tu*]** C.3.3: 18; **TA** II.1.4: 59; C.3.9: 40; C.3.10: 26, 31; D.1.1: 133, 180, 201; D.1.5: 13'; D.3.1: 6, 9, 11b; E.2.6: 16', 17'; **[T]A** B.1.1: 19; **⸢TA$^?$⸣** C.3.4: 19; ***ul-tu*** C.3.10: 7; D.3.1: 9, 11b; D.1.8: 6; ***ul-tú*** D.3.1: 9; ***ul-tú*$^!$** D.3.1: 6

išû G "to have; to exist": ***i*-[*ši*]** [G] D.1.1: 84; ***ti-šu*** [G] II.1.4: 45

itqu "wad, tampon": **ÀKA** B.2.4: 24'; C.1.9: 2, 5, 13; **⸢ÀKA$^?$⸣** A.2.2: 33; **À[KA]** B.2.4: 30'; **^{síg}ÀKA** A.1.1: 14'; A.2.2: 29, 38, 47, 69, 71, 73; A.2.3: 14'; B.1.1: 38; B.1.3: 10; B.2.2: 3, 4, 8, 10, 11, 12; B.2.4: 4', 10', 17'; C.1.1: 2, 17; C.1.2: 16; C.1.4: 25', 33', 34', 35', 36', 43', 45'; 160''', 161''', 162''', 163''', 164''', 165''', 166''', 167''', 168''', 169''', 173'''; C.1.7: 4'; C.2.2: 5, 6, 9; C.2.3: 6', 22'; D.1.1: 232; D.2.1: 53'; **^{síg}ÀKA$^!$** II.1.4: 12; **$^{síg?}$ÀKA** C.1.8: 10'; **^{síg}⸢ÀKA⸣** C.2.3: 7'; **⸢^{síg}ÀKA⸣** D.2.1: 68'; **^{síg}[ÀK]A** B.1.3: 7; **^{síg}À[KA$^?$]** A.2.2: 40; A.2.4: 14'; C.1.6: 4'; **^{síg}[ÀKA]** A.1.1: 21'; **⸢^{síg}⸣ÀKA** C.1.10: 18; **⸢$^{síg!}$ÀKA$^?$⸣** C.1.10: 15; **^{s}[^{íg}ÀKA]** A.2.2: 58; C.1.4: 138''; **[^{síg}À]KA$^?$** C.2.3: 5'

itqūru "spoon; salve bowl": **^{giš}DÍLIM** C.3.6: 16'

ittamir, *ittemir* (a stone): **^{na4}*it-ta-mir*** C.3.9: 8, 10, 22; **⸢^{na4}*it-ta-mir*$^?$⸣** C.3.9: 30; **[^{n}]^{a4}*it-te-mir*** A.1.3: 8'

itti "with": ***it-ti*** C.3.10: 1, 14; D.2.1: 7', 11'; ***it-ti-šú*** C.3.4: 19; ***it-ti-šú-nu*** D.3.1: 5; **KI** II.1.4: 28; A.1.3: 2'; A.2.5: 12'; B.1.6: 16'; C.3.4: 23; C.3.6: 58''''; C.3.9: 9, 13; D.1.1: 229; D.1.11: 11; D.2.1: 35', 53', 54'; F.1: 25, 30, 31; **K[I]** A.2.2: 10; **[K]I$^?$** B.2.4: 3'; **KI-*ka*** D.3.1: 25

ittī "on top of that; in addition to": ***it-ti-i*** C.3.10: 6

ittu "sign": **GISKIM** D.3.1: 25

ittû, *iṭṭû* "bitumen": ***it-tu-um-ma*** C.3.10: 25

izḫu "belt": ***iz-ḫa*** C.3.9: 7

izuzzu, *uzuzzu* G "to stand; to be present"; Š "to make someone stand; to set up; to provide; to make available": **GUB-*az-ma*** [G] D.3.1: 10b, 17; **GUB-*ma*** [G] D.3.1: 17; **⸢GUB⸣-*za*$^{?!}$** D.1.1: 99; **GUB-*za*-<<*ma*>>-*am-ma*** [G] II.1.4: 46; **GUB-*zu*** [G] C.1.4: 77''; H.1: 25'; **[GU]B-⸢*zu*⸣** [G] C.3.4: 49; **⸢GUB-*zu-ma*⸣** [G] D.3.1: 10b; ***iz-za*-⸢*az*⸣-*ma*** [G] D.3.1: 10b; ***iz-za-az-zu*** [G] C.3.4: 44; ***iz-zi-zu*** [G] B.2.2: 20', 25'; ***li-iz-zi-iz*** [G] B.2.6: 24; ***li-iz-ziz*** [G] D.1.8: 9, 10; ***t*[*a-az-za-az*$^?$]** [G] B.2.6: 16; ***tu-šá-zaz$_x$*** [Š] B.2.3: 14''; ***tuš-zaz-ma*** [Š] C.3.10: 85; ***uš-zi-is-su*** [Š] D.1.9: 39'

kabābu G "to burn"; D "to burn; scorch": ***ku-ub-bu*-[*bu*$^?$]** [D] B.2.5: 3; ***ku-ub-bu-ub*-[*bu*$^?$]** [D] A.2.6: 3; **⸢*ku-ub*⸣-*bu-ub-bu*** [D] A.2.6: 13

kabālu G "to be paralysed"; D "to constrict; to paralyse": ***kub-bu-lu$_4$*** [D] I.1.7: 12

kabāsu G "to step; to tread (on)"; D "to tread on; to trample"; N "to set the foot (on)": ***i-kab-ba*-[*as*$^?$]** [G] A.2.2: 46; ***ik-ka-ba*$^!$*-as*$^!$** [N] I.1.2: 4'; ***u-ka*-⸢*ba*⸣$^!$*-as*** [D] D.1.11: 13; ***ú-kab-bi-s*[*u*]** [D] C.3.10: 40; **ZUKUM** [G] I.1.2: 3'; **ZUKUM-*as*** [N] I.1.1: 72, 94, 95, 96, 97, 98

kabātu G "to be(come) heavy, aggravating, serious": **DU[GUD]** [G] I.1.2: 4'; **DUGUD-*at*** [G] I.1.1: 96; ***kab*-[*ta-at*]** [G] D.1.11: 7

kabbaru "very thick": ***kab-ba-ra*** B.2.2: 25', 28'; ***k*[*ab-ba-r*]*a*** B.2.2: 18'; **NÍG.GAL.GAL.LA** D.1.1: 175, 179

kabru "thick; fat": ***kab*$^{?!}$*-ri*** A.2.2: 19; ***kab*$^?$*-ri*$^?$** A.2.5: 9'

kabtu "heavy; eminent; important": **DUGUD** E.1.2: 10'

kadānu (a rush-like plant): ***ka-da-nu*** B.2.3: 17''

kadrayītu (epithet of Ištar): ***ka-ad-ra-a-a-i-tu$_4$*** C.1.4: 19'

kadrû "present; greeting gift": **⸢KÁDRA⸣** B.2.6: 5; **[KÁDR]A$^?$-*šú*** B.2.6: 14

KA.INIM.MA "wording" (in rubrics): **KA.INIM.MA** A.1.2: 7'; C.1.4: 17', 21', 65'', 80'', 91'', 137'', 141''; C.3.1: 29; C.3.9: 25; D.1.1: 53, 131, 161, 203; G.1: 26; H.1: 1, 22'; **KA.I[NIM.M]A** C.1.4: 86''; **K[A.INIM.MA]** C.1.4: 98''; **K[A.INIM.MA$^?$]** H.1: 15'; **⸢KA.INIM⸣.MA** B.1.1: 71; **[K]A.INIM.MA** C.1.1: 14; H.1: 9; **[KA].INIM.MA** C.1.2: 26'; **⸢KA⸣.[INIM].MA** B.2.1: 13; **[KA.INI]M.MA** C.1.4: 73''; C.1.5: 37; **[KA.INIM].MA** C.1.4: 131''

kakkabu "star": **[MU]L$^?$** B.2.1: 22; **MUL$_4$** A.1.1: 18'; A.2.2: 60; A.2.7: 30'; A.2.9: 4'; C.1.4: 28'; C.1.8: 58''; D.1.11: 9; **MU[L$_4$]** C.1.4: 75''

kakku "weapon; shaft; barb; thorn": **^{giš}TUKUL** C.1.1: 4; ***kak-ka*** A.2.2: 28; ***kak-ku*** I.1.7: 3

kakkû, *kakku'u* "lentil": **GÚ.TUR** B.1.1: 24; D.2.1: 12', 51'

kakkulti īni "iris": ***kak-kul-tu$_4$ i-ni-šú*** I.1.7: 9

kakkusakku (a stone): **^{na4}*kak-ku-sak-ku*** C.1.8: 54''; **[^{n}]^{a4}⸢*kak-ku*⸣*-sak-ku*** C.1.4: 24

kalab Bēlet-ilī "dog of Bēlet-ilī" (a plant?): ***ka-lab* DINGIR.MAḪ$^{!?}$** B.2.4: 21'

kalāma "all (of it); anything; everything; whole": **DÙ.A.BI** II.1.3: 39'''; A.2.2: 55; D.2.1: 55'; **[D]Ù$^?$.A.BI** B.2.6: 13; ***ka-la-ma*** C.1.4: 52''; ***ka-la-mu*** C.3.10: 53

kalbu "dog": **UR.GI$_7$** D.1.1: 209, 231; **⸢UR⸣.GI$_7$** D.1.1: 233

kal-damiq (a medicinal plant, lit. "it is good for everything"-plant): **^{ú}*kal-da-mi-iq*** A.2.8: 2

kalgukku a reddish mineral or pigment: **^{im}GÀ.LI.GUG** C.3.5: 6'; **^{im}KAL.GUG** C.1.5: 4; C.1.10: 3; D.1.1: 221; **^{im}KAL.GU[G]** A.2.1: 58'''; C.1.10: 6; **^{im}KAL.G[UG]** C.1.10: 1; **^{im}KAL.⸢GUG⸣** C.1.4: 1'; **^{im}KAL.⸢LA.GUG⸣** C.1.10: 16; **KAL.GUG** C.1.9: 22

kalîš "totally; everywhere": ***ka-liš*** C.3.10: 41, 48

kalītu "kidney": **ÉLLAG** A.2.2: 25; A.2.6: 19; D.2.1: 34'; **⸢ÉLLAG⸣** A.2.2: 23; **[ÉLL]AG$^?$** A.2.2: 27

kallātu "bride; daughter-in-law": ***kal-lat*** D.1.8: 5

kalû I "yellow ochre": ^{im}**GÀ.LI** C.3.5: 5'; ^{im}**KAL** A.2.1: 60'''; **[**^{im}**]KAL** C.1.4: 1'; **[**^{im}**KA]L** C.1.5: 4; ^{im}**KAL.LA** C.1.4: 148'''

kalû II "all; whole": **DÙ** D.1.3: 5'; **DÙ.A.BI** II.1.4: 61; **DÙ.A.BI-*šu-nu*** II.1.4: 27; D.1.1: 147; **DÙ-*šú-nu*** B.1.1: 14; ***ka-la*** D.1.1: 152, 154; ***ka-[la]*** B.1.1: 60; ***ka-li-šú-nu*** D.1.1: 147; ***kal*** A.2.2: 71; C.3.1: 33; C.3.10: 33; D.2.1: 9'; E.2.3: 12'

kalû III "lamentation priest": ^{lú}**GALA** G.1: 54

kalû IV G "to hold back; to stop; to block"; D "to hold back"; N pass. of G "to be held back": ***i-kal-la*** [G] D.2.1: 30'; ***ik-ka-li*** [N] D.1.1: 160; ***ik-kal-la*** [N] H.1: 35'; H.2: 4; ***ik-kal-lu-u*** [N] C.1.10: 9; ***ik-kal-lu-ú*** [N] A.2.7: 36'; ***ka-la-a*** [G] D.2.1: 71'; ***ka-lat*** [G] D.1.1: 31, 48, 49, 185, 186; ***[k]a-lat*** [G] D.1.1: 30; ***[k]a-le-e*** [G] H.1: 26', 31'; ***ka***$^{!}$***-lu-ú*** [G] II.1.4: 36; ***kul-lu-u*** [D] C.1.4: 57''; ***ta-kal-la*** [G] C.1.4: 76''; ***ta-ku-lu*** [G] C.1.4: 60''

kālû "dam; barrage": ***ka-lu-ú-šá*** C.1.4: 57''

kamādu G "to beat cloth": ***ka-ma-du*** [G] G.1: 45

kamantu (a medicinal plant): ⸢$^{šim?}$***ka***$^{?}$***-man***$^{?}$***-ti***$^{?}$⸣ C.2.3: 4'

kamāru (a fish): ***ka-ma-ru*** A.2.8: 38'

kamāsu, *kamāṣu*, *kamāšu*, *ḫamāšu* G "to kneel; to squat (down), to crouch"; Š "to have kneel down: ***ak-mis*** [G] D.3.1: 21; **DU$_{10}$.GAM-*si-ma*** [Š] C.3.10: 70; ***i-kam-mi-su*** [G] E.2.6: 15'; ***i-kam-mis-ma*** [G] C.1.4: 11'; ***ik-ta-mi-ṣi*** [G] D.1.1: 146; ***ka-an-ṣa*** [G] D.1.5: 6'; ***ta-aḫ-ti-me-iš*** [G] II.1.4: 57

kamkadu (a medicinal plant): ***[***^{ú}***k]a-am-kà-ta*** II.1.3: 48'''

kamû G "to bind": ***i-kam-ma-a*** [G] C.3.9: 19

kamūnu "cumin": ***ka-mu-nu*** A.2.2: 62; B.2.4: 7'; E.2.1: 2; E.2.5: 8'; ***[k]a-mu-nu*** A.2.2: 7, 11; ***ka-***⸢***mu***⸣***-nu*** A.2.8: 33'; ***ka-[mu-nu***$^{?}$***]*** II.1.3.1: 7'; ***k[a***$^{?}$***-mu-nu]*** A.1.4: 31''; ***ka-mun*** E.2.6: 38'; ^{ú}***ka-***⸢***mu***⸣***-nu*** B.2.4: 28'; ^{ú}***ka-m[u-nu]*** E.2.1: 2; ^{ú}***ka-mun*** D.1.11: 4, 7

kamūn bīni "tamarisk gall(s); gallnut": ***ka-mun*** ^{giš}**ŠINIG** C.1.4: 151'''

kanaktu (an aromatic tree and its gummy resin): ^{šim}**GIG** A.1.4: 13'; B.1.1: 26; C.1.4: 182'''; C.1.9: 7; C.1.10: 10, 11; E.2.5: 4'; **[**^{ši}**]**^{m}**GIG** A.2.1: 16'; **[**^{šim}**G]IG** C.1.9: 16, 30; E.2.2: 5'

kanāku G "to seal": ⸢***ak-nu-uk***$^{?}$⸣ [G] C.1.5: 47

kanānu G "to roll up; to wrap"; N "to contract", Ntn iter. of N: ***ta-kan-na-an*** [G] A.1.4: 27''; ***[i]t-ta-nak-n[a-na]*** [Ntn] I.1.4: 9'

kanku "sealed": ***kak-ka*** II.1.4: 48; ***ka-an-ga-tu***$_{4}$ D.1.1: 109, 122

kannu I "jar; large vessel": ***kan-nu*** G.1: 32

kannu II "band; loincloth; (menstrual) bandage": ***ka-an-ni*** C.3.5: 13'; ⸢***ka***$_{4}$⸣***-an-nu*** A.2.2: 38; ***[kan-na***$^{?}$***]-tú*** A.1.4: 27''; ***ka***$_{4}$***-an-ni-šú*** E.2.6: 15'; ***k[a***$_{4}$***-an-ni-šú]*** A.2.2: 11; ⸢***ka***$_{4}$$^{?}$⸣***-an-ni-šú*** A.2.8: 13; ***ka***$_{4}$***-ni-šú*** C.3.9: 40

kanû G "to care for"; D "to treat kindly; to care for; to look after": ***ú-ka-na-šá*** [D] D.1.1: 147; ***u-kan-ni-šú*** [D] D.1.9: 29'

kânu G "to be(come) permanent, firm, true"; D "to establish firmly; to fix, make firm; to set up (correctly)": **GIN**$^{!?}$ [D] B.2.6: 5; **G[IN]-*ma*** [D] B.2.6: 10; **GUB-*an*** [D] C.3.4: 39; **[G]UB-*an*** [D] C.3.4: 40; ⸢**GUB**⸣**-*[an]*** C.3.4: 42; **[GU]B-*an*** [D] C.3.6: 7'; **[GU]B**$^{?}$**-*an*** [D] C.3.4: 49; ***ku-na-at*** [D] II.1.4: 34, 35, 52; ***tu-ka-an*** [D] B.2.6: 8;

kaparru "shepherd-boy": ***ka-par-ri*** D.1.1: 143; ***ka-pár-ri*** D.1.1: 143; ***ka-par-ru*** D.1.1: 147; ***ka-pár-ru*** D.1.1: 147; ***ka-pár-ru***^{meš} D.1.1: 147

kapāru G "to wipe (up/clean)"; D "to wipe clean; to rub": ***ta-ká***$^{?}$***-pár-ma*** [G] II.1.3: 64'''; ***ta-kap-par*** [G] E.2.6: 7'; ***tu-kap-par***$_{5}$ [D] B.2.2: 19', 23'; ***tu-kap-pa-<ar>-šú*** [D] C.3.4: 26

kapāṣu (a shell or sea snail): ^{na4}***ka-pa-ṣa*** C.1.4: 5', 40'; ^{na4}***ka-pa-***⸢***ṣa***⸣ F.1: 33; ^{na4}***ka-pa-ṣu*** C.1.4: 44'; C.1.5: 21; C.3.6: 56''''; F.2: 24'; ^{na4}***ka-pa-***⸢***ṣu***⸣ F.1: 33

kappu "wing; feather": **PA.MEŠ-*šú*** A.2.7: 26'

karāku G "to roll up; collect; to block; to wrap; to entwine"; D "to wrap up": ***ka-ar-ka*** [G] A.2.6: 1; ***ta-kar-rik*** [G] C.3.10: 81; ***tu-kar-rak-šú*** [D] C.3.4: 5

karān īni "iris": ***ka-ra-an*** **IGI.MIN-*šú*** I.1.7: 8

karān šēlebi "fox grape" (an unidentified plant): **GEŠTIN.KA$_{5}$.A** C.3.3: 2; D.2.1: 19'; **GEŠTIN.KA$_{5}$.**⸢**E**⸣ C.3.5: 9'; ^{giš}**GEŠ.TIM.KA$_{5}$.A** A.2.7: 2; ^{giš}**GEŠTIN.KA$_{5}$.A** A.1.1: 45'''; D.1.1: 205, 213; D.1.4: 5'; ⸢$^{giš?}$**GEŠTIN.KA$_{5}$**⸣**.A** A.2.2: 10; ^{giš}⸢**GEŠTIN.KA$_{5}$**$^{?}$⸣**.A** A.1.1: 47'''; ⸢$^{giš?}$⸣**GE[ŠTIN.KA$_{5}$.A**$^{?}$**]** A.2.6: 24; **[**^{giš}**GEŠTIN.K]A$_{5}$.A** D.1.3: 3'; ^{ú}**GEŠTIN.KA$_{5}$.A** D.1.3: 8'; D.1.11: 5, 8; ^{ú}**GEŠTIN.KA$_{5}$.**⸢**A**⸣ A.1.1: 50'''; ^{ú}**<GEŠTIN>.KA$_{5}$.A** C.1.5: 16

karānu "wine; must; grape(s)": **GEŠ.TIN** E.2.6: 7'; **GEŠTIN** II.1.3: 37'''; A.2.2: 44; A.2.5: 18''; B.1.1: 33, 34, 35, 64; B.1.6: 6; C.3.9: 7; D.1.11: 14'; D.2.1: 6', 19'; E.2.5: 5'; **GEŠ[TIN**$^{?}$**]** A.2.2: 16; **[GEŠ]TIN**$^{?}$**-*nu*** B.2.2: 3; ^{giš}**[GEŠTIN**$^{?}$**]** E.2.8: 5'

karāru G "to put down; to discard": ***i-kar-ra-ár*** [G] D.1.5: 17'

karāṣu G "to pinch off; to break off"; N pass. of G: ***i-kar-ri-iṣ*** [N?] I.1.1: 1; ***ta-kar-ri-iṣ-ma*** [G] C.3.4: 81

karašu "leek": **GA.**⸢**RAŠ**$^{?}$⸣ A.2.7: 25'; ^{ú}**GA.RAŠ**^{sar} D.2.1: 64'

karā'u, *ka/erû* G "to bow down": ***i-ke-er-ri*** [G] D.3.1: 10b; ***i-ke-ri*** [G] D.3.1: 10b

karpatu "(clay) pot": **DUG** B.1.1: 15; D.1.2: 6

karû G "to be(come) short"; Gtn iter. of G: ***ik-te-ner-ra-a*** [Gtn] D.2.1: 67'

kāru "quay; harbour": **KAR** D.1.1: 48, 49, 90, 185, 186; ***kar*** D.1.1: 106, 107

kâru G "to rub": ***ta-ak-ra*** [G] D.2.1: 19'; ***ta-kar***$_{5}$$^{?}$***-aš*** [G] E.2.6: 39'

kaspu "silver (bead)": **[K]Ù.BABBAR** B.1.4: 12

kassibu, *kas(s)ipu*, *kusīpu* (a medicinal plant): ^{ú}***ka-si-bi*** A.2.6: 8

kasû I (a plant, probably *Cuscuta* dodder): **GAZI**^{sar} II.1.4: 23; A.1.2: 9'; B.1.1: 25; D.1.11: 12; D.2.1: 8', 20', 41', 43', 47', 50', 52', 56', 58', 60', 63', 65'; D.3.1: 15; **[GA]ZI**$^{?sar}$ A.2.1: 26'; **[GAZ]I**^{sar} E.2.6: 2'; **[GAZI**^{sa}**]**$^{r?}$ B.1.1: 4; **G[AZI**^{sa}^{r}**]** C.2.3: 4'; ^{ú}**[GAZ]I**^{sar} A.1.4: 34''

kasû II "bound; captive": ***ka-si-***⸢***i***⸣ E.2.3: 13'; ***ka-su-u*** D.3.1: 20; ***ka-su-ú*** D.3.1: 20

kasû III G "to bind"; D "to bind": ***ku-us-sà*** [D] II.1.2: 9

kaṣāru G "to tie; to make a knot; to constrict; to form"; D "to tie knots (for); to tie together"; N "to be tied": ***ik-[ka***$^{?}$***-ṣ]a-ru*** [N] D.2.1: 33'; **KÉŠ** [G] C.1.2: 28'; C.1.4: 7', 47', 100''; C.1.4: 22'; C.3.6: 53''''; D.3.1: 3, 4; E.1.1: 8; E.2.7: 16''; F.1: 27; H.1: 4, 24', 34'; **KÉ[Š**$^{?}$**]** [G] D.3.1: 36; **[K]ÉŠ** [G] D.3.1: 5; ⸢**KÉŠ**⸣ [G] H.1: 3; **KÉŠ-*ár*** [G] D.3.1: 3; C.1.8: 5'; F.1: 27; **KÉŠ-*ma*** [G] C.1.4: 186'''; **[KÉŠ]-*ma***$^{?!}$ [G] E.1.1: 8; **KÉŠ("SAR")-*ru*** [G] C.1.1: 16; **KÉ]Š**$^{?}$**-**⸢***ru***⸣ [G] H.1: 17';

ta-ka-ṣa-ar [G] C.1.4: 186'''; ***ta-ka-ṣar-ma*** [G] C.3.5: 14'; ***ta-kàṣ-ṣar*** [G] C.3.9: 12, 15; ***ta-kàṣ-[ṣar]*** [G] C.3.9: 32; ***tu-kàṣ-ṣar*** [D] F.1: 30; ***tu-ka-ṣar-ši*** [D] C.1.4: 184'''; ***tu-kàṣ-ṣar-ši*** [D] C.3.6: 55''''

kaṣû I "cold": **SED** C.1.4: 92''; ***ke***$^{?!}$***-ṣe-e-tú*** E.2.6: 5'

kaṣû II G "to be(come) cold/cool"; D "to cool down": **SED** [G] B.1.1: 18; ⸢**SED**⸣ [D] C.2.1: 5'; **SED-*ú*** [G] C.1.10: 9; ***tu-kàṣ-ṣa*** [D] A.2.5: 27''; D.2.1: 63'; ***[t]u***$^{?}$***-⸢kàṣ-ṣa⸣-[a***$^{?}$***]*** [D] A.2.2: 64; ***tu-kàṣ-ṣa-ma*** [D] D.2.1: 64'; ***ú-kàṣ-ṣa*** [D] C.1.10: 14

kâṣu G "to skin; to flay": ***ta-ka-aṣ*** [G] A.2.2: 78; ***ta-ka-ṣi*** [G] A.2.2: 78

kašādu G "to defeat; to reach; to obtain; to catch; to arrive; to approach": ⸢***ka***$^{?}$⸣***-š[a-di***$^{?}$***]*** [G] B.2.1: 29; ***ku-ul-da-a-ni*** [G] II.1.4: 47; ***kul-dan-ni*** [G] D.1.1: 101; **KUR-*ad-m[a]*** [G] D.1.6: 9; **KUR-*du*** [G] C.3.9: 37

kâši, *kâšu*, *kâša* "to you; for you": ***ka-a-šá*** D.3.1: 20; ***ka-a-šu*** D.3.1: 20; ***ka-<<šá>>-a-šú*** D.3.1: 20

kaššāptu "witch; sorceress": ***kaš-šá-pa-a-tú*** C.3.9: 16; ***kaš-šá-pa-a-tu***$_4$ C.3.9: 16; ***kaš-šap-tú*** C.3.10: 42, 59; ***k[aš-šap-tú]*** C.3.10: 44; ***[kaš-ša]p-⸢tú⸣*** C.3.10: 49; ***kaš-šap-tu***$_4$ C.3.10: 22, 24; ^{munus}**UŠ$_{11}$.ZU.MEŠ** C.3.9: 23

kaššāpu "sorcerer": ***ka-šap*** C.3.10: 22, 24; ***kaš-šap*** C.3.10: 42, 44, 49, 59

kašû, *kašā'u* G "to increase strongly": ***ki-šá-'a*** [G] H.1: 38'

kâšu G "to be late; to delay, linger"; Št "to be delayed, held up": ***i-ku-uš*** [G] A.2.1: 14'; ***ka-a-šú*** [G] G.1: 15; ⸢***uš***⸣***-[ta-kiš***$^{?}$***]*** [Št] A.2.1: 56'''

katāmu G "to cover; to overwhelm"; Gtn iter. of G; D "to cover": **DUL**$^{?}$***-ma*** [G] A.1.4: 31''; ***ik-ta-na-at-tam*** [Gtn] II.1.4: 43; ***ik-tùm*** [G] D.1.9: 18'; ***ka-at-ma*** [G] II.1.2: 10; II.1.4: 41; ***kut-tu-mu*** [D] G.2: 18''

katmu "covered": ***kat-me*** E.1.3: 4'

kayyamānu "regularly; repeatedly; constant": ***ka-a-a-ma-na-at-ma*** B.1.1: 75

kayyānu "constant; regular; repeatedly": ***ka-a-a-na*** D.1.1: 234; **SAG.ÚS** G.1: 15

kazābu G "to be attractive, alluring": ***kaz-bat*** [G] D.1.1: 137; G.2: 26''

kī "like; according to; just as; when": ***ki*** A.2.8: 22'; B.2.2: 5; D.1.6: 5; I.1.7: 6; ***ki***$^{?}$ B.2.2: 6; ***ki-i*** II.1.4: 38, 39, 40; A.2.5: 2'; B.2.2: 3, 4, 22', 24', 26', 27', 28'; C.1.10: 4, 12; D.1.11: 7, 14'; E.2.6: 6', 12'

kīam, *kâm* "thus; so": ***kam*** A.2.7: 39'; C.3.4: 19, 22, 26, 82; C.3.10: 63, 70; D.3.1: 10c; ***ki-a-am*** C.3.10: 27; D.1.1: 225; D.3.1: 10c; ***[k]i-a-am*** C.1.4: 187'''; ***ki-⸢am⸣*** C.3.4: 90; ***k[i-am]*** E.2.3: 8'; **UR$_5$.GIM** B.1.1: 56; C.3.4: 43, 47, 49, 51b; E.2.3: 20''; D.3.1: 10c; **U[R$_5$.GIM]** E.2.3: 9'

kibrītu "sulphur": ***[ki]b***$^{?}$***-ri-tu***$_4$ A.2.10: 4'; ***[k]ib-rit*** E.1.1: 1; **PIŠ$_{10}$.^{d}ÍD** C.1.4: 42'; D.1.3: 23''; F.1: 3; **PIŠ$_{10}$$^{!}$.Í[D]** E.2.2: 2'; **PIŠ$_{10}$.⸢$^{d?}$⸣[ÍD]** D.2.1: 34'; **[PIŠ$_{10}$.^{d}Í]D**$^{?}$ A.1.1: 40''

kibru "bank; world": ***kib-rat*** C.3.10: 41; ***kib***$^{!}$***-ra[t]-⸢ta⸣*** C.3.10: 48

kibsu "track; step; course; menses": ***ki-bís*** C.3.3: 19, 20; ***kib-si*** C.3.4: 65; ***kib-su*** A.2.6: 25; A.2.10: 2'; C.2.2: 13; C.3.9: 44

kibtu "wheat": **GIG**$^{!}$ B.1.1: 23; **GI[G]** B.1.2: 3'; **G[IG]** E.2.1: 5; **GIG.BA** A.2.4: 16'; **GIG.BA**$^{?}$ A.2.3: 11'; **ŠE.GIG** D.2.1: 41', 50'; ⸢**ŠE.GIG**$^{?}$⸣ A.2.3: 6'; **[ŠE].⸢GIG$^{?}$⸣** A.2.3: 8'; **Š[E.GIG$^{?}$]** A.2.1: 25'

KÌD.KÌD.BI (reading uncertain) "the ritual/procedure for it": **KÌD.KÌD.BI** B.2.1: 14; C.1.4: 81'', 92'', 138''; H.1: 2, 23'; **[K]ÌD.KÌD.BI** C.1.4: 142''; ⸢**KÌD**⸣**.KÌD.BI** C.1.4: 125''; ⸢**KÌD.KÌD.BI**⸣ B.1.1: 10; C.1.4: 74''; **KÌD.KÌD.B[I]** C.1.4: 66'', 87''; **KÌD.KÌD.[BI]** C.1.4: 132''; H.2: 3; **KÌ[D.KÌD.BI]** C.1.4: 99''

kīdu "countryside; outside": ***[ki]-di***$^{?}$ D.1.1: 78

kilallān "both": ***ki-la-la-⸢an⸣*** D.2.1: 72'; ⸢***ki-lal***⸣***-[la-an***$^{?}$***]*** B.2.6: 11; ***ki-lal-le-e*** C.3.10: 7

kīma (prep.) "like; according to; just as"; (conj.) "just as; as soon as; when; because": **GIN$_7$** A.2.7: 5, 37'; B.1.1: 28; B.2.1: 42; B.2.2: 9, 14; C.1.4: 12', 13'; C.1.8: 34'; C.3.1: 10; C.3.3: 12; C.3.4: 19, 43, 61; C.3.6: 37''; D.1.1: 23, 156, 171, 194; D.1.6: 8; D.2.1: 45'; I.1.1: 70, 117; **GIN$_7$**$^{?}$ C.3.4: 46; ⸢**GIN$_7$**$^{?}$⸣ B.2.2:19'; **[G]IN$_7$** B.1.1: 21; C.1.4: 59''; D.1.1: 35; **[GI]N$_7$** C.3.10: 92; **GI[N$_7$]** C.1.4: 57''; C.3.4: 20; ⸢**GIN$_7$**⸣ C.1.4: 58''; D.3.1: 37(f); **UR$_5$.GIM** C.3.4: 7, 9; **GIN$_7$-*ma*** II.1.4: 61; **[GI]N$_7$**$^{?}$**-⸢*ma*⸣** C.3.4: 22; ***ki-ma*** II.1.1: 33; C.3.1: 23; C.3.3: 42; C.3.4: 93; C.3.10: 73; D.1.1: 35, 45, 46, 94, 112, 113, 114, 125, 126, 158, 171, 172, 194; D.1.5: 13'; D.1.9: 18', 26'; G.1: 28, 29; ***[k]i-ma*** C.3.5: 23'; ⸢***ki***⸣***-ma*** A.2.4: 1'; C.3.4: 5; C.3.5: 24'; D.3.1: 38(b); ⸢***ki-ma***⸣ C.3.5: 25'; ⸢***ki***$^{?}$***-ma***$^{?}$⸣ D.1.1: 86; ***ki-[ma]*** D.1.1: 95; ***[ki-m]a*** D.1.2: 15

KI.MIN, DIŠ KI.MIN "ditto, alternatively": **KI.MIN** II.1.3:1', 35''', 36''', 37'''; A.1.4: 38'', 40''; A.2.1: 19'; A.2.2: 30, 31, 32; C.1.5: 5, 6, 7, 11, 12, 13, 14, 15, 16, 17, 18, 19, 20, 21, 22, 23, 28, 30; C.1.9: 4, 31, 33, 34, 35, 36, 37; D.1.1: 208, 209, 210, 212, 213, 214, 215, 216, 217, 218, 219, 220, 221, 222; I.1.1: 97, 107, 108, 109, 110, 111, 112, 113; I.1.3: 10; **KI.MIN**$^{!}$ A.1.1: 20'; **[K]I.MIN**$^{?}$ A.2.2: 15; **[KI].MIN**$^{?}$ A.2.2: 16, 17; ⸢**KI.MIN**⸣ A.2.4: 28''; C.1.5: 27; **K[I.MIN$^{?}$]** C.1.5: 31; **DIŠ KI.MIN** A.1.1: 6', 17', 19', 35''; A.1.2: 12'; A.1.4: 30''; A.2.1: 44'', 46'', 47'', 59''', 60''', 83'''''; A.2.2: 7, 15, 16, 17, 18, 24, 30, 32, 35, 36, 37, 40, 44, 45, 58; A.2.7: 27', 28', 29'; A.2.8: 5; A.2.9: 10''; B.2.2: 8, 10, 13; C.1.2: 12, 13, 14; C.1.4: 75'', 179''', 184'''; C.3.3: 5, 7; C.3.4: 58, 59; C.3.5: 5'; D.1.1: 208, 209, 210, 211, 213, 214, 215, 216, 217, 218, 219, 220, 221, 222, 223, 233, 234, 235; D.1.3: 23'', 25'', 27'', 28'', 30'', 36''; D.1.7: 4'; D.2.1: 23', 27', 31', 64'; D.3.1: 16; E.2.6: 27', 30', 33'; H.1: 23'; **[DIŠ] KI.MIN** C.1.8: 9'; **[DIŠ K]I.MIN** A.1.1: 16'; B.1.6: 18'; D.2.1: 2'; **[DIŠ KI.M]IN** A.2.2: 34; **[DIŠ KI.MI]N** C.1.2: 15; **DIŠ ⸢KI.MIN⸣** A.2.2: 21, 33; ⸢**DIŠ**⸣ ⸢**KI.MIN**⸣ A.2.1: 49''; A.2.7: 26'; C.1.8: 24'; **DIŠ K[I.MIN]** A.2.2: 6; **DIŠ [KI.MIN$^{?}$]** A.2.2: 5, 19; A.2.4: 12'; **D[IŠ KI.MIN$^{?}$]** A.2.2: 20

kimṣu, *kinṣu* "shin; lower leg": ***ki-i[n***$^{!}$***-ṣa-šá]*** D.1.5: 6'

kimtu "family; kin": ***kim-is-su*** C.3.10: 46, 47; ***kim-mit-su*** C.3.10: 61; ***kim-ti-ia***$_5$ C.3.4: 48, 52

kīmū "instead of": ***[ki-mu]-ú*** C.3.4: 20

kīniš "favourably; sincerely": ***ki-niš*** D.1.9: 29'

kīnu "reliable; true": ***ki-ni*** B.2.6: 24; ***ki-nu*** D.1.1: 129; ***ki-num*** D.1.9: 8'

kirbān eqli "field clod-plant": **LAG-A.ŠÀ.GA** C.1.4: 176'''; ^{ú}**LAG-A.ŠÀ** C.1.5: 28, 30; ^{ú}**LAG-[A.ŠÀ]** A.2.1: 83'''''

kirissu "needle; hairpin": ***ki-ri-is-su*** C.3.3: 35; G.1: 14; ***[ki-ri]s-su***$^{?!}$ C.3.4: 76

kirru I (a big jar): ^{dug}**KÍR**$^{!}$ II.1.4: 8

kirru, *kerru* II "throat; collarbone": ⸢***kir***⸣***-r[i***$^{?}$***-šá]*** A.2.7: 18

kirû "garden": ^{giš}**KIRI$_6$** C.3.10: 33; ^{giš}**KIRI$_6$.MEŠ** B.1.1: 10

kisibirru, *kissibirru*, *kisibirrītu*, pl. fem. *ki/usibirrātu* "coriander": ***kús-bir-rat-⸢tú⸣*** F.1: 4; ***kús-bir-r[at-tú]*** F.2: 3; **ŠE.LÚ** II.1.3: 65'''; **ŠE.LÚ**^{sar} D.2.1: 35'

kīsu "binding; bonds; constriction": ***ki-is***! A.2.2: 42

kiṣallu, *kiṣillu* "ankle": ***ki-ṣil-li-šá*** I.1.1: 93; ***[ki]-ṣil-li-šá*** I.1.1: 90; ***[ki-ṣil]-⸢li⸣-šá*** I.1.1: 92; **ZI.IN.GI.DIDLI-*šá*** I.1.1: 72

kiṣru "knot; bond; lump; nod; joint": **KA.KÉŠ** II.1.3: 33'''; C.1.2: 28'; C.1.4: 7', 8', 22', 23', 47', 100'', 110''; D.3.1: 3, 4; F.1: 23, 27, 29, 31; H.1: 3, 24', 34'; **KA.KÉ[Š]** C.1.4: 109''; H.1: 18'; **KA.⸢KÉŠ⸣** H.1: 4; **KA.K[ÉŠ]** F.1: 30; **[K]A.KÉŠ** C.1.2: 28'; **⸢KA.KÉŠ⸣** F.1: 24; **[K]A.⸢KÉŠ⸣** D.3.1. 36; F.1: 20; **[KA.KÉ]Š** C.3.6: 53''''; **KÉ[Š]** C.1.1: 15; **[KÉ]Š** C.1.4: 186'''; **KÉŠ.MEŠ** C.1.4: 186'''; **KÉŠ-*r[a*?*]*** II.1.3: 59'''; ***ki-iṣ-ri*** II.1.1: 29; ***ki-ṣi-ru*** C.1.4: 20'; ***ki-ṣir*** C.3.9: 12, 15, 32; D.3.1: 25; F.2: 30'; ***⸢ki*?*-ṣir*?⸣** C.1.10: 16; ***ki-ṣ[ir-šá]*** D.1.1: 119; ***[ki-ṣ]ir-ú-šá*** D.1.8: 15

kišādu "neck": **GÚ** C.3.4: 6; C.3.9: 13; D.1.4: 15''; F.1: 9; **GÚ-*ki*** C.3.3: 33; C.3.4: 74; C.3.9: 55; **GÚ-*šá*** B.1.4: 17; C.3.5: 3', 6'; F.1: 11; **⸢GÚ?⸣-*šá*** I.1.3: 26; **⸢GÚ-*šá*⸣** C.3.5: 1'; **GÚ-*šú*** B.1.5: 3'; C.3.9: 2, 13, 29; C.3.10: 3; D.1.1: 232; D.3.1: 3; F.1: 11; **⸢GÚ?-*šú*?⸣** B.1.5: 1'; **G[Ú-*šú*]** C.3.9: 33

kiškanû (a tree): **GIŠ.KÍN** C.1.4: 179'''

kišpū "witchcraft; sorcery": **UŠ$_{11}$.ZU** A.2.7: 1; C.3.3: 1; C.3.4: 56; ***kiš-pi*** B.1.1: 63; C.3.3: 6, 9; C.3.7: 11'', 16'', 23''; C.3.9: 21; ***⸢kiš⸣-pi*** A.2.2: 10; ***kiš-pi-ki-na*** C.3.9: 24; ***kiš-pu*** B.1.1: 48; C.3.5: 7', 15'; ***⸢kiš⸣-p[u]*** D.1.8: 20

kiššānu, *kiššēnu* (a legume, probably common vetch): ***kiš-še-ni*** B.1.1: 24

kiššatu "totality; world": ***kiš-šat*** I.1.2: 11'; **ŠÚ-*t[i*?*]*** D.1.2: 16

kittabru "arm; side": ***kit-tab-ra*** G.1: 44; ***kit-tab-ri*** G.1: 43; ***kit-tab-ri-šú*** G.1: 43; G.2: 21''; ***⸢kit-tab-ri-šú⸣*** D.1.1: 99; ***kit-tam-ri*** G.2: 22''

kittu "truth; righteousness; justice": ***kit-ti*** E.2.3: 10'; ***kit-[ti*?*]*** E.2.3: 14'; ***[ki]t-ti*** D.1.8: 9; ***kit-tú*** D.1.8: 9

kitû "flax; linen": **GADA** A.1.2: 10', 28'; A.2.1: 74''''; A.2.3: 9'; A.2.9: 6'; B.1.2: 2'; B.1.4: 16; D.1.9: 18'; D.2.1: 21', 51', 52'; D.3.1: 15; **GADA**? A.2.2: 41, 55; **⸢^{giš}GADA$^{sar?}$⸣** II.1.3: 61'''; ***k[i-ti-e]*** D.1.9: 18'; **^{ú}GADA** II.1.3.1: 6'

KU$_6$, Ú.KU$_6$ (reading uncertain), an aromatic plant, probably a variety of fennel: **[^{š}]^{im}KU$_6$** B.1.1: 6; **⸢^{šim}KU$_6$?⸣** A.2.4: 35''; **Ú.KU$_6$** C.1.4: 182'''; D.1.3: 25''

kukru, *kukuru* (an aromatic plant): **^{giš}GÚR.GÚR** D.2.1: 20', 33', 43', 47', 52', 55', 56', 62', 65'; **GÚR.GÚR** B.2.2: 6, 24', 28'; C.1.9: 19; D.3.1: 15; E.2.6: 37', 43'; **⸢GÚR.GÚR⸣** A.2.4: 18'; **^{šim}GÚR.GÚR** II.1.4: 3, 21; A.2.1: 72''''; A.2.2: 74; A.2.6: 21; B.1.1: 31; B.2.2: 18'; D.2.1: 41'; D.3.1: 15; E.2.6: 10'; **[^{š}]^{im}GÚR.GÚR** A.1.4: 5'; **⸢^{šim}⸣GÚR.GÚR** B.2.4: 11'; **⸢^{šim}GÚR.GÚR⸣** A.2.2: 8; **[^{ši}]^{m}⸢GÚR.GÚR?⸣** C.1.6: 11'; **[^{šim}GÚR.G]ÚR** A.1.2: 9'; **^{šim}G[ÚR.GÚR?]** D.1.7: 13'; **[^{šim}]⸢GÚR.GÚR?⸣** A.2.1: 94'''''', 101''''''''; **[^{ši}]^{m}GÚR.<GÚR>** C.1.9: 24; **^{ú}GÚR.GÚR** D.2.1: 25'

kulbābu "ant": **KIŠI$_9$** C.1.4: 180'''

kulīlītu "dragonfly": ***^{ú}ku-li-⸢li*?⸣*-[tú*?*]*** D.2.1: 75'

kulīlu "mayfly": ***ku-li-l[i]*** C.1.4: 182'''

kullatu I "clay pit": **KI.GAR** C.3.4: 81

kullatu II "totality; whole (world)": ***kul-lat*** I.1.2: 11'

kullu D "to hold (back); to grip": ***ú-kal*** [D] C.2.1: 15'; D.2.1: 45', 60'; ***ú-⸢kal⸣*** [D] A.2.2: 71; ***ú-k[al*?*]*** [D] D.2.1: 9'; ***ú-kal-la*** [D] I.1.1: 72; ***ú-kal-lu-šú*** [D] C.3.10: 44; ***⸢ú-kal⸣-ši-ma*** C.1.4.2: 5'

kullumu D "to show": **⸢IGI.LÁ!⸣.MEŠ** [D] B.2.1: 35; ***kul-lu-ma-tu$_4$*** [D] C.3.5: 3'; ***kul-lu-mu*** [D] A.2.1: 54''', 61'''; C.2.3: 21'; ***li-kal-lim*** [D] G.1: 38; ***li-⸢kal-lim⸣*** [D] A.2.6: 27; ***⸢li-kal-lim⸣*** G.2: 16''; ***mu-kal-lim***! [D] E.2.3: 14'; ***tu-kal-la-am*** [D] B.2.1: 36; ***tu-kal-lam*** [D] C.1.4: 170'''; ***t[u-kal-lam]*** [D] B.2.1: 27; ***ú-kal-la-mu-ši-ma*** [D] C.3.5: 4'

kulūlu "headband": ***ku-lu-lu-ša*** II.1.4: 44; G.2: 18''; ***⸢ku⸣-lu-lu-[šú]*** D.1.1: 83

kūm "instead of": ***ku-um*** E.2.6: 41'

kunāšu "emmer": **ZÍZ** A.2.5: 18''; **ZÍZ.ÀM** A.2.3: 6'; B.1.1: 23; D.2.1: 34', 36'; **ZÍZ.AN.NA** C.1.8: 18'

kuništu "strand, twist (made of hair)": ***ku-niš-tú*** H.1: 23'

kunukku "cylinder seal; cylindrical bead": **^{na4}KIŠIB** C.1.4: 61''; C.1.5: 44; C.3.9: 2; D.1.4: 17''; F.1: 9, 18, 19; F.2: 8, 16, 18

kupīrātu "wipings" (pl. tant.): ***ku-pi-ra-ti-šú*** C.3.4: 35

kupītu (a marsh-bird): ***ku-pi-ti*** C.1.4: 179'''

kupputu "conglomerated": ***ku-⸢pu-ut⸣*** A.2.1: 31'; ***kup-pu-tú*** C.3.9: 9; ***kup-pu-ut-⸢tu⸣*** F.1: 28

kupsu, *kuspu* "husk; bran; sesame pomace": **DUḪ.ŠE.GIŠ.Ì** A.1.4: 35''; D.2.1: 42', 51', 62'; ***ku-us-pu*** A.2.1: 27'; ***kus-pú***? A.2.4: 17'

KÚR (correction marker; reading uncertain): **KÚR** A.2.2: 11; C.3.5: 13'; **⸢KÚR?⸣** A.2.2: 13

kurinnu "necklace": ***ku-ri-nu-uš-šú*** C.3.9: 13

kurītu "shin": ***ku-ri-tú*** C.3.10: 5; ***ku-⸢rit⸣*** C.3.10: 77

kurkānû (a medicinal plant, probably an aromatic): ***⸢kur*?⸣*-<ka>-nam*** A.2.2: 7; ***^{ú}kur-ka-[na]-a*** B.1.1: 33; ***^{ú}kur-ka-nam*** B.1.1: 31; B.1.3: 8; B.2.1: 15; ***⸢^{ú}kur⸣-ka-nam*** B.2.1: 24; ***^{ú}k[u]-ur-ru-ka-nu*** A.2.8: 11

kurkû "goose": **KUR.GI^{mušen}** C.3.6: 52''''

kurû "short": ***ku-ri*** I.1.3: 16

kūru I "depression; daze; stupor": ***ku-ú-rum*** C.3.5: 26'

kūru II (a plant), see GI.ZÚ.LUM.MA

kurummatu "food offering; ration; provision": **KURUM$_6$** C.3.4: 90; **KURUM$_6$-*su*** B.2.6: 4

kurunnu a type of beer: **KURUN!.NAM** B.2.4: 4'; **[KURUN].⸢NAM⸣** A.2.3: 4'; **⸢KURUN.NAM⸣** B.2.6: 6; ***ku-ru-nu*** E.2.6: 36'

kuṣāru "amulet (necklace)": ***ku-ṣa-ri*** F.2: 34'

kuṣṣu I, *kūṣu* "cold; winter": ***ku-ṣu*** A.2.5: 14'; ***ku-uṣ-ṣu*** I.1.3: 8

kuṣṣu II "cooled": ***ku*?*-uṣ-ṣu*** E.2.6: 36'

KUŠ.TAB (reading uncertain) "tanned ox-hide": **KUŠ.TAB** I.1.1: 79, 80

kutallu "back(side); rear part; later time"; in prep. expression *ina kutal* "behind": ***ku-tal*** C.3.4: 97; ***ku-tal-la-tu$_4$*** E.2.1: 11; ***ku-tal-li-šú*** C.3.10: 11, 79; D.1.1: 172

kutimmu "goldsmith": **^{lú}KÙ.DIM** C.3.3: 31; C.3.4: 73; C.3.9: 54

kutmu "cover; covering": **⸢DUL?⸣** A.1.4: 29''

kutpû a black frit-like glass": ^{na4}**AN.ZAḪ.GI$_6$** C.1.4: 2', 42'

lā "not": **NU** II.1.3: 47''', 52'''; II.1.4: 18, 19, 26; A.1.1: 2'; A.1.4: 39''; A.2.1: 55'''; A.2.2: 8, 10, 64, 74; A.2.7: 1, 34', 38', 40'; B.1.2: 1'; B.2.2: 18', 20', 21', 22'; C.1.4: 12', 27', 175'''; C.1.5: 1; C.1.8: 15'; C.1.9: 21; C.2.1: 12', 14', 18'; C.2.2: 2; C.2.3: 2'; C.3.3: 1; C.3.4: 4, 23, 24, 36, 55, 56, 100; C.3.5: 7'; C.3.6: 5', 15'; C.3.7: 11'', 19''; C.3.8: 13'; C.3.9: 7, 14, 38; C.3.10: 82, 84, 93; D.1.1: 229, 231, 233; D.1.2: 7; D.1.4: 17''; D.1.10: 4', 11'; D.2.1: 70'; H.1: 25'; I.1.1: 30, 34, 54, 92, 102, 118; I.1.2: 15'; I.1.7: 11; ⸢**NU**⸣ A.1.1: 4'; A.2.2: 70; A.2.6: 27; C.3.3: 45; ⸢**NU**$^{!}$⸣ D.1.3: 7'; **N[U]** A.2.2: 61, 67; ***la*** II.1.2: 10; II.1.4: 32; A.1.3: 4'; A.2.1: 54'''; A.2.8: 10; A.2.6: 10'; B.2.1: 21, 27; B.2.2: 27', 28'; B.2.3: 7'; C.1.4: 57'', 58'', 59'', 63''; C.1.8: 14', 21'; C.1.10: 1, 7; C.3.1: 22; C.3.3: 10; C.3.4: 8, 45, 55, 60, 82, 94; C.3.5: 8', 17', 18'; C.3.9: 21, 22; C.3.10: 1, 9, 30, 31, 34, 36, 38, 39, 43, 46, 47, 72; D.1.1: 143; D.1.5: 3', 12', 20'; D.1.6: 3, 5, 7, 9, 11; D.1.11: 3, 11; D.2.1: 15', 30', 71'; D.3.1: 1, 32; E.2.6: 27', 29'; G.2: 18''; I.1.3: 8, 10; I.1.7: 13; ⸢***la***⸣ B.2.1: 36; C.3.6: 11'; ⸢***la***$^{?}$⸣ A.2.7: 36'; B.1.3: 4; B.2.1: 43; ⸢***la***$^{!}$⸣ D.1.1: 29; ***l[a]*** B.2.1: 30; C.3.10: 66; ***l[a***$^{?}$***]*** C.1.10: 8; C.3.1: 11; D.1.9: 6'; ***la-'*** G.1: 4

lā patān "on an empty stomach" (lit. "without eating"): ***la pa-tan*** A.1.2: 6'; C.1.4: 29', 93''; C.1.5: 10, 11, 35; C.2.1: 7'; D.1.1: 207, 208, 213; ***[la] pa-tan*** C.1.5: 39; **NU *pa-tan*** A.2.7: 33', 34'; A.2.9: 4'; B.1.6: 6, 9; C.1.4: 75'', 183'''; C.1.5: 41; D.1.1: 213, 214; D.1.3: 10'; D.1.7: 2'; E.2.2: 12''; **NU *pa-t[an]*** A.1.1: 18'; A.2.2: 12; **NU *pa-[tan]*** A.2.7: 30', 31'; **[N]U *pa-tan*** A.1.1: 11'; ⸢**NU**⸣ ⸢***pa-tan***⸣ B.1.6: 12; **[NU]** ⸢***pa-tan***⸣ C.1.8: 46''; **[NU *p]a-tan*** D.1.3: 12'

lā petītu "unmated" (of female animal): **GÌŠ.NU.ZU** D.2.1: 72'; **[G]ÌŠ.NU.ZU** C.1.4: 99''; **GÌŠ.NU.⸢ZU⸣** C.3.6: 49''''

labāku G "to be(come) soft, supple"; D "to soak; to soften; to absorb(?)": ***lu-ub-bu-ku*** [D] A.2.1: 10'; A.2.3: 11'; C.1.10: 2, 6; ***[l]u-ub-[b]u-k[u]*** [D] A.2.3: 26'''; ⸢***tu***⸣***-lab-bak*** [D] A.2.3: 4'; ***[tu]-lab-bak*** [D] B.2.3: 8'; ***[tu-la]b-bak*** [D] A.2.3: 29'''; ***t[u-lab-bak***$^{?}$***]*** [D] B.2.3: 4'; ***ú-lab-bak*** [D] C.1.10: 11, 14; ***ú-lab-bak-[ku***$^{?}$***]*** [D] C.1.10: 9

labanātu "frankincense": ⸢$^{\text{šim?}}$⸣***la-ba-***⸢***na***$^{!}$***-tú***$^{?}$⸣ A.2.2: 30

labāšu D "to clothe"; N "to clothe oneself": ***il-lab-ba-áš*** [N] C.3.10: 11; **MU$_4$.MU$_4$*-si*** [D] D.3.1: 30; **MU$_4$.MU$_4$*-su*** [D] C.3.4: 84; ⸢**MU$_4$.MU$_4$*-su***⸣ [D] D.3.1: 30; ***ú-lab-b[i-iš***$^{?}$***]*** [D] D.1.9: 42'

labiru "old": ***la-bi-ra*** D.2.1: 11'; ***la-bi-ri-šú*** D.1.2: 15; D.3.1: 37(A), 38(b); ***la-bi-ri-šú***$^{!}$ A.2.7: 5; ***la-bi-[ri-šú]*** C.3.3: 42; ***la-bir-ta*** D.2.1: 13'; **LIBIR.RA.BI.GIN$_7$** D.1.1: 237; **LIBIR.RA-*ša*** C.3.10: 92; **SUMUN** A.2.1: 52'''; A.2.2: 13; A.2.3: 9', 30'''; B.2.3: 4'; B.2.4: 4', 7', 15', 16'; C.1.6: 6'; C.1.7: 4'; C.1.9: 13; C.1.10: 12; C.2.2: 5; E.2.2: 5'; E.2.6: 20', 23', 31', 33', 34', 36', 37', 40', 42', 44'; ⸢**SUMUN**⸣ B.2.4: 26'; ⸢**SUMUN**$^{?}$⸣ E.2.1: 6; **[SUM]UN**$^{?}$ A.2.2: 29; **SUMUN-*šú*** B.2.1: 42; I.1.1: 117; **SUMUN-*š[ú]*** D.3.1: 37(f); **[SUMUN]-*šú*** C.2.1: 16'

labku "soft; moist": ***lab-ku*** A.2.2: 27

labtu "roasted (oven-parched) grain": **ŠE.SA.A** A.1.3: 2'; C.3.4: 12; D.1.1: 204; D.1.11: 1, 2, 11; **[ŠE.SA].⸢A**$^{?}$⸣ A.1.4: 7'

ladinnu (an aromatic or resin): ***la-di-ni-ia*** C.3.4: 45

laḫannu "bottle": ^{dug}**LA.ḪA.AN** B.2.6: 8, 9; C.3.4: 42, 95; D.1.1: 206; D.1.3: 9'; ⸢^{dug}⸣**LA.ḪA.AN** B.2.6: 7; ^{dug}**L[A.ḪA.AN]** B.2.6: 13; ^{d}[^{ug}**LA.ḪA.AN]** B.2.6: 12

laḫmu "hairy one": ***laḫ-mi*** C.3.9: 28

laḫru "ewe": **U$_8$** C.1.4: 47'; C.3.10: 70, 73, 74; ⸢**U$_8$**⸣ C.3.10: 69

lakû "weak: suckling (infant)": ⸢***la***$^{?}$⸣***-ke-e*** D.1.1: 93; ***la-ku***$^{!}$***-ú*** II.1.4: 53

lāma "before": ***la-am*** C.1.8: 37'; D.1.3: 6'; ⸢***la***⸣***-am*** D.1.6: 2; ***la-***⸢***am***⸣ C.1.8: 27'; ***la-<am>*** C.1.5: 35; ***la-ma*** C.3.10: 6; ⸢***lam***$^{?}$⸣ A.1.1: 18'; ***lam***$_5$ B.2.2: 6

lamādu G "to learn; to know; to recognise"; Gt "to learn": ***la-mad*** [G] D.1.1: 143; ⸢***la***⸣***-ma-di-šu*** [G] B.2.1: 40; ***lil-tan-du*** [Gt] D.1.8: 25; ***tal-ma-di-ma*** [G] C.3.3: 26; ***tal-ma-di-[ma]*** [G] C.3.4: 69; ***tal-ma-[di]-ma*** [G] C.3.9: 49

lamassu "(female) tutelary deity; protective spirit": ^{d}**LAMMA.MEŠ** D.1.1: 150; ***la-mas-sa-at*** D.1.1: 150

lamdu, fem. *lamittu* "experienced": ***la-mit-tu***$_4$ D.1.6: 9, 10; ***la-mit-t[u***$_4$***]*** D.1.6: 12; ***la-mit-[tu***$_4$***]*** D.1.6: 11

lamû G "to surround; to wrap up": ***la-a-ma-ku-ma*** [G] II.1.4: 47; ⸢***la-ma***⸣***-ku*** [G] D.1.1: 101; **NIGIN** [G] A.2.7: 38'; C.1.4: 25', 33', 34', 35', 36', 41', 43', 45', 94'', 110'', 147''', 160''', 161''', 162''', 163''', 164''', 165''', 166''', 167''', 168''', 169''', 173'''; ⸢**NIGIN**$^{?}$⸣ [G] C.1.8: 23', 34'; C.2.3: 22'; D.1.1: 232; D.2.1: 53'; **N[IGIN]** [G] C.1.9: 2; **N[IGIN$^{!}$]** [G] C.1.2: 18; **NIGIN-*ma*** [G] II.1.4: 12; **NIGIN**$^{?}$***-ma*** [G] A.2.2: 41; **NIGIN-*[m]a***$^{?}$ [G] C.1.2: 16; **[NIGIN-*m]a***$^{?}$ [G] A.2.4: 14'; **NIGIN-*mi*** [G] A.2.2: 29, 38, 47, 71; B.1.3: 7, 10; B.2.2: 8, 10; C.1.1: 2; C.1.4: 9', 23', 152'''; C.1.5: 3, 32, 38, 40; C.1.7: 6'; C.1.9: 5, 14; D.1.1: 232; E.2.7: 6'; ⸢**NIGIN-*mi***⸣ [G] C.1.8: 10'; C.2.3: 7'; D.2.1: 68'; **NIGIN-*m[i]*** [G] A.2.2: 21, 69; **[NIG]IN-*mi*** [G] A.2.1: 19'; C.1.5: 5; **[NIGIN]-*mi*** [G] A.2.2: 57; ⸢**NIGIN**⸣***-m[i]*** [G] A.2.3: 14'; **[NIGIN-*m]i*** [G] C.1.9: 25; **NIGIN-*ši*** [G] C.3.4: 14; ***ta-la-[am-mi]*** [G] B.1.1: 38; ***ta-[lam-mi***$^{?}$***]*** [G] II.1.3: 28'''; ⸢***ta***$^{?}$⸣***-***⸢***lam***$^{?}$⸣***-[mi]*** [G] A.2.10: 1'; ***t[a-lam-mi***$^{?}$***]*** [G] C.1.1: 17; ***ta-lam-mu*** [G] B.2.3: 13''

lānu "shape; form; figure": ***la-a-nu*** G.1: 19; ***la-ni-šu*** G.1: 19; ***la-ni-šú*** G.2: 4'; ⸢***la***$^{?}$***-nu***$^{?}$⸣ G.2: 4'

lapānu G "to be(come) poor": **ÚKU** [G] I.1.1: 36, 37

lapāpu G "to wrap around": ***ta-lap-pa-ap*** [G] C.3.10: 4; ***tála-pap*** [G] C.1.4: 8', 31', 39'; C.1.8: 4'; C.3.9: 6, 11, 29, 31, 32, 33; D.2.1: 44', 49'; F.1: 7, 14, 17, 27, 35, 38; ***[t]ála-pap*** [G] F.1: 3; ***[tál]a-pap*** [G] F.1: 23; ***[tála]-pap*** [G] F.1: 41

lapātu G "to touch; to smear; to apply; to rub; to hurt"; Gtn iter. of G; Gt "to smear"; D "to affect; to smear"; Dt pass. of D: ***il-pu-ut*** [G] II.1.4: 60; D.1.1: 151, 153; ***il-ta-nap-p[at***$^{?}$***-su-ma]*** [Gtn] A.2.1: 24'; ***la-pa-ti*** [G] D.1.1: 155; ***la-pat*** [G] C.3.10: 83; ***lu-pu-ut*** [G] G.1: 41; G.2: 21''; ***[lap-t]a***$^{?}$***-tu***$_4$ [G] D.1.9: 6'; **TAG.GA-*at*** [D] C.1.4: 87''; **TAG**$^{?}$***-ma*** [G?] A.2.9: 14''; **TAG.MEŠ** [Gtn?] C.3.6: 63''''; **TAG.MEŠ-*ši*** [Gtn] D.2.1: 17'; **TAG.TAG** [D?] A.2.3: 14'; **[TA]G.TAG** [D?] A.2.3: 12'; **TAG-*ši*** [G] I.1.3: 15; **TAG-*šú*** [G] A.2.2: 27; ***ta[l-t]a-nap-pat*** [Gtn] A.2.6: 23; ***tal-tap-pat*** [Gt] B.1.1: 29; ***tul-ta-nap-[pat***$^{?}$***]*** [Dtn] A.1.3: 11'; ***ú-lap-pat-ma*** [D] C.3.10: 88; ***ul-ta-a[p-pat***$^{?}$***]*** [Dt] A.1.3: 4'

larû "branch; twig": ***la-ri-ia*** C.3.4: 45

lasāmu G "to run": ***lu-us-ma*** [G] D.1.1: 194

lâšu G "to knead": **SILA$_{11}$** [G] B.2.2: 19'; **SILA$_{11}$*-aš*** [G] D.2.1: 63'; ***i-la-aš-šu-uš-ma*** [G] C.3.10: 89; ***ta-la-áš*** [G] II.1.3: 49'''

latāku G "to test": ***la-a-ti-ik*** [G] B.2.1: 34; ***ta-lat-tak*** [G] B.2.2: 29'

latku "tested; proven": ***la-tik-ta*** C.1.5: 185'''; ***[lat]-***⸢***ku***$^{?}$⸣ D.1.3: 5'; ***lat-***⸢***ku***⸣***-tu***$_4$ C.1.8: 29'

la'û "small child": ***la-a*** G.1: 10; ***la-i*** C.3.10: 36

lemnu , fem. *lemuttu* "bad; evil; wicked": **ḪUL** C.3.4: 24; ⸢**ḪUL**⸣ D.3.1: 25; **ḪUL.⸢A⸣.MEŠ-*šú*** A.2.6: 1; **ḪUL-*tì*** D.3.1: 25; ⸢***lem***$^{?}$***-ni***⸣ E.1.3: 1'; ***lem***$^{?}$***-***⸢***nim***⸣ D.1.3: 5'; ***lem-nu*** A.2.6: 21; C.3.4: 36; C.3.6: 15'; E.2.3: 22'', 23'', 24''; ***lem-n[u]*** D.1.1: 89; ***lem***$^{!}$***-nu*** D.1.3: 7'

lemuttu "evil; wickedness; misfortune": **ḪUL-*tú*** D.1.3: 33''

leqû G "to take; to accept"; Gtn iter. of G: ***[i-l]e***$^{?}$***-qé-ma*** [G] D.1.1: 23; ***il-te-ne[q***$^{?}$***-qé]*** [Gtn] C.1.10: 12; ⸢***li***$^{?}$⸣***-qa-am-ma*** [G] B.1.1: 57; ***le-qé*** [G] E.2.3: 25''; ***le-qí*** [G] I.1.3: 18; ***li-qé-e*** [G] C.3.10: 31; **ŠU.TI-*ma*** [G] C.3.5: 11'; **TI** [G] A.2.2: 40; A.2.7: 27; ⸢**TI-*qe***⸣ [G] C.1.4: 94''; **TI-*qé*** [G] A.2.7: 29'; B.1.1: 14, 28; B.2.1: 16; C.1.4: 9'; C.1.5: 29; C.1.8: 38'; H.1: 23'; **TI-*q[é***$^{?}$**]** [G] A.2.2: 32; **TI-**⸢***qé***⸣ [G] A.2.3: 27'''; **TI-*q[é***$^{?}$**]** [G] C.2.3: 8'; ⸢**TI**⸣**-[*qé*]** [G] A.2.7: 12; **[T]I-*qé*** [G] H.1: 18'; **TI-*qé-ma*** [G] C.3.3: 5; C.3.4: 58; **TI-*qé-m[a]*** [G] C.1.8: 40'

lētu "cheek; side": ***le-es-su*** C.3.10: 11; D.1.1: 172; ***[le-t]i*** C.1.4: 51''; ***let-su*** C.3.10: 79

le'û G "to be able (to do something); to be competent": ***i-la-'i*** [G] D.1.5: 20'; ***[i-l]a-u-ni*** [G] D.1.5: 20'; ***i-le-'e-e*** [G] D.2.1: 71'

lē'u "writing board; wax tablet": ^{giš}**DA** B.2.2: 29'; C.3.4: 99; ^{giš}***le-u***$_5$ D.3.1: 37(f); ^{giš}***le-u***$_5$***-um*** C.1.8: 30'; ^{giš}**ZU**$^{?}$ A.2.2: 41

libāru, *lipāru*, *lupāru* (a fruit tree): ***lu-pár*** E.2.6: 7'

liblibbi "offspring"; *ša liblibbīša* "(her) foetus": ***lìb-bìb-bi*** D.1.8: 3; **ŠÀ.ÁB.BA**$_4$**.ALLA** C.3.10: 93; **ŠÀ.BAL.BAL** G.1: 54; ***šà* ŠÀ-ŠÀ-*š[à]*** A.2.2: 50; ***[šà* ŠÀ-Š]À-*šú*** E.2.2: 1'; ***šá* ŠÀ-ŠÀ-ŠÀ-*šú*** A.2.2: 52

libbu "heart; inside; interior; womb; belly"; as prep. "from in(side)"; *ana libbi* (compound prep.; adv.) "in(to)"; *ina libbi* (compound prep.; adv.) "in"; *libbū* (loc.-adv.) "in the same way as; just like"; *ša libbīša* "(her) foetus": ***lìb-bi*** A.1.4: 31''; A.2.1: 56'''; B.1.1: 17; B.2.2: 4; C.3.5: 17'; C.3.9: 6, 37; C.3.10: 27; D.1.9: 22'; E.2.8: 11''; G.1: 40; I.1.3: 16; ***lìb-b[i]*** D.2.1: 73'; ⸢***lìb-bi***$^{?}$⸣ A.1.4: 17'; ***[lìb]-bi*** D.1.9: 12'; ***lìb-bi-ia*** C.3.10: 30, 31; ***lìb-bi-ka*** D.1.8: 8; ***lìb-bi-šu*** D.1.1: 162; ***lìb-bi-šú*** A.2.1: 14'; C.3.10: 28; D.1.1: 39; D.1.8: 17; D.1.9: 10'; ***lìb-bu-u*** G.1: 16, 18, 29, 41; ***lìb-bu-u***$^{?}$ C.1.10: 3; ***lìb-bu-ú*** G.2: 8', 20''; ⸢***lìb***⸣***-bu-ú*** G.2: 19''; **ŠÀ** II.1.4: 8, 12, 24, 25; A.1.2: 17''; A.1.3: 3', 12'; A.2.1: 75''''; A.2.2: 17, 48, 51, 63; A.2.4: 10', 15', 18'; A.2.7: 3; A.2.10: 11'', 13''; C.1.1: 2, 9; C.1.4: 3', 75'', 174''', 189'''; C.1.10: 9; C.3.4: 14, 19, 95; C.3.5: 17'; C.3.6: 50''''; C.3.9: 10; C.3.10: 39, 70, 73; C.4.1: 2'; D.1.1: 39, 52, 54, 55, 177, 178, 207; D.1.2: 3; D.1.3: 10'; D.2.1: 36', 39', 58'; E.2.6: 2', 8', 11', 16', 17', 18', 23', 24', 28', 31', 32', 35', 39', 44'; G.1: 38, 52; G.2: 16''; H.1: 17'; H.2: 4; I.1.1: 94; I.1.2: 3'; I.1.3: 24; **ŠÀ**$^{?}$ A.2.3: 28''; ⸢**ŠÀ**⸣ A.2.2: 51; A.2.10: 10''; B.2.1: 20; C.2.3: 14'; C.3.3: 4; D.1.1: 15; D.2.1: 71'; H.1: 16'; **Š[À]** D.1.4: 6'; **[Š]À**$^{?}$ D.1.2: 3; **ŠÀ-*ka*** C.3.10: 31; **ŠÀ-*ša*** C.3.5: 12'; I.1.1: 56; **ŠÀ-*šá*** D.1.1: 39, 179, 197, 201, 209, 212; D.1.3: 3'; D.1.7: 20'; D.2.1: 40'; I.1.1: 73; I.1.3: 18; **ŠÀ-[*šá*$^{?}$]** I.1.4: 8'; **ŠÀ-*šú*** A.2.2: 62, 78; ***šá***$^{!}$ **ŠÀ-*ía*** C.3.10: 87; ***šá* ŠÀ-*ia***$_5$ C.3.10: 87; ***ša* ŠÀ-*ki*** C.3.10: 86; ***ša* ŠÀ-*šá*** A.2.7: 1; C.3.4: 56; C.3.5: 8'; D.1.6: 7, 9, 12, 13; E.2.8: 4'; ***ša* [ŠÀ-*ša*]** I.1.1: 36; ⸢***ša***⸣ **[ŠÀ-*ša*$^{?}$]** I.1.1: 53; ***[š]a* ŠÀ-*šá*** C.3.7: 19''; ***[ša* Š]À-*šá*** C.3.7: 18''; ***šá* ŠÀ-*šá*** D.1.1: 227; ***šá***$^{?!}$ **ŠÀ-*šá*** D.1.3: 4'; ***šá* Š[À]-*šá*** C.3.3: 1; ***šá* Š[À-*šá*$^{?}$]** A.1.1: 48'''; I.1.6: 7'; ⸢***šá***⸣ ⸢**ŠÀ**⸣**-[*šá*$^{?}$]** D.1.6: 2; ⸢***šà***$^{?}$⸣ ⸢**ŠÀ-*šá***⸣ I.1.3: 28; ***[šà* Š]À-*šá*** A.2.7: 36'; ***[šà* ŠÀ]-**⸢***šá***$^{?}$⸣ A.2.7: 35', 37'; ***šà* ŠÀ-*šà*** A.2.2: 53; A.2.4: 3'; B.1.6: 1; C.3.2: 6';' I.1.1: 1, 2, 3, 4, 5, 6, 7, 8, 9, 10, 11, 12, 13, 15, 16, 17, 18, 19, 20, 21, 22, 23, 24, 25, 26, 27, 32, 36, 37, 38, 39, 40, 41, 46, 47, 48, 55, 56, 69, 77, 78, 79, 80, 83, 85, 86, 87, 88, 89, 103, 104, 105; ⸢***šà***⸣ **ŠÀ-*šà*** A.1.4: 41''; ⸢***šà***⸣ ⸢**ŠÀ-*šà***⸣ I.1.1: 14; ***šà* ŠÀ-<*šà*>** C.3.9: 7; ***[šà* Š]À-*šà*** A.1.4: 34''; B.1.6: 7, 10; ***š[à* ŠÀ-*šà*$^{?}$]** E.2.4: 11''; ***šà* ŠÀ-*šú*** C.3.9: 38

libittu "mudbrick": **SIG**$_4$ C.3.10: 68; ⸢**SIG**$_4$$^{?}$⸣ A.1.4: 24'', 27''; **[SI]G**$_4$$^{?}$ A.1.4: 31''; **SIG**$_4$**.ḪI.A** C.3.10: 68

li'bu (a type of fever/disease): ***li-'-ba*** D.2.1: 59'

līliātu, *līlâtu* (pl. tant.) "evening", *līliattam*, *līlâtan* "in the evening": ***li-i-li-[a-tam]*** D.1.11: 12; ***li-la-a-ti*** I.1.6: 15'

lillidu "offspring": ***li-li-da-am*** II.1.2: 4; ***lil-li-du*** G.1: 30; ***lil-li-d[u]*** D.1.10: 6'; ^{lú}***lil-lid-su*** D.1.11: 5, 8; G.1: 30, 35, 36

lilû "wind demon": **LÍL.LÁ.EN.NA** I.1.3: 11, 12, 13; **LÚ.LÍL.LÁ** D.1.1: 233

lippu "wad": ***li-ip-pi*** C.3.10: 4; ***lip-pa*** A.1.1: 30''; ***líp-pa*** D.2.1: 49'; F.1: 17; ***[lí]p-pa*** F.1: 14; ***líp-p[a]*** F.1: 11; ⸢***líp-pa***⸣ F.1: 22, 38; ⸢***líp-pa***$^{?}$⸣ F.1: 35; ***líp-pi*** C.3.9: 6, 11, 31, 33; F.1: 7, 11, 14, 35, 38; ⸢***líp***⸣***-[pi]*** C.3.9: 31; ***[lí]p-***⸢***pi***⸣ F.1: 27

lipû "tallow": **Ì.UDU** A.1.4: 9'; A.2.1: 4'; A.2.2: 7, 21, 25, 54, 79; A.2.3: 17', 30'''; A.2.4: 12'; A.2.6: 19; A.2.7: 35'; A.2.9: 14''; B.2.4: 7', 16', 26'; C.1.4: 171''', 180''', 182'''; C.3.4: 47; D.2.1: 7', 9', 34', 35'; E.2.2: 5'; E.2.8: 2'; ⸢**Ì**⸣**.UDU** A.1.4: 19'; C.1.6: 4'; D.2.1: 66'; ⸢**Ì.UDU**⸣ A.2.1: 52'''; A.2.3: 19''; B.1.1: 7; ⸢**Ì.UDU**$^{?}$⸣ A.2.6: 8; **Ì.[UDU]** C.3.4: 39; **[Ì].UDU** A.2.5: 11'; C.1.6: 6'; **[Ì].**⸢**UDU**$^{?}$⸣ A.1.4: 5'; ⸢**Ì**⸣**.[UD]U** B.2.4: 4'; **Ì.UD[U]** A.2.2: 27; **Ì.U[DU**$^{?}$**]** A.2.1: 66'''; A.2.3: 12'; **[Ì.UD]U**$^{?}$ A.2.3: 28'''; A.2.10: 9''

līpu "descendant; scion": ***li-pu*** C.3.6: 25'

liqtu "gathered materials; selection; gleanings; excerpt; (a quality of gold, textiles)": ***li-<iq>-ti***$^{?}$ A.2.7: 27'

līqu "palate": ***liq*** C.3.1: 8; C.3.9: 25

lišān ḫarriri "field mouse-tongue" (a medicinal plant?): **EME-PÉŠ.A.ŠÀ.GA** C.1.4: 2'

lišān kalbi "dog's tongue-plant" (a medicinal plant): ^{ú}**EME-UR.GI**$_7$ A.2.1: 35'; A.2.7: 37'; C.1.4: 156'''; C.2.1: 8'; D.1.1: 205, 213, 214, 216; D.1.3: 8'; D.2.1: 18', 31'; **EME-UR.[GI**$_7$**]** D.1.11: 8; ^{ú}⸢**EME**$^{?}$⸣**-U[R.GI**$_7$**]** A.2.2: 65

līšu "dough": **NÍG.SILA**$_{11}$**.GÁ** C.3.4: 26; **[N]ÍG.SILA**$_{11}$**.GÁ** C.1.8: 18'

littu "cow": **ÁB** A.2.2: 53; A.2.6: 19; C.1.4: 6', 22', 31', 41', 47'; D.1.1: 135, 144, 146, 164, 170; **ÁB**$^{!}$ II.1.4: 11; **[Á]B** C.1.4: 101''; **ÁB-*ia*** G.1: 21; **ÁB-*ia***$_5$ G.2: 6'; **ÁB.GAL** D.1.1: 181; **GU**$_4$**.ÁB** II.1.4: 55; D.1.1: 135, 144, 146, 152; ***[la]-***⸢***a-tim***⸣ G.2: 6'; ***la-a-tu***$_4$ G.1: 21; ***la-tu*** D.1.1: 140; ***lit-tu***$_4$ D.1.9: 9', 12'

lū I particle expressing wish or affirmation: ***lu*** C.3.3: 12: C.3.4: 50, 51a; D.1.9: 28', 38'; ***[l]u*** B.1.1: 75; ***lu-u*** C.3.4: 61; ***lu-ú*** C.3.10: 25, 32; G.1: 23; ***lu-[ú***$^{?}$***]*** C.1.4: 136'';

lū II "or": ***lu*** A.2.2: 40; 50; A.2.5: 6', 8', 9'; B.1.3: 9; B.2.2: 3, 23'; C.2.3: 5'; C.3.4: 37, 38, 79, 80, 85; C.3.6: 61''''; C.3.10: 90; H.2: 4; I.1.3: 20; ***lu***$^{!?}$ I.1.6: 36'; ⸢***lu***⸣ E.2.1: 13; ⸢***lu***$^{?}$⸣ A.2.3: 10'; A.2.5: 8'; ***[l]u***$^{?}$ A.2.5: 7'; ***lu-u*** A.2.3: 12'; ⸢***lu-u***⸣ A.2.1: 53''', 91''''''; ***lu-ú*** E.2.8: 5'; D.1.11: 10, 12; ⸢***lu***⸣***-ú*** A.2.10: 2'; ***[lu]-ú*** D.1.11: 13

lû, *lī'um* "bull": **G[U**$_4$$^{?}$**]** C.3.1: 10

lubāru "cloth; textile": **TÚG** II.1.3: 33'''; A.1.4: 27''; A.2.1: 29'; A.2.2: 68; A.2.9: 16''; C.1.4: 155'''; C.2.1: 11'; C.3.5: 13'; **TÚG**$^{?}$ D.2.1: 44', 63'; **T[ÚG]** II.1.3: 39'''; **TÚG.ḪI.A** II.1.4: 9, 15, 29; A.1.4: 28''; C.1.4: 177'''; C.3.4: 5; **TÚG.MEŠ-*šá*** II.1.3: 46'''

lubku "salve; lubricant": ***lu-ub-ki*** II.1.3: 50'''

lullû "primeval (hu)man": **LÚ-*la*** B.1.1: 50

lulû "antimony": **KÙ.GAN** C.1.4: 44'; C.3.5: 9'; **KÙ.GA[N]** C.3.3: 2; ***lu-lu-ú*** A.2.1: 82'''''

lummu D "to dissolve(?); to soften(?)": ***tu-lam*** [D] B.2.2: 23'; ***tu-***⸢***lam***$^{?}$***-ma***$^{?}$⸣ [D] A.2.4: 17'

lumnu "evil"; *lumun libbi* "misery": **ḪUL** E.2.3: 15'; I.1.1: 111; ⸢**ḪUL**⸣ D.3.1: 25; E.1.2: 11'; **ḪUL-*ši***$^{!}$***-na*** D.1.3: 34''; ***lum-ni*** D.3.1: 25; ***lum-ni-ia*** C.3.10: 16; ***lum-nu*** C.3.10: 14; ***lu-um-[n]i-šú*** C.3.10: 58; **ŠÀ.ḪUL** C.3.4: 8

lurmu "ostrich": **GA.NU$_{11}^{mušen}$** A.2.2: 28; **G[A.N]U$_{11}$⸢$^{mušen?}$⸣** A.2.5: 7'; **[G]A.NU$_{11}$[^{mušen}]** C.1.4: 168'''; **GA.[NU$_{11}^{mušen}$]** C.1.10: 11; **GA.⸢NU$_{11}^{mušen?}$⸣** C.1.6: 2'; ***lu-ur-mu*** A.2.1: 18'; A.2.10: 3'; C.1.9: 12; ***lu$^{!}$-ur-mu*** C.1.9: 23; ***⸢lu⸣-ur-mu$^{?}$*** A.2.5: 9'
lurmû "pomegranate": **^{giš}NU.ÚR.MA** C.1.4: 163'''; **[^{gi}]^{š}NU.ÚR.MA** A.2.9: 2'; **^{giš}[NU].⸢ÚR⸣.M[A$^{?}$]** A.1.4: 25''
lūtu, *lu'tu* "decay; debility": ***lu-'-tú*** C.3.4: 63; C.3.9: 42; ***lu-'-[tú]*** C.3.3: 16
lu''û "dirty": ***lu-'-a-ti*** I.1.3: 15
lu''û II D "to make dirty; to defile": ***lu-'a-[a$^{?}$-ni$^{?}$]*** [D] I.1.5: 7'; ***lu-'-at-ma*** [D] G.1: 2, 5; ***⸢lu⸣-ú$^{?}$-'-at-ma*** [D] A.2.2: 14

mādiš, *ma'diš* "much": ***ma-'-diš*** C.1.10: 14, 15; D.1.11: 7
mādu "many; numerous; plenty": ***ma-a-⸢da$^{?!}$-ti⸣*** A.2.2: 48; ***ma-a-du*** A.2.1: 86'''''; ***ma-da*** A.2.7: 27'
mâdu G "to be numerous; to increase": ***ma-a'-da*** [G] C.3.4: 38; ***ma-a'-du*** [G] C.3.4: 37, 38, 80; I.1.1: 68, 71, 75
magāgu G "to protrude; to have spasms"; N "to have cramps": ***[i-nam$^{?}$]-⸢ga$_5$$^{?}$-ag$^{?}$⸣*** [N] I.1.3: 23
magal "very (much); greatly": ***ma-gal*** C.1.4: 174'''; ***[m]a-gal*** A.1.4: 39''; ***m[a-gal$^{?}$]*** A.1.4: 23''; **UL$_4$.GAL** I.1.3: 8
magāru G "to be favourable; to find consent": ***mu-gur*** [G] D.3.1: 23
magarru "wheel": ***ma-gar-ri*** C.1.4: 28'
magru "favourable; auspicious": **ŠE** C.1.10: 8
maḫāḫu G "to soak; to steep (in a liquid); to dissolve (in a liquid)"; Gtn iter. of G; N "to be soaked, softened; to become fused"; Nt "to dissolve": ***li-taḫ-ḫi-ḫu-ma*** [Gtn] D.2.1: 11', 12', 13'; ***ta-at-tam-ḫa-ḫu*** [Nt$^{?}$] B.2.2: 26'
maḫāru G "to receive; to accept; to appeal; to befall; to encounter; to face; to confront": ***a-maḫ-ḫar-ka*** [G] D.1.1: 195; ***a-maḫ$^{!}$-ḫar-ka$^{!}$*** [G] D.1.1: 47; ***am-ḫu-ru*** [G] C.3.4: 20; ***am-ḫu-ur-ka*** [G] B.2.6: 22; ***am-ta-ḫar*** C.3.10: 78, 82, 84; ***i-maḫ-ḫar-ši-ma*** [G] C.3.4: 12; ***im-ḫur-ma*** [G] D.2.1: 69', 70'; ***in-da-ḫar-ú-'i-in-ni*** [G] C.3.10: 9; ***lim-ḫu-ra-an-ni*** [G] C.3.4: 10; ***lim-ḫu-ra-an-ni-ma*** [G] C.3.10: 65, 66; ***lim-ḫu-ru-in-ni*** [G] C.3.10: 78, 82, 84; ***lim-ḫu-ru-nin-ni*** C.3.4: 21; ***lim-ḫu-ru-n[in-ni]*** [G] C.3.4: 20; ***lim-ḫur*** [G] C.1.4: 72''; ***ma-ḫi-ir*** [G] C.3.4: 17, 93; ***maḫ-ra-ta*** D.1.1: 226; ***maḫ-rat*** [G] C.3.10: 32, 36; ***muḫ-ri-i[n-ni]*** [G] C.3.6: 3'; ***muḫ-ra-an-ni-ma*** [G] C.3.10: 13; ***mu-ḫur-an-ni-ma*** [G] C.3.10: 40; ***mu-uḫ-ra-an-ni-ma*** [G] C.3.10: 33; ***mu-uḫ-ri*** [G] C.3.4: 71, 72, 73, 74; C.3.9: 52, 53, 54, 55, 56; ***[mu-u]ḫ-ri*** C.3.4: 75; ***mu-úḫ-ri*** [G] C.3.3: 29, 31, 33, 34; ***[m]u-úḫ-ri*** [G] C.3.3: 30; ***mu-uḫ-ri-ni-ma*** [G] C.3.4: 49; ***ta-maḫ-ḫar*** [G] C.1.5: 9; D.1.1: 196
maḫāṣu G "to strike; to beat; to hit; to stir; to drive in (peg, bolt)"; D "to hurt; to smash, kill; to stir": ***in-d[aḫ-ṣu$^{?}$]*** [G] G.2: 11'; ***ma-ḫa-ṣu*** [G] I.1.7: 4; ***ma[ḫ-ṣ]a-at*** C.1.1: 4; **SÌG-*aṣ*** [G] D.1.1: 207, 209; D.1.3: 10'; I.1.3: 10; **SÌG-⸢*aṣ*⸣** [G] C.1.8: 26'; **SÌ[G-*at*$^{?}$]** [G] I.1.3: 26; **S[ÌG-*at*$^{?}$]** [G] I.1.3: 27; **SÌG-*át*** [G] I.1.3: 18; **SÌG.SÌG-*si*** [D] D.2.1: 65'; **ŠU.RA** [G] II.1.4: 35, 52; ***ta-ma-ḫa-[aṣ]*** [G] II.1.3: 37'''; ***ta-maḫ-ḫa-aṣ*** [G] D.1.1: 55; ***ta-maḫ-ḫa-a[ṣ]*** [G] D.2.1: 72'; ***ta-ma-[ḫa-aṣ]*** [G] C.1.4: 92''; ***ta$_5$-maḫ-aṣ*** [G] C.1.5: 35; ***tu-ma-ḫ[aṣ-m]a*** [D] C.1.4: 82''
māḫiru "opponent; rival; recipient; one who faces, withstands": ***ma-ḫi-ir*** B.1.1: 63; ***ma-ḫi-ra*** C.1.8: 14'; ***ma-ḫi-rat*** C.3.10: 33; ***ma-ḫi-r[u]*** B.1.1: 60; ***ma-ḫir*** C.3.9: 21
māḫiṣu "one to beats, strikes": ***ma-ḫi-iṣ*** C.3.9: 26; I.1.7: 6; ***⸢ma⸣-ḫi-ṣi*** C.3.1: 8
maḫru "front; past (time)"; *ana maḫar* (compound prep.) "before"; *ina maḫar* "before; in the presence of": **IGI** C.1.8: 35'; C.3.4: 81; C.3.6: 6'; C.3.10: 68, 70; **IGI-*ka*** D.3.1: 12; ***ma-ḫar*** D.1.8: 15, 18, 20; D.1.9: 27'; ***ma-ḫar-ka*** C.3.10: 55; ***maḫ-ri-ki*** C.3.4: 93
maḫrû "first; older; front"; U$_4$.1.KAM "first day of the month": **IGI-*ú*** I.1.1: I.1.1: 116; ***[m]aḫ-ri-i*** E.2.6: 16'; ***maḫ-ri-tu$_4$*** D.1.1: 173; **U$_4$.1.KAM** D.3.1: 6, 11b, 37(b); **U$_4$.1.KÁM** D.3.1: 6, 11b
makāku G "to extend; to spread out": ***i-ma-ak-ka-ak-ma*** [G] D.3.1: 10a
makkūru "property": **NÍG.GA** I.1.3: 37'
makû Š "to cause to go missing; to withhold": ***u-⸢ša⸣-am-àš*** [Š] C.3.10: 93
makurru "barge": **^{giš}MÁ.GUR$_8$** D.1.1: 31, 34, 49, 103, 107, 186, 189; **⸢^{giš}MÁ⸣.GUR$_8$** D.1.1: 88
mala "as much as; as many as; everything that; whatever": ***ma-la*** A.2.2: 37; A.2.4: 4', 10'; A.2.5: 26''; A.2.8: 31'; B.1.1: 10; B.2.2: 23'; C.1.10: 4, 12; C.3.4: 13, 87; C.3.10: 35; E.2.6: 17'; ***[m]a-la*** C.3.4: 88; ***[m]a-⸢la$^{?}$⸣*** A.2.5: 10'
malāsu G "to pluck (out); to tear out"; N "to be plucked": ***ma-la-su*** [G] G.1: 28; ***na-am-li-su*** [N] G.1: 28, 29; ***[na-a]m-[l]i-[su]*** [N] D.1.1: 45
malmališ "equally; correspondingly": ***m[al$^{?}$-ma-liš]*** E.2.8: 2'; ***mál-ma-liš*** A.2.2: 7; B.2.4: 9'; C.2.1: 4'; D.2.1: 31', 51'; ***[má]l-ma-liš*** A.2.1: 29'; ***mál-ma-liš$^{!}$*** C.1.9: 13
maltaktu, *maštaktu* "test": ***mál-tak-ta-šú*** B.2.2: 21'; ***⸢mál⸣-tak-tú*** A.2.1: 71''''; ***[mal-t]ak-tú*** B.2.2: 29'; ***maš-tak-ti*** A.2.2: 70; ***[maš-t]ak-⸢tu$_4$$^{?}$⸣*** A.1.1: 10'
malû I, fem. *malītu* "full": ***ma-li-ti*** D.3.1: 22; ***ma-li-tú*** D.3.1: 22; ***ma-lit*** D.3.1: 22
malû II G "to be(come) full; to be filled with"; D "to fill (up); to fulfil, reach fullness": **DIRI** [G] D.2.1: 29'; I.1.1: 6, 7, 33, 34, 35; **DIRI** [D] A.2.2: 78; D.1.3: 9'; **DIRI-*ma*** [D] C.3.4: 3; C.3.6: 58''''; D.1.1: 179, 206; D.3.1: 29; **⸢DIRI$^{?}$⸣-*ma*** [D] B.2.6: 8; **DIRI-⸢*ma*⸣** [D] C.3.6: 50''''; **⸢DIRI-*ma*$^{?}$⸣** [D] C.3.4: 42; **⸢DIRI$^{?}$⸣-*m[a$^{?}$]*** [G] I.1.3: 25; **DIRI.MEŠ** [G] I.1.1: 93; **DIRI$^{?!}$-*tú*** [G] B.2.2: 12; **DIRI-*ú*** [G] I.1.1: 80; ***im-ta-lu-ú*** [G] B.1.1: 21; ***im-tal-lu-[u]*** [G?] C.3.1: 23; ***lim-la-a'*** [G] C.3.10: 15; ***im-ma-lu-u*** [N] C.3.1: 21; ***ma-la-at*** [G] D.1.1: 23; ***ma-[lat$^{?}$]*** [G] D.1.1: 3; ***m[a-li$^{?}$]*** [G] A.2.8: 15; ***ma-lit*** [G] A.1.2: 8'; D.2.1: 20'; ***ma-lu-ú*** [G] G.1: 2; I.1.1: 79; ***ma-l[u-ú$^{?}$]*** [G] C.3.8: 8; ***mu-le-e*** [D] II.1.4: 56; ***ú-mal-l[i]*** [D] B.1.1: 41; ***ta-ma-al-le-⸢e⸣*** [G] C.3.10: 29
māmītu "oath; ban": **NAM.ÉRIM** C.3.4: 38, 55, 79, 97; I.1.1: 111; ***ma-mit*** C.3.4: 50, 51a; I.1.3: 6; I.1.4: 7'
mamma(n) "(any)body; somebody": **LÚ.NA.ME** D.1.1: 229; ***ma-am-m[a]*** B.2.1: 27; ***⸢ma⸣-am-ma*** B.2.1: 36; ***ma-a[m-ma]*** B.2.1: 28; ***mam-ma*** C.3.4: 94; I.1.5: 7'
MA.AN.DUL (a textile; reading uncertain): **MA.AN.DUL** D.3.1: 9; **^{túg}MA.AN.DUL** D.3.1: 10a; **^{túg}M[A].AN.DUL** D.3.1: 9; **[^{t}]^{úg}MA.AN.DUL** D.3.1: 30
mannu "who?; whoever": ***man-nu*** C.1.2: 22'; D.1.5: 21'; ***[man]-nu*** C.1.1: 12; ***man-nu-um-ma*** D.1.1: 167
manû I (a unit of weight) "mina": **MA.NA** E.2.6: 20'
manû II G "to count; to recite": **ŠID** [G] D.1.1: 197; **ŠID$^{!}$** [G] A.2.7: 14; **ŠID-*ma*** C.1.4: 8'; C.1.8: 20'; C.3.7: 16''; **ŠID-*nu*** [G] A.1.2: 6', 18''; C.1.2: 29'; C.1.4: 11', 93'', 104'', 187'''; C.1.5: 45; C.3.3: 39; C.3.4: 14, 55, 78; C.3.6: 55''''; C.3.9: 15; C.3.10: 19, 73; D.1.1: 39, 55, 178; D.3.1: 17; H.1: 17', 24', 34'; H.2: 4; **ŠID-*n[u]*** [G] C.1.1: 16; D.1.2: 4; **ŠID-*[nu]*** C.3.6: 9'; **⸢ŠID⸣-*nu*** [G] C.1.8: 6'; **Š[ID-*nu*]** [G] B.2.1: 20; **[ŠID]-*nu*** [G] C.3.1: 30; **ŠID-*nu-ma*** [G] C.1.4: 3',

16'; C.3.3: 4; C.3.9: 12; D.1.1: 201; D.1.2: 11; **ŠID-⌜*nu*⌝-*ma*** [G] C.3.3: 8; **ŠID-*nu-[ma]*** [G] C.1.4: 134''; **ŠID-*nu-[ma$^?$]*** [G] A.2.7: 3; **ŠID-*ú*** [G] C.3.10: 73; ***ta-man-nu*** C.3.10: 13

maqātu G "to fall; to befall"; Gtn iter. of G; Š "to cause to fall; to dispose of": ***im-qú-ut*** [G] D.1.1: 156; ***im-ta-qut*** [G] D.1.1: 156; ***lim-qu-ut-ma*** [G] D.1.1: 36; ***li-i[m]-taq-qú-ta-ak-ku*** [Gtn] C.3.5: 26'; ***li-ta-na-qu-ta*** [Gtn] D.1.5: 14'; ***ma-qit*** [G] D.2.1: 29'; **ŠUB-*ma*** [G] I.1.3: 8; **ŠUB-*uš-šú*** [Š] C.3.10: 90; ***ú-⌜šam-qàt-ma⌝*** [Š] I.1.6: 7'; ***⌜ú-šam-qàt-ma⌝*** [Š] I.1.6: 6'; ***[ú]-⌜šam$^?$-qàt$^?$-ma⌝*** [Š] I.1.6: 5'

maqqītu "libation": **BAL-*tú*** C.1.4: 13'; C.3.4: 43

maqtu "fallen": ***ma-qit*** D.1.1: 113, 126, 172; **ŠUB-*t[i]*** D.1.1: 132; **ŠUB-*tú*** G.1: 48, 50

marāqu G "to crush; to grind (down)"; D "to grind": ***i-mar-raq-ma*** [G] D.1.1: 222; ***ta-mar-raq*** [G] A.2.2: 30, 63; C.2.1: 7', 8'; ***ta-ma-⌜raq⌝*** [G] C.2.1: 13'; D.2.1: 5'; ***ú-mar-raq-ma*** [D] D.1.1: 222

marāṣu G "to be(come) sick": **GIG** [G] II.1.3: 38'''; C.1.4: 17', 154''', 160'''; I.1.4: 6'; **G[IG$^?$]** [G] A.1.4: 18'; **[GI]G** [G] II.1.3: 31'''; **GIG-*at*** [G] A.2.2: 42, 43, 47; C.1.4: 73'', 80'', 124'', 131''; **GIG-*a[t]*** C.1.4: 91''; **GIG-*[at]*** [G] C.1.4: 21', 137''; **G[IG-*at*]** C.1.4: 86'', 98''; **[GIG]-*at*** E.2.7: 15''; **GIG-*át*** [G] I.1.2: 7'; ⌜**GIG-*át***⌝ [G] I.1.3: 30'; **GIG-*ma*** [G] I.1.2: 13'; I.1.3: 1, 8, 9, 10, 11, 12, 17; **GIG-*m[a]*** [G] I.1.1: 116; **GIG-*ṣa-a[t$^?$]*** E.1.3: 5'; ***i-mar-ra-a[ṣ$^?$]*** [G] E.1.2: 10'; ***mar-ṣa-⌜at⌝*** [G] A.2.3: 6'

marḫaṣu "rinse; lotion; ablution": ***mar-ḫa-ṣi*** B.1.1: 19, 20, 72; ***mar-ḫaṣ*** E.2.6: 38'

markasu "rope; cable": ***mar-kas-sa*** D.1.1: 104; ***mar$^?$-⌜kas⌝-[s]a$^?$*** D.1.1: 98

marṣu "sick (person); patient": **LÚ.GIG** I.1.1: 117; I.1.3: 33'

martu "bile": **ZÉ$^?$** D.1.11: 14'

mārtu "daughter": **DUMU.MUNUS** II.1.4: 59; C.3.3: 15, 25; C.3.4: 13, 69, 91, 94; C.3.6: 14'; C.3.8: 7; C.3.9: 41, 49; C.3.10: 26; D.1.1: 227; D.1.10: 7'; D.3.1: 21; **DU[MU.MUNUS]** C.3.4: 62; **DUMU.MUNUS.MEŠ-*ki-na*** C.3.4: 68; C.3.9: 47, 48; **DUMU.<MUNUS>.MEŠ-*ki-na*** C.3.4: 67; **[DUMU.MUNUS].(-)MEŠ-*ki-na*** C.3.3: 23; **DUMU.[MUNUS.MEŠ-*ki-n*]*a*** C.3.3: 24; ***mar-ti*** D.1.8: 14

marû "fattened; fat": ***ma-ru-u-te*** D.1.5: 10'; ***ma-ru-u-t[e]*** D.1.5: 9'; **NIGA.MEŠ** D.1.5: 9', 10'

māru "son; child"; *mār māri* "descendant": **A** A.2.6: 29; D.3.1: 39(A); I.1.1: 118; **A-*šú*** C.2.1: 16'; C.3.3: 44; I.1.1: 118; I.1.3: 35'; **DUMU** A.2.6: 28; B.1.1: 51; C.3.4: 16, 100; D.1.1: 47; D.1.8: 1; D.1.10: 10'; D.3.1: 38(f); G.1: 53; I.1.3: 19, 20, 36'; **DUMU.A.NI** I.1.2: 14'; **DUMU.MEŠ** C.3.4: 94; I.1.1: 52; **DUMU.(-)MEŠ-*ki-na*** C.3.3: 22; C.3.4: 67; C.3.9: 47; **DUMU.MEŠ-*šá*** I.1.1: 42, 43, 44; **DUMU.MEŠ-*[šá]*** I.1.1: 45; **DUMU.MEŠ-*šú*** C.3.4: 17, 37, 80, 97; **DUMU.(-)MEŠ-<*šú*>** C.3.4: 80; **DUMU-*šú*** B.1.1: 55; C.3.4: 17, 86; **[DUMU$^?$]-*šu*** C.3.4: 86; ***ma-ra*** G.1: 40, 43; ***ma-ri*** B.1.1: 56; ***ma-ri-ia*** C.3.4: 23; **MAŠ** B.2.1: 38, 39

maruštu, *maruṣtu* "trouble; distress; menses": **GIG-*šá*** I.1.3: 24; **GIG-*te*** D.1.3: 5'; ***ma-ru-uṣ-ti-šú*** I.1.2: 3'; ***ma-ru-uš-ti-šá*** I.1.1: 94; **NÍG.GIG-*[šá]*** A.2.7: 28'; **NÍG.GIG-*šá*** C.2.1: 12'

masūktu "mortar": ^{na4}***ma-suk-tu$_4$*** A.2.1: 28'

maṣû G "to be equal; to be sufficient for; to be able to"; Š "to cause to suffice; "to let obtain": ***ta-máṣ-ṣi*** [G] B.2.2: 24'; ***šu-ta-am-ṣa-am-ma*** [Štn] G.1: 41; ***ú-šam-ṣu*** [Š] C.3.3: 40

maš'altu "questioning; interrogation": ***maš-'a-al-ti*** G.1: 52

mašku "skin; leather": **KUŠ** A.1.3: 9'; A.2.1: 32'; A.2.5: 9'; A.2.6: 3; C.2.3: 16'; C.3.5: 6'; C.3.10: 2; ⌜**KUŠ**⌝ C.3.5: 1'; ***maš-ku*** A.2.8: 27'

mašlu "half"; *ūmu mašlu* "midday": ***ma[š]-lu*** D.1.11: 13

mašmaššu, *mašmašu* "conjurer": ^{lú}**MAŠ.MAŠ** C.3.4: 99; D.3.1: 39(A); ⌜^{lú}**MAŠ**⌝**.MAŠ** C.3.4: 39; **MAŠ.MAŠ** I.1.3: 36'

mašqītu "(medicinal) potion; drink; watering place": ***maš-qa-a-[ti]*** D.1.11: 4; ***ma-áš-qi-sa*** C.1.4: 179'''; ***maš-qí-ti*** B.1.1: 73; ***[maš-q]í-ti*** B.1.1: 39; ***maš-q[í-tu$^?$]*** B.1.1: 74; ***maš-qit*** B.2.2: 6; C.1.10: 17

mašqû "watering place": ***maš-qé-e*** D.1.1: 142; ***m[aš-q]í$^?$*** II.1.4: 54; ***maš-qí-i*** D.1.1: 142

mašqûtu "potion; drink": ***[maš-q]u-tu$^?$*** C.1.4: 13'; ***maš-qut*** A.2.5: 4'

mašrû, *mešrû* "riches; wealth": **NÍG.TUK** I.1.1: 6

maššītu "carrying; ingredients; suppository": **ḪI-*tú*** A.2.1: 10'; A.2.2: 63; A.2.3: 11', 12'; ⌜**ḪI**⌝**-*tú*** A.2.2: 9; **[ḪI]-*tú$^?$*** A.2.1: 5'; ***maš-š[i$^?$-t]a$^?$*** A.1.4: 23''; ***maš-ši-ti*** A.2.1: 13'; C.1.10: 5; E.2.6: 17'; ***maš-ši-tú*** A.2.1: 52''', 90''''''; ***ma[š-ši-tú$^?$]*** B.2.3: 14''; ***maš-šit-tu$_4$*** C.1.9: 20; ***maš-šit*** A.2.3: 28'''; B.2.2: 6, 23', 25', 26', 27', 28'; C.1.10: 2, 6, 10, 16; D.1.11: 6; ***maš-šit*** A.2.2: 23; B.2.3: 14''

MAŠ.TAB.BA (a medicinal plant, probably *māštu* in Akkadian): ^{ú}**MAŠ.TAB.BA** B.2.4: 11'; C.1.10: 5; D.2.1: 48'

maštakal "soapwort": **I[N.NU.UŠ]** E.2.6: 10'; ^{ú}**IN.NU.UŠ** II.1.3: 62'''; C.1.4: 39', 40', 46', 158'''; C.1.9: 4, 27; D.1.1: 204, 216; ^{ú}**IN.NU.U[Š]** C.1.8: 42'; **[^{ú}IN].NU.UŠ** D.1.3: 9'; ^{ú}**I[N.NU.U]Š** C.1.4: 92''; ^{ú}**I[N.NU.UŠ]** C.1.8: 44'; ^{ú}**IN$_6$.ÚŠ** A.2.2: 33; A.2.5: 12'; C.1.2: 14; C.1.5: 19; C.1.10: 6, 11; D.1.11: 5, 8; **[^{ú}]IN$_6$.ÚŠ** C.1.2: 18; ^{ú}**IN$_6$.Ú[Š]** C.3.4: 49

māštu "(female) twin; twin sister": **MUNUS.MAŠ.TAB.BA** I.1.6: 28'

māšu "(male) twin; twin brother": **MAŠ.TAB.BA** I.1.1: 71, 92, 98; **NITA.MAŠ.TAB.BA** I.1.6: 27'

matqu "sweet": **KU$_7^?$** E.2.6: 35', 36'; ⌜**KU$_7^?$**⌝ E.2.6: 39'

mātu "land": **AŠ.AŠ** I.1.1: 118; **KUR** B.2.6: 3; C.3.9: 12, 16; D.1.4: 16''; I.1.1: 114; **KUR.[KUR]** D.1.10: 13'; ***ma-a-ti*** C.3.9: 16; ***ma-a-tú*** D.1.8: 12; ***ma-ta-ta*** D.1.8: 11

mâtu G "to die"; Gtn iter. of G: ***a-a-mu-ut*** [G] C.3.10: 35; **BA.UG$_7$** [G] I.1.1: 112; I.1.3: 18; I.1.6: 22'; I.1.7: 1; **GAM** [G] I.1.1: 79, 80, 83, 87, 88, 89; ***i-ma-at*** [G] D.1.11: 8; ***li-mut-ma*** [G] C.3.10: 86; ***mi-it*** [G] I.1.6: 31'; **UG$_7$** [G] I.1.1: 4, 17, 18, 21, 38, 77, 104, 105; I.1.3: 8, 9, 10, 17, 23; I.1.7: 11; **U[G$_7^?$]** [G] I.1.1: 16; **UG$_7$-*tu$_4$*** [G] C.3.4: 17, 80; **UG$_7$.UG$_7$-*tu$_4$*** [Gtn] C.3.4: 36

mayyālu "bed": **KI.NÁ-*šá*** I.1.3: 20

mazāqu G "to suck": ***i-man-za-qu*** [G] B.2.2: 26'; ***<i>-man-za-qu*** B.2.2: 27'

me'atu, *mât*, *mē* "(one) hundred": ***me*** C.3.9: 40; F.2: 33'

medû I, *madû* "to become visible; known": ***mi-du-ú*** [G] G.2: 24''

medû II "known": ***mi-di-ti*** G.2: 24''

meḫru, *miḫru* "equivalent; adversity": ***mi-ḫi-ir*** D.1.1: 138; ***mi-ḫi-ir-šú*** C.3.4: 24; ***mi-ḫir-ki*** C.3.10: 71; ***mi-iḫ-ri*** C.3.4: 17, 20

meḫû "storm": ***me-ḫu-ú*** D.1.1: 101; ***me-ḫu$^{?}$-⸢ú$^{?}$⸣*** D.1.1: 91

mêlu "(leather) bag": **<*me*>-⸢UGU$^{?}$⸣** C.1.10: 18; ***me-e-lu*** C.3.5: 2'; ***me-li*** C.3.9: 9

mēneštu "weakness": ***mi-niš-tu$_4$*** C.3.10: 14

mēreštu "wish; need": ***mé-re-eš-ta*** B.1.1: 22; ***[m]e-re-eš-ti*** C.3.10: 93

mersu, *mirsu* "honey cake": **NINDA.Ì.DÉ.A** D.2.1: 33'; **NINDA.Ì.⸢DÉ.A⸣** C.1.4: 12'; C.3.4: 89; **NINDA.Ì.D[É.A]** C.3.4: 41; **[NINDA.Ì.DÉ.À]M** C.3.6: 8'

mērû "pregnancy": ***⸢mé⸣-ra-a*** I.1.1: 103; ***[mé]-ra-a*** I.1.1: 104; ***mé-ra-a-a*** C.3.10: 65, 71; ***mé-ra-šú*** C.3.10: 66; ***me-re-e*** B.2.3: 16''; ***me-re-e-šú*** I.1.2: 8'; **PEŠ$_4$-*šú*** I.1.1: 82

mesû G "to wash; to rinse": ***⸢am-te$^{?}$-e$^{?}$- su$^{?}$⸣*** [G] C.3.10: 21; **LUḪ$^{?}$** [G] A.2.2: 31, 33; **LUḪ$^{!}$** [G] A.2.3: 29'''; **⸢LUḪ⸣-*ma*** [G] C.2.3: 7'; **LUḪ-*si*** [G] A.2.2: 34, 72; B.1.1: 15; B.2.2: 3, 11; D.3.1: 10c; **⸢LUḪ⸣-*s[i]*** [G] A.2.5: 20''

mešrêtu "limbs": ***meš-re-e-tu*** D.1.1: 108; ***meš-r[e-e-tu]*** D.1.1: 121; ***meš-[re-e-tu$_4$$^{?}$]*** D.1.10: 5'

miḫḫu (a type of beer): ***mi-iḫ-ḫa*** C.3.10: 63

miḫṣu, *meḫṣu* "blow; strike; attack": **SÌG-*iṣ*** I.1.3: 26, 27

mimma, *mimmu* "any(thing); whatever; everything": ***mim-ma*** B.1.1: 33; C.3.4: 13, 24, 36, 87; C.3.6: 15'; D.1.3: 7'; D.1.6: 1; E.2.3: 12'; ***⸢mim⸣-ma*** C.1.4: 64''; ***⸢mim$^{?}$-ma$^{?}$⸣*** D.1.3: 5'; ***[mim]-ma*** E.2.3: 22'', 23'', 24''; ***mím-ma*** B.2.2: 21'; ***mim-mu*** C.3.4: 18

mimmû "all (of); whatever; everything": ***mim-mu-ú*** C.1.4: 48'', 64''

MIN "ditto": **^{d}MIN** D.1.8: 5; D.1.9: 28'; G.1: 22; **MIN** B.1.1: 34, 35, 36; C.1.2: 13; C.1.4: 27', 30', 32', 33', 34', 35', 36', 37', 38', 39', 41', 43', 45', 47', 75'', 82'', 126''; C.1.4.2: 5'; C.3.9: 5; D.1.3: 13', 14', 15', 16', 17', 18', 19', 20', 21'; D.1.4: 6'; D.2.1: 43', 47', 50', 52', 54', 55', 56'; E.2.7: 12'', 21''; I.1.1: 38, 39, 40, 41, 42, 43, 45, 46, 47, 48; **MIN$^{?}$** A.2.2: 13; C.3.2: 1', 2'; D.1.1: 4; **⸢MIN⸣** B.1.1: 33; C.1.4: 31'; I.1.1: 30; **⸢MIN$^{?}$⸣** G.2: 25''; **MIN-*ma*** C.1.4: 126''; D.2.1: 30', 33', 34', 59', 65', 67'

minītu "measure; (normal) amount": ***mi-ni-[ti$^{?}$]*** A.2.8: 30'

mīnu, *mīnû* "what?"; *ina mīni* "with what?"; "how?": ***mi-ni-i*** B.1.1: 54; ***mi-nu*** D.1.5: 8'

minûtu "counting; calculation; recitation; form; physique": **ŠID-*tú*** C.3.6: 9'; ***mi-nu-ta*** D.1.1: 137; ***[m]i-nu-tú*** C.3.6: 28'

miqittu "dead (animal); carcass; collapse": **RI.RI.GA** C.1.4: 6', 22', 31', 41', 47', 101''

mīru "bull": ***mi-ru*** D.1.1: 144

misarru, *miserru* "belt": **^{kuš}E.ÍB** C.3.4: 84

mīšaru "justice": ***mi-ša-ri-im*** II.1.2: 13; ***mi-šá-ri*** D.1.8: 10

mišlu "half": **1/2** A.2.1: 11', 51''', 88''''', 89'''''; B.1.1: 29; B.2.4: 4'; C.4.1: 2', 4', 6', 8', 10'; E.2.1: 9; E.2.6: 23', 31', 33'; I.1.6: 17'; **1/2$^{?}$** E.2.2: 8'; **⸢1/2⸣** A.1.4: 12'; C.2.3: 16', 19'; ***mi-šil*** A.2.1: 44'', 45''; C.1.6: 11'; C.3.10: 90; ***mi-šil$^{!}$*** C.1.6: 10'

mitḫāru "corresponding (to one another); like (another one); proportionate; of the same size": ***mit-ḫar*** A.1.4: 35''

mû "water; (amniotic) fluid": **A** II.1.3: 49''', 59'''; B.1.1: 15; B.2.2: 11, 19', 23'; C.1.4: 9', 10', 92'', 138''; C.3.4: 25, 35, 40, 47, 54; C.3.10: 89; D.2.1: 8', 58', 60', 63', 67', 72'; I.1.3: 24; **A$^{?}$** E.2.5: 10'; E.2.6: 2'; **⸢A⸣** B.1.3: 9; B.2.6: 12; C.2.3: 4', 7'; D.1.11: 2; **⸢A$^{?}$⸣** A.2.1: 41''; A.2.2: 72; B.2.6: 8, 9; E.2.3: 2'; E.2.3: 20''; **A.A-*šá*** A.2.7: 35'; **A.ME** C.3.4: 61; **A.MEŠ** II.1.4: 59, 60; A.1.4: 24''; A.2.1: 25'; A.2.2: 51, 57, 77; B.1.1: 17, 18, 41; B.2.2: 26'; C.1.1: 11; C.1.4: 174'''; C.1.5: 41; C.2.3: 13', 19'; C.3.3: 12; C.3.4: 47, 49; C.3.9: 18; C.3.10: 10, 12, 21; D.1.1: 151; D.1.11: 9; E.2.6: 41'; **⸢A⸣.MEŠ** C.1.2: 22'; **A.M[EŠ]** A.2.5: 8'; **[A].MEŠ** II.1.4: 55; **A.⸢MEŠ$^{?}$⸣** A.2.5: 7'; **A.[MEŠ$^{?}$]** A.2.5: 27''; **[A.M]EŠ** C.1.4: 189'''; **A.MEŠ-*ka*** C.3.10: 14; **A.MEŠ-*ša*** II.1.4: 2; **A.MEŠ-*šá*** C.1.4: 26'; C.1.8: 12'; D.1.11: 8; **A.[MEŠ-*šá*]** C.1.4: 178'''; **[A].MEŠ-*šá*** C.1.4: 183'''; **A-*šá*** A.2.7: 36'; ***me-e*** A.2.1: 53''', 69'''', 91'''''; C.3.5: 23'; C.3.9: 18; D.1.1: 142, 151, 152, 154, 169; D.1.9: 26'; E.2.1: 6, 14; ***[m]e-e*** II.1.2: 1, 5; ***⸢me⸣-e*** A.2.8: 40'; ***⸢me$^{?}$-e⸣*** D.1.11: 4; ***[me]-⸢e$^{?}$⸣*** E.2.2: 12''; ***me$^{!}$-e$^{!}$*** D.1.11: 12; ***me*** B.2.2: 14; D.1.1: 154; ***me-[e-šá]*** C.1.4: 135''; ***mu-ka*** C.3.10: 13, 16; ***mu-ú-šá*** D.1.1: 114

muballiṭu "one who keeps alive": ***⸢mu⸣-balx-liṭ-ṭu$_4$*** D.1.10: 9'

mūdû "one who knows; knowledgeable (person)": **⸢ZU⸣** A.2.6: 27; **ZU.A** A.2.6: 27; B.2.1: 35

muḫḫu "skull; head; brain; top": as prep. "on, over"; *ana muḫḫi* (compound prep.) "upon; on; above; to"; *ina muḫḫi* "upon; on; to": ***mu-úḫ*** I.1.1: 2, 52; ***muḫ-ḫi*** C.3.1: 8; C.3.6: 55''''; C.3.9: 12, 15, 26; C.3.10: 26; D.2.1: 15'; D.3.1: 10b; I.1.7: 6; ***[mu]ḫ-ḫi*** C.3.6: 51''''; ***muḫ-ḫi-šá*** D.1.1: 169; ***muḫ-ḫi-šú*** C.3.4: 82; C.3.10: 13, 19; **UGU** II.1.4: 9, 15, 16; 55; A.1.4: 33''; A.2.5: 24''; C.1.4: 8', 26', 104'', 179'''; C.1.5: 28; C.3.3: 8; C.3.4: 47, 49, 55, 78; C.3.5: 12'; C.3.10: 7, 8, 68, 74; D.1.1: 39, 144, 179, 197; D.1.2: 13; D.3.1: 16; E.2.3: 6'; E.2.6: 21', 35', 36'; I.1.1: 1, 52; I.1.3: 32'; **U[G]U** C.3.1: 30; **U[GU]** A.1.4: 33''; **[UG]U$^{?}$** A.1.4: 28''; E.2.6: 36'; **UGU-[*šú*]** C.2.1: 15'; **UGU-⸢*šú-nu*$^{?}$⸣** C.3.4: 49

muḫru "presentation offering; gift; appeal; prayer": ***mu-ḫur*** C.3.10: 40

mullilu "purifier": ***mu-lil*** B.1.1: 61

mulmullu "arrow": ***mul-mul*** G.1: 33; ***[mul-m]ul*** G.2: 13'

munakkiru "one who changes, one who removes": ***mu-na-ki-ra*** C.3.9: 20

mundaḫṣu, *muttaḫṣu* "fighting, fighter": ***mu-ut-taḫ-iṣ*** II.1.4: 40; ***mut$^{!}$-taḫ-i[ṣ$^{?}$]*** D.1.1: 80

mundu "groats": ***mu-un-da*** D.2.1: 12'; **NÍG.ÀR.RA** B.1.2: 3'; D.2.1: 36'; **⸢NÍG$^{?}$⸣.ÀR.RA** D.2.1: 72'

mupaṭṭiru "one who releases": ***mu-paṭ-ṭir*** C.3.4: 8

muppiš(ū)tu "witchcraft; machinations": ***mu-up-pi-šá-a-tú*** C.3.9: 23

muqqalpītu "downstream": ***muq-qal-pi-ti*** D.1.1: 212; ***mu-qal-pi-tu$_4$*** C.3.10: 12

murru (an aromatic, probably not myrrh): **^{šim}ŠEŠ** II.1.4: 5; A.2.1: 86'''''; A.2.2: 24, 45, 78; C.1.6: 5', 7'; C.2.2: 11; E.2.5: 8'; **^{šim}⸢ŠEŠ⸣** A.2.2: 26, 30; A.2.6: 21; **⸢^{šim}⸣ŠEŠ** C.2.3: 4'; ***mur-ra*** II.1.3: 35'''; ***mur-[ru$^{?}$]*** A.2.10: 8'

murṣu "sickness; illness": **GIG** I.1.6: 18'; **[GI]G$^{?}$** E.1.2: 10'; **GIG.ME-*šú*** C.3.4: 37; **GIG.MEŠ-*šú*** C.3.4: 80; **GIG.MEŠ-*š[ú]*** C.3.4: 37; **GIG-*sa*** I.1.3: 13; **GIG-*sà*** I.1.3: 17, 23; **GIG-*šá*** I.1.3: 14, 15, 16, 19; **[G]IG-*šá*** I.1.5: 6'; ***mur-ṣ[i$^{?}$]*** A.2.1: 63'''; ***[m]ur-ṣu*** I.1.2: 9'; **NÍG.GIG-*ša*** C.1.4: 175'''

musakkiru "the one who blocks": ***mu-sak-ki-ru*** C.3.9: 20

musukkannu "rosewood", perhaps *Dalbergia sissoo*: **^{giš}MES.MÁ.GAN.NA** D.3.1: 3, 6a; **^{giš}MES.⸢MÁ⸣.GAN.NA** D.3.1: 2; **[^{giš}ME]S.MÁ.GAN.NA** D.3.1: 34

musukkatu "impure woman" (a woman who has recently given birth): ***ma-suk-ka-tu$_4$*** A.2.6: 19; **^{munus}⸢*ú*⸣-[*suk-k*]*at*** A.2.2: 11; ***[mu-suk$^{?}$]-ka-tu*** C.1.8: 13'

muṣa''irānu "frog": ⸢**BIL.ZA**?⸣**.ZA.MEŠ** C.3.9: 37

muṣiptu a garment: ***mu-ṣip-ti*** D.2.1: 13'; ***mu-ṣip-t[u$_4$]*** E.2.5: 7'

muṣlālu "noon": **AN.BIR$_9$** I.1.6: 16'

mūṣu (a stone): ^{na4}***mu-ṣa*** C.3.9: 4; D.1.1: 235; D.1.3: 29''; ^{na4}***mu-ṣu*** D.1.1: 235

mušallimtu "woman who delivers (her baby) soundly; who brings to term": ***mu-šal-in-d[u?]*** C.3.10: 43; ***mu-šal-li-mat*** I.1.1: 99; ***mu-šal-lim-ti*** C.3.10: 69; ***mu-šal-lim-tu*** C.3.4: 10

mušapšiqtu "woman having difficulty in delivery": **[^{munus}LA.R]A.AḪ** D.1.1: 36; ^{munus}**L[A.RA.AḪ.A.KAM?]** D.1.1: 37; ^{munus}**L[A.RA.AḪ.A.KAM?]** D.1.2: 2; ^{munus}**LA.RA.AḪ.A.KÁM** D.1.1: 37, 131, 53, 203; G.1: 26; ***mu-šap-ši-i[q-ti]*** D.1.1: 161; ***mu-ša-ap-ši-iq-tim*** II.1.1: 28; ***mu-šap-šiq-tu$_4$*** D.1.1: 159; ***mu-ša-ap-ši-iq-tum*** II.1.1: 30; ***mu-⸢ša⸣-a[p-ši-iq-tum?]*** II.1.1: 35

mušapširu "one who dispels": ***[mu-ša]p-⸢šir?⸣*** C.3.4: 8

mušāṭu "combed-out hair": **ḪAMANZER** E.1.1: 2; ***mu-šá-ṭa*** D.3.1: 15; ***mu-šá-ṭi*** D.3.1: 15; H.1: 18'; ***mu-šá-ṭi-šá*** H.1: 16', 23'; ***⸢mu⸣-šá-ṭí-šá*** H.1: 5, 17'; ***mu-šá-⸢ṭí-šá⸣*** H.1: 4; ***mu-šá-ṭi-šú*** H.1: 23'

mušēniqtu "wet-nurse": ***mu-še-ni-qé-ti-ka*** C.3.5: 20'; ***mu-še-niq-t[a]*** C.3.4: 92

mušēšertu, *mušēširtu*, *muštēšertu* "a woman who brings to term"; *lā muš(t)ēšertu* "a woman who does not bring to term": ***mu-še-šèr-tu$_4$*** C.3.10: 1; **NU SI.SÁ** C.3.10: 62; D.3.1: 5; **[NU S]I.SÁ** C.3.6: 6'; **NU SI.SÁ.KÁM** C.3.1: 7; **NU S[I].SÁ.[KÁM]** C.3.1: 29

mušēširūtu "ability to bring to term": ***mu-še-ši-ru-sa*** C.3.10: 67; ***mu-še-ši-ru-ti*** C.3.10: 66; ***mu-še-ši-ru-t[i]*** C.3.10: 72; ***mu-še-ši-ru-ut-ka*** C.3.10: 72; ***m[u-še-ši]-ru-ut-ki*** C.3.10: 72

mušīmu "one who determines; one who decrees": ***mu-šim*** D.3.1: 20

mušnammiru "illuminator": ***muš-na-mir*** D.1.8: 2

muššaru (a stone with red and white stripes, banded agate): ^{na4}**MUŠ.GÍR** F.2: 10; ⁿ**[**^{a4}**M]UŠ.GÍR** F.1: 39; ⸢^{na4}**MUŠ.GÍR**⸣ C.1.4: 132''; ^{na4}⸢**MUŠ**⸣**.[GÍR]** F.1: 9

muššu'u D "to rub; to massage": ***tu-ma-áš-šá-a'*** [D] D.1.5: 15'; ***tu-maš-šá-a'*** [D] D.1.1: 180; ***tu-maš-šá-a'-ma*** [D] D.1.1: 55, 134; ***tu-maš-šá-a'-ši*** [D] B.1.1: 18; ***ú-maš-šá-a'*** [D] D.2.1: 57'

muštapšiqtu, *multapšiqtu* "woman having difficulty in delivery": ^{munus}**LA.RA.AḪ.MEŠ** II.1.4: 62; ^{munus}**LA.<RA>.AḪ-*tu*** II.1.4: 33; ***mu-ul-tap-ši-iq-te*** II.1.4: 50

muštēpišu "sorcerer": ***muš-te-pi-šú*** C.3.10: 24

muštinnu "urethra": ***muš-tin-ni-ša*** C.1.4: 156''', 157'''; ***múš-tin-ni-šú*** A.2.2: 45

mušṭû "comb": ^{giš}**GA.RÍG** C.3.3: 34; C.3.4: 75; C.3.9: 56

mūšu "night": **GI$_6$** II.1.4: 13; C.3.4: 39, 85, 90; I.1.3: 11, 13, 17; I.1.6: 14'; **G[I$_6$]** I.1.6: 13'; ***mu-šu*** B.2.2: 2

muttappiḫtu (meaning uncertain): ***[mu-u]t-tap-pi-iḫ-tú*** A.2.1: 87''''''

muttarrītu "nurse": ***mu-ut-tar-ra-at*** C.3.4: 69; ***mu-ut-tar-ra-ta*** C.3.3: 26; ***mut!-tar-ra-tú*** C.3.9: 49

muterru "(re)turner"; *muter gimilli* "avenger; returning kindness": ***⸢mu-tir?⸣*** D.2.1: 69'

mutu "husband": ***mu-tu$_4$*** I.1.5: 5'

mūtu "death": ***mu-te*** II.1.4: 42; ***mu-ti*** D.1.1: 48, 86, 185; ***[mu]-ti*** D.1.1: 188; ***mu-tu$_4$*** C.3.4: 63; D.1.1: 48; ***mu-ú-te*** II.1.4: 37; ***[mu-ú]-ti*** D.1.1: 77; **ÚŠ** I.1.3: 14; **ÚŠ-*šá*** I.1.3: 26, 27

na'ādu G "to be attentive, concerned"; Gt "to watch carefully": ***it-mu-du*** [Gt] G.1: 46; ***it-ta-id*** [G] D.1.1: 116; ***it-ta-'i-id*** [G] G.1: 45; ***it-⸢ta?-'i?-du?⸣*** [G] C.3.4: 17; ***na-a'-da-át*** [G] I.1.3: 3, 4; I.1.5: 4'

nabalkutu N "to cross over; to roll (eyes)"; Ntn iter. of N; Š "to bring across; to overturn"; Štn iter. of Š; "to try repeatedly to move": **BAL.BAL.MEŠ** [Ntn] I.1.1: 89; ***na-bal-kut-ti-ka*** [N] D.1.8: 7; ***[u]š-ta-nab-l[ak-kát]*** [Štn] I.1.4: 3'

nablu "flash of fire; flame": ***nab-li*** D.1.5: 13'

nabnītu "creature": ***nab-ni-tu*** D.1.1: 109

nabruqqu, *namruqqu* (a medicinal plant): ***nam-ru-qu*** A.2.8: 12; ^{ú}***nab-rú-qi*** B.1.1: 31, 32; ⸢^{ú}⸣***nab-ruq-qu*** B.1.6: 4, 11; ***nam-ruq*** E.2.5: 6', 9'; E.2.6: 4'; ^{ú}***nam-ruq-qa*** E.2.4: 4'; ***[nam-ru]q?-qa*** A.1.4: 26''; ^{ú}***nam-ruq-qu*** A.1.4: 37'', 89''''''; ^{ú}***nam-ru-qu*** A.2.8: 2

nabû I "named; invoked": ***na-bu-ú*** C.3.10: 8, 9

nabû II G "to name": ***ib-bi*** [G] D.1.9: 41'; ***[i]b-bi*** [G] D.1.9: 35'

nadānu G "to give; to administer": ***ad-din-ka*** [G] C.3.4: 23, 52; E.2.3: 21''; ***id-di-nu*** [G] D.1.1: 130; ***i-din*** [G] A.2.5: 11'; ***id-nam-ma*** [G] D.1.1: 226; ***it-tan-nu-nu*** [G] C.3.10: 8; C.3.10: 8; ***lid-di-na*** [G] C.3.10: 66, 67; ***li-di-nu-ni-ki*** [G] D.1.5: 9'; ***li-di-n[u-ni-ki]*** [G] D.1.5: 8'; ***li-din-u-ni*** [G] D.1.5: 11'; ***na-da-nu*** [G] G.1: 44; **SUM?** [G] B.2.6: 14; **SUM-*in*** [G] A.2.5: 10', 12'; ⸢**SUM**⸣**-*in*** [G] A.2.5: 7'; **SUM-*nu-šú*** [G] E.2.6: 17'; **SUM-*su*** [G] B.2.2: 18', 21', 29'; C.1.10: 2, 3, 6, 7, 8, 9, 12, 13, 18; D.1.11: 7; E.2.6: 16'; **[SU]M-*su*** [G] D.1.11: 4; **SU[M?-*su*]** [G] C.1.10: 10; **SUM-*ši*** [G] C.1.10: 2; D.1.11: 8; **SUM-*šú*** [G] C.1.10: 12; **SUM-*šum-ma*** [G] B.2.2: 26'; ***ta-ad-da-áš-šum-ma*** [G] B.2.2: 25'; ***ta-nam-di-ma*** [G] A.2.4: 6'; ***ta-na-dín*** [G] E.2.6: 6'; ***⸢ta-nam-din⸣*** [G] B.2.6: 20; ***ta-nam-di-is-su*** [G] C.3.10: 6, 19

nādinu "giver": ***n[a?-din]*** D.1.1: 100

nadû I "thrown; placed; cast; deserted; uncultivated": **ŠUB-*i*** C.3.4: 22

nadû II G "to throw (down); to put; to set up; to cast (a spell); to pour; to discharge; to miscarry, abort"; Gtn iter. of G; Š caus. of G, "to cause to miscarry; N "to be thrown/laid down": ***ad-⸢di?⸣*** A.2.7: 9; ***[a]d-di*** [G] B.2.1: 12; ***ad-dú-ki*** [G] C.3.4: 93; ***id-di*** [G] D.1.1: 118, 172; ***id-di-ma*** C.3.5: 30'; ***i-di-ma*** [G] D.1.1: 169; ***i-na-an-di*** [G] C.3.10: 11; ***i-nam-di*** [G] C.3.10: 79; ***it-ta-nam-da-a*** [Gtn] C.3.9: 18; ***it-ta-<nam>-da-a*** [Gtn] C.3.9: 19; ***li-in-na-di-ma*** [N] B.2.1: 9; ***na!-de-e*** [G] C.3.4: 56; ***[na]-de?-e*** A.2.7: 37'; ***na-di*** [G] B.2.2: 28'; **ŠUB** [G] II.1.3: 51'''; A.2.2: 21, 47, 51; C.1.4: 28'; C.3.4: 43; C.3.9: 7; D.2.1: 30'; E.1.2: 6'; E.2.1: 10; E.2.4: 5'; E.2.5: 7'; E.2.6: 23', 24', 35', 41', 42', 44'; I.1.1: 32; ⸢**ŠUB**?⸣ [G] A.1.1: 7'; **ŠUB-*a*** [G] A.2.1: 15'; A.2.7: 35'; B.1.6: 7, 10; C.1.4: 63''; **ŠUB-⸢*a*⸣** [G] B.1.6: 17'; **ŠUB-*di*** [G] II.1.4: 8, 24; A.1.4: 31'', 41''; A.2.1: 9'; A.2.2: 17; A.2.4: 18'; A.2.5: 24''; A.2.7: 30'; C.1.4: 75''; C.1.8: 38'; C.3.4: 9; C.3.6: 50''''; C.3.10: 90; D.1.1: 177; E.2.6: 11', 32'; **ŠUB-*di*** [Š] B.1.6: 1; **ŠUB!-*di*** [G] A.1.1: 20'; **[ŠUB]-*di*** [G] A.2.4: 15'; ⸢**ŠUB**⸣**-*d[i?]*** [G] C.2.3: 14'; **Š[UB!-*di?*]** [G] C.3.4: 35; **ŠUB-*di-ma*** [G] C.3.5: 15'; D.3.1: 14; **[ŠUB?]-*di-ma*** [G] C.3.4: 51b; **ŠUB-*e*** [G] C.3.5: 8'; C.3.7: 19''; C.3.9: 38;

ŠUB-*e* [Š$^{?}$] A.1.4: 34''; **ŠUB-*[e]*** [G] C.3.3: 1; **ŠUB-*ma*** [G] C.3.7: 23''; C.3.10: 74; D.2.1: 35'; D.3.1: 14; E.2.6: 22', 36'; **ŠUB-*ma*$^{!}$** [G] E.2.6: 35'; **ŠUB-*m[a]*** [G] C.3.9: 13; **ŠUB-*ú*** [G] A.2.2: 39; I.1.1: 56, 62, 63, 69; **ŠUB.ŠUB-*a*** [Gtn] I.1.1: 83; **ŠUB.ŠUB-*[a]*** [Gtn] A.2.2: 77; **[ŠU]B.ŠUB-*a*** [Gtn] A.2.2: 50; **[ŠUB.ŠUB]-*a*** [Gtn] A.2.2: 52; **ŠUB.ŠUB-*di*** [Gtn] C.3.4: 43; I.1.3: 12; **ŠUB.ŠUB-*e*** [Š] C.3.7: 18''; **ŠUB.ŠUB-*ma*** [Gtn] A.2.2: 77; ***ta-n[a-ad-di$^{?}$]*** [G] A.1.4: 17'; ***ta*-ŠUB** [G] E.2.5: 9'

nādu "waterskin": **A.EDIN.⸢LÁ$^{?}$⸣** C.1.5: 43; ***na-a-di*** D.1.1: 23; ***na-a-a-du*** C.1.4: 59''

nâdu, *na'ādu* G "to praise; to celebrate": ***[ta-n]a$^{?}$-⸢ad$^{!}$-ki$^{?}$⸣*** [G] D.1.5: 1'

nagbu "underground water; source; (the) whole; totality": ***na-gab*** A.2.2: 35; ***na-[ga]b*** I.1.2: 11'

naggāru "carpenter": **^{lú}NAGAR** C.3.3: 34; C.3.4: 75; C.3.9: 56

nāgiru "herald": ***na-gi-ri*** G.1: 6, 7

naglabu "shoulder": **MAŠ.SÌL** C.3.4: 83

naḫīru "nostril": ***na-ḫi-ri-ša*** II.1.4: 17

naḫlaptu "cloak": **^{túg}GÚ.È** C.3.4: 83

naḫlu "sieved; strained": ***[n]a$^{?}$-aḫ-la*** D.1.2: 8

naḫšātu irregular bleeding (during pregnancy): ***na-aḫ-šá-te*** C.1.4: 17', 21'; ***na-aḫ-šá-a-ti*** C.1.4: 91'', 124''; ***na-aḫ-šá-a-[ti]*** C.1.4: 80''; ***na-aḫ-[šá-a-ti]*** C.1.4: 73''; ***[na-a]ḫ-šá-a-ti*** C.1.4: 98''; ***[n]a-aḫ-[š]á-a-ti*** C.1.4: 131''; ***na-[aḫ-šá-a-t]i*** C.1.4: 137''; ***na-⸢aḫ⸣-[šá-a-ti]*** C.1.4: 141''; ***[na-aḫ-š]a-a-ti*** C.1.4: 86''; ***na-[aḫ-š]á-a-tú*** I.1.2: 7'; ***na-aḫ-šá-ti*** I.1.1: 108; ***na-aḫ-šá-tú*** C.1.4: 24'; ***⸢na⸣-aḫ-šá-tu*** C.1.4: 29'; ***[na]-aḫ-šá-tu*** C.1.4: 74''

nāḫu "lard": **Ì.ŠAḪ** E.2.6: 14', 21', 26'; 32', 34'; **Ì.ŠAḪ$^{!}$** E.2.6: 26'; **Ì.Š[AḪ]** E.2.6: 39'

nâḫu, *nuāḫu* G "to calm down; to relent; to rest; to abate"; D "to calm (someone); to cool off; to extinguish": ***ina-aḫ*** [G] A.2.1: 37'; ***né-ḫe-e-ti*** [G] C.3.3: 11; C.3.4: 61; ***ne-e-ḫu*** [G] I.1.1: 78; ***ne-ḫu*** [G] I.1.1: 78; ***nu-uḫ-ḫi*** [D] D.2.1: 71'

nakādu G "to beat, throb; to be anxious, frightened; to be worrying": ***ik-kud*** [G] D.1.1: 116; G.1: 45; ***nak-da-a[t]*** [G] A.2.5: 13'; ***[na-ak-d]a-at*** C.1.9: 27

nakāpu G "to push; to thrust; to gore, to butt; to stab; to pierce"; D "to knock down; to butt": ***i[t$^{?}$-ta-kip$^{?}$]*** [G] B.1.1: 44; ***nu-uk-ku-pu*** [D] D.1.1: 182; ***ú-nak-kap*** [D] D.1.1: 182

nakāru G "to be different; to change"; Gtn "to keep changing"; D "to change; to remove; to expel"; Dt "to be changed": ***ik-ki-ru*** [G] I.1.1: 77; **KÚR.KÚR** [Gtn] D.2.1: 20'; ***ú-na-kar-ma*** [D] D.2.1: 45'; ***ú-na-ka-ru*** [D] I.1.1: 42; ***ú-ta-ak-⸢kàr⸣*** [Dt] A.2.8: 21'

nakāsu G "to cut (off); to slaughter": **KUD-*is*** [G] C.1.5: 8; C.3.4: 4

nākisu "cutter": ***na-ki-is*** G.1: 13

nakkaptu "temple; brow": **SAG.KI-*šá*** H.1: 4; I.1.1: 8, 13, 14; **[SAG].⸢KI$^{?}$⸣.MEŠ-*šá*** C.3.1: 1

nâku G "to copulate": ***na-ki$^{!}$-im*** II.1.1: 1

namāru I "clearing; path": ***na-ma-ra*** G.1: 37, 38; ***na-ma-ri*** G.2: 14''

namāru II G "to be(come) bright; to shine"; D "to illuminate; to make shine; to brighten": ***na-mir*** [G] I.1.1: 2; ***nam-ru*** [G] I.1.1: 102; **ZABAR$^{?}$** [G] A.2.7: 38'; **ZALAG** [D] C.3.10: 41

namru "bright; light": ***nam-ru*** D.1.1: 138; **ZALAG** F.1: 15; **⸢ZALAG$^{?}$⸣** F.1: 1; **ZAL[AG]** F.1: 37; **ZALAG.MEŠ** C.3.9: 1; F.1: 30; **ZALAG$^{?}$.⸢MEŠ$^{?}$⸣** F.1: 1

namurru "awe-inspiringly radiant": ***na-mur-rat*** C.3.4: 62; C.3.9: 41; ***na-mur-[rat]*** C.3.3: 14

namzītu "brewing vessel": **^{dug}NÍG.DÚR.BÙR** C.1.4: 58''; D.1.11: 12; **[^{d}]^{ug}NÍG.DÚR.BÙR** D.2.1: 37'; ***^{dug}nam-zi-tú*** A.2.1: 15'

nannāru "luminary; light (of the sky); moon": **$^{d+}$EN$^{!}$.ZU.KI-*ra*** D.3.1: 11a; **^{d}NANNA-*ra*** D.3.1: 11a; ***na-an-na-ar*** II.1.4: 58; ***⸢na-an-na-ar⸣*** B.2.6: 17; ***[na-a]n-na-ra*** D.3.1: 11a

napāḫu G "to blow; to light up; to become inflamed or swollen"; D "to become inflamed or swollen"; Dtn iter. of D; Ntn "to be inflamed/swollen repeatedly": **⸢KUR⸣** [G] C.1.5: 45; ***i-nap-paḫ-ma*** [G] D.2.1: 46'; ***i-nap-pa-⸢ḫu⸣*** [G] C.3.3: 13; ***it-tan-pa-ḫu*** [Ntn] D.2.1: 45'; ***na-pa-a-ḫu*** [G] C.3.10: 7; ***nap-ḫu*** [G] I.1.1: 67, 76; ***nu-up-pu-ḫa*** [D] I.1.1: 72; I.1.4: 8'; ***nu-up-[pu-ḫa]*** [D] I.1.4: 6'; **SAR-*aḫ*** [G] C.3.10: 68; **[S]AR-*ḫa*** [G] C.3.4: 25; ***ut-ta-tap-pi-iḫ*** [Dtn] A.1.2: 4'

napalsuḫu N "to fall to the ground; to squat": ***ne-pal-suḫ$_{4}$*** [N] D.1.1: 148

napālu G "to dig out, up; to demolish": ***i-na-⸢pal$^{?}$⸣*** [G] C.1.8: 19'; ***ta-n[ap-p]al$^{?}$*** [G] A.2.7: 38'; ***ta-nap-pa-al-ma*** [G] C.3.4: 18

napḫaru "total; entirety; all": ***nap-ḫar*** I.1.2: 9', 11', 12'; ***[n]ap-ḫa-rù*** I.1.2: 12'; **PAP** A.1.4: 7', 9'; B.1.4: 14; C.3.1: 7; F.1: 6, 10, 16, 22, 31, 34, 37; **⸢PAP$^{?}$⸣** A.1.4: 4'; **PAP-*ma*** F.2: 33'; **ŠU.NIGIN** B.1.1: 27

napištu "life; throat; person": **Z[I-*šú*]** I.1.3: 36'; **ZI-*te*** II.1.4: 35, 52; ***[nap-šá]-ti*** D.1.1: 100; ***nap-šá-a-tu$_{4}$*** G.1: 44; ***[nap$^{?}$]-⸢šá⸣-tu-šá*** D.2.1: 67'

nappāḫu "smith": **^{lú}SIMUG** C.3.4: 72; C.3.9: 53; **^{lú}⸢SIMUG⸣** C.3.3: 30

napṣu "damaged": ***[na]p-ṣu*** C.3.10: 38

napšaštu, napšaltu "ointment; salve": **EŠ** A.2.6: 18, 21, 24; ***nap-šal-ta*** B.1.1: 19; ***nap-šal-ti*** C.3.4: 78; ***nap-šal-t[i]*** B.1.1: 39; ***na[p-šal-ti]*** B.1.1: 72; ***[nap-šal-t]i*** C.3.3: 39; ***nap-šal-[tu$^{?}$]*** F.2: 43'; ***nap$^{?}$-ša-šu*** B.1.1: 74; ***nap*-ŠIL-*tu*** C.1.4: 14'

napṭu "naphtha": **⸢Ì$^{?}$⸣.ḪUL** A.2.2: 32

napû I "sifted": ***na-pi$_{5}$-tim*** A.2.2: 65

napû II G "to sift; to sieve": ***n[a-pu-ú$^{?}$]*** [G] B.2.3: 7'; **SIM** [G] A.2.1: 16', 75''''; A.2.2: 16; A.2.3: 7'; A.2.5: 11'; C.1.9: 5, 9; C.2.2: 6; **⸢SIM⸣** [G] A.2.3: 27'''; **S[IM]** [G] C.1.9: 31; **SIM$^{!}$-*pí*** [G] C.1.8: 25'; ***ta-[nap-pi$^{?}$]*** [G] A.2.3: 8'

naqbītu "recitation": ***na-aq-bi-ta*** C.3.10: 77, 81, 86; ***na-aq-bi-tú*** C.3.10: 83

naqû G "to sacrifice; to pour (a libation)": **BAL** [G] A.2.5: 15''; **BAL-*qí*** [G] C.1.4: 13'; C.3.4: 9, 12, 35; C.3.6: 9', 49''''; C.3.10: 63; D.3.1: 16; **BAL$^{!?}$-*qí*** [G] C.3.6: 29'; **BAL-*qí-ma*** [G] C.3.4: 43; D.3.1: 8

narāmu "beloved (one)": ***na-ram*** D.1.8: 5; ***na-ra-mi-[šá$^{?}$]*** D.1.9: 10'

narbu "soft; moist": ***nàr-bi*** A.2.2: 20

narbû "greatness; great deeds": ***nar-bi*** D.1.8: 25; ***nar-bi-ka*** D.1.8: 24; ***⸢nar⸣-bi-ka*** D.3.1: 27; ***nàr-bi-ka*** D.3.1: 13

narkabtu "chariot": **^{giš}GIGIR** II.1.4: 38; **^{giš}GIGIR-*ti*** C.1.4: 28'; **⸢^{giš}GIGIR$^{?}$⸣** D.1.1: 79

narmaktu "bath; washbasin": ***[nà]r-ma-ak-ti*** B.1.1: 39
nāru "river; canal": **ÍD** A.2.2: 33; C.1.8: 12'; C.3.4: 2, 6, 14, 15, 40, 43, 47, 48; C.3.10: 12, 16, 26; **ÍD**$^{!}$ C.3.4: 35; **[Í]D** C.1.1: 10; **ÍD.MEŠ** C.3.10: 15, 57
narūqu "leather bag": ^{kuš}**A.GÁ.LÁ** C.3.4: 19
nasāḫu G "to tear out; to pull out; to eradicate; to remove; to extract"; D "to tear out; to uproot; to extract; to copy"; N "to be removed; to be taken away": **ZI** [G] A.2.7: 29'; **ZI-*ḫi*** [G] B.2.2: 30'; C.2.2: 13; **ZI-*ḫu*** [N] B.2.2: 21'; **ZI-*ma*** [G] D.1.1: 228; **ZI.MEŠ-*ḫa*** [D?] D.1.4: 18''
nasāku G "to discard; to throw (down)"; Gtn iter. of G: ***[i]-⸢na⸣-[as]-suk*** [G] D.3.1: 7; ***i-na-suk*** [G] D.3.1: 7; **ŠUB** [G] C.3.4: 18; **ŠUB.ŠUB-*ši*** [Gtn] I.1.3: 20; ***ta-na-suk*** [G] C.1.8: 35'; ***ta-na-suk-ma*** [G] C.3.4: 18
nasāqu G "to select"; Št "to make ready, to prepare; to bring/keep in order": ***uš-ta-sí-iq-šu*** [Št] II.1.2: 12
naspuḫtu "dispersal; disintegration": **BIR-*ti*** C.3.4: 46
nasqu "chosen; select; precious": ***na-as-qa*** B.1.1: 50; ***na-[as-qa]*** B.1.1: 42
naṣāru G "to guard; to protect; to look over": ***ú-ṣur*** [G] B.2.1: 27; ***ú-ṣ[ur]*** [G] B.2.1: 36
naṣmattu "bandage; poultice": ***na-aṣ-ma-a[t-ta]*** B.1.1: 21; ***na-aṣ-ma-te*** B.1.1: 22; ***[na-aṣ-m]at$^{?}$-te-šá*** C.1.4.2: 4'
našāku G/D "to bite": ***ú-na-aš-šak*** [D] I.1.3: 15; ***ú-na-[aš-šak]*** [D] I.1.5: 6'
našallulu N "to slither": ***liš-šá-li-la*** [N] D.1.1: 171; ***li-i[š-ša-l]i-la-am*** [N] II.1.1: 33; ***na-šal-lu-lu-nim*** [N] I.1.1: 58, 59; ***na-áš-li-⸢la⸣*** [N] D.1.1: 46; ***⸢ni⸣-⸢šal$^{?}$⸣-[l]i-l[a]*** [N] D.1.1: 46
našāpu G "to pound; to pulverize?": ***ta$^{!}$-na$^{?}$-áš-šip*** [G] A.2.3: 8'
našāru G "to remove; to cut off": ***li-iš-šu-ra*** [G] C.3.4: 11
našpu (a type of beer): **SIG** D.2.1: 25', 43', 51', 56'; **SIG$_5$** A.2.4: 13'; B.2.4: 25', 48'; **SIG$_5^{?}$** A.2.1: 98''''''; **⸢SIG$_5$⸣** A.2.8: 23'; **⸢SIG$_5^{?}$⸣** A.1.1: 22'; **SIG$_5$.GA** A.1.3: 10'; **SIG.GA** B.1.1: 6; **SIG$_5$-*tú*** E.2.4: 7'
naštuq "(leather) bag": ^{kuš}***na-áš-tu-qa*** C.3.10: 2
našû I "carrying; holding; elevated": ***na-šu-ú*** C.3.10: 38
našû II G "to raise; to lift; to carry; to wear; to take away"; Gtn iter. of G; Š "to have someone raise/lift/wear"; N "to be carried; to be applied": ***aš-ši*** [G] C.3.5: 30'; **GUR$_{17}$** [G] I.1.1: 118; **ÍL** [G] C.2.3: 2'; D.2.1: 57'; I.1.1: 89; **ÍL-*ku*** [G] C.3.4: 20; **ÍL-*ma*** [G] A.2.9: 1'; B.2.2: 10; C.3.10: 85; D.2.1: 22', 45', 57'; D.3.1: 9; E.2.3: 8'; E.2.6: 14', 17'; **ÍL-*m[a]*** [G] II.1.3: 29'''; **ÍL-*ši*** [G] B.2.2: 26'; D.1.1: 144; **ÍL-*ši-ma*** [G] B.2.2: 8; **[Í]L$^{?}$-*ši-ma*** [G] A.2.9: 7'; **ÍL-*šú*** [Š] C.1.9: 28; E.2.6: 29'; **ÍL-*ú*** [G] C.1.10: 6; C.3.4: 21; ***i-na-áš-ši*** [G] C.1.2: 13; ***i-na-á[š-ši]*** [G] C.1.2: 14; ***ina-aš-ši*** [G] C.1.10: 4; ***i-na-áš-šu*** [G] C.3.10: 70; ***in-na-áš-šú*** [N] B.2.2: 6; ***iš-ši*** [G] D.1.1: 149; ***i-ta-na-aš-šá*** [Gtn] I.1.1: 105; ***⸢it-ta-na-šu$^{?}$⸣*** [G] C.2.3: 24'; ***liš-šá-a'*** [G] C.3.10: 57; ***liš-ši*** [G] D.2.1: 11'; 12', 13', 14'; ***na-šá-ku-ma*** [G] C.3.10: 78, 82, 84; ***na-šá-a*** [G] C.3.9: 18; ***na-ša-at*** [G] II.1.4: 59, 60; ***na-šá-at*** [G] D.1.1: 150; ***na-šá-⸢at⸣*** [G] D.1.1: 151; ***na-ši*** [G] D.1.1: 147; ***na-šu-ma*** [G] C.3.10: 78, 82, 84; ***ta-na-á[š-ši$^{?}$]*** [G] B.2.3: 15''; ***ú-šá-áš-šá*** [Š] C.3.10: 87
nâšu G "to rock; to shift; to become loose"; D "to move; to shift": ***ú-na-šá*** [D] D.1.6: 3
natāku G "to drip"; Gtn iter. of G; "to drip away": ***[i]t-ta-na-tuk*** [Gtn] C.1.4: 56''; ***[it-t]a-[na-tu-k]u*** [Gtn] C.1.4: 55''; ***it-tu-ku*** [G] C.1.4: 135''
naṭāpu D "to make drip(?)": ***t[u]-na-aṭ-ṭap*** [D] A.2.3: 7'; ***t[u-n]a-aṭ-ṭì-pu*** [D] A.2.3: 10'
naṭû G "to be suitable, proper": ***na-ṭa-at*** [G] G.1: 3, 4; ***na-ṭu-u*** [G] G.1: 4
nazāqu G "to creak; to be vexed, distressed": ***na-zaq*** C.3.4: 94
nēbeḫu "band; belt; sash": ***né-bè-eḫ*** C.3.4: 85
neḫelṣû, *neḫalṣû*, *naḫalṣû* N "to slip; to slide down; to make an error": ***na-ḫal-ṣu-u*** [N] G.1: 24
nēḫu "calm": ***né-ḫu-ú-ti*** C.3.5: 23'
nē'iru "one who strikes": ***né-'i-ir*** I.1.7: 6
nēmelu "success; thriving": ***ne-[mel$^{?}$]*** C.3.6: 2'; ***n[e-mel$^{?}$]*** C.3.8: 9; ***⸢né⸣-mel-šú*** C.3.10: 32
nēpešu "ritual": ***ne-pe-šá*** C.3.10: 91
nêru, *nâru* G/D "to strike; to kill": ***na-a-ra*** [G] I.1.7: 4, 5; ***nu-uḫ$_5$-ḫu-rat*** [D] I.1.7: 2; ***nu-ú-ú-ru*** [D] I.1.7: 3
nērubu, *nerrubu* N "to flee; to escape": ***né-er-ru-ba*** [N] D.1.1: 194
nesû G "to be off; to depart; to be distant"; D "to remove; to drive away": **BAD** [G] C.3.6: 17'; **BAD-*ši*** [G/D] I.1.3: 14
nešalpû, *nešelpû* N "to glide; to slither": ***na-šal-pú-u*** [N] G.1: 25; ***né-šal-pa-a*** [N] G.2: 7'; ***né-šal-pú-u*** [N] G.1: 24; ***né-šel-pa-a*** [N] D.1.1: 35; G.1: 23
nēšu "lion": **UR.MAḪ** C.3.4: 63; C.3.9: 42
nêšu G "to recover": ***ina-aš*** [G] C.1.2: 39'; ***ina-eš*** [G] A.2.2: 68; A.2.9: 7'; B.1.1: 37, 38; C.1.8: 8'; D.1.1: 230; D.2.1: 22', 25', 26', 27', 55', 57'; E.2.7: 17''; ***[i]na-eš*** [G] E.2.7: 19''; ***ina-[eš]*** [G] B.1.1: 30, 32; D.2.1: 46'; ***⸢ina-eš⸣*** [G] E.2.7: 1'; ***i[na-e]š$^{?}$*** [G] A.2.2: 20; ***ina-[i]š*** [G] C.1.4: 173'''
nê'u G "to turn back; to drive back; to flee": ***i-né-e'*** [G] D.1.1: 113, 126
nigkalagû (a bell): ^{urudu}**NÍG.KALA.GA** D.2.1: 26'; ^{urudu}**NÍG.KALA.GA-*e*** D.2.1: 28'
nignakku "censer": **NÍG.NA** B.2.1: 19; C.1.4: 10'; C.3.4: 6, 42, 55; C.3.10: 62; D.1.7: 4'; D.3.1: 8, 16; E.2.3: 4'
niḫlu (a disease): ***⸢ni-iḫ$^{?}$-lu$^{?}$⸣*** I.1.3: 30'
nikiptu I "blow; affliction": ***ni-k[i-ip$^{?}$]-⸢ti⸣*** B.1.1: 44
nikiptu II (an aromatic, gum-yielding plant, perhaps a *Euphorbia* shrub, spurge): $^{šim.d}$**MAŠ** A.2.2: 54; B.1.1: 26; $^{ú.d}$**MAŠ** B.1.1: 34
nīlu "wetness; moisture; flooding; semen": ***ni-il-š[u$^{?}$]*** D.1.10: 2'
nimšulu, *niššulu* "fish spawn(?)": ***ni-iš-šu-la-at*** II.1.1: 31
NI.NE (or Ì.KÚM; a disease; reading uncertain): **NI.NE** A.2.2: 42, 43
nīnû, pl. *nīnâtu* (a medicinal plant and spice, perhaps mint): ***ni-nu-ú*** A.1.4: 26''; B.2.4: 5'; ^{ú}**KUR.RA** A.1.2: 9'; B.1.1: 25; B.2.4: 27'; C.1.4: 146'''; C.1.5: 15; C.2.2: 4; D.2.1: 20'; E.2.6: 10'; ^{ú}**KUR.⸢RA$^{?}$⸣** II.1.3: 63'''; E.2.4: 1'; **[^{ú}KUR].RA** B.2.4: 13'; ⸢^{ú}⸣**[KUR.RA^{sar}]** A.2.7: 11; ^{ú}**KUR.RA^{sar}** B.2.1: 15; D.1.1: 214; ^{ú}***ni-na-a-tu$_4$*** E.2.1: 13; ***[^{ú}n]i-nu-ú*** A.1.4: 8'
nipiltu "something dug up": ***ni-pil-ti*** D.1.1: 209
nipṣu "smashing; shattering; twitch(?); (metal) filings: ***ni-i[p-ṣi$^{?}$]*** B.2.5: 4

nipšu I "combed wool; tuft (of wool)": ***ni-i[p]-še*** A.1.4: 35''
nipšu II "smell; stench": ***ni-ip-šú*** A.2.7: 18
niqû, nīqu "sacrifice": ***ni-qí-i*** G.1: 3; ***[ni]-qí$^{!}$-i*** D.1.1: 5; ***ni-qu-ú*** G.1: 5; **SISKUR**$^{!}$ A.2.5: 7'; **[S]ÍSKUR** C.3.4: 90
NI.RA (reading uncertain; a disease): **NI.RA** D.2.1: 18'
nirāḫu (a kind of snake): **MUŠ.TUR** D.1.1: 171, 194; **⸢MUŠ.TUR⸣** D.1.1: 46; ***ni-ra-ḫi*** D.1.1: 35, 46; ***ni-ra-ḫu*** G.1: 25
nīru "braided strings": ***⸢ni⸣-ri*** F.2: 38'
nisḫu "excerpt": ***nis-ḫu*** A.2.7: 41'; C.2.2: 1
niṣirtu "secret": ***ni-ṣir-tu*** D.1.1: 128
nīṣu "phlegm(?)": ***ni-ṣu*** D.1.5: 13', 17'
nišū "people": **UN.MEŠ** D.1.8: 25; **UN.MEŠ-*šá*** I.1.3: 14
nīšu "(oath on the) life": ***niš*** G.1: 22
nišūtu "relatives; kin": ***ni$^{?}$-š[u-ti-šú$^{?}$]*** C.3.1: 25
nuḫurtu (a medicinal plant): ***nu-ḫur-ti*** A.2.2: 59; C.1.6: 7'; ***nu-ḫur-tu$_4$*** A.2.8: 35', 36'; E.2.1: 1; ***n[u$^{?}$-ḫur-tu$_4$$^{?}$]*** A.2.10: 6'; ***⸢^{ú}nu-ḫur⸣-tú$^{?}$*** C.1.5: 27; **NU.LUḪ.ḪA** A.2.4: 45'''; B.2.2: 7; C.2.2: 4; E.2.6: 37', 44'; **^{ú}NU.LAḪ.ḪA** D.2.1: 47'; **^{ú}NU.LAḪ.Ḫ[A]** D.2.1: 43'; **^{ú}NU.LUḪ.ḪA** A.1.2: 12'; A.1.4: 34''; A.2.1: 73'''', 88''''''; C.1.4: 32', 75'', 149''', 158'''; D.2.1: 21', 23', 52'; E.2.6: 30'; **⸢^{ú}⸣NU.LUḪ.ḪA** II.1.3: 63'''; C.1.1: 5; **⸢^{ú}⸣NU.[LUḪ.ḪA]** C.1.2: 12; **[^{ú}NU.LUḪ].ḪA** C.1.4: 125''
NU.LUḪ (a drug): **NU$^{?}$.LUḪ$^{?}$** A.2.2: 40
nūnu "fish": **KU$_6$** D.1.11: 10; E.2.6: 26'
nurbu "soft place; tender part": ***nu-ru-ub*** II.1.4: 54; D.1.1: 141; G.2: 27''
nūru "light": **IZI.GAR** II.1.4: 49; ***nu-ru*** D.3.1: 13; G.2: 4'; ***⸢nu-ru$^{?}$⸣*** G.2: 16''; ***nu-u-ru*** D.3.1: 13; ***nu-ú-ru*** G.1: 19; ***[nu-ú-r]u$^{?}$*** G.2: 4'; ***nu-ú-rù*** G.1: 19, 38; ***nu-úr*** G.1: 35; ***nu-úr$^{?}$*** G.2: 27''; **ZALAG** D.1.1: 193; **ZALAG**$^{!}$ E.2.3: 14'; **ZÁLAG** C.3.3: 10; C.3.4: 60; D.1.1: 36, 52, 111; D.3.1: 18; **⸢ZÁLAG⸣** C.3.3: 11

PA.AN (reading uncertain): **PA.AN** I.1.1: 84
pa'āṣu G/D "to crush": ***<ta>-pa-aṣ-ma*** [G] D.1.11: 12; ***tu-pa-a[ṣ$^{?}$]*** [D] C.2.1: 11'; ***⸢tu⸣-pa-ṣa*** [D] A.2.2: 20; ***tu-pa-'-ṣú*** [D] A.2.5: 23''
padānu "way; path": ***pa-da-na-<am>*** II.1.2: 12
pagru "body; corpse": **ADDA-*šú*** I.1.3: 8; ***pa-gar-šá*** D.2.1: 45'; ***pag-ri*** II.1.4: 26; ***pag-ri-šá*** D.2.1: 46'
paḫāru I "potter": **BÁḪAR** B.2.6: 5; C.3.10: 26
paḫāru II G "to gather": ***⸢i$^{?}$-pa$^{?}$-aḫ$^{?}$-ḫar$^{?}$⸣*** [G] C.3.4: 18
palāḫu G "to fear; to revere; to respect": ***pal-ḫat*** [G] I.1.1: 103
palāsu N "to look (at); to see"; Ntn iter. of N: **IGI.BAR** [N] C.3.4: 23; D.1.1: 229; **[IGI$^{?}$].BAR.MEŠ** [Ntn] I.1.3: 22; ***ip-pal-la-su*** [N] C.3.10: 47; ***[na-a]p$^{?}$-li-sa*** [N] D.1.1: 45; ***nap-lu-su*** [N] G.1: 29
palāšu G/D "to pierce": ***pa-liš*** [G] I.1.1: 36, 37; ***[p]al-⸢šu⸣*** [G] C.1.4: 94''; ***tu-pa-la-áš*** [D] C.1.4: 185'''
palgu "ditch; canal": ***pal$^{?}$-ki$^{?}$*** C.1.5: 42
pāliḫu "one who reveres": **MUD** [G] C.3.4: 100; ***pa-liḫ*** [G] C.2.1: 18'; C.3.3: 45; I.1.1: 118; I.1.2: 15'
pannigu (a pastry of bread): **NINDA.DIM$_x$** C.3.4: 41
pānu "front; appearance; presence; face (pl.)"; (prep.) "before"; *ana pān* (compound prep.) "before"; *ina pān* "in front of": **IGI** II.1.3: 45'''; A.1.1: 8'; A.2.1: 10'; A.2.2: 62; B.2.1: 19; B.2.2: 26'; B.2.6: 15; C.1.4: 15', 87'', 108''; C.1.5: 9, 45; C.1.8: 17'; C.3.4: 12, 25, 43; C.3.6: 16', 20'; C.3.9: 42; D.1.11: 2; D.2.1: 30', 32', 61'; D.3.1: 8, 10c, 16; E.2.5: 7'; E.2.6: 24', 29', 35', 41'; H.1: 23'; I.1.3: 31'; I.1.6: 35'; **I[GI]** C.3.4: 40; **I[GI$^{?}$]** C.1.4: 110''; **IGI-*ka*** B.2.6: 23; **IGI.ME-*šú*** C.3.9: 42; **IGI.MEŠ-*šá*** I.1.1: 77, 78; **IGI.<MEŠ>-*šá*** I.1.1: 79, 80; **IGI.MEŠ-*šú*** C.3.10: 74; D.1.1: 233; I.1.1: 24, 25; **IGI-*šá*** I.1.1: 42; I.1.3: 27; **IGI-*šú*** A.2.6: 2; C.3.4: 87; E.2.6: 15'; I.1.1: 115; ***pa-an*** C.3.4: 63; D.1.1: 139; ***pa-na*** D.1.1: 154; ***pa-ni*** C.3.10: 32; ***pa-⸢ni$^{?}$⸣*** C.3.7: 9''; ***pa-ni-[šá]*** A.1.3: 5'; ***pa-nu*** D.1.1: 139; ***pa-nu-šá*** C.3.3: 17; D.1.1: 170; ***pa-n[u-šá]*** C.3.4: 63
papānu (a type of rush); *papān libbi* (a part of the body; belly): ***pa-pan*** D.1.1: 212; D.1.3: 3'
pappardilû (a stone; banded agate): **^{na4}BABBAR.DILI** C.3.9: 36; F.1: 15, 36, 39; F.2: 14; **^{na4}BABBAR.DI[LI]** C.1.4: 133''
pappasītu (a kind of sulphur): ***pa-pa-si-*^{d}ÍD** C.1.4: 182'''
pappāsu "porridge": ***pap-pa-su*** A.2.2: 18
paqādu G "to entrust; to hand over; to care for": ***ip-qid*** [G] E.2.3: 27''; ***pa-qid-m[a]*** [G] C.3.3: 41; ***piq-dan-ni*** [G] D.3.1: 12; ***piq-dan-ni-ma*** [G] D.3.1: 12
parāku G "to lie across; to obstruct"; D "to lie transversely"; N "to be blocked": ***i-pár-ri-ku*** [G] D.1.6: 7; ***ip-par-rik*** [N] D.1.1: 43; ***pur-ru-ku*** [D] I.1.1: 52, 53, 54, 55; ***ta-par-rik-ma*** [G] D.1.1: 197
parāmu G "to chop; to slice through": ***ta-par-ra-am*** [G] B.2.3: 6'
parāru G "to be dissolved, broken up; to be weak(?)"; Gtn iter. of G: ***lip-ru-ru*** [G] D.1.1: 33; ***[ip-ta-nar$^{?}$]-ra-ar*** [Gtn] I.1.1: 81
parāsu G "to cut (off); to decide; to stop; to halt; to isolate"; N pass. of G "to be stopped; to be separated; to be decided": **AL.[KUD]** [G] C.2.3: 11'; ***ip-pa-á[r-ra-as]*** [N] B.1.3: 4; ***ip-par-ra-su*** [N] C.1.10: 1, 7; **KUD** [G] C.3.1: 32; **⸢KUD$^{?}$⸣** [G] C.1.5: 11; F.1: 32; **[KU]D$^{?}$** F.1: 28; **KUD-*as*** [G] A.2.1: 13'; **⸢KUD⸣-*as*** [G] A.2.1: 20'; **KUD-*at*** [G] C.3.4: 40; **⸢KUD⸣-*at*** [G] B.1.2: 5'; **KUD-*á[t]*** [G] B.1.5: 5'; **KUD-*is*** [G] C.1.5: 3, 10; **⸢KUD-*is*$^{?}$⸣** [G] A.2.1: 17'; **KUD-*ma*** [G] C.2.1: 14'; **KUD-*ma*$^{?}$** [G] C.2.2: 2; **KUD-*sa*** [G] C.1.4: 24', 29', 74''; **KUD-*s[a]*** C.1.4.2: 4'; **KU[D-*sa*]** C.1.4.2: 2', 3'; **KUD-*sà-[at]*** [G] II.1.3: 43'''; **KUD-*si*** [G] A.2.1: 21'; A.2.2: 28, 29, 31, 39; C.1.2: 26'; C.1.3: 13'; C.1.5: 1, 36; C.1.8: 15', 32', 52''; C.1.9: 6, 10, 15, 20, 21, 25; C.1.10: 17; **KUD-*s[i]*** [G] B.2.4: 4'; **KUD-⸢*si*$^{?}$⸣** [G] C.1.8: 11'; **KUD-⸢*si*⸣** [G] C.1.9: 3; **KUD-*su*** [G] C.1.4: 27'; C.1.5: 30, 37; **KUD-*su*** [N] C.1.5: 1; C.1.8: 21'; **KUD-*su*$^{?}$** [G] C.2.2: 13; **KUD-*s[u]*** [G] C.1.4: 183'''; **KUD-*s[u$^{?}$]*** [G] C.2.3: 6'; **K[UD-*su*]** [G$^{?}$] C.1.1: 3; **KUD-*su*$^{!}$** [G] C.1.2: 17; **[KU]D-*su*** [G] C.1.4: 178'''; **KUD.MEŠ-*su*** [G] C.1.8: 28'; ***pa-ra-si*** [G] C.1.10: 1; ***par-sa-a-a[t]*** [G] C.1.5: 44; ***pár-sat*** [G] C.3.4: 40; ***pár-súm*** [G] C.1.4: 58''; ***tap-ru-su*** [G] A.2.6: 26; ***ta-pa-ra-as*** [G] C.3.10: 2; ***ta-pa-ar-ra-as*** [G] C.3.10: 42
parā'u, *parāḫu* I G "to cut off; to severe; to slit"; N pass. of G: ***i-par$^{?}$-ra-aḫ*** [N] A.2.2: 56
parā'u, *parāḫu* II G "to sprout; to ferment"; N "to become fermented(?)": ***ip-pa-ra-ḫu*** [N] A.1.2: 5'

pārisu "one who decides, stops, keeps away": ***pa-ri-is*** D.3.1: 19; ***⸢pa$^{?}$⸣-[r]i-is*** C.1.8: 13'
parištu "post-menopausal woman" (lit. cut off): **KUD** C.1.8: 13'; **KUD-*tu*$_4$** C.1.4: 22'
parku "blocked": ***pa-rik-tu*$_4$** C.3.10: 8
parsu "cut-off; secluded; stopped; weaned; determined": **KUD-*⸢si⸣*** C.3.6: 61''''; ***par-si*** C.1.4: 10'; ***pa-ar-su*** C.3.10: 7
parṣu (usually pl.) "rite(s); cultic ordinance(s)": ***par-ṣ[i-š]u*** D.1.9: 33'
parû I "mule": ***pa-ru-ka*** C.1.8: 36'
parû II G "to vomit"; Gtn iter. of G: ***⸢i$^{?}$⸣-pár-⸢rù$^{!?}$⸣*** [G] I.1.6: 9'; ***ip-ta-na-ar-ru*** [Gtn] I.1.1: 81
parzillu "iron (bead)": **AN.BAR** B.1.4: 13; C.1.4: 31', 44', 46'; **[^{na4}AN].BAR$^{?}$** C.1.5: 40
pasāmu, *pasānu*, *paṣānu* G "to cover; to conceal, hide"; D "to veil": ***pa-ṣu-na-at*** [D] II.1.4: 45; ***⸢pu-su-na⸣-[at]*** [D] D.1.1: 84; ***ta-pa-as-sà-am*** [G] A.1.4: 29''
pašāḫu G "to cool down; to calm down; to rest"; Š "to calm; to pacify; to assuage": ***šup-šú-ḫi*** [Š] D.2.1: 60'
pašāqu G "to be difficult, troublesome"; Š "to have difficulty (in delivery)"; Št "to have difficulty (in delivery): ***šap-šu-qa-at*** [Š] II.1.4: 33, 34, 51; ***šup-šu-qa*** [Š] G.1: 14; ***šup-šu-qat*** [Š] D.1.1: 22, 168; ***šup-š[u-qat]*** [Š] D.1.2: 1; ***⸢uš$^{?}$-tap$^{!}$⸣-áš-šaq*** [Št] D.1.3: 2'; ***uš-tap-pa-⸢áš⸣-ša[q]*** [Št] A.1.1: 46'''; ***uš-tap-šiq*** [Št] A.2.1: 58'''; D.1.1: 205, 221; D.1.3: 11'; ***u[š-tap-šiq$^{?}$]*** [Št] D.1.7: 12'; ***uš$^{!}$-tap-šiq$^{!}$-šú*** [Št] D.1.3: 8'
pašāru G "to release; to undo; to relax"; D "to release; to undo; to dispel"; Dt "to be undone; to be released"; Š "to bring about release"; N "to be released; to be relaxed; to be undone; to be appeased": **⸢BÚR⸣** [G] A.2.2: 49; **⸢BÚR$^{?}$⸣** [G] C.3.10: 1; **B[ÚR$^{?}$]** [G] D.1.3: 34''; **BÚR-*[i]r$^{!?}$*** [G] C.3.4: 55; **BÚR-*ni*** [G] C.3.4: 51a; **BÚR-*[n]i$^{?}$*** [G] C.3.4: 50; **DU$_8$-*ma*** [N] II.1.4: 26; ***ip-p[a$^{?}$-áš-šar]*** [N] A.2.8: 32'; ***lip-pa-áš-ru*** [N] D.1.8: 20; ***[lip-pa-š]ar*** [N] D.1.8: 20; ***lip-taš-ši-ra*** [Dt] D.1.1: 109; ***pa-šá-ri*** [G] C.3.5: 3'; ***pa-ši-ir*** [G] I.1.1: 85, 86; ***šup-šu-ri-ša*** [Š] II.1.4: 3; ***ú-pa-áš-šá-ru*** [D] C.3.9: 21, 23; ***up-taš-ši-ra*** [Dt] D.1.1: 122
pašāšu G "to anoint; to rub; to smear"; Gt "to rub oneself"; Gtn iter. of G; N "to be anointed": **EŠ** [G] A.1.1: 51'''; B.1.1: 7; D.2.1: 29'; **EŠ-*aš*** [G] D.2.1: 64'; **EŠ-*aš*** [N] C.3.6: 16'; **EŠ.MEŠ-*su-ma*** [Gtn] H.2: 4; **EŠ-*su*** [G] D.1.1: 235; ***ip-pa-áš-ši-⸢iš$^{?}$⸣*** [N] D.3.1: 14; ***ip-šu-us-su-ma*** [G] D.1.9: 37'; **ŠÉŠ** [G] II.1.4: 25; A.2.2: 62; C.1.4: 9'; D.1.1: 209, 210; D.2.1: 32'; D.3.1: 14; **ŠÉŠ-*aš*** [G] A.2.6: 20; C.1.4: 3'; **⸢ŠÉŠ⸣-*áš-ši-ma$^{?}$*** [G] A.2.8: 32'; **ŠÉŠ-*ma*** [G] C.3.3: 4; C.3.5: 13'; D.1.1: 212; D.1.3: 7', 17'; **ŠÉŠ-*m[a$^{?}$]*** [G] D.1.7: 30'; **[ŠÉ]Š-*ma*** [Gt] C.3.6: 31'; **[ŠÉŠ$^{?}$-*m]a$^{?}$*** D.1.3: 4'; **ŠÉŠ.ME-*su*** [Gtn] D.1.1: 234, 235; **ŠÉŠ.MEŠ** [Gtn] II.1.4: 18; **ŠÉŠ.MEŠ-*su*** [Gtn] D.1.1: 234, 235; **ŠÉŠ-*si*** [G] C.1.4: 14'; D.3.1: 14; **ŠÉŠ-*s[i]*** [G] B.1.1: 19; **[ŠÉ]Š-*si*** [G] D.3.1: 31; E.1.1: 4; **ŠÉŠ-*si-ma*** [G] B.1.1: 32; **ŠÉŠ-*su*** [G] D.3.1: 31; **[ŠÉ]Š-*su*** [G] A.2.2: 66; **⸢ŠÉŠ$^{?}$⸣-*su*** [G] A.2.6: 26; **Š[ÉŠ-*su*]** A.2.8: 3; **ŠÉŠ-*šú*** [G] A.2.2: 10; C.3.4: 54; ***ta-pa-šá-áš-ma*** [G] H.1: 35'; ***ta-pa-áš-ša-aš*** [G] D.1.9: 23'
pāširu "releaser": ***pa-šìr-[k]a*** C.3.3: 13
patānu G "to eat; to dine": ***pa-tan*** [G] C.1.8: 26'; E.1.2: 8'; ***pa-t[an$^{?}$]*** D.1.11: 2; ***p[a-tan]*** C.2.1: 2'; see also *lā patān*
paṭāru G "to loosen; to release; to undo; to remove"; D "to release; to undo; to dispel; to untie"; Dt "to be released"; N "to be loose; to be released": **DU$_8$** [G] A.2.5: 15''; H.1: 25'; **DU$_8$$^{!}$** [G] D.3.1: 25; **DU$_8$-*ár*** [G] B.2.6: 27; **DU$_8$-*at*** [G] D.2.1: 30'; **DU$_8$.DU$_8$** [D] C.3.4: 8; **DU$_8$-*ma*** [G] C.3.4: 54; E.2.3: 26''; **[D]U$_8$-*⸢ma$^{?}$⸣*** [G] A.2.1: 34'; **DU$_8$.M[E]** [G?] I.1.3: 26; **DU$_8$-*šú*** [G] C.3.9: 35; ***ip-ta-ṭar*** [G] D.1.1: 119; ***lip-pa-ṭir*** [N] D.1.1: 104; D.1.8: 15; ***lip-te-ṭi-ra*** [Dt] D.1.1: 108; ***lip-ṭu-ru*** [G] D.1.1: 188; ***pa-ṭa-r[i]*** [G] D.3.1: 25; ***pa-ṭi-ir*$_9$** [G] I.1.1: 27; ***paṭ-ra-at*** [G] E.2.6: 12'; ***paṭ-ri*** I.1.1: 57; ***pu-uṭ-ru*** [G] C.3.10: 56, 60; ***ta-pa-ṭú-ra-nim$^{?}$*** [G] B.2.6: 27; ***up-te-eṭ-ṭi-ra*** [Dt] D.1.1: 121
paṭīru "portable altar": **GI.DU$_8$** D.3.1: 8, 16; F.2: 39'; **GI.DU$_8$$^{!}$** C.3.4: 40
pāṭiru "one who releases": **DU$_8$** E.2.3: 13'
peḫû G "to close up; to seal; to block": ***te-pe$^{?}$-ḫ[i$^{?}$]*** [G] E.2.6: 27'; **ÚŠ** [G] B.2.2: 28'; **ÚŠ-*e*** [G] C.1.10: 2, 5, 10; **ÚŠ-*ḫi*** [G] C.3.4: 95; **ÚŠ$^{!}$-*ḫi*** [G] C.1.5: 43
pelû I "(bright) red": ***pe-lu-ti*** C.1.1: 7; ***pe-lu-[ti]*** C.1.1: 1
pelû II "egg": **NUNUZ** A.2.1: 18', 80'''''; A.2.2: 28; A.2.5: 9'; C.1.4: 34', 35', 180'''; C.1.5: 11; C.1.9: 12, 23; C.1.10: 11; **[NU]NUZ** A.2.10: 3'; **NU[NUZ$^{?}$]** C.1.4: 168'''; **[NUN]UZ$^{?}$** C.1.6: 2'
pelû III G "to be (bright) red": ***pe-lu-ú*** [G] I.1.1: 101
pēmtu, *pēntu* "charcoal": **DÈ** II.1.4: 7; C.1.4: 26', 154'''; D.1.1: 233; D.3.1: 15; E.1.1: 2, 3; **D[È$^{?}$]** D.1.7: 9'; ***pe-en-du*** A.2.4: 18'; **UDUB** A.1.4: 33''
pēmu, *pēnu* "upper thigh": ***pe-ni-šá*** B.1.1: 29; **ÚR** F.1: 33, 41; **ÚR-*šá*** F.1: 35; **ÚR-*šú*** I.1.7: 9; **^{uzu}ÚR** D.1.1: 230
pērtu "hair (of the head)": ***pe-re-es-s[u$^{?}$]*** D.1.1: 96; ***pe-ret*** I.1.7: 7; ***pe-ret-su*** C.3.4: 64; C.3.9: 43; ***pe-re[t-su]*** C.3.3: 18
peṣû, *paṣû* I "white; a light beer"; see also *šammu peṣû*: **BABBAR** A.2.2: 24; A.2.5: 11'; B.2.2: 3; C.1.1: 15, 27'; C.1.3: 10'; C.1.4: 39', 124'', 186'''; C.3.6: 52''''; C.3.9: 1, 30; D.1.7: 11'; F.1: 24, 30, 37, 41; F.2: 35'; H.1: 24'; **BAB[BAR]** C.1.4: 109''; **⸢BABBAR⸣** F.1: 30; H.1: 2; **BABBAR.MEŠ** I.1.1: 33, 54; ***pa-ṣu-ú*** A.2.4: 11'; A.2.5: 4', 24''
peṣû II G "to be white": **BABBAR** I.1.1: 2, 10, 30; **BABBAR$^{?}$** E.2.6: 18'; **BABBAR.DIDLI** I.1.1: 14; **BABBAR-*ma*** [G] A.2.2: 73; ***pe-ṣu-ú*** [G] E.2.6: 27'
petû G "to open"; D "to open"; N "to be opened": **BAD** [G] B.2.4: 26'; **BAD-*ma*** [G] A.1.4: 30''; A.2.2: 77, 78; **⸢BAD⸣-*m[a]*** [G] A.2.2: 78; **[BA]D$^{?}$-*ma*** [G] A.1.4: 26''; ***i-pét-ti*** [G] D.1.11: 7; ***ip-te-šu*** [G] II.1.2: 12; ***lip-pe-ti*** [N] D.1.1: 105; ***lip-pe-tu-ú*** [N] D.1.1: 170; ***⸢pa⸣-[ta-ni]*** [G] D.1.5: 7'; ***pa-te-e*** [G] A.2.8: 4, 36'; ***pa-t[e-e$^{?}$]*** [G] A.2.8: 18; ***pe-tu-u*** [G] G.1: 49; ***ta-pa-te*** [G] II.1.4: 42; ***up-[te-et-te]*** [D] D.1.1: 120; ***up-te-ti*** [D] H.1: 36'
pilaqqu "spindle": **^{giš}BAL** C.3.4: 75; C.3.9: 56; D.3.1: 2, 6; **^{giš}⸢BAL⸣** D.3.1: 6a; ***[pi]-laq-qí*** D.1.1: 12; ***^{giš}pi-laq-qu*** C.3.3: 34
pillû (a medicinal plant): **^{giš}NAM.TAL** C.1.4: 150'''; **^{giš}NAM.TAR** A.2.1: 62'''; A.2.6: 7; A.2.7: 29'; D.1.1: 211; **^{ú}NAM.TAR** B.1.1: 4
pilšu "breach; perforation": **BÙRU-*šu*** I.1.1: 36, 37, 38, 39, 40, 41, 42, 43, 44, 45, 46, 47, 48; ***pil-š[u]*** C.1.4: 94''
pinku, *pingu* "knob": ***pi-in-⸢gi⸣*** F.1: 31
piqannu "dung pellet": **A.GAR.GAR** B.1.5: 6'; D.2.1: 61'
pirištu "secret; mystery": ***pi-riš-ti*** B.1.1: 62
pišannu, *pisannu* "box; chest; drainpipe": **^{giš}PÍSAN** D.1.1: 127, 133; **PISAN** G.1: 51; ***pi-sa-an-ni*** D.1.1: 114, 174, 175; D.1.9: 26'; ***pi-sa-an-nu*** G.1: 51
pitiqtu "mud wall": ***pi-ti-iq-ti*** D.1.1: 224
pītu "opening; aperture": ***pi-it*** II.1.4: 36; B.2.2: 5
piṭru (a body part): ***pi-iṭ-ri-šú*** A.2.6: 23
pizallurtu "gecko": **[MUŠ.DÍM].GURUN.NA** A.1.1: 21'; **MUŠ.DÍM.GUR$_4$.RU.NU** C.1.4: 151'''; **AM.S[I.ḪA.RA.NA$^{?}$]** C.2.3: 16'

pizzer, *pizzir*, *penzer* "cobweb": ^{ú}**SUR.SUR** II.1.3: 66'''; $^{⌜ú?⌝}$***pi-i[n-ze-er]*** A.1.4: 15'

pû I "mouth; opening; oral lore": **KA** A.2.1: 15', 87'''''; A.2.2: 30; A.2.5: 26''; A.2.7: 5; B.2.1: 37; B.2.5: 7; C.1.10: 14; C.3.9: 39; C.3.10: 74; D.1.11: 12; E.2.6: 3'; G.1: 52; **KA**$^?$ D.1.7: 5'; **[K]A** D.3.1: 37(f); **KA-*ki-na*** C.3.9: 20; **KA.MEŠ-*šá*** II.1.4: 17; **KA-*ša*** II.1.4: 43; **KA-*šá*** D.1.1: 222; **KA-*šú*** C.3.4: 86; I.1.1: 82, 83; I.1.7: 11; **[KA$^?$]-*šú*** D.1.3: 7'; ***pa-šú*** A.2.6: 1; ***pi-i*** C.3.1: 17, 18; C.3.3: 24; C.3.4: 68; C.3.9: 26, 48; D.1.1: 54; D.2.1: 10'; ***p[i-i]*** B.2.1: 34; ***pi-ia*** C.3.1: 8; ***pi-[i-k]a*** D.1.1: 102; ***⌜pi⌝-i⌜i⌝-[k]a*** D.1.1: 103; ***[p]i-⌜i⌝-[ku]-nu*** C.3.10: 25; ***pi$^?$-ku-nu*** C.1.5: 47; ***pi-i-šú*** D.1.5: 16'

pû II "straw": ***pe-e*** C.1.5: 43

puḫādu "lamb": **SILA$_4$** C.3.4: 4, 9, 12; C.3.6: 34''

puḫālu "male animal; stud": ***pu-ḫa-li*** H.1: 24'

pūḫtu "substitute": ***pu-uḫ-tu$_4$*** G.1: 3

pūḫu "substitute": ***pu-ḫi-ia*** C.3.4: 52; ***[pu-ḫi$^?$]-ia*** E.2.3: 21''; ***[p]u-ḫu-šá*** A.2.5: 16''

puquddû "(formal) delivery; legal consignment": ***pu-qu-du-u*** B.1.1: 47

puquttu (a thorny plant): ^{ú}***pu-qut-te*** C.1.4: 153'''; ***pú-qut-te*** C.1.4: 159'''; ***pu-qut-ti*** A.2.2: 59; ^{ú}***pu-qut-ti*** C.1.5: 17

purkullu, *parkullu* "seal-cutter; lapidary": ^{lú}**BUR.GUL** C.3.4: 74; C.3.9: 55; ^{lú}**BUR.⌜GUL⌝** C.3.3: 33

purqa (adv.) (uncertain meaning): ***pur-qa*** D.2.1: 11', 12', 13'

pursītu "(offering) bowl": **[^{dug}BUR.Z]I** C.1.5: 9

pūru "jar; (stone) bowl": **BUR** D.1.1: 54, 133, 150, 151, 153; D.3.1: 31; G.1: 31; G.2: 11'; **[BU]R$^{?!}$** C.3.4: 18; ***pu-ú-ri*** II.1.4: 60

purussu "stopper; plug": ***⌜pu⌝-ru-⌜sa-šá⌝*** C.1.4: 58''

purussû "decision": **EŠ.⌜BAR⌝** D.3.1: 19; **EŠ.BAR-*šú-nu*** C.3.10: 42

pusummu, *puṣunnu* "veil": ***⌜pu⌝$^!$-su-um-m[i]*** D.1.1: 84; ***pu-ṣu-ni*** II.1.4: 45

pusumtu "veil": ***pa-su-um-tu$_4$*** G.2: 19''

pušikku "combed wool": ^{síg}**GA.RÍG.AK.A** C.1.4: 6'; C.3.9: 1; C.3.10: 81; F.1: 2, 13, 17; **[^{síg}G]A.RÍG.AK.A** A.2.9: 17''; ^{síg}***pu-šik-ki*** D.2.1: 14'

pušqu "narrowness; straits; hardship": ***pu-uš-qa*** G.1: 26; ***pu-uš-qí*** D.1.1: 30, 33

pūtu "forehead"; *ina pūt* (compound prep.) "opposite; in the presence of": ***p[u$^?$-t]am$^{?!}$*** D.1.1: 152; ***pu-us-sa*** D.1.1: 151, 153; ***pu-ut*** D.1.5: 7', 13'; **SAG.KI** F.1: 1; **SAG.KI.MEŠ-*sa*** II.1.4: 60; **SAG.KI-*šá*** F.1: 3; H.1: 4; I.1.1: 1, 2; I.1.3: 32'; **SAG.KI-⌜*šá*⌝** C.1.8: 7'; **ZAG** D.3.1: 37(A)

puzru "concealment": ***pu-zur*** D.1.1: 143

qablu I "middle part; waist; hips, loins": **ÍB-*šá*** C.1.4: 134''; **[Í]B-*šá*** C.1.4: 100''; **MURUB$_4$** C.1.4: 23', 102''; C.3.9: 8; F.1: 31; I.1.3: 8; **[MUR]UB$_4$** F.1: 30; **MURUB$_4$.MEŠ** D.3.1: 5; F.1: 31; **MURUB$_4$.MEŠ-*šá*** C.3.1: 5; **MU[RUB$_4$.M]EŠ-*šá*$^?$** A.2.1: 32'; **⌜MURUB$_4$.MEŠ-*šá*$^?$⌝** D.3.1: 6; **[MU]RUB$_4$$^?$.⌜MEŠ-*šú*$^?$⌝** A.2.10: 13''; **MURUB$_4$-*šá*** C.1.2: 29'; C.1.4: 8', 24', 31', 47'; F.1: 18, 25, 30; **MURUB$_4$-⌜*šá*⌝** F.1: 27; **[MURU]B$_4$$^?$-*šá*** I.1.3: 18; **⌜MURUB$_4$⌝-*šá*** B.1.1: 29; **MURU[B$_4$-*šá*]** C.1.3: 3'; **MUR[UB$_4$-*šá*]** C.1.1: 16; **M[URUB$_4$-*šá*]** C.1.3: 9'; **MURUB$_4$-*šú*** C.2.2: 12; C.3.9: 4, 35; F.1: 27; **MURUB$_4$-⌜*šú*⌝** A.1.4: 18'

qablu II "battle": **MURUB$_4$** C.3.10: 28

qabû G "to say; to speak; to order; to decree; to pray"; Š "to have someone say": **DU$_{11}$.GA** [G] A.2.7: 39'; C.1.8: 36'; C.3.4: 7, 9, 22, 43, 47, 49, 51b, 90; C.3.10: 63, 70, 77, 78, 81, 83; D.3.1: 10c; **DU$_{11}$.G[A]** C.3.4: 26; **D[U$_{11}$].GA** [G] C.3.10: 86; **D[U$_{11}$.GA$^?$]** C.3.4: 19; **DU$_{11}$.GA-*ma*** [G] B.2.6: 26; C.3.4: 9, 12, 23, 35, 47, 49, 95; C.3.10: 68, 82, 84; D.1.1: 225, 228; D.3.1: 14; **D[U$_{11}$.GA-*ma*]** [G] C.3.6: 44'''; **DU$_{11}$.GA-*šu*** [G] B.1.1: 56; **[D]U$_{11}$$^?$.[GA$^?$]-*šú*** [Š] B.2.6: 16; **[DU$_{11}$.GA$^?$]-*ú*** [G] E.2.3: 9'; **E** [G] B.2.2: 28'; **E-*u*** [G] G.1: 5, 50; **E-*ú*** [G] C.1.10: 5, 7, 13, 17; D.1.11: 14'; ***i-qab-bak-ka*** [G] D.1.11: 6; ***i-qab-bi*** [G] C.3.10: 9, 27; D.3.1: 10c; I.1.3: 16; ***⌜i⌝-qab-bi*** [G] D.3.1: 14; ***iq-bak-ka*** [G] A.2.5: 10', 13'; C.1.10: 4; ***iq-bak-k[a]*** [G] A.2.5: 7'; ***iq-ta-bi*** [G] G.1: 39; G.2: 16''; ***iq-ta-bu-ú*** [G] C.3.10: 9; ***liq-bi*** [G] C.1.1: 12; C.1.4: 64''; D.1.8: 8, 24; ***liq-b[i]*** [G] C.1.2: 22'; ***qí-bi-ma*** [G] D.1.1: 51; ***ta-qab-bi*** [G] C.3.10: 19

qadādu G "to bow down": ***qá-di-is-su*** [G] D.1.1: 147

qadāšu D "to purify": ***tu-qa-da-áš*** [D] C.3.4: 81; ***tu-qad-dáš*** [D] C.1.8: 33'

qaddadāniš "bowed down; bent over": ***qa-da-da-niš*** D.1.9: 16'; ***qa-d[a-da-ni]š*** D.1.9: 19'

qadum, *qadu* "together with; including": ***qá-du*** I.1.1: 80, 83

qalāpu G "to peel"; D "to strip of; to free (from husk, covering)"; Dt "to be peeled off"; N "to be peeled": ***[liq-q]a-⌜lip⌝*** [N] D.1.8: 22; ***tu-qal-l[ap]*** [D] A.2.3: 9'; ***uq-tal-la-pa*** [Dt] I.1.1: 24

qalātu (uncertain meaning): ***qa-la-tú*** D.1.5: 20'

qallalu "very small": ***qal-la-la*** I.1.2: 5'

qalliš "lightly; slightly": ***qal-liš*** C.1.4: 170'''

qalû I "roasted": **BIL** II.1.4: 28; **BÍL** D.2.1: 65'; **BIL.ME** E.2.6: 2'; **BÍL.MEŠ** D.2.1: 43', 44', 50'; **BÍ[L].MEŠ** D.2.1: 41'; **BÍL-*ti*** B.1.1: 4; ***qa-la-t[i$^?$]*** C.1.4: 126''; ***qa-li-tu$_4$*** E.2.6: 44'; ***qa-lu-tu*** A.2.1: 26'; ***[q]a$^?$-lu-tu$_4$*** A.1.2: 5'

qalû II G "to roast; to burn"; D "to roast; to burn": **BIL** [G] C.1.4: 38'; **BÍL** [G] B.2.2: 19'; **BÍL-*lu$_4$*** [G] D.2.1: 53'; ***iq-lu-ú*** [G] C.1.10: 15; ***qa-lu-ú*** [G] A.2.5: 11'; ***ta-qa-lu*** [G] C.1.4: 175'''; ***ta-qal-lu*** [G] H.1: 17'; ***ta-qàl-lu*** [G] C.1.4: 169'''; ***tu-qal-la*** [D] C.1.10: 3

qâlu G "to be silent": ***i-⌜qá$^?$⌝-a[l$^?$]*** [G] I.1.6: 33'

qan šalāli (a variety of reed): **GI.ŠUL.ḪI** B.1.1: 12

qannu "fringe; hem": ***qa-an-na-šú*** C.3.4: 71; C.3.9: 52

qanû "reed": **GI** II.1.1: 29; D.1.1: 175, 179; G.1: 12; **[G]I** B.1.1: 11; **[G]I$^?$** A.2.2: 19; **⌜GI.MEŠ$^?$⌝** C.4.1: 1'; ***qa-⌜né⌝-e*** D.1.1: 95; ***qa-nu-ú*** E.2.1: 3

qanû ṭābu "sweet reed" (perhaps sweet flag, *Acorus calamus*): **GI DU$_{10}$** D.2.1: 58'; **GI DU$_{10}$.GA** II.1.4: 4; D.1.1: 38; D.1.2: 9; **GI [DU$_{10}$.GA$^?$]** A.2.5: 21''; **G[I DU$_{10}$.GA]** D.1.2: 3

qâpu G "to fall down; to collapse": ***qa-a-pa*** [G] G.1: 50

qaqqadu "head": **SAG.DU** A.2.6: 2; C.3.1: 2, 6, 6a; H.1: 22', 36'; H.2: 3; I.1.7: 6; **⌜SAG.DU⌝** A.2.6: 12; **[SA]G.DU** C.3.1: 9; **SA[G.DU]** H.1: 9; **SAG.DU-*ia$_5$*** G.1: 37; **SAG.DU-*sa*** C.3.5: 12'; **SAG.DU-*su*** C.1.4: 62''; C.1.5: 8; C.1.8: 39'; C.3.4: 4; C.3.10: 80; **SAG.DU-*šá*** I.1.3: 10; **SAG.DU-*šú*** C.3.4: 85; C.3.9: 32; I.1.7: 2, 7; ***qaq-qa-da^{meš}*** A.2.8: 38'; ***qa-qa-di-šú*** D.1.9: 43'

qaqqaranû "Urukean" (the one from the Anu district"): ***^{lú}qaq-qar-^{d}anu^{ki}-ú*** C.3.4: 100
qaqqaru "ground; earth; netherworld": **KI** C.1.4: 10'; C.1.8: 27', 39'; C.3.4: 40; D.3.1: 9; E.2.3: 5'; **K[I$^{?}$]** A.1.4: 26''; **[K]I$^{?}$** E.2.6: 12'; ***qa-[aq-qa-ri]*** D.1.1: 156; ***qa-aq-qár-šu*** D.1.1: 156; ***⸢qaq⸣-qa-ra*** D.3.1: 14; ***[q]á$^{?}$-qá-ri*** B.2.1: 21; ***qaq-[qa-ri]*** D.3.1: 9; ***q[á-qá-ri$^{?}$]*** A.2.7: 14; ***qaq-qa-ri*** D.1.5: 14'; D.3.1: 14; ***qaq-qa-ru*** D.1.1: 183; D.3.1: 9, 14; ***[qaq]-qa-ru*** D.1.1: 24; ***qaq-qar*** E.2.6: 16'; G.1: 15; G.2: 1'; ***[q]aq-qàr*** C.1.5: 36; ***qaq-qar-šú*** D.1.1: 156; ***qaq$^{!}$-qar-šu*** D.1.1: 156
qardu "heroic (one); warrior": ***qar-du*** C.3.10: 28
qarnu "horn": ***[qar-ni]-šá*** G.2: 1'; ***qar-ni-šú*** G.1: 15; **SI** A.2.2: 53; B.1.5: 6'; C.1.4: 38', 111'', 113'', 159'''; C.1.5: 30; C.1.10: 15, 16; C.2.2: 5; **⸢SI⸣** D.2.1: 2'; **SI-*ia*$_5$** D.1.1: 183
qarrādu "warrior; hero": **UR.SAG** II.1.4: 40; **⸢UR.SAG$^{!}$⸣** D.1.1: 80
qaštu "bow": **⸢^{giš}⸣PAN$^{?}$** D.1.1: 54
qatāru G "to smoke; to be gloomy"; D "to burn incense; to fumigate": **SAR** [D] A.2.5: 25''; **SAR-*ši*** [D] A.1.2: 18''; D.3.1: 15; **SAR-*šú*** [D] D.1.1: 233; D.3.1: 15
qatû G "to come to an end; to finish"; D "to bring to an end; to finish": **AL.TIL** [G] I.1.1: 117; I.1.3: 34'; ***i-qát-tu-nim-ma*** [G] A.2.5: 3'; ***qa-tu-u*** [G] G.1: 20; ***qa-tu-ú*** [G] II.1.4: 35, 52; G.2: 5'; ***qu-ut-ti-i*** [D] D.1.1: 145; ***⸢qut$^{?}$⸣-ti-šá*** [D] D.1.9: 15'; ***qut-tu-ú*** [D] C.1.8: 12'; ***[t]u-qát-ta$_5$*** [D] C.3.10: 43; ***ú-qa-ta-ma*** [D] D.3.1: 32; ***ú-qat-ta-a*** [D] G.1: 19; ***ú-qé-et-ta-a*** [D] G.2: 4'
qātu "hand": ***qa-as-su*** D.1.1: 149; ***q[à-as-su]*** D.1.1: 149; ***qa-at-ka*** G.1: 41; ***qa-ta-šú*** I.1.5: 7'; ***qa-ti-šá*** I.1.5: 6'; **ŠU** A.2.7: 4; B.1.1: 28; C.1.8: 29'; C.3.3: 7; C.3.4: 79, 96; C.3.5: 14'; C.3.7: 13'', 20''; D.1.1: 147, 196, 200; F.1: 12, 14, 15, 17; I.1.3: 10, 16; **[Š]U** C.3.4: 79; **ŠU.MEŠ** I.1.3: 15; **ŠU.MEŠ-*šá*** C.1.4: 104''; **ŠU.MIN** C.3.1: 2, 3; C.3.4: 59, 96, 97; C.3.9: 3, 6, 39; C.3.10: 5; **ŠU.MIN-*⸢a-a⸣*** C.3.10: 21; **ŠU.MIN-*ia*** D.1.5: 12'; **ŠU.MIN-*ía*** C.3.4: 21; **ŠU.MIN-*ka*** G.2: 20''; **ŠU.MIN-*ki*** C.3.3: 30; C.3.4: 70, 72; C.3.9: 50; C.3.9: 53; **ŠU.MIN-*šá*** C.3.3: 16; C.3.4: 63; C.3.9: 42; D.3.1: 10c; I.1.1: 72, 84; I.1.3: 10, 15, 20; **ŠU.⸢MIN-*šá*⸣** C.3.3: 20; **ŠU+⸢MIN⸣-*šá*** D.3.1: 10c; **ŠU.MIN-*šú*** C.3.4: 84; C.3.9: 44; C.3.10: 80; D.1.9: 36'; D.3.1: 10c; E.2.3: 8'; **ŠU.MIN-*[šú]*** C.3.4: 65; **ŠU.MIN.MEŠ-*šú*** C.3.9: 34, 38; **ŠU-*su*** D.1.1: 149; **ŠU$^{?}$-*s[u$^{?}$]*** C.3.1: 12; **ŠU-*šá*** C.1.4: 105''; C.3.4: 3; I.1.3: 8
qebēru G "to bury": ***te-qeb-ber*** [G] C.3.4: 96; ***te-qeb-ber-ma*** [G] C.3.4: 97; ***te-qeb-ber-šú*** [G] C.3.4: 97; E.2.6: 12'
qēmu "flour; powder": **ZÌ** A.1.3: 2'; A.1.4: 31''; A.2.1: 27'; A.2.2: 31; A.2.3: 6', 29'''; A.2.6: 5; B.1.1: 23, 24; C.1.4: 126'', 164'''; C.3.4: 12; C.3.10: 75; D.1.1: 204; D.1.7: 7'; D.1.11: 1, 2, 11; D.2.1: 34', 41', 50', 62'; E.2.6: 1'; **ZÌ$^{?}$** E.2.6: 23'; **ZÌ$^{?!}$** A.2.3: 11'; **⸢ZÌ$^{?}$⸣** A.2.5: 18''; A.2.8: 34'; **ZÌ.DA** II.1.3.1: 4', 5', 6', 7', 8'; **ZÌ.D[A]** E.2.3: 6'; **⸢ZÌ⸣.DA** E.2.3: 5'; **Z[Ì.DA.ḪI.A$^{?}$]** B.1.1: 27
qerbēnu (adv.) "inside": ***qer-bé-nu*** D.2.1: 59', 65'
qerbītu "interior; womb": ***qer-bi-sa*** D.2.1: 69', 70'; ***qer-bi-s[a]*** D.2.1: 67'; ***⸢qer-bi-sà⸣*** D.2.1: 65'; ***⸢qer-bi-ti⸣*** C.3.6: 11'; ***qer-bit-si*** B.2.2: 21'
qerbu "centre; interior; belly; intestine": ***qer-bi*** B.1.1: 42, 50; ***qer-[bi$^{?}$]*** B.1.1: 16; **ŠÀ** E.2.5: 2'; **ŠÀ.ME-*šá*** I.1.1: 72; **ŠÀ.MEŠ-*ša*** II.1.4: 2; I.1.1: 57, 59, 76; **⸢ŠÀ⸣.MEŠ-*šá*** C.3.6: 59''''; **Š[À].M[EŠ-*šá*$^{?}$]** D.2.1: 4'
qerēbu G "to be close"; D "to bring; to draw near; to lead; to present": ***i-qar-ri-ba-am-m[a]*** [G] D.1.11: 5; ***i-qar-ru-ub*** [G] D.2.1: 15'; ***iq-ri-ba-am-ma*** [G] D.1.11: 3; ***iq-ri-bu-niš-šú*** [G] I.1.1: 106; ***iq-ri-bu-niš-ši*** [G] I.1.1: 106, 107, 108, 109, 110; I.1.3: 1; ***iq-ri-bu-niš-š[i]*** [G] I.1.1: 111, 112, 113; ***qé-ru-ub*** [G] D.1.11: 6; ***qer-bé-et-ma*** [G] C.3.10: 36; ***ú-qar-ra-bu*** [D] C.3.9: 22
qiāpu, *qâpu* G "to (en)trust; to believe": ***qa-a-pa*** [G] G.1: 44
qibītu "speech; command": ***qí-bi-ti*** G.1: 31
qiddatu "downstream": ***qid-da-tu$_4$*** C.3.10: 15
qilpu "rind; skin": **BAR** C.1.4: 163''', 179'''; **⸢BAR$^{?}$⸣** A.1.4: 25''; ***qí-lip*** D.2.1: 7'
qimmatu "crown; lock of hair; top": ***qim-ma-ti*** G.1: 42; ***qim-ma-ti-ia*** C.3.4: 46; **SUḪUR-*su*** D.1.1: 228
qinnāzu "whip": ***qin-na-zu*** D.1.9: 6'
qinnu "nest": ***qin-ni*** D.1.1: 210
qinû "envy; jealousy": ***qí-ne-e-šú*** C.3.4: 93
qīpu "entrusted": ***qí-ip*** G.1: 44; ***qí-i[p$^{?}$]*** D.1.1: 100
qiššû "cucumber": **⸢ÚKUŠ$^{?}$⸣** E.2.6: 40'
qištu "forest": **^{giš}TIR** G.1: 38
qīštu "gift; present": **[NÍG].BA** C.1.1: 6; **NÍG.BA-*ka*** D.1.1: 226
qitmu (a black paste/pigment): **IM.SAḪAR.GI$_6$.KUR** C.1.4: 36'; **IM.SAḪAR.GI$_6$.KUR.RA** A.1.3: 7'; C.1.2: 15; C.1.4: 42'; C.1.8: 9'; **SAḪAR.GI$_6$$^{?}$** A.2.2: 40
qû I "litre": **SÌLA** II.1.3: 31''', 32'''; II.1.3.1: 4'; A.2.4: 42'''; A.2.5: 19''; B.1.1: 29; C.1.4: 154'''; C.1.10: 18; C.2.3: 13'; C.3.10: 5; D.1.11: 11; D.2.1: 62'; E.2.1: 6, 8; E.2.6: 19', 21', 31', 33', 34', 37', 38', 40', 42'; **SÌLA$^{!}$** E.2.6: 23'; **[SÌ]LA** II.1.3.1: 6', 7', 8'; **⸢SÌLA$^{?}$⸣** A.1.4: 12'
qû II "thread; string; cord": **GU** F.2: 38'; **⸢GU⸣** D.1.4: 11''; **GU.MEŠ** I.1.1: 50; ***qé-e-ki*** C.3.3: 35; C.3.4: 76
qulqulliānu (a medicinal plant): ***^{ú}qúl-qúl-li-a-ni*** C.1.4: 176'''
qūltu "silence; despair": ***qu-lat*** C.3.9: 19; ***qu-la-⸢a⸣-[t]im*** C.3.9: 19
qūlu "silence; stillness": ***qú-lum*** C.3.10: 44
qunātā "woad": ***qu-na-a-ta*** B.2.3: 12''; ***qu-na-⸢a⸣-[ta]*** B.2.3: 20''
qunnabu "hemp": ***qu-un-nab*** E.2.5: 4'
quppû "sharp knife; scalpel": ***qú-pu-ú*** A.2.8: 35'
qutāru "incense, fumigant; fumigation": ***⸢qut-PA$^{?}$⸣^{ri}*** II.1.4: 16
qutrānu (a drug): ***qut-ra-nu*** A.1.4: 15'
qutru I "smoke": ***⸢qú-ut$^{?}$⸣-ru*** II.1.4: 16
qutru II (a plant): **^{ú}KI.^{d}IŠKUR** C.1.4: 165'''; ***^{ú}qut-ri*** B.2.4: 9'

rabāku G/D "to boil down; to make into a paste; to stir": ***tara-bak*** [G] A.1.1: 17'; A.2.1: 29'; A.2.2: 20; ***[t]u-rab-bak*** [D] E.2.6: 14'
rabīku, *ribīku* "paste": ***ri-bi-ku*** A.2.3: 4'; E.2.6: 16'; ***ri-b[i-ki$^{?}$]*** A.2.3: 3'; ***[ri-b]i-ku*** A.2.3: 6'
rābiṣu "lurker; a demon": **MAŠKIM** I.1.3: 10; **MÀŠK[IM$^{?}$]** C.3.1: 32

rabû I "great; big; large; old": **GAL.MEŠ** C.3.4: 51a; **GAL-*te*** C.3.6: 16', 20'; **GAL-*ti*** C.3.4: 51a; **[G]AL-*ti*** C.3.6: 16'; **GAL-*tú*** C.3.4: 50; C.3.6: 10'; **GAL-*tu*$_{4}$** C.3.6: 12'; ***ra-bi-i-[tu$_{4}$]*** C.3.6: 10'; ***ra-bi-tu$_{4}$*** C.3.10: 27; ***ra-bu-[ti]*** C.3.6: 27'

rabû II G "to be(come) large in size; to increase; to grow (up)"; D "to enlarge; to increase; to swell; to rear (children)"; Š "to make great; to enhance; to praise": ***lu-rab-bi*** [D] C.3.10: 60; ***tu-ra-bu-'u-šú-ma*** [D] A.2.4: 8'; ***ú-rab-bi-ka*** [D] C.3.10: 20; ***ú-rab-bu-ú*** [D] C.3.10: 46; ***ú-šar-bi*** [Š] D.1.1: 117

raḫāṣu G "to wash"; Gtn iter. of G: **RA-*si*** [G] II.1.4: 25; D.2.1: 61'; **RA.MEŠ** [Gtn] D.2.1: 60'; **RA.MEŠ-*si*** [Gtn] D.2.1: 58'; ***⸢ru⸣-ḫu-uṣ*** [G] A.2.2: 22

rakābu G "to ride": **⸢U$_{5}$⸣-*ma*** [G] D.1.11: 13

rakāsu G "to bind; to attach; to tie; to gird; to set up; to prepare; to arrange"; D "to tie on; to bind up": **KÉŠ** [G] A.2.2: 68; C.1.4: 8', 134'', 155'''; C.1.8: 53''; C.2.2: 12; C.3.4: 25, 59, 89; C.3.9: 3, 4, 33, 34, 36; D.3.1: 8; H.1: 4, 24'; **KÉ[Š]** [G] A.2.7: 4; C.1.4: 105''; **K[ÉŠ]** [G] A.2.2: 43; **K[ÉŠ$^{?}$]** [G] C.1.4: 104''; **⸢KÉŠ$^{?}$⸣** [G] D.3.1: 6; **⸢KÉŠ$^{?!}$⸣** [G] B.1.1: 30; **KÉŠ-*as*** [G] D.3.1: 8; H.1: 24'; **KÉŠ-⸢*as*⸣** [G] D.3.1: 16; **KÉ[Š]-*as*** [G] C.3.3: 7; **KÉŠ-*ma*** [G] C.1.2: 29'; C.1.4: 24'; C.3.9: 35, 36; C.3.10: 80; D.1.1: 230; **KÉŠ-*ma*$^{?}$** [G] A.2.2: 20; **KÉ[Š-*ma*]** [G] C.1.4: 100''; **KÉŠ-*si*** [G] C.1.4: 14'; D.3.1: 6; **KÉŠ-*su*** [G] C.3.4: 43; ***ru-ku-us*** [G] C.1.4: 62''; ***tara-kás*** [G] C.1.4: 47'; C.2.1: 11'; C.3.9: 2; D.1.1: 230; D.3.1: 8; E.2.3: 3'; E.2.6: 4'; F.1: 3, 8, 27; ***tara-⸢kás⸣*** [G] F.1: 11; ***⸢tara-kás⸣*** [G] F.1: 14; ***tara-k[ás]*** [G] F.1: 35; ***ta[ra-kás]*** F.1: 38; ***tara$^{!}$-⸢kàs⸣*** [G] C.3.4: 88; ***tara-kás-ma*** [G] C.3.6: 61''''; ***tu-[rak]-kas*** [D] C.1.4: 177'''

râku G "to pour out; to smear": ***[t]a$^{?}$-rak-ma*** [G] C.3.2: 6''; ***tara-ku*** [G] A.2.2: 23, 27; ***⸢tara-ku⸣*** [G] A.2.2: 25

ramāku G "to bathe; to wash; to steep"; D "to bathe; to wash": ***i-r[a-am-muk]*** [G] C.3.4: 47; ***ir-muk*** [G] A.2.3: 7'; ***[ta-ra]m-muk*** [G] A.2.3: 10'; ***tara-muk*** [G] C.1.5: 29, 31; **TU$_{5}$** [G] C.1.4: 9'; **TU$_{5}$$^{!}$** [G] C.3.4: 47; **T[U$_{5}$-*m*]*a*$^{?}$** [G] C.3.4: 49; ***tu-ra-am-ma-ak-šú*** [D] C.3.10: 10; **TU$_{5}$-*šú*** [D] E.2.3: 20''; **TU$_{5}$-*šú-ma*** [D] C.3.4: 54

ramānu "self": ***ra-man-šá*** D.3.1: 32; ***ra-man-šú*** E.2.8: 6'; ***[ra]-⸢man⸣-š[ú]*** D.3.1: 32

ramû I G "to slacken"; D "to loosen": ***li-ir-mu-ú*** [G] D.1.1: 108; ***[li]-ram-ma-a*** [D] D.1.1: 189; ***[ru-u]m-⸢mu⸣-'u*** [D] D.1.10: 5'; ***ú-ram-mi*** [D] D.1.1: 119

ramû II G "to set up; to establish": ***ir-mu-ú*** [G] C.3.10: 28

râmu G "to love": ***i-ra-'-ši*** [G] II.1.4: 54; ***i-ra-am-ši*** [G] D.1.1: 137; ***ta-ra-⸢am⸣-mi*** [G] C.3.6: 12'; ***ta-ra-am-mì*** [G] C.3.6: 12'

rapādu (a psychoactive, intoxicating plant): ***^{ú}ra-pad-du*** A.2.6: 4

rapaštu, *rapaltu* "loin; lower back; pelvic region": ***^{uzu}ra-pal-te-ša*** II.1.4: 31; ***ra-pa[l-ti-šá]*** B.1.1: 29

rapāšu G "to become wide; to expand"; D "to widen; to extend": ***lu$_{4}$-rap-pí-iš*** [D] C.3.10: 61; ***ú-rap-pa-šú*** [D] C.3.10: 46

rapšu "wide; broad; vast": **DAGAL-*tim*** C.3.9: 18

raqqu I "thin": ***raq-qat$_{7}$*** A.1.1: 7'

raqqu II "turtle; tortoise": **BA.AL.GI** C.1.4: 180'''

rasānu G "to soak; to steep": ***tàra-sà-an*** [G] D.2.1: 37'; ***[ta]ra-sà-an*** [G] C.2.1: 11'; ***⸢ta-ra⸣-sà-a[n$^{?}$]*** [G] A.2.3: 21''

rašû G "to get; to acquire; to have; to be affected by"; Gtn iter. of G; Š "to cause to get; to provide": ***lu-ur-ši*** [G] B.2.6: 24; ***šur-še-e*** [Š] C.3.6: 15'; ***[šu-u]r-ši-im-ma*** [Š] B.1.1: 9; **TUKU** [G] D.2.1: 34', 65'; I.1.3: 8; **T[UKU$^{?}$]** [G] D.2.1: 69'; **TUKU-*at*** [G] D.2.1: 71'; **⸢TUKU$^{!}$.MEŠ⸣** [Gtn] D.2.1: 59'; **TUKU-*ši*** [G] B.1.1: 40; **TUKU.[TUKU]-*ši*** [Gtn] D.2.1: 39'; **TUKU-*ú*** [G] C.1.4: 174'''; **⸢TUKU-*ú*⸣** C.1.8: 14'; ***tu-šár-ša*** [Š] B.2.6: 18; ***tu-šar-šú*** [Š] C.3.10: 38

raṭāpu G "to continue": ***ir-ṭú-pu-niš-ši*** [G] I.1.2: 13'; I.1.3: 1, 2, 3, 4, 5, 6, 7; ***⸢ir⸣-ṭ[ú-pu-niš-ši]*** [G] I.1.5: 1'

rebû "fourth"; *ina rebî ūmi* "on the fourth day": **4** C.1.4: 14'; I.1.1: 107; **4-*i*** C.4.1: 5'; E.2.6: 15'; I.1.1: 107; **4.KAM** I.1.3: 2; **U$_{4}$.4.KAM** A.2.5: 25''; **U$_{4}$.4.KÁM** I.1.1: 107

rebūtu "one fourth; quarter (of a shekel)": **4** A.1.4: 11'; **4-*tú*** A.2.1: 72'''', 73'''', 74'''', 89''''', 102''''''', 103'''''''; A.2.2: 19; B.2.2: 1; **[4]-*tú*** A.1.4: 11', 12'

redû G "to accompany; to pursue; to persecute; Š "to cause to overflow": **UŠ-*de*** [G] C.3.4: 65; ***i-red-de*** [G] C.3.9: 44; ***[i-red-d]e*** [G] C.3.3: 20; ***šur-du-ma*** [Š] C.1.4: 65''

rēḫtu, *rīḫtu* "remainder": **ÍB.TAG$_{4}$** H.1: 18'

reḫû G "to pour out; to inseminate; to impregnate": ***⸢i-ra⸣-ḫu-u*** [G] C.3.6: 11'; ***i-re-eḫ-ḫi-[ši$^{?}$]*** [G] A.1.3: 6'; ***ir-ḫi*** [G] I.1.1: 100, 101, 102

rēḫu "remaining; left over": **TAG$_{4}$.MEŠ** E.1.2: 9'

rēmēnû "merciful": ***re-ma-nu-ú*** II.1.4: 46; ***re-[me]-ni-[i]*** D.1.1: 23; ***re-mi-ni-i*** C.1.1: 12; ***[r]e-mi-ni-i*** C.1.2: 23'; ***reme-ni-⸢tu$_{4}$$^{!}$⸣*** C.3.10: 64; ***[re-me$^{?}$]-ni-tu$_{4}$*** D.1.10: 9'

rēmu "womb; mercy; pity": **ARḪUŠ** C.3.9: 29; **⸢ARḪUŠ⸣** D.1.1: 51; **ARḪUŠ-*mu*** II.1.4: 36; **ARḪUŠ-*šá*** E.2.6: 19', 25'; **ARḪUŠ-*š[á]*** B.1.1: 37; ***re-e-me*** D.1.1: 51; ***re-[mi$^{?}$]*** B.1.1: 43; ***[re$^{?}$]-mi*** B.1.1: 44

rêmu G "to have/show mercy; to be merciful": ***[r]e-man-né-e-ma*** [G] D.3.1: 23; ***re-man-ni*** [G] D.3.1: 23; ***[re]-⸢man-ni$^{?}$⸣-ma*** [G] D.3.1: 23; ***re-mi*** [G] D.1.1: 198

rēštû "foremost": ***reš-ti$^{!}$*** E.2.6: 42'

rēšu "head; top; beginning": ***re-e-eš*** D.1.1: 162; ***re-ši-šú*** C.3.10: 6; **SAG** C.3.4: 85; D.1.1: 201; I.1.1: 56, 73, 85; I.1.3: 18; **⸢SAG$^{?}$⸣** D.1.11: 14'; **S[AG]** I.1.1: 16; I.1.2: 1'

retû G "to drive in; to fix": ***te-ret-ti*** [G] C.3.4: 85

re'û G "to pasture; to tend (animals); (allow animals) to graze"; Gtn iter. of G: ***i-ra-'i-ši*** [G] D.1.1: 141; ***i-re-'i*** [G] D.1.1: 141; ***ir-ta-na-'i*** [Gtn] II.1.4: 54

rē'û "shepherd": ***re-é-a-šá*** D.1.1: 147; ***re-'-i*** D.1.1: 143, 196, 200; **^{lú}SIPA** D.1.1: 143, 147; **[^{lú}S]IPA** D.1.1: 147; **SIPA** G.1: 22

rē'ûtu "shepherdship": ***re-é-a-ú-tu*** D.1.1: 140; ***re-é-ú-tu*** D.1.1: 140

riāqu, *râqu* G "to be(come) empty"; Š "to empty; to unload": ***ta-ri-qa*** [G] C.3.10: 29; ***ú-šá-ra-qam-m[a]*** [Š] D.1.11: 8

rību "setting": ***ri-bi*** C.3.10: 1

ridût errī "diarrhoea": ***ri-du-ut ir-ri*** D.2.1: 34'; ***ri-du-u[t ir-ri]*** A.2.2: 59

ridûtu "pursuit; persecution": ***ri-du-ut*** D.1.6: 10

rigmu "voice; cry; noise": **GÙ.MEŠ** II.1.4: 58; ***[ri-g]i-im*** D.1.1: 148; ***ri-gim*** D.1.1: 148, 165; ***ri-gim-šá*** D.1.1: 149, 166; D.1.9: 17', 18'

riḫûtu "semen; progeny; spawn": ***ri-ḫu-tú*** D.2.1: 69', 70'; ***ri-ḫu-t[ú$^{?}$]*** D.1.9: 10'; ***ri-[ḫu-tu$_{4}$]*** C.3.6: 11'

rikibti arkabi "spur(?) of a bat" (a drug): **U$_{5}$ ARKAB^{mušen}** A.2.1: 59'''; D.1.1: 215; **U$_{5}$ ARK[AB^{mušen}]** A.1.4: 12'

riksu "bond; bandage; bundle; knot; ritual arrangement": **DUR** D.1.1: 119; **KEŠDA** A.2.2: 43; B.2.6: 7, 27; C.1.4: 59''; C.3.4: 25, 54, 89; E.2.3: 26''; E.2.6: 4'; **KEŠDA.MEŠ** C.1.4: 155'''; ***ri-kis*** C.3.10: 16, 58; ***ri-[kis]*** I.1.2: 9'; ***ri-ik-si*** G.1: 49; ***rik-sa*** D.1.1: 119; ***rik-si*** C.1.1: 8; G.1: 13

rīmu "wild bull": **AM**$^{?!}$ E.2.6: 20'

rinzu (a type of bewitchment): ***[r]i-in-zu*** B.1.1: 48

riqqi ḫīlī (a medicinal plant, lit. "aromatic for birth pangs"): **ŠIM** ***ḫi-i-li*** A.2.8: 3, 34'; **ŠIM** ***ḫi-i-l[i]*** A.2.8: 5

riqqu "aromatic plant": ***ri-qí*** D.1.1: 3; **ŠIM.ḪI.A** D.2.1: 55'; **ŠIM.⸢ḪI.A⸣** E.2.6: 40'; **ŠIM**$^{?!}$**.ḪI.A** A.2.2: 55; **ŠIM.MEŠ** II.1.3: 39'''; II.1.4: 27; **⸢ŠIM⸣.MEŠ** C.3.10: 75

rišûtu "itching (a skin disease)": ***ri-šu-[tú***$^{?}$***]*** A.2.3: 12'

rittu "hand; a handful": ***rit-tú*** A.1.4: 15'

rubṣu "lair; bedding; dung; womb": ***ru-bu-us-su*** B.2.2: 27'; ***[ru-bu-u]s-su*** B.2.2: 28'; **ŠURUN-*su*** B.2.2: 24', 26'

rubû "nobleman; prince; ruler": **NUN** D.3.1: 19

ruḫû "evil magic; sorcery": ***ru-ḫe-e*** C.3.9: 22; ***ru-ḫe-e-ki-na*** C.3.9: 24; ***ru-ḫu-ú*** B.1.1: 48

ruqqu "thinness; thin part": ***ruq-qí*** D.2.1: 63'

rūqu "distant": ***ru-qú-tim*** II.1.2: 7

ru'tītu "sulphur": **ÚḪ-*tú*** E.2.2: 2'

ru'tu "spittle; saliva": **ÚḪ-*su*** C.3.10: 74

ruṭibtu "dampness": ***ru-ṭib-ti*** C.1.10: 4; ***ru-ṭib-tú*** A.2.3: 6'

sābu (a red stone): ^{na4}***⸢sa***$^{?}$***⸣-[a]-⸢bu***$^{?}$***⸣*** F.1: 21

sābû "brewer": ^{lú}**KÚRUN** D.1.3: 9'; ^{lú}**KURUN.NAM** A.2.2: 65; ^{lú}**KÚRUN.NA** B.1.6: 5; D.1.1: 206

sadāru G "to set in a row; to do/occur regularly": ***i-sa-dir-ši-ma*** [G] I.1.3: 17; ***sa-ad-ru-ma*** [G] C.1.9: 26

sagû, *šagû* "(menstrual) flow; menses": ***sa-ge-⸢e⸣*** A.2.5: 4', 5'; ***sa-gu-šá*** A.2.1: 61''', 63'''; ***[s]a***$^{?}$***-gu***$_5$***-šá*** C.2.1: 10'; ***sa-gu-šú*** C.2.3: 9'; ***⸢sa⸣-gu-šú*** C.2.3: 6'; ***⸢sa⸣-⸢gu⸣-⸢šú***$^{?}$***⸣*** C.2.3: 8'; ***s[a-gu-šú]*** C.2.3: 15'; ***sa-gu-u*** I.1.2: 6'; ***⸢ša⸣-gu-šá*** A.1.1: 5'; ***⸢šá***$^{?}$***⸣-gu-šá*** C.1.1: 7; ***ša-gu***$_5$***-šá*** C.1.8: 15'; ***šá-g[u***$_5$***-šá]*** C.2.1: 6'; ***šu***$^{?}$***-gu-šá*** C.1.1: 1; **ŠÀ.KU.SA**(?) I.1.1: 100, 101, 102

saḫālu G "to prick; to pierce"; D "to cause a piercing pain": ***ú-sa-ḫal-ši*** [D] D.2.1: 17'

saḫāpu G "to envelope; to overwhelm; to spread; to overturn": ***saḫ-pa*** [G] B.2.2: 28'; ***saḫ-pu-ma*** [G] B.2.2: 24'

saḫāru G "to go around; to turn (to/around/away/back); to curve"; N "to turn back": ***as-ḫur-ka*** [G] D.3.1: 24; ***i-saḫ-ḫa-ru*** [G] C.3.9: 17; ***is-sa-ḫer*** [N] D.1.9: 26'; ***i-saḫ-ḫu-r[a]*** [G] C.3.9: 17; **NIGIN** [G] C.1.4: 38'; **NIGIN-*ma*** [G] C.3.10: 74; **NIGIN-*ra*** [G] C.3.7: 10''; ***saḫ-ru*** [G] I.1.1: 65

saḫḫu "meadow": ***sa-ḫi*** II.1.4: 54

saḫindu "yeast(?); sourdough(?)": ***sa***$^{!}$***-ḫ[i-in-du***$^{?}$***]*** B.1.2: 2'

saḫlû (a garden plant, probably garden cress): ***saḫ-le-e*** D.2.1: 9'; ***saḫ***$^{!}$***-le-e*** B.2.3: 7'; ***saḫ-l[e-e]*** A.1.4: 16'; ***[saḫ]-le-e*** A.1.4: 2'; ***saḫ-lé-e*** A.2.3: 9'; C.1.6: 10'; D.2.1: 21', 44', 55'; D.3.1: 15; E.2.6: 23'; ***saḫ-lé-[e]*** B.2.2: 18'; ***[saḫ]-lé-e*** A.2.3: 9'; ***[saḫ-l]é-e*** A.1.2: 10'; A.2.3: 15'; ***saḫ-lé-⸢e⸣*** A.2.3: 2'; ***⸢saḫ***$^{?}$***⸣-lé-e*** A.2.3: 29'''; **ZÀ.ḪI.LI** D.2.1: 5', 65'; D.3.1: 15; **ZÀ.ḪI.LI**^{sar} II.1.4: 11; D.3.1: 15

sakāpu G "to overthrow; to push away": ***i-sak***$_6$***-ki-pa*** [G] C.3.9: 19

sakikkû (a muscular illness); title of diagnostic omen series: **SA.GIG** I.1.1: 117; I.1.2: 9

sâku G/D "to pound; to pulverise": **SÚD** [G] A.1.1: 7'; A.2.1: 29', 57'''; A.2.2: 45, 50, 60, 62, 67, 79, 80; A.2.4: 14'; A.2.7: 2; B.1.1: 37; B.1.6: 8, 11, 18'; B.2.2: 23'; C.1.1: 2, 5; C.1.2: 9, 14, 18; C.1.4: 3', 25', 30', 32', 33', 34', 35', 36', 37', 40', 42', 45', 74'', 75'', 81'', 92'', 138'', 142'', 146''', 147''', 149''', 152''', 153''', 158''', 159''', 162''', 163''', 164''', 165''', 166''', 167''', 168''', 169''', 171''', 172''', 183'''; C.1.5: 4, 7, 11, 12, 13, 14, 15, 16, 17, 18, 19, 20, 21, 22, 26, 32, 38; C.1.8: 22', 51''; C.1.9: 24; C.2.2: 4, 5, 7, 8, 10, 11, 12; C.3.3: 3; D.1.1: 206, 208, 209, 210, 211, 213, 214, 215, 216, 220, 221; D.1.3: 9', 11'; D.2.1: 19', 25', 27', 30', 31', 33', 35', 42', 53', 54', 65', 66'; E.2.6: 8', 28'; **SÚD**$^{?}$ [G] C.1.8: 48''; **SÚD**$^{?!}$ [G] C.1.9: 11; **[S]ÚD** [G] B.1.6: 6; C.1.8: 50''; **[S]ÚD**$^{?}$ [G] A.1.1: 17'; A.2.2: 82; **[SÚ]D** [G] A.2.2: 58; C.1.8: 23'; **SÚ[D]** [G] A.1.4: 35''; **S[ÚD]** [G] A.1.1: 47'''; A.2.1: 59'''; C.1.5: 23, 24; **[SÚ]D**$^{?}$ [G] C.1.5: 6; C.1.9: 28; **⸢SÚD⸣** [G] A.2.2: 10; D.2.1: 51', 68'; H.1: 5; **⸢SÚD**$^{?}$**⸣** [G] D.1.3: 3'; **SÚD-*ma*** [G] A.2.5: 27''; D.1.11: 2, 9; ***ta-sà-ak*** [G] II.1.3: 44'''; ***ta-sàk*** [G] A.2.7: 20, 28', 34'; B.1.1: 33; C.1.4: 40', 125'', 150''', 156''', 157''', 160'''; C.1.5: 2; D.2.1: 3'; ***ta***$^{!}$***-sàk*** [G] C.3.5: 10'; ***[t]a-sàk*** [G] C.1.4: 161'''; ***⸢ta***$^{?}$***⸣-sàk*** [G] A.2.7: 21; ***⸢ta-sàk⸣*** [G] A.2.7: 33'; ***ta-s[ak***$_6$$^{?}$***]*** [G] II.1.3: 63'''; ***ta-sa-ka*** [G] A.2.8: 39'; ***⸢ta-sa⸣-[ka]*** [G] A.2.8: 31'; ***ta-s[a-ka***$^{?}$***]*** [G] A.2.8: 8; ***[t]a-sa-ku*** [G] A.2.2: 25; ***tu-sak*** [D] E.2.6: 28'

salāḫu G "to sprinkle (with)"; D "to sprinkle (with)": **SUD** [G] B.2.2: 19'; C.1.4: 39'; C.3.4: 25, 40; D.2.1: 49'; E.2.6: 26'; ***ta-sal-làḫ-ma*** [G] B.2.2: 19'; ***ta-sa-laḫ-ši*** [G] C.1.4: 10'; ***tu-sa-làḫ*** [D] II.1.4: 16

salāqu G "to boil": ***[t]a-sal-laq*** [G] E.2.6: 21'; ***⸢ta***$^{?}$***-sal***$^{?}$***⸣-laq*** [G] E.2.6: 23'

salātu I "relatives": ***sa-la-ti-ia*** C.3.4: 53; ***⸢sa-la⸣-[ti-ia***$_5$***]*** C.3.4: 48

salātu II G "to slit, slice through, split": ***is-li-it*** [G] E.2.6: 24'

salā'u G "to sprinkle; to infect; to be critically ill": **LÍL-*ma*** [G] E.2.6: 19'

samādu G "to grind (finely)": ***tasa-mud***$^{?}$ [G] A.2.3: 8'

samāḫu D "to mix": ***tu-sa-maḫ*** [D] II.1.4: 7; D.2.1: 35'; ***tu-sa-[ma]ḫ*** [D] A.2.4: 38'''; ***tu-sam-maḫ-ma*** [D] C.1.10: 13

samāne "eight": **8** B.1.6: 5; F.1: 34; I.1.1: 41; **⸢8⸣** F.1: 40

****samānēšeret*** "eighteen": **18** F.2: 12

samānû "eighth"; *ina samānî ūmi* "on the eighth day": **8** I.1.1: 111; **8-*i*** C.4.1: 9'; **8.KAM** I.1.3: 6; **U**$_4$**.8.KÁM** I.1.1: 111

samdu "ground": ***sa-an-du-tu*** E.2.6: 30', 33'; ***sa-an-du-tú*** E.2.6: 20'

samītu "battlement; parapet": ***sa-mit*** D.1.1: 132

sāmtu "redness; carnelian": **⸢GUG⸣** D.1.1: 1'; **G[UG**$^{?}$**]** C.1.3: 5'; ^{na4}**GUG** C.1.1: 10, 11, 13; C.1.4: 5', 40'; C.1.5: 44; C.3.3: 33; C.3.4: 74; C.3.9: 5, 55; F.1: 12, 28, 33, 36; F.2: 7; H.1: 3; ^{na4}**GUG**$^{?}$ C.2.2: 7; **[**^{n}**]**^{a4}**GUG** C.1.2: 24'; H.1:10; $^{⸢na4⸣}$**GUG** C.1.4: 185'''; **[**^{na4}**G]UG** C.1.2: 21'; ^{na4}**G[UG**$^{?}$**]** F.1: 5; $^{⸢na4}$**GUG⸣** F.1: 19; H.1: 33'; ***sa-'-mat*** C.1.4: 60''

samû G "to falter; to be inept": ***sa-ma-ta*** [G] I.1.7: 7; ***sa-mat*** [G] I.1.7: 7

sāmu "red; flushed": **SA$_5$** C.1.1: 15, 27'; C.1.4: 94'', 180'''; C.3.9: 6; D.2.1: 8'; F.1: 29, 30; F.2: 35'; H.1: 2; **S[A$_5$]** C.3.9: 30, 31; **SA$_5$.A** D.3.1: 3, 4; **SA$_5$.MEŠ** I.1.1: 7, 34, 52; **SA$_5$-*tim***$^{?!}$ F.1: 26; ***sa-mu-tú*** C.3.10: 4

sâmu G "to be red": **SA$_5$** [G] B.2.2: 16'; I.1.1: 4, 9, 18, 19, 25, 31, 45, 47, 51, 53; **S[A$_5$]** [G] A.1.1: 14'; ⸢**SA$_5$**$^?$⸣ [G] A.1.1: 23'; **SA$_5$-*at*** [G] A.2.2: 73; B.2.2: 3; **SA$_5$.DIDLI** [G] I.1.1: 13; **SA$_5$.M[EŠ]** [G] I.1.6: 21'; ***sa-a-mu*** [G] I.1.1: 100

sanāqu G "to check; to approach"; D "to check, control": **DIM$_4$** [G] C.3.4: 24; C.3.6: 15'; ⸢***i***⸣***-sa-***⸢***niq***⸣***-ši*** [G] B.1.3: 5; ***sa-an-qa-at*** [G] G.2: 18''; ⸢***sa***⸣***-an-q[a-at]*** [G] D.1.1: 83; ***sa-na-***⸢***aq***⸣ [G] C.3.6: 15'; ***sa-ni-iq*** [G] II.1.4: 36, 53; ***ú-sa-***⸢***niq***$^?$⸣ [D] E.1.3: 6'

sangû (uncertain meaning): ***sa-an-gi*** D.1.6: 5; ***sa-an-gu-u*** D.1.6: 4

sapādu G "to mourn": ***sa-ap-[du]*** [G] D.1.1: 147; ***sa-ap-du-ši*** [G] D.1.1: 147; ***sap-***⸢***du***⸣***-šú*** [G] D.1.1: 147

sapāḫu G "to scatter; to derange; to confound"; D "to scatter, disperse"; N "to be scattered, dispersed": ⸢**BIR**⸣ [N] I.1.3: 20; **BIR-*aḫ*** [G] I.1.3: 22; ***sa-ap-ḫa-at*** [G] I.1.7: 8; ***sà-pu-ḫu*** [D] II.1.4: 44; ***[s]a-pu-[ḫu]*** [D] D.1.1: 83

sapān(u), *sapannu* "soap(plant)" (an alkaline plant): ***sa-pan*** E.2.1: 4; E.2.6: 30', 43'; ⸢***sa***⸣***-[pan]*** B.2.3: 5'

sapānu G "to lay flat; to flatten; to drain(?)": ***ta-sa-pan*** [G] A.2.3: 7'; ***tas-pu-nu*** [G] A.2.3: 10'

saparru "cart": ^{giš}***sa-par-ri*** D.1.11: 13

sappartu "point, tip (of horn)": ***sap-pár-ti*** C.1.4: 111'''

sāqu "thigh (bone)": **GÌR.PAD.DU.GÍD.DA** D.2.1: 73'; **GÌR.PAD.DA.GÍ[D.DA]** D.2.1: 71'

sarāmu G "to cut open": ***ta-sar-ri-im*** [G] D.1.1: 176

sarāqu G "to strew; to scatter; to pour"; D "to strew": **DUB** [G] C.3.10: 75; **D[UB$^?$]** [G] D.1.11: 2; **DUB-*aq*** [G] A.1.4: 33''; C.1.10: 17; C.3.4: 41, 89; C.3.10: 69; **DU[B-*aq*]** [G] C.3.6: 7'; **DUB-*šú*** [G] D.1.11: 11; ***i-sar-raq*** [G] B.2.6: 6; ***ta-sa-raq*** [G] C.1.4: 15'; ***ta-sár-raq*** [G] C.1.4: 26'; D.2.1: 32'; ***tu-sar-ra-aq***$^!$ [D] C.3.4: 86

sartu, *ṣartu* "falsehood; dishonesty; crime": ***sar-tú*** I.1.1: 118; ***sar-tu$_4$*** D.1.10: 11'; ***ṣar-ti*** I.1.4: 7'

sar'u (meaning uncertain): ***sa-ra***$^?$***-'u***$^?$ A.2.3: 27'''

sasqû, *saskû* (a fine flour): **ZÌ.EŠA** C.3.4: 41, 89; C.3.6: 7'; ⸢**ZÌ.EŠA**⸣ C.3.6: 60''''

sebe "seven": **7** A.2.6: 6; B.2.1: 16; C.1.1: 15; C.1.3: 2'; C.1.4: 7', 46', 94'', 107'', 185''', 186'''; C.1.8: 35'; C.3.4: 39, 40, 42, 48; C.3.6: 56''''; C.3.9: 23; D.1.2: 7; D.1.4: 2'; E.2.6: 34'; F.1: 4, 27, 34; F.2: 2; H.1: 3, 4, 18', 24', 32', 34'; I.1.1: 40; ⸢**7**⸣ C.3.4: 49

sebîšu "seven times": **7-*šú*** II.1.3: 29'''; B.2.6: 12; C.1.1: 16; C.1.4: 93''; C.3.1: 29; C.3.4: 49, 95; D.1.1: 39, 178, 197, 201, 212; H.1: 17', 24'; ⸢**7**⸣**-*šú*** A.1.2: 6'; ⸢**7**$^?$⸣**-*šú*** C.1.4: 134''; **7-*š[ú***$^?$***]*** C.3.2: 5''; **7.TA.ÀM** C.3.6: 52''''; C.3.9: 11; F.1: 30; ⸢**7**⸣**.TA$^!$.ÀM** C.3.4: 41

sebû "seventh"; *ina sebî ūmi* "on the seventh day": **7** I.1.1: 110; **7-*i*** C.3.10: 74; C.4.1: 8'; **7-*ú*** D.1.4: 14''; **7.KAM** I.1.3: 5; **U$_4$.7.KÁM** I.1.1: 110

segû G "to roam; to wander"; Š caus. of G: ***tu-šá-as-ge-eš*** [Š] D.1.11: 10, 12; ***tu-šá-***⸢***as-ge-eš***⸣ [Š] D.1.11: 5

seḫû G (meaning uncertain): ***ta-se-ḫi*** [G] E.2.6: 24', 35'; ***te-se-eḫ-ḫi*** [G] E.2.6: 26'

sekēru G "to dam up; to close; to clog (canal); to enclose (in an oven); to heat"; Gtn iter. of G; N "to become blocked, dammed up"; Ntn iter. of N: ⸢***i***⸣***-te***$^!$***-en-né-es-ker*** [Ntn] B.1.1: 49; ***[it-te]-en-né-e[s***$^?$***-k]er*** [Ntn] B.1.1: 41; ***it-te-[es]-ki-ru*** [Ntn] D.2.1: 40'; ***li-is-ki-ru*** [G] C.1.2: 24'; ***se-kìr-ši*** [G] A.2.2: 39; ***[se-ek***$^?$***-r]a*** [G] C.1.5: 42; ***[se]k***$^?$***-re-et*** [G] C.1.8: 12'; ***s[ik***$^?$***-ru]*** [G] B.1.1: 53; ***te***$^!$***-se-kér*** [G] II.1.4: 29; **ÚŠ-*ir*** [G] D.2.1: 61'; ⸢**ÚŠ.MEŠ**⸣***-ra*** [Gtn] I.1.3: 26

semeru "ring": **ḪAR** C.3.4: 84; ***se-mer*** C.3.4: 72; ***se-me-ri*** C.3.9: 53; ***se-mé-ri*** C.3.3: 30

serdu "olive (tree)": ***sír-di*** D.3.1: 30

siāqu, *sâqu* G "to be narrow, tight": ***sa-qa-at*** [G] II.1.4: 44

sibbirru, *simbirru*, also *šibburratu* a medicinal plant, probably rue: ***si-im-bir-ri*** A.2.8: 35', 36'; ***sim-bar*** C.1.10: 6; ***sim-bir-ri*** C.1.9: 17; C.1.10: 5; ⸢^{ú}⸣***sim-bir-ri*** A.2.1: 11'; ^{ú}***sim-bi[r-ri]*** C.1.7: 7'; ⸢^{ú}⸣***sim-b[ir-ri]*** C.1.7: 9'; [$^{(ú)}$***šib-bur]-rat*** A.2.1: 86''''''

sīḫu (an aromatic plant/shrub and its resin): ^{giš}***si-ḫa*** II.1.4: 10; B.1.1: 13; C.1.4: 14'; ***si-ḫu*** A.2.1: 89''''''; ^{ú}***si-ḫa*** II.1.4: 22; ^{ú}***si-ḫu*** A.2.1: 97''''''

sikillu (a medicinal plant, lit. "pure herb", squill(?)): ^{ú}**SIKIL** D.2.1: 31'

sikkatu, *šiggatu* I "peg; nail; pock; pimple (a disease)": ***sik-kà-at*** A.2.3: 6'

sikkatu II a beer ingredient: ***sik-ka-tú*** D.2.1: 56'; ***sík-ka-tú*** B.1.2: 3'

sikkūru "(door) bolt": ^{giš}**SAG.KUL** II.1.4: 35; ***si-ku-rum*** II.1.4: 52; ***sik-kur-ru*** D.1.10: 5'

sīktu "powder": **KU** II.1.3.1: 9'; A.2.1: 26', 27'; A.2.9: 10'; A.2.10: 3'; B.1.1: 24, 25, 26, 27; B.2.5: 4, 5; C.1.6: 2'; C.1.10: 10, 12, 13; C.2.2: 5; D.2.1: 41', 50', 51', 62'; E.2.6: 9', 10', 43', 44'; ⸢**KU**⸣ II.1.3.1: 10'; A.2.2: 29; A.2.3: 4'; **[K]U** A.2.1: 28'; **KU**$^{?!}$ E.2.6: 40'; **KU$^?$.MEŠ** E.2.6: 12'; ***[si-ik***$^?$***]-ta***$^?$***-šú*** E.2.6: 11'; ***si-ik-ta-šú-nu*** E.2.6: 8'; ***si-ik-ti*** C.1.4: 39'; ***sík-te*** A.2.1: 36'

sili'tu, *silītu* "sickness; disease": **LÍL** C.3.6: 17'

silītu "placenta; afterbirth": ***[s]i-li-is-su*** A.2.1: 14'; ^{uzu}***si-lit-su*** A.2.1: 56'''; ⸢**ÙŠ**⸣***-sa*** B.1.6: 17', 19'

simdu, *sindu* (a cereal or flour): ***sim-di*** E.2.6: 33'; ***si-in-du*** E.2.1: 5

simmiltu "staircase": ***sim-mil-ti*** D.3.1: 9; ⸢***sim***⸣***-mil-ti*** D.3.1: 7

simmu "lesion": ***[s]im-mi*** I.1.3: 25

simtu "appropriate symbol; characteristic": ***si-mat*** C.3.3: 30, 32, 33; C.3.4: 72, 73, 74, 76; C.3.9: 53, 54, 55; ***si-[mat]*** C.3.3: 35

sinništu "woman; *zikar u sinniš* "male and female": **MUNUS** II.1.1: 34; II.1.3: 38''', 41''', 43''', 52'''; II.1.4: 1, 9, 15; A.1.1: 36'', 37''; A.1.2: 7'; A.1.4: 24'', 33''; A.2.1: 25', 53''', 56''', 58''', 61''', 79''''; A.2.2: 8, 11, 14, 23, 28, 29, 31, 42, 43, 47, 48, 49, 53, 56, 64, 67, 69, 74; A.2.3: 6', 28'''; A.2.4: 3', 24'', 40'''; A.2.5: 13'; A.2.6: 18, 21, 24, 25; A.2.8: 9, 13; A.2.9: 1', 12''; A.2.10: 5'; B.1.1: 20, 40, 53; B.1.2: 1', 5'; B.1.5: 2'; B.2.1: 30, 31; B.2.2: 4, 9, 14; B.2.3: 13''; B.2.6: 1; C.1.1: 4, 14; C.1.2: 26'; C.1.3: 12'; C.1.4: 4', 6', 11', 15', 17', 21', 22', 26', 63'', 73'', 80'', 86'', 137'', 141'', 154''', 174'''; C.1.4.1: 3'; C.1.8: 13', 32'; C.1.10: 1, 7, 17; C.2.1: 14'; C.2.2: 2; C.2.3: 2', 20', 24'; C.3.1: 7, 29; C.3.3: 7; C.3.4: 1, 9, 23, 59; C.3.5: 10'; C.3.6: 29', 55''''; 57''''; C.3.9: 2; C.3.10: 62, 85, 90; D.1.1: 134, 205, 221; D.1.3: 29''; D.1.4: 2'; D.1.5: 5'; D.1.6: 14; D.1.7: 12'; D.1.8: 23; D.1.11: 1, 14'; D.2.1: 4', 17', 18', 20', 25', 26', 28', 29', 30', 33', 34', 39', 40', 59', 65', 67', 69', 70', 71'; D.3.1: 1, 5, 28; E.2.1: 15; E.2.2: 1'; E.2.3: 7', 9'; E.2.4: 11''; E.2.6: 25'; E.2.8: 3'; F.1: 28, 34, 37; H.1: 1, 22', 31'; I.1.1: 2, 3, 10, 11, 23, 25, 29, 46, 48, 49, 52, 64, 67, 68, 70, 73, 75, 90, 95, 97, 114, 115; I.1.2: 5', 8'; I.1.3: 1, 2, 3, 4, 5, 6, 7, 8, 9, 10, 11, 12, 13, 14, 15, 16, 17, 18, 30'; I.1.5: 4', 10'; I.1.6: 7', 8', 9', 10', 12', 13', 14', 15', 18', 19', 20', 21', 22', 23', 24', 25', 26', 27', 28', 31', 32', 33', 34', 35', 36', 37', 38'; I.1.6: 26'; **MUNUS$^?$** C.1.9: 21; G.2: 20''; **[M]UNUS** C.1.4:

124''; ⸢**MUNUS**⸣ A.1.1: 2'; A.2.1: 91'''''; A.2.2: 50, 70, 72; A.2.8: 28'; B.2.1: 33; C.1.8: 21'; C.3.10: 75; D.2.1: 57'; E.2.3: 28''; F.1: 32; I.1.1: 14; I.1.6: 2', 3', 4', 6'; ⸢**MUNUS**$^{?}$⸣ A.1.2: 15'; D.1.11: 1; **MUNUS**$^{!}$ A.1.2: 4'; **MUN[US]** C.1.4: 65''; **MU[NUS]** A.2.1: 52'''; B.2.1: 32; D.1.5: 1'; I.1.3: 20, 21, 22, 23; I.1.6: 11'; **[MU]NUS** I.1.6: 29'; **[MUN]US** A.2.2: 73; A.2.7: 16; C.1.8: 15'; D.3.1: 16; I.1.6: 39'; **[MUNU]S** D.1.11: 3; I.1.6: 16', 17'; **[MUNU]S**$^{?}$ C.1.1: 1; **MUNUS.ME** I.1.1: 115; **MUNUS.MEŠ** A.2.2: 69; I.1.6: 30'; ⸢**MUNUS.MEŠ**$^{?}$⸣ A.2.2: 67; ***sin-niš-ti*** G.1: 34, 41; ***sin-niš-***⸢***ti***$^{?}$⸣ D.1.1: 85; ***sin-niš-tì*** G.1: 8, 11; ^{munus}***sin-niš-tú*** C.3.10: 56, 59; ^{munus}***sin-[niš-tu***$_4$***]*** C.3.10: 48; ^{munus}***sin-niš-t[u***$_4$***]*** C.3.10: 54; ***sin-niš-tú*** D.1.8: 16; ***sin-niš-tu***$_4$ C.3.10: 1; ⸢***sin-niš***⸣***-tu***$_4$ D.1.8: 14

siparru "bronze": **ZABAR** A.2.2: 45; C.1.4: 157'''; C.3.4: 84; C.3.9: 28; H.1: 33'

sīrāšû "brewer": ^{lú}**LUNGA** I.1.1: 118

sissiktu "(garment) hem": ^{túg}**SÍG-*ka*** D.3.1: 24

sisû "horse": **ANŠE.KUR.RA** H.1: 24'

suādu (an aromatic plant, probably yellow nutsedge, *Cyperus esculentus*): ^{giš}**MAN.DU** D.2.1: 47', 54', 56'; ^{šim}**MAN.DU** B.1.2: 2'; ⸢^{šim}**MAN.DU**⸣ C.2.3: 21'; ^{ú}**MAN**$^{?}$**.D[U**$^{?}$**]** A.1.1: 40''

sugbanda (Sum. loanword) lit. "little marsh": ***sug-bàn***$^{!}$***-***⸢***da***$^{?}$⸣ B.1.1: 11

sugullu, *sukullu* "herd; cattle": ***su-ku-li-ša*** D.1.1: 139; ***su-kul-lim*** D.1.1: 139

sukanninu "turtledove": **TU.KUR**$_4$^{mušen} C.1.4: 35'

sukkuku "deaf; mentally handicapped": ***šuk-ku-ku*** I.1.1: 61

suluppū "date(s)": **[**^{gi}**]**$^{š?}$**ZÚ.LUM.MA** A.2.5: 19''; **ZÚ.LUM** C.1.4: 25'; C.3.9: 4; **<ZÚ>.LUM** C.3.9: 9; **ZÚ.LUM.MA** A.1.4: 11'; A.2.5: 20''; A.2.8: 8; C.3.4: 41, 89; C.3.6: 7'; D.1.11: 11; D.2.1: 7', 23', 36'; **ZÚ.L[UM.MA]** E.2.8: 9''

summatu "dove": **TU**^{mušen} C.1.4: 34'; C.1.5: 11; D.2.1: 51'; **TU**$^{muš[en]}$ D.1.7: 8'; **TU**$^{m[ušen]}$ A.2.1: 80'''''; **[TU**$^{?m}$**]**^{ušen} C.1.5: 7; **TU**^{mušen}**.MEŠ** D.2.1: 42'

summunu "one-eighth"; one eighth of a *qû*-measure: ***su-u[m-m]u-nu*** E.2.1: 8

sunābu, *sunāpu* "loincloth": ***sun-*BAR*-ša*** A.2.2: 38

sunqu "famine": ***su-un-qam*** I.1.1: 114

sūnu "lap": ***su-un*** G.2: 20''; ***sú-un-šá*** D.2.1: 57'; **ÚR-*šá*** C.3.4: 13

supantu, *supandu* "powder": **KU.KU** C.1.4: 113''; C.1.5: 33, 34; C.1.8: 24'; **K[U**$^{?}$**.K]U**$^{?}$ A.2.5: 9'

supūru "sheepfold": ***sú-ú-pu***$^{!}$***-ur*** D.1.1: 24

sūq erbetti "crossroads": **E.SÍR.KA.LÍMMU** C.1.4: 9'; **E.SÍR.K[A.LÍMMU]** C.1.4: 99''; **[E.SÍR.KA.LÍM]MU** C.1.4: 102''; ⸢**E**⸣**.[SÍR].**⸢**KA.LÍMMU-*te***$^{?}$ F.1: 20; **SILA.LÍM.MA** A.2.2: 37; C.1.8: 17'; C.3.3: 5; C.3.4: 58, 97; C.3.10: 76, 81, 83, 88; D.1.1: 173; F.1: 30; **SI[LA.LÍM.MA**$^{?}$**]** A.1.1: 19'; **[SI]LA.LÍM.MA** F.1: 20; ⸢**SILA**⸣**.LÍM.MA** D.1.1: 38; **SILA.LÍMMU** C.1.4: 180'''; **SILA.LÍMMU.BA** F.2: 31'; **[SILA**$^{?}$**.LÍMMU]-*te***$^{?}$ F.1: 30; **SILA.LÍMMU-*ti*** C.3.1: 6

sūqu "street": **SILA** C.3.4: 22, 23; C.3.6: 5'; C.3.9: 18; C.3.10: 82, 84, 90; ⸢**SILA**⸣ C.3.4: 19; C.3.8: 13; **SILA.MEŠ** C.3.9: 18

sūtu "seah container": ^{dug}**BÁN** II.1.4: 28; ^{giš}**BÁN** C.3.6: 50''''

ṣabāru G "to bend; twist": ***taṣ-bu-ru*** [G] C.3.4: 45

ṣabātu G "to seize; to take"; Gtn iter. of G; D "to enclose, bind, set; to fasten"; Š "to cause to seize/take": ***aṣ-bat*** [G] D.3.1: 24; **DAB** [G] A.2.2: 47; D.2.1: 28'; **DAB-*bat*** [D?] C.3.9: 38, 40; D.1.4: 15''; F.1: 30; **DAB**$^{?}$**-*b[at***$^{?}$***]*** [D?] F.1: 25; **DAB.DAB** [D] I.1.1: 50; **DAB.DAB-*si*** [Gtn] I.1.3: 11, 12, 13; **DAB-*si*** [G] D.2.1: 18', 36'; I.1.3: 6; **DAB-*si*** [Š] C.3.10: 80; **D[AB-*si***$^{?}$**]** [G] I.1.4: 7'; **[DAB**$^{?}$**-*s]i*** [G] I.1.3: 21, 22; **DAB-*su*** [G] I.1.1: 111; **DAB-**⸢***su***⸣ [G] C.3.4: 38; **DAB-*ši*** [G] A.1.3: 6'; ***iṣ-b[a***$^{?}$***-a]s***$^{?}$***-su*** [G] B.2.2: 6; ***[iṣ-ba]t***$^{?}$ D.1.1: 25; ***iṣ-bat-ka*** [G] C.3.1: 15; ***ṣa-bat*** [G] D.3.1: 38(A); ***ṣa-bit*** [G] I.1.3: 18; ***ul-ta-aṣ-bi-si*** [Š] D.1.1: 139; ***ú-ṣa-***⸢***bi-ta***⸣***-ši*** [D] I.1.3: 20; ***uš-te-eṣ-bi-is-si-ma*** [Š] D.1.1: 139

ṣabbaru "sheaf(?)": ***ṣab-bar*** C.3.10: 88

ṣabītu "gazelle": **MAŠ.DÀ** B.1.5: 6'; C.1.3: 7'; C.1.4: 6'; C.3.3: 12; C.3.6: 52''''; D.1.1: 45, 194; G.1: 29; **M[AŠ.DÀ]** C.1.5: 30; ***ṣa-bi-ti*** D.1.1: 45; ***ṣa-bi-tim*** C.3.5: 24'; ***ṣa-bi-tu***$_4$ G.1: 28

ṣabtu "seized (one)": ***ṣab-ta*** D.3.1: 20; ***ṣab-tu*** D.3.1: 20

ṣabû, *ṣapû* G "to soak; to drench; D "to soak; to bathe; to irrigate (field)": ***[t]u-ṣa-ab-ba-ma*** [D] B.1.1: 30

ṣadānu (a fruit-bearing bush): ^{giš}***ṣa-da-ni*** C.1.4: 176'''

ṣadāru G "to be (placed) askew"; D "to twitch": ***ṣu-un-du-ru*** [D] I.1.7: 12

ṣaḫātu G "to press out; to squeeze": **SUR-*at*** [G] B.2.4: 3'; ***ta-ṣa-ḫat*** [G] E.2.6: 8'; ⸢***ta***⸣***-ṣáḫ-***⸢***ḫat***⸣ [G] B.2.3: 3'

ṣāḫitu "oil presser": ^{lú}**Ì.SUR** G.1: 32

ṣaḫtu "pressed": **SUR.RA** A.2.2: 44; D.2.1: 6'

ṣâḫu, *ṣiāḫu* G "to laugh; cry"; Gtn iter. of G: ***iṣ-ṣe-né-eḫ*** [Gtn] A.1.3: 5'

ṣalālu G "to lie (asleep); to sleep": **NÁ** [G] I.1.1: 5; ***ṣa-la-la*** [G] C.3.10: 34; ⸢***ṣal-la***⸣***-a-t[a]*** [G] C.3.3: 12; ***ṣal-la-ta*** [G] C.3.4: 61

ṣalāmu G "to be(come) dark/black"; D "to blacken; to darken": **GI**$_6$ [G] I.1.1: 3, 16, 17, 28, 46, 48; I.1.3: 24, 31'; ⸢**GI**$_6$⸣ [G] A.2.8: 9; ***tu-ṣa-lam*** [D] C.3.6: 35''

ṣalā'u G "to throw, lay (down); to lie; to miscarry, abort (a foetus)": ***ṣa-la-at*** [G] II.1.4: 40; ***[ṣa]-***⸢***lat***$^{?}$⸣ [G] D.1.1: 80; ***ṣal-tu***$_4$ [G] D.1.10: 4'

ṣālilu "sleeping; one who sleeps": **NÁ** I.1.1: 94

ṣallālû "sleepy": ***ṣal-la-li-i*** C.3.5: 24'

ṣallūtu "(state of) sleep": ***ṣal-lu-ti-šú*** A.2.2: 48

ṣalmāt qaqqadi "black-headed ones": ***ṣal-mat qaq-qa-du*** D.1.8: 13

ṣalmu I "figurine; image": **NU** C.3.4: 13, 39, 47, 48, 95; C.3.10: 89, 90; **NU**$^{!}$ E.2.3: 6'; **NU.MEŠ** C.3.4: 48

ṣalmu II "black; dark": **GI**$_6$ A.2.6: 3, 19; C.1.4: 109'', 164'''; C.2.2: 12; C.3.9: 8; D.1.1: 231; E.2.5: 10'; F.1: 30; F.2: 35'; ⸢**GI**$_6$$^{?!}$⸣ F.1: 26; **GI**$_6$**.MEŠ** I.1.1: 35, 53; ***ṣa-a[l-m]u***$^{?}$ B.1.1: 35

ṣamādu G "to bind; to harness; to tie on (bandage); attach; apply"; Gtn iter. of G: **LÁ** [G] C.1.4.2: 3', 4'; D.1.7: 11'; D.2.1: 51'; **LÁ-*id*** [G] D.2.1: 32', 63'; **LÁ-*id-ma*** [G] A.2.1: 37'; **L[Á**$^{?}$**-*i]d***$^{?}$***-ma*** [G] A.2.1: 29'; **LÁ-*ma*** [G] D.2.1: 25'; **LÁ-*si*** [G] D.2.1: 18'; **LÁL-*id-ma*** [G] II.1.4: 31; ***[t]a-aṣ-ṣa-mid*** [G$^{!}$] A.2.1: 33'; ***ta-ṣa-m[id]*** [G] D.3.1: 5; ***[t]a-ṣa-***⸢***na***⸣***-mi-id-m[a]*** [Gtn] II.1.3.1: 3'

ṣânu, *ṣênu* G "to fill up; to bloat": ***⸢i$^{?}$⸣-ṣa-nu*** [G] B.1.1: 43; ***ṣa-na*** [G] G.1: 2; ***ṣa-na-at*** [G] G.1: 1; ***⸢ṣe-en⸣*** H.1: 39'

ṣapāru, *ṣepēru* G "to press down; to be flat, depressed; to strand, plait (hair, linen)": ***ṣa-pa-ru*** [G] I.1.7: 12, 13; ***ṣa-pir*** [G] I.1.1: 15; I.1.7: 11; ***ta-ṣa-pir*** [G] H.1: 23'; ***ta-ṣap-pir*** [G] H.1: 23'

ṣapû G/D "to soak; to drench": ***⸢tu-ṣap⸣-p[a$^{?}$]*** [D] A.2.5: 28''

ṣarbatu "(Euphrates) poplar": ^{giš}**ÁSAL** C.1.4: 113'', 154'''; ^{giš}**ÁS[AL]** C.1.4: 166'''; C.1.10: 13; ***ṣar-bat*** A.2.2: 43; A.2.5: 9'; ***[^{giš}ṣar-ba]-ti*** II.1.3: 32'''

ṣarḫu "burning": **ÚḪ** I.1.3: 8

ṣarpu "burned; fired; baked": **[A]L.ŠEG$_{6}$.GÁ** D.1.2: 7

ṣaṣumtu, *ṣaṣuntu* (a medicinal plant): ***^{ú}ṣa-ṣu-um-tú*** D.1.1: 235; ***^{ú}ṣa-ṣu-un-tu*** B.1.1: 35; ***^{ú}ṣa-ṣu-un-tú*** C.2.1: 13'; ***^{ú}[ṣ]a-ṣu-un-tú*** D.1.1: 235; ***^{ú}ṣa-ṣu-tú*** D.1.1: 235

ṣeḫēru G "to be small, young": **TUR** [G] I.1.2: 5'; **TUR.MEŠ** [G] I.1.1: 99

ṣeḫru, fem. *ṣeḫertu* "little; young; child; infant": **LÚ.TUR** C.3.4: 5, 25, 36; C.4.1: 2'; D.1.1: 231, 233; **LÚ$^{?}$.TUR** D.1.7: 30'; **LÚ.TU[R]** C.3.4: 36; **[LÚ.TU]R$^{?}$** D.1.1: 43; **MUNUS.TUR** C.3.10: 89; ***ṣa-ḫar*** G.1: 9, 10, 51; ***ṣa-aḫ-ri*** G.1: 9; **TUR** I.1.1: 118

ṣemēru G "to be swollen, bloated": ***ṣe-em-rat*** [G] D.2.1: 26'

ṣēnu "flock; sheep (and goats)": **⸢U$_{8}$$^{?}$⸣.[UDU.ḪI].⸢A$^{?!}$⸣** A.2.3: 27'''

ṣerḫu "feverish heat": ***[ṣer$^{?}$]-ḫi*** E.2.6: 19'

ṣerpu "fired (clay)": ***ṣe-er-pi*** B.2.1: 37

ṣerrāniš "like a snake": ***ṣe-ra-niš*** C.3.4: 66; C.3.9: 45; ***[ṣ]e-ra-niš*** C.3.3: 21

ṣerri karāni "(grape)vine snake": **MUŠ** ***ka-r[a-ni-im$^{?}$]*** II.1.1: 33

ṣerru "snake": **MUŠ** D.1.1: 35, 171

ṣēru "back; steppe; wilderness": **EDIN** C.3.10: 74; **[ED]IN** A.2.7: 37'; **EDIN-*ia*** C.3.10: 35; **EDIN.NA** A.1.1: 21'; ***ṣe-ri*** D.1.1: 93

ṣētu "bright (sun)light; heat; open air; weather": **UD.DA** E.2.3: 7'

ṣiātu, *ṣâtu* "distant time"; commentary (on words of an excerpted text)": ***ṣa-a-ti*** G.1: 52

ṣibtu "seizure": **DAB-*it*** I.1.3: 11, 12, 13; **DAB-*sa*** I.1.3: 11, 12

ṣidītu "travel provisions": ***ṣi-di-is-su*** C.3.3: 29; ***ṣi-di-is-[su]*** C.3.4: 71; ***ṣi-di-is$^{!}$-su*** C.3.9: 52

ṣillatu see *išqillatu*

ṣillu "shade": **GISSU** C.3.4: 96; ***ṣil-lu*** A.2.2: 79

ṣimdu "binding; bandage": ***[ṣ]i-im-⸢du⸣*** B.1.1: 74

ṣīru "exalted; supreme": **⸢MAḪ$^{?}$⸣-*ti*** E.2.3: 15'; ***ṣi-rim*** D.1.8: 12; ***ṣ[i-r]im*** D.1.8: 13; ***ṣir-tu$_{4}$*** D.1.9: 9'

ṣīt šamši "sunrise; east": ^{d}**UTU.È** C.1.8: 37'; **[^{d}U]TU.È** E.2.3: 2'

ṣītu "exit; loss; sprouting": **ZI.GA** C.3.4: 37; ***⸢ṣi⸣-it*** C.3.10: 35

ṣubātu "garment; textile; cortex(?) of the date palm": ***ṣu-ba-tú*** D.1.9: 18'; **TÚG** H.1: 23'; **TÚG-*sa*** I.1.3: 12; **TÚG-*su*** C.3.10: 10, 11

ṣulû, *ṣullû* "supplication; prayer": ***ṣu-le-e*** G.1: 5, 6

ṣulūlu "protection; aegis": ***ṣu-lu-lu*** D.1.8: 4

ṣumlalû (a spice and aromatic plant): **⸢^{giš}GAM⸣.[MA$^{?}$]** A.1.1: 29''**GAM.M[A]** II.1.3.1: 10'; A.2.5: 22''; **⸢GAM⸣.M[A$^{?}$]** E.2.2: 8'; **GAM$^{!}$.<MA>** E.2.6: 43'; ^{šim}**GAM.MA** B.1.1: 27; C.1.10: 5; **[^{šim}G]AM.M[A]** C.2.3: 1'; ^{šim}**GAM.ME** II.1.4: 4, 21

ṣurāru "lizard"; *ṣurār igāri* "wall-lizard": **EME.DIR** C.1.4: 151'''; **EME.DIR IZ.ZI** B.1.6: 8; D.1.3: 11'; **[EME.D]IR IZ.ZI** B.1.6: 2; D.1.1: 208

ṣurrānītu (a stone): ^{na4}**GUG.ZÚ** C.1.4: 40'

ṣurru "obsidian; flint": ^{na4}**ZÚ** A.2.6: 15; F.1: 1, 12, 15, 30, 37; F.2: 11; ^{na4}**Z[Ú]** F.2: 1; **ZÚ** C.3.9: 1, 10

ša "of; that; which; who; what": ***ša*** II.1.1: 29, 34; II.1.4: 50, 61; A.2.7: 31', 40'; B.2.1: 11, 15, 30, 34, 38; C.1.4: 17', 20', 21', 38', 57'', 62'', 63'', 73'', 80'', 94'', 105'', 107'', 124'', 137'', 141'', 175''', 180''', 185'''; C.1.8: 31'; C.2.1: 12'; C.3.1: 7; C.3.4: 45; C.3.5: 13'; C.3.6: 10', 12', 13', 14', 34''; C.3.9: 22; D.1.1: 117, 118, 129, 142; D.1.5: 11', 12', 18'; D.2.1: 61'; D.3.1: 2, 37(f); F.1: 11, 14; F.2: 39'; I.1.1: 87, 88, 108, 109, 110, 111, 112, 113; I.1.3: 2, 3, 4, 5, 6, 7; ***ša$^{!}$*** C.1.4: 64''; ***ša$^{?!}$*** E.2.6: 3'; ***⸢ša⸣*** C.3.6: 42'''; D.1.11: 1; I.1.1: 107; ***š[a]*** C.1.4: 86''; ***[š]a*** B.1.1: 22; C.1.4: 91''; I.1.1: 106; ***š[a$^{?}$]*** C.1.4: 133''; C.3.6: 11'; ***šá*** II.1.3: 33'''; II.1.4: 51; A.1.1: 48'''; A.1.4: 27'', 35''; A.2.1: 5', 10', 13', 15', 48'', 52''', 53''', 63''', 71'''', 91''''''; A.2.2: 11, 13, 18, 23, 29, 30, 40, 50, 53, 59, 63, 76, 84; A.2.3: 3', 5', 6', 10', 11', 12', 27''', 28'''; A.2.4: 4', 9', 10', 44'''; A.2.5: 4', 5', 6', 7', 8', 26''; A.2.6: 1, 3, 11, 13, 17, 18, 21, 24, 25, 28; A.2.7: 26', 28'; A.2.8: 4, 13, 36', 38', 40'; A.2.10: 2', 4', 11''; B.1.1: 11, 31, 53; B.1.5: 2'; B.2.2: 21', 24', 25', 28'; B.2.3: 7', 15'', 17''; B.2.4: 4', 8', 10', 26'; B.2.5: 2, 7; B.2.6: 24; C.1.3: 2', 12'; C.1.4: 6', 46', 54'', 58'', 59'', 60'', 63'', 155''', 185'''; C.1.8: 16', 29'; C.1.9: 1, 3; C.1.10: 2, 5, 6, 7, 8, 9, 10, 13, 14, 15, 17; C.2.1: 16'; C.2.2: 13; C.2.3: 3'; C.3.3: 12, 29, 30, 31, 33, 34; C.3.4: 15, 44, 45, 48, 71, 72, 73, 74, 75, 92, 94, 100; C.3.5: 2', 3'; C.3.6: 56''''; C.3.9: 6, 7, 10, 11, 15, 20, 21, 22, 23, 28, 30, 31, 37, 38, 40, 52, 53, 54, 55, 56; C.3.10: 1, 14, 22, 23, 24, 27, 30, 31, 41, 42, 43, 44, 45, 48, 49, 55, 65; C.4.1: 2'; D.1.1: 52, 54, 95, 117, 118, 128, 129, 135, 138, 152, 164, 170, 181, 196, 200, 208, 211, 224, 226, 227; D.1.4: 4'; D.1.5: 2'; D.1.6: 4, 5, 14; D.1.8: 12, 17; D.1.9: 6', 8'; D.1.10: 7'; D.1.11: 1, 2, 3, 6, 10, 12, 14'; D.2.1: 10', 12', 16', 18', 40'; D.3.1: 1, 2, 5, 6, 6a, 11b, 22, 31, 38(A); E.2.1: 15; E.2.3: 6', 7', 22'', 23'', 24''; E.2.5: 10'; E.2.6: 2', 5', 6', 11', 14', 15', 16', 18', 21', 22', 23', 24', 26', 29', 31', 34', 36', 37', 38', 40'; E.2.8: 3'; F.1: 4, 7, 8, 14, 17, 27, 30, 31, 32, 35, 38; F.2: 34', 38'; G.1: 1, 5, 7, 10, 12, 13, 19, 20, 30, 32, 36, 38, 39, 41, 47, 50, 52, 54; G.2: 5'; H.1: 3, 6, 23', 32'; H.2: 4; I.1.2: 1', 7', 8', 13'; I.1.3: 1, 8, 35'; I.1.5: 7'; I.1.6: 23'; I.1.7: 9', 10', 11', 17'; ***⸢šá⸣*** C.3.4: 61, 91; E.2.3: 28''; G.2: 4', 11', 16'', 18'', 27'', 30''; ***[š]á*** E.1.3: 4'; ***[š]á$^{?}$*** C.3.4: 52; ***⸢šá$^{?}$⸣*** A.2.6: 14; B.1.1: 59; C.1.3: 1'; C.3.4: 51a; C.3.10: 53; ***⸢šá$^{?!}$⸣*** C.3.3: 44

šabāšu, *šabāsu* G "to gather": ***ta-šab-bu-uš*** [G] D.1.1: 223

šabāṭu G "to beat; to sweep (away)": ***iš$^{?}$-biṭ*** [G] A.2.9: 5'; ***iš-biṭ-ma*** [G] A.1.2: 8'; D.2.1: 20'; **SAR** [G] C.3.4: 25, 40, 88; E.2.3: 2'; ***ta-ša-biṭ*** [G] C.1.4: 10'

šabsû "male midwife; accoucheur": ***šab-sa-ku*** D.1.1: 195; ***⸢šab-sa-ku⸣*** D.1.1: 47

šabsūtu "midwife": ^{munus}**ŠÀ.ZU** A.2.5: 1'; B.2.2: 21'; D.1.11: 6; ***šab-su-ta-šá-ma*** D.1.1: 199; ***šab-su-tu$_{4}$*** D.1.1: 160; ***šab-šu-tu$_{4}$*** D.1.1: 160

šadādu G "to stretch; to draw (curtain); to drag off; to move away": ***i-šad-da-ad-ma*** [G] D.3.1: 9; ***šad-du*** [G] I.1.7: 8

šadânu "haematite": **KA.GI** A.2.7: 31'; ^{na4}**KA.G[I.NA]** C.1.1: 18; **KUR-*ni*** F.2: 18, 19; **KUR-*nu*** F.1: 18

šadânu ṣābitu "magnetite": **^{na4}KA.GI.NA DAB.BA** C.1.4: 44', 138''; **^{na4}KA.GI.NA DAB.B[A]** C.3.5: 8'; **^{na4}KA.GI.NA ⸢DAB.BA⸣** C.1.4: 2'; **^{na4}KUR-*nu* DAB** A.2.1: 20'; A.2.2: 38, 56; C.1.5: 32, 33; C.1.8: 24'; C.1.9: 7; C.2.2: 12; C.3.3: 2; C.3.9: 9; **^{na4}KUR-*nu* [DAB]** E.1.1: 6; **[^{n}]^{a4}KUR-*nu* DAB** C.1.1: 2; C.1.8: 22'; **[^{na4}KU]R-*nu* DAB** C.1.5: 38; **⸢^{na4}KUR⸣-*nu* DAB** C.1.10: 17; **[^{na4}]KUR$^{!}$-*nu* DAB** C.1.9: 2; **[^{n}]^{a4}KUR-*nu* D[AB]** C.1.9: 29; **^{na4}KUR-*nu* DAB.BA** C.3.1: 5; **^{na4}*šá-da-nu* DAB.BA** C.3.10: 3

šadû "mountain(s)": **KUR** A.2.2: 13; A.2.7: 35'; B.2.1: 15; C.3.4: 15; H.1: 6; **KUR-*e*** B.1.1: 31; **KUR-⸢*e*⸣** B.1.1: 37; **KUR-*i*** C.1.4: 180'''; **K[UR.RA]** H.2: 3; ***šá-da-a*** H.1: 33'; ***šá-du-u*** D.1.8: 7

šagāšu G "to kill; to murder": ***i-šag-gi-šá*** [G] C.3.9: 19; ***i-šag-gi-šú*** [G] C.3.9: 19

šaḫāḫu G "to become loose; to fall out": ***i-šaḫ-ḫu-uḫ*** [G] H.1: 22'

šaḫālu G "to sieve; to filter": ***ta-šá-ḫal*** [G] II.1.4: 24; D.1.7: 18'; D.2.1: 19'; ***[ta]-⸢šá-ḫal⸣*** [G] A.2.4: 21'; ***[ta]-⸢šá$^{?}$⸣-ḫal*** [G] C.2.3: 17'; ***ta-šá-ḫal-ma*** [G] D.1.11: 9

šaḫarru "porous": **SÁḪAR** A.2.2: 30; B.2.1: 18; C.1.4: 168'''; C.1.10: 14; C.3.4: 95; **SÁḪAR.MEŠ** C.3.4: 42; **SÁḪAR-*ra*** C.1.4: 112''

šaḫāru D "to heat(?)": ***tu-šaḫ-ḫi-ru*** [D] E.2.6: 14'

šaḫātu G "to wash; to rinse (off)"; D "to rinse off": ***uš-taḫ-ḫi-it*** [D] C.3.10: 22, 23, 24

šaḫāṭu I G "to jump; to attack; to escape; to mount"; D "to attack": ***il-[ta-ḫi-iṭ]*** [G] D.1.1: 144; ***il-ti-ki-iṭ*** [G] II.1.4: 55; ***iš-ta-ḫi-iṭ*** [G] D.1.1: 144; ***šá-ḫa-ṭu*** [G] G.1: 26; ***ú-šá-[aḫ-ḫi-iṭ$^{?}$]*** [D] C.3.1: 10

šaḫāṭu II G "to strip off; to remove": ***i-šaḫ-ḫaṭ-ma*** [G] C.3.10: 10; ***⸢iš-ḫu⸣-ṭu*** [G] G.2: 19''

šaḫittu "verdigris; patina(?)": ***ša-ḫi-it-tu$_4$*** B.2.4: 15'; ***⸢šá$^{?}$⸣-ḫi-tú*** E.2.4: 5'

šaḫû "pig": **ŠAḪ** D.1.1: 218, 231, 235

šakāku G/D "to harrow; to thread on a string": **È** [G] B.1.4: 16; C.3.6: 57''''; C.3.9: 1, 6; D.1.4: 11''; F.1: 6, 17, 24, 29, 30, 34, 38; **⸢È⸣** [G] F.1: 13; **È-*ak*** [G] C.1.4: 7', 47'; C.1.8: 3'; C.3.9: 8, 10; D.3.1: 3; F.1: 38; **È-*a[k]*** [G] C.1.3: 8'; D.3.1: 4; **È-⸢*ak*$^{?}$⸣** [G] F.1: 10, 34; **È-*ma*** [G] C.3.9: 31, 33, 34, 35; **GIŠ.ÙR$^{!}$.MEŠ** [D$^{?}$] II.1.4: 39; ***ta-šak-kak*** [G] C.3.10: 4; ***tu-šá-kak*** [D] C.1.4: 186'''

šakānu G "to place; to put; to set up; to provide with; to cause"; Gtn iter. of G; N "to be placed; to be equipped (with); to be inflicted": ***áš-šak-ka-na-ki-na-šim-ma*** [N] C.3.9: 20; **GAR** [G] A.2.2: 38; B.2.2: 8, 10; C.1.4: 35', 36', 39'; C.1.7: 6'; C.1.9: 3; C.3.4: 3, 90; D.2.1: 67'; D.3.1: 16; E.2.4: 7', 8'; **⸢GAR$^{?}$⸣** [G] B.1.5: 5'; **GA[R]** [G] C.1.7: 8'; **GAR-*an*** [G] A.1.1: 23'; A.1.4: 39''; A.2.3: 21''; A.2.2: 55, 58, 69; B.1.4: 17; B.2.2: 2, 20'; B.2.6: 7; C.1.1: 6, 9; C.1.4: 13', 25', 33', 41', 43', 45', 138'', 147''', 152''', 155''', 160''', 161'''; C.1.5: 36, 38, 40; C.1.7: 5'; C.1.8: 23'; C.3.4: 3, 6, 41, 42, 87; C.3.6: 9', 51'''', 59''''; C.3.7: 20''; C.3.9: 2, 10, 29, 42; C.3.10: 62, 76, 79, 81; D.1.1: 232; D.2.1: 49', 53', 54', 64', 65', 68', 74'; D.3.1: 3, 8, 16; E.2.5: 7'; E.2.6: 13', 21'; E.2.7: 5'; F.1: 11, 31; I.1.4: 5'; **GAR-*an*$^{?}$** [G] C.1.5: 45; **GAR-⸢*an*⸣** [G] F.1: 14; **⸢GAR⸣-*an*** [G] A.1.4: 25''; C.3.6: 60''''; **⸢GAR-*an*⸣** [G] A.2.2: 47, 57; A.2.3: 23'''; **⸢GAR$^{?}$-*an*⸣** [G] C.3.4: 49; **[GA]R$^{?}$-*an*** [G] II.1.3: 59'''; **⸢GAR⸣-*a[n]*** F.1: 17; **G[AR]-*a[n]*** [G] C.3.4: 90; **[GAR]-*an*** [G] A.1.4: 36''; C.3.6: 49''''; E.2.7: 20''; **GAR-*a[n]*** [G] C.1.2: 19; C.3.6: 8'; **GAR-*an-ma*** [G] A.2.1: 19'; C.1.2: 17; C.1.4: 178'''; C.3.4: 13, 14; C.3.10: 83, 88; **GAR-*an-m[a]*** [G] II.1.3: 34'''; C.3.5: 3'; **GAR-⸢*an*⸣-*ma*$^{!}$** [G] A.2.2: 68; **GAR-*a[n-ma]*** [G] C.1.4: 23'; **GAR-*[an-ma]*** [G] A.2.2: 77; **GAR-*a[n-(ma)]*** [G] C.2.3: 7'; **GAR-*an-ši*** [G] C.1.4: 10', 11'; C.3.5: 6'; **[GAR]-*an-ši*$^{!}$** [G] C.3.4: 4; **GAR-*an-š[i]*** [G] C.3.7: 13''; **GAR-*an-[ši]*** [G] C.3.5: 1', 14'; **GAR-*an-šú*** [G] C.3.4: 84, 96; **GAR.GAR-*ma*** [Gtn] II.1.4: 12; **GAR-*ma*** [G] A.1.1: 21'; A.2.1: 17', 86''''''; A.2.2: 29, 77, 79; B.1.1: 38; C.1.5: 3; C.1.8: 11'; C.1.9: 5, 9, 14, 25; C.2.3: 6'; C.3.4: 19, 22, 95; C.3.10: 77; D.1.1: 232; D.1.7: 20'; D.2.1: 9'; **GAR-*m[a]*** [G] A.2.5: 16''; **⸢GAR-*ma*⸣** [G] A.2.2: 71; **⸢GAR$^{?}$-*ma*⸣** [G] A.2.1: 92''''''; **[GA]R$^{?}$-*ma*** [G] A.2.3: 11'; **[GAR$^{?}$]-*ma*** [G] C.3.4: 47; **GAR-*na-ma*** [G] I.1.3: 10; **GAR-*ni*** [G] D.1.3: 7'; **GAR-*nu*** [G] A.1.1: 8'; C.1.8: 27'; G.2: 5'; I.1.1: 61; **⸢GAR-*nu*$^{?}$⸣** D.1.1: 15; **GAR-*ši*** [N] I.1.3: 31'; **GAR-*šú*** [G] C.3.4: 37; **GAR-*š[ú$^{?}$]*** [G] D.1.3: 33''; ***i-šak-kan*** [G] G.1: 20; ***il-ta-kan*** [G] D.1.1: 157; ***[i]š-ku-na$^{?}$*** [G] D.1.10: 2'; ***iš-kun*** [G] D.1.9: 44'; ***[iš-k]un*** [G] D.1.9: 43'; ***iš-ta-kan*** [G] D.1.1: 157; ***iš-ta-kan-ši*** [G] D.1.1: 138; ***iš-ta-nak-ka-na*** [Gtn] C.3.9: 19; ***li-iš-ku-<un>-ka*** [G] II.1.2: 13; ***lu-uš-tak-ka-na*** [Gtn] C.3.4: 68; C.3.9: 48; ***lu-uš-ti-kan*** [Gtn] C.3.3: 24; ***šá-ka-ni*** [G] I.1.7: 10; ***šá-kín*** [G] A.2.2: 43; ***šak-na*** [G] C.3.3: 27; C.3.4: 70; ***[šak-n]a*** [G] C.3.3: 20; ***ša-ak-nu*** [G] C.3.4: 63; ***šak-nu*** [G] C.3.9: 44, 50; ***šak-[nu]*** [G] C.3.3: 17; ***šu-kun*** [G] D.1.5: 12'; ***ta-aš-tak-⸢na⸣*** [G] C.3.5: 22'; ***ta-šak-kan*** [G] C.3.10: 3, 5, 8; ***ta-šak-k[an]*** [G] A.2.8: 24'; ***ta-⸢šak-kan⸣*** [G] C.3.10: 42; ***[t]a-⸢šak-kan⸣*** [G] B.2.3: 11''; ***ta-[šak-kan$^{?}$]*** [G] E.2.6: 5'; ***ta-šak-kan-ma*** [G] C.3.10: 8; ***taš-ku-nu*** [G] C.3.4: 13

šākinu "one who places; provider": **GAR$^{?!}$** E.2.3: 14'

šakirû (a plant, possibly henbane): **^{ú}ŠAKIRA** A.2.2: 58; C.1.4: 153'''; D.2.1: 31'; ***[^{ú}š]á-ki-ru-ú*** A.2.5: 14'

šalāmu G "to be healthy, well, favourable; to succeed"; D "to keep well, sound; to preserve; to bring (pregnancy, foetus) to term; to carry out in full": ***⸢i⸣-šal-la-mu-u*** [G] A.2.4: 10'; ***i-šal-lim*** [G] A.2.1: 92''''''; A.2.4: 39'''; A.2.5: 2'; I.1.1: 103; ***i-šal-[lim]*** C.2.3: 10'; ***liš-li-ma*** [G] D.1.1: 102; ***liš-lim-ma*** [G] C.3.10: 32; ***lu-uš-lim*** [G] D.3.1: 12; **⸢SILIM$^{?}$⸣** [G] D.1.3: 4'; **SILIM-*im*** [G] I.1.1: 3; **SILIM-*[im$^{?}$]*** [G] C.3.6: 65''''; **⸢SILIM$^{?}$⸣-*ma*** [G] D.1.1: 36; **SILIM-*mi*** [D] C.3.7: 12''; ***šal-ma-ti-ma*** [G] C.3.10: 28; ***šal-mu*** [G] C.3.10: 29; ***⸢šal⸣-mu*** [G] C.3.10: 31; ***tuš-tál-li-mu*** [D] C.1.4: 12'; ***ú-šal-lam*** [D] A.2.7: 36'; I.1.1: 43, 44, 78, 81, 85; ***ú-[š]al-lam*** [D] C.3.10: 30; ***[ú]-šal-[lam]*** [D] A.2.2: 12; ***ú-šal-lim*** [D] C.3.4: 10

šalāš "three"; *šalāšat ūmī* "three days": **3** A.1.4: 39''; A.2.1: 64''', 65''', 66'''; A.2.2: 23, 50, 53; A.2.3: 2'; A.2.4: 6', 37'''; A.2.5: 19'', 22''; B.1.1: 20; B.2.2: 8, 10; B.2.4: 7'; C.1.4: 13'; C.1.10: 8; C.2.3: 13', 21', C.3.10: 4, 91; C.4.1: 7', 8', 12'; E.2.5: 5'; E.2.6: 4', 23', 24', 31', 34', 36', 37', 39', 42'; F.1: 7, 11, 14, 17, 19, 30, 35, 38; F.2: 5, 13; I.1.1: 36; **⸢3$^{?}$⸣** F.2: 10; **3-*aš*** B.2.4: 24', 27', 30'; **3-*ta*** E.2.1: 10; **U$_4$.3.KAM** B.2.1: 23; **U$_4$.3.KA[M]** B.2.1: 22; **U$_4$.3.K[AM]** A.2.5: 24''; **[U$_4$].⸢3⸣.KAM** I.1.3: 31'; **U$_4$.3.KAM-*ma*** I.1.3: 9; **U$_4$.3.KÁM** H.1: 25'

šalāšā "thirty": **30** B.2.4: 20', 23', 25', 26', 17', 28'; C.3.9: 37; D.3.1: 2, 3, 4; F.2: 33'; **⸢30⸣** D.3.1: 34; **⸢30$^{?}$⸣** B.2.4: 19'; **[3]0$^{?}$** B.2.4: 21'

šalāšīšu "thrice": **3-*šú*** A.2.2: 51; A.2.4: 38'''; A.2.7: 9; B.2.2: 7, 20'; B.2.6: 6, 26; C.1.4: 3', 8', 11', 12', 16'; C.1.8: 20'; C.1.9: 28; C.3.3: 8; C.3.4: 9, 12; C.3.6: 9', 28', 62''''; C.3.9: 12; C.3.10: 12, 19, 68, 78, 79, 86, 87; D.1.1: 55; D.3.1: 14, 17, 28; H.2: 4; **3-*šú*$^{?}$** D.1.7: 29'; **⸢3⸣-*šú*** C.1.5: 45; **⸢3⸣-*[šú]*** B.2.1: 20; **3.TA.ÀM** C.3.10: 73

****šalaššer*** "thirteen": **13** F.2: 30'

šalāšû "thirtieth day of the month": **U$_4$.30.KAM** D.3.1: 37(b); **U$_4$.⸢30.KAM⸣** D.3.1: 6; **U$_4$.30.KÁM** D.3.1: 6, 11b

šallu "(taken) captive": ***šal-la*** D.3.1: 20

šalmiš "well; safely": ***šal-míš*** A.2.2: 46; D.1.8: 16, 18, 19

šalmānūtu "sound condition": ***šal-ma-nu-ut-ka*** C.3.10: 30; ***šal-ma-nu-ta-ma*** C.3.10: 30

šalšiš "thirdly": ***šal-šiš*** G.1: 42; G.2: 17''; I.1.7: 5

šalšu "third (in rank, quality); one third"; *ina šalši ūmi* "on the third day": **3** I.1.1: 106; **3.KAM** I.1.2: 13'; I.1.3: 1; **3.⸢KÁM$^{?}$⸣** A.1.4: 44''; **3-*šú*** A.1.4: 32''; ***šal-šá-a-tú*** E.2.6: 22', 31', 37', 40'; ***šal-šá-a-[tú]*** E.2.6: 19'; ***šal-[šá-a-tú]*** E.2.6: 34'; ***šal-ši*** D.1.1: 155; ***ša-a[l-ši]*** D.1.1: 155; ***šal-šú*** A.2.1: 61'''; A.2.4: 11'; A.2.6: 18; B.2.2: 11; C.1.9: 18; C.4.1: 4'; ***š[al-š]ú*** A.2.4: 11'; **U$_{4}$.3.KÁM** I.1.1: 106

šalšūti "for the third time": ***šal-šu$^{!}$-ti-iš-šu*** D.1.1: 155

šamallû "(scribal) apprentice": **^{lú}ŠÁMAN.LÁ** I.1.3: 36'

šamāmū "heavens; sky": ***šá-ma-me*** D.1.1: 149

šamāru G "to rage": ***šam-rat*** [G] A.2.7: 3; C.3.3: 4, 14; C.3.4: 62; C.3.9: 41

šamaššammū "sesame": ***[šá-maš$^{?}$]-šá$^{?}$-mi*** E.2.6: 7'; **ŠE.GIŠ.Ì** A.2.2: 75; A.2.3: 15'; E.2.6: 4', 7'; **⸢ŠE.GIŠ.Ì⸣** E.2.6: 25'; **⸢ŠE.Ì.GIŠ$^{?}$⸣** A.2.1: 8'

šambaliltu "fenugreek": **SULLIM^{sar}** A.2.3:9'; B.2.2: 8, 9; ***šam-ba-lil-[tu$_{4}$]*** A.2.2: 75; **^{ú}SULLIM^{sar}** A.2.3: 8'

šammaru "very furious; impetuous": ***ša-am-ma-rat*** C.3.9: 27

šammi ašî "*ašû*-disease-plant": ***Ú a-ši-e*** D.2.1: 21', 52', 55', 56'; **Ú *⸢a⸣-ši-⸢i⸣*** A.1.2: 10'

šammi balāṭi "plant of life" (unidentified medicinal plant): **Ú.NAM.TI.LA** A.1.4: 6', 17'; **Ú.NAM.TI.L[A]** A.1.4: 3'; **Ú.NAM.TI.⸢LA⸣** A.1.4: 8'; **Ú.NAM.T[I.LA]** A.1.1: 16'; **[Ú.NAM.T]I.LA** A.2.10: 6'; **Ú.NA[M].⸢TIN⸣** A.2.5: 6'; **Ú.NAM.TIN** B.2.4: 24', 29'

šammi eqli "field (clod)-plant": **Ú A.ŠÀ** A.2.6: 18

šammi ḫursāni "mountain-plant": **Ú.ḪUR.SAG.GÁ** A.1.4: 14'

šammi qišti "forest-plant": **Ú ^{giš}TIR** B.1.1: 14

šammu "plant; drug": ***šam-me*** D.1.1: 141; ***šam-[me]*** G.2: 27''; ***šam-mi*** D.1.1: 141; ***[šam-m]i$^{?}$*** D.1.9: 10'; **Ú** A.1.2: 10'; A.2.2: 84; A.2.6: 18; A.2.7: 40'; B.1.1: 62; D.1.1: 226; D.2.1: 24'; **⸢Ú⸣** B.1.1: 35; **<Ú>** A.2.6: 5; **Ú.ḪI.A** II.1.3: 67'''; II.1.4: 6, 23; A.1.2: 13'; A.1.4: 17'; A.2.1: 4', 67'''', 75''''; A.2.2: 74; A.2.7: 12; B.1.6: 5; C.1.4: 174''', 183'''; D.1.1: 207; D.2.1: 22'; **Ú.<ḪI.A>** II.1.4: 8; **Ú.⸢ḪI⸣.A** B.2.1: 16; H.1: 6; **Ú.⸢ḪI.A⸣** C.1.4: 2'; **Ú.[ḪI.A]** C.1.4: 176'''; **[Ú].ḪI.A** A.1.2: 11'; D.1.3: 10'; **⸢Ú.ḪI.A⸣** A.2.1: 42''; **[Ú].⸢ḪI.A⸣** A.2.6: 11; **[Ú.ḪI].⸢A⸣** E.1.1: 3; **Ú-*⸢ka⸣*** A.2.7: 39'; **Ú.MEŠ** II.1.4: 54; A.1.4: 4', 18'; B.1.1: 57; C.1.10: 4, 5, 9; D.1.1: 141; D.1.4: 15''; **⸢Ú⸣.MEŠ** E.1.1: 9; **[Ú$^{?}$].MEŠ** A.1.2: 17''; **⸢Ú⸣.[ME]Š** A.1.4: 7'

šammu ēdu see *ēdu*

šammu peṣû "white drug" (resin of *ṣarbatu*-poplar): **Ú BABBAR** A.1.4: 12'; A.2.1: 2', 88''''''; A.2.2: 44, 81; B.2.2: 1, 10; B.2.4: 9'; C.1.4: 157'''; D.2.1: 22', 52'; E.2.4: 3'; **Ú$^{?}$ BABBAR** E.2.6: 20'; **Ú BABBAR$^{?}$** A.2.10: 12''; **⸢Ú⸣ BABBAR** A.1.2: 13'; **[Ú] BABBAR** A.2.1: 96''''''

šamnu "oil; fat": **Ì** II.1.3: 35''', 56''' II.1.4: 11, 18, 60; A.1.2: 5', 11'; A.2.2: 45, 51, 56, 62; A.2.3: 1', 10', 12'; B.2.2: 19', 23'; C.1.4: 3', 9'; C.2.1: 13'; C.3.6: 16', 20', 30', 58''''; D.1.1: 133, 150, 151, 232, 234, 235; D.1.3: 7', 22''; D.1.7: 15', 29'; D.1.11: 11; D.2.1: 22', 29', 49', 53', 54', 61', 66'; E.2.2: 3'; E.2.6: 21', 24', 26', 32', 34', 39', 41', 42', 44'; F.2: 41'; G.1: 31, 32; G.2: 29''; **Ì$^{?}$** A.2.3: 6'; **Ì$^{!}$** A.2.4: 11'; **⸢Ì⸣** A.2.2: 58; C.3.4: 57; C.3.6: 58'''', 59''''; F.2: 41'; **⸢Ì$^{?}$⸣** A.2.2: 30; A.2.4: 26''; D.1.3: 3'; **Ì.GIŠ** II.1.1: 28; II.1.4: 25; A.1.3: 3'; A.2.6: 20, 23, 26; B.1.1: 29; B.1.3: 7, 9; B.2.5: 8; C.1.4: 157'''; C.3.3: 3; D.1.1: 38, 54, 150, 151, 153, 177, 204, 209, 210, 211, 234; D.1.2: 10; D.1.4: 9'; D.2.1: 32'; D.3.1: 14, 30, 31; E.2.6: 11', 14', 41'; G.2: 11'; **Ì.GIŠ$^{?}$** B.1.6: 16'; **Ì.GI[Š]** C.3.4: 54; **Ì.GI[Š]$^{!}$** B.1.1: 32; **Ì.GI[Š$^{?}$]** G.2: 29''; **⸢Ì.GIŠ⸣** B.2.4: 3'; C.3.6: 59''''; **[Ì.G]IŠ** E.2.7: 7'; **Ì+GIŠ** A.1.1: 51'''; C.3.4: 54; C.3.5: 11'; C.3.6: 16'; D.3.1: 14; **Ì+GIŠ$^{!}$** D.1.1: 153; **⸢Ì⸣.GIŠ** A.2.2: 21; **Ì.MEŠ** D.1.5: 15'; ***šá-am-nu*** G.1: 11, 12, 31; ***šam$^{!}$-ni*** E.2.1: 8

šamru "wild, furious, raging, violent": ***ša-am-⸢ru⸣-tim*** II.1.2: 5

šamšu "sun": **^{d}UTU** C.3.10: 6; **^{d}UTU-*ši*** C.3.4: 60; C.3.10: 1; D.1.1: 52, 111, 193; **^{d}UTU-*š[i]*** C.3.5: 18'; **[^{d}U]TU-*ši*** C.3.3: 10; **⸢^{d}UTU⸣-*[ši]*** C.3.3: 11; ***šam-ši*** C.3.4: 13

šamû "sky; heaven": **AN** C.3.4: 15; D.1.1: 149; **AN-*e*** II.1.4: 58, 59; B.1.1: 69; B.2.6: 17; C.1.4: 20', 61''; C.3.2: 4''; C.3.4: 98; C.3.10: 83; D.1.1: 112, 125, 132, 149, 150; D.1.5: 13'; D.1.8: 5, 6; D.1.9: 18'; G.1: 46, 48; G.2: 25''; **AN-*⸢e⸣*** D.3.1: 11a; **⸢AN⸣-*[e]*** D.1.9: 8'; **[A]N-*e*** E.2.3: 10'

šâmu G "to decree; to determine": ***⸢i⸣-šim-šú*** [G] D.1.9: 34'; ***[i-š]im-šú*** [G] D.1.9: 46'

šanîš "alternatively; secondly": ***šá-niš*** G.1: 11, 15, 16, 18, 29, 31, 32, 34, 36, 42; G.2: 17''; I.1.7: 4; ***šá$^{?}$-niš$^{?}$*** G.2: 15''; ***⸢šá$^{?}$-niš$^{?}$⸣*** D.3.1: 33

šanû I, fem. *šanītu* "second; (an)other; next": **2** II.1.4: 14; **2-*i*** C.4.1: 3'; D.1.11: 11; E.2.6: 6'; **2.KAM** I.1.3: 32'; **2-*ú*** C.3.10: 11; **⸢2⸣-*ú*** D.1.2: 6; **MAN** A.2.2: 41; **⸢MAN$^{?}$⸣-*nu$^{?}$*** C.1.10: 10; ***šá-na-a*** D.1.1: 153; ***šá-ni-i*** C.4.1: 3' ***ša-⸢ni-i⸣*** D.1.1: 153; ***[šá-n]im$^{?}$-ma*** A.1.2: 4'; ***ša-ni-tu*** II.1.4: 59; ***šá-ni-tu$_{4}$*** D.1.1: 151

šanû II G "to do twice, for a second time; to repeat": ***iš-ni-m[a]*** [G] D.1.1: 153

šanû III G "to change; to be(come) different": ***iš-nu-ú*** [G] I.1.7: 11

šapāḫu, *šabāḫu* G/D "to sprinkle": ***ta-šab-bàḫ*** [G] C.3.6: 58''''; ***u[š-tap-pi-ḫa]*** [D] D.1.1: 152; ***ú-šap-pi-ḫa*** [D] D.1.1: 152, 154; ***ú-<šap>-pi-<ḫa>*** [D] II.1.4: 60

šapāku G "to pile up; to pour out": **DUB-*ak*** [G] C.1.4: 156''', 157'''; ***ta-ša-ap-pa-ak-m[a]*** [G] II.1.1: 29

šapālu G "to be(come) deep, low"; D "to dig deep; to bring down": ***šá-pil-ma*** [G] E.2.2: 1'; ***tu-ša[p$^{?}$-pal]*** [D] A.1.4: 30''; ***ú-šap-pa-la*** [D] D.1.1: 151

šapāru G "to send": ***[lu-uš]-pur*** [G] D.1.1: 32; ***[lu-uš-pu]r$^{?}$*** [G] D.1.1: 187

šaplāniš "underneath; below": ***šap-la-niš*** D.1.1: 134

šaplānu "below; bottom": **KI.TA** C.1.4: 23'; **KI.TA-*nu*** I.1.1: 11, 12, 18, 19, 20, 21, 22, 23; ***šap-la-an*** C.3.10: 73; D.1.1: 55, 201; ***[ša]p$^{?}$-la-an*** D.1.1: 70; ***šap-[la]-an*** C.1.4: 108''; ***šap-la-a-nu*** A.2.1: 30', 32'; ***šap-la-nu*** D.1.1: 55, 180; ***šap-la-nu$^{?!}$*** A.2.6: 25

šapliš "below": ***šap-liš*** C.3.10: 41; **KI.TA** I.1.1: 65

šaplītu "lower part": **KI.TA.MEŠ** D.3.1: 18; E.2.3: 11'; ***šap-la-a-ti*** C.3.4: 98; ***šap-lit*** D.1.8: 12

šaplu "bottom; underside"; (*ina*) *šapal* (prep.) "below": **KI.TA** C.3.6: 51''''; D.1.1: 223; ***šá-pal-ka*** D.3.1: 21

šaplû, *šiplû* "lower; lower-lying": ***ši-ip-li-i*** D.1.1: 174

šaptu "lip": **[N]UMDUM.MEŠ-*šá*** I.1.1: 24; **⸢NUMDUM⸣.MEŠ-*šú*** I.1.1: 24; ***šap-ta-šá*** II.1.4: 41; ***[šap-ta-š]ú$^{?}$*** D.1.1: 81

šapû I G "to be dense, thick, loud; to be obscured; to cloud over; to billow": ***i-šá-pi*** [G] D.1.1: 95; ***ša-pa-a*** [G] II.1.4: 42

šapû II G "to wrap; to fasten with laces, thongs": **DÙ.DÙ-*p[i]*** [G] A.1.3: 9'

šaqālu G/D "to weigh, pay; to balance; to suspend": ***tu-ša-qal-la-al-šú*** [D] C.3.10: 7

šaqû I G "to give to drink"; Gtn iter. of G: ***i-šaq-qu-ši*** [G] D.1.1: 142; ***iš-ta-qí-ka*** [G] C.3.10: 21; **NAG.MEŠ-*[ši]*** [Gtn] II.1.4: 55; **NAG-*ši*** [G] A.2.7: 30'; C.1.1: 5; C.1.4: 13'; D.2.1: 19', 66'; **NAG$^{?}$-*ši*** [G] A.1.2: 6'; **⸢NAG$^{?}$⸣-*ši*** [G] A.1.1: 3'; **[NA]G$^{?}$-*ši*** [G] A.1.1: 9'; **NAG-*ši-ma*** [G] A.1.3: 4'; B.1.6: 6; C.1.4: 74'', 75'', 93''; D.1.1: 204, D.1.3: 10'; D.1.7: 3'; D.2.1: 27', 38'; **NAG-*ši-m[a]*** [G] C.1.4: 183'''; **[NA]G-*ši-ma*** [G] B.1.6: 19'; **NAG-*šú*** [G] A.2.2: 5, 60; A.2.4: 12'; B.2.2:

6; C.1.2: 11; C.1.5: 39, 41; D.1.11: 5, 10, 12; **NAG$^!$-*šú*** [G] D.1.11: 2; **NAG-*šú-ma*** [G] A.2.2: 51; **NAG-⸢*šú*⸣-*ma*** [G] A.2.2: 6; ***ta*-⸢*šaq*⸣-*qí-iš*** [G] A.2.8: 12; ***ta-š*[*aq*$^?$*-qí-iš*]** [G] A.2.8: 17

šaqû II G "to grow high; to rise; to increase;"; D "to lift up; to raise; to elevate; to promote": **⸢*tu*⸣*-šá-aq-qá-a-šú*** [D] B.2.6: 12

šarḫu "splendid, radiant, proud": ***ša-ru-uḫ-tim*** II.1.2: 6

šarku "pus": **LUGUD** D.2.1: 60', 65'; I.1.1: 83

šarmadu (a medicinal plant): **^{ú}GUR$_5$.UŠ** D.2.1: 68'

šarru "king": **LUGAL** D.1.2: 16; D.1.10: 13'; I.1.1: 118

šārtu "hair": **[*s*]*a-ra-as-sa*** I.1.5: 9'; **SÍG** D.1.1: 233; H.1: 1, 35'; H.2: 4, 22'; **⸢SÍG⸣** C.3.6: 51''''; H.1: 9; **[SÍ]G** H.1: 31'; **SÍG-*šá*** H.1: 24', 25'; **SÍG-*šú*** H.1: 24'; **⸢*šá*⸣*-ra-as-sa*** I.1.5: 10'

šarû G "to be(come) rich": ***i-šár-rù*** [G] I.1.1: 2; ***i$_{11}$-šár-rù*** [G] I.1.1: 7

šāru "wind": **LÍL$^?$** B.2.2: 6; ***šá-a-ri*** C.3.10: 33; **TU$_{15}$** A.1.4: 18'; A.2.9: 5'; C.3.9: 24; D.2.1: 20', 25', 26', 28'; E.2.6: 29'; I.1.3: 18; **[T]U$_{15}$** A.1.2: 8'; **⸢TU$_{15}$$^?$⸣** A.2.3: 28'''; A.2.10: 13''

šarūru "brilliance; rays": ***ša-ru-ri*** C.3.5: 18'; ***ša-ru-ru*** C.3.5: 18'

šassūru "womb; uterus": **ŠÀ.SUR-*šá*** C.2.3: 7'; ***šà-su-ri-šá*** II.1.3: 34''', 36'''; ***šà-su-ri-*[*šá*]** II.1.3: 40'''; ***šá-su-*⸢*ri-šú*⸣** A.2.8: 24'; **ŠÀ.TÙR** A.2.2: 77; D.1.1: 130; D.2.1: 53'; **ŠÀ.TÙR-*šá*** A.2.1: 17', 19'; A.2.2: 29; B.2.2: 10, 20'; C.1.4: 25', 33', 34', 35', 36', 39', 41', 43', 45', 138'', 147''', 152''', 155''', 160''', 161''', 173'''; C.1.5: 3; C.1.6: 3', 9'; C.1.7: 6', 8'; C.2.1: 6'; D.1.2: 13; D.2.1: 9', 24', 49', 53', 61', 64', 65', 68'; E.2.4: 8'; **ŠÀ.TÙR-[*šá*]** C.1.8: 43'; **ŠÀ.T[ÙR]-⸢*šá*⸣** A.1.1: 23'; **ŠÀ.T[ÙR-*šá*]** C.2.1: 11'; **[ŠÀ].TÙR-*šá*** B.2.2: 8; C.1.8: 11'; **[ŠÀ].TÙR-<*šá*>** A.1.1: 21'; **[ŠÀ.T]ÙR-*šá*** B.2.2: 2; E.2.7: 5'; **⸢ŠÀ.TÙR-*šá*⸣** D.2.1: 8'; **ŠÀ.TÙR$^!$-*šá*** C.1.8: 23'; D.2.1: 54'; **[ŠÀ].⸢TÙR$^?$⸣-*šá*** C.1.2: 17; **[ŠÀ.TÙ]R$^!$-*šá*** C.1.2: 19; **Š[À.TÙR-*šá*]** B.1.3: 10; D.2.1: 44'; **ŠÀ.TÙR-*šú*** A.2.2: 73, 77, 79, 82; C.1.5: 38, 40; C.1.9: 5, 14, 25; C.2.3: 6'; E.2.5: 2'; **ŠÀ.TÙR<-*šú*>** C.1.9: 9; **ŠÀ$^!$.TÙR-*šú*** B.2.2: 4; **ŠÀ.TÙR-⸢*šú*⸣** A.2.2: 47; **ŠÀ.TÙR-*š*[*ú*]** A.2.2: 80; C.1.9: 32; **⸢ŠÀ.TÙR-*šú*⸣** A.2.2: 57; **[Š]À.TÙR-*šú*** C.1.9: 3; **[Š]À.⸢TÙR⸣-*šú*** A.2.2: 69; **[ŠÀ.T]ÙR-*šú*** A.1.4: 36''; **[ŠÀ.TÙ]R-*šú*** A.2.2: 58; **ŠÀ.⸢TÙR⸣-[*šú*]** A.2.2: 79; **⸢ŠÀ.TÙR⸣-[*šú*]** A.2.2: 68; **⸢ŠÀ⸣.[TÙR-*šú*]** C.1.5: 32; **[Š]À.T[ÙR-*šú*]** E.2.2: 3'; **Š[À.TÙR]-⸢*šú*⸣** A.2.4: 15'; **Š[À.TÙR-*šú*]** C.2.3: 22'

šasû G "to call (upon/out); to cry out; shout"; Gtn iter. of G: ***al-si-ka*** [G] D.3.1: 21; I.1.7: 7; **DUG$_4$.GA.MEŠ-*si*** [Gtn] II.1.4: 46; **GÙ.DÉ-*šú*** [Gtn] I.1.1: 118; **GÙ.G[Ù-*si*]** [Gtn] I.1.4: 2'; I.1.6: 34'; **[G]Ù.⸢GÙ$^?$⸣-*s*[*i*$^?$]** [Gtn] I.1.3: 28; **[*i*]*l*$^?$*-su-ni*** [G] C.1.4: 52''; ***i-šá-as-sa-a*** [G] C.3.9: 17; ***i-ša-si*** [G] C.1.4: 15', 16'; ***i-šá-si*** [G] C.1.4: 12'; ***i-šá-si-m*[*a*]** [G] C.1.1: 6; **⸢*i*⸣-[*šá-as-si*$^?$]** [G] B.1.1: 52; ***i-šá-as-si-ka*** [G] D.3.1: 20; **[*i-šá*]-⸢*as-su*⸣*-ka*** [G] D.3.1: 20; ***i-še-su-ka*** [G] D.3.1: 20; ***iš-ta-*[*na-as-sa-a*]** [Gtn] I.1.3: 23; ***iš-ta-na-as-si*** [Gtn] D.1.9: 16'; G.1: 7; ***iš-t*[*a-n*]*a-as-si*** [Gtn] D.1.9: 19'

šâši "(to) her": ***šá-a-ši*** B.1.1: 22; ***ša-ši*** B.1.1: 20; ***šá-ši*** II.1.4: 9

šâšunu "them; those": ***šá-šu-nu*** II.1.4: 8

šatānu G "to urinate": ***iš-tin*** [G] A.2.2: 48

šâti "(of) him; that; this": ***ša-ti*** II.1.4: 48

šattišam "annually": ***šat-ti-šam-ma*** C.3.4: 92

šattu "year"; *šat*(*ta*) *ana šat*(*ti*) "year by year": **MU** D.1.10: 12'; I.1.1: 118; **MU.AN.NA** D.2.1: 61'; ***šat*** C.3.10: 29

šâtunu "those; these same": ***šá-tu-nu*** B.1.1: 17

šatû G "to drink"; Gtn iter. of G: **NAG** [G] II.1.3: 42'''; A.2.9: 4'; B.1.1: 33, 34; B.2.2: 7; C.1.2: 12; C.1.4: 29', 30', 32', 37', 38', 40', 126'', 132'', 138'', 148''', 149''', 150''', 153''', 158''', 159'''; C.1.8: 47'', 48'', 49'', 50'', 51'', 56'', 57'', 58''; C.2.3: 20'; D.2.1: 29'; E.2.7: 2', 3'; **⸢NAG⸣** [G] A.2.2: 44; C.1.8: 46''; C.2.3: 17'; **NA[G]** [G] D.2.1: 6'; E.2.2: 12''; **NA[G$^?$]** [G] D.1.7: 2'; **N[AG]** [G] B.1.1: 35, 36; C.2.1: 8'; C.2.2: 3, 4, 7, 8, 12; **NAG-*ma*** [G] II.1.3: 46'''; A.2.7: 25', 33', 34', 35'; B.1.6: 9; C.1.5: 10, 36; C.1.8: 27'; C.2.3: 15'; D.1.1: 207, 208, 213, 214, 220, 221; D.1.3: 12'; **NAG-*ma*$^?$** [G] A.2.1: 15'; **NAG-*m*[*a*]** [G] C.1.5: 11; **⸢NAG⸣*-ma*** [G] D.2.1: 55'; **⸢NAG-*ma*⸣** [G] B.1.6: 12; **⸢NAG$^?$⸣*-ma*** [G] B.1.6: 17'; **N[AG-*ma*]** C.1.4: 87''; **[NAG-*m*]*a*** C.1.4: 82''; **NAG.M[EŠ$^?$]** [Gtn] C.2.1: 7'

šaṭāru G "to write": **AB.SAR-*ma*** [G] D.1.1: 237; **DU-*ma*** [G] I.1.1: 118; **⸢IN$^?$⸣.[SAR$^?$]** [G] A.2.2: 41; **IN.SAR-*ma*** [G] C.2.1: 17'; **[*iš-ṭ*]*ù-ur*** [G] B.2.1: 41; **SAR** [G] A.2.5: 14'; D.1.4: 17''; **SAR-*ár* [G]** C.3.4: 82, 83; **SAR-*ma*** [G] C.3.4: 99; D.3.1: 37(A); **⸢SAR-*ma*⸣** D.3.1: 37(f); ***ša-ṭ*[*è-er-ma*]** [G] C.3.10: 92; ***ša-*[*ṭir*]** [G] A.2.7: 5; ***šà-ṭír*** [G] C.3.1: 31; **<*šá*>*-ṭir-ma*** [G] D.3.1: 38(b); **[*ša-ṭi-ir-m*]*a*$^{!?}$** [G] B.2.1: 34; ***šà-*[*ṭir-ma*$^?$]** [G] D.1.2: 15

šebû G "to be full, satisfied"; D "to fill; to satisfy": ***šub-be*** [D] D.1.1: 142; ***šub-bé-e*** [D] D.1.1: 142

šediš, fem. *šeššet* "six": **6** A.1.2: 13'; A.1.4: 9'; B.2.1: 16; C.1.4: 176'''; F.1: 6, 37; I.1.1: 39; I.1.6: 23'; **⸢6⸣** A.2.7: 12; **⸢6$^?$⸣** A.2.4: 7'

šēdu protective deity; protective spirit: **^{d}ALAD** C.3.1: 32; **^{d}ALAD$^?$** C.3.1: 11

šegušša "millet": **ŠE.MUŠ$_5$** A.2.6: 5; C.3.6: 50'''', 60''''; C.3.10: 88; D.2.1: 50'

šēḫu "wind; draft": ***še-ḫa*** II.1.4: 18, 26

šēlebūtu "vixen": **MUNUS.KA$_5$.A** D.1.1: 219

šeleppû "turtle": **NÍG.BÚN.NA^{ku6}** D.1.1: 217

šelû G "to be neglectful; to neglect": ***še-la-at*** [G] I.1.1: 104

šemû G "to hear; to listen": ***i-še*[*m*$^?$]*-me-ma*** [G] B.1.1: 54; ***i-šem-mu-ú*** C.3.4: 94; ***iš-mé*** C.3.4: 94; ***iš-me-ši-ma*** [G] C.3.4: 68; C.3.9: 49; ***iš-mé-ši-m*[*a*]** C.3.3: 25; ***iš-ta-ma-a*** [G] D.1.1: 149; ***iš-tam-me*** [G] D.1.1: 149; ***iš-te-mi*** [G] D.1.1: 166; **ŠE.GA-*a*** [G] II.1.4: 43; **[*š*]*e*-⸢*ma-a*⸣$^{!}$** [G] D.1.1: 82; ***še-mé-e-šu*** [G] D.1.1: 115; ***še-mu-ú*** [G] G.1: 46; ***ši-man-ni*** [G] D.3.1: 23

šēpu "foot"; *šēpānuššu* "on foot; feet first": **GÌR** B.2.2: 5; C.3.4: 40; F.1: 38; **⸢GÌR$^?$⸣** F.1: 39; **GÌR-*šá*** C.1.8: 27'; C.3.4: 63; I.1.1: 96; **GÌR.DIDLI-*ša*** I.1.1: 72; **GÌR.MEŠ-⸢*šá*⸣** C.3.6: 51''''; **GÌR.MIN** C.3.9: 4, 5, 6; **⸢GÌR⸣.MIN** C.3.1: 3; **[G]ÌR.MIN** C.3.1: 4; **GÌR.MIN-*ki*** C.3.3: 31; C.3.9: 53; **GÌR.MIN-*k*[*i*]** C.3.4: 72; **GÌR.MIN-*šá*** I.1.1: 84, 99; I.1.3: 20; **GÌR.MIN$^?$-*šá*** I.1.1: 6'; **[G]ÌR$^{?!}$.MIN$^?$-*šá*** C.1.8: 53''; **GÌR.MIN-*šú*** C.3.4: 63, 84; C.3.9: 42; I.1.2: 4'; **GÌR.MIN.MEŠ** C.3.9: 36; **GÌR.MIN.MEŠ-*šú*** C.3.9: 38; **GÌR-*šú*** I.1.2: 5'; **GÌR-[*šú*]** C.1.5: 35; ***še-pa-nu-uš-šu*** I.1.6: 24', 25', 26'

šer'ānu "muscle; sinew; tendon; vein": **SA** C.1.3: 7'; C.1.4: 6', 22', 31', 41', 47', 59''; C.3.6: 52''''; I.1.1: 9, 49, 90, 93; **⸢SA$^?$⸣.DIDLI** I.1.1: 13; **SA-*ia*$_5$** E.2.3: 24''; **SA.MEŠ** D.1.1: 108; I.1.1: 52, 56; **SA.MEŠ-*šá*** D.2.1: 59'; I.1.1: 73; ***šér-a-ni*** I.1.7: 13; ***še*$_{20}$*-er-ḫa*-⸢*nu*⸣*-ú*** II.1.2: 3; **^{uzu}SA-*ni*** C.3.1: 9

šerru "baby; (young) child": **GENNA** C.3.4: 87; **⸢GENNA⸣** D.1.6: 2, 7; **LÚ.TU[R]** A.2.5: 2'; **⸢LÚ⸣.TUR** D.3.1: 37(b); **⸢LÚ.TUR⸣** A.2.5: 3'; **⸢LÚ.TUR-*šá*⸣** C.3.6: 65''''; ***še-er-ra*** II.1.4: 34, 35, 51, 52; C.3.10: 35; ***še-er-ri*** C.3.10: 45, 60; G.1: 9; **[*š*]*e-er-ri*** C.3.10: 52; ***še-er-<ri>-šu-ma*** C.3.10: 46; ***še*$_{20}$-⸢*er-ru*⸣*-um*** II.1.2: 8; ***še-er-*[*ru*$^?$]** A.2.4: 1'; ***šèr-ra*** D.3.1: 13; ***šèr-ri*** D.3.1: 13; **[*šè*]*r-ri*** D.1.1: 39; ***šèr-r*[*i*]** D.1.1: 55; ***šer-ru*** D.1.2: 5, 14; ***šèr-ru*** D.1.1: 36, 39

šērtu I "fault": **[*š*]*e-er-tu*$_4$** B.1.1: 47; ***šèr-ti*** I.1.3: 17; ***šèr-tú*** C.3.10: 14, 34

šērtu II "morning": ***šèr-t*[*i*]** D.1.6: 1

šēru "morning": **[A.GÚ].ZI.GA** A.1.1: 8'; ***še-e-ri*** II.1.3: 51'''; C.3.10: 6; ***še-rim*** A.1.1: 18'; A.2.1: 84'''''; A.2.2: 60; A.2.7: 30', 38'; A.2.9: 4'; B.1.1: 16; C.1.4: 29', 75''; C.1.5: 10, 35; C.1.8: 26', 37'; C.3.4: 39; D.1.11: 9; ***š*[*e-r*]*im*** C.3.10: 68; ⸢***še-rim***⸣ C.3.10: 76

šeššer "sixteen"; *šeššer ūmī* "sixteen days": **16** I.1.1: 46; **U$_4$.16.KAM** II.1.3: 52'''

šeššīšu "six times": ***6-šú*** E.2.6: 24'

šeššu "sixth; one-sixth"; *ina šešši ūmi* "on the sixth day": **1/6**(ŠÚ) C.1.10: 18; **6** I.1.1: 109; ***6-šú*** D.1.4: 12''; ***6$^{!}$-šú*** C.4.1: 7'; **6.KAM** I.1.3: 4; ⸢**U$_4$**⸣**.6.KÁM** I.1.1: 109

šêtu, *sêtu* G "to be/leave remaining": ***i-se-tu*** [G] D.1.1: 114, 127

šêṭu G "to despise; to neglect": ***i-šiṭ*** [G] I.1.5: 11'

še'u "barley; grain; seed(s)": **ŠE** A.2.1: 27'; A.2.3: 9'

še'û G "to seek out": ***a-š*[*e*]*-e-ka*** [G] D.3.1: 24; ***eš-e-ka*** [G] D.3.1: 24; ⸢***eš$^{?}$-šim$^{?}$-ka***⸣ [G] D.3.1: 24

šī "she; that; this same": **BI** A.1.1: 14'; 15'; A.2.1: 25'; A.2.2: 43, 49, 73; A.2.9: 1'; B.1.1: 40; B.2.2: 4, 9, 14; C.1.4: 11', 15', 26'; C.2.3: 20', 24'; C.3.4: 9; D.1.1: 134; D.2.1: 18, 40', 67'; D.3.1: 16, 28; E.2.3: 9'; I.1.3: 1, 2, 3, 4, 5, 6, 7, 30'; I.1.5: 4', 10'; ⸢**BI**⸣ A.1.1: 23'; A.2.2: 72; C.3.6: 29'; **B[I]** A.1.1: 37''; C.2.3: 2'; ⸢**BI$^{?}$**⸣ A.1.2: 15'; **[B]I** B.2.2: 27'; ***ši-i*** A.2.7: 16; B.2.1: 33; C.3.4: 62; C.3.9: 41; C.3.10: 36; D.2.1: 8', 45'; D.1.8: 16, 23; G.1: 3, 13; ⸢***ši***⸣***-*[*i$^{?}$*]** B.2.1: 31; H.1: 18'; ***š*[*i-i*]** D.1.8: 14

šibburratu see *sibbirru*

šibirtu "piece; block; lump": **LAGAB** B.1.1: 5; **[*ši*]*-bìr-ti$^{?}$*** A.2.2: 69

šibītu "suture; seam": ***ši-bit*** I.1.7: 2

šibsātu "(divine) wrath; anger": **[*š*]*ib$^{!}$-sa-at*** B.1.1: 46 ***šib-sat*** D.2.1: 70'

šibṭu "blow; blast; epidemic": ***ši-biṭ*** C.3.1: 10

šiddu "side; edge; curtain; cloth bale": ***šid-di*** C.3.4: 75

šigû, *šegû* a cry of lamentation; a type of prayer: ***še-gu-ú*** C.1.1: 6; C.1.4: 12', 15', 16'; ***ši-gu-ú*** I.1.7: 6

šiḫṭu "strike; attack; rising": ***š*[*i$^{?}$-ḫi*]*-iṭ$^{?!}$*** C.3.1: 10

šikaru "beer": **KAŠ** II.1.3: 37'''; II.1.4: 16; A.1.1: 7', 17'; A.1.4: 7'; A.2.1: 29', 40'', 75''''; A.2.2: 5, 6, 20, 60; A.2.3: 7', 9', 29''', 17'; A.2.4: 42'''; A.2.5: 20''; A.2.7: 25', 28', 30', 31', 33', 35'; B.2.6: 4; C.1.1: 5; C.1.2: 11, 12; C.1.4: 30', 32', 37', 38', 126'', 146''', 148''', 149''', 150''', 153''', 158''', 159''', 183'''; C.1.5: 11, 29, 31, 35; C.1.8: 26', 47'', 48'', 49'', 49'', 50'', 51''; C.2.1: 5', 7', 8'; C.2.2: 3; 4, 7, 8, 10, 11, 12; C.3.4: 9, 35, 90; C.3.6: 9', 49''''; D.1.1: 151, 204, 206, 208, 213, 214, 220, 221; D.1.2: 6; D.1.3: 9'; D.1.11: 9; D.2.1: 6', 19', 29', 49', 54', 55', 57', 61', 66'; D.3.1: 8, 16; E.1.2: 6'; E.2.6: 23', 31', 34', 36', 37', 40', 42'; **KA[Š]** II.1.3: 44'''; A.1.3: 2'; **K[AŠ]** A.2.7: 12, 34'; A.2.9: 11''; ⸢**KAŠ**⸣ A.2.2: 15; C.1.8: 46''; C.2.1: 13'; C.3.6: 29'; **[KA]Š** B.1.6: 9, 12; E.2.1: 6; **[KA]Š$^{?}$** B.1.6: 5; C.1.8: 57''; **KAŠ.ḪI.A** B.2.3: 4'; **KAŠ.SAG** A.1.2: 11'; B.1.1: 65; C.1.4: 28', 40', 74'', 75''; C.3.4: 12; D.2.1: 22', 24', 27'; D.3.1: 16; **KAŠ.**⸢**SAG**⸣ A.2.8: 17; **KAŠ.SA[G]** C.1.4: 81''; **KAŠ.S[AG]** C.3.4: 42; **KAŠ.S[AG$^{?}$]** A.2.7: 20; **KA[Š.SAG]** A.1.2: 13'; **[K]AŠ.SAG** B.1.1: 17; ⸢**KAŠ$^{?}$.SAG$^{?}$**⸣ E.2.6: 27'; ⸢**KAŠ**⸣**.[SA]G** B.2.1: 17; **[KAŠ].SAG** C.1.4: 87''; **[KAŠ.S]AG** C.1.4: 132''

šikittu "figure; shape": ***ši-ik-na-te*** D.1.1: 136

šikkû "mongoose": ***šik-ke-e*** A.2.1: 7'

šiknu "appearance; form; nature (of an illness); deposit; sediment; silt": ***ši-ki-in*** A.2.8: 37'; ***ši-kín*** A.1.3: 5'; ***ši-kin-šú$^{!}$*** I.1.7: 11

šiltāḫu "arrow": **^{gi}GAG.U$_4$.TAG.GA** G.2: 11'; ⸢^{gi}⸣**GAG.U$_4$.TAG.GA** G.2: 12'; **^{giš}GAG.U$_4$.TAG.GA** D.1.1: 54; **^{urudu}GAG.U$_4$.TAG.GA** C.1.8: 37'; **[^{urud}]^{u}GAG.U$_4$.TAG.(-)GA** C.1.4: 81''; **^{urudu}GAG.U$_4$.TAG.E** G.1: 32; ***šil-ta-ḫu*** G.1: 33; G.2: 12', 13'

šimeššalû (a tree, possibly box): **ŠIM.ŠAL** B.1.2: 6'; **[ŠI]M.ŠAL** A.2.3: 7'; **[ŠIM].ŠAL** C.1.6: 5'; **[ŠIM.ŠAL]-*e$^{?}$*** A.2.3: 9'; **ŠAL** A.2.5: 21''

šimētān "(in the) evening": **AN.USAN** I.1.3: 12; ***ši-mi-tan*** D.2.1: 37'

šimtu "paint; mark(ing)": ***ši-mat*** II.1.4: 42

šīmtu "fate; destiny": **NAM.MEŠ** D.3.1: 20; ***ši-ma-ta*** II.1.4: 42; ***šim-tú*** D.1.9: 34'

šina I "they (fem.); these": ***ši-na***

šina II, fem. *šitta* "two"; *šina ūmī* "two days": **2** II.1.4: 59; A.1.4: 14', 15', 16', 30''; A.2.2: 26, 50; A.2.5: 20'', 21'', 22''; A.2.8: 26'; C.3.9: 9, 34, 36; C.3.10: 5, 70; C.4.1: 5', 6'; D.1.1: 150; D.1.11: 1; E.2.1: 4, 6; E.2.6: 1', 9', 21', 23', 24', 30', 31', 32', 36', 38', 39'; F.1: 1; F.2: 8, 11, 17, 18, 20; I.1.1: 114, 115; I.1.6: 29', 30'; ⸢**2**⸣ B.2.1: 35; B.2.4: 3', 5', 6', 7', 27'; E.2.1: 8; E.2.4: 4'; ⸢**2$^{?}$**⸣ A.1.4: 13'; B.2.1: 15; D.3.1: 6; ***2-ta*** D.1.1: 150; ⸢**2**⸣**.TA.ÀM** C.3.10: 76; **U$_4$.2.KAM** B.2.2: 20'; I.1.3: 9

šīnātu "urine": **KÀŠ** A.1.4: 39''; A.2.2: 9, 42, 46, 49; E.2.6: 5', 6', 33'; KÀŠ$^{?}$ A.2.2: 18; ⸢**KÀŠ$^{?}$**⸣ A.2.1: 72''''; A.2.2: 22; **KÀŠ$^{!}$** A.2.2: 47; **KÀŠ.ḪI.A** B.2.5: 6; **KÀŠ$^{!}$.MEŠ** A.2.2: 48; **KÀŠ-*šú*** A.2.2: 48

šinipu, fem. *šinipât* "two-thirds": **2/3** E.2.6: 20'

šinīšu "twice": ***2-šú*** B.2.2: 7, 20'; C.1.9: 28

šinnu "tooth": **ZÚ** C.1.4: 164'''

šinšer "twelve": **12** A.2.1: 4'; A.2.4: 5'; C.3.1: 7

šinūnūtu "(type of) swallow": **SIM.MAḪ^{mušen}** D.1.1: 210

šipassu "clay sealing; sealed bulla": ***ši-pat-su*** C.1.4: 63''

šīpātu "wool; hair": **SÍG** A.2.2: 21; B.2.3: 20''; C.1.1: 15, 27'; C.1.3: 10'; C.1.4: 39', 94'', 109'', 134'', 186'''; C.1.5: 38; C.3.6: 57''''; C.3.9: 1, 6, 8, 30, 31, 33, 34, 35, 36, 37; D.1.7: 11'; D.3.1: 3, 4; F.1: 6, 10, 13, 22, 24, 26, 29, 30, 34, 37, 41; F.2: 35'; H.1: 2; ⸢**SÍG**⸣ B.2.3: 12''; ⸢**SÍG$^{?}$**⸣ F.1: 1; **[S]ÍG** C.3.6: 52''''; **SÍG.ḪI.A** B.2.3: 15''; **SÍG.MEŠ** C.3.6: 51''''; ⸢**SÍG$^{?!}$**⸣**.MEŠ** F.1: 22

šipru "work; task; skill; (characteristic) activity; affliction": ***ši-pir*** A.2.2: 67, 69; ***šip-ru-šú*** B.2.2: 5

šiptu "incantation; spell": **ÉN** A.2.7: 3; B.1.1: 67, 71, 73; B.2.1: 20; C.1.1: 16; C.1.4: 8', 11', 16', 18', 64'', 93'', 187'''; C.1.4.1: 1'; C.1.5: 45, 48; C.3.1: 8, 26, 28; C.3.3: 4, 8, 10, 38, 39; C.3.4: 14, 55, 59, 60, 62, 77, 98; C.3.5: 15', 16', 27'; 28', 29'; C.3.6: 53'''', 54''''; C.3.7: 22''; C.3.9: 12, 15, 16, 21, 24, 26, 41; C.3.10: 13, 17, 18, 19, 20, 25, 32, 40, 41, 61, 78; D.1.1: 47, 48, 55, 118, 128, 129, 135, 161, 163, 172, 178, 181, 187, 193, 194, 195, 197, 198, 199, 201, 202, 236; D.1.2: 11; D.1.4: 6', 7'; D.1.10: 9'; D.3.1: 11a, 17, 18, 28; G.1: 1, 53; H.1: 17', 19', 21', 24', 34', 39'; H.2: 1, 2; **ÉN$^{?}$** E.2.7: 14''; ⸢**ÉN**⸣ A.2.7; B.1.1: 67, 70: 6; B.2.1: 12;

C.1.4: 3'; C.1.8: 6', 20'; C.3.1: 27; C.3.3: 4; C.3.7: 15''; D.1.8: 1; H.1: 18'; **É[N]** C.3.3: 14; C.3.4: 57; C.3.5: 30'; **É[N$^{!}$]** C.1.4: 100''; **[É]N** B.1.1: 72; C.1.2: 30'; C.1.4: 48''; C.3.1: 29; C.3.3: 13; C.3.4: 52; C.3.7: 23''; C.3.9: 27; C.3.10: 53; H.2: 4; **[É]N$^{!}$** D.1.5: 18'; ***ši-pa-at*** II.1.1: 28; II.1.2: 15; ***ši-pat*** D.1.1: 100; ***ši-i[p$^{?}$-ti]*** C.3.5: 29'; ***ši-ip-tu*** II.1.4: 50; ***[ši]-⸢ip⸣-tu$_4$*** B.2.1: 11

šiqdu "almond (tree)": **EŠ$_{22}$** B.2.4: 5'

šiqittu "almond (tree)": ***ši-qit-tú*** A.2.2: 76

šiqlu "shekel": **GÍN** A.1.4: 10', 19', 20'; A.2.1: 3', 16', 64''', 65''', 66''', 88''''', 90'''''; A.2.2: 23, 24, 25, 26, 27, 63, 70, 75, 76; A.2.4: 9', 45'''; A.2.5: 21'', 22''; A.2.7: 35'; A.2.8: 25', 26', 33'; B.2.3: 5'; B.2.4: 1', 2', 4', 5', 6', 7', 11', 12', 13', 14', 16', 25', 27', 32'; C.1.9: 7; C.2.3: 16'; E.2.1: 1, 2, 3, 4, 9; E.2.4: 2', 3', 6'; E.2.6: 9', 10', 20', 23', 24', 25', 26', 30', 31', 33', 35', 37', 38', 39'; **[G]ÍN** A.2.1: 1'; B.2.3: 2'; **[GÍ]N** A.2.1: 2'; B.2.4: 15'; **[G]ÍN$^{?}$** E.2.4: 6'; **⸢GÍN⸣** A.2.1: 8'; A.2.4: 9', 36'''; B.2.4: 14'; A.2.7: 11; B.2.1: 15; B.2.4: 3'; **G[ÍN$^{?}$]** A.2.5: 20''; **⸢GÍN$^{?}$⸣** A.2.4: 35'''; E.2.6: 42'

šiqqu "fish sauce": **⸢AL$^{?}$⸣.[Ú]S.SA$^{?}$** II.1.3: 58'''

šīru "flesh; body": ***ši-ru-ú*** II.1.2: 3; **UZU** A.2.2: 26; C.3.3: 20, 27; C.3.4: 65, 70; C.3.9: 44, 50; C.3.10: 8, 39; D.1.1: 218, 219; E.2.6: 20'; **⸢UZU⸣** D.1.1: 217; **UZU-*ia$_5$*** E.2.3: 23''; **UZU.MEŠ-*šá*** D.2.1: 59'; **UZU.MEŠ-*šú*** I.1.6: 19', 20', 21'; **[U]ZU-*šá*** E.1.3: 3'; **UZU-*šú*** C.1.10: 9; C.3.10: 5; **[U]ZU-⸢*šú*⸣** A.2.2: 61

šīt "she; this; that": ***ši-it*** II.1.4: 32

šītu, šētu "escaping": ***ši-<ta>-tu*** A.2.2: 49

šizbu "milk": **GA** A.2.1: 46''; A.2.2: 11; A.2.3: 29'''; A.2.5: 5'; A.2.6: 19; B.1.1: 66; B.2.6: 7, 9; C.3.4: 86; D.1.1: 157; D.2.1: 12', 13'; E.2.6: 11', 12', 35', 36'; **⸢GA⸣** E.2.6: 39

šittu "excrement": ***šit-t[u]-š[a$^{?}$]*** II.1.4: 1

šuḫḫu "buttock": ***^{uzu}šu-ḫe-e-ša*** II.1.4: 30

šū "he; that; this same": **BI** B.2.6: 4, 10; C.3.4: 19; I.1.1: 115; **⸢BI⸣** C.3.4: 18; **[B]I$^{?}$** D.3.1: 1; ***šu-u*** G.1: 20; ***šu-ú*** C.3.4: 87; G.2: 5'; ***š[u$^{?}$-ú]*** E.2.3: 15'; ***šú-ú*** C.4.1: 2', 3', 4', 5', 6', 7', 8', 9', 10', 11', 12', 13'

šû (a stone or shell): ***^{na4}šu-a*** C.1.4: 44'; ***^{na4}šu-u*** C.1.4: 4'; F.1: 36; ***⸢^{na4}⸣šu-u*** A.1.1: 32''; ***^{na4}š[u-u]*** C.1.4: 67''; ***<^{na4}>šu-u*** C.3.6: 57''''

šû sinniš "female *šû*-stone": ***^{na4}šu-u* MUNUS** A.2.7: 4; F.1: 40; F.2: 15; **⸢^{na4}⸣[*šu-u* MU]NUS$^{?}$** A.1.1: 33''; ***^{na4}šu-u* ⸢MUNUS$^{?!}$⸣** F.1: 15

šû zikar "male *šû*-stone": ***^{na4}šu-u* NITA** C.1.4: 4'; F.2: 12; ***^{na4}šu-u* NÍTA** A.2.7: 4; C.3.3: 7; C.3.4: 59; C.3.5: 14'; C.3.6: 57''''; C.3.9: 2; F.1: 12, 21, 29, 34; ***⸢^{na4}šu⸣-u* NÍTA** F.1: 36-37; **[^{n}]^{a4}⸢*šu*⸣-*u* NÍTA** C.3.7: 20''; ***^{na4}šu-u* NÍTA.MEŠ** F.1: 29; ***šu-u* NITA** D.1.4: 2'

šuāti, *šuātu* "him; her; it; that; the same": **BI** A.1.4: 33''; C.3.4: 15, 95; C.3.6: 55'''', 59''''; ***šú-a-ti*** C.3.4: 25; ***šu-a-tim*** C.3.4: 54; ***šu-a-tú*** D.1.11: 14'; ***[š]u$^{?}$-a-tú*** B.2.2: 29'; ***[šu]-⸢a⸣-tu$_4$*** E.2.3: 4'

šubāḫu (uncertain meaning): ***šu-ba-ḫi*** D.1.1: 138

ŠU.BI.AŠ.ÀM (reading uncertain) "ditto": **ŠU.BI.AŠ.ÀM** C.3.7: 12'', 19''; I.1.1: 62

šubtu "dwelling; seat; shrine": ***šu-bat-su*** C.3.10: 28

šubû (a stone or shell): **^{na4}ŠUBA** C.3.3: 2; C.3.5: 9'; F.1: 18; F.2: 17; **ŠUBA** C.1.3: 5'; C.3.9: 2; F.1: 18; F.2: 16; ***^{na4}šu-bu-u*** C.3.1: 4, 5

šubû imittu "right *šubû*-stone": **^{na4}ŠUBA Á.ZI.DA** C.1.4: 4', 184''; C.1.5: 23, 34; C.3.9: 3; **[^{na4}]ŠU[BA] ⸢Á.ZI⸣.DA** B.1.4: 2

šūbû seḫru "bent/convoluted *šubû*-stone": **[^{na4}ŠUBA]** ***síḫ-ru*** C.1.8: 54''

šubû šumēlu "left *šubû*-stone": **^{na4}ŠUBA Á.GÙB.BA** C.1.4: 4'; **^{na4}ŠU[BA] ⸢Á⸣.[GÙB.BA]** C.1.4: 184'''; **^{na4}ŠUBA Á.GÙB.BU** C.3.9: 3; **[^{na4}ŠUBA 2],30** C.1.8: 54''

šubû zikar "male *šubû*-stone": **⸢^{na4}⸣ŠUBA$^{!}$ NITA** C.1.8: 25'; **[^{na4}ŠUB]A ⸢NITA⸣** C.1.8: 7'

šuburru "anus; rectum": **DÚR-*šá*** D.2.1: 29'; **DÚR-*šú*** A.2.4: 43'''

šudingirakku "hand of a god (disease)": **ŠU.DINGIR.RA** D.1.1: 231

šugallītu lit. "she with big hands" (designation of a goddess): ***šu$^{!}$-gal-l[i-tu$_4$]*** C.1.4: 18', 19'

šugarruru Š "to roll": ***tu-šag-r[a-ar$^{?}$]*** [Š] D.1.2: 12; ***tuš-ga-ra-ár*** [Š] D.1.1: 201

šukbusu "ramp": ***šuk-bu-si*** D.3.1: 17

šukênu Š "to prostrate oneself": ***tuš-ken*** [Š] D.3.1: 8; ***tuš-^{ki}ken*** [Š] D.3.1: 8; ***tuš-ken-ma*** [Š] D.3.1: 28; ***tuš-⸢ken-ma$^{?}$⸣*** [Š] D.3.1: 8; ***uš-ke-en*** [Š] B.2.6: 27; ***uš-kìn*** C.1.4: 12', 13'

šukkallu, *sukkallu* "vizier": ***suk-kal-li*** D.1.8: 8; ***[su]k-kal-⸢lum⸣*** D.1.8: 8

šuklulu Š "to perfect; to complete": ***ú-šak-lal*** [Š] I.1.1: 69; ***⸢ú⸣-šak-lil*** [Š] D.1.9: 33'

šulmu "well-being; health": ***šul-me*** D.1.1: 106, 151; ***šul-m[e]*** D.1.1: 118

šuluḫḫu "purification rite": ***šu-luḫ-[ḫi]*** D.1.9: 32'

šumēla "on the left": **150** I.1.1: 19, 21, 23; **GÙB** I.1.1: 12, 17

šumēlu "left": **150** C.3.9: 3, 34, 36; F.1: 8, 15, 39; I.1.3: 8; **⸢150$^{!?}$⸣** F.1: 3; **150-*šá*** D.1.1: 230; **⸢150⸣-[*šá$^{?}$*]** F.1: 17, 41; **150-*šú*** B.2.6: 10; C.3.4: 83; C.3.9: 5; **GÙB** C.1.4: 105''; E.1.2: 6'; I.1.1: 71, 88, 91, 92, 95, 97, 98; **GÙB-*šá*** C.3.1: 3, 4; C.3.5: 14'; D.1.1: 230; **GÙB-⸢*šá*⸣** C.3.7: 13'', 20''; ***šu-me-li-ka*** D.1.8: 10

šumerû "a Sumerian": ***šu-me-ru-u*** G.1: 55

šumma "if": **BAD** A.2.2: 10; B.2.6: 1; E.1.2: 6'; **DIŠ** A.1.1: 36'', 44'''; A.1.4: 18', 24''; A.2.1: 56''', 58''', 61''', 79'''''; A.2.2: 8, 11, 42, 47, 48, 53, 56, 57, 61, 64, 67, 69, 74; A.2.4: 3', 24'', 40'''; A.2.4: 40'''; B.1.2: 1', 5'; C.1.4: 154''', 174'''; C.1.10: 1; C.2.1: 14', 15'; C.2.2: 2; C.3.3: 40, 41; D.1.1: 205, 221; D.1.3: 32''; D.1.4: 3'; D.1.7: 12'; D.2.1: 4', 17', 20', 25', 26', 25', 28', 33', 34', 39', 43', 47', 50', 52', 54', 55', 56', 59', 64', 65', 67', 69', 70', 71'; E.2.4: 11''; E.2.6: 25'; E.2.8: 3', 8''; I.1.1: 2, 3, 4, 5, 6, 7, 8, 9, 10, 11, 12, 13, 14, 15, 16, 17, 22, 23, 24, 25, 26, 27, 28, 29, 30, 31, 32, 33, 34, 35, 36, 37, 38, 39, 40, 41, 42, 43, 44, 45, 46, 47, 48, 49, 50, 51, 52, 53, 54, 55, 56, 57, 58, 59, 60, 61, 62, 63, 64, 65, 66, 67, 68, 69, 70, 71, 72, 73, 74, 75, 76, 77, 78, 79, 80, 81, 82, 83, 84, 85, 86, 87, 88, 89, 90, 91, 92, 93, 94, 95, 96, 97, 98, 99, 100, 101, 192, 103, 104, 105, 106, 107, 108, 109, 110, 111, 112, 113, 114, 115, 116; I.1.2: 13'; I.1.3: 1, 8, 9, 10, 11, 12, 13, 14, 15, 16, 17, 18, 19, 20, 21, 22, 32', 33'; I.1.6: 2', 3', 4', 5', 7', 8', 9', 10', 11', 12', 13', 14', 15', 16', 17', 18', 19', 20', 21', 22', 23', 24', 25', 26', 27', 28', 31', 32', 33', 34', 35', 36', 37', 38'; **⸢DIŠ⸣** A.2.2: 50, 59; A.2.7: 35'; A.2.9: 9'', 12''; C.1.8: 21'; D.2.1: 36'; D.3.1: 1; I.1.6: 1', 30'; I.1.7: 1; **⸢DIŠ$^{?}$⸣** D.1.11: 1; ***šum-ma*** A.1.1: 14'; A.1.2: 4'; B.2.1: 31; C.1.4: 27'; C.2.3: 3'; C.3.4: 96; F.1: 28; I.1.2: 13'; I.1.3: 1, 2, 3, 4, 5, 6, 7; ***⸢šum⸣-ma*** B.2.1: 32; ***šum$_4$-ma*** II.1.4: 19; A.2.2: 22, 72, 73; A.2.4: 16'; A.2.5: 25''; B.2.2: 9, 11, 12; C.1.8: 41'; C.3.4: 86, 87, 96, 97; D.1.7: 11'; E.2.6: 35'; I.1.1: 1, 116; I.1.3: 32'; ***šum$_4$-[ma]*** F.1: 28

šumšû Š "to spend the night": ***ú-šam-šá*** [Š] I.1.3: 19; ***⸢ú$^{?}$-šam$^{?}$⸣-<šá>-ma$^{?}$*** [Š] I.1.6: 10'

šumu "name; offspring; line (in text)": **MU** B.1.1: 40; **[M]U** B.2.1: 10; **MU-*ia*** C.3.8: 8; **MU-*ki*** C.3.9: 57; **MU.ŠID.BI** I.1.1: 116; I.1.3: 34'; ***šu-ma*** B.2.6: 24; ***šu-mi-ia*** B.2.6: 22; ***šum-šá*** D.1.1: 135, 164; ***šum-šu*** D.1.1: 117; ***šum-šú*** D.1.9: 35'; E.2.3: 12'; ***šu-um*** D.1.1: 157; ***šu-ú-um*** D.1.1: 157
šūmū "garlic (bulb)": **SUM**^{sar} D.1.11: 10; **[S]UM**^{sar} D.1.4: 13''
šumuttu (a field and garden plant): ^{ú}***šu-mut-tu***$_4$ C.2.2: 3
šum'uttu "(textual) addition; oral lore(?)": ***šum-'u-ut-tu*** D.2.1: 16'
šunḫu (a bulbous plant): ^{ú}***šu-un-ḫu*** A.2.2: 34; D.2.1: 48'
šunu "they; those; these": ***šú-nu*** D.1.11: 9
šunû "chaste tree(?)": ^{giš}**ŠE.NÁ.A** D.2.1: 23', 50', 58'; ^{giš}**ŠE.NU** C.1.4: 166'''; D.2.1: 41'; ^{giš}***šu-ni-i*** A.2.1: 26'; ***šu***$^{\text{!}}$***-nu-ú*** E.2.6: 10'
šūnuḫu "exhausted (one)": ***šu-nu-ḫu*** B.2.6: 21
šunūti "them; those; the same": ***šu-nu-ti*** D.1.1: 177; ***šú-nu-ti*** C.3.4: 47; D.2.1: 44', 73'; ***šú-nu-tu*** C.2.3: 19'
šupālītu "undergarment": ^{túg}**KI.TA** A.2.2: 36
šupālu "depression"; (*ina*) *šupāl* (prep.) "below": ***šu-pal*** C.3.10: 87; ***šu-⸢pal⸣*** C.3.10: 85
šuparruru Š "to spread out": ***⸢uš⸣-par-r[i-ir]*** [Š] D.1.9: 18'
šuplu "depth": ***šup-li*** E.2.5: 10'
šupšuqtu "woman labouring, having difficulty (in childbirth)": ***šup-šuq-ta*** D.1.1: 198; ***šu[p-šuq-ti***$^{?}$**]** A.2.1: 70''''; ***šup-šuq-tùm-ma*** G.1: 14
šupuḫru a variety of cedar: **EREN.BAD** C.1.10: 10, 11; ^{giš}**EREN.BAD** A.1.4: 13'; A.2.1: 16'; D.2.1: 47'; **[**^{giš}**ER]EN**$^{?}$**.BAD** A.2.1: 104'''''''
šuqallulu Š "to hang (down); cause to be suspended": ***tu-ša-qal-la-al-šú*** C.3.10: 7
šurbû "very great; eminent": ***šur-bu-u*** C.3.4: 98; D.3.1: 17, 18; ***šur-bu-ú*** C.3.4: 98; D.3.1: 17, 18; ***[šu]r-bu-tu*** C.3.10: 64
šurdû "leaking; overflowing": ***šur-di-i*** D.1.1: 114, 127, 133; G.1: 51
šurdunû (a medicinal plant, perhaps rocket): ^{ú}**SI.⸢SÁ⸣** H.1: 5
šurmēnu "cypress": **ŠUR.MÌN** C.3.5: 11'; ⸢^{giš}⸣**ŠUR.MIN** A.1.1: 42''; ^{giš}**ŠUR.MÌN** C.3.3: 3; C.3.4: 57; ^{šim}**ŠUR.MÌN.NA** II.1.4: 20; **ŠUR.MÌN** A.2.2: 31; ^{giš}**ŠUR.MÌN-*ni*** A.2.6: 5, 20; ^{giš}**ŠU.Ú[R.MÌN]** II.1.3: 67'''
šuršu "root": **SUḪUŠ** II.1.4: 6; A.2.1: 62'''; A.2.6: 4, 6; A.2.7: 29', 37'; B.1.6: 4; C.1.4: 147''', 150''', 176''', 181''', 182'''; C.3.6: 18'; D.1.1: 211; **SUḪU[Š]** C.2.1: 12'; **SUḪ[UŠ]** B.1.3: 8; **SU[ḪUŠ]** A.2.1: 1'; **⸢SUḪUŠ⸣** C.3.6: 19'; **[S]UḪUŠ** B.1.1: 12; **SUḪUŠ-*su*** A.2.7: 29'; C.1.8: 38', 40'; D.1.1: 228; **SUḪUŠ-*šú*** C.1.8: 38'; ***šur-ši-šu*** A.2.7: 38'
šuršummu "sediment; dregs": ***⸢šur***$^{?}$***-šum***$^{?}$***⸣-mi*** E.2.6: 42'
šuššān, *šulšān* "one third": ***šú-šá-na*** A.2.8: 16
šūši, *šūš*, *šūša*, *šuššu* "sixty": **60+*šu*** D.3.1: 2, 3; **UŠ** I.1.1: 116; I.1.3: 34'; ***šu-ši*** D.3.1: 2, 3
šūšu "liquorice": ^{giš}***šu-še*** D.2.1: 62'; ***šu-ši*** II.1.4: 23; ^{giš}***šu-šum*** C.1.4: 149'''; C.3.6: 18'; D.2.1: 58'; ^{giš}***šu-⸢šum⸣*** A.2.6: 18; ^{giš}***š[u-šum]*** B.1.2: 5'
šūt "he; it; that; this": ***šu-ut*** A.2.1: 87'''''; A.2.3: 11'; C.3.9: 39; G.1: 52
šuttu "dream": **MÁŠ.G[I**$_6$**.MEŠ]** D.1.3: 32''

tabāku G/D "to pour (out); to spill": **DUB** [G] D.2.1: 24', 53'; **DUB-*ak*** [G] D.2.1: 61'; **DUB-[*ak*$^{?}$]** [G] A.2.2: 45; **DUB-*ma*** [G] C.2.1: 6'; **DUB-*m[a]*** [G] A.2.4: 43'''; ***i-ta-b[a-ak]*** [G] II.1.3: 36'''; ***i-tab-ba-ka*** [G] D.2.1: 8'; ***ta-tab-bak*** C.3.6: 5'; D.1.1: 38, 224; ***ta-t[ab-bak]*** [G] B.2.1: 18; ***⸢ta***$^{?}$***-tab-bak⸣*** [G] A.2.7: 13; ***⸢ta***$^{?}$***⸣-[tab-ba-ak***$^{?}$**]** [G] B.2.6: 14; ***t[u-tab-bak]*** [D] B.1.1: 17
tabālu G "to take away; to carry off": **TÙM** [G] C.3.4: 100; I.1.2: 15'; **TÙM**$^{?}$ [G] D.1.10: 11'; **⸢TÙM⸣** [G] C.3.3: 45; ***⸢i***$^{?}$***⸣-tab-bal*** [G] E.1.2: 4'; ***i***$_{11}$***-ta***$_8$***-áb-bà-alla*** [G] C.3.10: 93; ***i***$_{11}$***-t[a***$_8$***-áb-bà-alla***$^{?}$**]** C.2.1: 18'; ***ta-bal*** [G] C.3.10: 15; ***tab-li-ma*** C.3.10: 71, 72
tabarru "red wool": ^{síg}**ḪÉ.ME.DA** C.1.4: 6', 8', 9', 22', 23', 31', 39', 40', 109'', 110'', 152''', 186'''; C.1.5: 32; C.1.9: 24; C.3.10: 4; D.3.1: 29; F.1: 7, 38; ^{síg}**ḪÉ.<ME>.DA** C.1.5: 40; ^{síg}**ḪÉ.ME.D[A]** C.3.5: 13'; F.1: 17, 35; **[**^{sí}**]**^{g}**ḪÉ.ME.<DA>** II.1.3: 28'''; **[**^{síg}**]ḪÉ.ME.DA** F.1: 11; ^{síg}**Ḫ[É.M]E.DA** C.1.2: 18; ^{síg}**HÉ.[ME.DA]** C.1.3: 6'; ^{síg}**Ḫ[É.ME.DA]** E.1.1: 10; ^{s}**[**^{íg}**ḪÉ.M]E.DA** C.1.4: 106''; ^{síg}**⸢ḪÉ.ME.DA⸣** F.1: 27; ⸢^{síg}**ḪÉ.ME.DA⸣** C.1.8: 23'; F.1: 14; ⸢^{síg}**ḪÉ⸣.[ME.DA]** F.1: 22; ^{síg}**ḪÉ.MID** F.1: 11, 14
tabribu, *tabrimu* "red-dyed wool": ***tab-ri-bu*** F.2: 37'; ***tab-ri-mu*** F.2: 36'
taḫapšu "felt": ***ta-ḫap-šá*** D.2.1: 11'
tāḫāzu "battle": ***ta-ḫa-zi*** II.1.4: 38; ***[ta-ḫa-z]i***$^{?!}$ D.1.1: 79
taḫsistu "memorandum; note; aide-mémoire": ***[t]aḫ-sis***$_x$***-tu***$_4$ A.2.4: 16'
takāku G "to oppress; to suffer" (a physical feature or defect): ***ta-a-ka*** [G] I.1.7: 9
takālu G "to trust in": ***⸢tak***$^{?}$***⸣-lu***$^{?}$***-[ma]*** [G] D.1.2: 17
takāpu G "to prick; to puncture; to be dotted; to impress"; N "to be dotted": ***i-tak-kip*** [N] E.2.6: 19', 25'; ***[ta]k-pu*** [G] C.1.4: 108''
takkussu "reed stem; tube": ^{gi}**SAG.KUD** D.1.1: 38; D.1.2: 3, 9
taklu "trustworthy, reliable": ***tak-lu*** C.1.4: 59''
takpītu "pearl": **⸢ÉLLAG**$^{?}$**⸣** B.2.2: 9; $^{\text{na4}}$**ÉLLAG-*tu*$_4$** A.2.2: 37; ***ták-pít*** A.2.2: 54
takṣâtu "cold (season); frost; cooling(?)": ***tak-ṣa-⸢a⸣-[tú]*** E.2.6: 21'
takṣīru "string of amulet stones": ***tak-ṣi-ri*** F.1: 32; ***tak-ṣi-ru*** F.1: 32; ***tak-ṣir*** C.3.9: 7, 38, 40
takullû "pain": ***[t]a-kul-la*** E.2.1: 16; ***ta-kul-lu-ú*** E.2.1: 16
taltallû "pollen, stamen (of date palm)": ***tál-tál*** E.2.5: 3'
tamirtu (a type of) meadow: ***[t]a-mir-ti*** C.1.1: 12; ***[ta***$^{?}$***]-mir-ti*** C.1.1: 11; ***⸢ta-mir-ti⸣*** C.1.4: 57''
tamkāru "merchant": ^{lú}**DAM.GÀR** C.3.4: 71; C.3.9: 52; ^{lú}**DAM.[GÀ]R** C.3.3: 29
tâmtu "sea": ***tam-tim*** C.3.9: 18; G.2: 15''; ***ta-<am>-tim*** C.3.9: 18; ***[t]a-ma-ti*** C.3.4: 15; ***t[a-ma-a-tim]*** II.1.1: 31
tamû G "to swear"; D "to put someone under an oath": ***at***$^{\text{!}}$***-mu-u*** [G] C.3.4: 51; ***at-mu-ú*** [G] C.3.4: 51; ***ta-ma-at*** [G] G.1: 23; ***tum-ma-ta*** [D] C.3.4: 16; ***ú-tam-mi-ki*** [D] C.3.3: 36, 37, 38; C.3.4: 76, 77; C.3.9: 57
tangussu, *tamgussu* (a metal cooking vessel): **ŠEN** E.2.5: 10'; **ŠEN.TUR** B.1.1: 28; ^{urudu}**ŠEN.TUR** B.1.2: 4'; B.2.1: 17; C.2.1: 5'; ^{urudu}**⸢ŠEN.TUR⸣** A.2.7: 19
tankittu "worry; anxiety(?)": ***ta-an-ki-tu***$_4$ G.1: 45

tappinnu (a kind of flour): **DABIN** D.2.1: 51'
tappû "companion; partner; friend": **⸢tap-pá⸣-a-am** B.2.6: 18
taqānu D "to adorn": **tuq-qù-na-at** [D] D.1.1: 136
taqnu "good; safe; in order": **taq-né-e-ti** E.2.6: 5'
tarāku G "to beat; to be dark": **tar-[ku]** [G] I.1.6: 19'
tarāpu G "to be covered with colour"; D "to be discoloured": **tur-ru-pa** [D] I.1.1: 80
tarāṣu I G "to be(come) in order, correct, alright; to succeed, prosper": **i-tar-ra-aṣ** [G] A.2.1: 87'''''
tarāṣu II G "to stretch out; to point at; to spread; to straighten": **ta-at-tar-ṣu-uš** [G$^{?}$] B.2.2: 24'; **ta-ra-ṣu** [G] I.1.7: 13
tarbaṣu "(cattle) pen; courtyard": **TÙR-šá** D.1.5: 18'
tārītu "nursemaid; nanny": **ta-ra-ti-ka** C.3.5: 19'; **ta-ri-ta** C.3.4: 92; **ta-ri-[it-ka]** C.3.5: 19'
tarmuš (unidentified plant): **tar-muš** C.2.2: 10; **^{ú}tar-muš** A.2.2: 63, 70; A.2.8: 5; C.1.4: 142''; **^{ú}tar-⸢muš⸣** B.2.1: 14; D.3.1: 30; **^{ú}⸢tar-muš⸣** A.2.7: 11; **^{ú}tar-m[uš]** C.3.8: 14'; **^{ú}tar-[muš]** B.1.3: 6; **[^{ú}tar-m]uš** A.2.2: 80, 81; **^{ú}tar-muš$_{8}$** A.1.1: 17'; C.1.5: 14; D.1.3: 27''; D.3.1: 30
tarû G "to lift up"; Gtn iter. of G: **lu-tar-ri** [Gtn] C.3.3: 23; **lu-ut-tar-ra** [Gtn] C.3.9: 47; **lut-t[ar-ri]** [Gtn] C.3.4: 67
târu G "to return; to turn back; to send back; to bring back; to turn into; to reduce (to); to do again"; D "to bring back; to return; to regurgitate; to turn around; to (b)lock; to repeat; to retreat": **GUR** [G] C.3.4: 55; E.2.1: 8; E.2.6: 21', 31', 38'; **GUR$^{!}$** [G] E.2.6: 34', 41'; **GUR-át** [D] A.1.4: 24''; **GUR.GUR-ár** [D] C.1.4: 13'; **GUR-ma** [G] C.1.4: 27'; **GUR$^{?!}$-ma** [D] B.2.2: 5; **GUR.GUR-ši-ma** [D] B.1.1: 30; **GUR.MEŠ-ru** [D] II.1.4: 3; **GUR.RU** [D] B.2.2: 22'; **GUR-[šú]** [D] I.1.2: 15'; **i-ta-[r]i** [G] C.3.10: 36; **i-tur** [G] D.1.1: 112, 125; **ta-tar-ma** [G] A.2.7: 17; **tur-rat** [D] A.2.1: 25'; **⸢tur⸣-rat** [D] C.3.3: 6; **[tur]-rat** [D] A.2.1: 30'; **tur-ra-tú** [D] A.2.1: 53''', 91'''''; **ú-tar** [D] C.1.4: 11'; C.3.9: 24; **ú-tar-ra-ši-ma** [D] D.1.6: 11
taskarinnu "boxwood": **^{giš}TASKARIN** C.3.6: 58''''; **[^{giš}tas-k]a$^{?}$-rin-na** A.2.2: 13
tašriḫtu "splendour": **taš-ri-iḫ-ti** G.1: 17
tattīku, *tattīktu* "dribble; dripping; leakage": **ta-ti-ka-at** II.1.3: 38'''
tebû G "to rise; to get up"; Š caus. of G: **i-te-eb-<be>-e-ma** [G] C.3.10: 10; **i-teb-bé-e-ma** [G] D.3.1: 10b; **i-teb-bi-ma** [G] D.3.1: 10b; **it-te-bi** [G] I.1.3: 17; **li-še-et-ba** [Š] D.1.11: 13; **te-bi** [G] I.1.1: 11, 12, 22, 23; **ZI-bi** [G] I.1.1: 22, 23, 90; **ZI-b[i]** [G] I.1.1: 91; **⸢ZI-bi⸣** [G] I.1.1: 92; **ZI-ma** [G] I.1.1: 16, 17
telītu "very competent one" (epithet of goddesses): **te-li-t[u$_{4}$]** C.1.4: 19'
tēnīqu "suckling (infant)": **ti-nu-qí** II.1.4: 36; **ti$^{!}$-nu$^{!}$-qí** II.1.4: 53
temēru G "to cover (in earth); to bury": **te-te-mer-ma** [G] C.3.3: 6
tēnû "substitute": **te-nu-ú** C.3.10: 36
terku, *tirku* "blow; dark spot": **ter-ku** D.2.1: 59'
teslītu "prayer; appeal": **tés-li-ti** D.3.1: 23; **tés-l[iti]** D.3.1: 23; **tés-li-tú** D.3.1: 23; **tés-li-t[u$_{4}$]** D.3.1: 23
tēšû "confusion": **te-šu-ú** II.1.4: 47
tigilû "colocynth; squash": **⸢^{ú}⸣ÚKUŠ.[TI.GI.LI$^{?}$]** C.1.4: 87''
tikku "neck": **ti-ik-ka-šá** H.1: 25'; **ti-ik-ku** G.1: 47
tikpu "dot; spot": **G[ÙN.MEŠ]** C.1.7: 107''; **GÙN.MEŠ-šá** C.3.6: 56''''; H.1: 3, 32'; **⸢GÙN⸣.MEŠ-⸢šá⸣** F.1: 4; **GÙN-šá** C.1.4: 46'; **[GÙN]-šá$^{?!}$** C.1.4: 133''; **ti-ik-pi** E.2.6: 19', 22', 25', 29'
tīku "rain shower; raindrop": **ti-ik** D.1.1: 112, 125, 132; **ti-ki** G.2: 25''; **ti-ik-ku** G.1: 46
tillatu "vine": **te-e[l-la]-tú$^{?}$** A.2.5: 8'
tinūru "(bread) oven": **^{im}<ŠU>.RIN.NA** II.1.4: 29; **NINDU** D.2.1: 61'; **⸢NINDU$^{!}$⸣** E.2.6: 28'; **TINUR** A.1.4: 25''; **T[INUR]** A.1.4: 26''
tiqnu "proper equipment; ornament": **tíq-nu** A.2.2: 40; **ti-iq-na-a-te** D.1.1: 136; **⸢ti⸣-iq-na-a-[t]i** D.1.1: 136
tiskur (a plant): **^{ú}ti-is-kur** C.3.9: 20
tiše "nine": **9** C.1.4: 5'; I.1.1: 42
tišû, *tešû* "ninth"; *ina tišî ūmi* "on the ninth day": **9** I.1.1: 112; **9-i** C.4.1: 10'; **9.KAM** I.1.3: 7; **[U$_{4}$].⸢9⸣.KÁM** I.1.1: 112
titāpū "beer mash": **BÁRA.MUNU$_{6}$** B.1.1: 5
tittu "fig": **PÈŠ** B.2.2: 15; **PÈŠ$^{?}$** C.2.3: 4'
tīyatu (a medicinal plant and spice): **KU.NU.LUḪ** B.2.4: 6'; **KU.NU.LUḪ.ḪA** A.2.5: 6'; B.2.4: 27'; **^{ú}KU.NU.LUḪ.ḪA** A.2.1: 65'''; **[^{ú}]KU.NU.LUḪ.ḪA** A.2.1: 3'; **^{ú}KU.NU.[LUḪ.ḪA]** A.2.1: 61'''; **ti-ia-a-t[i]** A.2.2: 25; A.2.8: 29'; **^{giš}ti-ía-tú** D.2.1: 47'; **^{ú}ti-iá$^{!?}$-t[u$_{4}$$^{?}$]** C.1.6: 5'
tû "spell; incantation": **TU$_{6}$** B.2.1: 12; C.1.4: 20', 90'', 123'', 130''; C.3.1: 28; C.3.4: 77; C.3.5: 30'; C.3.7: 15''; C.3.10: 17; D.1.1: 37, 172, 193, 195, 199, 202; **⸢TU$_{6}$⸣** C.1.5: 48; H.1: 21'; **T[U$_{6}$]** C.1.4: 79''; D.3.1: 27; **[T]U$_{6}$** C.1.4: 136''; **TU$_{6}$-ka** B.1.1: 64, 65, 66; **te** C.1.4: 64''; C.3.9: 24; C.3.10: 18, 25, 32, 40, 61; D.1.10: 9'; **tu-ú** D.1.1: 118
tūʾamtu "(female) twin; twin sister": **MUNUS.MAŠ.TAB.BA** I.1.6: 28'
tūʾamu "(male) twin; twin brother": **NITA.MAŠ.TAB.BA** I.1.6: 27'
tubqu "corner": **UB** C.3.4: 96
tuḫḫu "residue, waste product; bran, draff": **DUḪ** A.1.4: 7'; E.2.6: 7'; **tu-ḫu^{me}** A.2.3. 29'''
tuḫlu (a medicinal plant): **^{ú}tuḫ-lam** D.1.1: 206
tukultu "trust": **NIR-su** D.3.1: 38(A)
tullal lit. "you purify" (a soap plant): **^{ú}tu-lal** C.1.4: 7'; **⸢^{ú}⸣tu-lal** B.1.1: 61
tulû "breast; nipple": **UBUR** I.1.1: 36, 52; **UBUR$^{!?}$** D.1.3: 6'; **UBUR.MIN-a-a** C.3.3: 24; **UBUR-šá** I.1.1: 26, 49, 52; **tu-la-a** C.3.3: 24; C.3.4: 68; C.3.9: 48; **tu-le-šú** C.3.4: 9; **tu-lu-ša$^{!?}$** E.2.1: 15
tuppu "tablet": **DUB** I.1.1: 117; I.1.3: 32', 33'; **⸢DUB⸣** C.2.1: 15'; **[DU]B$^{?}$** A.1.4: 44''; E.2.3: 30''; **DUB$^{?}$.ḪI.A** B.2.1: 35; **IM** A.2.5: 14'; A.2.6: 28; C.2.1: 17'; **⸢IM⸣** D.1.11: 15'; **tup-pi** A.2.7: 41'; C.3.4: 99; C.3.3: 43; I.1.1: 116; **tup-p[i]** D.2.1: 10'; **tup-pu** II.1.4: 32
turbuʾtu, *turbuʾu* "dust; dust heap; sand dune": **tur-bu-ʾ-i** D.1.1: 184

turminabandû (a stone, a kind of breccia): **[^{na4}D]ÚR.MI.NA.BÀN.DA** A.2.6: 10
turru "turned; locked": ***tur-re-ti*** D.2.1: 67'
tūrtu "reversion; retribution; (magical) undoing of an oath": ***tur-tu$_4$*** B.1.1: 47; ***tu-uš-tu$_4$*** A.2.8: 40'
tūšaru "desert; flat land; battlefield": ***tu-šá-r[i$^?$]*** B.1.1: 61

ṭabāḫu G "to slaughter": ***t[a-ṭa-ba-aḫ$^?$]-⸢ma⸣*** [G] C.3.10: 76
ṭābat emesalli (a type of salt): **MUN *eme-sal-lim*** C.1.6: 8', 11'; F.2: 29'; **⸢MUN$^{?!}$⸣ *[eme-sal-lim]*** D.1.3: 35''
ṭābātu "vinegar": **A.GEŠTIN.N[A]** A.2.1: 57'''; C.2.1: 13'
ṭābtu "salt": **MUN** A.2.2: 32; B.2.4: 12'; D.2.1: 55'; **MUN$^!$** II.1.3: 63'''; **⸢MUN⸣** A.2.4: 16'; **[MU]N$^?$** A.1.4: 6'; **MUN.ḪI.A** A.2.2: 27; **[M]UN.ḪI.A** A.2.2: 23; **⸢MUN$^?$⸣-*tú*** C.2.3: 21'
ṭâbu, *ṭiābu* G "to be good, pleasant; to be content; to please": **DU$_{10}$.GA** [G] C.1.10: 14, 15; **DU$_{10}$-*ta*** [G] A.2.2: 64
ṭābu "good; pleasant; sweet; aromatic": **DU$_{10}$** E.2.6: 28'; **⸢DU$_{10}$⸣** A.2.5: 7'; **DU$_{10}$.GA** II.1.4: 18; B.1.1: 3; C.3.6: 16', 30'; D.1.1: 38; F.2: 41'; **DU$_{10}^!$.GA** C.3.6: 20'; **DU$_{10}$.G[A$^?$]** C.3.1: 11; **DU$_{10}$.[GA]** A.2.5: 18''; **⸢DU$^{?!}$10.GA$^?$⸣** E.2.7: 7'; ***[ṭa-ab-t]u$_4$*** D.1.9: 10'
ṭamû G "to twist; to spin": **NU.NU** [G] C.1.1: 15, 27'; C.1.4: 7', 22', 31', 99'', 101'', 103'', 109''; C.1.8: 2'; C.3.6: 52''''; H.1: 4, 18', 24', 32'; **NU.NU-*ú*** [G] D.1.1: 230
ṭâpu, *dâpu* G "to churn": ***li-ṭe-e-pi*** [G] C.3.10: 15; ***li-ṭe-pi*** [G] C.3.10: 57
ṭarādu G "to drive away"; D "to drive, chase away": ***ṭur-da$^!$*** [G] D.1.1: 106, 107; **DUR$^{⸢ṭu⸣\text{-}ur}$-*da*** [G] G.2: 22''; ***ṭú-ur-da*** [G] G.2: 22''; ***⸢ṭú⸣-ri-di*** [D] G.2: 23''
ṭardu "driving away": ***ṭa-ri-du-ti*** C.3.5: 25'
ṭebû G "to sink; to drown; to submerge; D "to cause to sink; to settle; to clear up"; Dt pass. of D: ***uṭ$^?$-ṭa-ab-ba*** [Dt] D.1.1: 42
ṭeḫû G "to be near; to approach"; D "to present; to bring": **⸢TE⸣** [G] D.1.3: 7'; **TE-*e*** [G] C.3.4: 24; C.3.5: 7'; C.3.7: 11''; D.1.1: 231, 233; **⸢TE$^?$-*e*$^?$⸣** [G] A.2.2: 10; **TE.G[Á]** [G] C.3.4: 36; **TE-*ma*** [G] A.2.7: 1; C.3.3: 1; **TE-*ši*** [G] C.3.5: 4'; C.3.7: 16'', 23''; I.1.3: 19, 20; **T[E-*ši*]** [G] C.3.5: 15'; **TE-*šú*** [G] B.2.2: 20'; **TE.⸢MEŠ⸣-*šú*** [G] C.3.3: 9; ***tu-ṭaḫ-ḫa-áš-šú*** [D] C.3.4: 88
ṭēmu "mind; reason; (fore)thought; planning; instruction; report; opinion; decision": ***ṭé-mi-šá*** D.2.1: 15'
ṭēnu "ground; milled": ***[ṭ]e$_4$-né-e-tì*** A.2.9: 6'
ṭênu G "to grind": **ÀR** [G] A.2.2: 50, 79; **ÀR-*en*** [G] A.2.3: 8'; ***i-ṭe$_4$-en-ma*** [G] C.3.10: 89; ***te-ṭe$_4$-en*** [G] II.1.3: 64'''; D.2.1: 49'; ***te-ṭe$_4$-e[n]*** [G] II.1.3.1: 2'; ***⸢te⸣-[ṭe$_4$-en$^?$]*** [G] A.2.8: 23'
ṭepû G "to apply; to add"; D "to apply (drugs as plaster)": ***[te$^?$]-ṭe-pi*** [G] A.2.2: 34, 35, 36; ***t[a-[ṭ]e$_4^?$-pi*** [G] A.2.2: 21; ***tu-ṭa-pí*** [D] E.2.6: 26'
ṭerû I G "to extract liquid; to squeeze; to spread": **SUR** C.3.2: 5''; **SUR.RA** [G] A.2.1: 29', 32'; **SUR-*ri*** [G] D.2.1: 63'; **SUR-*r*[*i*]** [G] A.2.9: 16''; ***te-ṭe$_4$-ri*** [G] II.1.4: 30; ***⸢te-ṭe$^?$⸣-[ri]*** [G] A.2.8: 27'
ṭerû II G "to pierce": ***ṭa-ru-u*** [G] G.1: 15, 16; ***ṭe-ra-ku*** [G] D.1.1: 183; ***ṭe-ra-at*** [G] D.1.1: 24; G.1: 15, 16; ***ṭe-r[a-at]*** [G] G.2: 1'
ṭīdu "clay": **IM** C.1.5: 43; C.3.4: 2, 81; **⸢IM⸣** A.2.4: 34'''; **I[M]** C.3.4: 3
ṭīpu "poultice; wrapping": ***ṭi-pi*** A.2.2: 35; A.2.5: 26''
ṭūbtu "remedy": ***ṭu-ub-tú*** A.2.1: 63'''
ṭūbu "goodness; well-being; improvement"; *ṭūb libbi* "mental well-being; happiness"; *ṭūb šīri* "physical well-being": **DU$_{10}$-*ba*** II.1.4: 13, 19; **DU$_{10}$-*ub*** D.2.1: 70'; ***ṭu-ub*** C.3.10: 39; ***ṭ[u-ub]*** A.2.5: 17''
ṭūdu "way; path": ***ṭù-dam*** II.1.2: 12
ṭulīmu "spleen": **BI.RI** C.1.4: 170'''
ṭurru I "cord; rope; string; thread": **DUR** B.1.4: 16; C.3.9: 1, 8; D.1.1: 230; D.1.4: 12''; F.1: 24, 26, 30; H.1: 18'; **⸢DUR$^?$⸣** F.1: 1; ***ṭú-ur-ru*** D.1.4: 14''
ṭurru II "rectum; anus": ***ṭúr-⸢ru⸣-šú*** E.2.1: 11; ***ṭúr-ri-šú*** E.2.1: 11
ṭūru (a resin/gum, probably opopanax): **^{šim}ḪAB** II.1.4: 5; A.1.4: 10', 32''; A.2.1: 6', 74''''; A.2.2: 26; A.2.3: 16', 18'; A.2.8: 6; A.2.9: 2'; D.2.1: 12', 21', 55', 56'; E.2.6: 13', 24', 26', 31', 35', 39', 48'; **^{šim}ḪA[B]** A.2.2: 8; **[^{š}]^{im}ḪAB** A.2.2: 24; **[^{ši}]^{m}ḪAB** E.2.6: 43'

u "and; but; or": ***u*** II.1.4: 2, 17, 31, 42; A.1.4: 23'', 32'; A.2.1: 30', 70''''; A.2.2: 39, 73, 77; A.2.3: 10', 16', 17', 30'''; A.2.4: 2'; A.2.5: 8', 15''; A.2.6: 25; A.2.10: 9'; B.1.1: 29; B.2.2: 7, 21', 22', 24', 26', 27', 29'; B.2.4: 26'; B.2.6: 2, 22, 24; C.1.4: 3', 4', 6', 7', 8', 54'', 56'', 87'', 126''; C.1.5: 48; C.1.8: 19', 32'; C.1.10: 2, 3, 6, 9, 14, 16; C.2.1: 13'; C.3.3: 7; C.3.4: 11, 13, 14, 15, 35, 37, 53, 59, 62, 65, 67, 70, 71, 72, 84, 100; C.3.5: 2'; C.3.6: 57'''', 59''''; C.3.7: 4'; C.3.9: 2, 6, 9, 10, 24, 28, 29, 34, 36, 38, 41, 44, 47, 50, 52, 53, 56; C.3.10: 5, 13, 17, 18, 24, 29, 31, 34, 35, 36, 39, 43, 44, 47, 65, 71, 74, 79, 83, 87; D.1.1: 39, 163, 204, 228; D.1.2: 17; D.1.3: 5', 29''; D.1.4: 2', 15''; D.1.6: 4; D.1.8: 3, 12, 25, 26; D.1.11: 4, 7, 8, 10, 12, 16'; D.2.1: 22', 26', 28', 49', 61', 66'; D.3.1: 11a, 18, 20; E.2.3: 3'; E.2.6: 26'; F.1: 3, 34, 37; G.1: 9, 38, 52; H.1: 18', 24', 34'; I.1.1: 16, 17, 24, 25, 72, 84, 92, 96, 97, 98, 99; I.1.2: 15'; I.1.3: 12, 19, 23; I.1.7: 1, 10; ***u$^?$*** A.2.3: 6'; A.2.7: 37'; A.2.8: 17; C.3.10: 4, 8, 11, 13, 24, 41, 42, 47, 57, 77; E.1.2: 11'; E.2.3: 7', 10', 11'; E.2.6: 14', 29'; ***u$^!$*** C.3.4: 49; ***ù*** II.1.1: 36; A.1.2: 8', 11'; A.2.7: 2, 35'; A.2.8: 3; B.2.1: 35; B.2.2: 7; B.2.5: 3; C.1.4: 20', 110''; C.3.3: 20, 35; C.3.5: 9', 12', 15', 21', 28'; C.3.6: 35''; C.3.10: 19, 70, 75, 76; D.1.1: 86, 105, 147, 174, 176; D.2.1: 20'; D.3.1: 6a, 20; I.1.1: 45, 46, 47, 48, 80; I.1.3: 7; ***⸢ù⸣*** A.2.7: 9; B.2.1: 11; C.3.10: 90; ***⸢ù$^?$⸣*** A.1.1: 5'; C.3.10: 76; ***⸢ù$^{?!}$⸣*** C.3.4: 15
ū'a, *ūya* "woe; alas": ***ú-ia*** II.1.4: 43; ***u$_8$-ú-a*** C.3.10: 34
ubānu "finger": **ŠU.SI** A.1.4: 30''; A.2.4: 5'; C.3.9: 2; C.4.1: 12'; F.1: 2; **Š[U.SI]** A.2.4: 6'; **$^{[u]zu}$ŠU.SI-*šá*** D.1.5: 16'; ***ú-ba-nu*** G.1: 14
Ú.BÍL.LÁ (reading uncertain; a drug/plant): **Ú.BÍL.LÁ** B.1.1: 12
udû "ware; tools": ***ú-de-e*** E.2.6: 5', 11', 27', 13'; ***ú-de-e-ka*** C.3.10: 29; ***ú-du-ú*** C.3.10: 31
ūdu "distress; difficulties": ***ú-da*** C.3.10: 36
ugāru "grassland; meadow; arable land": ***ú-ga-ri*** B.1.1: 41; ***ú-g[a-r]i*** B.1.1: 49
uḫinnu "fresh date(s)": **^{giš}U$_4$.ḪI.IN** H.2: 3; ***u$_4$-ḫi-nu*** E.2.5: 3'
uḫūlu "potash; soda-ash" (salt-plant and their alkaline ashes): **NAGA** C.3.10: 20; **⸢NAGA$^?$⸣** A.2.4: 34'''; **[NAG]A** C.3.10: 19

uḫūlu qarnānû "salicornia" (lit. 'horned salt-plant'): **NAGA.SI** A.1.4: 12'; A.2.1: 3', 7'; A.2.2: 17; B.1.5: 7'; B.2.2: 10; B.2.4: 12'; B.2.4: 22', 28'; C.1.7: 7'; **NAGA.SI**$^{?!}$ B.2.2: 15; **[NAG]A.⸢SI⸣** A.1.4: 9'; **[NAGA].SI** A.2.1: 88''''''; **[NAGA].⸢SI⸣**$^{?}$ A.2.1: 95''''''; **NAG[A**$^{?!}$**.SI]** A.2.4: 41'''; ^{ú}**NAGA.SI** A.1.4: 6'; ⸢^{ú}⸣**[NAGA.S]I**$^{?}$ C.1.9: 17

ukullû "provisions; subsistence; fodder": ***ú-kul-li*** D.1.9: 10'

ukultu "food; fodder": **NÍG.⸢GU$_7$⸣**$^{?}$ E.2.6: 23'; ***[uk***$^{?}$***]-la-ti-šú*** C.3.4: 19

ul "not": **NU** A.2.5: 14'; B.2.2: 4; C.3.3: 9; C.3.5: 4', 15'; C.3.7: 16'', 23''; I.1.1: 39, 44, 82, 86, 117; I.1.3: 7, 34'; **N[U]** A.2.2: 72; ***ul*** II.1.4: 41, 42, 43, 44, 45; A.1.1: 46'''; B.1.1: 67; B.2.1: 28; B.2.2: 27'; C.1.10: 13; C.3.4: 10; C.3.5: 27'; C.3.8: 10; C.3.9: 29, 35, 40; C.3.10: 11, 17, 30, 40, 79; D.1.1: 5, 84, 125, 126, 127; D.1.5: 10'; G.1: 3, 4, 6; I.1.1: 26, 81; ***u[l]*** C.3.1: 26; ***[u]l*** D.1.1: 83; D.1.2: 2'; G.2: 18''

ulû "best oil": ***ul-la*** G.1: 31

ūlū, *ū lū* "or": ***ù-lu*** D.1.6: 8; ⸢***ù***⸣***-lu*** D.1.6: 12; ***[ù]-lu*** D.1.6: 13

ulḫaḫ (a type of acacia or thornbush): ^{giš}**KIŠI$_{16}$**-***ḫa-[a]ḫ*** C.1.4: 81''

ulla "well; now" (interjection): ***ul-la*** G.1: 30; G.2: 10'; ***ul-la***$^{!}$ D.1.1: 50; ***u[l-la***$^{?}$***]*** D.1.1: 87

ūma "today; on this day; for one day": ***u$_4$-ma*** A.2.7: 28'

ūmakkal "for one day": **U$_4$.1.KAM** A.2.2: 61; C.2.3: 20'

umma "thus; saying": ***um-ma*** D.1.1: 225; D.1.11: 6; G.1: 5, 6; G.2: 23''

ummânu "expert; scholar": ***um-ma-nu*** G.1: 52; **UM.ME.⸢A⸣** C.1.8: 31';

ummu I "mother"; *ummi ummi* "grandmother": **AMA** C.3.4: 50; C.3.10: 64; ⸢**AMA**⸣$^{?}$ C.3.4: 15; ⸢**AMA**⸣***-ia$_5$*** C.3.4: 50; **AMA**-⸢***ka***⸣ C.3.9: 57; **AMA**-***[ka]*** C.3.5: 17'; **AMA**-***ki*** C.3.3: 37; **[AM]A**-***ki*** C.3.4: 77; **AMA**$^{!}$-***šú*** C.4.1: 2'; **A[M]A**-***šú*** C.3.1: 25; ***um-mi*** G.2: 17''; ***um-mi-ka*** C.3.5: 21'; ***um-m[i-ka]*** C.3.5: 17'; ***um-mu*** D.1.9: 31'

ummu II "fever; heat"; pl. fem. "summer (heat)": ⸢**É**⸣**.[MEŠ**$^{?}$**]** D.1.7: 11'; **KÚM** A.2.6: 18, 21, 24; D.2.1: 39', 59'; I.1.3: 8; **[K]ÚM** C.2.1: 15'; ***um-ma*** D.1.6: 8

umṣatu "mole; birthmark": **SAMAG.MEŠ** I.1.1: 33, 34, 35

ūmu "day": **U$_4$** II.1.3: 52'''; A.2.2: 61; B.2.2: 8, 10; C.1.4: 13'; C.3.4: 88; D.1.10: 12'; D.3.1: 6; E.1.3: 5'; I.1.1: 106, 107, 108, 109, 110, 111; I.1.3: 9; ⸢**U$_4$**⸣ II.1.3: 29'''; A.2.5: 7'; **U$_4$.MEŠ** C.3.9: 37; C.4.1: 12'; ⸢**U$_4$**⸣$^{?}$**.MEŠ** E.1.2: 9'; ⸢**U$_4$**⸣**.[MEŠ**$^{?}$**]** A.2.4: 7'; **U$_4$.MEŠ**-***ša*** II.1.4: 56; D.1.1: 145; **U$_4$.MEŠ**-***šá*** B.1.1: 21; D.1.1: 145; **U$_4$**$^{?}$**.(-)[MEŠ**-***šá***$^{?}$**]** E.1.2: 6'; ***u$_4$-me*** II.1.4: 14; A.1.4: 39''; B.1.1: 20; B.2.2: 11; C.1.4: 14'; D.2.1: 9'; ***u$_4$-mi*** C.3.6: 62''''; I.1.1: 106, 107, 108, 109, 110, 111, 112, 113; I.1.6: 17'; ***u$_4$-mu*** A.2.2: 71; A.2.3: 5'; C.1.10: 8; C.3.9: 40; C.4.1: 2', 3', 4', 5', 6', 7', 8', 9', 10', 11'; D.1.11: 1, 11; D.3.1: 6; E.2.5: 5'; E.2.6: 15', 16'; ***u$_4$-[mu]*** E.2.6: 17'; ⸢***u$_4$-mu***⸣ D.1.8: 24; ***u$_4$-um*** B.2.6: 2; C.3.6: 63''''; C.3.10: 89; ***um*** D.1.11: 13

ūmussu "daily": ***u$_4$-mu-us-sú*** A.2.8: 12

unīqu "female kid": ^{munus}**ÁŠ.GÀR** C.3.6: 49'''; D.2.1: 72'; ***ú-ni-***⸢***i***⸣***-[qí]*** D.1.1: 29

upnu "cupped hand": ***[up-na]-šá*** D.1.5: 7'; ***up-ni-šú*** C.3.10: 85

uppu "tube, pipette": MUD A.2.2: 45; C.1.4: 157'''; D.2.1: 46'; ***up-pí*** II.1.3: 36'''

uppulu "late": **SIG** A.2.1: 27'; ***up-ul*** C.3.10: 37

upšāšû "(magical) procedure(s); machinations": ***[u]p-šá-še-e*** C.3.6: 15'; ***up-šá-su***$^{!}$***-u*** D.1.8: 20; ***up-šá-[šu-ú]*** B.1.1: 48

uqnâtu, *uqniātu* "blue wool; woad": **[**^{síg}**]ZA.GÌN** A.1.4: 35''; ⸢^{síg}**ZA.GÌN**⸣ F.1: 16; ^{síg}**ZA.GÌN.NA** A.1.4: 40''; C.1.4: 6', 147'''; C.3.9: 6, 11; F.1: 13, 16, 37; F.2: 36'; H.1: 2; ⸢^{síg}⸣**ZA.GÌN.NA** F.1: 34; **[**^{síg}**]ZA.GÌN.NA** F.1: 30; ^{síg}**ZA.G[ÌN.NA]** F.1: 41; ^{síg}⸢**ZA**⸣**.[GÌN.NA]** F.1: 26; ⸢^{ú}⸣**ZA.GÌN** A.2.1: 8'; ^{ú}**ZA.GÌN**-***tu$_4$*** A.2.8: 11

uqnû "lapis lazuli": ^{na4}**ZA.GÌN** A.2.2: 40; C.3.1: 2; C.3.6: 56''''; C.3.9: 5; C.3.10: 3; F.1: 9, 12, 33; F.2: 9; H.1: 33'; ⸢^{na4}⸣**ZA.GÌN** F.1: 15; ^{na4}**ZA.GÌ[N]** C.1.2: 24'; ^{na4}**Z[A.GÌN**$^{?}$**]** H.1: 10; ***uq-na-a*** G.1: 1; ***[uq]-na***$^{?}$***-[a]*** D.1.1: 4; ⸢**ZA.GÌN**⸣ D.1.4: 1'

urânu, *urannu* (a medicinal plant, probably fennel): ***[u$_5$-r]a-an-na*** C.1.8: 48''; ***u$_5$-ra-nu*** A.2.6: 4; ***u$_5$-r[a-nu***$^{?}$***]*** A.2.2: 83

urbatu (a type of rush): ^{ú}**NINNI$_5$** C.1.4: 22'; ^{ú}**NÚMUN** C.1.1: 8; C.1.4: 38', 167'''; ***ur-bat*** A.2.2: 43; ***ur-ba-te*** C.1.2: 13; ^{ú}***ur-ba-te*** C.1.4: 175'''

urgulû "lion": **UR.GU.LA** D.1.1: 233

urḫu "road; path": ***ur-ḫu*** D.1.1: 52

urīṣu "billy goat": **MÁ[Š**$^{?}$**]** C.1.5: 25; **UDU.MÁŠ** C.1.4: 111''

uriyāḫu (a stone): ^{na4}***u$_5$-ri-ia-<ḫu>*** C.2.2: 7

urīzu, *ḫurīzu* (a stone): ^{na4}***u$_5$-ri-za*** C.1.4: 44'; ^{na4}***u$_5$-ri-zu*** C.1.8: 22'; ^{na4}***u$_5$***$^{!}$***-ri-zu*** C.1.5: 33; ^{na4}***ḫu-rí-zu*** C.1.5: 22

urnû (a medicinal plant): ***ú[r-né-e]*** A.2.1: 26'; ***[u]r-nu-ú*** E.2.6: 10'

urpatu "cloud": ***ur-pe-e-ti*** C.3.10: 21

urqu "yellow-green colour": **SIG$_7$** B.2.2: 12; I.1.1: 69; **SIG$_7$.MEŠ** I.1.1: 56; ***ur-q[a]*** I.1.1: 55

urru "daytime; early morning": **U$_4$** C.3.4: 85; **U$_4$.ZAL** I.1.6: 14'; **[U$_4$.ZA]L**$^{?}$ I.1.6: 13'; ***ur-ra*** II.1.4: 13

urruru D "to parch": ***li-ir-ri-<ru>-ma*** [D] D.2.1: 14'; ***tur-ár*** [D] C.1.4: 25', 38', 147''', 152''', 164''', 165''', 166''', 175'''; C.1.10: 11; D.2.1: 30'; H.1: 5; ***tur-***⸢***ár***⸣ A.2.2: 28; C.1.7: 3'; ***[t]ur-ár*** A.2.2: 67; ⸢***tur***⸣***-ár*** A.2.6: 22; ***tur-<ár>*** C.1.9: 11; ***tur-á[r]*** E.1.1: 3; ***tur-á[r***$^{?}$***]*** C.2.3: 21'; ***ú-ru-ru*** [D] C.3.2: 17'''

urṣu "mortar": ***ur-ṣa*** E.2.6: 28'; ^{na4}**NA.ZÀ.ḪI.LI** D.2.1: 42'

urṭû "fibre; dyed wool": ***ur-ṭe-e*** H.1: 23'

urû "cut branch; palm frond": ***ú-ru-ú-a*** C.3.4: 45

ūru I "vulva; vagina": **GAL$_4$.LA**-***ša*** II.1.4: 12; **GAL$_4$.LA**-***šá*** B.1.1: 38; C.1.1: 9; C.1.4: 3', 54'', 63'', 174''', 178''', 189'''; D.2.1: 19', 25', 74'; **GAL$_4$.LA**$^{!?}$-***[šá]*** D.1.1: 97; **GAL$_4$.[LA**-***šá*]** A.1.3: 12'; ⸢**GAL$_4$**⸣$^{?}$.***<LA-šú>*** A.2.2: 48; **GA[L$_4$.LA**$^{?}$-***ša]*** E.2.1: 16; **G[AL$_4$**$^{!}$**.LA**-***šá]*** C.1.1: 2; **[GAL$_4$.LA**$^{?}$**]**-***šú***$^{?}$ B.2.2: 5; ***ú-ri-ša*** II.1.3: 38'''; ***u-ri-šá*** D.2.1: 17'; ***ú-ri-š[á]*** D.1.1: 97; ***ú-ru-u*** G.1: 40

ūru II "roof": **ÙR** B.2.6: 4; C.3.4: 25, 88; D.3.1: 8, 9; E.2.3: 2'; I.1.3: 10; **Ù[R]** A.2.7: 13; B.2.1: 19; ***ú-ri*** D.3.1: 8; ⸢***ú***⸣***-[ri]*** D.3.1: 9

uruḫḫu "hair (of the head)": ***ú-ru-úḫ-šá*** I.1.3: 9; ***ú-ru-uḫ-šá*** I.1.5: 8'

URUxKEŠDA (reading uncertain; a body part): **URUxKEŠDA**-***šú-nu*** I.1.1: 45

uruttu (a stone): ⸢^{na4}⸣***ú-ru-ut-tu$_4$*** A.2.6: 9

usābu, *usāpu* (a plant): ^{ú}***ú-sa-bu*** B.2.2: 22'

ušallu "(fields) along river valley": ***ú-šal-li*** C.3.4: 40; ***ú-šal$^{!}$-li*** C.3.4: 2
ušaru "penis": **[G]IŠ** C.1.4: 180'''
ušburrudû "ritual to undo witchcraft": **UŠ$_{11}$.BÚR.RU.D[A.KAM]** C.3.9: 25
ušû (a hard wood and a tree, perhaps ebony): **^{giš}ESI** C.1.4: 169'''
ušummu "dormouse": **⸢PÉŠ⸣.GIŠ.GI** A.2.2: 78
utullu "herdsman": ***ú-tul-la-a-tú*** G.1: 23
utūnu "kiln; oven": **UDUN** A.2.2: 30; C.1.10: 14; C.3.4: 97; ***a-tu-nu*** C.3.10: 26; ***⸢a⸣-tu-nu*** C.3.10: 27
uṭṭatu "barley; grain(s); seeds (of plants)"; unit of weight (1/180 of a shekel); a wart: **ŠE** A.2.2: 54; B.2.4: 22', 24', 29'; C.1.8: 35'; C.4.1: 2', 3', 4', 5', 6', 7', 8', 9', 10', 11'; D.3.1: 3; E.2.6: 23', 31', 34', 36', 37', 40', 42'; **Š[E]** B.2.4: 21'; **⸢ŠE⸣** D.3.1: 34; **⸢ŠE$^{?}$⸣** C.1.8: 38'; **ŠE.BAR** B.1.1: 23; C.3.10: 85, 87; D.1.11: 9; **ŠE.B[AR$^{?}$]** A.2.4: 42'''; **⸢ŠE⸣.BAR** E.2.1: 6; **ŠE.BAR-*tú*** E.2.6: 39') ***uṭ-ṭe-ti*** I.1.1: 6, 7
uzālu see *ḫuzālu*
uznu "ear; attention; understanding": **GEŠTU.MEŠ-*šá*** II.1.4: 44; **GEŠTU.MIN** C.3.10: 70; **GEŠTU.MIN-*ki*** C.3.3: 32; C.3.9: 54; **GEŠTU.MIN-*k[i]*** C.3.4: 73; **GEŠTU.MIN.MEŠ** C.3.10: 73; **GEŠTU.MIN.MEŠ-*šá*** D.3.1: 29; **[GEŠTU.MI]N$^{?}$-*šá*** I.1.3: 23; **GEŠTU.MIN-*šú*** D.3.1: 29; **GEŠTU.[MIN$^{?}$]-*šú*** D.1.1: 82

yānibu, *nibu* (a shell or cowrie snail): ***^{na4}ia-ni-ba*** H.1: 32'; ***^{na4}ía-ni-ba*** C.1.4: 5'; ***^{na4}ni-ba*** C.3.9: 4
yaraḫḫu (a kind of high-quality barley): **ŠE.S[AG$^{?}$]** B.1.1: 2
yaruttu (a bush and its spice or aromatic substance): ***ia-a-ru-tú*** A.2.5: 22''
yâši "to me; from me": ***a-a-ši*** D.1.5: 11'
yā'u, *yû*, fem. *yuttu(n)*, *yattu(n)* "my; mine": ***⸢ia-a⸣-tú-⸢nu⸣*** C.3.1: 26; ***ia-a-tu-un*** C.3.10: 17; ***iu-ut-tu*** C.3.5: 27'; ***iu-⸢ut$^{?}$⸣-tu*** B.1.1: 67

zabālu G "to bear"; Š "to have someone carry": ***ú-šá-az-ba-lu-uš*** [Š] C.3.10: 45
zakāru G "to speak; to pronounce; to invoke; to name"; N "to be pronounced; to be called": ***li-iz-za-ki-ir-ma*** [N] B.2.6: 23
zakû G "to be(come) clean/clear": ***i-zak-ku-ú*** [G] A.2.5: 17''
zalāqu (a light-coloured stone): **^{na4}ZÁLAG** C.3.9: 4; **^{na4}ZÁ[LAG$^{?}$]** F.1: 19
zamar "quickly; immediately; suddenly": ***za-mar*** D.2.1: 8'; ***⸢za⸣-<<a>>-mar*** C.2.2: 13
zamāru G "to sing": ***za-ma-ra*** [G] C.3.9: 17; ***za-ma-ru*** [G] C.3.9: 17
zappu "bristle": ***zap-pi*** H.1: 24'; ***zap$^{!}$-pi*** C.1.9: 23
zaqāpu G "to set up; to erect; to install": ***za-qip*** [G] I.1.1: 70
zaqāru G "to project; to stick up; to protrude": ***za-qir*** [G] I.1.: 15; ***zaq-ru*** [G] I.1.1: 58, 60, 64, 65, 73, 74
zaqpu "erect(ed); standing upright": **GUB.BA** C.1.4: 9'; ***za-qip-ti*** C.3.4: 58; ***za-qip-tu*** C.1.4: 102''; ***za-qip-tú*** C.1.8: 17'; ***za-qip-tu$_4$*** C.3.3: 5; ***zaq$^{!}$-pi*** D.1.1: 179
zaqru "high": ***zaq-ra-ti*** C.3.4: 15
zarû G "to winnow; to sow; to scatter": **MAR** [G] A.1.4: 26''; **MAR-*ru*** [G] A.2.2: 36; ***[i$^{?}$]-za-ra-ma*** [G] B.2.6: 11; [G] ***ta-az-za-ru*** [G] A.2.1: 10'; ***ta-za-ru*** [G] D.1.7: 5'
zâru G "to twist": ***zi-i-ir$_9$*** [G] I.1.1: 26, 86
zaytu, *zā'itu* "olive": ***za-a'-it*** A.2.8: 11
zâzu G "to divide into parts/shares": **Ì.BA** [G] C.1.4: 177'''
zerru "reed fence": ***ze-ri*** G.1: 34
zēru I "seed; offspring; descendant": **NUMUN** II.1.3: 65'''; II.1.4: 23; A.1.2: 10'; A.2.1: 28', 57''', 74''''; A.2.3: 9'; A.2.5: 12'; A.2.6: 6; A.2.7: 8; A.2.8: 16; A.2.9: 6'; B.1.2: 2'; B.1.6: 2; B.2.1: 8; C.1.2: 14; C.1.4: 7', 40', 46', 92'', 146''', 149''', 150''', 153''', 156''', 159''', 165''', 166''', 169''', 172'''; C.1.5: 17; C.1.8: 42', 44'; C.1.9: 4; C.1.10: 16; C.3.4: 91; C.3.6: 12', 15'; D.1.3: 36''; D.2.1: 21', 51', 52'; D.3.1: 15, 30; E.1.1: 1; G.1: 12, 30; **NUMUN$^{?}$** D.1.10: 4'; **⸢NUMUN⸣** A.1.4: 1'; A.2.2: 7; C.1.5: 18; **NU[MUN$^{?}$]** A.2.3: 7'; **NUMUN$^{?}$-*ia$_5$*** C.3.4: 48, 52; **⸢NUMUN$^{?}$⸣-*rù*** B.2.4: 8'; **NUMUN-*šú*** A.2.2: 33; **ŠE.NUMUN** C.3.10: 5, 8; **ŠE.NUMUN-*šú*** C.3.6: 43'''; ***ze-er*** G.2: 30''; ***ze-ri*** G.1: 10, 11, 25, 33, 48; ***ze-rù*** G.1: 39, 47
zēru II "hated; hateful": ***[ze]-ru-ti*** C.3.6: 3'
zērūtu, *zīrūtu* "hatred": ***ze-ru-te*** C.1.4: 174'''
zibbatu "tail": **KUN-*ia$_5$*** D.1.1: 184; **⸢KUN⸣-*ša*** D.1.1: 24; ***<zib>-ba-tuš-šá*** D.1.1: 144
zibītu (a mineral or shell): ***^{na4}zi$^{!}$-bi-tú*** C.3.10: 4; ***^{na4}zi-É*** C.3.1: 3; F.1: 21, 33, 36; ***[^{n}]^{a4}zi-É*** F.1: 39; ***[^{na4}z]i-É*** C.3.6: 57''''
zibtu (a stone or shell): ***[^{n}]^{a4}zíb-tú*** H.1: 33'; ***^{na4}zib-tu$_4$*** C.1.4: 5'; ***^{na4}zíb-tu$_4$*** C.1.4: 46'
zibû "black cumin": ***^{ú}zi-bu-ú*** B.2.4: 6', 23', 27'; ***[zi]-bu-u*** E.2.4: 4; ***⸢zi⸣-bu-ú*** B.2.4: 13'
zidubdubbû (a small, apotropaic heap of flour): **ZÌ.DUB.DUB.BU** C.3.4: 43
zikaru "man; male"; *zikar u sinniš* "male and female": **MU.PA** I.1.1: 58; **MU.TIN** I.1.1: 59; **NITA** A.2.1: 62''', 81''''; A.2.2: 11; A.2.6: 7; C.1.4: 4', 6', 7', 22', 62''; C.1.5: 8; C.3.4: 1, 59; C.3.10: 89; D.1.1: 211; E.2.3: 7'; H.1: 2; H.2: 4; I.1.1: 1, 4, 6, 8, 9, 12, 13, 15, 19, 22, 24, 28, 31, 35, 45, 47, 50, 53, 57, 63, 65, 66, 72, 74, 76, 93, 96, 100, 101, 114; I.1.6: 25'; **NITA.ME** I.1.1: 114; **NITA.MEŠ** I.1.6: 29'; **NITA-*š[a$^{?}$]*** A.1.1: 9'; **[NI]TA-*š[a]*** A.1.1: 3'; **NITA-*šú*** B.2.2: 20'; **NÍTA** A.2.7: 29; C.1.4: 150''''; C.3.3: 3, 7; C.3.4: 57; C.3.6: 57''''; C.3.9: 2; D.1.3: 29''; F.2: 26'; H.2: 3; I.1.1: 52
zikru "utterance; name": ***zik-ri*** D.1.1: 117
zīmu "countenance": ***⸢zi-mi⸣-šá*** C.3.6: 59''''; ***zi-mu*** D.1.5: 11'
zisurrû "(magic) flour circle": **ZÌ.SUR.[R]A** C.3.4: 14; ***$^{⸢be⸣-pí}$*** **SUR.RA** A.2.7: 38'; ***zi-sur-ra-a*** C.1.8: 34'
zittu "share; portion; division": ***zi-⸢it⸣-tu$_4$*** E.2.1: 10, 12
zû "excrement; refuse": **ŠE$_{10}$** C.1.4: 151'''; D.1.1: 208, 231; D.1.3: 11', 26''; D.1.7: 8'; D.1.11: 4, 6, 7; D.2.1: 42', 51'; **ŠE$_{10}$$^{?!}$** C.3.2: 5''; ***ze-e*** A.2.1: 7'
zukku "cleansing": ***zuk-ku*** A.2.4: 11'

zumru “body”: **NÍ** D.1.6: 9; **SU** I.1.3: 14; ***SU-ia***$_{5}$ E.2.3: 22''; ***SU.MEŠ-ša*** II.1.4: 61; ***SU-šá*** D.2.1: 20', 29'; ***S[U-šá***$^{?}$**]** A.1.2: 4'; ***SU-šu*** D.1.1: 154; ***SU-šú*** B.2.2: 16'; ***zu-mur-ri-šú*** C.3.10: 60; ***zu-ru*** C.3.9: 22; ***zu-um-ri-i-ia*** C.3.10: 14; ***zu-um-ri-šá*** D.1.1: 152, 154; ***zu-ur-šú*** A.2.8: 15
zūtu, *zu'tu* “sweat”: **IR** D.2.1: 30'; **⸢IR**$^{?}$**⸣*-sú*** A.2.2: 64; ***zu-'u-tú*** A.2.1: 34'
zūzu “half (unit); half a shekel”: **1/2 GÍN** A.1.4: 19'; A.2.1: 2', 6', 7', 16'; A.2.2: 15, 74, 81; A.2.4: 41'''; A.2.10: 6', 7', 8'; B.2.2: 1; B.2.5: 4, 5; C.1.9: 8, 16, 18, 30; E.2.6: 26'; **1/2**$^{?}$ **GÍN** E.2.6: 25'; **⸢1/2**$^{?}$**⸣ ⸢GÍN⸣** B.2.4: 3'; **⸢1/2⸣ ⸢GÍN**$^{?}$**⸣** A.2.1: 3', 12'; **1/2 GÍ[N]** A.2.1: 38''; **1/2 G[ÍN]** A.2.1: 51'''; **1[/2**$^{?}$ **GÍN]** A.1.4: 10'; **⸢1/2**$^{?}$**⸣ [GÍN]** A.2.4: 45'''

Sumerian Words

a I “arm; side”: **á** C.3.4: 29; D.1.8: 9, 10
a II “water; fluid; semen; progeny”; **a ri** “to impregnate”: **a** II.1.1: 1, 2, 3, 4; D.1.1: 236; D.1.9: 3', 10', 26'; G.1: 40, 51; **é** II.1.3: 7''; **a-k[a**$^{?}$**]** C.3.2: 15''; **an** G.1: 25, 48
a'abak “sea; seawater”: **a-ab-ba** C.3.4: 55
ab “cow”: **áb** D.1.9: 5', 9', 12', 13', 15', 16'; **⸢áb⸣** D.1.9: 14'
abzu “subterranean ocean”: **abzu-ke**$_{4}$ C.1.4: 77''; **[ab]zu-ke**$_{4}$ D.1.1: 21; **[ab]zu-ta-a** C.1.4: 83''
ad “voice; cry; noise”: **ad** C.1.4: 119''
aguba “holy water vessel”: **a-gúb-ba** D.1.9: 36'
ak “to do; to act; to perform”: **ì-ak-a** D.1.9: 15'
ala I (a demon): **ú-la-a** II.1.3: 19''
ala II “exuberance”: **⸢a**$^{?}$**⸣-la** C.3.2: 15'''
alan “image; form; statue; figurine”: **alan-bi** II.1.3: 19''
ama “mother”: **ama** C.3.4: 55; D.1.9: 30', 31'
amaš “sheepfold”: **a[maš]** D.1.9: 9'
ambar “marsh”: **ap-pa-ar** II.1.1: 19; **èn-bar** G.1: 8
an “heaven; sky”: **an** C.3.2: 23'''; G.1: 48; **an-e** D.1.9: 17'; **an-na** C.3.4: 27, 28; **an-na-kam** D.1.9: 14'; **⸢an⸣-na-ke**$_{4}$ D.1.9: 7'; **[an]-⸢na⸣-ke**$_{4}$ D.1.9: 8'
andul “shade; protection”: **an-dùl** D.1.8: 4
ane “he; she; it”: **e-ne** II.1.3: 23''
anki “heaven (and) earth”: **an-k[i]** H.1: 13'; **an-ki-bi-da-ke**$_{4}$ C.1.4: 18'; **an-ki-bi-[da-ke**$_{4}$**]** D.1.8: 2; **an-⸢ki⸣-⸢kam**$^{?}$**⸣-m[a**$^{?}$**]** II.1.3: 16''
ana “what?”: **a-na-àm** II.1.1: 14; **[a]-na-àm** II.1.1: 15
anšag “heaven's interior”: **an-šà** D.1.8: 6
antašuba “epilepsy”: **an-ta-šub-ba** II.1.3: 13''
anur “horizon”: **an-úr-ra** D.1.9: 18'
ara “times (with numbers)”: **a-rá** H.1: 29'
ašag “field”: **a-šà** C.1.4: 77''
ašbala “curse, insult”: **áš-bala**$^{!}$ C.1.4: 117''
ašuĝiri “limbs”: **á-šu-<<bi>>-ĝìri-bi** II.1.3: 21''; **a-zu-<<bi-šè>>- ĝìri-b[i]** II.1.3: 22''
aya “father”: **[a]-⸢a⸣** D.1.8: 13; **a-a-ni** II.1.1: 11

bad “to open”: **bad** G.1: 49
bad “wall, fortification”: **bàd** G.1: 49
bala “to turn; to cross; to transfer; to pour out”: **bal-dè-zu-ne** D.1.8: 7
balak “spindle”: ^{ĝiš}**bala** D.1.1: 12
banda “(to be) junior, small; child”: **ba-an-du** II.1.1: 19; **bàn-da** G.1: 8
bar “outside(r); outer form; body; to place outside; to set aside; to split; to send away; to peel away”: **bar** C.3.2: 23'''; G.1: 8; **bar**$^{\text{ba-ár}}$ G.1: 30; **bar-gin**$_{7}^{?}$ II.1.3: 7''; **bar-šè** H.1: 30'; **ḫé-en-bar-ra** D.1.8: 22
barag I “dais; seat; ruler; king”: **⸢bara⸣-ga-ni** D.1.9: 13'
barag II “to spread; to be spread out”: **⸢mi-ni-in-bàra⸣** D.1.9: 18'
bisaĝ “basket; drainpipe”: **⸢bísaĝ⸣** D.1.9: 26'; $^{\text{ma-a}}$**ĝá** G.1: 51
bur “bowl”: **bur** G.1: 32; **[b]ur** D.1.9: 37'
bur II “to release; to undo; to unravel”: **[ḫé-e]n-búr-ra** D.1.8: 20; **ḫé-en-búr-re** D.1.8: 20, 21

dab “to seize”: **⸢mu**$^{?}$**⸣-ra-dab** C.3.7: 15''; **[x]x-dab-ba** II.1.1: 10; **[x]-⸢x⸣-dab-e-da** C.1.4: 130''
dadag “(to be) pure; to purify”: **⸢dadag-ge⸣** D.1.9: 36'; **dadag-ge-ta** II.1.3: 24''; **dad[ag-ge-ta]** II.1.3: 23''; **[ḫé]-en-dadag** H.1: 30'
daĝal “(to be) wide”: **dam-gal-la** C.1.4: 188'''
de I “to pour”; **gu de** “to say; to cry out”: **gù mu-un-na-de-e** II.1.1: 12; **íb-dè** C.1.2: 30', 31'
de II “to carry; to bring”: **de**$_{6}$ C.1.2: 31'
diĝir “god”: **diĝir** D.1.9: 13'; **⸢diĝir⸣-ra-⸢na⸣** D.1.9: 45'; **[diĝir]-ra-na** D.1.8: 14; **diĝir-re-e-ne** C.3.4: 55; **diĝir-zu** D.1.8: 18, 20; **diĝir**$^{!}$**-zu** D.1.8: 20; **diĝir-⸢zu⸣** D.1.8: 15

dikud "judge": **di-ku$_5$** D.1.8: 13; ⸢**di-ku$_5$**⸣ D.1.8: 12
dili "single; sole; alone": **dili** C.1.2: 31'
dim I "post; binding; bond; knot": **dím-ma** H.1: 20'
dim II "to create": **dím$^?$** II.1.3: 7''; **dím-dím** C.1.4: 114'', 115'', 116''; **dím-[dím]** C.1.4: 114'', 115''
dirig "to fall down, collapse": **dirig** G.1: 50; **ù-me-e-⸢ta$^?$⸣-⸢dirig$^?$⸣** II.1.1: 25
du I "to build; to make": **bí-in-dù-a** II.1.1: 42'
du II "to go; to walk about": **ba-du** C.1.4: 127''; **du-du** II.1.3: 15''; **ḫé-en-du-du** D.1.8: 18; **mu-du** C.1.4: 69''; **nu-du-du** C.1.4: 120''
du'a "(with) young; child": $^{du-u}$**dù** G.1: 30, 35, 36
dug I "(to be) good; (to be) sweet": **ba-du$_{10}$-ga** C.1.4: 79''; **du$_{10}$-ga** D.1.9: 10'; **[d]u$_{10}$-ga** C.1.4: 85''; **du$_{10}$$^?$** II.1.3: 17''; **du-g[a]** II.1.1: 19; **nu-du$_{10}$-ga** II.1.3: 16''; **nu-d[u$_{10}$-du$_{10}$-da]** II.1.3: 18''
dug II "to speak; to proclaim; to perform": **du-du** C.1.4: 118''; **du$_{11}$-ga** D.1.9: 29'; ⸢**du$_{11}$**⸣**-du$_{11}$-ga** C.1.4: 117''; **du$_{11}$-ga-ab** D.1.8: 8; **ḫé-im-mi-íb-⸢du$_{11}$$^?$⸣** C.1.4: 123''
duga "command": **[d]u$_{11}$-ga-bi** C.3.4: 33
duḫ "to loosen; to release; to undo": ⸢**du$_8$-ù**⸣**-[d]a** D.1.8: 15
dul "to cover; to overwhelm": **mi-ni-in-dul** D.1.9: 18'
dumu "son": **dumu** D.1.8: 1
dumuga "suckling": ⸢**dumu$^?$-ga$^?$**⸣ C.3.4: 31
dun "to lay the warp": $^{tu-un}$**dun$_x$**(DÚB) G.1: 45

e I "house; temple": **é** II.1.1: 12; A.2.7: 32'; D.1.9: 28', 38'; G.1: 18
e II "to leave; to come out": **e-ti-a-zu-ne** D.1.8: 6; **ḫé-em-ma-ra-è** C.3.4: 30, 31, 33; D.1.9: 27'; **nam-ta-è** II.1.3: 4''; **i** G.1: 12; **ia$_4$** G.1: 39
e III "to speak": **ḫé-éb-bé** D.1.8: 24
egar "form; figure": **é-gar$_8$** G.1: 19; ⸢**é**⸣**-gar$_8$** G.2: 4'; **é-gar$_8$-bi** G.1: 18; G.2: 3'
egia "bride": **é-gi$_4$-a** D.1.8: 5
egir "back": **egir-bi** C.1.4: 120''
eme "tongue": **eme** H.1: 30'
en "lord": **en** D.1.8: 4; **en-**⸢**e**⸣ D.1.8: 24; ⸢**en$^?$**⸣**-e** D.1.9: 31'
endur "navel; umbilical cord": **[èn-d]ur** D.1.9: 34'
enenuru, enuru "enuru-incantation": **en-ni-in-nu-**ra II.1.2: 14; **én-[é-nu-ru]** II.1.1: 27
eren "cedar": ^{giš}**ere[n]** D.1.1: 3; ^{giš}**eren-na** II.1.1: 7; ^{giš}**eren-na-ke$_4$** II.1.1: 7
eria "wasteland": **a-ri-a-[ta$^?$]** II.1.3: 5''
eššadu "trap": **èš-sa$^!$-du** H.1: 20'

ga "milk; suckling": **ga-ta** C.3.4: 31
gab "left (hand, side)": **gùb-bu** C.3.4: 29; **gùb-bu-zu** D.1.8: 10
gaba "chest; breast; surface": **[gab]a** D.1.9: 19'
gabari "copy; equal; opponent": **gaba-ri** C.3.4: 30, 31; **gaba-ri-bi-šè** C.3.4: 30
gada "flax; linen (cloth)": **gada-gin$_7$** D.1.9: 18'
gal "great": **gal** D.1.9: 7', 9', 10', 13'
gala "vulva": **gal$_4$-la** II.1.1: 21
galanzu "wise; knowing": **gal-zu** C.1.4: 77''
gaz "to kill; to beat; to break; to smash; to crush": **gaz** I.1.7: 5
gi I "reed": **gi** G.1: 8; **[g]i** II.1.1: 19
gi II "to turn; to return; to answer; to entrust": **gi** H.2: 1; **mu-un-na-ni-íb-gi$_4$-gi$_4$** II.1.1: 13; **[nam-ba$^?$]-ra-an-gi** A.2.7: 32'
gi III "(young) woman" (Emesal): **gi** G.1: 34; I.1.2: 6'
gib "to block; to lie crosswise": **gi-ba-a** II.1.1: 10; **im-me-gi-bi** II.1.1: 10
gid "(to be) long; to lengthen; to extend": **gíd-gíd** C.3.2: 19'''
gidim "ghost": **gidim** II.1.3: 11''
gig "(to be) sick; to hurt; to be troublesome, painful; "sickness": **gig-bi** II.1.3: 20''; **gig-ga** C.3.4: 32; **gig-**⸢**ga**⸣ G.2: 8'; **gig-ga-a-ta** II.1.3: 8''; **[g]ig-ga-ta** II.1.3: 5''; **ki** II.1.3: 24''; ⸢**lú-gig**⸣ C.3.4: 31
gi'izila "torch": **gi-izi-lá** D.1.9: 36'
gilim "to lie across; to block": **gi-li-ib** A.2.7: 32'
gir "to slip; to slide; to glide": **gir$_5$-gir$_5$** G.1: 24, 25
gu I "thread; cord": **gu** H.1: 20'
gu II "neck; bank": **gú** II.1.1: 42'; D.1.9: 17'; **gú$^!$** D.1.9: 16', 19'; **u-gu$_4$** G.1: 47
gu III "voice; cry; noise": **gù** II.1.1: 12; D.1.9: 16'; **gù-bi** D.1.9: 17', 18'
gu IV "entirety, sum, total": **gú** I.1.2: 10', 12'
gu V "to eat; to feed": **[ka-muš]-**⸢**ì**⸣**-gu$_7$** II.1.3: 14''
gu de "to say; to cry out": **gù mu-un-na-de-e** II.1.1: 12; **gù mu-un-na-an-dé-dé-e** D.1.9: 16'; **gù m[u-u]n-na-an-dé-[dé-e]** D.1.9: 19'
gu la "to embrace": **gú$^!$-lá** G.1: 17

gub "to stand; to set up": **al-gub-b[a]** D.1.8: 9, 9; **al-gub-bu** D.1.8: 9, 10; **gub-ba** C.3.4: 28, 29; **ḫé-em-ta-gub** H.1: 30'; **mu-ni-in-gub** D.1.9: 39'; **mu-ra-an-gub** H.2: 2
gud I "ox": **gu$_4$** D.1.9: 9'
gud II "to jump": **gud** G.1: 26
guda ri "to embrace one another": **gú-da ri** G.1: 16
gug "carnelian": **gug** G.1: 2, 3; **gug$^!$** D.1.1: 5; **gu-ki** II.1.1: 5; **[^{n}]$^{a4?}$ku$^?$-ug** II.1.1: 9
guĝiri "breach": **gu-ĝar-ra$^{?!}$** II.1.3: 6''
gula "totality: **gul-la** I.1.2: 10'
gur "to turn (back), return; bring back; turn away from; avoid": **gur-⸢ra$^?$⸣** C.3.4: 33
gurum "to bend; to curve; to (make) bow": **⸢gurum$^?$⸣** II.1.3: 24''
gusa "totality": **gú-sa-a** I.1.2: 10', 11'

ĝa'e "I": **ĝá** D.1.8: 26
ĝar "to place; to put": **ba-ni-in-ĝar** D.1.9: 16'; **[b]a-ni-in-ĝar** D.1.9: 19'; **bí-in-ĝar** D.1.7: 24'; **ḫé-em-ma-ni-in-ĝar** D.1.9: 26'; **mu-ni-in-ĝar** C.3.4: 33; **mu-ni-in-[ĝar]** D.1.9: 44'; **[mu-ni]-i[n-ĝar$^?$]** D.1.9: 43'; **nu-ga** II.1.3: 18''
ĝen "to go; to flow; to come": **ĝá** G.1: 51; **ba-ta-ĝen-na-ta** D.1.1: 236; **[ḫ]é-em-ma-an-ĝen** D.1.9: 25'
ĝeš "wood; tree; weapon": **ĝiš** I.1.7: 4
ĝi "night": **gi** II.1.3: 15''
ĝi'unak "night(time)": **ĝi$_6$-ù-na** II.1.3: 16''
ĝurušlil "young men wind-demon": **ĝuruš-líl-lá** II.1.3: 12''

ḫal (a basket): **^{gi}ḫal** C.1.2: 30'
ḫalam "to forsake; to destroy; to forget": **mu-ni-in-ḫa-la[m]** D.1.9: 40'
ḫarran "road; path; passage; caravan": **[ḫar$^?$]-ra-an-na** II.1.3: 11''
ḫaš "thigh; crotch": **ḫu-us-ḫu-us-ta** II.1.1: 25
ḫaza "to hold": **bí-ḫa-za** D.1.7: 25'
ḫazin "axe": **ḫa-zí-in** C.3.2: 20''', 21'''
ḫe'am "so be it!": **[ḫé]-a** D.1.1: 12
ḫuĝ "to calm (down); pacify": **⸢ḫuĝ-ĝá⸣** C.3.4: 33
ḫulu "(to be) bad, evil": **ḫul** C.1.4: 118''; H.1: 8; **ḫul$^!$** C.3.4: 31; **[ḫ]ul** A.1.2: 19'; **ḫul-a** C.1.4: 118'', 119''; C.3.2: 22'''; H.1: 26'; **ḫul-bi** H.2: 2; **ḫul-gin$_7$** C.1.4: 89''; **ḫul-ḫul** H.1: 8; H.2: 2; **ḫul-lu-bi** C.3.4: 29; **ḫu-ul** H.1: 26', 27'
ḫulugig "hate": **ḫul-gig** II.1.3: 7''
ḫuluĝal "evil": **ḫul-ĝál** II.1.3: 10''; H.1: 30'
ḫuš "(to be) furious, angry; to be reddish": **ḫuš** C.1.4: 77'', 139'', 140''; H.1: 19'

i "oil": **ì** II.1.1: 20; **⸢ì⸣** G.1: 11; **ì$^{i\text{-}'u\text{-}u}$** G.1: 31
ib "(to be) angry; to curse; anger": **⸢íb$^?$⸣** C.3.4: 31
ibi "eye; face" (Emesal): **i-bi** H.2: 1
ibila "heir; descendant": **ibila** D.1.8: 2
id "river": **íd** C.3.2: 19'''
idim "source; spring; underground water": **idim-ta** D.1.1: 236
igi I "eye": **igi** C.3.2: 22'''; **igi-da** C.1.4: 127''; **igi-ni** II.1.1: 11
igi II "front; face; before": **igi** II.1.1: 24; C.1.2: 32'; D.1.8: 15, 18, 20; D.1.9: 27'; **⸢igi⸣** D.1.9: 20'; **igi-bi** II.1.3: 20''
igi sig "to see"; see also **sig** I
iginim "upper land": **igi-nim** D.1.8: 12
igisig "lower land": **igi-sig** D.1.8: 12
il "to raise; to lift; to support": **ḫé-em-⸢íl$^?$⸣** H.1: 19'
imin "seven": **imin** H.1: 29'
inim "word; command; spell": **inim** C.1.4: 118''
inun "ghee": **ì-nun** II.1.1: 20
iškila "shell": **^{na4}iškila** G.1: 39
itud "month; moon": **iti$^!$-da** D.1.9: 15'

kag "mouth": **ka** C.1.4: 119''; **⸢ka$^?$⸣** C.1.2: 30'
kalam "land (Sumer)": **kalam-ma-ke$_4$** D.1.9: 30'
kan "gate": **^{ĝiš}ká** C.1.2: 32'
Kamadduru (a demon): **^{d}kamad-duru$_5$** II.1.3: 17''
Kamad-LAGAB (a demon): **^{d}⸢kamad⸣-[LAGAB$^?$]** II.1.3: 17''
Kamadme (a demon): **^{d}kamad-me** II.1.3: 17''
KA.muš "(disease-causing) worm": **[ka-muš]-⸢ì⸣-gu$_7$** II.1.3: 14''

katar “praise; glory”; **katar sil** “to praise”: **ka-tar-zu** C.3.4: 34; D.1.8: 19, 26
kešda “binding; ritual assemblage”: **kéš** G.1: 49
kešed “to bind”: **kéš** C.1.4: 76'', 187'''; **ké[š]** C.1.4: 83''; **⸢kéš-da⸣** G.2: 8'; **ke-še-da-ni** H.1: 28'; **ke-še-da-nu** H.1: 28'; **nu-k[éš]** C.1.4: 120''
ki “earth; netherworld”: **ki** C.1.4: 77''; D.1.7: 22'; H.1: 19'; **ki-na** C.3.2: 16'''; **ki-šè** D.1.9: 16', 19'; **ki-⸢šè⸣** D.1.9: 17'
ki’aĝ “to love”: **ki-⸢a?⸣-ga** II.1.3: 15''; **ki-áĝ** D.1.8: 5; **ki-áĝ-ĝá-[né]** D.1.9: 10'
kiĝ “(to) work; message”: **kin** H.1: 11'
kiri “orchard (garden)”: **kiri$_6$** C.1.4: 76''
kirid “hairpin”: **^{giš}[$^{ki-ri-is}$]kirid** G.1: 14
kisikillil “maiden wind-demon”: **ki-sikil-[líl-lá]** II.1.3: 12''-13''
kišar “the whole earth; totality”: **ki-šá-ra** I.1.2: 10'
kituš “dwelling”: **ki-tuš** D.1.8: 5
kud “to cut (off); to uproot; to separate; to clear; to decide”: **⸢kud?⸣** C.1.2: 30'; **ku$_5$-da** D.1.9: 34'
kug “(to be) pure”: **kù** D.1.9: 9'; **kù-ga** D.1.9: 16'; **kù-g[a]** D.1.8: 5; **kù-ga-ta** D.1.8: 6; **[kù-ga]-ta** D.1.9: 9'
kur I “mountain(s); land; netherworld”: **kur** C.1.4: 76'', 187'''; D.1.8: 7, 12; **kur-kur** C.3.2: 18'''; **⸢kur-kur?⸣-ra** C.3.4: 31; **kur-kur-ra-k[e$_4$]** C.3.4: 27; **kur-kur-ra-me-en** D.1.8: 11; **kur-ra** II.1.3: 6'', 22''; C.3.2: 19'''; **kur-ra-ke$_4$** D.1.9: 19'
kur II “to enter”: **ba-ši-in-ku$_4$** II.1.1: 12; **kur-ra-a** II.1.3: 18''

lal “to be little, small; to diminish; to reduce”: **ma-al-lal** H.2: 2
laraḫ “dire straits; difficult labour (in childbirth)”: **la-ra-aḫ** D.1.1: 40, 41; G.1: 26; G.2: 8'; **la-[ra-aḫ]** G.2: 7'
lil, lulil “wind-demon”: **[lú]-líl-lá** II.1.3: 12''
limmu “four”: **lam$_4$-ma** G.1: 10, 18
lu I “(hu)man; person”: **lú** II.1.1: 26; C.1.2: 32'; C.3.4: 31, 33; **[l]ú** C.1.2: 31'; **lú-ba** D.1.9: 36'; **nu** II.1.3: 15''; **saĝ-lú-ti-la** II.1.1: 24
lu II “to disturb; to stir up; to cover; to mix”: **u-me-ni-lù** D.1.9: 22'
lumumun “exorcist”: **lú-⸢mu$_7$-mu$_7$⸣** D.1.8: 26
lutur “child; youth”: **⸢lú-tur⸣** C.3.4: 33; **⸢lú?⸣-tur-bi** C.3.4: 33

ma “ship; boat”: **[$^{(ĝiš)}$m]á** D.1.1: 3; **[m]á** II.1.1: 6, 7; **mi-ki** II.1.1: 1, 2, 3, 4
mada “land”: **ma-da** A.1.2: 19''; H.1: 8, 27'
magur “cargo boat; barge”: **[m]á-gur$_8$** II.1.1: 5
maḫ “great; mighty; exalted”: **maḫ** D.1.8: 12, 13; **maḫ-e** D.1.9: 5', 9'
maššaĝ “foremost”: **máš-saĝ** D.1.8: 11
me “divine properties; rites; prayer”: **me-bi** D.1.9: 33'
mi dug “to care for; to treat well, kindly”: **mí** D.1.9: 29'
min “two; ditto”: **min** II.1.3: 5'', 6'', 7'', 8'', 9'', 10'', 11'', 12'', 13'', 14''; **⸢min?⸣** II.1.3: 4''
mu I “year”: **⸢mu⸣** II.1.1: 41'
mu II “name”: **mu-ni** D.1.9: 35'
mu III “to grow”: **mú** D.1.9: 10'
mul “star; to shine; to radiate”: **mul** C.3.4: 29; **mul-mul** G.1: 33
mulmul I “arrow”: **mul-mul** G.1: 33
mulmul II “reed fence”: **^{gi}mul-mul** G.1: 34; **⸢mul⸣-m[ul]** G.2: 13'
munus “female; woman”: **mu-nu-ús** II.1.1: 22; **munus** C.1.4: 70''; C.3.7: 21''; C.3.9: 15; G.1:1, 53; **⸢munus?⸣** A.2.7: 6; **⸢munus⸣** C.1.4: 49''; **munus-bi!** D.1.8: 16; **munus-⸢bi⸣** D.1.8: 14; **⸢munus⸣-[bi]** D.1.8: 23
mur “to clothe oneself; to wear; to put on clothing”: **mi-ni-in-[mu$_4$?]** D.1.9: 42'
muš “snake”: **[mu-u]š?-gin$_7$** II.1.1: 25

nam “destiny; fate”; **nam tar** “to decree (destiny)”: **nam** D.1.9: 34'
nammaḫ “greatness”: **nam-maḫ** D.1.8: 25; **nam-maḫ-zu** D.1.8: 24
namlulu “humankind; (hu)man”: **nam-lú-u$_{18}$-lu** C.3.4: 32
namtaga “sin”: **[na-á]ĝ?-tag** II.1.3: 9''
namtar “fate; destiny”: **nam-tar** II.1.3: 8''
nigru “snake charmer; exorcist”: **nigru** G.1: 7
niĝ “thing”: **níĝ** C.3.4: 32
niĝdim “manufactured object”: **níĝ-dím** C.3.4: 32
niĝdimdima “magical procedures”: **níĝ-dím-dím-[ma]** C.3.4: 32
niĝgig “that which is bad, evil”: **níĝ-gig** C.3.4: 33
niĝḫuludima “evil machinations”: **níĝ-ḫul-dím-ma** D.1.8: 20
niĝin “total; sum; entirety”: **niĝin** C.3.4: 31
niĝnam “everything”: **níĝ-nam** C.3.4: 29
niĝsisa “justice”: **^{d}níĝ-si-sá** D.1.8: 10
niĝzid “truth”: **[^{d}níĝ-z]i-da** D.1.8: 9

nin “lady”: **nin** C.3.4: 27; D.1.9: 31'; $^{\text{ni-ig}}$**níĝ** G.1:11
nita “male; man”: **ni-in-ta** II.1.1: 22
nu I “not”: **nu** C.1.4: 72''; G.1: 4
nu II “male genitalia”: **nu** G.1: 11
nud “to lie down”: **ná** C.1.4: 70'; **in-nú** C.3.4: 34
numun “seed”: **⸢numun**$^{?}$**⸣** A.2.7: 6

pa e “to (cause to) appear”: **pa-è** C.1.4: 123''; **[p]a ḫé**$^{!}$**-è**$^{!}$**-a-⸢ke**$_4$**⸣** D.1.1: 19
pad “to swear; to adjure”: **ḫé-pàd** G.1: 22
paḫal “distressed; troubled”: **⸢pa**$_4$**-ḫal⸣-l[a]** D.1.8: 14
pana “bow”: **pa-na-gin**$_7$ II.1.1: 26
pešturzi “offspring”: **⸢peš⸣-tur-zi** D.1.8: 3
piriĝ “lion”, var. for **ka-piriĝ** “conjurer; incantation priest”: **piriĝ** C.1.4: 77'', 78'', 84''
pisaĝ *see* **bisaĝ**

raḫ “to beat; to strike; to kill; to break”: **ra** I.1.7: 4
ri “to cast; to place; to throw down; to pour out; to release; to walk along; to ride; to lead away”: **ba-ni-[in-ri**$^{?}$**]** D.1.9: 10'; **mi-ni-ri** II.1.1: 2, 3, 4; **mi-ni**$^{!}$**-ri** II.1.1: 1; **ri-a** II.1.1: 21; D.1.9: 3'; **ra-a** II.1.3: 21''; **ri-r[i**$^{?}$**]** II.1.3: 26''

sa I “muscle; sinew; vein”: **sa** II.1.3: 24''; C.1.4: 78''; I.1.7: 13; **⸢sa⸣** C.3.4: 33
sa II “bundle”: **sa** I.1.2: 12'
sa’adnim (a disease): **sa-ad-nim** II.1.3: 22''
sag “(to be) good, sweet, favourable; goodness”: **sa**$_6$**-ga** D.1.1: 21
saĝ “head; person; first; top”: **saĝ** I.1.7: 3; **[sa]ĝ** II.1.3: 20''; **[sa]ĝ-bi** II.1.3: 19''; **saĝ-ĝá-na** D.1.9: 43'; **saĝ-lú-ti-la** II.1.1: 24
saĝ ĝeš raḫ “to kill”: **saĝ ĝiš ra** I.1.7: 2; **[saĝ ĝiš ra-r]a-e-dè** II.1.3: 10''; **saĝ ĝiš ra-ra** II.1.3: 11''
saĝamaḫ a priest: **[sáĝa]-maḫ** D.1.9: 36'
saĝgig “headache”: **saĝ-gig** II.1.3: 23'', 24''
saĝgiga “black-headed people”: **saĝ-gi**$_6$**-ga** C.3.4: 32; D.1.8: 13
saḫar “dust”: **saḫar** G.1: 9; **sa-ḫar** G.1: 9
si I “to fill”: **a-am-mi-íb-si** II.1.1: 6, 7, 8; **a-mi-íb-si** II.1.1: 5; **s[a**$_5$$^{?}$**]** D.1.1: 4
si II “light”: **si** G.1: 18, 19; G.2: 3'
sig I “to put”; **igi sig** “to see”: **[im-ma**$^{?}$**]-⸢an**$^{?}$**⸣-sig**$_{10}$**-g[e]** D.1.9: 20'; **im-ma-an-zi** II.1.1: 11
sig II “(to be) weak”: **sìg** C.1.2: 32'
sil “to split; to expel”; **katar sil** “to praise”: **ḫé-si-il** D.1.8: 19, 26; **ḫé-en-si-il-lá** D.1.8: 19; **ḫé-en-si-il-[e-en]** C.3.4: 34
sila “street”: **sila**^{la} G.1: 9; **sila** G.1: 10
silim “(to be) healthy, well, favourable, safe”: **silim-ma** D.1.8: 16, 17, 18, 19
sipad I “shepherd”: **sipa** G.1: 22
sipad II (a bird): **si-pa-ad-da** II.1.1: 21; **sipa** D.1.9: 8', 14'
sisa “to straighten; to put in order; to set straight”: **ḫé-em-ma-rab-si-sá-e-dè** D.1.8: 12; **ḫé-em-ma-an-si-sá-e-dè** D.1.8: 12; **[s]i ḫé-en-si-sá-e** D.1.1: 20; **si-sá-⸢e⸣-[dè]** II.1.1: 26; **si-s[á]** C.1.4: 72''; **si-sá-e** D.1.9: 32'; **si** G.1: 10, 36, 50
siškur “prayer; offering; sacrifice”: **siskur** G.1: 5
su I “flesh; body”: **⸢su-ni-ta**$^{?}$**⸣** G.2: 8'
su II “red; blood”: **sa** I.1.2: 6'
sug “marsh”: **sú-gu** II.1.1: 19
sukkal “vizier”: **sukkal** D.1.8: 8
sur “canal; ditch; (burial) pit”: **sùr**$^{?}$ II.1.3: 26''

šag “heart; interior; insides; in(side)”: **šà** G.1: 40; H.1: 28'; **šà-bé** D.1.9: 10'; **[š]à-bé** D.1.9: 22'; **šà-bi** D.1.8: 17
šag ḫul “to be happy”: **šà-ḫú[l]** D.1.9: 12'; **šà-ḫúl-la-zu-šè** D.1.8: 8
saĝki “forehead; brow; front”: **saĝ-ki** H.2: 1
šagtur “womb”: **šà-tùr** C.1.4: 79''
še I “to call by name”: **bi-[in-s]a**$_4$**-a** D.1.9: 35'; **bí-in-s[a**$_4$**]** D.1.9: 41'; **sa**$_4$**-a** D.1.9: 41'
še II “tip(?); side(?)”: **še** G.1: 43, 44
šeg I “brick”: **sig**$_4$ A.2.7: 32'
šeg II “(to be) favourable; to agree”: **še-ga** C.1.4: 128''; **še-g[a**$^{?}$**]** C.1.4: 119'', 128''
šer “(to be) bright; brilliance”: **še-er** H.2: 2
šerda “crime”: **šu-re-dè** II.1.3: 9''
šeš “to rub; to anoint; to smear”: **šéš-š[éš]** D.1.9: 37'; **[u]-me-ni-šéš** D.1.9: 23'
šid “to recite; to utter”: **[u]-me-ni-šid** D.1.9: 24'

šim "aromatics": **še-em-ma** II.1.1: 6; **še-em-ma-ak-ke$_4$** II.1.1: 6
šu "hand": **šu** II.1.3: 15''; **šu-n[é$^?$]** D.1.9: 36'; **šu-za-a** D.1.7: 24'
šu de "to carry": **šú tum** C.1.2: 30'
šu du "to perfect; to complete": **šu du$_7$** D.1.9: 33'
šu kuku "to withstand, approach": **<šu> nu-gu** II.1.3: 11''
šu teĝ "to accept; to receive": **šu u-me-ti** G.1: 8; **[šu] ù-me-ti** D.1.9: 21'
šuluḫ "handwashing rite": **šu-luḫ-[ḫa]** D.1.9: 32'
šum "garlic": **šúm$^{\ulcorner\text{sar}\urcorner}$-gin$_7$** D.1.8: 22
šusar "palm fibre cord": **šu-sa[r]-gin$_7$** D.1.8: 21

tag "to touch; to inflict": **[t]ag$^?$-ga** D.1.9: 6'
taḫ "to add": **a-ra-ab-daḫ-ḫe-e** II.1.1: 14, 15
taka "to leave behind; to abandon; to reject; to divorce; to save": **tag-ga** G.1: 35
tar "to cut; to decree"; **nam tar** "to determine (destiny)": **[m]i-ni-in-[tar$^?$]** D.1.9: 46'; **⸢tar⸣-tar-re** D.1.9: 34'
teĝ "(to be) near; to approach": **ba-te** D.1.9: 17'; **i-te** C.3.2: 23'''; **al-ti** C.1.2: 32'; **nam-ba-ti** C.1.4: 119''
til I "to be complete(d)": **saĝ-lú-ti-la** II.1.1: 24; **til** G.1: 19, 20; G.2: 5'; **til-la** G.1: 18; G.2: 3'; **ti-la-šè** H.1: 20'
til II "(to be) alive; to live; to recover": **al-ti-la** D.1.1: 202; D.1.8: 24; **ḫé$^!$-en$^!$-ti-la** D.1.8: 23; **ḫé-ti** C.3.4: 33, **ti-la** D.1.8: 17
tu "incantation; spell": **tu** II.1.2: 14; **[t]u$_6^!$** II.1.1: 27
tug "textile; garment": **túg** G.1: 45; **túg-⸢gin$_7$⸣** D.1.9: 19'
tuḫul, tugul "thigh/hip (bone)": **tu-ḫul** A.1.2: 19''; **tu-ḫu-ul** H.1: 7, 26'
tuku "to acquire; to get; to have": **nu-tuku** II.1.3: 15''
tukumbi "if": **tu-ku-ub-bi** II.1.1: 22, 23, 24
tur I "(to be) ill, sick; sickness": **tu-ra** II.1.3: 16''
tur II "(to be) small, young, narrow": **tur-ra** D.1.7: 22'
tur III "animal stall": **tùr** D.1.9: 9'

u I "and": **u** D.1.8: 26; **ù** II.1.1: 16; D.1.1: 5; G.1: 2
u II "sleep": **ù** II.1.3: 18''
u III "plant(s); herb; grass; food": **ú** C.1.2: 30'; C.3.2: 22'''; D.1.9: 11'
u ku "(to) sleep": **ù ⸢ku$^?$⸣** D.1.7: 23'; **ù ku-uk-ku** II.1.3: 21''
ubila "charcoal": **ú-bil-lá** C.1.2: 31'
ud "day; sun": **⸢u$_4$⸣** II.1.1: 40'; **u$_4$-da** D.1.8: 24; **u$_4$-da-a-ni** D.1.9: 15'; **[u$_4$-d]a-a-ni** D.1.9: 36'
udiliya "fifteen": **15.kam** II.1.1: 40'
udul "herdsman": **ú-dúl** D.1.9: 7', 13'; **udul$_{10}$-lu-ú-a** G.1: 22
udug (a demon): **udug** II.1.3: 10''
ugu I "skull": **ag-ga-ab** II.1.1: 10
ugu II "to bear; to give birth": **gu** G.1: 48
uĝ "people": **ùĝ-bi** D.1.8: 25
ur I "root; trunk; base; limb(s); lap; loin": **ú-ra** II.1.1: 10
ur II "roof": **⸢ùr-ra-gin$_7$⸣** D.1.9: 26'
urdu "servant": **[urd]u-zu** D.1.8: 26; **uru$^{?\text{rù}}$-du-zu** D.1.8: 26
ursaĝ "hero; warrior": **[ur$^?$]-saĝ** C.3.4: 28
urud "copper": **urudu** G.1: 34
us "to lean on; to follow; to lead; to flow copiously": **mu-un-da-ús-sa** D.1.1: 236
usan "whip": **^{kuš}ùsan** D.1.9: 6'
ušušru "debility, decay": **uš-šú-uš-ru** II.1.3: 14''; **uš-šú-uš-ru-a** II.1.3: 19''
ušzu "witchcraft": **⸢uš$_{11}$⸣-z[u]** D.1.8: 20
utud "to bear (a child); to give birth": **du-da-an-ni** II.1.1: 1, 2, 3, 4; **ḫé-ù-tu-du** D.1.9: 28'; **ḫé-ù-tu-ud-d[a]** D.1.9: 38'; **mu-un-ù-tu-ud** C.1.4: 71''; **ù-tu-ud** D.1.9: 31'; **ù-tu-ud-da** D.1.8: 16, 17, 19; **⸢ù⸣-tu-ud-da** D.1.9: 3', 4'; **⸢ù⸣-tu-ud-⸢da⸣** D.1.9: 5'; **ù-tu-ud-da-a-ni** G.1: 1, 53
uzusa'umbin "nerve(?)": **<uzu>-⸢sa$^?$⸣-umbin-⸢a-ni$^?$⸣** II.1.3: 25''

za'e "you; yours": **za-a-kám** D.1.1: 21; **ze-e** II.1.1: 16
zag "side": **zag** C.1.4: 139'', 140''
zagin "lapis lazuli": **[$^{\text{na4}}$za]-gìn$^?$** D.1.1: 4; **$^{\text{na4}}$za-gìn-na** II.1.1: 8; **za-gi-in** II.1.1: 8, 9
zalag "(to be) pure; (to be) bright; to shine; to illuminate; light": **hé-en-zálag-ga** H.2: 29'; **ḫé-en-zálag-ge** H.2: 1, 2; **$^{\text{za-al}}$zalag** G.1: 35; **zálag** D.1.8: 2
zalaḫ "to slip through an opening": **iz-za-la-aḫ** D.1.1: 202; **za-la-aḫ** D.1.1: 202; D.1.4: 6', 7'
zi I "life": **zi** G.1: 22
zi II "to cut; to remove; to pluck": **zí** G.1: 28
zid "right; right hand": **zi** D.1.9: 8', 14'; **[zi-d]a** C.3.4: 29; **zi-da-zu** D.1.8: 9; **zi-dè-eš** D.1.9: 29'

zig "to rise; to remove": **zi** H.2: 2; **zí** H.2: 1; **zi-z[i]** C.1.4: 122''; **zi-ga** C.1.4: 129''; **iz** H.2: 1
zil "(to be) good, beneficent": **zíl-zíl-le-bi** D.1.1: 21
zu I "tooth; barb; blade": **⸢^{gi}⸣z[ú$^{!?}$]** D.1.9: 34'
zu II "to know": **ḫé-[e]n-zu-zu** D.1.8: 25; **in-ga-ra-e-zu** II.1.1: 16; **nu-me-e-zu** II.1.1: 14, 15; **nu-uz-zu** II.1.1: 9; **nu-zu** G.1: 2; **n[u-zu]** D.1.1: 5; **zu** G.1: 4; **zu-zu** II.1.3: 12''
zukešed "bond; binding; knot": **zú-kéš** C.3.7: 21''; C.3.9: 15; **[z]ú-kéš** C.3.7: 22''; **⸢zú⸣-kéš-bi** D.1.8: 15; **zú-kéš-da** C.3.7: 21'', 22''; C.3.9: 15; **zú-kéš-da-šè** H.1: 29'

Personal Names

Ammiditana: **a[m]-m[i]-di-ta-na** II.1.1: 41'
Anu-ikṣur: **^{md}60-*ik-ṣur*** C.2.1: 16'; **[^{m}AN.Š]ÁR-ZÚ.KÉŠ** C.3.10: 92
Anu-[...]: **⸢^{m}⸣^{d}60-x-x** D.1.11: 15'
Artaḫšassu (Artaxerxes): **^{m}*ar*** I.1.1: 118; **[^{m}*ar-taḫ*]*-šá-as-su*** D.1.10: 13'
Aššur-bāni-apli (Ashurbanipal): **^{m}*Aš-šur*-DÙ-A** D.1.2: 16; **^{m}AN.ŠÁR-[DÙ-IBILA]** D.1.6: 16''
Arad-nubatti: **^{m}ÌR-⸢*nu*$^{!}$*-ba*⸣*-at-ti*** B.2.1: 41
Banītu'a: **[^{munus}*ba-ni-t*]*u*$^{?}$*-ú-a*** D.1.10: 7'
Bāštī-Bābili: **[^{m}TÉŠ$^{?}$]-⸢TIN⸣.TIR^{ki}** B.2.1: 42
Bēl-erība: **^{md}EN-SU** I.1.1: 118
Bullussa-rabi: ***bu-luṭ-sa*$^{?}$-GA[L]$^{?}$** D.1.1: 129
Dāda: **U.U** C.3.9: 7
Ea-[...]: **^{md}IDIM-[x-x]** D.1.10: 7'
Egi-Suena: ***e-gi-*^{d}EN.ZU.NA** D.1.1: 170
Egizinītu: ***e-gi-zi-ni-ti*** G.1: 37; **⸢*e*⸣*-gi-zi-ni-tu*$_{4}$** D.1.1: 181
Enlil-kāṣir: **^{d}50-KÁD** G.1: 54
Enlil-šuma-imbi: **^{md}*en-líl*-MU-*im-bi*** G.1: 54
Ēṭiru: **^{m}*e-ṭi-ru*** A.2.6: 29; D.3.1: 38(f)
Gaḫul-Tutu: **^{m}GA.ḪÚL-^{d}*tu-tu*** B.2.1: 38; **[^{m}GA.ḪÚL$^{?}$-^{d}]*tu-tu*** B.2.2: 30'
Geme-Sîn: **GÉME-^{d}EN.ZU.NA** D.1.1: 135, 158; **GÉME-^{d}30** D.1.1: 135, 158, 164; G.1: 37
Gī-Sîn: ***gi-se-en*** II.1.4: 51; ***gi-i-*^{d}30** II.1.4: 61
Gula-balāssu-iqbi: **^{md}*g[u]-la-*⸢TI⸣*-su-iq-bi*** B.2.1: 39
Ḫuṣābi: **^{m}*ḫu-ṣa-bi*** I.1.1: 118
Iprā'ya: ŠE.BA-*'-ia* A.2.6: 28; **⸢^{m}ŠE⸣.B[A$^{?}$-*'a-a*]** D.3.1: 37(f)
Ištar-[...]: **^{md}KÁR.ŠUL-*id*-[...]** I.1.2: 14'
Ištarāya: **⸢^{d}INNIN⸣*-a-a*** D.1.10: 10'
Itti-Marduk-balāṭu: **^{m}KI-AMAR.UTU-TIN** I.1.3: 35; **^{m}*it-ti-*^{d}A[MAR.UTU-*balāṭu*]** C.3.3: 43
Kiṣir-Nabû: **^{m}*ki-ṣir-*^{d}AG** D.3.1: 38(A)
Ludumununna: **^{m}LÚ-DUMU-NUN.NA** G.1: 55
Marduk-[...]: **⸢^{d}AMAR.UTU⸣-[...]** E.2.3: 30''
Mušallim-Marduk: **⸢GI⸣-⸢^{d}AMAR⸣.[UTU]** I.1.3: 35'
Nabû-iddina: **⸢$^{md+}$AG$^{?}$⸣*-i-din-*⸢*nam*⸣** E.2.3: 30''
Nabû-kuṣuršu: **^{md}AG-*ku-ṣur-šú*** I.1.1: 118
Nādinu: **^{m}*na-di-nu*** C.3.4: 100
Ninurta-nāṣir-šumi: **^{md}MAŠ-PAP-MU** B.2.1: 42
Nūr-Marduk: **^{m}*nu-úr-*^{d}AMAR.UTU** C.1.8: 31'
Sîn-iddina: **^{md}30-SUM-*n[a]*** C.3.1: 31; **^{md}*ša-máš*-SUM-*na***
Sîn-multēšir: **^{md}30-*mu-ul-te-ši-ir*** B.2.1: 38
Šamaš-aḫa-iddina: **^{md}20-PAP-MU** I.1.2: 14'
Šamaš-ibni: **^{m}⸢^{d}⸣UTU-*ib-ni*** D.3.1: 39(A)
Šamaš-iddina: **^{md}UTU-SUM-*na*** C.3.4: 99; **^{md}UTU-MU-*n[a]*** C.2.1: 17'; **^{m}[^{d}UTU-MU-*na*]** C.2.1: 16'
Šangû-Ninurta: ^{lú}SANGA-^{d}*nin-urta* C.3.4: 100; **^{lú}SANGA-^{d}[*nin-urta*]** C.3.10: 93
Šangû-parakki: **^{lú}SANGA-BARAG-*ki*** I.1.3: 36'
Zababa-pir'u-uṣur: **^{md}*za-ba*$_{4}$*-ba*$_{4}$-NUNUZ-ÙRU** A.2.6: 28; **^{md}*za-ba*$_{4}$*-ba*$_{4}$-NUNUZ-Ù[R]U** D.3.1: 38(f)

Geographical Names

Bābili (Babylon): **KÁ.DINGIR.⸢RA^{ki}⸣** C.1.8: 31'; **TIN.TIR^{ki}** C.3.9: 39

Borsippa: **BÁR.SIPA^{ki}** I.1.1: 117

Dūr-Ammiditana: **bàd-am-mi-di-ta-na^{ki}** II.1.1: 42'

Eanna: ***é-an-na*** I.1.3: 37'

Ebabbar (temple of Šamaš): ***é-babbar-r[a]*** D.1.8: 4; **é-bab[bar-ra-ke$_{4}$]** D.1.8: 4

Ekur (temple of Enlil): **é-[ku]r-ra-ke$_{4}$** D.1.9: 31'

Eridu: ***eri$^{!}$-dù$^{!}$-ke$_{4}$*** B.1.1: 11; ***eri-[du$_{10}$^{ki}]*** D.1.1: 128

Gutû "Gutean": ***gu-ti-tú*** H.1: 33'

Ḫašur: ***ḫa-šur*** D.1.8: 7; **ḫa-šur-ra-ta** D.1.8: 7

Hatti: ***ḫat-ti*** A.2.4: 9'

Kār-bēl-mātāti: **^{uru}KAR-EN-KUR.KUR** C.3.10: 91

Keš: **kèš^{ki}-ke$_{4}$** D.1.9: 28'; **[kèš^{ki}-k]e$_{4}$** D.1.9: 38'

Māt Aššur "Assyria": **KUR AN.ŠÁR^{ki}** D.1.4: 16''

Me-Enlil (canal): **⸢íd⸣-me-en-líl-lá-ke$_{4}$** II.1.1: 42'

miṣrāyu, *muṣrāyu* "Egyptian": ***mi-ṣir-a-a*** B.2.2: 13; ***mi-[ṣir-a-a$^{?}$]*** A.1.1: 31''

Sippar: *sip-par* D.1.8: 4; **zimbir^{ki}** D.1.8: 4

Uruk: **UNUG^{ki}** I.1.3: 35'; **⸢UNUG^{ki}⸣** C.2.1: 16'

Deities, Demons and Star Names

Adad: ^{d}*ad-da-a* C.3.10: 21; **^{d}IŠKUR** D.1.5: 7'

An: **an-na-k[e$_{4}$]** D.1.8: 1

Antu: ***an-tum*** C.3.9: 57; ***an-[tum]*** C.3.3: 37; ***an-⸢tum⸣*** C.3.4: 15; **^{d}KI.ŠÁR** C.3.10: 93

Anu: **^{d}60** C.3.4: 100; C.3.9: 57; I.1.2: 15'; **^{d}*a-nim*** II.1.4: 59; C.3.3: 25; C.3.9: 49; C.3.10: 27; D.1.8: 1; **^{d}*a-[n]im*** C.3.4: 62; **^{d}*a-nu*** C.1.4: 61''; C.3.4: 13, 62, 69, 76; C.3.9: 41; **^{d}*a-n[u]*** C.2.1: 18'; C.3.3: 15; **^{d}*a-⸢num$^{?}$⸣*** C.3.4: 15; **^{d}*a-num*** C.3.3: 36; **[AN.ŠÁ]R** C.3.10: 93

Anzû: ***an-ze-e*** A.2.6: 16; ***an-zu-ú*** C.3.9: 42; ***an-[zu]***-*ú* C.3.4: 63

Ardat-lilî: **⸢KI$^{?}$⸣.SIKIL.[L]ÍL.LÁ$^{?!}$** C.3.1: 32

Aruru: **^{d}*a-ru-ru*** D.1.1: 87; **[^{d}*a-r*]*u$^{?}$-ru*** D.1.10: 4'

Asalluḫi: **^{d}*a-sa-lu-ḫa*** II.1.2: 11; **^{d}asal-lú-ḫi** II.1.1: 17; C.1.4: 121''; **^{d}*asal-lú-ḫi*** B.1.1: 51, 55; B.2.1: 11; C.1.5: 48; C.3.1: 26; C.3.5: 28'; C.3.10: 17; D.1.1: 47, 115, 128, 195; E.2.3: 3'; **⸢^{d}⸣*asal-lú-ḫi*** A.2.7: 9; D.1.8: 25; **[^{d}]asal-lú-ḫi** II.1.1: 13; **[^{d}as]al-⸢lú-ḫi⸣** D.1.9: 20'; **^{d}*as[al-lú-ḫi$^{?}$]*** C.3.7: 3'; **^{d}*[asal-lú-ḫi]*** B.1.1: 56

Aššur: **AN.ŠÁR** C.1.4: 136''; D.3.1: 39(A); **⸢AN.ŠAR⸣** D.1.2: 17

Aya: **^{d}a-a** D.1.8: 5; **^{d}*a-a*** D.1.8: 5

Bau, Baba: **$^{d?}$*[ba]-ba$_{6}$$^{?}$*** B.1.1: 7

Bēlet-ēkalli: **^{d}NIN.É.GAL$^{!}$** D.1.5: 18'

Bēlet-ilī: **DINGIR.MAḪ** C.1.4: 53''; **[DINGIR.M]AḪ** C.1.4: 49''; **^{d}*be-let*-DINGIR.MEŠ** D.1.5: 18'; **^{d}*be-let-ì-lí*** D.1.1: 51; **^{d}GAŠAN-DINGIR** G.1: 6

Bunene: **[^{d}*b*]*u-ne-ne*** D.1.8: 8

Damu: **^{d}*da-mu*** B.1.1: 68; C.3.1: 27; C.3.10: 18

Dingirmaḫ: **diĝir-maḫ** C.3.4: 34; **⸢diĝir-maḫ⸣** C.3.4: 32

Dumuzi: **⸢^{d}⸣*dumu-zi*** C.3.10: 71; **[^{d}]*dumu-zi*** C.3.10: 65; **^{d}d[umu-zi$^{?}$]** D.1.9: 8'; **^{d}dumu-zi-da** D.1.9: 14'

Ea: ^{d}40 D.1.1: 187; **[^{d}]⸢40⸣** C.1.5: 48; ***é-a*** II.1.2: 11; **^{d}*é-a*** B.1.1: 52, 55; B.2.1: 11; C.3.4: 77; C.3.5: 28'; D.1.1: 117, 129; **⸢^{d}*é*⸣*-a*** D.1.8: 25; **^{d}*é-[a]*** C.3.4: 68; **^{d}⸢*é*⸣*-[a]*** B.1.1: 51, 67; **[^{d}]⸢*é*⸣*-a*** E.2.3: 3'; **[^{d}*é*]-⸢*a*⸣** C.3.1: 26; **^{d}*[é-a]*** C.3.3: 38; **^{d}IDIM** C.1.4: 50''; C.3.7: 3'; C.3.9: 49, 57; C.3.10: 17; D.1.1: 47; **^{d}I[DIM]** C.3.10: 53

Ea-šarru: **^{d}40-LUGAL** D.1.1: 130

Ella(m)-mê (a name of the moon god): ***el-la-me-e*** G.1: 17; ***[el-l]am-me-e*** G.2: 2'; ***el-lam-mu-u*** G.1: 18; ***el-lam-mu-ú*** G.2: 3'; ***i-il-la-a-me-e*** D.1.1: 26; ***i-il-la-a-⸢me⸣-e*** D.1.1: 27

Enbilulu: **^{d}en-bi-lù-l[ù]** C.1.4: 121''

Enki: **^{d}en-ki** C.1.4: 115''; **⸢$^{d+}$en⸣-ki** D.1.8: 25; **^{d}en-ki-ke$_{4}$** C.1.4: 116''; **^{d}en-ki-k[e$_{4}$]** C.1.4: 115''; **⸢^{d}⸣en-ki-[ke$_{4}$]** C.1.4: 117''; **^{d}en-ki-ra** II.1.1: 11

Enlil: **^{d}*en-líl*** G.1: 54; **$^{d+}$*en-líl*** C.3.8: 5; **^{d}en-líl-lá-ke$_{4}$** D.1.9: 36'

Enzu Lyra ("Goat star"): **^{mul}ÙZ** C.1.5: 9; **^{mul4}Ù[Z$^{?}$]** C.1.5: 29

Ereqqu Ursa Major ("Wagon star"): **^{mul}MAR.GÍD.DA** II.1.3: 45'''; **⸢^{mul}⸣MAR.GÍD.D[A]** C.3.8: 2; **[^{mul}]MAR.GÍD.DA** C.3.4: 89; **^{mul}MAR.GÍD.D[A]** C.3.8: 3, 4

Girra: ^{d}*gíra* C.3.10: 28
GUD: ^{d}**GU$_4$** G.1: 25
Gula: ^{d}***gu-la*** B.1.1: 70; C.1.4: 53''; C.3.4: 79, 96; C.3.5: 30'; C.3.10: 18, 62; ⸢^{d}⸣ ***gu-la*** C.1.8: 14'; ^{d}⸢***gu***⸣***-la*** C.3.6: 41'''; ^{d}***g[u-l]a*** A.1.1: 8'; ^{d}***g[u-la]*** C.3.1: 27

Igigi: ^{d}**i-gi$_4$-gi$_4$** C.3.4: 31; ⸢**i$^{?}$-gi-gi**⸣ C.3.4: 31; ^{d}***í-gì-gì*** D.3.1: 19
Inanna: ^{d}**inanna** C.1.4: 79''; [^{d}**inan]na$^{?}$** C.1.4: 69''; ⸢^{d}⸣**inanna** C.1.4: 70''; [^{d}**inann]a-ke$_4$** II.1.1: 2
Ištar: ^{d}**INANNA** C.1.4: 18'; ^{d}15 C.1.4: 53''; C.2.1: 18'; C.3.4: 100; I.1.3: 16; $^{d+}$**INANNA** I.1.2: 15'; ^{d}***iš-tar*** B.2.1: 3; ⸢^{d}***iš***⸣***-[tar]*** C.1.4: 15'; ^{d}⸢***iš$_8$-tár***⸣

Kamadduru (a demon): ^{d}**kamad-duru$_5$** II.1.3: 17''
Kamad-LAGAB (a demon): ^{d}⸢**kamad**⸣**-[LAGAB$^{?}$]** II.1.3: 17''
Kamadme: ^{d}**kamad-me** II.1.3: 17''; see also Lamaštu
Kiririša: **ki-ri-ri-šá** H.1: 21'; ***[ki]-ri-ri-[šá]*** D.1.1: 42; ***ki-ri-ri-šú*** D.1.1: 42

Lamaštu: ^{d}**DÌM.ME** C.3.4: 41, 79; ^{d}⸢**DÌM**⸣**.ME** C.3.4: 96; **DIM$_{10}$.ME** D.2.1: 28'
Lillu: ^{d}***lil-lum*** C.3.1: 20, 24
Lugal-amaš-pa'e: **lugal-maš-pa-è-a** II.1.3: 9''
Lugal-nam-en-na: **[^{d}lugal]-nam-me-en-na** II.1.3: 22''-23''

Mami: ^{d}***ma-mi*** C.1.4: 51''; D.1.1: 129; ^{d}***ma-***⸢***mi***⸣ D.1.1: 88; ⸢^{d}***ma-mi$^{?}$***⸣ D.1.1: 91; ^{d}***ma-***⸢***mi$^{?}$***⸣ D.1.1: 97
Marduk: ^{d}**AMAR.UTU** II.1.4: 46; C.1.2: 23'; D.1.1: 23, 99, 198; D.1.8: 25; ^{d}**A[MAR.UTU]** C.1.1: 12

Nabû: ^{d}**AG** D.3.1: 38(A); I.1.1: 118; ^{d}**MUATI** C.3.3: 45
Naḫḫunte: ^{d}**na-ḫu-un-d[i]** A.1.2: 3'; ***na-ḫu-un-di*** D.1.1: 163, 167; G.1: 27; G.2: 9'; ***[na-ḫ]u-un-di*** D.1.1: 44; ***na-ḫu-un-du*** D.1.1: 44
Nanamgišir: ***na-nam-gi-ši-ir*** D.1.1: 163
Nanna: ^{d}**NANNA** D.1.1: 25; ^{d}**[NANNA]** D.1.1: 26; ^{d}**NANNA-*ru*** D.1.1: 149, 166
Napiriša: **nap-ri-šá** H.1: 21'; ***nap-ri-šá*** D.1.1: 42; ***nap-ri-šú*** D.1.1: 42
Narunde: ***na-ru-un-di*** D.1.1: 44, 163, 167; G.1: 27; ***na-ru-un-du*** D.1.1: 44; G.2: 9'
Nindara: ^{d}**nin-dar-a** G.1: 22, 23
Ningal, Nikkal: ^{d}**NI[N.GAL]** D.1.8: 3; ^{d}**ni[n-gal-la-ke$_4$]** D.1.8: 3
Ningirima: ^{d}***nin-gìrima*** C.3.5: 29'; C.3.10: 18; ⸢^{d}⸣***nin-gìrima*** C.3.1: 27
Ninḫursaĝa: **[^{d}nin-hur]-saĝ-ĝá-ke$_4$** II.1.1: 4
Ninisina: ⸢^{d}⸣**nin-ì-si-in-na** D.1.9: 30'
Ninkarrak: ^{d}***nin-kar-ra-a[k]*** B.1.1: 68; ^{d}***nin-kar-ra-ak-a*** C.3.10: 64
Ninlil: ^{d}***nin-líl*** C.3.8: 6
Ninmaḫ: ^{d}***nin-maḫ*** C.3.4: 90; [^{d}**n]in-maḫ** C.3.4: 27; [^{d}**ni]n$^{?}$-maḫ** C.3.4: 32; [^{d}***n]in-maḫ*** C.3.6: 10'
Ninšubur: **[^{d}NIN.ŠU]BUR$^{?}$** B.1.1: 69
Nintinuga: ^{d}**nin-tin-ug$_5$-ga** D.1.9: 29'
Nintur: ^{d}**nin-tu-ra-ke$_4$** D.1.9: 28', 38'
Niraḫ: **ni-ra-aḫ** G.1: 25

Papnuna: **[^{d}]**⸢**pap-nun**⸣**-[na]** D.1.8: 8
Pazuzu: ***pa-zu-zu*** C.3.9: 28

Sîn, Suen: **30** D.3.1: 11a; ^{d}**30** II.1.4: 51, 53, 58, 61; B.2.6: 2, 5, 6, 15; C.3.10: 20; D.1.1: 135, 137, 138, 149, 164, 166, 181; D.1.8: 3; D.3.1: 8, 10c, 11a; G.1: 20, 21, 23, 27; G.2: 9', 27''; ⸢^{d}⸣**30** D.3.1: 14; ^{d}⸢**30**⸣ B.2.6: 17; ⸢^{d}⸣**[30]** G.2: 6'; ⸢^{d}**EN**⸣**.ZU** B.2.1: 19; $^{d+}$**suen-na** D.1.8: 3
Sukku: ⸢^{d}⸣**sú-uk-ku** A.1.2: 2'

Šakkan: ^{d}**ŠÁKKAN** C.3.4: 45; C.3.10: 65, 71; D.1.1: 24
Šamaš: <^{d}>**20** C.3.10: 70; ^{d}**UTU** II.1.2: 13; A.2.7: 39'; B.2.6: 2, 5, 6; C.1.4: 53'', 82'', 87''; C.1.8: 35', 36'; C.3.3: 13; C.3.4: 12, 81; C.3.6: 61''''; C.3.10: 6, 20, 41, 48, 68, 70; D.1.1: 18; D.1.8: 1, 2, 6, 13; D.1.9: 27'; D.3.1: 16, 17, 23; E.2.3: 3', 9', 15'; G.1: 27; G.2: 10'; ⸢^{d}⸣**UTU** D.1.1: 50; ^{d}**U[TU]** G.2: 9'; ^{d}**[UTU]** C.3.5: 18'; ⸢^{d}**UTU**⸣ D.3.1: 18; ^{d}*šá-maš* C.3.1: 14, 24
Šarrat-kidmuri: ^{d}**GAŠAN-*k[id-mu-ri$^{?}$]*** C.3.1: 20, 24
Šazu (a name of Marduk, lit. divine midwife): ⸢^{d}⸣**šà-zu** C.1.4: 85''; ^{d}⸢**ŠÀ$^{!}$.ZU**⸣ D.1.1: 199
Šukudu Sirius ("Arrow-Star"): ^{mul}**KAK.SI.SÁ** G.1: 37
Šulpae'a: ^{d}**šul-pa-è-a** C.3.4: 28

Utu: ^{d}**utu** D.1.8: 1, 2, 6, 13; ^{d}**utu-šè** D.1.9: 27'

Month Names

Abu (fifth month): ^{iti}**AB** A.2.6: 29
Ayyāru (second month): ^{iti}**GU$_4$** D.3.1: 6, 11b
Nisannu (first month): ^{iti}**BÁRA** D.3.1: 1, 6, 11b, 23, 32, 37(b), 38(f); ^{iti}**BÁRA.ZAG.GAR** B.2.6: 2
Simānu (third month): [^{it}]^{i}**SIG$_4$** D.1.10: 12'

Text Concordances

Museum No.	Joins to	Previous Publication	CDLI No.	Text No.	Plate
Anadolu Medeniyetleri Müzesi, Ankara					
372/f		KUB 37, 189	P445909	I.1.1	
SU 51/13		STT 254	P338573	C.3.4	
SU 52/83 (+) 52/83A (+) 52/111 (+) 52/130 (+) 52/130A (+)	SU 52/137	STT 98	P338419	A.1.1	
SU 52/99 + 149		STT 241	P338560	C.3.1	
SU 52/137 (+)	SU 52/83 (+) 52/83A (+) 52/111 (+) 52/130 (+) 52/130A (+)	STT 284	P338602	A.1.1	
SU 52/146 + 173 + 338		STT 278	P338596	F.1	
Vorderasiatisches Museum, Berlin					
VAT 8004		KAR 223 Hätinen 2021, pl. 11–12	P369187	D.3.1	
VAT 8007 +	VAT 13875 + VAT 14099 (+) VAT 16457	KAR 266 BAM 244	P285330	B.1.1	
VAT 8577 +	VAT 13655 + VAT 13671 + VAT 13706 + VAT 13707 + VAT 13708 + VAT 13828 + VAT 14177 + VAT 14185 (+)	KAR 194 BAM 237	P285323	C.1.4	
VAT 8809		KAR 247 CMAwR 3, pl. 9	P369211	C.3.6	
VAT 8869		KAR 196 BAM 248	P285333	D.1.1	
VAT 8881		KAR 195 BAM 240	P285326	D.2.1	
VAT 8943		KAR 205 BAM 183	P285275	D.1.1	
VAT 9029		KAR 202 BAM 3	P285108	H.1	
VAT 9543 (+) → VAT 10757			P285327	II.1.3	7–8
VAT 10476		BAM 247	P285332	B.1.3	
VAT 10575 (+)	VAT 9543	BAM 241	P285327	II.1.3	
VAT 11415		BAM 245	P281822	A.1.3	
VAT 13628 → BAM 14151+					
VAT 13629 +	VAT 13866	KAL 2, No. 41	P480934	C.3.7 F.1	
VAT 13724		BAM 235	P285321	C.1.1	
VAT 13896		BAM 246	P285331	B.1.6	
VAT 13897		BAM 251	P285336	E.1.1	
VAT 13972		BAM 249	P285334	D.1.1 D.1.3	
VAT 14123 (+)	VAT 8577 +	BAM 238	P285324	C.1.4.1	
VAT 14145 (+)	VAT 8577 +	BAM 239	P288325	C.1.4.2	
VAT 14150 +	VAT 14156 (+)	KAL 2, No. 36	P480948	C.3.9	
VAT 14151 +	VAT 14152 + VAT 14153 + VAT 13628 (+)	KAL 2, No. 36 KAL 7, No. 11	P480948	C.3.9	
VAT 14389		BAM 242	P285328	II.1.3.1	
VAT 14528		LKU 55 BAM 408	P285479	A.2.9	
VAT 14587		LKU 126	P414257	I.1.6	

https://doi.org/10.1515/9781501506475-014

(continued)

Museum No.	Joins to	Previous Publication	CDLI No.	Text No.	Plate
VAT 16446		BAM 386	P285457	C.1.4	
VAT 20785		KAL 7, No. 16		C.1.3	
Iraq Museum, Baghdad					
–		UET 7, No. 123		B.2.2	
IM 67636 → ND 5590					
IM 74452 → W. 23311					
IM 76830 → W. 23262					
IM 76849 → W. 23287					
IM 76998 → W. 22649					
IM 77020 → W. 22668/0					
ND 5590		CTN 4, No. 105	P363519	C.3.6	
W. 22307/23 + 74		SpTU 1, No. 39	P348460	I.1.2	
W. 22307/50 + 54 + 62 + 69 + 76		SpTU 1, No. 59	P348480	C.2.1	
W. 22649		SpTU 4, No. 153	P348746	C.1.10 D.1.11	26
W. 22668/0		SpTU 5, No. 253		E.2.6	
W. 23262		SpTU 5, No. 248	P348835	C.3.10	
W. 23279		SpTU 4, No. 129	P348723	C.1.4	
W. 23281		SpTU 4, No. 173	P348766	C.4.1	
W. 23287		SpTU 3, No. 84	P348688	C.3.4	
W. 23311		SpTU 1, No. 40		I.1.7	
Institute for the Study of Ancient Cultures, Chicago (formerly Oriental Institute)					
A. 3438		TDP II, pl. LVII		I.1.3	
A. 3461				A.1.2	9
Arkeoloji Müzeleri, Istanbul					
A 37		LKA 9		C.3.5	
A 177		LKA 142	P414051	C.3.4	
A 203		BAM 236	P285322	C.1.2	
A 218		BAM 250	P285335	B.1.4	
A 265		BAM 363	P285434	F.2	
A 624		BAM 346	P285418	F.1	
A 2732		BAM 243	P285329	B.1.2	
Bo 4822		KUB 4, No. 13		D.1.1	
British Museum, London					
BM 34208			P562539	D.1.9	40–41
BM 36339			P562979	D.1.1	35
BM 37014			P557508	C.4.1	34
BM 37476			P563325	D.1.9	42
BM 38624 +	BM 38828 + BM 45414			A.2.1	12–13
BM 40152			P564810	C.1.8	28–29
BM 42313 +	BM 42427 + BM 42585 + BM 43174 + BM 43215 + BM 43274 + BM 43279 + BM 43281 + BM 43439 + BM 43483 + BM 43595 + BM 43766 + BM 43803		P564872	A.2.2	14–15
BM 42327 +	BM 42410 + BM 42604 + BM 42628 + BM 43474 + BM 43523	Farber 1989a, pl. 14–15	P480131	C.3.3	
BM 42333 +	BM 42453 + BM 43602	Finkel, *FS Lambert*, Fig. 24		A.2.2	
BM 42507		Finkel, *FS Lambert*, Fig. 9		E.2.1	

(continued)

Museum No.	Joins to	Previous Publication	CDLI No.	Text No.	Plate
BM 42450 +	BM 43809	Finkel, *FS Lambert*, fig. 23		B.2.3	
BM 42587 +	BM 42640 + BM 43217 + BM 43287 + BM 43475 + BM 43812	Finkel, *FS Lambert*, Fig. 22		B.2.4	
BM 43110 +	BM 43291 + BM 43470	Finkel, *FS Lambert*, Fig. 25		E.2.2	
BM 43229		Finkel, *FS Lambert*, Fig. 11		E.2.1	
BM 43268	(+) F 238	Finkel, *FS Lambert*, Fig. 10		E.2.1	
BM 45559 +	BM 45574		P564929	A.2.4	17
BM 45736			P564931	A.2.5	18
BM 47459				D.3.1	
BM 47491				A.2.6	19
BM 47578			P564970	C.2.2	31
BM 47770 +	BM 47904			F.1	52
BM 47801				E.2.3	48
BM 48030		CMAwR 3, pl. 3		C.3.8	
BM 48557			P565013	A.2.10	
BM 48710			P565025	E.2.4	
BM 48997			P480868	E.2.7	
BM 49133			P565063	E.2.8	
BM 50700				A.2.3	16
BM 51246 +	BM 53217 + BM 53744		P480873	A.2.7	20
BM 54587 +	BM 73802			C.2.3	32
BM 54846				D.1.10	43
BM 57853		CT 55, No. 377	P314769	E.2.5	
BM 59710				B.2.5	26
BM 61975				C.2.4	33
BM 65450 +	BM 76497			I.1.1	1–2
BM 68458 +	K. 11550	*NABU* 2019/3, 139 Figs. 1–2		D.3.1	
BM 73802 +	BM 54587				
BM 79061				A.2.8	21–22
BM 92694		TDP II, pl. LII–LVI	P273373	I.1.1	
BM 97093			P527479	II.1.1	4–5
BM 115745				II.1.2	6
F 238	(+) BM 43268	Finkel, *FS Lambert*, Fig. 10		E.2.1	
K. 54		BAM 497	P393731	H.1	
K. 879 +	K. 2769 + K. 10527	CMAwR 3, pl. 8	P237921	D.1.8	
K. 1930 +	K. 11752	AMT 65/2 CT 28, No. 40	P238115	D.1.7	39
K. 263 +	K. 10934	*Sudhoffs Archiv* 96, 93–94	P237802	C.1.5	
K. 2354+	K. 2412 + K. 2453 + K. 2491 + K. 3237 + K. 6774 + K. 7086 + K. 8356 + K. 8800 + K. 8842 + K. 9828 + K. 10428 + K. 11868 + K. 13398 + K. 13399 + K. 16541 +? K. 17155 +? K. 17315 +? K. 17359 +? K. 20138 + Sm. 637 + Sm. 1156 (+?) K. 13417	CT 23, 23–38 + AMT 92/3 BAM 480	P365742	H.2	
K. 2413 +	K. 16363 + K. 18482	AMT 67/1	P394413	D.1.1	

(continued)

Museum No.	Joins to	Previous Publication	CDLI No.	Text No.	Plate
K. 2416 +	+ K. 9224 + K. 10624 + K. 11172 + K. 16402 + DT 215 + Rm. 254 (+) K. 2424 + 7016 (+?) K. 6206 + K. 16449 (+) K. 20128 (+?) K. 18178	BAM 498 BAM 499 BAM 500 AMT 3/2 AMT 4/1 AMT 26/4 AMT 16/4 AMT 25/8 AMT 46/3	P394416	H.1	
K. 2424 + → K. 2416 +	K. 7016 (+)	BAM 498	P394424	H.1	
K. 3025 +	K. 5982 + K. 8917	CMAwR 3, pl. 6–7	P238249	D.1.8	
K. 3304 +	K. 7698 + K. 8785 + K. 9217		P238268	C.1.4	
K. 3485 +	K. 10443	Geers, Folio J93	P395046	D.1.1	36
K. 4727 +	K. 9426 + 81-2-4, 386 (+)	Geers, Folio D93	P395702	F.1	49–50
K. 6206 + → K. 2416+	K. 16449 +	AMT 16/4	P396382	H.1	
K. 6688 (+)	K. 4727+	Geers, Folio G16	P396732	F.1	49–50
K. 7016 + → K. 2416+	K. 2424	BAM 498	P394424		
K. 7071			P397007	I.1.1	3
K. 7698+ → K. 3304+			P238698	C.1.4	
K. 8112 +	K. 9666 (+)	CMAwR 1, pl. 31	P397495	C.3.9	
K. 8210			P397536	D.1.1	37
K. 8666		Hätinen 2021, pl. 13–14	P238752	D.3.1	44–45
K. 8678 +	K. 10567 + K. 13901 + K. 16461 + K. 19344	Geers, Folio A21	P238756	A.1.4	10–11
K. 8893		Geers, Folio A32	P238816	C.1.6	27
K. 9071		Geers, Folio D95	P397891	F.1	51
K. 9224 + → K. 2416+		AMT 3/2 AMT 4/1 BAM 499	P394416	H.1	
K. 10507		AMT 66/4	P398722	D.1.1 D.1.4	
K. 10567 → K. 8678+		AMT 81/9 Geller, *BAM* 7, pl. 28	P238756	A.1.4	10–11
K. 10624 +	K. 11172 +	BAM 500	P398787	H.1	
K. 11172 + → K. 2416 +	K. 10624 +	BAM 500	P398787	H.1	
K. 11530		ABRT 2, 19	P334932	D.1.5	
K. 11550 +	BM 68458	Geers, Folio N95 *NABU* 2019/3, 139 Figs. 1–2	P239012	D.3.1	
K. 11647		AMT 66/3	P399372	C.3.2	
K. 11939		Heeßel 2019, 1	P3995329	I.1.5	
K. 11956 +	K. 14200	Geers, Folio A135	P399540 P400683	D.1.2	38
K. 13315		Geers, Folio M117	P239201	D.3.1	47
K. 13366		BAM 526	P400259	A.1.2	
K. 13901 → K. 8678+		AMT 58/1 Geller, *BAM* 7, pl. 28	P238756	A.1.4	10–11
K. 14028		Geers, Folio A164	P400591	E.1.2	37
K. 14032		AMT 66/9	P400593	B.1.5	

(continued)

Museum No.	Joins to	Previous Publication	CDLI No.	Text No.	Plate
K. 14200 + → K. 11956+					
K. 16363 → K. 2413+			P404833	D.1.1	
K. 16402 + → K. 2416+		AMT 46/3 BAM 499	P394416		
K. 16449 (+) → K. 2416 +		AMT 25/8	P402032	H.1	
K. 16461 → K. 8678+		AMT 62/5	P238756	A.1.4	10–11
K. 17499		Lambert, Folio 11281	P420836	E.1.3	53
K. 17663			P402974	I.1.1	
K. 18178 (+) → K. 2416+			P403424	H.1	
K. 18482 → K. 2413+			P403690	D.1.1	
K. 19344 → K. 8678+			P238756	A.1.4	10–11
K. 19506			P239871	C.3.10	27
K. 20128 (+) → K. 2416 +			P418607	H.1	
K. 20138 + → K. 2354+			P418615		
K. 20254		Lambert, Folio 14148	P239949	C.1.7	34
Rm. 254 (+) → K. 2416 +		AMT 26/4 BAM 498	P424664	H.1	
Rm. 376		*AS* 16, 287–288	P282433	D.1.1	
Sm. 123 (+)	Sm. 1138 (+) Sm. 1991	Geers, Folio D82	P240236	C.3.10	
Sm. 157 +	Sm. 1134	Thompson 1930, pl. 54 *Iraq* 31, pl. III	P426420	D.1.6	
Sm. 637 + → K. 2354+		AMT 92/3			
Sm. 1138 → Sm. 123 (+)		Geers, Folio B140	P240343	C.3.10	
Sm. 1991 → Sm. 123 (+)		AMT 66/5	P240436	C.3.10	
DT 28		Geers, Folio G18	P237716	F.1	53
DT 215 + → K. 2416+	K. 2424 +	AMT 3/2 AMT 4/1 BAM 499	P394416	H.1	
79-7-8, 95		Geers, Folio Ab 54	P236879	D.3.1	46
U. 30654		UET 6/3, 897	P346934	G.2	
Louvre, Paris					
AO 4425A+B				B.2.6	24–25
AO 6473		TCL 6, 49 Thureau-Dangin, *RA* 18, 162–163		C.3.9	
University of Pennsylvania, Philadelphia					
11N-T3				G.1	
N. 1568		*NABU* 2019/3, 141	P276694	D.1.1	
N. 4001				B.2.1	23
National Museum, Damascus					
RS 25.436		AuOr Suppl. 23, pl. 11		D.1.1	
Free Library Philadelphia					
FLP 1306			P459867	C.1.9	30
Department of Near Eastern Studies, Cornell University, Ithaca					
CUNES 52-15-029		CUSAS 30, No. 448	P326684	C.3.5	

(continued)

Museum No.	Joins to	Previous Publication	CDLI No.	Text No.	Plate
Giancarlo Ligabue Collection, Venice					
–		*Iraq* 31, Pl. V–VI	P282478	II.1.4 D.1.1	
Other Texts (Unclear Location)					
W. 17360f		TDP II, pl. LXVI		I.1.1	
W. 17360i		TDP II, Pl. LXVII		I.1.4	
W. 17360q		TDP II, pl. LXVIII		I.1.3	

Plates

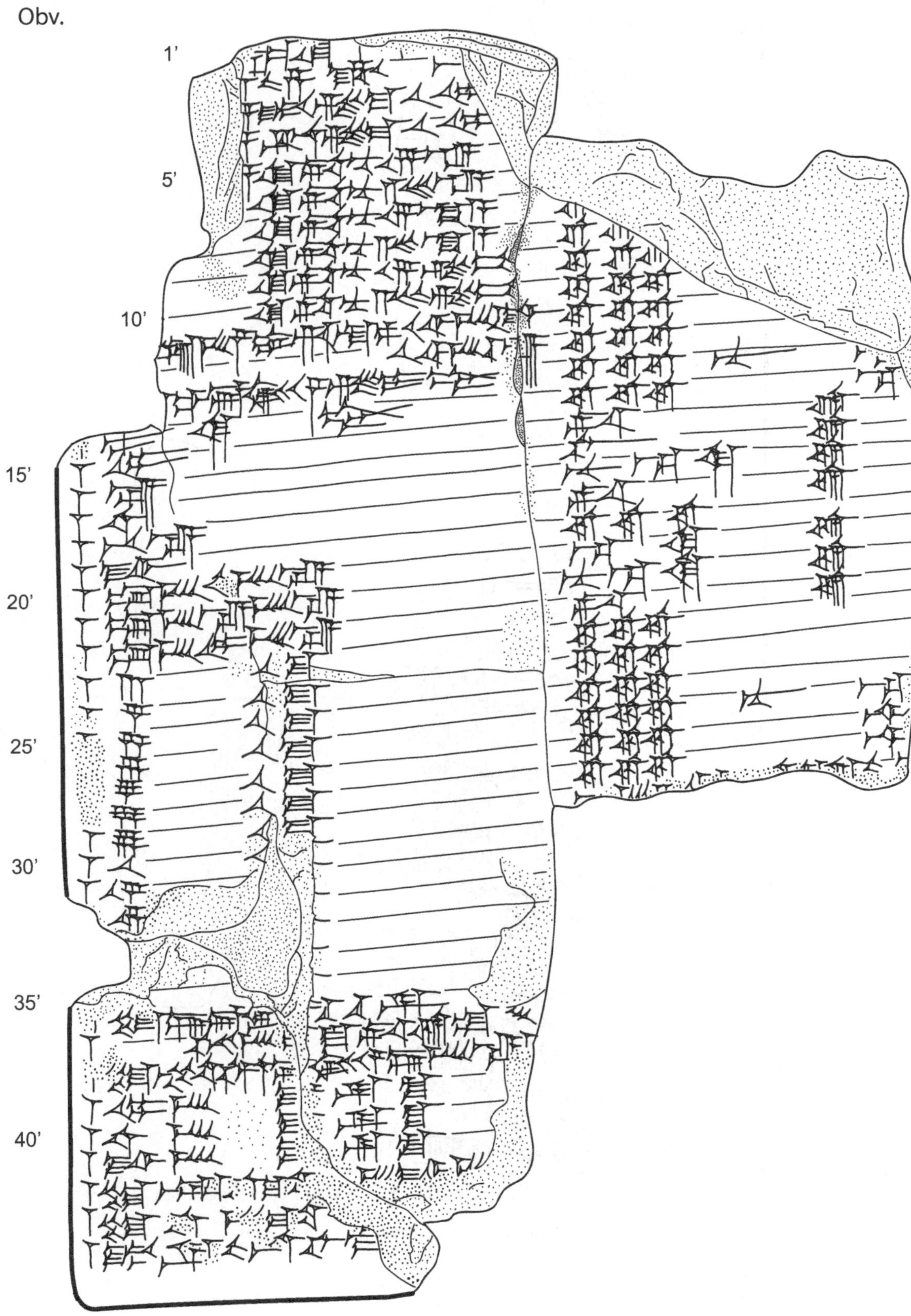

Plate 1: BM 65450 + 76497.

https://doi.org/10.1515/9781501506475-015

Rev.

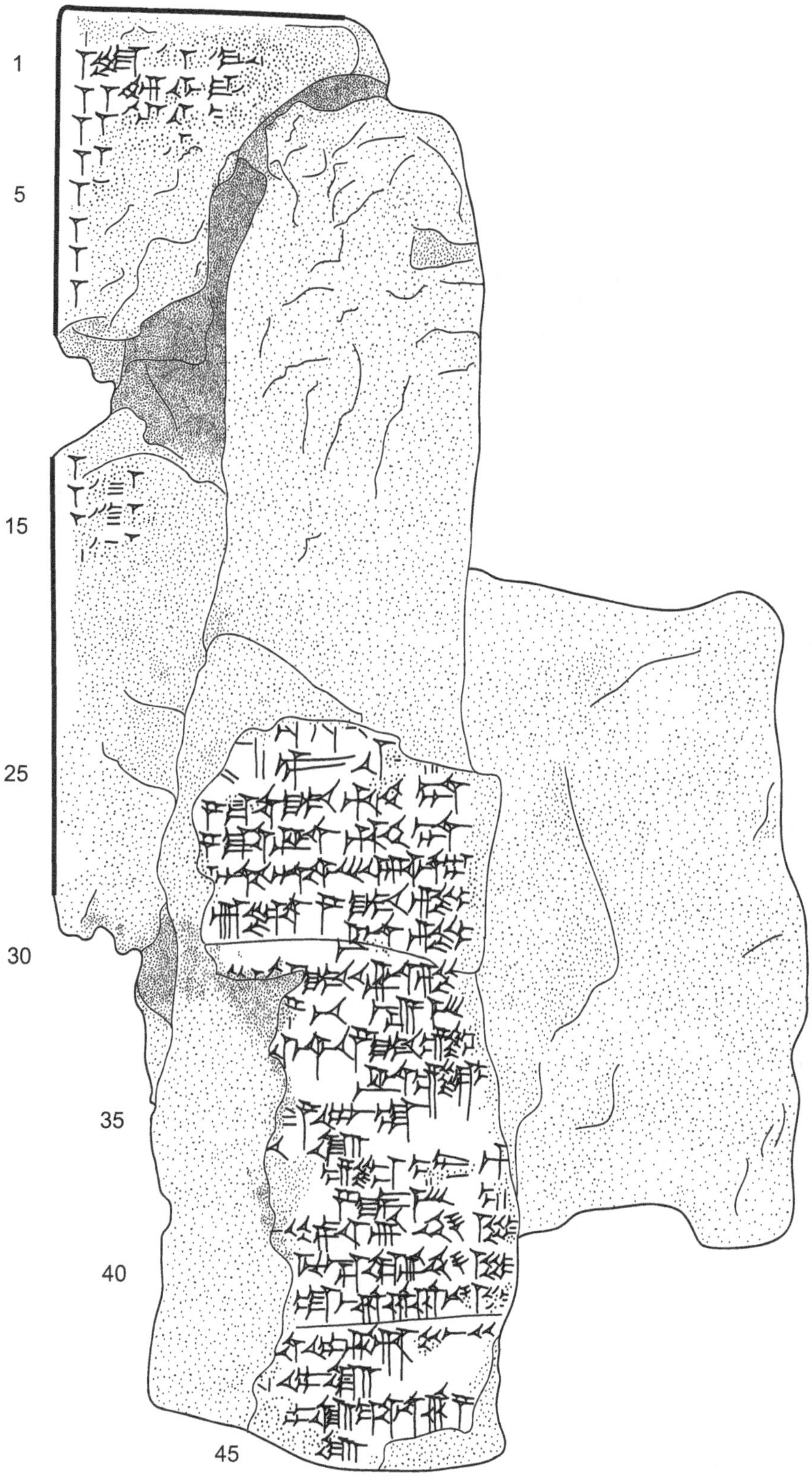

Plate 2: BM 65450 + 76497.

Rev.(?)

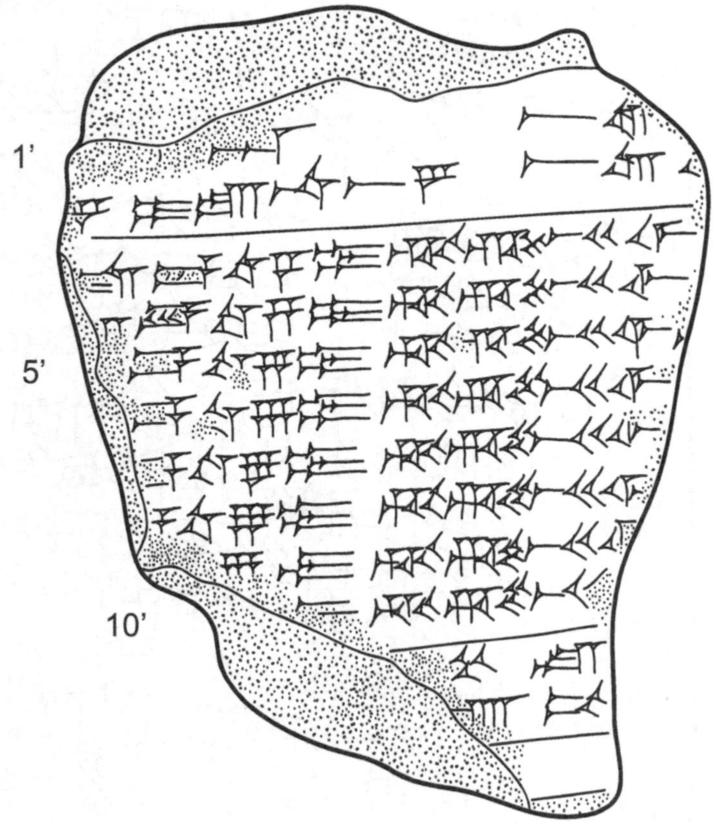

Plate 3: K. 7071.

Obv.

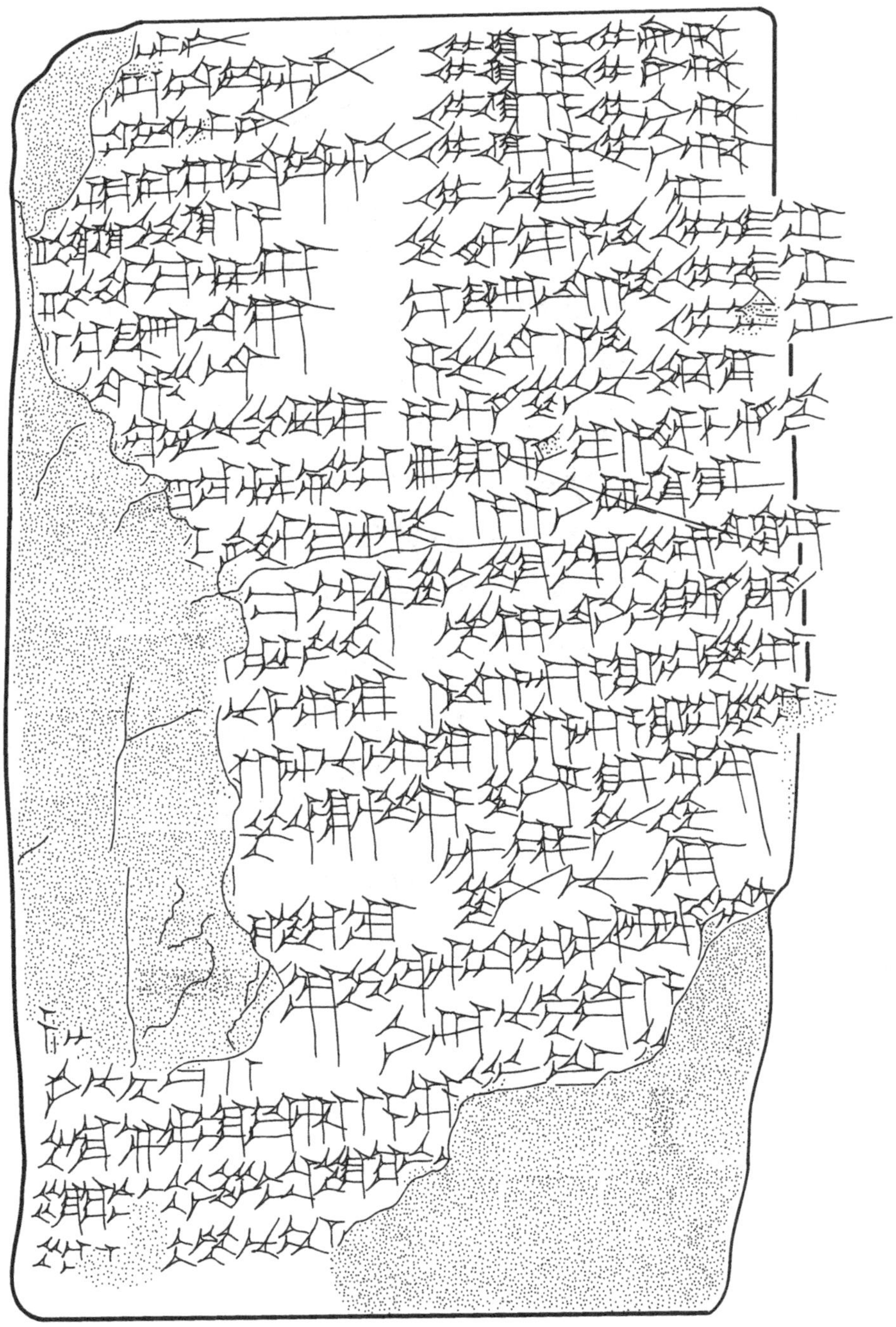

Lower edge

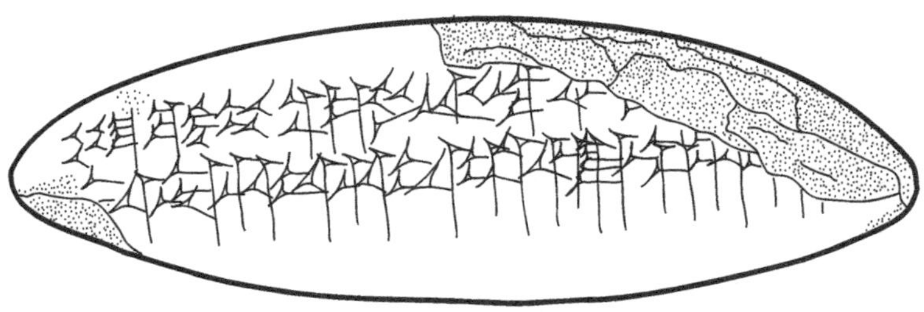

Plate 4: BM 97093.

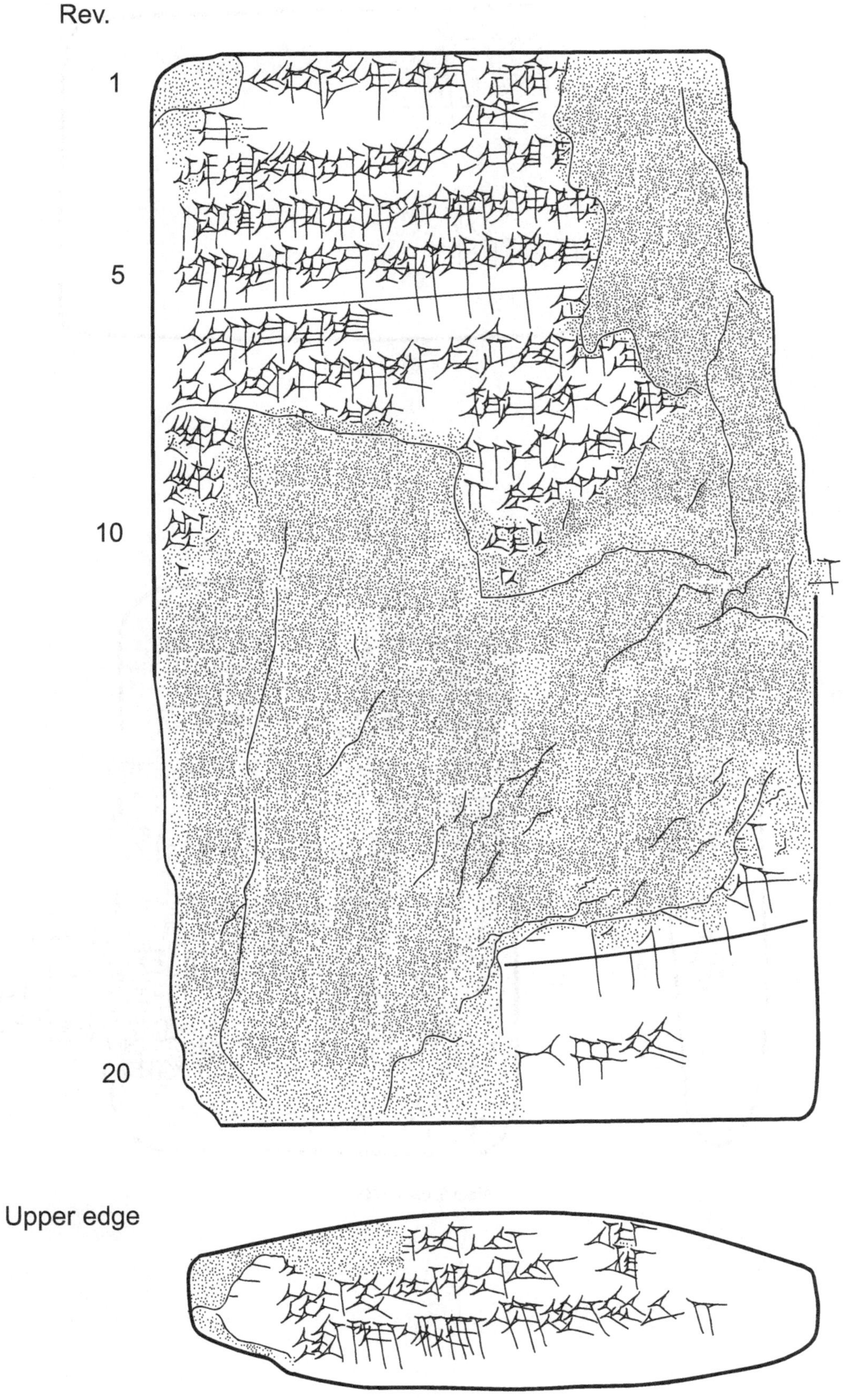

Plate 5: BM 97093.

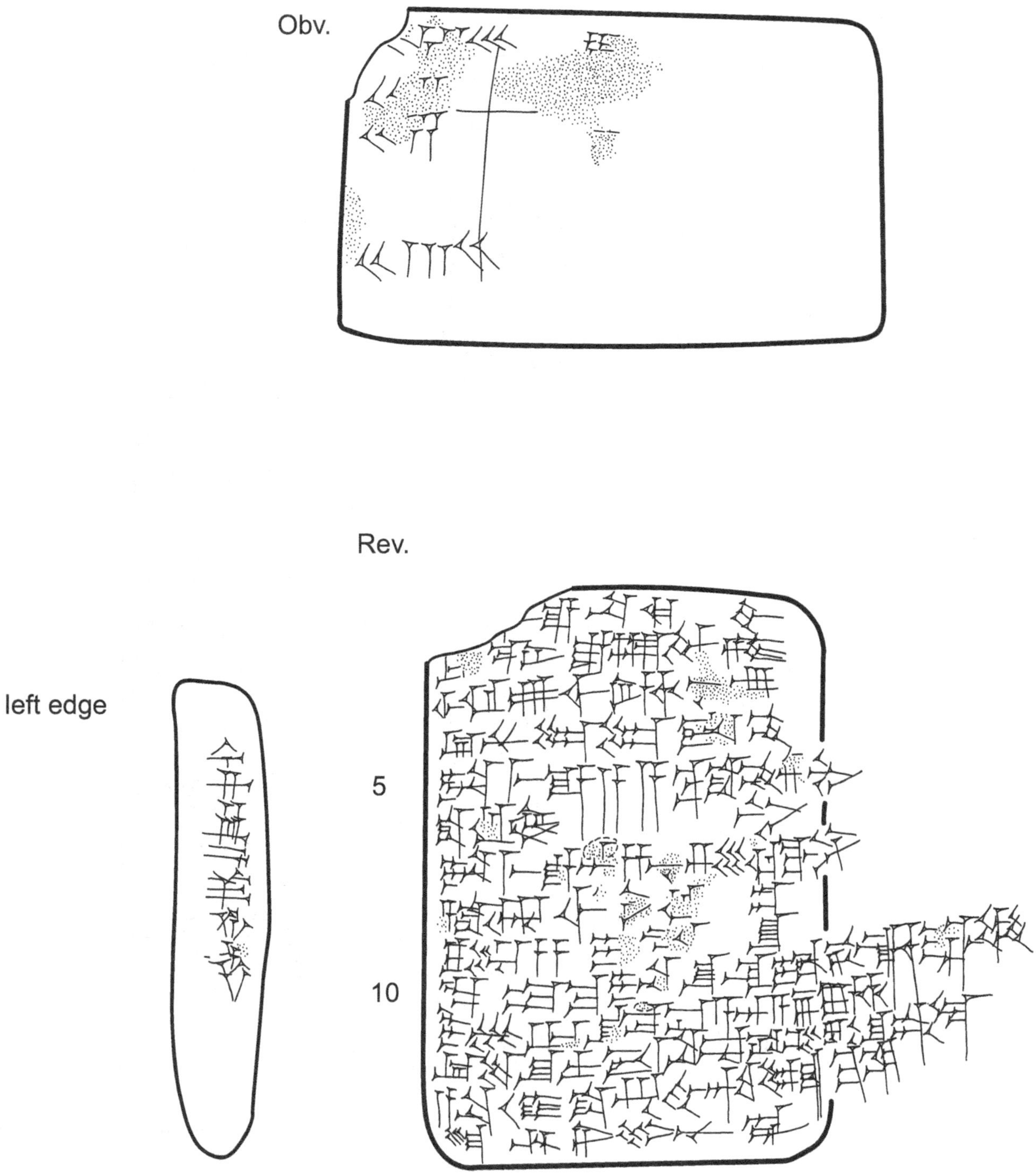

Plate 6: BM 115745.

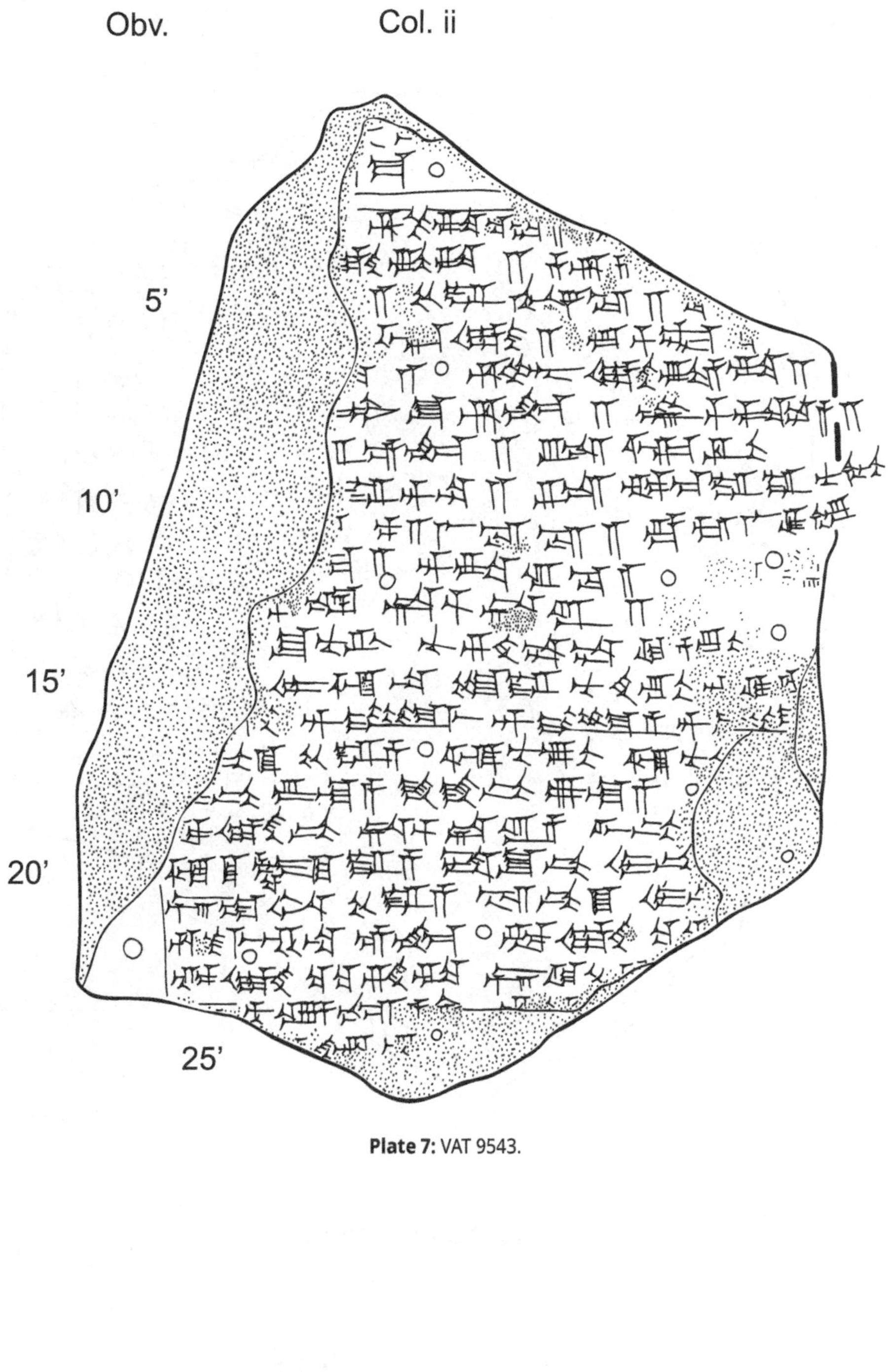

Plate 7: VAT 9543.

Rev. Col. iii

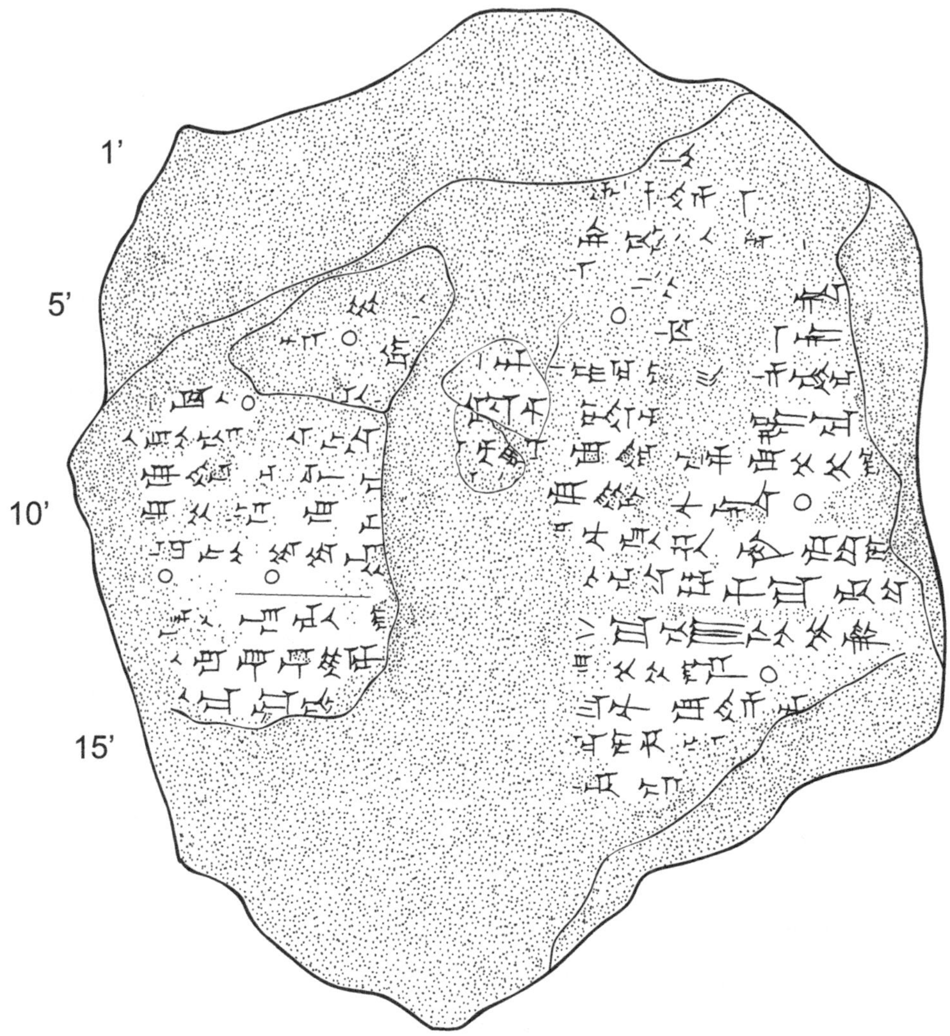

Unplaced Fragments

No. 1 No. 2

Plate 8: VAT 9543.

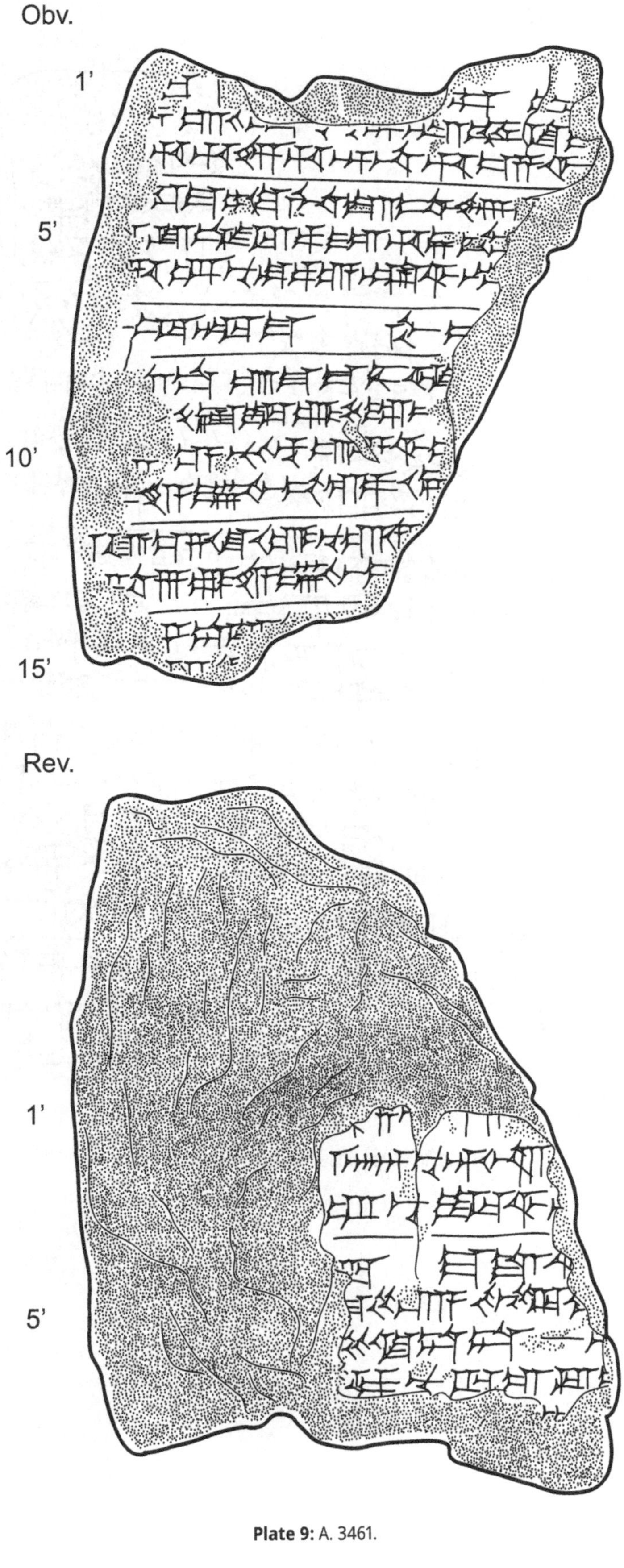

Plate 9: A. 3461.

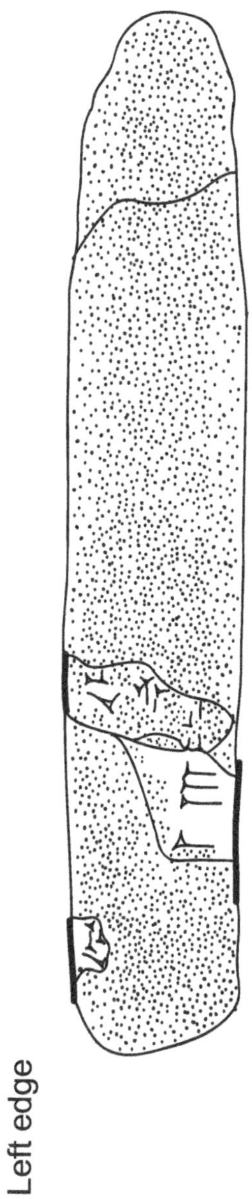

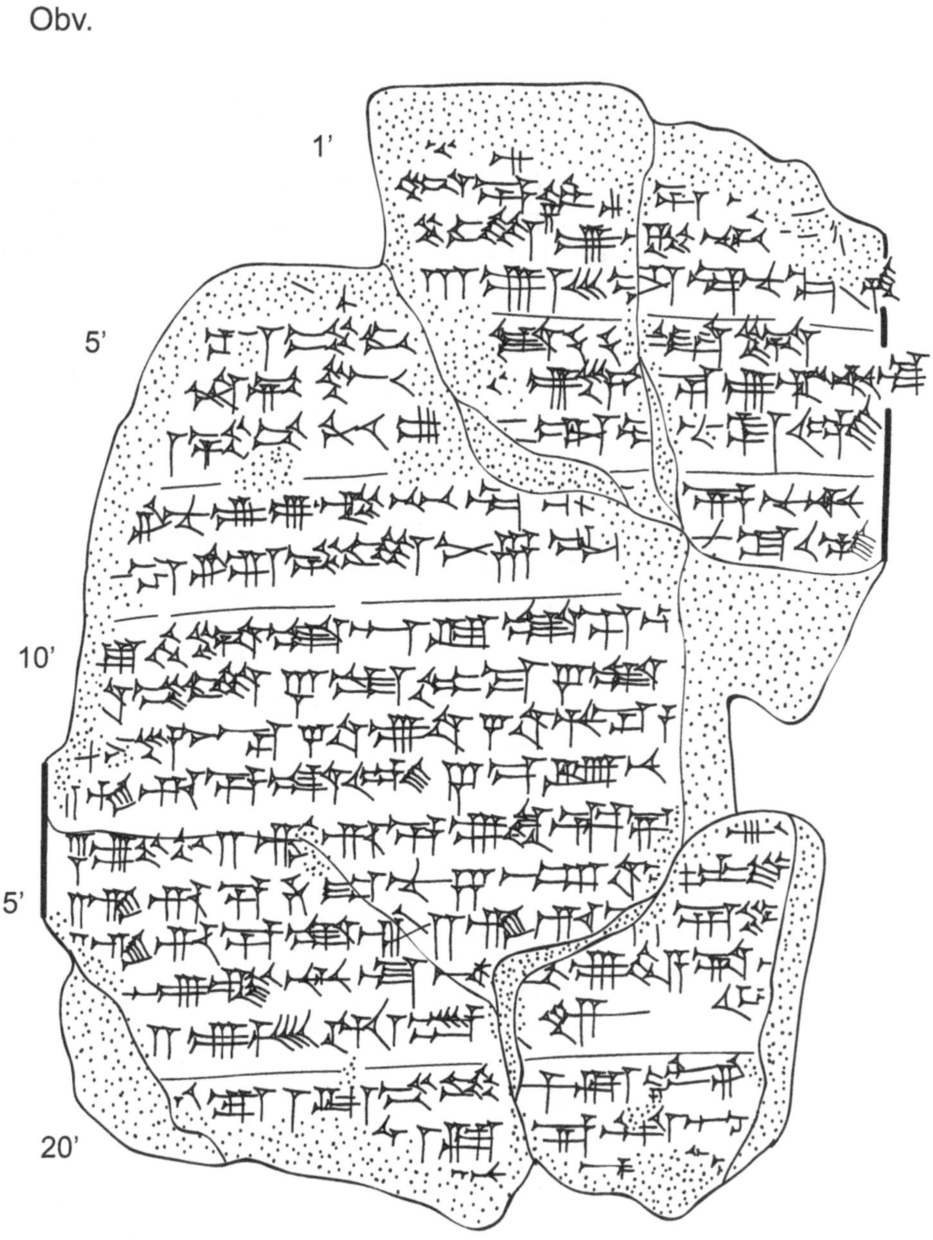

Plate 10: K. 8678 + 10567 + 13901 + 16461 + 19344.

Rev.

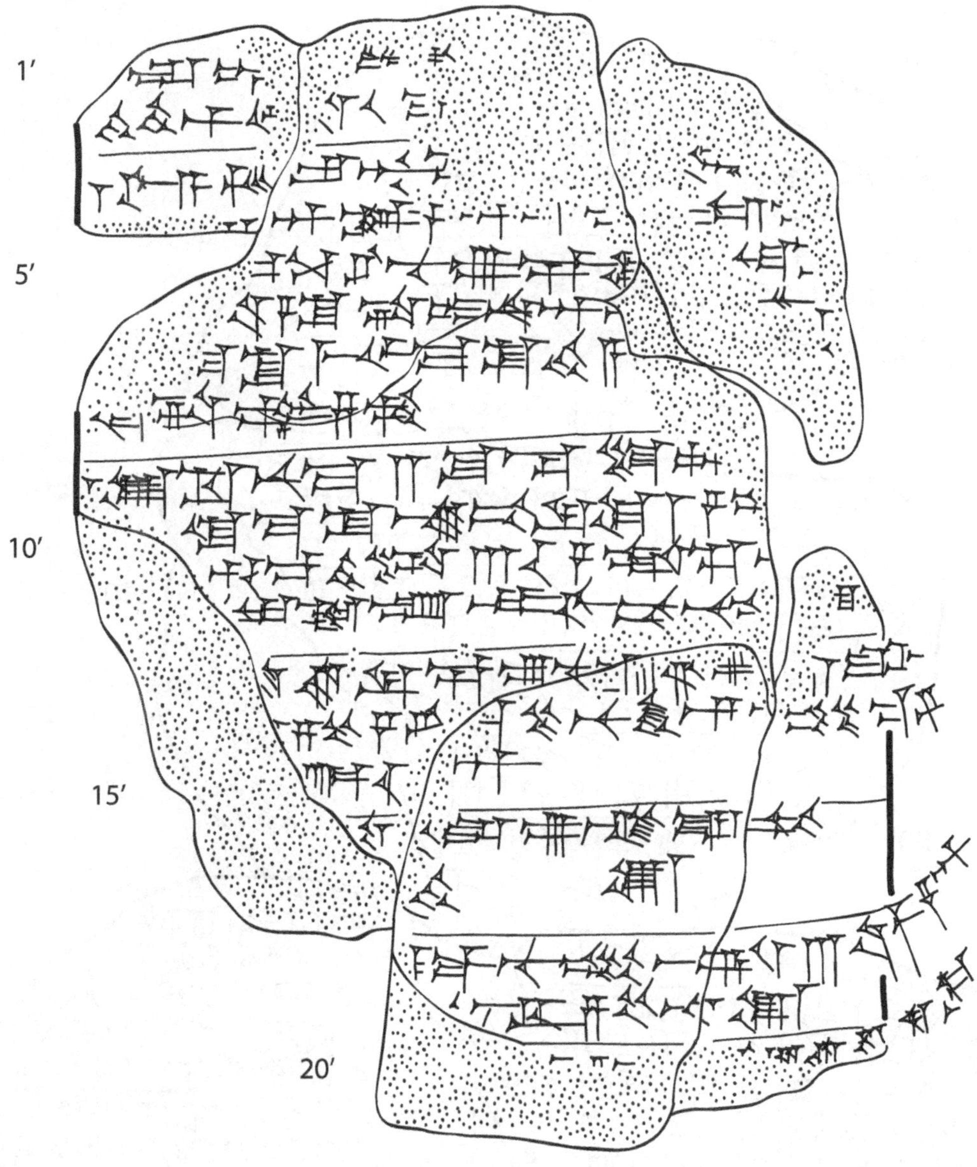

Plate 11: K. 8678 + 10567 + 13901 + 16461 + 19344.

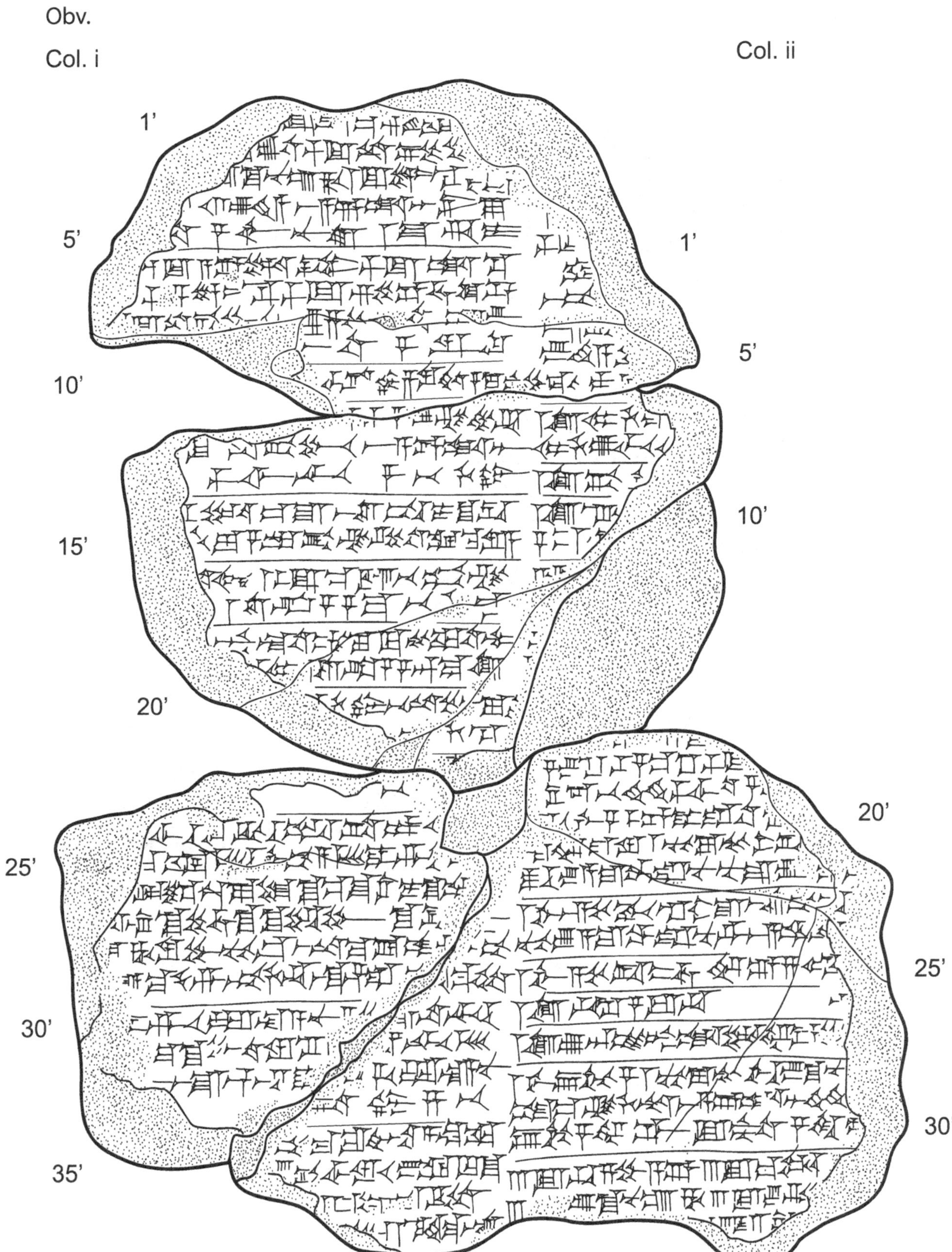

Plate 12: BM 38624 + 38828 + 45414.

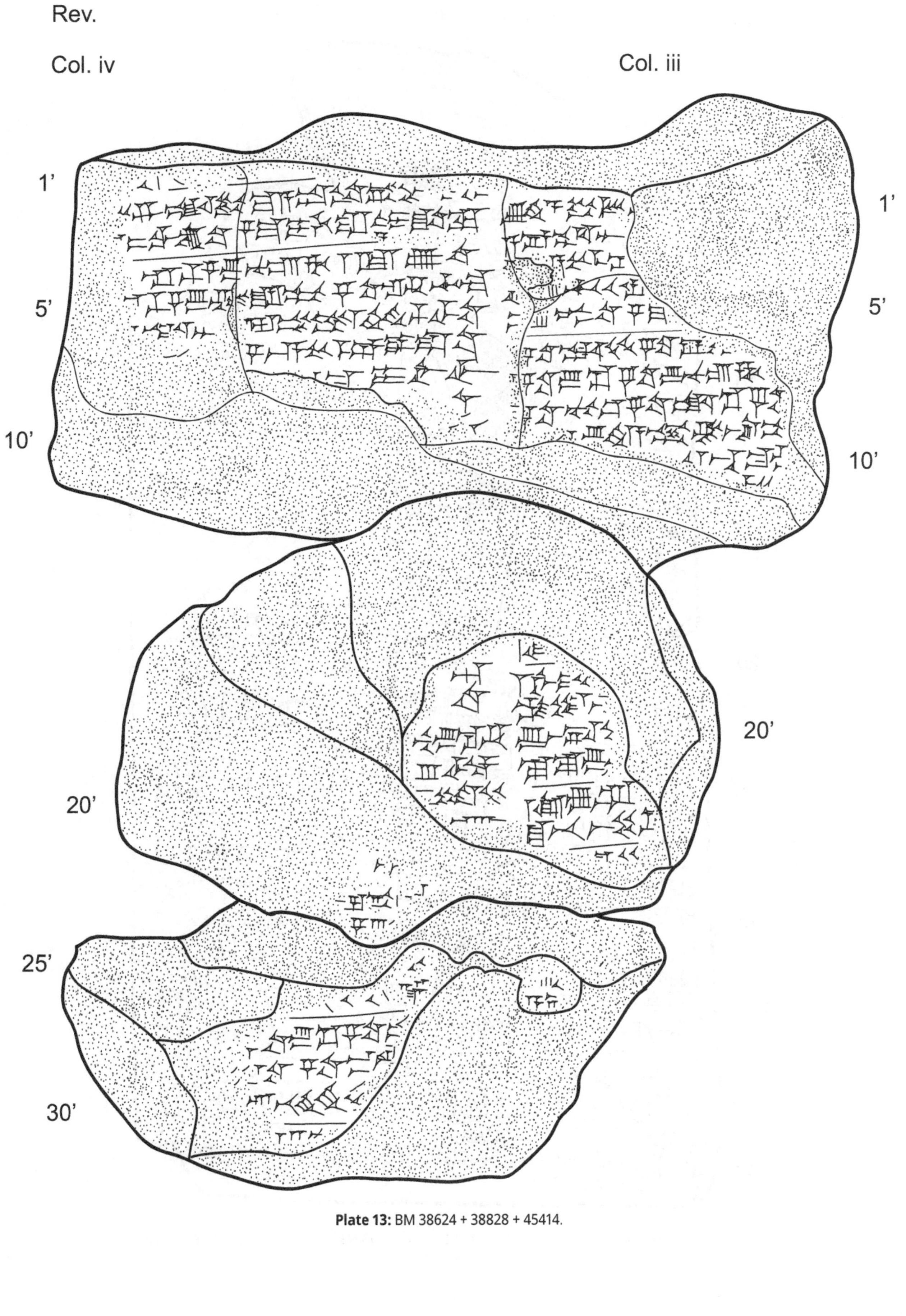

Plate 13: BM 38624 + 38828 + 45414.

Obv.

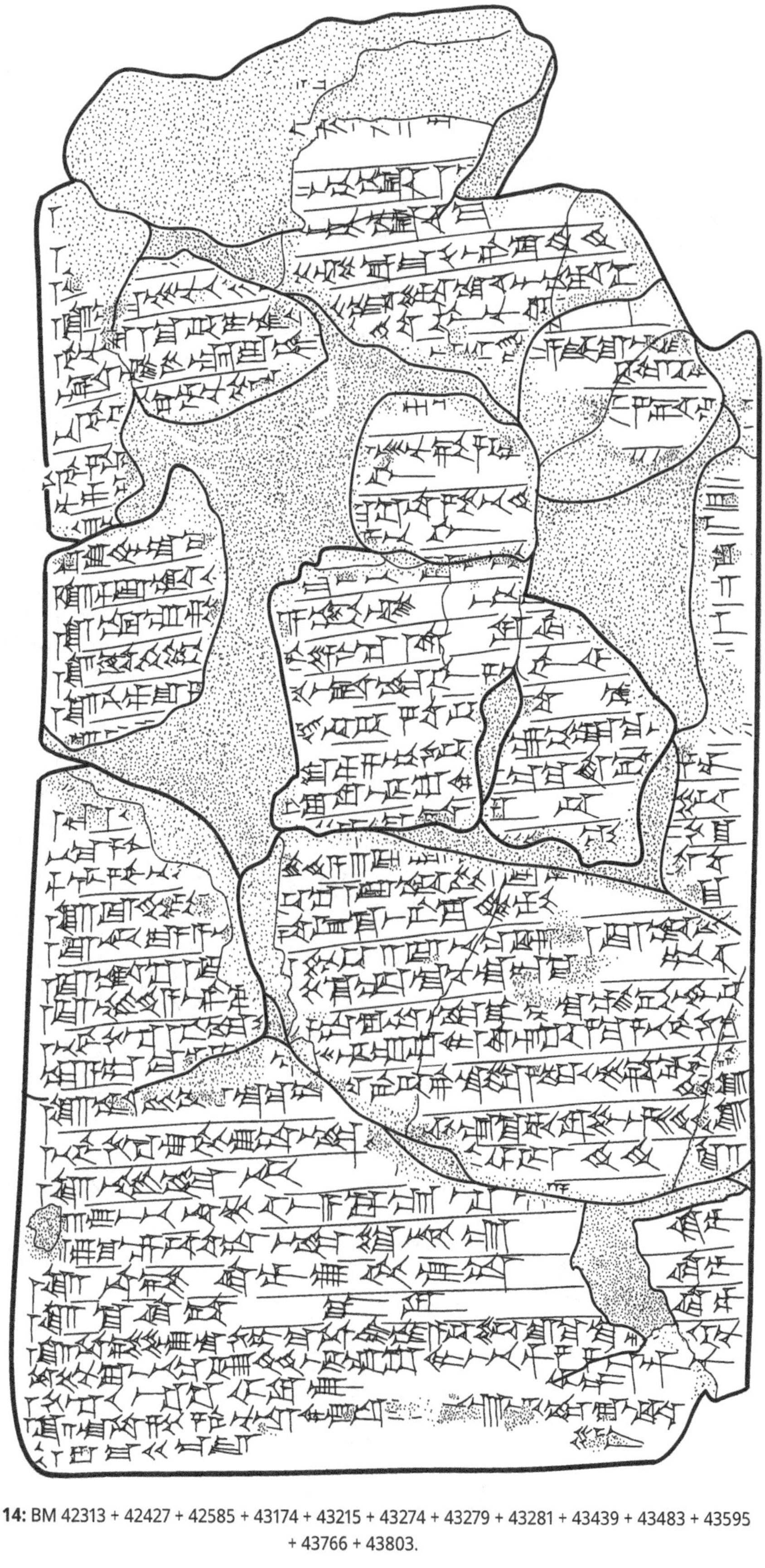

Plate 14: BM 42313 + 42427 + 42585 + 43174 + 43215 + 43274 + 43279 + 43281 + 43439 + 43483 + 43595 + 43766 + 43803.

Rev.

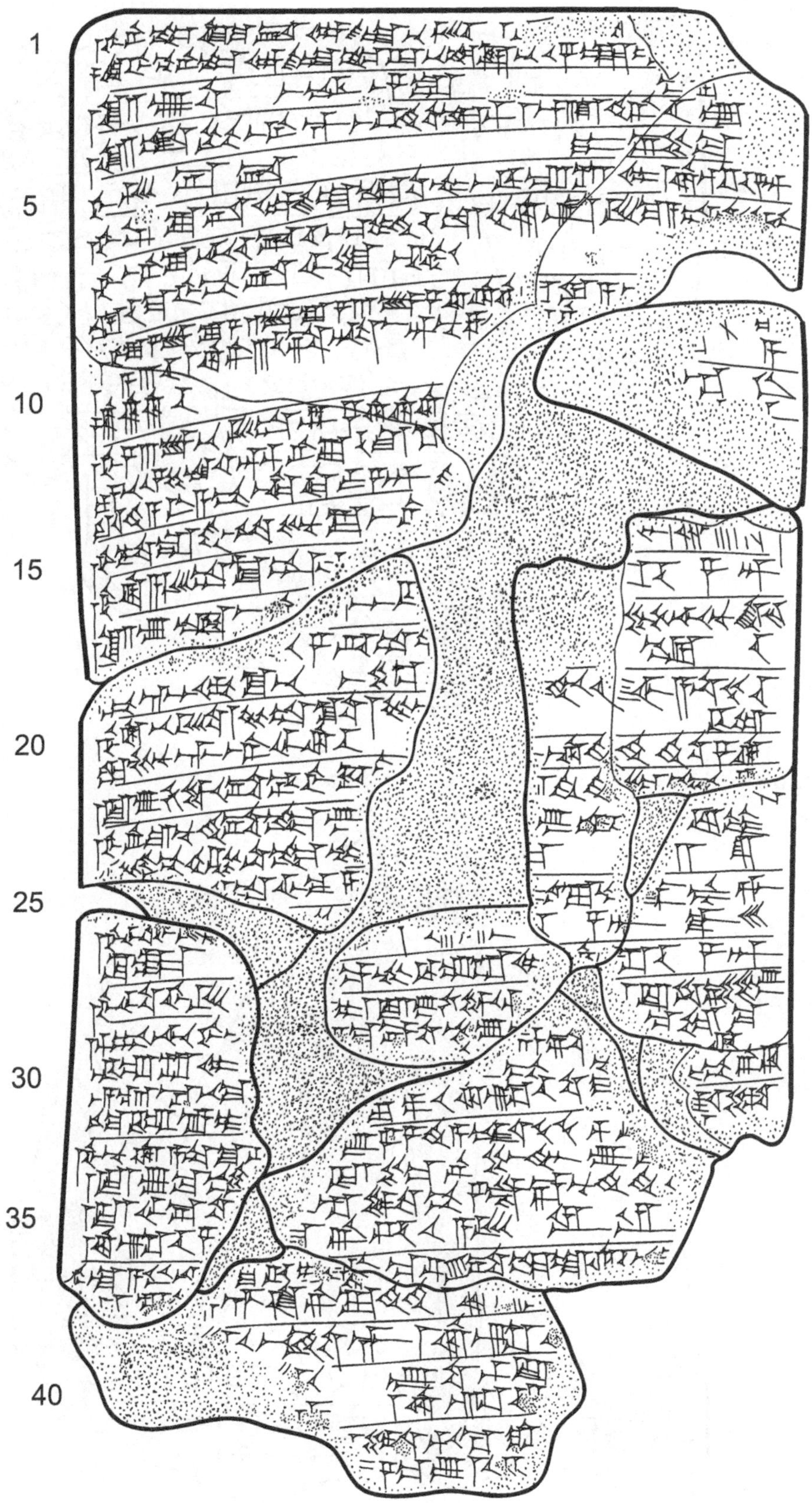

Plate 15: BM 42313 + 42427 + 42585 + 43174 + 43215 + 43274 + 43279 + 43281 + 43439 + 43483 + 43595 + 43766 + 43803.

Obv.

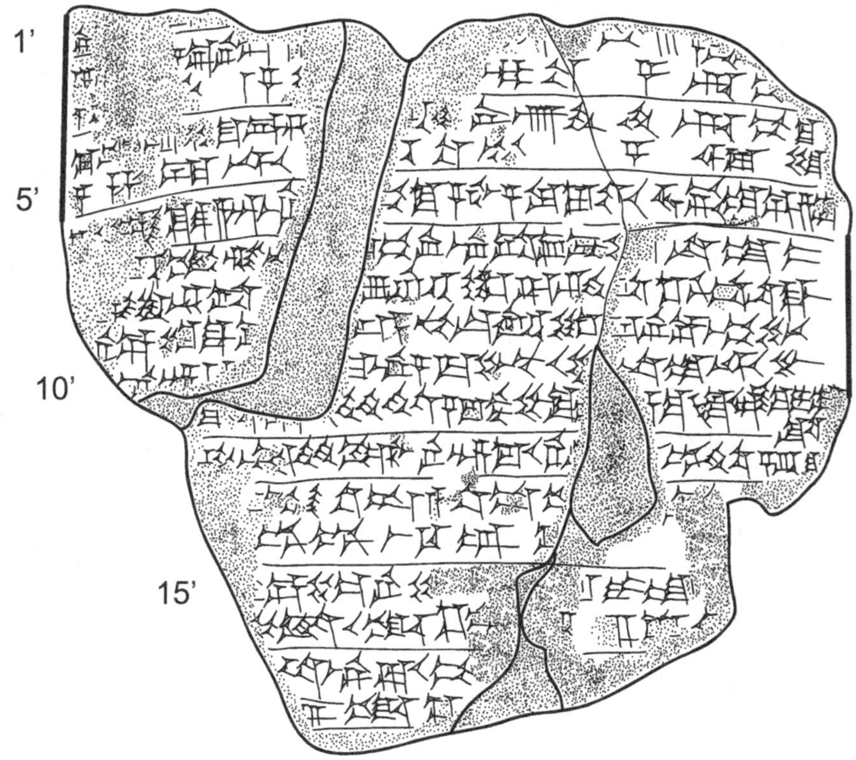

Rev.

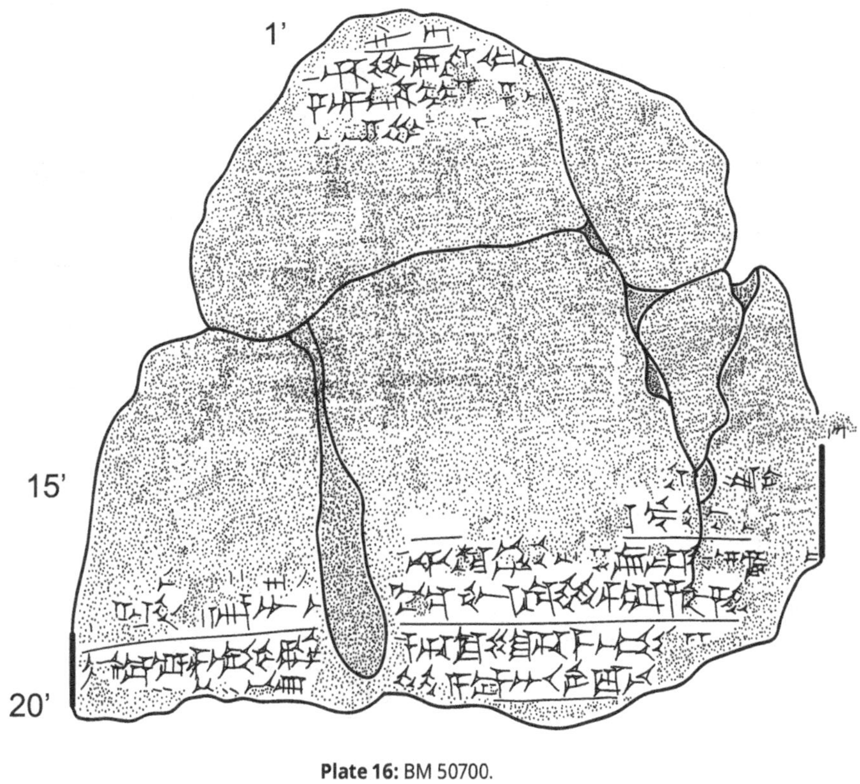

Plate 16: BM 50700.

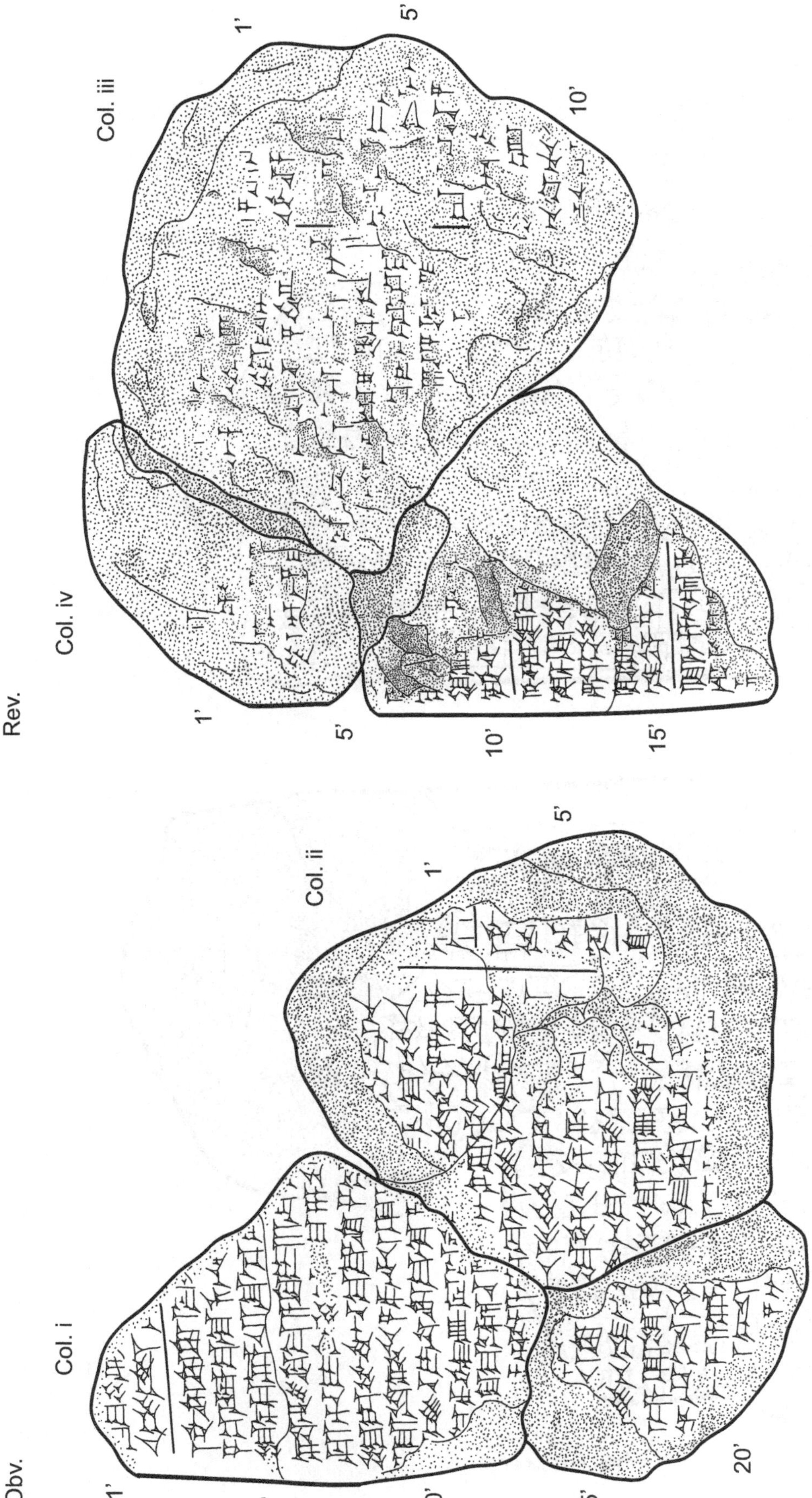

Plate 17: BM 45559 + 45574.

Obv. Col. i

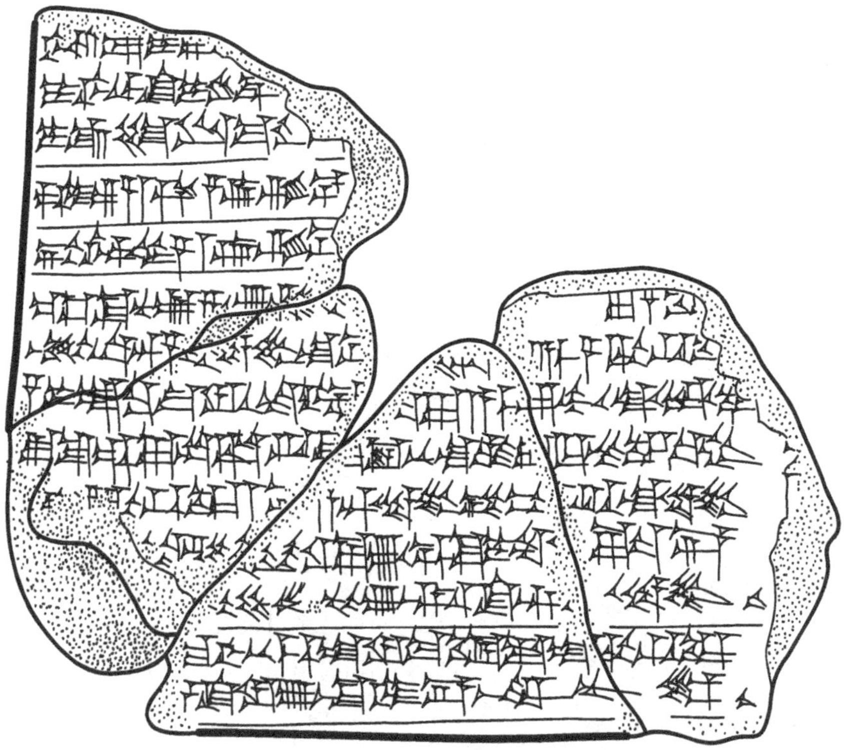

Rev. Col. iv

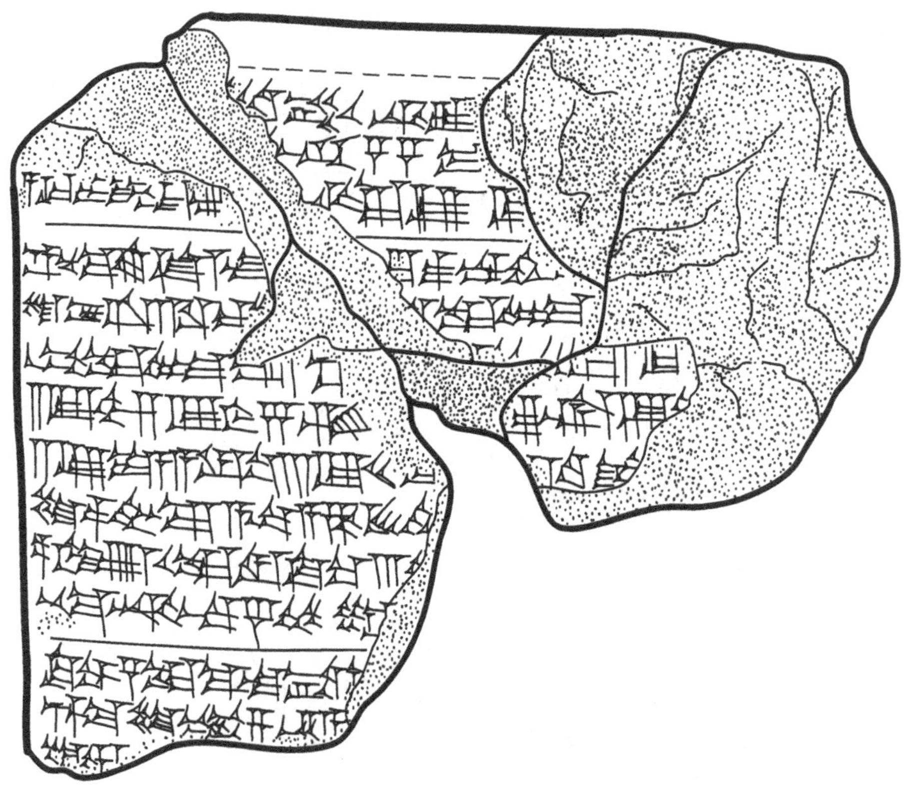

Plate 18: BM 45736.

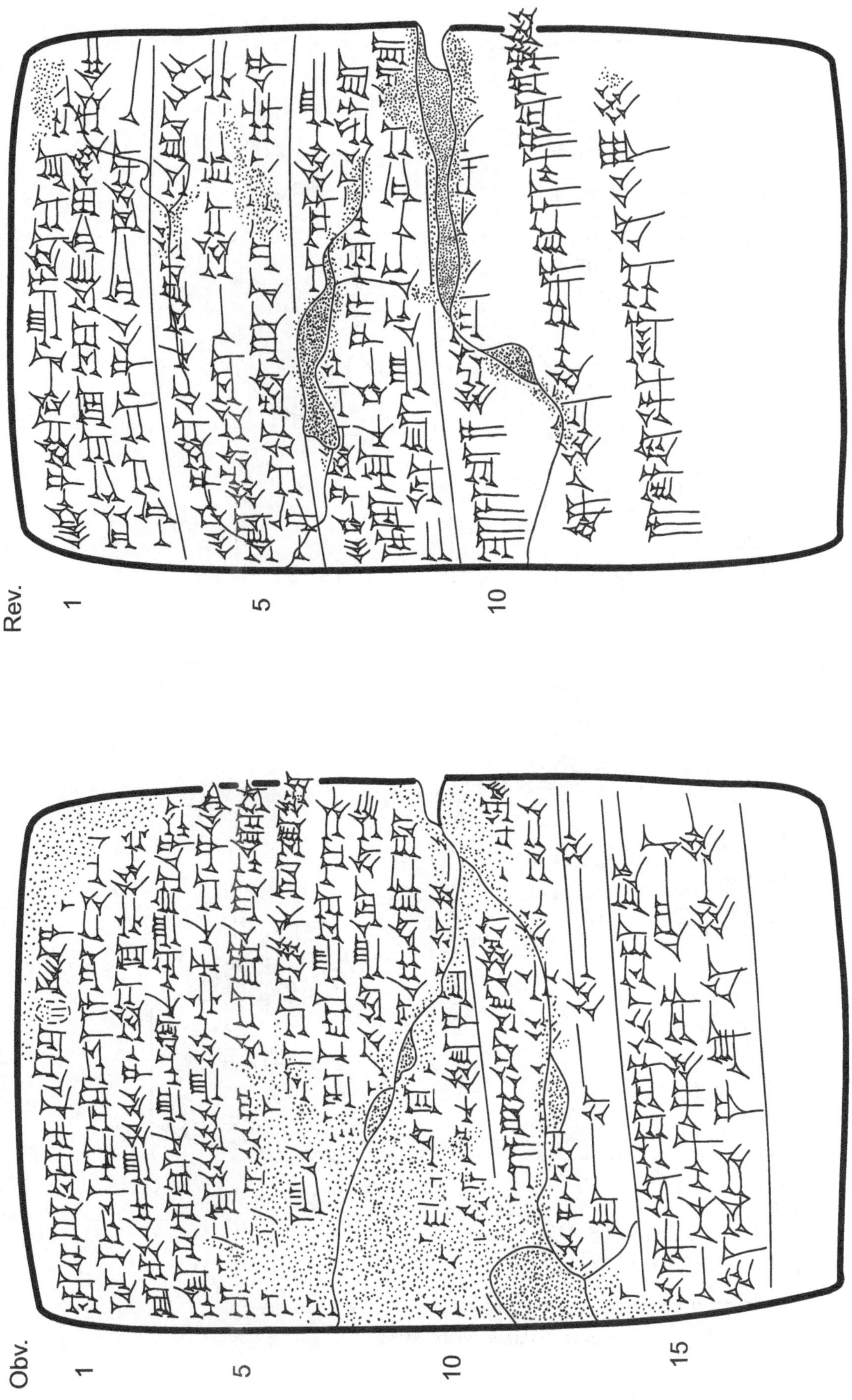

Plate 19: BM 47491.

Obv.

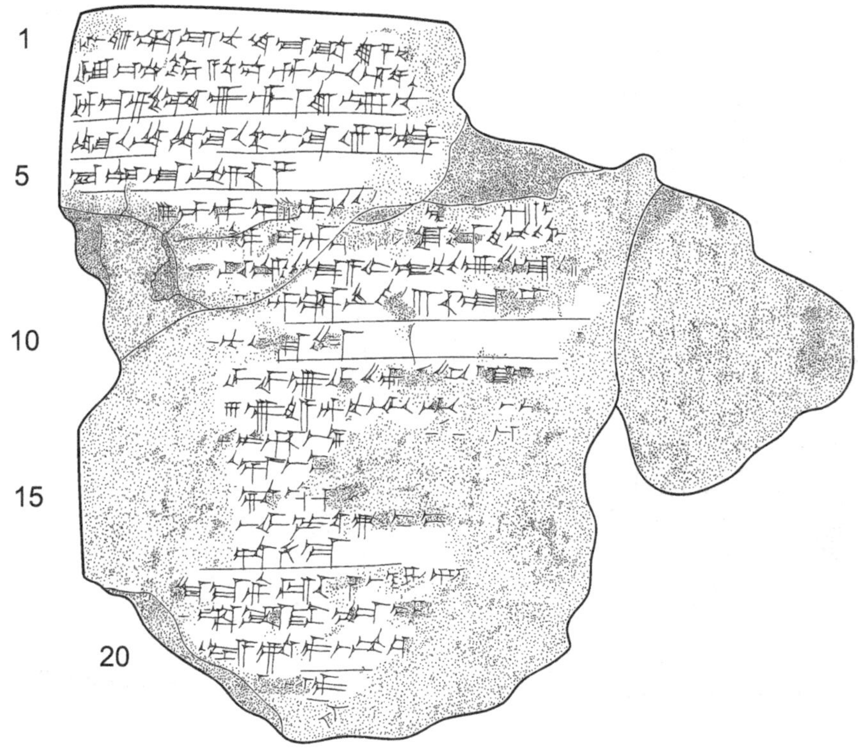

Rev.

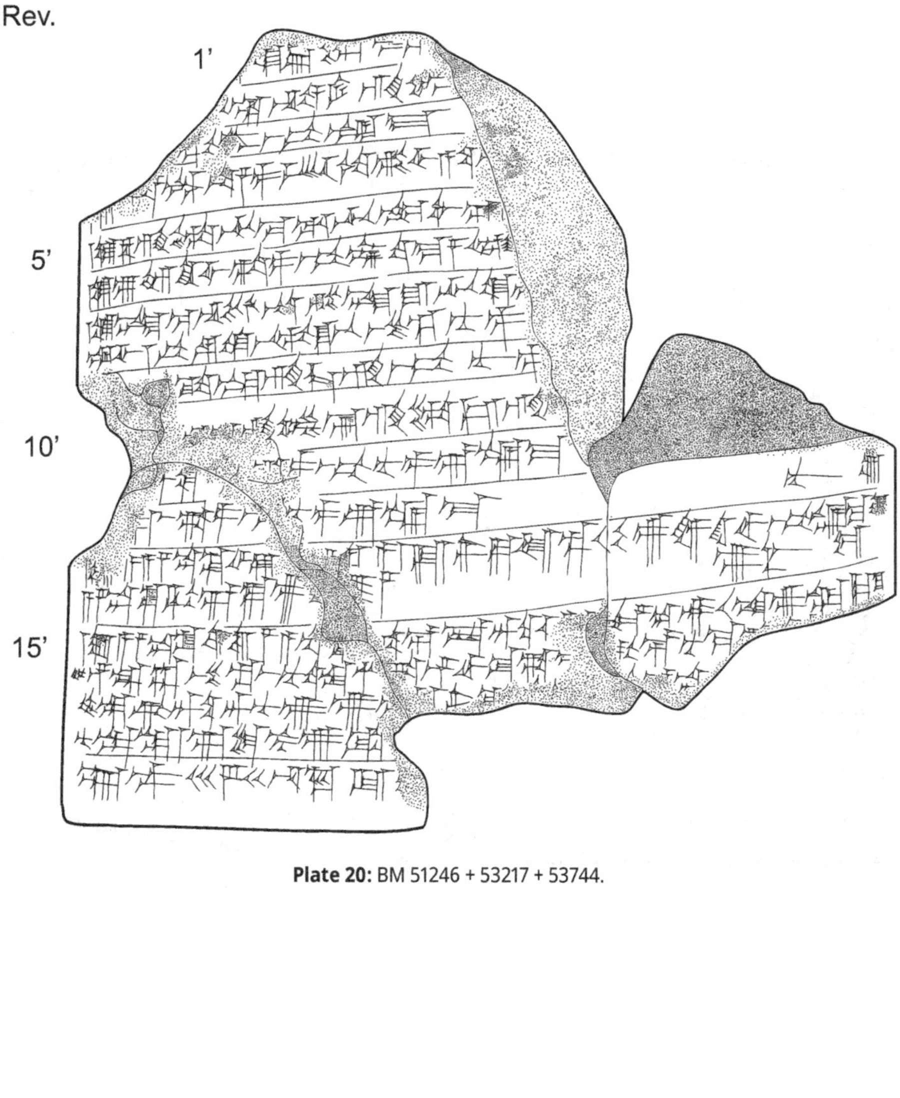

Plate 20: BM 51246 + 53217 + 53744.

Obv.

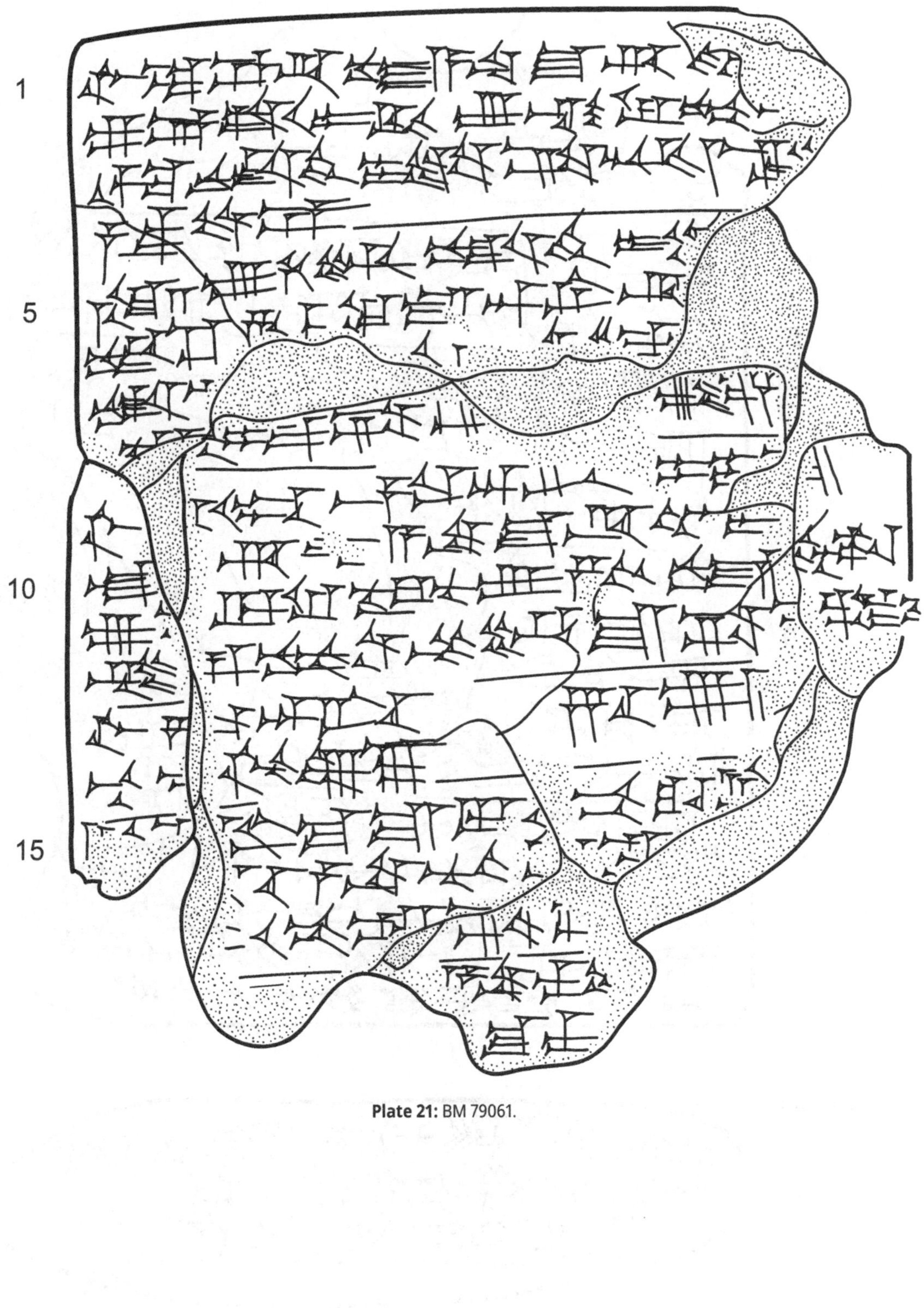

Plate 21: BM 79061.

Rev.

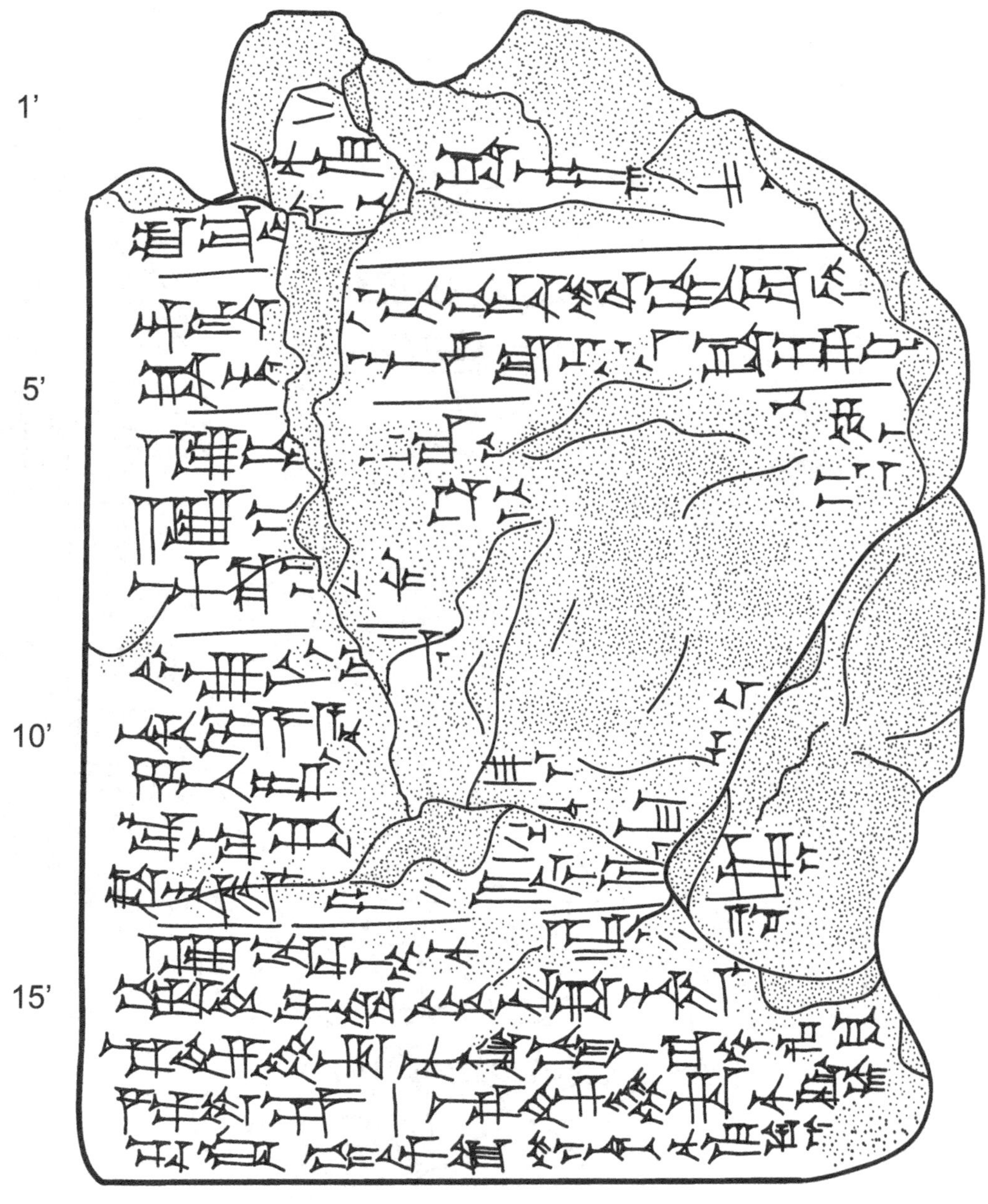

Upper edge

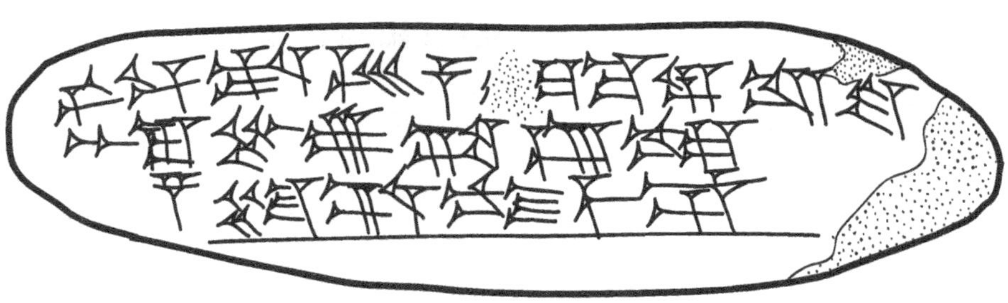

Plate 22: BM 79061.

Obv.

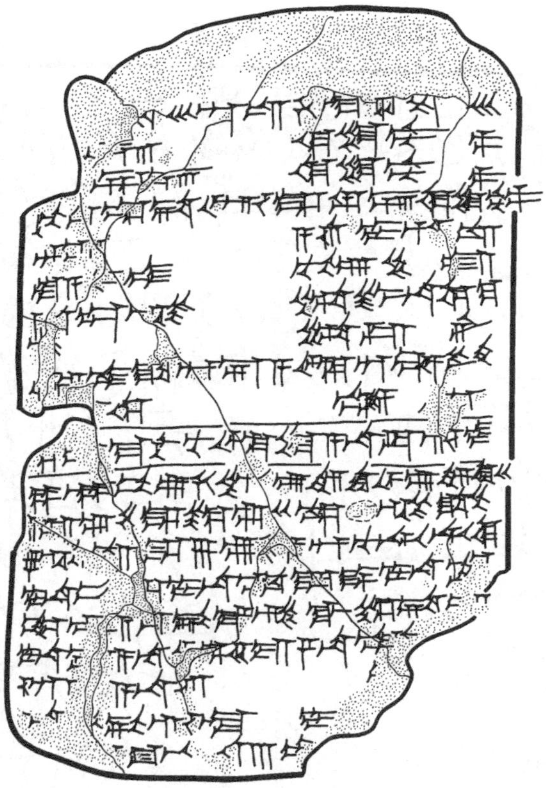

Rev.

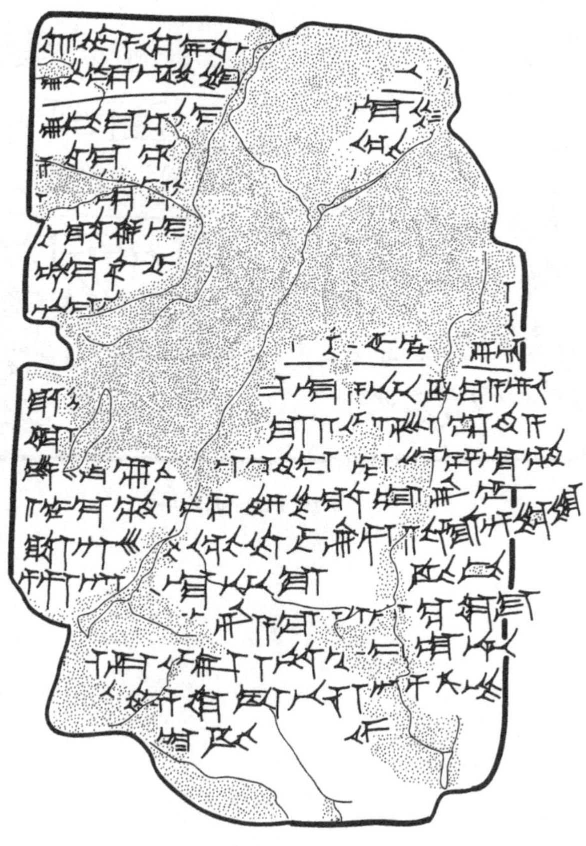

Plate 23: N. 4001.

Obv.

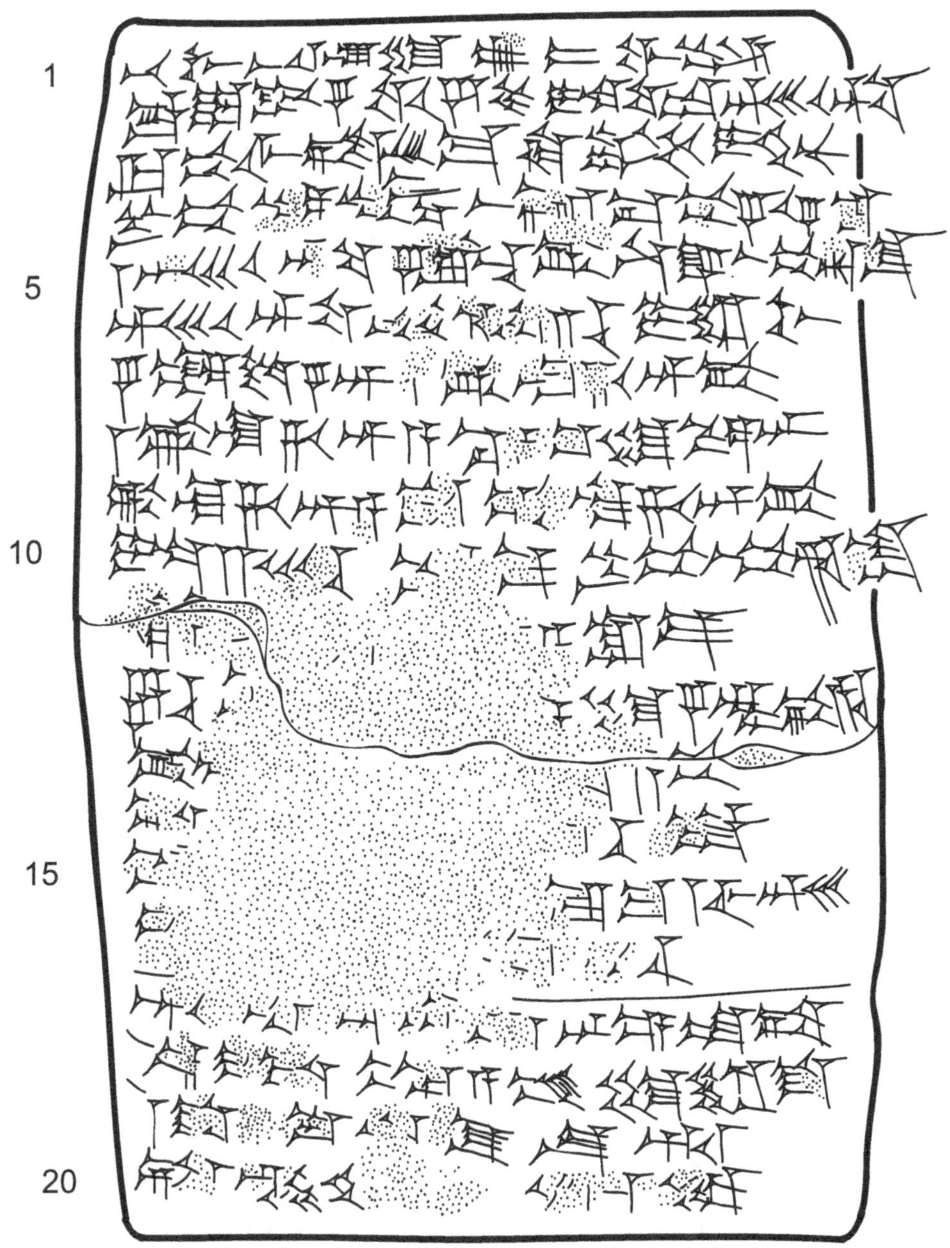

Plate 24: AO 4425 A+B.

Rev.

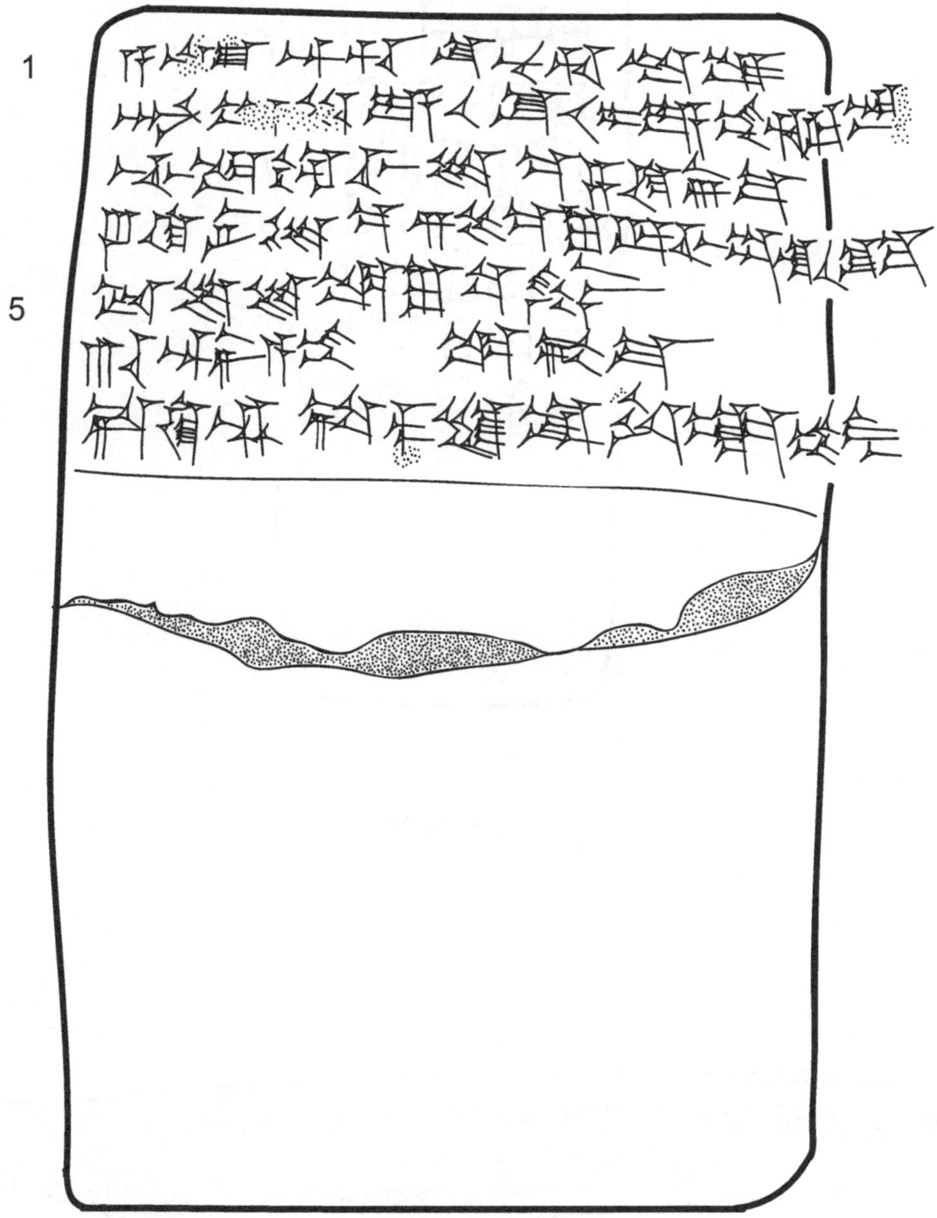

Plate 25: AO 4425 A+B.

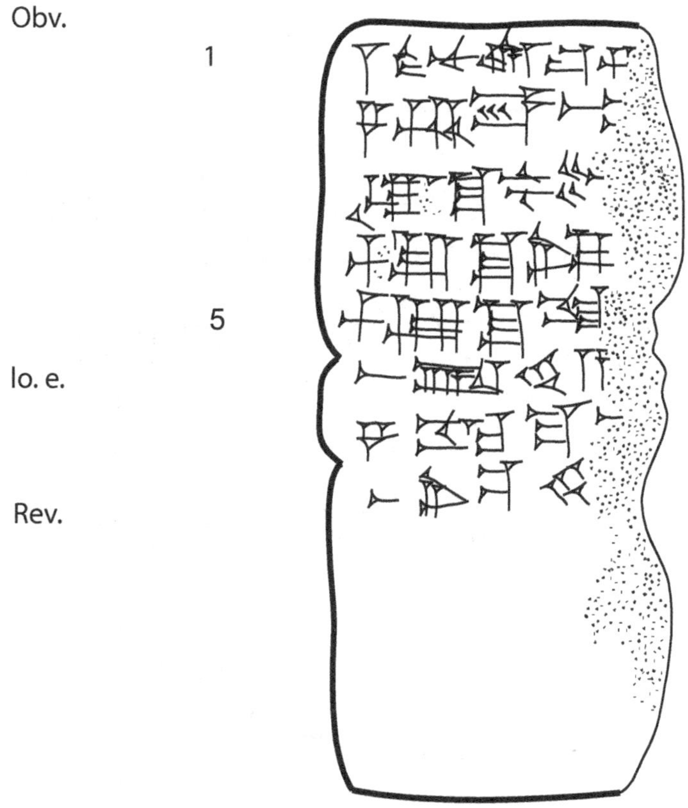

BM 59710

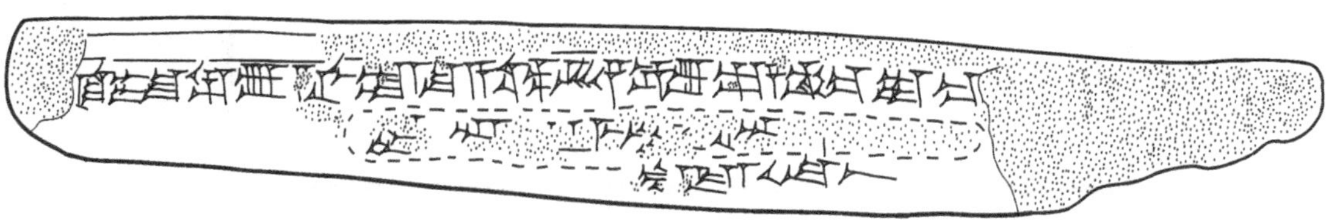

SpTU 4, 153 upper edge

Plate 26: BM 59710 and SpTU 4, 153 upper edge.

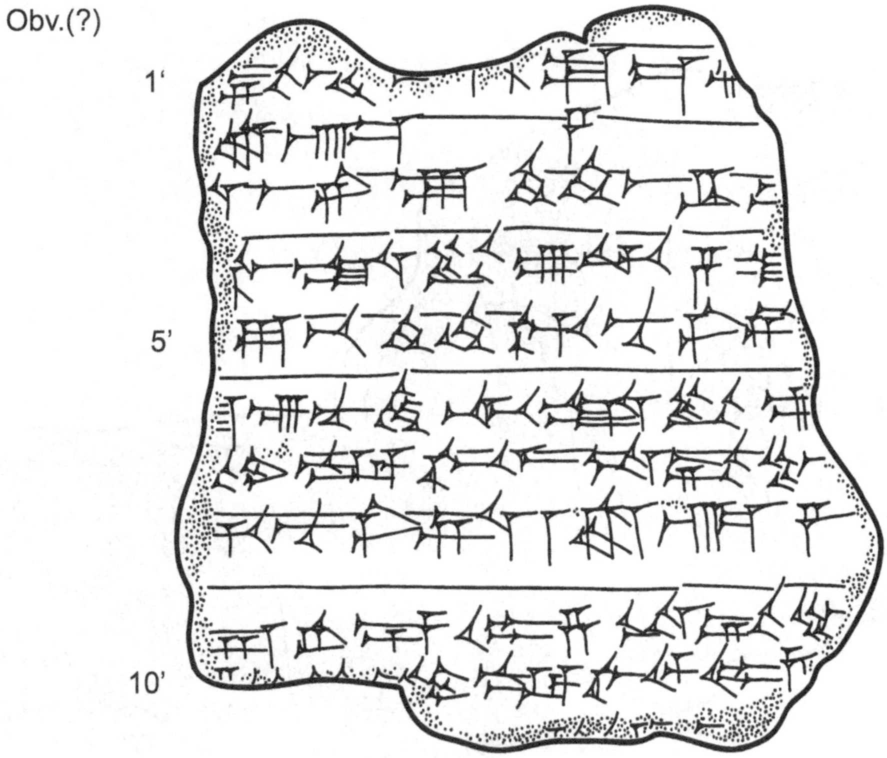

K. 8893

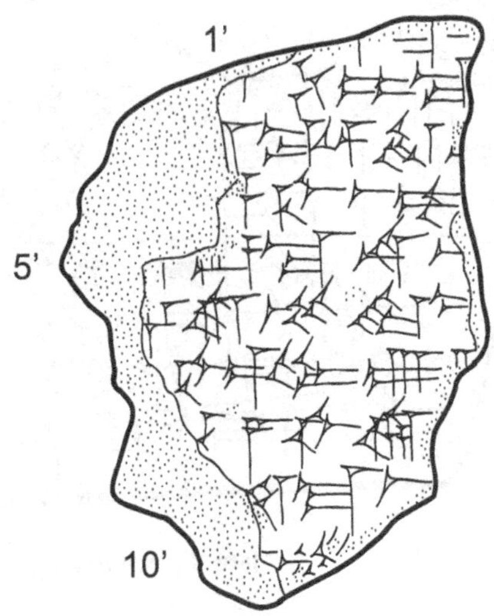

K. 19506

Plate 27: K. 8893 and K. 19506.

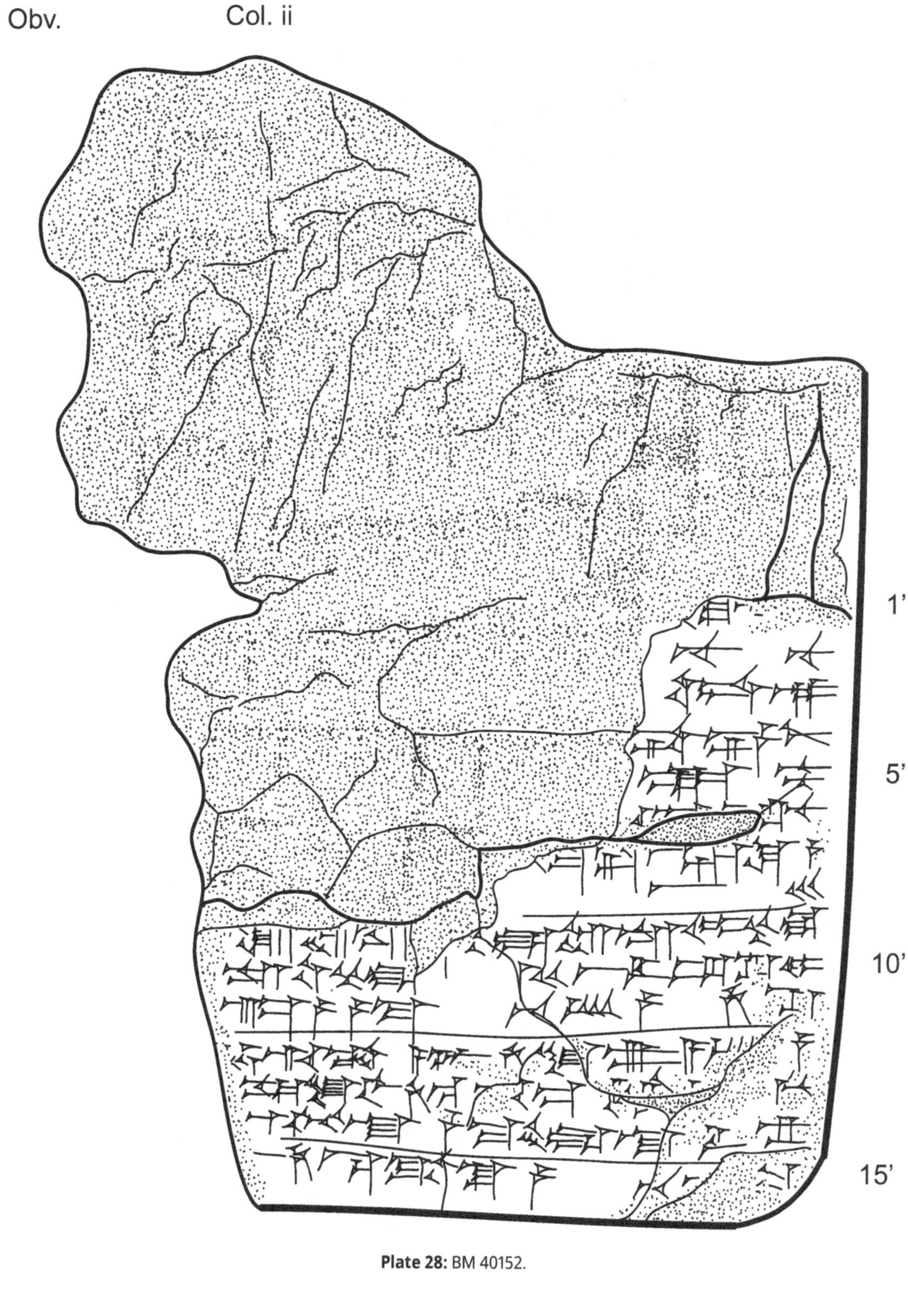

Plate 28: BM 40152.

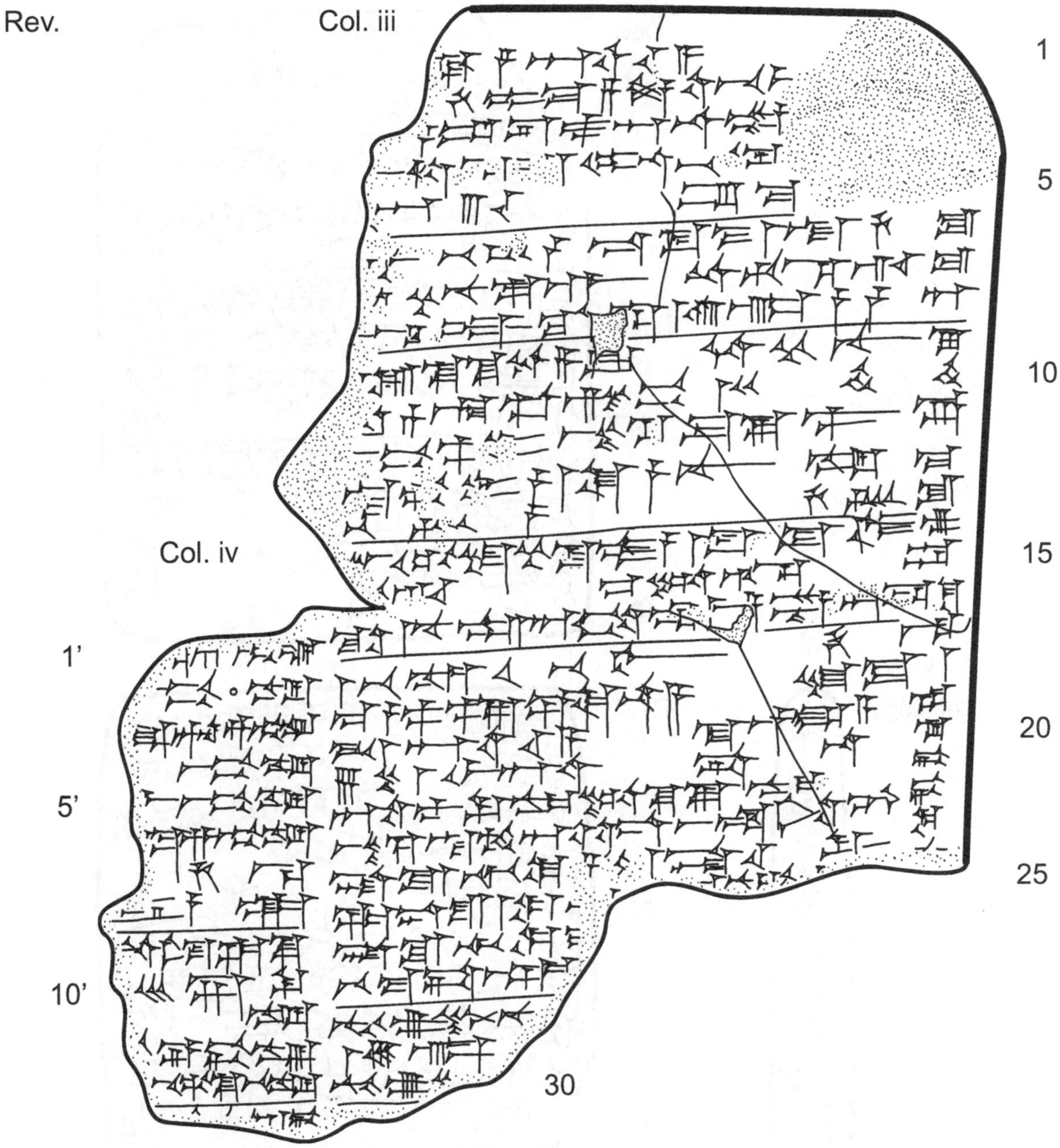

Plate 29: BM 40152.

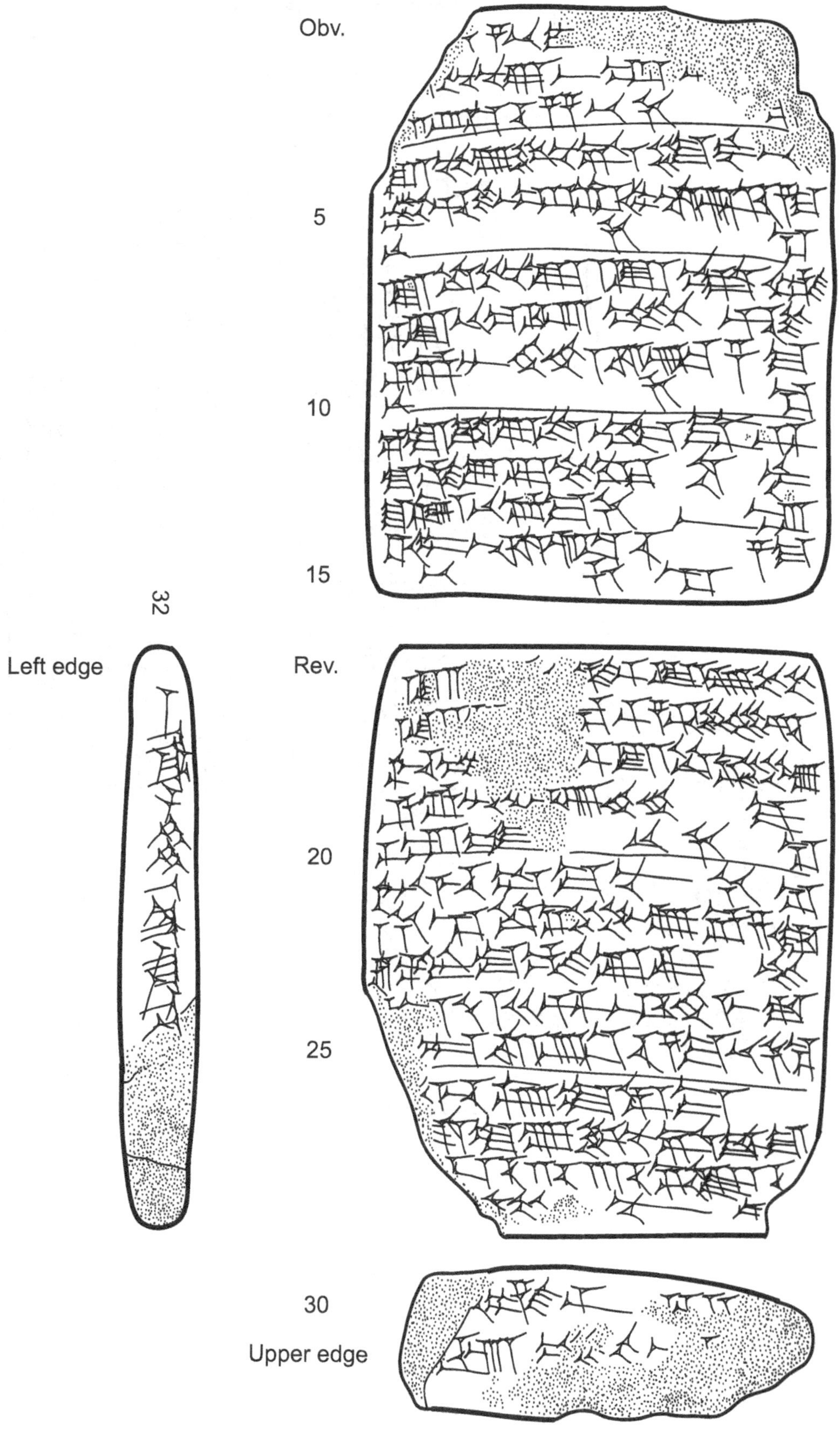

Plate 30: FLP 1306.

Obv.

1

5

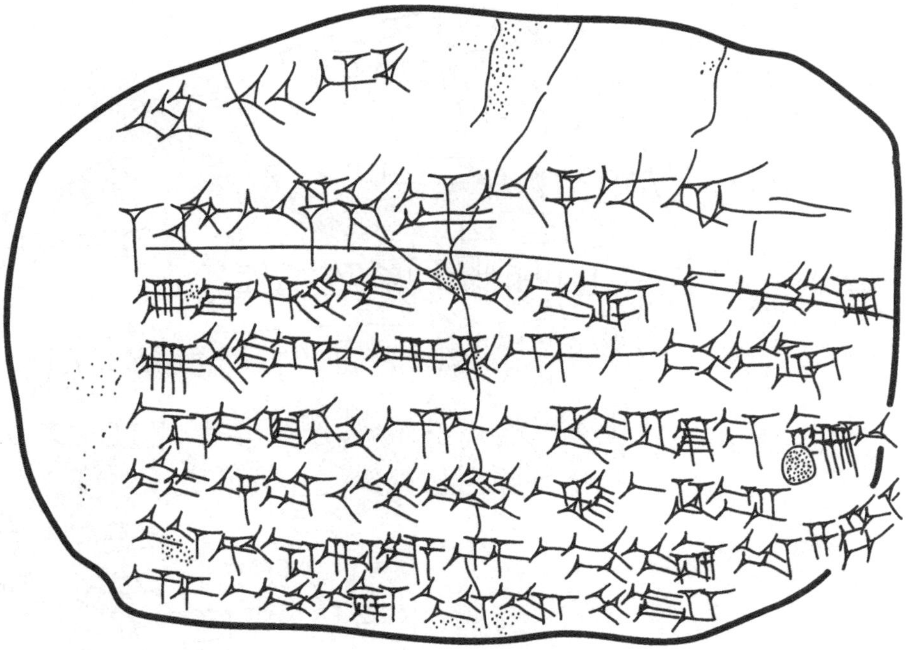

Lower edge

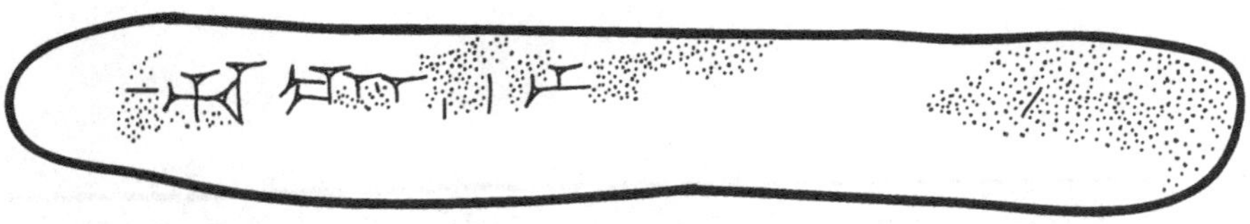

Rev.

1

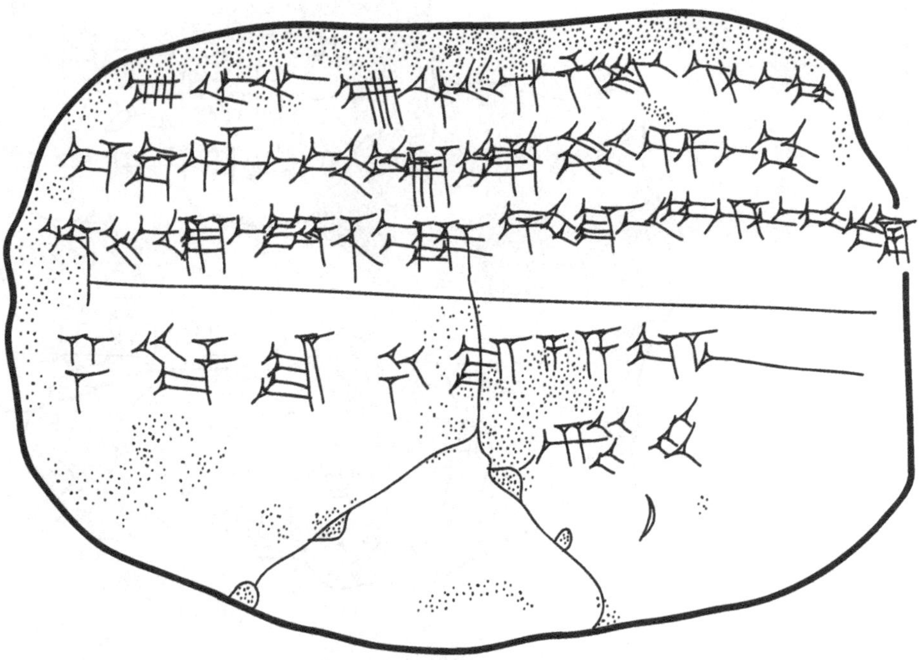

Plate 31: BM 47578.

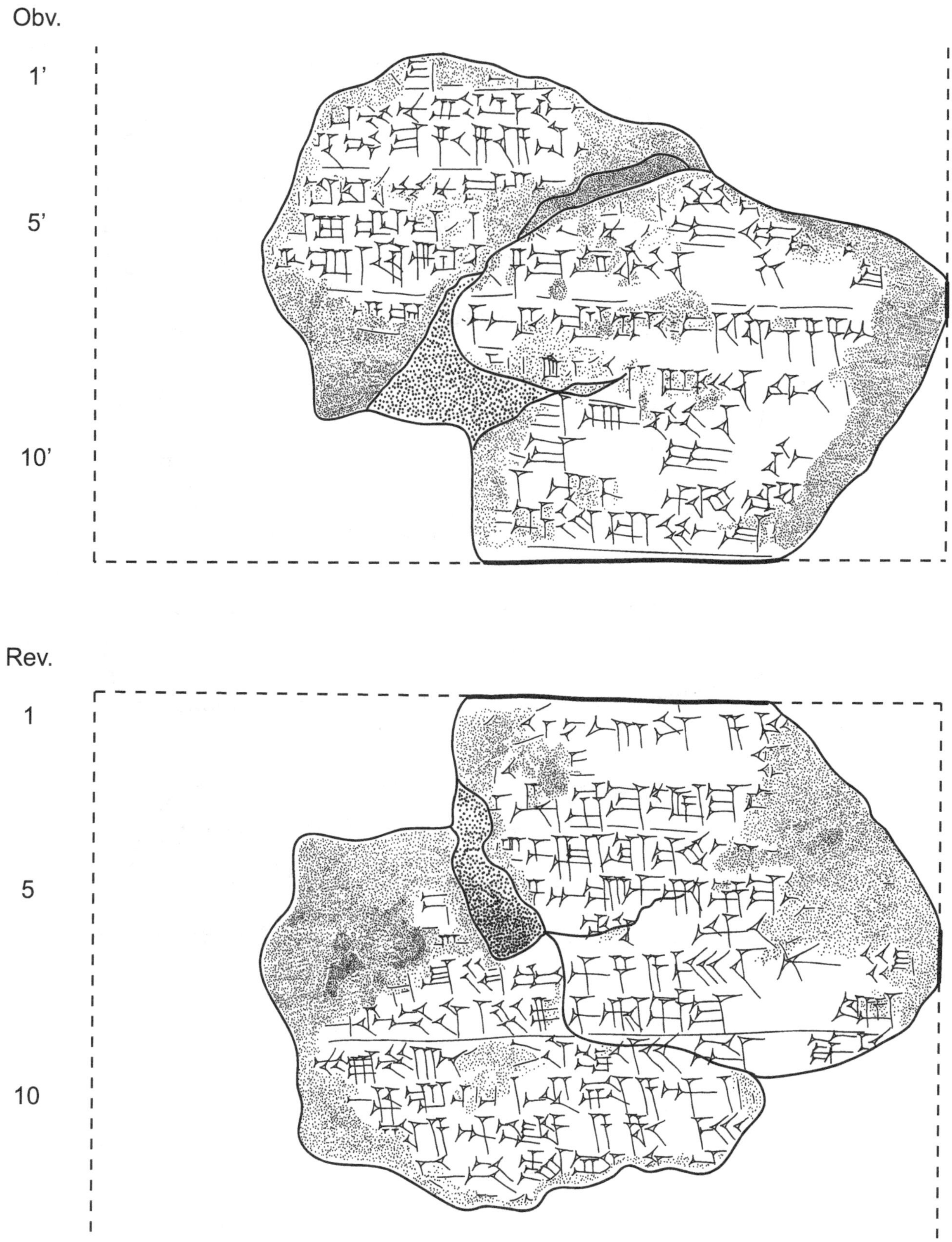

Plate 32: BM 54587 + 73802.

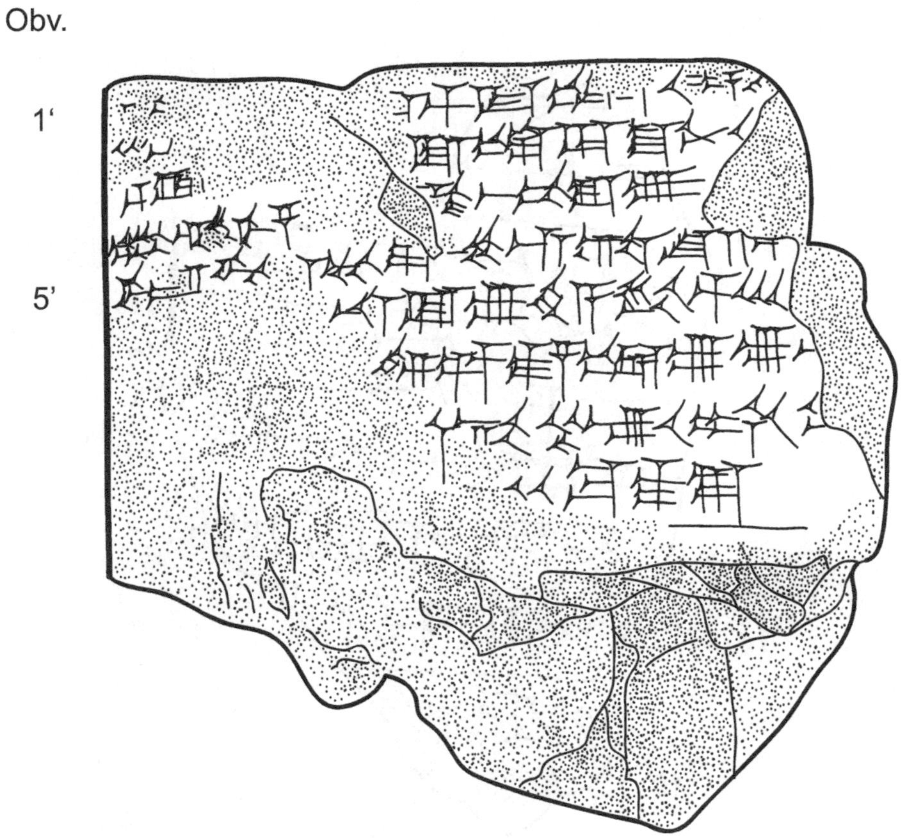

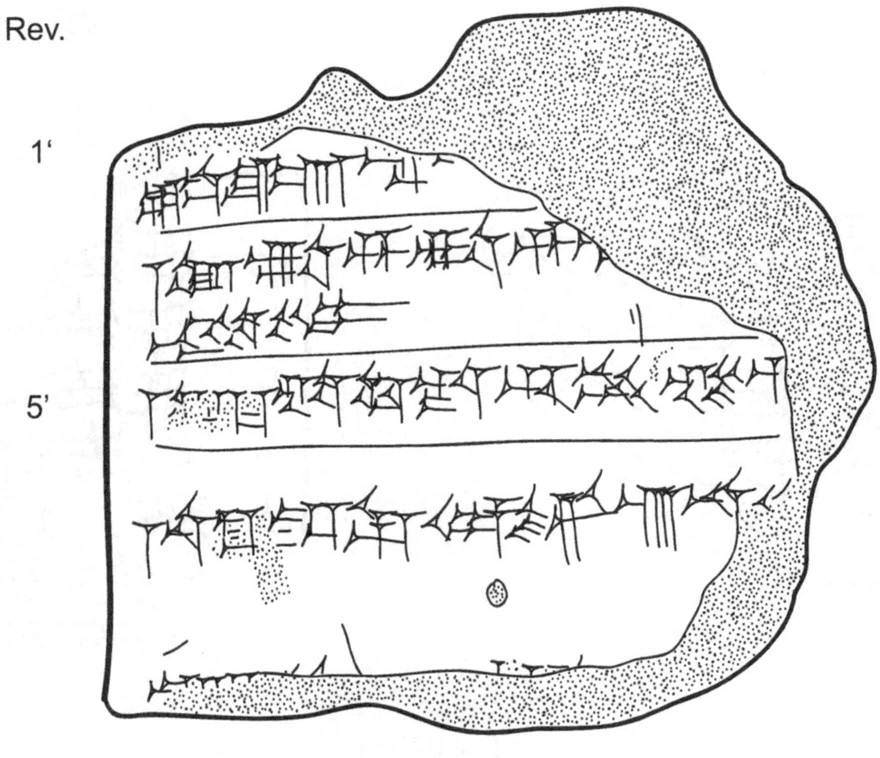

Plate 33: BM 61975.

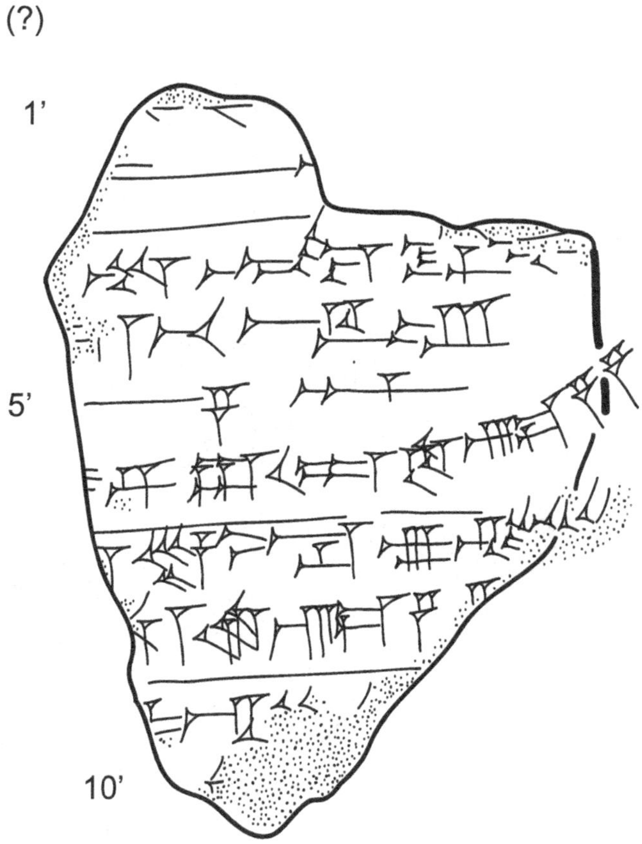

K. 20254

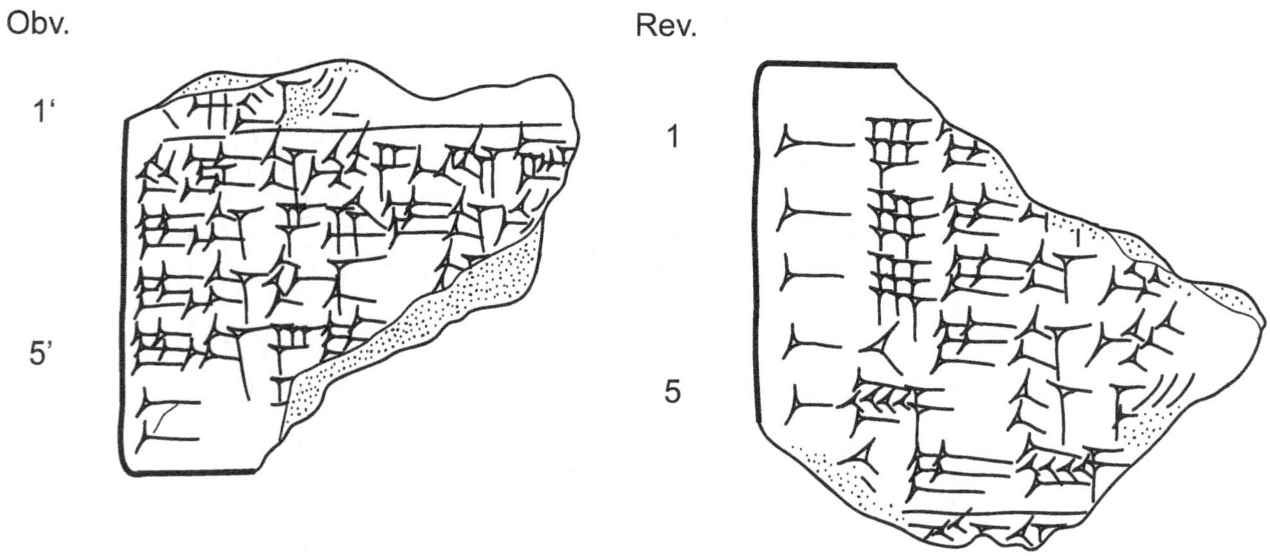

BM 37014

Plate 34: K. 20254 and BM 37014.

Obv.

Rev.

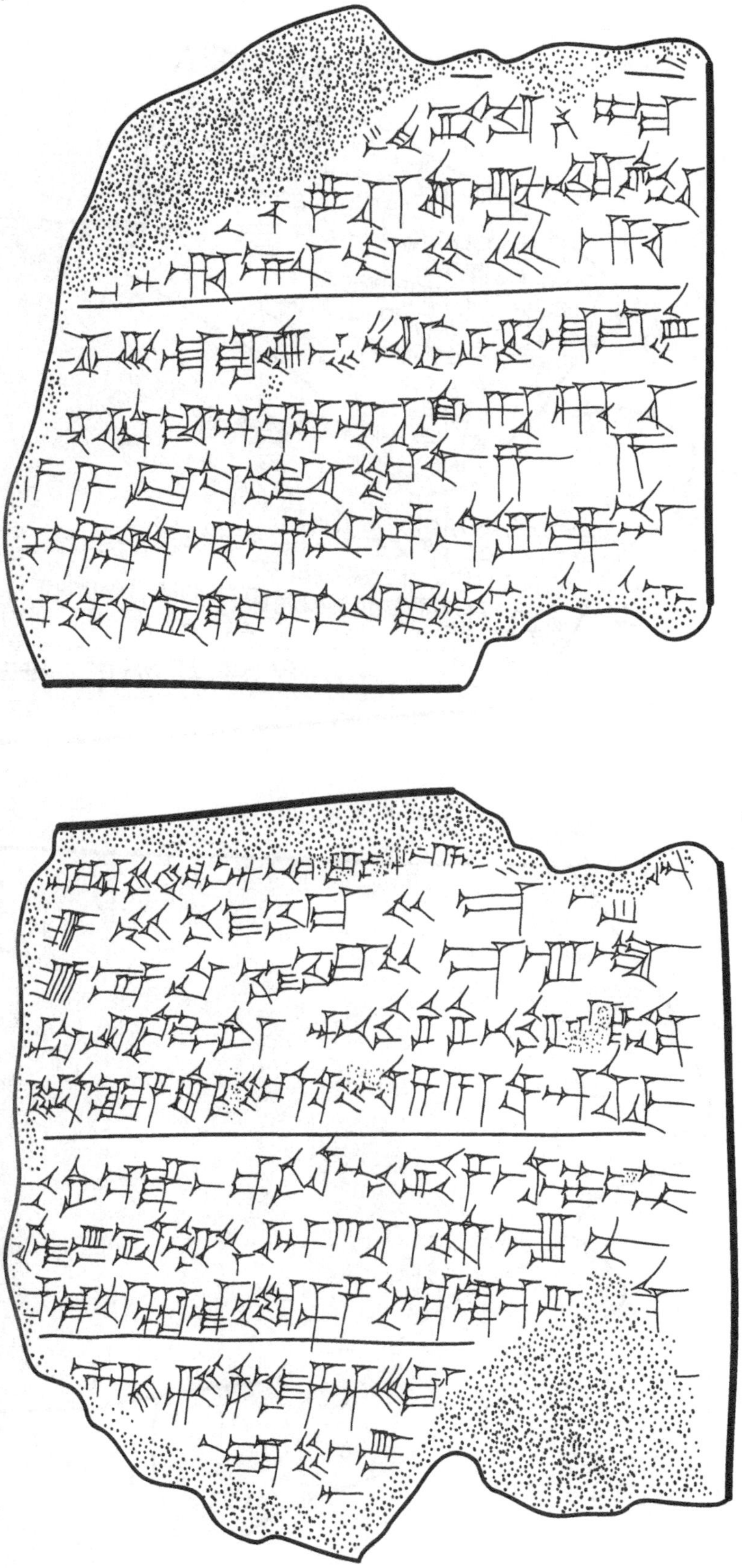

Plate 35: BM 36339.

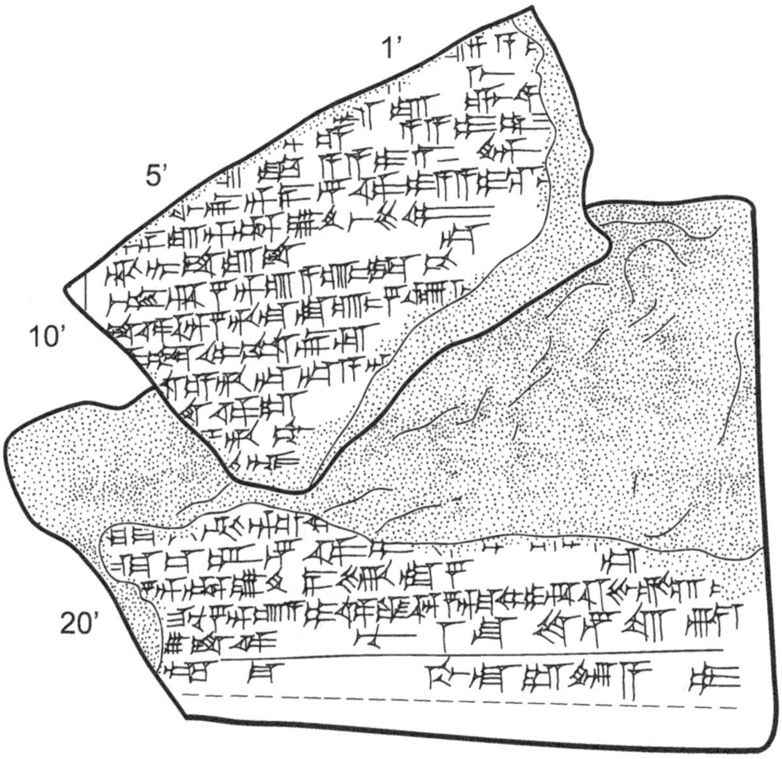

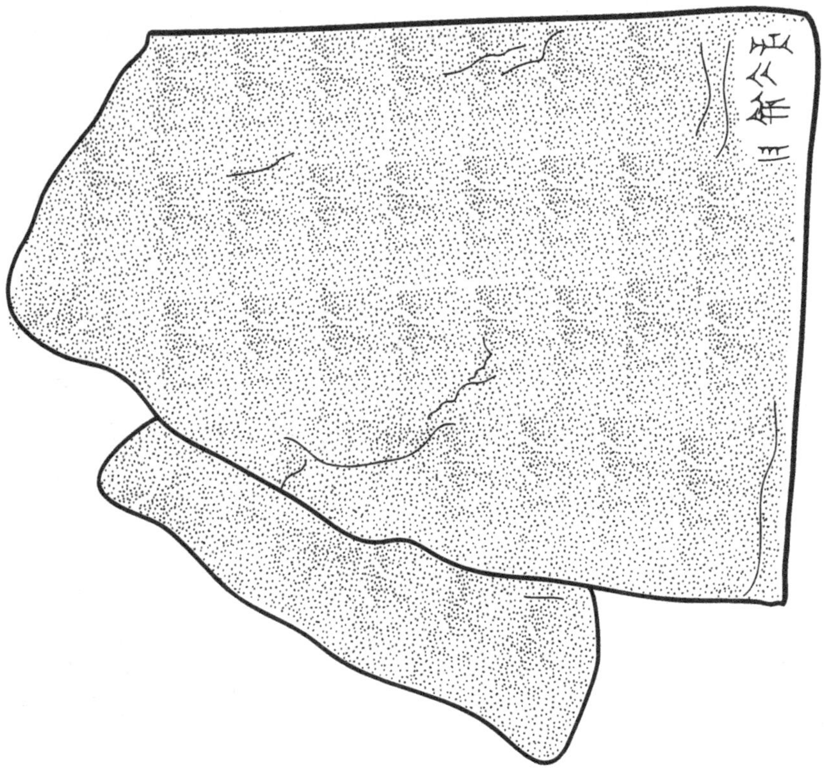

Plate 36: K. 3485 + 10443.

Obv.

Col. i Col. ii

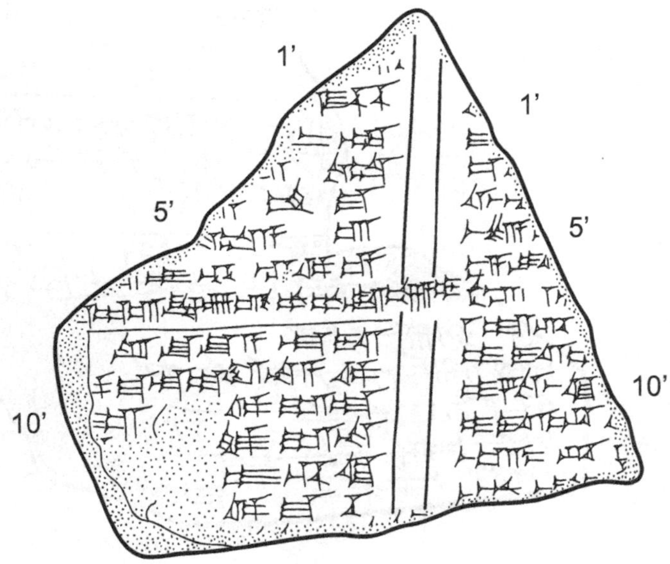

K. 8210

Obv. (?)

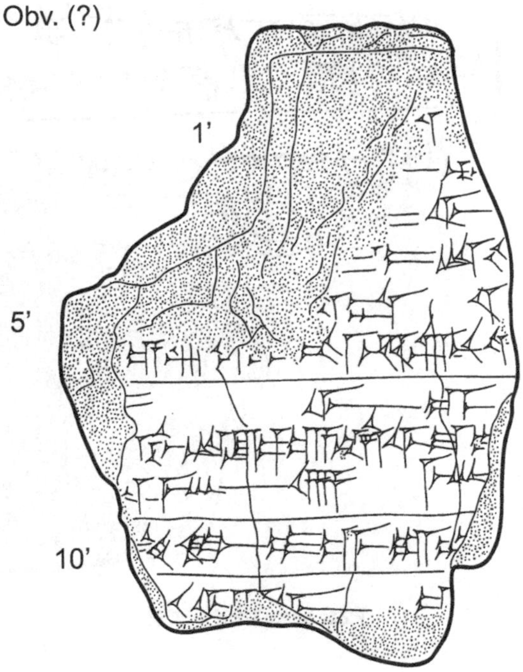

K. 14028

Plate 37: K. 8210 and K. 14028.

Obv.

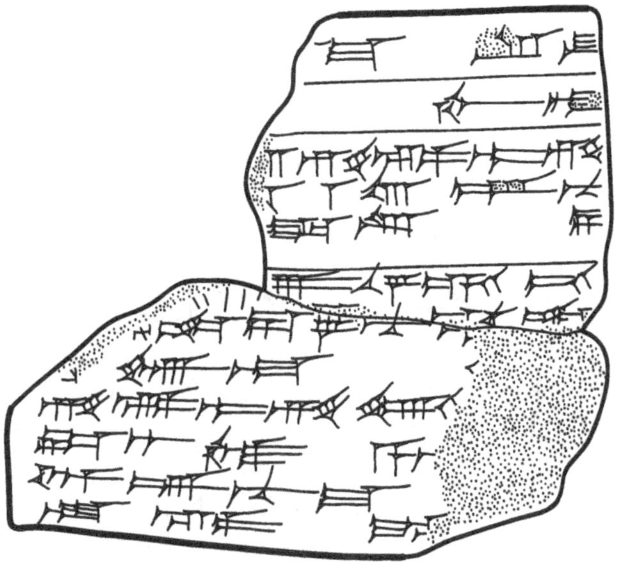

Rev.

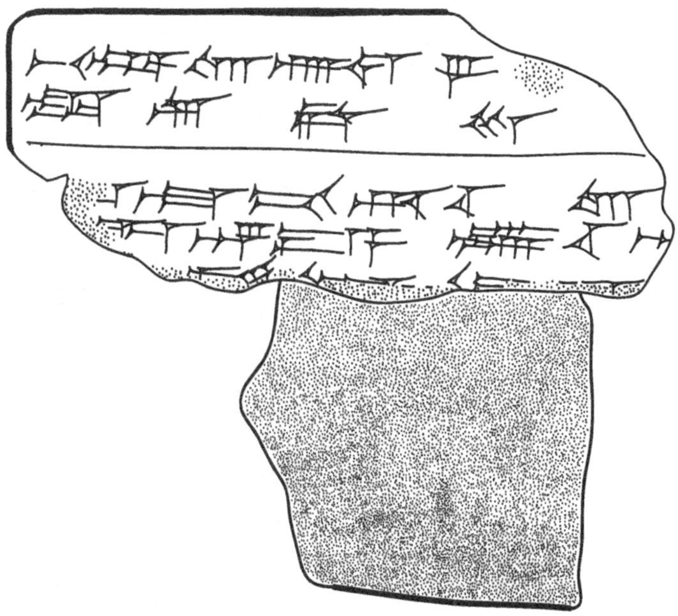

Plate 38: K. 11956 + 14200.

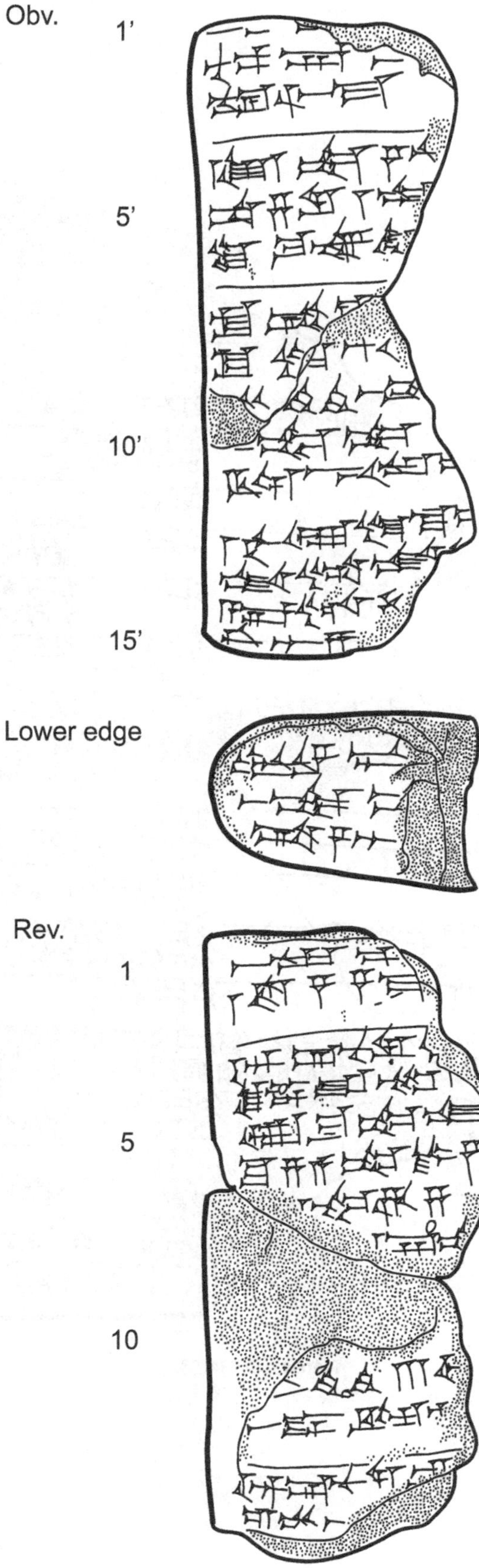

Plate 39: K. 1930 + 11752.

Obv.

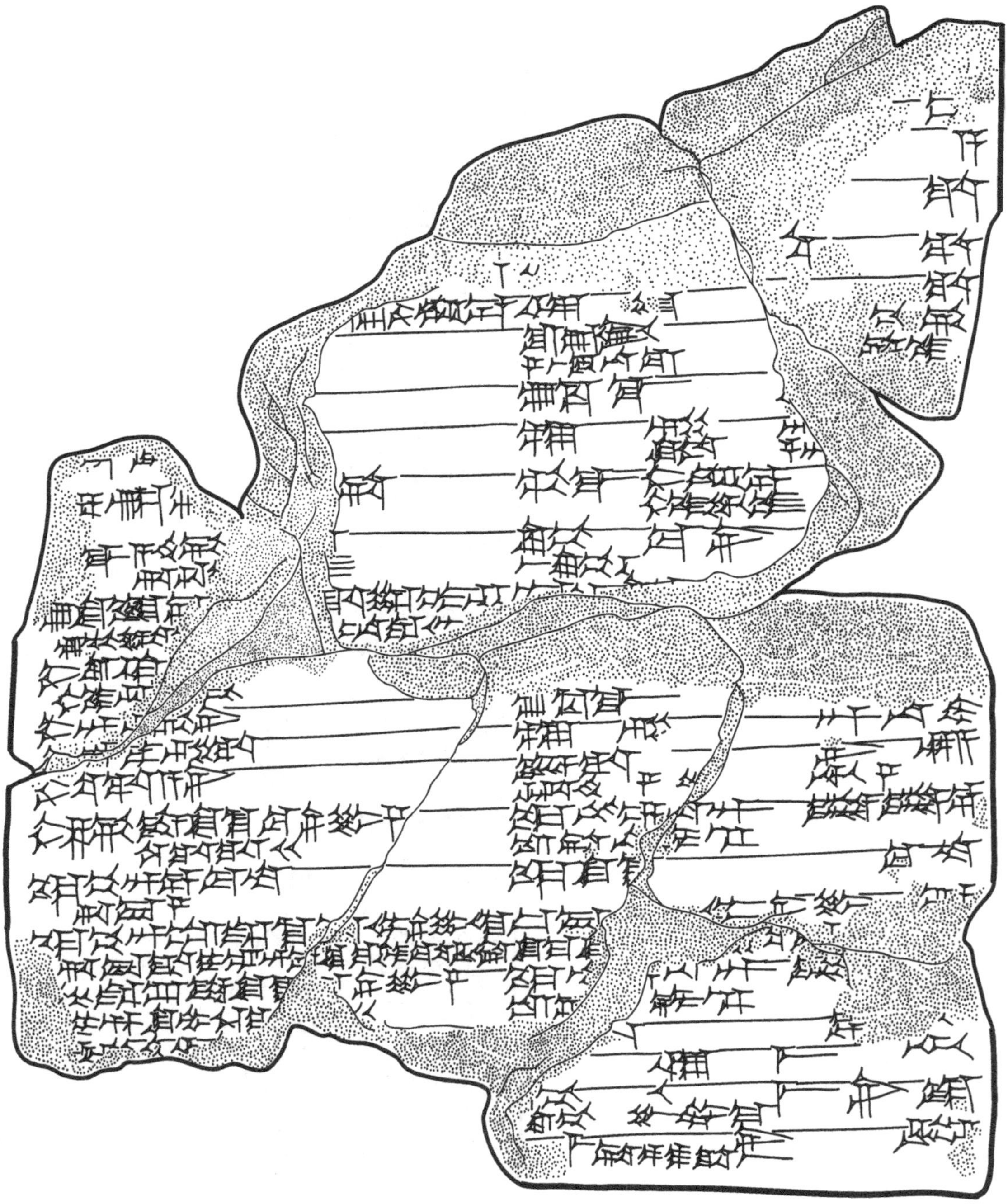

Plate 40: BM 34208.

Rev.

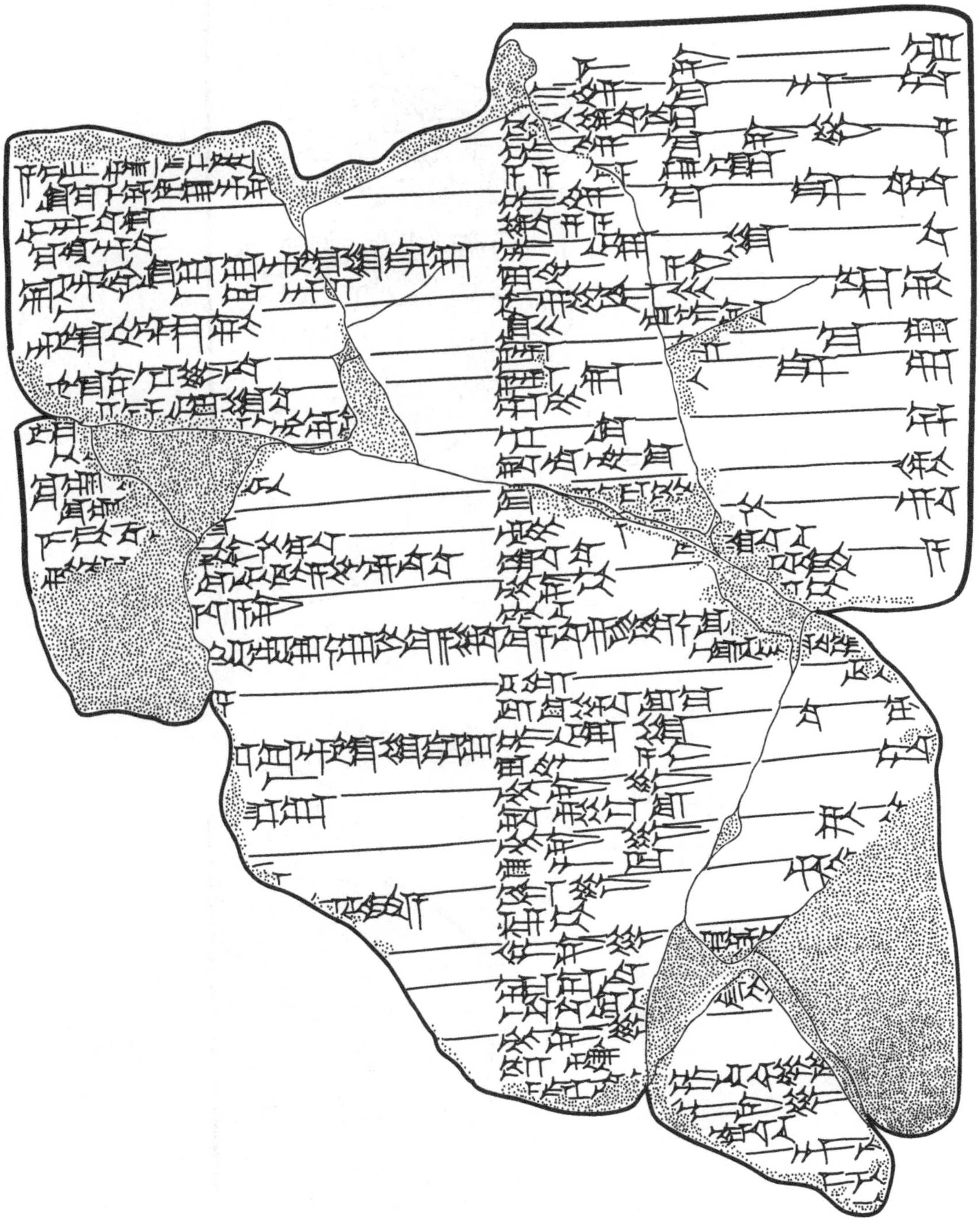

Plate 41: BM 34208.

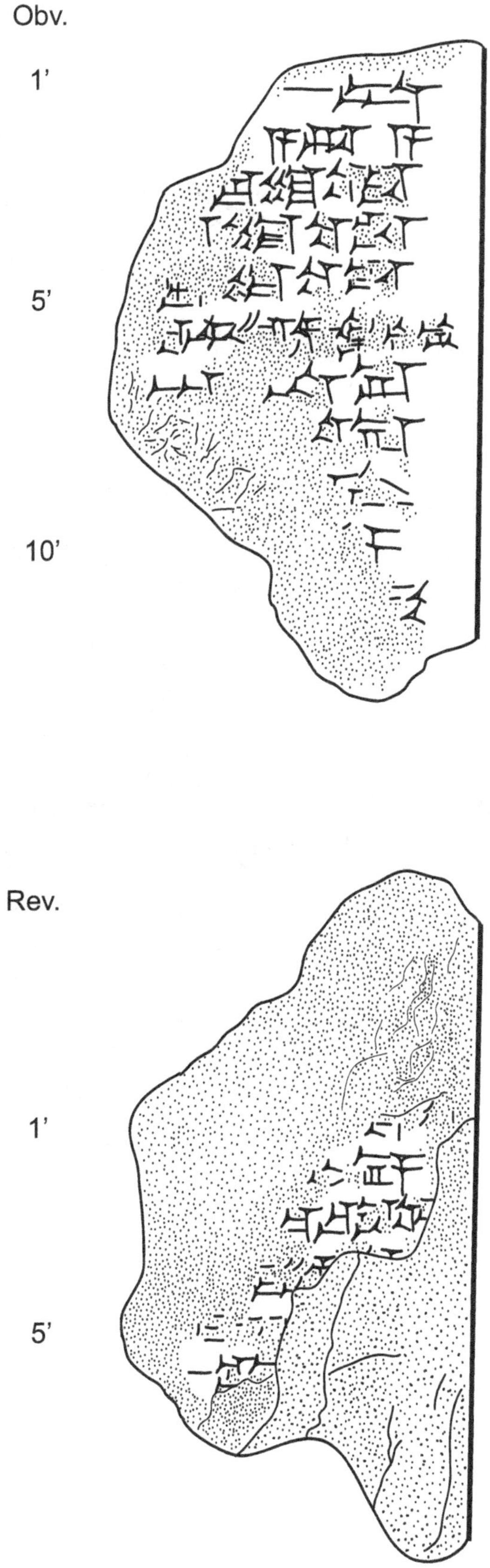

Plate 42: BM 37476.

Obv.

1'

5'

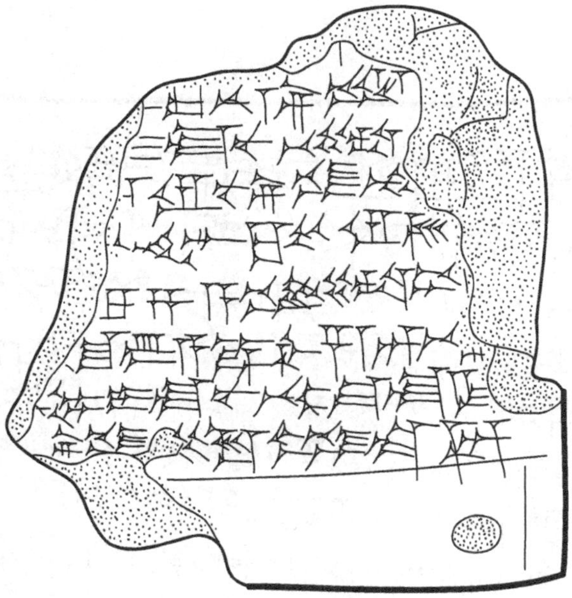

Rev.

1

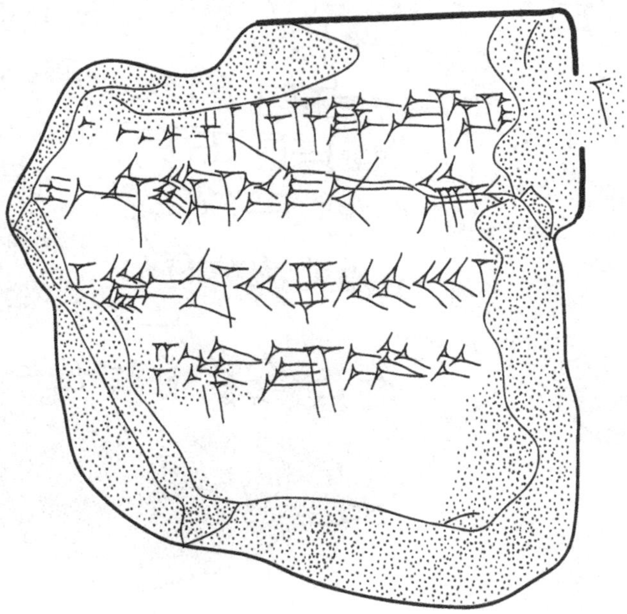

Plate 43: BM 54846.

Obv.

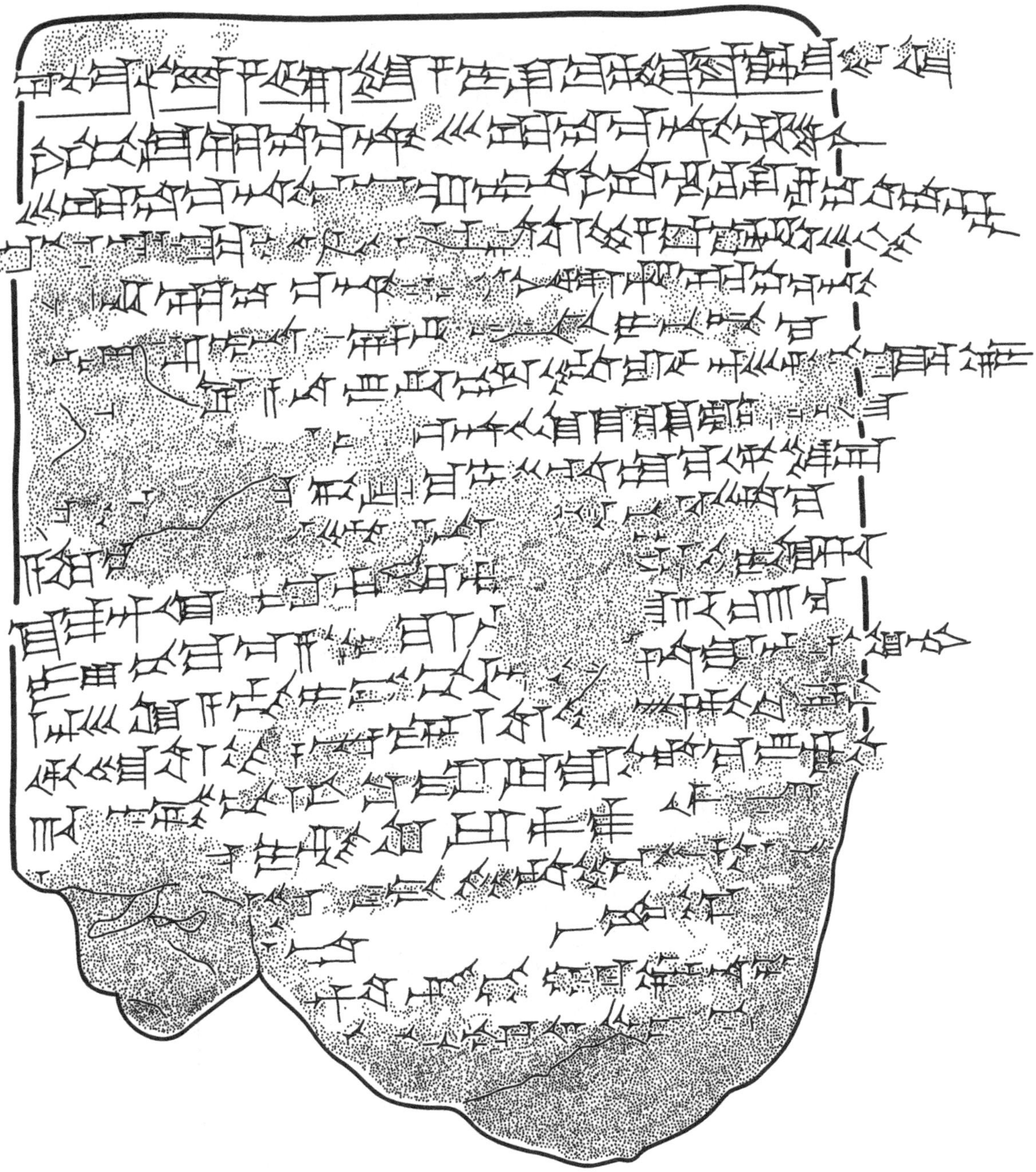

Plate 44: K. 8666.

Rev.

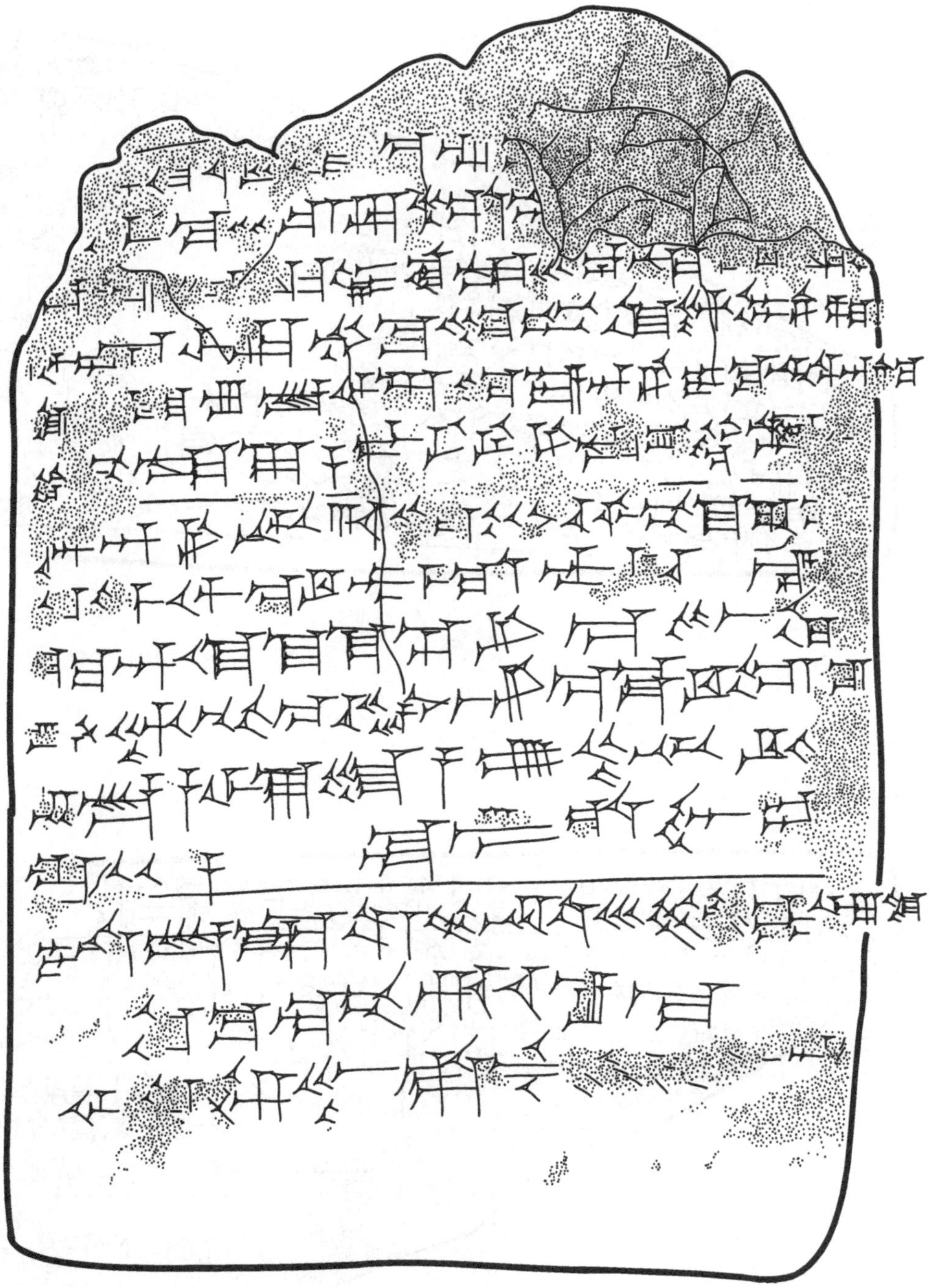

Plate 45: K. 8666.

Obv.

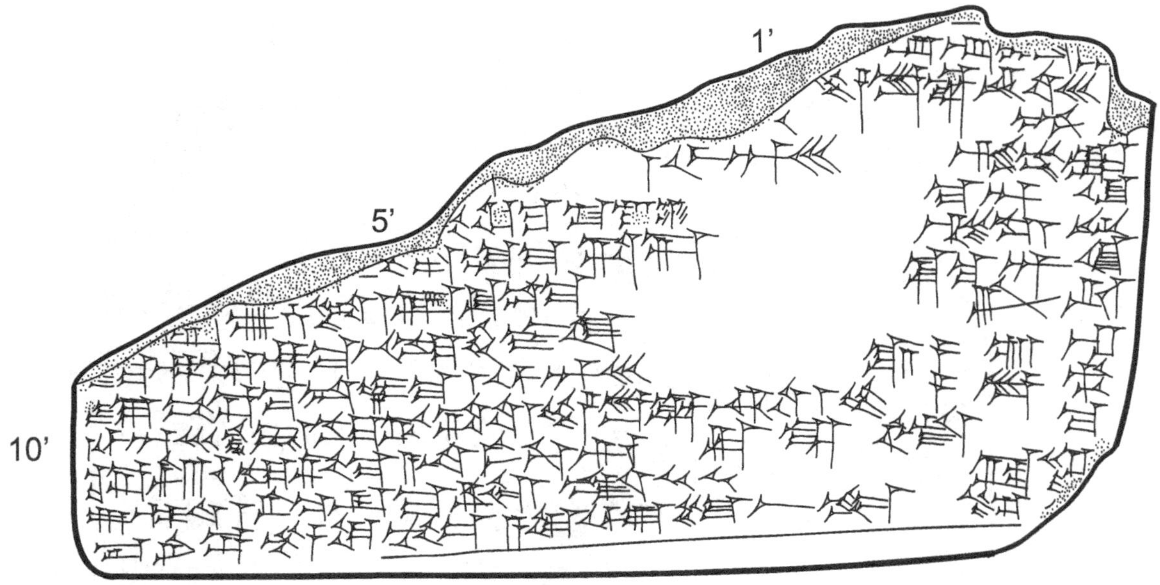

Rev.

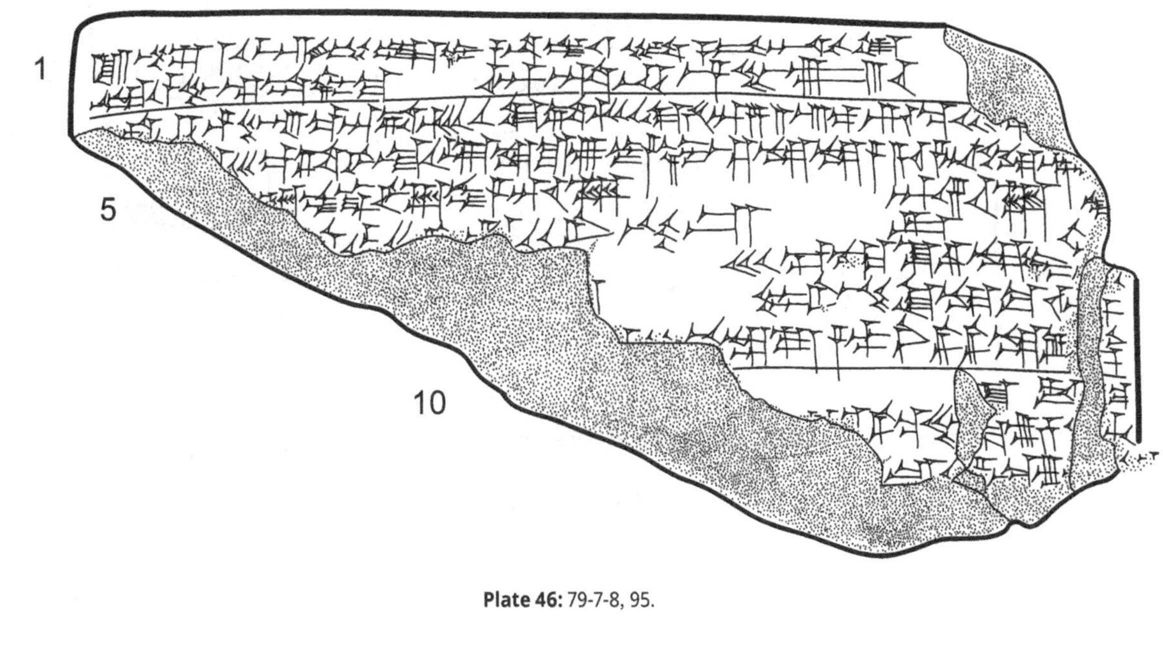

Plate 46: 79-7-8, 95.

Obv.

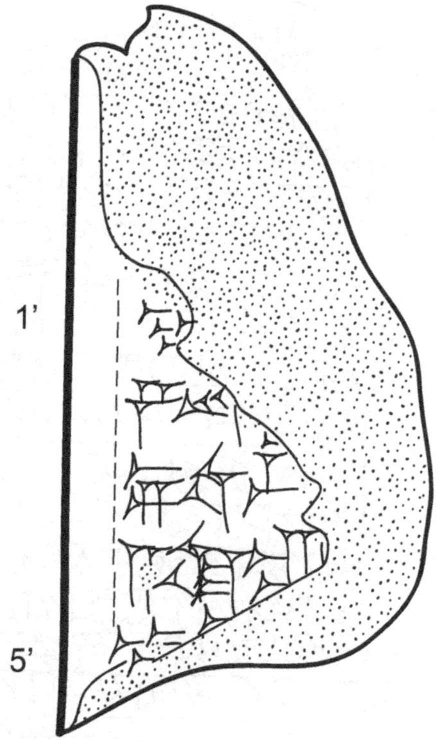

Rev.

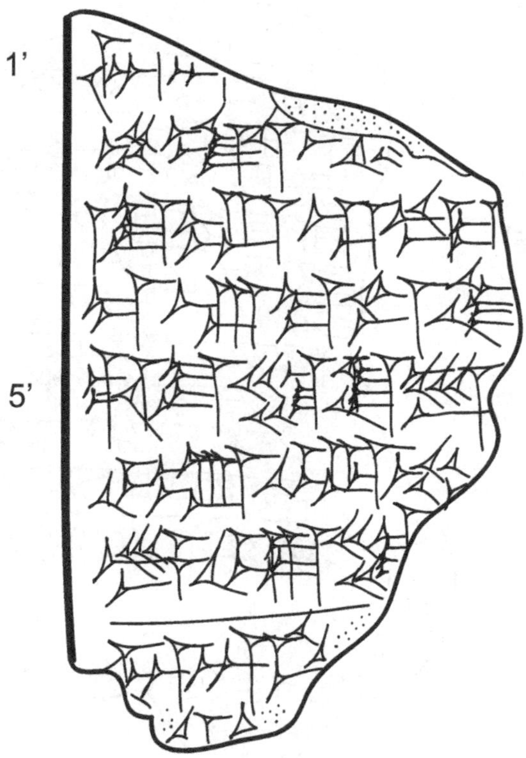

Plate 47: K. 13315.

Obv.

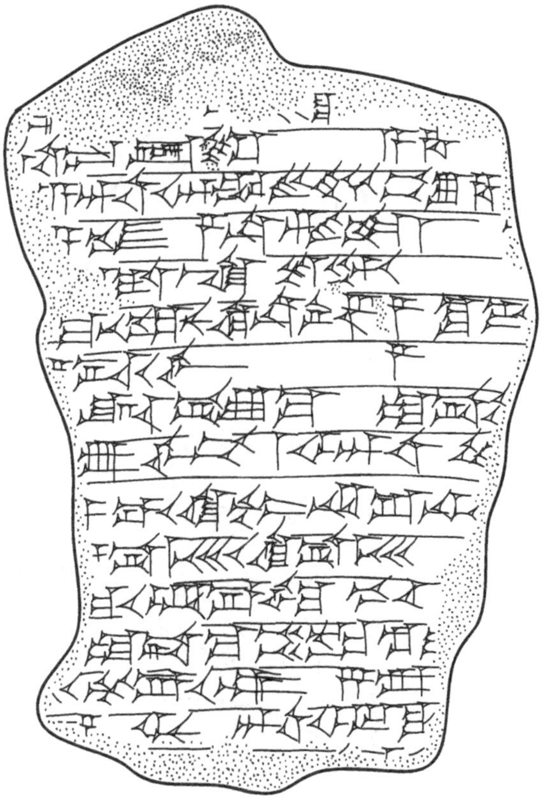

Rev.

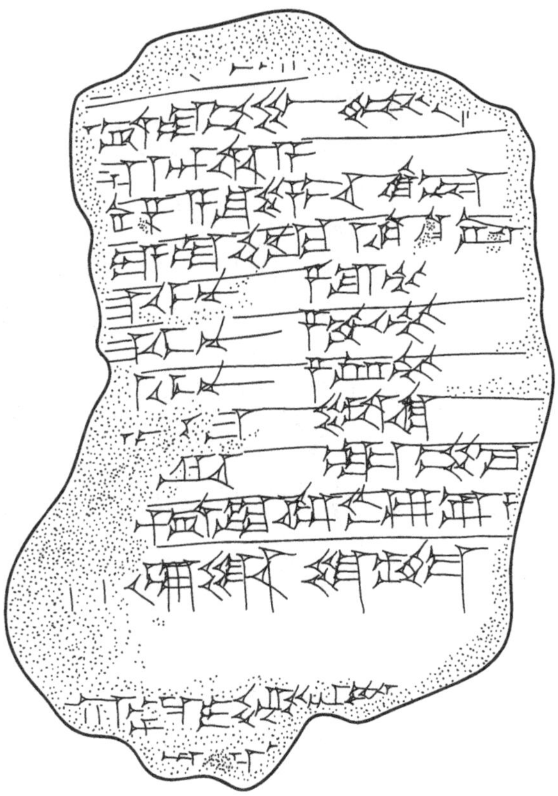

Plate 48: BM 47801.

Obv.

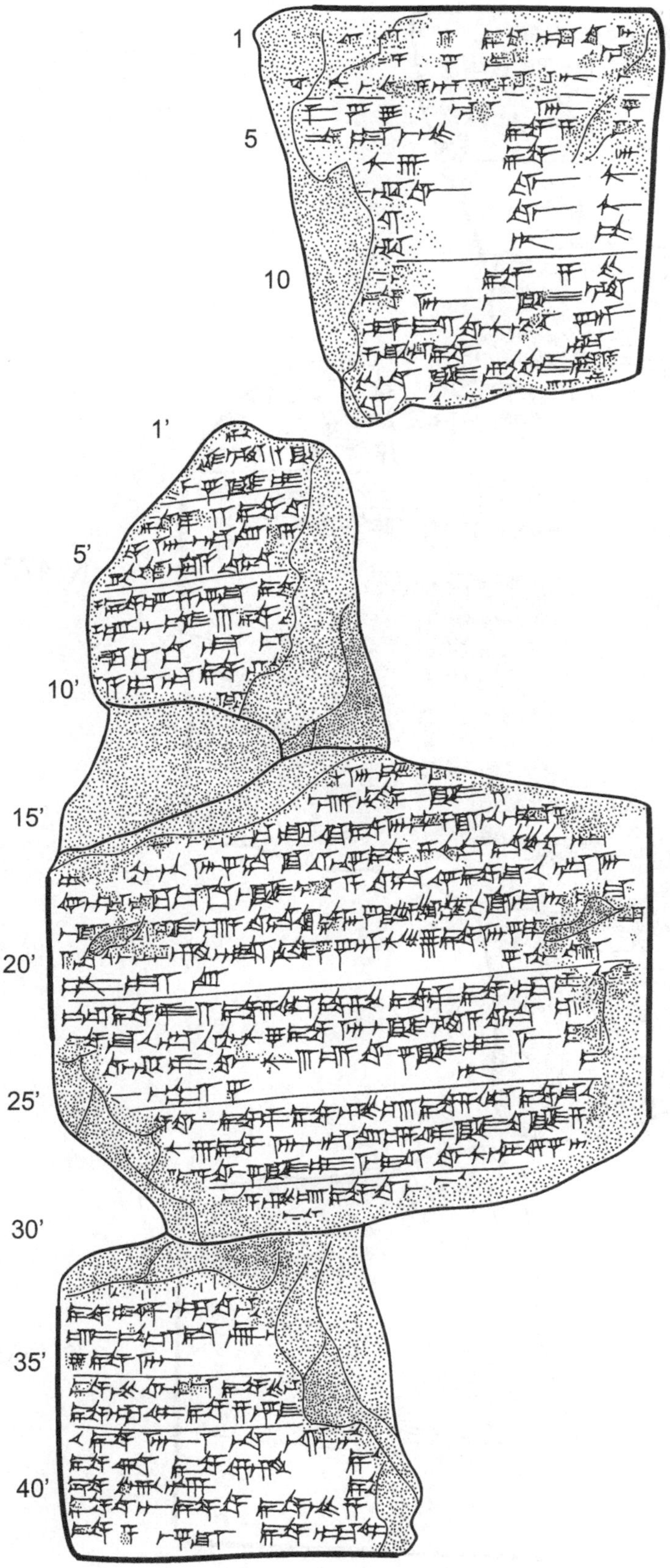

K. 6688

K. 4727 +

Plate 49: K. 4727 + K. 9426 + 81-2-4, 386 (+) K. 6688.

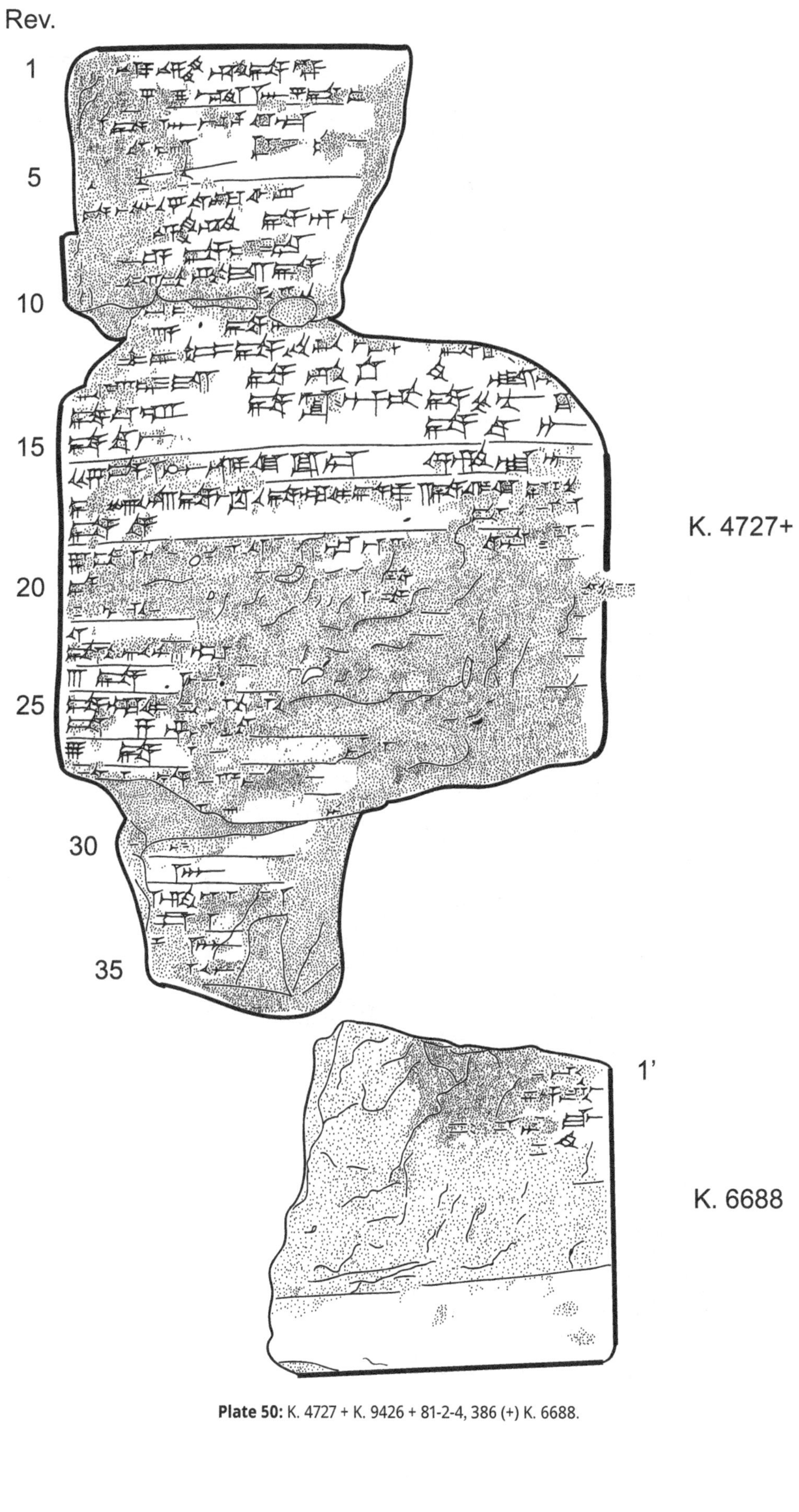

Plate 50: K. 4727 + K. 9426 + 81-2-4, 386 (+) K. 6688.

Obv.

1’
5’
10’
15’

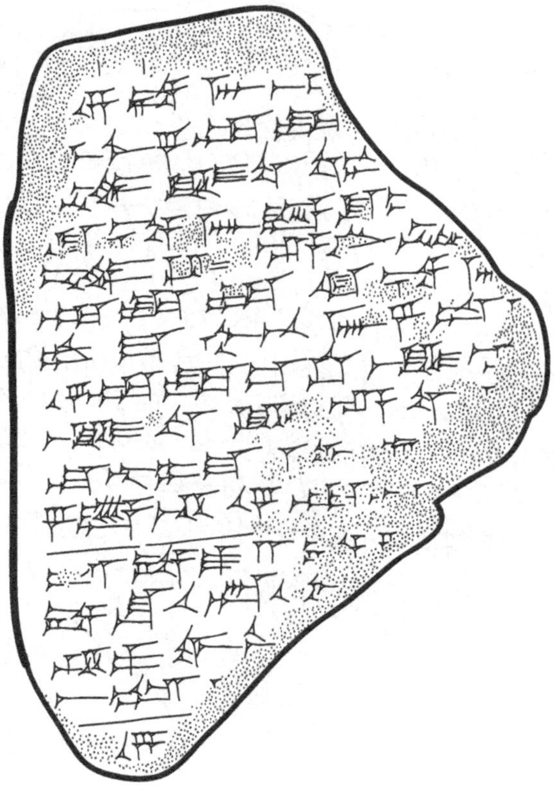

Rev.

1’
5’
10’

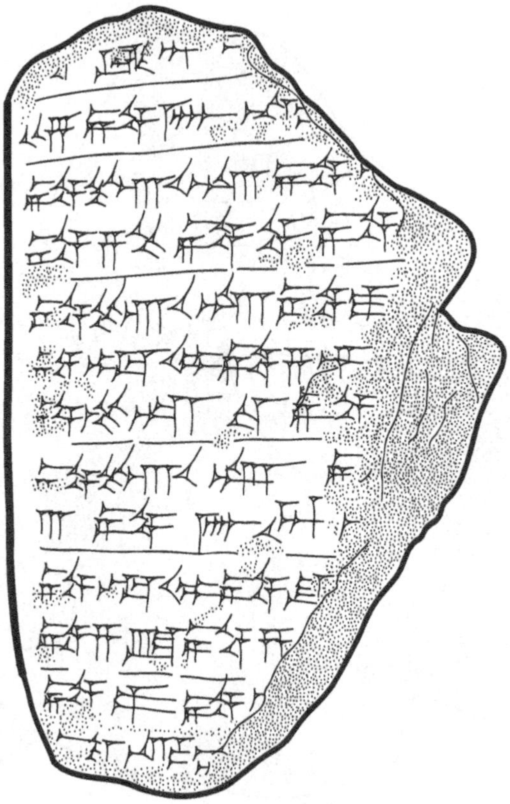

Plate 51: K. 9071.

Obv.

1‘

5‘

10‘

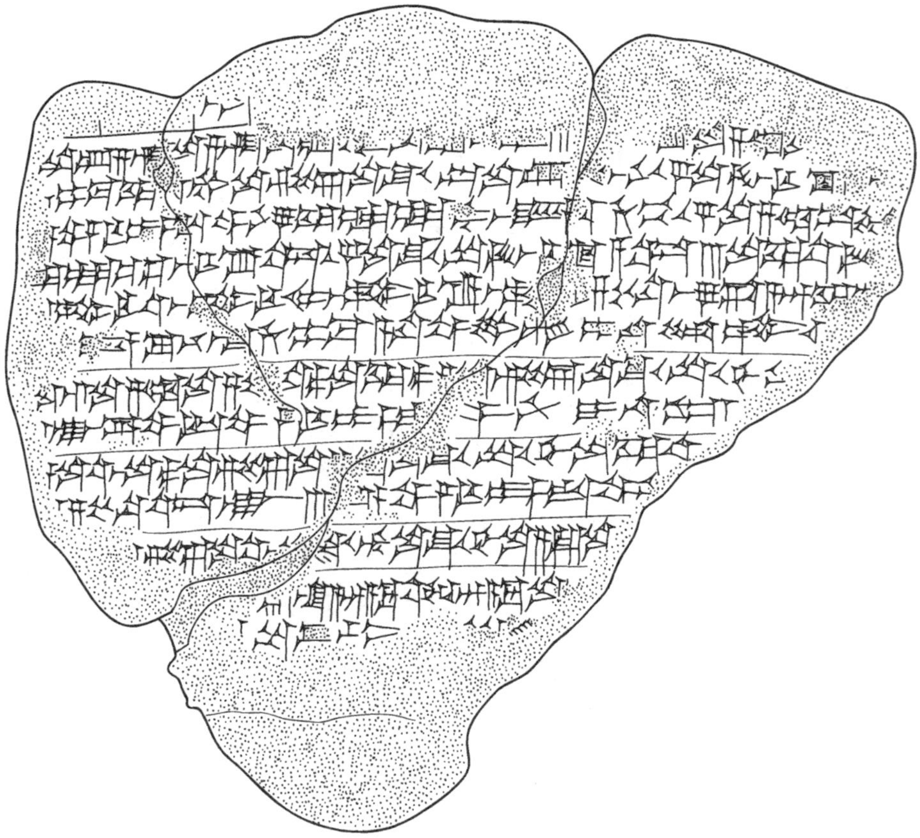

Rev.

1‘

5‘

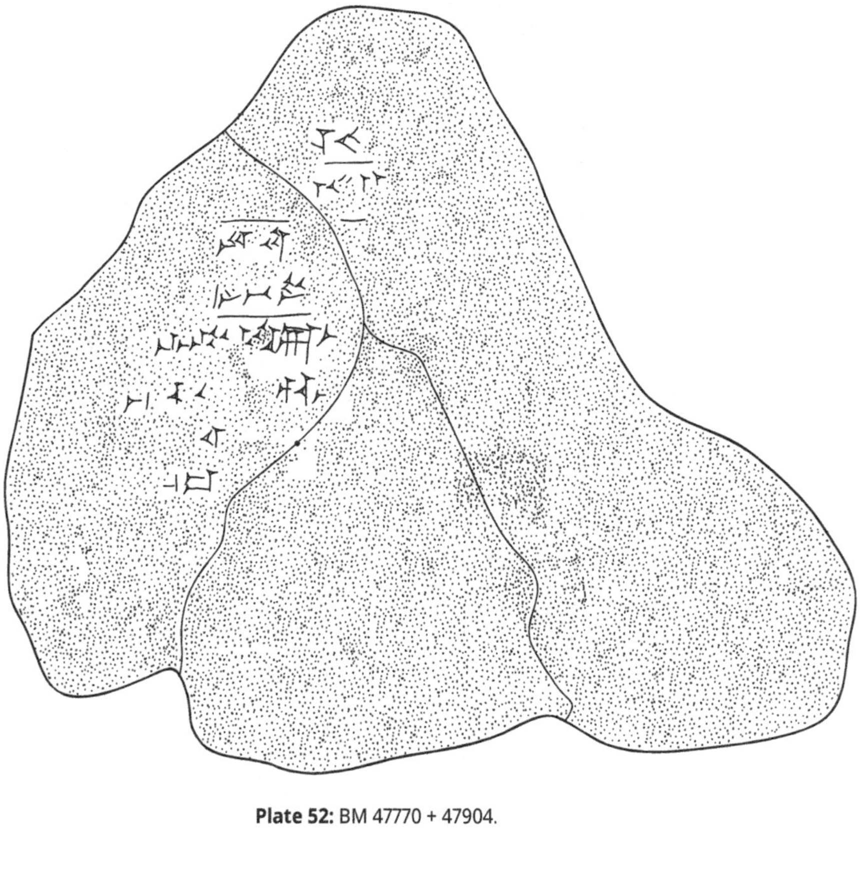

Plate 52: BM 47770 + 47904.

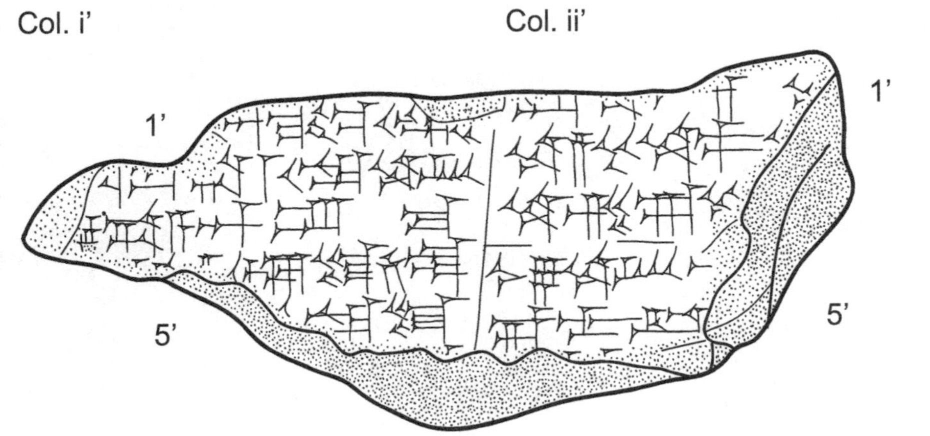

DT 28

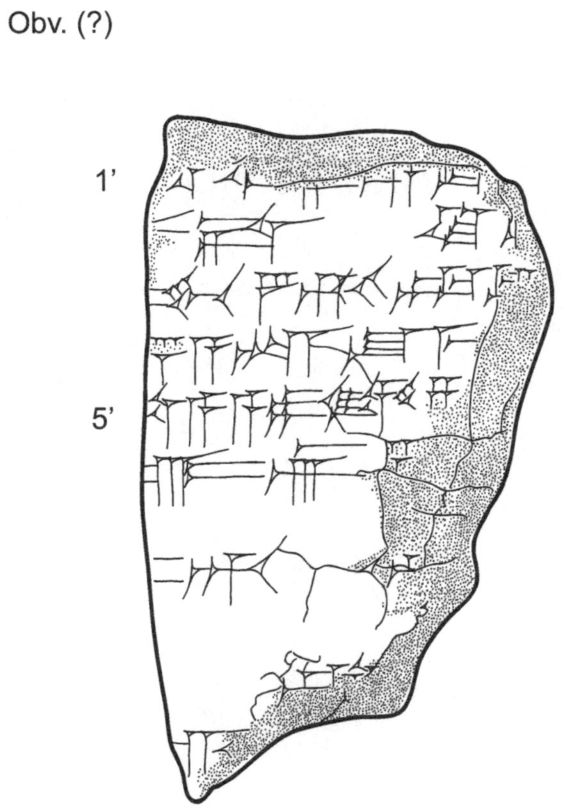

K. 17499

Plate 53: DT 28 and K. 17499.

Indices

Subject Index

https://doi.org/10.1515/9781501506475-016

Divine Names

Personal Names

Geographical Names

Selective Index of Texts